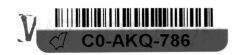

C0-AKQ-786

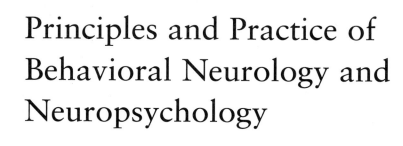

Principles and Practice of Behavioral Neurology and Neuropsychology

Principles and Practice of Behavioral Neurology and Neuropsychology

Edited by

Matthew Rizzo, MD
Professor of Neurology, Engineering, and Public Policy;
Director, Division of Neuroergonomics,
Senior Faculty Member, Division of Behavioral
Neurology and Cognitive Neuroscience,
Attending Physician, Memory Disorders Clinic,
Department of Neurology,
Roy J. and Lucille A. Carver College of Medicine
University of Iowa
Iowa City, IA

Paul J. Eslinger, PhD
Professor, Departments of Neurology, Neural and
Behavioral Science, and Pediatrics
(Division of Developmental Pediatrics and Learning);
Director, Clinical Neuropsychology and
Cognitive Neuroscience
Penn State University College of Medicine
Hershey, PA

Foreword by

Arthur Benton, PhD

SAUNDERS
An Imprint of Elsevier

W.B.Saunders Company
An Imprint of Elsevier
The Curtis Center
Independence Square West
Philadelphia, Pennsylvania 19106

Copyright © 2004, Elsevier Inc. (USA). All Rights Reserved

No part of this publication may be reproduced or transmitted in any form or by any means, electronic or mechanical, including photocopy, recording, or any information storage and retrieval system, without permission in writing from the publisher.

Notice

Neurology is an ever-changing field. Standard safety precautions must be followed but as new research and clinical experience broaden our knowledge, changes in treatment and drug therapy may become necessary or appropriate. Readers are advised to check the most current product information provided by the manufacturer of each drug to be administered to verify the recommended dose, the method and duration of administration, and contraindications. It is the responsibility of the treating physician, relying on experience and knowledge of the patient, to determine dosages and the best treatment for each individual patient. Neither the Publisher nor the author assumes any liability for any injury and/or damage to persons or property arising from this publication.

The Publisher

Library of Congress Cataloging-in-Publication Data

Principles and practice of behavioral neurology and neuropsychology / Matthew Rizzo,
    Paul J. Eslinger, [editors].
        p. ; cm.
    Includes bibliographical references.
    ISBN 0-7216-8154-9
    1. Clinical neuropsychology. I. Rizzo, Matthew. II. Eslinger, Paul J.
    [DNLM: 1. Brain Diseases—diagnosis. 2. Neurobehavioral Manifestations. 3. Cognition
    Disorders—diagnosis. 4. Forensic Psychiatry—methods. 5. Neurologic
    Examination—methods. 6. Neuropsychology—methods. WL 340 P957 2003]
    RC386.6.N48P75 2004
    616.8—dc21

                                                                    2003041530

Executive Publisher: Susan Pioli
Developmental Editor: Jennifer Ehlers

Printed in the United States of America

Last digit is the print number: 9 8 7 6 5 4 3 2 1

Contents

CONTENTS

Contributing Authors

Ralph Adolphs, PhD
Associate Professor, Division of Behavioral Neurology and Cognitive Neuroscience, Department of Neurology, Roy J. and Lucille A. Carver College of Medicine, University of Iowa, Iowa City, IA

Vicki A. Anderson, MA, PhD
Professor, Behavioral Sciences, University of Melbourne, Victoria, Australia; Director, Psychology, Royal Children's Hospital, Parkville, Victoria, Australia

Zoe Arvanitakis, MD
Assistant Professor, Rush Alzheimer's Disease Center, Rush University Department of Neurological Sciences, Rush-Presbyterian-St. Luke's Medical Center, Chicago, IL

Joan K. Austin, DNS, MNS, RN
Distinguished Professor, Indiana University School of Nursing, Indianapolis, IN

Karlene K. Ball, PhD
Professor of Psychology and Director, Center for Research on Applied Gerontology, University of Alabama at Birmingham, Birmingham, AL

Anna M. Barrett, MD
Assistant Professor, Neurology and Behavioral Science, Penn State College of Medicine, Hershey, PA

Jason J. S. Barton, MD, PhD, FRCP(C)
Assistant Professor of Neurobiology, Harvard Medical School, Boston, MA; Adjunct Professor of Bioengineering, Boston University, Boston, MA; Associate Physician, Neurology and Ophthalmology, Beth Israel Deaconess Medical Center, Boston, MA

H. Richard Beresford, MD, JD
Professor of Neurology, University of Rochester School of Medicine, Rochester, NY; Adjunct Professor of Law, Cornell Law School, Ithaca, NY; Attending Neurologist, Strong Memorial Hospital, Rochester, NY; Chief of Neurology, Canandaigua Veterans Administration Medical Center, Canandaigua, NY

Gregg L. Caporaso, MD, PhD
Associate Research Scientist, Skirball Institute of Biomolecular Medicine, Molecular Neurobiology Program, New York University; Adjunct Clinical Assistant Professor of Neurology, Weill Medical College, Cornell University; Assistant Attending Neurologist, Department of Neurology and Neuroscience, New York Presbyterian Hospital; New York, NY

Lance W. Carluccio, PhD
Dean of Graduate Studies and Continuing Education, Salve Regina University, Newport, RI

Richard J. Caselli, MD
Professor of Neurology, Mayo Medical School, Rochester, MN; Chairman, Department of Neurology, Mayo Clinic, Scottsdale, AZ

Freeman Chakara, PsyD
Licensed Psychologist, Providence Behavioral Health Services, Leola, PA

Stanley L. Chapman, PhD
Associate Professor, Emory University School of Medicine, Atlanta, GA

Lawrence Charnas, MD, PhD
Assistant Professor of Pediatrics and Neurology, University of Minnesota, Minneapolis, MN; Director, Child Neurology Residency Program, University of Minnesota Medical School, Minneapolis, MN

Dawn Cisewski, PsyD
Neuropsychology Fellow, Department of Anatomy and Neurobiology, Boston University School of Medicine, Boston, MA

Edward David, MD, JD
Deputy Chief Medical Examiner, State of Maine, Augusta, ME

Debora A. Davidson, MS, OTR/L
Associate Professor, Occupational Therapy Program, Marysville University School of Health Professions, St. Louis, MO

John DeLuca, PhD
Professor, Departments of Physical Medicine and Rehabilitation and Neurosciences, University of Medicine and Dentistry of New Jersey – New Jersey Medical School, Newark, NJ; Director of Neuroscience Research, Kessler Medical Rehabilitation Research and Education Corporation, West Orange, NJ

Ricardo de Oliveira Souza, MD, PhD
Researcher, Cognitive Neuroscience and Behavioral Neurology Group LABS, D'Or Hospitals, Rio de Janeiro, Brazil; Professor of Neurology, Neurology Department, University of Rio de Janeiro, Rio de Janeiro, Brazil

Ashok Devasenapathy, MD
Assistant Professor of Neurology, Division of Cerebrovascular Diseases, Penn State College of Medicine, Hershey, PA

David W. Dunn, MD
Associate Professor, Departments of Psychiatry and Neurology, Indiana University School of Medicine, Indianapolis, IN; Director of Child and Adolescent Clinics, Riley Hospital for Children, Indianapolis, IN

Jerri D. Edwards, PhD
Postdoctoral Trainee, Center for Research on Applied Gerontology,
University of Alabama at Birmingham, Birmingham, AL

Philip S. Fastenau, PhD
Associate Professor, Department of Psychology, Indiana University—Purdue
University Indianapolis, Indianapolis, IN; Adjunct Assistant Professor of
Clinical Psychology, Department of Psychology, Indiana University School
of Medicine, Indianapolis, IN

Deema Fattal, MD
Assistant Professor, Neurology Department, and Director, Balance
Disorders Clinic, Neurology Department, Roy J. and Lucille A. Carver
College of Medicine, University of Iowa, Iowa City, IA

Christopher M. Filley, MD
Director, Behavioral Neurology Section and Professor of Neurology and
Psychiatry, University of Colorado School of Medicine, Denver, CO;
Attending Neurologist, University of Colorado Hospital, Denver Veterans
Affairs Medical Center, Denver, CO

Anne L. Foundas, MD
Associate Professor, Department of Psychiatry and Neurology, Tulane
University School of Medicine, New Orleans, LA; Neurology Service,
Department of Veterans Affairs Medical Center, New Orleans, LA

Clare J. Galton, MB BS, FRCP, MD, F Med Sci
Professor of Behavioural Neurology, University of Cambridge, Cambridge,
UK; Professor of Behavioural Neurology, MRC Cognition and Brain
Sciences Unit, Cambridge, UK

Joseph T. Giacino, PhD
Clinical Assistant Professor, Robert Wood Johnson Medical School, New
Brunswick, NJ; Associate Director of Neuropsychology, JFK Johnson
Rehabilitation Institute, Edison, NJ

Neill R. Graff-Radford, MBBCh, FRCP (London)
Chair, Department of Neurology, Mayo Clinic, Jacksonville, FL

Robert C. Green, MD
Associate Professor of Neurology, Genetics Program and Alzheimer's
Disease Center, Boston University School of Medicine, Boston, MA

Jeremy D. W. Greenlee, MD
Chief Resident, Department of Neurosurgery, Roy J. and Lucille A. Carver
College of Medicine, University of Iowa, Iowa City, IA

Mark Guttman, MD, FRCPC
Assistant Professor, Division of Neurology, Department of Medicine (cross
appointment with Department of Psychiatry), University of Toronto,
Toronto, Ontario, Canada; Director, Centre for Movement Disorders,
Markham, Ontario, Canada

Vladimir Hachinski, MD, FRCP(C), DSc
Professor of Neurology, Department of Clinical Neurological Sciences,
University of Western Ontario, London, Ontario, Canada

Sylvie Hébert , PhD
Assistant Professor, Faculté de médicine, Ecole d'Orthophonie et
Audiologie, Université de Montréal, Montréal, Quebec, Canada;
Researcher, Centre de Recherche, Institut Universitaire de Gériatrie de
Montréal, Montréal, Quebec, Canada

Peter Herscovitch, MD, FACP, FRCPC
Chief, PET Imaging Section, PET Department, The Warren Grant
Magnuson Clinical Center, National Institutes of Health, Bethesda, MD

David J. Hewitt, MD
Director, Neuroscience/Analgesia Research, Ortho-McNeil Pharmaceutical
Inc., Raritan, NJ

Jacqueline J. Hinckley, PhD
Assistant Professor, Department of Communication Sciences and Disorders,
University of South Florida, Tampa, FL

John R. Hodges, MD, FRCP
MRC Professor of Behavioral Neurology, MRC Cognition and Brain
Sciences Unit, Cambridge, UK

Stephen R. Hooper, PhD
Professor, University of North Carolina School of Education, University of
North Carolina School of Medicine Department of Psychiatry, and
University of North Carolina Department of Psychology, Chapel Hill, NC;
Associate Director, Clinical Center for the Study of Development and
Learning, Chapel Hill, NC

Matthew A. Howard III, MD
Professor of Neurosurgery and Head, Department of Neurosurgery, Roy J.
and Lucille A. Carver College of Medicine, University of Iowa, Iowa City, IA

Linda Hunt, PhD, OTR/L
Instructor, Flathead Valley Community College, Kalispel, MT

Todd J. Janus, PhD, MD
Assistant Professor, Departments of Neurological Sciences and Internal
Medicine (Oncology), Rush Medical College, Chicago, IL; Attending
Physician, Community Hospital, Munster, IN

R. D. Jones, PhD
Associate Professor, Clinical Neurology, Division of Behavioral Neurology
and Cognitive Neuroscience, Department of Neurology, Roy J. and
Lucille A. Carver College of Medicine, University of Iowa, Iowa City, IA

Douglas I. Katz, MD
Associate Professor, Neurology, Boston University School of Medicine,
Boston, MA; Medical Director, Brain Injury Programs, Healthsouth
Braintree Rehabilitation Hospital, Braintree, MA

Walter E. Kaufmann, MD
Associate Professor of Pathology, Neurology, Pediatrics, Psychiatry, and
Radiology, Johns Hopkins University School of Medicine, Baltimore, MD;
Pediatric Neuropathologist, Department of Pathology, Johns Hopkins
Hospital, Baltimore, MD; Neurologist, Division of Neurology and
Developmental Medicine, Kennedy Krieger Institute, Baltimore, MD

Howard S. Kirshner, MD
Professor and Vice Chair, Department of Neurology, Vanderbilt University
School of Medicine, Nashville, TN; Director, Vanderbilt Stroke Center,
Vanderbilt University Medical Center, Nashville, TN

Karl J. Kreder, MD
Professor of Urology, University of Iowa, Iowa City, IA; Vice Chair,
Department of Urology, University of Iowa Hospitals and Clinics,
University of Iowa, Iowa City, IA

Michelle V. Lambert, MBChB, MRCPsych, MSc
Honorary Clinical Lecturer, Department of Psychiatry, Newcastle
University, Newcastle, UK; Consultant Neuropsychiatrist, Neurobehavioral
Service, Hartside Clinic, St. Nicholas Hospital, Newcastle, UK

Jean Lengenfelder, PhD
Assistant Professor, Department of Physical Medicine and Rehabilitation,
University of Medicine and Dentistry of New Jersey – New Jersey Medical
School, Newark, NJ; Clinical Research Scientist, Neuropsychology and
Neuroscience Laboratory, Kessler Medical Rehabilitation Research and
Education Corporation, West Orange, NJ

Fern Leventhal, PhD
Neuropsychologist, Department of Neurology, New York University
Medical Center, New York, NY

Alicia G. Lischinsky, MD
Staff Psychiatrist, Cognitive and Behavioral Neurology Section, Department
of Neurology, Raul Carrea Institute for Neurological Research, Buenos
Aires, Argentina

Mark W. Mahowald, MD
Professor, Department of Neurology, University of Minnesota Medical
School, Minneapolis, MN; Director, Minnesota Regional Sleep Disorders
Center, Hennepin County Medical Center, Minneapolis, MN

Nigel V. Marsh, PhD
Reader in Clinical Psychology Research, School of Health and Social Care,
University of Teesside, Middlesbrough, United Kingdom

Michael F. Martelli, PhD, DAAPM
Clinical Associate Professor, Department of Rehabilitation Medicine,
University of Virginia, Charlottesville, VA; Clinical Associate Professor,
Departments of Psychiatry and Psychology, Virginia Commonwealth
University Health Sciences Center, Richmond, VA; Commissioner of
Psychology, Commission for Disability Examiner Certification, Midlothian,
VA; Director, Medical Psychology and Rehabilitation Neuropsychology,
Concussion Care Center of Virginia, Ltd., Glen Allen, VA

Catherine A. Mateer, PhD, ABPP/CN
Professor and Chair, Department of Psychology, University of Victoria,
Victoria, British Columbia, Canada

David J. McGonigle, PhD
Postdoctoral Fellow, Department of Radiology, University of California,
San Francisco, San Francisco, CA

Scott R. Millis, PhD
Associate Professor, Department of Physical Medicine and Rehabilitation, University of Medicine and Dentistry of New Jersey – New Jersey Medical School, Newark, NJ; Director, Office of Clinical Trials, Kessler Medical Rehabilitation Research and Education Corporation, West Orange, NJ

Jorge Moll, MD, PhD
Researcher, Cognitive Neuroscience and Behavioral Neurology Group LABS, D'Or Hospitals, Rio de Janeiro, Brazil; Visiting Professor, Department of Anatomy, Federal University of Rio de Janeiro, Rio de Janeiro, Brazil

Lidia M. Nagae-Poetscher, MD
Postdoctoral Fellow, School of Medicine, Kennedy Krieger Institute; Research Fellow, Radiology and Radiologic Science, Johns Hopkins University, Baltimore, MD

Ruth Nass, MD
Professor of Clinical Neurology, Department of Neurology, New York University Medical Center, New York, NY

Carissa Nehl, BS
Graduate Research Assistant, University of Iowa, Iowa City, IA

Jane S. Paulsen, PhD
Professor of Psychiatry, Neurology, Psychology, and Neuroscience, The University of Iowa Department of Psychiatry, Iowa City, IA; Director, Predict Huntington's Disease Research Program, Roy J. and Lucille A. Carver College of Medicine, University of Iowa, Iowa City, IA

Isabelle Peretz, PhD
Professor, Départment de Psychologie, Université de Montréal, Montréal, Quebec, Canada; Researcher, Centre de Recherche, Institut Universitaire de Gériatrie de Montréal, Montréal, Quebec, Canada

Jonathan H. Pincus, AB, MD, MA
Professor, Neurology and Chairman Emeritus, Neurology, Georgetown University, Washington, DC; Chief of Neurology, Veterans Administration Medical Center, Washington, DC

Thomas C. Pritchard, PhD
Associate Professor, Department of Neural and Behavioral Sciences, Penn State College of Medicine, Hershey, PA

Jeanette C. Ramer, MD
Associate Professor of Pediatrics and Medical Director of Pediatric Rehabilitation, Penn State College of Medicine and Children's Hospital, Hershey, PA

Satish S-C. Rao, MD, PhD, FRCP
Professor and Director, Neurogastroenterology and GI Motility, Roy J. and Lucille A. Carver College of Medicine, University of Iowa, Iowa City, IA

Mehrdad Razavi, MD
Clinical Associate, Division of Behavioral Neurology and Neuropsychology, Department of Neurology, Roy J. and Lucille A. Carver College of Medicine, University of Iowa, Iowa City, IA

Norman R. Relkin, MD, PhD
Associate Professor of Clinical Neurology and Neuroscience, Weill Medical College, Cornell University, New York, NY; Associate Attending Neurologist, New York Presbyterian Hospital, New York, NY; Director, Cornell Memory Disorders Program, New York Presbyterian Hospital, New York, NY

Timothy P. L. Roberts, PhD
Associate Professor, Director of Research, and Deputy Chair, Department of Medical Imaging, University of Toronto, Toronto, Ontario, Canada

Mary J. Roman, PhD
Clinical Neuropsychologist, Family Development Services, Camp Hill, PA

Karen L. Roos, MD
John and Nancy Nelson Professor of Neurology, Indiana University School of Medicine, Indianapolis, IN

Gail Ross, PhD
Associate Professor of Psychology in Pediatrics and Psychiatry, Weill Medical College of Cornell University, New York, NY; Director, Pediatric Psychology Program and Associate Attending in Pediatrics and Psychiatry, New York Presbyterian Hospital-Cornell Medical Center, New York, NY

Jeremy D. Schmahmann, MD
Associate Professor, Harvard Medical School, Boston, MA; Director, Ataxia Unit, Cognitive/Behavioral Neurology Unit, Massachusetts General Hospital, Boston, MA

Meryl A. Severson III, MD
Human Brain Research Laboratory Resident, Department of Neurosurgery, Roy J. and Lucille A. Carver College of Medicine, University of Iowa, Iowa City, IA

Elsa G. Shapiro, PhD
Professor of Pediatrics and Neurology, Director of Pediatric Neuropsychology Unit, Division of Pediatric Clinical Neuroscience, University of Minnesota Medical School, Minneapolis, MN

Sergio E. Starkstein, MD, PhD
Associate Professor, School of Psychiatry and Clinical Neurosciences, University of Western Australia, Fremantle Hospital, Fremantle, Western Australia, Australia

Pamela J. Thompson, PhD
Head of Psychological Services, National Society for Epilepsy, Gerrards Cross, Bucks, UK; Consultant Neuropsychologist, Department of Clinical and Experimental Epilepsy, Institute of Neurology, London, UK

Jon Tippin, MD
Assistant Professor (Clinical), Department of Neurology, Roy J. and Lucille A. Carver College of Medicine, University of Iowa, Iowa City, IA; Private practice, Medford Neurological Clinic, Medford, OR

Daniel Tranel, PhD
Chief, Benton Neuropsychology Laboratory and Professor of Neurology, Department of Neurology, Roy J. and Lucille A. Carver College of Medicine, University of Iowa, Iowa City, IA

Michael Trimble, BSc; M Phil; MD; FRCP; FRCPsych
Professor of Behavioral Neurology, The Institute of Neurology, University College, Queen Square, London, UK

David E. Vance, PhD
Postdoctoral Trainee, Center for Research on Applied Gerontology, University of Alabama at Birmingham, Birmingham, AL

Shaun P. Vecera, PhD
Associate Professor, Department of Psychology, University of Iowa, Iowa City, IA

Virginia G. Wadley, PhD
Res. Assistant Professor of Psychology and Assistant Director, Center for Research on Applied Gerontology, University of Alabama at Birmingham, Birmingham, AL

JianLi Wang, MD, PhD
Postdoctoral Scholar, Department of Radiology (Center for NMR Research), Penn State College of Medicine, Hershey, PA

Jeffrey S. Wefel, PhD
Neuropsychology Fellow, Department of Neuro-Oncology, University of Texas M.D. Anderson Cancer Center, Houston, TX

Michael Weinrich, MD
Director, National Center for Medical Rehabilitation Research, National Institute of Child Health and Human Development, NIH, Bethesda, MD

Kathleen A. Welsh-Bohmer, PhD
Associate Professor, Department of Psychiatry, Duke University Medical Center, Durham, NC

Ernest W. Willoughby, MBChB, FRACP
Consultant Neurologist, Auckland Hospital, Auckland, New Zealand

Qing Yang, PhD
Associate Professor, Department of Radiology (Center for NMR Research), Penn State College of Medicine, Hershey, PA

Nathan D. Zasler, MD, FAAPM&R, FAADEP, DAAPM, CIME
CEO and Medical Director, Concussion Care Centre of Virginia, Ltd.; CEO and Medical Director, Tree of Life Services, Inc.; Medical Consultant, Pinnacle Rehabilitation, Inc.; Glen Allen, VA

Richard Ziegler, PhD
Assistant Professor of Pediatrics and Neurology, Director of Training, Pediatric Neuropsychology, Division of Pediatric Clinical Neuroscience, University of Minnesota Medical School, Minneapolis, MN

PLATE 1

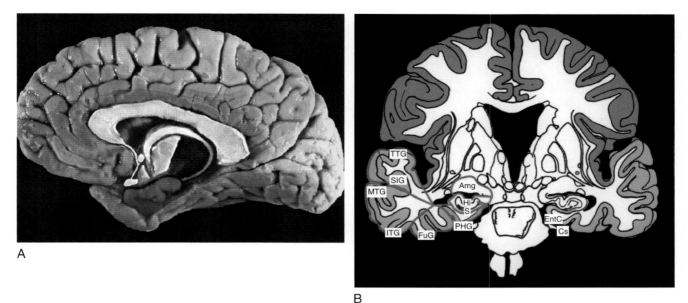

FIGURE 4-1. *A,* Distribution of Alzheimer-type pathology. Tangle and plaque density are highest in the medial temporal lobe (*red*) and spread out to decreasing color intensity areas. *B,* Illustration of the anatomy of the temporal lobe. Amg, amygdala; CS, collateral sulcus; EntC, entorhinal cortex; FuG, fusiform gyrus; Hi, hippocampus; ITG, inferior temporal gyrus; MTG, middle temporal gyrus; PHG, parahippocampal gyrus; S, subiculum; STG, superior temporal gyrus; TTG, transverse temporal gyrus. (*A,* Adapted from Braak H, Braak E: Neuropathological stages of Alzheimer's disease, in DeLeon MJ [ed]: An Atlas of Alzheimer's Disease. London: Parthenon Publishing Group, 1991. *B,* Adapted from Assheur J, Mai JK, Paxinos G: Atlas of the Human Brain. San Diego, CA: Academic Press, 1998.)

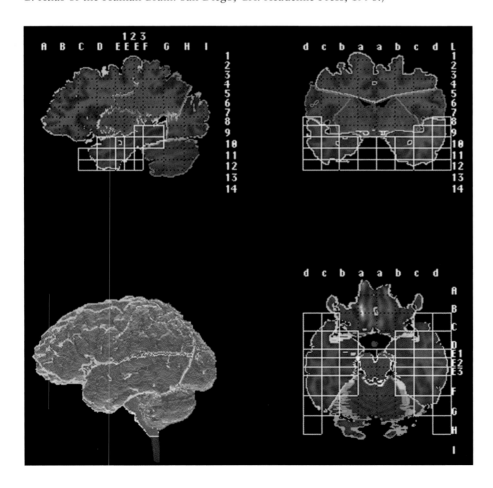

FIGURE 5-6. Talairach coordinate system. The brain has been positionally normalized, and Talairach sectors designated as representing the temporal lobe are shown superimposed (as white boxes), in the three orthogonal views, over manually derived sulcal-based "gold standard regions" (in color). In this example, the temporal lobe (yellow) volume would be calculated by adding the temporal lobe-designated voxels in all slices. (Reprinted from Kates WR, Warsofsky IS, Patwardhan A, et al: Automated Talairach atlas-based parcellation and measurement of cerebral lobes in children. Psychiatry Res 91:11–30, 1999, by permission of Elsevier Science B. V.)

PLATE 2

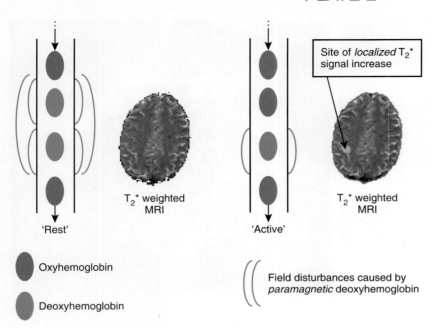

FIGURE 7-1. Schematic representation of how differences in the ratio of (paramagnetic) deoxyhemoglobin to oxyhemoglobin in blood vessels leads to differences in T2* shortening effects in surrounding tissue. These can be detected using the appropriate MR pulse sequences (see text) and is the basis of the blood oxygenation level dependent (BOLD) contrast mechanism, widely used in fMRI.

FIGURE 7-2. A more detailed examination of the link between neuronal function and BOLD fMRI. The uppermost figure shows the typically conceptualized concept of baseline activity, where a low local rate of firing in the neurons whose axonal terminals lie in the region served by the arteriole and venule does not lead to any changes in the local concentration of deoxyhemoglobin (although it is still unknown if spontaneous discharge of this kind from a given region will cause a detectable BOLD effect or not). When these neurons undergo a net increase in activity (which may translate as an increase in the firing rate or firing synchrony), the accompanying increase in local CBF causes an increase in the ratio of oxyhemoglobin to deoxyhemoglobin (seen in the figure as the increase in red in the venule). This effect is thought at present to underlie the increase in MR signal seen in BOLD fMRI studies.

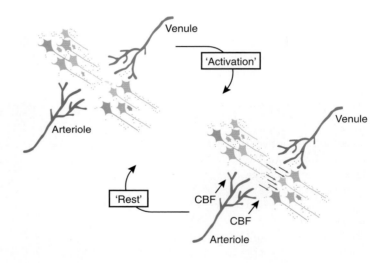

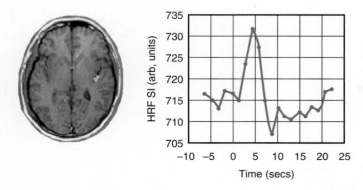

FIGURE 7-3. The temporal form of MR signal changes to an isolated stimulus—the hemodynamic response function (hrf). In this example, acquired at 1.5 T using 1.5-second temporal resolution in an event-related paradigm, BOLD signal changes were observed in a few highlighted pixels of auditory cortex (left). Interrogating these pixels for the time course of their signal change (right), it is apparent that the BOLD signal changes achieve a peak approximately 4.5 to 6 seconds after the stimulus, and this is followed by a signal undershoot before eventual recovery to baseline after approximately 15 to 20 seconds.

PLATE 3

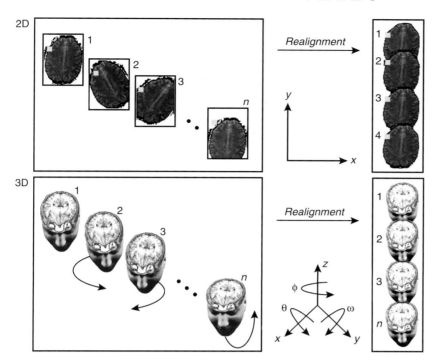

FIGURE 7-6. Subject movement and realignment. The top panel illustrates how subject movement can be problematic when movement is limited to within the axial imaging plane (i.e., a two-dimensional [2D] problem). Even in this simplified case, it is obvious that subject movement has an impact on the tissue content of the example voxel (in yellow). The inferior panel shows the more familiar case with humans, in which movement is truly a three-dimensional (3D) problem (modeled with six parameters by most rigid-body realignment algorithms).

FIGURE 7-7. The effect of using different correlation thresholds on activation maps. Two successive single axial slices (5 mm thick) are shown coregistered with the result of a correlation analysis using a simple shifted 'boxcar' as the regressor of interest (active voxels are shown in yellow). It is evident that, though it is possible to lower one's threshold to get "activated" voxels, doing so will, of course, increase the false-positive rate of the experiment. The large amount of voxels identified as "active" in the figure, even at "high" correlation thresholds, points to the importance of using a correction factor that takes into account the number of statistical tests being performed across the imaging volume.

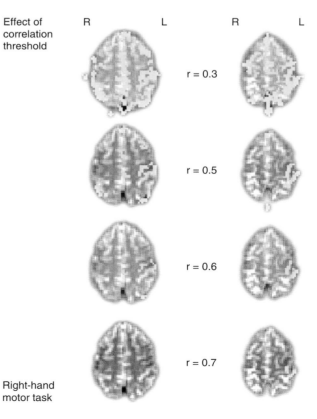

Effect of correlation threshold

Right-hand motor task

PLATE 4

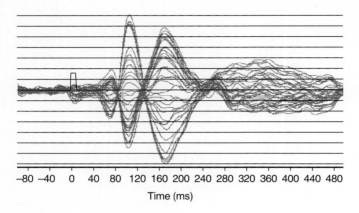

FIGURE 7-11. A neuromagnetic evoked field. In this representation the magnetic field detected by a 37-channel array biomagnetometer in response to presentation of 1-kHz sinusoidal auditory stimulus is shown collapsed onto a common axis. The time-domain duration of the displayed evoked response is 500 msec, with 100 msec of "baseline" sampled prior to stimulus onset. The peak amplitude of the evoked field occurs approximately 100 msec after the stimulus (the M100 component) and has an amplitude of approximately 100 fT (root mean square across sensor channels).

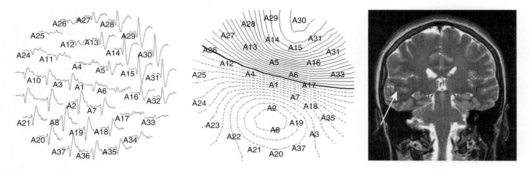

FIGURE 7-12. Magnetic source imaging. *Left,* The time-domain representation of 37 spatially distinct sensor channel signals in response to auditory stimulation (1 kHz sinusoid). *Center,* At the M100 peak (determined by maximum root mean square signal), the instantaneous magnetic field across the sensor array can be plotted in contour form. *Right,* Single equivalent current dipole modeling of this magnetic field distribution, combined with coregistration (via external landmarks) with MRIs allows the creation of an MSI, combining anatomic and functional information in a single image.

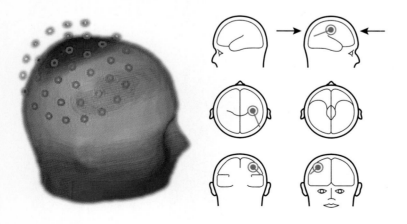

FIGURE 7-13. *Left,* An alternative representation of evoked response data is to plot the instantaneous magnetic field distribution at the peak of an evoked response (in this case contralateral somatosensory stimulation of the thumb) over the three-dimensional reconstructed surface of the head. This representation invites comparison with some typical EEG topographic descriptions. *Right,* A single current source (vector shown in various planes) describes approximately 90% of the measurement variance. In this software package (BESA2000, MEGIS Software GmbH, Gräfelfing, Germany), additional focal current sources can be introduced to account for residual variance.

PLATE 5

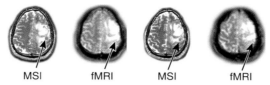

MSI fMRI MSI fMRI

FIGURE 7-14. Similarity of fMRI and MSI sources of right sensorimotor activation in a patient with a large left hemisphere glioma. In this subject, despite underlying neurophysiologic differences between MSI and fMRI and despite the presence of the mass lesion, both fMRI and MSI indicate the encroachment of the posterior margin of the tumor on functional eloquent cortex.

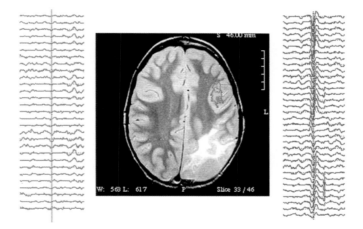

FIGURE 7-15. Application of MEG to spontaneous recording of interictal discharges in patients with seizure disorders. In this patient with nevus syndrome, an interictal event is detected in the sensor array positioned over the left hemisphere; no abnormal activity is detected over the right hemisphere. Single equivalent dipole modeling of this event and other similar spontaneous recordings point to a focal left frontal source (*yellow area*). This was found to correlate with the modeled source of seizure onset itself.

PLATE 6

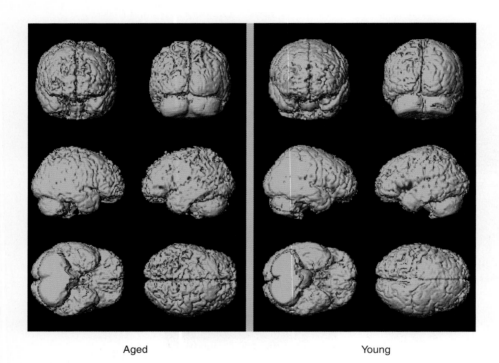

Aged   Young

FIGURE 15-3. Functional magnetic resonance image (fMRI) of aged (*left*) and young (*right*) normal volunteers showing areas of brain activation (red areas) after exposure to odorants. Significant areas of activation included the primary olfactory cortex (anterior olfactory nucleus, olfactory tubercle, frontal and piriform cortex, and amygdala), the insula, and prefrontal regions.

PLATE 7

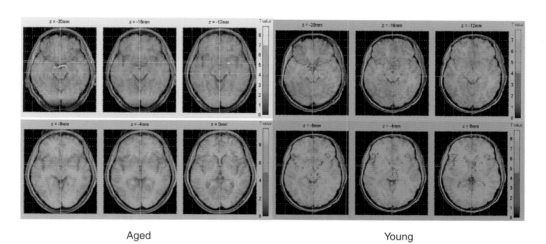

Aged   Young

FIGURE 15-4. Olfactory fMRI maps in the axial plane from aged (*left*) and young (*right*) groups showing areas of statistically significant activation ($P < 0.001$). Stronger activation was observed in the major olfactory-related structures of the young group compared to the aged group ($P = 0.035$).

PLATE 8

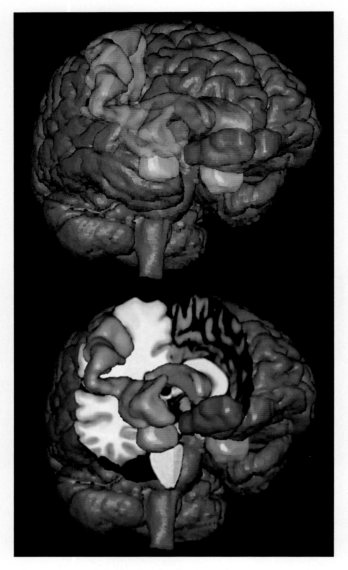

FIGURE 21-2. Neuroanatomy of a few of the structures implicated in processing emotion. Three-dimensional renderings of the amygdala (yellow), ventromedial prefrontal cortex (red), right somatosensory cortices (S-I, S-II, and insula; green) and for orientation the lateral ventricles (light blue) were obtained from segmentation of these structures from serial magnetic resonance images of a normal human brain. The structures were corendered with a three-dimensional reconstruction of the normal brain (top) and a reconstruction of the brain with the anterior right quarter removed to clearly show location of the internal structures (bottom). Images prepared by Ralph Adolphs, Hanna Damasio, and John Haller, Human Neuroimaging and Neuroanatomy Laboratory.

PLATE 9

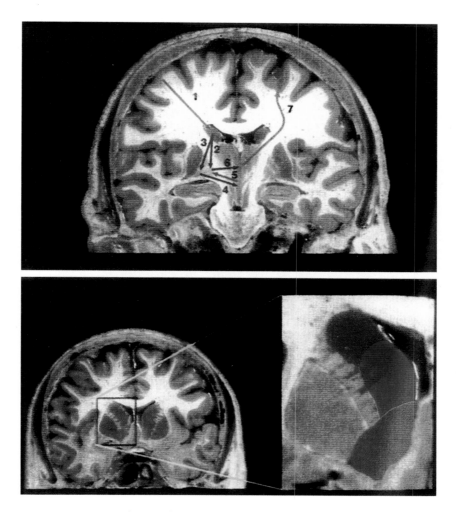

FIGURE 24-1. Frontal-striatal projections. Brain sections illustrating the frontal-subcortical circuits. Top, The direct and indirect circuits (red arrows indicate excitatory connections and blue arrows indicate inhibitory connections). (1) Excitatory gultamatergic corticostriatal fibers. (2) Direct inhibitory g-aminobutyric acid (GABA)/substance P fibers (associated with D1 dopamine receptors) from the striatum to the globus pallidus interna/substantia nigra pars reticulata. (3) Indirect inhibitory GABA/enkephalin fibers (associated with D2 dopamine receptors) from the striatum to the globus pallidus externa. (4) Indirect inhibitory GABA fibers from the globus pallidus externa to the subthalamic nucleus. (5) Indirect excitatory glutamatergic fibers from the subthalamic nucleus to the globus pallidus interna/substantia nigra pars reticulata. (6) Basal ganglia inhibitory outflow via GABA fibers from the globus pallidus interna/substantia nigra pars reticulata to specific thalamic sites. (7) Thalamic excitatory fibers returning to the cortex (shown in the contralateral hemisphere for convenience). Bottom, The general segregated anatomy of the oculomotor (purple), dorsolateral prefrontal (blue), orbitofrontal (green), anterior cingulated (red), and motor (yellow) circuits in the striatum. (From Litvan I, Paulsen JS, Mega MS, et al: Neuropsychiatric assessment of patients with hyperkinetic and hypokinetic movement disorders. Arch Neurol 55:1313–1319, 1998. Copyright 1998 by the American Medical Association. Reprinted by permission.)

PLATE 10

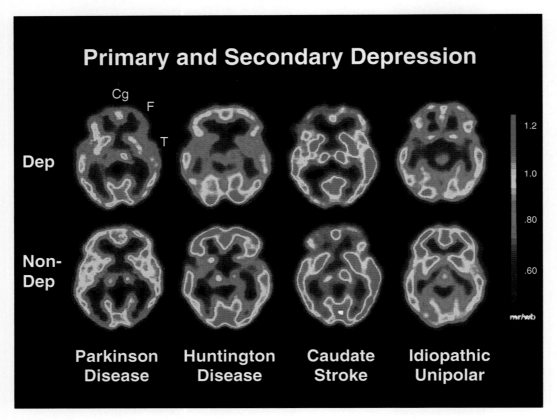

FIGURE 24-5. Depression in movement disorders. Paralimbic hypometabolism common to patients with primary and secondary depression. ^{18}F-fluoro-2-deoxyglucose (FDG) positron emission tomography (PET) studies of patients with secondary depression identify the bilateral ventral frontal (F), anterior temporal (T), and anterior cingulated (Cg) hypometabolism that characterizes the depressive syndrome, independently of underlying disease etiology. Images are individual patients. (From Mayberg HS: Depression and frontal-subcortical circuits: Focus on pre-frontal-limbic interactions, in Lechter DG, Cummings JL [eds]: Frontal-Subcortical Circuits in Psychiatric and Neurological Disorders. New York: Guilford Press, 2001, pp. 177–206. Copyright 2001 by The Guilford Press. Reprinted by permission.)

PLATE 11

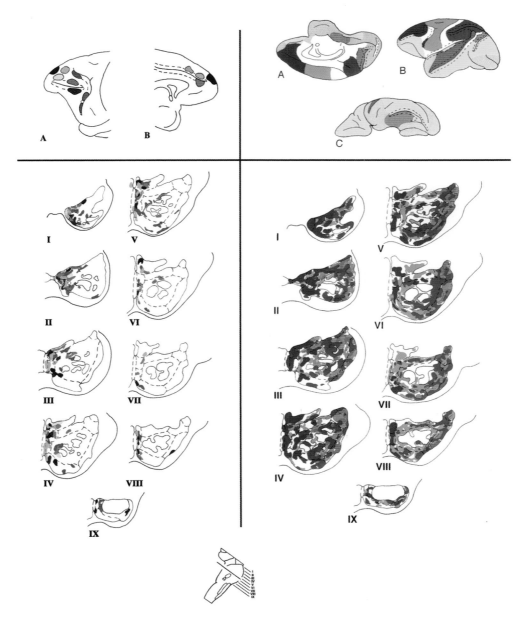

FIGURE 25-11. Color-coded summary diagrams of the corticopontine projections from associative, paralimbic, and motor cortices in the rhesus monkey. *Left,* Tract tracers (tritiated amino acids) were injected into selected architectonic regions of the prefrontal cortices of rhesus monkeys, and the termination patterns of the anterogradely transported label in the nuclei of the basilar pons were identified. Each color represents a single case. Terminations are mostly in the medial part of the pons, and each cortical area has its own unique set of terminations in the basilar pontine nuclei. Lateral prefrontal cortex in *A,* medial surface in *B.* Levels I (rostral) through IX (caudal) of the basilar pons are shown, as seen in the schematic of the brainstem below. *Right,* In this composite diagram, corticopontine projections are seen from the prefrontal cortices (purple), posterior parietal area (blue), superior temporal region (red), posterior parahippocampal and parastriate cortices (orange), and motor and supplementary motor cortices (green). Each cortical area has its own region of termination in the pons. The associative and paralimbic projections are not overshadowed by the motor projections. Areas in the cerebral hemispheres in yellow and gray do not project to the pons (yellow, as shown by anterograde and retrograde techniques; gray as shown by retrograde techniques). Medial surface of the rhesus monkey brain is shown in *A,* lateral surface in *B,* orbital surface in *C.* (*Left* From Schmahmann JD, Pandya DN: Anatomic organization of the basilar pontine projections from prefrontal cortices in rhesus monkey. J Neurosci 17:438−458, 1997. *Right* From Schmahmann JD: From movement to thought: Anatomic substrates of the cerebellar contribution to cognitive processing. Hum Brain Mapping 4:174−198, 1996).

PLATE 12

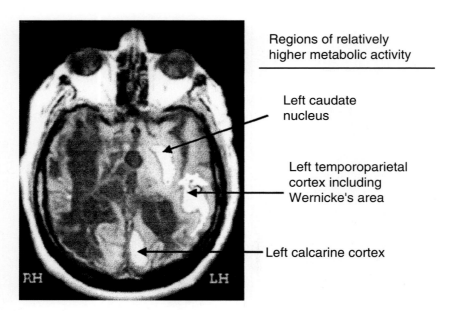

Regions of relatively higher metabolic activity

Left caudate nucleus

Left temporoparietal cortex including Wernicke's area

Left calcarine cortex

RH   LH

FIGURE 30-2. Coregistered image of positron emission tomography with ^{18}fluorodeoxyglucose (FDG-PET) with magnetic resonance imaging (MRI) of a woman in a vegetative state for more than 20 years after arteriovenous malformation hemorrhages. The patient had no evidence of command following, communication, or other purposeful behavior, but she displayed intelligible verbalization of single words every 24 to 72 hours. The FDG-PET study indicated that average global cerebral metabolism was reduced to 43% of normal; however the left frontal operculum, left superior temporal gyrus, and left basal ganglia remained active at 50% to 60% of normal. Regions of relatively higher metabolism are bright areas (*arrows*). The patient's capacity to generate words may represent a "fixed motor action pattern" mediated by remnant circuits of the speech module but unrelated to intentional language function (Reproduced with permission from Schiff ND, Ribary U, Plum F, et al: Words without mind. J Cogn Neurosci 11:650–656, 1999.)

Preface

Principles and Practice of Behavioral Neurology and Neuropsychology seeks to present a pragmatic and evidence-based approach to cognitive, behavioral, and adaptive impairments caused by neurologic, traumatic, and medical disorders. Neurobehavioral and neuropsychological impairments generate huge global costs in terms of medical bills, suffering, disability, and death. In addition to reducing these human burdens, recognition and management of symptoms and signs associated with these disorders also provide clues to the operations of the human mind.

The book begins with an overview of key issues in behavioral neurology and neuropsychology, and covers many specific topics in 55 subsequent chapters. The subject matter is comprehensive and wide ranging, and required the input of specialists with a variety of insights on medicine, human factors engineering, psychology, radiology, pediatrics, public health, public policy, and law. Effective response to these issues requires coordinated efforts of primary care providers and relevant specialists, utilizing shared knowledge, and the cross-fertilization of ideas. We hope this book contributes to these ends.

M.R.
P.J.E.

Acknowledgments

We wish to express our gratitude to Dr. Arthur Benton for his knowledge, encouragement, and sage advice over many years. The breadth and depth of this volume, as described in his Foreword, would not have been possible without his steady influence and vision for our fields and our training. We are extremely indebted to the chapter authors for their creative contributions and timely responses to our extensive editorial advice.

We thank Dr. Daniel Tranel for his early discussion of this project and Mrs. Anita Makuluni for her initial conversations on format and didactic devices. We are grateful to several of our colleagues for taking time to review and advance some of the materials in this volume, including Dr. Steven Anderson, Dr. Richard Hichwa, Dr. Daniel Bonthius, Dr. Ergun Uc, Dr. Richard Tenser, Dr. George Blackall, Ms. Ida Kellison, Mrs. Nicole Skaar, Dr. Stefanie Griffin, Dr. Sonya Mehta, Ms. Janell Behnke, Ms. Jennifer Taylor, and Mr. Nathan Salinas.

We thank our many colleagues in the University of Iowa Department of Neurology and its Head, Dr. Antonio Damasio, as well as colleagues at Penn State University/Hershey Medical Center in the Neurology Department and especially the Developmental Pediatrics and Learning Division, and its Director, Dr. Keith Verner, for fostering collaborative and productive academic environments and making available departmental resources necessary for completing this work. We are especially indebted to Dr. Carol Devore for her tireless and patient assistance in all phases of this project, from contact and communication between authors, editors, and publishers, to content and quality of the material.

Many mentors and colleagues have also been critical to the formation and completion of this project, including Dr. Paul Eslinger, Dr. Frank Terrell, the late Dr. H. Wayne Ludvigson, Dr. Ray Remley, and Dr. Rusty Gage, who nurtured and supported the earliest stirrings of brain-behavior curiosity and science methods. Dr. Antonio Damasio, Dr. Hanna Damasio, and Dr. Gary W. Van Hoesen have been instrumental in melding our clinical and scientific approaches to the difficult questions about brain and behavior that continue to drive our investigations and the search for solutions. Dr. Mark Nawrot, Dr. Warren Darling, Dr. Randall Blake, Dr. Robert Sekuler, Dr. Karlene Ball, and Dr. Cynthia Owsley have been constant friends and advisors to Dr. Matthew Rizzo on a wide range of research matters of relevance to this book. Dr. Rizzo also thanks Dr. David Forkenbrock, Director, Public Policy Center; Dean P. Barry Butler, College of Engineering; Dr. Craig Zwerling, Director, Injury Prevention Research Center; and their respective faculty and staff.

We thank the individuals at Elsevier/Saunders including Susan Pioli, Joan Sinclair, Jennifer Ehlers, Laurie Anello, and Faith Voit, and at P. M. Gordon Associates, including Peggy M. Gordon, Denise Bracken, and Janine White for their help along the road to publication. Thanks to Allan Ross who helped us get started.

This work was supported by NIA AG15071 (MR), NIA AG17177 (MR), and NIH PONS 19632 (MR); NIH 1-EB00454-01A1 (PJE); and the Children, Youth and Family Consortium/Division of Developmental Pediatrics and Learning of Penn State University (PJE).

Dr. Matthew Rizzo is deeply grateful to Michael and Evelyn for nurturing his curiosity and to Annie, Ellie, and Frannie for their enduring support. Dr. Paul Eslinger is deeply grateful to Vicki, Alicia, Ryan, and Luke for their enduring support, and dedicates this volume to Fran, Bill, and Ken, his best friends.

Foreword

Behavioral neurology/neuropsychology is concerned with the reciprocal relationships of the nervous system: *reciprocal* because two issues are addressed—the question of which alterations in nervous function and structure influence mentation and behavior, and the question of the effects of experience on the functioning, and indeed the structure, of the nervous system itself. That is to say, studies of brain-behavior relationships must consider the human brain as an outcome, as well as a cause, as a dependent, as well as an independent, variable.

Although there are recognized specialists in behavioral neurology/neuropsychology, the field is not a conventional discipline but rather a broad sphere of interest to which experts in different disciplines, medical and nonmedical, have made important contributions—neurologists and psychologists, anatomists and physiologists, neonatologists and gerontologists, engineers and physicists, as well as experts in the fields of industrial management and public policy. The editors of this work, both of whom are well-known productive investigators in the field, know this very well. That is why their treatise is so far-reaching and comprehensive, dealing with issues such as problems in the assessment of driving competence and the elderly, criminal behavior, and legal questions.

The nature of the relationships between brain and behavior has been the subject of serious empirical study since the 1600s, when the brain definitively displaced the heart as the organ of mentation. Over the centuries, neuroscientists have generated a large mass of interesting and useful findings about these relationships. The radical technological advances of the past 25 years, reflected largely (but not exclusively) in the remarkable neuroimaging approaches at our disposal, have opened the way to ever more incisive empirical studies of the basic questions. There is every reason to expect that this development will continue. The result must be a broader, deeper, and more fruitful field of normal and abnormal brain function in relation to thinking and conduct. In this comprehensive, forward-looking volume, Matt Rizzo and Paul Eslinger have given us a vision of what is likely to be the new approach to the longstanding "mind-brain" question.

Arthur Benton, PhD
Professor Emeritus,
Departments of Neurology
and Psychology and
Founder,
Benton Neuropsychology Laboratory,
Roy J. and Lucille A.
Carver College of Medicine,
University of Iowa,
Iowa City, Iowa

Overview and Introduction

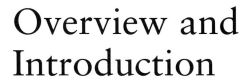

Overview and Introduction

Matthew Rizzo

Paul J. Eslinger

SCOPE OF THE PROBLEM

Neurologic disease, aging, trauma, and stress provoke a broad spectrum of brain pathophysiology that causes deficits in human behavior. The recognition and treatment of these deficits can relieve human suffering and disability and also provide unique clues to the organization and operations of the human mind. Neurobehavioral impairments also generate incalculable costs due to medical bills, insurance premiums, legal fees, taxes, lost work and wages, disability, pain, suffering, and family disruption, and fuel global debates in medical ethics, philosophy, public health policy, legislation, and research agendas.

The magnitude of neurobehavioral-related problems is a world wide health concern. Millions of people suffer stroke, traumatic brain injury (TBI), Alzheimer disease (AD) and other dementias, brain infections, tumors, and epilepsy every year. In the United States alone, there are almost 10 million stroke and TBI survivors, with an associated economic burden that approaches 90 billion dollars annually (Thurman & Guerrero, 1999; American Heart Association, 2000a,

2000b). Each year two million more people in the United States suffer stroke or TBI. The recent World Health Report 2002 from the World Health Organization (WHO, 2002), sounded a startling wake-up call to global communities about reducing the risks for illness and promoting healthy lifestyles as well as human environments. Not surprisingly, brain-based disorders were found to be the leading cause of disability worldwide, covering the spectrum of neuro-psychiatric disorders, injuries, stroke, infections, neoplasms, and nutritional and maternal/perinatal conditions. The latter contribute to the rising number of neurobehavioral disorders and add to the burden due to increasing adult-onset illness, trauma, and disabilty. (See URL: http://www.who.int/whr/2002, where a summary and further information are available in English, French, Chinese, Arabic, Russian, and Spanish.) The report emphasizes that reducing risks to health has been a human undertaking dating back at least 5,000 years to some of the earliest civilizations. Reducing such risks today is more vital than ever. This is accomplished through national and international health policies, and the one-to-one patient-provider contact that takes place in millions of offices, clinics, and hospitals every day. The most effective health policies and practices depend upon scientific research and translation of scientific findings into the daily tasks and activities that promote healthy lives and environments. The evidence assembled in this book is geared toward improving the recognition, diagnosis, and treatment of many brain-based disorders that occur in children and adults and that cause disability and death.

In this regard, many pathfinders in behavioral neurology and neuropsychology deserve much credit, such as Geschwind (1965), Benton (1975), Damasio and Damasio (1989), Grant and Adams (1996), Taylor (1999), Mesulam (2000), Kirshner (2002), Feinberg and Farah (2003), Heilman and Valenstein (2003), Pincus and Tucker (2003). Their textbooks have helped define and shape current understanding of the breadth and depth of brain-based disorders and their effects on human behavior. Naturally, new scientific and practical issues continue to emerge and new problems must be solved. For example, what is the best treatment approach to neurologic patients with comorbid psychiatric disorders (e.g., AD, Huntington chorea, attention-deficit/hyperactivity disorder [ADHD], TBI), and how should such services be provided? What is the role of neurology and neuropsychology in primary psychiatric disorders whose neural substrates are finally coming to light (e.g., schizophrenia, obsessive-compulsive disorder)? Which specialty referrals or tests are appropriate? What treatments are effective, when should they conclude, and how should we track improvement? When should a patient return to work, or is he or she disabled, and if so, how much and in what ways?

Tragic outcomes in children and adult patients may result within evolving health care delivery systems (such as managed care/managed cost) due to inadequate time, resources, training, and insensitivity to the complexities of these cognitive and behavioral cases. Restricted access to specialty care, in addition to inadequate training and resources applied to these behavioral cases, may lead to medical errors caused by misdiagnosis, overmedication, and inadequate or wrong test selection. Inaccurate predictions regarding a patient's functioning at work, in school, and in key activities such as automobile driving may lead to further suffering, doctor shopping, family and social problems, and costs to society. Effective responses to these issues require coordinated efforts from primary providers together with relevant specialists, a shared body of knowledge, and better cross-fertilization of ideas. We hope this book contributes to these ends.

Principles and Practice of Behavioral Neurology and Neuropsychology seeks to present a pragmatic and evidence-based approach to cognitive and behavioral impairments caused by neurologic, traumatic, and medical disorders. The primary aim of the volume is to advance the care of patients who present with perceptual, cognitive, language, memory, emotional, and many other behavioral symptoms associated with these disorders. Materials are presented at a scientific level that is appropriate for a wide variety of providers including neurologists, psychiatrists, psychologists, physiatrists, geriatricians, neuropsychologists, other primary caregivers who care for patients in routine and specialty practices, and students, interns, residents, and fellows.

BRAIN-BASED AND BRAIN-RELATED DISORDERS

Primary Brain Disorders

Common causes of primary brain disorders and acquired cognitive deficits include cerebrovascular disease, cancer, head trauma, demyelinating disorders, infection, toxins, epilepsy, aging, and age-related diseases including AD, Parkinson disease, and related neurodegenerative disorders. The massive burden of these conditions is a function of sheer patient numbers, age of onset, and misery (Bergen & Silberberg, 2002; Grann & Neugut, 2003). Brain pathophysiology affects not only cognition and behavior, but also emotion, personality, and vegetative functions including eating, sleeping, procreation, and elimination. Patients may complain of pain, urinary incontinence, sexual dysfunction, and depression; they may fail to meet personal, professional, and social responsibilities, become unable to conduct key daily activities such as automobile driving, or fail to render self-care. Neurodegenerative disorders represent a growing burden, given current demographic projections of an aging population. Compounding the problem, some patients are completely unaware they have any impairments (i.e., anosognosia).

Acquired brain lesions are more common in the elderly. These patients may already have neural decline resulting in decreased memory and processing speed due to normal aging mechanisms (see Chapters 36 and 22) that may be amenable to cognitive training interventions (Ball et al., 2002). These cognitive changes may be the result of aging in the endocrine system, with potentially treatable declines in estrogen (in menopause), androgen (e.g., testosterone deficiency in andropause), and growth hormone/insulin-like growth factor (in "somatopause") (Lamberts, 2002).

Secondary Brain-Related Disorders

Brain-related disorders can result from impaired and altered functioning of the body's many systems (i.e., immune, endocrine, and visceral-autonomic) that, in turn, exert abnormal influence back upon the brain. For example, damage to the hypothalamic-pituitary axis caused by tumor or trauma can disrupt production of psychoactive hormones (such as thyroxine, cortisol, androgens, growth hormone, and prolactin) or cause systemic electrolyte disturbances (as in diabetes insipidus). Metabolic, cardiovascular, respiratory, and gastrointestinal diseases undermine the complex bodily environment that provides crucial support for the brain (Table 1). Although only 3% of body weight on average, the brain requires up to 20% of the oxygenated blood supply to function normally, indicating its exquisite sensitivity to bodily functioning.

Common medical conditions often impair cognitive functioning by several mechanisms at once. For instance, a diabetic patient may be confused as a result of hypoglycemia, cerebrovascular disease, and side effects of analgesic medicine for painful neuropathy. An alcoholic patient may be cognitively impaired due to

TABLE 1. Medical Conditions Associated with Cognitive Impairments

Cancer: chemotherapy, radiation, immunologic gastrointestinal
Cardiac: watershed infarctions, cardiac arrest
Organ transplantation
Chronic pain syndromes
Endocrine
Hepatic
Renal
Toxic
Pulmonary (e.g., sleep apnea)
Autoimmune
Other metabolic (delirium)

acute intoxication, stroke (e.g., caused by atrial fibrillation and cardiomyopathy with "holiday heart"), meningitis, sepsis, thiamine deficiency (causing Wernicke-Korsakoff syndrome), seizures, anticonvulsant toxicity, liver failure, subdural hematoma, and alcohol-induced dementia. Cancer patients may have cognitive decline associated with depression, side effects of chemotherapy and radiation, opportunistic brain infections, brain metastases, or limbic encephalitis. Acquired immune deficiency syndrome (AIDS) patients may develop encephalitis due to human immunodeficiency virus (HIV) or opportunistic infections, central nervous system (CNS) lymphoma, and other causes. Interest in behavioral effects of general medical conditions has had positive effects, including renewed efforts at understanding the quality of life and the level of suffering caused by varieties of disease.

Mind-Brain-Body Interactions

In addition to primary brain and primary body systems, *mind-brain-body interactions* have a significant effect on health risks, disease onset, and health outcomes. These important interactions depend on and contribute to a patient's mood, personality, self-perception, situational awareness, and reaction to environmental stress, including disease. Mental and emotional stresses may pathologically alter mind-brain-body interactions. Chronic stress from environmental, interpersonal, vocational, and intrapsychic causes (including depression, illness, anxiety, panic, and obsessive-compulsive disorders [OCD]) may increase gastric acid secretion, leading to development of ulcers (in stomachs that carry *Helicobacter pylori*). Chronic stress may also lead to irritable bowel syndrome, menstrual cycle disorders, sexual dysfunction, toxic effects on brain structures, psychosocial dwarfism and related neurodevelopmental disturbances, cardiac disease, fatigue, dysphoria, pain, and other somatic complaints, nightmares, and sleep disturbances. Sleep disorders reduce cognitive performance, as in depression, obstructive sleep apnea syndrome, and Parkinson disease (PD). Extreme fright may result in chronic behavioral complaints as in post-traumatic stress disorder, or might even prove acutely fatal (Sylvester, 2002). These are health issues that we clearly cannot afford to ignore and on which we all should be better informed.

The Special Case of Neurodevelopmental Disorders

Cognitive and behavioral impairments are also prevalent in childhood and affect learning and development in children with a variety of conditions, including Down syndrome and other causes of mental retardation, autism, Asperger and Rett syndromes; epilepsy; and chronic diseases including cancer, diabetes, neurodegenerative disorders, muscular dystrophy; and chronic infection including HIV. Understanding the natural history of these childhood conditions is beneficial to managing these conditions into adulthood. Some children have subtle and relatively specific cognitive defects in the context of normal intellect, and would fare better with early diagnosis and intervention, as in children with developmental dyslexia who present with slow reading, word transpositions, and reduced reading comprehension. Others, with autism or forms of mental retardation, may never function independently, yet can perform satisfying and meaningful activities with educational accommodations (see Chapters 43 and 44). A patient with Down syndrome may develop behavioral changes in adulthood due to depression, psychoactive medication used to mitigate conduct problems, or superimposed neurodegenerative impairment (see Chapter 22).

Gender-Brain Interactions

Behavioral differences between men and women are driven by culture, politics, and biology. Gender determination in mammals is coordinated by the endocrine system: XX is female; XY is male. A hypothetic gene on the Y chromosome, the TDF (testes-determining factor), drives testes formation in the undifferentiated gonad in the first couple of months of gestation. Leydig cells inside the testes begin making testosterone, which binds to androgen receptors and activates male-specific gene expression. Embryos without Y chromosomes have no TDF, no Leydig cells, and no testosterone; therefore no receptors are activated, and the default pathway is female (see Chapter 32). Men's and women's brains do differ slightly in organization, which may be reflected in the differing prevalence of common conditions such as migraine in females (see Chapter 33) and attention-deficit disorder in males (see Chapter 42), and cognitive disturbances and patterns of discovery that men and women display after brain lesions.

PRINCIPLES

Klein and Mayer-Gross (1957) observed that "the study of disorders after cerebral lesions is beset with difficulties." Identical lesions are rare and clinical presentations vary considerably, even with lesions of similar localization and extent, foiling comparisons, deductions, and discovery of general rules. It has also been suggested that the neurobehavioral effects of acquired brain injuries "defy any unified global description" because of varying symptoms, complicating factors and differential outcomes (Grimm & Bleiberg, 1986, p. 499). Hence, "the statistical approach which facilitates conclusions in other branches of medicine is almost inapplicable" (Klein & Mayer-Gross, 1957,

p. xi), and reigning theories and generalizations relied mainly on case studies (such as Broca's description of motor aphasia with damage of the frontal operculum, Harlowe's description of the crowbar case of Phineas Gage, and Scoville and Milner's report on HM). The ideas of *localization of function* and focal representation of cognitive functions seemed to conflict with theories of the wholeness of cerebral functions that were related to Gestalt psychology (Koffka, 1934) and applied to clinical material by the famous psychologist Karl Lashley (1890–1958). Lashley studied learning and memory in laboratory animals and challenged notions of cortical localization of function, forming a holistic approach in his notions of "mass action" and "equipotentiality" (Beach et al., 1960).

Holmes (1945) asserted that behavior cases were rarely "simple or clean cut" and key observations could only be assembled by sifting through the "irregular rubble" of clinical material. In contrast, neurophysiologic and neuroanatomic observations (such as the delineation of cytoarchitectonic areas in the brains of monkeys and humans by Brodmann [1909]) were "built in ashlar or hewn stones which can be easily fitted together." Yet, conceptual, methodological, taxonomic, and philosophical debates pervade modern cognitive neuroscience and fundamental assumptions continue to be questioned.

For instance, neuroscientists and computer scientists often attribute key information-processing significance to cytoarchitectonic layers identified on cross-sections of cortex. Yet, pyramidal neurons traverse layer boundaries, and layers may simply be a way to nourish vast numbers of highly active neurons in a small, protected space: the skull. Lobe demarcations such as frontal, temporal, parietal, and occipital lobe may reflect folding of the brain to allow it to fit into the skull, not clear-cut functional differentiation.

The cortex can be divided into many areas based on histochemical properties and patterns of degeneration following lesions. Yet, the cortex of each hemisphere is a continuous sheet and generally has no separate sections with distinct borders. Maps defined by electrophysiologic techniques may differ in spatial location by as much as a centimeter from corresponding maps defined by functional neuroimaging techniques (Wandell & Wade, 2003). Brain metabolic activity measured by these techniques may reflect glial more than neuronal activity. Perhaps Holmes' assertion above was a case of "the grass is greener."

Current interpretations of human cognition and its disorders often draw from information-processing paradigms and computational models, yet computer architectures and human brains differ in scale of connections and type and complexity of processes. Concepts of "automatic" or parallel processing and the idea of an information-processing bottleneck have been applied to describe processes of vision and attention, yet parallel processing might simply reflect fast or efficient processing, or inhibition of interference between connected areas rather than parallel streams (see Chapter 10). Along these lines, the idea of two visual streams can help describe and organize aspects of vision and visual dysfunction in animals and humans, yet there are clearly rich interconnections between neuronal streams and in many directions. How exactly do maps fit into streams?

Distinctions have been made between simple, complex, and hypercomplex neurons in visual cortex (e.g., Hubel, 1988), perhaps the best understood region of the brain, but these distinctions may simply reflect differences among connections, not neurons. The idea that neuronal connections are shaped after birth by Darwinian competition between neurons (Edelman, 1987) runs against Darwin's requirement of changes over successive reproductive generations: no such reproductive process is going on between pairs or parts of brain neurons.

The "binding problem" has been considered a fundamental problem in cognitive neuroscience and refers to the idea that different perceptual features (e.g., color, shape, movement, depth) are processed in separate modules and must be "bound" or "glued" together (e.g., by attention; Treisman, 1996) to give a unified representation of objects at the level of conscious experience. Electric oscillations in the cortex (of about 40 Hz) have been advanced as an essential mechanism in the binding process. A skeptic might argue that the brain is an integrated system without modular representations to bind; there is no binding problem. Oscillations may simply be an epiphenomenon not serving any particular mental function. An essential question remains: How can we link the psychometric performance of patients with models of the underlying neurophysiological processes? (See Brindley, 1970; Teller, 1984, on "linking propositions"; and Bub, 2000).

Regarding taxonomy and classification, there seem to be few unambiguous definitions of seemingly basic concepts such as attention and consciousness, language, memory, and executive functions, all of which should probably not be regarded as unitary entities, but as umbrella or "folk" terms comprising multiple processes. Lumping and splitting debates also arise in other domains, as in studies of learning and memory. Findings of preserved learning in some cases of amnesia have lead to hypotheses of multiple anatomically discrete memory systems (such as procedural, semantic, episodic, and working memory). Yet working memory, the process of maintaining information (for a separate system so that it is available for use) may reside within each cortical region that processes primary sensory signals (Super, 2003), rather than depend on a special committed system (often attributed to the prefrontal areas).

Despite these essential difficulties, knowledge of human behavioral disorders has grown enormously since the second half of the 20th century. Even with the diverse and seemingly idiosyncratic nature of neurobehavioral deficits, research data and observations consistently support specified cognitive, behavioral, and emotional deficit patterns in brain-based disorders. Advances have also been related to modern research strategies that employ new experimental tools and favorable allocation of resources through public policy initiatives such as the Decade of the Brain initiative in the 1990s and the approximate doubling of the National Institutes of Health [NIH] budget between 1997 and 2003. The Human Genome Project has identified most, if not all, the genes on human chromosomes, including several associated with brain and behavioral disorders (see the National Human Genome Research Institute website; see also U.S. Department of Energy, Office of Science website).

The emerging results continue to generate new hypotheses for further investigation and questions such as what are the relationships between genes, cognitive processes, neurotransmitters, and behavior? These are issues that will likely interest science and the public for centuries.

EVOLUTION OF UNDERSTANDING

Humans have probably long wondered about relationships among the mind, body, and the environment. Prehuman primates evolved in trees, developing binocular vision, eye-hand coordination and, perhaps, a primitive apprehension of basic physics. Prehuman hominids such as *Australopithecus* roamed African savannas at least 5 million years ago, hands freed for tool- and weapon-making, hunting, and gathering (Jones et al., 1992). Animals such as *Homo erectus* migrated from Africa to Eurasia, and had fire and a "Rubicon" brain mass of 1250 cc, perhaps large enough to support modern human mental qualities. *Homo sapiens* emerge in the fossil record from at least 125,000 years ago, with a brain mass of about 1350 cc and highly developed neocortex (especially the frontal lobes). Humans became better able to inhibit habitual and stereotypic responses, maintain and link disparate data to make tactical and strategic plans, and respond to altered contingencies of action based on previous experience. We became able to use abstract and symbolic language and sustain working relationships in agrarian societies, tribes, kingdoms, and then nations, subject to guns, germs, steel (Diamond, 1999), ethics, philosophy, and the scientific method.

The ancient Greeks speculated on the innateness of mental functions (as today; Pinker, 2002) and localization of mental functions in the brain and its ventricles. Pre-19th–century psychologists pondered the metaphysical and ontologic problem of how the mind could interact with the body (as in Cartesian dualism) and the epistemologic problem of how a mind can know an object, but favored speculation and introspection over empirical studies of laws governing psychological and behavioral phenomena.

The scientific revolution that had advanced the physical sciences in the 17th century reached the brain by the 19th century. Gall (1758–1828) argued that the brain is the organ of the mind and that its structure and function could be observed. He favored observation over simple introspection and emphasized mind-brain homologies between humans and animals before Darwin's theory of evolution. Gall's idea of a 1:1 correspondence between mental function and cerebral regions proved to be incorrect, and the flawed technique of phrenology gave way to early experimental neuroscience practiced by anatomists, physiologists, psychologists, and physicians. Timelines of breakthroughs, ideas, theories, and experiments that influence modern neurology, psychology, psychiatry, and philosophy, as well as investigators, are outlined in a number of sources (e.g., Spillane, 1981; Damasio, 1994; Churchland, 1995; Benton, 2000).

Modern approaches to behavioral disorders have combined theories, methods, and evidence from neurology, neuropsychology, pathology, brain imaging, physiology, psychiatry, and cognitive psychology. Heuristic frameworks and specific theories from cognitive, social, personality, and developmental psychology have been applied to a range of brain disorders, encompassing most cerebral systems. Intensively studied systems include vision, audition, motor control, attention, memory, language, executive function, and emotion as discussed throughout Section III (Disorders of Higher Brain Functions) of this book.

The lesion method continues to successfully address the nature of mental representations and organization of brain processes ("psychoanatomy") in animals and humans with brain lesions. The informative approach of Dr. Hanna Damasio and Dr. Antonio Damasio at the University of Iowa and other investigators has been to develop and maintain a registry of patients with lesions in virtually every cerebral area (Damasio & Damasio, 1989; Palca, 1990; Damasio, 1995). Many lesion patients show behavioral "dissociations," which means performance in one experimental task changes much less than performance on a second. A double dissociation is evident when damage to another area affects performing the first task but not the second, and suggests the two tasks are mediated by separate systems or differing sets of neurons within the

same system. Resulting patterns of cognitive deficits are sometimes described using information-processing metaphors including serial processing, parallel processing, feedback, feedforward, and distributed processing.

Complementary methods can reflect normal patterns of regional cerebral activity during cognitive tasks in neurologically normal volunteers and alterations of these patterns in brain-damaged individuals. The main techniques used to measure functional brain activity include positron emission tomography (PET), functional magnetic resonance imaging (fMRI), and related techniques such as electrical brain evoked potentials (EPs) and magnetoencephalography (MEG). Although informative about spatial and temporal aspects of functional brain activity, a weakness of these techniques is their inability to settle issues concerning mechanisms. In some studies the approach seems not so far from Gall's phrenology (Uttal, 2001). Identifying that a specific area is active during a specific task does not provide sufficient evidence that it is critical or that there is a point-to-point map of task to brain area; rather, various activity may be an epiphenomenonon and hence require cross-validation with other sources of scientific evidence.

EVIDENCE-BASED APPROACH

An evidence-based approach has advanced behavioral medicine beyond its customary realms (of neurology, psychiatry, and psychology) and into new fields (including general medicine and subspecialties such as gastroenterology, urology, oncology, endocrinology, and pain medicine). Evidence-based analysis seeks to extend an individual or single-case experience of health care providers with identification of the relative merit of particular patient care practices that have been evaluated according to objective criteria. Signs of maturity in evidence-based medicine include decreased reliance on single case descriptions, expert consensus, introspection, appeals to authority and common sense, and increased reliance on a hierarchy of data from the level of clinical trial and single randomized clinical trial to meta-analysis of randomized clinical trials across multiple institutions (Geyman et al., 2000) (Table 2). There have also been commensurate gains in science-based diagnosis and treatment.

Behavioral neurology and neuropsychology have gained from intellectual approaches and techniques from cognitive science, psychophysics, psychophysiology, philosophy, physics, radiology, and other disciplines. Computational models have provided information processing metaphors for reframing and interpreting cognitive disorders. Pharmacologic developments have improved treatment of disorders of decision making, attention, memory, mood, and somatic state, including depression, anxiety, mania, psychosis,

TABLE 2 . Levels of Evidence (Agency for Health Care Policy and Research [AHCPR], 1992)

Ia	Evidence obtained from meta-analysis of systematic reviews of randomized control trials (RCTs)
Ib	Evidence obtained from at least one RCT
IIa	Evidence obtained from at least one well-designed, individual controlled study without randomization
IIb	Evidence obtained from other types of well-designed, quasi-experimental studies
III	Evidence obtained from well-designed, nonexperimental, descriptive studies, such as comparative studies, correlation studies, case-control studies
IV	Evidence obtained from expert committee reports or opinions or clinical experience of respected authorities or study groups

pain, and addiction. Genetic developments (e.g., sequencing of the human genome; genetic "knockouts") have provided fundamental clues to hereditary and molecular bases of neural development and disease (as in Huntington disease, inborn errors of metabolism, autism spectrum disorder, triplet repeat disease, forms of parkinsonism, certain learning disabilities such as from neurofibromatosis-1, developmental dyslexia, and other diseases that affect cognition). Animal models have enhanced the understanding of neurotransmitters, drug effects, neural representations, maps, plasticity, and rehabilitation. Ideas from philosophy, sociology, and public opinion have led to development of legal and ethical frameworks for addressing key issues from brain death, consciousness, and cognitive competency, to free will.

Effective practitioners of behavioral neurology, neuropsychology, and neuropsychiatry can assemble data and apply scientific principles to diagnose and understand data patterns in single patients, while adhering to principles of logic and avoiding fallacies such as *post hoc ergo propter hoc* (after this therefore because of this). For example, just because a patient complains of memory or word-finding problems some time after a new carpet installation does not mean that the carpet was the cause. Practitioners understand how diagnostic certainty is increased after applying a diagnostic test (as in Bayes's theorem) and are able to decide which tests to order to test diagnostic hypotheses among differential diagnoses.

Specific tests help rule in (support) a hypothetical diagnosis—if a specific test is positive, a patient likely has the condition. Sensitive tests help rule out (reject) a diagnosis—if a sensitive test is negative, the hypothesized condition is not likely. There are pros and cons of using very specific versus not-so-specific tests. The apoliprotein E epsilon-4 allele has been linked to AD (see Chapter 22 on Neurodegenerative Disease), yet is present in about 15% of the general population, many of whom will not develop AD. It is not useful to test for this allele in a patient who shows no evidence of dementia, but in persons who already have dementia, a possible test result favors AD over other conditions. Nonspecific electroencephalogram (EEG), MRI, or PET scan changes in an older patient with whiplash or uncomplicated minor head injury associated with a Glasgow Coma Scale Score of 15 at the scene of injury (see Chapter 27 on Head Trauma) are unlikely to specify traumatic brain damage. In contrast, the presence of the Huntington allele (located on chromosome 4) in a person with a family history of Huntington disease has a reliable grave prognosis.

From probabilistic or causal association between clinical findings and test results, rules can be derived and applied in the behavior clinic. Rule-based reasoning goes by "if-then" structure (Wickins & Holland, 2000). Diagnostic or treatment rules can be organized as a stepwise set of instructions and presented as algorithms. Algorithms, however, are not well suited to patients with multiple behavioral problems, may not allow clinicians to bypass low-yield steps in the clinical workup, and can become a complicated hindrance. The Centers for Medicare and Medicaid Services (CMS), formerly the Health Care Financing Administration (HCFA), recognizes that keeping track of these cognitive processes for reimbursement, as it mandates, is a difficult exercise. A better understanding of the rules of clinical reasoning may partly ease this difficulty.

TERMINOLOGY, TAXONOMY, AND OPERATIONAL DEFINITIONS OF BEHAVIORAL DISORDERS

Taxonomy and nomenclature of disease are key issues in behavioral neurology and neuropsychology. Use of euphemisms, name changes, or reclassifications of conditions may imply new mechanisms, or acceptance of conceptualizations that are not warranted (Payer, 1994; Satel, 2000). Examples include loose substitution of the term post-traumatic stress disorder for "fear," fibromyalgia or myofascial pain syndrome for "neurasthenia, rheumatism, or muscle aches," chronic fatigue syndrome for "depression" or "laziness," somatoform disorder for "hypochondriac" or "hysteric." Some longstanding terms lose popular usage (e.g., organic brain syndrome, hardening of the arteries, minimal brain dysfunction), usually due to vagueness and lack of explanatory value, while others are coined for current clinical vocabulary (e.g., dysphoria, multiple chemical sensitivity syndrome, self-regulatory disorder).

The *Diagnostic and Statistical Manual of Mental Disorders, 4th edition* (DSM-IV) and *International Classification of Diseases, 9th Revision* (ICD-9) have

TABLE 3. ICD-9 Diagnosis Codes Typically Not Covered on an Outpatient Basis by Medicare.

Aphasia	784.3
Apraxia	784.69
Alzheimer disease	331.0
Brain hemorrhage	431
Brain infarction	434.91
Brain injury	854.30
Epilepsy	345-10–345.91
Late effect of stroke/cerebral vascular disease with residual cognitive deficits	438.0
Mental retardation	317–319
Memory loss, unspecified	780-99
Multi-infarct/arteriosclerotic dementia	290.40–290.42
Multiple sclerosis	340
Parkinson disease	332.0
Primary progressive aphasia	784.3

ICD-9, International Classification of Diseases, 9th Revision.
In reference to the Cahaba GBA–Medicare Part A Policy 00011, although coverage may vary depending on the carrier (APA, 1994).

provided operational definitions of disease with some predictive value (and will be succeeded by newer-generation classification schemata (e.g., DSM-V and ICD-10 [WHO]). However, these schemata are not specific to neurologic disease and are often inadequate for classifying related behavioral disorders. For additional information on policy see URL http://www.noridianmedicare.com/provider; for definitions see URL http://www.cdc.gov/nchs/datawh/nchsdefs/medicare.htm. Moreover, there are as yet no specific plans by important organizations such as the American Academy of Neurology to develop such a schema. Administrative coding requirements are a pitfall for diagnosticians. Several common ICD diagnosis codes in behavioral neurology are not covered by Medicare (Table 3). Federal interpretations of diagnoses are sometimes incorrect (as when the CMS decided for a brief time that an ischemic stroke is not a cerebral infarction). It is it often helpful if the clinician documents associated cognitive findings in these cases (specific and general) and secondary problems such as anxiety or depression. These can be coded (e.g., according to DSM criteria) and reimbursed.

Behavioral neurology and neuropsychology has often lacked operational definitions for its terms, which are loosely applied and used differently by different investigators. Consider the term simultanagnosia, which refers to difficulty perceiving more than one object at a time, no matter what size. First of all, the term has nothing to do with term agnosia, which is understood as the inability to recognize previously familiar items or to learn new items that is not explained by perceptual difficulties alone. The varied impairment was reframed as dorsal and ventral simultanagnosia, the latter referring to severe cases of pure alexia, an acquired reading defect in which patients may resort to letter-by-letter reading. Furthermore, the term simultanagnosia has been confused with visual disorientation in which patients have trouble judging the relative distance and location of objects. Increasing precision of terminology and agreement on their meaning are essential dimensions of advancing the recognition, diagnosis, treatment, and research of brain-based behavioral disorders. The key terms enumerated for each chapter and the glossary section at the end of this book are meant to identify and clarify this common vocabulary with working definitions. (These issues are further addressed in "Assembling the Evidence" below.)

SCOPE AND CHALLENGES OF CLINICAL PRACTICE

Patients with cognitive deficits present at all health care levels with complaints that are often poorly articulated. They may arrive in primary care, emergency room, or general medical and surgical settings before being referred to the care of a behavioral specialist. Patients, family members, legal guardians, and health care professionals may misunderstand and be unable to disentangle the patient's symptoms. Additional hurdles to diagnosis and treatment include patient poverty, poor education, and culture and language differences (in the United States, there are immigrant speakers of a hundred native tongues besides English and Spanish). In addition to patient variables, health providers are increasingly hampered by the confusing mix of administrative flux, funding, and public policies that drive federal and other organized health care programs. Escalating malpractice rates add to the increasing administrative burden of clinical practice. Many children and adults with behavioral and cognitive disorders cannot afford to see a health care provider, let alone purchase prescription medicines within current Medicare and Medicaid structures. Provider groups and hospitals often lose money on visits to "cognitive" subspecialties such as neurology, neuropsychology, and psychiatry that spend a large amount of face-to-face time diagnosing and treating cognitive disorders. Established neurorehabilitation units provide an important model of multidisciplinary care that is well integrated and focused on functional goals for recovery, but more often are being limited to a defined recovery period (e.g., first 60 days after stroke). As a consequence, such pressure has spurred more research on optimizing outcomes and evidence-based practice. The situation in long-term care is much less clear, where access to behavioral specialists may be quite difficult.

APPROACH TO COGNITIVE AND BEHAVIORAL IMPAIRMENTS

Effective care of children and adults with cognitive impairments depends on many factors related to practice site and resources, referral patterns, support staff, and reimbursement issues. For the individual provider, effective care depends on learning to:

- Recognize clinical and historical signs in different categories of disease
- Apply and interpret appropriate tests (such as neuroradiologic, electrophysiologic, and neuropsychological)
- Use psychoactive medications
- Refer to other experts, including medical, surgical, psychiatric, psychological, and rehabilitative
- Estimate likely outcomes of disease

Comprehensive evaluation includes thorough review of the patient's current complaints and medical, psychological, social, and family history. The examiner inquires about specific mental functions, such as alertness, attention, concentration, perception, memory, language, judgment, planning and decision making, and self-awareness. The behavioral neurologist conducts a detailed neurologic examination, including mental status screening tests, appropriate rating scales, and knowledge of key aspects of the clinical neurologic examination (such as visual, somatosensory, motor, and cognitive) as addressed within the chapters of this book. The neuropsychologist can assess behavioral, cognitive, and emotional abilities in detail using a variety of clinical interviews, standardized cognitive tests, and inventory procedures.

In addition to neuropsychological testing, key diagnostic tests may include:

1. Brain computed tomography (CT) and/or magnetic resonance imaging (MRI) with its diverse scan sequences
2. Functional imaging with MRI, single photon emission computed tomography (SPECT), and/or positron emission tomography (PET)
3. Electroencephalography and evoked potentials, with brief, ambulatory, and long-term monitoring
4. Specialized laboratory tests including immunologic, hormonal, blood panel, spinal fluid, and even brain biopsy examinations

To properly interpret and apply the results, providers must understand the principles and pitfalls of these tests, including their indications, sensitivity, specificity, validity, and reliability. Test results, history, and physical findings may trigger referrals to experts in several fields. Multidisciplinary management includes neurologists, neuropsychologists, psychiatrists, internists, neurosurgeons, radiologists, physiatrists, ophthalmologists, otolaryngologists, speech and language pathologists, occupational and physical therapists, clinical psychologists, pain experts, social workers, vocational rehabilitation counselors, and others.

Subsequent hospitalizations, treatment, and long-term planning and care depend on a clear understanding of the underlying pathophysiology and time course of disease. Accurate appraisals of deficits are needed for rehabilitation and counseling of patients and their families on what to expect following illness, including determinations of cognitive competency at work, school, and home. This includes ability to conduct activities such as driving an automobile, giving informed consent (e.g., on health care options), making a will, and knowing right from wrong. A person who shows the ability to discriminate what is right from what is wrong may still not be able to do what is right. These appraisals may be needed for legal purposes.

Neuropsychologists can plan and manage cognitive interventions, behavior modification, and cognitive-behavioral therapies that involve patients, families, teachers, and employers. Behavioral physicians prescribe medications and may enroll some patients in clinical drug studies. Neurobehavioral drug treatments have targeted specific neurotransmitter system deficiencies, such as dopamine in Parkinson disease, acetylcholine in AD, and serotonin in depression, as well as specific neurotransmitter system excesses such as dopamine in schizophrenia and attention deficit disorders. Effective drugs for pain, epilepsy, depression, and psychosis have overlapping pharmacologic profiles and behavioral indications. However, overprescription and side effects are a costly cause of patient morbidity and, sometimes, death. Optimal clinical practice requires a clear understanding of scientific principles underlying diagnosis and treatment.

Throughout all aspects of health care delivery for brain-based disorders, it is incumbent upon providers to *demystify* the disease(s), terms, tests, treatments, and outcome possibilities for patients and families. It is unfair to expect patients and families to make decisions based on something they cannot understand (e.g., recovery curves, differential diagnosis, half-life, aphasia, etc.). Educational materials can be prepared and provided through a number of services. These can be critical aspects of treatment that help prevent pessimism, loss of hope, and decompensation in patients and families.

NEUROLOGIC HISTORY AND EXAMINATION

The patient's narrative allows comparisons of behavior with verbal descriptions of actual inner experience. The verbal self-report provides the dominant clues to diagnosis in certain conditions, such as "dizziness," anxiety, hallucinations, mental inefficiency, memory problems, mood disturbances, pain, phantom limb syndrome, and other abnormal sensory phenomena. Further, this information motivates diagnostic studies that can identify or exclude potential etiologies such as stroke, migraine, epilepsy, traumatic brain injury, neurodegenerative disease, and specific drug effects.

Not all patients convey a lucid account of their symptoms. Some have acquired damage in language-related brain structures and cannot express their ideas verbally. Others have amnesia or anosognosia and do not report their impairment because they are unaware of it, as in denial of left-sided paresis or visual loss by a patient who has left spatial hemineglect due to a right parietal lobe lesion. Conversely, some patients with cerebral lesions show preserved residual capacities, but deny them. They are not malingerers and do not have conversion disorders: rather, they are unaware of their residual capacities. The phenomenon of *knowledge without awareness* has been demonstrated in prosopagnosia. Patients who no longer identify previously familiar faces or learn new faces following bilateral lesions in the inferior visual association cortex may still discriminate between familiar and unfamiliar faces under certain conditions of forced choice tasks and by electrodermal responses (Tranel & Damasio, 1985). Other patients with occipital lobe lesions perform better than expected on simple forced choice reading and detection tasks and on localization tasks in which accuracy of finger pointing or eye movements provides an index of perception of targets presented in their scotoma. However these patients appear to have no experience of the items they localize or detect, and have been described under the oxymoron "blindsight" (Weiskrantz, 1986; see Chapter 12).

Another puzzling but important distinction must be made in patients who appear to be entirely intact during office and clinic exams; nevertheless, family members insist that they cannot function adequately and independently in the real world. Even after patients receive extensive neuropsychological testing, they may still perform entirely normally, even well above average, yet not be able to maintain their job, exercise sound judgment, and handle their interactions with others in the real world, sometimes leading to legal and criminal complications. Neurologic patients can present with such a pattern, with diagnoses that range from frontal lobe syndromes and early AD to progressive frontotemporal dementia (e.g., Eslinger & Damasio, 1985; Grossman, 2002). Such patients can make sophisticated judgments on a gamut of test procedures and surveys (e.g., Kihlstrom et al., 2000); unlike animals in experimental situations, they are not limited to lever pressing or orienting responses on simple detection and discrimination tasks as the main expression of their cognitive abilities.

Accurate diagnosis in patients with diverse cognitive and behavioral disorders requires a clear understanding of the historical evidence and relevant pathologic mechanisms, which vary considerably depending on the referral sources (which include neurologists, psychiatrists, neurosurgeons, psychologists, insurance companies, law firms, and others). The patient's history of present illness, past medical history, and psychological history can be enhanced by information from the patient's family members or friends. The examiner should focus upon what these lay informants observed more than on their interpretations or diagnoses. Other sources of collateral data include medical records and associated laboratory studies preceding and following the current complaint, teachers, school and employment records, coworkers, and employers. In forensic cases, there may be testimony from the patient and other witnesses (disinterested or not) to evaluate.

Attempts to standardize data collection in behavior cases can include questionnaires, surveys, and other measurement tools. Health measurement scales in neurology are reviewed in the *Handbook of Neurologic Rating Scales* (Herndon, 1997; see also Chapter 1 on Mental Status Screening and Chapter 2 on Neuropsychological Assessment). Scale development involves item generation, refinement, and reduction; reliability testing between subjects and raters; test/retest design; internal consistency; and validity testing (see section titled "Assembling the Evidence"). A tool that is reliable, valid, and sensitive in one population or culture might not be valid in another.

Premorbid Status

Academic, psychological, occupational, and psychiatric histories all aid the assessment of cognitive and behavioral disorders. Academic performance can be recorded by education level, grades, honors, awards, and standardized test scores (e.g., Iowa Tests, ACT, SAT) and may be the best predictor of premorbid cognitive status in children, teenagers, and young adults who still attend school. Military records and written evaluations by job supervisors may provide similar evidence on achievements. Occupational history is a key factor in estimating a patient's capability and future success in returning to work. Key issues should address if the patient held a steady job, job demands, how current performance deviates from past (i.e., there is defined disability), and which levels of modifications and allowances are required for the impaired employee. The Barona index provides a standardized algorithm for estimating premorbid intelligence quotient (IQ) (Spreen & Strauss, 1991). Social history should address work, friendships, and family life. For example, husbands and wives may bicker, children's grades may suffer, and homemakers may fail to conduct customary activities of cooking, cleaning, shopping, or paying bills and taxes. Some patients abandon reading, hobbies, or even television watching, and simply sit and stare all day. There are many strategies for inquiring into these issues, including detailed instruments for assessing the activities of daily living (ADL) (e.g., see Chapters 1, 2, 36, and 44).

Physical Examination

The neurologic examination is a cornerstone in the evaluation of patients with behavioral disturbances, yet may be underappreciated or misunderstood by nonphysicians. Like a general medical examination, the neurologic examination takes a head-to-toe approach aimed at: (1) mental status, (2) cranial nerves, (3) coordination, (4) motor functions, (5) reflexes, and (6) sensory functions. Like neuropsychological test protocols, the neurologic examination strategy relies on administering a core set of procedures (see Chapters 2 and 27). The examiner instructs the patient, marks the outcome on core tasks, asks additional questions, repeats and varies the sequence of tasks, and administers additional tests, based on the pattern of findings. The findings depend on examiner expertise, training, sensitivity and response criteria, variability in patient effort and ability, and fluctuation in physiologic state, yet provide a source of diagnostic data (Van Allen & Rodnitzky, 1988; Haerer, 1992; Gilman, 2000) not available from any other source.

Without proper history of understanding of neurologic findings, a neuropsychologist might conclude: (1) reduced finger tapping in the right hand indicates a left hemisphere brain lesion when it is really reflects carpal tunnel syndrome or arthritis; (2) reduced left ear performance on a dichotic listening task is due to cerebral damage when it is really due to sensorineural hearing loss, compression of the auditory nerve by an acoustic neuroma, or just cerumen impaction; (3) intermittent tingling in the extremities indicates seizure activity when it is actually the symptom of neuropathy in a patient with absent reflexes; and so on.

In the neurologic exam, there is an assessment of the 12 cranial nerves. The first cranial (olfactory) can be screened using aromatic substances (such as orange or clove oil) and tested in detail on a standardized smell identification tests (Sensonics). Reduced olfaction may be due to damage to the olfactory nerve, or the pyriform (olfactory) cortex may be damaged by an olfactory groove meningioma or head injury, but reduced olfaction is much more likely to be due to tobacco smoking, congestion, age, medications, psychiatric disorders, or sinus disease (see Chapter 15). Examinations relevant to vision (CN 2) and eye movements (CN 3, 4, and 6) are covered in Chapter 12. For examination of

vestibular and auditory components of CN 8, see Chapters 13 and 16. Aspects of the examination of the muscles of the face, jaw, tongue, and palate relevant to speech, swallowing, and facial movement are reviewed in Chapter 51.

Motor examination should include testing of muscle strength, tone, station, and gait and the ability to conduct functional maneuvers such as hopping and toe, heel, and tandem walking. Coordination testing comprises several maneuvers including rapid alternating movement of the hands such as finger-on-thumb tapping, alternating pronation and supination of the hand, pointing movements between the examiner's finger and the patient's nose, and heel-to-knee-to-shin testing. Tendon reflexes and the presence of pathologic reflexes (Babinski, glabellar, snout, root, suck) should be assessed as usual.

A 3–6-Hz pill-rolling tremor may help distinguish a patient with idiopathic Parkinson disease from patients with overlapping signs, such as hypomimia, slow gait, small steps, and trouble rising from a chair (see Chapters 24 and 32). These findings may be obtained in other basal ganglionic disorders, depression, Lewy body disease, or depression. A patient with Creutzfeldt-Jakob disease may show startle myoclonus to an unexpected loud stimulus, but so might a patient with hypoxic brain damage. Liver failure (e.g., resulting from alcoholism or other causes), renal disease, or even stroke may show asterixis, a brief "flap" (loss of tone) of the extended wrists. Aspects of these examinations are reviewed in Chapters 24, 25, 29, and 35. The sensory examination (reviewed in Chapter 14) asks the patient to detect, discriminate, identify, and report on different sensory stimuli (e.g., sharp, dull, vibration, joint position); it is susceptible to error in patients without optimal cooperation.

The mental status screening assessment is of central importance in behavioral neurology and is reviewed in detail in Chapters 1 and 2. The examiner can make useful observations throughout the interview and examination and even in waiting areas. Mental status screening tests are often employed for semi-formal assessment of perception, attention, language, memory, reasoning, judgment, decision making, and implementation. The Mini-Mental State Examination (MMSE) is an easily administered 30-point scale screening test (Folstein et al., 1975). Recent follow-up study of independent, community dwelling older persons over 6 years indicated that a drop of 3 or more points on the MMSE may signify a significant departure from healthy functioning (Eslinger et al., 2003). However, a drop of 3 to 4 points per year on serial MMSE administration a year apart is not uncommon in AD. The findings may help direct a referral for a detailed cognitive assessment by a neuropsychologist, when questions about patients' abilities to live independently and make financial and other decisions arise, and whether various forms of assisted living services may be needed. Screening assessment of patient's mood, anxiety, and general psychological adjustment are also important in neurologic and neuropsychological examinations. Screening tests are available for self-report and examiner-rated symptoms that must be carefully combined with clinical interview, history, and exam. It is important to note that most cognitive test results are sensitive to debilitating effects of depression, fatigue, drug side effects, sleep disturbance, and chronic pain and require expert interpretation.

Also, depending on the pattern of complaints, the patient may warrant evaluation by a specialist in psychiatry, otolaryngology, neuro-ophthalmology, pain management, or other specific area. Application of a few basic screening tests can help guide referrals to other specialists. The practical challenge is to coordinate care so that different specialists function cooperatively as a team. Blood pressure readings and auscultation of carotid bruits can uncover risk factors for stroke or causes of headache. Assessment of chronic headache should also check for dental caries, tenderness over frontal and maxillary sinuses, point tenderness and restricted movement of the neck, and reduced visual acuity. A neuro-ophthalmologic screen for papillary, ocular motility, or visual field defects can be performed using a flashlight, Snellen card or magazine, and ophthalmoscope (see Chapter 12). The Dix-Hallpike maneuver can be used to screen for a neuro-otologic disturbance (see Chapter 16). A general medical examination will help identify treatable systemic factors that could be causing malaise. For example, a patient who is underweight or wasting may have an occult malignancy, metabolic disorder, or depression (see Chapters 28 and 38).

Use of Diagnostic Procedures

As behavioral neurology, neuropsychology, and neuropsychiatry have grown, so have the number of evaluation procedures and diagnostic tests. Procedures employed currently include neuropsychological testing batteries, diverse MRI methods, electrophysiologic studies, and functional neuroimaging techniques along with other special procedures and techniques outlined in Section II (Methods of Assessment) and throughout this book. Deciding when to apply such procedures can be difficult, particularly in this era of managed cost health care. Few have been subjected to strict evidence-based analysis in relationship to behavioral and cognitive complaints. Another consideration regards the use of nonstandardized tests and procedures that have not been fully validated. For example, most neuropsychological examinations report standardized test results that have both high reliability and validity and also informal observations that are based on clinical and process-oriented impressions of the examiner. The latter

may prove very valuable for patient care but should not be confused with validated or diagnostic tests. Some tests have research value (e.g., fMRI), but are prematurely applied to clinical issues. Their value remains to be established with respect to sensitivity, specificity, diagnostic impact, and therapeutic impact (in replacing more costly or risky tests, or identifying who would benefit from treatment). Other tests are well accepted (e.g., EEG, nerve conduction studies) but may have technical problems or lack standards and controls for the laboratory or population in which they are being used. Long-term EEG monitoring in epilepsy monitoring units can be used to discriminate between epileptic and nonepileptic episodes but may be expensive and time intensive. It is also not clear whether the use of PET, SPECT, MR spectroscopy, quantitative EEG, and P300 evoked potentials improve diagnosis and treatment outcomes, reduce morbidity and mortality, provide useful or incremental information, or save money. It is not recommended that these tests be used routinely at this time. In a continuing effort to identify practice guidelines, the American Academy of Neurology has adopted positions on the use of certain tests, including thermography and EEG brain mapping (also termed computerized or quantitative EEG). Such guidelines should be carefully followed. This is an evolving landscape that requires ongoing clinical research to identify new applications, procedures, and guidelines for brain-based behavioral disorders.

Assembling the Evidence

To provide effective care for patients with behavioral and cognitive disorders, clinicians typically need to undertake the following steps:

- Locate all relevant case data and critically assess the reliability and biases of the sources
- Undertake direct clinical examination of patients
- Consider appropriate tests and referrals for specialty opinions regarding medical, neurologic, psychological, psychiatric, and other issues
- Be aware of valid diagnostic categories and classifications and not propose new ones without ample justification
- Locate and evaluate relevant scientific literature and apply those data to individual cases
- Select treatment and evaluate efficacy and side effects, decide on alternative therapies, and determine satisfaction and concerns of the patient, family, and referring physician
- Educate patients, families, and referral sources all along the way

A hypothesis-based, deductive approach to behavioral diagnoses is probabilistic. Clinical neuroscientists gather clinical observations, historical and collateral data, and results of tests that have varying sensitivity and specificity for behavioral conditions. This combined evidence triggers differential hypotheses regarding diagnoses that are operationalized as working diagnoses. Working diagnoses are probed with further tests and follow-up care to provide explanation, validation, verification, decision making, therapeutic actions, and prognosis. If the test data do not support or validate a hypothesis, they are combined with clinical data to generate new hypotheses. The ability to distinguish a behavioral disorder from a neurologically normal state can be described using receiver operator characteristic (ROC) curves. ROC curves plot true positives (detecting a disease when disease is present) versus false positives (making a diagnosis in a patient with no disease). Criteria for diagnosis (i.e., ruling in or ruling out a condition) depend on the costs and benefits of making or missing a diagnosis. For example, a neurologist may be sensitive to diagnosing and treating bacterial meningitis in a patient with headache and fever because the benefits of treatment are great and the risk relatively low. However, it pays to be cautious in diagnosing AD in a middle-aged person with complaints of memory difficulty in the context of depression and psychosocial stress, because treatment with anticholinesterase inhibitors is relatively expensive and unlikely to produce clear improvement, while the premature diagnosis of AD may create undue distress.

Many behavioral clinicians work in academic settings and conduct behavioral research using techniques from experimental psychology, psychophysics and psychophysiology, motor control, neuroimaging, pharmacology, and neuroepidemiology (Batchelor & Cudkowicz, 2001). They benefit from understanding differences between main elements of clinical design including Phase 1, Phase 2, Phase 3, and Phase 4 trials; elements of experimental design including sample size; and clinicometric methods including principles and development of cognitive instruments. It is important for behavioral clinicians to understand the fundamental issues that underlie accuracy of behavioral assessment and diagnosis. These include: (1) reliability, the extent that a test instrument yields the same result on repeated trials under identical circumstances, with different examiners, and with different forms; (2) internal consistency, the correlation of items within a test; (3) sensitivity of tests to change; and (4) validity, the extent that a test measures what it is theoretically supposed to measure (construct validity), correlates with other validated measures (concurrent validity), provides additional information beyond available measures (incremental validity), and measures something that has functional implications for the person's life (ecological validity) (Table 4).

A practitioner who adheres to rigorous standards of medical evidence has a better chance of drawing fair and accurate conclusions in difficult cases. Clinical data may be incomplete or biased, test results may be nonspecific, and the underlying scientific evidence may be unproven beyond anecdote. Anecdotal evidence abounds in cognitive complaints associated with chronic Lyme disease and no proven rickettsial infection; Gulf War syndrome; post-traumatic stress disorder; fibromyalgia; and severe brain damage from low-level exposure to carbon monoxide, cell-phone use, living near radio stations, working in "sick buildings," "junk food" ingestion, mild "whiplash" without head trauma, and related conditions. The behavioral clinician has a pivotal role in dispelling popular myths about brain, behavior, cognition, and emotion in healthy development and aging and in various disease conditions.

TABLE 4. Aspects of Validity

Criterion validity	The extent a test instrument correlates with an accepted external criterion that measures the construct of interest (like a gold standard).
Content validity	Degree to which an instrument represents the domain of content for the construct of interest.
Face validity	Related to the sensibility of the construction of the measurement and refers to the simple concept that the instrument appears to measure what it should. For example, a road test would appear to measure real-world driving behavior.
Construct validity	The extent a measure is consistent with theoretically derived hypotheses concerning anticipated associations between the construct of interest and other assumed related and unrelated constructs. This is assessed by testing hypotheses on the relative degree of association between the instrument and instruments of other related and other unrelated constructs.
Incremental validity	The extent to which a new measure provides additional or novel information beyond that from available measures.
Ecological validity	The extent to which a measure reflects or predicts an individual's functioning in real-world settings contexts or tasks.

A clinical neuroscientist must be able to critically evaluate the evidence on which treatment and policy decisions are made. Quantitative evidence is generally preferable (especially "double-blind" experiments in which the experimenter is not aware of the case and control subjects or treatments). Negative studies seem less likely to get published, leading to observational selection (counting the hits and forgetting the misses), which is especially relevant in fields that rely on case reports. Small sample sizes in rare behavioral disorders do not allow valid statistical conclusions. Strategies and principles for evaluating data fairly are outlined in popular sources (e.g., Sagan, 1996; Shermer, 2001) and can be applied to clinical data. Briefly, for a clinical argument to hold, all of the steps must work. If two hypotheses explain the behavioral data equally well, the simpler (that requires the fewest assumptions) is more likely to be correct ("Occam's razor"). Are the data reliable? Does a diagnosis fit the data and can it be explained by plausible mechanisms that fit within existing theoretical frameworks? A clinical hypothesis has no meaning unless it can in principle be rejected (falsified) by some reliable tests. Are there confounding factors and alternative diagnoses? Occasionally, a patient's complaints will defy expected physiology, as in dense amnesia with convenient islands of recall or forgetting one's own name. In such cases, alternative diagnostic possibilities should be explored. These include psychological or psychiatric conditions such as somatoform, conversion, or personality disorders and malingering. Mark Twain (1894) observed that truth is stranger than fiction because fiction has to make sense. In behavioral neurology and neuropsychology, it is critical to keep an open mind and initially accept a patient's complaints at face value, strange as the complaints may sometimes seem.

USING DRUGS

Drug options for treating behavioral neurology patients continue to grow in number and efficacy, and include a wide variety of agents such as antipsychotics, analgesics, sedatives, hypnotics, antianxiety agents, antidepressants, cognitive activators, hormones, antiepileptics, and psychostimulants. The choice to treat must be weighed against specific expected benefits, Food and Drug Administration–approved indications, problem severity, patient attitude toward treatment, side effects, and interactions with other drugs the patient may be taking. Drugs are generally not covered by Medicare or Medicaid, and many are restricted by private third-party payers. Some of the drugs used in patients with behavioral disorders are prohibitively expensive for patients of moderate means.

Actions of drugs for behavioral, cognitive, and emotional brain-based disorders occur at the neuro-

biologic level, but are evaluated at the level of patient impairments and handicaps. Most drugs act at the neurotransmitter level that influences the functional expression of numerous brain networks mediating a wide variety of processes. Thus, it would be naïve to expect that we will have an armamentarium of effective drug treatments for specific cognitive, behavioral, and emotional impairments (Eslinger & Oliveri, 2002; Whyte, 2002). Medicines intended to treat behavioral or cognitive problems can actually worsen behavior and cognition and cause constitutional complaints. For instance, cholinesterase inhibitors for memory disorders, dopamine agonists for Parkinson disease, and psychostimulants for attention deficit disorders may all cause psychosis. Drugs for behavioral disorders also have wide effects on other systems: for instance, antidepressants can cause fatigue, lethargy, and weight gain; antipsychotics can have marked cardiac side effects. Overtreatment can be fatal.

A wide range of prescription drugs have neurotoxic side effects (Brust, 1996). These include antibacterials; cardiovascular drugs; antihypertensive drugs; drugs for gastrointestinal and respiratory disorders, immunosuppressants; anticoagulants; hypolipemics; drugs for diabetes; hormones; neuroleptics; drugs for depression, mania, and obsessive-compulsive disorders; sedative and hypnotic drugs; opioids; psychostimulants; anorectics; drugs for drug dependence; anticonvulsants; anti-Parkinsonian drugs; migraine and cluster headache drugs; urology drugs; dermatology drugs; vitamins; enzymes; cognitive activators; drugs for multiple sclerosis; and metal antagonists.

Despite these cautions and constraints, medication trials are becoming an increasingly effective tool for mitigation and management of some cognitive, behavioral, and emotional impairments that are associated with brain-based disorders. These issues are discussed throughout many chapters.

MAPPING PROGRESS IN BEHAVIORAL DISCIPLINES

Key points, key references, key words, and glossary terms are mechanisms for making the material in each chapter of this book more transparent and accessible to the reader. Key words provide hooks to the literature in behavioral neurology, neuropsychology, and neuropsychiatry. These fields have grown as a reflection of their own success. This growth is attributable to favorable health care policy such as the Decade of the Brain initiative (promulgated by the late Representative Silvio Conte—D, MA), growth of support through the NIH between 1998 and 2002, public exposure and fascination with research findings amplified through the modern news media, and general desire to understand and cure disorders of brain and behavior.

Quantifying research progress in behavioral neurology is difficult because behavioral neurology is not really a consistent enough search term to quantify this growth in publication databases. However, the field of neuroscience is multidisciplinary, is well represented in the medical literature, and can provide a surrogate source for evaluating progress that includes that of behavioral neurology.

To assess current activity surrounding behavioral neurology we used a variety of search and evaluative tools, bibliographic and citation databases, and health care websites, including the Institute of Scientific Information's (ISI) *Web of Science* and the National Library of Medicine's MEDLINE. Information retrieval strategies included manipulation of data and compiled statistics from the ISI's *Web of Science* family of indexes, and evaluation and analysis tools (*Current Contents Connect, Journal Citation Reports [JCR], ISI Essential Science Indicators*), informed searches of journal publications based on guidelines provided by individual journals, and more targeted searching of MEDLINE, using the key words *behavioral neurology* in conjunction with relevant MeSH (Medical Subject Headings) descriptor hierarchies that produce MEDLINE. We were then able to visualize the parameters of behavioral neurology within the greater body of medical and neurologic literature. Guided by the results of this search, we extracted the high-impact journals within the "neuroscience and behavior" category, one of ISI's main classification domains (Tables 5 through 7). Description of the technical factors involved in these types of numbers is a field unto itself (i.e., bibliometrics) and beyond the scope of this review. Nevertheless, it appears that the evidence in behavioral neurology and neuropsychology and related areas has grown due to greater public interest, federal support, and scientific activity.

NEW DIRECTIONS

Behavioral Neurology, Neuropsychology, and Neuropsychiatry

One of the most important professional issues in the clinical fields of behavioral and cognitive neuroscience entails the interrelationships among behavioral neurology, neuropsychology, and neuropsychiatry. A number of factors are influencing these professional and practice developments. Foremost among these are:

1. The recognition of *neurologic* pathophysiology in conditions previously classified as *psychiatric,* such as attention-deficit/hyperactivity disorder (see Chapter 42), autism, obsessive-compulsive disorder and Tourette syndrome (see Chapter 43), disorders involving emotion processing (see Chapter 21), and "personality changes" from underlying frontal lobe disease (see Chapters 20 and 22) and in epilepsy (see Chapter 34).
2. The advances in drug treatment options for behavioral, cognitive, and emotional

TABLE 5. Top Neuroscience Journals Ranked by Article Count and Journal's Total Citation Count (2001)*

Rank	Journal title	2001 articles	2001 total citations
1	*Brain Research*	1,187	59,622
2	*Journal of Neuroscience*	1,083	70,894
3	*Neuroscience Letters*	958	23,123
4	*Neuroreport*	804	14,800
5	*Journal of Neurochemistry*	648	30,358
6	*Neuroscience*	567	27,130
7	*Journal of Neurophysiology*	531	28,881
8	*European Journal of Neuroscience*	469	11,119
9	*Journal of Comparative Neurology*	438	31,718
10	*Journal of Neuroscience Research*	339	9,124
11	*Experimental Brain Research*	338	13,343
12	*Psychopharmacology*	324	13,638
13	*Neuron*	313	34,720
14	*Vision Research*	302	10,997
15	*Clinical Neurophysiology*	277	1,298

* Total cites are listed for purposes of noting ranking differences when different measures are used to evaluate a journal. For instance, *Neuron*, ranked as 13th by article count, would be ranked 3rd by total citation count.
(Data courtesy of Thomson ISI; ISI's *Journal Citation Reports*® 2001, JCR Science Edition, category: "Neurosciences").

TABLE 6. Top 10 Journals in the Neuroscience Category: 1991–2001*

Journal of Neuroscience

Brain Research

Neuron

Journal of Neurochemistry

Neurology

Neuroscience

Neuroscience Letters

Journal of Comparative Neurology

Journal of Neurophysiology

Annals of Neurology

*Based on ranking of citations (i.e., total citations to indexed papers during the 10-year indexing period). (Data courtesy of Thomson ISI; ISI's *Web of Knowledge, Essential Science Indicators*®).

impairments that require increasingly specialized knowledge of behavioral neuropharmacology.

3. Treatment of affective disorders such as depression and anxiety may soon include brain stimulation techniques such as vagal nerve stimulation, deep brain stimulation, and transcranial magnetic stimulation heretofore used to treat neurologic diseases such as epilepsy and Parkinson disease (Bolwig, 2003).

4. The increasing recognition of secondary psychiatric symptoms in patients who have neurologic disease. Studies of poststroke depression, psychosis in AD and Huntingon chorea, mood, and adjustment disorders in epilepsy and multiple sclerosis provide good examples. There is also greater recognition of frank psychiatric presentations that can be a primary result of certain neurologic disease, particularly involving the frontal lobe and limbic system (e.g., hypersexuality, impulsivity, aggression, mood disorders, etc.).

5. The complexity of certain behavioral, cognitive, and emotional symptomatology, their precise etiology (e.g., premorbid combined with disease and postmorbid factors), and management approaches that require multidisciplinary team effort. An example of a multidisciplinary memory disorders clinic is presented in Chapter 11.

6. The increasing use of functional neuroimaging and neuropsychological testing in psychiatric disorders.

All these factors are fostering closer collaboration among neurology, neuropsychology, and neuropsy-

TABLE 7. Top 15 Journals Publishing "High-Impact" Articles (1989–1998)*

Rank	Journal	Citations	Articles
1	*Neuron*	65,515	292
2	*Journal of Neuroscience*	30,207	163
3	*Trends in Neuroscience*	29,985	125
4	*Annual Review of Neuroscience*	21,452	68
5	*Archives of General Psychiatry*	15,523	56
6	*Annals of Neurology*	12,717	60
7	*Neurology*	9,382	43
8	*Journal of Neurochemistry*	8,381	37
9	*Neuroscience*	8,218	29
10	*Psychological Review*	7,563	24
11	*Psychological Bulletin*	7,371	26
12	*American Journal of Psychiatry*	6,301	30
13	*Journal of Computational Neuroscience*	5,689	23
14	*Journal of Cerebral Blood Flow & Metabolism*	5,047	19
15	*Brain Research*	4,193	14

*This ranking does not consider the three journals from the category "Multidisciplinary" that are also searched for inclusion in the "Neuroscience and Behavior" category. If included here, two of those journals, *Nature* (with 73,0505 citations) and *Science* (with 70,843 citations) would assume the 1st and 2nd positions. (Data courtesy of Thomson ISI; *Web of Science*, category: "Neuroscience and Behavior," 1989–1998, high-impact papers ranked by total citations; accessed 9.2002).

chiatry. This clinical imperative may eventually prove to be cost effective as well, because targeted treatment and preventive care can be marshaled much more effectively toward patients who are at highest risk. These increasing collaborations are also being reflected in research protocols, scientific journals, and books that naturally draw upon expertise from all three approaches (e.g., *The Human Frontal Lobes*, Miller & Cummings, 1999). This collaboration was evident in the bold NIH initiative for establishing Alzheimer disease research centers in the late 1980s, when several were located in departments of psychiatry as well as neurology. This collaboration is being revitalized by the current functional neuroimaging era and the development of affective and social-cognitive neuroscience (e.g., *Foundations in Social Neuroscience*, Cacioppo et al., 2002). Revision of this text in the future might well need a larger section devoted to neuropsychiatric disorders.

Neuroergonomics

As the study of brain-behavior relationships increases, new specialty fields continue to emerge. An example of a new behavioral discipline is neuroergonomics (Parasuraman, 2003). This multidisciplinary field dovetails with behavioral neurology, neuropsychology, and neuropsychiatry and addresses neural substrates of perception, cognition, and performance in human operators interacting with real-world systems, technologies, and machines. An overarching goal is to identify cognitive processes in the performance of real-world tasks and to use this information to optimize safety and efficiency at the levels of individuals and systems. Areas of interest include interactions with entities such as computers, automobiles, and health care organizations by humans in health and disease states. The field aims to better understand how the organization of human cognitive processes constrain our interactions with real-world tasks. Patterns of performance and error in operators with abnormalities of specific mental function (e.g., perception, attention, working memory, emotion, decision making and implementation, awareness) can reveal how these functions map to real-world tasks.

Neuroergonomics addresses how human operators perform in real-world tasks and has implications for safety, productivity, and design in a range of key systems from transportation to health care to the power industry. Examples of potential research questions relevant to neurologic patients include: (1) cognitive predictors of injurious crashes in drivers with age-related cognitive impairments; (2) optimal design features for presentation of information streams in user devices such as "smart cars"; (3) design of health care systems or nuclear plants to minimize errors and maximize safety; (4) neurotransmitter effects (of prescription drugs or drugs of abuse) on man-machine interactions; (5) optimization of human-machine systems based on evidence of cerebral metabolic activity during mental workload in complex tasks; (5) control of computer interfaces and devices using eye movement or brainwave signals of the physically disabled; (6) use of desktop simulation assessment and virtual reality paradigms to probe and quantify more real-world aspects of cognitive performance (e.g., strategic management simulation, gambling tasks, Theory of Mind).

GUIDE TO THE BOOK

This opening chapter provides a brief introduction and overview to the issues in behavioral neurology and neuropsychology. Specific topics are covered in the other 55 chapters of the book. The subject matter is far ranging, and required the input of specialists with a variety of insights on medicine, safety engineering, psychology, radiology, pediatrics, public health, public policy, and the law.

Section II (Methods of Assessment) covers mental status screening, neuropsychological and neuropsychiatric assessment, and brain imaging—including Morphometric Brain Analysis in Disorders of Dementia; Structural Brain Imaging in Neurodevelopmental Disorders; Functional Neuroimaging with PET, fMRI, and Related Techniques; Electrophysiology; and Assessment of Automobile Driving. For the most part, the text is presented at a general scientific level, although occasionally, it was necessary to outline a few technical details. Many of these techniques are critical to the assessment of conditions discussed in the remainder of the book.

Section III (Disorders of Higher Brain Function) includes chapters on attention and concentration, memory and learning, perceptual systems (visual, auditory, somatosensory, olfactory, gustatory, and vestibular), language (aphasia, alexia, agraphia, and acalculia), apraxia, disconnection syndromes, executive functions, and emotion. We have taken care to avoid overlap so that, for example, alexia without agraphia is covered primarily in the chapter on language (Chapter 17) as opposed to vision (Chapter 12).

Section IV (Cognition/Behavior and Disease) covers multiple topics and is the largest section of the book. This section covers degenerative disease, brain infections, movement disorders, subcortical deficits, cerebrovascular disease, closed head trauma and brain injury, encephalopathies, neurosurgical perspectives, coma, altered consciousness, delirium, disorders of sleep and arousal, urinary and fecal incontinence and sexual dysfunction chronic pain, epilepsy, multiple sclerosis, aging and the brain, and cancer. A number of complementary approaches are developed here. For example, the chapter on neurodegenerative conditions dovetails with the chapter on aging, and the chapter on Parkinson disease dovetails with the chapter on subcortical disorders, without redundant overlap. The latter chapter is an example of the systems approach.

Section V (Pediatric/Developmental Behavioral Neurology & Neuropsychology) focuses on special problems in childhood regarding neuropsychological assessment; head trauma and brain injury; learning disabilities; ADD/ADHD; autism spectrum disorders including Asperger syndrome, obsessive-compulsive disorder, and Tourette syndrome; mental retardation; cerebral palsy; epilepsy; and chronic disease, ranging from storage disorders to leukemia and HIV.

Section VI (Rehabilitation and Treatment) provides an Overview by Michael Weinrich, Director of the NIH's National Center for Medical Rehabilitation Research, National Institute of Child Health and Human Development, with sections on the emerging fields of cognitive rehabilitation, speech and language therapy, occupational therapy and vocational rehabilitation, and ratings of impairment and disability.

The final section, VII (Forensics, Competence, Legal Issues), includes competency, capacity, wills, power of attorney, and informed consent; malingering, somatization disorder, and hysteria; Legal Proceedings and Crime. Included here are the Victorian era's McNagton Rule (not guilty by reason of insanity), the Durham rule (not guilty if the unlawful act was due to a mental disease or defect), and the 1984 U.S. Comprehensive Crime Control Act that supplanted it (not guilty if there is clear evidence a defendant could not appreciate the wrongfulness of his or her acts at the time of the commission due to a severe mental disease or defect). This section is highly relevant because health care personnel are frequently called on to advise the court in behavioral matters.

REFERENCES

American Heart Association: Economic cost of cardiovascular diseases. Dallas, TX: Author, 2000a.

American Heart Association: Stroke statistics. Dallas, TX: Author, 2000b.

American Psychiatric Association: Diagnostic and Statistical Manual of Mental Disorders (DSM-IV). Washington, DC: American Psychiatric Press, 1994.

Ball K, Berch DB, Helmers KF, et al: Effects of cognitive training interventions with older adults: A randomized controlled trial. JAMA 288:2271–2281, 2002.

Batchelor T, Cudkowicz ME (eds): Principles of Neuroepidemiology. Boston: Butterworth-Heinemann, 2001.

Beach FA, Hebb DO, Morgan CT, et al (eds): Neuropsychology of Lashley: Selected Papers of K. S. Lashley. McGraw-Hill Series in Psychology. New York: McGraw-Hill, 1960.

Benton A: Neuropsychological assessment, in Tower DB (ed): The Nervous System, Vol. 2: The Clinical Neurosciences. New York: Raven Press, 1975.

Benton A: Exploring the History of Neuropsychology. New York: Oxford University Press, 2000.

Bergen DC, Silberberg D: Nervous system disorders: A global epidemic. Arch Neurol 59:1194–1196, 2002.

Bolwig TG: Putative common pathways in therapeutic brain stimulation for affective disorders. CNS Spectrums 8:490–495, 2003.

Brindley GS: Introduction to sensory experiments, in Physiology of the Retina and Visual Pathway, ed 2. Baltimore: Williams and Wilkins, 1970, pp. 133–138.

Brust JCM: Neurotoxic Side Effects of Prescription Drugs. Boston: Butterworth-Heinemann, 1996.

Bub DN: Methodological issues confronting PET and fMRI studies of cognitive function: With special reference to Human Brain Function (1997). Cogn Neuropsychol 17:467–484, 2000.

Cacioppo JT, Bernston GG, Adolphs R, et al: Foundations in Social Neuroscience. Cambridge MA: MIT Press, 2002.

Churchland P: Neurophilosophy: Toward a Unified Science of the Mind-Brain. Cambridge, MA: MIT Press, 1995.

Damasio AR: Descartes' Error: Emotion, Reason and the Human Brain. New York: Putnam, 1994.

Damasio H: Human Brain Anatomy in Computerized Images. New York: Oxford University Press, 1995.

Damasio H, Damasio AR: Lesion Analysis in Neuropsychology. New York: Oxford University Press, 1989.

Diamond J: Guns, Germs, Steel: The Fate of Human Societies. New York: Norton, 1999.

Edelman GM: Neural Darwinism: The Theory of Neuronal Group Selection. New York: Basic Books, 1987.

Eslinger PJ, Damasio AR: Severe disturbance of higher cognition after bilateral frontal lobe ablation: Patient EVR. Neurology 35:1731–1741, 1985.

Eslinger PJ, Oliveri MV: Approaching interventions clinically and scientifically, in Eslinger PJ (ed): Neuropsychological Interventions. New York: Guilford, 2002, pp. 3–15.

Eslinger PJ, Swan GE, Carmelli D: Changes in the mini-mental state exam in community-dwelling older persons over 6 years: Relationship to health and neuropsychological measures. Neuroepidemiology 22:23–30, 2000.

Feinberg TE, Farah MJ (eds): Behavioral Neurology and Neuropsychology. New York: McGraw-Hill, 2003.

Folstein MF, Folstein SE, McHugh PR: Mini-Mental State: A practical method for grading the cognitive status of patients for the clinician. J Psychol Res 12:189–198, 1975.

Geschwind N: Disconnexion syndromes in animals and man: Part I. (Part II), 237–234; (Part III), Brain 88, 585–644, 1965.

Geyman JP, Deyo RA, Ramsey SD: Evidence-based Clinical Practice: Concepts and approaches. Boston: Butterworth-Heinemann, 2000.

Gilman S (ed): Clinical Examination of the Nervous System. New York: McGraw-Hill, 2000.

Grann VR, Neugut AI: Lung cancer screening at any price? JAMA 289:357–358, 2003.

Grant I, Adams K (eds): Neuropsychological Assessment of Neuropsychiatric Disorders. New York: Oxford University Press, 1996.

Grimm BH, Bleiberg J: Psychological rehabilitation in traumatic brain injury, in Filskov SB, Boll TJ (eds): Handbook of Clinical Neuropsychology. New York: Wiley, 1986, pp. 495–560.

Haerer A: DeJong's The Neurologic Examination, ed 5. New York: Lippincott, 1992.

Heilman KM, Valenstein E: Clinical Neuropsychology, ed 4. New York: Oxford University Press, 2003.

Herndon RM: Handbook of Neurologic Rating Scales. New York: Demos, 1997.

Holmes G: The organization of the visual cortex in man. Proc R Soc Lond B Biol Sci 132:348–361, 1945.

Hubel D: Eye, Brain, and Vision. New York: Freeman, 1988.

Jones S. Martin RD, Pilbeam DR (eds): The Cambridge Encyclopedia of Human Evolution. Cambridge, UK: Cambridge University Press, 1992.

Kihlstrom J, Eiche, Sandbrand D, et al: Emotion and memory: Implications for self-report, in Stone AA, Jaylan S, Turkkan

CA, et al. (eds): The Science of Self-Report: Implications for Research and Practice. Mahwah, NJ: Lawrence Erlbaum Associates, 2000.

Kirshner HS: Behavioral Neurology: Practical Science of Mind and Brain, ed 2. Boston: Butterworth-Heinemann, 2002.

Klein R, Mayer-Gross W (eds): The Clinical Examination of Patients with Organic Cerebral Disease. London: Cassell, 1957.

Koffka K: Principles of Gestalt psychology. London: Lund Humphries, 1934.

Lamberg L: Mind-body medicine explored at APA meeting. JAMA 288:435–440, 2002.

Lamberts SWJ: The endocrinology of aging and the brain. Arch Neurol 59:170911, 2002.

Mesulam M-M (ed): Principles of Behavioral and Cognitive Neurology, ed 2. New York: Oxford University Press, 2000.

Miller BL, Cummings JL: The Human Frontal Lobes. New York: Guilford, 1999.

National Human Genome Research Institute (NHGRI). Available at: http://genome.gov/. Accesssed May 7, 2003.

Palca J: Insights from broken brains. Science 248:812–814, 1990.

Parasuraman R: Neuroergonomics: Research and practice, in Karwowski W (ed): Theoretical Issues in Ergonomics Science, 2003, pp. 5–20.

Payer L: Disease-Mongers : How Doctors, Drug Companies, and Insurers Are Making You Feel Sick. New York: Wiley, 1994.

Pincus JH, Tucker GJ: Behavioral Neurology, ed 4. New York: Oxford University Press, 2003.

Pinker S: The Blank Slate: The Modern Denial of Human Nature. New York: Viking, 2002.

Rao G, Fisch L, Srinivasan S, et al: Does this patient have Parkinson disease? JAMA 289:347–356, 2003.

Sagan C: The Demon-Haunted World: Science as a Candle in the Dark. New York: Random House, 1996.

Satel S: PC M.D.: How Political Correctness Is Corrupting Medicine. New York: Basic Books, 2000.

Shermer M: Baloney detection: How to draw boundaries between science and pseudoscience. Part I (November, 2001); Part II. More baloney detection (December 2001). Accessible at URL: http://www.sciam.com.

Spillane JD: The Doctrine of the Nerves. New York: Oxford University Press, 1981.

Spreen O, Strauss E: A Compendium of Neuropsychological Tests: Administration, Norms, and Commentary. New York: Oxford University Press, 1991.

Super H: Working memory in the primary visual cortex. Arch Neurol 60:809–812, 2003.

Sylvester B: Scared to death? Maybe. CNS News 38, March 2002.

Taylor MA: The Fundamentals of Clinical Neuropsychiatry. New York: Oxford University Press, 1999.

Teller DY: Linking propositions. Vision Res 10:1233–1246, 1984.

Thurman DJ, Guerrero J: Trends in hospitalization associated with traumatic brain injury. JAMA 282:954–957, 1999.

Tranel D, Damasio AR: Knowledge without awareness: An autonomic index of facial recognition by prosopagnosics. Science 228: 351–352, 1985.

Treisman A: The binding problem. Current Opinion in Neurobiology 6:171-178, 1996.

Twain M: Following the Equator: Pudd'nhead Wilson's New Calendar [1894].

U.S. Department of Energy [DOE] Office of Science. DOEgenomes.org. Available at: http://www.ornl.gov/TechResources/Human_Genome/. Accessed May 7, 2003.

Uttal WR. The New Phrenology: The limits of localizing cognitive processes in the brain. Cambridge, MA: MIT Press, 2001.

Van Allen MW, Rodnitzky RL: Pictorial Manual of Neurologic Tests: A Guide to the Performance and Interpretation of the Neurologic Examination. Chicago: Yearbook Medical Publishers, 1988.

Wandell A, Wade AR: Functional imaging of the visual pathways, in Barton JJS, Rizzo M (eds): Vision and the Brain, Vol. 21. Neurol Clin N Am. Philadelphia: Saunders, 2003.

Weiskrantz L: Blindsight: A Case Study and Implications. Oxford, UK: Clarendon Press, 1986.

Whyte J: Pharmacological treatment of cognitive impairments: Conceptual and methodological considerations, in Eslinger PJ (ed): Neuropsychological Interventions. New York: Guilford Press, 2002, pp. 59–79.

Wickins CD, Holland JG: Decision making, in Engineering, Psychology and Human Performance, ed 3. Upper Saddle River, NJ: Prentice-Hall, 2000, p. 293.

World Health Organization (WHO). World Health Report 2002. Geneva, Switzerland: WHO, 2002. Available: http://who.int/whr/2002.

PART

II

Methods of Assessment

Mental Status Evaluation in the Neurologic Examination of Dementia

Dawn Cisewski

Robert C. Green

Kathleen A. Welsh-Bohmer

Clock Drawing Test
Mental Status Questionnaire
Mini-Mental State Examination
Orientation-Memory-Concentration Test
Seven-Minute Screen

INTRODUCTION

The mental status evaluation of cognitive function is a standard part of the neurologic examination and it forms a critical piece of the evaluation of memory disorders and dementia (Strub & Black, 1985; Weintraub & Mesulam, 1985). In the latter situation, it permits an objective assessment of cognitive function from which initial clinical decisions are made regarding the presence (or absence) of dementia and the need for additional diagnostic procedures. Despite its importance, there is tremendous variability across medical practices in the form of the mental status assessment conducted to detect dementia. Many neurologists perform an informal and relatively unstructured clinical or "bedside" evaluation of mental status, whereas others employ a more formal approach with standardized (often paper and pencil) mental status instruments. These variations emerge from differences in theoretical orientation in clinical evaluation of dementia, lack of familiarity with screening methods available and their merit, as well as time and resource demands (Doraiswamy et al., 1998; Sternberg et al., 2000; Valcour et al., 2000). Importantly, until recently the use of standardized tests of cognition within the neurologic examination has not been viewed as necessary for either the effective diagnosis of dementia or for patient management and care (Besdine et al., 1995). However, with the recent advances in early diagnosis and treatment of dementia, the situation is changing. The ability to reliably detect prodromal states of Alzheimer disease (AD) and other dementias benefits substantially from a quantification of cognition and a comparison of performance to normative standards (Geldmacher, 2002). Additionally, the ability to track subtle improvement in function over short treatment intervals requires a reliable metric with sensitivity to small effects (Ferris et al., 1997; Oremus et al., 2001; Schneider, 2001). Consequently there is a growing need to apply quantifiable, validated scales in the neurologic examination of dementia.

Deciding on when it is appropriate to screen for dementia and when referral for more detailed neuropsychological evaluation is necessary depends on the clinical situation. To assist the neurologist in this type of clinical decision making, the Quality Standards Subcommittee of the American Academy of Neurology (AAN) recently proposed guidelines and recommendations for cognitive screening in the evaluation of dementia (Knopman et al., 2001) and milder forms of memory problems (Petersen et al., 2001). These evidence-based reviews emphasize the careful documentation of mental status changes for the diagnosis of dementia and underscore the particular utility of screening tests for the detection of milder forms of memory dysfunction and early-stage neurodegenerative diseases. Neuropsychological evaluation is recommended in situations in which the diagnosis is ambiguous or confounded by conditions that interfere with mentation, such as depression.

The selection of instruments to use for screening purposes is not always a straightforward decision and is frequently influenced by practical considerations including brevity, flexibility, and general utility for the local clinical population. In this chapter, we review briefly the role of mental status screening tests within the neurologic assessment of dementia and consider in some detail the many different screening approaches available for this purpose. We also consider some of the standardized screening batteries that might be used by other specialists, such as neuropsychologists or speech pathologists, to whom the neurologist may routinely refer patients within their settings. The goal of this discussion is to present a balanced overview of the strengths and limitations of the various standardized mental status screening tests currently available to clinicians and to underscore directions for continuing research and development. Consideration is given to current accepted standards of care for dementia screening and to newer emerging trends that use computerized testing and telephone screening.

MENTAL STATUS TEST CONSIDERATIONS IN CLINICAL PRACTICE

History of symptoms is an essential part of the geriatric assessment, particularly in the determination of mild prodromal states of dementia. Following that, mental status tests or "cognitive screening examinations" as they are sometimes referred to, form a necessary step of the diagnostic process. These tests are intended to briefly assess an individual's overall global cognitive capacities and typically they examine areas of higher-order behavior relevant to disturbances of the central nervous system (CNS) that are easily observable in a clinical setting. Commonly, the areas tapped in such screening measures are aspects of language production, aural and reading comprehension, repetition, time orientation, attentional capacity, recent memory, and nonverbal constructional abilities. The information from the assessment is used to generate a diagnostic impression and to guide decisions regarding the need for further diagnostic assessment and laboratory studies. Routine use of mental status screening measures also allows an objective, quantitative baseline of behavior for purposes of tracking change over time and confirming the presence or absence of a progressive condition. It is important to realize that, by itself, a mental status test is not diagnostic of any condition, including dementia. These tests are simply benchmarks of cognition. When considered in the context of the overall neurologic examination, the results of a mental status test can guide the clinician's decisions regarding the need for ordering additional laboratory tests or a more extensive medical work-up for dementia. More detailed neuropsychological testing is often ordered to verify the presence of dementia (when the situation is ambiguous), provide objective information for competency and driving decisions, and contribute additional information for differential diagnosis and management purposes.

Numerous instruments are available, any of which can be appropriately incorporated into the neurologic examination of mental status (Table 1-1). However, because very few of these methods were developed specifically for dementia screening purposes, the instruments vary a great deal in terms of their brevity, the training requisites for administration, and their suitability to elderly populations. Each instrument has limitations, particularly if used in isolation. The fundamental performance characteristics of a test will depend on its basic construction (e.g., items included) and demonstrated psychometrics, including test reliability (i.e., reproducibility or consistency) and validity (i.e., measures what it is intended to measure). Particularly relevant are the properties of the test within populations of interest (e.g., elderly patients with memory complaints) under differing patient conditions (e.g., low education). Additional considerations when judging test utility are construct validity and predictive validity. *Construct validity* refers to the relationship between the test of interest and the underlining theoretical construct it is intended to measure. To determine construct validity a test is examined in relationship to a "gold standard" such as an indisputable established measure of the same construct. For example, in the case of mental status measures, construct validity might be determined by comparing test concordance with other common measures of mental status (Mini-Mental State Examination, Folstein et al., 1975) or with longer measures of global cognitive function (e.g., the impairment index of the Halstead Reitan battery; Reitan & Wolfson, 1993). *Predictive validity* refers to how well the test predicts a future outcome in the domain of interest. In the case of dementia screening, predictive validity would be measured by the extent to which the test effectively captures cognitive decline over time.

Other principal considerations in selection of an instrument are its sensitivity (reliable detection of cases of disease) and specificity (correct identification of cases without disease). The sensitivity of brief mental status tests is frequently a limitation of brief mental status screens, largely due to insufficient information for reliable distinctions between early pathologic processes and normal aging. Sensitivity is also more limited when detecting mild dementia in which neuropsychological deficits are subtle. This situation is particularly problematic in young, high-functioning, and educated individuals who may score in the normal range on these instruments, even when they are clearly suffering decrements in cognitive performance. In addition, because some questionnaires sample only a limited range of behaviors and do not necessarily control for confounding factors, such as low education, minority or cultural background, poor health status, and advanced age, they frequently have limited specificity and false-positive errors are a common problem. Classification errors can be avoided when using screening tests by understanding the limitations of the instruments selected and through the application of appropriate correction factors, when available, for the modifying effects of age, education, gender, and race. As the various instruments are considered in the text that follows, the psychometric information available on each is reviewed and the limitations discussed.

COMMON SCREENING INSTRUMENTS

Numerous screening instruments are available to assist the clinician in the assessment of mental status. The list continues to grow with advances made in neuropsychology and test development, and full consideration of all available tools is beyond the scope of this text to review (see Nelson et al., 1986; Ogrocki & Welsh-Bohmer, 2000, for a review). Of the available measures, eight tests are highlighted in this chapter because these instruments are among the most promising and commonly used methods available to rapidly screen for the presence of memory impairments or dementia. These screening tests include the Mini-Mental State Examination (MMSE), the modified MMSE—the 3MS, the Blessed Orientation-Memory-Concentration (OMC) test, the Mental Status Questionnaire (MSQ), the Short Portable Mental Status Questionnaire (SPMSQ), the Seven-Minute Screening Instrument (7MSI), the Memory Impairment Screen (MIS), and the Clock Drawing Test.

Mini-Mental State Exam

By far the most common measure used for briefly assessing mental status is the MMSE, developed in the mid-1970s (Folstein et al., 1975). The MMSE has been extensively used in both the clinical and epidemiologic literature (Nelson et al., 1986; Fillenbaum et al., 1990; Fratiglioni et al., 1993; Ganguli et al., 1993; Ganguli, 1997). As a consequence it is the most widely used brief cognitive screening instrument. Because it takes on average only 5 minutes to administer, is generally available, and has until recently involved no cost, the MMSE has enjoyed popular use in clinical samples for the evaluation of memory impairment and as a metric to stage the progression of dementia. The instrument is now commercially supplied and involves minimal cost for purchase of the standardized forms, clinical user guides, and normative information (Folstein et al., 2001).

The MMSE is comprised of items assessing six principal domains of mentation: orientation, language, attention/concentration, mental flexibility (working memory), short-term memory, and constructional copy. The original standardization sample was comprised of a group of hospitalized psychiatry inpatients and a group of normal elderly community residents (Folstein et al.,

TABLE 1-1. Comparison of Mental Status Screening Tools

Test name	Low expense	Minimal personnel	Alternate forms	Sensitive to mild AD	Norms available	Ed info	Spanish version	Test-retest reliability	Construct validity	Predictive validity for dementia	Other unique features
PAPER & PENCIL TESTS											
MMSE*	•	•	•	–	++	++	•	•	•	•	Extensive psychometric information
3MS	•	•	•	+	•	•	•	•	•	•	Longitudinal validity for high and low functioning
MSQ	•	•	–	–	•	•	•	•	•	•	Very brief
SPMSQ	•	•	–	–	•	•	•	•	•	•	Very brief
OMC	•	•	–	–	•	•	•	•	•	•	Very brief
7MSI†	•	•	•	+	nr	nr	nr	•	•	•	Very brief
MIS	•	•	•	++	•	•	nr	•	•	++	Good discriminant validity
Clock Drawing	•	•	–	+/–	•	•	•	•	•	–	Very brief
EXTENDED SCREENING TESTS											
Mattis DRS*	–	–	–	+++	•	•	•	•	+++	+++	Psychologist administered
CERAD	–	–	•	+++	•	•	•	•	+++	+++	Psychologist administered
RBANS*	–	–	+++	+++	•	•	nr	•	+++	+++	Psychologist administered
NCSE* (Cognistat)	–	–	–	–	•	•	nr	•	+++	–	Psychologist administered
COMPUTERIZED TESTS											
Microcog	–	•	+++								Computer expenses
CANTAB‡	–	•	+++	+++	+++	+++	nr	+++	+++	+++	Computer expenses
Neurocognitive Scan	–	•	+++								Computer expenses

TABLE 1-1. Comparison of Mental Status Screening Tools (*Continued*)

Test name	Low expense	Minimal personnel	Alternate forms	Sensitive to mild AD	Norms available	Ed info	Spanish version	Test-retest-reliability	Construct validity	Predictive validity for dementia	Other unique features
TELEPHONE SCREENING TESTS											
TICS/TICSm	•	•	–	•	•	•	•	•	•	•	Efficient/human subject issues
3MS	•	•	•	•	•	•	•	•	•	•	Efficient/human subject issues
MIS	•	•		•							Efficient/human subject issues
Blessed IMC	•	•									Efficient/human subject issues

Key
•   present
–   not a feature
+/–   good
++   very good
+++   excellent
nr   not reported
*Commercial supplier: Psychological Assessment Resources
†Supplied by Janssen Pharmaceutica or contact www.7minutescreen.com
‡Commercial supplier: Cambridge Cognition UK
Acronyms are defined in the text.

1975). The dementia patients from the psychiatric sample scored significantly lower than the normal elderly individuals and lower than a group of age-matched patients with affective disorders, leading to a recommended cut-point of 20 of a possible 30 points. Test-retest reliability over short (24 hours) and longer (28 days) time intervals was reported as r = 0.887 and r = 0.98, respectively. Inter-rater reliability was also high (0.827). Subsequent study in a series of consecutively hospitalized patients to a general medical ward led to a revision in the recommended cut-point to 23/24 to optimize discrimination performance in patients with either dementia or delirium (Anthony et al., 1982). At this cut score, the sensitivity was 87%, the specificity was 82%, the false-positive rate was 39%, and the false-negative rate was 5%. Analyses of possible modifying factors suggested that age, education, race, and gender significantly influenced performance. In those individuals for whom age and education were known, the specificity was particularly low in individuals with 8 years of formal education or less (63%) and in subjects who were older than 60 years of age (65.2%). Test sensitivity and specificity are even more restricted when used in unselected elderly outpatients and in community samples (Robins et al., 1984; Escobar et al., 1986; Fillenbaum et al., 1988). Here the application of the traditional cut-point of 23/24 may overestimate cognitive impairment in older individuals, those with low education, and in minority groups. Additionally, the same cut-point will also underestimate decline in individuals with high premorbid function. To this end, it is common for individuals with high educational attainment to score above the cut-point of 24 in the early stages of diagnosable AD (Welsh et al., 1992). Consequently, to control for the modifying effects of education and cultural/ethnic differences on performance, adjustments of one point or more may be needed for some low education and minority groups (Wells et al., 1992; Fratiglioni et al., 1993). It must be also noted that normative studies in diverse cultural and racial groups suggest that these adjustments may not be entirely adequate in non-English speakers or in those with little formal schooling (Katzman et al., 1988; Anzola-Perez et al., 1996). To offset this problem, clinical decision making in all groups may be facilitated by attention to the history of functional change, and to the types of items failed on the examination rather than the absolute cutting score. Patients with AD and early-stage dementias tend to fail memory items (e.g., poor savings scores—percentage retained over time), and these items are not influenced by age, education, or cultural variables to a large extent (Fillenbaum et al., 1998).

Beyond the psychometric limitations noted above, the MMSE has been criticized for its emphasis on orientation questions (10 questions) and its abbreviated coverage of other important cognitive domains, such as executive functioning, memory, and visuospatial ability. This imbalance in the items can limit the utility of the MMSE in detecting frontotemporal dementias and other forms of cognitive impairment (Schwamm et al., 1987; Mendez et al., 1996), although some studies report utility in differentiating subcortical and cortical dementias (Brandt et al., 1988a). The restriction in range on the memory items also renders the MMSE less than ideal in measuring treatment effects in clinical drug trials for dementia (Summers et al., 1990). For repeated measurement, it was also criticized for the absence of alternative forms, but this limitation has been remedied recently (Folstein et al., 2001).

A complication when comparing studies using the MMSE is the lack of uniformity in the different tests of attention and concentration used (serial 7s and WORLD backward). This problem has been largely mitigated with the commercial publication of a standardized version of the MMSE and appropriate interpretative norms (Folstein et al., 2001). The original instruction required the use of serial 7s and the alternative procedures only if subjects were unable or unwilling to do the backward subtraction tests. The two items are not equivalent (Ganguli et al., 1990) and administration of the items across studies has been inconsistent. Because the item serves as an interference task for the later delayed recall procedures, some studies administer only the WORLD backward item to ensure the same brief delay period for all subjects (e.g., CERAD; Morris et al., 1989). A number of alternative scoring procedures have also been developed for the item, which complicate the application of suggested cut-points and interpretation of performance (Ganguli et al., 1990). As noted, the new commercially available norms serve to mitigate this problem (Folstein et al., 2001). As such and despite criticism, the MMSE is still the most highly used test of cognitive status in both clinical and research settings. The problems noted are generally offset in the minds of the many users by the ease of administration, the brevity of the test, the wealth of psychometric data available for diverse patient populations, widespread familiarity with the test, and the ability to augment the MMSE easily with other forms of complementary data (informant reports) to clarify the diagnostic picture when ambiguities exist.

Modified Mini-Mental State Exam

The 3MS is a revision of the MMSE designed to address some of the latter's limitations as a screening instrument for dementia (Teng & Chui, 1987). The 3MS retains essentially all of the items of the original MMSE but has expanded coverage of a broad range of cognitive functions, including aspects of memory encoding, storage, retrieval, verbal fluency, abstraction, and constructional praxis. The scaling is expanded as a result, from 30 to 100 points. The new items allow for partially correct responses and are of varying levels of difficulty to permit more reliable assessment of cognitive loss in individuals with low levels of education. Despite the additional items, the 3MS remains a very brief screening tool. The average administration time is approximately 7 to 8 minutes, although assessment of demented individuals will often require longer administration time. Preliminary studies suggest a cut-off score of 79 for dementia (Teng et al., 1987). More recent epidemiologic work suggests that by using higher cut-points (86/87) an improved detection rate for mild cognitive syndromes can be achieved (Khachaturian et al., 2000).

The 3MS has gained its widest popularity in epidemiologic and community-based studies as opposed to clinical settings (e.g., Canadian Study of Health and Aging, 1994; Breitner et al., 1999). Its slightly longer administration time and complexity compared to the original MMSE may be reasons for its slowness to gain popularity in clinical use. Additionally, some initial training in administration and scoring is required for correct use of the test. Because the 3MS, like the MMSE, is somewhat insensitive to the detection of mild cognitive disorders and is influenced by the same educational and cultural biases (McDowell et al., 1996; Tombaugh et al., 1996), the selection of it over the MMSE may appear to offer few advantages to a busy clinician.

Nevertheless, the 3MS has robust psychometric properties that provide an advantage in detecting a broad range of disorders even in the very old and that facilitate its ability to track disease progression. In one study involving a very elderly population with a range of cognitive syndromes, the sensitivity of the 3MS was reported at nearly 96% with specificity at 79% for the detection of prevalent cases of dementia (Khachaturian et al., 2000). Further investigation in the detection of incident cases of dementia within the same elderly population has suggested that using a cut-point of 82/83 improves the specificity to over 90% while only modestly reducing the sensitivity to 92% (Hayden et al., in press). This cut-point may be the optimal solution for clinical practice where the cost of false-positive errors would be high. Normative studies are also available to provide information for applying selected cut-points to older age ranges and to persons with low education (Tschanz et al., 2000). Telephone adaptations of the 3MS permit surveillance at a distance, where in person assessment is not feasible (Norton et al., 1999). Telephone application of the 3MS (or of any other screening instrument) is discouraged for clinical use but is a useful option for research studies in which subjects may be geographically dispersed.

Another strength of the 3MS is that there are no commercial restrictions on its use, so the expenses associated with its use are minimal. The memory items include semantic cuing and recognition procedures, which allows some distinction between amnesic disorders and conditions with partial forgetting such as normal aging. There is also an expanded assessment of language and other cognitive functions. Partial credit is awarded on many items including those assessing memory, constructional praxis, and language repetition. These facets of the test make it an attractive choice in the differential diagnosis of neurologic disorders (e.g., stroke versus neurodegenerative disease) in which neurobehavioral distinctions between cognitive profiles may be relevant (Grace et al., 1995). As in the MMSE, the 3MS is not highly sensitive to right hemisphere syndromes may still be a limitation, as it is with the MMSE (Suhr et al. 1999).

Mental Status Questionnaire and Short Portable Mental Status Questionnaire

Other traditional cognitive screening instruments include the MSQ (Kahn et al., 1960) and its revision, the SPMSQ (Pfeiffer, 1975). The MSQ predates the development of the MMSE and was based largely on an institutionalized sample. It is a 10-item measure assessing orientation to personal information (age, date of birth), time (date), place (location), and recent events (celebrities, president, previous president). All items carry the same weight, and performance is judged by number of errors committed, the range extending from 0 to 10. The final score is trichotimized, with a low number of errors suggesting no cognitive impairment (0–2); scores in an intermediate range (3–8) raise the possibility of impairment; and higher error scores (9–10) indicate the likelihood of significant impairment. Because the normative properties have been determined for the MSQ on a substantial institutional sample, the instrument has proven inadequate in unselected community-based samples in which the memory symptoms are of a milder nature (Nelson et al., 1986; Fillenbaum et al., 1990).

The SPMSQ is a 10-item psychometric tool designed to be a revision of the MSQ and to be more difficult (Pfeiffer, 1975). Many of the same test items of the MSQ are retained and new items of serial subtraction and personal memory (age, birth date, mother's maiden name) are added. Administration requires approximately 5 to 10 minutes and is easily accomplished by an appropriately trained health care professional. The normative studies, conducted in a random sample of 997 community residents (age 65 and older), provide cut-off scores with adjustments for race/ethnicity and education (nonwhite, low educated allowed more errors; Pfeffer et al., 1981, 1982). Test-retest reliability is high (r = 0.82) and validation studies suggest that this scale relates well to clinical diagnosis of organic brain syndrome (Pfeiffer, 1975). However, a significant limitation of the instrument is the inherent difficulty that accompanies the verification of the personal information items. Without a knowledgeable informant or some other objective means of verifying this information, the reliability of the items is indeterminant. Like the MMSE, the MSQ and SPMSQ are dominated by items related to orientation and both neglect broader coverage of other cognitive domains including episodic memory recall. As a consequence, there are limitations in terms of sensitivity to dementia. In a reanalysis of the original data, the sensitivity of the SPMSQ was quite low (55%) despite quite respectable specificity (96%; Fillenbaum, 1980).

The MSQ and SPMSQ are not as commonly used in current practice as they once were in the 1960s and 1970s, in large part due to the introduction and popularization of the MMSE in community-based studies. However, both the MSQ and SPMSQ remain appropriate choices for assessing either community-based or institutionalized patients, particularly when a very brief screen is desired. One particularly attractive feature is the availability of Spanish translations and cross-cultural validation studies in groups of varying levels of literacy (Gornemann et al., 1999). These studies suggest that the SPMSQ can be used reliably in diverse populations for detecting cognitive disorders and that missing items due to illiteracy do not pose a serious threat to the test properties.

Orientation-Memory-Concentration Test

The OMC test, also known as the Short Blessed, the Modified Blessed Test, and the Blessed Information-Memory-Concentration test (BIMC), is a popular brief screening tool developed by Katzman and colleagues in 1983. Derived from a longer screening tool, the 26-item BIMC, the OMC is confined to six items and therefore is exceptionally brief, taking no more than 5 minutes to complete. The OMC correlates highly with the longer BIMC version (0.96) and has equally strong psychometrics, justifying the utility of this briefer version (Katzman et al., 1983). The OMC assesses orientation to current year, current month, and current time (within 1 hour). There is a single item requiring repetition of a phrase, and there are two items assessing mental control and flexibility (counting backward from 20 to 1; saying the months of the year in reverse order). One point is awarded for each incorrect response with a weighted maximum total score of 28. Weighted error scores greater than 10 are reported to be consistent with the presence of dementia. The repetition item and the recitation of months backward have been found to be the most sensitive items in detecting early dementia.

Reliability of the OMC in several small studies ranges from 0.77 to 0.82. Correlation between the MMSE and the OMC is consistently high, ranging from −0.73 (Thal et al., 1986) to −0.83 (Fillenbaum et al., 1987). Because the MMSE correlates well with the OMC in patients with probable AD (Fillenbaum et al., 1987), the briefer OMC may be the preferred choice in some settings, such as epidemiologic studies or busy clinical practices in which time demands are high. To this end, the OMC is easy to administer, requires minimal training, and has little cost associated with its use. However, because of the limited information provided by either screen and the relative absence of information regarding the performance of the OMC in diverse dementias and demographic segments, some caution must be exercised when using the OMC test in clinically and ethnically diverse populations.

Seven-Minute Screening Instrument

The 7MSI is a relatively new screening test for dementia developed in part with pharmaceutical company support (Solomon et al., 1998). The 7MSI is a paper-and-pencil test that can be administered by a health care professional. It is very brief, taking between 7 and 8 minutes on average to administer, and consists of four component processes of cognition typically affected by AD—time orientation, memory, visuospatial ability, and verbal fluency. The test specifically requires subjects to (1) identify the current day of the week, month, and year; (2) recall with the help of reminder cues 16 pictures presented on flash cards; (3) draw a clock with hands set to 20 minutes to 4 o'clock; and (4) generate words on a category (e.g., vegetables). Scoring is determined by entering errors directly into an automated electronic scoring device, from which a probability of impairment is determined. An individual's likelihood of impairment is rated as either "hi," "lo," or indeterminate "re" with suggested retest at a later time.

Initial validation studies of the 7MSI were conducted in a clinical sample of 60 patients with AD and an equal number of volunteer controls. The reliability of the test appears excellent. Reported test-retest reliability ranged from 0.83 to 0.93 for the various components, with an overall reliability of 0.91. Inter-rater reliability was 0.92. Discrimination between patients with AD and normal elderly controls was also high. The sensitivity and specificity in this sample were each reported at 100%. There has not been additional validation in other samples; overall sensitivity and specificity are likely to be lower when applied to unselected populations with greater diversity of cognitive impairments.

Memory Impairment Screen

The MIS is a new instrument developed to fill the need for a very brief memory assessment that might be applied in clinical practice to screen for memory impairments (Buschke et al., 1999). The test consists of a four-item delayed free- and cued-recall test that uses a structured learning procedure to facilitate initial encoding and later retrieval. Participants read four words from four distinct categories off a stimulus card (e.g., potato, nickel, table, lion). They are then asked to recall the four words when given a category prompt (e.g., vegetable, money, furniture, animal). A nonsemantic interference task follows (counting from 1 to 20 and backward), after which the individual is asked to recall the four items in any order. Category cues are provided following this free-recall procedure, if the individual is unable to recall some or all of the items. The number of items recalled under free and cued-recall procedures is recorded. The MIS score is calculated as $2 \times$ (no. of items on free recall) + (no. of items on cued recall), giving a possible range of 0 to 8.

The original study sample of 522 community-residing adults (ages 66–97) included 89 subjects with dementia (29 with AD) and 433 normal controls. Alternative forms of the MIS were assessed in a subset of dementia cases and nondemented participants (n = 429) who had been administered both forms of the test, one at the beginning of a neuropsychological evaluation and the other at the end of the testing session. The intraclass correlation between forms was high (0.69), indicating a high level of reliability between alternative forms. Internal consistency of both forms was also respectable (0.67). Validation studies were conducted in a criterion sample of 483 and were geared toward construct and discriminative validity. The MIS showed a strong association with memory impairment (kappa = 0.62) as measured by a longer traditional test of memory, the Buschke Free and Cued Selective Reminding Test (FCSRT; Buschke, 1984). Identification of clinically diagnosed dementia was also very good. Using receiver operating characteristic curves, which permit an assessment of sensitivity and specificity at all possible cut-points, the MIS had an area under the curve of 0.94 for dementia in general and 0.97 for AD in particular. Using a cut-point score of 4, the MIS had a high level of sensitivity (0.80), specificity (0.96), positive predictive value (PPV = 0.69), and negative predictive value (NPV range of 0.95–0.99, depending on base rate used). Finally, analyses of demographic variables including age, education, and gender and their interaction showed no influence of any of these factors on performance. Ethnicity/race also appeared unrelated to false-positive results. Two of the 17 nondemented subjects screening positive were African American individuals, a number that is less than expected given the sample composition (16.2% African Americans in sample). Twelve of the subjects had Clinical Dementia Rating (CDR; Hughes et al., 1982) scores of 0.5, indicating questionable dementia. Four of these individuals went on to develop a fulminant dementia by the next assessment wave 18 months later.

On balance, the initial psychometric work with the MIS is very encouraging. Additional field validation in other samples is required to be assured that these properties hold in other diverse groups. Additionally, the original validation sample was not aimed at the identification of ambiguous cases of dementia. Thus, the sensitivity of the MIS to the detection of mild and preclinical AD remains unclear at present and will require further investigation.

Clock Drawing Test

The drawing of clocks is a common procedure in neurobehavioral examinations (Goodglass & Kaplan, 1983; Freedman et al., 1994) and has been adopted by some examiners as a quick screening test for dementia and other neurologic disorders (Wolf-Klein et al., 1989; Shulman, 2000; Richardson & Glass, 2002). Briefly, an individual is required to draw the face of a clock on command, putting in all the numbers in the correct order, and placing the hands at a requested time typically either "10 after 11" or "20 after 3." Because the test requires conceptualization and abstraction, planning, organization, visuospatial judgment, and motor abilities, it constitutes a broad screen for diverse cognitive problems (Table 1-2).

To establish the utility of the clock drawing as a screening test for cognitive disorders in elderly patients of diverse backgrounds, considerable psychometric work has been done over the last 19 years since the original publication by Goodglass and Kaplan (see Shulman, 2000, for a review). Overall, these studies suggest reasonable sensitivity and specificity (each 85% on average) for the detection of probable dementia (see Shulman, 2000). Additional validation studies in poorly educated, non-English speakers have suggested it is superior to the MMSE in predicting dementia (Borson et al., 1999); however, its overall specificity is not optimal (79%). A number of expanded scoring systems and detailed criteria for detecting impaired performance have been suggested to improve overall discrimination performance in patients with neurologic and neuropsychiatric impairments (e.g., Rouleau et al., 1996; Royall et al., 1998). These systems vary in terms of their complexity, range of values assigned, and normative data available. The method used in the Consortium to Establish a Registry for Alzheimer's Disease (CERAD) study uses a 3-point scoring system (0 = normal; 1–3 abnormal); no normative data, per se, are available using this approach (Borson et al., 1999). Another method provides detailed information on the types of errors committed and provides a range of scores from 0 to a maximum correct of 10 (Rouleau et al., 1996). Again normative information is not available. Although these approaches do afford better characterization and detection of various forms of dementia (e.g., frontotemporal dementia, AD, Huntington disease [HD]), the main limitation of the clock drawing test is

TABLE 1-2. Clock Drawing Scoring Method

Clock Drawing—Command Condition			
INSTRUCTION IS TO: "Draw the face of a clock, showing all the numbers, and set the hands to read ten after eleven."			
Command condition scores	*Error type*	Score 1 point if...	Score 1 or more points if...
	Size	Face <34 mm or >102 mm	
	Distortion	(longest diameter) ÷ (diameter perpendicular to longest diameter) >1.26	
	Segmentation	>1 stroke used to complete clock face	
	Multiple attempts	>1 initial attempt at drawing circumference of clock face	
	Numbers missing		Count omission(s) of numbers 1 through 12 on clock face
	Correction time	Incorrect time is indicated OR failure to indicate any time.	
	Indication of time	Hour and minute are indicated without using hour and minute hands OR hands do not originate from center of clock face	
	Number outside the clock face		Count numbers placed outside of clock face
	Anchor location		Count misplaced anchor numbers (12, 3, 6, 9) on clock face
	Circular format		Count numbers that do not touch the circle of best fit
	Hyperkinetic perseverations	Clear instance of overwriting; subject was unable to desist from executing a repeated graphomotor response	
	Interminable perseverations		Count instances of interminable perseverations defined as continued output of a response
	Pull to stimulus	Time is indicated in words or numerically outside the clock face	
	Counterclockwise sequence	Numbers were placed on the clock face in counterclockwise order	
	Conceptual	Misrepresentation of clock OR misrepresentation of the time on the clock	

The scoring method used here (from the Cache County Study of Memory and Aging, unpublished; courtesy K. Garrett-Davis & K. A. Welsh-Bohmer) combines the scoring of Wolf-Klein et al (1989) and Rouleau et al (1996) and illustrates the complexity of behaviors underlying performance on the task including motor function, organization, and planning.

that it lacks a screen for memory, and therefore by itself is not considered a sensitive indicator for mild dementia. More recent studies show that the addition of memory items to the clock drawing task improves overall psychometric performance in the detection of dementia in a heterogeneous sample of elderly community residents. A composite screening test, the "Mini-Cog," comprised of a three-item recall test with a clock drawing test, has been developed as a result. This version of the clock drawing test is simple to administer and score, and it shows excellent performance in a demographically heterogeneous sample of community dwelling elderly subjects (Borson, et al., 2000). The sensitivity is reported at 99%, specificity at 93%, and an overall correct detection rate of 96%.

EXTENDED COGNITIVE SCREENING TESTS

Gaining in popularity are somewhat longer screening measures of cognitive function, which permit more detailed assessment of key cognitive domains (see Table 1-1). These batteries are generally commercially supplied and sometimes require verification of psychology licensure for their purchase. Consequently, tests of this nature are not typically practical for a routine neurologic or psychiatric examination of dementia. However, when used as part of a neuropsychology referral, the extended screening battery may offer an alternative to a comprehensive and more costly neuropsychological examination. For example, in cases in which dementia is already established the use of an extended screening battery affords more extensive baseline information for tracking reliable changes over time. The extended screening battery may also be preferred when screening high-risk populations for dementia before making decisions regarding the need for more extensive laboratory studies. Instruments developed specifically for use with elderly and dementia populations include the Mattis Dementia Rating Scale (Mattis, 1976), the neuropsychological battery from the CERAD (Morris et al., 1989), the Alzheimer's Disease Assessment Scale (ADAS; Rosen et al., 1984), and the Repeatable Battery for the Assessment of Neuropsychological Status (RBANS; Randolph, 1998). For more general neurologic populations, the Neurobehavioral Cognitive Status Examination (NCSE; also known as the Cognistat) allows a more in-depth assessment of global cognitive functions (Schwamm et al., 1987) than conventional short screening measures of dementia and is useful for documenting impairment and tracking change across a diversity of neurologic conditions (Schwamm et al., 1998). Each of these extended screening batteries is considered in this chapter to provide a general overview of these neuropsychological screening approaches and their utility as an adjunct to the neurologic evaluation of dementia.

Mattis Dementia Rating Scale

The Mattis Dementia Rating Scale (Mattis DRS) and its revision (DRS-2) were developed as brief but comprehensive measures of neuropsychological functions affected by neurodegenerative diseases (Mattis, 1973; Jurica et al., 2002). In contemporary neuropsychological practices, the DRS is commonly used as a screen for dementia symptoms and as an efficient metric for tracking changes in mentation over time. In other settings, such as specialty clinics or research studies, the instrument also finds similar utility. It provides rich information well suited to detection of preclinical dementias (Salmon et al., 2002), to diagnosis and characterization of geriatric depression (Alexopoulos et al., 2000), and for longitudinally tracking change in cognition over time, such as patient response to treatment (Jurica et al., 2002). However, because of the test emphasis on sampling a broader range of cognitive functions, it is lengthier and technically more difficult to administer and score than traditional brief mental status tests. Consequently, its practical utility is limited as a screening measure for routine use in the neurologic examination. This caveat holds true for the other extended neuropsychological screening batteries discussed later. Each of these batteries finds particular use as a brief neuropsychological screening examination, allowing the neurologist to track patient change over time and response to treatment in a highly sensitive manner while maintaining relatively low costs compared to full neuropsychological evaluations.

The DRS consists of 36 items presented in a fixed order. Items comprise five basic scales: attention/concentration (8 items), initiation/perseveration (11 items), visuo-construction (6 items), conceptualization (6 items), and memory (5 items). Item order within a scale begins with the most difficult item. If passed, the subsequent easier items can be prorated as correct without actual administration. Total scores possible range from impaired to intact (0–144). The recommended cut-off score for dementia is generally 127. Test-retest reliability, as well as both sensitivity and specificity, are reported as reasonable at this cut-point (Mattis, 1973, 1976); however, more recent studies suggest that a degree of higher sensitivity and specificity can be attained using a cut-off score of 133 (Green et al., 1995). Additionally, considerable empirical work with the DRS indicates sensitivity to age and education effects (e.g., Jurica et al., 2002). As a consequence, the scale has been recently revised. This new version, the DRS-2, provides norms for an expanded age range and has age corrections and education adjustments for the DRS total score. With either version, a carefully trained technician or a nurse can administer the scale. However, it requires some skill in interpretation, making it ideally suited for neuropsychologists or neurologists with neurobehavior training. The total administration time ranges from 20 to 45 minutes depending on severity of cognitive deficits and whether items are prorated. This renders the instrument less than ideal for settings in which rapid screening is preferred.

The major strengths of the DRS are its broad assessment of a wide range of cognitive abilities, allowing for distinctions between forms of cognitive disorders and the ability to track the progression of dementia. It is also sensitive to early dementia if an appropriate cut-point is used (Green et al., 1995) and for this reason is often an instrument of choice among neuropsychologists when screening for cognitive disorders in clinically ambiguous situations, such as potential early-stage AD or so-called Mild Cognitive Impairment (MCI; Petersen et al., 2001; Salmon et al., 2002). Another distinct advantage of the DRS over any other mental status screen is the inclusion of subscales, which directly assess executive functions. Because assessment of executive functions have frequently been overlooked or minimized in traditional brief mental status screens, the DRS has enjoyed considerable application in the assessment of geriatric depression and schizophrenia, and in the differential diagnosis of dementing disorders (Salmon et al., 1989; Lukatela et al., 2000). In some studies the initiation/perseveration subscale is used in isolation to reduce total administration time (e.g., Alexopoulos et al., 2000).

Consortium to Establish a Registry for Alzheimer Disease Battery

The neuropsychological battery developed for the CERAD battery is an expanded battery designed specifically for the assessment of symptoms associated with AD (Morris et al., 1989). The instrument borrows heavily from its predecessor, the ADAS-cog (Mohs et al., 1983; see text below) and also from other available psychometric tests (e.g., Boston naming test, animal fluency). The CERAD battery is comprised of (1) a standardized version of the MMSE, (2) an animal fluency test, (3) a 15-item version of the Boston naming test, (4) a 10-item word list learning test, and (5) a constructional praxis test, the latter two tests adapted from the ADAS (Rosen et al., 1984). Each of the individual subtests in the CERAD battery has high reliability (Morris et al., 1989). The battery is widely accepted at specialty clinics evaluating memory disorders in the elderly and is used at many of the AD centers sponsored by the National Institutes of Health (NIH). It has aided in the identification of cognitive characteristics of the different stages of AD (see Welsh-Bohmer & Mohs, 1997, for a review). Total administration time ranges from 25 to 30 minutes, and a trained technician or nurse can administer it, with oversight from a neuropsychologist for clinical interpretation.

The CERAD neuropsychological battery has much more detailed memory and language tests than most other conventional brief screening exams. This factor contributes to its sensitivity to detecting early-stage AD and its effectiveness in staging the course of illness (Welsh et al., 1992; Chen et al., 2000). There are two alternative forms, and both test-retest and alternative forms reliability are high (Morris et al., 1989). Longitudinal validity and discriminant validity between cases and controls have both been demonstrated (Morris et al., 1989). Normative studies are available for older adults with low (<12 years) and high (>12 years) education (Welsh et al., 1994), and for racial or ethnic minorities (Fillenbaum et al., 2001). There is also information on performance of African American patients with AD (Welsh et al., 1995) and in the oldest examined in epidemiologic studies of dementia (Tschanz et al., 2000). The wealth of empirical data along with other published information in some non-AD contexts (e.g., schizophrenia; Davidson et al., 1996) facilitate CERAD's widespread use in neuropsychology practices. Of note, the CERAD battery has been applied in a variety of different cultural contexts and is one of the few screening devices for dementia that has very good translations available (Spanish, French, Dutch, Portuguese, Japanese, and Chinese, to name a few). The battery is considered public domain and is available to licensed psychologists with permission from the CERAD study at Duke University Medical Center.

The major limitation of the CERAD battery is the absence of a set metric score for the entire battery. Consequently, there is no set cut-point that can be applied for determining likelihood of impairment or dementia. Interpretation rests on the application of normative values and requires neuropsychological appreciation for inferential judgments of differential diagnosis. In many clinical neurology practices this may require referral to a neuropsychology specialist, thereby defeating the purpose of a brief routine examination. Another limit is the relatively brief assessment of executive functioning, which can limit application to non-AD dementias and was never the intention of the original battery design (Welsh-Bohmer & Mohs, 1997).

Alzheimer Disease Assessment Scale

The ADAS was developed to provide a global measure of cognitive and noncognitive functioning in individuals with dementia of the Alzheimer type for application in geriatric psychopharmacological research (Rosen et al., 1984; Mohs & Cohen, 1988). The instrument is divided into cognitive and noncognitive scales. The cognitive measure (ADAS-cog), in particular, has met with considerable success as a metric of AD dementia severity. As a consequence, the ADAS-cog has been used in all U.S. Food and Drug Administration pharmaceutical trials for AD dementia to date (see Doraiswamy et al., 2001, for a review). The ADAS-cog is comprised of 15 items assessing orientation, language, memory, constructional ability, and ideational praxis. Orientation to time and place is assessed by questions that parallel the items in the MMSE. For language assessment there are tasks to document comprehension (ability to follow 1- to 5-step commands) and expression (naming fingers and 12 real objects). Assessment of constructional praxis involves the copying of four increasingly complex geometric figures (circle, diamond, overlapping rectangles, and cube). Ideational praxis is assessed through a five-part task requiring the patient to fold a piece of paper, place it in an envelope, address the letter to himself or herself, seal it, and indicate the location for stamp placement. Memory is assessed with a 10-item word-learning test administered over three trials. Recognition for a separate word list is assessed with three-trial immediate recognition task. The maximum composite score on the cognitive subscale is 70. Total administration time varies from 30 to 45 minutes.

Considerable psychometric research has been conducted on the ADAS-cog (see Dorwaiswamy et al., 2001, for a review). The initial work with the scale demonstrated high test-retest reliability at 1 month (0.918 Spearman rank order correlation in AD patients) and high inter-rater agreement for the cognitive subscale (0.989; Mohs et al., 1983; Rosen et al., 1984). Compared to the MMSE, the ADAS-cog appears to be less influenced by demographic factors such as educational level (Burch & Andrews, 1987). More recent work reports that the ADAS-cog may be useful for the detection of dementia and its staging over time (Zec et al., 1992). Similar to reports with the CERAD battery, which is patterned after the ADAS-cog (Welsh et al., 1992), the ADAS word list learning test has been reported as the most sensitive in detecting a change from normal to mild dementia (Zec et al., 1992). However, unlike the CERAD battery, the ADAS includes immediate recall only and does not include delayed recall of the word list.

The disadvantages of the ADAS-cog are its limited assessments of attention, concentration, and aspects of executive functions. Additionally, the absence of a delayed recall of the word list test or any visual memory procedures limit its utility in dementia screening to some extent. Consequently, the test may miss some individuals with cognitive impairment and may not be ideally suited for early AD detection (Mohs et al., 1997). Another problem with the test is the overlap between the word recall and the word recognition procedures. This appearance of redundancy can lead to confusion and poor patient compliance. Specialized training is needed for administration, scoring, and interpretation of test results. The test is not readily available to individuals not involved in pharmaceutical trials, which limits widespread use. Because the test is not commercially available, the stimuli for naming are not necessarily uniform from battery to battery. This may be a limitation in standardizing the battery across multiple sites.

Repeatable Battery for the Assessment of Neuropsychological Status

The RBANS is a relatively new assessment battery that permits screening for cognitive impairment. The battery is comprised of 12 subtests that assess attention, immediate and delayed memory, language, and visuospatial/constructional abilities (Randolph, 1998). The measures include a word list learning procedure, story memory, figure copy, line orientation, digit span, coding, picture naming, fluency, and then recall and recognition for the word list, story recall, and figure recall. The RBANS is considered brief by neuropsychological standards, taking 30 to 40 minutes to complete. The instrumentation and scoring require training and oversight by a psychologist, which limits its more general application in general neurology practices. However, the battery has advantages in that it provides a solid "core" battery useful for detecting and fully characterizing cognitive disorders in young and elderly patients. The norms cover ages 20 to 89, and it can be used in individuals with diverse neurologic disorders from stroke, head injury, and dementia. Its greatest advantage is the availability of two parallel forms, which permits assessment of patient change over time while reducing the potential confounding influences of practice effects. Used in the elderly, this tool can provide information regarding progression of symptoms, response to treatment interventions, and recovery from acute events such as stroke.

The basic psychometrics are respectable. The reliability coefficient for the total scale score is reported to be 0.94, and test-retest reliability is 0.88. The intraclass correlation coefficient is 0.85. Validation studies have found that it is effective in detecting and characterizing dementia of different etiologies (Randolph et al., 1998). In one study, the RBANS showed good performance in distinguishing 60 patients with AD from 32 patients with diagnosed vascular dementia according to standard clinical criteria (Fink & Randolph, 1998). The strengths of this instrument include testing across a broad range of cognitive domains and providing a more in-depth evaluation of verbal and visual memory than is the case with brief mental status screening tools. The availability of parallel forms is another distinct advantage over many other short and longer screening approaches. The main limitations are greater time demands and the need for specialized training. Because the instrument is commercially available, it has a purchasing fee associated with its use. It also is supplied, in general, only to "qualified users," that is, licensed psychologists or other professionals with appropriate levels of training in assessment, for test security reasons.

Neurobehavioral Cognitive Status Examination

The NCSE or "Cognistat," as it is currently called, was designed to provide a brief cognitive assessment of patients with cognitive disorders (Kiernan et al., 1987; Schwamm et al., 1987). A fundamental goal in its design is to provide information that allows detection and characterization of cognitive impairment. The intention is to provide sufficient information to allow distinctions between confusional states, dementia, and the consequences of stroke and other disorders. To be useful in general office and acute care settings, the instrument is designed to be relatively brief. It accomplishes this aim by using a "screen and metric" approach to allow streamlined administration. Cognitively intact individuals can skip portions of the test, resulting in an administration time of approximately 5 minutes. For individuals who are cognitively impaired, the test allows more in-depth evaluation of problem areas. Administration times in these instances range from 15 to 20 minutes. The NCSE assesses a broad range of functioning, including level of consciousness, orientation, attention, language, memory, calculation, constructional praxis, and high-level reasoning. The test provides norm-referenced scores for each cognitive domain, with scores determined to fall within the average range or in the mild, moderate, or severe impairment range.

The original normative studies were completed in a group of well-characterized normal volunteers (n = 60), a sample of geriatric subjects ranging in age from 70 to 92 (n = 59), and in a small group (n = 30) of neurosurgical patients (Kiernan et al., 1987). The instrument suffers from ceiling effect in healthy individuals. As a consequence, it does not perform well in detecting subtle defects. Because of the limited range of values in normal individuals on nearly all subtests, the usual reliability criteria do not apply well to this instrument. Test-retest scores are high but are not informative because subjects are scoring nearly perfectly on all tests.

A subsequent study in a large psychiatric inpatient sample (n = 886) ranging in age from 15 to 92 supports the instrument's construct validity in patient populations. Expected age-related effects have been demonstrated, with poorer performance associated with advancing age, particularly on the subtests typically sensitive to aging (e.g., memory). Subtest intercorrelations, however, do not yield expected patterns of differential validity. Some of the highest correlations are reported in theoretically independent cognitive domains (e.g., repetition, similarities, naming, construction), whereas weak relationships were found within similar neuropsychological domains (e.g., similarities and judgment, language tests: comprehension, repetition, naming; Logue et al., 1993). The major strengths of the NCSE are efficiency of use and broad coverage of diverse cognitive domains often overlooked in screening examinations. The limitations particularly in screening normal and community-residing elderly populations are ceiling effects in normal subjects and inadequacies in memory

assessment. These factors combined with some expense, personnel needs, and requisite training make it a less attractive option for either routine neurologic practice or for neuropsychological screening of elderly populations. It has enjoyed some popular use in rehabilitation settings and in other contexts, such as in speech and language evaluations, as a general cognitive metric.

Other Extended Screens for Dementia

Other approaches to cognitive screening used by neuropsychologists and researchers alike are empirically based. One method builds on a literature suggesting memory is the most powerful discriminator of early-stage AD (Welsh et al., 1991) and uses a focused assessment of memory, such as aspects of the Hopkins Verbal Learning Test, California Verbal Learning Test, or the Buschke Selective Reminding Test (Grober et al., 1988; Buschke et al., 1999; Hogervorst et al., 2002) for screening purposes. Another method is the use of relatively brief subsets of neuropsychological tests that are most discriminating based on regression-based methods. Examples of this approach include the Iowa Screening Battery (Eslinger et al., 1985) and the battery advocated by Storandt and colleagues (1984), both developed in geriatric patient population settings.

COMPUTER-BASED COGNITIVE SCREENING

Computerized testing is gaining attention in dementia research as new technologies become more common in everyday life and in the practice of medicine (Thrall & Boland, 1998; Murdoch, 1999). There are a number of potential advantages offered by computerized methods that might be implemented in the future either for routine screening of patient populations or applied more selectively as an adjunct to the mental status examination (see Green et al., 1994, for a review). First, computerized methods allow a high degree of control over important stimulus parameters for memory screening (e.g., timing of stimulus presentation, delay intervals). Second, in contrast to paper-and-pencil methods, the computerized method can reduce the possibility of errors that arise in the complex data-handling procedures required by paper-and-pencil methods. The mechanics of test administration can be simplified, the transcription of scores to record forms eliminated, and the interpretation of outcomes facilitated by automatic comparison to computer-based normative tables (Gur et al., 2001a, 2001b). A third advantage of computerized screening is the minimal demand the method places on staff time. As such, this approach permits an efficient means for objective evaluation of cognitive status and for tracking this information from visit to visit. Finally, from a patient perspective, screening memory with computerized methods can be relatively nonthreatening and engaging, leading to reductions in some forms of test-taking anxiety (Gur et al., 2001a). As computerized technologies continue to improve, this approach is likely to become more common. But as is the case with any clinical or laboratory test, it will form only one component of the examination for dementia and will require clinical oversight, as discussed below, to avoid misinterpretation.

Among the measures that have shown the most merit in current research applications are the MicroCog battery published by the Psychological Corporation (Kane & Kay, 1992; Green et al., 1994) and the Cambridge Neuropsychological Test Automated Battery (CANTAB; Robbins et al., 1994). Both have considerable developmental work to support their validity and general clinical utility in the evaluation of neurologic patients. Each assesses a number of cognitive domains; consequently, when used in its entirety, either instrument takes 1 hour or more to complete. However, for screening purposes the judicious selection of specific subtests can reduce the testing time and enhance detection of memory disorders. Two subtests of the CANTAB (paired associate learning and delayed matching to sample) have been shown to be particularly sensitive to early-stage dementia and appear to be comparable to traditional paper-and-pencil approaches (Fowler et al., 1997), although direct comparisons of delayed memory measures using these methods have not yet been reported.

Currently the commercially available computer-based tests and the newly emerging tools, such as the neurocognitive scanning approach of Gur and colleagues (2001a,b), show particular promise within research settings as opposed to clinical practice. The main limitations that restrict broader clinical appeal include: (1) overall diagnostic utility, (2) loss of qualitative information regarding the testing session and patient approach to the tasks at hand (e.g., role of confounding influences such as distractions), (3) ease of implementation in busy clinical practices, (4) patient perception of this method (e.g., artificial nature and face validity), (5) the availability of technical support when needed, and (6) the associated expenses involved in maintaining a computerized setup. For use in neurologic settings, the rather narrow range of behavioral functions assessed and the strong emphasis on visual presentations of stimuli further limit the current computerized methods. Consequently, computerized screening may be of limited clinical utility in individuals with sensory compromise or in patients in whom language disorders are a concern. Because the methods do not allow a direct assessment of factors that can influence cognitive performance (e.g., sensory loss, motivation, cheating), reliance on the method without direct examination of the patient is not advised (Letz et al., 1996).

TELEPHONE SCREENING INSTRUMENTS FOR DEMENTIA

Telephone screening for cognitive status has been suggested as an economical alternative to in-person assessment. The approach has been used with great success in large-scale epidemiologic studies of dementia where in-person assessment is not feasible (Kent & Plomin, 1987; Nesselroade et al., 1988; Breitner et al., 1995, 1999). One of the first instruments developed for this purpose was the Telephone Interview of Cognitive Status (TICS; Brandt et al., 1988b). This test has been revised, eliminating items difficult to verify and adding a delayed-memory procedure (TICS-m; Welsh et al., 1993). There are also telephone versions of conventional mental status screening tests including a telephone version of the MMSE (Roccaforte et al., 1992), the 3MS (Norton et al., 1999), the SPMSQ (Roccaforte et al., 1993), the Blessed IMC test (Kawas et al., 1995), and the MIS (Lipton et al., in press). All of these various instruments have received considerable empirical validation and are generally equivalent in their overall reliability and validity. Spanish translations are available for both the TICS and the 3MS. Two large-scale epidemiologic studies, the MIRAGE study (Multi-Institutional Research in Alzheimer's Genetic Epidemiology) of Boston University and the SALSA study (Sacramento Area Latino Study of Aging) at the University of California–Davis, have both utilized these translated tools (Mungas et al., 2000; Guo et al., 2000). The advantages of the telephone tests that also have a parallel in-person version (e.g., MMSE, OMC, 3MS, SPMSQ) is that comparisons can be readily made between telephone and in-person versions. For longitudinal research studies, in which frequent testing visits with lengthy psychometric batteries can lead to subject attrition, the telephone assessment method offers an alternative strategy with minimal subject demands (Plassman et al., 1994). Used as an interim time point, the telephone screening approach facilitates the collection of multiple data points and the ability to model change in cognition over time.

Although the telephone screening method finds some utility in research studies where large geographically dispersed samples are to be screened, it is not advised for clinical purposes. The method has serious psychometric limitations and raises other serious human subject concerns. The reliability and validity of the method in everyday practice can vary substantially from published studies. This is due to the lack of examiner control over a multitude of external influences that contaminate performance and contribute to test variance. Coaching by spouses or other observers, the use of written notes, and subject referral to other auxiliary aids (e.g., clock, calculator, dictionary) can be used to enhance performance despite examiner attempts to restrict these practices. The ease of the approach also makes it attractive to nonclinicians. An example of this type of application is the use of telephone screening for dementia adopted by some private insurance companies as a mechanism for screening out subjects with likely cognitive disorders (Vinzant, 2002). The use of telephone screening in this manner and broad dissemination of the item information compromises the reliability of the tool. Even in the hands of well-trained professionals, the approach is discouraged as a poor substitute for a clinical, face-to-face evaluation of a memory complaint (Alzheimer's Association 2002, Fact Sheet 3/8/02).

Continued research into the use of telephone and computer automation has some appeal as an effective means of monitoring the follow-up status of geriatric patients at a distance. These methods when combined may be particularly attractive. In the future new advances in the technology may conceivably allow clinicians to monitor their established clinical patients for new cognitive complaints and functional changes over the interval since last seen in clinic. Some studies have begun to examine the utility of telecommunication systems that use interactive voice response options with computerized processing systems to monitor cognitive function in the elderly (Mahoney et al., 1999; Mundt et al., 2001). These approaches appear promising, particularly in detecting early-stage dementing disorders. However, similar to office computerized testing and other telephone methodologies, the new automated approaches suffer disadvantages. Most notably, there is a loss of information regarding how patients approach the task. As a consequence, the reliability of the results can be challenged because there is no way to verify the use of mnemonic aids or to determine the presence of distractions and situational confounds during the session. Because the potential for disease misidentification is large, which may lead to high emotional burden and financial costs, extreme caution is urged at the present time in applying telephone methods as a routine clinical screening approach.

RATING SCALES OF COGNITION

Complementing the psychometric approach to measuring cognitive change in older adults, a number of clinician-based and informant-based rating scales of cognition have also been developed and are worth mentioning here. Among the most commonly used clinician rating scales for dementia, the Clinical Dementia Rating Scale (CDR; Hughes et al., 1982; Berg, 1988) and the Global Deterioration Scale (GDS; Reisberg et al., 1982) are the best developed and validated for measuring cognitive change from normal aging to advanced dementia (Fig. 1-1 and Table 1-3). Both these scales were developed for purposes of staging severity of cognitive

change in the context of dementia research. They combine clinician observations of patient behavior with some clinical testing and take into account family or informant report of changes in function. The CDR covers six categories (box scores) of cognitive and functional ability: memory, orientation, judgment and problem solving, community affairs, home and hobbies, and personal care. From this a global rating is derived along a 5-point scale, defining no impairment as CDR score of 0, questionable impairment (0.5), mild dementia (1.0), moderate dementia (2.0), severe dementia (3.0), profound (4.0), terminal (5.0).

The GDS also stages severity of dementia in a manner similar to the CDR. The GDS is a 7-point scale with larger numbers indicating more severe levels of functional and cognitive impairment as well as emotional changes. As can be seen in Table 1-3, the rating begins with no evidence or complaints of cognitive decline (1) and becomes progressively more involved with ratings including: very mild cognitive decline (2), mild cognitive decline (3), moderate cognitive decline (4), moderately severe cognitive decline (5), severe cognitive decline (6) and very severe cognitive decline (7). Because clinician ratings of behavior require some judgment, the reliability of the CDR and GDS have been somewhat lower than psychometric assessments of cognition, although in the hands of well-trained clinicians the inter-rater reliability and test-retest reliability are quite good (range, 0.82–0.92 for GDS, Reisberg et al., 1988; 0.87 for CDR, Berg 1988). Factors such as the nature of the clinician examination, the extent of formal cognitive evaluation, and the reliability of informants influence the quality of the data received and subsequent rating. To enhance reliability, considerable work has been devoted to the development of systematic, structured instructions for both tools. The results of this effort are the Brief Cognitive Rating Scale (BCRS; Reisberg & Ferris, 1988) for the GDS, and a very carefully developed interview for the CDR available from the developer (Morris, 1993). Both of these staging systems and interviewer-enhanced materials are primarily used in research settings and are not generally applicable to the routine clinical practice.

Informant-based rating scales include the Informant Questionnaire on Cognitive Decline in the Elderly (IQCODE; Jorm & Jacomb, 1989) and rating scales of functional ability such as the Blessed Dementia Rating Scale (Blessed et al., 1968), the Katz Activities of Daily Living Scale (ADL; Katz et al., 1970), and the Lawton Instrumental Activities of Daily Living Scale (IADL; Lawton & Brody, 1969). These measures provide useful information regarding a patient's functional ability from an informant's perspective and provide a starting point for determining the history of symptoms and patient complaints. However, because

	Memory	Orientation	Judgment and Problem Solving	Community Affairs	Home and Hobbies	Personal Care
None (0)	No memory loss or slight, inconstant forgetfulness	Fully oriented	Solves everyday problems well; judgment good in relation to past performance	Independent function at usual level in job, shopping, business and financial affairs, volunteer and social groups	Life at home, hobbies intellectual interests well maintained	Fully capable of self-care
Questionable (0.5)	Consistent slight forgetfulness; partial recollection of events; "benign" forgetfulness	Fully oriented except for slight difficulty with time relationships	Slight impairment in solving problems, similarities, differences	Slight impairment in these activities	Life at home, hobbies, intellectual interests slightly impaired	Fully capable of self-care
Mild (1)	Moderate memory loss; more marked for recent events; defect interferes with everyday activities	Moderate difficulty with time relationships; oriented for place at examination; may have geographic disorientation elsewhere	Moderate difficulty in handling problems, similarities, differences; social judgment usually maintained	Unable to function independently at these activities though may still be engaged in some; appears normal to casual inspection	Mild but definite impairment of function at home; more difficult chores abandoned; more complicated hobbies and interests abandoned	Needs prompting
Moderate (2)	Severe memory loss; only highly learned material retained; new material rapidly lost	Severe difficulty with time relationships; usually disoriented in time, often to place	Severely impaired in handling problems, similarities, differences; social judgment usually impaired	No pretense of independent function outside home. Appears well enough to be taken to functions outside family home	Only simple chores preserved, very restricted interests, poorly sustained	Requires assistance in dressing, hygiene, keeping of personal effects
Severe (3)	Severe memory loss; only fragments remain	Oriented to person only	Unable to make judgments or solve problems	No pretense of independent function outside home. Appears too ill to be taken to functions outside family home	No significant function in home	Requires much help with personal care; frequent incontinence
Subitem scores	[ ] 1	[ ] 2	[ ] 3	[ ] 4	[ ] 5	[ ] 6

Although rules for assigning CDR stages beyond CDR 3 have not been established, the following have been proposed to distinguish additional levels of impairment in advanced dementia

Profound (4)	Speech usually unintelligible or irrelevant; unable to follow simple instructions or comprehend commands; occasionally recognizes spouse or caregiver. Uses fingers more than utensils, requires much assistance. Frequently incontinent despite assistance or training. Able to walk a few steps with help; usually chair bound; rarely out of home or residence; purposeless movements often present.
Terminal (5)	No response or comprehension. No recognition. Needs to be fed, may have nasogastric tube and/or swallowing difficulties. Total incontinence. Bedridden, unable to sit or stand, contractures.

Current staging of dementia: (Computer will score if desired)

0	=>	No dementia	2	=>	Moderate dementia
0.5	=>	Uncertain or deferred dx	3	=>	Severe dementia
1	=>	Mild dementia	4	=>	Profound dementia
			5	=>	Terminal dementia

FIGURE 1-1. CDR staging. (Reproduced with permission from Berg L: The Clinical Dementia Rating Scale [CDR]. Psychopharmacol Bull 24:637–639, 1988.)

the reliability of these ratings can be colored by a number of factors including symptom ambiguity, comorbid conditions leading to functional decline (e.g., arthritis, sensory limitations of age), availability of an informed observer, and a variety of environmental and social situational factors, a clinical examination and physician interview are almost always required for verification of any endorsed problems (Jorm, 1996). A full discussion of this topic is not possible within this chapter. For a more comprehensive review, the reader is referred to other sources, Besdine et al., 1995.

CONCLUSIONS AND FUTURE DIRECTIONS

Mental status testing in the evaluation of memory complaints allows a brief and objective assessment of cognitive function. Many different instruments are available for this purpose, only a portion of which were reviewed here. All of these tests, whether a brief assessment or a more expanded screening battery conducted by a neuropsychologist, have their own limitations in terms of sensitivity, specificity, and predictive power. None of

TABLE 1-3. Global Deterioration Scale

Ratings of patient's level of cognitive function	
1	
No cognitive decline	No subjective complaints and no evidence of memory problems on interview.
2	
Very mild cognitive decline	Subjective complaints (e.g., forgetfulness for object placement, forgetting names of individuals known well). No objective deficits in employment or social situations. Appropriate concern with respect to symptom severity.
	Subjective complaints (e.g., forgetfulness for object placement, forgetting names of individuals known well). No objective deficits in employment or social situations. Appropriate concern with respect to symptom severity.
3	
Mild cognitive decline	Earliest clear deficits by history and evident after careful examination on clinical evaluation. Decreased performance in demanding employment and social settings. May include some decreased appreciation of deficit and anxiety may accompany the symptoms.
4	
Moderate cognitive decline	Clear-cut deficit on examination. Frequently no deficit in orientation to time or person, familiarity with persons and faces, or ability to travel to familiar locations. Inability to perform complex tasks. Denial common as is a flattening of affect and/or social withdrawal.
5	
Moderately severe cognitive decline	Patient now requires assistance for day-to-day needs. Frequent time disorientation.
6	
Severe cognitive decline	Clearly impaired to the extent that may be largely unaware of recent events and experiences in their lives. Requires assistance in ADLs and may have incontinence. Diurnal rhythm may be disturbed. Personality and emotional changes common.
7	
Very severe cognitive decline	All verbal abilities lost. Loss of basic psychomotor skills (e.g., walking). Generalized and cortical neurologic signs and symptoms are frequently present.

(From Reisberg B, Ferris SH, de Leon MJ, et al: Global Deterioration Scale [GDS]. Psychopharmacol Bull 24:661–663, 1988.)

these tests are "diagnostic of dementia" and cognitive screening, as such, should never be used in isolation for this purpose.

Future directions include improving the instruments available to further assist the neurologist in the identification of dementia patients. One approach to improving instrumentation is the inclusion of some brief quantifiable assessment of functional ability, which would enhance the psychometric screening process in complicated medical conditions and detection of early dementia (Mackinnon & Mulligan, 1998). Combining any of a number of brief functional rating scales with cognitive testing provides information about the patient's cognition and ability to manage ADL (i.e., bathe, dress, and cook). Preliminary work using both sources of quantified information suggests more enhanced diagnostic reliability in the detection of dementia cases than is possible using either brief cognitive screening or structured functional assessment

scales alone (Khatchaturian et al., 2000). Another encouraging direction is the development of direct assessment approaches of functional ability, which would permit a more reliable determination of the effects of cognitive change on function. Until such metrics are forthcoming for the neurologist's use, the method that would appear optimal for screening at this point in time is one that uses combined sources of quantifiable information including in-person, objective cognitive assessment measures (e.g., MMSE) complemented by either informant or self-reported rating scales of function in ADL, including measures of mood and depression. With limited information on cognition, function, and mood the clinician is able to make some preliminary inferences about the likelihood of a cognitive disorder and the influence of major medical comorbidity in the elderly, such as late-life depression. This approach is also most likely to capture early-stage dementias, which may manifest with differing degrees of memory impairment and functional change (Morris et al., 2001; Petersen et al., 2001).

■ KEY POINTS

☐ Psychometric screening tests augment the mental status examination in the neurologic evaluation of dementia by providing objective, quantifiable information from which a patient's status can be interpreted and tracked over time.

☐ A host of different short and long screening tools are available that provide quantifiable assessment of a variety of cognitive domains. The utility of these tools will vary depending on the needs and resources of the individual clinical settings. The MMSE is the most extensively used and researched instrument for screening purposes.

☐ The most efficient "screening" for dementia across the continuum of clinical presentations (e.g., early-stage illness, complicated medical conditions) is likely to include both quantifiable functional and cognitive assessments.

KEY READINGS

Doody RS, Stevens JC, Beck C, et al: Practice parameter: Management of dementia (an evidence-based review). Report of the Quality Standards Subcommittee of the American Academy of Neurology. Neurology 56:1154–1166, 2001.

Knopman DS, DeKosky ST, Cummings JL, et al: Practice parameter: Diagnosis of dementia (an evidence-based review). Report of the Quality Standards Subcommittee of the American Academy of Neurology. Neurology 56:1143–1153, 2001.

Petersen RC, Stevens JC, Ganguli M, et al: Practice parameter: Early detection of dementia: Mild cognitive impairment (an evidence-based review). Report of the Quality Standards Subcommittee of the American Academy of Neurology. Neurology 56:1133–1142, 2001.

REFERENCES

Alexopoulos GS, Meyers BS, Young RC, et al: Executive dysfunction and long-term outcomes of geriatric depression. Arch Gen Psychiatry 57:285–290, 2000.

Anthony JC, LeResche L, Niaz U, et al: Limits of the Mini-Mental State as a screening test for dementia and delirium among hospital patients. Psychol Med 12:397–408, 1982.

Anzola-Perez E, Bangdiwala SI, Barrientos de Llano G, et al: Towards community diagnosis of dementia: Testing cognitive impairment in older persons in Argentina, Chile, and Cuba. Int J Geriatr Psychiatry 11:429–438, 1996.

Berg L: The Clinical Dementia Rating Scale (CDR). Psychopharmacol Bull 24:637–639, 1988.

Besdine RW, Butler RN, Cassel CK, et al: Merck Manual of Geriatrics, ed 2. Whitehouse Station, NJ: Merck Research Laboratories, 1995, pp. 1129–1159.

Blessed G, Tomlinson B, Roth M: The association between quantitative measures of dementia and senile change in the cerebral grey matter of elderly subjects. Br J Psychiatry 114:797–811, 1968.

Borson S, Brush M, Gil E, et al: The Clock Drawing Test: Utility for dementia detection in multiethnic elders. J Gerontol Biol Sci Med Sci 54A:M534–540, 1999.

Borson S, Scanlan J, Brush M, et al: The Mini-Cog: A cognitive "vital signs" measure for dementia screening in multi-lingual elderly. Int J Geriatr Psychiatry 15:1021–1027, 2000.

Brandt J, Folstein S, Folstein MF: Differential cognitive impairment in Alzheimer's disease and Huntington's disease. Arch Neurol 23:555–561, 1988.

Brandt J, Spencer M, Folstein M: The telephone interview for cognitive status. Neuropsychiatry Neuropsychol Behav Neurol 1:111–117, 1988.

Breitner JCS, Welsh KA, Gau BA, et al: Alzheimer's disease in the National Academy of Sciences–National Research Council Registry of Aging Twin Veterans. III. Detection of cases, longitudinal results, and observations on twin concordance. Arch Neurol 52:763–771, 1995.

Breitner JCS, Wyse BW, Anthony JC, et al: APOE e4 predicts age when prevalence of Alzheimer's disease increases—then declines. Neurology 53:321–331, 1999.

Burch EA, Andrews SR: Comparison of two cognitive rating scales in medically ill patients. Int J Psychiatry Med 17:193–200, 1987.

Buschke H: Cued recall in amnesia. J Clin Neuropsychol 6:433–440, 1984.

Buschke H, Kuslansky G, Katz M, et al: Screening for dementia with the Memory Impairment Screen. Neurology 52:231–238, 1999.

Canadian Study of Health and Aging. The Canadian study of health and aging: Risk factors for Alzheimer's disease in Canada. Neurology 44:2073–2080. 1994.

Carr AC, Wilson SL, Ghosh A, er al: Automated testing of geriatric patients using a microcomputer-based system. Int J Man-Machine Studies 17:297-300, 1982.

Chen P, Ratcliff G, Belle SH, et al: Cognitive test that best discriminate between presymptomatic AD and those who remain non-demented. Neurology 55:1847–1853, 2000.

Collie A Maruff R, Shafiq-Antonacci M, et al: Memory decline in healthy older people: Implications for identifying mild cognitive impairment. Neurology 56:1533–1538, 2001.

Davidson M, Harvey P, Welsh KA, et al: Cognitive functioning in late-life schizophrenia: A comparison of elderly schizophrenic patients and patients with Alzheimer's disease. Am J Psychiatry 153:1274–1279, 1996.

Doraiswamy KL, Bieber F, Garman RL: The Alzheimer's Disease Assessment Scale: Evaluation of psychometric properties and patterns of cognitive decline in multicenter clinical trials of mild to moderate Alzheimer's disease. Alzheimer Dis Assoc Disord 15:174–183, 2001.

Doraiswamy KL, Steffens DC, Pitchumoni S, et al: Early recognition of Alzheimer's disease: What is consensual? What is controversial? What is practical? J Clin Psychol 59:S6–18, 1998.

Escobar JI, Burnam A, Karno M, et al: Use of the Mini-Mental State Examination in a community population of mixed ethnicity: Cultural and linguistic artifacts. J Nerv Ment Dis 174:607–614, 1986.

Eslinger PJ, Damasio AR, Benton AL, et al: Neuropsychological detection of abnormal mental decline in older person. JAMA 253:670–674, 1985.

Ferris SH, Lucca U, Mohs R, et al: Objective psychometric tests in clinical trials of dementia drugs. Position paper from the International Working Group on Harmonization of Dementia Drug Guidelines. Alzheimer Dis Assoc Disord 11(Suppl. 3):34–38, 1997.

Fillenbaum GG: A comparison of two brief tests of organicity: The Mental Status Questionnaire and the Short Portable Mental Status Questionnaire. J Am Geriatr Soc 28:381–384, 1980.

Fillenbaum GG, Heyman A, Huber MS, et al: Performance of elderly African American and white community residents on the CERAD neuropsychological battery. J Int Neuropsychol Soc 7:502–509, 2001.

Fillenbaum GG, Heyman A, Wilkinson WE, et al: Comparison of two screening tests in Alzheimer's disease: The correlation and reliability of the Mini-Mental Status Examination and the modified Blessed tests. Arch Neurol 44:924–927, 1987.

Fillenbaum GG, Heyman A, Williams K, et al: Sensitivity and specificity of standardized screens of cognitive impairment and dementia among elderly black and white community residents. J Clin Epidemiol 43:651–660, 1990.

Fillenbaum GG, Hughes DC, Heyman A, et al: Relationship of health and demographic characteristics to Mini-Mental State Examination score among community residents. Psychol Med 18:719–726, 1988.

Fillenbaum GG, Peterson B, Welsh-Bohmer KA, et al: Progression of Alzheimer's disease in African-American and White patients: The CERAD experience, Part XVI. Neurology 51:154–158, 1998.

Fink JW, Randolph C: Semantic memory in neurodegenerative disease, in Troster AI (ed): Memory in Neurodegenerative Disease: Biological, Cognitive, and Clinical Perspectives. New York: Cambridge University Press, 1998, pp. 197–209.

Folstein MF: Mini-mental and son. Intl J Geriatr Psychiatry 13:290–294, 1998.

Folstein MF, Folstein SE, Fanjiang G: Mini-Mental State Examination (MMSE™) Clinical Guide. Odessa, FL: Psychological Assessment Resources, 2001.

Folstein MF, Folstein SE, McHugh PR: Mini-Mental state: A practical method for grading the cognitive state of patients for the clinician. J Psychiatr Res 12:189–198, 1975.

Fowler KS, Saling MM, Conway EL, et al: Computerized neuropsychological tests in the early detection of dementia: Prospective findings. J Intl Neuropsychol Soc 3:139–146, 1997.

Fratiglioni L, Jorm AF, Grut M, et al: Predicting dementia from the Mini-Mental State examination in an elderly population: The role of education. J Clin Epidemiol 46:281–287, 1993.

Freedman M, Kaplan E, Delis D, et al: Clock Drawing: A neuropsychological analysis. New York: Oxford University Press, 1994.

Ganguli M: The use of screening instruments for the detection of dementia. Neuroepidemiology 16:271–280, 1997.

Ganguli M, Belle S, Ratcliff G, et al: Sensitivity and specificity for dementia of population based criteria for cognitive impairment: The MoVies Project. J Gerontol Med Sci 48:M152–M161, 1993.

Ganguli M, Ratcliff G, Huff J, et al: Serial sevens versus world backwards: A comparison of the two measures of attention from the MMSE. J Geriatr Psychiatry Neurol 3:203–207, 1990.

Geldmacher DS: Cost-effective recognition and diagnosis of dementia. Semin Neurol 22:63–70, 2002.

Goodglass H, Kaplan E: The Assessment of Aphasia and Related Disorders, ed 2. Philadelphia, PA: Lea & Febiger, 1983.

Gornemann I, Zunzunegui MV, Martinez C, et al: Screening for impaired cognitive function among the elderly in Spain: Reducing the number of items in the Short Portable Mental Status Questionnaire. Psychiatry Res 89:133–145, 1999.

Grace J, Nadler JD, White DA, et al: Folstein vs Modified Mini-mental State Examination in geriatric stroke: Stability, validity and screening utility. Arch Neurol 52:477–484, 1995.

Green RC, Green J, Harrison JM, et al: Screening for cognitive impairment in older individuals: Validation of a computer-based test. Arch Neurol 51:779–786, 1994.

Green RC, Woodard JL, Green J: Validity of the Mattis Dementia Rating Scale for detection of cognitive impairment in the elderly. J Neuropsychiatry Clin Neurosci 7:357–360, 1995.

Grober E, Buschke H, Crystal H, et al: Screening for dementia by memory testing. Neurology 38:900–903, 1988.

Guo Z, Cupples LA, Kurz A, et al: Head injury and the risk of AD in the MIRAGE study. Neurology 54:1316–1323, 2000.

Gur RC, Ragland JD, Moberg PJ, et al: Computerized neurocognitive scanning: I: Methodology & validation in healthy people. Neuropsychopharmacology 25:766–776, 2001a.

Gur RC, Ragland JD, Moberg TH, et al: Computerized neurocognitive scanning: II: The profile of schizophrenia. Neuropsychopharmacology 25: 777-788, 2001b.

Hayden KA, Khachaturian AS, Tschanz JT, et al: Characteristics of a two-stage screen in a population survey of incident dementia: The Cache County Study. J Clin Epidemiol, in press.

Hogervorst E, Combrinck M, Lapuerta P, et al: The Hopkins Verbal Learning Test and screening for dementia. Dement Geriatr Cogn Disord 13:13–20, 2002.

Hughes CP, Berg L, Danziger WL, et al: A new clinical scale for the staging of dementia. Br J Psychiatry 140:566–572, 1982.

Jorm AF: Assessment of cognitive impairment and dementia using informant report. Clin Psychol Rev 16:51–73, 1996.

Jorm AF, Jacomb PA: The Informant Questionnaire on Cognitive Decline in the Elderly (IQCODE): Socio-demographic correlates, reliability, validity and some norms. Psychol Med 19:1015–1022, 1989.

Jurica PJ, Leitten CL, Mattis S: Dementia Rating Scale 2- Professional Manual. Odessa, FL: Psychological Assessment Resources, 2002.

Kahn RL, Goldfarb AI, Pollack M: Brief objective measures for the determination of mental status in the aged. Am J Psychiatry 117:326–328, 1960.

Kane RL, Kay GG: Computerized assessment in neuropsychology: A review of tests and test batteries. Neuropsychol Rev 3:1–117, 1992.

Katz S, Downs TD, Cash HR, et al: Progress in the development of the index of ADL. Gerontologist 10:20–30, 1970.

Katzman R, Brown T, Fuld P, et al: Validation of a short orientation-memory-concentration test of cognitive impairment. Am J Psychiatry 140:734–739, 1983.

Katzman R, Zhang M, Ouang Y-Q, et al: A Chinese version of the Mini-Mental State Examination: Impact of illiteracy in a Shanghai dementia survey. J Clin Epidemiol 41:971–978, 1988.

Kawas C, Karagiozis H, Reseau L, et al: Reliability of the Blessed Telephone Information-Memory-Concentration Test. J Geriatr Psychiatry Neurol 8:238–242, 1995.

Kent J, Plomin R: Testing specific cognitive abilities by telephone and mail. Intelligence 11:391–400, 1987.

Khachaturian A, Gallo JJ, Breitner JCS: Performance characteristics of a two-stage dementia screen for a population sample. J Clin Epidemiol 53:531–540, 2000.

Kiernan RJ, Mueller J, Langston JW, et al: The Neurobehavioral Cognitive Status Examination: A brief but differentiated approach to cognitive assessment. Ann Intern Med 107:481-485, 1987.

Knopman DS, DeKosky ST, Cummings JL, et al: Practice parameter: Diagnosis of dementia (an evidence based review). Report of the Quality Standards Subcommittee of the American Academy of Neurology. Neurology 56:1143–1153, 2001.

Lawton M, Brody E: Assessment of older people: Self-maintaining and instrumental activities of daily living. Gerontologist 9:179–186, 1969.

Letz RL, Green RC, Woodard JL: Development of a computer-based battery designed to screen adults for neuropsychological impairment. Neurotoxicol Teratol 18:365–370, 1996.

Logue PE, Tupler LA, D'Amico CJ, et al: The Neurobehavioral Cognitive Status Examination: Psychometric properties in use with psychiatric inpatients. J Clin Psychol 49:80–89, 1993.

Lukatela KA, Cohen RA, Kessler HA, et al: Dementia rating scale performance: A comparison of vascular and Alzheimer's dementia. J Clin Exp Neuropsychol 22:445–454, 2000.

Mackinnon A, Mulligan R: Combining cognitive testing and informant report to increase accuracy in screening for dementia. Am J Psychiatry 155:1529–1535, 1998.

Mahoney D, Tennstedt S, Friedman R, et al: An automated telephone system for monitoring the functional status of community residing elders. Gerontologist 39:229–234, 1999.

Mattis S: Dementia Rating Scale Professional Manual. Odessa, FL: Psychological Assessment Resources, 1973.

Mattis S: Mental status examination for organic mental syndrome in the elderly patient, in Bellak L, Karasu TB (eds): Geriatric Psychiatry. New York: Grune & Stratton, 1976, pp. 77–122.

McDowell I, Kristjansson B, Hill GB, et al: Community screening for dementia: The Mini-Mental State Exam (MMSE) and Modified Mini-Mental State Exam (3MS) compared. J Clin Epidemiol 50:377–383, 1997.

Mendez MF, Cherrier M, Perryman KM, et al: Frontotemporal dementia versus Alzheimer's disease: Differential cognitive features. Neurology 47:1189–1194, 1996.

Mohs, RC, Cohen L: Alzheimer's Disease Assessment Scale. Psychopharmacol Bull 24:627–628, 1988.

Mohs RC, Knopman D, Petersen RC, et al: Development of cognitive instruments for use in clinical trials of antidementia drugs: Additions to the Alzheimer's Disease Assessment Scale that broaden its scope. Alzheim Dis Assoc Disord 11(S2):S13–S21, 1997.

Mohs RC, RosenWG, Davis KL: The Alzheimer's Disease Assessment Scale: An instrument for assessing treatment efficacy. Psychopharmacol Bull 19:448–450, 1983.

Morris JC: The Clinical Dementia Rating Scale: Current version and scoring rules. Neurology 43:2412–2414, 1993.

Morris JC, Heyman A, Mohs RC, et al: The consortium to establish a registry for Alzheimer's disease (CERAD): Part 1. Clinical and neuropsychological assessment of Alzheimer's disease. Neurology 39:1159–1165, 1989.

Morris JC, Storandt M, Miller JP, et al: Mild cognitive impairment represents early-stage Alzheimer disease. Arch Neurol 58:397–405, 2001.

Mundt JC, Ferber KL, Rizzo M, et al: Computer-automated dementia screening using a touch-tone telephone Arch Intern Med 161:2481–2487, 2001.

Mungas D, Reed BR, Marshall SC, et al: Development of psychometrically matched English and Spanish language neuropsychological tests for older persons. Neuropsychology 14:209–223, 2000.

Murdoch I: Telemedicine. Br J Ophthalmol 83:1254–1256, 1999.

Nelson A, Fogel BS, Faust D: Bedside cognitive screening instruments. A critical assessment. J Nerv Ment Dis 174:73–83, 1986.

Nesselroade JR, Pederson NL, McClearn GE, et al: Factorial and criterion validities of telephone assessed cognitive ability measures. Res Aging 10:220–234, 1988.

Norton MC, Tschanz JT, Fan X, et al: Telephone adaptation of the Modified Mini-Mental State Examination (3MS): The Cache County Study. Neuropsychiatry Neuropsychol Behav Neurol 12:270–276, 1999.

Ogrocki PK, Welsh-Bohmer KA: Assessment of cognitive and functional impairment in the elderly, in Clark C (ed): Neurodegenerative Dementia: Clinical Features and Pathological Mechanisms. New York: McGraw-Hill, 2000, pp. 15–32.

Oremus M, Perrault A, Demers L, et al: Review of outcome measurement instruments in Alzheimer's disease drug trials: Psychometric properties of global scales. J Geriatr Psychiatry Neurol 13:197–205, 2001.

Petersen RC, Stevens JC, Ganguli M, et al: Practice parameter: Early detection of dementia: Mild cognitive impairment (an evidence-based review). Report of the Quality Standards Subcommittee of the American Academy of Neurology. Neurology 56:1133–1142, 2001.

Pfeffer RI, Kurosaki TT, Harrah C, et al: A survey diagnostic tool for senile dementia. Am J Epidemiol 114:515–527, 1981.

Pfeffer RI, Kurosaki TT, Harrah CH, et al: Measurement of functional activities in older adults in the community. J Gerontol 37:323–329, 1982.

Pfeiffer E: A short portable mental status questionnaire for the assessment of organic brain deficit in elderly patients. J Am Geriatr Soc 23:433–441, 1975.

Plassman BL, Newman TT, Welsh KA, et al: Properties of the telephone interview for cognitive status. Neuropsychiatry Neuropsychol Behav Neurol 7:235–241, 1994.

Randolph C: Repeatable Battery for the Assessment of Neuropsychological Status manual. San Antonio, TX: The Psychological Corporation, 1998.

Randolph C, Tierney MC, Mohr E, et al: The Repeatable Battery for the Assessment of Neuropsychological Status (RBANS): Preliminary clinical validity. J Clin Exp Neuropsychol 20:310–319, 1998.

Reisberg B, Ferris SH: Brief Cognitive Rating Scale (BCRS). Psychopharmacol Bull 24:629–636, 1988.

Reisberg B, Ferris SH, deLeon MJ, et al: The Global Deterioration Scale (GDS) for the assessment of primary degenerative dementia. Am J Psychiatry 139:1136–1139, 1982.

Reisberg B, Ferris SH, deLeon MJ, et al: Global Deterioration Scale (GDS). Psychopharmacol Bull 24:661–663, 1988.

Reitan RM, Wolfson D: The Halstead-Reitan Neuropsychological Test Battery: Theory and Clinical Interpretation. Tucson, AZ: Neuropsychology Press, 1993.

Richardson HE, Glass JN: A comparison of scoring protocols on the Clock Drawing Test in relation to ease of use, diagnostic group, and correlations with Mini-Mental State Examination. J Am Geriatr Soc 50:169–173, 2002.

Robbins T, James M, Owen A, et al: The Cambridge Neuropsychological Test Automated Battery (CANTAB): A factor analytic study in a large number of normal elderly volunteers. Dementia 5:26–281, 1994.

Robins LN, Helzer JE, Weissman MM, et al: Lifetime prevalence of specific psychiatric disorders in three sites. Arch Gen Psychiatry 41:949–958, 1984.

Roccaforte WH, Burke WJ, Bayer BL, et al: The reliability of a phone version of the Mini-Mental State Examination. J Am Geriatr Soc 40:697–702, 1992.

Roccaforte WH, Burke WJ, Bayer BL, et al: Reliability and validity of the Short Portable Mental Status Questionnaire administered by telephone. J Geriatr Psychiatry Neurol 6:33–38, 1993.

RosenWG, Mohs RC, Davis KL: A new rating scale for Alzheimer's disease. Am J Psychiatry 141:1356–1364, 1984.

Rouleau I Salmon DP, Butters N: Longitudinal analysis of clock drawing in Alzheimer's disease patients. Brain Cogn 31:17–34, 1996.

Royall DR, Cordes JA, Polk M: CLOX: An executive clock drawing task. J Neurol Neurosurg Psychiatry 64:588–594, 1998.

Salmon DP, Kwo-on-Yuen PF, Heindel WC, et al: Differentiation of Alzheimer's disease and Huntington's disease with the Dementia Rating Scale. Arch Neurol 46:1204–1208, 1989.

Salmon DP, Thomas RG, Pay MM, et al: Alzheimer's disease can be accurately diagnosed in very mildly impaired individuals. Neurology 59:10022–1028, 2002.

Schneider LS: Assessing outcomes in Alzheimer disease. Alzheim Dis Assoc Disord 15(Suppl. 1):S8–18, 2001.

Schwamm LH, Van Dyke C, Kiernan RJ, et al: The Neurobehavioral Cognitive Status Examination: Comparison with the Cognitive Capacity Screening Examination and the Mini-Mental State Examination in a neurosurgical population. Ann Intern Med 107:486–491, 1987.

Shulman KI: Clock drawing: Is it the ideal cognitive screening test? Intl J Geriatr Psychiatry 15:548–561, 2000.

Solomon PR, Hirschoff A, Kelly B, et al: A 7 minute neurocognitive screening battery highly sensitive to Alzheimer's disease. Arch Neurol 55:349–355, 1998.

Sternberg SA, Wolfson C, Baumgarten M: Undetected dementia in community-dwelling older people: The Canadian Study of Health and Aging. J Am Geriatr Soc 48:1430–1434, 2000.

Storandt M, Botwinick J, Danziger WL, et al: Psychometric differentiation of mild senile dementia of the Alzheimer type. Arch Neurol 41:497–499, 1984.

Strub R, Black F: The Mental Status Examination in Neurology. Philadelphia, PA: Davis, 1985.

Suhr JA, Grace J: Brief cognitive screening of right hemisphere stroke: Relation to functional outcome. Arch Phys Med Rehabil 80:773–776, 1999.

Summers WK, DeBoynton V, Marsh GM, et al: Comparison of seven psychometric instruments used for evaluation of treatment effect in Alzheimer's dementia. Neuroepidemiology 9:193–207, 1990.

Teng EL, Chui HC: The Modified Mini-Mental State (3MS) Examination. J Clin Psychiatry 48:314–318, 1987.

Teng EL, Chui HC, Schneider LS, et al: Alzheimer's dementia: Performance on the Mini-Mental State Examination. J Consult Clin Psychol 55:96–100, 1987.

Thal LJ, Grundman M, Golden R: Alzheimer's disease: A correlational analysis of the Blessed Information-Memory-Concentration Test and the Mini-Mental State Examination. Neurology 36:262–264, 1986.

Tombaugh TN, McDowell I, Kristjansson B, et al: Mini-mental State Examination (MMSE) and the Modified MMSE (3MS): A psychometric comparison and normative data. Psychol Assess 8:48–59, 1996.

Thrall JH, Boland G: Telemedicine in practice. Semin Nucl Med 28:145–157, 1998.

Tschanz JT, Welsh-Bohmer KA, West N: Identification of dementia cases derived from a neuropsychological algorithm: Comparisons with clinically derived diagnoses. Neurology 54:1290–1296, 2000.

U.S. Department of Health and Human Services. Clinician's Handbook of Preventive Services. Washington, DC: Department of Health and Human Services, 1998.

Valcour VG, Masaki KH, Curb JD, et al: The detection of dementia in the primary care setting. Arch Intern Med 160:2964–2968, 2000.

Vinzant CX: Dialing for dementia: A long distance Alzheimer's screen? Hold the phone. The Washington Post, February 19, 2002.

Weintraub S, Mesulam M: Mental state assessment of young and elderly adults in behavioral neurology, in Mesulam M (ed): Principles of Behavioral Neurology. Philadelphia, PA: Davis, 1985, pp. 71–85.

Wells JC, Keyl PM, Chase GA, et al: Discriminant validity of a reduced set of Mini Mental State Examination items for dementia and Alzheimer's disease. Acta Psychiatr Scand 86:23–31, 1992.

Welsh KA, Breitner JCS, Magruder-Habib KM: Detection of dementia in community volunteers using telephone screening of cognitive status. Neuropsychiatry Neuropsychol Behav Neurol 6:103–110, 1993.

Welsh KA, Butters N, Hughes JP: Detection of abnormal memory decline in mild Alzheimer's disease using CERAD neuropsychological measures. Arch Neurol 48:278–281, 1991.

Welsh KA, Butters N, Hughes JP, et al: Detection and staging of dementia in Alzheimer's disease: Use of the neuropsychological measures developed for the Consortium to Establish a Registry of Alzheimer's Disease (CERAD). Arch Neurol 49:448–452, 1992.

Welsh KA, Butters N, Mohs RC, et al: The Consortium to Establish a Registry of Alzheimer's disease (CERAD) Part V: A normative study of the neuropsychological battery. Neurology 44:609–614, 1994.

Welsh KA, Fillenbaum G, Wilkinson W: Neuropsychological performance of black and white patients with Alzheimer's disease. Neurology 45:2207–2211, 1995.

Welsh-Bohmer KA, Mohs RC: Neuropsychological assessment of Alzheimer's disease. Neurology 49:S11–S13, 1997.

Wolf-Klein GP, Silverstone FA, Levy AP, et al: Screening for Alzheimer's disease by clock drawing. J Am Geriatr Soc 37:730–734, 1989.

Zec RF, Landreth ES, Vicari SK, et al: Alzheimer Disease Assessment Scale: A subtest analysis. Alzheim Dis Assoc Disord 6:164–181, 1992.

Neuropsychological Assessment

Ricardo de Oliveira Souza

Jorge Moll

Paul J. Eslinger

Cognitive impairments

Neuropsychological testing

Psychometrics

Reliability

Validity

INTRODUCTION

The term neuropsychology was formally used by Donald Hebb in his 1949 book *Organization of* *Behavior: A Neuropsychological Theory* (Bruce, 1985). Up to the 1970s, neuropsychology consisted mainly of a set of theories primarily devoted to the nature of the mind-brain problem and other philosophical quests (Dimond, 1978). The recognition that neuropsychology could provide a set of clinical diagnostic and assessment tools grew slowly from the application of statistical techniques to the standardization of psychological tests and scales in normal and patient samples (Green, 1981; Hess & Hart, 1990). This growth was particularly apparent after World War II, with the need for extensive clinical services for many young veterans and through successive decades has grown alongside related fields of clinical psychology, behavioral neurology, neuroscience, neuropsychiatry, and neurorehabilitation.

Although the art and science of clinical neuropsychology should not be viewed as simply test administration and scoring, the psychometrics of human behavior continues to play a pivotal role in the development and validation of it as a branch of clinical practice. *Psychometrics* refers to the quantitative measurement of behavior. Its main parameters include measurement reliability and validity, each with multiple components of *how repeatable* such measurement can be (reliability) and *what* such measurement may be reflecting about processes of human behavior in relationship to brain function (validity). Neuropsychological assessment refers to standardized procedures that act as stimuli for the elicitation of behavioral responses under specific controlled conditions (Benton, 1994; Levin, 1994). Neuropsychological tests differ from rating scales and inventories in that the latter result from the subjective attachment of arbitrary numerical values (often on an ordinal scale) to naturalistic observations, for example, ankle swelling, confusion, or paranoid delusions (Stevens, 1946). Tests and scales are used routinely in the assessment of varied clinical problems. The essential distinction is that neuropsychological tests conform to the classical stimulus-response paradigm for evaluation of neurocognitive processes, whereas rating scales sample general impressions about symptom occurrence and frequency. These approaches can be illustrated further within the context of a diagnostic work-up.

In the first place, we wonder whether a presenting patient has a diagnosis. Most often it is complaints from patients, family members, or a third party (such as employer or teacher) or referral because of another clinician's concerns that prompts a comprehensive history and medical evaluation. This often outlines the nature and extent of the presenting problems. For example, an older person is brought for evaluation because of concerns by family members about failing memory. Yet, mental status screening and medical evaluation can be unrevealing or only minimally revealing of a problem (e.g., mild cerebral atrophy, an average or slightly low score on a mental status screening test). (See Chapter 1 for strengths and limits of such screening tests.) Despite the negative objective findings, questions may nevertheless be raised about early stages of a degenerative or other dementia, possible effects of depression or other psychological maladies, or age-associated memory

changes that are not necessarily pathologic. Detailed neuropsychological testing may then be in order to sort out and evaluate each of these possibilities. In other patients, history and medical evaluation may already support a specific diagnosis such as postconcussive syndrome after traumatic brain injury, multiple sclerosis, stroke, or cardiac arrest with cerebral hypoxia. These diagnoses rely on a *categorical decision* after proper criteria are applied, and this stage of the evaluative process may suffice for certain clinicians in their practice to decide on prognosis and management. When we wish to know how much of the diagnosed condition is present, we proceed to a *dimensional* evaluation (McHugh & Slavney, 1998). Certain rating scales and inventories may be suited to this aim and can be helpful initially, but these are impressionistic and subjective. For purposes of confirming diagnosis, planning rehabilitation, determining disability, and establishing baseline functioning, we may also need to document and clarify which cognitive domains are impaired and to what degree. For all of these situations, neuropsychological testing is the ideal process to illuminate and even settle outstanding questions about brain and behavior capacities and profiles. Given its quantitative and standardized nature, neuropsychological testing is more objective and precise than the qualitative clinical examination and also allows for gauging changes along definite time frames.

Although clinical neuropsychology has strong working and historical affiliations with other fields of clinical practice, particularly neurology, neurosurgery, and psychiatry, it should not be confused either in purpose or in method. The critical notion is that neuropsychological assessment is an examination process that addresses behavioral, cognitive, and emotional issues within combined neurologic and psychological frameworks. As such, it entails certain methodological virtues and limitations as do other quantitative and clinical assays of neurobiology and behavior.

THE CLINICAL CONCEPT OF BEHAVIOR AND NEUROBEHAVIORAL DISORDER

Mental life expresses itself outwardly as verbal and gestural actions and somatic changes that are collectively referred to as behavior. Gestural action in this context encompasses most kinds of nonverbal and motor behaviors (Goodglass & Kaplan, 1963). Because behavior is the only manifestation of another person's mind that can be overtly observed and measured, we infer the occurrence of normality and abnormality in mental processing and its underlying neural substrate from patterns of behavioral change. This inference is made on the basis of (1) information often gathered with the patient, relatives, nurses, or physicians; (2) systematic observation, during which qualitative data, such as symptoms and signs, are probed by a trained professional; (3) semiquantitative data extracted from standardized inventories and scales; and (4) quantitative data generated from standardized neuropsychological tests that are validated in diverse neurologic samples with structural brain lesions and other forms of neurologic pathophysiology.

Cognition, emotion, and motivation comprise the foundation of normal mental life (Hilgard, 1980; Fisher, 1993). Cognition refers to information processing by which knowledge is acquired, stored, manipulated, retrieved, and used by the individual for instrumental and adaptive functioning within complex environments (Neisser, 1967). It is composed of multiple domains, such as attention, memory, language, perception, visuospatial abilities, and executive performance, which are themselves comprised of more elementary processes. Mind and behavior are the product of complex interactions involving regional and widely projecting neural systems. The former are composed of cortico-cortical and cortico-subcortical networks that engender emotion, motivation, and cognition, whereas the latter are composed of brainstem and basal forebrain-hypothalamic projecting systems that set behavioral states, such as wakefulness and sleep, and modify the level and quality of the activity of the regional systems.

The mental state exam is often an initial office or bedside assessment that probes neurobehavioral impairments. It is incorporated into most clinical neurologic and psychiatric consultations and addresses the major compartments of the normal and abnormal mind (see Chapter 3 for further description and details). As part of the clinical examination, it centers on the following qualitative aspects of patient presentation:

- The ability to sit, stand, and walk
- General appearance and behavior
- The ability to define long-term goals and handle the daily challenges of life
- Social skills and style of interpersonal interactions, including emotional expression
- The form of thought, language, and nonverbal behavior
- The content of thought, speech and language, and nonverbal behavior
- Delusions and hallucinations
- Screening of cognitive abilities, in particular orientation, memory, and general reasoning skills

In most cases skillful clinicians can identify gross mental status abnormalities related to the above-mentioned items during office and bedside consultation.

WHEN TO ORDER NEUROPSYCHOLOGICAL TESTING: AIMS, SCOPE, INDICATIONS, AND LIMITS

The need for neuropsychological assessment usually becomes evident when a patient presents with or is referred for known or suspected behavioral/cognitive changes that may have a neurologic or other biologic basis. Indications for assessment can arise from several fields of medical practice, including neurology, neurosurgery, and psychiatry most frequently but also from internal medicine, cardiology, family practice, rheumatology, and gerontology. Clinical neuropsychologists are typically accessible through departments of neurology and psychiatry of major medical centers and medical schools, sometimes in neurosurgery departments, psychology or rehabilitation medicine departments, in graduate university settings where clinical psychology training programs (and training clinic) are offered, and in some private practice settings. Common indications for referral are summarized in Table 2-1.

To accomplish diagnostic testing, clinical neuropsychologists must rely on background data from several sources that typically include the patient himself, relatives, the referral source, and in certain circumstances the patient's colleagues, teachers, and friends. This stage of assessment is based on informal conversations, review of medical records, and structured interviews from which semiquantitative data may be adduced through ordinal scales such as behavioral inventories. Many patients referred for neuropsychological assessment may bring along the results of ancillary exams, such as clinical neurologic exam, brain computed tomography scan, other neuroimaging, and blood biochemistry, that may inform and help sharpen the focus of assessment. Collateral information and test data as summarized in a referral letter or through available records are helpful in guiding the type of neuropsychological testing to be used in individual patients. Such information is often critical to frame the type of questions neuropsychological assessment is expected to pose and answer and hence what kind of assessment approach to use.

There are two general types of neuropsychological assessment approaches. Fixed batteries are composed of established assemblies of tests that have general sensitivity to varied brain diseases. Examples include the Wechsler scales for general intelligence and the Halstead-Reitan battery (e.g., Reitan & Wolfson, 1993; Wechsler, 1997). The reliability and validity of such measures depend on the fixed presentation of specific stimulus materials, with no flexibility for variation or modification, at least if the available normative data are to be accurately referenced. In contrast, flexible batteries are composed through the selection of independent

TABLE 2-1. Common Indications for Ordering Neuropsychological Testing

- To determine if some apparently minor deviations from usual behavior should be valued as harbingers of a serious illness. This is especially important for the early diagnosis of several kinds of dementia, such as HIV-related dementia, Alzheimer disease, and other primary degenerative and vascular dementias
- To characterize the effects of neurologic and psychiatric disease in cognitive and behavioral terms, both qualitative and quantitative aspects
- To monitor progression of disease
- To monitor recovery or the effects of treatment
- To diagnose and scale mental retardation
- To estimate premorbid intelligence
- To understand the underlying structure of behavioral symptoms
- To define the impact of abnormality or change on real-world activities, which encompass the major domains of family, social, and occupational life (i.e., identifying impairments, functional limitations, and disabilities), at times to qualify for disability, vocational, and other services
- To plan rehabilitation
- To tailor rehabilitation programs to the needs of individual patients
- To assess mental competency in forensic settings
- To distinguish "organic," "psychiatric," and "functional" conditions
- To establish the cognitive, behavioral, and emotional effects/consequences of suspected neurologic illness or injury, such as chemical and toxic exposures, and in systemic medical disease (cardiac arrest, liver failure)
- To assess the cognitive and sensory-motor skills that are needed for the adequate performance of diverse and risky activities of civilian life, such as driving and piloting

tests. The specific choice of tests depends on the particular presenting symptoms and history of the patient as well as the training, experience, and judgment of the examiner. For example, complaints of "lapses of attention" versus "short-term memory loss" versus "reading comprehension difficulties" versus "poor and impulsive decision making" will prompt quite different test selections to address the specific questions and concerns raised in consultation. Other substantial differences can exist between the two approaches. These often revolve around the amount of testing hours (often longer with fixed batteries), costs of testing, type of description and interpretation of neuropsychological test results the examiner strives for, and the examiner's view of what role the assessment should play in evaluation and management processes. (Further discussion of the pros and cons of fixed and flexible batteries can be found in Tranel [1992], Lezak [1995], and in Chapter 27.) Obvious frail, ill, agitated, hyperactive, and inattentive patients may be able to participate in very limited neuropsychological testing; hence, a flexible approach is imperative. The flexible battery approach is the predominant mode of training and practice in the field and we recommend it for all neuropsychological consultation needs. To initially establish rapport with patients, help them acclimate to

the testing process, and encourage their best efforts, clinical neuropsychologists typically begin with a general screening approach to survey major cognitive domains and abilities. This sampling method helps define problem areas that can then be investigated in depth with more specific instruments.

The clinical practice of neuropsychological assessment depends not only on characteristics of one's patient population (e.g., acutely ill, rehabilitation setting, outpatient neurology, psychiatry, or gerontology clinic), but also on one's institutional or private practice resources (e.g., space, materials, computers, technical assistance), health insurance/financial reimbursement requirements (e.g., preauthorization for services, limitations to provider services and payments, self-pay, etc.), and other consultative demands. Those constraints aside, neuropsychological consultation should, at a minimum, endow the referring health care provider and patient with fresh insights into the processes underlying the patient's profile of spared and impaired cognitive capacities, their relationship to the patient's history, presentation and other exam findings, diagnostic possibilities, prognosis and recommendations for further evaluation, intervention options, rehabilitation planning, management, occupational, and educational recommendations, and follow-up care.

TABLE 2-2. Examples of Relating Neuropsychological (Np) Tests to Patient Presentations and Larger Constructs About Behavior and the Brain

Neuropsychological construct	Symptoms or syndromes	Examples of tests useful in diagnosis and follow-up
Wakefulness	Stupor and coma	Not applicable
	Acute confusional states	Not applicable
Attention	Acute confusional states	Digit and spatial span
	Neglect syndromes	Trailmaking, A and B
		Stroop interference task
		Double simultaneous stimulation
		Cancellation tasks
Psychomotor agility	Acute confusional states	Wechsler Digit Symbol Subtest
		Wechsler Block Design Subtest
Orientation	Acute confusional states	Temporal orientation
	Certain dementia syndromes, such as Alzheimer disease	Mini-Mental State Exam
Global cognitive state	Acute confusional states	Mini-Mental State Exam
	Certain dementia syndromes, such as Alzheimer disease	Cognitive Capacity Screening Exam
		Cognistat
Language	Aphasia	Multilingual Aphasia Exam
		Boston Diagnostic Aphasia Exam

See Lezak (1995), Spreen & Strauss (1998), and Weintraub (2000) for test details.

STRUCTURE AND RATIONALE OF NEUROPSYCHOLOGICAL ASSESSMENT

In this section we discuss the rationale and neurobehavioral bases of neuropsychological assessment. We have organized it to present the general scientific principles underlying neuropsychological assessment, the contents of a neuropsychological report, and its implications for management (Caplan, 1990). Emphasis is placed on the neuropsychological counterparts of both the observable and qualitative aspects of behavior. Details of individual test administration, norms, and interpretation can be found in sources including Lezak (1995) and Spreen and Strauss (1998).

Fundamental and Regulatory Neurobehavioral States

In considering the epistemology of contemporary neuropsychiatry, Cummings (1999) proposed that brain dysfunction arises from two general types of changes: "fundamental" and "instrumental." Fundamental changes result from disorders in brain mechanisms that permit behavioral and mental states to occur. These mechanisms exert regulatory influences on brain networks mediating specific instrumental or goal-directed behaviors such as praxis, language, and decision making (Mesulam, 1987). Such regulation revolves around the initiation, inhibition, and maintenance of neurobiologic activity and depends on the physiologic effects of ascending projection systems from specific nuclei in the upper brainstem, hypothalamus, and basal forebrain. The main syndromes resulting from impairments of regulatory mechanisms are typically described as diffuse or multifocal brain disease and include:

- Acute confusional states and delirium (Victor et al., 2001)
- Stupor and coma (Plum, 1991)
- Catatonia, with or without catatonic stupor (Barnes et al., 1986)

At the bedside, neuropsychological assessment is useful to follow worsening or improving symptoms in patients with impairments of regulatory brain systems. Table 2-2 illustrates some of the relationships among neuropsychological constructs, neurobehavioral syndromes, and some neuropsychological tests commonly used in their assessment. Note that neuropsychological constructs cut across a wide range of clinical diagnoses, a phenomenon often observed when dimensional are compared with categorical analyses (Andreasen, 1999).

Instrumental and Goal-Directed Behaviors

Impairments of instrumental and goal-directed behaviors usually result from dysfunction and disease in functional cortical and subcortical networks. Behavioral neurology and neuropsychology are historically linked to classical neurology (Geschwind, 1965a, 1965b; Luria, 1980) where forms of neuropsychological assessment were implicitly exerted by neurologists with personal interests in the behavioral syndromes resulting from cortical damage (e.g., Marie, 1911; Dejerine, 1914; Liepmann, 1980). By the beginning of the 20th century, restricted injuries to the cerebral cortex were already known to give rise to "the syndromes of the 4A's": *aphasias, agnosias, apraxias, and amnesias* (American Psychiatric Association [APA], 1994). The recognition of the clinical relevance of cortical syndromes required that the neurologic exam be eventually refined to account for the evaluation and description of symptoms of far greater complexity than damage to the pyramidal tract or visual pathways (Bouchard & Brissaud, 1904). This created the need for new techniques of examination that have continued to multiply ever since. In this volume alone, there are chapters devoted to aphasia (see Chapter 17), apraxia (see Chapter 18), amnesia (see Chapter 11), as well as agnosias (see Chapters 12 and 13). Pioneer efforts were closely followed by conceptual shifts in how the brain functioned, its organization, and the relationships between brain and behavior. Questions about "localization of function" have persisted ever since. Nevertheless, the clinical-anatomic concepts of the 4A's syndromes fostered major advances in the practice of neurology and particularly neuropsychology in the 1970s and 1980s when neuropsychology eventually became firmly established as a clinically useful procedure (Benton, 1994).

Aphasias, agnosias, apraxias, and amnesias have more recently been supplemented by emphasis on the frontal lobe and dysexecutive syndromes, disorders of awareness, emotion and the brain, and the key roles of cortical-subcortical networks (e.g., frontal-striatal, thalamo-cortical in adaptive behavior; Eslinger & Damasio, 1985; Tranel et al., 1994; Grafman & Litvan, 1999; Rolls, 1999). These broadened approaches provide solid ground on which new syndromes have been described, departing from simply the fractionation and recombination of the classical ones. They have also defined some of the main lines of reasoning that pervade contemporary concepts of brain-behavior relationships and how the human brain is organized not only in anatomic terms but also in functional networks that subserve people's adaptation to complex social and physical environments. Recent emphasis on integrating cognition and emotion has been particularly refreshing because some have perceived that the convexity of the cerebral hemispheres were the province of the neurologist, whereas the mediobasal parts were the province of the psychiatrist (Papez, 1937; Luria, 1980). No matter how simplistic this formulation may appear today, it has framed some of the ways medicine is practiced and how we think about normal and abnormal human behavior, its diagnostic evaluation, treatment, and management.

The domains discussed in this section represent those underlying processes and observable actions of the individual on his environment for the purpose of achieving goals (i.e., goal-directed behavior). Goal-directed behaviors depend on internally represented mental models, expectations, and working memory capacities and are often expressed through instrument means, be it words, gestures, tool use, reading, or grocery shopping (Yakovlev, 1948; Vygotsky, 1978). Goal-directed instrumental actions must be organized within the spatial-temporal constraints of our environment and finely coordinated so that behavior is adjusted to both physical and sociocultural frameworks.

The syndromes of amnesia, apraxia, aphasia, agnosia, and executive dysfunction broadly define the field of "instrumental and goal-directed neuropsychology." Much information can be informally obtained about these functions by observing the patient's behavior with an inquiring and trained mind. Several neuropsychological instruments also exist to provide the clinician with data extracted from systematic and quantitative methods of analysis.

NEUROPSYCHOLOGICAL DOMAINS AS TARGETS OF NEUROPSYCHOLOGICAL ASSESSMENT

A classification of neuropsychological domains appears in Table 2-3. There are now many tests designed to assess each domain, though psychometric properties, normative observations, and clinical utility are still highly variable and often incomplete (Barton et al., 1981; Lezak, 1995; Spreen & Strauss, 1998; Weintraub, 2000). The task of establishing the reliability and validity of neuropsychological instruments is difficult and challenging, given the tremendous diversity of human abilities and the influence of age, language, and culture, as well as diseases of the central nervous system. Thus, extensive graduate training and supervised clinical experience are critical to the accurate recognition of the possibilities and limitations of neuropsychological testing. The recent association of neuropsychology and neuroimaging has refined our understanding of some of the neural correlates of widely used tests (Damasio & Damasio, 1989; Kertesz, 1994). The introduction of *functional* brain imaging is providing the impetus for the development of novel instruments that reliably activate discrete cerebral areas and circuits involved in higher-order cognitive processes.

Abnormality on group I tests in Table 2-3 (Regulatory and Fundamental Neurobehavioral Systems) reflects impairment in functional systems across to large extensions of the cerebral hemispheres. Normal performance on such tests is hardly compatible with a diffuse or multifocal pathophysiology, whether arising locally or resulting from systemic disease. Such sensitivity to brain dysfunction is counterbalanced by a low anatomic and functional localizing value. Functional localization and

TABLE 2-3. Neuropsychological Domains

Group I. Regulatory and fundamental neurobehavioral systems

- Wakefulness

  The ability to keep the eyes open for extended periods; spontaneous blinking is also a feature of normal wakefulness
- Attention-concentration

  Involuntary: reflex orientation of head and eyes to sudden and/or unexpected stimuli

  Voluntary: the ability to concentrate attentional resources and resist distraction by extraneous stimuli (e.g., focused, divided, and sustained attention; shifts of attention)

  Inhibition

  Behavioral comportment (speech, actions)

  Inhibition of impulsive and prepotent responses
- Psychomotor agility

  Global: locomotor and gestural

  Visuomanual (pegboard, finger tapping)

  Audioverbal
- Orientation to place and time
- Global cognitive status

Group II. Instrumental and goal-directed neurobehavioral systems

- Executive behavior

  Flexibility

  Planning/organization

  Strategy application

  Set alternation and response shifting

  Working memory
- Auditory perception and language

  Expressive naming and discourse

  Aural comprehension and reading

  Repetition of words, numbers, sentences

  Written expression (copy, dictation, composition)

  Calculations

  Prosody—emotional intonation and comprehension of speech

  Nonverbal auditory recognition (environmental sounds, music)
- Praxis

  Ideomotor

      Execution of actions in response to verbal commands

      Execution of actions in response to visual commands (visuoimitative)

  Ideational or conceptual

      Performance of sequential actions (e.g., serving coffee and mailing a letter, use of tools and utensils)

  Tactile and body schema

  Discrimination, recognition, and localization of tactile stimuli

  Finger localization

  Right-left discrimination

  Tactile memory

Continued

TABLE 2-3. Neuropsychological Domains—cont'd

Group II. Instrumental and goal-directed neurobehavioral systems

- Visual perception and construction
  - Object perception, such as faces, animals, and tools
  - Perception of spatial relationships, such as line angles and depth
  - Color perception
  - Motion perception
  - Constructional praxis
  - Recognition of familiar environments and landmarks
- Learning, memory, and recall
  - Encoding, consolidation, and retrieval/recognition of verbal and nonverbal materials including:
    - Verbal list learning and memory
    - Story recall—immediate and delayed
    - Digit sequence learning
    - Paired associate learning and memory
    - Geometric figure learning and memory
    - Faces, pictures—immediate and delayed recall and recognition

Group III. Interhemispheric asymmetries and laterality effects

- Object naming with nonpreferred hand
- Nonpreferred hand praxis to verbal commands
- Dichotic listening
- Tachistoscopic testing
- Sensory extinction and spatial allocation of attention

Group IV. Neuropsychological tasks under research scrutiny with potential clinical utility in the near future

- The gambling task family
- Complex planning and managerial tasks
- Probes for complex social cognition and behavior (e.g., theory of mind tasks)
- Cognitive simulation
- Emotion perception and processing

lateralization are best accomplished by applying tests of groups II (Instrumental and Goal-Directed Neurobehavioral Systems) and III (Interhemispheric Asymmetries and Laterality Effects). The latter tests are specifically directed at evaluation of how accurately and efficiently the two cerebral hemispheres communicate and coordinate cognitive and motor processes, principally through the corpus callosum but also other subcortical pathways as well (see Chapter 19). Examples of some of the tests that may be used to assess these neuropsychological domains are listed in Table 2-4.

Interpretation of performance on specific neuropsychological tests is accomplished by first establishing that the administration of the procedure was valid and that the results likely represent the best efforts of the patient. Second, scoring the test follows a specified algorithm that may provide "correction" factors for educational background, sex, and even age. Third, comparison is made to tables of normative observations that permit identification of the patient's score relative to their peer group, usually in the form of a percentile rank or performance range (e.g., low average, superior, etc.).

Importantly, it is not only the test score that is of interest, but also the actual performance of patients. Performance is often accomplished by tracking the kinds of errors that patients commit, whether a prompt or a cue is helpful, whether patients are aware of their errors, and how they process and react to task demands. Some tests permit probing of errors and benefit of cues, whereas others are standardized for very specific instructions and feedback by the examiner. For example, a patient who experiences difficulties in generating names of objects may verbalize a paraphasic type of error (e.g., "chair," "shable," or "wooden top with

TABLE 2-4. Examples of Neuropsychological Tests

Group I. Regulatory and fundamental neurobehavioral systems	
Wakefulness	Epworth Sleepiness Scale (Johns, 1991)
Attention-concentration	Tests of Everyday Attention (Robertson et al., 1994)
	Continuous Performance Test (Conners, 2000)
	Brief Test of Attention (Schretlen, 1997)
	Wechsler Digit and Spatial Span (Wechsler, 1997)
Inhibition	Go/No Go Tasks
	Stroop Color-Word Test
	Antisaccade Task
	Continuous Performance Test (Conners, 2000)
	Motor Impersistence (Benton et al., 1994)
Psychomotor agility	Purdue Pegboard (Tiffin, 1968)
	Timed tests from UPDRS and CAPIT (Fahn et al., 1987)
	Wechsler Digit Symbol Subtest (Wechsler, 1997)
	Symbol Digit Modalities Test (Smith, 1982)
Orientation to place and time	MMSE (Crum et al., 1993)
	Temporal Orientation (Benton et al., 1994)
Global cognitive status	Wechsler Adult Intelligence Scale III (Wechsler, 1997)
	Cognistat (Kiernan et al., 1983)
	Mattis Dementia Rating Scale (Mattis, 1988)
Group II. Instrumental and goal-directed neurobehavioral systems	
Executive functions	Wisconsin Card Sorting Test (Heaton et al., 1993)
	Tower tests: London, Hanoi, Toronto (Goldberg et al., 1990; Krikorian et al., 1994)
	Strategy Application Test–Revised (Levine et al., 2002)
	Trailmaking Test, part B (Reitan & Wolfson, 1993 1993), 1993)
	Paced Auditory Serial Addition Test (Gronwall & Wrighston, 1975)
	Verbal Associative Fluency (Benton, 1968)
Language and auditory perception	Multilingual Aphasia Examination (Benton & Hamsher, 1989)
	Boston Diagnostic Aphasia Examination (Goodglass & Kaplan, 1987)
	Boston Assessment of Severe Aphasia Examination (Helm-Estabrooks et al., 1989)
	Sound Recognition Test (Benton & Hamsher, 1989)
Praxis	Florida Apraxia Battery (Heilman & Rothi, 1993)
Tactile and body schema	Finger Localization (Benton et al., 1994)
	Right Left Discrimination (Benton et al., 1994)
	Tactile Form Perception (Benton et al., 1994)
Visual perception, spatial and construction	Visual Form Discrimination (Benton et al., 1994)
	Benton Facial Recognition Test (Benton et al., 1994)
	Judgment of Line Orientation Test (Benton et al., 1994)
	Visual Object and Space Perception Battery (Warrington & James, 1991)
	3-D Block Construction (Benton et al., 1994)
	Copy of Rey Complex Figure (Lezak, 1995)
	Clock Drawing Test (Royall et al., 1998)

Continued

TABLE 2-4. Examples of Neuropsychological Tests—cont'd

Group II. Instrumental and goal-directed neurobehavioral systems	
Learning, memory, and recall	California Verbal Learning Test (Delis et al., 1987)
	Enhanced Cued Recall Test (Grober et al., 1988)
	Wechsler Memory Scale III (Wechsler, 1997)
	Serial Digit Learning (Benton et al., 1994)
	Benton Visual Retention Test (Sivan, 1992)
	Recall of Rey Complex Figure (Lezak, 1995)
	Rivermead Behavioural Memory Test (Wilson et al., 1991)
Group III. Interhemispheric asymmetries and laterality effects	
	Dichotic listening
	Tachistoscopic presentation
	Tactile naming with nonpreferred hand
	Praxis to verbal command with nonpreferred hand
Group IV. Neuropsychological tasks under research scrutiny with potential clinical utility in the near future	
Gambling tasks	Siegel (1978); Bechara et al. (1994)
Strategic management simulation	Satish et al. (1999)
Theory of Mind tasks	Happé (1994); Baron-Cohen et al. (2001)

legs" for table), a nonsense word (neologism), or simply say "I don't know" and refuse to guess. The examiner can probe whether phonemic cues ("the word starts with ta…"), semantic cues ("It is used when you eat a meal" or "It is a piece of furniture") or a visual cue ("It has four legs and a hard top") are helpful for the patient. If so, retrieval and perceptual types of deficits can be investigated alongside visual and verbal knowledge representations. These qualitative observations are useful in identifying disturbed and preserved cognitive *processes* and subsequent development of remediation options and possible interventions that can be implemented by the patient, family members, or other therapists. Similar analyses can be undertaken for learning and memory, problem solving, perceptual tasks, attention, and many other domains of processing. Learning and memory are perhaps the most common areas of neuropsychological investigation. Learning processes are broadly defined as *encoding* and encompass an array of attention-concentration, learning strategy, working memory, and associative mechanisms for registration, maintenance, manipulation, and integration of new information. Any or all of these underlying mechanisms may be affected and produce impaired learning. Specialized tests can tease apart several of these components to help delineate the specific nature of the learning impairment. After it is encoded, new information undergoes an extended consolidation period that entails neurobiologic mechanisms of protein synthesis for receptor growth, potentiation of synaptic connections, and stabilization of memory traces that can endure in long-term storage. Although the behavioral components of consolidation are not well understood, rehearsal, review, and utilization of the new information likely contribute to consolidation. Amnesic patients may show relatively normal encoding but rapid forgetting (deficient consolidation), leading to loss of recent information and experiences. It is possible to generate "forgetting curves" through several neuropsychological tests, evaluating the rate and characteristics of forgetting and remembering. Other patients with memory disorders show normal levels of encoding, consolidation, and long-term memory but exhibit a retrieval deficit that essentially interferes with *access* to long-term memory. Still other patients with memory disorders will exhibit material-specific memory deficits (i.e., verbal or visuospatial), autobiographical amnesia, or fractionated forms of knowledge loss. These many possibilities must be investigated through a careful selection of neuropsychological tests along with comprehensive history, interview, and review of the patient's medical test data.

LOCALIZATION IN NEUROPSYCHOLOGY

"Localization" in neuropsychology should be understood in both functional and anatomic terms. In addition to the anatomic correlates of various neuropsychological impairments, there has been increasing interest in the relationship between real-life outcomes and neuropsychological performance (Mesulam, 1990; Eslinger, 2002b). Such functional analyses are advancing understanding of localization of nervous function in essential ways (Zangwill, 1963; Gazzaniga, 2000). Several factors influence the clinical expression of the symptoms produced by brain damage in decisive ways (e.g., Geschwind, 1982). Important among them are the size and multiplicity of lesions, as well as their rate of growth ("momentum"), histopathologic nature, age at onset, and the integrity of brain systems that might provide compensatory support. The recognition of these factors is important for the solution to several apparent paradoxes and for the development of a valid theory of localization that accounts for the variability of clinically observed facts. The following case illustrates this point.

CASE STUDY

Nearly Normal Language Coexistent with Gross Destruction of the Left Hemisphere Language Areas

A 59-year-old engineer presented to consultation after a first generalized seizure. During the preceding few months he occasionally mixed words of the three languages he spoke. He had some word-finding difficulties, which were easily corrected by lexical or phonemic cues. Magnetic resonance imaging (MRI) showed an invasive tumor in the superior and middle sectors of the left temporal lobe with mass effects on the frontal and parietal lobes and subcortical structures. Wernicke's area seemed to be destroyed, yet he understood what was said to him and expressed himself fluently and meaningfully (Fig. 2-1). He could repeat words and sentences of varying length without hesitation. He was not apraxic to gestural or verbal commands. A functional MRI (fMRI) protocol was undertaken to visualize his language areas. Dynamic T2* echo-planar images were acquired with a 1.5 T scanner during alternating periods of rest and while he listened to the news from a newspaper. Language comprehension activated the temporal and parietal areas surrounding the tumor (arrow), the cingulate gyrus, and the right superior temporal gyrus, including the primary auditory cortex (Fig. 2-2). The patient became aphasic after surgical removal of the tumor. Histopathologic analysis confirmed the hypothesis of glioblastoma multiforme.

Comment. This patient showed spared ability to understand and produce spoken language despite gross destruction of the left hemisphere posterior language areas as revealed on structural MRI. Such a lesion typically is associated with significant aphasia. fMRI revealed that language activation still occurred in areas around the tumor and was not displaced to the right hemipshere since aphasia developed after subsequent tumor resection. The slow, progressive nature of the lesion may have permitted the compensatory language processing.

Damage to Different Neural Sites May Present as Similar Behavioral Syndromes

The organization and continuity of behavior depends on the dynamic interplay of discrete brain regions in

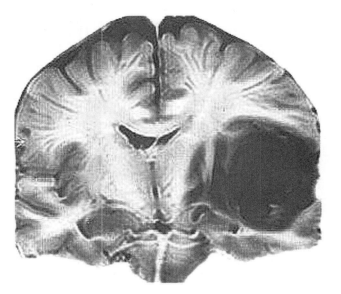

FIGURE 2-1. Brain MRI showing tumor.

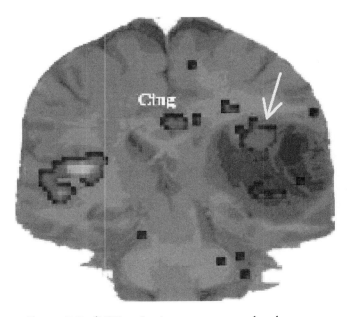

FIGURE 2-2. fMRI activation pattern to spoken language.

space and time (Friston, 1996). Each node of the neural circuitry that mediates a given process contributes with a specific dimension to the accomplishment of various tasks (Crowe, 1998). Test scores represent the output of a functional system and, as such, convey clues only about the overall quality of a particular neuropsychological process operations. Accordingly, damage to different regions that are typically recruited during the execution of a test may lead to similar low scores. This point is illustrated in normal humans executing a verbal adaptation of the Trailmaking Test (TMT; Oliveira-Souza et al., 2000). In comparison to part A, which does not involve cognitive shifting, part B of the TMT recruits activity in a network encompassing the lower middle frontal gyrus

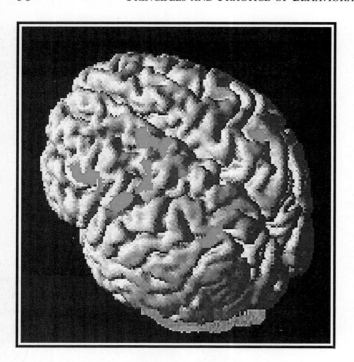

FIGURE 2-3. fMRI study showing the combined activation in prefrontal and premotor cortices as well as the parietal lobe related to cognitive set-shifting, motor switching, and visuospatial attention, respectively.

and premotor cortex of the left hemisphere as well as the intraparietal sulcus bilaterally (Moll et al., 2000a) (Fig. 2-3). The lower middle prefrontal activation is critically related to set-shifting (Konishi et al., 1999a), whereas activation of the premotor cortex is involved in switching between motor programs (Moll et al., 2000b). Activation of the intraparietal sulcus probably reflects the visuoattentional discriminative demands of the task (Sohn et al., 2000). Another illustration of this principle comes from comparisons of the performance of patients with lesions of the frontal or parieto-occipital cortex on block design (Luria & Tsvetkova, 1964). Patients with damage to the parieto-occipital cortex score in the normal range if they are allowed to look at a real model of the structure they are supposed to construct. What is at fault is their ability to mentally make spatial transformations of objects in two- and three-dimensional space. In contrast, patients with frontal damage do not profit from the real model of the structure they must construct. They lack the ability to apply strategies that lead them toward their goals, in this case to reproduce the visually presented model. These patients perform normally if they are guided by explicit instructions at each step of the constructional process. In short, whereas lesions in the frontal and in the parieto-occipital cortex lead to low scores on block designing, these low scores are traceable to rather different underlying neuropsychological mechanisms.

The above findings account for the some of the low anatomic localizing value of neuropsychological instruments in general. They show that symptoms are not always predictive of the anatomic localization of brain damage because lesions seated throughout the extended neural circuitry that mediates the execution of a given task can impair performance on that task. This is not to say that cerebral networks are equipotential with respect to functional localization (Chapman & Wolff, 1959). Actually, this impression of low specificity results from the reasons stated above, from the large units of behavior being assessed (e.g., memory, problem solving), and from the size and multiplicity of brain lesions, which surpass the dimension of the functional units in the brain by several orders of magnitude (Raichle, 1997; Grinvald et al., 2000).

The clinical syndrome produced by a circumscribed brain lesion often reflects damage to critical nodes in functionally heterogeneous systems traversing the compromised area. Because, as a rule, different neural systems are damaged by a focal lesion in the cerebral hemispheres, the emerging clinical picture usually represents a collection of apparently disparate symptoms.

Damage to Discrete Neural Sites May Present as Diverse Behavioral Symptoms

Although several brain areas commonly participate in the execution of a complex task, for example, auditory cortex and hippocampus in a verbal list learning task, it is also the case that each of these brain areas will participate in multiple functional networks. Neither auditory cortex nor hippocampus is devoted exclusively to verbal list learning. The lower middle prefrontal area that is active during execution of the TMT is also recruited by a card-sorting task (Moll et al., 2002). Although card sorting pertains to an entirely different family of tasks than the TMT, processes underlying both tasks draw on the neural substrate that mediates switching among cognitive sets (Konishi et al., 1999b). The frontal poles have been shown to participate in such diverse tasks as moral judgment (Moll et al., 2001) as well as complex planning (Koechlin et al., 2000). A corollary of this phenomenon is that damage to a particular neural site, as a rule, will give rise to a variety of behavioral symptoms. Whether discrete areas ultimately contribute with unique functions to every behavioral and mental function is still a matter of conjecture without clear practical implications. It should be noted, however, that a few discrete areas in the prefrontal cortex are indeed activated by a broad range of disparate cognitive functions, which favors the hypothesis that some of them may be responsible for the organization of "behavioral universals" (Duncan & Owen, 2000).

PROSPECTS

The Neuropsychology of Emotion and Will

Since its inception, neuropsychology has been heavily biased by its cognitive orientation. More recently, the practice and thinking of cognitive neuropsychology have been broadened by a wealth of tasks designed for tapping emotional behavior (Borod et al., 2000). This search for reliable instruments for assessing the various aspects of emotional behavior is an old one (Penfield & Evans, 1935). It grew out of the recognition that cognitive tasks were largely ineffective at detecting the correlates of behavioral disturbances that were otherwise noisily perceived in real life (Eslinger & Damasio, 1985; Flynn et al., 1988).

Emotional behavior is a generic label for perceptive and expressive processes that are intimately related to the visceral and endocrine systems (Gellhorn, 1967; Ekman et al., 1983; Bowers et al., 1993; Tranel & Damasio, 1994; Heilman, 1997). The neuropsychology of emotional and cognitive behavior is structurally identical despite their differences in content. Neuropsychological emotional probes must be grounded in instruments devised to elicit emotional experiences and behaviors in controlled settings. To be considered reliable, valid, and clinically useful, they must pass the same rigorous procedures that are required for conventional cognitive tests. Finally, they are open to analogous brain-behavior relationships and may give rise to equally sound predictions concerning functional localization in normal individuals as well as in patients with neurobehavioral disorders (Ross et al., 1994; Eslinger, 1998; Perry et al., 2001). Part of the bodily impact of emotional experiences elicited by patterned stimuli can be gauged by psychophysiologic probes (Mesulam & Perry, 1972; Tranel & Damasio, 1994; Bauer, 1998).

Of the three pillars of mental life, motivation or will has been the most difficult to quantify. By "motivation or will" we refer specifically to the energizers of thought and behavior, providing them with spontaneity and strength against opposing inner psychic or outer environmental forces. The word *motivation* has strong psychophysiologic roots (Stellar, 1954), whereas *will* was used by clinicians until the first quarter of the 20th century (Berrios & Gili, 1995). Although spontaneity and strength are intensive factors that lie at the core of all voluntary behaviors, voluntary behavior cannot be reduced to them. Cognitive operations are structured on the will to provide behavior with strategy, directionality, and foresight. These "surface" elements, which lend themselves to classical neuropsychological analysis, are currently subsumed under the concept of "executive behavior" (Tranel et al., 1994).

Disorders of motivation and will stand out among the most disabling in clinical practice. There is much evidence in favor of the notion that, like cognition and emotion, the disorders of will comprise a heterogeneous family of symptoms and abnormal behaviors with discrete neural correlates (Lhermitte, 1986; Laplane, 1990; Northoff et al., 1999; Eslinger, 1999, 2002a). They have been variously described under the rubric of "abulia" (Fisher, 1984) or "avolition" (Andreasen et al., 1995) and may result from many different diseases affecting the body or the brain (Habib, 2000). Kraepelin wrote a particularly vivid account of the clinical picture that emerges when the power of the will is pathologically weakened (Kraepelin, 1971):

> In the first place we have commonly to do with a general *weakening of volitional impulses*. The patients have lost every independent inclination for work and action; they sit about idle, trouble themselves about nothing, do not go to their work, neglect their most pressing obligations, although they are perhaps still capable of employing themselves in a reasonable way if stimulated from the outside.
>
> As the inner activity of volition fails, the resistance which outside influences meet within us is also easily lost. The patients are therefore usually docile, let themselves be driven as a herd, so that they form the necessary nucleus of those crowds which conform willingly to the monotonous daily round in large institutions. A not inconsiderable number join without resistance the crowds of vagabonds which chance leads to-day hither, to-morrow thither (p. 37, italics in the original).

Several instruments for assessing the executive components of voluntary behavior have been developed in the past decades. The challenge for the future is to devise psychometric tests that tap the energizers of behavior so that we can measure and understand the structure of the fuel of the mind and manage it more efficiently (Richards & Ruff, 1989; Cohen et al., 1999).

The Neuropsychology of Daily Life: Strategy Application, Theory of Mind, and Theory of Context

Structural neuroimaging provides a rapid and flexible means of localizing anatomic lesions suspected on the basis of neuropsychological testing. With the rise of neuroimaging in the past decades, neuropsychology migrated to other fields of clinical practice and has focused more on ecological correlates of neuropsychological test scores (Siris, 1991; Burgess et al., 1998; Channon & Crawford, 1999). Currently, a major challenge of experimental neuropsychology is to expand beyond laboratory measurement to understand better how specific sectors of life in real contexts can be sampled by standardized and quantitative tests. Answering this challenge could aid in predictions relevant to rehabilitation and functional reinsertion of patients with a variety of neurobehavioral disorders (see Table 2-1). Frontal lobe mechanisms are likely to play a key role in recovery and reorganization of independent, productive, and successful life. Classical concepts of frontal lobe functions including problem solving and executive behavior have been extended to naturalistic settings under the rubric of "strategy application" (Shallice & Burgess, 1991; Levine et al., 1999). Patients with impaired strategy application disorder may perform normally, or nearly so, in several neuropsychological tasks in the laboratory, yet fail in real life due to gross mistakes in instrumental and social functioning (Eslinger & Damasio, 1985; Shallice & Burgess, 1991; Satish et al., 1999). Drawing on the documented experiences of astronaut Jerry Linenger aboard the Mir space station, Burgess (2000) identified the characteristics that pervade most everyday situations demanding strategy application:

- Multitasking: a number of discrete and different tasks that have to be simultaneously tracked and completed
- Interleaving: to be time effective, performances need to be dovetailed
- Organization to undertake one task at a time
- Interruptions and unexpected behavioral outcomes
- Working memory: the time to return to a task that is already running is not signaled directly by the situation and must be kept in mind

The development of tasks that tap the intricacies of multitasking of real life has only begun to be actively pursued by neuropsychologists (e.g., Sivak et al., 1981). Their role in diagnosis and prognosis has begun to be demonstrated in individual cases and in selected samples of patients with neurobehavioral disorders (Satish et al, 1999; Levine et al., 2000). One potentially fruitful approach is cognitive simulation testing, such as placing an individual in a simulated position in which the person must make realistic decisions under varying circumstances over a period of time (see Satish et al., 1999, for a description of such an approach).

Complementary to strategy application is a domain of neurobehavioral mechanisms related to the judgment of other people's feelings and intentions ("Theory of Mind" processes; see also Chapter 43), the evaluation of the meaning and possible outcomes of social contexts ("Theory of Context"), and the role of the self as an active character in the social chess game (Leakey, 1996). These complex attitudes and behaviors are broadly subsumed under the label of social cognition. Though closely linked to cognitive processes, social cognition also includes elaborate emotional, motiva-

tional, and interpersonal factors that are typically human (Rozin et al., 1999). The neuropsychology of social behavior, both instrumental and interpersonal, is a fruitful area of research with many clinical implications for neuropsychological assessment and interventions.

SUMMARY

Neuropsychological assessment entails careful psychological and medical history, clinical interview, and administration of standardized cognitive tests. More importantly, it encompasses the formulation of hypotheses regarding the etiology of known or suspected neurobehavioral impairments from interpretation of objective test findings in relationship to the patient's background, presentation, and other test results such as brain imaging. Prospectively, neuropsychological assessment also delineates possible interventions, rehabilitation options, prognosis, management of day-to-day neurobehavioral problems, and plan for follow-up care. In addition to test scores, neuropsychological assessment should encompass analysis of important patient behaviors such as initiation, motivation, error patterns, use of feedback, and handling of stressful tasks. Many different neuropsychological tests are available that can assess the impact of diverse pathophysiology on both fundamental, regulatory mechanisms of brain function and on the instrumental and goal-directed competencies essential to everyday adaptation. There are clear limits to what neuropsychological assessment can identify and define, particularly with regard to complex cognitive functioning, motivation, emotion, and the fine aspects of cognitive and behavioral change in nonnormal samples (such as autism, severe retardation), and those with low education and diverse language and cultural backgrounds who have not been studied sufficiently with psychometric methods. However, clinical neuropsychology is an evolving specialty with more practice standards being developed, more test procedures being validated, and more integration occurring with diverse medical and neurobiologic approaches to health, disease, and rehabilitation. We expect that future developments will emphasize greater normative observations of individuals of low educational level and diverse cultural and language backgrounds, and hence provide neuropsychological tests that are more ecologically valid for a wider number of patients and more sensitive and specific to the pathophysiology of the nervous system.

■ KEY POINTS

☐ Neuropsychological assessment refers to standardized test procedures that act as a stimulus for the elicitation of behavioral responses under specific controlled conditions. Neuropsychological tests generate a profile of specific test scores, whereas rating scales and inventories sample general impressions about symptom occurrence and frequency. Given its quantitative and standardized nature, neuropsychological testing is more objective and precise than the qualitative clinical examination and also allows for gauging changes along definite time frames.

☐ The need for neuropsychological assessment usually becomes evident when a patient is referred for suspected behavioral/cognitive changes that may have a neurologic or other biologic basis. Indications for assessment can arise from several fields of medical practice, including neurology, neurosurgery, and psychiatry, but also from internal medicine, cardiology, family practice, rheumatology, and gerontology. Clinical neuropsychologists are typically accessible through departments of neurology and psychiatry of major medical centers and medical schools, sometimes in neurosurgery departments, medical psychology, and rehabilitation medicine departments, in graduate university settings where clinical psychology training programs (and training clinics) are offered, and in some private practice settings.

☐ Neuropsychological consultation should, at a minimum, endow the referring health care provider and patient with fresh insights into several matters. These include processes underlying the patient's profile of spared and impaired cognitive capacities; their relationship to the patient's history, presentation, and other exam findings; diagnostic possibilities; prognosis and recommendations for further evaluation; intervention options; rehabilitation planning; management; occupational and educational recommendations; and follow-up care.

☐ The task of establishing the reliability and validity of neuropsychological instruments is difficult and challenging, given the tremendous diversity of human abilities and the influence of age, language, and culture, as well as diseases of the central nervous system. Interpretation of performance on specific neuropsychological tests is accomplished by first establishing that the administration of the procedure was valid and that the results likely represent the best efforts of the patient. Second, scoring the test follows a specified algorithm that may provide "correction" factors for educational background, sex, and even age. Third, comparison is made to tables of normative observations that permit identification of the patient's score relative to a peer group, usually in the form of a percentile rank or performance range (e.g., low average, superior etc.). Thus, extensive graduate training and supervised clinical experience are critical to the accurate recognition of the possibilities and limitations of neuropsychological testing. The recent association of neuropsychology and

neuroimaging has refined our understanding of some of the neural correlates of widely used tests. The introduction of functional brain imaging is providing the impetus for the development of novel instruments that reliably activate discrete cerebral areas and circuits involved in higher-order cognitive processes.

☐ It is not only the neuropsychological test score that is of interest, but also the actual performance of the patient. This is often accomplished by tracking the kinds of errors committed, whether a prompt or a cue is helpful, whether the patient is aware of errors, and how the individual processes and reacts to task demands. Some tests permit probing of errors and benefit of cues, whereas others are standardized for very specific instructions and feedback by the examiner. Qualitative observations are useful in identifying disturbed and preserved cognitive processes and subsequent development of remediation options and possible interventions that can be implemented by the patient, family members, or other therapists.

☐ Aphasias, agnosias, apraxias, and amnesias have more recently been supplemented by emphasis on the frontal lobe and dysexecutive syndromes, disorders of awareness, emotion and the brain, social cognition and Theory of Mind processing, and the key roles of cortical-subcortical networks (e.g., frontal-striatal, thalamocortical). These broadened approaches provide solid ground on which new syndromes have been described, departing from simply the fractionation and recombination of the classical ones.

☐ Currently, a major challenge in neuropsychological assessment is to expand beyond laboratory measurement with isolated tests in an attempt to delineate how specific sectors of life in real contexts can be sampled by standardized and quantitative tests. This program could set, among other things, the limits and opportunities for rehabilitation and functional reinsertion of patients with a variety of neurobehavioral disorders. Although the neurobehavioral mechanisms of an independent, productive and successful life are still largely unknown, it cannot be achieved without the participation of critical regions of the frontal lobes.

KEY READINGS

Benton AL, Sivan AB, deS Hamsher K, et al: Contributions to Neuropsychological Assessment. A Clinical Manual, ed 2. Oxford, UK: Oxford University Press, 1994.

Levin HS: A guide to neuropsychological testing. Arch Neurol 51: 854–859, 1994.

Tranel D: Neuropsychological assessment. Psychiatr Clin 15:283–299, 1992.

REFERENCES

American Psychiatric Association: Diagnostic and Statistic Manual of Mental Disorders, ed 4 (DSM-IV). Washington, DC: Author 1994.

Andreasen NC: Changing boundaries in psychiatry. Lancet 354(Suppl):SIV56, 1999.

Andreasen NC, Arndt S, Alliger R, et al: Symptoms of schizophrenia: Methods, meanings, and mechanisms. Arch Gen Psychiatry 52:341–351, 1995.

Barnes MP, Saunders M, Walls TJ, et al: The syndrome of Karl Ludwig Kahlbaum. J Neurol Neurosurg Psychiatry 49:991–996, 1986.

Baron-Cohen S, Wheelwright S, Hill J, et al: The "Reading the Mind in the Eyes" test revised version: A study with normal adults, and adults with Asperger syndrome or high-functioning autism. J Child Psychol Psychiatry 42:241–251, 2001.

Bauer RM: Physiologic measures of emotion. J Clin Neurophysiol 15:388–396, 1998.

Bechara A, Damasio AR, Damasio H, et al: Insensitivity to future consequences following damage to human prefrontal cortex. Cognition 50:7–15, 1994.

Benton AL: Neuropsychological assessment. Ann Rev Psychol 45:1–23, 1994.

Benton AL, Hamsher deS K: The Multilingual Aphasia Examination. Iowa City, IA: AJA Associates, 1989.

Benton AL, Eslinger PJ, Damasio AR: Normative observations on neuropsychological test performances in old age. J Clin Neuropsychol 3:33–42, 1981.

Benton AL, Sivan AB, Hamsher deS K, et al: Contributions to Neuropsychological Assessment. A Clinical Manual, ed 2. Oxford, UK: Oxford University Press, 1994.

Berrios GE, Gili M: Will and its disorders: A conceptual history. Hist Psychiatry 76:87–104, 1995.

Borod J, Tabert MH, Santschi C, et al: Neuropsychological assessment of emotional processing in brain-damaged patients, in Borod J (ed): The Neuropsychology of Emotion. New York: Oxford University Press, 2000, pp. 80–105.

Bouchard C, Brissaud É: Traité de Médecine, deuxième édition. Tome IX. Paris: Masson et Cie, 1904.

Bowers D, Bauer RM, Heilman KM: The nonverbal affect lexicon: Theoretical perspectives from neuropsychological studies of affect perception. Neuropsychology 7:433–444, 1993.

Bruce D: On the origin of the term "neuropsychology." Neuropsychologia 23:813–814, 1985.

Burgess PW: Strategy application disorder: The role of the frontal lobes in human multitasking. Psychol Res 63:279–288, 2000.

Burgess PW, Alderman N, Evans J, et al: The ecological validity of tests of executive function. J Int Neuropsychol Soc 4:547–558, 1998.

Caplan LR: The Effective Clinical Neurologist. Cambridge, MA: Blackwell Scientific, 1990.

Channon S, Crawford S: Problem-solving in real-life-type situations: The effect of anterior and posterior lesions on performance. Neuropsychologia 37:757–770, 1999.

Chapman LF, Wolff HG: The cerebral hemispheres and the highest integrative functions of man. Arch Neurol 1:357–424, 1959.

Cohen RA, Kaplan RF, Zuffante P, et al: Alteration of intention and self-initiated action associated with bilateral anterior cingulotomy. J Neuropsychiatry Clin Neurosci 11:444–453, 1999.

Conners CK: Conners Continuous Performance Test (CPT II). North Tonawanda, NY: MHS, 2000.

Crowe SF: The differential contribution of mental tracking, cognitive flexibility, visual search, and motor speed to performance on parts A and B of the Trail Making Test. J Clin Psychol 54:585–591, 1998.

Crum RM, Anthony JC, Bassett SS, et al: Population-based norms for the Mini-Mental State Examination by age and educational level. JAMA 269:2386–2391, 1993.

Cummings JL: Principles of neuropsychiatry: Towards a neuropsychiatric epistemology. Neurocase 5:181–188, 1999.

Damasio H, Damasio AR: Lesion Analysis in Neuropsychology. New York: Oxford University Press, 1989.

Dejerine J: Sémiologie des Affections du Système Nerveux. Paris: Masson et cie, 1914.

Delis DC, Kramer JH, Kaplan E, et al: The California Verbal Learning Test. San Antonio, TX: The Psychological Corporation, 1987.

Dimond SJ: Introducing Neuropsychology. The Study of Brain and Mind. Springfield, Ill: Charles C Thomas, 1978.

Duncan J, Owen AM: Common regions of the human frontal lobe recruited by diverse cognitive demands. Trends Neurosci 23:475–483, 2000.

Ekman P, Levenson RW, Friesen WV: Autonomic nervous system activity distinguishes among emotions. Science 221:1208–1210, 1983.

Eslinger PJ: The neurological and neuropsychological bases of empathy. Eur Neurol 39:193–199, 1998.

Eslinger PJ: Orbital frontal cortex: Historical and contemporary views about its behavioral and physiological significance. Neurocase 5:225–229, 1999.

Eslinger PJ: The anatomical basis of utilization behavior: A shift from frontal-parietal to intra-frontal mechanisms. Cortex 38:–, 2002a, pp. 273–276.

Eslinger PJ (ed): Neuropsychological Interventions. Clinical Research and Practice. New York: Guilford Press, 2002b.

Eslinger PJ, Damasio AR: Severe disturbance of higher cognition after bilateral frontal lobe ablation: Patient EVR. Neurology 35:1731–1741, 1985.

Fahn S, Elton RL, Members of the UPDRS Development Committee: The Unified Parkinson's Disease Rating Scale, in Fahn S, Marsden CD, Calne DB, et al (eds): Recent Developments in Parkinson's Disease. Florham Park, NJ: Macmillan Healthcare Information, 1987, pp. 153–163.

Fisher CM: Abulia minor vs. agitated behavior. Clin Neurosurg 31:9–31, 1984.

Fisher CM: Concerning mind. Can J Neurol Sci 20:247–253, 1993.

Flynn F, Cummings JL, Tomiyasu U: Altered behavior associated with damage to the ventromedial hypothalamus: A distinctive syndrome. Behav Neurol 1:49–58, 1988.

Friston KJ: Statistical parametric mapping and other analyses of functional imaging data, in: Toga AW, Mazziota J (eds): Brain Mapping. The Methods. New York: Academic Press, 1996, pp. 363–386.

Gazzaniga MS (ed): The New Cognitive Neurosciences, ed 2. Cambridge MA: MIT Press, 2000.

Gellhorn E: Principles of Autonomic-Somatic Integrations. Physiological Basis and Psychological and Clinical Implications. Minneapolis: University of Minnesota Press, 1967.

Geschwind N: Disconnexion syndromes in animals and man. Part I. Brain 88:237–294, 1965a.

Geschwind N: Disconnexion syndromes in animals and man. Part II. Brain 88:585–652, 1965b.

Geschwind N: Disorders of attention: A frontier in neuropsychology. Philos Trans R Soc Lond B Biol Sci 298:173–185, 1982.

Goldberg TE, Saint-Cyr JA, Weinberger DR: Assessment of procedural learning and problem solving in schizophrenic patients by Tower of Hanoi type tasks. J Neuropsychiatry Clin Neurosci 2:165–175, 1990.

Goodglass H, Kaplan E: Disturbance of gesture and pantomime in aphasia. Brain 86:703–720, 1963.

Goodglass H, Kaplan E: The Boston Diagnostic Aphasia Examination. Philadelphia: Lea & Febiger, 1987.

Grafman J, Litvan I: Importance of deficits in executive functions. Lancet 354:1921–1922, 1999.

Green BF: A primer of testing. Am J Psychol 36:1001–1011, 1981.

Grinvald A, Slovin H, Vanzetta I: Non-invasive visualization of cortical columns by fMRI. Nat Neurosci 3:105–107, 2000.

Grober E, Buschke H, Crystal H, et al: Screening for dementia by memory testing. Neurology 38:900–903, 1988 .

Gronwall D, Wrighston P: Cumulative effect of concussion. Lancet 2:995–997, 1975.

Habib M: Disorders of motivation, in Bogousslavsky J, Cummings JL (eds): Behavior and Mood Disorders in Focal Brain Lesions. Cambridge, UK: Cambridge University Press, 2000, pp. 261–284.

Happé FGE: An advanced test of Theory of Mind: Understanding of story characters' thoughts and feelings by able autistic, mentally handicapped, and normal children and adults. J Autism Dev Disord 24:129–154, 1994.

Heaton RK, Chelune GJ, Talley JL, et al: Wisconsin Card Sorting Test Manual. Revised and Expanded. Odessa, FL: Psychological Assessment Resources, 1993.

Heilman KH: The neurobiology of emotional experience, in Salloway S, Malloy P, Cummings JL (eds): The Neuropsychiatry of Limbic and Subcortical Disorders. Washington, DC: American Psychiatric Press, 1997, pp. 133–142.

Heilman KM, Rothi LJG: Apraxia, in Heilman KM, Valenstein E (eds): Clinical Neuropsychology, ed 3. New York: Oxford University Press, 1993, pp. 141–163.

Hess AL, Hart R: The specialty of neuropsychology. Neuropsychology 4:49–52, 1990.

Hilgard ER: The trilogy of mind: Cognition, affection, and conation. J Hist Behav Sci 16:107–117, 1980.

Johns MW: A new method for measuring daytime sleepiness: The Epworth Sleepiness Scale. Sleep 14:540–545, 1991.

Kertesz A (ed): Localization and Neuroimaging in Neuropsychology. San Diego, CA: Academic Press, 1994.

Koechlin E, Corrado G, Pietrini P, et al: Dissociating the role of the medial and lateral anterior prefrontal cortex in human planning. Proc Natl Acad Sci U S A 97:7651–7656, 2000.

Konishi S, Nakajima K, Uchida I, et al: Transient activation of inferior prefrontal cortex during cognitive set shifting. Nat Neurosci 1:80–84, 1999a.

Konishi S, Nakajima K, Uchida I, et al: Common inhibitory mechanism in human inferior prefrontal cortex revealed by event-related functional MRI. Brain 122:981–991, 1999b.

Kraepelin E: Dementia Præcox and Paraphrenia (originally published 1919). Translated by R. Mary Barclay. Huntington, NY: Robert E. Krieger Publishing, 1971.

Krikorian R, Bartok J, Glay N: Tower of London procedure: A standard method and developmental data. J Clin Exp Neuropsychol 16:840–850, 1994.

Laplane D: La perte d'auto-activation psychique. Rev Neurol (Paris) 146:397–404, 1990.

Leakey RD: The Origin of Humankind. New York: Basic Books, 1996.

Levin HS: A guide to clinical neuropsychological testing. Arch Neurol 51:854–859, 1994.

Levine B, Dawson D, Boutet I, et al: Assessment of strategic self-regulation in traumatic brain injury: its relationship to injury severity and psychosocial outcome. Neuropsychology 14:491–500, 2000.

Levine B, Freedman M, Dawson D, et al: Ventral frontal contribution to self-regulation: Convergence of episodic memory and inhibition. Neurocase 5:263–275, 1999.

Levine B, Katz DI, Dade L, et al: Novel approaches to the assessment of frontal damage and executive deficits in traumatic brain injury, in Stuss DT, Knight RT (eds): Principles of Frontal Lobe Function. New York: Oxford University Press, 2002, pp. 448–465.

Lezak M: Neuropsychological Assessment, ed 3. New York: Oxford University Press, 1995.

Lhermitte F, Pillon B, Serdaru M: Human autonomy and the frontal lobes. Part I: Imitation and utilization behavior: A neuropsychological study of 75 patients. Ann Neurol 19:326–334, 1986.

Liepmann H: The left hemisphere and action, in Kimura D (ed): Translations of Liepmann's Essays on Apraxia. London, ON: DK Consultants, 1980, pp. 17–50.

Luria AR: Higher Cortical Functions in Man, ed 2. New York: Basic Books, 1980.

Luria AR, Tsvetkova LS: The programming of constructive activity in local brain injuries. Neuropsychologia 2:95–107, 1964.

Marie P: La Pratique Neurologique. Paris: Masson et Cie, 1911.

Mattis S: Dementia Rating Scale. Odessa, FL: Psychological Assessment Resources, 1988.

McHugh PR, Slavney PR: The Perspectives of Psychiatry, ed 2. Baltimore, MD: The Johns Hopkins University Press, 1998.

Mesulam MM: Asymmetry of neural feedback in the organization of behavioral states. Science 237:537–538, 1987.

Mesulam MM: Large-scale neurocognitive networks and distributed processing for attention, language, and memory. Ann Neurol 28:597–613, 1990.

Mesulam M-M, Perry J: The diagnosis of love-sickness: Experimental psychophysiology without the polygraph. Psychophysiology 9:546–551, 1972.

Moll J, Oliveira-Souza R, Bramati IE, et al: Functional MRI of cognitive set-shifting using an oral version of the Trail Making Test. Neuroimage 11:S-41, 2000a.

Moll J, Oliveira-Souza R, Passman LJ, et al: Functional magnetic resonance imaging of pantomimes of tool use. Neurology 54:1331–1336, 2000b.

Moll J, Eslinger PJ, Oliveira-Souza R de: Frontopolar and anterior temporal cortex activation in a moral judgment task. Arq Neuropsiquatr 59:657–664, 2001.

Moll J, Oliveira-Souza R, Moll FT, et al: The cerebral correlates of set-shifting: An fMRI study of the Trail Making Test. Arq Neuropsiquatr 2002, p. 60.

Neisser U: Cognitive Psychology. Englewood Cliffs, NJ: Prentice-Hall, 1967. (Cited in: Kandel ER, Schwartz JH, Jessell TM (eds): Principles of Neural Science, ed 4. New York: McGraw-Hill 2000, p. 381.)

Northoff G, Koch A, Wenke J, et al: Catatonia as a psychomotor syndrome: A rating scale and extrapyramidal motor symptoms. Mov Disord 14:404–416, 1999.

Oliveira-Souza R, Moll J, Passman LJ, et al: Trail making and cognitive set-shifting. Arq Neuropsiquatr 58:826–829, 2000.

Papez J: A proposed mechanism of emotion. Arch Neurol Psychiatry 38:725–744, 1937.

Penfield W, Evans J: The frontal lobe in man: A clinical study of maximum removals. Brain 58:115–133, 1935.

Perry RJ, Rosen HR, Kramer JH, et al: Hemispheric dominance for emotions, empathy and social behavior: Evidence from right and left handers with frontotemporal dementia. Neurocase 7:145–160, 2001.

Plum F: Coma and related global disturbances of the human conscious state, in Peters A, York N (eds): Normal and Altered States of Function. Cerebral Cortex, Vol. 9. New York: Plenum, 1991, pp. 359–425.

Raichle ME: Food for thought: The metabolic and circulatory requirements of cognition. Ann N Y Acad Sci 835:373–385, 1997.

Reitan RM, Wolfson D: The Halstead-Reitan Neuropsychological Battery, ed 2. Tucson, AZ: Neuropsychology Press, 1993.

Richards PM, Ruff RM: Motivational effects on neuropsychological functioning: Comparison of depressed versus nondepressed individuals. J Consult Clin Psychol 57:396–402, 1989.

Robertson I: The Test of Everyday Attention. Suffolk, UK: Thames Valley Test Company, 1994.

Rolls ET: The Brain and Emotion. Oxford: Oxford University Press, 1999.

Ross E, Homan RW, Buck R: Differential hemispheric lateralization of primary and social emotions. Implications for developing a comprehensive neurology for emotions, repression, and the subconscious. Neuropsychiatry Neuropsychol Behav Neurol 7:1–19, 1994.

Royall DR, Cordes JA, Polk M: CLOX: An executive clock drawing task. J Neurol Neurosurg Psychiatry 64:588–594, 1998.

Rozin P, Loewry L, Imada S, et al: The CAD Triad Hypothesis: A mapping between three moral emotions (contempt, anger, disgust) and three moral codes (community, autonomy, divinity). J Pers Social Psychol 76:574–586, 1999.

Satish U, Streufert S, Eslinger PJ: Complex decision making after orbitofrontal damage: Neuropsychological and strategic management simulation assessment. Neurocase 5:355–364, 1999.

Schretlen D: Brief Test of Attention. Odessa, FL: Psychological Assessment Resources, 1997.

Shallice T, Burgess PW: Deficits in strategy application following frontal lobe damage in man. Brain 114:727–741, 1991.

Siegel RA: Probability and punishment and suppression of behavior in psychopathic and nonpsychopathic offenders. J Abnorm Psychol 87:514–522, 1978.

Siris SG: Is life a Wisconsin Card Sorting Test? Am J Psychiatry 148:1413–1414, 1991.

Sivak M, Olson PL, Kewman DG, et al: Driving and perceptual/cognitive skills: Behavioral consequences of brain damage. Arch Phys Med Rehabil 62:476–483, 1981.

Sivan AB: Benton Visual Retention Test, ed 5. San Antonio, TX: The Psychological Corporation, 1992.

Smith A: Symbol Digit Modalities Test Revised. Los Angeles, CA: Western Psychological Services, 1982.

Sohn M-H, Ursu S, Anderson JR, et al: The role of the prefrontal cortex and posterior parietal cortex in task switching. Proc Natl Acad Sci U S A 97:13448–13453, 2000.

Spreen O, Strauss E: A Compendium of Neuropsychological Tests. Administration, Norms, and Commentary, ed 2. New York: Oxford University Press, 1998.

Stellar E: The physiology of motivation. Psychol Rev 61:5–22, 1954.

Stevens SS: On the theory of scales of measurement. Science 103:667–680, 1946.

Tiffin J: Purdue Pegboard Examiner's Manual. Rosemont, IL: London House, 1968.

Tranel D: Neuropsychological assessment. Psychiatr Clin 15:283–299, 1992.

Tranel D, Anderson SW, Benton AL: Development of the concept of "executive behavior" and its relationship to the frontal lobes, in Boller F, Grafman J (eds): Handbook of Neuropsychology, Vol. 9. Amsterdam: Elsevier, 1994, pp. 125–148.

Tranel D, Damasio H: Neuroanatomical correlates of electrodermal skin conductance responses. Psychophysiology 31:427–458, 1994.

Victor M, Ropper AH, Adams RD: Adams and Victor's Principles of Neurology, ed 7. New York: McGraw-Hill, 2001.

Vygotsky LS: Mind in Society. The Development of Higher Psychological Processes. Cambridge, MA: Harvard University Press, 1978.

Warrington EK, James M: The Visual Object and Space Perception Battery. Bury St. Edwards, UK: Thames Valley Test Company, 1991.

Wechsler D: Wechsler Adult Intelligence Scale, ed 3. San Antonio, TX: Harcourt Brace Jovanovich, 1997.

Weintraub S: Neuropsychological assessment of mental state, in Mesulam M-M (ed): Principles of Behavioral and Cognitive Neurology, ed 2. New York: Oxford University Press, 2000, pp. 121–173.

Wilson B, Cockburn J, Baddeley A: The Rivermead Behavioural Memory Test, ed 2. Bury St. Edwards, UK: Thames Valley Test Company, 1991.

Yakovlev PI:. Motility, behavior, and the brain. J Nerv Ment Dis 107:313–335, 1948.

Zangwill OL: The cerebral localisation of psychological function. Adv Sci 20:335–344, 1963.

Neuropsychiatric Assessment

Alicia G. Lischinsky
Sergio E. Starkstein

Anxiety
Apathy
Delirium
Depression
Dysthymia
Mania
Psychosis

of life, highlighting the importance of making an accurate diagnosis of this disorder (Robinson, 1999).

This chapter begins by addressing methodological problems that complicate the diagnosis of psychiatric and behavioral disorders among patients with neurologic disease. We then discuss the main structured psychiatric interviews and standardized diagnostic criteria that are currently used to generate diagnoses of psychiatric disorders, and we review the most useful instruments to rate the severity of psychiatric and behavioral problems in neurologic disease.

INTRODUCTION

Cognitive impairments and physical deficits are the most prominent consequences of brain injury, but psychiatric symptoms and behavioral disturbances are also frequent and may cause great distress to patients and caregivers. Moreover, psychiatric disorders after brain injury or dysfunction are associated with a worse recovery in activities of daily living (ADL), increased mortality, significant cognitive decline, and decreased quality

METHODOLOGICAL ISSUES

The diagnosis of psychiatric and behavioral disorders in neurologic disease should be made after a thorough mental status examination, with a specific evaluation of signs and symptoms of psychiatric disorders. One initial dilemma is how to diagnose psychiatric disorders such as depression and anxiety among patients with neurologic disease when symptoms of the putative psychiatric disorder may be produced by the neurologic disease itself. For instance, insomnia, psychomotor retardation, loss of energy and libido, and poor appetite may be understandable findings in patients with acute brain lesions (e.g., stroke, traumatic brain injury) or neurodegenerative diseases (e.g., Parkinson disease [PD], dementia); but are also cardinal symptoms of "primary" depression (i.e., no known brain injury). We will discuss this issue with depression as the main example because this is the most frequent psychiatric disorder among the neurologically ill.

Cohen-Cole and Stoudemire (1987) proposed four different approaches to assess depression among individuals with physical illnesses: (1) the "inclusive approach," which considers all depressive diagnostic symptoms, regardless of their relationship to the physical illness (Rifken et al., 1985); (2) the "etiological approach," which considers symptoms only if the examiner believes they are not caused by the physical illness (Rapp & Vrana, 1985); (3) the "substitutive approach," which replaces vegetative or autonomic symptoms of depression with psychological symptoms (Table 3-1; Endicott, 1984); and (4) the "exclusive approach," which removes symptoms from the diagnostic criteria for depression whenever they are not more frequent among depressed than nondepressed patients (Bukberg et al., 1984).

The relative usefulness of these strategies to diagnose depression in stroke was examined by Paradiso and colleagues (1997), who assessed a series of 142 patients who had acute stroke lesions and were followed for examination at 3, 6, 12, or 24 months after stroke. Throughout this follow-up period, those patients reporting a depressed mood during the acute stroke hospitalization (n = 60, 42% of the sample) showed a significantly higher frequency of all autonomic and psychological symptoms of depression (see

TABLE 3-1. Phenomenology of Depression

Psychological symptoms

Worrying
Brooding
Loss of interest
Hopelessness
Suicidal tendencies
Social withdrawal
Self-deprecation
Ideas of reference

Autonomic symptoms

Autonomic anxiety
Loss of appetite
Initial insomnia
Middle insomnia
Early morning awakening
Anergia and retardation
Loss of libido

Table 3-1) as compared to the group without in-hospital depressed mood, except for the symptoms of early morning awakening, loss of libido, weight loss, suicide plans, and pathologic guilt. Paradiso and colleagues (1997) calculated the frequency of patients meeting the criteria of the *Diagnostic and Statistical Manual of Mental Disorders,* 4th edition (DSM-IV; American Psychiatric Association [APA], 1994) for a major depression using some of the different diagnostic strategies described above and found that frequencies of major depression at the initial evaluation were 18% for the inclusive strategy (i.e., depressive symptoms were counted regardless of their presumed cause), and 22% for the substitutive approach (i.e., all autonomic symptoms were eliminated, and major depression was diagnosed based on the presence of at least four psychological symptoms plus depressed mood). Another important finding was that three autonomic symptoms (autonomic anxiety, morning depression, and subjective anergia) were significantly more frequent in stroke patients with in-hospital depressed mood as compared to patients without a depressed mood at all times throughout the 2-year period. Moreover, the specificity of unmodified DSM-IV criteria had a sensitivity of 100% and a specificity that ranged from 95% to 98% as compared to criteria that included only specific symptoms. Based on these findings, Robinson (1999, p. 72) suggested that "modifying DSM-IV criteria because of the existence of an acute medical illness is probably unnecessary."

Fedoroff and colleagues (1991) assessed the frequency of depressive symptoms in 205 patients with acute stroke, who were divided into those who reported a depressed mood (41% of the sample) and those patients who reported no mood change (the remaining 59%). The main finding was that patients with depressed mood had a significantly higher frequency of every autonomic and psychological symptom of depression, except for early morning awakening, as compared to patients without depressed mood. Patients with depressed mood had an average of four autonomic and four psychological symptoms of depression as compared to an average of one autonomic and one psychological symptom of depression in patients without a depressed mood. Based on additional findings, Fedoroff and colleagues estimated that the use of standardized diagnostic criteria (such as the DSM-III) might falsely elevate the frequency of major depression by 1% to 2% and concluded that both autonomic and psychological symptoms of depression were significantly related to the presence of a depressed mood among patients with acute stroke.

Starkstein and colleagues (1990) examined the frequency of autonomic and psychological symptoms of depression in 33 patients with PD who reported a depressed mood and 33 patients with PD who reported no mood change. The main finding was that patients with a depressed mood had a significantly higher frequency of all psychological and autonomic symptoms of depression (see Table 3-1), except for early morning awakening, loss of energy, and psychomotor retardation.

Chemerinski and colleagues (2001) assessed autonomic and psychological symptoms of depression in Alzheimer disease (AD) in a study that included 92 AD patients with a depressive mood, 62 AD patients without a depressed mood, 47 patients with primary depression (i.e., without dementia), and 20 healthy age-comparable individuals. The main finding was that depressed AD patients had significantly more frequent autonomic and psychological symptoms of depression than AD patients without a depressed mood. Moreover, the profile of depressive symptoms for AD patients with depressed mood and patients with primary depression was similar. Finally, AD patients without a depressed mood and healthy controls had a similar frequency of depressive symptoms, demonstrating that dementia does not "produce" symptoms of depression in the absence of depressed mood, and that the symptoms of depression are not rampant among AD patients without depressed mood.

In conclusion, the diagnosis of depression should be made only after a thorough mental status examination. Findings in patients with stroke lesions, traumatic brain injury, PD, or AD suggest that diagnostic criteria for depressive disorders should be determined specifically for each condition, but most studies show a high concordance of autonomic and affective symptoms of depression. Depressive symptoms are not rampant among patients with neurologic disease, but usually point to an underlying depression.

IMPACT OF LANGUAGE AND COGNITIVE DEFICITS ON PSYCHIATRIC EVALUATION

A psychiatric evaluation requires a verbal report with the patient, which may be an important limitation in those with moderate or severe language or cognitive deficits. Several authors (e.g., Ross & Rush, 1981) suggested that depression in aphasic patients should be diagnosed based on the presence of specific behavioral signs, such as decreased sleep or decreased food intake, but to our knowledge, a set of criteria to diagnose depression based on behavioral observation has not been validated. Gainotti and colleagues (1999) designed the Post-Stroke Depression Rating Scale, which rates a number of nonverbal behaviors such as vegetative symptoms, apathy, loss of interest, anxiety, catastrophic reactions, hyperemotionalism, anhedonia, and diurnal mood variations. However, the validity of these signs for the diagnosis of a depressive syndrome using standardized diagnostic criteria, and whether this idiosyncratic type of depressive construct is valid, have not

been demonstrated. Several studies examined the usefulness of biologic "markers" of primary depression to diagnose depression in neurologic disease, such as the dexamethasone suppression test and the growth hormone response to desipramine, but none of these laboratory assessments showed adequate sensitivity and specificity (Robinson, 1998).

Before a structured psychiatric interview could be attempted, Robinson and colleagues required in their initial studies that the patient should score within 10 points following readministration of the Zung Depression Scale, approximately 30 minutes apart (for a review, see Robinson, 1993). In later studies, these investigators required their patients to perform part 1 of the Token Test without error (this test examines the patient's ability to comprehend and follow verbal instructions of increasing complexity; Robinson, 1993). This strategy, although including patients who can be reliably assessed with a psychiatric interview, does not permit the examination of psychiatric disorders in patients with moderate to severe comprehension deficits, and alternative strategies should be designed for those patients in whom verbal interviews are not feasible.

Whether cognitive deficits are an important limitation to the diagnosis of depression was examined by Chemerinski and colleagues (2001), who compared Hamilton Depression Scale ratings obtained from AD patient interviews with those obtained from their respective caregivers. The main finding was that caregivers rated patients as significantly more depressed than the AD patients themselves. On the other hand, only 3% of the patients with AD rated as depressed by their respective caregivers denied having a depressed mood. These findings suggest that the presence of cognitive deficits does not impair the patient's ability to provide valid information about the mood state, but may impair the patient's ability to rate the severity of depression.

In conclusion, language and cognitive deficits are important limitations to the diagnosis of depression in neurologic disease. Whereas several strategies have been proposed to diagnose depression in aphasic patients, no specific diagnostic instrument or criteria was validated, and biologic markers of primary depression did not demonstrate adequate sensitivity and specificity in neurologic disease. Patients with cognitive deficits are aware of their depressive mood, but may not report the full extent of their depressive symptoms.

STANDARDIZED PSYCHIATRIC INTERVIEWS IN NEUROLOGIC DISEASE

Ideally, the presence of psychiatric signs and symptoms should be assessed with a semistructured or structured psychiatric interview that includes questions for a variety of behavioral and emotional disorders and items to rate observed abnormal behaviors. In their initial studies, Robinson and colleagues used the Present State Exam (PSE), which was developed by Wing and colleagues (1974) and has been administred in epidemiologic studies of psychiatric disorders throughout the world. The PSE incorporates a "probe and question" structure that allows both examiner and subject to develop, interpret, and elaborate on inquires about symptoms, with a glossary of symptom definition. Reliable symptom clusters may be generated based on the mental status information derived from the PSE; however, items about personal psychiatric history need to be added to make diagnoses based on diagnostic criteria, such as in the DSM-IV (APA, 1994) or *International Classification of Diseases*, 10th edition (ICD-10; World Health Organization [WHO], 1994a). The 10th edition of the PSE (PSE-10) is divided into two parts: part I assesses somatoform, dissociative, anxiety, depressive disorders, bipolar disorders, eating disorders, and abuse of substances, and part II assesses psychotic and cognitive disorders and observed abnormalities of speech, affect, and behavior.

The Schedules for Clinical Assessment in Neuropsychiatry (SCAN) is a set of instruments that assess, measure, and classify the major psychiatric disorders of adult life (WHO, 1994b). The SCAN includes the full PSE-10, an Item Group Checklist (IGC), which permits the rating of information obtained from case records or informants other than the proband, and a Clinical History Schedule, which is completed with information obtained from the proband, informants, and clinical records. The SCAN allows the use of different algorithms to generate diagnoses, such as in ICD-10 and DSM-IV. This instrument should be used by trained psychiatrists who have taken a specific course at a WHO training center.

The Structured Clinical Interview for DSM-IV (SCID) is a semistructured interview for making the major Axis I and Axis II diagnoses (Spitzer et al., 1992). Specific sections of the SCID may be used by a clinician who after the usual mental status evaluation wants to confirm a DSM-IV diagnosis. Alternatively, the whole SCID may be assessed with the aim of making a diagnosis of all Axis I or II disorders present in the patient. For those patients with a known neurologic disorder it is better to use the Non-Patient edition (SCID-NP), which includes an overview section that inquires about a history of psychopathology. The SCID starts with an overview of the present psychiatric complaint and past episodes of psychopathology. This is followed by specific sections with open-ended questions to obtain symptom description from the patient. These questions are worded in such a way that allows the assessment of every criterion on the DSM-IV for specific psychiatric disorders. It is important to stress that the examiner should use all sources of information available at the time of the evaluation (e.g., notes, reports from relatives

or caregivers, etc.), and use one's own judgment about the absence or presence of a specific symptom. The SCID usually takes from 60 to 90 minutes to be completed.

In conclusion, the best strategy to diagnose a psychiatric disorder among individuals with neurologic disease is to use a standardized psychiatric interview, such as the SCID, the PSE, or the SCAN. We will now review the most frequent emotional and behavioral disorders reported in patients with neurologic disease, and review the most useful diagnostic criteria and rating instruments.

EMOTIONAL AND BEHAVIORAL DISORDERS

Depression

A high frequency of depression has been consistently reported among patients with a variety of neurologic disorders, such as acute brain lesions (e.g., traumatic brain injury, stroke) and neurodegenerative disorders (e.g., PD, dementia) (Starkstein & Robinson, 1993). Standardized diagnostic criteria for depression in neurologic disease may be found in the DSM-IV (APA, 1994) and the ICD-10 (WHO, 1994a). The DSM-IV includes the category of "Mood Disorder Due to a General Medical Condition" (Table 3-2). This category consists of 2 subtypes: one with depressive features, whenever the predominant mood is depressed but the full criteria for a major depressive episode are not met, and a second with major depressive-like episode, whenever the full criteria for a major depressive episode are met. The DSM-IV criteria for a major depressive episode are provided in Table 3-3.

The ICD-10 (diagnostic criteria for research) includes criteria for "Mental Disorders Due to Brain Damage and Dysfunction, and to Physical Disease" (Table 3-4). If these criteria are met, mood disorders may be diagnosed whenever the criteria for specific affective disorders are also met. Table 3-5 shows the ICD-10 criteria for a Depressive Episode, and Table 3-6 the ICD-10 criteria for a Mild Depressive Episode (F32.0). The ICD-10 criteria for a Moderate Depressive Episode (F32.1) require the presence of six of the symptoms from criteria C (see Table 3-6), whereas the ICD-10 criteria for a Severe Depressive Episode (F32.2) require the presence of eight of the symptoms from criteria C. Organic affective disorders may be specified using the following codes: F06.30 for organic manic disorder, F06.31 for organic bipolar disorder, F06.32 for organic depressive disorder, and F06.33 for organic mixed affective disorder.

In their early studies on poststroke depression Robinson and colleagues (1983) described the syndromes of major and minor (dysthymic) depression. They used the DSM criteria for dysthymia (Table 3-7), excluding the criterion that requires the syndromic

TABLE 3-2. Diagnostic Criteria for a Mood Disorder Due to a General Medical Condition

A. A prominent and persistent disturbance in mood predominates in the clinical picture and is characterized by either (or both) of the following:
  1. Depressed mood or markedly diminished interest or pleasure in all, or almost all, activities
  2. Elevated, expansive, or irritable mood
B. There is evidence from the history, physical examination, or laboratory findings that the disturbance is the direct physiologic consequence of a general medical condition.
C. The disturbance is not better accounted for by another mental disorder.
D. The disturbance does not occur exclusively during the course of a delirium.
E. The symptoms cause clinically significant distress or impairment in social, occupational, or other important areas of functioning.

Adapted from American Psychiatric Association: Diagnostic and Statistical Manual of Mental Disorders (DSM-IV). Washington, DC: American Psychiatric Press, 1994.

TABLE 3-3. Criteria for Major Depressive Episode

A. Five (or more) of the following symptoms have been present during the same 2-week period and represent a change from previous functioning; at least one of the symptoms is either (1) depressed mood or (2) loss of interest or pleasure.
  1. Depressed mood most of the day, nearly every day, as indicated by either subjective report or observation made by others
  2. Markedly diminished interest or pleasure in all, or almost all, activities most of the day, nearly every day
  3. Significant weight loss or decrease or increase in appetite nearly every day
  4. Insomnia or hypersomnia nearly every day
  5. Psychomotor agitation or retardation nearly every day
  6. Fatigue or loss of energy nearly every day
  7. Feelings of worthlessness or excessive or inappropriate guilt nearly every day
  8. Diminished ability to think or concentrate, or indecisiveness, nearly every day
  9. Recurrent thoughts of death, recurrent suicidal ideation without a specific plan, or a suicide attempt or a specific plan for committing suicide

Adapted from American Psychiatric Association: Diagnostic and Statistical Manual of Mental Disorders (DSM-IV). Washington, DC: American Psychiatric Press, 1994.

TABLE 3-4. Criteria for Other Mental Disorders Due to Brain Damage and Dysfunction and to Physical Disease

G1. Objective evidence and/or history of cerebral disease, damage, or dysfunction, or of systemic physical disorder known to cause cerebral dysfunction, including hormonal disturbances (other than alcohol or other psychoactive substance-related) and nonpsychoactive drug effects
G2. A presumed relationship between the development of the underlying disease, damage, or dysfunction and the mental disorder
G3. Recovery from or significant improvement in the mental disorder following removal or improvement of the underlying presumed cause
G4. Insufficient evidence for an alternative causation of the mental disorder
If criteria G1, G2, and G4 are met, a provisional diagnosis is justified; if, in addition, there is evidence of G3, the diagnosis can be regarded as certain.

Adapted from World Health Organization: The ICD-10 Classification of Mental and Behavioral Disorders. Geneva, Switzerland: Author, 1994.

cluster of depressive symptoms to be present most of the time for more than 2 years. The DSM-IV defines poststroke major depression as "a mood disorder due to stroke with major depressive-like episode," and also provides research criteria for minor depression, which require depression or anhedonia with at least one but fewer than four additional symptoms of major depression.

The diagnosis of any psychiatric disorder should be based on a systematic mental status examination leading to a psychiatric diagnosis based on the presence of a syndromic symptom cluster. Depression rating scales are useful to rate the severity of depressive disorders and may also be used as screening instruments to determine the likelihood of the presence or absence of a given psychiatric diagnosis. Several widely used

TABLE 3-5. Depressive Episode

G1. The depressive episode should last for at least 2 weeks.

G2. There have been no hypomanic or manic symptoms sufficient to meet the criteria for hypomanic or manic episode at any time in the individual's life.

G3. The episode is not attributable to psychoactive substance use or to any organic mental disorder.

Somatic Syndrome

Some depressive symptoms, widely regarded as having special clinical significance, are called "somatic." To qualify for the somatic syndrome, four of the following symptoms should be present:

1. Marked loss of interest or pleasure in activities that are normally pleasurable
2. Lack of emotional reactions to events or activities that normally produce an emotional response
3. Waking in the morning 2 hours or more before the usual time
4. Depression worse in the morning
5. Objective evidence of marked psychomotor retardation or agitation
6. Marked loss of appetite
7. Weight loss (5% or more of body weight in the past month)
8. Marked loss of libido

Adapted from World Health Organization: The ICD-10 Classification of Mental and Behavioral Disorders. Geneva, Switzerland: Author, 1994.

TABLE 3-6. Mild Depressive Episode

A. The general criteria for a depressive episode (see Table 3-5) must be met.
B. At least two of the following three symptoms must be present:
   1. Depressed mood to a degree that is definitely abnormal for the individual, present for most of the day and almost every day, largely uninfluenced by circumstances, and sustained for at least 2 weeks
   2. Loss of interest or pleasure in activities that are normally pleasurable
   3. Decreased energy or increased fatigability
C. An additional symptom or symptoms from the following list should be present, to give a total of at least *four*:
   1. Loss of confidence or self-esteem
   2. Unreasonable feelings of self-reproach or excessive and inappropriate guilt
   3. Recurrent thoughts of death or suicide, or any suicidal behavior
   4. Complaints or evidence of diminished ability to think or concentrate, such as indecisiveness or vacillation
   5. Change in psychomotor activity, with agitation or retardation (either subjective or objective)
   6. Sleep disturbance of any type
   7. Change in appetite (decrease or increase) with corresponding weight change

Adapted from World Health Organization: The ICD-10 Classification of Mental and Behavioral Disorders. Geneva, Switzerland: Author, 1994.

TABLE 3-7. Diagnostic Criteria for a Dysthymic Disorder

A. Depressed mood for most of the day, for more days than not, as indicated by either subjective account or observations by others, for at least 2 years
B. Presence, while depressed, of two (or more) of the following:
   1. Poor appetite or overeating
   2. Insomnia or hypersomnia
   3. Low energy or fatigue
   4. Low self-esteem
   5. Poor concentration or difficulty making decisions
   6. Feelings of hopelessness

Adapted from American Psychiatric Association: Diagnostic and Statistical Manual of Mental Disorders-DSM-IV. Washington, DC: American Psychiatric Press, 1994.

depression scales are the Hamilton Depression Scale (HAM-D; Hamilton, 1960), Beck Depression Inventory (BDI; Beck et al., 1961), Zung Depression Scale (ZDS; Zung, 1965), General Health Questionnaire (GHQ; Goldberg & Hiller, 1979), Montgomery-Asberg Depression Rating Scale (Montgomery & Asberg, 1979), and the Center for Epidemiological Scales for Depression (CES-D; Radloff, 1977). The HAM-D is a 17-item interviewer-rated scale that measures psychological and autonomic symptoms of depression. This scale assesses, for instance, the individual's interest in daily life activity and work productivity; rating this item in a patient with a neurologic disorder requires some judgment. Other HAM-D items, such as those rating sleep problems; psychomotor retardation; loss of appetite, weight, energy, and libido; and hypochondriasis may be difficult to assess in patients with neurologic conditions. Based on findings on the specificity of depressive symptoms for depression in neurologic disease (Starkstein & Robinson, 1993), the HAM-D should be adapted to each specific condition to account for the influence of neurologic disease. The BDI is a self-rated questionnaire, which may be impossible to answer by patients with moderate to severe comprehension problems. Several items on the scale, such as self-appeareance, capacity to work, and worries about health may be clearly influenced by symptoms of neurologic disorders. Thus, scoring of these items based on their relationship with the neurologic condition may increase or decrease the score on the BDI based on the judgment made.

Several studies examined the proportion of "false positives" (i.e., individuals over the cut-off score criterion on a depression rating scale but not meeting diagnostic criteria for a depressive disorder after formal mental status evaluation) and "false negatives" (i.e., individuals under the cut-off score criterion on the depression rating scale but meeting diagnostic criteria for a depressive disorder after a semistructured psychiatric interview). Parikh and colleagues (1988) compared the CES-D with DSM-III criteria for depressive disorder based on a semistructured psychiatric interview in a series of 180 stroke patients. Using a cut-off score of 16 or higher on the CES-D, Parikh and colleagues found a specificity for major or minor depression of 90%, a sensitivity of 86%, and a positive predictive value of 80%. This study demonstrated that 14% of stroke patients with either major or minor depression are misdiagnosed as nondepressed when using a cut-off score of 17 or higher on the CES-D. Schramke and colleagues (1998) examined the validity of different depression rating scales for the diagnosis of depression based on DSM-III-R criteria for anxiety and mood disorders. A series of stroke patients and healthy controls were assessed using the SCID, CES-D, HAM-D, and the Beck Anxiety Inventory (Beck et al., 1998), and the main finding was that the frequency and severity of depressive symptoms varied greatly depending on the rating instrument used. Many patients had abnormal scores on depression rating scales but did not meet a DSM diagnosis, demonstrating that rating scales were highly sensitive but not specific.

Gainotti and colleagues (1999) examined the phenomenology of poststroke depression using the Poststroke Depression Rating Scale. They found two profiles of depression after stroke: an "endogenous" type, with higher scores on suicide and anhedonia, and a "reactive" type, with higher scores on catastrophic reaction, hyperemotionalism, and diurnal mood variation. Both catastrophic reaction and hyperemotionalism (also known as "pathological affective display") were reported by other authors to be significantly associated with depression in stroke patients (Robinson, 1993), and many depressed stroke patients may lack those "endogenous" and "reactive" constructs.

In conclusion, the diagnosis of depression in patients with neurologic disorder requires a thorough mental status assessment for specific symptoms of mood disorders. Depression rating scales are useful to screen patients for depressive disorders, to determine the relative severity of depressive symptoms, and to quantify changes in depression after specific treatment, but should not be used to make psychiatric diagnoses.

Anxiety

Anxiety disorders are among the most frequent psychiatric problems in the general population (Regier et al., 1988) and in neurologic disease. About 40% of patients with PD were reported to show at least one clinically significant anxiety symptom (Marsh, 2000). Among patients with acute stroke, about 11% may show generalized anxiety disorder, whereas in community-based samples about 3% of stroke patients were reported to have anxiety "neurosis" (Robinson, 1998).

Symptoms of anxiety may be normal emotional responses to specific situations, whereas anxiety disorders specifically refer to pathologic states in which the intensity and duration of anxiety produces impairment in social, occupational, and other areas of functioning (Marsh, 2000). The spectrum of anxiety disorders includes panic attacks, phobias, obsessive-compulsive disorders (OCDs), posttraumatic stress disorder, and generalized anxiety disorder (GAD). The DSM-IV (APA, 1994) defines GAD as characterized by at least 6 months of persistent and excessive anxiety and worry, and three or more of the symptoms listed in Table 3-8. Early studies of GAD in neurologic disease used DSM-III criteria for GAD, which were slightly modified so that the time constraint (i.e., symptoms present during 1 month in DSM-III and 6 months in DSM-IV) was not fulfilled whenever patients were studied early in their illness (e.g., within the first 2 weeks after an acute cerebral lesion), and criterion F (i.e., that GAD was not due to a general medical condition), were not considered. The DSM-IV also includes the diagnosis of Anxiety Disorder Due to a General Medical Condition, which is defined as clinically significant anxiety that is considered to be due to the direct physiologic effects of a general medical condition. The ICD-10 includes the category of "Organic Anxiety Disorder" (F06.4), which consists of the generic criteria for a "mental disorder due to brain damage and dysfunction, and due to physical disease" (see Table 3-4), and the specific criteria for Panic Disorder (F41.0; Table 3-9) or Generalized Anxiety Disorder (F41.1).

One limitation of the above criteria is the potential overlap with symptoms of physical illness, stressing the importance of examining the specificity of anxiety symptoms for each neurologic condition. Chemerinski and associates (1998) compared the profile of anxiety symptoms in AD between 18 patients meeting DSM-III-R criteria for GAD and 36 AD patients without GAD, matched for age, duration of illness, and severity of dementia. The AD-GAD group had higher scores on the Hamilton Anxiety Scale (Hamilton, 1959) items of anxious mood, tension, fears, insomnia, muscular symptoms, somatic symptoms, and autonomic symptoms. On the other hand, there were no significant between-group differences on the items of concentration and memory, depressed mood, genitourinary symptoms, and behavior at interview, suggesting that these criteria should not be considered for the diagnosis of GAD among demented patients.

In conclusion, anxiety disorders in patients with neurologic disease should be diagnosed after semistructured psychiatric interviews such as the SCAN or SCID, and standardized criteria of either the DSM-IV or the ICD-10. Once a diagnosis of a GAD is made, its severity is usually measured with the Hamilton Anxiety Scale (Hamilton, 1959), although some of the symptoms of anxiety may not be specific to the psychiatric condition.

Apathy

Apathy is a term coined by the Greek stoic philosophers to refer to the condition of being free from emotions and

Table 3-8. Diagnostic Criteria for Generalized Anxiety Disorder

A. Excessive anxiety and worry (apprehensive expectation), occuring more days than not for at least 6 months, about a number of events or activities.
B. The person finds it difficult to control the worry.
C. The anxiety and worry are associated with three (or more) of the following six symptoms.
   1. Restlessness or feeling keyed up or on edge
   2. Being easily fatigued
   3. Difficulty concentrating or mind going blank
   4. Irritability
   5. Muscle tension
   6. Sleep disturbance (difficulty falling or staying asleep, or restless unsatisfying sleep)

Adapted from American Psychiatric Association: Diagnostic and Statistical Manual of Mental Disorders-DSM-IV. Washington, DC: American Psychiatric Press, 1994.

TABLE 3-9. Panic Disorder (Episodic Paroxysmal Anxiety)

A. The individual experiences recurrent panic attacks that are not consistently associated with a specific situation or object and that often occur spontaneously. The panic attacks are not associated with marked exertion or with exposure to dangerous or life-threatening situations.
B. A panic attack is characterized by all of the following:
   1. It is a discrete or intense fear or discomfort
   2. It starts abruptly
   3. It reaches a maximum within a few minutes and lasts at least some minutes
   4. At least four of the symptoms listed below must be present, one of which must be from items (a) to (d):

Autonomic arousal symptoms

(a) Palpitations or pounding heart, or accelerated heart rate
(b) Sweating
(c) Trembling or shaking
(d) Dry mouth (not due to medication or dehydration)

Symptoms involving chest and abdomen

(e) Difficulty in breathing
(f) Feeling of choking
(g) Chest pain or discomfort
(h) Nausea or abdominal distress

Symptoms involving mental state

(i) Feeling dizzy, unsteady, faint, or light-headed
(j) Feeling that objects are unreal (derealization), or that the self is distant or "not really here" (depersonalization)
(k) Fear of losing control, "going crazy," or passing out
(l) Fear of dying

General symptoms

(m) Hot flashes or cold chills
(n) Numbness or tingling sensations

Adapted from World Health Organization: The ICD-10 Classification of Mental and Behavioral Disorders. Geneva, Switzerland: Author, 1994.

passions, such as fear, pain, desire, and pleasure. In the psychiatric nomenclature, the concept of apathy was subsumed under different terms such as the amotivational syndrome, emotional blunting, negative psychomotor symptoms, retardation, flat affect, withdrawal, or avolition. Among neurologic disorders, apathy was reported to be highly prevalent in patients with stroke, PD, AD, and traumatic brain injury (TBI), but whether apathy is a specific syndrome or just a symptom of another disorder such as depression or dementia has been examined only recently. We review below the main phenomenological aspects of apathy and the most useful diagnostic and rating instruments.

Diagnosis of Apathy in Dementia

Marin (1991) defined apathy as the absence of feeling, emotion, interest, or concern, and suggested that apathy should be construed as a syndrome, given that a group of symptoms characterized by deficits in overt behavioral, cognitive, and emotional concomitants of goal-directed behavior are consistently present in a variety of neurologic and psychiatric disorders. Whereas there is recognition that apathy is an important behavioral change in patients with dementia, to our knowledge there are no standardized diagnostic criteria for this condition. Moreover, it has not been clearly established whether apathy is always related to syndromal or subsyndromal depressive states or cognitive deficits. Symptoms of apathy such as loss of interest and psychomotor retardation are included within the DSM-IV diagnostic criteria for depression, and a large overlap of apathy and depression was reported in patients with different neurologic disorders (Starkstein et al., 1995). Several studies demonstrated a lack of association between depression and apathy in dementia. Levy and colleagues (1998) examined the relationship between apathy and depression in patients with AD, frontotemporal dementia, PD, Huntington disease (HD), and progressive supranuclear palsy, and found nonsignificant correlations between apathy and depression, suggesting that apathy and depression may be separate phenomena. Marin and colleagues (1991) reported data on a group of patients with either AD or stroke lesions with high apathy and low depression scores. Reichman and colleagues (1996) examined whether negative symptoms in AD (defined as affective withdrawal) were distinct from depression. They found a group of nondepressed AD patients with significantly higher scores of avolition, apathy, and social and emotional withdrawal than age-comparable normal controls. Taken together, these findings suggest that apathy is a behavioral problem separate from depression in dementia, although the above studies were limited by the lack of clinical diagnoses and different assessment techniques.

Several instruments were developed to measure the severity of apathy. Marin and colleagues (1991) developed an 18-item scale with self-, informant-, and clinician-rated versions based on the assessment of the subject's thoughts, emotions, and activities during the 4 weeks prior to the interview. Starkstein and colleagues (1992) developed the Apathy Scale based on Marin's scale (Table 3-10). The Apathy Scale includes 14 items that can be assessed with the patient and caregivers. Each question has four possible answers, which are scored from 0 to 3, and final scores range from 0 to 42 points,

TABLE 3-10. Apathy Scale

Questions	Not at all	Slightly	Some	A lot
Are you interested in learning new things?				
Does anything interest you?				
Are you concerned about your condition?				
Do you put much effort into things?				
Are you always looking for something to do?				
Do you have plans and goals for the future?				
Do you have motivation?				
Do you have the energy for daily activities?				
Does someone have to tell you what to do each day?				
Are you indifferent to things?				
Are you unconcerned with many things?				
Do you need a push to get started on things?				
Are you neither happy nor sad, just in between?				
Would you consider yourself apathetic?				

For questions 1–8, the scoring system is the following: not at all = 3 points; slightly = 2 points; some = 1 point; a lot = 0 points. For questions 9–14, the scoring system is the following: not at all = 0 points; slightly = 1 point; some = 2 points; a lot = 3 points.

Adapted from Starkstein SE, Migliorelli R, Manes F, et al: The prevalence and clinical correlates of apathy and irritability in Alzheimer's disease. Eur J Neurol 2:540–546, 1995.

with higher scores indicating more severe apathy. Starkstein and colleagues (2000) demonstrated the reliability and validity of this scale in different samples of patients with neurologic disease, such as AD, PD, stroke, and HD (Starkstein, 2000).

One major limitation in diagnosing apathy is the lack of a specific structured interview, and apathy has usually been diagnosed based on either the rater's own subjective impression, or using cut-off scores on ad hoc apathy scales. In a recent study, Starkstein and colleagues (2001) examined the usefulness and clinical correlates of specific diagnostic criteria for apathy in a study that included a consecutive series of 319 patients with AD and 36 age-comparable healthy controls. Diagnoses of apathy were generated using a specific diagnostic scheme (Table 3-11), with the important provision that diagnoses were always based on caregiver's ratings on the Apathy Scale. The main findings of the study were that apathy was present in 37% of the 319 patients with AD as compared to none of the controls. In 24% of the AD group apathy coexisted with depression, whereas the remaining 13% of patients had apathy only. Apathy was significantly correlated with more severe impairments in activities of daily living and poor awareness of behavioral and cognitive deficits. Another important finding was that the AD group with apathy only had similar depression scores as the nondepressed nonapathetic AD group, supporting the validity of apathy as a behavioral syndrome independent from depression.

In conclusion, whereas apathy is frequently reported in patients with neurologic disease, it is not yet clear whether this is a syndrome or just a symptom, and whether this is a specific behavioral change or just a symptom of other psychiatric syndromes. Several scales are used to rate apathy in neurologic disease, but there are no structured interviews or specific diagnostic criteria.

Psychosis

The concept of psychosis in neurologic disease primarily includes delusions and hallucinations. Delusions are defined as erroneous beliefs that usually involve a misinterpretation of perceptions or experiences. Hallucinations are sensory perceptions in the absence of identifiable external stimuli and should be distinguished from illusions, which are misperceptions or misinterpretations of real external stimuli. An individual with hallucinations may recognize that she or he is having a false sensory experience (a phenomenon known as hallucinosis), whereas another person may be convinced of the reality of the sensory experience (i.e., a "true" hallucination). Delirium is usually included within the spectrum of psychotic behaviors. Delirious episodes have an acute onset and relatively brief duration and are characterized by impaired awareness of self and surroundings, impairment of direct thinking, disorder of attention with hypoalertness or hyperalertness, impairment of memory, diminished perceptual discrimination, disturbance of psychomotor behavior with hypoactivity or hyperactivity, disordered sleep-wake cycle with drowsiness during the day and insomnia at night, and fluctuations in alertness and in severity of cognitive impairment (Lipowski, 1990).

Assessment of psychotic symptoms may be adequately carried out with a semistructured psychiatric interview (e.g., SCID, SCAN). The DSM-IV includes several entries for psychotic disorders in neurologic disease

---

TABLE 3-11. Diagnostic Criteria for Apathy

A. Lack of motivation relative to the patient's previous level of functioning or the standards of his or her age and culture as indicated either by subjective account or observation by others.

B. Presence, with lack of motivation, of at least one symptom belonging to each of the following three domains:

Diminished goal-directed behavior

1. Lack of effort
2. Dependency on others to structure activity

Diminished goal-directed cognition

3. Lack of interest in learning new things, or in new experiences
4. Lack of concern about one's personal problems

Diminished concomitants of goal-directed behavior

5. Unchanging affect
6. Lack of emotional responsivity to positive or negative events

C. The symptoms cause clinically significant distress or impairment in social, occupational, or other important areas of functioning.

D. The symptoms are not due to diminished level of consciousness or the direct physiologic effects of a substance (e.g., a drug of abuse, a medication).

Adapted from Marin RS: Apathy: A neuropsychiatric syndrome. J Neuropsychiatry Clin Neurosci 3:243–254, 1991.

such as "Psychotic Disorder Due to a General Medical Condition" (293.8x; Table 3-12), and "Delirium Due to a General Medical Condition" (293.0; Table 3-13). The ICD-10 includes specific criteria for "Delirium, Not Induced by Alcohol and Other Psychoactive Substances" (code F05; Table 3-14), which are further subdivided into the categories of "Delirium, Not Superimposed on Dementia" (code F05.0), "Delirium, Superimposed on Dementia" (code F05.1), "Other Delirium" (code F05.8), and "Delirium, Unspecified" (code F05.9). The ICD-10 criteria for "Organic Hallucinosis" (code F06.0) includes the general criteria listed in Table 3-14, and the provisions that the clinical picture is dominated by persistent or recurrent hallucinations, and hallucinations occur in clear consciousness. The ICD-10 criteria for "Organic Delusional (Schizophrenia-like) Disorder (code F06.2) include the general criteria listed in Table 3-14 and the provisions that the clinical picture is dominated by delusions (of persecution, body change, disease, death, jealousy), and intact memory and clear consciousness.

Assessment of severity of psychosis and other behavioral disorders in neurologic disease may be carried out with rating instruments that are frequently used in patients with primary psychiatric disorders. A variety of instruments were specifically designed to assess the presence of psychotic and other abnormal behavior in neurologic disease. The BEHAVE-AD (Reisberg et al., 1987) is a useful instrument used in dementia to rate abnormal behaviors such as delusions, hallucinations, abnormal motor behaviors, aggressive behavior, agitation, mood, anxiety, and phobias. The Neuropsychiatric Inventory (NPI; Cummings et al., 1994) is a relatively brief interview assessing the following behavioral disturbances: delusions, hallucinations, dysphoria, anxiety, agitation/aggression, euphoria, disinhibition, irritability/lability, apathy, and aberrant motor behavior. Severity and frequency of abnormal behaviors are independently assessed. The NPI demonstrated good concurrent validity and adequate inter-rater reliability. The Manchester and Oxford Universities Scale for the Psychopathological Assess-

TABLE 3-12. Diagnostic Criteria for a Psychotic Disorder Due to a General Medical Condition

A. Prominent hallucinations or delusions
B. There is evidence from the history, physical examination, or laboratory findings that the disturbance is the direct physiologic consequence of a general medical condition.
C. The disturbance is not better accounted for by another mental disorder.
D. The disturbance does not occur exclusively during the course of a delirium.

Adapted from American Psychiatric Association: Diagnostic and Statistical Manual of Mental Disorders-DSM-IV. Washington, DC: American Psychiatric Press, 1994.

TABLE 3-13. Diagnostic Criteria for Delirium Due to a General Medical Condition

A. Disturbance of consciousness with reduced ability to focus, sustain, or shift attention
B. A change in cognition (such as memory deficit, disorientation, language disturbance) or the development of a perceptual disturbance that is not better accounted for by a preexisting, established, or evolving dementia
C. The disturbance develops over a short period of time (usually hours to days) and tends to fluctuate during the course of the day.
D. There is evidence from the history, physical examination, or laboratory findings that the disturbance is caused by the direct physiological consequences of a general medical condition.

Adapted from American Psychiatric Association: Diagnostic and Statistical Manual of Mental Disorders-DSM-IV. Washington, DC: American Psychiatric Press, 1994.

ment of Dementia (MOUSEPAD; Allen et al., 1996) is a 59-item instrument that is rated by an experienced clinician during a 15- to 30-minute interview with the patient's caregivers. This instrument measures the presence of hallucinations; delusions; misidentifications; reduplications; problems with walking, eating, and sleeping; sexual behavior; and aggression in the last month and since the onset of the neurologic illness. Trzepacz (1999) designed the Delirium Rating Scale (DRS) as a clinician-rated instrument to assess the severity of delirium. This scale contains 10 items that rate the presence of hallucinations and delusions, temporal onset of symptoms, perceptual disturbances, psychomotor behavior, cognitive status, sleep-wake cycle disturbances, lability of mood, and variability of symptoms. Lischinsky and colleagues (in preparation) developed the Disinhibition Scale, which consists of 26 questions rating abnormal behaviors over the preceding 4 weeks. Items rate abnormal motor behaviors (e.g., hyperactivity, wandering, utilization behavior), stereotyped routines (e.g., verbal stereotypes, motor routines, obsessive ideas and rituals), delusions, hallucinations, hypomanic behavior (e.g., pressured speech, euphoria, irritability, hyperphagia, hypersexuality, overspending, grandiose ideas, inappropriate social behavior), and poor self-care (e.g., poor hygiene, careless dressing, poor insight about own deficits, distractibility, excessive sleep, and poor awareness of danger). The Disinhibition Scale demonstrated high inter-rater and intrarater reliabilities and adequate validity for disinhibited behaviors in AD.

Manic behaviors are frequently reported in patients with TBI and more rarely among those with stroke lesions or neurodegenerative disorders, such as PD or AD. The presence of manic symptoms may be assessed with structured psychiatric interviews, such as the SCID or the SCAN. Several diagnostic criteria may apply to

TABLE 3-14. Delirium, Not Induced by Alcohol or Other Psychoactive Substances

A. There is clouding of consciousness (i.e., reduced clarity of awareness of the environment, with reduced ability to focus, sustain, or shift attention).

B. Disturbance of cognition is manifest by both:

   1. Impairment of immediate recall and recent memory, with relatively intact remote memory

   2. Disorientation in time, place, or person

C. At least one of the following psychomotor disturbances is present:

   1. Rapid, unpredictable shifts from hypoactivity to hyperactivity

   2. Increased reaction time

   3. Increased or decreased flow of speech

   4. Enhanced startle reaction

D. There is disturbance of sleep or of the sleep-wake cycle, manifested by at least one of the following:

   1. Insomnia, which in severe cases may involve total sleep loss, with or without daytime drowsiness, or reversal of the sleep-wake cycle

   2. Nocturnal worsening of symptoms

   3. Disturbing dreams and nightmares, which may continue as hallucinations or illusions after awakening

E. Symptoms have rapid onset and show fluctuations over the course of the day.

There is objective evidence from history, physical and neurologic examination, or laboratory tests of an underlying cerebral or systemic disease (other than psychoactive substance-related) that can be presumed to be responsible for the clinical manifestations in criteria A–D.

Adapted from World Health Organization: The ICD-10 Classification of Mental and Behavioral Disorders. Geneva, Switzerland: Author, 1994.

patients with manic behavior and neurologic disease. The DSM-IV criteria for a Mood Disorder Due to a General Medical Condition with manic features are used whenever the patient meets the qualifier for having developed the mood change due to a general medical condition, and whenever the mood disturbance is judged to be the direct physiologic consequence of a medical illness. However, the relationship between the mood disturbance and a medical disorder may be difficult to establish. Another related DSM-IV category is "Personality Change Due to a General Medical Condition, Disinhibited or Aggressive Type," but one limitation of these criteria is that no specific definitions for disinhibition or aggressiveness are provided. Starkstein and Robinson (1996) have used the DSM criteria for a "Manic Episode" (excluding the organic condition; Table 3-15), given that these criteria are more clearly defined and more restrictive than the other two alternatives described above. The ICD-10 includes the related categories of Organic Manic Disorder (F06.30) and Organic Personality Disorder (F07.0; Table 3-16).

Pathologic Affective Display

Patients with acute or chronic neurologic disease, such as stroke or dementia, may present with sudden episodes of crying or laughing that are generically termed pathologic affective display. This entity is subdivided into two different categories: (1) "Emotional lability," which is defined as the sudden onset of laughing or crying that the patient is unable to suppress, which generally occurs in appropriate situations and is accompanied by a congruent alteration of mood (e.g., depression in patients with crying episodes); and (2) "Pathological laughing and/or crying," which is the sudden onset of laughing or crying episodes that do not correspond to an underlying emotional change (e.g., crying episodes in the context of normal mood). Robinson and colleagues (1993) developed the Pathologic Laughter and Crying Scale (PLACS), an interviewer-rated scale that quantifies aspects of pathologic affect, including the duration of the episodes, their relation to external events, degree of voluntary control, inappropriateness in relation to emotions, and degree of resultant distress. Among stroke patients, this scale demonstrated both high test-retest reliability and validity. There were no significant correlations between PLACS scores and scores of depression, cognitive impairment, deficits in activities of daily living, or social functioning, indicating that the PLACS was assessing a factor other than the factors being measured by these instruments.

Newsom-Davies and colleagues (1999) developed the Emotional Lability Questionnaire (ELQ) that includes a self-rated version assessed as a structured interview and a caregiver version. They found a good association between both subscales, demonstrating its internal validity.

TABLE 3-15. Diagnostic Criteria for Manic Episode

A. A distinctic period of abnormality and persistently elevated, expansive, or irritable mood, lasting at least 1 week

B. During the period of mood disturbance, three (or more) of the following symptoms have persisted (four if the mood is only irritable) and have been present to a significant degree:
   1. Inflated self-esteem or grandiosity
   2. Decreased need for sleep
   3. More talkative than usual or pressure to keep talking
   4. Flight of ideas or subjective experience that thoughts are racing
   5. Distractibility (i.e., attention too easily drawn to unimportant or irrelevant external stimuli)
   6. Increase in goal-directed activity or psychomotor agitation
   7. Excessive involvement in pleasurable activities that have a high potential for painful consequences (e.g., engaging in unrestrained buying sprees, sexual indiscretions, or foolish business investments)

Adapted from American Psychiatric Association: Diagnostic and Statistical Manual of Mental Disorders—DSM-IV. Washington, D.C.: American Psychiatric Press, 1994.

TABLE 3-16. Organic Personality Disorder

A. The general criteria for "Personality and Behavioral Disorders Due to Brain Disease" must be met.

B. At least three of the following features must be present over a period of 6 months or more:
   1. Consistently reduced ability to persevere with goal-directed activities, especially those involving relatively long periods of time and postponed gratification
   2. One or more of the following emotional changes:
      (a) Emotional lability (uncontrolled, unstable, and fluctuacting expression of emotions)
      (b) Euphoria and shallow, inappropriate jocularity, unwarranted by the circumstances
      (c) Irritability and/or outbursts of anger and aggression
      (d) Apathy
   3. Disinhibited expression of needs or impulses without consideration of consequences or of social conventions
   4. Cognitive disturbances, typically in the form of:
      (a) Excessive suspiciousness and paranoid ideas
      (b) Excessive preocupation with a single theme such as religion, or rigid categorization of other people's behavior in terms of "right" and "wrong"
   5. Marked alteration of the rate and flow of language production, with features such as circumstantiality, overinclusiveness, viscosity, and hypergraphia
   6. Altered sexual behaviour (hyposexuality or change in sexual preference)

Adapted from World Health Organization: The ICD-10 Classification of Mental and Behavioral Disorders. Geneva, Switzerland: Author, 1994.

Anosognosia

Anosognosia is defined as the lack of awareness of the physical, cognitive, or behavioral problems produced by a neurologic illness. The term was coined by Babinski (1914), who used it to refer to patients who did not recognize their hemiplegia. It is also a well-known finding among patients with dementia, who may deny the presence of cognitive deficits.

Starkstein and colleagues (1992) developed the Anosognosia Questionnaire to be used in patients with stroke lesions (Table 3-17). This instrument was constructed using questions identified by other investigators as indicative of anosognosia for motor and visual deficits. The main purpose of this scale is to diagnose the presence of anosognosia (i.e., the full denial of a deficit) or anosodiaphoria (i.e., the emotional indifference to the deficit). To measure the severity of anosognosia among patients with stroke lesions Starkstein and colleagues (1993) also developed the Denial of Illness

Scale (DIS). The DIS is an abridged and modified version of the Hackett-Cassem Denial Scale (Hackett & Cassem, 1974) and includes 10 questions. Severity is assessed on each item using a 0 to 1 or 0 to 2 scale, with higher scores indicating greater denial. The DIS showed high inter-rater and intrarater reliabilities and adequate validity.

To assess the phenomenon of anosognosia in dementia, Migliorelli and colleagues (1995) developed the Anosognosia Questionnaire-Dementia (AQ-D), which consists of 30 questions divided into two sections. The first section assesses intellectual functioning, whereas the second section examines changes in interests and personality. Higher scores indicate more severe impairments. Form A is answered by the patient alone (with clarifications by the examiner if needed), whereas form B (a similar questionnaire written in the third person) is answered by the patient's caregiver blind to the patient's answers in form A. The final score is

TABLE 3-17. Anosognosia Questionnaire

1. Why are you here?
2. What is the matter with you?
3. Is there anything wrong with your arm or leg?
4. Is there anything wrong with your eyesight?
5. Is your limb weak, paralyzed, or numb?
6. How does your limb feel?

If denial is elicited, ask the following:

a. (arm picked up) What is this?
b. Can you lift it?
c. You clearly have some problem with this?
d. (asked to lift both arms) Can't you see that the two arms are not at the same level?
e. (asked to identify finger movements in and out of the abnormal visual field) Can't you see that you have a problem with your eyesight?

Scoring

0: The disorder is spontaneously reported or mentioned following a general question about the patient's complaints.
1: The disorder is reported only following a specific question about the strength of the patient's limb or about visual problems.
2: The disorder is acknowledged only after its demonstration through routine techniques of neurologic examination.
3: No acknowledgment of the disorder.

obtained by subtracting the scores on form B from those on form A. Thus, positive scores indicate that the caregiver rated the patient as more impaired than the patient's own evaluation. The AQ-D showed both high intrarater and inter-rater reliabilities, high internal consistency, and adequate validity.

One limitation to most studies on anosognosia is that diagnoses were generated based on either subjective impressions or arbitrary cut-off scores on ad hoc scales, and to our knowledge, there are neither structured interviews to elicit signs or symptoms of anosognosia nor clinical criteria to diagnose this phenomenon.

CONCLUSIONS

Psychiatric disorders are frequently found among patients with acute or chronic neurologic disease and were reported to have an impact on patients' recovery, cognitive ability, general functioning, and quality of life. Thus, it is important to readily diagnose those disorders to begin early treatment. There are several limitations to the diagnoses of psychiatric disorders among patients with neurologic disease, such as the presence of neurologic symptoms that may overlap with symptoms of psychiatric disease and the presence of language and cognitive deficits that may complicate the obtention of reliable information. Recent efforts were devoted to producing valid and reliable diagnostic criteria for psychiatric disorders in patients with neurologic disease, which were primarily developed in the DSM-IV and ICD-10. Structured psychiatric interviews for neurologic disease have been specifically designed (e.g., SCAN) or adapted to be used among these patients (e.g., SCID). Rating scales were also developed to rate frequent behavioral problems in patients with neurologic disease, such as apathy, irritability, pathologic affective display, and anosognosia, whereas other scales frequently used in psychiatric populations demonstrated to be valid and reliable among those with neurologic disease.

■ KEY POINTS

☐ The diagnosis of psychiatric and behavioral disorders in neurologic disease should be made after a thorough mental status examination with a specific evaluation of signs and symptoms of psychiatric disorders.

☐ Language and cognitive deficits are important limitations to the diagnosis of depression in neurologic disease.

☐ Psychiatric signs and symptoms should be assessed with a psychiatric interview that includes questions for a variety of behavioral and emotional disorders and items to rate observed abnormal behaviors.

☐ The diagnosis of depression in patients with neurologic disorder requires a thorough mental status assessment for specific symptoms of mood disorders.

☐ Depression rating scales are useful to screen patients for depressive disorders, to determine the relative severity of depressive symptoms, and to quantify changes in depression after specific treatment.

KEY READINGS

Cohen-Cole SA, Stoudemire A: Major depression and physical illness: Special considerations in diagnosis and biologic treatment. Psychiatr Clin North Am 10:1–14, 1987.

Fedoroff JP, Starkstein SE, Parikh RM, et al. Are depressive symptoms non-specific in patients with acute stroke? Am J Psychiatry 148:1172–1176, 1991.

Schramke CJ, Stowe RM, Ratcliff G, et al: Poststroke depression and anxiety: Different assessment methods result in variations in incidence and severity estimates. J Clin Exp Neuropsychol 20:723–737, 1998.

REFERENCES

Allen NHP, Gordon S, Hope T, et al: Manchester and Oxford Universities Scale for Psychopathological Assessment of Dementia (MOUSEPAD). Br J Psychiatry 169:293–307, 1996.

American Psychiatric Association: Diagnostic and Statistical Manual of Mental Disorders-DSM-IV. Washington, DC: American Psychiatric Press, 1994.

Babinski J: Contribution a l'etude des troubles mentaux dans l'hemiplegic organique cerebrale (anosognosie). Rev Neurol (Paris) 27:845–848, 1914.

Beck AT, Epstein N, Brown G, et al: An inventory for measuring clinical anxiety: Psychometric properties. J Consult Clin Psychol 56:893–897, 1998.

Beck AT, Ward C H, Mendelson M: An inventory for measuring depression. Arch Gen Psychiatry 4:551–571, 1961.

Bukberg J, Pernan D, Holland JC: Depression in hospitalized cancer patients. Psychosom Med 46:199–212, 1984.

Chemerinski E, Petracca G, Manes F, et al: Prevalence and correlates of anxiety in Alzheimer's disease. Depress Anxiety 7:166–170, 1998.

Chemerinski E, Petracca G, Sabe L, et al: Specificity of depressive symptoms in Alzheimer's disease. Am J Psychiatry 158:68–72, 2001.

Cummings JL, Mega M, Gray K, et al: The Neuropsychiatric Inventory: Comprehensive assessment of psychopathology in dementia. Neurology 44:2308–2314, 1994.

Endicott J: Measurement of depression in patients with cancer. Cancer 53:2443–2248, 1984.

Gainotti G, Azzoni A, Marra C: Frequency, phenomenology and anatomical-clinical correlates of major poststroke depression. Br J Psychiatry 175:163–167, 1999.

Goldberg DP, Hiller VF: A scaled version of the General Health Questionnaire. Psychol Med 9:139–198, 1979.

Hackett TP, Cassem NH: Development of quantitative rating scales to assess denial. J Psychosom Res 18:93–100, 1974.

Hamilton M: The assessment of anxiety states by rating. Br J Med Psychol 32:50–55, 1959.

Hamilton MA: A rating scale for depression. J Neurol Neurosurg Psychiatry 23:56–62, 1960.

Levy ML, Cummings JL, Fairbanks LA, et al: Apathy is not depression. J Neuropsychiatry Clin Neurosci 10:314–319, 1998.

Lipowski ZI: Delirium: Acute Confusional States. Oxford, UK: Oxford University Press, 1990.

Marin RE, Biedrzycki RC, Firinciogullari SF: Reliability and validity of the Apathy Evaluation Scale. Psychiatry Res 38:143–162, 1991.

Marin RS: Apathy: a neuropsychiatric syndrome. J Neuropsychiatry Clin Neurosci 3:243–254, 1991.

Marsh L: Anxiety disorders in Parkinson's disease. Int Rev Psychiatry 12:307–318, 2000.

Migliorelli R, Teson A, Sabe L, et al: Anosognosia in Alzheimer's disease: A study of associated factors. J Neuropsychiatry Clin Neurosci 7:338–344, 1995.

Montgomery SA, Asberg M: A new depression scale designed to be sensitive to change. Br J Psychiatry 134:382–389, 1979.

Newsom-Davis IC, Abrahams S, Goldstein LH, et al: The emotional lability questionnaire: A new measure of emotional lability in amyotrophic lateral sclerosis. J Neurol Sci 31:22–25, 1999.

Paradiso S, Ohkubo T, Robinson RG: Vegetative and psychological symptoms associated with depressed mood over the first two years after stroke. Int J Psychiatry Med 27:137–157, 1997.

Parikh RM, Eden DT, Price TR, et al: The sensitivity and specificity of the Center of Epidemiologic Studies depression scale as a screening instrument for post-stroke depression. Int J Psychiatry Med 18:169–181, 1998.

Radloff LA: The CES-D Scale, a self-report depression scale for research in the general population. Appl Psychol Measures, 1:385–401, 1977.

Rapp SR, Vrana S: (1989). Substituing nonsomatic for somatic symptoms in the diagnosis of depression in elderly male medical patients. Am J Psychiatry 146:1197–1200, 1989.

Regier DA, Boyd JH, Burke JD, et al: One-month prevalence of mental disorders in the U.S.: Based on five epidemiologic catchment sites. Arch Gen Psychiatry 45:977–986, 1988.

Reichman WE, Coyne AC, Amirneni S, et al: Negative symptoms in Alzheimer's disease. Am J Psychiatry 153:424–426, 1996.

Reisberg B, Borenstein J, Salob SP, et al: Behavioral symptoms in Alzheimer's disease: Phenomenology and treatment. J Clin Psychiatry 48:9–15, 1987.

Rifken A, Reardon G, Siris S, et al: Trimipramine in physical illness with depression. J Clin Psychiatry 46:2, 4–8, 1985.

Robinson RG: The Clinical Neuropsychiatry of Stroke. Cambridge, UK: Cambridge University Press, 1999, p. 72.

Robinson RG, Parikh RM, Lipsey JR, et al: Pathological laughing and crying following stroke: Validation of a measurement scale and a double-blind treatment study. Am J Psychiatry 150:286–293, 1993.

Robinson RG, Starr LB, Kubos KL, et al: A two year longitudinal study of poststroke mood disorders: Findings during the initial evaluation. Stroke 14:736–744, 1983.

Ross ED, Rush AJ: Diagnosis and neuroanatomical correlates of depression in brain damaged patients. Arch Gen Psychiatry 38:1344–1354, 1981.

Spitzer RL, Williams JBW, Gibbon M, First MB: The structured clinical interview for DSM-III-R (SCID). I: History, rationale, and description. Arch Gen Psychiatry 49:624–629, 1992.

Starkstein SE: Apathy and withdrawal. Int Psychogeriatr 12:135–138, 2000.

Starkstein SE, Fedoroff JP, Price TR, et al: Anosognosia in patients with cerebrovascular lesions: A study of causative factors. Stroke, 23:1446–1453, 1992.

Starkstein SE, Fedoroff JP, Price TR, et al: Denial of illness scale: A reliability and validity study. Neuropsychiatry Neuropsychol Behav Neurol 6:93–97, 1993.

Starkstein, SE, Mayberg HS, Preziosi TJ, et al: Reliability, validity and clinical correlates of apathy in Parkinson's disease. J Neuropsychiatry Clin Neurosci 4:134–139, 1992.

Starkstein SE, Migliorelli R, Manes F, et al: The prevalence and clinical correlates of apathy and irritability in Alzheimer's disease. Eur J Neurol 2:540–546, 1995.

Starkstein SE, Petracca G, Chemerinski E, et al: The syndromic validity of apathy in Azheimer's disease. Am J Psychiatry 158:872–877, 2001.

Starkstein SE, Preziosi TJ, Forrester AW, et al: Specificity of affective and autonomic symptoms of depression in Parkinson's disease. J Neurol Neurosurg Psychiatry 53:869–873, 1990.

Starkstein SE, Robinson RG: Mechanism of disinhibition after brain lesions. J Nerv Ment Dis 185:108–114, 1995.

Starkstein SE, Robinson RG: Depression in Neurologic Disease. Baltimore, MD: The Johns Hopkins University Press, 1993.

Trzepacz, PT: The Delirium Rating Scale. Its use in consultation-liaison research. Psychosomatics, 40:193–204, 1999.

Wing JK, Cooper JE, Sartorius N: Measurement and Classification of Psychiatric Symptoms. Cambridge, UK: Cambridge University Press, 1974.

World Health Organization: The ICD-10 Classification of Mental and Behavioral Disorders. Geneva, Switzerland: Author, 1994a.

World Health Organization: Schedules for Clinical Assessment in Neuropsychiatry, version 2.0. Geneva, Switzerland: Author, 1994b.

Zung WWK: A self-rating depression scale. Arch Gen Psychiatry 12:63–70, 1965.

Morphometric Brain Analysis in the Dementias

Clare J. Galton and John R. Hodges

INTRODUCTION
Measurement of Brain Structures
Normal Variation
Pathologic Correlates of Atrophy

NEUROIMAGING IN EARLY ALZHEIMER DISEASE
CT Studies
MRI Cross-sectional Studies
MRI Longitudinal Studies

NEUROIMAGING AND DIFFERENTIAL DIAGNOSIS OF ALZHEIMER DISEASE
Introduction
Frontotemporal Dementia

RELATIONSHIP OF IMAGING AND COGNITION IN NEURODEGENERATIVE DISEASE
Introduction
Episodic Memory
Semantic Memory

CONCLUSIONS

Alzheimer disease (AD)
Episodic memory
Frontotemporal dementia (FTD)
Hippocampus
Medial temporal lobe
Magnetic resonance imaging (MRI)
Mild cognitive impairment (MCI)
Volumetry

INTRODUCTION

There have been huge technological developments in the ability to image and measure the living brain over recent decades. In this chapter, we review the impact of these advances in the diagnosis and understanding of neurodegnerative dementias. We focus primarily on the use of magnetic resonance imaging (MRI), with volumetric assessment, in the early and differential diagnosis of Alzheimer disease (AD) and frontotemporal dementia

(FTD). Structural neuroimaging is a rapidly moving research area with new imaging techniques and software being developed; however, we have confined ourselves to the more widely available and clinically relevant techniques. The role of these techniques for exploring the brain structure-function relationships in these dementias is also an exciting area that is explored in this review.

Measurement of Brain Structures

Computed tomography (CT) scanning is fast, well tolerated by patients, and widely available. The ability to visualize the temporal lobe is, however, hampered by bone-hardening artifact, limited view angle, and partial voluming. MRI, in contrast, has excellent soft tissue resolution and flexible image orientation, and is less limited by artifact obscuring the temporal lobes, but suffers from poor patient tolerance and more limited availability. Different methods of quantifying atrophy can be applied to both structural imaging modalities. Rating scales have been used as semiquantitative measures of atrophy, usually based on qualitative criteria of structural appearance and a categorical scale. The assessment is rapid and can be performed on CT and MRI, but precision is limited by the range of the scoring scale, and poor inter-rater reliability is exacerbated by scale complexity (Sullivan et al., 1998). Measurement of a structure in two dimensions (i.e., on a single CT or MRI slice) can be undertaken using linear or area measures (planimetry). These are quantitative measures which provide more sensitivity, but there are several methodological issues. The technique is sensitive to head alignment and the orientation of acquision resulting in sampling bias. Measuring a brain structure in three dimensions has become possible because software improvements have enabled many thin slices to be obtained in MRI imaging. Volumetric techniques, of tracing anatomically defined regions over many slices and multiplying the area by slice thickness to calculate a volume measurement, have enabled accurate quantitative assessment of structures as small as the hippocampus or entorhinal cortex. Volumetric-based measurements are likely to provide the best estimate of the size of a structure but are time-consuming and still prone to inter-rater variation. These methods were pioneered in the diagnosis and assessment of temporal lobe epilepsy, but have been extensively used in the assessment of neurodegenerative diseases, especially AD. More recently, highly sensitive automated methods of image coregistration have been developed, which avoid operator bias but are technically very demanding and require serial imaging (Fox et al., 1996a, 1999b).

Normal Variation

When assessing brain structures by these methods, the variation in the normal population has to be considered. General brain size varies with size and age of a person, with smaller brains occurring in smaller individuals (including women) and older people. CT studies have shown increasing brain atrophy and ventricular enlargement with increasing age, creating difficulty in distinguishing AD from controls (see below). The same is true for hippocampal size with similar relationships described for gender and age. Researchers have adjusted for normal population variation with three main methods in cross-sectional imaging studies: (1) adjusting for intracranial volume (Jack et al., 1992); (2) adjusting for cross-sectional intracranial area (Ikeda et al., 1994; Laasko et al., 1995); and (3) regression when large numbers of controls are available (Fama et al., 1997; Sullivan et al., 1998). In longitudinal studies where rate of change is measured these adjustments are not required (Fox et al., 1996b).

Pathologic Correlates of Atrophy

Pathologic validation of volumes measured with neuroimaging techniques has also been undertaken. The Consortium to Establish a Registry for Alzheimer's Disease (CERAD) used ratings of temporal lobe atrophy before and after death to establish a positive relationship between CT and MRI scanning and pathologic atrophy (Davis et al., 1995). Postmortem studies have also shown that MRI hippocampal volumes are equivalent to histologically derived volumes (Bobinski et al., 2000), and both volumes are strongly associated with neuronal counts and numbers of neurofibrillary tangles (DeLeon et al., 1997a) suggesting that MRI atrophy does reflect pathology in vivo. The Oxford Project to Investigate Memory and Aging (OPTIMA) has also demonstrated that measures of neurofibrillary tangles, neuritic plaques, and amyloid load in the hippocampus at postmortem examination were inversely correlated with the medial temporal lobe measure on CT imaging (Nagy et al., 1996).

NEUROIMAGING IN EARLY ALZHEIMER DISEASE

In the absence of biomarkers of AD, the diagnosis remains clinically based. There is, however, still much controversy regarding the earliest detectable stages of the disease. The initial focus of neuroimaging in AD was to exclude treatable structural causes of dementia, such as subdural hematomas, tumors, and normal pressure hydrocephalus. Subsequently, research efforts concentrated on the characterization of more specific abnormalities on structural (MRI and CT) imaging. More recently, imaging studies have attempted to diagnose AD earlier in the disease course and to monitor progression of the disease. Much of this effort has concentrated on patients with isolated memory impairment, so-called mild cognitive impairment (MCI), who are known to be at high risk of conversion to AD. Most studies show a conversion rate of 25% to 40% over 2 to 4 years (Petersen, 1999).

CT Studies

Early CT studies demonstrated generalized brain atrophy with ventricular enlargement in patients with AD compared to controls (for a review, see DeCarli et al., 1990). More recent studies have focused on brain areas known to be involved pathologically early in the course of AD, namely, the medial temporal lobe (Braak & Braak, 1991; Fig. 4-1A).

OPTIMA has examined extensively CT atrophy of the medial temporal lobe in AD with the advantage of histologic confirmation of the diagnosis. They reported a reduction in thickness of the medial temporal lobe, as measured linearly on temporal lobe angulated CT scans, in 44 histologically confirmed AD cases (Jobst et al., 1992). This measure separated AD from controls with a sensitivity of 92% and specificity of

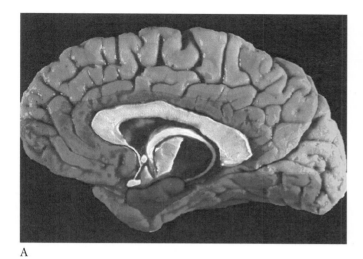

A

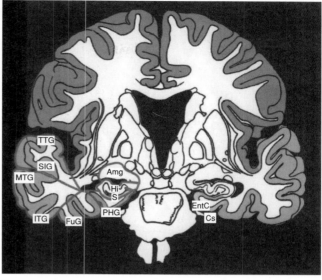

B

FIGURE 4-1. *A,* Distribution of Alzheimer-type pathology. Tangle and plaque density are highest in the medial temporal lobe (*red*) and spread out to decreasing color intensity areas. *B,* Illustration of the anatomy of the temporal lobe. Amg, amygdala; CS, collateral sulcus; EntC, entorhinal cortex; FuG, fusiform gyrus; Hi, hippocampus; ITG, inferior temporal gyrus; MTG, middle temporal gyrus; PHG, parahippocampal gyrus; S, subiculum; STG, superior temporal gyrus; TTG, transverse temporal gyrus. (*A,* Adapted from Braak H, Braak E: Neuropathological stages of Alzheimer's disease, in DeLeon MJ [ed]: An Atlas of Alzheimer's Disease. London: Parthenon Publishing Group, 1991. *B,* Adapted from Assheur J, Mai JK, Paxinos G: Atlas of the Human Brain. San Diego, CA: Academic Press, 1998.) (See Color Plate 1)

95%. In a subsequent report, Jobst and colleagues (1994) demonstrated that the rate of atrophy as measured by the minimum width of the medial temporal lobe was accelerated in 61 AD patients (20 confirmed pathologically), with rates in the AD group of 15% compared to 1.5% per year in the control group.

DeLeon and colleagues (1993) used a visual rating scale based on the quantity of cerebrospinal fluid (CSF) in the parahippocampal regions on temporally oriented CT scans to address the value of CT scanning in predicting conversion of MCI to AD. They assessed the scans of 54 controls and 32 elderly subjects with MCI and followed them clinically for 4 years; 29% progressed to a diagnosis of AD, which was predicted by the medial temporal lobe measure with 91% specificity and 89% sensitivity. Thus, both CT-based linear measures and visual ratings of medial temporal lobe atrophy, in cross-sectional and longitudinal studies, appeared helpful in distinguishing controls from incipient AD.

MRI Cross-sectional Studies

Initial Studies

Early MRI reports confirmed the CT data demonstrating ventricular enlargement and general cortical atrophy; however, MRI technology enabled the medial temporal lobe to be assessed more thoroughly than

was possible with CT imaging, as shown in Figure 4-2. The early MRI studies used manually based volumetric analysis (Kesslak et al., 1991; Killiany et al., 1993; Ikeda et al., 1994) and visual rating scales (Scheltens et al., 1992; O'Brien et al., 1994) in small groups of AD patients with well-established AD (mean minimental status examination [MMSE] <24) compared with controls. Several measures of the medial temporal lobe, typically including the hippocampus plus the amygdala (Killiany et al., 1993), total temporal lobe (Ikeda et al., 1994), parahippocampal gyrus, or entorhinal cortex (Kesslak et al., 1991) were used. In general, the hippocampus emerged as the best measure differentiating AD from controls, with around 85% of AD patients significantly below the control group range (Jack et al., 1992) and a 52% to 82% reduction of volume of the hippocampus, compared to controls (Kesslak et al., 1991; Killiany et al., 1993; Ikeda et al., 1994). More recent larger-scale studies have essentially confirmed these observations (Jack et al., 1997).

Although hippocampal measures are clearly best at distinguishing AD from the control groups and depressed elderly patients (O'Brien et al., 1994), several caveats should be made. First, the overlap between groups is such that a volume measure has little individual predictive value, as illustrated in Figure 4-3. Second, the patient groups studied were well advanced at the

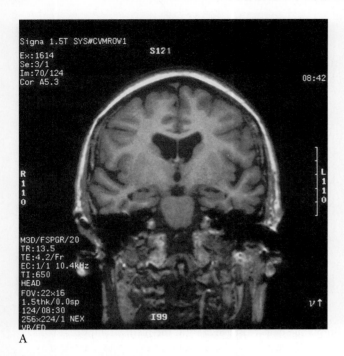
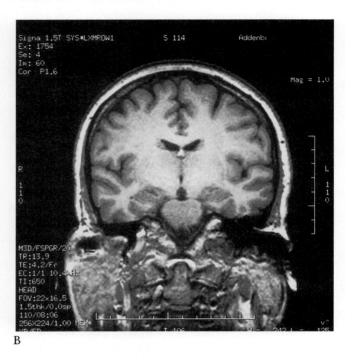

FIGURE 4-2. Cross-sectional T1-weighted MR image demonstrates hippocampal atrophy in Alzheimer's disease (A) compared with age-matched control (B).

time of scanning so there was little diagnostic uncertainty regarding the diagnosis of dementia. Third, there has been little attempt to separate AD from other dementing disorders. Finally, patient groups in all studies have been carefully selected to screen out comorbidity such as vascular disease and head injury, so results from these studies cannot be generalized to the community population.

Imaging in Incipient Dementia: Hippocampal Measures

More recent studies have addressed these problems by including patients in the earliest stages of disease with MCI (Convit et al., 1997; DeLeon et al., 1997b; DeToledo-Morrell et al., 1997; Jack et al., 1999; Convit et al., 2000; Xu et al., 2000). The problems with positive prediction of a diagnosis of AD are amplified in this group. Although the hippocampi are smaller in the MCI than the control groups, by about 14% (Convit et al., 1997), the discrimination of the controls and MCI groups is hampered by overlap between the groups. For example, in the study by DeLeon and colleagues (1997a), based on visual rating of MRIs, involving 405 subjects, hippocampal atrophy was present in 29% of the controls, 78% of the MCI group, and 96% of the severe AD group. In a study using more sensitive volumetric measures (Jack et al., 1999), 80 MCI patients were followed up for an average of 3 years; of the patients who converted from MCI to AD, 92.5% had hippocampal atrophy, but of subjects with hippocampal atrophy (between 0 and −2.5 w scores), only 40% converted to AD, giving a relative risk of 0.70 (Fig. 4-4).

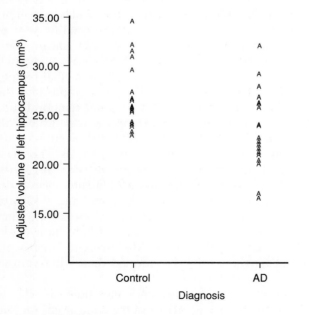

FIGURE 4-3. Scatter plot demonstrates overlap of hippocampal volumes between controls and AD subjects (Adapted from Galton C, Patterson K, Graham K, et al: Differing patterns of temporal atrophy in Alzheimer's disease and semantic dementia. Neurology 57:216–225, 2001b.)

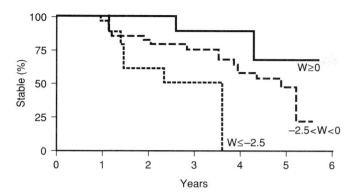

FIGURE 4-4. Kaplan-Meier curves of progression to AD from MCI prediction by hippocampal volume. (Reproduced with permission from Jack CR, Petersen RC, Xu YC, et al: Prediction of AD with MRI-based hippocampal volume in mild cognitive impairment. Neurology 52:1397–1403, 1999.)

Entorhinal Cortex Measurements

Other studies have concentrated on volumetric measurements of the entorhinal cortex, which is thought to be involved at the earliest stages of AD pathology (Juottonen et al., 1998a; Bobinski et al., 1999; DeToledo-Morrell et al., 2000b). Bobinski and colleagues (1999) demonstrated that a measure of the entorhinal cortex was better than hippocampal volume in distinguishing patients with AD from controls, although the numbers in this study were small. Not all studies have, however, concurred with this result (Juottonen et al., 1999; Xu et al., 2000). Other investigators have argued that the hippocampal and entorhinal volume measures are equivalently useful in the early discrimination of AD. In the cross-sectional study of Xu and colleagues (2000), an MCI group was included, and there was a relatively low sensitivity/specificity (60%/80%, respectively) in distinguishing controls from MCI. A follow-up study of an MCI group found that entorhinal volume was better than hippocampal volume in predicting decline to AD with a sensitivity of 83% and specificity of 72% (DeToledo-Morrell et al., 2000a).

Imaging and Genetic Markers

In attempts to improve the diagnostic sensitivity of MR volumetrics, some studies have stratified AD subjects by apolipoprotein E4 allele and demonstrated more severe entorhinal, hippocampal, and amygdala atrophy in the patients homozygous for the e4 allele (Lehtovirta et al., 1996; Juottonen et al., 1998b).

In summary, there is good evidence that the medial temporal lobe can be measured accurately with MRI volumetric techniques and that AD is associated with medial temporal lobe atrophy in the earliest stages of the disease. These findings support the pathologic literature, which point to initial involvement of the medial temporal lobe in AD (Braak & Braak, 1999) and the neuropsychological work, which suggests that the first cognitive deficit in AD is impaired episodic memory. It is also clear that MRI volumetric analysis of the temporal lobe structures is limited in clinical application. The measures are extremely time-consuming and the positive predictive value is relatively low. Measurement of the entorhinal cortex might have greater discriminating power, but the results, to date, are conflicting.

MRI Longitudinal Studies

As outlined above, the results of studies using CT measures have suggested that the rate of atrophy may be able to separate the groups with greater sensitivity than the actual volume of the structure (Jobst et al., 1994). This finding has been explored further with more sensitive MRI techniques in AD subjects (Fox et al., 1996a) and those at high risk of conversion to AD (Fox et al., 1996b). There remains, however, the problem that such methods are time-consuming, and there are limits to the minimal rate of atrophy that can be detected by volumetric assessment. Fox and colleagues have adopted a radical approach to the problem by developing a coregistration technique to subtract one image from another. Using this technique they have been able to quantify the whole brain atrophy over time in AD and at-risk subjects (Fox et al., 1996a, 1999). Patients with very early stage AD show a 10 times greater rate of brain volume loss compared to matched controls. Brain atrophy can also be detected several years before patients fulfill clinical criteria for a diagnosis of AD. Perhaps the most interesting result from this technique is that the atrophy in the earliest cases is not limited to medial temporal lobe structures but involves instead a global loss of brain substance. This finding supports the early imaging studies that demonstrated generalized brain atrophy, particularly expansion of the ventricular system. These data present an interesting challenge to current pathologic models of AD (Braak & Braak, 1999). One interpretation is that the initial transentorhinal stages of Braak and Braak (1999) represent a much earlier preclinical stage of AD. Supporting this view is evidence that the transentorhinal stage (Braak stage I and II) peaks, in population studies of accidental deaths, in the fourth decade, whereas the earliest clinical manifestations of AD relate to the limbic stages of pathology (III and IV) when the disease had already spread from the medial temporal lobe (Braak et al., 1998).

In conclusion, examining rates of change of atrophy is still the most promising, and technically demanding, way to distinguish early AD from normal elderly subjects. Two questions remain: How do rates of atrophy (or volumetric measures cross-sectionally) differentiate AD from other dementias, and is imaging better than neuropsychological assessment in the early diagnosis of AD?

NEUROIMAGING AND DIFFERENTIAL DIAGNOSIS OF ALZHEIMER DISEASE

Introduction

Compared to the large body of work comparing controls to AD and MCI, there has been a paucity of studies comparing AD patients with those with other neurodegenerative diseases. Some researchers have suggested that there is less medial temporal lobe atrophy in patients with dementia with Lewy bodies compared to AD based on volumetric analysis and rating scales (Hashimoto et al., 1998; Harvey et al., 1999). Laakso and colleagues (1996) compared hippocampal volumes in AD, vascular dementia, and Parkinson disease; in the AD group the mean volume (as a percentage of the control volume) was 68% on the right and 65% on the left, for vascular dementia the values were 86% and 75%, for Parkinson disease with dementia, 62% and 63%, and in Parkinson disease without dementia 74% and 75%. Thus, there is some tentative evidence that hippocampal atrophy is not specific to AD. MRI studies have also been undertaken in other dementias; for example, volumetric analyses demonstrate caudate atrophy in Huntington disease, which correlates with the CAG repeat (Rosas et al., 2001).

Frontotemporal Dementia

Frontotemporal dementia (FTD) is now preferred to the older term Pick disease to describe patients with focal frontal or temporal focal atrophy or both. There have been several nomenclatures to describe the differing clinical presentations, which reflect the sites of pathology. At least in the earliest stages of disease there are two main clinical syndromes: frontal variant FTD in which patients present with features of a frontal dementia, and the temporal variant (or semantic dementia) in which patients present with a form of progressive fluent aphasia. FTD is being increasingly recognized as a common cause of early onset dementia (for review of disease concepts, see Hodges & Miller, 2001).

Early reports of CT imaging findings in FTD all demonstrated frontal and temporal lobe atrophy (Cummings et al., 1981; Knopman et al., 1989). Several studies have now compared the patterns of lobar brain atrophy in groups of subjects with FTD and AD (Kitagaki et al., 1998; Fukui & Kertesz, 2000). Although the methodology differed in these reports, the major finding was of asymmetrical widespread general

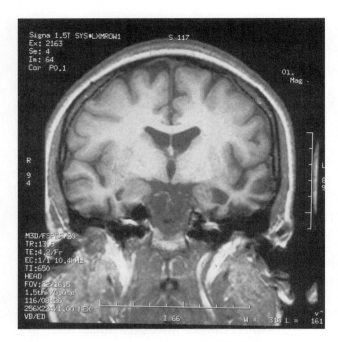

FIGURE 4-5. Cross-sectional T1-weighted MR image demonstrating asymmetrical hippocampal and temporal lobe atrophy in a patient with semantic dementia.

atrophy with more predominant frontal and temporal atrophy in FTD compared with the AD cases (Fig. 4-5).

Medial Temporal Lobe Atrophy in FTD

Several studies have compared the medial temporal lobe structures in FTD and AD, but excluded semantic dementia cases (Frisoni et al., 1996, 1999; Laasko et al., 2000). Using linear measures, Frisoni and colleagues (1996) found greater frontal atrophy in the FTD group compared to AD patients, but the medial temporal lobe structures were equivalently involved in FTD and AD. Frisoni and colleagues extended this work by showing that whereas the entorhinal cortex was equivalently atrophied in the AD and FTD groups, the hippocampi were less atrophied in FTD than AD (Frisoni et al., 1999), with an anterior predominance of atrophy in the FTD group (Laasko et al., 2000). Our recent study (Galton et al., 2001a) compared medial and lateral temporal lobe atrophy in 30 probable AD subjects and 13 frontal and 17 temporal variant (semantic dementia) FTD patients. The temporal lobe was assessed using a modification of the visual rating of Scheltens and colleagues (1992), which included the hippocampus, the parahippocampal gyrus, and other temporal lobe regions. The frontal FTD group was very similar to the AD group in terms of the pattern of temporal lobe atrophy; 50% of the AD group showed severe bilateral hippocampal atrophy versus 54% of the frontal variant FTD group. The temporal FTD (semantic dementia) group showed a distinct pattern with severe atrophy of the temporal pole and medial and inferolateral temporal lobe structures, which was worse on the left.

There are few quantitative imaging studies of semantic dementia patients. In a study of six patients with semantic dementia using voxel-based morphometry, an automated technique in which individual subjects' gray matter volumes are compared with a normalized template, the left temporal pole was the most significantly and consistently area affected, with additional involvement of the inferolateral temporal lobe on the left, right temporal pole, and ventromedial frontal lobe (Mummery et al., 2000). This study commented on the sparing of the hippocampus and parahippocampal structures, although the authors were cautious in their conclusions regarding the resolution of voxel-based morphometry to detect changes in small medial temporal lobe structures. Two recent studies have examined in detail specific temporal lobe regions using volumetric analysis in semantic dementia and AD patients (Chan et al., 2001; Galton et al., 2001b). Both studies found significant hippocampal and medial temporal lobe atrophy in both the semantic dementia and AD groups, especially on the left; additionally, the semantic dementia group had asymmetrical polar and inferolateral atrophy.

In summary, studies that have looked at the pattern of atrophy in FTD have consistently demonstrated involvement of the polar and inferolateral temporal lobe compared to AD. It appears that hippocampal atrophy is equally likely to occur in FTD and AD, although it is typically symmetrical in AD and left-sided in semantic dementia.

RELATIONSHIP OF IMAGING AND COGNITION IN NEURODEGENERATIVE DISEASE

Introduction

Despite the large number of studies identifying differences between AD and controls on structural imaging, few studies have attempted to correlate cognitive performance with cerebral atrophy. Although several studies (e.g., Stout et al., 1996; Fox et al., 1999b) have reported the expected relationship between measures of total brain atrophy and general neuropsychological measures, such as the MMSE (Folstein et al., 1975), there are inherent problems in attempting to further define these structure-function relationships. The main concerns are small sample sizes and a priori selection of limited brain regions, because correlational analysis is particularly susceptible to sample selection. For example, an association may be shown between a brain area (such as the hippocampus) and a measure of episodic memory, but the a priori selection of only one

brain region may overlook additional relationships between episodic memory and other brain areas (or total brain atrophy) that were not measured (Golomb et al., 1993). Moreover, several studies have used global nonspecific neuropsychological tests, which depend on many cognitive modalities (Stout et al., 1996; Fox et al., 1999b). Other issues regarding the validity of results include the mixing of samples (e.g., AD and normal controls) in the correlational analysis (Mizuno et al., 2000), and floor and ceiling effects on cognitive test performance may affect the observed relationship. Nevertheless, bearing these technical problems in mind, the investigation of brain-behavior relationships in the degenerating brain is of great interest and potentially complements functional imaging studies of cognition.

Episodic Memory

Alzheimer disease provides a useful experimental model to examine the anatomic regions that subserve episodic memory. Many studies have looked specifically at the association between medial temporal lobe atrophy and episodic memory in AD. These studies can be divided into (1) those in which there was a control brain region, such as the caudate nucleus (Deweer et al., 1995), frontal region (Laakso et al., 1995), whole brain volume (Mori et al., 1999), and regional gray matter (Fama et al., 1997), and (2) those that used medial temporal lobe measurements only (Soininen et al., 1994; Mori et al., 1997; Kohler et al., 1998; DeToledo-Morrell et al., 2000a; Mizuno et al., 2000).

Reviewing the studies where control regions were used, the hippocampal volume correlated with immediate and delayed verbal and visual memory scores (Deweer et al., 1995; Laasko et al., 1995; Fama et al., 1997), whereas memory scores for emotional events correlated better with amygdala volumes than with hippocampal volumes (Mori et al., 1999). Deweer and colleagues (1995) investigated the structure-function relationship in 18 AD subjects, measuring the hippocampal formation, amygdala, and caudate nucleus. The neuropsychological examination was thorough, including the MMSE, Dementia Rating Scale (DRS; Mattis, 1988), verbal and visual episodic memory tasks, and tests of executive functions, language, and praxis. All memory measures (except long-term recall on the California Verbal Learning Task) and the MMSE correlated with the hippocampus specifically. Fama and colleagues (1997) correlated the five subscales of the DRS with measurements of hippocampal volume, regional cortical gray matter, and lateral ventricles in 50 AD subjects. The memory subtest correlated specifically with the size of the left and right hippocampus and not with other cerebral regions, whereas the attention subtest correlated with the right anterior and bilateral posterior superior temporal regions and the size of the lateral ventricles. Perseveration and initiation were the only nonmemory subtests to correlate with the hippocampus. Using multiple regression analyses, hippocampal volume predicted the memory scale score from the DRS (Fama et al., 1997). The relationship of the hippocampus to episodic memory scales was supported further by a study of 32 patients with mild AD (Laasko et al., 1995). The MMSE score and immediate and delayed story recall all correlated with the hippocampal measures, whereas the executive tasks correlated with the frontal lobe measures specifically (Laasko et al., 1995). By contrast, several studies have not found a relationship between the hippocampus and episodic memory (Mori et al., 1997; Mizuno et al., 2000). Mori and associates (1997) found that delayed recall of verbal material correlated with the left subiculum and both amygdala in very mild AD subjects and controls, whereas Mizuno and colleagues (2000) found a correlation between visual and verbal delayed recall and the amygdala rather than the hippocampus. It should be noted that these studies did not have independent control brain areas outside the medial temporal lobe.

Examining the medial temporal lobe structure further, DeToledo-Morrell and colleagues (2000a) found a laterality effect with the left hippocampus correlating with verbal recall and the right hippocampus with spatial recall. Several studies have looked at the cognitive correlates of parahippocampal gyrus atrophy (Mori et al., 1997; Kohler et al., 1998; DeToledo-Morrell et al., 2000a; Mizuno et al., 2000), but the results have also been contradictory. Kohler and colleagues (1998) found that delayed recall of visual material correlated with the parahippocampal gyrus and verbal delayed recall with the hippocampus, whereas other studies showed no relationship between the parahippocampal gyrus and performance on episodic memory tests (Mori et al., 1997; DeToledo-Morrell et al., 2000a; Mizuno et al., 2000).

There are a couple of possible explanations for these contradictory findings. First, pathologic involvement of other nontemporal lobe structures, such as the basal forebrain cholinergic system or posterior cingulated, may be critical for the genesis of episodic memory deficits found in AD. Second, there is considerable heterogeneity in the cognitive deficits found in AD (Hodges & Patterson, 1995).

Semantic Memory

Patients with FTD syndromes may prove a more informative testing ground for exploring brain structure-function relationships. In a first attempt to address these issues, we recently correlated the cognitive profiles in semantic dementia and AD subjects with the volumes of temporal lobe subregions (Galton et al., 2001b). Performance on tests of semantic memory association (the pyramids and palm trees test) was strongly correlated with the size of the left fusiform gyrus, whereas tasks requiring name production also correlated with the inferior and middle temporal gyri, and the left temporal pole, in both the AD and semantic dementia subjects. These findings highlight the role of the left fusiform region in semantic processing. Episodic memory measures, however, with the exception of recognition memory for faces, did not correlate with any of the temporal measures in either the AD or semantic dementia groups.

In summary, a number of rigorous structural MRI studies have supported pathologic data in showing a relationship between the medial temporal lobe and episodic memory. The finer discrimination of verbal and visual recall, and recognition in episodic memory have not been clearly addressed. The structural basis of semantic memory has been addressed in our one study, which suggested a pivotal role of the left fusiform gyrus in semantic memory.

CONCLUSIONS

Structural MR imaging is an excellent tool to examine brain structures in neurodegenerative disease. In the early and differential diagnosis of AD, volumetric studies of the medial temporal lobe demonstrate, unfortunately, that the techniques are not sufficiently discriminating to be of clinical use at the present. New developments in technology may, in time, provide the ability to distinguish between differing dementias and normal aging.

There is also considerable potential for investigating the structure-function relationships in the diseased brain, which could complement functional imaging studies. The detailed analysis of patients with semantic dementia and other forms of FTD is likely to be the most informative.

■ KEY POINTS

☐ Medial temporal lobe atrophy can be accurately measured with MRI volumetry.

☐ AD is associated with medial temporal lobe atrophy in the very earliest stages of disease. However, these measurements are currently of limited clinical application.

☐ Longitudinal measures of rates of atrophy are promising but time-consuming at present.

☐ Medial temporal lobe atrophy is not specific for AD, and the differing patterns of brain atrophy in other neurodegenerative disorders have only recently started to be elucidated.

☐ MRI studies have supported the pathologic data in suggesting a relationship between the medial temporal lobe and episodic memory. This area of research may provide further insights into the anatomic basis of memory.

KEY READINGS

Braak H, Braak E: Neuropathological stages of Alzheimer's disease, in DeLeon MJ (ed): An Atlas of Alzheimer's Disease. London: The Parthenon Publishing Group, 1999, pp. 57–74.

Hodges JR, Miller B: The classification, genetics and neuropathology of frontotemporal dementia. Introduction to the special topic papers: Part I. Neurocase 7:31–35, 2001.

Jack CR, Petersen RC, Xu YC, et al: Prediction of AD with MRI-based hippocampal volume in mild cognitive impairment. Neurology 52:1397–1403, 1999.

REFERENCES

Bobinski M, DeLeon M, Convit A, et al: MRI of entorhinal cortex in mild Alzheimer's disease. Lancet 353:38–39, 1999.

Bobinski M, DeLeon MJD, Wegiel J, et al: The histological validation of post mortem magnetic resonance imaging-determined hippocampal volume in Alzheimer's disease. Neuroscience 95:721–725, 2000.

Braak H, Braak E: Neuropathological staging of Alzheimer-related changes. Acta Neuropathol (Berlin) 82:239–259, 1991.

Braak H, Braak E: Neuropathological stages of Alzheimer's disease, in DeLeon MJ (ed): An Atlas of Alzheimer's Disease. London: Parthenon Publishing Group, 1999, pp. 57–74.

Braak H, Braak E, Bohl J, et al: Evolution of Alzheimer's disease related cortical lesions, in Gertz HJ, Arendt T (eds): Alzheimer's Disease—From Basic Research to Clinical Applications. Vienna: Springer-Verlag, 1998, pp. 97–106.

Chan D, Fox NC, Scahill RI, et al: Patterns of temporal lobe atrophy in semantic dementia and Alzheimer's disease. Ann Neurol 49:433–442, 2001.

Cummings JL, Duchen LW: Kluver-Bucy syndrome in Pick disease: Clinical and pathological correlations. Neurology 31:1415–1422, 1981.

Convit A, deAsis J, DeLeon MJ, et al: Atrophy of the medial occipitotemporal, inferior, and middle temporal gyri in nondemented elderly predict decline to Alzheimer's disease. Neurobiol Aging 21:19–26, 2000.

Convit A, DeLeon M, Tarshish C, et al: Specific hippocampal volume reductions in individuals at risk for Alzheimer's disease. Neurobiol Aging 18:131–138, 1997.

Davis PC, Gearing M, Gray L, et al: The CERAD experience, part VIII: Neuroimaging-neuropathology correlates of temporal lobe changes in Alzheimer's disease. Neurology 45:178–179, 1995.

DeCarli C, Kaye JA, Horwitz B, et al: Critical analysis of the use of computer assisted transverse axial tomography to study human brain in aging and dementia of the Alzheimer type. Neurology 40:872–883, 1990.

DeLeon M, Convit A, DeSanti S, et al: Contribution of structural neuroimaging to the early diagnosis of Alzheimer's disease. Int Psychogeriatr 9:183–190, 1997a.

DeLeon M, George A, Golomb J, et al: Frequency of hippocampal formation atrophy in normal aging and Alzheimer's disease. Neurobiol Aging 18:1–11, 1997b.

DeLeon J, Golomb J, George A, et al: The radiologic prediction of Alzheimer's disease: The atrophic hippocampal formation. AJNR Am J Neuroradiol 14:897–906, 1993.

DeToledo-Morrell L, Dickerson B, Sullivan MP, et al: Hemispheric differences in hippocampal volume predict verbal and spatial memory performance in patients with Alzheimer's disease. Hippocampus 10:136–142, 2000a.

DeToledo-Morrell L, Goncharova I, Dickerson B, et al: From healthy aging to early Alzheimer's disease: In vivo detection of entorhinal cortex atrophy. Ann N Y Acad Sci 91:240–254, 2000b.

DeToledo-Morrell L, Sullivan MP, Morrell F, et al: Alzheimer's disease: In vivo detection of differential vulnerability of brain regions. Neurobiol Aging 18:463–468, 1997.

Deweer B, Lehericy S, Pillon B, et al: Memory disorders in probable Alzheimer's disease: The role of hippocampal atrophy as shown with MRI. J Neurol Neurosurg Psychiatry 58:590–597, 1995.

Fama R, Sullivan E, Shear P, et al: Selective cortical and hippocampal volume correlates of Mattis Dementia Rating Scale in Alzheimer's disease. Arch Neurol 54:719–728, 1997.

Folstein MF, Folstein SE, McHugh PR: "Mini-mental state": A practical method for grading the cognitive state of patients for the clinician. J Psychiatr Res 12:189–198, 1975.

Fox NC, Freeborough PA, Rossor MN: Visualization and quantification of rates of atrophy in Alzheimer's disease. Lancet 348:94–97, 1996a.

Fox NC, Warrington E, Freeborough P, et al: Presymptomatic hippocampal atrophy in Alzheimer's disease: A longitudinal study. Brain 119:2001–2007, 1996b.

Fox NC, Scahill RI, Crum WR, et al: Correlation between rates of brain atrophy and cognitive decline in Alzheimer's disease. Neurology 52:1687–1689, 1999a.

Fox NC, Warrington EK, Rossor MN: Serial magnetic resonance imaging of cerebral atrophy in preclinical Alzheimer's disease [letter]. Lancet 353:2125, 1999b.

Frisoni GB, Beltramello A, Geroldi C, et al: Brain atrophy in frontotemporal dementia. J Neurol Neurosurg Psychiatry 61:157–165, 1996.

Frisoni GB, Laakso MP, Beltramello A, et al: Hippocampal and entorhinal cortex atrophy in frontotemporal dementia and Alzheimer's disease. Neurology 52:91–100, 1999.

Fukui T, Kertesz A: Volumetric study of lobar atrophy in Pick complex and Alzheimer's disease. J Neurol Sci 174:111–121, 2000.

Galton CJ, Gomez-Anson B, Antoun N, et al: The temporal lobe rating scale: Application to Alzheimer's disease and frontotemporal dementia. J Neurol Neurosurg Psychiatry 70:165–173, 2001a.

Galton CJ, Patterson K, Graham K, et al: Differing patterns of temporal atrophy in Alzheimer's disease and semantic dementia. Neurology 57:216–225, 2001b.

Golomb J, Leon MD., Kluger A, et al: Hippocampal atrophy in normal aging: An association with recent memory impairment. Arch Neurol 50:967–973, 1993.

Harvey GT, Hughes J, McKeith IG, et al: Magnetic resonance imaging differences between dementia with Lewy bodies and Alzheimer's disease: A pilot study. Psychol Med 29:181–187, 1999.

Hashimoto M, Kitagaki H, Imamura T, et al: Medial temporal and whole-brain atrophy in dementia with Lewy bodies. Neurology 51:357–362, 1998.

Hodges JR, Miller B: The classification, genetics and neuropathology of frontotemporal dementia. Introduction to the special topic papers: Part I. Neurocase 7:31–35, 2001.

Hodges JR, Patterson K: Is semantic memory consistently impaired early in the course of Alzheimer's disease? Neuroanatomical and diagnostic implications. Neuropsychologia 33:441–459, 1995.

Ikeda M, Tanabe H, Nakagawa Y, et al: MRI-based quantitative assessment of the hippocampal region in very mild to moderate Alzheimer's disease. Neuroradiology 36:7–10, 1994.

Jack C, Petersen R, Xu YC, et al: Medial temporal atrophy on MRI in normal aging and very mild Alzheimer's disease. Neurology 49:786–794, 1997.

Jack CR, Petersen RC, O'Brien PC, et al: MR-based hippocampal volumetry in the diagnosis of Alzheimer's disease. Neurology 42:183–188, 1992.

Jack CR, Petersen RC, Xu YC, et al: Prediction of AD with MRI-based hippocampal volume in mild cognitive impairment. Neurology 52:1397–1403, 1999.

Jobst K, Smith A, Szatmar, M, et al: Detection in life of confirmed Alzheimer's disease using a simple measurement of medial temporal lobe atrophy by computer tomography. Lancet 340:1179–1183, 1992.

Jobst K, Smith A, Szatmari M, et al: Rapidly progressing atrophy of medial temporal lobe in Alzheimer's disease. Lancet 343:829–830, 1994.

Juottonen K, Laakso M, Insausti R, et al: Volumes of the entorhinal and perirhinal cortices in Alzheimer's disease. Neurobiol Aging 19:15–22, 1998a.

Juottonen K, Laakso MP, Partanen K, et al: Comparative MR analysis of the entorhinal cortex and hippocampus in diagnosing Alzheimer disease. Am J Neuroradiol 20:139–144, 1999.

Juottonen K, Lehtovirta M, Helisalmi S, et al: Major decrease in the volume of the entorhinal cortex in patients with Alzheimer's disease carrying the apolipoprotein E e4 allele. J Neurol Neurosurg Psychiatry 65:322–327, 1998b.

Kesslak JP, Nalcioglu O, Cotman CW: Quantification of magnetic resonance scans for hippocampal and parahippocampal atrophy in Alzheimer's disease. Neurology 41:51–54, 1991.

Killiany R, Moss MB, Albert MS, et al: Temporal lobe regions on magnetic resonance imaging identify patients with early Alzheimer's disease. Arch Neurol 50:949–954, 1993.

Kitagaki H, Mori E, Yamaji S, et al: Frontotemporal dementia and Alzheimer's disease: Evaluation of cortical atrophy with automated hemisphere surface display generated with MR images. Radiology 208:431–439, 1998.

Knopman DS, Christensen KJ, Schut LJ, et al: The spectrum of imaging and neuropsychological findings in Pick's disease. Neurology 39:362–368, 1989.

Kohler S, Black S, Sinden M, et al: Memory impairments associated with hippocampal versus parahippocampal-gyrus atrophy: An MR volumetry study in Alzheimer's disease. Neuropsychologia 36:901–914, 1998.

Laasko M, Frisoni G, Kononen M, et al: Hippocampus and entorhinal cortex in frontotemporal dementia and Alzheimer's disease: A morphometric MRI study. Biol Psychiatry 47:1056–1063, 2000.

Laakso M, Partanen K, Riekkinen P, et al: Hippocampal volumes in Alzheimer's disease, Parkinson's disease with and without dementia, and in vascular dementia. Neurology 46:678–681, 1996.

Laakso MP, Soininen H, Partanen K, et al: Volumes of hippocampus, amgydala and frontal lobes in the MRI-based diagnosis of early Alzheimer's disease: Correlation with memory functions. J Neural Transm 9:73–86, 1995.

Lehtovirta M, Soininen H, Laasko MP, et al: SPECT and MRI analysis in Alzheimer's disease: Relation to apolipoprotein E epsilon4 allele. J Neurol Neurosurg Pyschiatry 60:644–649, 1996.

Mattis S: Dementia Rating Scale. Windsor, Ontario: NFER Nelson, 1998.

Mizuno K, Wakai M, Takeda A, et al: Medial temporal atrophy and memory impairment in early stage of Alzheimer's disease: A MRI volumetric and memory assessment study. J Neurol Sci 173:18–24, 2000.

Mori E, Ikeda M, Hirono N, et al: Amygdalar volume and emotional memory in Alzheimer's disease. Am J Psychiatry 156:216–222, 1999.

Mori E, Yoneda Y, Yamashita H, et al: Medial temporal structures relate to memory impairment in Alzheimer's disease: An MRI volumetric study. J Neurol Neurosurg Psychiatry 63:214–221, 1997.

Mummery CJ, Patterson K, Price CJ, et al: A voxel based morphometry study of semantic dementia: The relation of temporal lobe atrophy to cognitive deficit. Ann Neurol 47:36–45, 2000.

Nagy Z, Jobst KA, Esiri MM, et al: Hippocampal pathology reflects memory deficit and brain imaging measures in Alzheimer's disease: Clinicopathological correlations using three sets of pathological diagnostic criteria. Dementia 7:76–81, 1996.

O'Brien J, Desmond P, Ames D, et al: The differentiation of depression from dementia by temporal lobe magnetic resonance imaging. Psychol Med 24:633–640, 1994.

Petersen RC: Mild cognitive impairment: Clinical characterization and outcome. Arch Neurol 56:303–308, 1999.

Rosas HD, Goodman J, Chen YI, et al: Striatal volume loss in HD as measured by MRI and the influence of the CAG repeat. Neurology 57:1025–1028, 2001.

Scheltens P, Leys D, Barkhof F, et al: Atrophy of medial temporal lobes on MRI in "probable" Alzheimer's disease and normal aging: Diagnostic value and neuropsychological correlates. J Neurol Neurosurg Psychiatry 55:967–972, 1992.

Soininen HS, Partanen K, Pitkanen A, et al: Volumetric MRI analysis of the amygdala and the hippocampus in subjects with age-associated memory impairment: Correlation to visual and verbal memory. Neurology 44:1660–1668, 1994.

Stout JC, Jernigan TL, Archibald SL, et al: Association of dementia severity with cortical gray matter and abnormal white matter volumes in dementia of the Alzheimer type. Arch Neurol 53:742–749, 1996.

Sullivan EV, Cahn DA, Fama R, et al: Structural neuroimaging correlates of memory dysfunction in neurodegenerative disease, in Troster AI (ed.): Memory in Neurodegenerative Disease: Biological, Cognitive, and Clinical Perspectives. Cambridge, UK: Cambridge University Press, 1998, pp. 100–127.

Xu Y, Jack CR, O'Brien PC, et al: Usefulness of MRI measures of entorhinal cortex versus hippocampus in AD. Neurology 54:1760–1767, 2000.

Structural Brain Imaging in Neurodevelopmental Disorders

Walter E. Kaufmann

Lidia M. Nagae-Poetscher

Diffusion-weighted imaging (DWI)

Image analysis

Magnetic resonance imaging (MRI)

Magnetic resonance spectroscopy (MRS)

Morphometry

The structural evaluation of the developing brain has been a subject of scientific interest for a long time. Fundamental questions about human nature, behavior, and cognition are linked to the study of the extraordinary morphologic process that leads to the complex structure of the adult human brain. Recent advances in developmental neurobiology and genetics, including the introduction of transgenic animals technology, have further increased the relevance of examining changes in brain structure during development. However, it is the medical field, with the incorporation of high-resolution imaging techniques, that has been one of the most important driving forces behind the renewed interest in the macroscopic anatomy of the normal and abnormal developing brain.

As in the case of adult neurologic and psychiatric disorders, the introduction of quantitative neuroimaging to the study of neurodevelopmental disorders was initially carried out by investigators in the field of child psychiatry. These early studies focused on conditions such as attention deficit/hyperactivity disorder (ADHD), autism, and schizophrenia (Eliez & Reiss, 2000). Later, developmental disorders with a predominant neurologic component (e.g., Down syndrome) were examined by quantitative magnetic resonance imaging (MRI) methods (Jernigan et al., 1993; Reiss et al., 1993). The development of high-resolution MRI techniques in the 1990s had probably a greater impact on neurodevelopmental disorders than on adult neurodegenerative conditions because of their safety advantages (when compared with x-ray- and isotope-based neuroimaging methods). Increasing restrictions and regulations on children and control subject participation in biomedical research, in recent times, have only emphasized the unique role of quantitative MRI as an investigational tool in the pediatric field. An additional advantage of MRI, of particular relevance to pediatric populations, is the ability to perform longitudinal evaluations. Considering our limited knowledge about the structural changes occurring in the human brain during postnatal life (Kaufmann, 2002), longitudinal pediatric assessments not only provide critical *noninvasive* information about the dynamics of a particular developmental disorder, but also on the final stages of brain development (Zametkin & Liotta, 1997; Giedd et al., 1999a). Finally, pediatric neuroimaging has become the main approach for characterizing the macroscopic neuroanatomy/neuropathology of a number of developmental disorders (e.g., ADHD, fragile X syndrome). The latter is due to the fact that, in contrast to neurodegenerative conditions, limited postmortem material is available for even some relatively frequent developmental disorders (Kaufmann et al., 2002). Although structural MRI does not provide information about chemical composition or fine anatomy of the brain, novel MR-based techniques such as MR spectroscopy (MRS; Van Zijl & Barker, 1997) and diffusion-weighted imaging (DWI; Mori & Barker, 1999) contribute valuable insights into tissue organization.

Despite the aforementioned advantages, MRI studies of children have inherent complications. The first is the need for sedation or behavioral modification for young or cognitively or behaviorally impaired subjects. There is also an agreement among institutional review boards of biomedical research institutions that sedation of control subjects, including children, is unacceptable. In our experience, behavioral training strategies are quite effective in normal children older than 7 years. However, even under these circumstances slight motion artifacts may be appreciated. Although low-level motion has a relatively modest impact on delineating and measuring many brain structures, it can substantially affect more complex MR sequences (e.g., DWI). Consequently, normative MR data as well as that obtained from individuals with milder conditions (e.g., ADHD), considered in the same situation as controls with regard to sedation, have potential technical limitations. Advances in fast acquisition techniques may reduce these limitations in the not-so-distant future. For recent reviews on structural pediatric neuroimaging, we refer the reader to articles by Kates and colleagues (1997b), Eliez and Reiss (2000), Rivkin (2000), Paus and associates (2001), and Huppi and Inder (2001).

Structural pediatric neuroimaging has evolved from the early quantification of clinical imaging sequences (e.g., digitization of scans) to the current highly sophisticated acquisition and quantitative analysis methods. This chapter presents an overview of structural brain imaging in disorders affecting brain development from a strategic perspective. Following a brief review of MRI principles, we cover different approaches to measuring different brain tissue components and regions along with examples of their application to normal brain development and neurodevelopmental disorders. Quantifications of structure size include manual and automatic methods as well as area versus volume measurements. The chapter closes with a discussion of novel morphometric strategies (e.g., mechanical tensors) and MR analyses that evaluate tissue composition (i.e., T1 and T2 maps, DWI, and MRS), and their relationship with more strictly morphometric MR methods.

PRINCIPLES OF MAGNETIC RESONANCE IMAGING

Tissues are composed of molecules whose atomic nuclei may have an odd number of either protons or neutrons or both (Anderson & Gore, 1997; Inder & Huppi, 2000). These odd-numbered nucleons have magnetic and angular momenta, which can be influenced by a magnetic field. The angular momentum or spin of these nuclei makes them behave as *de facto* magnetic dipoles. The hydrogen nuclei are the most abundant among these magnetic-susceptible nuclei of use in MRI, with their main sources being body water and fat.

For structural and functional MRI applications, individuals are exposed first to a strong static magnetic field, typically 1.5 T (15,000 G), although magnets of larger strength are becoming available for research purposes. This process aligns the spins along the direction of the field. A second step is spin excitation by radiofrequency (RF) pulses, which are selected on the bases of the target nuclei and magnetic field, and that changes and further realigns the position of the spins. The recording of this process (i.e., resonance), specifically the "relaxation" of the spins to their original axes/positions, by an RF coil appropriately located, generates information about the structure and composition of the examined tissues. MR images reflect these diverse tissue properties, including the density of proton or hydrogen nuclei (i.e., water content), the content of other atoms and molecules (e.g., iron, lipids), and the overall tissue organization (e.g., axon bundle packing). Besides proton density, two relaxation times that are influenced by the other aforementioned factors are used: T1 that represents the spins realignment in the longitudinal plane (recovery of longitudinal magnetization) and T2 that reflects transverse relaxation and the influence of inhomogeneities in the local tissue magnetic fields (local rate of decay or de-phasing) (Inder & Huppi, 2000; Paus et al., 2001). Figure 5-1, from the review by Paus

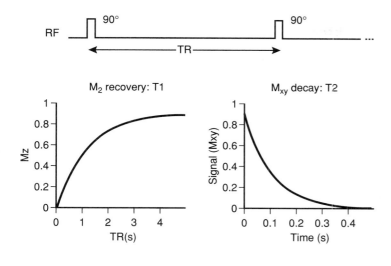

FIGURE 5-1. Illustration of longitudinal relaxation time (T1) and transverse relaxation time (T2). Radiofrequency (RF) excitations are applied with a repetition time (TR) (*top*) with each excitation producing a magnetic resonance signal (Mxy) that exponentially decays with a time constant T2 (*bottom right*). Between excitations, the magnetization also exponentially returns to its equilibrium state, pointing along the direction of the main magnetic field, with a time constant T1 (*bottom left*). By manipulating the TR and TE (time delay after excitation before the signal is measured; *bottom right*), the relative contributions of T1 and T2 can be manipulated to produce T1- and T2-weighted images. If the effects of both T1 and T2 are minimized (long TR and short TE), the remaining contrast is simply the proton density weighted. (Reprinted from Paus T, Collins DL, Evans AC, et al: Maturation of white matter in the human brain: A review of magnetic resonance studies. Brain Res Bull 54:255–266, 2001, by permission of Elsevier Science B. V.)

and colleagues (2001), illustrates the processes of longitudinal relaxation time (T1) and transverse relaxation time (T2). Because for image acquisition, repeated measures of MR signal are needed, tissue contrast is obtained by differentially weighting T1 and T2 properties (repetition time [TR], time-to-echo [TE]) during these repeated measures. For instance, degree of tissue organization is inversely related to T1 time (and recovery). Similarly, more structured brain regions have faster de-phasing and, therefore, shorter T2. Consequently, on T1-weighted images, the highly organized (short T1) white matter appears bright, and on T2-weighted sequences, it is the gray matter (long T2) that shows bright signal.

In clinical practice and research, T1-weighted sequence images have been considered the prototypical anatomic images. The gray matter appears gray, the white matter looks white, and the cerebrospinal fluid (CSF), because of the long T1 of water, appears black. T2-weighted images, in which white matter is darker than both gray matter and CSF, are currently not being used as a primary morphometric sequence. However, they continue to be a choice for diagnostic purposes. If T1- and T2-dependent effects are reduced, the image contrast is mainly proton density–weighted; this sequence is frequently used in combination with T2-weighted images for delineating lesions (Ito et al., 1994). Inversion recovery sequences are acquisitions that allow a combination of T1- or T2-weighting, with resulting advantages in terms of delineating gray and white matter. This is possible because during the complex process of measuring signal recovery, certain tissue compartment signals (e.g., CSF) can be suppressed depending on the time of inversion. Clinically,

inversion recovery sequences such as fluid-attenuated inversion recovery (FLAIR) have been incorporated into the diagnostic repertoire because of their high sensitivity for detecting focal pathologic processes (Yamanouchi et al., 1995).

The relationship between paramagnetic molecules, such as deoxyhemoglobin, and T2 signal is discussed in the context of functional MRI in Chapter 7.

The most widely currently used sequence for high-resolution anatomic studies is the T1-weighted three-dimensional volumetric RF spoiled gradient-echo (SPGR), which also receives other terms depending on the MR scanner manufacturer. SPGR has progressively replaced other T2 or lower resolution sequences that were initially applied for structural analyses. In addition to being a three-dimensional type of acquisition that covers the entire structure, due to its T1-type of contrast, SPGR images provide an atlas-like view of the brain. Furthermore, SPGR and other higher-resolution sequences, with their relatively thin slices, allow more precise structural analyses. Despite these features, the gray-white matter delineation on SPGR is relatively poor. The latter particularly affects structures of small size, because of partial volume effects, or complex composition. Some examples include the thalamus, the basal ganglia, and the mesial temporal structures. The search for better-contrasted high-spatial resolution sequences (Magnotta et al., 2000; Song et al., 2000) has led to magnetization-prepared rapid gradient-echo (MP-RAGE), an inversion recovery sequence, which possesses both high anatomic resolution and high contrast (Insausti et al., 1998; Deichmann et al., 2000). In the case of pediatric neuroimaging, achieving fast acquisition (<10 minutes) of high-contrast volumetric

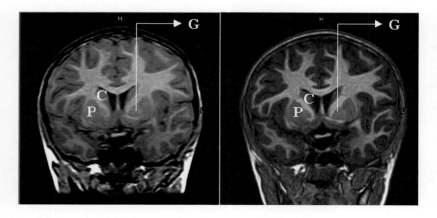

FIGURE 5-2. Volumetric sequences applied to a 6-year-old boy, who was prenatally exposed to drugs of abuse. The image on the right (*B*) shows a three-dimensional Inversion Recovery (IR) fast gradient-echo sequence acquired in the coronal plane, also known as MP-RAGE. Note the better delineation of the basal ganglia, particularly of the globus pallidus (G; dorsal to the anterior commissure), when compared with (*A*) a conventional SPGR sequence depicting the same level. C, caudate; G, globus pallidus; P, putamen. (Images courtesy of Xavier Golay, PhD, F. M. Kirby Research Center for Functional Brain Imaging, and Margaret Pulsifer, PhD, and Harolyn Belcher, MD, Johns Hopkins University School of Medicine and Kennedy Krieger Institute, Baltimore, MD.)

sequences has represented a tremendous advance that is allowing more accurate measurements in many developmental conditions. Other recently published inversion recovery sequences include cortex-attenuated inversion recovery (CAIR; Magnotta et al., 2000). Figure 5-2 depicts a comparison between SPGR and an inversion recovery sequence, currently under development at our imaging center. Table 5-1 summarizes the most frequently used structural MRI sequences, including their research and clinical applications.

Finally, the recent advances in MRI acquisition can only be interpreted in the context of parallel progress in image data analysis. These more precise methods have also been possible because of advances in computer hardware and software (Barta et al., 1997; Giedd et al., 1999a). Implementation of thin-slice, gapless, volumetric sequences has been conducted in conjunction with the application of protocols for higher-resolution manual delineation of brain structures (Crespo-Facorro et al., 1999, 2000). Moreover, better anatomic resolution and identification of anatomic landmarks has allowed the development of more precise automatic and semiautomatic measurement techniques (Andreasen et al., 1996; Kates et al., 1999, 2001). The following sections review different processes and strategies for in vivo measurement of brain structures, with emphasis on pediatric populations. A review of morphometry of the aged brain, with emphasis on dementias, is provided in Chapter 4. In general terms, the brain can be divided into its main tissue constituents (tissue segmentation) or into specific regions (region parcellation). The term segmentation is also used for referring to partitioning the brain into discrete entities.

Tissue Segmentation

To carry out quantitative analyses following acquisition by volumetric sequences, MRIs are processed electroni-

cally. This procedure includes importation of the raw images from the scanner into appropriate computer programs, including configuration into specific formats compatible with the software; correction of shading, and other artifacts, due to signal intensity inhomogeneity between slices; removal of nonbrain material, by typically semiautomatic methods; and conversion of the stacks of images into cubic volumetric units (i.e., voxel) datasets. Because of their three-dimensional nature, these sets of images can be visualized and analyzed in any one, or a combination of the three, orthogonal planes. They can also be reoriented and positioned according to landmarks, a process that is essential for data normalization across subjects.

Differences in signal intensity among discrete brain regions, which reflect their distinct tissue composition, cannot only be used to better delineate or separate structures but also for tissue comparisons between groups of subjects. The process of segmentation assigns each voxel to a tissue class, namely gray matter, white matter, and CSF. As expected, segmentation strongly depends on image contrast and spatial resolution. For instance, the tissue composition of large voxels is usually mixed and, therefore, not quite informative. Although segmentation is commonly performed on the volumetric sequences mentioned in the preceding section, T2-weighted sequences can also be segmented. The latter sequences are particularly useful for quantifying lesions (e.g., unidentified bright objects in neurofibromatosis type 1 [NF-1]), which are better distinguished on these types of sequences (Moore et al., 2000). Tissue classification can be done either manually or automated by two different approaches: categorical and probabilistic. In the former approach, each voxel is assigned according to its range of signal intensity to mutually exclusive tissue categories. It is typically done by establishing signal intensity/scale thresholds for tissue classification. Although this method gives origin

TABLE 5-1. Frequently Used Magnetic Resonance Imaging Sequences

Imaging sequence	Technique	Visualization	Applications
T1	Short TR (500–600 ms), short TE (≤20 ms)	Gray matter is gray; white matter is white; CSF is black	General anatomy; evaluation of myelination in the first 6–8 mo of life; detection of paramagnetic contents (bright)
T2	SE: long TR (3000 ms), long TE (120 ms) Other techniques as fast spin-echo and gradient-echo are also used.	White matter is darker than gray matter; CSF is bright	Lesion detection; myelination after 6–8 mo of life; ferromagnetic content (dark)
Proton density	Long TR (3000 ms), intermediate TE (60 ms) It reflects the density of protons in the tissue.	White matter is darker than gray matter; CSF is darker than on T2	Lesion detection; in most centers, it has been substituted by FLAIR
FLAIR	T2-weighted inversion-recovery sequence, attenuating CSF (fluid) signal	White matter is darker than gray matter; CSF is black	More conspicuous lesion detection than with T2; advantageous also in depicting lesions close to CSF spaces
SPGR	T1-weighted inversion recovery; use of gradient pulse to "spoil" transverse magnetization; fast 3-D acquisition with thin slices	As T1-weighted (see above); contrast is better between gray and white matter	Research/clinical volumetric studies; myelination; malformations; atrophy
MP-RAGE	T1-weighted inversion-recovery sequence followed by a 3-D RF-spoiled gradient-echo sequence with small flip angles	As T1-weighted (see above); highest (available) contrast between gray and white matter	Research volumetric studies; tissue segmentation analyses; other studies requiring high-resolution/contrast anatomic images
CAIR	Inversion-recovery sequence, attenuating cortical gray matter signal	Higher gray-white contrast to better delineate mixed tissues (e.g., thalamic nuclei)	Research: proposed for delineation of thalamic nuclei

CAIR, cortex-attenuated inversion recovery; CSF, cerebrospinal fluid; 3-D, three-dimensional; FLAIR, fluid-attenuated inversion recovery; MP-RAGE, magnetization prepared rapid gradient-echo; RF, radiofrequency; SE, spin-echo; SPGR, radiofrequency spoiled gradient-echo; TE, time-to-echo; TR, repetition time.

to datasets that are relatively easy to analyze, it does not recognize the fact that distinction between tissue classes at the histologic level is extremely difficult and that transitions between tissue types are continuous rather than abrupt. An example of this problem is the cortical gray-white matter junction, in which the border between these two compartments is in general imprecise. For these reasons, probabilistic or "fuzzy" segmentation methods permit the evaluation of the signal intensity of a given voxel as belonging to "pure" or "mixed" tissue classes, as well as in the context of its neighborhood (Fig. 5-3). In this way, a voxel can be defined in terms of percentages of tissue classes or type of adjacent voxels. Regions that, at present, are not systematically evaluated by high-resolution protocols (e.g., globus pallidus) may, in the future, be evaluated in a more precise manner by the incorporation of these probabilistic tissue segmentation methods. For more details about data acquisition and initial processing, including tissue segmentation, see Kaplan and colleagues (1997), Kates and colleagues (1999), and Figure 5-3.

Principles of Brain Parcellation

The process by which brain MR images are divided into discrete regions is usually termed tissue parcellation. Because quantification of the size of brain regions has been one of the primary objectives of neuroimaging, brain parcellation has evolved dramatically in the course of the last decade. Two different strategies, with

distinct advantages and disadvantages, have been continuously applied in MRI morphometric protocols. Manual delineation of "regions of interest" (ROIs) dates back to the tracing of brain regions on films of MRI scans, following through the period of evaluation of "incomplete" or noncontiguous electronic datasets, to the current volumetric acquisition era. Currently, it is the method of choice for precise measurements of structures, particularly using high-resolution scans. In this regard, the manual outlining of an ROI allows its complete inclusion in any evaluation; in this way, individual variations or unusual anatomic features will be taken into account in the process and will be reflected in the measurements. A major disadvantage of manual delineation-based protocols is the fact that they are quite time-consuming. Another problem with these manual protocols is that because they are based on the identification of usually many anatomic landmarks, they require a high level of knowledge or training for their reliable application. Therefore, this type of study includes only a few subjects per group, preventing the analysis of samples with larger statistical value. Automatic methods, on the other hand, rely on the standardization of the anatomic data. Methods as those based on the Talairach atlas, for instance, involve the identification and alignment of the brain according to landmark/anchor points, followed by transformations of the images to fit into a stereotactic coordinate system. These data transformations eliminate some of the individual features, which may better describe the characteristics of a condition under study. Standard

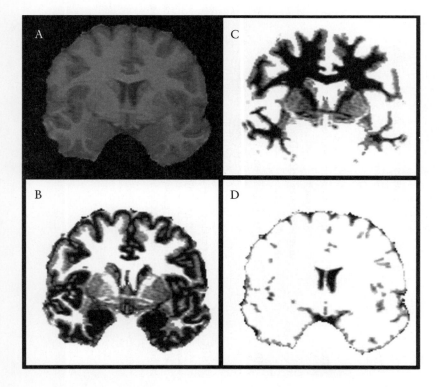

FIGURE 5-3. Fuzzy tissue segmentation. *A,* Gray scale image of a coronal slice through the posterior portion of the frontal lobe. *B-D,* Gray matter, white matter, and CSF tissue "fractions," respectively, resulting from segmentation of the same image. Note the partial gray and white voxels corresponding to subcortical nuclei and along the boundary of the cortical gray-white matter compartments. (Reprinted from Reiss AL, Hennessey JG, Rubin M, et al: Reliability and validity of an algorithm for fuzzy tissue segmentation of MRI. J Comput Assist Tomogr 22:471–479, 1998, by permission of Lippincott-Raven Publishers.)

frameworks also need to be adequate for application to different populations, including some with substantial volumetric reductions, and to different age groups. These issues make automatic and semiautomatic (i.e., requiring more input from evaluator) methods ideal as first examinations of a particular situation, to be followed by more detailed evaluations by manual methods. In our opinion, the strategy for measuring, for instance, the volume of the frontal lobe in a particular disorder should include as initial step an atlas- or framework-based automatic assessment in a relatively large population. The resulting data will guide higher-resolution measurements, by manual protocols, in a carefully selected group of representative subjects. Finally, the last duality in terms of parcellation analyses is whether the determination of size should be done through area (usually cross-sectional area) or volume measurements. Currently, only brain regions with ill-defined boundaries (e.g., corpus callosum) or challenging location (e.g., cerebellar vermis) or shape (e.g., planum temporale) should be measured in terms of area. Even in these cases, new methodologies are beginning to make possible their volumetric evaluations, which are essential to adequately assess their size in the context of their shape and localization. The following sections review the most common area measurements still used in pediatric neuroimaging, as well as fundamental automatic and manual morphometric approaches.

Area Measurements

Area measurement methods in pediatric neuroimaging are among the earliest. However, MRI studies using linear measurements, such as width and length of representative slices of a brain region, were still being reported in recent years. With the advent of volumetric acquisitions, cross-sectional area measurements combining all the acquired slices of a given ROI were replaced by stacks of contiguous images as the morphometric technique of choice. Nevertheless, cross-sectional areas are presently used to describe a number of structures in individuals with developmental disorders. The best examples are the midsagittal measurements of the corpus callosum, whose medial aspect is reliably identifiable in contrast to its ill-defined lateral borders, and the cerebellar vermis, a region that has become the surrogate of the entire cerebellum. Availability of an atlas for neuroanatomic and neuroimaging studies of the cerebellum (Schmahmann et al., 2000) brings the promise of replacing vermis area measurements for more comprehensive (i.e., including the cerebellar hemispheres) and precise (i.e., not depending of arbitrary definition of midline) evaluations of this brain region. In the case of the corpus callosum, rather than protocols or software, new acquisitions such as inversion recovery techniques, which may better delineate the cerebral

white matter, and diffusion tensor-weighted imaging (DTI) appear to be the advances needed for more complete analyses of this structure. Few brain regions are defined as a two-dimensional structure; the most important example is the planum temporale. This area of cortical tissue, which corresponds to the plane immediately behind the Heschl gyrus (or gyri, in some cases) in the superior temporal region, has been functionally linked to comprehensive aspects of language as a component of the so-called Wernicke area. Because most neuroanatomic/neuropathologic data about the planum are based on area measurements, only recently have investigators incorporated the three-dimensional aspects of this structure and have begun to measure the gray matter underlying the plane. This reevaluation has also been extended to more recent neuroimaging studies.

Considering the need for fast and reliable morphometric approaches, which can evaluate large number of subjects, the question about the accuracy of area measurements has been periodically reformulated. In a recent publication, Whalley and Wardlaw (2001) have shown high intra- and inter-reliability and accuracy for area measurements of several major brain regions. There was a good correlation between area and volume for the caudate and lentiform nuclei, and lateral and third ventricles. In contrast, such correspondence was not present for the amygdalo-hippocampal complex and the thalamus. This study also demonstrated, as expected, that area-volume agreement is low for small structures and for area measurements, typically performed along the main axis of an ROI.

As stated above, important features of several neurodevelopmental disorders have been characterized by area measurements. Here we present a selection, which does not intend to be inclusive, of some significant publications in this area.

Corpus Callosum

The medial surface of this commissure has been divided into five to seven regions. Using this midsagittal approach, Baumgardner and colleagues (1996) have demonstrated that the corpus callosum is larger in children with Tourette syndrome (TS). In contrast, in ADHD, the area is reduced, at expense of its rostral region. Emphasizing the importance of gender differences not only for understanding normal development, but also neurodevelopmental disorders, Mostofsky and colleagues (1999) in a follow-up study of girls found no significant differences in total or subdivision corpus callosum area in girls with TS or ADHD and controls. Another developmental disorder associated with callosal abnormalities is prenatal alcohol exposure. Sowell and colleagues (2001b) added to area measurements, analyses of shape and location in a wide range of individuals prenatally exposed to alcohol, including exposure to alcohol and the more severe fetal alcohol syndrome that presents with facial dysmorphia. These authors showed that in fetal alcohol syndrome, and to a lesser extent in fetal alcohol exposure, in addition to decrease in size particularly in the isthmus and splenium, there was also an anterior and inferior displacement of the corpus callosum affecting these posterior regions. The latter data were obtained by mapping and assigning coordinates to the callosal boundaries, which were used for reconstructing the shape and location of the commissure. Anatomic-behavioral correlations further emphasized the importance of the novel callosal measures, because displacement but not size reduction was correlated to impairment in verbal learning. A recent study on adult dyslexic subjects also examined callosal displacement; Robichon and colleagues (2000) developed a four-angle measurement-based system to demonstrate that in dyslexia there is an inferior displacement of the posterior regions of the commissure. In summary, midsagittal measurements are a valuable strategy for characterizing functionally relevant developmental anatomic abnormalities of the main cerebral commissure. Size evaluations can be complemented by analyses of shape and location. Additional information about callosal measurements can be found in Chapter 19.

Cerebellar Vermis

Most neuroanatomic approaches subdivide the vermis into 10 lobules (Carpenter, 1976). Lobules I to V correspond to the medial aspect of the anterior lobe (paleocerebellum), whereas lobules VI to IX are part of the posterior lobe or neocerebellum. Lobule X, or nodulus, is the vermian component of the flocculonodular lobe (archicerebellum). Additional information about cerebellar anatomy and dysfunction can be found in Chapter 25. Some of the most significant yet controversial findings include the reports of selective lobules VI to VII hypoplasia in children and young adults with idiopathic autism (Courchesne et al., 1994). This initial finding was later expanded to both hypo- and hyperplasia affecting the same vermian lobules in autism.

Although issues related to study design remain a concern in these reports, the methodology for measuring midsagittal vermian area, in particular the criteria for establishing the appropriate midsagittal plane, was carefully addressed by the authors (Courchesne et al., 1994). Another condition showing selective vermian hypoplasia is fragile X syndrome (reviewed by Kates et al., 2002). (See also Chapter 44.) Several studies have reported a relative decrease in the size of the posterior vermis, more severe in affected boys. However, still unclear is whether it affects more severely some regions of the lobules VI to X. The specificity of these findings was demonstrated by comparisons with a group of cognitively impaired matched boys. Figure 5-4 illustrates the posterior vermian hypoplasia in boys with fragile X.

Another developmental disorder in which vermian hypoplasia has been reported is ADHD (reviewed by Eliez & Reiss, 2000). Several groups have shown that, in boys with this condition, there is a reduction in inferior posterior lobe (lobules VIII-X) area. One of these studies also found agreement between area and (semiautomatic) volume measurements of the vermian hypoplasia. Interestingly, a recent investigation that also incorporated manual volumetric determinations did not find changes in the vermis in girls with ADHD (Castellanos et al., 2001), further emphasizing the gender effect in developmental anomalies. Posterior inferior reductions are apparently nonspecific because they have also been demonstrated in childhood-onset schizophrenia (Jacobsen et al., 1997).

Finally, the issue of correspondence between area and volume measurements in the posterior fossa, which has been reported in some of the aforementioned publications with regard to the vermis, was directly addressed for other structures by Aylward and Reiss (1991). These authors found high correlation between midsagittal area measurements and axial slice-based volumetric determinations for the pons, medulla, and fourth ventricle, but not for the cerebellum. As recently shown by Whalley and Wardlaw (2001), only the largest axial area measure of the cerebellum correlated with the volume of this region.

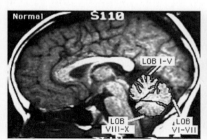 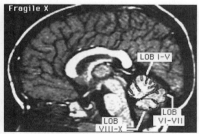

FIGURE 5-4. Midsagittal MR images of (A) a male control patient and (B) a male patient with fragile X. Borders are drawn around the anterior cerebellar vermis (lobules I-V), and lobules VI to VII and lobules VIII to X of the posterior cerebellar vermis. The area of the lobules comprising the posterior vermis appears smaller in the patient with fragile X syndrome. (Reprinted from Reiss AL, Aylward E, Freund LS, et al: Neuroanatomy of fragile X syndrome: The posterior fosse. Ann Neurol 29:26–32, 1991, by permission of John Wiley and Sons.)

Planum Temporale

Few studies have measured this surface area in pediatric populations, although several publications have discussed this region in adults with developmental disorders. Most of the reports deal with developmental dyslexia, in which initial neuropathologic and neuroimaging studies of either adult males had shown a lack of the normal leftward asymmetry. Several MRI investigations had challenged this view, demonstrating the standard pattern of asymmetry in dyslexic subjects and controls (Rumsey et al., 1997; Heiervang et al., 2000). These findings are puzzling considering the relationship between dyslexia and developmental language disorders. In the latter group, Gauger and colleagues (1997) found a reduction in the area of the left planum and an increase in rightward asymmetry. The complicated nature of the subject is underscored by a recent study on planum temporale asymmetry in normal children (Preis et al., 1999); these authors found that the adult pattern of the planum is already present by age 3 years and that girls demonstrate a stronger leftward asymmetry than boys. The latter finding was intriguing considering that neuroanatomic studies had suggested that stronger lateralization was a "male feature." Other developmental disorders in which the planum temporale has been assessed by MRI include schizophrenia and Down syndrome. Although it is unclear whether in children or adults with schizophrenia there is any planum anomaly (Shapleske et al., 2001), a single evaluation of the volume of the planum temporale in Down syndrome showed a selective reduction in contrast to the proportional decrease of the volume of the superior temporal gyrus (Frangou et al., 1997).

VOLUMETRICS OF THE CEREBRUM: AUTOMATIC AND SEMI-AUTOMATIC METHODS

Automatic or semi-automatic methods for quantifying brain volumes are based on the capacity to delineate gray and white matter compartments on the basis of tissue class or easy-to-identify (reliable) landmarks. In other words, the different brain regions are parcellated by their distinct tissue composition or tissue interphases or by identifying and registering external (e.g., sulci, gyri) or internal (e.g., commissures) landmarks. An example of the tissue class segmentation-based approach is the assessment of total cerebral gray or white matter volumes (Swayze et al., 1997; Castellanos et al., 2001). Nonetheless, tissue intensity methods are still also used to outline and parcellate cortical and subcortical regions, which can be further delineated by manual tracing protocols (Alarcon et al., 2000). Current automated techniques generally include the placement of the brain in a standardized or normalized framework. This allows the registration of appropriate landmarks for atlas-based (Kates et al., 2001) or template-based transformations (Giedd et al., 1999a) and facilitates the application of manual delineation protocols (Archibald et al., 2001).

The selection of surface or internal landmarks involves structures that are both easy to recognize and relatively consistent among individuals. Methods that rely on surface landmarks have evolved in parallel with advances in MRI sequences and image analysis-rendering techniques. The most influential anatomic frameworks for early cerebral parcellation were published by Zipursky and associates (1992), Filipek and colleagues (1997), and Rademacher and colleagues (1992). Reiss and colleagues (1993) introduced the first model to the volumetric assessment of individuals with developmental disorders. It consists of a set of coordinates or planes that divides the cerebrum into 16 regions (8/hemisphere): (1) a midsagittal plane along the interhemispheric fissure, (2) a transaxial plane along the anterior commissure (AC)/posterior commissure (PC) or AC/PC line, (3) a coronal plane perpendicular to no. 2 and passing through the most anterior point of the genu of the corpus callosum, (4) a coronal plane perpendicular to no. 2 and passing through the most posterior point of the splenium of the corpus callosum, and (5) a coronal plane perpendicular to no. 2 and passing through a point midway between no. 3 and no. 4 (Fig. 5-5). The resulting subhemispheric regions are prefrontal, posterior frontal, orbital-frontal, parietal, superior parietal-occipital, inferior parietal-occipital, anterior temporal, and mid/posterior temporal. The early application of this coordinate system, using two-dimensional 5-mm-thick T2-weighted MRI sequences, included normal development (Reiss et al., 1996) as well as conditions such as Rett syndrome (Reiss et al., 1993), fragile X syndrome (Eliez et al., 2001), and Turner syndrome (Reiss et al., 1995). In the first study by Reiss and colleagues (1996), these authors found that, in the 5- to 17-year age range, independent of gender differences (cerebral gray matter was 10% larger in boys), there is little change in cerebral volume during the examined period (Reiss et al., 1996). Despite the modest volumetric changes, gray matter tends to decrease over time while white matter volumes become larger in both sexes. These authors also found that prefrontal gray matter is the main contributor to IQ variance. In Rett syndrome, the predominant reduction in cerebral gray matter was mainly due to volumetric decreases in frontal (Reiss et al., 1993; Subramaniam et al., 1997) and anterior temporal (Subramaniam et al., 1997) ROIs. Similar applications of this parcellation scheme to Turner syndrome (Reiss et al., 1995) and fragile X syndrome (Eliez et al., 2001) demonstrated selective parietal reductions and abnormal rates of cerebral (cortical) gray matter decreases, respectively.

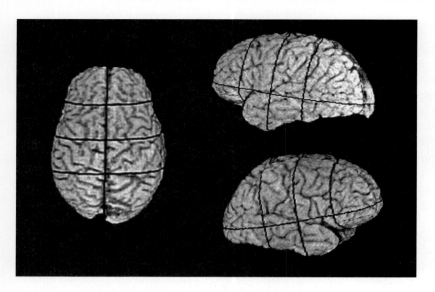

FIGURE 5-5. Lateral (left and right) and dorsal (superior) view of the coordinate system that divides the cerebral cortex into eight regions in each hemisphere. The lines represent either the plane or the projection of the plane on the cerebral surface. (Reproduced with permission from Reiss AL, Faruque F, Naidu S, et al: Neuroanatomy of Rett syndrome: A volumetric imaging study. Ann Neurol 34:227–234, 1993.) See text for explanation.

The use of commissures, including the corpus callosum, as major points of reference for either spatial standardization or delineation of planes, has become a common practice due to their reliable identification. In this line, Giedd and colleagues (1996a) used a similar method to the one described in the preceding paragraph for studying in a semiautomatic way changes in cerebral volume during normal development. However, these authors applied this method to higher-resolution images, specifically 2-mm-thick volumetric SPGR sequences, than those analyzed by Reiss and colleagues. The cerebrum was parcellated into five regions: I or prefrontal sector containing all of the brain in front of the anterior-most point of the corpus callosum; II or premotor/temporal sector between the coronal plane intersecting the anterior-most point of the corpus callosum and the coronal plane intersecting the AC; III or precentral/temporal sector between the AC and PC; and the posterior regions, IV or parietal/temporal sector and V or occipital sector, that were arbitrarily divided by a plane 1.5 times the region III length, posterior to the PC. This strategy was applied extensively to normal development and to neurodevelopmental disorders; in their normative study of children aged 4 to 18, Giedd and colleagues (1996a) confirmed the larger absolute and relative cerebral volumes in boys. As for Reiss and colleagues, this cross-sectional investigation showed no significant volumetric changes across the age range and a right-to-left cerebral asymmetry. With regard to cerebral sectors, all of them were larger in boys and only prefrontal and premotor/temporal showed the same global right > left asymmetry (Giedd et al., 1996a). Considering the hypothesized role of frontostriatal pathways in attentional and inhibitory mechanisms, Castellanos and colleagues (1996) used the same parcellation method to assess cerebral changes in ADHD. They found that

boys with ADHD had smaller total cerebral (~5%) and right anterior frontal region volumes. The most recent version of a commissural-based parcellation method is the protocol reported by Peterson and colleagues (2000, 2001), in which these authors also divided the cerebrum into eight regions per hemisphere using a combination of axial and coronal planes: an axial plane containing the AC/PC line and three limiting coronal planes—one tangent to the genu of the corpus callosum, one tangent to the anterior border of the AC, and one through the PC. The sectors were termed dorsal prefrontal, orbitofrontal, premotor, subgenual, sensorimotor, parieto-occipital, midtemporal, and inferior occipital. Five of the eight sectors, in particular the sensorimotor one, were reduced in children (age 8 years) who were born prematurely. Volumes of sensorimotor and midtemporal cortices were also correlated with IQ scores in the preterm subjects (Peterson et al., 2000). Application of this approach to a large, wide age-range sample of individuals with TS demonstrated that they had larger dorsal prefrontal and parieto-occipital volumes, whereas inferior occipital volumes were reduced. There was also an inverse association between cerebral volume and age in those with TS, particularly children with TS. Orbitofrontal, midtemporal, and parieto-occipital region volumes were also significantly associated with the severity of tics (Peterson et al., 2001).

Another automated approach that has gained considerable acceptance is the use of reference frameworks. In this case, landmarks are used not only to standardize position but also to transform the anatomic data to a standard set of coordinates, which represents specific brain regions, or to a template brain. The stereotactic atlas-based technique of Talairach was initially proposed by Andreasen and colleagues in 1996. We have implemented and standardized this method to pediatric populations as follows. After the identification of three landmarks/anchor points, the AC, the PC, and a mid-sagittal point above the axis created by the first two points, the six faces of the brain "cube" or volume are located and a proportional stereotactic grid is overlaid onto the brain. Grid placement is accomplished by a linear interpolation of areas anterior to AC, posterior to PC, and between these two commissures (Kaplan et al., 1997). This process normalizes the position of the brain and parcellates the brain into 1232 "volumetric" sectors, which are grouped and assigned to a particular ROI (Kaplan et al., 1997; Kates et al., 1999). Because each voxel is also segmented, the protocol can determine automatically gray matter, white matter, and CSF volumes for each ROI. In comparative analyses with manually delineated lobar "gold standards" from adult and pediatric controls and a group of girls with Rett syndrome, we demonstrated the high sensitivity and specificity of this method for volumetric determinations of the total cerebrum and cerebral lobes (Kaplan et al., 1997; Kates et al., 1999). Although its adequacy for cerebral measurements has been documented, the Talairach method has relatively low sensitivity and specificity for subcortical structures, including the brainstem and cerebellum (Kates et al., 1999). For this reason, we have restricted the application of the Talairach method to cerebral lobes (Kates et al., 2001, 2002) and, more recently, we have developed sublobar ROI parcellation strategies (Kaufmann, 2001). As

depicted in Figure 5-6, availability of software with multiplanar visualization and rendering capabilities is essential for ensuring the rapid and accurate application of this parcellation protocol.

The Talairach atlas-based method has been used for examining lobar volumetric abnormalities, either as technical validation or direct analysis, in several neurodevelopmental disorders. As with the method reported by Giedd and colleagues (1996a), these studies are not only of interest because of the validity of the technique (i.e, high correspondence with manual delineation) but also due to the fact that they use high-resolution MRI sequences in parallel to more robust segmentation algorithms. In fragile X syndrome, we found larger cerebral (Kaplan et al., 1997; Kates et al., 2002) and parietal white matter (in relationship with gene dosage; Kates et al., 2002) volumes. In a preliminary study in Rett syndrome, contrary to a previous report using the Zipursky strategy (Reiss et al., 1993), there was a marked reduction affecting similarly all four lobes and not preferentially the frontal region. Reiss and colleagues have continued applying the Talairach method, reporting that in velocardiofacial syndrome (VCFS), in addition to a greater global cerebral white matter decrease, there was a selective parietal gray matter reduction (Eliez et al., 2000a). Our own investigation of VCFS showed a rather relative decrease in the volume of nonfrontal white matter (Kates et al., 2001); issues related to study design may explain the discrep-

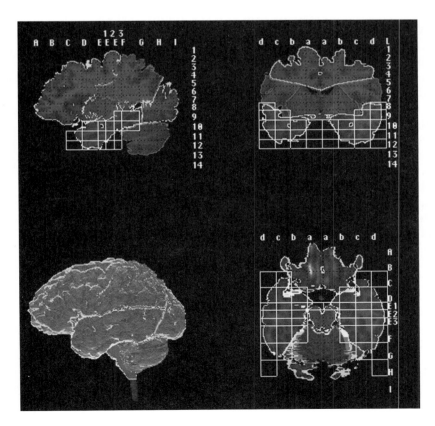

FIGURE 5-6. Talairach coordinate system. The brain has been positionally normalized, and Talairach sectors designated as representing the temporal lobe are shown superimposed (as white boxes), in the three orthogonal views, over manually derived sulcal-based "gold standard regions" (in color). In this example, the temporal lobe (yellow) volume would be calculated by adding the temporal lobe-designated voxels in all slices. (Reprinted from Kates WR, Warsofsky IS, Patwardhan A, et al: Automated Talairach atlas-based parcellation and measurement of cerebral lobes in children. Psychaitry Res 91:11–30, 1999, by permission of Elsevier Science B. V.) (See Color Plate 1)

ancies with the earlier publication. In Williams syndrome, Reiss and colleagues (2000) found a reduction in cerebral volume, mainly affecting the white matter, which was associated with a greater ratio of frontal to posterior (parietal plus occipital) tissue. In Klinefelter syndrome, Patwardhan and colleagues (2000) found that there is a selective reduction in left temporal gray matter, which can be "prevented" by exogenous administration of testosterone. Finally, in young men with dyslexia, Eliez and colleagues (2000b) found a selective reduction in temporal lobe gray matter volume that affected more the left side. Additional preliminary data on other developmental disorders were reported in our study on young men with fragile X mentioned above (Kates et al., 2002). An evaluation of two contrast groups, nonspecific language delay and Down syndrome, demonstrated that, as in fragile X, there were temporal lobe gray matter reductions. The group with Down syndrome also showed marked global cerebral decreases, as well as selective parietal reductions. These data suggested that temporal lobe gray matter reductions are characteristic, and relatively nonspecific, of disorders associated with impaired language development.

An example of a second approach, using a reference framework, is the one reported in several publications by the neuroimaging group at the Child Psychiatry Branch of National Institute of Mental Health (NIMH). These investigators have applied templates for determinations of total cerebral volume, as well as of cerebral lobar volumes. The former application is based on an original study by Snell and colleagues (1995), which uses an active surface template of the brain. This technique considers the cerebral surface a deformable structure within certain constraints of shape and topology, and complements tissue segmentation (i.e., signal intensity) data. In this way, for instance, Alaghband-Rad and associates (1997) showed that the smaller brain size of children and adolescents with childhood-onset schizophrenia associates inversely with a scale of symptoms. An extension of this method, for measuring lobes and sublobar regions, uses a template brain in which regions have been manually delineated (Giedd et al., 1999b) after nonlinear registration of the images. One of its first applications consisted of a longitudinal normative study; cerebral lobe volumes were measured on SPGR scans from 145 subjects aged 4 to 21 years. The data show that white matter of all four lobes increased linearly, more pronouncedly in male subjects. In contrast, frontal and parietal gray matter volumes increased to a peak, at 12 years in boys and 10 to 11 in girls, respectively, which was followed by a decline during adolescence. Temporal and occipital gray matter volumes increased steadily until late adolescence in a more similar pattern for both sexes (Giedd et al., 1999a). These results do not correspond with previous cross-

sectional studies mentioned above (Castellanos et al., 1996; Eliez et al., 2001), which indicate declines in gray matter. Discrepancies appear to be related to the true longitudinal nature of the more recent study. Template-based lobar measurements include progressive frontal, parietal, and temporal gray matter reductions in adolescents with childhood-onset schizophrenia (Rapoport et al., 1999) and mild left frontal decreases in girls with ADHD (Castellanos et al., 2001). An additional investigation restricted evaluations to the anterior frontal region (anterior to the corpus callosum), in adolescents with psychotic disorder not otherwise specified and childhood-onset schizophrenia, and showed mild reductions in both groups with psychotic disorder (Kumra et al., 2000).

The most recent automated approach for brain parcellation, voxel-based morphometry, applies analytic protocols pioneered in functional MRI (to high-resolution MRIs). The principle of this system is that each voxel can be analyzed as an independent unit, in terms of gray matter, white matter, or CSF "density." As for any of the aforementioned methods, the brain is reoriented and scaled to a standard space. Voxel signal intensity analyses are done, by determining specific thresholds, according to the statistical parametric mapping (SPM) technique, comparing sets of voxels for each tissue class separately. One of the first pediatric applications of voxel morphometry was conducted by Sowell and colleagues (1999), who examined the differences between the brains of normal children and adolescents. These investigators used categorical segmentation thresholds to analyze the tissue content of each voxel. In this and other studies, voxel-based data are used to construct statistical maps of significant differences, which could be analyzed in terms of anatomic regions. For instance, in the normative study by Sowell and colleagues (1999) there were reductions in gray matter (i.e., voxels that initially were labeled as gray were then segmented as white matter) from childhood to adolescence, mainly in dorsal parietal and frontal areas. The accuracy of voxel-based morphometry for determining changes in brain composition and size, particularly in developmental disorders, is still unknown. Recent publications on juvenile myoclonic epilepsy (Woermann et al., 1999) and temporal lobe epilepsy (Woermann et al., 2000), early-onset schizophrenia (Sowell et al., 2000), prenatal alcohol exposure (Sowell, et al., 2001c), and dyslexia (Brown et al., 2001) reveal the possibility of detecting abnormal proportions of gray and white matter in multiple cortical and subcortical regions in several of these conditions. Woermann and colleagues (1999) found an increase in mesial frontal gray matter in adolescents with juvenile myoclonic epilepsy, whereas reductions in left frontal gray matter characterized patients with temporal lobe epilepsy and aggressive episodes when compared with controls and with patients with the epileptic syndrome but not aggressive behavior (Woermann et al., 2000). Brown and colleagues (2001) showed in young adults with dyslexia decreases in gray matter affecting the left temporal lobe, and bilaterally the temporoparieto-occipital juncture and the frontal lobe, as well as other subcortical regions. Finally, Sowell and colleagues (2000) demonstrated that in subjects with early onset schizophrenia lateral ventricles were larger, predominantly in the posterior horns, and that midcallosal and posterior cingulate voxels were abnormal. In their study of children and adolescents with histories of prenatal alcohol exposure, SPM analyses revealed relative increase in gray matter, and reductions in white matter, in left perisylvian cortices of the temporal and parietal lobes (Sowell et al., 2001c).

Lastly, a strategy that combines automated segmentation-parcellation with manual delineation for measuring cerebrocortical regions was reported by the Neurology/Massachusetts General Hospital (MGH) group (Filipek et al., 1992). In terms of regional subdivisions, it is based on the concept that each one of the volumetric units, which constitute the cerebral cortex, corresponds to all or a portion of an individual gyrus. In addition to AC/PC axis, the corpus callosum and several prominent gyri and sulci helped to delineate cortical regions. The initial steps included positional normalization and segmentation/parcellation using algorithms for signal intensity evaluation and mapping ("intensity contour mapping" and "differential intensity contour") and definition of commissural landmarks (for more information, see also section on tissue segmentation). This is followed by manual drawings of surface landmarks; in this way, the cerebrum is parcellated into precallosal (prefrontal), retrocallosal, and anterior and posterior pericallosal blocks. The latter are further divided into superior, inferior, and temporal sections. The validity of this protocol was assessed by its application to SPGR scans from a group of children and adolescents with ADHD (Filipek et al., 1997). As postulated, frontal regions were abnormal; there was a reduction in the volume of the right anterior-superior, mainly involving the white matter. A global (gray plus white matter) decrease was also detected in the anterior-inferior region bilaterally. However, there was also a reduction in white matter volume in the parieto-occipital region (Filipek et al., 1997). A complementary and extended analytical strategy reported by the same group, based on an anatomic scheme by Rademacher and colleagues (1992), further (with respect to the protocol described above) subdivides the cerebral cortex into a total of 48 units per hemisphere. This parcellation scheme was designated by the authors as "gyri analysis" (Kennedy et al., 1998). In addition to the automated methods for orientation and tissue and region segmentation, manual editing was included for

gray-white matter delineation. Following this, the cortical ribbon was separated from the rest of the brain, then parcellated by coronal planes determined by 42 surface landmarks, the trajectory of 31 fissures, and visual recognition and labeling (Kennedy et al., 1998). The application of this protocol to a sample of 10 male and 10 female normal young adults revealed that there was a 10% variability for total cerebral volume and approximately twice as much variability for individual cortical sectors. Despite the effects of cerebral size and gender, the most important factors contributing to gyral variability were subject and specific gyrus. Further refinements of this mixed automated/manual cortical parcellation have been reported by these investigators (Goldstein et al., 1999, 2001); however, none of these studies involves normal or developmentally disabled children.

In summary, automated and semiautomated parcellation strategies for the cerebrum continue evolving. They have been greatly influenced by advances in MRI acquisition, currently mainly volumetric type, image-processing algorithms, and hardware and software capabilities that allow combination of automated segmentation and manual drawing approaches. Automated strategies have their obvious limitations, which relate to "discarding" information about individual neuroanatomy that is particularly critical in the case of the cerebral cortex. However, they provide a fast way to examine potentially informative ROIs, in a particular condition, which can be studied in more detail with manual techniques (e.g., Talairach-followed manual delineation of a specific lobe). Moreover, automated methods should not be seen as opposite to manual delineation. They constitute the current preferred strategy for calculating total cerebral volume and for preparing data (e.g., spatial normalization) for higher-resolution parcellation protocols. The next section represents a continuation of this one, focused on manual delineation techniques for the cerebral cortex.

MANUAL DELINEATION OF THE CEREBRAL CORTEX

As mentioned, cerebral parcellation strategies that require manual drawing date back to the early 1990s, prior to the systematic implementation of volumetric MRI acquisitions. This section deals exclusively with the few studies that evaluated cortical volumes in children or developmental disorders. The first protocol for a comprehensive evaluation of the cerebral cortex, by manual delineation in a pediatric population, was recently published by Jernigan and colleagues (2001). It represents a refinement of protocols previously reported by this group (Jernigan et al., 1990), adding an interactive tissue segmentation (classification) strategy that uses tissue-type sampling. Parcellation is accomplished by delineating standard boundaries on spatially normalized image sets. The frontal lobe is tissue (gray and white matter) anterior to the central sulcus and superior to the sylvian fissure (including cingulate, but excluding the insula). The parietal lobe is defined as posterior to the central sulcus and anterior to the sylvian fissure, and the temporal lobe as inferior to the sylvian fissure (excluding the insula). The posterior borders of both parietal and temporal lobes were defined stereotactically as the coronal plane anterior to the occipital notch. All cortices posterior to this plane were defined as occipital (Archibald et al., 1991). Application of this protocol to children exposed prenatally to alcohol demonstrated that in the most severe situation, fetal alcohol syndrome, there is a marked reduction in cerebral volumes mainly affecting the white matter and the parietal lobe. Individuals exposed to alcohol, but without facial dysmorphia, showed milder parietal changes (Archibald et al., 1991). A pediatric normative study, aiming at establishing frontal lobe structure-behavioral correlations, revealed that in children between 7 and 16 years of age, the age-dependent reduction in frontal gray matter strongly predicted delayed verbal memory. A weaker association was found for measures of visuospatial memory and frontal lobe volume (Sowell et al., 2001a).

Using a combination of tissue signal intensity thresholds and manual delineation, according to standard anatomic landmarks that excluded the insular cortex, Carper and Courchesne (2000) developed a protocol for frontal lobe volumetrics on T2-weighted images. Their application to boys with autism demonstrated a relative frontal enlargement, which is inversely related to the cerebellar vermis (lobules VI-VII) area. Matsuzawa and colleagues (2001) have recently published a method for determining the volume of the frontal and temporal lobes not only in children, but also in infants with relatively less myelination. These authors used an axial SPGR volumetric sequence, with emphasis on robust segmentation using an algorithm (i.e., cubic B-spline function) that, among other features, reduces shading and bias against small regions. Parcellation was done by an adaptation of a protocol by Gur and colleagues (1991). They implemented the protocol to normal children between ages 1 month and 10 years and found growth spurts of whole brain and frontal and temporal lobes during the first 2 postnatal years. During this active period, the frontal lobes grew more rapidly than the temporal lobes, with relatively more increase in gray matter. As reported by other studies cited in this chapter, after age 2 years the volume of the cerebral white matter increased at a higher rate throughout childhood (Matsuzawa et al., 2001).

Several studies have reported measurements of the temporal lobe in pediatric populations. A number of these studies restrict the measurements to the superior temporal gyrus (STG). A global temporal lobe volumetric assessment for interpreting hippocampal measurements (see more detail in section on limbic structures), in children ranging in age from 3 weeks to 14 years, with variable positive histories but normal MRI and neurologic examinations, was communicated by Utsunomiya and colleagues (1999). These investigators used MP-RAGE and a combined automated thresholding tissue segmentation and manual delineation in the AC/PC axis protocol. They reported that, as for the hippocampus, there was a right > left asymmetry for the anterior temporal lobe since early infancy (Utsunomiya et al., 1999). Although several studies have evaluated the STG in adults with developmental disorders (e.g., Down syndrome, Williams syndrome, dyslexia), few reports are available on children with these conditions. Eliez and colleagues (2000a) found that children with VCFS have a proportional reduction in temporal and STG volumes. Nonetheless, contrary to controls, children with VCFS have an age-dependent reduction in temporal lobe volume, particularly affecting the gray matter. Investigations on adults have shown that although dyslexic men have whole left temporal lobe reductions (2000b), individuals with Williams syndrome have relative preservation of cerebellar, cerebral gray matter, and STG volumes (Reiss et al., 2000). Finally, in adults with Down syndrome the STG is smaller but in proportion to the overall cerebral volumetric reduction (Frangou et al., 1997). The latter study should be interpreted in the context of older data, using two-dimensional thick-slice acquisitions and less precise parcellation approaches, indicating that cortices posterior to a midcallosal point, which include posterior temporal lobe, are more preserved than regions anterior to this plane in Down syndrome (while the opposite was found for Williams syndrome). The only direct temporal region assessment, in this study, was that of the "temporal limbic" structures, which were selectively involved in Down syndrome (Jernigan et al., 1993).

So far, no pediatric and very few adult studies have examined volumetric changes affecting components of any cerebral lobe, by manual delineation. Detailed high-resolution cortical measurement protocols, applying advanced neuroanatomic methods, have recently been developed (Insausti et al., 1998; Andreasen et al, 1999; Frederikse et al., 1999; Crespo-Facorro et al., 1999, 2000; Andreasen et al., 2000; Kim et al., 2000). We expect to see their application to pediatric neuroimaging in the next few years. They are a necessary complement and extension of the increasing number of semiautomated protocol-based volumetric determinations in developmental disorders.

Manual Parcellation of Subcortical Nuclei

The basal ganglia are among the first structures to be evaluated morphometrically in pediatric neuroimaging. Most of the early studies measured single thick slices, T2-weighted sequences, or linear variables (e.g., bicaudate ratio) instead of volume (Aylward et al., 1991; Hynd et al., 1993; Mattson et al., 1994; Mataro et al., 1997). Although image contrast was relatively good, measurements were affected by partial volume effects and incomplete sampling of the structure. The issue of partial volume is specifically important considering that the basal ganglia and the thalamus are nuclei with a complex mixture of gray and white matter. Nonetheless, before the SPGR era, valuable data were obtained by these early approaches. Studies focused on developmental disorders in which clinical or neuropathologic information suggested basal ganglia involvement. For instance, Reiss and colleagues (1993), using 5-mm-thick axial (paralleled to the AC/PC axis) T2-weighted images, and Singer and colleagues (1993), using 3-mm-thick axial T2-weighted inversion recovery slices, measured caudate and lenticular nucleus volumes in Rett syndrome and TS, respectively. In Rett syndrome, there was a selective reduction in the caudate that contrasted with a proportional (to brain size) volumetric decrease of other subcortical structures. In the second study, which compared males with TS only and TS plus ADHD with controls, it was found that in TS plus ADHD there is a reversal of the asymmetry of the lenticular nucleus with a greater right-sided predominance due to a smaller left globus pallidus. A follow-up publication by Aylward and colleagues (1996), which included boys with TS and ADHD or ADHD and controls, concluded that the smaller globus pallidus was a feature related to ADHD. Despite the spatial resolution limitations, the application of T2-weighted or inversion recovery sequences in the aforementioned studies provided adequate contrast for delineating, in particular, the globus pallidus, a structure with poor distinction on SPGR images.

One of the first studies introducing volumetric sequences (i.e., SPGR) to the morphometry of the basal ganglia was the normative investigation by Giedd and colleagues (1996a), which surveyed a large number of brain regions in approximately 100 boys and girls, between ages 4 and 18 years. As most SPGR-based studies, the measurements were done in the coronal plane. The caudate and putamen were manually traced, in every other 2-mm-thick coronal slice, and the volume was calculated as the sum of the areas measured multiplied by 4 mm (thickness). The globus pallidus was traced in every 2-mm-thick coronal slice, beginning 2 mm anterior to the AC and extending for 14 mm posteriorly. Putamen and globus pallidus were found to be larger in boys, even after adjusting for total cerebral volume. Caudate, on the other hand, was shown to be larger in girls after adjusting for total cerebral volume. Right caudate volumes were larger than the left, whereas left putamen volumes were larger than the right, with no gender differences. Caudate and putamen volumes were shown to decrease with age only in boys. The same group applied this methodology for examining the basal ganglia in boys with ADHD (Castellanos et al., 1996); these authors expanded and confirmed their previous work (Castellanos et al., 1994) demonstrating loss of right > left asymmetry due to a smaller right caudate. Other studies using similar MRI sequences and morphometric methodology have further contributed to the abundant evidence supporting abnormalities in right caudate size and symmetry in boys, but not in girls, with ADHD (Casey et al., 1997; Filipek et al., 1997; Semrud-Clikeman et al., 2000; Castellanos et al., 2001). Other basal ganglia volumetric abnormalities in developmental disorders include basal ganglia reductions in fetal alcohol syndrome (Mattson et al., 1996) and preterm children (Peterson et al., 2001), and enlargements in idiopathic autism (Sears et al., 1999), childhood-onset schizophrenia (Frazier et al., 1996), and in children with obsessive-compulsive disorder (OCD) or tics associated with streptococcal infection (Giedd et al., 2000), changes that affected in the same direction all three basal ganglia components. Despite these studies, the delineation and measurement of the globus pallidus, which has a relatively larger proportion of white matter than the striatum (Carpenter, 1976), is particularly difficult on SPGR sequences. Similar problems affect basal ganglia delineation in conditions with hypomyelination, such as in infants with periventricular leukomalacia (Lin et al., 2001). The use of either T2-weighted or volumetric inversion recovery sequences (Magnotta et al., 2000; Lin et al., 2001) has been proposed as an alternative for improving contrast between these subcortical ROIs.

The thalamus is another structure of great interest, which represents a challenge for MRI morphometry. First, as the globus pallidus, the thalamus has a complex tissular mix that may be difficult to delineate on SPGR scans. In addition, the thalamus is not a discrete nucleus but rather a conglomerate of nuclei with complex neuroanatomic borders (i.e., nuclear delineation requires a combination of cytoarchitectonic and histochemical stains; Carpenter, 1976). Because the medial aspect of the thalamus is easily identified, one of the strategies for measuring this structure has been to delineate the area on a midsagittal slice (Giedd et al., 2000). Attempts at manually tracing and measuring the thalamus on T2- or T1-weighted (SPGR) images have been made by Reiss and colleagues (1993), Subramaniam and colleagues (1997), and Gilbert and associates (2000, 2001), respectively. The first two publications reported only proportional reductions in thalamic size in groups of patients with Rett syndrome, when compared to controls. Gilbert and colleagues (2000) provided more detailed information about their protocol. The boundaries of the thalamus were: anteriorly, the mamilary bodies and interventricular foramen; laterally, the internal capsule; medially, the third ventricle; inferiorly, the hypothalamus; and posteriorly, the crux fornix. These authors found that although in untreated patients with obsessive-compulsive disorder the thalamic volume is larger, in patients receiving the serotonin reuptake inhibitor paroxetine the volume of the thalamus had decreased. In a more recent investigation, Gilbert and colleagues (2001) found that the thalamic volumes were smaller in adolescents and young adults with first-episode schizophrenia. Further subdivision of the thalamus demonstrated that several subdivisions were more reduced, among them the central medial subdivision that comprises the dorsomedial nucleus (postulated to be affected in this disorder). Although as specified in previous sections area measurements tend to be less accurate, in the case of the thalamus they are important because of the reliability of midsagittal evaluations and the scarcity of data on this structure. Frazier and colleagues (1996) found that in children and adolescents with childhood-onset schizophrenia total cerebral volume and thalamic area were reduced, contrasting with the enlargements of the basal ganglia mentioned above. In preterm infants (mean age, 29.6 weeks) with moderate to severe periventricular leukomalacia, ratios of cerebral-cerebellar areas and thalamic-cerebellar areas were decreased, whereas those of basal ganglia-cerebellum were preserved (Lin et al., 2001).

In conclusion, volumetric measurements of the basal ganglia and thalamus are inherently difficult due to the intrinsic constitution of these brain regions, with a complex mixture of gray and white matter, and ill-defined borders. Their deep location also makes difficult their approach by automated or semiautomated methods. Development of new higher-contrast volumetric techniques, such as MP-RAGE and other inversion recovery techniques (Magnotta et al., 2000), such as the previously mentioned CAIR, as well as automated registration algorithms for using atlas-based (Iosifescu et al., 1997) or voxel-based strategies, promise significant improvements in the analyses of these subcortical nuclei (see Table 5-1).

MORPHOMETRIC ANALYSES OF THE MESIAL TEMPORAL LOBE

Although several studies have reported either area (Saitoh et al., 1995) or automated volumetric measurements of the hippocampus and amygdala (Peterson et al., 2001) in a variety of developmental disorders, the method of choice for morphometric assessment is manual delineation of these structures. As in the case of diseases affecting the mature brain, the interest in the limbic regions of the temporal lobe has focused on epilepsy and disorders characterized by psychiatric manifestations or severe cognitive deficit. Early volumetric studies examined hippocampal volumes in different forms of epilepsy, mainly intractable temporal lobe seizures (Cascino et al., 1991; Cendes et al., 1993; Kim et al., 1994). The investigations that showed "atrophy" and abnormal asymmetry of hippocampus and amygdala used clinically oriented sequences (e.g., T2-weighted) or material and were limited, therefore, for not using volumetric acquisitions. In addition, these reports as well as a normative study by Filipek and colleagues (1994) included mainly adolescents or young adults. The first volumetric evaluation of children with a neurodevelopmental disorder was the study by Reiss and colleagues (1994) on fragile X syndrome. In a group of children and young adults of both genders with this condition, these authors found a moderate increase in hippocampal volume. Technical limitations of the study were related to the type of sequence (i.e., T2-weighted) and slice thickness (the control data also included images with gaps). In 1996, Giedd and colleagues (1996b) published the first pediatric study using SPGR sequences; this investigation was aimed at characterizing the development of the temporal lobe between ages 4 and 18. These authors found variable volume for all temporal lobe structures (not only mesial). After adjusting for total cerebral volume, there were no gender differences. However, in boys the left amygdala volume increased over time, whereas the same was true for the right hippocampus in girls. Related studies by the same group found no abnormalities in the temporal lobe of children and adolescents with childhood-onset schizophrenia (Jacobsen et al., 1996) and in boys with ADHD (Castellanos et al., 1996). Amygdala and hippocampus were manually traced and their separation, acknowledged to be difficult by both authors, included criteria such as the most anterior view of the mammillary bodies as amygdalo-hippocampal border and the posterior hippocampal boundary as the most posterior slice displaying the fornix (Giedd et al., 1996b). Another study describing gender differences in normal brain development in children aged 7 to 11 years reported that, although there was proportionality between total brain and region volumes, some structures did not follow this "uniform scaling" (Caviness et al., 1996). These regions included the caudate, hippocampus, and pallidum, which were disproportionately larger in brains of girls than boys, and the amygdala, which was disproportionately smaller in the brains of girls. The discrepancy between these results and those communicated by Giedd and colleagues (1996b) may be due to the narrower age range of the latter study; however, methodological differences could also play a role. As described in the section on automated cerebral measurements, the Neurology/MGH group used an "anatomic segmentation" approach, based on signal intensity, for parcellating 3-mm-thick SPGR slices (Caviness et al., 1996).

We developed a manual tracing protocol for both amygdala and hippocampus, which took into account brain (or temporal lobe) position and fine anatomic borders (Kates et al., 1997a). We compared the reliability of coronal (SPGR, 1.5-mm thick) slices perpendicular to the AC/PC axis with coronal slices perpendicular to the long axis of the hippocampus. Both approaches were comparable (no significant difference), although amygdala measurement was slightly more reliable when the brain was rotated parallel to the AC/PC plane, whereas hippocampal volume was slightly more consistent along the main axis of the structure. The validity of the method was tested in a sample of children with fragile X; the study replicated the previous finding of a relatively larger hippocampus, in this case the right side. Figure 5-7 illustrates our amygdala/hippocampus protocol in the two examined orientations. Other important data on these mesial lobe structures include progressive reduction in hippocampal volume during adolescence in childhood-onset schizophrenia (Giedd et al., 1999b); decrease in hippocampal volume and persistence of right > left hippocampal asymmetry in young children with complex febrile seizures (Szabo et al., 1999); asymmetry of hippocampal volume as a more sensitive, but not specific (in terms of type of epilepsy), measure in intractable epilepsy (Lawson et al., 2000); reduction in hippocampal volume with preservation of amygdala size in Down syndrome (Pinter et al., 2001); and absence of abnormalities in children with idiopathic autism (Piven et al., 1998). In contrast with the latter publication, a recent study of adolescents and adults with idiopathic autism found an absolute and, particularly, relative decrease in the volume of the amygdala and hippocampus (Aylward et al., 1999). This investigation applied another SPGR-based, manual delineation protocol that shares many features with ours (Kates et al., 1997a). However, this method by Honeycutt and colleagues (1998) also measures the entorhinal cortex. To date, virtually no data have been reported on the latter mesial temporal lobe component in pediatric populations.

Morphometric assessments of the limbic temporal lobe have been greatly advanced in the last 2 years by

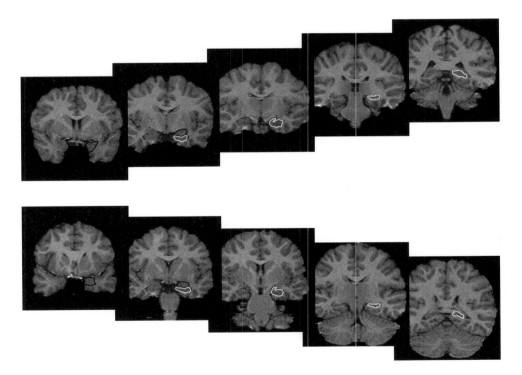

FIGURE 5-7. Coronal sections of the same brain in the anterior commissure-posterior commissure rotation (*top*) and the long axis of the hippocampus rotation (*bottom*). The amygdala has been outlined in black and the hippocampus in white, in both sets of images. (Reprinted from Kates WR, Abrams MT, Kaufmann WE, et al: Reliability and validity of MRI measurement of the amygdala and hippocampus in children with fragile X syndrome. Psychaitry Res 75:31–48, 1997, by permission of Elsevier Science B. V.)

new measurement protocols and new higher-contrast MRI sequences. As mentioned in previous sections, SPGR sequences have relatively low gray-white matter definition, which represents a particular limitation for delineating the hippocampus and adjacent structures (e.g., fimbria). For this reason, recent publications have incorporated MP-RAGE as the main volumetric sequence, in addition to new protocols for segmenting, quantifying, and spatially and volumetrically normalizing hippocampal volumes in children. With these novel approaches, Obenaus and colleagues (2001) demonstrated feasibility and reliability of hippocampal measurements in controls 13 to 60 months of age, and Scott and colleagues (2000) showed that children with mesial temporal lobe sclerosis and a history of prolonged febrile seizures had smaller and more asymmetrical hippocampi than those without such a history. Other new protocols for amygdala and hippocampus include an SPGR-based one that relies on spatial standardization and multiplanar high-resolution visualization (Prussner et al., 2000), and another method using a combination of multiplanar visualization and T1- and T2-weighted images, and tissue class-segmented data, for delineating the entire hippocampus (Pantel et al., 2000). The last two techniques have not yet been applied to pediatric populations. Finally, two other studies have expanded the age range of available normative data, which will facilitate assessments of neurodevelopmental disorders. Utsunomiya and colleagues (1999) measured the hippocampus in children 3 weeks to 14 years of age using an MP-RAGE-like sequence and found that after a sharp increase in hippocampal volume, before the third postnatal year, there is a slower period of growth that leads to a smaller hippocampal proportion of the total temporal lobe volume. As in previous studies, these authors reported a right > left asymmetry that was observed since early infancy. Pfluger and colleagues (1999), using another three-dimensional sequence and a stereologic method, found similar results to the aforementioned study; however, these authors also examined gender differences demonstrating that hippocampal growth is faster in girls.

COMPLEMENTARY MAGNETIC RESONANCE APPROACHES

As mentioned in the section on MRI sequences, T1 and T2 MRI properties cannot only be used for defining image contrast but also for measuring neural tissue properties. Maps of T1 and T2 relaxation times, typically named 1/T1 and 1/T2, reflect factors such as brain water content, degree of myelination, and mineral concentration (Steen et al., 1994; Baratti et al., 1999). Clinically, reduced T1 values have been associated with dysplastic myelination, remyelination, and calcifications (Steen et al., 2001). The precise and accurate technique

for measuring T1 relaxation, developed by Steen and colleagues (1997), consists of a single-slice inversion recovery sequence acquisition. In their application to normal development, these authors showed an age-dependent decrease in T1 in subcortical nuclei, cortical gray matter, and cerebral white matter, with the exception of the occipital white matter, maintaining a relatively constant T1 gray-white matter ratio from childhood to adulthood. Studies of patients with sickle cell disease have demonstrated widespread longer T1 that paralleled clinical severity, particularly in the thalamus (Steen et al., 1996). A more recent study evaluating relatively mildly affected subjects with sickle cell disease found lower gray matter T1 values that, as cognitive measures, were correlated with hematocrit (Steen et al., 1999). In NF-1, neurologically asymptomatic children showed low T1 values in multiple gray and white matter regions, which were associated with macrocephaly, enlarged brain structures, and cognitive deficit (Steen et al., 2001).

Changes in T2 values are less obvious on imaging and more difficult to measure; there is still controversy about the components of T2 maps and the methodology to evaluate them. In white matter, a long T2 component is attributed to axonal and extracellular water, whereas a short T2 component appears to reflect water present between the myelin bilayers (Baratti et al., 1999). Experimental studies have shown similar reductions in T2 to those in T1 values during brain development; however, they affect all type of structures, whereas T1 changes are less pronounced in gray matter (Baratti et al., 1999). T2 relaxometry has been mainly applied to examine temporal limbic structures in epilepsy and other conditions. Longer T2 relaxation times in hippocampus have been correlated to reduced hippocampal volume (Scott et al., 2001) and specific impairments in verbal memory (Wood et al., 2000) in hippocampal sclerosis, whereas prolonged T2 (postulated to reflect blood volume) in the putamen has been shown to be reversed by methylphenidate in boys with ADHD (Teicher et al., 2000). T2 maps promise to be valuable complementary tools to white matter volumetric assessments because different fiber bundles have characteristic T2 profiles, as Stieltjes and colleagues (2001) recently reported in the brainstem (Fig. 5-8).

Several strategies using conventional volumetric MRI sequences (e.g., SPGR) have been proposed for analyzing the architecture of the cerebral white matter, including the parcellation of specific fiber bundles. The Neurology/MGH group described a semiautomatic method for parcellating central cerebral white matter (Makris et al., 1999; Meyer et al., 1999), which constitutes a substantial upgrade of previous cerebral parcellation schemes (Reiss et al., 1996) and has been applied, so far, only to young adult subjects. A collaboration between the Montreal Neurological Institute and the

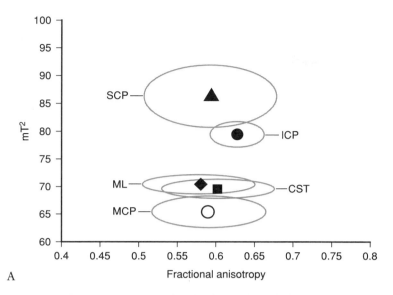

A

FIGURE 5-8. Correlation between fractional anistropy (FA) and T2 of each tract at the pons level (*A*) and images of FA (*left*) and T2 (*right*) maps at a slice of the pons level (*B*). CST, corticospinal tract; ICP, inferior cerebellar peduncle; MCP, middle cerebellar peduncle; ML, medial lemniscus; SCP, superior cerebellar peduncle. (Reprinted from Stieltjes B, Kaufmann WE, van Zijl PC, et al: Diffusion tensor imaging and axonal tracking in the human brainstem. Neuroimage 14:723–735, 2001, by permission of Academic Press.)

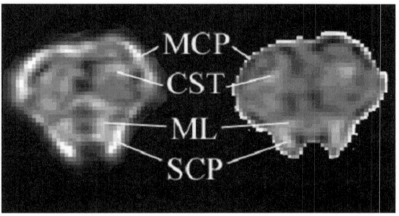

B

NIMH Child Psychiatry Branch led to an in-depth analysis of the white matter of the pediatric normative data reported by Giedd and associates (1996a). The SPGR scans were subjected, after spatial normalization and tissue class segmentation, to blurring of white matter binary masks. The latter generated three-dimensional maps (of voxels) of white matter "density" that were correlated with the subject's age, revealing age-related increases in white matter density in putative corticospinal (bilateral) and frontotemporal (left) pathways (Paus et al., 2001). Another strategy for analyzing volumetric MRI data, termed tensor mapping, provides spatially complex, four-dimensional quantitative maps of growth patterns for longitudinal evaluations. The maps take into account spatial topography and distribution of volumetric changes along time, by using deformation field principles. The process creates a template of the first imaged brain, and then, a tensor model is used to calculate local pattern of changes in relation to the template. The study focused on the corpus callosum and demonstrated, at age 3 to 6 years, growth of the ante-rior corpus callosum, corresponding to frontal networks involved in action planning. Between 6 and 15 years of age, the isthmus was the corpus callosum region with most prominent growth, consistent with temporoparietal fibers related to language function and associative processes (Thompson et al., 2000).

Finally, two MR techniques have emerged as a natural extension and complement to quantitative structural neuroimaging. Magnetic resonance spectroscopy (MRS), particularly proton MRS (^{1}H MRS), is an MR-based method that can detect and measure the concentration of important neurometabolites (Van Zijl & Barker, 1997). These include: *N*-acetyl-aspartate (NAA), a neuronal marker; choline (Cho), a glial and membrane turnover marker; creatine, an index of metabolic activity; and myoinositol, an organic osmolyte that is also an astrocytic marker. Data on concentrations of most of these compounds can be put in the format of "metabolic" map or image, when using the MRS modality termed MRS imaging (MRSI). Numerous MRS studies have evaluated normal development

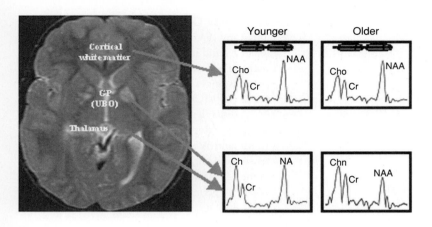

FIGURE 5-9. Diagrammatic representation of MRSI findings in NF-1. For more details, see text and Wang and colleagues (2000).

and specific disorders; the purpose of this review is to emphasize the complementary nature of MRS to MRI morphometry. Complementation not only includes correlations between changes in NAA (or another metabolite) concentrations and volumes in the same region but also, as an extension of MRI morphometry, as a higher-resolution assessment of structure. Although integration between MRS and MRI data depends on the development of coregistration and segmentation strategies, the importance of MRS for morphometric evaluations is underscored by our recent study on NF-1. In this investigation, we intended to both characterize the chemical composition of the characteristic T2 hyperintense lesions (unidentified bright objects [UBOs]) and to see whether the tissue abnormality was confined to the boundaries of the lesion. We found that although the metabolic changes were rather mild in the UBOs, there were marked abnormalities in the adjacent regions. For instance, for the typically globus pallidus-located UBOs the decrease in NAA/Cho ratio was more severe in the nearby thalamus and intermediate, with respect to the normally appearing tissue, in the basal ganglia (Wang et al., 2000; Fig. 5-9).

Diffusion tensor- or weighted-imaging (DWI or DTI) is an MRI technique that is based on the principle that water diffusion in the white matter occurs in a restricted and directional way (anisotropy) that is determined by the white matter components, namely, axonal fibers and their myelin sheaths. DWI/DTI can provide information about the magnitude of water diffusion (average diffusion constant [ADC]), affected in brain edema; extent of restriction of water diffusion (degree of diffusion anisotropy), which appears to reflect axonal preservation; and degree of alignment of water diffusion (coherence or organizational index), a postulated measure of axonal bundling (Mori & Barker, 1999). Based on high-resolution anisotropy maps, it is also possible to delineate specific fiber bundles. Although some early DTI studies have examined normal white matter development (Klingberg et al., 1999) and developmental disorders, such as dyslexia (Klingberg et al., 2000) and Rett syndrome (Naidu et al., 2001), the widespread application of this technique, as well as its integration with other morphometric assessments of the white matter, is at early stages. Figure 5-10 illustrates our preliminary studies in Rett syndrome.

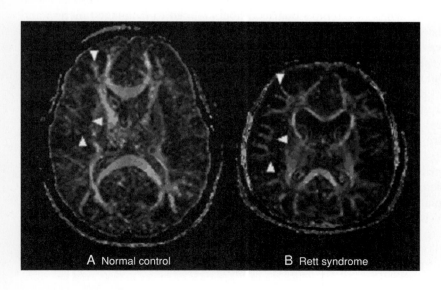

FIGURE 5-10. Color-coded anisotropy maps displaying axial slices, at the level of the dorsal basal ganglia, in Rett syndrome (B) and age/gender-matched normal control (A). The white arrowheads show longitudinally oriented (in green) dorsolateral frontal fibers. The yellow arrowheads indicate laterally oriented (in red) insular/posterior frontal fibers. Fibers running preferentially in the dorsoventral plane are shown in blue. (Reprinted from Naidu S, Kaufmann WE, Abrams MT, et al: Neuroimaging studies in Rett syndrome. Brain Dev 23(Suppl. 1):S62–S71, 2001, by permission of Elsevier Science B. V.)

CONCLUDING REMARKS

Structural pediatric neuroimaging has progressed considerably in the last decade. Advances in MRI acquisition, image analysis (software), computer hardware, and study design have contributed to this success. The current challenges include, among others, the integration of multimodality MR data, improvement of high-resolution morphometric analyses, and expansion of normative datasets. At present, we can begin to outline schemes for structural neuroimaging analyses of specific neurodevelopmental disorders that depend on the neurobiologic knowledge of the condition. The future includes the work on the aforementioned areas, as well as integration of morphometric methods and data with the emerging field of functional MRI.

■ KEY POINTS

☐ Pediatric neuroimaging is the main approach for characterizing the neurobiology of many developmental brain disorders.

☐ Longitudinal MRI studies are critical for understanding normal and aberrant brain development.

☐ Advances in MRI acquisition, image analysis (software), computer hardware, and study design have contributed to the rapid development of pediatric neuroimaging.

☐ Initial focus on psychiatric conditions has expanded to a wide spectrum of developmental disorders.

☐ Current challenges include integration of morphometric and other MR modalities (e.g., functional MRI), development of high-resolution morphometry, expansion of normative datasets, and MRI acquisition without sedation.

Acknowledgments

Supported in part by National Institutes of Health grants HD 24061, HD 24448, and HD 33175.

KEY READINGS

Kates WR, Kaufmann WE, Reiss AL: Neuroimaging of developmental and genetic disorders. Child Adolesc Psych Clin N Am 6:283–303, 1997b.

Rivkin MJ: Developmental neuroimaging of children using magnetic resonance techniques. Ment Retard Dev Disabil Res Rev 6:68–80, 2000.

Paus T et al: Maturation of white matter in the human brain: A review of magnetic resonance studies. Brain Res Bull 54:255–266, 2001.

REFERENCES

Alaghband-Rad J, Hamburger SD, Giedd JN, et al: Childhood-onset schizophrenia: Biological markers in relation to clinical characteristics. Am J Psychiatry 154:64–68, 1997.

Alarcon M, Pennington BF, Filipek PA, et al: Etiology of neuroanatomical correlates of reading disability. Dev Neuropsychol 17:339–360, 2000.

Anderson W, Gore JC: The physical basis of neuroimaging techniques—Neuroimaging—Child psychiatry. Child Adolesc Psychiatr Clin N Am 6:213–264, 1997.

Andreasen NC, Rajarethinam R, Cizadlo T, et al: Automated atlas-based volume estimation of human brain regions from MR images. J Comput Assist Tomogr 20:98–106, 1996.

Archibald SL, Fennema-Notestine C, Gamst A, et al: Brain dysmorphology in individuals with severe prenatal alcohol exposure. Dev Med Child Neurol 43:148–154, 2001.

Aylward EH, Harris GJ, Hoehn-Saric R, et al: Normal caudate nucleus in obsessive-compulsive disorder assessed by quantitative neuroimaging. Arch Gen Psychiatry 53:577–584, 1996.

Aylward EH, Minshew NJ, Goldstein G, et al: MRI volumes of amygdala and hippocampus in non-mentally retarded autistic adolescents and adults. Neurology 53:2145–2150, 1999.

Aylward EH, Reiss A: Area and volume measurement of posterior fossa structures in MRI. J Psychiatr Res 25:159–168, 1991.

Aylward EH, Schwartz J, Machlin S, et al: Bicaudate ratio as a measure of caudate volume on MR images. Am J Neuroradiol 12:1217–1222, 1991.

Baratti C, Barnett AS, Pierpaoli C: Comparative MR imaging study of brain maturation in kittens with T1, T2, and the trace of diffusion tensor. Radiology 210:133–142, 1999.

Barta PE, Dhingra L, Royall R, et al: Improving stereological estimates for the volume of structures identified in three-dimensional arrays of spatial data. J Neurosci Methods 75:111–118, 1997.

Baumgardner TL, Singer HS, Denckla MB, et al: Corpus callosum morphology in children with Tourette syndrome and attention deficit hyperactivity disorder. Neurology 47:447–482, 1996.

Brown WE, Eliez S, Menon V, et al: Preliminary evidence of widespread morphological variations of the brain in dyslexia. Neurology 56:781–783, 2001.

Carpenter MB: Human Neuroanatomy. Baltimore, MD: Williams & Wilkins, 1976.

Carper RA, Courchesne E: Inverse correlation between frontal lobe and cerebellum sizes in children with autism. Brain 123:836–844, 2000.

Cascino GD, Jack CR Jr, Parisi JE, et al: Magnetic resonance imaging-based volume studies in temporal lobe epilepsy: Pathological correlations. Ann Neurol 30:31–36, 1991.

Casey BJ, Castellanos FX, Giedd JN, et al: Implication of right frontostriatal circuitry in response inhibition and attention-deficit/hyperactivity disorder. J Am Acad Child Adolesc Psychiatry 36:374–383, 1997.

Castellanos FX, Giedd JN, Berquin PC, et al: Quantitative brain magnetic resonance imaging in girls with attention-deficit-hyperactivity disorder. Arch Gen Psychiatry 58:289–295, 2001.

Castellanos FX, Giedd JN, Eckburg P, et al: Quantitative morphology of the caudate nucleus in attention deficit hyperactivity disorder. Am J Psychiatry 151:1791–1796, 1994.

Castellanos FX, Giedd JN, Marsh WL, et al: Quantitative brain magnetic resonance imaging in attention-deficit hyperactivity disorder. Arch Gen Psychiatry 53:607–616, 1996.

Caviness VS Jr, Kennedy DN, Richelme C, et al: The human brain age 7–11 years: A volumetric analysis based on magnetic resonance images. Cereb Cortex 6:726–736, 1996.

Cendes F, Andermann F, Gloor P, et al: MRI volumetric measurement of amygdala and hippocampus in temporal lobe epilepsy. Neurology 43:719–725, 1993.

Courchesne E, Saitoh O, Yeung-Courchesne R, et al: Abnormality of cerebellar vermian lobules VI and VII in patients with infantile autism: Identification of hypoplastic and hyperplastic subgroups with MR imaging. Am J Roentgenol 162:123–130, 1994.

Crespo-Facorro B, Kim JJ, Andreasen NC, et al: Human frontal cortex: An MRI-based parcellation method. Neuroimage 10:500–519, 1999.

Crespo-Facorro B, Kim J, Andreasen NC, et al: Cerebral cortex: A topographic segmentation method using magnetic resonance imaging. Psychiatry Res 100:97–126, 2000.

Deichmann R, Good CD, Josephs O, et al: Optimization of 3-D MP-RAGE sequences for structural brain imaging. Neuroimage 12:112–128, 2000.

Eliez S, Blasey CM, Freund LS, et al: Brain anatomy, gender and IQ in children and adolescents with fragile X syndrome. Brain 124:1610–1618, 2001.

Eliez S, Reiss AL: MRI neuroimaging of childhood psychiatric disorders: A selective review. J Child Psychol Psychiatry 41:679–694, 2000.

Eliez S, Rumsey JM, Giedd JN, et al: Morphological alteration of temporal lobe gray matter in dyslexia: An MRI study. J Child Psychol Psychiatry 41:637–644, 2000a.

Eliez S, Schmitt JE, White CD, et al: Children and adolescents with velocardiofacial syndrome: A volumetric MRI study. Am J Psychiatry 157:409–415, 2000b.

Filipek PA, Richelme C, Kennedy DN, et al: The young adult human brain: An MRI-based morphometric analysis. Cereb Cortex 4:344–360, 1994.

Filipek PA, Semrud-Clikeman M, Steingard RJ, et al: Volumetric MRI analysis comparing subjects having attention-deficit hyperactivity disorder with normal controls. Neurology 48:589–601, 1997.

Frangou S, Aylward E, Warren A, et al: Small planum temporale volume in Down syndrome: A volumetric MRI study. Am J Psychiatry 154:1424–1429, 1997.

Frazier JA, Giedd JN, Hamburger SD, et al: Brain anatomic magnetic resonance imaging in childhood-onset schizophrenia. Arch Gen Psychiatry 53:617–624, 1996.

Frederikse ME, Lu A, Aylward E, et al: Sex differences in the inferior parietal lobule. Cereb Cortex 9:896–901, 1999.

Gauger LM, Lombardino LJ, Leonard CM: Brain morphology in children with specific language impairment. J Speech Lang Hear Res 40:1272–1284, 1997.

Giedd JN, Blumenthal J, Jeffries NO, et al: Brain Development during childhood and adolescence: A longitudinal MRI study. Nat Neurosci 2:861–863, 1999a.

Giedd JN, Jeffries NO, Blumenthal J, et al: Childhood-onset schizophrenia: Progressive brain changes during adolescence. Biol Psychiatry 46:892–898, 1999b.

Giedd JN, Rapoport JL, Garvey MA, et al: MRI assessment of children with obsessive compulsive disorder or tics associated with streptococcal infection. Am J Psychiatry 157:281–283, 2000.

Giedd JN, Snell JW, Lange N, et al: Quantitative magnetic resonance imaging of human brain development: Ages 4–18. Cereb Cortex 6:551–560, 1996a.

Giedd JN, Vaituzis AC, Hamburger SD, et al: Quantitative MRI of the temporal lobe, amygdala, and hippocampus in normal human development: Ages 4–18 years. J Comp Neurol 366:223–230, 1996b.

Gilbert AR, Moore GJ, Keshavan MS, et al: Decrease in thalamic volumes of pediatric patients with obsessive-compulsive disorder who are taking paroxetine. Arch Gen Psychiatry 57:449–456, 2000.

Gilbert AR, Rosenberg DR, Harenski K, et al: Thalamic volumes in patients with first-episode schizophrenia. Am J Psychiatry 158:618–624, 2001.

Goldstein JM, Goodman JM, Seidman LJ, et al: Cortical abnormalities in schizophrenia identified by structural magnetic resonance imaging. Arch Gen Psychiatry 56:537–547, 1999.

Goldstein JM, Seidman LJ, Horton NJ, et al: Normal sexual dimorphism of the adult human brain assessed by in vivo magnetic resonance imaging. Cereb Cortex 11:490–497, 2001.

Gur RE, Mozley PD, Resnick SM, et al: Magnetic resonance imaging in schizophrenia. I. Volumetric analysis of brain and cerebrospinal fluid. Arch Gen Psychiatry 48:407–412, 1991.

Heiervang E, Hugdahl K, Steinmetz H, et al: Planum temporale, planum parietale and dichotic listening in dyslexia. Neuropsychologia 38:1704–1713, 2000.

Honeycutt NA, Smith PD, Aylward E, et al: Mesial temporal lobe measurements on magnetic resonance imaging scans. Psychiatry Res 83:85–94, 1998.

Huppi PS, Inder TE: Magnetic resonance techniques in the evaluation of the perinatal brain: Recent advances and future directions. Semin Neonatol 6:195–210, 2001.

Hynd GW, Hern KL, Novey ES, et al: Attention deficit-hyperactivity disorder and asymmetry of the caudate nucleus. J Child Neurol 8:339–347, 1993.

Inder TE, Huppi PS: In vivo studies of brain development by magnetic resonance techniques. Ment Retard Dev Disabil Res Rev 6:59–67, 2000.

Insausti R, Juottonen K, Soininen H, et al: MR volumetric analysis of the human entorhinal, perirhinal, and temporopolar cortices. Am J Neuroradiol 19:659–671, 1998.

Iosifescu DV, Shenton ME, Warfield SK, et al: An automated registration algorithm for measuring MRI subcortical brain structures. Neuroimage 6:13–25, 1997.

Itoh T, Magnaldi S, White RM, et al: Neurofibromatosis type 1: The evolution of deep gray and white matter MR abnormalities. Am J Neuroradiol 15:1513–1519, 1994.

Jacobsen LK, Giedd JN, Berquin PC, et al: Quantitative morphology of the cerebellum and fourth ventricle in childhood-onset schizophrenia. Am J Psychiatry 154:1663–1669, 1997.

Jacobsen LK, Giedd JN, Vaituzis AC, et al: Temporal lobe morphology in childhood-onset schizophrenia. Am J Psychiatry 153:355–361, 1996.

Jernigan TL, Archibald SL, Fennema-Notestine C, et al: Effects of age on tissues and regions of the cerebrum and cerebellum. Neurobiol Aging 22:581–594, 2001.

Jernigan TL, Bellugi U, Sowell E, et al: Cerebral morphologic distinctions between Williams and Down syndromes. Arch Neurol 50:186–191, 1993.

Jernigan TL, Press GA, Hesselink JR: Methods for measuring brain morphologic features on magnetic resonance images. Validation and normal aging. Arch Neurol 47:27–32, 1990.

Kaplan DM, Liu AM, Abrams MT, et al: Application of an automated parcellation method to the analysis of pediatric brain volumes. Psychiatry Res 76:15–28, 1997.

Kates WR, Abrams MT, Kaufmann WE, et al: Reliability and validity of MRI measurement of the amygdala and hippocampus in children with fragile X syndrome. Psychiatry Res 75:31–48, 1997a.

Kates WR, Burnette CP, Jabs EW, et al: Regional cortical white matter reductions in velocardiofacial syndrome: A volumetric MRI analysis. Biol Psychiatry 49:677–684, 2001.

Kates WR, Folley BS, Lanham DC, et al: Cerebral growth in Fragile X syndrome: Review and comparison with Down syndrome. Microsc Res Tech 57:159–167, 2002.

Kates WR, Kaufmann WE, Reiss AL: Neuroimaging of developmental and genetic disorders. Child Adolesc Psych Clin North Am 6:283–303, 1997b.

Kates WR, Warsofsky IS, Patwardhan A, et al: Automated Talairach atlas-based parcellation and measurement of cerebral lobes in children. Psychiatry Res 91:11–30, 1999.

Kaufmann WE: Cortical development in Rett syndrome: Molecular, neurochemical, and anatomical aspects, in Kerr A, Engertrom IW (eds): The Rett Disorder and the Developing Brain. Oxford: Oxford University Press, 2001, pp. 85–110.

Kaufmann WE. Cortical histogenesis, in Aminoff MJ, Daroff RB (eds): Encyclopedia of the Neurological Sciences. Section on Neuroanatomy & Clinical Localization (Masdeu JC, ed). New York: Academic Press, 2003.

Kaufmann WE, Cohen S, Sun H-T, et al: The molecular phenotype of Fragile X syndrome: FMRP, FXRPs, and protein targets. Microsc Res Tech 57:135–144, 2002.

Kennedy DN, Lange N, Makris N, et al: Gyri of the human neocortex: An MRI-based analysis of volume and variance. Cereb Cortex 8:372–384, 1998.

Kim HI, Palmini A, Choi HY, et al: Congenital bilateral perisylvian syndrome: Analysis of the first four reported Korean patients. J Korean Med Sci 9:335–340, 1994.

Kim JJ, Crespo-Facorro B, Andreasen NC, et al: An MRI-based parcellation method for the temporal lobe. Neuroimage 11:271–288, 2000.

Klingberg T, Vaidya CJ, Gabrieli JD, et al: Myelination and organization of the frontal white matter in children: A diffusion tensor MRI study. Neuroreport 10:2817–2821, 1999.

Klingberg T, Hedehus M, Temple E, et al: Microstructure of temporo-parietal white matter as a basis for reading ability: Evidence from diffusion tensor magnetic resonance imaging. Neuron 25:493–500, 2000.

Kumra S, Giedd JN, Vaituzis AC, et al: Childhood-onset psychotic disorders: Magnetic resonance imaging of volumetric differences in brain structure. Am J Psychiatry 157:1467–1474, 2000.

Lawson JA, Vogrin S, Bleasel AF, et al: Cerebral and cerebellar volume reduction in children with intractable epilepsy. Epilepsia 41:1456–1462, 2000.

Lin Y, Okumura A, Hayakawa F, et al: Quantitative evaluation of thalami and basal ganglia in infants with periventricular leukomalacia. Dev Med Child Neurol 43:481–485, 2001.

Magnotta VA, Gold S, Andreasen NC, et al: Visualization of subthalamic nuclei with cortex attenuated inversion recovery MR imaging. Neuroimage 11:341–346, 2000.

Makris N, Meyer JW, Bates JF, et al: MRI-based topographic parcellation of human cerebral white matter and nuclei II. Rationale and applications with systematics of cerebral connectivity. Neuroimage 9:18–45, 1999.

Mataro M, Garcia-Sanchez C, Junque C, et al: Magnetic resonance imaging measurement of the caudate nucleus in adolescents with attention-deficit hyperactivity disorder and its relationship with neuropsychological and behavioral measures. Arch Neurol 54:963–968, 1997.

Matsuzawa J, Matsui M, Konishi T, et al: Age-related volumetric changes of brain gray and white matter in healthy infants and children. Cereb Cortex 11:335–342, 2001.

Mattson SN, Riley EP, Jernigan TL, et al: A decrease in the size of the basal ganglia following prenatal alcohol exposure: A preliminary report. Neurotoxicol Teratol 16:283–289, 1994.

Mattson SN, Riley EP, Sowell ER, et al: A decrease in the size of the basal ganglia in children with fetal alcohol syndrome. Alcohol Clin Exp Res 20:1088–1093, 1996.

Meyer JW, Makris N, Bates JF, et al: MRI-based topographic parcellation of human cerebral white matter. Neuroimage 9:1–17, 1999.

Moore BD 3rd, Slopis JM, Jackson EF, et al: Brain volume in children with neurofibromatosis type1: Relation to neuropsychological status. Neurology 54:914–920, 2000.

Mori S, Barker PB: Diffusion magnetic resonance imaging: Its principle and applications. Anat Rec 257:102–109, 1999.

Mostofsky SH, Wendlandt J, Cutting L, et al: Corpus callosum measurements in girls with Tourette syndrome. Neurology 53:1345–1347, 1999.

Naidu S, Kaufmann WE, Abrams MT, et al: Neuroimaging studies in Rett syndrome. Brain Dev 23(Suppl. 1):S62–S71, 2001.

Obenaus A, Yong-Hing CJ, Tong KA, et al: A reliable method for measurement and normalization of pediatric hippocampal volumes. Pediatr Res 50:124–132, 2001.

Pantel J, O'Leary DS, Cretsinger K, et al: A new method for the in vivo volumetric measurement of the human hippocampus with high neuroanatomical accuracy. Hippocampus 10:752–758, 2000.

Patwardhan AJ, Eliez S, Bender B, et al: Brain morphology in Klinefelter syndrome: Extra X chromosome and testosterone supplementation. Neurology 54:2218–2223, 2000.

Paus T, Collins DL, Evans AC, et al: Maturation of white matter in the human brain: A review of magnetic resonance studies. Brain Res Bull 54:255–266, 2001.

Peterson BS, Staib L, Scahill L, et al: Regional brain and ventricular volumes in Tourette syndrome. Arch Gen Psychiatry 58:427–440, 2001.

Peterson BS, Vohr B, Staib LH, et al: Regional brain volume abnormalities and long-term cognitive outcome in preterm infants. JAMA 284:1939–1947, 2000.

Pfluger T, Weil S, Weis S, et al: Normative volumetric data of the developing hippocampus in children based on magnetic resonance imaging. Epilepsia 40:414–423, 1999.

Pinter JD, Brown WE, Eliez S, et al: Amygdala and hippocampal volumes in children with Down syndrome: A high-resolution MRI study. Neurology 56:972–974, 2001.

Piven J, Bailey J, Ranson BJ, et al: No difference in hippocampus volume detected on magnetic resonance imaging in autistic individuals. J Autism Dev Disord 28:105–110, 1998.

Preis S, Jancke L, Schmitz-Hillebrecht J, et al: Child age and planum temporale asymmetry. Brain Cogn 40:441–452, 1999.

Pruessner JC, Li LM, Serles W, et al: Volumetry of hippocampus and amygdala with high-resolution MRI and three-dimensional analysis software: Minimizing the discrepancies between laboratories. Cereb Cortex 10:433–442, 2000.

Rademacher J, Galaburda AM, Kennedy DN, et al: Human cerebral cortex: Localization, parcellation and morphometry with magnetic resonance imaging. J Cogn Neurosci 4:352–374, 1992.

Rapoport JL, Giedd JN, Blumenthal J, et al: Progressive cortical change during adolescence in childhood-onset schizophrenia: A longitudinal magnetic resonance imaging study. Arch Gen Psychiatry 56:649–654, 1999.

Reiss AL, Abrams MT, Singer HS, et al: Brain development, gender and IQ in children: A volumetric imaging study. Brain 119:1763–1774, 1996.

Reiss AL, Eliez S, Schmitt JE, et al: IV. Neuroanatomy of Williams syndrome: A high-resolution MRI study. J Cogn Neurosci 12(Suppl. 1):65–73, 2000.

Reiss AL, Faruque F, Naidu S, et al: Neuroanatomy of Rett syndrome: A volumetric imaging study. Ann Neurol 34:227–234, 1993.

Reiss AL, Lee J, Freund L: Neuroanatomy of fragile X syndrome: The temporal lobe. Neurology 44:1317–1324, 1994.

Reiss AL, Mazzocco MM, Greenlaw R, et al: Neurodevelopmental effects of X monosomy: A volumetric imaging study. Ann Neurol 38:731–738, 1995.

Rivkin MJ: Developmental neuroimaging of children using magnetic resonance techniques. Ment Retard Dev Disabil Res Rev 6:68–80, 2000.

Robichon F, Bouchard P, Demonet J, et al: Developmental dyslexia: Re-evaluation of the corpus callosum in male adults. Eur Neurol 43:233–237, 2000.

Rumsey JM, Donohue BC, Brady DR, et al: A magnetic resonance imaging study of planum temporale asymmetry in men with developmental dyslexia. Arch Neurol 54:1481–1489, 1997.

Saitoh O, Courchesne E, Egaas B, et al: Cross-sectional area of the posterior hippocampus in autistic patients with cerebellar and corpus callosum abnormalities. Neurology 45:317–324, 1995.

Schmahmann J, Doyon J, Petrides M, et al: MRI Atlas of the Human Cerebellum. Orlando, FL: Academic Press, 2000.

Scott RC, Gadian DG, Cross JH, et al: Quantitative magnetic resonance characterization of mesial temporal sclerosis in childhood. Neurology 56:1659–1665, 2001.

Sears LL, Vest C, Mohamed S, et al: An MRI study of the basal ganglia in autism. Prog Neuropsychopharmacol Biol Psychiatry 23:613–624, 1999.

Semrud-Clikeman M, Steingard RJ, Filipek P, et al: Using MRI to examine brain-behavior relationships in males with attention deficit disorder with hyperactivity. J Am Acad Child Adolesc Psychiatry 39:477–484, 2000.

Shapleske J, Rossell SL, Simmons A, et al: Are auditory hallucinations the consequence of abnormal cerebral lateralization? A morphometric MRI study of the sylvian fissure and planum temporale. Biol Psychiatry 49:685–693, 2001.

Singer HS, Reiss AL, Brown JE, et al: Volumetric MRI changes in basal ganglia of children with Tourette's syndrome. Neurology 43:859–861, 1993.

Snell JW, Merickel MB, Ortega JM, et al: Boundary estimation of complex objects using hierarchical active surface templates. Pattern Recognit 28:1599–1609, 1995.

Song CJ, Kim JH, Kier EL, et al: MR imaging and histologic features of subinsular bright spots on T2-weighted MR images: Virchow-Robin spaces of the extreme capsule and insular cortex. Radiology 214:671–677, 2000.

Sowell ER, Delis D, Stiles J, et al: Improved memory functioning and frontal lobe maturation between childhood and adolescence: A structural MRI study. J Int Neuropsychol Soc 7:312–322, 2001a.

Sowell ER, Levitt J, Thompson PM, et al: Brain abnormalities in early-onset schizophrenia spectrum disorder observed with statistical parametric mapping of structural magnetic resonance images. Am J Psychiatry 157:1475–1484, 2000.

Sowell ER, Mattson SN, Thompson PM, et al: Mapping corpus callosum morphology and neurocognitive correlates: The effects of severe prenatal alcohol exposure. Neurology 57:235–244, 2001b.

Sowell ER, Thompson PM, Holmes CJ, et al: Localizing age-related changes in brain structure between childhood and adolescence using statistical parametric mapping. Neuroimage 9:587–597, 1999.

Sowell ER, Thompson PM, Mattson SN, et al: Voxel-based morphometric analyses of the brain in children and adolescents prenatally exposed to alcohol. Neuroreport 12:515–523, 2001c.

Steen RG, Gronemeyer SA, Kingsley PB, et al: Precise and accurate measurement of proton T1 in human brain in vivo: Validation and preliminary clinical application. J Magn Reson Imaging 4:681–691, 1994.

Steen RG, Langston JW, Reddick WE, et al: Quantitative MR imaging of children with sickle cell disease: Striking T1 elevation in the thalamus. J Magn Reson Imaging 6:226–234, 1996.

Steen RG, Ogg RJ, Reddick WE, et al: Age-related changes in pediatric brain: Quantitative MR evidence of maturational changes during adolescence. Am J Neuroradiol 18:819–828, 1997.

Steen RG, Taylor JS, Langston JW, et al: Prospective evaluation of the brain in asymptomatic children with neurofibromatosis type 1: Relationship of macrocephaly to T1 relaxation changes and structural brain abnormalities. Am J Neuroradiol 22:810–817, 2001.

Steen RG, Xiong X, Mulhern RK, et al: Subtle brain abnormalities in children with sickle cell disease: Relationship to blood hematocrit. Ann Neurol 45:279–286, 1999.

Stieltjes B, Kaufmann WE, van Zijl PC, et al: Diffusion tensor imaging and axonal tracking in the human brainstem. Neuroimage 14:723–735, 2001.

Subramaniam B, Naidu S, Reiss AL: Neuroanatomy of Rett syndrome: Cerebral cortex and posterior fossa. Neurology 48:399–407, 1997.

Swayze VW II, Johnson VP, Hanson JW, et al: Magnetic resonance imaging of brain anomalies in fetal alcohol syndrome. Pediatrics 99:232–240, 1997.

Szabo CA, Wyllie E, Siavalas EL, et al: Hippocampal volumetry in children 6 years or younger: Assessment of children with and without complex febrile seizures. Epilepsy Res 33:1–9, 1999.

Teicher MH, Anderson CM, Polcari A, et al: Functional deficits in basal ganglia of children with attention-deficit/hyperactivity disorder shown with functional magnetic resonance imaging relaxometry. Nat Med 6:470–473, 2000.

Thompson PM, Giedd JN, Woods RP, et al: Growth patterns in the developing brain detected by using continuum mechanical tensor maps. Nature 404:190–193, 2000.

Utsunomiya H, Takano K, Okazaki M, et al: Development of the temporal lobe in infants and children: Analysis by MR-based volumetry. Am J Neuroradiol 20:717–723, 1999.

Van Zijl PC, Barker PB: Magnetic resonance spectroscopy and spectroscopic imaging for the study of brain metabolism. Ann N Y Acad Sci 820:75–96, 1997.

Wang PY, Kaufmann WE, Koth CW, et al: Thalamic involvement in neurofibromatosis type 1: Evaluation with proton magnetic resonance spectroscopic imaging. Ann Neurol 47:477–484, 2000.

Whalley HC, Wardlaw JM: Accuracy and reproducibility of simple cross-sectional linear and area measurements of brain structures and their comparison with volume measurements. Neuroradiology 43:263–271, 2001.

Woermann FG, Free SL, Koepp MJ, et al: Abnormal cerebral structure in juvenile myoclonic epilepsy demonstrated with voxel-based analysis of MRI. Brain 122:2101–2108, 1999.

Woermann FG, van Elst LT, Koepp MJ, et al: Reduction of frontal neocortical grey matter associated with affective aggression in patients with temporal lobe epilepsy: An objective voxel by voxel analysis of automatically segmented MRI. J Neurol Neurosurg Psychiatry 68:162–169, 2000.

Wood AG, Saling MM, O'Shea MF, et al: Components of verbal learning and hippocampal damage assessed by T2 relaxometry. J Int Neuropsychol Soc 6:529–538, 2000.

Yamanouchi H, Kato T, Matsuda H, et al: MRI in neurofibromatosis type I: Using fluid-attenuated inversion recovery pulse sequences. Pediatr Neurol 12:286–290, 1995.

Zametkin A and Liotta W: Future of brain imaging—Neuroimaging—Child psychiatry. Child Adolesc Psychiatr Clin N Am 6:447–460, 1997.

Zipursky RB, Lim KO, Sullivan EV, et al: Widespread cerebral gray matter volume deficits in schizophrenia. Arch Gen Psychiatry 49:195–205, 1992.

Functional Neuroimaging

Peter Herscovitch

Cerebral blood flow
Fluorodeoxyglucose
Functional brain mapping
Neuronal activation
Positron emission tomography
Radiotracer
Single photon emission computed tomography

INTRODUCTION

The term *functional brain imaging* refers to methods that provide images of the brain related to its physiology or biochemistry rather than structure. There are two nuclear medicine-based approaches to functional brain imaging, positron emission tomography (PET) and single photon emission computed tomography (SPECT). Both use compounds that are labeled with radioactive atoms, or radionuclides. These compounds,

All material in this chapter is in the public domain, with the exception of any borrowed figures or tables.

termed radiotracers, are administered in very small quantities, so that they have no effect on the underlying process being studied. Specialized devices provide tomographic images of the distribution of the radiotracer in brain, from which physiologic information can be obtained. These tomographic images are views of "slices" or planes through the body. X-ray computed tomography (CT) uses radiation from a source of x-rays external to the body to provide cross-sectional images that represent the relative tissue density in the slice. Tomographic methods in nuclear medicine use radiation that is emitted from within the body, from radiotracers administered to the subject. These methods, referred to as "emission computed tomography," provide images of the distribution of radioactivity in tissue slices. Tomographic planes are typically obtained perpendicular to the long axis of the body and are two-dimensional in nature. However, a set of such images can be assembled to provide a three-dimensional representation of the distribution of radioactivity in the body.

Methods to measure cerebral blood flow (CBF) and metabolism in humans are the most common applications of functional brain imaging. They have been progressively refined over several decades, becoming more regional and less invasive. These methods were developed synergistically with extensive research that showed that CBF and metabolism are related to local neuronal activity and that the brain needs an uninterrupted supply of oxygen and glucose to maintain tissue integrity. In the 1940s, Kety and Schmidt (1948) pioneered a method for calculating CBF from measurements of the arterial and cerebral venous concentrations of inhaled nitrous oxide gas. These CBF values, combined with measurements of brain arterial-venous differences for glucose and oxygen, permitted the determination of the metabolism of the brain as well. The Kety-Schmidt technique, however, did not provide regional measurements. The need for regional data led to methods to measure CBF with radiotracers and external radiation detectors. They were used to record the clearance from different brain regions of diffusible radioactive gases such as xenon-133 (^{133}Xe) that were administered by inhalation or by injection into the internal carotid artery (Obrist et al., 1967; Lassen & Ingvar, 1972). Subsequently, techniques using intracarotid injection of tracers labeled with positron-emitting radioactivity were developed to measure not only CBF, but also cerebral blood volume and metabolism (Welch et al., 1975). These methods were limited, however, by their invasiveness and poor spatial resolution.

While these methods were being developed for use in humans, major advances were made to measure regional CBF (rCBF) and glucose metabolism in laboratory animals with radiotracers. These methods used tissue autoradiography to record local radioactivity from brain slices applied to photographic film and mathematical models to describe the in vivo behavior of

the radiotracer. rCBF was measured with diffusible radiotracers (Kety, 1951; Kety, 1960; Sakurada et al., 1978) and regional cerebral glucose metabolism (rCMRglc) with deoxyglucose labeled with carbon-14 (Sokoloff et al., 1977). Because of the ability to label similar radiotracers with positron-emitting atoms, PET could be used to extend these methods to humans, to permit truly regional measurements throughout the brain.

The PET scanner provides tomographic images of the distribution of positron-emitting radiotracers in the body. From these images, physiologic measurements can be obtained. PET has been widely used as a research tool to study normal brain function and the pathophysiology of neurologic and psychiatric disease. Its role in the management of patients with brain disorders is at an earlier stage. Conceptually, PET consists of three components: (1) tracer compounds labeled with radioactive atoms that emit positrons; (2) scanners that provide tomographic images of the concentration of positron-emitting radioactivity in the body; and (3) mathematical models that describe the in vivo behavior of radiotracers, so that the physiologic process under study can be quantitated from the images. The first tomographs for quantitative PET imaging were developed in the mid 1970s (Ter-Pogossian et al., 1975). Subsequent advances resulted in instruments with improved spatial resolution and sensitivity. Radiotracer techniques have been developed to study a wide variety of physiologic variables, including rCBF and blood volume; glucose, oxygen, and protein metabolism; blood-brain barrier (BBB) permeability; neuroreceptor-neurotransmitter systems; and tissue pH.

SPECT is another nuclear medicine technique that provides tomographic images of radioactivity. It is simpler than PET because it uses radiotracers labeled with radionuclides that are available in clinical nuclear medicine departments, such as technetium-99m (^{99m}Tc); a cyclotron is not required for radionuclide production. However, its quantitative accuracy is less than that of PET, and the variety of radiopharmaceuticals for studying the brain is more limited. It has been used primarily to map cerebral perfusion. Improvements in instrumentation and radiopharmaceuticals are being actively pursued, especially in the development of radiotracers to image neuroreceptors, and there is a strong interest in clinical SPECT brain studies.

This chapter provides an overview of PET instrumentation, radiotracers, and mathematical modeling, emphasizing methods to measure cerebral hemodynamics and metabolism, the most commonly used methods. These methods have resulted in fundamental contributions to our understanding of the normal and diseased brain, especially in the areas of neuropsychology and behavioral neurology. They remain important research tools and are also being applied in the clinical environment. In addition, SPECT instrumentation and radiotracer methods are reviewed. The analysis and interpretation of functional brain images obtained with both PET and SPECT are discussed.

COUPLING OF CEREBRAL BLOOD FLOW AND METABOLISM TO NEURONAL ACTIVITY

A fundamental premise underlying functional brain imaging is that CBF and metabolism are intimately related to the activity of neurons. The concept that local CBF and metabolism could reflect local brain function was anticipated over 100 years ago. In a remarkably prescient paper, Roy and Sherrington (1890; Friedland & Iadecola, 1991, p. 10) hypothesized that:

(There is) an automatic mechanism by which the blood-supply of any part of the cerebral tissue is varied in accordance with the activity of the chemical changes which underlie the functional action of that part. Bearing in mind that strong evidence exists of localisation of function in the brain, . . . an automatic mechanism . . . is well fitted to provide for a local variation of the blood supply in accordance with local variations of the functional activity.

It was only many decades later that methodological advances made it possible to test the Sherrington hypothesis. Experiments in both animals and humans have demonstrated proportional relationships, termed coupling, between neuronal activity and both rCBF and rCMRglc (Sokoloff, 1981; Yarowsky & Ingvar, 1981; Jueptner & Weiller, 1995; Villringer & Dirnagl, 1995; Clarke & Sokoloff, 1999).

Under normal conditions, virtually all of the brain's energy needs are met by glucose (Clarke & Sokoloff, 1999). At rest, about 85% of brain glucose consumption is used to provide energy for functional metabolism via the production of the energy-containing molecule, adenosine triphosphate (ATP); the remainder is used for synthesis of macromolecules (Jueptner & Weiller, 1995). Because there are minimal stores of glucose in brain, increased energy demands must be met by increased glucose extraction from arterial blood. Several fundamental experiments demonstrated that rCMRglc is *coupled* or linearly related to local neuronal activity. Increased rCMRglc due to increased neuronal firing was demonstrated in animal models in the superior cervical ganglion, the dorsal horn of the spinal cord, and the visual system. Decreased rCMRglc was also observed with interventions that decrease neuronal activity. In humans, PET experiments with [^{18}F]fluorodeoxyglucose (FDG) demonstrated graded increases in rCMRglc in visual cortex with increasing neuronal activity due to more complex visual stimuli (Phelps et al., 1981).

Several studies demonstrated that the increase in rCMRglc reflects the activity in synapses where nerve cells communicate. Most of the additional glucose consumption during functional activation is required by the ATP-dependent Na$^+$-K$^+$ pump to maintain ionic gradients across cell membranes (Yarowsky & Ingvar, 1981; Sokoloff, 1999). These gradients must be restored after depolarization. The site of largest metabolic demand is not the neuronal cell body. Rather, it is in the neuropil, where axons terminate and synapse with dendrites (Schwartz et al., 1979; Kadekaro et al., 1985). This is where neurons have the greatest surface area-to-volume ratio, and therefore where ions pumping across cell membranes is the greatest. These observations are important for the interpretation of rCMRglc measurements. A local increase in rCMRglc is not necessarily due to increased firing of neuronal cell bodies locally; rather, it can reflect increased activity in the terminal fields of neurons projecting to the region (Wooten & Collins, 1981) or a change in the activity of local interneurons. Inhibitory activity of axon terminals also increases energy consumption, so that increases in rCMRglc may represent neuronal activity that is, at least in part, inhibitory.

Recent work has implicated a biochemical mechanism involving astrocytes in the coupling of glucose utilization to neuronal activity (Magistretti & Pellerin, 1999). Astrocytes take up the excitatory neurotransmitter glutamate that is released by activated neurons. The energy for glutamate uptake and its subsequent conversion to inactive glutamine is provided by increased glucose uptake and utilization in the astrocyte. Lactate is subsequently produced and may support the increased energy demand of neurons.

These considerations of the relationship between local neuronal activity and metabolism provide the background for discussing two other physiologic "couplings," between rCBF and metabolism, and between rCBF and neuronal activity. In the resting state, there is a tight correlation between rCBF and rCMRglc in both the awake and anesthetized rat (Sokoloff, 1981). Dynamic coupling of rCBF and rCMRglc occurs during somatosensory activation in the rat. Coupling between rCBF and rCMRglc is present in human brain at rest and during increased neuronal activity (Fox et al., 1988).

Several studies demonstrated that rCBF is coupled to functional activity. Sokoloff observed an increase in rCBF in visual pathways in the rat during photic stimulation, anticipating the use of rCBF measurements to map human brain function (Sokoloff, 1961). Leniger-Follert and Hossman (1979), using hydrogen clearance to monitor cortical flow in animals, demonstrated a flow response in somatosensory cortex during sensory stimulation that was related to the stimulus frequency and the amplitude of the cortical electrical response. Flow coupling was demonstrated in humans with PET. For example, there is a linear relationship between the rate of pattern-flash visual stimulus and rCBF in visual cortex (Fox & Raichle, 1984) and between the presentation rate of words and rCBF in the primary auditory cortex (Price et al., 1992).

The vascular response to activation is fast, occurring within seconds of the change in neuronal activity. The underlying vascular event appears to be local dilation of arterioles, rather than recruitment of previously unperfused capillaries (Villringer & Dirnagl, 1995). Despite extensive research, however, the physiologic mechanism underlying the flow response to neuronal activation is not known. The classical teaching was that oxidative metabolism of glucose supported increased neuronal activity. Local depletion of oxygen and accumulation of metabolites would dilate blood vessels and increase rCBF to maintain local homeostasis (Lou et al., 1987). This mechanism has not been demonstrated, however. Furthermore, although rCMRglc substantially increases during activation, there is only a small increase in regional cerebral oxygen metabolism (rCMRO$_2$); this implies *nonoxidative* metabolism of glucose. For example, during somatosensory or visual stimulation in humans, there is a minimal increase in rCMRO$_2$, despite large increases in rCBF and rCMRglc (Fox & Raichle, 1986; Fox et al., 1988). The increase is so much greater in rCBF than in rCMRO$_2$ that the percent extraction of oxygen from blood substantially *decreases*. (The resultant increase in local blood oxygenation is the basis for the blood oxygen level dependent [BOLD] signal in functional magnetic resonance imaging; see Chapter 7.)

This observation challenged the hypothesis that oxidative glucose metabolism regulates rCBF during activation. Both a reexamination of earlier reports as well as subsequent work have provided additional evidence supporting this observation (Raichle, 1998). Several chemical mediators have been proposed to control rCBF during activation, including pH, adenosine, potassium ions, and nitric oxide, but none proven. The need for increased metabolic substrate per se does not drive the flow response; there is no increase in the rCBF response to activation during either hypoglycemia or hypoxia (Powers et al., 1996; Mintun et al., 2001). The cerebral microvasculature is densely innervated with nerves that release vasoactive neurotransmitters, and these have been postulated to regulate acute flow changes, but a specific mechanism has not been demonstrated.

APPLICATIONS OF METHODS TO MEASURE REGIONAL CEREBRAL BLOOD FLOW AND METABOLISM

Measurements of rCBF and metabolism are widely used to study the pathophysiology of neurologic and psychiatric disease (Fulham & Di Chiro, 1996; Drevets, 1998). Abnormalities in specific brain regions, in comparison to data from an appropriate control group, reflect abnormal neuronal activity. The degree of the abnormality can be correlated with disease severity, and the effect of treatment can be studied over time. Often, several brain areas are affected, implying an abnormality in underlying brain networks. The effects of drugs on rCBF and metabolism can provide insight into their mechanism of action, especially when correlated with changes in symptoms. Tissue damage or loss, either gross or due to loss of neurons, decreases flow and metabolism. In addition, decreases can occur *distant* to a lesion. This phenomenon, called *diaschisis*, is attributed to decreased neuronal activity in a brain structure due to loss of projections from a damaged region. For example, flow and metabolism often are decreased in the cerebellum contralateral to a cerebral hemispheric infarct.

Studies of cerebral hemodynamics and oxygen metabolism with PET and oxygen-15 labeled tracers have been particularly useful to study cerebrovascular disease (Baron, 2001; Grubb & Powers, 2001). A CBF image alone, however, is inadequate to characterize a patient's physiologic status. It does not show whether flow is reduced due to decreased metabolic needs of brain tissue versus decreased perfusion pressure in carotid disease. In diaschisis, for example, decreased flow reflects decreased local metabolic demand rather than impaired circulation. Distal to a narrowed or occluded carotid artery, blood flow can be decreased, or it can be maintained by autoregulatory vasodilation in response to the decrease in perfusion pressure. This can be detected with measurements of regional cerebral blood volume (rCBV). Tissue integrity distal to a carotid lesion can be maintained not only by vasodilation but also by increased extraction of oxygen from blood. Measuring oxygen metabolism as well as CBF gives information about the adequacy of oxygen delivery in relation to tissue needs. Combined measurements of rCBF, rCBV, and rCMRO$_2$ have provided insights into the evolution of acute cerebral infarction, the flow levels required to maintain tissue integrity, the physiologic abnormalities that predict increased risk for stroke, and the effect of medical and surgical therapies.

One of the most common uses of rCBF imaging with PET is mapping brain function in humans (Herscovitch, 1995; Jueptner & Weiller, 1995). rCBF is imaged while subjects perform different neurobehavioral tasks—cognitive, motor, or sensory. Because of the coupling between flow and neuronal activity, changes in rCBF reflect changes in local brain activity during the task. Typically, one task is a control condition, with the others being specific tasks of interest. The ability to perform many brief measurements of rCBF in one scan session (see below) has made this a very powerful approach. Sophisticated methods of data analysis are used to localize the areas of significant rCBF change and identify those brain areas involved in task performance.

POSITRON EMISSION TOMOGRAPHY

PET Physics

Formation of the PET Image

PET provides tomographic images of the distribution of positron-emitting radioactivity using rings of radiation detectors that are arrayed around the body. Because of the nature of the positron and the techniques used for image reconstruction, it is possible to obtain *absolute* radioactivity measurements from these images (Daube-Witherspoon & Herscovitch, 1996).

Certain radioactive atoms, such as oxygen-15 or fluorine-18, decay by emitting a positron from their nucleus. Positrons are the "antimatter" particles to electrons; they have the same mass, but are positively charged. After emission from the nucleus, positrons travel up to a few millimeters in tissue, losing kinetic energy. When almost at rest, they interact with atomic electrons, resulting in the "annihilation" of both particles. Their combined mass is converted into two high-energy (511-keV each) photons or gamma rays that travel in opposite directions from the annihilation site at the speed of light. (Gamma rays or photons have the same physical properties as x-rays, but arise from subatomic processes.) Positrons from a specific radionuclide do not all have the same energy. Rather, they have a range of energies. The greater the positron energy, the farther it travels from the nucleus before annihilation. The term *positron range* refers to the net distance away from the decay site that the positron travels.

Detection of these annihilation photon pairs is used to measure both the location and the amount of radioactivity in the brain. The two annihilation photons are detected by two opposing radiation detectors that are connected by an electronic coincidence circuit (Fig. 6-1). This circuit records a decay event only when both detectors sense the almost simultaneous arrival of both photons (the time window for coincidence detection is typically 5–20 ns). The site of the decay event is therefore localized to the volume of space between the two detectors.

Several rings of radiation detectors are used. Opposing detectors in each ring are connected by coincidence circuits. With each decay event, the two resulting annihilation photons are detected as a coincidence line, so that the number of coincidence lines sensed by any detector pair is proportional to the amount of radioactivity between them. A computer records the coincidence events from each ring. The coincidence lines are sorted into parallel groups, each group representing a view or projection of the radioactivity from a different angle. Tomographic images of the underlying distri-

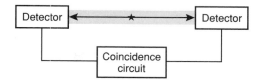

★   Site of annihilation
→   Annihilation photon path
▨   Volume in which annihilation events are detected

FIGURE 6-1. The two high-energy photons resulting from a positron emission and annihilation are detected by two radiation detectors that are connected by an electronic coincidence circuit. A radioactive decay event, that is, a positron emission, is recorded as a coincidence line between the detectors only when both photons are detected almost simultaneously. A very short time window for photon arrival, typically 5 to 20 nsec, called the coincidence resolving time, is allowed for registration of a coincidence event. This coincidence requirement localizes the site of the annihilation to the space between the detectors.

bution of radioactivity are then reconstructed with the same mathematical technique used in conventional x-ray CT (Fig. 6-2). The intensity of each point or pixel in the reconstructed PET image is proportional to the concentration of radioactivity at the corresponding location in the brain. To calibrate the scanner to obtain absolute radioactivity measurements, a cylinder filled with a uniform solution of known radioactivity concentration is imaged. The calibration factor is calculated to convert the counts in the PET image to units of radioactivity concentration (e.g., nCi/cc).

Limitations to Quantification of the PET Signal

A variety of physical processes, such as attenuation, deadtime losses, scatter, and random coincidences, affect the PET image and are accounted for during image reconstruction. Other factors such as image noise and spatial resolution also affect image quality and are important considerations when using PET (Daube-Witherspoon & Herscovitch, 1996).

A key step is a correction for the absorption or attenuation of annihilation photons that occurs when they interact with tissue. This substantially decreases the number of coincidence counts detected. The amount of attenuation can be estimated using an assumed value for the attenuating properties of tissue, but actual measurements are more accurate. Before the administration of radiotracer, a separate "transmission scan" is performed with a source of positron-emitting radioactivity positioned between the subject's head and the detector rings. The rod-shaped source is rotated around the head. A similar measurement is made with nothing in the scanner field of view. The ratio of the two

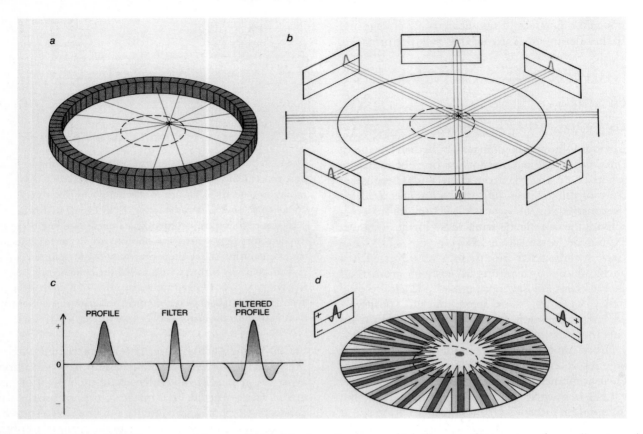

FIGURE 6-2. The steps in PET reconstruction are depicted in these diagrams, which illustrate the imaging of a small region of uniform radioactivity in a single tomographic plane. *A,* Multiple coincidence lines are recorded by opposing detector pairs in the ring. Each line results from a positron emission and annihilation, so that the number of coincidence lines recorded by any detector pair is proportional to the amount of radioactivity between them. *B,* After the "scan," the coincidence lines are sorted into parallel groups representing the profile or projection of the radioactivity distribution viewed from a different angle. These projections are then combined using the same mathematical technique as in x-ray CT to obtain the PET image. *C,* Each projection is mathematically processed by means of a special function called the filter function. *D,* The modified projections are then combined by "back-projection" to reconstruct an image of the radioactivity distribution. Note that there are several other steps in reconstruction, for example, corrections for attenuation, deadtime, and random and scattered coincidence counts, as described in the text. (From "Positron-Emission Tomography," M. M. Ter-Pogossian et al. Copyright © October 1980 by SCIENTIFIC AMERICAN, Inc. All rights reserved. By permission of SCIENTIFIC AMERICAN.)

measurements gives the amount of attenuation between each detector pair by the head and is used in the image reconstruction process to correct for attenuation.

The PET image has statistical noise because of the random nature of radioactive decay. The disintegration rate of a radioactive sample undergoes moment-to-moment variation. The resultant uncertainty in measuring the amount of radioactivity decreases as the number of counts recorded increases. Similarly, the statistical reliability of a PET measurement depends on the number of counts. The situation is more complex, however, because the value of radioactivity in any brain region is obtained from an image reconstructed from multiple views of the radioactivity in the entire brain slice. Thus, the noise in a brain region is increased by noise in other brain regions. Excessive noise gives the PET image a grainy appearance and decreases the ability to quantitate radioactivity accurately. Image noise depends on the number of counts collected, which in turn depends on scanner sensitivity, the duration of the scan, and the concentration of radioactivity in the field of view. Sensitivity (the number of decay events detected in relation to the number that occur) is determined by scanner design features, such as the nature, size, and arrangement of the radiation detectors. Although increasing scan duration increases counts, this is often not possible, because of the short half-life of the radiotracer or because it is not compatible with the tracer-kinetic model being used. Administering more radioactivity is limited by radiation safety considerations and also by the inability of tomographs to operate accurately at high count rates, that is, by count rate performance.

Count rate performance refers to the level of radioactivity that can be accurately measured. It is limited by deadtime loss and by random coincidences. Deadtime loss is the decreasing ability to register counts as the count rate increases, because of the time required by the detectors and electronic circuitry to process each count. Deadtime causes a reduction in measured coincidences with increasing radioactivity. This reduction can be predicted for a given count rate so that a correction factor can be applied. This correction however, does not compensate for the loss in statistical accuracy that occurs because fewer counts were collected. Random coincidences also limit count rate performance. These occur when two photons from two *different* positron annihilations are sensed by a detector pair within the coincidence resolving time, so that a false or random coincidence count is collected. The fraction of total coincidences recorded that are random increases linearly with radioactivity. Random coincidences add noisy background to the image. Although corrections can be made that subtract an estimate of these false counts, the contribution to image noise persists. Thus, the amount of radioactivity administered must be carefully selected to balance the competing effects of improved counting statistics with the "diminishing returns" due to deadtime and random coincidences.

Another source of background noise is Compton scattering. Scattering occurs when an annihilation photon traveling in tissue is deflected in a collision with an electron, so that its direction changes. This results in incorrect positioning of the coincidence line. Not only is information lost from the affected coincidence line, but also a noisy background level is added to the image. This leads to an overestimation of radioactivity, especially in areas with low radioactivity. It is necessary to correct for scatter, because it can contribute 20% or more of the counts in an image.

A critical issue in interpreting PET (and SPECT) images is the concept of image resolution. Image resolution is the minimum distance by which two points of radioactivity must be separated to be perceived independently in the reconstructed image. Limited resolution, which is visually apparent as blurring of the image, has a major effect on the ability to quantify radioactivity accurately, especially in small structures. The resolution of a PET image depends on the accurate localization of positron-emitting nuclei. This is affected by the physics of positron annihilation and by detector design. Annihilation photons are produced only after the positron has traveled up to several millimeters from the nucleus. This limits the accuracy of localizing the nucleus. The distance the positron travels before annihilation varies, depending on the radionuclide; average positron range is 1.2 mm for ^{18}F, 2.1 mm for ^{11}C. In addition, the angle between the two annihilation photons deviates slightly from 180 degrees, causing a slight misplacement of the coincidence line. These effects result in a 1- to 3-mm resolution loss. Detector size and shape determine how accurately the position of each coincidence line is recorded; smaller detectors provide better resolution. Resolution is measured by imaging a thin line-source of positron-emitting radioactivity (Fig. 6-3). The resolution of current scanners is about 4 to 5 mm in the image plane. Small-animal scanners specially designed to image rats and mice have achieved resolutions better than 2 mm.

PET Instrumentation

A PET system consists of many components. Several rings of radiation detectors are mounted in a gantry. Each detector consists of a small scintillation crystal that gives off light when the energy of an annihilation photon is deposited in it. The detector is coupled to a photomultiplier tube, an electronic device that converts the light pulse to an electrical signal that is fed into the coincidence circuitry. Scanners have numerous rings, each containing up to several hundred detectors, with a tomographic slice provided by each ring. In addition, "cross-slices" halfway between the detector rings are derived from coincidences between opposing detectors in adjacent rings. Lead septa or shields between detector rings block photons that originate in more distant tissue slices. In a state-of-the-art system with 32 rings of detectors, 63 contiguous slices are obtained simultaneously. A dedicated computer is used to control the scanning process, collect the coincidence count information, and reconstruct the images. A major advance in scanner design permits coincidence counts to be collected by opposing detectors that are not in the same or adjacent rings (Bailey et al., 1998). These scanners operate without lead septa between slices. Because more coincidence lines are collected by this "three-dimensional" imaging approach, scanner sensitivity is increased about fourfold. This permits the same number of image counts to be obtained with shorter scans or less administered radioactivity. The number of scattered events that are detected substantially increases as well, increasing the need for accurate scatter correction.

During the scan, the subject lies on a special table that is fitted with a head holder that restrains head movement. The gantry has low-powered lasers that project lines onto the subject's head to aid in positioning. Some gantries can be tilted from the vertical to obtain slices in specific planes, for example, parallel to the canthomeatal line.

Positron-Emitting Radiotracers

The second requirement for PET is a radiotracer of physiologic interest that is labeled with a positron-emitting radionuclide. A radiotracer can be a naturally

FIGURE 6-3. This figure shows how the resolution of a PET scanner is defined and measured. Thin line sources of positron-emitting radioactivity perpendicular to the image plane are scanned (*upper panel*). Because of resolution limitations, the radioactivity in each source appears blurred or spread over a larger area (*middle panel*) than the small dot one would expect. Scanner resolution is defined by the amount of spreading that occurs. A plot of the image intensity along a line through the center of the images (*lower panel*) shows that this spreading approximates a bell-shaped or gaussian curve. The width of this curve at one half of its maximum height (termed the full-width-at-half-maximum, or FWHM) is the measure of resolution. Here the resolution is 1.2 cm. (Reproduced with permission from Ter-Pogossian MM, Phelps ME, Hoffman EJ, et al: A positron-emission transaxial tomograph for nuclear imaging [PETT]. Radiology 114:89–98, 1975.)

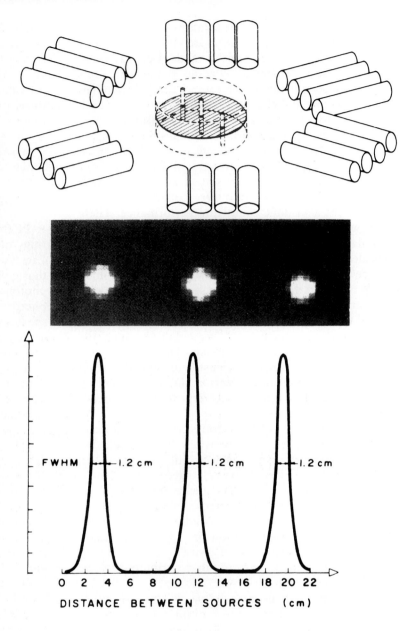

occurring compound such as glucose, in which one of the atoms is replaced with its radioactive counterpart, or it can be a labeled analog with in vivo behavior similar to that of the natural substance. Alternatively, it can be a synthetic compound, such as a radiolabeled drug, which interacts with a specific biologic system.

The positron-emitting nuclides most commonly used to label PET radiotracers and their half-lives are oxygen-15 (^{15}O; 2.04 minutes), nitrogen-13 (^{13}N; 9.97 minutes), carbon-11 (^{11}C; 20.3 minutes), and fluorine-18 (^{18}F; 109.8 minutes). The half-life is the time required for radioactivity to decay to one half of its original value; after five half-lives, less than 2% of the original radioactivity remains. The chemical nature of ^{15}O, ^{13}N, and ^{11}C is identical to that of their nonradioactive counterparts, which are basic constituents of living matter as well as of most drugs. Thus, they can be incorporated into radiotracers with the same in vivo behavior as the corresponding nonradioactive compound. ^{18}F is used to substitute for hydrogen or hydroxyl (OH) groups to synthesize analogs with characteristics similar to those of the unsubstituted compound. In addition, some drugs contain fluorine, so that ^{18}F-labeled counterparts can be synthesized. Because of their short half-lives, relatively large amounts of these radionuclides can be administered to provide good-quality images, but because of rapid decay, the radiation exposure is acceptable. The short half-lives, especially of ^{15}O, permit repeat studies in the same subject in one experimental session because of rapid physical decay after each administration.

The short half-life of PET nuclides imposes demands on the synthesis of PET radiotracers. On-site production of radionuclides by means of a cyclotron is typically required, although regional distribution of ^{18}F-labeled tracers from a central facility is becoming common. Rapid techniques for radiotracer synthesis and quality control are necessary. These must yield products that are pure, sterile, and nontoxic. An important consideration is specific activity, the amount of radioactivity per unit weight of compound. It is not possible to remove all traces of nonradioactive elements, for example, carbon or fluorine, from the chemical apparatus. When these atoms are incorporated in the synthesis rather than radioactive atoms, some of the compound is produced in its nonradioactive form, lowering specific activity. Radiotracers must have high enough specific activity so that the amount administered produces good quality images without causing physiologic or toxic effects. The required specific activity depends on the potential for the compound to cause such effects. For example, this potential exists for ^{15}O or ^{11}C carbon monoxide used to measure blood volume (see below), and for tracers that bind to neuroreceptors.

A radiotracer must have properties that permit the desired physiologic measurement to be made. Important factors include how well it enters the brain across the BBB, its metabolism in the body to radioactive metabolites and whether these metabolites enter brain, and the ability to develop a mathematical model to calculate the physiologic measurement of interest. There are several other considerations for radiotracers designed to image neuroreceptors. These include how well the tracer binds to the receptor type of interest, whether it binds to other receptors, and the degree of "nonspecific binding" in tissue. This refers to uptake and retention in tissue because of physicochemical properties such as solubility that is unrelated to the presence of neuroreceptors. Nonspecific binding obscures the PET signal that comes from radiotracer that is specifically bound to receptors.

Preclinical experiments are required to characterize a potential radiotracer before human use. These use tissue sampling or autoradiography in small animals or PET studies in large ones. The recent development of PET scanners designed to image small animals such as rats will facilitate the assessment of new PET tracers (Myers, 2001). A wide variety of positron-emitting radiopharmaceuticals have been synthesized (Table 6-1) (Wagner et al., 1995).

Radiotracer Modeling

A mathematical model is required to calculate the value of the physiologic variable of interest from measurements of radiotracer concentration in brain and blood.

The model describes the in vivo behavior of the radiotracer, that is, the relationship over time between the amount of tracer delivered to a brain region in its arterial input and the amount of tracer in the region. The use of models allows PET to be a quantitative physiologic technique rather than just an imaging modality (Carson, 1996).

Compartmental models are generally used. It is assumed that there are entities called compartments, which have uniform biologic properties and in which the tracer concentration is uniform at any instant in time. The compartments can be physical spaces such as the extravascular space, or biochemical entities such as neuroreceptor-binding sites. The number and nature of the compartments in a model depend on knowledge of the system being studied. Rate constants describe the movement of the tracer between compartments. The amount of tracer that leaves a compartment per unit time is proportional to the amount that is in the compartment; the rate constant is the constant of proportionality. The model is described by one or more equations that contain measurable terms, that is, the brain and blood radiotracer concentrations over time, and unknowns of interest such as blood flow or neuroreceptor concentration. Several factors must be considered in developing a model. These include tracer transport across the BBB, the behavior of the tracer in brain, the presence of labeled metabolites in blood, the changes in tracer behavior in abnormal tissue, and the ability to solve the model for the unknown parameters. The number of unknowns cannot be so large that is impossible to solve the model accurately from the measured data.

Methods to assess receptor binding are often complicated (Ichise et al., 2001). They can require complex mathematical equations, extended measurements of blood and tissue radioactivity, and determination of radioactive metabolites in blood so they can be subtracted from total blood radioactivity to obtain the level of parent radiotracer. For clinical research and diagnostic applications, it is desirable to have simpler methods of data collection and analysis. These methods involve achieving an equilibrium distribution of radiotracer in brain, either by waiting for an appropriate period after bolus tracer injection or by using a constant infusion of tracer. When the tracer has achieved equilibrium, the radioactivity in a structure of interest reflects the binding of the radiotracer to the receptor (specific binding) as well as nonspecific uptake. Receptor binding is measured by comparing the radiotracer concentration in the area of interest to that in an area devoid of the receptor. For example, with dopamine D2 receptor radioligands, the ratio of activity in striatum to cerebellum is used.

Error analysis and model validation are important in developing a model. Error analysis consists of

TABLE 6-1. Representative PET Radiotracers

Physiologic process or system	Radiotracer
Cerebral blood flow	[^{15}O]water, [^{15}O]CO$_2$, [^{15}O]butanol, [^{11}C]butanol
Cerebral blood volume	[^{15}O]CO, [^{11}C]CO
Cerebral energy metabolism	
Oxygen metabolism	[^{15}O]oxygen
Glucose metabolism	[^{18}F]fluorodeoxyglucose, [^{11}C]glucose
Glucose transport	[^{11}C]-3-O-methylglucose
Neuroreceptor systems	
Dopamine	
Presynaptic dopamine pool	[^{18}F]fluoro-L-DOPA, [^{18}F]fluoro- L -m-tyrosine
D2 dopamine receptors	[^{11}C]N-methylspiperone, [^{11}C]raclopride, [^{18}F]spiperone, [^{18}F]N-methylspiperone
D1 dopamine receptors	[^{18}F]fallypride
Dopamine reuptake sites	[^{11}C]nomifensine, [^{11}C]cocaine
Vesicular monoamine transporter	[^{11}C]dihydrotetrabenazine
Opiate receptors	[^{11}C]carfentanil, [^{11}C]diprenorphine, [^{18}F]cyclofoxy
Acetylcholine	
M2 muscarinic receptors	[^{18}F]TZTP
Acetylcholinesterase enzyme	[^{11}C]PMP
Benzodiazepine receptors	[^{11}C]flumazenil
Serotonin	
5-HT$_{1A}$ receptors	[^{11}C]WAY100635
5-HT$_{2A}$ receptors	[^{11}C]MDL100907, [^{18}F]altanserin, [^{18}F]setoperone
Serotonin reuptake sites	[^{11}C]DASB, [^{11}C]McN5652
Monoamine olidase-B enzyme	[^{11}C]deprenyl
Amino acid transport, protein synthesis	[^{11}C]methionine, [^{11}C]leucine, [^{11}C]tyrosine
Tissue pH	[^{11}C]CO$_2$

This is a partial listing of radiotracers that have been used to study physiologic processes or systems in the brain with PET. The most commonly used radiotracer methods are those to measure CBF and metabolism.

mathematical simulations to determine the sensitivity of the model to potential sources of measurement error, such as inaccurate measurement of brain radioactivity. Validation experiments are usually performed to demonstrate that the method provides reproducible, accurate, and biologically meaningful measurements. With indirect validation, the experimental environment is manipulated and one determines whether the PET measurement varies as expected. For example, one can determine whether CBF measurements follow changes in flow produced by varying arterial pCO$_2$. Direct validation consists of comparing the PET measurement to the same measurement determined in an accepted but usually more invasive manner. A method to measure cerebral oxygen metabolism was validated in baboons by comparison to the brain's uptake of oxygen meas-

ured from arterial and jugular venous blood samples (Altman et al., 1991). Often, though, a "gold standard" reference technique does not exist.

CEREBRAL GLUCOSE METABOLISM
The [^{14}C]Deoxyglucose Method

One of the most widely used PET methods is the measurement of rCMRglc with FDG. It is based on the deoxyglucose (DG) method developed by Sokoloff to measure rCMRglc in laboratory animals with [^{14}C]deoxyglucose and tissue autoradiography (Sokoloff et al., 1977). DG is a glucose analog that differs from glucose by the substitution of a hydrogen atom for the hydroxyl group on the second carbon atom (Fig. 6-4). It

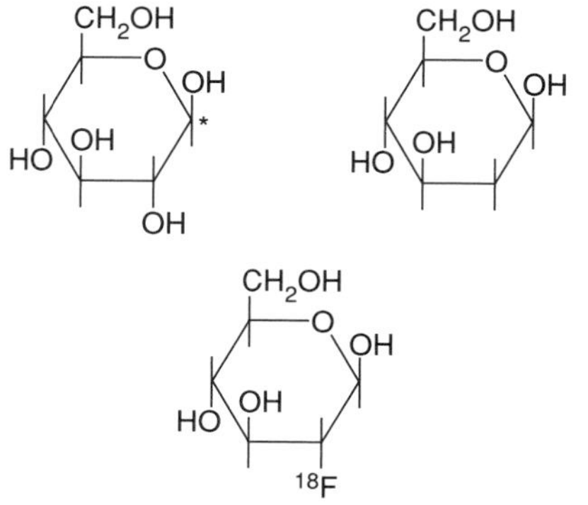

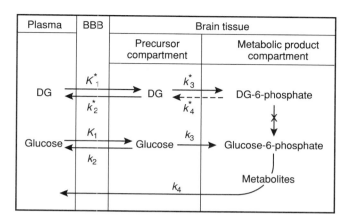

FIGURE 6-4. Glucose and glucose analogs. *A,* Glucose molecule. The asterisk denotes the 1-carbon position, which is labeled with ¹¹C to produce [1-¹¹C]glucose. *B,* Deoxyglucose molecule, in which a hydrogen atom has been substituted for the hydroxyl group on the 2-carbon atom of glucose. *C,* [¹⁸F]Fluorodeoxyglucose molecule.

FIGURE 6-5. Sokoloff's three-compartment model to measure rCMRglc with deoxyglucose (DG). The lower portion of the figure shows the metabolic fate of glucose in brain; the upper portion, that of DG. The three compartments consist of DG in plasma, DG in brain tissue, and DG-6-phosphate in tissue. Rate constants describe the movement of DG between compartments: K_1^* and k_2^* for the bidirectional transport of DG across the blood-brain barrier, and k_3^* for the phosphorylation of DG to DG-6-P. Once phosphorylated, DG does not proceed further down the metabolic pathway for glucose. In the original method for use with autoradiography in animals, DG is labeled with ¹⁴C; in the adaptation to PET, ¹⁸F-labeled DG is used and a fourth rate constant, k_4^* is added to account for dephosphorylation of FDG-6-P back to FDG. The asterisks distinguish rate constants for DG from those for glucose.

is transported bidirectionally across the BBB by the same transport system as that for glucose. In tissue, DG is phosphorylated by hexokinase as is glucose, to form [¹⁴C]deoxyglucose-6-phosphate (DG-6-P). Because of its anomalous structure, however, DG-6-P cannot be further metabolized. Also, there is little dephosphorylation of DG-6-P back to DG due to low glucose-6-phosphatase activity in brain. As a result of this "metabolic trapping" and its low membrane permeability, there is negligible loss of DG-6-P from tissue. This facilitates the calculation of rCMRglc from measurements of local tissue radioactivity.

A three-compartment mathematical model describes the behavior of DG. The compartments consist of DG in the plasma of brain capillaries, free DG in tissue, and DG-6-P in tissue (Fig. 6-5). Three rate constants describe the movement of tracer between these compartments. An operational equation was derived from the tracer model to calculate rCMRglc (Fig. 6-6). It contains terms readily measured in laboratory animals: the time course of DG concentration in plasma after pulse intravenous administration of DG, the plasma glucose concentration, and the local radioactivity concentration measured at a single time point after tracer injection from tissue autoradiographs. The equation also contains the three rate constants and a factor termed the lumped constant (LC), all of which must be specified. Neither the rate constants nor the LC can be routinely measured in each experimental animal. It was found possible, however, to use standard values that can be determined once in separate groups of animals.

The rate constants are estimated from measurements of tissue and plasma radioactivity obtained at different times after DG administration. Average rate constants for gray matter and white matter are used.

Because the rate constants can vary in different experimental conditions, a strategy was developed to minimize the error associated with using standard values. A 45-minute delay between DG injection and animal sacrifice was chosen. By this time, plasma DG values have fallen to very low levels. The terms in the operational equation containing the rate constants approach zero with increasing time and have little effect on calculated rCMRglc. A longer period was avoided to reduce loss of DG-6-P from tissue due to the small amount of glucose-6-phosphatase activity in brain, which would convert DG-6-P back to DG.

The LC corrects for the use of a glucose analog rather than glucose as the tracer. It accounts for differences between glucose and DG in transport across the BBB and in phosphorylation. It combines several physiologic parameters related to transport and phosphorylation of glucose and DG. The LC is uniform throughout brain under normal physiologic conditions. It can be measured from the ratio of the brain arterial-venous extraction fraction of DG to that of glucose. The DG method has been widely applied to study animal models of disease, brain development, pharmacologic interventions, and effects of functional activity in motor, visual, sensory, and other systems.

FIGURE 6-6. Operational equation of the deoxyglucose (DG) method to measure rCMRglc. The equation is also expressed in words (lower panel) to aid in its understanding. $C(T)$ is the tissue radioactivity concentration measured at time T, typically 45 minutes after pulse intravenous administration of DG. The concentration of free DG in tissue at time T is calculated from the plasma concentration of DG over time $[C_p^*(t)]$ and the rate constants. The difference between the two terms in the numerator equals the local DG-6-P that has been formed. The denominator represents the amount of DG delivered to tissue. Therefore, the ratio on the right-hand side equals the fractional rate of phosphorylation of DG. Multiplying this by the plasma glucose concentration (Cp) would give the rate of glucose phosphorylation if DG and glucose had the same behavior. Because this is not the case, the lumped constant (LC) is included to account for the difference. In the adaptation of the model to PET with FDG, a fourth rate constant (k_4^*) is included, and the operational equation is more complex.

$$rCMRGlc = \frac{C_p}{LC} \cdot \frac{C(T) - K_1^* \exp[-(k_2^* + k_3^*)T] \int_0^T C_p^*(t) \exp[(k_2 + k_3)t] dt}{\int_0^T C_p^*(t) dt - \exp[-(k_2^* + k_3^*)T] \int_0^T C_p^*(t) \exp[(k_2 + k_3)t] dt}$$

$$= \frac{\text{Plasma glucose concentration}}{\text{Lumped constant}} \cdot \frac{\text{Tissue radioactivity at time T} - \text{Free DG in tissue at time T}}{\text{Total amount of DG entering tissue up to time T}}$$

The [¹⁸F]Fluorodeoxyglucose Method

The DG method was adapted for PET by labeling DG with ^{18}F to produce FDG (see Fig. 6-4) (Phelps et al., 1979; Reivich et al., 1979; Huang et al., 1980). In tissue, FDG is phosphorylated to FDG-6-P, which is metabolically trapped. To obtain PET images from several brain levels with the single-slice tomographs in use in the early 1980s, it was necessary to scan well beyond the 45-minute tracer uptake period used in laboratory animals. Because there was felt to be a greater possibility for dephosphorylation of FDG-6-P and loss of labeled metabolic products from tissue, a fourth rate constant, k_4^*, was added to account for this (see Fig. 6-5). Average values for the rate constants were estimated from plasma and brain time-activity curves after FDG administration in normal subjects. A value for the LC (0.42) was selected so that the average whole brain glucose metabolic rate would equal that determined with the Kety-Schmidt technique. The operational equation is used to convert images of FDG concentration to images of rCMRglc using the values of the rate and lumped constants, and measurements of plasma glucose and FDG concentration over time.

The accuracy of using standard values for the rate constants and LC has been the subject of considerable investigation (Baron et al., 1989; Schmidt et al., 1996). The originators of the method noted that these parameters might change in abnormal conditions (Sokoloff et al., 1977). Although the form of the operational equation lessens the impact of errors in the rate constants, incorrect rCMRglc values can be obtained in pathologic conditions, such as ischemia or tumor. Investigators have developed alternative formulations of the operational equation to further decrease its sensitivity to the rate constants. In addition to providing more accurate estimates of rCMRglc, measured rate constants are of physiologic interest. K_1^* reflects glucose transport across the BBB, and k_3^* glucose phosphorylation. Decreases in these parameters have been reported in Alzheimer disease (Piert et al., 1996).

Reivich (1985) measured the LC in man. The value, 0.52, has been widely used, but is now felt to be an underestimate because of technical difficulties with the experiments. Recent work has provided LC values of 0.81 to 0.86 (Spence et al., 1998; Hasselbalch et al., 2001). The use of an incorrect value for the LC is not as critical as it might seem. This is because in the neuropsychiatric diseases typically studied with FDG, it is very unlikely that the LC changes. Because the LC appears as a scale factor in the calculation of rCMRglc (see Fig. 6-6), differences in rCMRglc between patients and control subjects will be maintained. Also, investigators frequently "normalize" rCMRglc values to the average brain metabolic rate to decrease the variability of regional measurements. This approach cancels out the LC value. The LC does change in some pathologic states. It is increased in acute cerebral ischemia, recent cerebral infarction, brain tumor (Spence et al., 1998), and hypoglycemia and is decreased in hyperglycemia. It is necessary to redetermine the lumped and rate constants in such pathologic conditions, where there is a gross abnormality of tissue or an imbalance between glucose supply and demand.

Implementation of the FDG Method

PET images are obtained 30 to 45 minutes after intravenous injection of about 5 to 10 mCi FDG. The subject fasts for several hours prior to the study, to maintain constant plasma glucose levels. Blood samples are collected through an indwelling arterial catheter (Jons et al., 1997) to measure the plasma concentration of glucose and FDG over time. Measurements of plasma glucose are averaged to reflect the mean value during the procedure. With current three-dimensional multislice scanners that have high sensitivity, scan data from the entire brain can be obtained in 5 to 15 minutes. The operational equation is then used to generate rCMRglc images. Typical normal values of rCMRglc are 6 to 7 mg/(min-100 g) in gray matter and 2.5 to 3 mg/(min–100 g) in white matter. To avoid arterial catheterization, some investigators perform venous sampling from a hand heated to 44°C to "arterialize" venous blood (Phelps et al., 1979). This approach is less accurate, however (Schmidt et al., 1996). Some investigators have proposed using a "population-based" input curve obtained by averaging arterial data from many subjects. The standard input function is then calibrated for individual subjects by using one or two blood samples. Another alternative is to image the heart to determine the activity in the left ventricular blood pool from the time of tracer injection to just prior to brain imaging.

The FDG tracer-kinetic model assumes that rCMRglc is constant throughout the procedure. If it changes, the measured rCMRglc is approximately a weighted average of the metabolic values during the study, with the weightings proportional to the plasma FDG concentrations at the corresponding times (Huang et al., 1981). Because the plasma FDG level soon declines to relatively low values, rCMRglc measurements reflect the state of the subject during the first 20 minutes or so after tracer injection. During the FDG uptake period, before a constant distribution of FDG in brain has been reached, it is necessary to keep the subject in a controlled behavioral state. Subjects are often maintained with eyes closed and ears occluded. Some investigators prefer to have subjects perform a simple cognitive task to control the subjects' cognitive status.

The ability to perform a transmission scan *after* tracer injection has simplified FDG studies. Previously, subjects had to be positioned in the scanner with the head restrained throughout the transmission scan, the 30- to 45-minute uptake period, and the emission scan. Instead, subjects can be placed in the scanner *after* the uptake period, at which time both transmission and emission scan data can be obtained (Carson et al., 1988). The fact that the distribution of FDG is fixed after the uptake period coupled with the ability to perform postinjection transmission scans increases the flexibility of FDG studies. Patients, including children, who cannot tolerate a head restraint can be sedated after the uptake period, before emission scanning. It is also possible to obtain FDG studies in awake, behaving nonhuman primates. After task performance during the uptake period, the animal is placed under general anesthesia for brain imaging (Blaizot et al., 2000).

The 110-minute half-life of ^{18}F precludes multiple repeat studies in the same experimental session. It is possible to perform two sequential scans, however, using a "split" FDG method in which residual activity from the first scan is subtracted from the second (Chang et al., 1987). Therefore, the same subject can be studied in one session during both a baseline and an experimental condition, for example, before and after the administration of a drug.

The FDG method has been a powerful tool in clinical research. It has been used in numerous applications, including studies of postnatal brain development, healthy aging, dementia, movement disorders, epilepsy, and psychiatric diseases such as schizophrenia and affective disorder (Fulham & Di Chiro, 1996; Drevets, 1998).

Use of [^{11}C]Glucose

An alternative approach for measuring rCMRglc uses glucose labeled with ^{11}C (Blomqvist et al., 1990; Powers et al., 1995; Spence et al., 1998). [^{11}C]Glucose is transported and metabolized in the same fashion and at the same rate as glucose. Therefore, a correction factor such as the LC is not required to account for differences between radiotracer and glucose. This is a decided advantage, because, as noted above, the LC can change in pathologic conditions. A disadvantage is that the labeled metabolites of glucose, such as [^{11}C]CO_2, are not trapped in tissue. Therefore, tracer kinetic models must account for the formation and egress from tissue of radiolabeled metabolites. The use of [^{11}C]glucose selectively labeled in the 1-carbon position (see Fig. 6-4), rather than uniformly labeled glucose, decreases the production of labeled metabolites. This is because the 1-position carbon is incorporated into glucose metabolites later in the metabolic pathway. A four-compartment model has been used, consisting of the intravascular compartment of the brain, unmetabolized [1-^{11}C]glucose in brain tissue, [^{11}C]-labeled metabolites of glucose, and a compartment for the loss of these metabolites from tissue (see Fig. 6-5).

Scan data and the arterial plasma time-activity curve following [1-^{11}C]glucose administration are used to calculate the rate constants. In addition to the glucose metabolic rate, other physiologic parameters can be calculated from the rate constants, including the concentration of free glucose in brain and the rate of glucose transport into brain. [1-^{11}C]glucose has been used when the standard FDG approach is not valid because of changes in the LC, such as brain tumor and hyperglycemia and hypoglycemia.

CEREBRAL BLOOD VOLUME

The measurement of rCBV, the amount of blood per unit mass of brain tissue, requires a tracer that remains confined to the intravascular space. Because there are no appropriate radiotracers that label both the cellular and plasma components of blood, the most common approach is to label red blood cells with [^{11}C]- or [^{15}O]carbon monoxide (CO) administered in trace amounts in air by inhalation (Grubb et al., 1978; Martin et al., 1987). The labeled CO binds avidly to hemoglobin and remains in the intravascular space. Scanning is begun about 2 minutes after CO inhalation, when labeled carboxyhemoglobin has equilibrated throughout the blood. Scan data are collected over approximately 5 minutes with [^{15}O]CO; longer scan times can be used with [^{11}C]CO. Blood samples are drawn, typically one per minute, to measure blood radioactivity. The use of [^{15}O]CO has practical advantages over [^{11}C]CO. The 2-minute half-life of ^{15}O permits other PET studies to be performed with little delay and lowers radiation exposure.

rCBV is calculated from the ratio of the radioactivity in brain to that in peripheral blood. Due to the behavior of blood in the cerebral microvasculature, the concentration of red cells in blood, that is, the hematocrit, is less in brain than in peripheral large vessels. This difference must be taken into account because the radiotracer is bound to red cells. Equation 1 or a modification (Videen et al., 1987) is used to calculate rCBV:

$$rCBV = \frac{\text{tissue radiotracer concentration}}{R \bullet \text{ average blood radiotracer concentration}}$$
(1)

R is the ratio of cerebral hematocrit to peripheral hematocrit. A value of 0.85 has been used, based on the average of values obtained in several animal and human studies. Normal values for rCBV measured with PET are approximately 4 to 6 mL/100 g in gray matter and 2 to 3 mL/100 g in white matter. The measurement of rCBV is of interest in cerebrovascular disease because it reflects vasodilation in response to decreased perfusion pressure, as may occur distal to a narrowed internal carotid artery (Grubb & Powers, 2001). rCBV data are also used to correct other PET measurements for radiotracer in the intravascular space, so that one can determine the amount of radiotracer that actually entered brain tissue.

CEREBRAL BLOOD FLOW

The conventional concept of fluid flow is the volume that passes a particular point per unit time. A more meaningful physiologic concept, however, is that of tissue perfusion, the volume of blood flowing through a particular volume or weight of tissue per unit time. Perfusion flow has units of milliliters per minute per milliliter or gram of tissue. (For historical reasons, rCBF is typically quoted in units of milliliters per minute per 100 g tissue: mL/(min – 100 g).)

The Kety Tissue Autoradiographic Method

Methods for measuring rCBF with PET are based on a one-tissue compartment model developed by Kety to measure rCBF in laboratory animals with diffusible radiotracers and tissue autoradiography (Kety, 1951; Landau et al., 1955). Important to an understanding of the model are the concepts of tracer diffusibility and partition coefficient. Diffusibility refers to the ability of the tracer to cross the BBB. An ideal flow tracer is freely diffusible across the BBB. The brain capillaries are highly permeable to the tracer, so that it equilibrates between tissue and blood in a single capillary transit. The amount of tracer entering tissue depends only on its delivery, that is, the local flow. A second concept is that of partition coefficient. If the concentration of tracer in blood is held constant, the concentration in tissue ultimately becomes constant as well. The partition coefficient, λ, is the ratio of the tissue-to-blood tracer concentrations at equilibrium. It can be measured experimentally from this definition or it can be calculated as the ratio of the solubility of the tracer in tissue and blood.

The Kety model describes the in vivo behavior of freely diffusible tracers. Although initially implemented with [^{131}I]trifluoroiodomethane, [^{14}C]iodoantipyrine is now used (Sakurada et al., 1978). The tracer is infused intravenously over 1 minute and the animal is then killed. Frequent blood samples are obtained to determine the arterial time-radioactivity curve. The regional brain radioactivity present the end of the experiment is measured by quantitative tissue autoradiography. An equation was derived to calculate rCBF, based on several assumptions: rCBF is constant during the experiment; the tracer is not metabolized; the tracer is freely diffusible across the BBB; the tissue region is a single compartment that is uniform in density, flow, and tracer solubility; and the tracer uniformly and instantaneously distributes in this region.

The rate of change of tracer concentration in a brain region equals the rate at which the tracer is transported to tissue in the cerebral arterial circulation, minus the rate at which it is washed out into the venous drainage:

$$\frac{dC_t}{dt} = fC_a - fC_v \qquad (2)$$

where f is the tissue blood flow, C_t is the tissue radiotracer concentration, and C_a and C_v are the time-varying radiotracer concentrations in the arterial input and venous drainage respectively. The time-activity curve measured from a peripheral artery is used to obtain C_a. It is not possible to measure C_v regionally. For a freely diffusible tracer, however, the radiotracer in the local venous drainage is in equilibrium with radiotracer in tissue, so that $\lambda = C_t/C_v$. C_v can be replaced by C_t/λ:

$$\frac{dC_t}{dt} = f\left(C_a - C_t/\lambda\right) \qquad (3)$$

This equation can be integrated and rearranged to give

$$C_t(T) = f\int_0^T C_a(t)\exp\left[-f/\lambda(T-t)\right]dt \qquad (4)$$

Equation 4 states that at time T after onset of tracer administration, the value of the local brain radiotracer concentration $C_t(T)$ depends on the flow f, the arterial time-activity curve $C_a(t)$, and λ. The unknown parameter in this equation, f, can be determined numerically from measurements of $C_t(T)$ and $C_a(t)$. The tissue autoradiographic method has been widely used in animals during physiologic and pharmacologic manipulations, and in experimental models of disease, such as seizures and cerebral ischemia.

Measurement of Regional Cerebral Blood Flow with PET

Kety's model is the basis for methods used to measure rCBF with PET. These methods share many features, including the use of a diffusible, positron-emitting tracer, blood sampling to determine the time-activity curve in arterial blood, and modifications of equations 3 and 4 to calculate rCBF from PET images of tissue radioactivity.

The most commonly used flow tracer is [^{15}O]water. It can be administered by intravenous injection, or alternatively, scan subjects can inhale [^{15}O]carbon dioxide ([^{15}O]CO$_2$). The catalytic action of carbonic anhydrase in red blood cells in the pulmonary vasculature results in rapid transfer of the ^{15}O label to water. [^{15}O]Water has several useful characteristics as a flow tracer. Water is a biologically inert, chemically

stable compound that occurs naturally in the body and has no undesirable physiologic effects. [^{15}O]Water and [^{15}O]CO$_2$ are easily synthesized. Because of the short half-life of ^{15}O (2 minutes), relatively large amounts of radioactivity can be used to obtain PET images over brief time periods with acceptable radiation exposure to the subject. Rapid decay of the radioactive background permits further PET measurements to be performed. A value of λ for [^{15}O]water can be calculated from the ratio of the water contents of brain and blood (Herscovitch & Raichle, 1985); the average value in human brain is 0.90 mL/g.

Steady-State Regional Cerebral Blood Flow Method

The steady-state or equilibrium method was the earliest widely used method for measuring rCBF with PET (Frackowiak et al., 1980). The subject inhales trace amounts of [^{15}O]CO$_2$, which is delivered continuously in air at a fixed rate. [^{15}O]Water is generated in the lungs through the action of carbonic anhydrase and circulates throughout the body. After approximately 10 minutes, a steady state is reached in which the blood radioactivity remains constant. Also, the radioactivity delivered to a brain region in its arterial input becomes equal to that leaving the region by physical decay and by washout of [^{15}O]water into venous blood. The distribution of radioactivity in the brain therefore remains constant, and because the rate of change of regional radioactivity is zero, equation 3 may be reformulated as:

$$\frac{dC_t}{dt} = f\left(C_a - C_t/\lambda\right) - \alpha C_t = 0 \qquad (5)$$

where α is the decay constant of ^{15}O (i.e., ln 2/half-life of ^{15}O, 0.34/min), and αC_t is the loss of radiotracer due to physical decay. Solving for flow gives:

$$f = \frac{\alpha}{C_a/C_t - 1/\lambda} \qquad (6)$$

C_a, the arterial radiotracer concentration, is determined from arterial blood samples, and C_t, the tissue radiotracer concentration, is measured with PET. The steady-state method was especially convenient with early, single-ring tomographs, because multiple tomographic slices could be obtained by repositioning the patient during continued [^{15}O]CO$_2$ inhalation. Because these tomographs operated most accurately at low count rates, the rate of radiotracer delivery was adjusted to suit the count rate capability. Validation studies in animals showed that measured rCBF changed appropriately in response to variations in arterial pCO$_2$ and was similar to measurements obtained with a reference microsphere technique.

The advantages and limitations of the steady-state method have been extensively studied (Lammertsma et al., 1981; Lammertsma et al., 1982; Herscovitch & Raichle, 1983). Most of the limitations arise from the nonlinear relationship in equation 6 between rCBF and tissue radiotracer concentration C_t. At higher flow levels, a large change in rCBF produces a relatively smaller change in brain concentration of ^{15}O. Thus, small errors in measurement of C_t produce proportionately larger errors in measured rCBF. Calculated flow values are also sensitive to measurement errors in C_a and to any difference between the value of λ used in equation 6 and its true value, which may vary in pathologic conditions. Although there are other approaches to measure rCBF, the steady-state method is still popular, especially when combined with measurements of $rCMRO_2$ in studies of cerebrovascular disease.

PET/Autoradiographic Method

An alternative approach is to measure rCBF after bolus intravenous injection of $[^{15}O]$water. Kety's tissue autoradiographic method cannot be used in its original form (equation 4) because scanners cannot accurately measure the instantaneous brain radiotracer concentration $C_t(T)$. A scan must be performed over many seconds, summing enough counts to obtain a satisfactory PET image. Therefore, equation 4 was modified by an integration of the instantaneous radiotracer concentration, from the scan start time T_1 to the scan end time T_2, to correspond to the summing process of tomographic data collection. It is necessary to account for physical decay of ^{15}O during the study. Tissue and blood radioactivity measurements can be decay-corrected to the time of tracer administration. It is more convenient and accurate, however, to include radioactive decay explicitly in the model (Herscovitch et al., 1983; Raichle et al., 1983; Videen et al., 1987):

$$C = \int_{T_1}^{T_2} C_t(T)dt = f\int_{T_1}^{T_2}\int_{0}^{T} C_a(t)\exp\left[-(f/\lambda+\alpha)(T-t)\right]dt\,dT$$

(7)

C is the local number of counts per gram of tissue recorded during the scan. The relationship between tissue counts and rCBF is almost linear. This has several advantages. Errors in measurement of tissue radioactivity result in approximately equivalent errors in rCBF; there is no amplification of error. Inaccuracy in the value of λ used in equation 7 results in minimal error.

$[^{15}O]$Water is administered by bolus intravenous injection, and a brief scan, typically 1 minute or less, is obtained after arrival of radiotracer in the head. Blood is rapidly sampled through an indwelling arterial catheter to determine $C_a(t)$. Once a value for λ is specified, equation 7 can be solved numerically for flow. This equation is applied pixel-by-pixel to the image of tissue counts to obtain an image in quantitative blood flow units, mL/(min − 100 g). With earlier-generation scanners, 30 to 80 mCi $[^{15}O]$water was used, depending on scanner performance characteristics. Current three-dimensional scanners require as little as 10 mCi (Sadato et al., 1997). rCBF measurements obtained with this technique were validated in the baboon. Average values for rCBF in normal subjects obtained with either the steady-state or the PET/autoradiographic method are in the range of 50 to 60 mL/(min − 100 g) in gray matter and 20 to 30 mL/(min − 100 g) in white matter.

Dynamic Methods

Other approaches using the Kety model have been developed to measure rCBF and are referred to as dynamic methods. Scan data are collected in multiple sequential images for 4 to 6 minutes after tracer administration, so that tissue time-activity curves can be constructed. Equation 7 is used to describe the relationship between tissue counts and flow for each image. A parameter estimation method using least-squares fitting is used to calculate both f and λ from scan data and measurements of arterial radioactivity. Not having to specify a value for λ may increase the accuracy of the rCBF estimate. Estimated values for λ, 0.83 to 0.88 mL/g, are similar to or somewhat lower than those calculated from tissue water content.

Determination of the Arterial Time-Activity Curve

With rCBF techniques that use bolus administration of radiotracer, it is assumed that the time-activity curve sampled from a peripheral artery, usually the radial artery, equals the arterial input to the brain. If this is not true, the rCBF calculation will be inaccurate. In fact, the radiotracer arrives at the radial artery several seconds later than in brain because the distance between heart and artery is greater than that between heart and brain. In addition, there is dispersion or smearing of the curve as the tracer bolus traverses the arterial system. Because the bolus travels farther to the artery, more dispersion occurs in the sampled curve. Different rCBF methods vary in their sensitivity to time delay and dispersion; the PET/autoradiographic method is more sensitive than dynamic methods. Approaches have been developed to correct for these effects by estimating the time delay and the dispersion time constant from blood and tissue time-activity curves. To simplify blood sampling, automated systems have been designed to draw blood continuously through tubing past a radiation detector (Eriksson & Kanno, 1991). They produce a finely sampled blood curve and reduce the radiation exposure to personnel that occurs during manual sampling.

Flow Tracers for PET

rCBF methods based on the Kety model assume that the radiotracer is freely diffusible across the BBB. However, [^{15}O]water does not exhibit this ideal behavior. There is a limitation to diffusion, so that it does not freely equilibrate with tissue. With increasing CBF, there is a progressive decline in the extraction of [^{15}O]water from blood. This results in less tracer entering tissue than would be predicted by the flow model and leads to an underestimation of rCBF at higher flows (Raichle et al., 1983). There are, however, PET flow tracers that are not diffusion limited. [^{11}C]Butanol is freely diffusible at whole brain CBF values as high as 170 mL/(min − 100 g) in the nonhuman primate (the average whole brain CBF in humans is 50 mL/(min − 100 g)). In comparison to [^{11}C]butanol, [^{15}O]water underestimates whole brain CBF by approximately 15% (Herscovitch et al., 1987). The 20-minute half-life of ^{11}C is inconvenient, however. A rapid synthesis of [^{15}O]butanol has been developed (Berridge et al., 1991). This tracer has several advantages, including absence of diffusion limitation, a short half-life, and intravenous method of administration. A value of 0.77 mL/g for λ was measured with dynamic scanning in humans (Herzog et al., 1996). [^{15}O]Butanol has been used in functional brain mapping studies; its ability to reflect higher blood flows more accurately is an advantage.

Regional Cerebral Blood Flow Imaging for Functional Brain Mapping

One of the most common applications of rCBF imaging has been functional brain mapping studies (Herscovitch, 1995; Jueptner & Weiller, 1995). Subjects perform different neurobehavioral tasks during a scan session, with rCBF mapped during each task. Because of the coupling between neuronal activity and flow, changes in local activity during the task are reflected in rCBF changes. Typically, one task is a control or baseline condition, with the others being cognitive, sensory, or motor tasks of interest.

These studies were originally performed with [^{15}O]water and absolute quantitation of rCBF, which required arterial sampling. However, the linear relationship between tissue counts and rCBF with the PET/autoradiographic approach was subsequently used to advantage in these studies. The image of tissue counts collected over a brief time period after bolus injection of [^{15}O]water closely reflects relative differences in flow. Therefore, the same information about changes in relative rCBF can be obtained without arterial blood sampling. Tissue count images rapidly replaced absolute rCBF measurements. Relative changes in rCBF during different tasks are determined by comparing tissue count images that have been normalized for total brain radioactivity. The introduction of high-sensitivity three-dimensional scanners made it possible to use smaller doses of [^{15}O]water (Bailey et al., 1998). It was necessary to determine the dose to maximize signal-to-noise ratio and the ability to detect rCBF changes. Although increasing the dose increases useful counts, it also increases scattered and random counts and leads to increasing deadtime losses. Ultimately, a point is reached at which further increases in activity add more noise than useful counts. One should scan somewhat below this level. Optimal performance is achieved at doses of 10 to 15 mCi of [^{15}O]water. The data collection period could extend over several minutes. However, after a bolus tracer injection, the relationship between flow and accumulated counts becomes increasingly nonlinear as scan duration increases, and the sensitivity to local flow changes decreases. The gain due to increased counts is counterbalanced by the loss of flow information. The optimal scan duration is about 1 minute (Sadato et al., 1997).

The number of scans that can be performed during an experimental session depends not only on the dose per scan but also on the limits for radiation exposure to research subjects. Using 10 mCi [^{15}O]water per scan, one can administer up to 540 mCi per study session (i.e., 54 scans), and 1620 mCi/yr under the authority of a Radioactive Drug Research Committee of the U.S. Food and Drug Administration. Thus, the limiting factor is not radiation exposure, but rather the tolerance of the experimental subject. Typically, no more than 10 to 15 scans are performed per session. The ability to perform scans with only 10 mCi makes brain-mapping experiments possible in single subjects. Enough scans can be obtained in different task conditions to perform a meaningful statistical comparison and detect local flow changes in an individual.

The physical half-life of ^{15}O is 2 minutes, so typically one waits 10 to 12 minutes, that is, 5 or 6 half-lives, between scans for the radioactive background to decay. However, scans can be repeated more rapidly, for example, every 6 to 8 min, by correcting each scan for residual radioactivity from the previous scan. The rapid production of [^{15}O]water doses for activation studies is facilitated by equipment designed to synthesize the tracer in the scan room from [^{15}O]oxygen that is continuously pumped from the cyclotron.

An important consideration is the temporal resolution of [^{15}O]water scans. The duration of a scan is typically 1 minute for tissue count imaging. However, because of the kinetics of [^{15}O]water in tissue, the images obtained after bolus administration reflect the rCBF pattern during the first 15 to 20 seconds after the tracer reaches the head (Hurtig et al., 1994), resulting in much better temporal resolution than would be anticipated. This must be taken into account in the design of brain-mapping studies; changes in task performance after this 20-second window will not be reflected in the rCBF images. This CBF sensitivity window may be too short for some complex activation paradigms. In these cases, a slow infusion rather than a bolus injection of tracer can be used. Infusions of 90 seconds with scan lengths of 90 to 120 seconds extend the window of sensitivity to flow changes with little effect on signal-to-noise ratio (Sadato et al., 1997). It is also possible to capture brief, randomly occurring neuropsychological events during PET data collection (Silbersweig et al., 1994). For each scan, the amount of [^{15}O]water entering the brain during these timed events is calculated from the tracer model, and a score is derived that reflects the contribution of the events to the image. Then, a statistical analysis is performed to find the voxels in which the intensity covaries with the scan score; these are the ones involved in the neuropsychological event.

CEREBRAL OXYGEN METABOLISM

rCMRO$_2$ is measured using inhaled [^{15}O]oxygen gas. One method for measuring rCMRO$_2$ was developed in conjunction with the steady-state rCBF technique and uses continuous inhalation of [^{15}O]oxygen (Frackowiak et al., 1980). Another uses a brief inhalation of [^{15}O]oxygen and is a companion to the PET/autoradiographic rCBF method (Mintun et al., 1984). Average normal values for gray matter rCMRO$_2$ with these methods are 2.5 to 3.5 mL O$_2$/(min – 100 g).

The principles underlying these methods are similar. Only a fraction of the oxygen delivered to brain, approximately 0.40, is extracted by tissue and metabolized. Both methods measure this fraction, termed the oxygen extraction fraction (OEF). There are essentially no stores of oxygen in brain, and all extracted oxygen is metabolized. Therefore, rCMRO$_2$ can be calculated from the product of rOEF and the rate of oxygen delivery to brain, which equals rCBF multiplied by arterial oxygen content.

The tracer model must describe the fate of the ^{15}O label. [^{15}O]Oxygen extracted from arterial blood is metabolized, producing ^{15}O-labeled water of metabolism, which washs out of brain. Labeled water of metabolism is also produced by the rest of the body. It recirculates to brain and diffuses into and out of tissue. Therefore, the tracer model must take into account several sources that contribute to the measured ^{15}O activity in brain: extracted [^{15}O]oxygen that is metabolized to [^{15}O]water and washed out of brain, intravascular [^{15}O]oxygen, and recirculating [^{15}O]water. A large component of the measured radioactivity consists of intravascular, unextracted [^{15}O]oxygen. It is necessary to account for this component, so that it is not attrib-

uted to radioactivity in tissue. This would lead to an overestimation of OEF. Determination of the intravascular component requires an independent measurement of rCBV. Therefore, both the steady-state and brief inhalation methods require three separate scans to measure rCMRO$_2$: an rCBF scan, an rCBV scan, and a scan obtained with [^{15}O]oxygen. In addition, arterial blood samples are required to measure the components of radioactivity in blood: [^{15}O]oxygen bound to hemoglobin and [^{15}O]water of metabolism in plasma and red blood cells.

With the steady-state method, scanning is performed during continuous delivery and inhalation of [^{15}O]oxygen, after a constant distribution of radiotracer is reached in brain. In the same scan session, rCBF is measured with continuous inhalation of [^{15}O]CO$_2$ and rCBV with [^{15}O]CO. rOEF is computed from data obtained during these three scans and from measurements of blood radioactivity. Indirect validation experiments showed that when arterial pCO$_2$ was increased, rCBF increased, and rOEF decreased while rCMRO$_2$ remained constant, as would be expected. Studies in baboons demonstrated an overestimation of rOEF, most likely because the tracer model did not account for intravascular [^{15}O]oxygen (Lammertsma et al., 1983). The steady-state method finds continuing use in the study of cerebrovascular disease in humans and in animal models (Yamauchi et al., 1999). It has an advantage when studying patients with impaired cognition or sensorium, because it does not require patient cooperation to inhale the radiotracers.

rOEF and rCMRO$_2$ can also be measured following a brief inhalation of [^{15}O]oxygen (Mintun et al., 1984; Videen et al., 1987). A 40-second emission scan is obtained following inhalation, and frequent arterial blood samples are collected for measurements of blood radioactivity. The method also involves measurement of rCBF with intravenous [^{15}O]water and of rCBV with inhaled [^{15}O]CO. It takes approximately 30 minutes to perform the three required scans, because one must wait for decay of the radioactive background between scans. The method was validated in baboons. In these experiments, because rOEF was varied by changing arterial pCO$_2$, rCMRO$_2$ changed little. Subsequent validation experiments showed that the method is accurate when rCMRO$_2$ is low (Altman et al., 1991). This is important because it is frequently used to study cerebrovascular disease, in which reduced rCMRO$_2$ can occur.

Although the brief inhalation method has been successfully applied in research studies, its technical demands could limit clinical utility. In patients with symptomatic carotid artery occlusion, a count-based estimate of rOEF using the ratio of tissue counts in the [^{15}O]oxygen image to those in an [^{15}O]water image, identified patients at risk of stroke with the same accuracy as the full quantitative method (Derdeyn et al.,

1999). This approach could simplify research and clinical applications.

Both the steady-state and brief inhalation methods require data from three separate scans obtained over 30 to 60 minutes. Methods have been sought to estimate rCMRO₂ from a single dynamic scan after [¹⁵O]oxygen administration. Because such scans contain information not only about CMRO₂, but also about CBF (from the delivery of [¹⁵O]oxygen and the wash-in and wash-out of labeled water of metabolism) and CBV (from intravascular [¹⁵O]oxygen), it has been hypothesized that all three parameters could be estimated from dynamic scan frames obtained after a single [¹⁵O]oxygen inhalation. Although this has not been feasible, estimates of rCMRO₂ alone can be obtained from data collected over 1 to 3 minutes (Ohta et al., 1992).

SINGLE PHOTON EMISSION COMPUTED TOMOGRAPHY

SPECT Principles

SPECT is widely used in clinical nuclear medicine with radiopharmaceuticals designed to demonstrate areas of disease, for example, local tumor deposits in bone or inflammation associated with infection. Many SPECT radiotracers have been developed for brain imaging, with the goal of introducing methods useful to manage patients with specific conditions or to study the pathophysiology of neuropsychiatric disease.

SPECT uses radionuclides that decay by emitting a photon or gamma ray. The radionuclides most commonly used to label SPECT radiotracers for brain imaging are radioactive forms of technetium (^{99m}Tc; half-life 6 hours) and iodine (^{123}I; half-life 13 hours). ^{123}I is produced commercially in large cyclotrons. ^{99m}Tc is more convenient to use because it is easily obtained from generators that are regularly delivered to nuclear medicine departments. A generator contains a "parent" radionuclide that is produced in a nuclear reactor and has a long half-life. It decays to a desired shorter-lived "daughter" nuclide that is separated from the parent on the basis of their chemical differences.

The most commonly used SPECT systems have one or more gamma camera "heads." Each head of a SPECT system consists of a large scintillation crystal, an array of photomultiplier tubes, and a collimator (Fig. 6-7). The scintillation crystal is made of sodium iodide containing a small amount of thallium and is in the shape of a large, relatively thin slab or disk (e.g., 3/8 in. by 12–20-in. diameter). The crystal gives off a localized flash of visible light when it absorbs a gamma ray. A bank of photomultiplier tubes packed closely together covers the back surface of the scintillation crystal. The tubes produce a pulse of electricity in response to the light flash. The size of the pulse pro-

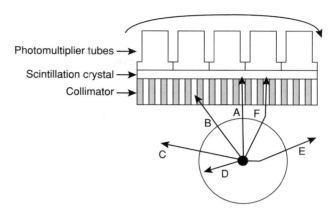

FIGURE 6-7. Diagram of a SPECT camera head. The head has three components: (1) a large scintillation crystal which senses the arrival of gamma rays; (2) an array of photomultiplier tubes that determines where gamma rays strike the crystal; and, (3) a collimator in front of the crystal to allow gamma rays only from a certain direction to enter the crystal. An emitted photon can undergo several possible interactions in tissue and with the camera head (see text). Modern SPECT systems consist of two or three heads in a gantry, which is rotated around the body.

duced by each tube depends on its location in relation to the flash of light. Position logic circuits use this information to determine the location of each gamma ray interaction in the crystal.

Gamma rays leaving the body can strike the crystal from any angle. To select the rays that represent a view of the radioactivity in the body from one direction, the front of the crystal is covered with a collimator, a sheet of absorbing material such as lead, perforated by closely spaced small holes. Only those rays traveling parallel to the holes, that is, perpendicular to the crystal face, can pass; others are absorbed. Therefore, one obtains a two-dimensional view of the radioactivity in the body from one direction. The camera head is rotated around the body to obtain multiple views. These views are combined to reconstruct tomographic images of the distribution of radioactivity in the body.

Several physical factors relating to the interaction of photons with tissue and with the camera head affect image quality. A photon escaping the body in a straight line perpendicular to the collimator face will be detected by the camera (see photon A in Fig. 6-7). Many photons, however, have different paths. Photon B strikes the collimator and is not detected. Neither is photon C, because it does not travel toward the camera head. Many photons interact with tissue. Some are completely absorbed (D). Others are deflected by Compton scattering. They may escape the body without being detected (E). If detected, they will appear to have come from a different direction (F). As a result of scattering away from the camera head (E) and absorption (D), the number of photons reaching the head is reduced or attenuated. Attenuation is not uniform; it depends on the properties of the tissue and the distance through which the photon travels. Mathematical methods to correct for attenuation are imprecise. Newer SPECT devices can measure attenuation directly and more accurately using a source of gamma rays outside the body, but this method is not widely used. Scattered photons that are detected by the camera (F) decrease image contrast and resolution; electronic and mathematical techniques are used to correct for this effect.

To increase the number of detected photons (A) and thereby improve sensitivity and image quality, modern SPECT systems have two heads facing each other or three heads in a triangular arrangement, mounted in a gantry that rotates around the body. Sensitivity is still low, however, because of the need for collimators, which block many of the photons, so that imaging time is typically many minutes. Therefore, radiotracers that provide a static or slowly changing radioactivity distribution are preferred. Typically, radioactivity is not quantitated in absolute terms, but rather the tomographic images are used to obtain information about the relative amount of radioactivity in different brain regions.

The resolution of SPECT systems is defined and measured in a fashion similar to that for PET. SPECT cameras with single heads have a spatial resolution of about 15 mm; resolution is 6 to 9 mm with multiple heads. Resolution is determined primarily by collimator design; smaller collimator holes provide better resolution, but decrease camera sensitivity. The resolution of a camera head worsens as the distance between the collimator and the source of radioactivity increases. This effect is taken into account in the reconstruction method used for multihead systems to provide more uniform resolution.

Formal procedures have been devised to test the performance characteristics of both SPECT and PET scanners. These are performed when a scanner is delivered from the manufacturer to ensure that it meets specifications and are repeated at regular intervals to verify that it continues to operate within these specifications.

SPECT Radiotracer Methods

Radiotracers for SPECT imaging fall into two broad categories, those for imaging rCBF, and those for imaging neuroreceptors (Table 6-2). It is also possible to measure rCBV with SPECT and ^{99m}Tc-labeled red cells. There are no SPECT radiotracers, however, to study brain glucose or oxygen metabolism. The most common application of SPECT is to map CBF with radiotracers administered intravenously. The radiotracer strategy is based on the microsphere method, a technique used to measure local flow in experimental animals. With that method, radioactive microspheres of a size appropriate to be trapped in capillaries are introduced into the left side of the animal's heart. They are distributed and trapped in tissue in proportion to flow and then local radioactivity is measured in samples of tissue. To use this approach for mapping brain perfusion with SPECT, one requires a "chemical microsphere," a radiotracer with microsphere-like behavior. The tracer should diffuse freely across the BBB, be completely extracted by tissue so that its initial distribution is proportional to local flow, and be retained in brain in an unchanged pattern. The stable distribution permits image acquisition over 20 to 30 minutes to obtain images of good quality. Several SPECT perfusion agents are based on these principles, although their extraction or retention is not necessarily complete.

The first widely used SPECT CBF tracer was [^{123}I]iodoamphetamine, which is retained by interaction with nonspecific binding sites. It must be prelabeled by a commercial supplier, however, which is logistically difficult. Tracers using ^{99m}Tc are preferable. ^{99m}Tc is more convenient to use, because it is obtained from generators that are delivered regularly to nuclear medicine departments; thus on-site labeling is possible. In addition, the physical characteristics of its radioactive decay are more favorable for SPECT imaging. ^{99m}Tc-tracers are converted in tissue to hydrophilic compounds that are retained. [^{99m}Tc]hexamethylpropylene amine oxime ([^{99m}Tc]HMPAO) has been widely used. [^{99m}Tc]Ethyl cysteinate dimer [^{99m}Tc]ECD) provides better quality images because of more rapid clearance from blood and is easier to use because of greater in vitro chemical stability. It remains stable for several hours after constitution, so it does not need to be prepared immediately before administration. Although there are methods to measure rCBF in absolute terms with these tracers, they are rarely used. They require arterial blood sampling, and depending on the tracer, analysis of the metabolites of the tracer in blood and correction for incomplete extraction by brain. In fact, it is the ease with which SPECT provides a map of relative cerebral perfusion that is its strong point. Therefore, SPECT studies typically are used to provide information about relative CBF.

SPECT perfusion studies are relatively easy to perform, because the scanners are widely available and an in-house cyclotron is not required to produce the radiotracer. The distribution of radiotracer in brain reflects the blood flow during the first few minutes after injection of the tracer and remains relatively stable. Therefore, scanning can start up to a half-hour after tracer injection and it is not necessary to inject the tracer with the subject in the scanner. Repeat SPECT studies cannot be performed rapidly because of the

TABLE 6-2. Representative SPECT Radiotracers

Physiologic process or system	Radiotracer
Cerebral blood flow	[123I]iodoamphetamine
	[99mTc]hexametazime ([99mTc]HMPAO)
	[99mTc]ethyl cysteinate dimer ([99mTc]ECD)
Cerebral blood volume	[99mTc] red blood cells
Neuroreceptor systems	
Dopamine	
D2 dopamine receptors	[123I]IBZM, [123I]IBF, [123I]epidepride
Dopamine reuptake sites	[123I]β-CIT, [99mTc]TRODAT-1
Benzodiazepine receptors	[123I]iomazenil
Acetylcholine	
Muscarinic receptors	[123I]QNB, [123I]iododexetimide
Acetylcholine vesicular transporters	[123I]iodobenzovesamicol
Serotonergic 5-HT$_{2A}$ receptors	[123I]R93274
Amino acid transport	[123I]iodo-α-methyl tyrosine

This is a partial listing of radiotracers that have been used to study physiologic processes or systems in the brain with SPECT. The most commonly used radiotracers are those used to image CBF.

6-hour half-life of ^{99m}Tc, unless methods are used to subtract residual radioactivity.

Several SPECT radiotracers have been developed to image neuroreceptors. The radiotracer properties that are required are similar to those for PET. Simple methods of data collection and analysis have been developed that involve achieving an equilibrium, constant distribution of radiotracer in brain, either by waiting for a long period after bolus tracer injection, for example, 1 day, or by using a constant infusion of tracer over several hours. These imaging protocols match the relatively long half-lives of ^{123}I and ^{99m}Tc. When the tracer has achieved equilibrium, the ratio of radioactivity in a structure of interest to that in an area devoid of the receptor is used as a measure of receptor binding.

Radioligands used for clinical research include [123I]iodobenzamide for imaging postsynaptic D2 receptors, [123I]iomazenil for central benzodiazepine receptors, [123I]β-CIT and [99mTc]TRODAT-1 for presynaptic dopamine transporters (DATs), and [123I]iodobenzovesamicol for acetylcholine transporters in presynaptic cholinergic vesicles. These tracers have been used to study receptor changes in neurologic and psychiatric disease. [123I]β-CIT has been widely used to study movement disorders (Emami-Avedon et al., 2000). It binds to presynaptic DATs and can demonstrate decreased striatal DATs caused by degeneration of dopaminergic neurons of the nigrostriatal pathway. Patients with Parkinson disease have decreased binding in striatum that correlates with disease severity and decreases that are asymmetrical and greater contralateral to the more affected side of the body. [123I]β-CIT is sensitive to neu-

ronal loss over time and could be used to evaluate the effects of neuroprotective treatments. It has potential for use in the early diagnosis of Parkinson disease and for the differential diagnosis of movement disorders.

DATA ANALYSIS

General Principles

After a PET study has been completed, the relevant tracer model is applied to calculate the physiologic variable of interest. For the methods to measure cerebral hemodynamics and metabolism, the model is applied on a point-by-point basis and the intensity of the resultant image reflects the value of the physiologic measurement. Although visual inspection of images may reveal abnormalities, quantitative analysis and appropriate statistical techniques are required for clinical research. Data reduction, analysis, and interpretation are very demanding. Newer scanners acquire up to 63 slices simultaneously, each containing data from many brain structures. Several scans of the same or different types may be obtained in one session, for example, multiple rCBF scans, or rCBF and rCMRglc scans, and subjects may have repeat studies on different days. The analysis of functional brain imaging data is greatly facilitated by interactive computer programs. These programs permit regions of interest (ROIs) of arbitrary size and shape to be placed over different structures for which the physiologic variable is then computed. Also, whole brain measurements can be obtained by averaging over several PET slices.

PET measurements must be related to the underlying anatomy. Early approaches to data analysis used PET images obtained in standard planes, for example, parallel to the canthomeatal line. The images were visually compared to corresponding anatomic sections in a brain atlas and ROIs manually drawn. This method, however, is subjective and liable to observer bias. A refinement uses a template of standard regions to sample brain structures of interest, with visual adjustment to fit the template to the images. Alternative approaches have been developed that relate PET images to anatomy more accurately and objectively. A popular approach uses the principles of stereotactic localization to establish a correspondence between structures in a brain atlas and specific regions or pixels in the PET image (Fox et al., 1985; Friston et al., 1989). Other methods are required, however, if structural abnormalities are present. An approach widely used for both normal and abnormal brain is to obtain anatomic images with CT or magnetic resonance imaging (MRI) in the same planes as the PET slices. Methods to achieve this include head holders transferable between imaging modalities, fiducial markers affixed to the head, and most conveniently, automated computer techniques to register and reslice PET and MR or CT images (Woods et al., 1993). After coplanar anatomic and PET images have been obtained, ROIs identified on the anatomic image can be transferred to the functional image. These automated techniques have also been used to register SPECT images with CT or MR images.

There is variability in both regional and global PET measurements. The coefficient of variation (i.e., the ratio of the standard deviation to the mean value) for measurements of rCBF, rCMRglc, and rCMRO$_2$ is 10% to 20% in groups of normal subjects, although the variability in repeat measurements in the same subject is less. This may reflect normal physiologic variation or methodological inaccuracies. Approaches have been developed to facilitate detecting regional changes despite this variability. These adjust for the effect of global variations by "normalizing" regional data, thereby decreasing their variance. This can be done by dividing regional values by the global average value or by the value in a structure presumed to be minimally involved in the disease being studied. Such techniques, however, can result in a loss of the information contained in the absolute values, especially if widespread changes occur. If both the denominator and numerator differ between groups, erroneous conclusions may be drawn. For example, in a study of Alzheimer disease, normalized rCMRglc in thalamus was significantly *increased* because of a *decrease* in global metabolism. In other words, the metabolism in the thalamus was relatively spared. Therefore, normalized data must be carefully interpreted. Despite the variability of PET measurements, it is possible to demonstrate meaningful physiologic abnormalities with absolute data, for example, in cerebrovascular disease (Grubb & Powers, 2001).

SPECT perfusion studies typically do not involve quantitation of absolute rCBF. Although the image intensity is proportional to flow, it also depends on the amount of tracer reaching the brain, which can vary among patients and even in the same patient due to variations in the peripheral circulation as well as body size. In clinical research studies, a normalization procedure is performed if regional tissue count data are to be averaged in a patient group or compared to data from normal subjects. This is accomplished by dividing the count data in individual ROIs by the average whole brain value or by the value in the cerebellum, assuming that it is not involved in the disease process. There are potential ambiguities with this approach, as with normalized PET data. In clinical applications of SPECT and PET, images are visually assessed for symmetry of radiotracer concentration and for continuity of radiotracer distribution in the cortical rim. Visual analysis of images requires a rigorous approach. The criteria for defining an abnormality are often subjective, however, and care should be taken to define the sensitivity and specificity for detecting abnormalities (Juni, 1994).

Data from control subjects are required to interpret PET or SPECT measurements obtained in patients. Quantitative data obtained in appropriately selected normal subjects are used. Depending on the nature of the study, selection criteria must control for variables such as age, gender, handedness, and condition of general health. Average data from patients are statistically compared to the same regional measurements made in a group of normal subjects. It is also possible to analyze regional data obtained in an individual patient, for example, by determining whether they are outside the range of normal. In comparing measurements obtained from many brain regions, it is possible that some regions will be found to be significantly different by chance because of the large number of comparisons being made. One approach to avoid this error, which is rather conservative, is to adjust the study P value (typically .05) by dividing it by the number of measurements being made (the Bonferroni correction). One must also consider the possibility of a drift in measurements in the case of longitudinal studies. Usually, these changes over time can be corrected by covariance analysis. This stresses the importance of rigorous quality control of scanners and the interleaving of patients and controls over the duration of a study.

A variety of sophisticated methods have been developed to extract information from functional brain images. One approach consists of calculating the relationship between CBF or metabolism in multiple pairs of brain regions. A high degree of correlation or covariance between the activities in two brain regions indicates a high level of functional connectivity during a particular condition. This implies that the regions work together, influence each other, or are affected in a similar fashion by a third region. In a refinement of this approach called path analysis, knowledge of the neuroanatomic connections between brain areas is included in the computation of interregional correlations, and functional networks consisting of several brain regions can be identified (McIntosh et al., 1994).

Effect of Limited Spatial Resolution

Artifactual abnormalities of CBF and metabolism can be observed with PET or SPECT because of the limited spatial resolution of the imaging devices. Limited resolution affects the accuracy of radioactivity measurements (Fig. 6-8) (Mazziotta et al., 1981). Because the radioactivity appears spread out over a larger area, a brain region in the image contains only a portion of the radioactivity that was in the corresponding brain structure. In addition, some of the radioactivity in surrounding structures appears to be spread into the region. Because of this effect, called partial volume averaging, a regional measurement contains a contribution from both the structure of interest and surrounding structures. High radioactivity levels surrounded by lower values will be underestimated, whereas low radioactivity surrounded by high activity will be overestimated. These errors are less when the size of the structure of interest is large with respect to scanner resolution. In a circular, uniform structure with a diameter twice the resolution, the radioactivity concentration will be accurately represented in the center. However, statistical considerations limit obtaining a measurement with a very small ROI. In general, it is not possible to measure pure gray matter radioactivity, especially in thin cortical regions.

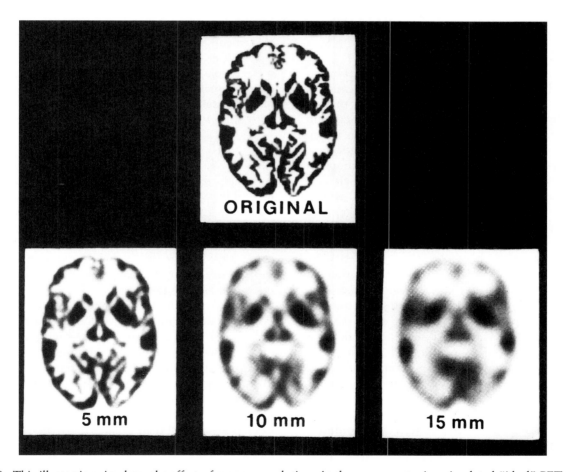

FIGURE 6-8. This illustration simulates the effect of scanner resolution. At the upper center is a simulated "ideal" PET image of regional radioactivity, reflecting the higher metabolic activity in gray matter. Subsequent images simulate the effect of obtaining this image with tomographs of varying spatial resolution, from 5 to 15 mm FWHM. Note the blurring or spreading out of radioactivity, with gray matter structures appearing paler. As a result, radioactivity in cortical and subcortical gray matter regions is underestimated. Similar considerations hold for SPECT images. (Reproduced with permission from Mazziotta JC, Phelps ME, Plummer D, et al: Quantitation in positron computed tomography: 5. Physical-anatomical effects. J Comput Assist Tomogr 5:734–743, 1981.)

Partial volume averaging with cerebrospinal fluid in sulci or ventricles can lead to an underestimation of tissue blood flow and metabolism. If there is cerebral atrophy, for example, as occurs in Alzheimer disease, PET and SPECT measurements will be further reduced because of partial volume averaging with enlarged, metabolically inactive, cerebrospinal fluid spaces (Videen et al., 1988). Recently, decreased CBF and metabolism in the subgenual prefrontal cortex in patients with familial depression was found to be associated with a focal reduction in gray matter volume of the affected cortical structure. This intriguing observation indicates that altered PET measurements can be found due to partial volume averaging in conditions with an unsuspected anatomic abnormality (Drevets et al., 1997). Methods have been developed to correct for partial volume averaging and recover a more accurate radioactivity measurement from small brain structures (Meltzer et al., 1996; Iida et al., 2000).

Analysis of Functional Brain-Mapping Studies

The detection of significant changes in functional brain-mapping studies with [^{15}O]water is complex because of the large amount of data. Several different tasks may be performed by many subjects, and the images contain thousands of voxels, small volume elements in which rCBF can change. Specialized software packages have been developed to analyze the data. Statistical parametric mapping (SPM), developed at Hammersmith Hospital, London, has become a standard, widely applied method (Frackowiak et al., 1997; Acton & Friston, 1998). It is used to determine the differences, on a voxel-by-voxel basis, between sets of rCBF images obtained in different study conditions.

The method conceptually consists of three steps. The first is image normalization, in which each voxel from each rCBF scan in all subjects is mapped into the same stereotactic space. All voxels in the entire data set are transformed into a common reference brain in a three-dimensional coordinate system of a brain atlas (Tailarach & Tournoux, 1988). This permits the second step, averaging images obtained from different subjects during the same condition. Typically, one first adjusts for differences in global flow or tissue counts among subjects that may obscure focal changes. These differences may reflect physiologic differences in tracer delivery due to variations in arterial pCO_2, cardiovascular dynamics, or body size. This adjustment for global differences can be done with an analysis of covariance (ANCOVA), or by a ratio normalization in which all voxels are divided by the whole brain average counts. Averaging count-normalized images across subjects reduces image noise and facilitates the detection of differences between study conditions. Because noise in

PET images is random, it decreases when images are averaged, whereas the rCBF pattern, which should be consistent across subjects, remains. The final step is to perform statistical tests on a voxel-by-voxel basis between data sets from different tasks to identify clusters of voxels with significant rCBF change. This is a complex statistical procedure because of the large number of multiple comparisons that are made. The results of an SPM analysis are displayed as three-dimensional maps or views of the reference brain on which voxels with a significant change and the level of significance are highlighted. The stereotactic coordinates of voxels with significant rCBF changes are available, so that these areas can be precisely localized.

SPM was originally designed to determine the changes in local CBF measured with [^{15}O]water in subjects studied during different neurobehavioral tasks. It can also be applied in a parametric analysis to see which brain regions covary in a systematic fashion with some parameter related to the performance of a cognitive, sensory, or motor task, for example, the rate of hand movement. SPM has subsequently been applied to both [^{15}O] water and FDG images in other types of studies, for example, before and after administration of a drug, or to compare a group of patients to a control group. It has also been used to analyze perfusion images obtained with SPECT.

RADIATION EXPOSURE

Although the short half-lives of PET radionuclides favorably affect radiation exposure, it is not negligible. Radiation from PET and SPECT is an important consideration when they are used for research rather than diagnostic purposes (Huda & Scrimger, 1989; Ernst et al., 1998). Limits on radiation exposure to research subjects are set by regulatory bodies such as the U.S. Food and Drug Administration and institutional radiation safety committees. A potential risk associated with low levels of radiation such as those received from PET and SPECT is carcinogenesis. Although the risk is very low, the smallest amount of radiotracer necessary to perform a study should be administered. Genetic effects in future generations have never been observed in humans. The use of newer, three-dimensional PET scanners has made it possible to decrease radiation exposure in PET. Because of their greater sensitivity, it is possible to administer smaller doses of radiotracer and maintain image quality.

There are standard methods to calculate radiation exposure from internally administered radiopharmaceuticals (Loevinger et al., 1988; Stabin, 1996). One first determines the distribution of the radiotracer in the body as a function of time. This information can be calculated using physiologic models of in vivo tracer behavior, extrapolated from measurements in animals, or measured in a small group of human subjects. Then the radiation exposure to each organ is calculated using a model of the body that simulates the size, shape, and properties of body organs. The effective dose (ED) is a measure of the radiation exposure to the whole body. The ED from 5 mCi FDG is 0.34 rem, and for 10 rCBF scans with 10 mCi [^{15}O]water each, 0.59 rem. In comparison, the average person in the United States receives an annual radiation exposure of 0.30 rem from natural background sources such as the sun, outer space, and radioactive materials occurring naturally in the air and soil.

USE OF FUNCTIONAL BRAIN IMAGING IN PATIENT MANAGEMENT

A final consideration is the use of SPECT or PET brain studies in the clinical management of individual patients. The use of functional brain imaging in patient care is not as developed as its use in research. This may seem surprising, because SPECT and PET provide physiologic information that is qualitatively different from the structural information provided by CT and MRI. However, physicians are experienced in dealing with anatomic and neuropathologic information (e.g., brain slices, surgical visualization) that CT and MRI provide noninvasively. There is no equivalent knowledge base for dealing with physiologic images, and little empirical support for using them in clinical decision making. Most studies using functional brain imaging were not designed to examine its role in the diagnosis or management of the condition under investigation. Rather, they were performed to learn about disease pathophysiology. Thus, extrapolation of this information into the clinical arena is not justified. For example, many studies report the differences between a group of well-characterized patients and normal control subjects. An abnormality identified in patients with a specific disease cannot be applied directly to the assessment of an individual patient who is suspected of having the disease. To establish diagnostic accuracy, one must compare patients with the full spectrum of the disease to control subjects with the full spectrum of conditions with which the disease may be confused in clinical practice (Powers et al., 1991).

The clinical value of functional brain imaging can be rigorously assessed in the same way that new treatments can be evaluated and compared to existing treatments in a randomized, controlled trial. Such studies should be prospectively designed to evaluate PET or SPECT in a specific clinical setting, so as to establish its diagnostic accuracy, its efficacy in patient management, or its effect on outcome. There should be a comparison to a standard of "truth," for example, pathology or long-term follow-up. Bias must be avoided (Ransohoff & Feinstein, 1978). Selection bias occurs if the study is not performed in a consecutive series of predefined patients, or is unrandomized if comparing the course of patients treated with or without the test. Spectrum bias occurs when the study population is not the same as the one in which the procedure will be used. Work-up bias refers to using the new test to help decide who receives the "gold standard" test, whereas review bias occurs when the new test is not reviewed independently of the "gold standard" test and other information. Papers reporting on a new test should meet several criteria (Reid et al., 1995). They should describe the characteristics of the study population, for example, age and sex distribution, and presenting clinical symptoms or disease stage. Data from pertinent subgroups should be analyzed. The confidence intervals or standard errors for the test sensitivity and specificity should be given. It is important that indeterminate test results are included in the analysis, including nondiagnostic or equivocal results. Information of test reproducibility should be provided to indicate reader variability when the same or different readers review a set of images.

Kent and Larson (1992) have listed criteria for assessing the potential clinical contribution of a diagnostic imaging procedure. These are (1) technical capacity, that is whether it measures a phenomenon with precision; (2) diagnostic accuracy, the accurate detection and classification of pathology, including information about disease detection (sensitivity) and exclusion (specificity); (3) diagnostic impact, that is, a judgment of the test's accuracy and clinical value compared with existing alternatives; (4) therapeutic impact, the effect of the test on patient care, for example, replacing a more costly, uncomfortable or risky test, or identifying patients who would not benefit from treatment; and, finally, (5) patient outcome, that is, will the use of the test in a patient group prolong life, relieve suffering, or improve functional status? As put more succinctly, the ultimate criterion is for a test to reduce morbidity and mortality or to save money (Powers et al., 1991). The utility of PET or SPECT in managing most patients with neuropsychiatric disease has not been demonstrated using these criteria. In fairness, it must be said that there is still controversy about the role of more widely used tests, such as MRI, in specific clinical situations (Kent et al., 1994). However, appropriate studies must be performed before functional brain imaging is routinely used in patients. This is not only a question of cost containment, but also an issue of ensuring that the decisions made using these tests will actually help rather than harm patients.

The role of clinical functional brain imaging is gradually expanding. Both PET and SPECT are used in the presurgical evaluation of patients with epilepsy of focal onset that is refractory to medical therapy, especially in patients with temporal lobe epilepsy and when scalp electroencephalographic (EEG) recordings do not localize the seizure focus (Theodore, 1996). Interictal

PET scans with FDG show hypometabolism in the area of the focus. Although the physiologic basis for this finding is not completely understood, the finding is useful in patient evaluation. SPECT rCBF scans are used to demonstrate the brief focal increase in blood flow at the site of seizure origin. It is important to inject the tracer as soon as possible after seizure onset. This requires the tracer to be available at the patient's bedside during EEG monitoring, which is possible with ^{99m}Tc-ECD. The sensitivity of ictal SPECT is further increased by comparison with interictal images.

In patients with malignant brain tumors who present with recurrent focal symptoms after receiving radiation therapy, FDG PET is used to differentiate radiation necrosis from recurrent tumor (Langleben & Segall, 2000). Tumors have a high rate of glucose metabolism and FDG uptake, whereas areas of necrosis typically have low uptake. The sensitivity of PET for recurrent malignancy is about 80%, although the specificity is lower.

It might seem that CBF images would be useful to manage patients with cerebrovascular disease. As discussed above, however, relative or even absolute CBF measurements with PET or SPECT are inadequate on their own to characterize the underlying pathophysiology in cerebrovascular disease. Measurements of tissue oxygen metabolism are also required. Increased rOEF measured with PET, a compensatory mechanism for decreased cerebral perfusion pressure, is an independent predictor of stroke in patients with symptomatic carotid artery occlusion (Grubb & Powers, 2001). A clinical trial using PET to measure rOEF is planned to determine whether it can identify patients who would benefit from surgical revascularization.

In patients with Alzheimer disease, PET scans typically demonstrate a pattern of bilateral hypometabolism in temporal and posterior parietal lobes. SPECT changes of hypoperfusion in these areas appear to be somewhat less sensitive than the PET findings. The role of these modalities in the assessment and management of patients with dementia or early cognitive impairment is under active investigation (Hoffman et al., 2000; Silverman et al., 2001). Many SPECT studies have been reported in patients with head trauma, either in the acute or chronic phase of injury. Although there are broad correlations between local CBF decreases and neurologic or cognitive deficits, such studies have not shown aid in the management of individual patients.

Mayberg (1992, p. 18N) discussed the use of functional brain imaging data in criminal trials and noted that it has "not reached the level of sophistication to predict any neurologic or psychiatric deficit." Juni (1994, pp. 1894–1895), in a critical review of brain SPECT, noted that "while it may be possible in a given case to state that a particular scan defect is consistent with certain behavioral abnormalities, it is generally not possible to state with certainty that the two are causally related." Thus, the presence of a SPECT or PET abnormality does not prove it is causing a specific behavior, nor does its absence prove that the behavior is not due to organic illness. It also follows that functional brain images cannot be used to prove or exclude malingering.

In conclusion, PET provides unique quantitative measurements of rCBF and metabolism. Although SPECT studies of cerebral perfusion are more limited in scope, they can also be informative. Both modalities play an important role in clinical research studies designed to understand normal brain function and pathophysiology of neuropsychiatric disease. Their role in patient management will expand as careful studies define their role in specific clinical situations.

■ KEY POINTS

☐   Functional brain imaging refers to methods that provide images of the brain related to its physiology or biochemistry rather than to its structure.

☐   PET and SPECT are functional brain imaging techniques that provide cross-sectional images of the distribution of radioactivity in the brain and other parts of the body. These images represent physiologic or biochemical processes on a regional basis.

☐   Methods to measure CBF and metabolism in humans are the most common applications of functional brain imaging.

☐   A fundamental premise underlying functional brain imaging is that CBF and metabolism are intimately related to the activity of neurons.

☐   Functional brain imaging has been widely used as a research technique to map normal brain function and to study the pathophysiology of diseases affecting the brain.

☐   The role of clinical functional brain imaging is gradually expanding. Both PET and SPECT are used in the presurgical evaluation of patients with epilepsy of focal onset that is refractory to medical therapy, especially in patients with temporal lobe epilepsy and when scalp EEG recordings do not localize the seizure focus.

KEY READINGS

Daube-Witherspoon ME, Herscovitch P: Positron emission tomography, in Harbert JC, Eckelman WE, Neumann RD (eds): Nuclear Medicine. New York: Thieme, 1996, pp. 121–143.

Herscovitch P: Functional mapping of the human brain, in Wagner HN Jr, Szabo S, Buchanan JW (Eds): Principles of Nuclear Medicine. Philadelphia: Saunders, 1995, pp. 514–531.

Herscovitch P, Raichle ME, Kilbourn MR, et al: Positron emission tomographic measurements of cerebral blood flow and permeability-surface area product of water using [^{15}O]water and [^{11}C]butanol. J Cereb Blood Flow Metab 7:527–542, 1987.

Huang S-C, Phelps ME, Hoffman EJ, et al: Error sensitivity of fluorodeoxyglucose method for measurement of cerebral metabolic rate of glucose. J Cereb Blood Flow Metab 1:391–401, 1981.

Raichle ME: Behind the scenes of functional brain imaging: A historical and physiological perspective. Proc Natl Acad Sci U S A 95:765–772, 1998.

Silverman DH, Small GW, Chang CY, et al: Positron emission tomography in evaluation of dementia: Regional brain metabolism and long-term outcome. JAMA 286:2120–2127, 2001.

Villringer A, Dirnagl U: Coupling of brain activity and cerebral blood-flow—Basis of functional neuroimaging. Cerebrovasc Brain Metab Rev 7:240–276, 1995.

REFERENCES

Acton PD, Friston KJ: Statistical parametric mapping in functional neuroimaging: Beyond PET and fMRI activation studies. Eur J Nucl Med 25:663–667, 1998.

Altman DI, Lich LL, Powers WJ: Brief inhalation method to measure cerebral oxygen extraction with PET: Accuracy determination under pathologic conditions. J Nucl Med 32:1738–1741, 1991.

Bailey DL, Miller MP, Spinks TJ, et al: Experience with fully 3D PET and implications for future high- resolution 3D tomographs. Phys Med Biol 43:777–786, 1998.

Baron JC: Perfusion thresholds in human cerebral ischemia: Historical perspective and therapeutic implications. Cerebrovasc Dis 11(Suppl. 1):2–8, 2001.

Baron JC, Frackowiak RSJ, Herholz K, et al: Use of PET methods for measurement of cerebral energy metabolism and hemodynamics in cerebrovascular disease. J Cereb Blood Flow Metab 9:723–742, 1989.

Berridge MS, Adler LP, Nelson AD, et al: Measurement of human cerebral blood flow with [^{15}O]butanol and positron emission tomography. J Cereb Blood Flow Metab 11: 707–715, 1991.

Blaizot X, Landeau B, Baron JC, et al: Mapping the visual recognition memory network with PET in the behaving baboon. J Cereb Blood Flow Metab 20:213–219, 2000.

Blomqvist G, Stone-Elander S, Halldin C, et al: Positron emission tomographic measurements of cerebral glucose utilization using [1-^{11}C]D-glucose. J Cereb Blood Flow Metab 11:467–483, 1990.

Carson RE: Mathematical modeling and compartmental analysis, in Harbert JC, Eckelman WE, Neumann RD (eds): Nuclear Medicine. New York: Thieme, 1996, pp. 167–193.

Carson RE, Daube-Witherspoon ME, et al: A method for postinjection PET transmission measurements. J Nucl Med 29:1558–1567, 1988.

Chang JY, Duara R, Barker W, et al: Two behavioral states studied in a single PET/FDG procedure: Theory, method, and preliminary results. J Nucl Med 28:852–860, 1987.

Clarke DE, Sokoloff L: Circulation and energy metabolism of the brain, in Siegel GJ, Agranoff BW, Albers RW, et al (eds): Basic Neurochemistry. Philadelphia: Lippincott, Williams & Wilkins, 1999, pp. 637–669.

Daube-Witherspoon ME, Herscovitch P: Positron emission tomography, in Harbert JC, Eckelman WE, Neumann RD (eds): Nuclear Medicine. New York: Thieme, 1996, pp. 121–143.

Derdeyn CP, Videen TO, Simmons NR, et al: Count-based PET method for predicting ischemic stroke in patients with symptomatic carotid arterial occlusion. Radiology 212:499–506, 1999.

Drevets WC: Functional neuroimaging studies of depression: The anatomy of melancholia. Annu Rev Med 49:341–361, 1998.

Drevets WC, Price JL, Simpson JR, et al: Subgenual prefrontal cortex abnormalities in mood disorders. Nature 386:824–827, 1997.

Emami-Avedon SS, Ichise M, Lang AE: The use of SPECT in the diagnosis of Parkinson's disease. Can Assoc Radiol J 51:189–196, 2000.

Eriksson L, Kanno I: Blood sampling devices and measurements. Med Prog Technol 17:249–257, 1991.

Ernst M, Freed ME, Zametkin AJ: Health hazards of radiation exposure in the context of brain imaging research: Special consideration for children. J Nucl Med 39:689–698, 1998.

Fox PT, Perlmutter JS, Raichle ME: A stereotactic method of anatomical localization for positron emission tomography. J Comput Assist Tomogr 9:141–153, 1985.

Fox PT, Raichle ME: Stimulus rate dependence of regional cerebral blood flow in human striate cortex, demonstrated by positron emission tomography. J Neurophysiol 51:1109–1120, 1984.

Fox PT, Raichle ME: Focal physiological uncoupling of cerebral blood flow and oxidative metabolism during somatosensory stimulation in human subjects. Proc Natl Acad Sci U S A 83:1140–1144, 1986.

Fox PT, Raichle ME, Mintun MA, et al: Nonoxidative glucose consumption during focal physiologic neural activity. Science 241:462–464, 1988.

Frackowiak RSJ, Friston KJ, Frith CD, et al (eds): Human Brain Function. San Diego, CA: Academic Press, 1997.

Frackowiak RSJ, Lenzi G-L, Jones T, et al: Quantitative measurement of regional cerebral blood flow and oxygen metabolism in man using ^{15}O and positron emission tomography: Theory, procedure and normal values. J Comput Assist Tomogr 4:727–736, 1980.

Friedland RP, Iadecola C: Roy and Sherrington (1890): A centennial reexamination of "On the Regulation of the Blood Supply to the Brain." Neurology 41:10–14, 1991.

Friston KJ, Passingham RE, Nutt JG, et al: Localisation in PET images: Direct fitting of the intercommissural (AC-PC) line. J Cereb Blood Flow Metab 9:690–695, 1989.

Fulham MJ, Di Chiro G: Neurological PET and SPECT, in Harbert JC, Eckelman WE, Neumann RD (eds): Nuclear Medicine. New York: Thieme, 1996, pp. 361–385.

Grubb RL Jr., Powers WJ: Risks of stroke and current indications for cerebral revascularization in patients with carotid occlusion. Neurosurg Clin N Am 12:473–487, 2001.

Grubb RL Jr., Raichle ME, Higgins CS, et al: Measurement of regional cerebral blood volume by emission tomography. Ann Neurol 4:322–328, 1978.

Hasselbalch SG, Holm S, Pedersen HS, et al: The ^{18}F-fluorodeoxyglucose lumped constant in human brain from extraction fractions of ^{18}F-fluorodeoxyglucose and glucose. J Cereb Blood Flow Metab 21:995–1002, 2001.

Herscovitch P: Functional mapping of the human brain, in Wagner HN Jr, Szabo S, Buchanan JW (eds): Principles of Nuclear Medicine. Philadelphia: Saunders, 1995, pp. 514–531.

Herscovitch P, Markham J, Raichle ME: Brain blood flow measured with intravenous H$_2$^{15}O. I. Theory and error analysis. J Nucl Med 24:782–789, 1983.

Herscovitch P, Raichle ME: Effect of tissue heterogeneity on the measurement of cerebral blood flow with the equilibrium $C^{15}O_2$ inhalation technique. J Cereb Blood Flow Metab 3:407–415, 1983.

Herscovitch P, Raichle ME: What is the correct value for the brain-blood partition coefficient of water? J Cereb Blood Flow Metab 5:65–69, 1985.

Herscovitch P, Raichle ME, Kilbourn MR, et al: Positron emission tomographic measurements of cerebral blood flow and permeability-surface area product of water using [^{15}O]water and [^{11}C]butanol. J Cereb Blood Flow Metab 7:527–542, 1987.

Herzog H, Seitz RJ, Tellmann L, et al: Quantitation of regional cerebral blood flow with ^{15}O-butanol and positron emission tomography in humans. J Cereb Blood Flow Metab 16:645–649, 1996.

Hoffman JM, Welsh-Bohmer KA, Hanson M, et al: FDG PET imaging in patients with pathologically verified dementia. J Nucl Med 41:1920–1928, 2000.

Huang S-C, Phelps ME, Hoffman EJ, et al: Error sensitivity of fluorodeoxyglucose method for measurement of cerebral metabolic rate of glucose. J Cereb Blood Flow Metab 1:391–401, 1981.

Huang SC, Phelps ME, Hoffman EJ, et al: Non-invasive determination of local cerebral metabolic rate of glucose in man. Am J Physiol 238:E69–E82, 1980.

Huda W, Scrimger JW: Irradiation of volunteers in nuclear medicine. J Nucl Med 30:260–264, 1989.

Hurtig RR, Hichwa RD, O'Leary DS, et al: Effects of timing and duration of cognitive activation in [^{15}O]water PET studies. J Cereb Blood Flow Metab 14:423–430, 1994.

Ichise M, Meyer JH, Yonekura Y: An introduction to PET and SPECT neuroreceptor quantification models. J Nucl Med 42:755–763, 2001.

Iida H, Law I, Pakkenberg B, et al: Quantitation of regional cerebral blood flow corrected for partial volume effect using O-15 water and PET: I. Theory, error analysis, and stereologic comparison. J Cereb Blood Flow Metab 20:1237–1251, 2000.

Jons PH, Ernst M, Hankerson J, et al: Follow-up of radial arterial catheterization for positron emission tomography studies. Hum Brain Mapp 5:119–123, 1997.

Jueptner M, Weiller C: Review: Does measurement of regional cerebral blood flow reflect synaptic activity? Implications for PET and fMRI. Neuroimage 2:148–156, 1995.

Juni JE: Taking brain SPECT seriously: Reflections on recent clinical reports in *The Journal of Nuclear Medicine*. J Nucl Med 35:1891–1895, 1994.

Kadekaro M, Crane AM, Sokoloff L: Differential effects of electrical stimulation of sciatic nerve on metabolic activity in spinal cord and dorsal root ganglion in the rat. Proc Natl Acad Sci U S A 82:6010–6013, 1985.

Kent DL, Haynor DR, Longstreth WT Jr., Larson EB: The clinical efficacy of magnetic resonance imaging in neuroimaging. Ann Intern Med 120:856–871, 1994.

Kent DL, Larson EB: Disease, level of impact, and quality of research methods. Three dimensions of clinical efficacy assessment applied to magnetic resonance imaging. Invest Radiol 27:245–254, 1992.

Kety SS: The theory and applications of the exchange of inert gas at the lungs and tissues. Pharmacol Rev 3:1–41, 1951.

Kety SS: Measurement of local blood flow by the exchange of an inert diffusible substance. Methods Med Res 8:228–236, 1960.

Kety SS, Schmidt CF: The nitrous oxide method for the quantitative determination of cerebral blood flow in man: Theory, procedure, and normal values. J Clin Invest 27:476–483, 1948.

Lammertsma AA, Heather JD, Jones T, et al: A statistical study of the steady state technique for measuring regional cerebral blood flow and oxygen utilization using ^{15}O. J Comput Assist Tomogr 6:566–573, 1982.

Lammertsma AA, Jones T, Frackowiak RSJ, et al: A theoretical study of the steady-state model for measuring regional cerebral blood flow and oxygen utilization using oxygen-15. J Comput Assist Tomogr 5: 544–550, 1981.

Lammertsma AA, Wise RJS, Heather JD, et al: Correction for the presence of intravascular oxygen-15 in the steady-state technique for measuring regional oxygen extraction ratio in the brain: 2. Results in normal subjects and brain tumor and stroke patients. J Cereb Blood Flow Metab 3:425–431, 1983.

Landau WM, Freygang WH Jr, Rowland LP, et al: The local circulation of the living brain: Values in the unanesthetized and anesthetized cat. Trans Am Neurol Assoc 80:125–129, 1955.

Langleben DD, Segall GM: PET in differentiation of recurrent brain tumor from radiation injury. J Nucl Med 41:1861–1867, 2000.

Lassen NA, Ingvar DH: Radioisotopic assessment of regional cerebral blood flow. Progr Nucl Med 1:376–409, 1972.

Leniger-Follert E, Hossman K-A: Simultaneous measurements of microflow and evoked potentials in the somatomotor cortex of rat brain during specific sensory activation. Pflügers Arch 380:85–89, 1979.

Loevinger R, Budinger TF, Watson EE: MIRD Primer: Absorbed Dose Calculations. New York: Society of Nuclear Medicine, 1988.

Lou HC, Edvinsson L, MacKenzie ET: The concept of coupling blood flow to brain function: Revision required? Ann Neurol 22:289–297, 1987.

Magistretti PJ, Pellerin L: Cellular mechanisms of brain energy metabolism and their relevance to functional brain imaging. Philos Trans R Soc Lond B Biol Sci 354:1155–1163, 1999.

Martin WRW, Powers WJ, Raichle ME: Cerebral blood volume measured with inhaled $C^{15}O$ and positron emission tomography. J Cereb Blood Flow Metab 7:421–426, 1987.

Mayberg HS: Functional brain scans as evidence in criminal court: An argument for caution. J Nucl Med 33:18N–25N, 1992.

Mazziotta JC, Phelps ME, Plummer D, et al: Quantitation in positron computed tomography: 5. Physical-anatomical effects. J Comput Assist Tomogr 5:734–743, 1981.

McIntosh AR, Grady CL, Ungerleider LG, et al: Network analysis of cortical visual pathways mapped with PET. J Neurosci 14:655–666, 1994.

Meltzer CC, Zubieta JK, Links JM, et al: MR-based correction of brain PET measurements for heterogeneous gray matter radioactivity distribution. J Cereb Blood Flow Metab 16:650–658, 1996.

Mintun MA, Lundstrom BN, Snyder AZ, et al: Blood flow and oxygen delivery to human brain during functional activity: Theoretical modeling and experimental data. Proc Natl Acad Sci U S A 98:6859–6864, 2001.

Mintun MA, Raichle ME, Martin WRW, et al: Brain oxygen utilization measured with O-15 radiotracers and positron emission tomography. J Nucl Med 25:177–187, 1984.

Myers R: The biological application of small animal PET imaging. Nucl Med Biol 28:585–593, 2001.

Obrist WD, Thompson HK, King CH, et al: Determination of regional cerebral blood flow by inhalation of 133-xenon. Circ Res 20:124–135, 1967.

Ohta S, Meyer E, Thompson CJ, et al: Oxygen consumption of the living human brain measured after a single inhalation of positron emitting oxygen. J Cereb Blood Flow Metab 12:179–192, 1992.

Phelps ME, Huang SC, Hoffman EJ, et al: Tomographic measurement of local cerebral glucose metabolic rate in humans with (F-18) 2-fluoro-2-deoxy-D-glucose: Validation of method. Ann Neurol 6:371–388, 1979.

Phelps ME, Mazziotta JC, Kuhl DE, et al: Tomographic mapping of human cerebral metabolism: Visual stimulation and deprivation. Neurology 31:517–529, 1981.

Piert M, Koeppe RA, Giordani B, et al: Diminished glucose transport and phosphorylation in Alzheimer's disease determined by dynamic FDG-PET. J Nucl Med 37:201–208, 1996.

Powers WJ, Berg L, Perlmutter JS, et al: Technology assessment revisited: Does positron emission tomography have proven clinical efficacy? Neurology 41:1339–1340, 1991.

Powers WJ, Dagogo-Jack S, Markham J, et al: Cerebral transport and metabolism of 1-^{11}C-D-glucose during stepped hypoglycemia. Ann Neurol 38:599–609, 1995.

Powers WJ, Hirsch IB, Cryer PE: Effect of stepped hypoglycemia on regional cerebral blood flow response to physiological brain activation. Am J Physiol 270(2 Pt 2):H554–559, 1996.

Price C, Wise R, Ramsay S, et al: Regional response differences within the human auditory cortex when listening to words. Neurosci Lett 146:179–182, 1992.

Raichle ME: Behind the scenes of functional brain imaging: A historical and physiological perspective. Proc Natl Acad Sci U S A 95:765–772, 1998.

Raichle ME, Martin WRW, Herscovitch P, et al: Brain blood flow measured with intravenous H$_2$^{15}O. II. Implementation and validation. J Nucl Med 24:790–798, 1983.

Ransohoff DF, Feinstein AR: Problems of spectrum and bias in evaluating the efficacy of diagnostic tests. N Engl J Med 299:926–930, 1978.

Reid MC, Lachs MS, Feinstein AR: Use of methodological standards in diagnostic test research. Getting better but still not good. JAMA 274:645–651, 1995.

Reivich M, Alavi A, Wolf A, et al: Glucose metabolic rate kinetic model parameter determination in humans: The lumped constants and rate constants for [^{18}F]fluorodeoxyglucose and [^{11}C]deoxyglucose. J Cereb Blood Flow Metab 5:179–192, 1985.

Reivich M, Kuhl D, Wolf A, et al: The [^{18}F]fluorodeoxyglucose method for the measurement of local cerebral glucose utilization in man. Circ Res 44:127–137, 1979.

Roy CS, Sherrington CS: On the regulation of the blood supply of the brain. J Physiol Lon 11:85–108, 1890.

Sadato N, Carson RE, Daube-Witherspoon ME, et al: Optimization of noninvasive activation studies with ^{15}O-water and three-dimensional positron emission tomography. J Cereb Blood Flow Metab 17:732–739, 1997.

Sakurada O, Kennedy C, Jehle J, et al: Measurement of local cerebral blood flow with iodo[^{14}C]antipyrine. Am J Physiol 234:H59–H66, 1978.

Schmidt KC, Lucignani G, Sokoloff L: Fluorine-18-fluorodeoxyglucose PET to determine regional cerebral glucose utilization: A re-examination. J Nucl Med 37:394–399, 1996.

Schwartz WJ, Smith CB, Davidsen L, et al: Metabolic mapping of functional activity in the hypothalamo-neurohypophysial system of the rat. Science 205:723–725, 1979.

Silbersweig DA, Stern E, Schnorr L, et al: Imaging transient, randomly occurring neuropsychological events in single subjects with positron emission tomography: an event-related count rate correlational analysis. J Cereb Blood Flow Metab 14:771–782, 1994.

Silverman DH, Small GW, Chang CY, et al: Positron emission tomography in evaluation of dementia: Regional brain metabolism and long-term outcome. JAMA 286:2120–2127, 2001.

Sokoloff L: Local cerebral circulation at rest and during altered cerebral activity induced by anesthesia or visual stimulation, in Kety SS, Elkes J (eds): Regional Neurochemistry. New York: Pergamon Press, 1961, pp. 107–117.

Sokoloff L: Relationships among local functional activity, energy metabolism, and blood flow in the central nervous system. Fed Proc 40:2311–2316, 1981.

Sokoloff L: Energetics of functional activation in neural tissues. Neurochem Res 24:321–329, 1999.

Sokoloff L, Reivich M, Kennedy C, et al: The [^{14}C]deoxyglucose method for the measurement of local cerebral glucose utilization; theory, procedure, and normal values in the conscious and anesthetized albino rat. J Neurochem 28:897–916, 1977.

Spence AM, Muzi M, Graham MM, et al: Glucose metabolism in human malignant gliomas measured quantitatively with PET, 1-[C-11]glucose and FDG: Analysis of the FDG lumped constant. J Nucl Med 39:440–448, 1998.

Stabin MG: MIRDOSE: Personal computer software for internal dose assessment in nuclear medicine. J Nucl Med 37:538–546, 1996.

Tailarach J, Tournoux P: Co-planar Stereotactic Atlas of the Human Brain. New York: Thieme, 1988.

Ter-Pogossian MM, Phelps ME, Hoffman EJ, et al: A positron-emission transaxial tomograph for nuclear imaging (PETT). Radiology 114:89–98, 1975.

Theodore WH: Positron emission tomography and single photon emission computed tomography. Curr Opin Neurol 9:89–92, 1996.

Videen TO, Perlmutter JS, Herscovitch P, et al: Brain blood volume, flow, and oxygen utilization measured with ^{15}O radiotracers and positron emission tomography: Revised metabolic computations. J Cereb Blood Flow Metab 7:513–516, 1987.

Videen TO, Perlmutter JS, Mintun MA, et al: Regional correction of positron emission tomography data for the effects of cerebral atrophy. J Cereb Blood Flow Metab 8:662–670, 1988.

Villringer A, Dirnagl U: Coupling of brain activity and cerebral blood-flow—Basis of functional neuroimaging. Cerebrovasc Brain Metab Rev 7:240–276, 1995.

Wagner HN Jr, Szabo S, Buchanan JW (eds): Principles of Nuclear Medicine. Philadelphia: Saunders, 1995.

Welch MJ, Eichling JO, Straatman MG, et al: New short-lived radiopharmaceuticals for CNS studies, in De Blanc HJ Jr, Sorenson JA (eds): Noninvasive Brain Imaging: Computed Tomography and Radionuclides. New York: Society of Nuclear Medicine, 1975, pp. 25–44.

Woods RP, Mazziotta JC, Cherry SR: MRI-PET registration with automated algorithm. J Comput Assist Tomogr 17:536–546, 1993.

Wooten GF, Collins RC: Metabolic effects of unilateral lesions of the substantia nigra. J Neurosci 1:285–291, 1981.

Yamauchi H, Fukuyama H, Nagahama Y, et al: Significance of increased oxygen extraction fraction in five-year prognosis of major cerebral arterial occlusive diseases. J Nucl Med 40:1992–1998, 1999.

Yarowsky PJ, Ingvar DH: Neuronal activity and energy metabolism. Fed Proc 40:2353–2362, 1981.

fMRI and Related Techniques

Timothy P. L. Roberts

David J. McGonigle

Blood oxygenation level dependent (BOLD)

Functional MRI (fMRI)

Functional mapping

Magnetoencephalography (MEG)

Neuronal activity

Neurovascular coupling

Presurgical planning

NONINVASIVE BRAIN IMAGING

In the quest to understand the functioning of the human brain, many insights have been obtained from the careful study of patients suffering from neurologic deficits. This approach has proved extremely useful; by observing the behavioral consequences of spatially discrete lesions, researchers have been able to draw conclusions about the functional roles of brain regions. Yet a reliance on lesion studies alone may have its limitations. First, certain regions of the brain may rarely be damaged in isolation in humans, and second, the dense and reciprocal connectivity of the brain often makes it difficult to infer the function of a region by observing the deficits caused after its removal or injury (see Young et al., 2000, for a discussion of these issues).

These factors explain the attractiveness of *noninvasive* imaging methods. A number of these techniques are now in common use in the neurologic clinic. In addition to human electroencephalography (EEG), the analogous (magnetic) technique of magnetoencephalography (MEG) is now routinely used. Brain mapping methods that use metabolic-based measures to indirectly study neuronal activity are also common; in the last decade, positron emission tomography (PET) has been joined by functional magnetic resonance imaging (fMRI). However, although each of these techniques professes to measure "neuronal function," the means by which they do so vary considerably. It is therefore important to recognize the relative strengths and weaknesses of each technique, especially before interpreting results in a clinical setting. The purpose of this chapter is to focus on the methodology and application of two of these techniques, fMRI and MEG, representing hemodynamic (or metabolic) methods and neuroelectrical approaches, respectively.

MEASUREMENT OF NEURONAL ACTIVITY

The Electrical Activity of Neurons

Whatever metric neuroimaging techniques ultimately rely on to measure brain function, it is worthwhile remembering that information transfer in the human brain involves the production and processing of *electrical* signals. These signals are generated by changes in the potential difference across the neuronal cell membrane and comprise two broad categories: *action potentials* and *local potentials*. Action potentials are brief, explosive electrochemical events that are characterized by a transient depolarization of the neuronal membrane potential (Kuffler et al., 1984). This change propagates along the neuron's axon to the presynaptic terminal. Local potentials occur at a neuron's dendrites, typically as a consequence of neurotransmitter action.

As a result of these events the brain is almost constantly electrically active. Caton (1875) was the first to formally demonstrate this by applying a galvanometer to the exposed brains of rabbits and monkeys. However, the magnitude of current flow across a single neuronal membrane is small, about 1 mA/cm^2 during depolarization. To produce a signal that can be detected by an *external* recording device, many neurons must be "active" at the same time. The first widely used device to monitor the brain's electrical activity was the *electroencephalogram,* or EEG, first demonstrated on humans by Hans Berger (1929). Berger showed that EEG could be used to measure human cognitive processing by showing a decrease in the amplitude of the "α rhythm" during mental calculation. Although crude, this demonstrated that it was possible to "eavesdrop" on the normal functioning of the human brain with a remote device, circumventing the need to expose the actual cortical surface.

From Neuron to Vein

Using the electrical activity of the brain to monitor synaptic function is one possible noninvasive method. The relationship between synaptic function and neuronal *metabolism* offers another route. All organs of the body that perform "work" must be fueled. These processes require adenosine triphosphate (ATP), produced from glucose by oxidative phosphorylation and the Kreb cycle (Guyton & Hall, 1996). The brain is no exception to this rule: synaptic processes require energy. However, the metabolism of the brain is characterized by a number of unique features when compared with other physiologic systems of the body. The brain has a high "energy demand-to-weight" ratio (in humans, the brain takes up only 2% of the body's weight, yet requires roughly 20% of its oxygen and 15% of its blood flow). In addition, it appears to lack a "functional reserve" or store of energy. Finally, *an*aerobic metabolism is rarely, if ever, observed in the healthy primate brain. These qualities mean that the brain is almost completely reliant on oxygen delivered via blood to drive the biochemical processes vital for synaptic transmission. Oxygen must therefore be delivered to neurons via a locally regulated mechanism, targeted to those regions that need it most. Tracking these local changes in neuronal hemodynamics offers a window to noninvasively image brain function.

The existence of the link between cerebral blood flow and local function has been appreciated for over a century. One of the first papers to relate blood flow to local cerebral metabolism was published by Roy and Sherrington in 1890. Their work on animals led them to postulate that the brain's blood supply was locally regulated, so that the areas that required energy would receive the highest proportion of the global flow. They concluded ". . . the chemical products of cerebral metabolism contained in the lymph which bathes the walls of the arterioles of the brain can cause variations of the caliber of the central vessels: that in this reaction the brain possesses an intrinsic mechanism by which its vascular supply can be varied locally in correspondence with local variations of functional activity" (Roy & Sherrington, 1890, p. 105). This remarkably prescient statement is a precise summary of the main assumptions underlying metabolism-based functional brain imaging techniques.

Since this pioneering work, evidence has steadily accrued supporting a link between local blood flow and local oxidative metabolism (Villringer, 2000) and, by extension, local neuronal activity. The assumption underlying this link is that "the energetic requirements associated with synaptic function represent the indicators detected with functional brain imaging techniques" (Magistretti & Pellerin, 1999, p. 1156). Thus an increase in neuronal activity is accompanied by stereotypical changes in local neuronal glucose consumption, local cerebral blood flow (CBF), and the oxygen content of local blood. Knowing something about the nature of these changes in cerebral *vascular* parameters allows one to make inferences about local changes in *neuronal* activity.

Although the link between metabolism and function was appreciated at an early stage in the development of modern neurology, the technology to exploit this relationship did not exist. The earliest attempts to produce standardized instruments and methodologies that could be used to link local flow and metabolism were carried out by Kety and Schmidt in the 1940s (Kety & Schmidt, 1945). However, application of these techniques to the study of human functional neuroanatomy was largely unsuccessful because a disadvantage of this method was that only global flow could be measured. Animal studies using autoradiographic techniques were more successful (for a review, see Sokoloff et al., 1977). However, these techniques relied on sacrificing the subject at the end of the experiment. For obvious reasons, the procedure did not lend itself to (ethical) human experimentation.

Yet this situation did not persist for long. The experiments of Ingvar, Lassen, and colleagues in the 1960s and 1970s (reviewed in Lassen et al., 1991) led to the development of methods that allowed the measurement of regional CBF in humans, using nuclear medicine techniques such as single photon emission computed tomography (SPECT) and PET. These techniques demonstrated that it was possible to image the *local* metabolic consequences of the synaptic transmission of information in the human brain, in effect, to directly observe the mechanisms that Roy and Sherrington had proposed.

Magnetic Resonance Imaging

Although both PET and SPECT have been used extensively in experimental neuroscience, they have relatively low spatial and temporal resolution (e.g., blood flow PET studies of cerebral activation require the summation of signal over several seconds/minutes). To overcome these problems, it is common practice in functional neuroimaging studies to "coregister" PET "functional" images to higher-resolution images of brain structure. These "structural" or "anatomic" images are typically acquired using either computed tomography (CT) or, more commonly, magnetic resonance imaging (MRI). MRI is based on the principles of nuclear magnetic resonance (NMR), a spectroscopic technique used to obtain microscopic chemical and physical information about atoms and molecules. Most MRI methods specifically probe the hydrogen nuclei of the water molecule, present at very high concentrations in the human body. MR structural images of the brain are three-dimensional volume images in which the signal intensity at each voxel (or *volume element*) represents the value of an MR parameter reflecting the underlying composition of the tissue and in particular the physicochemical microenvironment of water within the voxel. However, MRI is not limited to the production of an anatomic backdrop for the analysis of flow-based images from other imaging techniques. A variety of MRI techniques exist that can produce tomographic images containing both structural and functional information. These techniques are known collectively as *functional* magnetic resonance imaging, or fMRI.

In a broad sense, fMRI can be used to study a wide range of pertinent physiologic parameters. Local or global blood flow changes can be imaged by using contrast agents (e.g., lanthanide chelates, such as gandolium-diethylene-triamine-pentaacetic acid [GdDTPA]) or by "tagging" or labeling arterial blood using the magnetic fields produced by the MR scanner, for subsequent tracking. Fractional blood volume changes can be examined in a similar fashion, whereas some metabolic activity can be studied using in vivo magnetic resonance spectroscopy (MRS), which focuses not on the hydrogen nuclei of water molecules, but of metabolites, such as N-acetyl aspartate (NAA). However, over the last decade one of the most widely used contrast mechanisms in fMRI of the human brain has been the ratio of oxygenated blood to deoxygenated blood. This particular contrast is known as the blood oxygenation level dependent (BOLD) contrast mechanism; BOLD fMRI has rapidly evolved into one of the most extensively used imaging techniques in both clinical and experimental neuroscience.

To BOLDly Go Where No Contrast Has Gone Before?

The ultimate goal of most BOLD fMRI experiments is to use the coupling between metabolism and neuronal information transmission to map brain function. In this fashion, fMRI is similar to PET and SPECT. But what do experiments performed with BOLD fMRI actually measure? PET and SPECT measure regional cerebral blood flow (rCBF) directly and quantitatively (in units of mL/100 g/min). By contrast, the signal at each voxel in a BOLD fMRI experiment is weighted by rCBF, but is not a direct measure of it, being also dependent on other factors. This can be explained by examining the mechanisms underlying the BOLD contrast in more detail.

All BOLD fMRI experiments rely on the different intrinsic magnetic properties of hemoglobin (the primary oxygen-carrying molecule in blood) and deoxyhemoglobin (Pauling & Coryell, 1936) as a means by which changes in local neuronal metabolism can be indexed. In the human body there are a number of molecules that have endogenous magnetic properties. Some of these molecules are termed *paramagnetic* (the antonym is *diamagnetic*) because they will magnetize (positively) to a slight degree when exposed to an externally applied field (e.g, the static or "B_0" field of the MR scanner). A high concentration of paramagnetic molecules at a given point in the brain will produce a local magnetic field disruption. This will reduce (shorten) the value of T2*, an MR parameter that measures how quickly an induced NMR signal will decay due to the spatial variation (heterogeneity) of the local magnetic field. Areas in the brain with a greater concentration of a paramagnetic moiety (such as deoxyhemoglobin) will have a shorter T2* value, reflecting the locally disrupted or heterogeneous magnetic field (Fig. 7-1). Conversely, if the concentration of deoxyhemoglobin is lowered (usually by a relative increase in oxyhemoglobin), T2* values will increase. The use of appropriate imaging pulse sequences (such as gradient recalled echo imaging, or echo planar imaging [EPI]) and parameters (long echo time, TE) can make MR images sensitive to the value of T2* and thus, by interpretation, to the ratio of oxyhemoglobin to deoxyhemoglobin.

How does the change in T2* and subsequent change in image intensity in the MR image assist in the study of neuronal function? The ability to use T2* values to image blood oxygenation was first demonstrated empirically in vivo by animal work carried out by the research groups of Ogawa (Ogawa & Lee, 1990a; Ogawa et al., 1990b) and Turner (Turner et al., 1991). Both groups showed that by experimentally manipulating the ratio of deoxyhemoglobin to oxyhemoglobin (usually by the induction of hypoxia) one could image contrast changes around blood vessels using MRI. Of pivotal importance, the signal intensity changes occurred not only in blood water, but also in the tissue water around vessels. This effect was subsequently demonstrated in humans by Kwong and colleagues (1992) and Ogawa and colleagues (1990c). These experiments showed that local changes in deoxyhemoglobin concentration under normal physiologic conditions could be detected. The signal increase seen in BOLD fMRI experiments is therefore produced by a vascular embodiment of a *disinhibitory* effect: a decrease in the local deoxyhemoglobin concentration at a voxel reduces its shortening effect on T2*, causing a net increase in this parameter, and thus an increase in signal intensity on an image acquired with T2* sensitivity. The increase in rCBF delivered in response to functional activation results in more oxygenated blood in local capillaries and venous vascular beds, which in turn results in less magnetic field disruption around the vascular beds and increased local signal intensity. Although Belliveau and colleagues (1991) had already used an exogenous (paramagnetic) contrast agent to examine blood volume changes in human visual cortex during simple photic stimulation, the work by Kwong and Ogawa demonstrated the potential of BOLD fMRI as a truly noninvasive imaging technology using *intrinsic* contrast.

Flow, Firing, and False Positives? BOLD Contrast and Neurophysiology

In a typical neuroimaging experiment using PET or fMRI, investigators design an experiment, scan a number of subjects, and analyze the resulting maps of signal change at each voxel to find "activated" regions in the brain. The ease with which such experiments can now be performed means that it is easy to forget that

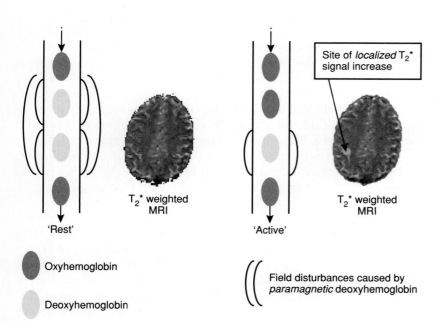

FIGURE 7-1. Schematic representation of how differences in the ratio of (paramagnetic) deoxyhemoglobin to oxyhemoglobin in blood vessels leads to differences in T2* shortening effects in surrounding tissue. These can be detected using the appropriate MR pulse sequences (see text) and is the basis of the blood oxygenation level dependent (BOLD) contrast mechanism, widely used in fMRI. (See Color Plate 2)

the link between changes in neuronal firing within an imaging voxel, and the resulting hemodynamics, are not yet fully understood.

Although few would deny, in general, the existence of a relationship between BOLD signal increase and neuronal metabolism in the healthy brain, it is fair to say that at the time of writing (autumn 2001), the exact nature of this relationship is still unknown. Although rCBF and glucose consumption increase locally and colocalize with the site of increased neuronal metabolism in a robust fashion, the local metabolic rate of oxygen ($CMRO_2$) does not change correspondingly (Fox & Raichle, 1986). Since the first demonstration of this effect in 1986, different investigative groups have shown varying relationships between oxygen consumption and flow/glucose consumption, either confirming (Madsen et al., 1995) or contradicting (Hyder et al., 1996) the findings of Fox and Raichle (1986). Although at present this remains a controversial topic, it is widely accepted that the delivery of oxygen to functionally activated neuronal tissue *overcompensates* for initial oxygen demand. In other words, there will be a local surplus of oxygenated hemoglobin (Fig. 7-2). The uncoupling (or weak link) between the changes in rCBF and $rCMRO_2$, with the rCBF changing more than local oxygen uptake, leads to a decrease in deoxyhemoglobin concentration in local capillaries.

As discussed above, this is the basis of the BOLD effect; BOLD signal changes result from differences in the ratio of deoxygenated to oxygenated hemoglobin within a voxel, producing an increase in T2* signal intensity within the voxel. However, until now we have tacitly assumed that neurons constitute the majority of the brain's metabolic load. This is not necessarily the case. On average, neurons occupy only 50% of the cerebral cortical volume (Kimelberg & Norenberg, 1989). The remainder is populated by glial cells and vascular

endothelial cells. In addition to the energetic requirements of neurons, the process of cerebral metabolism must support these cells.

It is now thought that glial cells may play an active role in cerebral metabolism by acting as a buffer between the "sources and sinks" of energy (Magistretti & Pellerin, 2000). Astrocytes occupy a strategic position between synaptic terminals and capillaries, and in vitro data suggest that they sense local synaptic activity at glutamatergic synaptic terminals via the activation of glutamate receptors. This initial event is thought to trigger the uptake of glutamate from the synaptic cleft by astrocytes, where it is converted to glutamine and transported back into neurons. In addition, the release of glutamate stimulates glucose uptake in astrocytes. These observations suggest an essential role for glia, particularly astrocytes, in coupling neuronal activity to cerebral metabolism.

These observations appear to present a problem for the interpretation of functional neuroimaging data. If it is *glial* metabolism that is being studied instead of *neuronal* metabolism, what are PET and fMRI signal changes actually indexing? The existence of other metabolically active cells may only be minimally important for current metabolically based imaging techniques, however. Although the distinction between neuronal and glial metabolism is important at the cellular level, this distinction does not invalidate functional neuroimaging methods. First, the changes in glial metabolism occur in the local vicinity of the changes in neuronal firing and are well within the spatial resolution of all current neuroimaging modalities. The two events (increases in glial and neuronal metabolism) are, at a first approximation, spatially concurrent. In fact, if, as some investigators have suggested, glucose is processed glycolytically in astrocytes, the mismatch of oxygen supply and demand that produces the BOLD effect may rely on astrocyte metabolism for its existence. Yet the somewhat inexact

FIGURE 7-2. A more detailed examination of the link between neuronal function and BOLD fMRI. The uppermost figure shows the typically conceptualized concept of baseline activity, where a low local rate of firing in the neurons whose axonal terminals lie in the region served by the arteriole and venule does not lead to any changes in the local concentration of deoxyhemoglobin (although it is still unknown if spontaneous discharge of this kind from a given region will cause a detectable BOLD effect or not). When these neurons undergo a net increase in activity (which may translate as an increase in the firing rate or firing synchrony), the accompanying increase in local CBF causes an increase in the ratio of oxyhemoglobin to deoxyhemoglobin (seen in the figure as the increase in red in the venule). This effect is thought at present to underlie the increase in MR signal seen in BOLD fMRI studies. (See Color Plate 2)

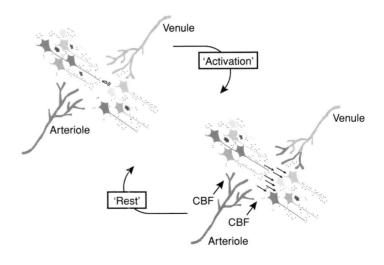

link between metabolic measures and local neuronal activity should always be kept in mind by functional neuroimagers. For example, in some clinical situations (such as where the subject has suffered a vascular insult), the reliance on a hemodynamic "reporting" mechanism (and thus the interpretation of BOLD contrast fMRI) remains controversial.

The relationship between neuronal metabolism and neuronal activity remains an active area of research. A number of studies have used optical imaging techniques to study the process of neurovascular coupling. These techniques record reflectance changes from the exposed cortical surface caused by a number of optically active processes. However, it is difficult to separate out these different sources when using traditional optical imaging. A series of experiments performed by Arminen Grinvald and colleagues has provided crucial insights (Grinvald et al., 1986; Malonek & Grinvald, 1996; Vanzetta & Grinvald, 1999) into both the spatiotemporal limitations of fMRI and the sources underlying responses to local increases in neuronal activity. Expanding on early work in cat visual cortex, Grinvald and colleagues (1986) used optical imaging spectroscopy (Malonek & Grinvald, 1996) to obtain detailed information on the temporal pattern of oxyhemoglobin and deoxyhemoglobin changes in active tissue after simple visual stimulation. Finally, they used an oxygen-sensitive dye method (Vanzetta & Grinvald, 1999) to study with greater temporal resolution the oxygen uptake during stimulation.

The results from this series of papers support a triphasic model of hemodynamic changes subsequent to neuronal activation. According to Grinvald and colleagues' results, there is an initial increase in oxygen consumption, caused by an increase in oxygen metabolism in "active neurons." This results in an increase in local deoxyhemoglobin concentrations and begins around 100 msec after initial sensory stimulation (the so-called initial dip). This component is well localized to the actual site of neuronal activity (Grinvald and colleagues used columnar-specific visual stimuli and were able to resolve columnar-specific patterns), and the existence of this "initial dip" in humans was confirmed by high-magnetic-field (4 T) fMRI studies (Hu et al., 1997). This phase is followed by an increase in blood volume caused by capillary dilation beginning around 300 to 500 msec later, which is less well colocalized with the site of electrical activity. Finally, there is an increase in local blood flow that begins around 500 msec to 1 second after stimulation. This process decreases deoxyhemoglobin concentration and increases oxyhemoglobin concentration and is thought to be the primary cause of the BOLD effect. This third phase of the neurovascular response causes a much larger decrease in deoxyhemoglobin concentration than the initial increase (on the order of ×4 difference). The cat experiments of Grinvald and colleagues

(1986) suggest that this late response is not localized to the activated cortical columns but is spread over neighboring columns as well.

Quite apart from the relationship between the BOLD signal and neuronal activation is the spatial veracity of BOLD fMRI signal increase. This problem is typified by the "brain or vein" question (Kleinschmidt & Frahm, 1997) because the BOLD signal can also be detected in the macrovasculature surrounding areas of activation (Lai et al., 1993; Segebarth et al., 1994; Disbrow et al., 2000). How confident can one be that BOLD signal in voxels truly represents activation of the underlying cortex and not the oxygen content of nearby vessels? One possible solution to this problem is to increase the strength of the scanner's B_0 field. Work carried out by Ogawa and colleagues (1993) demonstrated that the BOLD signal is proportional to B_0 for large vessels (i.e., with a diameter of >10 mm), yet in smaller vessels (diameter <10 mm), it is proportional to B_0^2. Thus at higher field strengths the signal from smaller vessels is weighted proportionally higher. In addition, as the B_0 field increases, the T2 value of blood shortens dramatically, to about 7 msec at 7 T in humans (Yacoub et al., 2001), when compared to tissue T2. The use of echo times that are optimally weighted toward the T2 time of neural tissue at high field should therefore allow the intravascular component of the BOLD signal to be virtually eliminated. However, the (field strength dependent) increases in magnetic field–induced susceptibility artifacts in some anatomic areas and the lack of general availability of ultrahigh (>7 T) MR scanners suggest that this solution may not be appropriate, in general.

The high-resolution images of ocular dominance columns produced at high field strengths suggest that (at least in visual cortex) the use of the initial dip will also assist in distinguishing between brain and vein as possible sources of changes in BOLD signal. However, other solutions exist. Using spin-echo (SE) rather than gradient-echo (GE) pulse sequences can significantly change the underlying vascular specificity of the BOLD signal at clinical field strengths (for a review, see Kennan, 2000). SE sequences should be more sensitive to signal changes in small vessels than GE sequences are; however, this increase in the specificity of the source of BOLD signal change is offset by the worse sensitivity of SE sequences at 1.5 T. Some studies have suggested a compromise approach afforded by the asymmetrical spin-echo (ASE) sequence.

To summarize, the problems associated with imaging the initial dip exemplify the problems of imaging small signal changes in MRI, in general. Because the vascular compartment occupies only a small fraction of a gray matter voxel, BOLD signal changes at clinical field strengths (i.e., 1.5 T) are small. Even the positive-going component of the BOLD response produces signal changes of the order of only 2% to 4% in primary sensory areas at 1.5 T (Cohen, 1996). Imaging the BOLD response to neuronal stimulation is further complicated by the dynamics of the neurovascular response. The BOLD signal is a temporally delayed response to neuronal activity; whereas neuronal dynamics are measured on the order of milliseconds, the BOLD response takes a number of seconds to evolve. This means that although one can theoretically acquire several MR images in a second, the temporal smoothing of the underlying neuronal signal by the mechanism of the BOLD response ultimately defines the effective temporal resolution (Fig. 7-3). Determining the *temporal point spread function* (Friston et al., 1994) of fMRI data is therefore important, if the hemodynamic changes detected using BOLD are to be related to the neuronal dynamics underlying and preceding them. These issues, and others, mean that sophisticated image processing and analysis techniques must be used to ensure that neurophysiologically relevant MR signal changes are being interpreted. This had led to the development of software suites of processing tools of ever-increasing sophistication, targeted on extracting neurophysiologically specific information from dynamic MRI data, while recognizing (and compensating for or discarding) contributions from extraneous irrelevant, or *noise*, sources. In such terms, "noise" may include any signal fluctuation that is not of neurophysiologic interest, including not only the random image noise inherent to MR, but also physiologic signal changes (associated with arterial or cerebrospinal fluid [CSF] pulsations, respiration, etc.) as well as time-varying subject movement. Thus, multiple components of signal change must be considered when describing the observed signal changes, and statistical means must be used to eliminate signal changes of no immediate interest, preserving only those changes relating to the question under study.

PREPROCESSING AND ANALYSIS OF fMRI DATA

The rapid improvement in the sophistication and ease with which BOLD fMRI data can now be acquired means that a dedicated researcher with access to an MRI scanner can formulate an experimental question, acquire data from a group of subjects, and analyze the dataset in little more than a month. However, each new advance in acquisition technology brings with it new challenges. A less positive aspect of the swift advances in the field has been the struggle faced by new researchers to come to grips with the sheer volume of practical issues involved in designing a good BOLD fMRI experiment, that is, one that has sufficient power to reject a null hypothesis (Aguirre & D'Esposito, 2000). The methodology underlying experimental design in fMRI is not remarkably different from that used in all good expositions of experimental design, of which the design of Box and colleagues (1978) is a good reference. However, other issues must be addressed. Raw BOLD fMRI data consist of a complex assembly of different signal sources, both interesting and confounding to the experimental design, and, as such, it is typical for a number of preprocessing steps to precede the actual analysis. Because these steps typically involve filtering in the temporal or spatial domains to improve signal-to-noise ratio (SNR), it is important to be aware of them a priori, i.e. before beginning the experiment. Figure 7-4 summarizes the main steps involved in the acquisition and analysis of a simple fMRI dataset.

At the heart of BOLD fMRI experimental methodology is the concept of the "subtraction experiment." This idea is little changed from its initial introduction to experimental psychology in the 19th century by Franz Donders. In reaction time experiments, Donders claimed he could isolate the time that subjects needed to perform the "differentiation" inherent in a complex task by subtracting the time subjects took to respond to a simple stimulus from the time subjects took to respond to a more complex stimulus. In its simplest form, an fMRI experiment can be conceptualized in a similar manner; two images are acquired during different experimental conditions and are subtracted to isolate the "sensory or cognitive component of interest," the particular cognitive operation that the investigator is interested in studying and ultimately localizing (Fig. 7-5).

In practice, however, it is rare to subtract only two images; in BOLD fMRI, as in other neurobiologic disciplines, a number of observations of each experimental condition are made. Because these are typically acquired

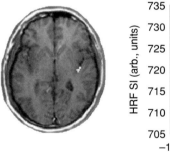
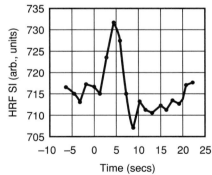

FIGURE 7-3. The temporal form of MR signal changes to an isolated stimulus—the hemodynamic response function (hrf). In this example, acquired at 1.5 T using 1.5-second temporal resolution in an event-related paradigm, BOLD signal changes were observed in a few highlighted pixels of auditory cortex (left). Interrogating these pixels for the time course of their signal change (right), it is apparent that the BOLD signal changes achieve a peak approximately 4.5 to 6 seconds after the stimulus, and this is followed by a signal undershoot before eventual recovery to baseline after approximately 15 to 20 seconds. (See Color Plate 2)

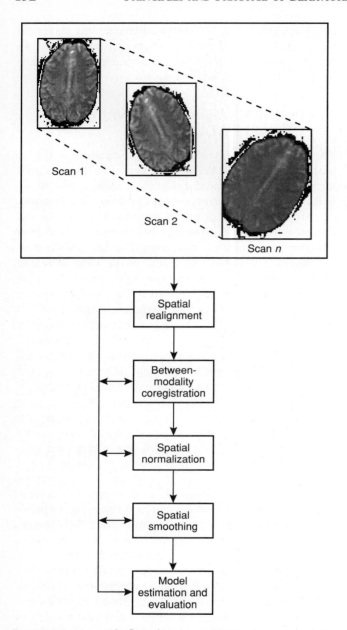

FIGURE 7-4. A simple flow diagram outlining the major steps involved in the postprocessing of fMRI data. Although the diagram here represents a typical SPM99 analysis flow chart, most contemporary software packages for fMRI analysis carry out similar steps. However, some aspects of preprocessing, such as the spatial smoothing carried out to allow the use of gaussian random field theory to correct for multiple comparisons, tend to be exclusive to SPM.

in sequence during a single experimental session, and the BOLD response is delayed by several seconds in time from its neuronal source, BOLD fMRI data are nonindependent time series data, typically acquired over a period of several minutes. A number of confounding factors can arise when subjects are asked to lie

still for a long period of time, each of which may potentially affect the experimenter's ability to draw meaningful conclusions from his or her dataset. The first of these that we will examine is subject movement.

Movement and Realignment

Effective data analysis in functional imaging experiments relies on the ability of the experimenter to compare "like with like" over a series of scans acquired over a period of time. It is easy for this assumption to be violated, for example, if the subject moves between the acquisitions of successive images. This can produce changes in signal intensity within the image, mainly arising from different areas being sampled in successive scans (e.g., think of how movement will affect signal intensity in a voxel lying on the white matter/ventricular boundary, if it moves so that in successive scans it is located over either white matter or gray matter). In situations such as this, it can be difficult to unambiguously interpret the data. Indeed, it was common for early fMRI studies to be viewed with suspicion due to the problems caused by subject motion (e.g., Hajnal et al., 1996). Although every physical attempt is generally made to limit subject head motion during the MR acquisition itself, it is now standard in functional neuroimaging experiments for researchers to subsequently use a "realignment" algorithm to ensure that the confounding effects of movement are reduced (Fig. 7-6).

Typically, realignment algorithms move all images into a standard space. This space is usually defined by the first image in the series (after images with T1 saturation effects have been discarded), and so realignment can be conceptualized as a problem in which the differences between subsequent images and the first image in the series must be minimized. Most current approaches (Ashburner & Friston, 1997; Woods, 2000) treat each image as a *rigid body* or an object in which the relationship between each element (voxel) of the body remains constant under all possible motions. This simplifies the problem, allowing the differences between images to be describable by a set of simple geometric parameters. Six parameters are typically used in fMRI realignment: three translations (in the x-, y-, and z-axes) and three rotations (q, f, and w, respectively). Typically, the transformations described by these parameters are applied iteratively until the sum-of-squares difference between the two images is minimized (Ashburner & Friston, 1997).

It is simple to appreciate the problems of movement when it is of a large enough magnitude to be observable by eye, but even subvoxel movement is a serious problem. As well as introducing potential false-positive activations at tissue boundaries, movement can reduce the signal to noise ratio (SNR) of the image.

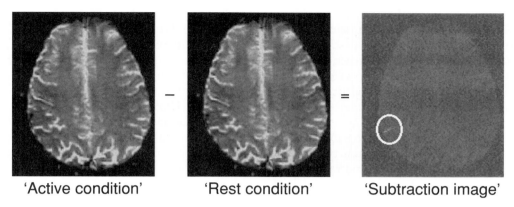

'Active condition'   'Rest condition'   'Subtraction image'

FIGURE 7-5. A basic subtraction experiment in BOLD fMRI. The first image is acquired while the subject is performing the task being studied (here, finger opposition with the digits of the left hand). The second image is acquired at rest. The third image represents what is left when the second image (rest) is subtracted from the first (activation). Some evidence for localized signal increase in the left motor cortex can be observed, although the subtraction of only two images will invariably yield overwhelming image noise.

Perhaps most significantly, motion introduces an unmodeled source of variance into voxel time series. In addition, the rigid-body assumptions of most realignment algorithms can fail quite spectacularly in brain areas where fast MR volume acquisition sequences (such as echo planar imaging [EPI]) induce geometric distortions that have a different form between subsequent scans (for a new approach addressing this problem, see Andersson et al., 2001). It is therefore important to remember that there is much scope for the future improvement of approaches to realignment.

Coregistration

Realignment attempts to minimize the differences between subsequent imaging acquisitions of the same imaging modality. But what if it is necessary to compare data acquired using different imaging sequences in fMRI or from a different neuroimaging modality? It is common practice to acquire a "T1-weighted" or structural image of subjects during a typical fMRI scanning session. These images are used to localize the fMRI activity to the underlying anatomic structures because

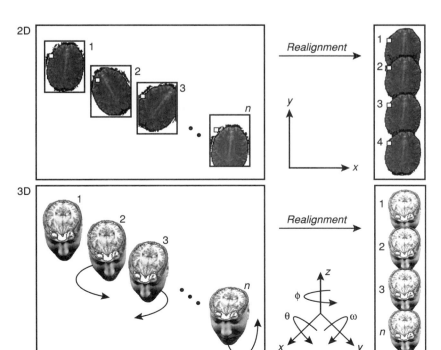

FIGURE 7-6. Subject movement and realignment. The top panel illustrates how subject movement can be problematic when movement is limited to within the axial imaging plane (i.e., a two-dimensional [2D] problem). Even in this simplified case, it is obvious that subject movement has an impact on the tissue content of the example voxel (in yellow). The inferior panel shows the more familiar case with humans, in which movement is truly a three-dimensional (3D) problem (modeled with six parameters by most rigid-body realignment algorithms). (See Color Plate 3)

the T1-weighted images typically have higher spatial resolution and better gray/white matter contrast. However, this means that the functional data must somehow be "overlaid" onto the higher-resolution structural image. This problem is conceptually similar to realignment, i.e. two images are not spatially contingent, and the researcher wishes to minimize the differences between them. However, the assumptions that any differences between images are now merely down to subject movements are no longer tenable, because the two images have been generated using different contrast mechanisms, having different spatial resolutions and potentially suffering from different geometric distortions.

At present, a number of methods are used in medical imaging to coregister data of the same structure acquired using different methodologies, including heuristic voxel intensity measures (Woods et al., 1993) and mutual information registration schemes (Collignon et al., 1995). One approach to this problem is to preprocess the images from both modalities, as suggested by Ashburner and Friston (1997). After the images have been segmented into maps of different tissue constituents, a rigid-body transformation is used to coregister the images. Whichever method is used, it is appropriate to examine both images after the transformation to assess the success (or otherwise) of the algorithm.

Linear and Nonlinear Spatial Normalization

The need to combine sequential observations on the same subject to increase statistical power in BOLD fMRI begat the process of image realignment. A similar situation occurs when a number of different subjects are scanned under the same experimental protocol. The researcher would like to combine these separate samples. Yet, at a gross level, individual brains can look very dissimilar. How can this problem be overcome? Just as realignment algorithms were developed to allow the comparison of like with like over a scanning session, spatial *normalization* algorithms have been developed that address the problem of comparisons between different subjects. Note that this process is of particular importance in cognitive neuroscience research, in which common areas and patterns of activity across a population are investigated, and of lesser importance in the clinical investigation of an individual patient, especially in the presence of intracranial structural lesions, disturbing anatomic relationships.

The process of normalization seeks to transform individual subject data into a common reference space. However, affine or other classes of linear spatial transformations are not powerful enough for this task, due to the nonstationary variation in local shape between different brains. The nonlinear "warping" algorithms used in neuroimaging are spatial transformations that act to change the global shape of the subject's brain while preserving the spatial relationships of local structures (see Thompson & Toga, 2000, for an extensive review of different warping algorithms).

The uncertain relationship between gross anatomic structure and function in the human brain, elegantly illustrated by the studies of Zilles and colleagues (1995) and Geyer and colleagues (1999, 2000), means that investigators should be aware that even a perfect normalization might not allow them to make the kind of comparisons they require because matching gross structure is not equivalent to matching local function. Yet normalization approaches are constantly subject to improvements. If warping performs its task efficiently, that is, by minimizing the global shape differences between different subjects, multisubject analysis techniques can be used.

Analysis of fMRI Data: The General Linear Approach and Statistical Parametric Mapping

The preprocessing steps outlined above are relatively standard approaches, performed by the majority of neuroimaging research groups, at the time of writing. The rest of this section will concentrate on the use of a widely used and readily available neuroimaging software package, Statistical Parametric Mapping, or SPM99 (downloadable from http://www.fil.ion.ucl.ac.uk) to infer the presence of significant effects in the dataset.

Statistical Parametric Mapping

The concept of SPM was introduced by Friston and colleagues (1995a), and although the approach owes much to the work on change distribution analysis pioneered by members of the St. Louis neuroimaging group (Fox & Mintun, 1989), there are significant differences. SPMs are three-dimensional images of *statistical* values, such as ts or Fs, recorded over a volume of interest that can range from the entire brain to a single plane through a structure of interest. The intensity of each voxel represents the value of the statistic (and not the effect size) in question under the particular hypothesis being examined. The underlying philosophy of SPM as summarized by Friston and colleagues (1995a), is that ". . . one proceeds by analyzing each voxel using any (univariate) statistical parametric test. The resulting statistics are assembled into an image that is then interpreted as a spatially extended statistical process" (p. 189). SPMs can efficiently summarize a vast body of data in a form that is easier to examine and interpret.

Gaussian Fields and Nonindependence

Before detailing a typical SPM fMRI analysis, it is important to discuss some issues that frequently arise in the analysis of neuroimaging data. In a typical single fMRI volume there can be hundreds of thousands of voxels. At the standard rejection rate of $P < .05$, we would expect, by chance, to reject the null hypothesis (H_0) of no experimental effects in a 20th of our sample (note, for a dataset of 200,000 voxels, 5% of 200,000 is 10,000 voxels!). One can therefore obtain a large number of activated voxels in the imaging volume by simply testing one's hypothesis enough times. Thus the probability of rejecting H_0 at each voxel must take into account the number of times H_0 is tested. Obviously, setting this criterion too low will cause an increase in type I errors (false positives). Changing the significance level at which H_0 is rejected without acknowledgment of this fact can lead to confusion (Fig. 7-7).

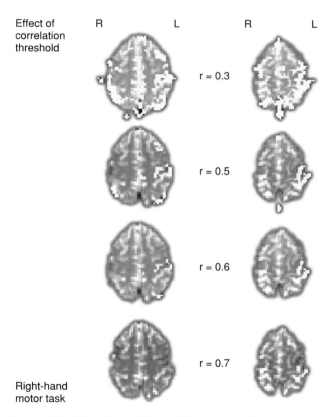

Effect of correlation threshold

R   L   R   L

r = 0.3

r = 0.5

r = 0.6

r = 0.7

Right-hand motor task

FIGURE 7-7. The effect of using different correlation thresholds on activation maps. Two successive single axial slices (5 mm thick) are shown coregistered with the result of a correlation analysis using a simple shifted "boxcar" as the regressor of interest (active voxels are shown in yellow). It is evident that, though it is possible to lower one's threshold to get "activated" voxels, doing so will, of course, increase the false-positive rate of the experiment. The large amount of voxels identified as "active" in the figure, even at "high" correlation thresholds, points to the importance of using a correction factor that takes into account the number of statistical tests being performed across the imaging volume. (See Color Plate 3)

The standard solution to this problem is to use Bonferroni correction, which simply adjusts the P value at which H_0 is rejected. For example, in the above case one would divide the usual P value of .05 by 200,000, to get a corrected P value of 25×10^{-7}. However, the Bonferroni correction is widely criticized as being too conservative because it assumes independent data (which translates to a requirement for spatially independent data in fMRI).

As an alternative to Bonferroni correction, the SPM software uses *gaussian random field* (GRF) theory to determine the critical value of the statistic at which to reject H_0. GRF theory deals with "the behavior of stochastic processes defined over a space of D dimensions" (Poline et al, 1997, p. 86). Knowing about the behavior of gaussian fields under certain constraints (Adler, 1981; Worsley, 1994) means that it is possible to determine the probability of a given local excursion of the gaussian field at any location. For the purposes of BOLD fMRI, the local excursions can be conceptualized as local peaks within the statistical map, signifying high statistical values (and thus significant local patterns of signal change). GRF theory allows the correct significance to be assigned to these values.

However, preprocessing of neuroimaging data is necessary before GRF theory can be used. Spatial smoothing is used to ensure that the smoothness of the fMRI data is greater than the resolution of the fMRI data (Fig. 7-8).

The full-width at half-maximum (FWHM) of the smoothing kernel should typically be at least two or three times larger than the initial voxel size; for example, it is common practice to smooth fMRI data with a raw resolution of $2 \times 2 \times 2$ mm with a gaussian kernel of 6-mm FWHM. Although this may appear to defeat the purpose of acquiring high-resolution functional data, it is necessary for the application of GRF theory and the benefits thereof. It is also worthwhile remembering that the *effective* resolution of the data is determined in any case by the spatial congruence between metabolic demand and vascular supply, not merely by digital, or prescribed, voxel size.

The General Linear Model

The vast majority of currently available software packages for neuroimaging analysis use univariate linear tests at each and every voxel to attempt to reject the H_0. All parametric versions of these tests, ranging from simple correlation tests of a single stimulus vector, for example, STIMULATE (Strupp, 1996), to more sophisticated analysis frameworks using ANCOVAs, can be thought of as special cases of a unifying analysis framework, the general linear model (GLM). The GLM lies at the heart of the SPM package.

The GLM allows for a great deal of flexibility in the design and analysis of experiments. Variation in the

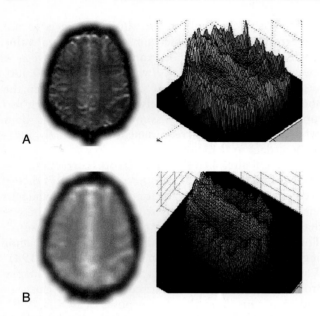

FIGURE 7-8. Spatially smoothing images. To use GRF theory to acquire corrected P values the individual volume scans must be spatially smoothed. A, A single slice through an EPI image, with a "mesh plot" of the voxel intensity values shown on the right. B, This is the same slice after spatial smoothing with an 8-mm FWHM isotropic gaussian kernel. Note that the previously "spiky" mesh plot now approximates a smooth, continuous function.

dependent variable Y (rCBF or BOLD contrast for PET and fMRI, respectively) is modeled as a linear combination of a number of explanatory variables, plus an error term. In other words, the signal at a particular voxel is assumed to consist of a mixture of different effects, some of interest (those following the time course of the experiment) and some that are not (i.e., low-frequency drifts in scanner signal, or signal changes resulting from the cardiac and respiratory cycles). If all of these components are included in the experimental model, the GLM allows one to investigate signal change resulting from each in turn.

The GLM formulation for a single observation (i.e., a single data point) (j) at a voxel is:

$$Y_j = \beta_1 \, x_{j1} + \dots + \beta_l \, x_{jl} + \dots + \beta_L \, x_{jL} + \varepsilon_j \quad (1)$$

The errors (ε_j) are assumed to be independent and normally distributed with zero mean and variance σ^2. The xs are the independent or *explanatory* variables, and can take two forms: *covariates* ("real" levels of a particular variable, such as time or the concentration of a pharmacologic agent) and *indicator* variables (so called because they *indicate* the presence or absence of an experimental factor) (Friston et al., 1995a). We wish to solve Equation 1 and estimate the parameters of the model (the βs, which can be thought of as the size of the contribution of each explanatory variable to the variation

in Y). Although in neuroimaging experiments there are usually more than one x to fit to Y (i.e., we do not think that there is only one process underlying signal change in a particular voxel), it is useful to consider that for one continuous explanatory variable, (x_{j2}), Equation 1 reduces to:

$$Y_j = \mu x_{j1} + \beta_2 \, x_{j2} + \varepsilon_j \quad (2)$$

which is simply linear regression (in this form, "y = c + mx" plus an error term). The μx_{j1} term is the Y-axis intercept, and introduces the use of a "dummy" variable (x_{j1}) whose value is unity for all J scans. This allows mean or "constant" offset terms to be included in the GLM formulation, and so explicitly model condition, subject, or even population means in the design matrix. In this manner, changes in BOLD signal intensity can be examined that reflect *relative* increases across subjects or groups. For example, when studying two groups, it is important to account for the possible difference in the group means before examining relative increases in BOLD. In Equation 2, it is evident that a simple way to think about the βs is as "regression slope" coefficients, describing the size and sign of the relationship between Y and the xs. However, it is rare for a neuroimaging experiment to reduce to simple linear regression. Similarly, it is rare for only one observation to be taken of each voxel, and so for every scan j there is a corresponding Equation 2. The following expansion of Equation 2 represents the typical form of a single subject neuroimaging analysis using SPM:

$$
\begin{aligned}
Y_1 &= \beta_1 \, x_{11} + \dots + \beta_l \, x_{1l} + \dots + \beta_L \, x_{1L} + \varepsilon_1 \\
&\;\;\vdots \\
Y_j &= \beta_1 \, x_{j1} + \dots + \beta_l \, x_{jl} + \dots + \beta_L \, x_{jL} + \varepsilon_j \\
&\;\;\vdots \\
Y_J &= \beta_1 \, x_{J1} + \dots + \beta_l \, x_{Jl} + \dots + \beta_L \, x_{JL} + \varepsilon_J \quad (3)
\end{aligned}
$$

This rather cumbersome formulation can be summarized by:

$$\mathbf{Y} = X \, \beta + \varepsilon \quad (4)$$

which is the vector form of the GLM: $\mathbf{Y}$ is a column vector of observations, β is a column vector of parameter estimates, and ε is a column vector of error terms. X represents a concept that is essential in the application of the GLM in neuroimaging analysis: the *design matrix*.

To summarize the above, to test for experimental effects at a given voxel the data $\mathbf{Y}$ are collected over J scans, the experimental model of explanatory variables X is fitted to the data, and the column vector of parameters β is estimated. The "goodness-of-fit" of the model to the data is indexed by the errors ε. Maximizing the fit of the model to the data will increase subsequent calculations of statistical significance. Intelligent formulation of the experimental model (i.e., consideration of all the possible influences that might in part account for observed signal changes) is therefore extremely important. Note that in the absence of explicitly stated expectation regressors, or for the purposes of unbiased "hypothesis generation," a number of groups have proposed the use of variations of independent component analysis (ICA) for the identification of features in the signal time series data (Calhoun et al., 2001). Although this has the appeal of being unconstrained by requirements of specific regressor definition and offers the possibility of identifying novel aspects to the response time course, unambiguous interpretation of the resultant component waveforms themselves is somewhat limited. It is perhaps useful at this stage to demonstrate the GLM formulation of a simple two-condition fMRI experiment on a single subject. The experimental design is summarized in Figure 7-9. Briefly, a number of volumes (in this example, 36) are acquired under two different states: stimulation (in this example, 8 Hz reversing checkerboard "visual" stimulation) and rest (in this example, passive fixation). In this simple experiment there is only one experimental manipulation—the effect of visual stimulation contrasted against rest, or vice versa. Thus the model contains only a single explanatory variable, representing the stimulus time course (convolved with the expected hemodynamic response function). The session-specific mean is also modeled to ensure that any comparisons between subjects or sessions are corrected for the main effects of session/subject, although this is less relevant in our single-subject example.

Figure 7-9 shows the graphic representation of the design matrix in SPM99. It is important to note that the graphic grayscale representations of the model used

within SPM are merely the lower plots turned on their side, so that the expected voxel signal value for each successive scan (or TR interval) is represented by each new row of the matrix. The model itself (here, the two columns that make up the matrix **X** in the figure) is again just the plot shown at the bottom of Figure 7-9, turned on its side and represented using grayscale values.

To solve the above equation involves estimating the βs that produce the best fit between the model and the data. The best values of βs are those that minimize the total distance between the model and the data. This quantity is formulated as the *sum of squared error (S)* or the sum of the squared distances between each Y_j (data) and (model). This process of fitting the model to the data such that S is minimized is an example of *least squares* fitting.

Modeling of fMRI Time Series: Signal Processing Issues

As discussed above, BOLD fMRI data are *time series* data. In PET and SPECT each scan is treated as an independent observation, but fMRI scans occur in a continuous series, sampled at a high enough rate to render each observation nonindependent; formally, as ". . . the sampling interval of . . . [f]MRI . . . is typically much shorter than the time-constants of hemodynamic changes, the resulting timeseries can show substantial autocorrelation" (Friston et al., 1994, p. 153). The hemodynamic response smooths the fMRI signal so that signal in the *n*th scan will contain a contribution from patterns of BOLD signal change to events that occurred in previous (e.g., n-2, n-1th) scans. This smoothing is problematic. As eloquently summarized by Aguirre and D'Esposito (2000, p. 375), the 1/f noise spectrum and the smoothness of the hemodynamic response function (hrf) are the ". . . Scylla

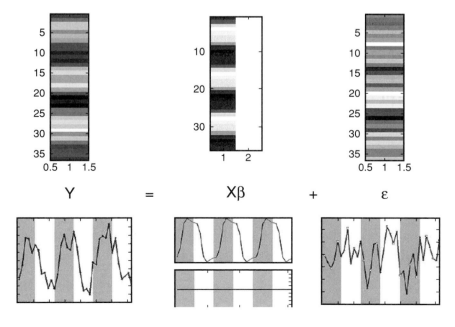

FIGURE 7-9. A graphic representation of the relationship between the different components of the general linear model (GLM). The top row of images shows the typical SPM representations of the GLM at each voxel: the data (**Y**), the model or *design matrix* (**X**), and the error vector (e). By comparing these columns vectors with the plots at the bottom of the figure, it is easier to appreciate that the design matrix produced by SPM99 is merely a grayscale plot of the different regressors (i.e., the vectors within *X*, the experiment model). When *X* is fitted to *Y*, the sizes of each experimental effect are estimated (the βs), and the significance of the fit is assessed by the error vector (ε).

and Charybdis of fMRI experimental design: experimental variance must be present at sufficiently low frequencies to pass through the hemodynamic transfer function but at sufficiently high frequencies to avoid the elevated noise range." The 1/f (frequency) noise spectrum means that, in fMRI, the noise spectrum (the distribution of signal across frequencies under the null hypothesis) is not uniform (i.e., not "white"). A number of empirical studies (Boynton et al., 1996; Zarahn et al., 1997a) have shown that fMRI noise is colored under the null hypothesis, violating the assumptions of the GLM. Although the exact shape of fMRI noise spectrum is contentious, the 1/f model proposed by Zarahn and colleagues (1997) is accepted as a good approximation. As one can appreciate, because of the approximate 1/f form the power of the noise is highest at low frequencies. The causes of these low-frequency components include both periodic physiologic noise (Jezzard et al., 1993) and scanner drift. Whatever the underlying cause, low-frequency noise presents two problems for the analysis of fMRI data. As mentioned above, it violates the assumptions of traditional parametric statistics. In addition, it reduces the sensitivity of fMRI designs where the frequency of the experimental effects are similar to the intrinsic noise spectrum, as the experimental model will end up fitting noise as well as signal. As such, the researcher is stuck between a rock and a hard place.

However, the fMRI researcher has two (not mutually exclusive) means by which to circumvent these problems. The first is effective experimental design, ensuring that the fundamental frequency of the experimental paradigm is high enough to escape the high-power (low-frequency) elements of the 1/f spectrum, yet low enough so that its power is not reduced by the hrf. The second approach is temporal filtering, analogous to the spatial smoothing used to ensure that the data conform to GRF assumptions. Filtering fMRI data before the experimental model is estimated and inference is made is an effective way to regularize the temporal autocorrelation structure. The approach implemented in the current version of the SPM software is to use bandpass filtering. Although the raw errors ε are autocorrelated, by choosing a kernel of a larger size than the endogenous autocorrelation it is assumed that these serial correlations are swamped (Friston et al., 1995b). It is then possible to determine the effective degrees of freedom of the ensuing t or F statistic. The approach above is by no means the only way to solve this problem; a variety of other methods to model or remove the serial correlations in fMRI have been proposed (Bullmore et al., 1996; Aguirre et al., 1997; Zarahn et al., 1997a).

The Main Event—Event-Related fMRI

The use of event-related fMRI (efMRI) is becoming increasingly prevalent in fMRI; yet the technique itself is still relatively immature. Demonstrations of detectable fMRI signal changes in response to relatively brief stimulus (~2 seconds) presentations were made as early as 1992 (Blamire et al., 1992). Subsequent studies demonstrating the ability of fMRI to detect neurovascular events of shorter duration (Savoy et al., 1995) showed that fMRI has the power to resolve the neurovascular correlates of transient stimuli. Based on this initial work, Dale and Buckner (1997), following an empirical example in Buckner and colleagues (1996), proposed an analysis framework influenced by techniques commonly in use to analyze event-related potentials (ERPs) for the analysis of transient hemodynamic events. Thus, efMRI was born.

Subsequent to the Dale and Buckner formulation, a number of analytical frameworks for the analysis of efMRI were published (Josephs et al., 1997; Zarahn et al., 1997b). The approach used by SPM is that described by Josephs and colleagues (1997), which is an extension of the basic GLM framework to encompass the modeling of single events or "transients/delta functions/stick functions" as they are variously described (Fig. 7-10) and each with a concomitant BOLD response, or hrf. Although, at heart, the SPM implementation of efMRI can be simplified for those familiar with the block-mode fMRI by considering a design matrix with an extremely brief block, efMRI demands that a number of additional issues be addressed.

efMRI is extremely useful from an experimental design perspective as it allows ". . . new *genres* of fMRI experiment" (Josephs et al., 1997, p. 243). An oft-quoted example is the oddball paradigm, in which the experimental effects of interest are the subject's responses to transient, infrequently presented stimuli that break the set of the context established by preceding stimuli (e.g., AAAABAA). It also allows an opportunity to circumvent undesired auditory "stimulation" arising from the noise of the scanner itself (Le et al., 2001). Similarly, efMRI is extremely useful for stimuli over which the experimenter has no control, for example, any form of pathologic episode or spontaneous shifts in perception (Kleinschmidt et al., 1998). In addition, most experimenters would agree that modeling subject responses to stimuli over a protracted period of time as is done in block-mode fMRI is often not the most sensitive way to proceed; effectively, the assumption is that the subject's responses are invariant over the time of the block, ignoring effects of fatigue, habituation, and short-term learning. Modeling each trial as a separate event and thus allowing for within-block or trial-to-trial variation in response will be a more sensitive way to model the experimental variance (Price et al., 1999).

As well as increasing the number of possible fMRI paradigms, efMRI experiments present an opportunity

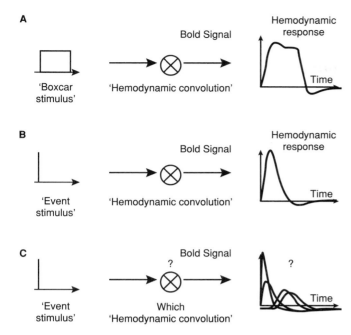

FIGURE 7-10. Modeling event-related responses in SPM99. Panel *A* shows the usual assumption typified by the "boxcar" study, in which trains of stimuli are given in blocks. The blue plot in panel *A* shows the expected hemodynamic response to a stimulation epoch of this sort (assuming that the response exhibits saturation, producing the tonic response exemplified by the boxcar). Panel *B* shows how the hemodynamic response in SPM99 to a brief event can be thought of as that to a very brief block/boxcar. Panel *C* demonstrates what happens when the hemodynamic convolution kernel is not known a priori, and it becomes difficult to successfully model the "family" of hemodynamic responses that result due to the possible spatial and temporal nonstationarity of the hemodynamic response functions.

to explicitly test some of the assumptions of the GLM, namely, the linear transform assumptions. The study by Boynton and colleagues (1996) was one of the first to address the linear assumptions underlying the transfer of neuronal activity to the vascular response. While showing that the response was approximately linear over a range of stimulus-onset asynchronies (SOAs), this study demonstrated that some nonlinearities in the hrf exist at short SOAs, which the authors thought may be due to neuronal adaptation. At present it is unknown whether nonlinearities in efMRI signal are due to the BOLD response itself or the underlying neuronal response (Friston et al., 1998) or both.

Assumptions of Linear Modeling of BOLD Signal Changes

fMRI studies using counterbalanced or randomized experimental designs with brief stimulus presentations

(efMRI) have become increasingly popular. In practice, the majority of these designs use some form of linear modeling; the expected BOLD signal to a given sensory stimulus, or cognitive or motor event, is estimated to be a convolution of the time course of the event with a hemodynamic kernel, or hrf. Thus the hrf is seen to be the mathematical description of the sequential BOLD changes observed in the optical experiments of Malonek and Grinvald (1996), and is the source of the indirectness linking fMRI with underlying neuronal activity. With the assumption of linearity, the response to any stimulus can be predicted if the response to a very short stimulus (called the impulse response) is known. In addition, any changes in the latency or amplitude of the BOLD fMRI response can be attributed to changes in the underlying neuronal activity over the time course of the stimulus. Determining, or estimating, the form of the hrf under conditions of rapid stimulus presentation (challenging linearity assumptions) and across individuals, anatomic substrates, and systemic physiologic perturbations is a critical step in relating the patterns of activity observed with fMRI to underlying neuronal events.

Although linear methods have been used with some success, they may be less useful when the measured signal has high spectral complexity, such as the evoked hemodynamics that occur in response to neuronal activity (Mayhew et al., 1998). There are a number of reasons why the assumption of linearity may not be tenable over some temporal and spatial scales. A number of studies have found that for short stimulus durations (<3 seconds, Boynton et al., 1996; 1 and 2 seconds, Vazquez & Noll, 1998; <6 seconds, Friston et al., 1998; Robson et al., 1998) a better model fit was obtained using nonlinear regression, or that the recorded hemodynamic response departed significantly from linear predictions of its amplitude or duration. In addition, the form of the hrf has been estimated to be different between different cortical regions (Bullmore et al., 1996; Lange & Zeger, 1997). These observations have prompted some authors to use nonlinear regression (Kruggel & Von Cramon, 1999) to obtain better estimates of the hemodynamic response across different cortical areas and subjects.

However, although many studies have focused on attributing the source of the nonlinearity in the observed BOLD fMRI response to the hemodynamic component, an equally plausible contributor is the underlying neuronal activity itself. For example, single-cell responses in visual cortex show departures from linearity when short stimuli are used (Tolhurst et al., 1980), and evoked field potentials show amplitude and latency nonlinearities in both visual and auditory cortex as interstimulus intervals (ISIs) are shortened. In addition, the decrease in amplitude of the visual evoked potentials going from an ISI of 2 seconds to 1 second is substantially different from the decrease seen when comparing ISIs of 1 second and

0.5 second. Furthermore, the majority of BOLD fMRI studies assume that the time course of the underlying neuronal activity evoked by a given stimulus can be equated with the time course of the stimulus itself. In a landmark study, Logothetis and colleagues (2001) have claimed that the duration of fMRI echoes the duration of field potentials but not unit activity. Thus, though not ruling out a vascular influence on BOLD fMRI nonlinearities, using the time course of some metric of neuronal activity in defining the "event" may result in a better model fit to the fMRI data. Whether this is practical to use in typical fMRI studies or not, future work addressing this issue should determine how nonlinearities in the neuronal event relate to the nonlinearities in the BOLD fMRI response, and are likely to indicate that there is an interaction between both the event and the hemodynamic reporting mechanism that compounds the nonlinearities in the observed response. Overall, nonlinearities in observed responses can be considered to be potentially attributable to nonlinear effects in either or both the underlying neuronal activity and the hemodynamic reporting system. Practically, the ability to resolve functional hemodynamics in a meaningful fashion is limited by the spatial coupling between neuronal activity and hemodynamic change. This can be thought of as the neurovascular point-spread function (PSF; Engel et al., 1997), perhaps the spatial manifestation of the indirect link between fMRI and neuronal activity, analogous to the hrf convolution that leads to indirectness in the temporal domain. As discussed earlier, optical imaging studies (Malonek & Grinvald, 1996) have suggested that the spatial pattern of changes in deoxyhemoglobin concentration are not tightly coupled to sites of ongoing neuronal activity.

The delayed yet transient form of the hrf presents challenges when performing efMRI experiments. One significant problem to models using phase-dependent variables (or regressors) is the nonsimultaneous acquisition of imaging data in a single volume. During most multislice (typical) imaging acquisitions, the last slice is acquired up to several seconds after the first slice. Yet each fMRI volume is often treated as though each slice is acquired simultaneously. The relatively long (20-30 seconds) state-related designs used for block-mode fMRI will be minimally affected by this fact. However, it may significantly bias efMRI results because the experimental model will fit some slices better than others (Price et al., 1999). In addition, if the experimental stimulus is time-locked to a slice consistently throughout the experiment, the hrf will be sampled very sparsely. Josephs and colleagues (1997) proposed a way to circumvent both problems by "jittering" the phase of data acquisition relative to the stimulus. This provides greater *effective* temporal resolution and also goes some way toward reducing the effects of nonsimultaneous slice acquisition. To effectively overcome different slice-timing problems, it is often necessary to use a temporal interpolation algorithm (Josephs & Henson, 1999). In the absence of such schemes, the choice of *basis functions* for modeling the hrf can help to overcome slice-timing issues (e.g., using a Fourier set of basis functions, or allowing systematically time-shifted functions for each slice). Basis functions are defined formally as a set of vectors that span a space such that each element of the space can be uniquely expressed by a linear combination of the functions. In the current context the space is defined as containing all possible expressions of the shape of the hrf to a transient event. However, when the dimensions of the space are not known in advance, it becomes difficult to choose the most efficient basis set.

When considering the choice of basis functions, the single Poisson function suggested by Friston and colleagues (1994) to model the hrf may not be as efficient as other possible formulations. For example, Boynton and colleagues (1996) showed that the time constant chosen by Friston for the Poisson response was several seconds slower than the form suggested by data from primary visual cortex, V1. Using multiple basis functions to form a more intricate hemodynamic response function considerably reduces variance in the model/data fit. Consequently many groups use a "canonical" hrf as one basis function and its temporal derivative as a second. As with any multiparametric fitting, whereas the model/data fit improves (in terms of residual variance) unambiguous inference becomes harder, as each basis function is associated with an amplitude and latency coefficient, with little direct neurophysiologic interpretation on their own. As an alternative to estimation of the form of the hrf, Aguirre and colleagues (1998) suggested that because between-subject variance in efMRI responses was greater than within-subject variance, empirically derived subject-specific hrfs would be the most efficient basis functions. However, although it makes intuitive sense to obtain a good estimate of each subject's hrf for use in subsequent analyses, the Aguirre group's results remain to be confirmed across different brain areas and cognitive paradigms. Other analysis frameworks (Lange & Zeger, 1997; Kruggel & Von Cramon, 1999) allow for a more complete specification of the hrf, and can model spatially nonstationary hrfs well. Although the use of multiple basis functions in the GLM allows for good approximations to these more complicated specifications, it is important to appreciate that, although computationally expensive, nonlinear modeling of the hrf is essential if one wishes to analyze amplitude and latency differences independently.

Despite the above complications in ultimate interpretation, efMRI looks set to open up new vistas of insight into the neural substrates, networks, and, importantly, time courses of complex cognitive processes, with clinical application to behavioral neurology, psychology, and psychiatry, as well as neuroscience.

MAGNETOENCEPHALOGRAPHY (MEG) AND MAGNETIC SOURCE IMAGING (MSI)

Much of the conceptual underpinning of early event-related BOLD fMRI analyses emerged from the related field of event-related potentials (ERPs). Broadly speaking, ERPs allow the researcher to study the evoked neuroelectrical responses to a broad array of experimental paradigms, in a similar manner to efMRI. However, the use of ERPs and their magnetic-field analogs, event-related fields (ERFs), recorded using magnetoencephalography (MEG; for a review, see Hämäläinen et al., 1993) has a number of distinguishing characteristics when compared to efMRI. First and foremost, these techniques *directly* record the electrical and magnetic activity generated by the membrane depolarization and ion flux secondary to neuronal information processing. Thus, in one important sense, these techniques can be considered more directly related to the activity of neurons because they do not have to rely on the more indirect hemodynamic coupling mechanism underlying the BOLD response of fMRI. Secondly, electrical activity detected using EEG and MEG has intrinsically higher temporal resolution than indirect metabolic techniques. This temporal resolution is limited largely by analog-to-digital converter circuitry; sampling rates of several kHz (and thus sub-millisecond temporal resolution) are commonly available. Treated simply, EEG and MEG offer temporal insight into the time course, or "temporal signature," of neuronal activity that is deficient in the coarsely sampled, hemodynamically convolved, fMRI response. However, the integrated use of both types of technology may allow the neuroscience researcher to build up a multidimensional spatiotemporal description of brain function (e.g., Dale & Halgren, 2001). We now address the conceptual similarities and differences between EEG and MEG methods and provide a primer to the considerably less prevalent, more expensive, but potentially more powerful technique of MEG.

Comparison of EEG and MEG

The neuronal origin of the signal detected in the MEG is similar to that underlying the EEG (Hämäläinen et al., 1993; Lewine & Orrison, 1995). Consequently, MEG and EEG share obvious physical similarities. In a sense, MEG can be considered the magnetic counterpart of EEG, and the raw data from both techniques appear quite similar at first inspection. Despite these similarities, important fundamental differences exist between EEG and MEG. These differences arise from the physical properties of the signal (electrical versus magnetic), the instrumentation used for signal detection, the sensitivity of each modality, and the available approaches for analysis. A fundamental and obvious difference is that EEG measures electrical potentials, whereas MEG senses the obli-

gate magnetic field. The electrical signal has its origin in extracellular currents that are conducted through many layers of tissue before reaching the scalp recording electrodes. The scalp tissues possess varying electrical conductivities and can be substantially altered by the effect of lesions, craniotomy defects, or surgery (Lewine & Orrison, 1995). This makes it hard for EEG models to account for these regional variations, demanding both realistic head shapes as well as volumetric estimates of electrical conductivity. In the absence of such detailed knowledge, a craniotomy defect could allow current to pass preferentially through one margin, leading to false EEG-based estimation of source localization. MEG, in contrast, records magnetic flux that passes through these tissue layers with much less spatial distortion, due to the similar magnetic permeabilities of skull, CSF, and brain soft tissues. Thus the MEG signal may be more amenable to source modeling than its electrical counterpart.

As well as the obvious differences in the ultimate sources of the EEG and MEG signals, the two techniques differ in their sensitivity to the orientation and depth of neuronal activity. EEG is in general more sensitive to radially oriented currents, and MEG is better suited to the detection of tangentially oriented sources. Furthermore, MEG is in general less sensitive than EEG to deep sources of brain activity. This differential sensitivity has important implications for experimental design. In epilepsy, for example, the depth of mesial temporal spikes may render MEG detection difficult or impossible, whereas they may be readily seen on EEG. In contrast, the activity of tangential electrical currents in the lateral temporal lobe (e.g., auditory cortex) is easily seen and localized by MEG, but may be poorly characterized by EEG.

EEG and MEG have also been used in different ways in the clinical environment. EEG has been established for over 70 years and is a relatively inexpensive test to perform. MEG, however, is emerging as a clinical modality; has a limited, but rapidly increasing, installation base; and is somewhat less standardized. MEG is also more expensive due to the usual requirement for magnetic shielding, superconducting electronics, and the use of liquid helium. However, the technical advantages offered by MEG in terms of improved source localization opportunities and reduced contamination from distant electrical sources provide compelling motivation for its use for the remote sensing of neuronal electrical activity. Although the remainder of this chapter will focus on the application of MEG technology, many of the points raised are equally applied to the EEG method (given the intrinsic and practical differences discussed above).

An MEG Primer

Neuronal Underpinnings of the MEG Signal

Although we have acknowledged that MEG is in many ways a more direct technique than fMRI, it is not without its caveats. Although intracranial neuronal currents generate the extracranial magnetic fields detected by MEG, it would be wrong to regard MEG as being exquisitely sensitive to all forms of neuroelectrical activity. For example, MEG will be most sensitive when large numbers of neurons (see below) are sufficiently synchronous to allow adequate summation of the magnetic fields associated with each neuron. This will allow a resolvable signal (on the order of femtotesla) to be detected. Thus, MEG and EEG are biased toward the detection of certain forms of macroscopic neuronal dynamics. To satisfy the condition of synchrony defined above, it seems likely that the signals detected by MEG arise from postsynaptic ionic current flow in the pyramidal cells of layers III and IV of the cerebral cortex, because these possess the appropriate spatial organization (elongated shape and columnar layering) and temporal synchrony to allow superposition of the current elements (Lewine & Orrison, 1995). It has been estimated that at least 30,000 neurons need to be simultaneously activated for the detection of extracranial fields (Williamson & Kaufman, 1990).

It is probable that MEG is not sensitive to the action potentials generated at the output of a cortical area because they may not be sufficiently synchronous to allow detection (see Logothetis et al., 2001, for a recent suggestion that fMRI may be similarly insensitive to the output, i.e., layer V of a given cortical region). Instead, due to their longer duration, the excitatory and inhibitory postsynaptic currents of apical dendrites are the most likely electrophysiologic source of signals detected by MEG. In summary, as with fMRI, MEG is but one technique out of several, each offering a slightly different metric on the underlying neuronal activity.

Technology Required to Record MEG

Recording the minute neuromagnetic fields generated by the brain (typical fields have peak amplitudes of 10–100 fT, some 10 log orders of magnitude less than the earth's magnetic field) is not a trivial challenge. The required sensitivity is provided by SQUID (superconducting quantum interference device) technology. Briefly, the SQUID acts as a low-noise amplifier connected to a primary pick-up coil. The voltage output of the SQUID can be made proportional to the magnetic field detected through the use of appropriate feedback electronics. In practice, the detector coil may take several forms, from a simple single-coil magnetometer, through axial or planar two-coil gradiometers to high-order multicoil gradiometers (Flynn, 1994; Vrba, 1996). In general, a compromise must be achieved between sensitivity (maximum for magnetometers) and rejection of distant sources (most effective for high-order gradiometers). Most contemporary biomagnetometer systems, consisting of over 100 detector channels

arranged in a helmet-style configuration, however, require housing in a magnetically shielded room (MSR), typically constructed of alternating layers of aluminum and mu-metal, to provide electric and magnetic field shielding.

Components of the MEG Waveform

Some features in the time-domain of the neuromagnetic evoked response are sufficiently robust over related experimental paradigms and across subjects that they are termed "components" and can be used to define aspects of the evoked response. The tacit assumption in adapting such an approach to the analysis of MEG/EEG data (describing an entire high temporal resolution evoked response in terms of the amplitude and latency of a few well-chosen peaks) is that the use of these features allows a parsimonious reduction of the original waveform (Fig. 7-11). This analysis can be compared to similar approaches in EEG, and even in fMRI when the hemodynamic response is modeled by a canonical function that is scaled along a single dimension, usually height, to fit the data. These forms of analysis can be regarded as the simplest possible approaches to characterizing neuroimaging data; however, this does not deny their utility. Indeed there are intrinsic features of these measured components that relate to processes of sensation, perception, and cognitive processing, revealed as modulation of the component amplitudes or latencies, or as the occurrence of

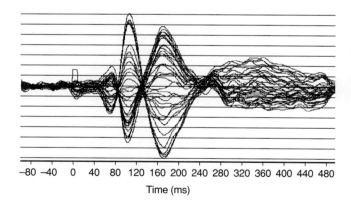

FIGURE 7-11. A neuromagnetic evoked field. In this representation the magnetic field detected by a 37-channel array biomagnetometer in response to presentation of 1-kHz sinusoidal auditory stimulus is shown collapsed onto a common axis. The time-domain duration of the displayed evoked response is 500 msec, with 100 msec of "baseline" sampled prior to stimulus onset. The peak amplitude of the evoked field occurs approximately 100 msec after the stimulus (the M100 component) and has an amplitude of approximately 100 fT (root mean square across sensor channels). (See Color Plate 4)

novel components, specifically elicited by a particular experimental paradigm or condition. Restricting attention to a few "measurable" quantities, namely, the amplitude and latency of such peaks or components in MEG and EEG, allows the researcher to use univariate statistical methods and the hypothesis-testing framework that underlies them.

Indeed, some features of evoked responses, in particular the poststimulus latency of particular components, have been described as constituting a time-domain signature, revealing properties of the stimulus and the subject's perception thereof. An example can be found in the 100-msec component of the auditory evoked field (termed N1m or M100). Whereas the latency of this component is approximately 100 msec, it has been shown to vary with stimulus properties (such as intensity, pitch, and timbre), as well as with developmental age (in children and teenagers) (Roberts & Poeppel, 1996; Roberts et al, 2000a). Although such temporal variation in an evoked response component does not necessarily imply "temporal encoding" of stimulus feature information at a neuronal level, it is tempting to speculate that these readily observed "reflections" of neuronal activity correspond to identification and discrimination of stimuli according to their physical attributes, and may form a "temporal signature" of the neuronal activity involved.

A special type of context-dependent response that has proven to be a valuable research tool is the mismatch negativity (MMN) and its magnetic counterpart, MMNm (Näätänen, 1995; Koyama et al., 2000). The MMN, or difference wave, in evoked potentials elicited by a rare stimulus is attributed to a cortical change detection mechanism whereby a mismatch in the sensory memory trace representing the features of the standard occurs when a deviant is presented. The MMN and MMNm can thus be considered as observable correlates of "change" or "feature difference" detection processes. MMN paradigms typically involve a series of identical stimuli ("standard") being presented interspersed with a rare stimulus ("deviant") differing along a physical dimension such as duration, intensity, and frequency (Näätänen & Picton, 1987). The responses to rare (10%–20%) and frequent (80%–90%) tokens are separately sorted and selectively averaged. The MMN may also be elicited in the absence of explicit attention; most MMN paradigms, in fact, use experimental designs where subjects are instructed to ignore stimuli or to perform an unrelated (distractor) task. Analysis of physical attributes (e.g., frequency) in stimuli that produce an MMN provides information relating to the just noticeable differences (JNDs) in features that invoke change detection mechanisms, which in turn provides insight into the nature of central (cortical) sensory representation of stimuli.

Frequency Analysis: Bands, Evoked versus Induced

The increased temporal resolution of MEG and EEG when compared to fMRI and PET offers the ability to study stimulus-locked waveforms in the time domain. In addition, the high sampling rates of the two techniques allow researchers to examine the frequency content of the electrical or magnetic fields recorded. It is typical to use sophisticated digital signal processing (DSP) techniques to analyze these data, because techniques such as signal averaging may disguise the true frequency content of the signal. For example, the waveforms of interest may not be phase-locked, and thus may disappear on signal averaging (for a review, see Pfurtscheller & Lopes-da-Silva, 1999).

An increasingly popular application of time-domain analyses lies in the evaluation of frequencies within the γ band range (usually taken as 25–50 Hz). Oscillations in this frequency band have been cited as a potential substrate for the "binding together" of spatially discrete unimodal representations within the brain to form a coherent and integrated whole (Ribary et al., 1991; Engel & Singer, 2001). It is important to make the distinction between *evoked* responses of a particular frequency (that are phase-locked to a particular trigger) and *induced* responses that have a variable offset with respect to the trigger (Tallon-Baudry & Bertrand, 1999). To study the induced responses it is necessary to use time-frequency analysis techniques. This can involve the use of "sliding window" transforms such as the Gabor transform (e.g., Makeig, 1993) that allow estimates of the instantaneous spectral density at each time point to be computed. Performing time-frequency analyses of single trials and then averaging the results allows one to examine the induced frequency spectrum.

Source Modeling: Magnetic Source Imaging

Until now we have treated the evoked fields from MEG or EEG as intrinsically interesting. However, in many functional neuroimaging studies the investigator may have a hypothesis relating to the contribution of a certain brain area to the task being examined. It is therefore necessary to relate how changes seen in the evoked field pattern may relate to the actual neuronal sources that ultimately produce the fields. Thus, although there is a great deal of intrinsic temporal data available in the evoked response, this information is rendered more useful when the origin of the observed field is estimated. Source estimation is not, however, trivial.

The inverse problem, which relates the observed magnetic field data to the source current distributions (and thus the neuronal generators), does not have a unique solution. To render this problem more tractable, it is common to adopt two strategies: the

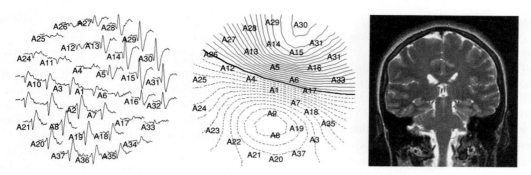

FIGURE 7-12. Magnetic source imaging. *Left,* The time-domain representation of 37 spatially distinct sensor channel signals in response to auditory stimulation (1 kHz sinusoid). *Center,* At the M100 peak (determined by maximum root mean square signal), the instantaneous magnetic field across the sensor array can be plotted in contour form. *Right,* Single equivalent current dipole modeling of this magnetic field distribution, combined with coregistration (via external landmarks) with MRIs allows the creation of an MSI, combining anatomic and functional information in a single image. (See Color Plate 4)

incorporation of prior data to reduce the search space of possible solutions, or to simplify the model with which sources of electrical activity are estimated. Following from early biomagnetic investigations of cardiac function, it is common to model the generators of the evoked fields as equivalent current dipoles. The simplest possible implementation of this (Fig. 7-12) and that which has received the most extensive experimental and practical implementation is the "single equivalent current dipole" (SECD) description (Sarvas, 1987; Scherg et al., 1989).

The SECD model assumes that the neuronal current distribution at each time point can be adequately approximated as a single-current dipole element enclosed within a sphere of uniform conducting medium (of course, when this assumption is wrong the model can fail quite spectacularly). The assumption of spherical symmetry allows so-called volume return currents to be neglected and thus obviates the requirement for measurement or estimation of regional electrical conductivities. In addition, the source is assumed to be tangential to the skull surface. It is common to model the dipole with a number of free parameters, such as the

amplitude (current dipole moment), location, and orientation of the dipole. These parameters are estimated using any one of a number of iterative optimization algorithms. Based on the computed parameters, the corresponding magnetic field at each sensor location is computed using the Biot-Savart law, or magnetic "forward" equations (Fig. 7-13).

The results from an SECD analysis will produce parameter estimates for the spatial location of the dipole, its strength (current dipole moment or "Q"), and orientation. It is common to use confidence limits along each orthogonal plane to represent the goodness-of-fit of the data to the model, and consequently the "ellipsoid of 95% confidence," or confidence volume. To place the current "point source" in an anatomic context, the source localization coordinate can be overlaid on high spatial resolution images, such as MRI, yielding the magnetic source image (MSI), combining, in a single image, descriptions of anatomy and function. When quantifying the amplitude of the neuronal response indicated by the peak of the MEG recorded signal, two considerations compete. First, the modeled current dipole moment, Q (measured in nAm), is relatively independent

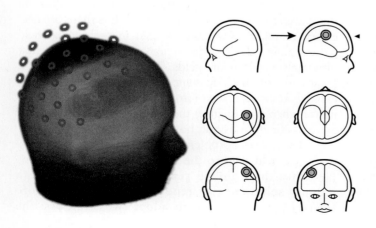

FIGURE 7-13. *Left,* An alternative representation of evoked response data is to plot the instantaneous magnetic field distribution at the peak of an evoked response (in this case contralateral somatosensory stimulation of the thumb) over the three-dimensional reconstructed surface of the head. This representation invites comparison with some typical EEG topographic descriptions. *Right,* A single current source (vector shown in various planes) describes approximately 90% of the measurement variance. In this software package (BESA2000, MEGIS Software GmbH, Gräfelfing, Germany), additional focal current sources can be introduced to account for residual variance. (See Color Plate 4)

of acquisition confounds, such as exact sensor position in relation to the head. However, compared to evoked field amplitude, measured at the sensor array, uncertainty is introduced into the quantity, Q, by the very process of mathematical modeling. When the model and the data are highly consistent, Q tracks with evoked field amplitude and is potentially better suited for *inter*session comparisons, whereas the measured quantities such as evoked field amplitude might be considered superior (because they obviate the requirement for model assumptions) for the purposes of *intra*session comparisons. Especially in situations in which the model fails to adequately describe the data, large errors in Q are likely. In practice, system variations (primarily sensor placement) are relatively insignificant (*inter*session variations in a single subject are comparable to variations found in repeated measurements within a single recording session). Thus, the measured quantity, evoked field amplitude, provides a reasonably robust basis for estimating neuronal activity. In a study comparing Q and evoked field amplitude measures of extent of activation in response to stimulation of one, two, three, or four fingers of the left hand, both Q and evoked field amplitude showed comparable efficacy for resolving different numbers of stimulated digits, although Q tended to fail in situations with low SNR, for example, in the comparison of one finger versus two fingers, because the modeling process is sensitive to measurement noise (Roberts et al., 2000b). Additionally, because the modeling process invokes an assumption of a single focal source of activity, it might be expected to be less appropriate when used to describe activation arising from stimulation of multiple digits, where an extended cortical area is involved.

However, while we have so far dealt with MEG's separate abilities to perform sophisticated analyses of the temporal features or frequency content of the evoked field and its usefulness in inferring the spatial location of the underlying generators of such, it is also possible to combine these two capabilities. Approaches to harness the spatiotemporal information present in the data and also to allow the possibility of multiple and extended simultaneous sources of activity are both under constant development (Mosher et al., 1992; Sekihara et al., 1997). In addition, strategies for improving MEG source estimation by inclusion of spatial activity estimates drawn from other modalities such as fMRI (Liu et al., 1998; Dale & Halgren, 2001) are receiving increasing attention. Furthermore, a feature of the sensitivity of MEG is that it is capable of capturing the extremely transient magnetic fields associated with spontaneous electrical discharges. Interestingly, this has a specific clinical relevance in patients with seizure disorders. Interictal (subclinical) spontaneous electrical discharges can be detected using MEG, and using source-modeling techniques it is possible to localize the epileptogenic zone (Knowlton et al., 1997), for example, see Figure 7-14. This example succinctly demonstrates the usefulness of the MEG technique in a clinical environment.

SUMMARY

This chapter has focused on the application of two different techniques, BOLD fMRI and MEG, as tools for the noninvasive study of human brain function. These do not exist in a vacuum, of course; other techniques such as PET, SPECT, EEG, and transcranial magnetic stimulation (TMS) also play a role. As the number of techniques has grown, so has the expectation of health professionals and neuroscience researchers surrounding their abilities. To conclude this chapter we will focus on some of the exciting possibilities that await users of these techniques in the future, but we also note the caveats that must accompany their use.

Multimodal Imaging: Combining Direct (MEG/EEG) and Indirect (PET/fMRI) Measures

It should now be evident from the body of this chapter that MEG and fMRI provide different metrics of neuronal activity. The reasons for this may be obvious (the vastly different sensitivities of the two techniques in the temporal domain, for example) or more subtle (MEG is reliant on synchrony in neuronal populations to produce signal of sufficient magnitude to be detectable; it is still unclear how this neuronal synchrony or lack thereof impact the BOLD contrast mechanism). Yet accepting these differences, it is hard not to be swayed by the potential that exists for complementary fMRI and MEG experiments (Roberts & Rowley, 1996).

Most combinations of EEG/MEG and PET/fMRI data to date (reviewed in Dale & Halgren, 2001) have used fMRI/PET data as seeds or weights for subsequent localization algorithms. By using the metabolic data as starting estimates for source fitting in this manner, it may

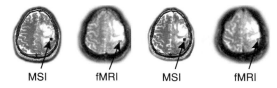

FIGURE 7-14. Similarity of fMRI and MSI sources of right sensorimotor activation in a patient with a large left hemisphere glioma. In this subject, despite underlying neurophysiologic differences between MSI and fMRI and despite the presence of the mass lesion, both fMRI and MSI indicate the encroachment of the posterior margin of the tumor on functional eloquent cortex. (See Color Plate 5)

be possible to circumvent some of the problems associated with the nonlinear estimation of the underlying generators of the observed electrical or magnetic field. Yet it is also important to realize that it may be undesirable to combine MEG and fMRI data in this manner. For example, MEG is insensitive to radial signal sources, and as such, using fMRI data that reflect signal from such a source as prior information for dipole estimation may be unwise (fMRI visible/MEG invisible). Conversely, there are some anatomic substrates to which fMRI may be particularly insensitive (e.g., due to magnetic susceptibility artifacts in areas of temporal lobe), in which case fMRI may underspecify the number of putative neuronal sources (fMRI invisible). In addition, the low temporal resolution of fMRI may hamper the integration of the two modalities. The temporal smoothing caused by the hemodynamic response function makes the consideration of a single fMRI cluster or "blob" as analogous to a source detected using MEG or EEG somewhat contentious. Nevertheless, combining information from separate imaging modalities in this fashion may overcome the limitations posed by using one alone.

An emerging possibility, which in combination with the above approaches bridges structure and function, can be found in subcortical fiber-tracking techniques becoming available with diffusion tensor imaging. In these analyses, pixel-by-pixel determination of diffusion anisotropy (directional preference) allows mapping of structural connectivity between brain regions (Mori et al, 2000).

Clinical Considerations: MEG/fMRI Use in Neurologic Patients

Since the development of large-array (>37 channel) biomagnetometer hardware, clinical adoption of MEG technology has been gradually advancing. There are two primary recognized indications: presurgical mapping of eloquent cortex prior to neurosurgical procedures and the estimation of the epileptogenic zone in patients with seizure disorders. It is beyond the scope of this chapter to discuss these clinical aspects in detail (see, however, Orrison et al., 1992; Gallen et al., 1993; Sobel et al., 1993; Lewine & Orrison, 1995; Roberts et al., 1995a;). However, such clinical procedures are routinely performed by MEG centers and have been recognized by the American Medical Association (AMA) with the recent issue of three Current Procedural Terminology (CPT) codes for spontaneous and evoked MEG mapping.

Indeed, the clinical utility of MSI for presurgical planning and intraoperative guidance of neurosurgical procedures has been underscored by many groups, who have attempted validation of the MSI source estimates with intraoperative direct cortical stimulation mapping, the neurosurgical gold standard for the definition of eloquent cortex. In particular, for the identification of the central sulcus, and localization of primary somatosensory and motor cortices, concordance has been extremely encouraging (Roberts et al., 1995b, 2000c; Ganslandt et al., 1999; Schiffbauer et al., 2001) with spatial displacements of the order of 1 cm with no evidence of systematic bias, other than the generally deeper sources found using the MSI approach, compared to the superficial sites identified intraoperatively by stimulation at the cortical surface. These findings have led to the suggestion that MSI be used not only for the presurgical planning of surgical approach and evaluation of surgical risk (Hund et al., 1997), but also for guidance of the intraoperative mapping procedure, reducing the time taken for such invasive determination of functional organization, with presumed associated reductions in morbidity and cost.

Beyond sensorimotor function, a neurosurgical concern is the avoidance of essential language areas during resection, to minimize chances of postoperative aphasia. Hemispheric dominance for language may be assessed using the Wada test (Wada & Rasmussen, 1960), an invasive estimator of language lateralization, using selective catheterization of alternate carotid arteries and administration of sodium amytal. This effectively suppresses activity in each cerebral hemisphere alternately. Language impairment as a function of anesthetized hemisphere allows elucidation of the hemispheric distribution of the language faculties. However, cost and morbidity are high and this procedure is increasingly challenged by noninvasive alternatives, such as fMRI and MEG. Using MEG, Papanicolaou and associates have pioneered analysis of later (>200 msec) components of the evoked neuromagnetic activity during tasks accessing language and memory functions (Breier et a.l, 1999a, 1999b, 2000, 2001; Papanicolaou et al., 1999; Simos et al., 1999). Szymanski and colleagues (2001) have adapted this methodology to use a simple passive stimulation paradigm, appropriate for the noncooperative or pediatric patient. In general, this application highlights an interesting opportunity offered by the high temporal resolution of MEG recordings, namely, the restriction of analysis to specific latency windows, to allow focus, for example, on "sensory" versus "subsequent/cognitive" processing.

Future clinical opportunities for MEG will likely further exploit its high temporal resolution and will therefore focus on disorders of timing and temporal processing as well as localization of abnormal rhythmic activity, for example, in transient ischemic attack (TIA), trauma (Lewine et al., 1999), and Parkinson disease (PD).

Due to the prevalence of MRI scanning technology, a number of studies have reported the successful use of fMRI for preoperative identification of eloquent cortex (primarily sensorimotor and language areas; Jack et al., 1994; Puce et al., 1995; Lee et al., 1999). Beisteiner and colleagues (2000) have defined "functional risk maps" based on repeated fMRI and areas of reproducible activation, with the aim of identifying essential cortex and accounting for fMRI spatial localization variability. Although considerable successes have been documented, as shown in Figure 7-15 (Jack et al., 1994; Schulder et al., 1998; Kober et al., 2001), some potential caveats remain when exploiting the hemodynamic response methodology inherent to fMRI to identify active cortex in the vicinity of mass lesions, and especially lesions with compromised vascular function, such as arteriovenous malformations (AVMs). If vessels are unable to react to vascular challenges (i.e., compensatory autoregulation is impaired), or if they are maximally vasodilated (perhaps consequent to slow flow or ischemia), or indeed if they are physically compressed by a neighboring mass, it seems plausible that the BOLD mechanism may not remain intact and the ability of fMRI to report functionally active areas may be compromised (Inoue et al., 1999). In such cases, it is perhaps prudent to consider alternative brain mapping strategies (such as MEG) that are not reliant on hemodynamic or vascular reactivity.

The Neuronal Generators of Noninvasive Imaging Measures

As mentioned briefly above, a number of studies have suggested that the initial dip, the negative-going component of the BOLD fMRI response, may be better spatially related to the underlying neuronal generators than the delayed positive-going component. It may be that studies with spatially specific hypotheses, based on knowledge of the underlying cytoarchitecture, will

require the use of the negative component to achieve unambiguous results (Duong et al., 2000). However, to date, only one study has reported the presence of the initial dip at 1.5 T, which remains the standard field strength for clinical MR scanners. And, although studies that use subject-invariant neuroanatomic features such as ocular dominance columns (Menon & Goodyear, 1999) may overcome the inherent problems of the neurovascular point-spread function, as noted by Zarahn (2001) in his recent review, ocular dominance columns remain one of the few examples of this kind of feature. Perhaps with the current trend toward high-field MRI scanner availability, more studies will be able to adequately address the spatial concordance between BOLD fMRI observed signal changes and underlying neuronal activity.

A related issue in noninvasive functional neuroimaging is whether increases in local BOLD fMRI signal or MEG reflect excitatory or inhibitory synaptic transmission. The majority of cortical neurons are spiny neurons (70%–85%, mainly pyramidal; Fairen et al., 1984), whereas the rest are inhibitory interneurons. It has been suggested that the relative balance between inhibition and excitation is essential for normal cortical function, and may underlie many "emergent" properties of local cortical circuits such as plasticity within topographical maps (Buonomano & Merzenich, 1998). Thus, both classes of neurons are important for cortical function, and excitatory and inhibitory transmissions are, at least at the level of the individual synapse, metabolically active processes (Nudo & Masterton, 1986). However, despite much debate, it is currently unclear if decreases in the BOLD fMRI signal at a voxel can be interpreted as a decrease in the *net* neuronal activity over that region, or, in a related fashion, if voxel-wide activation of inhibitory synapses would cause an increase or decrease in BOLD signal (see Waldvogel et al., 2000, for an examination of the latter hypothesis).

As these hypotheses in functional neuroimaging become more focused and more reliant on information from contemporary neurophysiology, this point will become increasingly important. A proper resolution of this debate will allow functional neuroimaging techniques to take their place as experimental neuroscientific tools, generating data that can be combined with other techniques to provide a richer image of human brain function in both health and disease.

Overall the techniques of fMRI and MEG exploit different neurophysiologic routes to probe neuronal function. Consequently, each is conferred with a different combination of spatial and temporal resolutions, sensitivities, and limitations. However, appropriately interpreted, each allows significant insights into the neural operations of the human brain and, indeed, mind. Approaches to use the two recording modalities synergistically promise a spatiotemporal description of

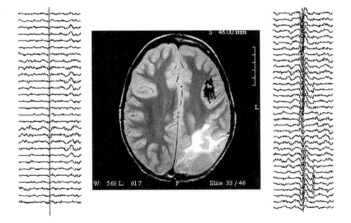

FIGURE 7-15. Application of MEG to spontaneous recording of interictal discharges in patients with seizure disorders. In this patient with nevus syndrome, an interictal event is detected in the sensor array positioned over the left hemisphere; no abnormal activity is detected over the right hemisphere. Single equivalent dipole modeling of this event and other similar spontaneous recordings point to a focal left frontal source (*yellow area*). This was found to correlate with the modeled source of seizure onset itself. (See Color Plate 5)

brain function at a neuronal and vascular level, offering the tools for both clinical and research development, opportunity, and progress.

Acknowledgments

The authors would like to thank Dr. Howard A. Rowley for his insights and collaboration and Susanne Honma, Jeff Walker, and Mary Mantle for excellent technical assistance. Dr. Jesper Andersson is gratefully acknowledged for his review of and comments on the manuscript.

■ KEY POINTS

☐   Magnetic resonance imaging (MRI) can be used to localize brain function by exploiting regional changes in blood oxygenation that accompany neuronal electrical activity.

☐   Magnetoencephalography (MEG) can identify the temporal characteristics of neuronal activity by direct recording of the tiny extracranial magnetic field that accompanies neuronal electrical activity.

KEY READINGS

Frackowiak RSJ, Friston KJ, Frith C, et al (eds): Human Brain Function. San Diego, CA: Academic Press, 1997.

Friston KJ, Holmes AP, Worsley KJ, et al: Statistical parametric maps in functional imaging: A general linear approach. Hum Brain Mapp 2:189–210, 1995.

Holmes AP, Friston KJ: Gereralisability, random effects and population inference. Neuroimage 7:S754, 1998.

Josephs O, Turner R, Friston KJ: Event-related fMRI. Hum Brain Map 5:243–248, 1997.

Kwong KK, Belliveau JW, Chesler DA, et al: Dynamic magnetic resonance imaging of human brain activity during primary sensory stimulation. Proc Natl Acad Sci U S A 86:5675–5679, 1992.

Moonen CTW, Bandettini PA (eds): Functional MRI. Berlin, Germany: Springer Verlag, 2000.

REFERENCES

Adler RJ (1981). The Geometry of Random Fields. New York: Wiley, 1981.

Aguirre GK, D'Esposito M. Experimental design for brain fMRI, in Moonen CTW, Bandettini PA (eds): Functional MRI. Berlin: Springer Verlag, 2000, pp. 369–380.

Aguirre GK, Zarahn E, D'Esposito M: Empirical analyses of BOLD fMRI statistics: II. Spatially smoothed data collected under null-hypothesis and experimental conditions. Neuroimage 5:199–212, 1997.

Aguirre GK, Zarahn E, D'Esposito M: The variability of human BOLD hemodynamic responses. Neuroimage 8:360–369, 1998.

Andersson JLR, Hutton C, Ashburner J, et al: Modeling geometric deformations in EPI time series. Neuroimage 13:903–919, 2001.

Ashburner J, Friston KJ: Spatial transformation of images, in Frackowiak RSJ, Friston KJ, Frith C, et al (eds): Human Brain Function. San Diego, CA: Academic Press, 1997, pp. 43–58.

Beisteiner R, Lanzenberger R, Novak K, et al: Improvement of presurgical patient evaluation by generation of functional magnetic resonance risk maps. Neurosci Lett 290:13–16, 2000.

Belliveau JW, Kennedy DN, McKinstry RC, et al: Functional mapping of the human visual cortex by magnetic resonance imaging. Science 254:716–719, 1991.

Berger H: Über das Elektrenkephalogramm des Menschen. Arch Psychiatr Nervenkr 87:527–570, 1929.

Blamire AM, Ogawa S, Ugurbil K, et al: Dynamic mapping of the human visual cortex by high-speed magnetic resonance imaging. Proc Natl Acad Sci U S A 89:11069–11073, 1992.

Box GEP, Hunter WG, Hunter JS: Statistics for Experimenters. New York: Wiley, 1978.

Boynton GM, Engel SA, Glover GH, et al: Linear systems analysis of functional magnetic resonance imaging in human V1. J Neurosci 16:4207–4221, 1996.

Breier JI, Simos PG, Zouridakis G, et al: Lateralization of cerebral activation in auditory verbal and non-verbal memory tasks using magnetoencephalography. Brain Topogr 12:89–97, 1999a.

Breier JI, Simos PG, Zouridakis G, et al: Language dominance determined by magnetic source imaging: A comparison with the Wada procedure. Neurology 53:938–945, 1999b.

Breier JI, Simos PG, Zouridakis G, et al: Lateralization of activity associated with language function using magnetoencephalography: A reliability study. J Clin Neurophysiol 17:503–510, 2000.

Breier JI, Simos PG, Wheless JW, et al: Language dominance in children as determined by magnetic source imaging and the intracarotid amobarbital procedure: A comparison. J Child Neurol 16:124–130, 2001.

Buckner RL, Bandettini PA, O'Craven KM, et al: Detection of cortical activation during averaged single trials of a cognitive task using functional magnetic resonance imaging. Proc Natl Acad Sci U S A 9:14878–14883, 1996.

Bullmore E, Brammer M, Williams SC, et al: Statistical methods of estimation and inference for functional MR image analysis. Magn Reson Med 35:261–277, 1996.

Buonomano DV, Merzenich MM: Cortical plasticity: From synapses to maps. Annu Rev Neurosci 21:149–186, 1998.

Calhoun VD, Adali T, Pearlson GD, et al: Spatial and temporal independent component analysis of functional MRI data containing a pair of task-related waveforms. Hum Brain Mapp 13:43–53, 2001.

Caton R: The electrical currents of the brain. Br J Med 2:278, 1875.

Cohen MS: Rapid MRI and functional applications, in Toga AW, Mazziotta JC (eds): Brain Mapping: The Methods. San Diego, CA: Academic Press, 1996.

Collignon A, Maes F, Delaere D, et al: Automated multi-modality image registration based on information theory, in Bizais YY, Barillot C, Di Paola R (eds): Information Processing in Medical Imaging: 14th International Conference. Dordrecht, NL: Kluwer Academic Publishers, 1995.

Dale AM, Buckner RL: Selective averaging of rapidly presented individual trials using fMRI. Hum Brain Mapp 5:329–340, 1997.

Dale AM, Halgren E: Spatiotemporal mapping of brain activity by integration of multiple imaging modalities. Curr Opin Neurobiol 11:202–208, 2001.

Disbrow EA, Slutsky DA, Roberts TP, et al: Functional MRI at 1.5 Tesla: A comparison of the blood oxygenation level-dependent signal and electrophysiology. Proc Natl Acad Sci U S A 97:18–23, 2000.

Duong TQ, Kim DS, Ugurbil K, et al: Spatiotemporal dynamics of the BOLD fMRI signals: Toward mapping submillimeter cortical columns using the early negative response. Magn Reson Med 44:231–242, 2000.

Engel SA, Glover GH, Wandell BA: Retinotopic organization in human visual cortex and the spatial precision of functional MRI. Cereb Cortex 2:181–192, 1997.

Engel AK, Singer W: Temporal binding and the neural correlates of sensory awareness. Trends Cognitive Sci 5:16–25, 2001.

Fairen JD, DeFelipe J, Regidor J: Nonpyramidal neurons: General account, in Peters A, Jones EG (eds): Cerebral Cortex. New York: Plenum Press, 1984, pp. 201–253.

Flynn E: Factors which affect spatial resolving power in large array biomagnetic sensors. Rev Sci Instrum 65:922–935, 1994.

Fox PT, Mintun MA: Non-invasive functional brain mapping by change distribution analysis of averaged PET images of H15O2 tissue activity. J Nucl Med 30:141–149, 1989.

Fox PT, Raichle ME: Focal physiological uncoupling of cerebral blood flow and oxidative metabolism during somatosensory stimulation in human subjects. Proc Natl Acad Sci U S A 83:1140–1144, 1986.

Friston KJ, Holmes AP, Worsley KJ, et al: Statistical parametric maps in functional imaging: A general linear approach. Hum Brain Mapp 2:189–210, 1995a.

Friston KJ, Holmes AP, Poline J-B, et al: Analysis of fMRI time-series revisited. Neuroimage 2:45–53, 1995b.

Friston KJ, Jezzard P, Turner R: Analysis of functional MRI time-series. Human Brain Mapp 1:153–171, 1994.

Friston KJ, Josephs O, Rees G, et al: Nonlinear event-related responses in fMRI. Magn Reson Med 39:41–52, 1998.

Gallen CC, Sobel DF, Waltz T, et al: Noninvasive presurgical neuromagnetic mapping of somatosensory cortex. Neurosurgery 33:260–268, 1993.

Ganslandt O, Fahlbusch R, Nimsky C, et al: Functional neuronavigation with magnetoencephalography: Outcome in 50 patients with lesions around the motor cortex. J Neurosurg 91:73–79, 1999.

Geyer S, Schleicher A, Zilles K: Areas 3a, 3b, and 1 of human primary somatosensory cortex. Neuroimage 10:63–83, 1999.

Geyer S, Schormann T, Mohlberg H, et al: Areas 3a, 3b, and 1 of human primary somatosensory cortex. Part 2. Spatial normalization to standard anatomical space. Neuroimage 11(6 Part 1): 684–696, 2000.

Grinvald A, Lieke E, Frostig RD, et al: Functional architecture of cortex revealed by optical imaging of intrinsic signals. Nature 324:341–364, 1986.

Guyton AC, Hall JE (eds): Textbook of Medical Physiology. Philadelphia, PA: Saunders, 1996.

Hajnal JV, Bydder GM, Young IR: Stimulus-correlated signals in functional MR of the brain. Am J Neuroradiol 17:1011–1012, 1996.

Hämäläinen H, Hari R, Ilmoniemi LJ, et al: Magnetoencephalography: Theory, instrumentation, and application to noninvasive studies of the working human brain. Rev Mod Physics 65:413–497, 1993.

Hu X, Le TH, Ugurbil K: Evaluation of the early response in fMRI in individual subjects using short stimulus duration. Magn Reson Med 37:877–984, 1997.

Hund M, Rezai AR, Kronberg E, et al: Magnetoencephalographic mapping: Basics of a new functional selection of patients with cortical brain lesions. Neurosurgery 40:936–942, 1997.

Hyder F, Chase JR, Behar KL, et al: Increased tricarboxylic acid cycle flux in rat brain during forepaw stimulation detected with 1H[13C]NMR. Proc Natl Acad Sci U S A 93:7612–7617, 1996.

Inoue T, Shimizu H, Nakasato N, et al: Accuracy and limitation of functional magnetic resonance imaging for identification of the central sulcus: Comparison with magnetoencephalography in patients with brain tumors. Neuroimage 10:738–748, 1999.

Jack CR Jr, Thompson RM, Butts RK, et al: Sensory motor cortex: Correlation of presurgical mapping with functional MR imaging and invasive cortical mapping. Radiology 190:85–92, 1994.

Jezzard P, LeBihan D, Cuenod C, et al: An investigation of the contribution of physiological noise in human functional MRI studies at 1.5 Tesla and 4 Tesla. Abstracts of the 12th Meeting of the Society of Magnetic Resonance in Medicine, New York, 3, 1392, 1993.

Josephs O, Henson RN: Event-related functional magnetic resonance imaging: Modeling, inference and optimization. Philos Trans R Soc London.B Biol Sci 354:1215–1228, 1999.

Josephs O, Turner R, Friston KJ: Event-related fMRI. Hum Brain Mapp 5:243–248, 1997.

Kennan RP: Gradient echo and spin echo methods for functional MRI, in Moonen CTW, Bandettini PA (eds): Functional MRI. Berlin, Germany: Springer Verlag, 2000, pp. 127–136.

Kety SS, Schmidt CF: The determination of cerebral blood flow in man by the use of nitrous oxide in low concentrations. Am J Physiol 143:53–66, 1945.

Kimelberg HK, Norenberg MD: Astrocytes. Sci Am 260:66–72, 1989.

Kleinschmidt A, Buchel C, Zeki S, et al: Human brain activity during spontaneously reversing perception of ambiguous figures. Proc R Soc London B Biol Sci 265:2427–2433, 1998.

Kleinschmidt A, Frahm J. Linking cerebral blood oxygenation to human brain function, in Villringer A, Dirnagl U (eds): Optical Imaging of Brain Function and Metabolism II. New York: Plenum Press, 1997, pp. 221–234.

Knowlton RC, Laxer KD, Aminoff MJ, et al: Magnetoencephalography in partial epilepsy: Clinical yield and localization accuracy. Ann Neurol 42:622–631, 1997.

Kober H, Nimsky C, Moller M, et al: Correlation of sensorimotor activation with functional magnetic resonance imaging and magnetoencephalography in presurgical functional imaging: A spatial analysis. Neuroimage 14:1214–1228, 2001.

Koyama S, Gunji A, Yabe H, et al: The masking effect in foreign speech sounds perception revealed by neuromagnetic responses. Neuroreport 11:3765–3769, 2000.

Kruggel F, Von Cramon DY: Modeling the hemodynamic response in single-trial functional MRI experiments. Magn Reson Med 42:787–797, 1999.

Kuffler SW, Nichols JG, Martin AR: From Neuron to Brain. Sunderland, MA: Sinauer, 1984.

Kwong KK, Belliveau JW, Chesler DA, et al:. Dynamic magnetic resonance imaging of human brain activity during primary sensory stimulation. Proc Natl Acad Sci U S A 89:5675–5679, 1992.

Lai S, Hopkins AL, Haacke EM, et al: Identification of vascular structures as a major source of signal contrast in high resolution 2D and 3D functional activation imaging of the motor cortex at 1.5T: Preliminary results. Magn Reson Med 30:387–392, 1993.

Lange N, Zeger S. Non-linear Fourier time series analysis for human brain mapping by functional magnetic resonance imaging. J R Stat Soc 46:1–29, 1997.

Lassen NA, Ingvar DH, Raichle ME, et al (eds): Brain Work and Mental Activity. Copenhagen, Denmark: Munksgaard, 1991.

Le T-H, Patel S, Roberts TPL: Functional MRI of human auditory cortex using block and event-related designs. Magn Reson Med 45:254–260, 2001.

Lee CC, Ward HA, Sharbrough FW, et al: Assessment of functional MR imaging in neurosurgical planning. Am J Neuroradiol 20:1511–1519, 1999.

Lewine JD, Davis JT, Sloan JH, et al: Neuromagnetic assessment of pathophysiologic brain activity induced by minor head trauma. Am J Neuroradiol 20:857–866, 1999.

Lewine JD, Orrison WW Jr:. Magnetoencephalography and magnetic source imaging, in Orrison WW Jr, Lewis D, Saunders J, et al (eds): Functional Brain Imaging. St. Louis, MO: Mosby, 1995, pp. 369–417.

Liu AK, Belliveau JW, Dale AM: Spatiotemporal imaging of human brain activity using functional MRI constrained magneto-encephalography data: Monte Carlo simulations. Proc Natl Acad Sci U S A 95:8945–8950, 1998.

Logothetis NK, Pauls J, Augath M, et al: Neurophysiological investigation of the basis of the fMRI signal. Nature 412:150–157, 2001.

Madsen PL, Hasselbalch SG, Hagemann LP, et al: Persistent resetting of the cerebral oxygen/glucose uptake ratio by brain activation: Evidence obtained with the Kety-Schmidt technique. J Cereb Blood Flow Metab 15:485–491, 1995.

Magistretti PJ, Pellerin L: Cellular mechanisms of brain energy metabolism and their relevance to functional brain imaging. Philos Trans R Soc London B Biol Sci 354:1155–1163, 1999.

Magistretti PJ, Pellerin L: The astrocyte-mediated coupling between synaptic activity and energy metabolism operates through volume transmission. Prog Brain Res 125:229–240, 2000.

Makeig S: Auditory event-related dynamics of the EEG spectrum and effects of exposure to tones. Electroencephalogr Clin Neurophysiol 86:283–293, 1993.

Malonek D, Grinvald A. Interactions between electrical activity and cortical microcirculation revealed by imaging spectroscopy: Implications for functional brain mapping. Science 272:551–554, 1996.

Mayhew J, Hu D, Zheng Y, et al: An evaluation of linear model analysis techniques for processing images of microcirculation activity. Neuroimage 1:49–71, 1998.

Menon RS, Goodyear BG: Submillimeter functional localization in human striate cortex using BOLD contrast at 4 Tesla: Implications for the vascular point-spread function. Magn Reson Med 41:230–235, 1999.

Mori S, Kaufman WE, Pearlson GD, et al: In vivo visualization of human neural pathways by magnetic resonance imaging. Ann Neurol 47:412–414, 2000.

Mosher JC, Lewis PS, Leahy RM: Multiple dipole modeling and localization from spatio-temporal MEG data. IEEE Trans Biomed Eng 39:541–557, 1992.

Näätänen R: The mismatch negativity: A powerful tool for cognitive neuroscience. Ear Hearing 16:6–18, 1995.

Näätänen R, Picton T: The N1 wave of the human electric and magnetic response to sound: A review and analysis of the component structure. Psychophysiology 24:375–425, 1987.

Nudo RJ, Masterton RB: Stimulation-induced [14C]2-deoxyglucose labeling of synaptic activity in the central auditory system. J Comp Neurol 245:553–565, 1986.

Ogawa S, Lee TM: Magnetic resonance imaging of blood vessels at high fields: In vivo and in vitro measurements and image simulation. Magn Reson Med 16:9–18, 1990a.

Ogawa S, Lee TM, Nayak AS, et al: Oxygenation sensitive contrast in magnetic resonance image of rodent brain at high magnetic fields. Magn Reson Med 14:68–78, 1990b.

Ogawa S, Lee TM, Kay AR, et al: Brain magnetic resonance imaging with contrast dependent on blood oxygenation. Proc Natl Acad Sci U S A 87:9868–9872, 1990c.

Ogawa S, Menon RS, Tank DW, et al: Functional brain mapping by blood oxygenation level-dependent contrast magnetic resonance imaging: A comparison of signal characteristics with a biophysical model. Biophys J 64:803–812, 1993.

Orrison WWJ, Rose DF, Hart BL, et al: Noninvasive preoperative cortical localization by magnetic source imaging. Am J Neuroradiol 13:1124–1128, 1992.

Papanicolaou AC, Simos PG, Breier JI, et al: Magnetoencephalographic mapping of the language specific cortex. J Neurosurg 90:85–93, 1999.

Pauling L, Coryell CD: The magnetic properties and structure of hemoglobin, oxyhemoglobin and carbonoxyhemoglobin. Proc Natl Acad Sci U S A 22:210–216, 1936.

Pfurtscheller G, Lopes-da-Silva FH: Event-related EEG/MEG synchronization and desynchronization: Basic principles. Clin Neurophysiol 110:1842–1857, 1999.

Poline JB, Holmes AP, Worsley KJ, et al: Making statistical inferences, in Frackowial RSJ, Friston KJ, Frith C, et al (eds): Human Brain Function. San Diego, CA: Academic Press, 1997, pp. 85–106.

Price CJ, Veltman DJ, Ashburner J, et al: The critical relationship between the timing of stimulus presentation and data acquisition in blocked designs with fMRI. Neuroimage 10:36–44, 1999.

Puce A, Constable RT, Luby ML, et al: Functional magnetic resonance imaging of sensory and motor cortex: Comparison with electrophysiological localization. J Neurosurg 83:262–270, 1995.

Ribary U, Ioannides AA, Singh KD, et al: Magnetic field tomography of coherent thalamocortical 40-Hz oscillations in humans. Proc Natl Acad Sci U S A 88:11037–11041, 1999.

Roberts TPL, Disbrow EA, Roberts HC, et al: Quantification and reproducibility of cortical extent of activation with functional magnetic resonance imaging and magnetoencephalography. Am J Neuroradiol 21:1377–1387, 2000b.

Roberts TPL, Ferrari P, Perry D, et al: Presurgical mapping with magnetic source imaging: Comparisons with intraoperative findings. Brain Tumor Pathol 17:57–64, 2000c.

Roberts TPL, Ferrari P, Stufflebeam SM, et al: Latency of the auditory evoked neuromagnetic field components: Stimulus dependence and insights toward perception. J Clin Neurophysiol 17:114–129, 2000a.

Roberts TPL, Poeppel D: Latency of auditory evoked M100 as a function of tone frequency. Neuroreport 7:1138–1140, 1996.

Roberts TPL, Rowley HA: Multimodal functional imaging of the sensorimotor cortex with fMRI and magnetic source imaging (MSI). In Proceedings of the Tenth International Conference on Biomagnetism, Santa Fe, NM. New York: Springer, 1996.

Roberts TPL, Rowley H, Kucharczyk J: Applications of magnetic source imaging to presurgical brain mapping. Neuroimaging Clin N Am 5:251–266, 1995a.

Roberts TPL, Zusman E, McDermott M, et al: Correlation of functional magnetic source imaging with intra-operative cortical stimulation in neurosurgical patients. J Image Guided Surg 1:339–347, 1995b.

Robson MD, Dorosz JL, Gore JC: Measurements of the temporal fMRI response of the human auditory cortex to trains of tones. Neuroimage 7:185–198, 1998.

Roy CS, Sherrington CS: On the regulation of the blood supply of the brain. J Physiol (Lond) 11:85–108, 1890.

Sarvas J: Basic mathematical and electromagnetic concepts of the biomagnetic inverse problem. Physics Med Biol 32:11–22, 1987.

Savoy RL, Bandettini PA, O'Craven KM, et al: Pushing the temporal resolution of fMRI: Studies of very brief visual stimuli, onset variability and asynchrony, and stimulus-correlated changes in noise. In Proceedings of the 3rd Annual Meeting of ISMRM, Nice, France, 1995.

Scherg M, Vajsar J, Picton T: A source analysis of the late human auditory evoked potentials. J Cognitive Neurosci 1:336–355, 1989.

Schiffbauer H, Ferrari P, Rowley HA, et al: Functional activity within brain tumors: A magnetic source imaging study. Neurosurgery 49:1313–1320, 2001.

Schulder M, Maldjian JA, Liu WC, et al: Functional image-guided surgery of intracranial tumors located in or near the sensorimotor cortex. J Neurosurg 89:412–418, 1998.

Segebarth C, Belle V, Delon C, et al: Functional MRI of the human brain: Predominance of signals from extracerebral veins. Neuroreport 5:813–816, 1994.

Sekihara K, Poeppel D, Marantz A, et al: Noise covariance incorporated MEG-MUSIC algorithm: A method of multiple-dipole estimation tolerant of the influence of background brain acitivity. IEEE Trans Biomed Eng 44:839–847, 1997.

Simos PG, Papanicolaou AC, Breier JI, et al: Localization of language-specific cortex by using magnetic source imaging and electrical stimulation mapping. J Neurosurg 91:787–796, 1999.

Sobel DF, Gallen CC, Schwartz BJ, et al: Locating the central sulcus: Comparison of MR anatomic and magnetoencephalographic functional methods. Am J Neuroradiol 14:915–925, 1993.

Sokoloff L, Reivich M, Kennedy C, et al: The [14C]deoxyglucose method for the measurement of local cerebral glucose utilization: Theory, procedure, and normal values in the conscious and anesthetized albino rat. J Neurochem 28:897–916, 1977.

Strupp JP: STIMULATE: A GUI based fMRI software analysis package. Neuroimage 3:S660, 1996.

Szymanski MD, Perry DW, Gage NM, et al: Magnetic source imaging of late evoked field responses to vowels: Toward an assessment of hemispheric dominance for language. J Neurosurg 94:445–453, 2001.

Tallon-Baudry C, Bertrand O: Oscillatory gamma activity in humans and its role in object representation. Trends Cognitive Sci 3:151–162, 1999.

Thompson PM, Toga AW: Warping strategies for intersubject registration, in Bankman IN (ed): Handbook of Medical Imaging. San Diego, CA: Academic Press, 2000, pp. 569–602.

Tolhurst DJ, Walker NS, Thompson ID, et al: Non-linearities of temporal summation in neurones in area 17 of the cat. Exp Brain Res 38:431–435, 1980.

Turner R, LeBihan D, Moonen CTW, et al: Echo-planar time course MRI of cat brain oxygenation changes. Magn Res Med 22:159–166, 1991.

Vanzetta I, Grinvald A: Increased cortical oxidative metabolism due to sensory stimulation: Implications for functional brain imaging. Science 286:1555–1558, 1999.

Vazquez AL, Noll DC: Nonlinear aspects of the BOLD response in functional MRI. Neuroimage 7:108–118, 1998.

Villringer A: Physiological changes during brain activation, in Moonen CTW, Bandettini PA (eds): Functional MRI. Berlin: Springer Verlag, 2000, pp. 3–14.

Vrba J: SQUID gradiometers in real environments, in Weinstock H (ed): SQUID Sensors: Fundamentals, Fabrication and Applications. Dordrecht, The Netherlands: Kluwer Academic Publishers, 1996, pp. 117–178.

Wada J, Rasmussen T. Intracarotid injection of sodium amytal for the lateralization of cerebral speech dominance. J Neurosurg 17:266–282, 1960.

Waldvogel D, van Gelderen P, Muellbacher W, et al: The relative metabolic demand of inhibition and excitation. Nature 406:995–998, 2000.

Williamson SJ, Kaufman L: Evolution of neuromagnetic topographic mapping. Brain Topogr 3:113–127, 1990.

Woods RP: Spatial transformation models, in Bankman IN (ed): Handbook of Medical Imaging. San Diego, CA: Academic Press, 2000, 465–490.

Woods RP, Mazziotta JC, Cherry SR: MRI-PET registration with automated algorithm. J Comput Assist Tomogr 17:536–546, 1993.

Worsley KJ: Local maxima and the expected Euler characteristic of excursion fields of c2, f and t fields. Adv App Prob 26:13–42, 1994.

Yacoub E, Shmuel A, Pfeuffer J, et al: Imaging brain function in humans at 7 Tesla. Magn Reson Med 45:588–594, 2001.

Young MP, Hilgetag CC, Scannell JW: On inputing function to structure from the behavioural effects of brain lesions. Philos Trans R Soc Lond B Biol Sci 355:147–161, 2000.

Zarahn E: Spatial localization and resolution of BOLD fMRI. Curr Opin Neurobiol 11:209–212, 2001.

Zarahn E, Aguirre GK, D'Esposito M: Empirical analyses of BOLD fMRI statistics: I. Spatially unsmoothed data collected under null-hypothesis conditions. Neuroimage 6:179–197, 1997a.

Zarahn E, Aguirre GK, D'Esposito M: A trial-based experimental design for fMRI. Neuroimage 6:122–138, 1997b.

Zilles K, Schlaug G, Matelli M, et al. Mapping of human and macaque sensorimotor areas by integrating architectonic, transmitter receptor, MRI and PET data. J Anat 187:515–537, 1995.

Electrophysiology

Jon Tippin

Alzheimer disease
Anoxic encephalopathy
Dementia
Electroencephalography
Evoked potentials
Head trauma

INTRODUCTION

The use of electrophysiologic technology to explore human behavior has a rich history in the development of the electroencephalogram (EEG). Hans Berger, a German neuropsychiatrist, began exploring the human EEG in 1924 and 5 years later was the first to record the alpha rhythm and blocking response (Berger, 1929). It is interesting to note that Berger's interest in EEG was based on questionable scientific grounds. His primary goal was to find a physiologic correlate of what he termed "psychische Energie," a fundamental psychic force that connected all human minds. Among the powers that he believed this force controlled was telepathic communication. These unconventional views, as well as his falling-out with the Nazi regime, led to his forced early retirement from the Psychiatric Hospital of the Alma Mater Jenensis in 1938. Despondent over this personal loss, and more importantly, the loss of access to his laboratory and further research, he committed suicide in 1941 (Niedermeyer, 1993). Further development of the EEG was actively pursued by other laboratories, both in Europe and North America, often within psychology or psychiatry departments. However, by the mid-1930s following the work of Fredric and Erna Gibbs and William Lennox, the effectiveness of EEG in the evaluation of patients with epilepsy was established and EEG ultimately became firmly entrenched as a neurodiagnostic procedure (Grass, 1984). The discovery of the delta wave by Walter (1936) showed that the EEG was capable of recording electrophysiologic evidence of disturbed cerebral function caused by underlying structural pathology. In fact, until computed tomography (CT) and magnetic resonance imaging (MRI) became available in the 1970s and 1980s, the EEG was one of the primary noninvasive means of "imaging" the brain. In recent decades, the development of digital technology has led to the emergence of new applications based on the routine EEG, including computer-assisted or quantitative EEG (QEEG) and evoked potentials (EPs).

PHYSIOLOGIC BASIS OF THE EEG

The potential usefulness of the EEG in the evaluation of disordered behavior is based on the fact that it is fundamentally a test of brain function. Pyramidal cells in the cerebral cortex generate all EEG potentials recorded at the surface. Postsynaptic potentials of cortical pyramidal cells are responsible for producing most of the activity commonly recorded in the routine, scalp EEG (Creutzfeldt & Houchin, 1974). Although pyramidal cell action potentials are of higher amplitude, resting postsynaptic potentials are the major generator of the EEG because they are of longer duration, involve a much larger membrane surface area, and result from synchronous firing of thousands of pyramidal neurons. However, burst firing of cortical neurons, in which there are clusters of action potentials followed by prolonged hyperpolarization, probably contributes a small amount of activity to the recordable scalp EEG. Postsynaptic potentials result from changes in the resting potential caused by transmembrane ion fluxes (Creutzfeldt & Houchin, 1974; Speckmann et al, 1984). Excitatory postsynaptic potentials (EPSPs) occur when the membrane potential is depolarized, bringing it closer to the threshold for generating an action potential. EPSPs are caused by an influx of Na^+ or Ca^{++} or both. The major excitatory neurotransmitter in the brain leading to EPSPs is glutamate acting at kainate, quisqualate, and N-methyl-D-aspartate (NMDA) receptors. Contrariwise, inhibitory postsynaptic potentials (IPSPs) result from hyperpolarization of the membrane potential due to increased membrane permeability to Cl^- or K^+ or both. γ-Aminobutyric acid (GABA) is the major inhibitory neurotransmitter in both the brain and spinal cord. An EPSP leads to membrane depolarization with a resultant inward flow of positive charges ("sink"). Figure 8-1A shows an ESPS-induced depolarization occurring at the apical dendrites of a cortical pyramidal cell that is compensated by an outward positive current flow from deeper portions of the cell body and basal dendrites ("source"). This current flow produces a dipole in which the *extracellular* potential is more negatively charged near the surface than that recorded deeper. An EEG electrode on the scalp over this neuron would record a negative potential (by convention, an upward pen deflection). Just the opposite would be expected from an IPSP occurring in the same part of the neuron (Fig. 8-1B). However, because pyramidal cell dendrites extend through most cortical layers, both ESPSs and IPSPs may appear either positive or negative

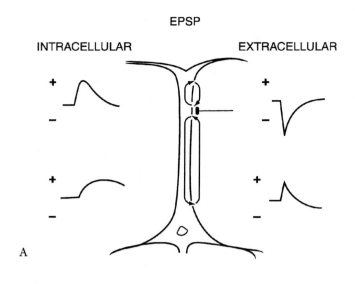

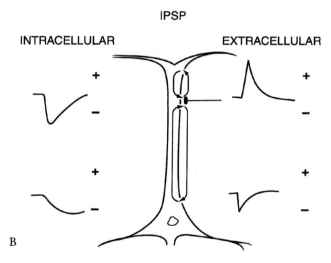

FIGURE 8-1. Cortical pyramidal cells showing the presence of an EPSP (*A*) and IPSP (*B*) at the apical dendrites. Note that an EPSP produces an influx of positive charges at the dendritic membrane, with localized intracellular positivity and extracellular negativity in that region. At the soma, an intracellular recording shows a lesser and more delayed positivity. The opposite is seen with an IPSP.

at the surface depending on which parts of the cell body or its dendrites are affected.

Cortical pyramidal cells are closely packed into functional vertical columns containing several hundred cells arranged in parallel with their apical dendrites at right angles to the surface of the cortex. This allows for greater spatial summation of currents generated by these neurons. Also, groups of pyramidal cells receive collateral afferent input that permits synchronous firing of a fairly large area of the cortex (Freeman, 1975). Synchronously firing cortical neurons with a surface area of 6 cm^2 are required to allow detection by a single

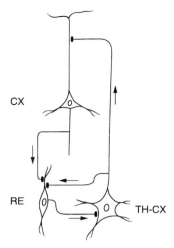

CX

RE   TH-CX

FIGURE 8-2. Relationship between cells of the thalamic reticular nucleus (RE), thalamocortical projections (TH-CX), and cortex (CX) leading to rhythmic activity of the scalp-recorded EEG. (Reproduced with permission from Striade M, Deschenes M: Intrathalamic and brainstem-thalamic networks involved in resting and alert states, in Bentivoglio M, Spreafico R (eds): Cellular Thalamic Mechanisms. Amsterdam: Elsevier, 1988, pp. 37–62.

scalp electrode (Abraham & Ajmone-Marsan, 1958). One might expect that the electrical activity recorded at the scalp would consist of irregular, asynchronously occurring potentials given the myriad of relatively independent activities of cortical pyramidal cells. Although it is true that the EEG of a hyperalert subject shows *desynchronized* activity, the EEG recorded in relaxed wakefulness and nonrapid eye movement (NREM) sleep is characterized by synchrony and rhythmicity. This rhythmicity is determined in large part by input to the cortex from the thalamus. Thalamic influence leads to synchronous activity of a large area of cortex because one thalamocortical neuron innervates many thousands of cortical neurons, and many of these fire simultaneously due to intrathalamic synchronizing mechanisms (Fig. 8-2). Rather than a single nuclear structure in the thalamus acting as the pacemaker, it appears that multiple neuronal populations interact with one another by means of recurrent inhibition leading to rhythmic activity of cortical neurons. Cells of the nucleus reticularis (RE) have been shown to have the ability to spontaneously release GABA in rhythmic bursts and the thalamocortical neurons (TH-CX) that are influenced by them produce pulses of depolarization as a rebound response to these inhibitory stimuli (Striade & Deschenes, 1988). Branches of the thalamocortical neurons then feed back onto the inhibitory cells of the nucleus reticularis. This activity ultimately leads to row on row of synchronized dipoles in the cortex generating potentials large enough to be recorded at the scalp. In the healthy, quietly awake adult, rhythmic activity in the

posterior quadrants of the scalp consists of *alpha activity* (frequency range 8–13 Hz) and is designated the posterior dominant or *alpha rhythm*. Another rhythmical activity seen in most normal adults is *beta* (frequency >13 Hz), which is maximal in the frontal and central regions. Dysfunction of neurons in the cortex, thalamus, ascending reticular activating system (which contributes input to the thalamus), or thalamocortical projections (providing output from the thalamus) may produce changes in these normal rhythms or lead to the appearance of abnormal slow activity that falls into either *theta* (4–7.5 Hz) or *delta* (<3.5 Hz) frequency bands.

ROUTINE EEG

As one considers the usefulness of the EEG in evaluating patients with cognitive impairment, it should be borne in mind that EEG abnormalities are, for the most part, nonspecific; a variety of pathologic conditions may produce largely identical changes. Certain changes may be highly suggestive of a particular diagnosis but are almost never "pathognomonic." Nevertheless, interpreted within the clinical context of the patient, the EEG may provide unique, useful clinical information. For example, the EEG may identify a potentially treatable cause of cognitive decline, such as nonconvulsive status epilepticus (Granner & Lee, 1994). It is fundamentally important to recall that the degree to which the EEG is clinically useful is largely determined by the accuracy of its interpretation. This accuracy depends heavily on the competency and experience of the electroencephalographer; those with board certification, more full-time EEG training, and more time spent in an active EEG laboratory interpret EEGs more accurately (Williams et al., 1985). In addition, EEG tracings typically include electrical activities of noncerebral origin that may mimic genuine cerebral activity and easily mislead the less experienced electroencephalographer. These artifacts can be either of physiologic or nonphysiologic origin (e.g., eye movements and electrode artifacts, respectively). Head and body movements occasionally create artifacts that resemble abnormal slow activity or epileptiform discharges. Technical modifications, such as filter and sensitivity (amplifier gain) changes, can alter EEG patterns; for example, muscle twitch artifacts may be mistaken for spikes when a low-pass (high-frequency) filter of 15 Hz is used (Tyner et al., 1983). Experienced electroencephalographers distinguish these variables by visually characterizing a given EEG event by its waveform, potential field distribution, polarity, and timing in relation to the patient's level of consciousness. As will be discussed in a later section, digital technology has been used to produce what has been referred to as "quantitative EEG" in an attempt to enhance the usefulness of EEG. However, proper interpretation of these computer-assisted studies still requires a firm understanding of the visually inspected, routine

EEG, inattention to which may only confuse the interpretation of these studies (Nuwer, 1990).

In the following sections, a review will be presented of some common clinical situations in which the EEG has been used in the evaluation of cognitively impaired patients.

Alzheimer Disease

The EEG is usually normal, or nearly so, in the early stages of Alzheimer disease (AD). As the disease progresses, however, one typically sees a deterioration in the EEG characterized by a reduction in the amount of the posterior dominant (alpha) rhythm, slowing of the background frequency, a reduction in beta activity, and the appearance of generalized, predominantly bianterior delta bursts and series (Rae-Grant et al., 1987; Brenner et al., 1988). Several of these abnormalities are demonstrated in the EEG shown in Figure 8-3. Slowing of the posterior dominant rhythm may be the earliest, most subtle sign of EEG deterioration but may be difficult to differentiate from the changes caused by normal aging (Fig. 8-4). Past the age of 60 there is a normal reduction in alpha frequency at a rate of about 0.08 Hz/yr (Wang & Busse, 1969). However, even most healthy centenarians have a background frequency of 8 to 9 Hz (Hubbard et al., 1976). It has been generally accepted that the alpha frequency recorded in full wakefulness should exceed 8.5 Hz even in the very elderly. Therefore, only a value less than this can be clearly identified as abnormal in any one individual, although one should be aware of the fact that a considerable decline in background frequency may have occurred that has not yet fallen into an abnormal range. If premorbid studies are available for comparison, which is unfortunately not often the case, interval deterioration may be appreciable. Strikingly focal abnormalities are not usually seen in AD, but asymmetrical slowing in the temporal areas (maximal on the left) is not uncommon (Obrist, 1976). Here again care should be exercised in considering this finding as abnormal because temporal slowing is often found in healthy elderly individuals, as shown in Figure 8-5. This finding also increases with normal aging with up to 45% of normal volunteers over the age of 60 having temporal slowing (Kazis et al., 1982; Torres et al., 1983). There has been some speculation that the EEG changes described in AD may reflect a deficiency of acetylcholine in the basal forebrain and cortex, because similar findings have been recorded in subjects demonstrating memory disturbances following administration of the centrally active anticholinergic agent scopolamine (Sannita et al., 1987). However, it seems unlikely that the scopolamine model completely explains either the EEG changes or the cognitive impairments of AD. Although the EEG frequency changes seen after administration of this agent are similar to those

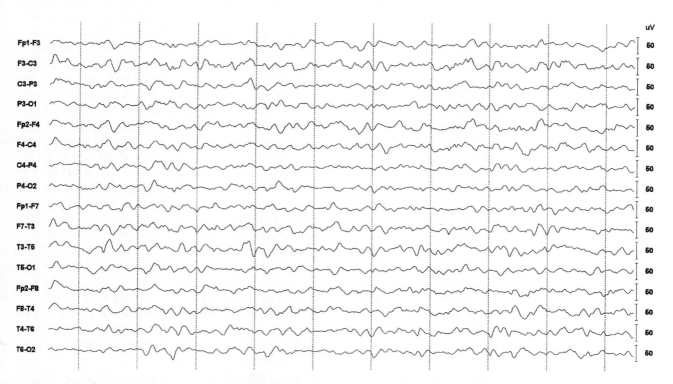

FIGURE 8-3. EEG from an 81-year-old patient with AD showing slowing of the posterior dominant rhythm to 5 to 6 Hz and diffuse, irregular theta-delta activity. Calibration marking shows 50 μV; bandpass is 1.6 to 35 Hz.

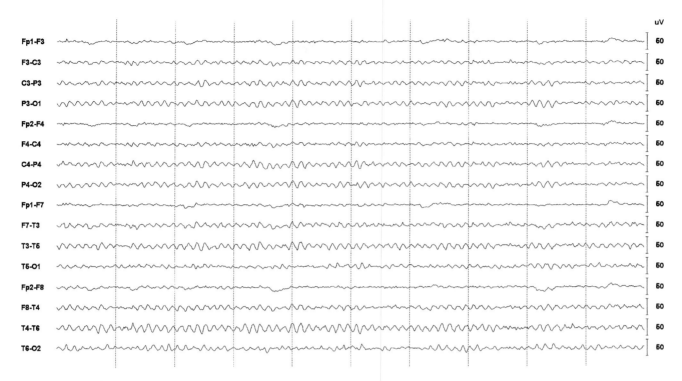

FIGURE 8-4. EEG from a 77-year-old patient with mild, early AD. Note that the posterior dominant rhythm in full wakefulness falls just below the lower limit of normal for frequency at 7 to 7.5 Hz in the absence of abnormal slow activity. Calibration marking shows 50 μV; bandpass is 1.6 to 70 Hz.

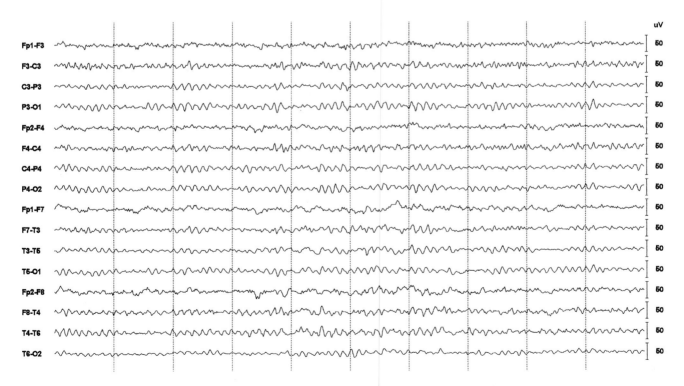

FIGURE 8-5. This EEG shows a 3- to 4-second long series of irregular delta activity in the midtemporal regions, more on the right. This 77-year-old patient had no complaints of memory loss or other cognitive difficulties. Temporal slow activity such as this is a common finding in normal elderly patients. Calibration marking shows 50 μV; bandpass is 1.6 to 70 Hz.

found in AD (decreased alpha, increased theta and delta), the cognitive impairments do not closely mimic what is found in AD, where abnormalities of attention, learning, and memory show a much greater magnitude of impairment (Ebert & Kirch, 1998).

Periodic discharges, such as the triphasic waves seen in Figure 8-6, are usually only seen in the most advanced cases of AD (Blatt & Brenner, 1996). Rae-Grant and colleagues (1987) noted them in only 6% of the 268 demented patients with a wide range of cognitive impairment. Typical triphasic waves, such as those more commonly seen in metabolic disorders, tend to be maximal in the anterior electrodes (Bickford & Butt, 1955), whereas those seen in AD may be more posteriorly located (Blatt & Brenner, 1996). It should be recalled, however, that periodic discharges in a patient with dementia may suggest another diagnosis, such a Creutzfeldt-Jakob disease (see below), a toxic-metabolic process, or anoxia (Brenner & Schaul, 1990). Hence, these discharges are nonspecific and may be seen in many different causes of dementia. Epileptiform discharges are rarely seen in AD (Markland, 1990).

There is a rough correlation between EEG findings and clinical severity and disease progression in AD; marked abnormalities are generally seen only late in the course of AD. Because of this, the EEG may assist in pointing toward the correct diagnosis if one considers the severity of EEG abnormalities in light of disease duration (Rae-Grant et al., 1987; Brenner et al., 1988). A strikingly abnormal EEG early in the course of a dementing illness would be very unusual for AD and would strongly suggest another, potentially reversible process, such as a toxic-metabolic or infectious disease (Harner, 1975). On the other hand, a patient who has had a significant decline in cognitive function but whose EEG is relatively normal or only mildly abnormal most likely has a degenerative cortical dementia. An alternative explanation in this setting is, however, that the patient may have a depressive pseudodementia because no EEG abnormalities would be anticipated in that situation (Benson, 1983). Because the routine EEG usually does not become abnormal until fairly late in the disease, it is not very useful for differentiating mild AD from normal aging.

The EEG's utility in determining prognosis in patients with AD is probably limited. Although there is usually progressive deterioration in the EEG as the disease worsens, this is not always the case (Rae-Grant et al., 1987). Patients with abnormal EEGs associated with psychotic symptoms of hallucinations and delusions appear to deteriorate more rapidly than those without (Lopez et al., 1991). Helkala and coworkers (1991) showed that AD patients with abnormal EEGs tend to have more evidence of apraxia, hallucinations,

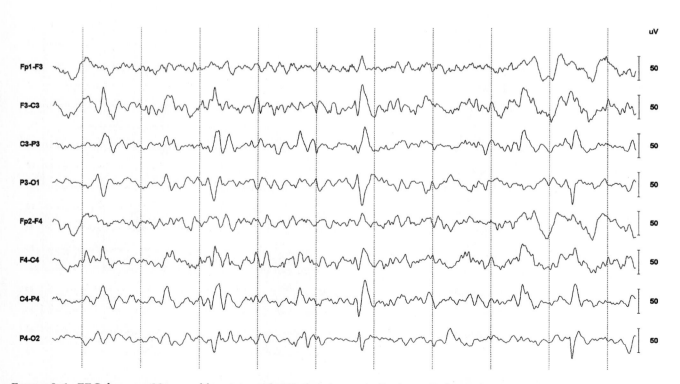

FIGURE 8-6. EEG from an 80-year-old patient with AD showing periodic sharp discharges. In contrast to typical triphasic waves, the periodic discharges occasionally seen late in the course of AD tend to be more posteriorly located than the typical triphasic waves of metabolic encephalopathies. Bandpass is 1.6 to 70 Hz.

and extrapyramidal signs. Also, the rate of institutionalization for their group increased if serial EEGs showed evidence of worsening over the preceding year. However, the clinical description of their patients suggests that they may not have had AD, but instead diffuse Lewy body disease (DLBD), in which psychosis and parkinsonism appear early in the disease along with evidence of cortical dysfunction (Simard et al., 2000). Supporting the notion that these patients probably had DLBD rather than classical AD, Crystal and colleagues (1990) showed that the patients they studied with DLBD had more strikingly abnormal EEGs early on than those patients who were felt to have AD. Further discussions regarding prognosis in AD are found in the sections concerning quantitative EEG and evoked potentials.

Creutzfeldt-Jakob Disease

Creutzfeldt-Jakob disease (CJD) is one of the prion protein diseases. Histologically, spongiform changes are seen primarily in the cortex but may also occur in the hippocampus, striatum, thalamus, and cerebellar cortex (De Armond & Prusiner, 1997). The EEG in patients with this disease typically shows periodic sharp discharges (PSDs) at some point in the course of their illness. These discharges are characterized by sharply contoured, biphasic or triphasic waves recurring repetitively at a rate of around 1 Hz (Brenner & Schaul, 1990). The topographic distributions of the PSDs are usually generalized, although striking asymmetry or unilaterality may be seen in some patients early on (Au et al., 1980). An example of unilateral PSDs is shown in Figure 8-7. As the disease progresses, the background, which is usually abnormal even before PSDs appear, tends to drop in amplitude and become attenuated while periodic discharges persist (Chiofalo et al., 1980). Although PSDs may be seen even late in the course of the disease, the frequency with which these discharges repeat tends to decline (Lee & Blair, 1973). Despite the fact that PSDs are not pathognomonic for CJD, their presence in a patient who has a rapidly evolving dementia, myoclonus, and ataxia should cause the clinician to be suspicious of the diagnosis. PSDs are not commonly seen at the time clinical symptoms begin but are found in about 90% of patients after 12 weeks of disease progression (Levy et al., 1986). The absence of PSDs at the end of 3 months in a patient with suggestive clinical

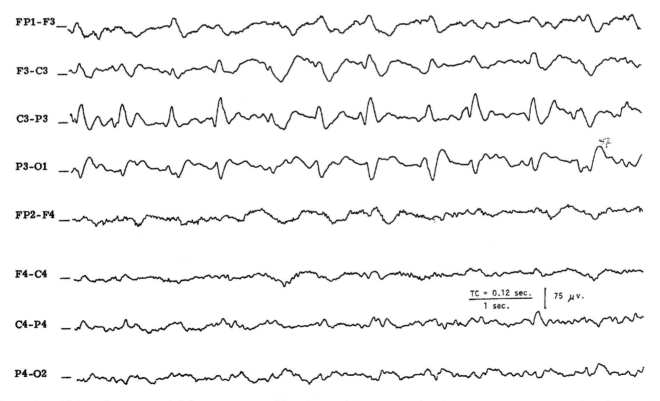

FIGURE 8-7. This EEG was recorded from a 63-year-old patient with CJD 2 months after symptom onset. Note that the periodic discharges are seen exclusively over the left hemisphere. However, an EEG performed 2 weeks later (not shown) demonstrated generalization of the periodic discharges. (Reproduced with permission from Au WJ, Gabor AJ, Viyan N, et al: Periodic lateralized epileptiform complexes [PLEDs] in Creutzfeldt-Jakob disease. Neurology 30:611–617, 1980.)

features strongly militates against the diagnosis. On the other hand, the presence of PSDs does not guarantee that a patient has CJD, even if there has been a rapid decline in mental status and involuntary movements are present. As mentioned earlier, PSDs with a triphasic waveform may be seen in a variety of metabolic (Bickford & Butt, 1955) and toxic encephalopathies (Smith & Kocen, 1988). Although EEG findings may be highly suggestive of the diagnosis, detection of the 14-3-3 protein in the cerebrospinal fluid (CSF) of these patients has been found by some investigators to more accurately discriminate CJD from other rapidly progressive dementias than either EEG or MRI (Poser et al., 1999).

Human Immunodeficiency Virus-1 Dementia

Dementia is probably the most frequent neurologic disorder seen in patients with acquired immunodeficiency syndrome (AIDS) (Gabuzda & Hirsh, 1987). In those demented patients without opportunistic infections, central nervous system neoplasms, neurotoxic effects of medications, or other toxic-metabolic aberrations, this condition is usually due to direct invasion of the brain, especially subcortical structures, by human immunodeficiency virus-1 (HIV-1) (Shaw et al., 1985). Likely due to the predominant subcortical pathology seen in these patients, the EEG generally shows only nonspecific changes with mild, diffuse slowing as the most commonly reported finding (Goodin et al., 1990). Neurologically asymptomatic, HIV seropositive patients have been reported by some investigators to have abnormal EEGs. Koralnik and colleagues (1990) found slowing of the posterior dominant rhythm and bianterior theta activity in 30% of the seropositive patients they initially studied. After a period of 6 to 9 months, the figure rose to 40%. Similar findings have been reported by others (Parisi et al., 1989). However, Goodin and co-investigators (1990) found no EEG abnormalities in the 41 asymptomatic seropositive patients they studied, and Harrison and co-investigators (1998) failed to detect an increase in EEG abnormalities in their cohort of seropositive patients with a CD4 count greater than 350. If EEG abnormalities are encountered, they should not be attributed to the patient's serostatus but, instead, lead to a search for other, potentially treatable causes (Nuwer et al., 1992).

Other Dementias

Pick disease, a subcategory of what is now referred to as frontotemporal dementia (FTD), typically presents differently from AD, with personality and executive function abnormalities that are out of proportion to memory disturbances, and a more rapidly deteriorating course (Binetti et al., 2000). The EEG in these patients

is usually normal (Stigsby, 1988). This is not surprising because the anterior involvement of cortex that is characteristic of this condition would not be expected to be associated with changes in the posterior dominant alpha rhythm. Also, subcortical involvement that leads to theta and delta activity only occurs late in the disease. However, as the disease progresses, diffuse slowing and epileptiform discharges may be seen (Sperfeld et al., 1999).

Patients with multi-infarct dementia (MID) commonly show more focal abnormalities on their EEGs than do those with AD (Bucht et al., 1984). This is especially true if the infarcts are in the territory of large pial arteries, such as the middle cerebral artery; subcortical lacunar infarcts caused by occlusion of small penetrating arteries lead to EEG abnormalities in only a small percentage of patients (Macdonell et al., 1988). Mild, largely nonspecific abnormalities are occasionally seen in patients with progressive supranuclear palsy and Parkinson disease (PD), and only then late in the disease (Fowler & Harrison, 1986; Soikkeli et al., 1991). Few abnormalities have been described in patients with normal pressure hydrocephalus (Brown & Goldensohn, 1973). A pattern of generalized low amplitude EEG activity has been seen in some patients with Huntington disease (HD). However, as pointed out by Pedley and Miller (1983), this pattern is almost never seen early in the course of the disease when the diagnosis may be unclear, and with the ready availability of genetic testing, the EEG adds little to the diagnostic evaluation of these patients.

Head Trauma

Shortly after a head injury, the EEG will show a large variety of patterns depending on the severity of the injury, depth of coma, age of the patient, and time between trauma and recording of the EEG. In cases of mild head trauma, in which there has been little or no alteration of consciousness, the EEG is typically normal or shows subtle, nonspecific abnormalities; fewer than 20% of such patients have an abnormal record (Dow et al., 1944; Yoshii et al., 1970). Hypersomnolence is common in this type of injury, and the EEG typically shows normal sleep patterns as these patients drift from wakefulness into drowsiness and sleep (Stockard et al., 1975). As the severity of head trauma increases, the EEG shows a greater degree of worsening and a more varied set of patterns. As a rule, there is good correlation between the EEG and depth of coma; progressive worsening of the EEG is associated with rostrocaudal deterioration (Hockaday et al., 1965; Rumpl et al., 1979). The EEG recorded in the acute post-traumatic period has been shown by several authors to be useful in the prognostication of outcome of head-injured patients (Karnaze et al., 1982; Rae-Grant et al., 1991).

EEG reactivity (desynchronization, attenuation, appearance of widespread delta or theta activity) is generally associated with a better outcome (Synek, 1990), whereas a record showing persistent delta slowing usually portends a poor one (Dusser et al., 1989). Gutling and coworkers (1995), in fact, found EEG reactivity to be highly predictive of outcome; 92% of their patients were correctly classified into good or bad outcome groups based on the presence or absence and type of reactivity.

In those patients who recover from their head injury, the EEG generally shows a gradual increase in frequencies and the ultimate development of a reactive, posterior dominant alpha rhythm (Stockard et al., 1975). In contrast, those patients who make a poor recovery and are left in an apallic state typically have EEGs that show a monotonous pattern with a predominance of theta and delta activity, a loss of normal sleep patterns, and occasionally, markedly attenuated records (Rumpl et al., 1983; Strnad & Strnadova, 1987). Prognostication based on the EEG is characteristically problematic in this group, but patients whose EEG shows an increase in frequency to faster rhythms and an alpha-like coma generally improve. Patients who show no improvement in their EEGs by 3 years typically show no further improvement in later recordings (Strnad & Strnadova, 1987). For reasons that are not entirely clear, there appears to be less correlation between EEG abnormalities and the clinical examination in this later stage of recovery than is seen in the acute period. Except in the most severely injured, abnormal EEGs tend to normalize regardless of clinical outcome (Courjon & Scherzer, 1972). The explanation for this discrepancy may be that the EEG is relatively insensitive in detecting pathology in subcortical structures, where trauma-induced diffuse axonal injury (DAI), a major cause of persisting disability, predominates (Gennarelli et al., 1982).

Some patients who recover from the acute injury develop symptoms of the postconcussive syndrome: headache, disequilibrium, sleep disturbances, depression, and complaints of cognitive impairment (Binder, 1986; Jacome & Risko, 1984). Early EEG studies of patients with the postconcussive syndrome reported frequent abnormalities. Denker and Perry (1954) found that 50% of their patients who had their EEGs within 3 months after trauma were abnormal. In those whose EEG was recorded more than 3 months later, 58% were abnormal, with a mixture of focal slow activity, diffuse symmetrical and asymmetrical abnormalities, and amplitude asymmetries. Torres and Shapiro (1961) studied 90 patients with either head trauma or whiplash injuries without head injury or loss of consciousness. The frequency of postconcussive symptoms was similar in these two groups. They found EEG abnormalities (either generalized or focal) in 44% of the patients with head injury and in 46% of those with only whiplash. Rather difficult to explain is the finding that epileptiform discharges were seen more frequently in the whiplash group than in those who had suffered a direct blow to the head. Also, in contrast to the well-described pattern of improvement that has been documented in most EEG studies of head trauma, the follow-up studies of their patients were frequently more abnormal than those performed initially. Both this study, and the one by Denker and Perry (1954), had several methodological limitations; they were done before the era of CT, none of the patients had corroborating neuropsychological testing, and the results were not compared with those of a matched control group.

Using more rigidly defined criteria for abnormality than earlier investigators and recording both standard and 24-hour ambulatory EEGs, Jacome and Risko (1984) found no significant abnormalities in 54 patients with the postconcussive syndrome. They did note nonspecific paroxysmal abnormalities in three patients and focal or generalized epileptiform discharges in two. However, the EEG pattern in these patients was judged to be chronic in nature and probably predated the head injuries. Haglund and Persson (1990) studied 47 amateur boxers and compared the EEG findings in this cohort with a group of 50 soccer players and track and field athletes. Not only did they fail to find a significant difference in the frequency of EEG abnormalities in the two groups, but they were also unable to find a correlation between EEG abnormalities and such indirect measures of repetitive trauma as the numbers of lost fights and knockouts and the duration of boxing careers. Sulg and Dencker (1968) studied monozygotic twins discordant for head injury and found a high concordance rate in the twin pairs regardless of whether the EEG was abnormal or not. In addition, they were unable to find a correlation between EEG normalities and the twin who had suffered a blow to the head. Hence, it appears that the routine EEG is probably of little benefit in evaluating patients with remote mild head injuries or the postconcussive syndrome.

Anoxia

Not dissimilar from what is seen after head trauma, EEG patterns following an anoxic event vary depending on the nature of the insult, its duration, and timing of the study. In situations in which there has been complete cessation of brain perfusion, such as after a cardiac arrest, EEG abnormalities tend to be generalized and severe (Gurvitch & Ginsberg, 1977). However, focal changes in the parieto-occipital regions superimposed on more generalized slowing may be seen in cases of profound, but incomplete, systemic hypotension resulting in pancerebral hypoperfusion and associated "watershed" infarcts (Malone et al., 1981). In addition, periodic complexes and epileptiform discharges may be seen in some patients (Janati et al., 1986). Generalized polyspike-slow wave complexes, burst suppression, and generalized pseudoperiodic repetitive sharp transients associated with generalized myoclonic status epilepticus have been described following cardiac arrest, usually portending a poor outcome (Celesia et al., 1988). Prognostication based on EEG findings may be useful, especially if one attends to the presence or absence of reactivity and sleep spindles (Synek, 1990) and the pattern of change in serial recordings (Jorgensen & Malchow-Moller, 1981). However, in a series of 40 patients reported by Rothstein and colleagues (1991), the EEG correctly predicted a poor outcome primarily when unequivocal "malignant" patterns were recorded. In those with "uncertain" patterns, the EEG was unable to distinguish those patients ultimately making a good recovery from those left with neurologic impairment, such as the persistent vegetative state (PVS). There are few published data concerning routine EEG in the late, postanoxic state. However, one series has reported markedly attenuated activity largely obscured by electromyographic (EMG) artifact and poorly differentiated sleep-wake cycles in three apallic patients 4 to 28 months after severe anoxic-ischemic insults (Matsuo, 1985). The electrophysiologic evaluation of patients in the late postanoxic phase is further discussed in the section on evoked potentials.

QUANTITATIVE EEG

The term *quantitative EEG* (QEEG) refers to a technique by which EEG activity is either displayed or analyzed following conversion of the raw EEG signal into a series of numerical values. The process is accomplished by feeding the amplified EEG analog signals into a digital converter, the output of which may be kept in its digital form for additional mathematical analysis or may be displayed graphically. The techniques discussed in this section are frequency spectral analysis by compressed spectral array (CSA) and topographic brain mapping (TBM). In the former process, the digitized EEG activity is displayed as a power spectrum showing the absolute or relative amplitudes of various frequencies of which the recorded EEG is composed. The mathematical process used to accomplish this is fast Fourier transformation. The displayed activity shows the distribution of frequencies in a prescribed period of time (e.g., 8 seconds), with each subsequent epoch stacked vertically to produce the CSA. The process by which brain mapping is produced is essentially the same, but an additional step is taken in which the amplitudes of the recorded EEG for a specific frequency band are displayed graphically as a topographic map. Blocks of amplitude ranges are displayed as different colors over a representation of the scalp.

The purported benefits of these procedures include the ability to detect abnormalities not apparent with other techniques (particularly the routine EEG) and the improvement of long-term monitoring. The latter is accomplished by eliminating seemingly unnecessary information, making the information of interest clearer by reducing the amount of data to be analyzed and stored (Nuwer, 1990). However, a word of caution is needed. QEEG recordings must be interpreted along with the routine EEG for accurate detection of common artifacts (electrocardiographic, EMG, eye blinks, and the like) that may not be obvious when looking at CSA or brain mapping alone. Also, CSA is unable to recognize transient phenomena such as spikes or bursts. Therefore, rather than making analysis easier, there is an additional level of complexity inherent in the interpretation of these studies, and a firm understanding of routine EEG interpretation is still required of those reading EEGs (Nuwer, 1990). Also, as pointed out in an editorial by Epstein (1994), the routine clinical use of these techniques should be discouraged. The medicolegal cases he reviewed were frequently flawed by poor technique; by misinterpretation of drowsiness, sleep, and medication effects as evidence of abnormality; and by misapplication of statistical analyses. The role of QEEG in the routine evaluation of patients with cognitive disturbances has yet to be established.

Alzheimer Disease

CSA, like the routine EEG, is able to demonstrate a shift to lower frequencies in patients with AD relative to healthy elderly controls. In patients with milder disease, there is a reduction in beta, while theta power increases (Coben et al., 1983; Coben et al., 1985; Brenner et al., 1986). As cognitive function declines further, alpha power begins to drop and delta increases, as shown in Figure 8-8 (Coben et al., 1985, 1990; d'Onofrio et al., 1996). A progressive shift in power spectra toward increasing theta and delta activity has been shown to occur over a period of more than 2 years in patients with AD (Coben et al., 1985). It has been suggested that this technique may differentiate presenile- from senile-onset dementias with earlier, more severe slowing seen predominately in the former group (Miyauchi et al., 1994). Whether or not this technique adds any unique information in the evaluation of demented patients is unsettled. Brenner and colleagues (1988) did not find that CSA was superior to standard EEG in being able to differentiate demented AD patients from normal elderly. Perhaps most importantly, CSA did not add any advantage over routine EEG in detecting evidence of cerebral dysfunction in patients with mild dementia, at a time when the clinical diagnosis may be difficult. However, Jordan and co-investigators (1989) reported that CSA more correctly identified mildly demented

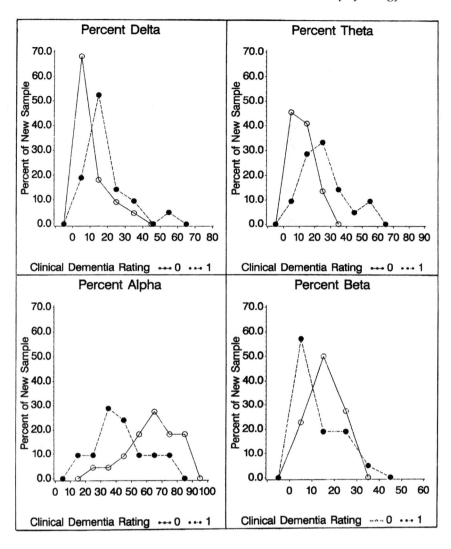

FIGURE 8-8. Percentage of subjects (ordinate) who had a given percentage of delta, theta, alpha, or beta score (abscissa) in a sample of 21 patients with AD compared to 22 healthy controls. Clinical Dementia Rating scale score of 0 and 1 correspond to *normal* and *mildly demented*, respectively. Note that the demented patients show increased theta and delta activity, whereas the controls have a higher percentage of alpha activity. (Reproduced with permission from Coben LA, Chi D, Snyder AZ, et al: Replication of a study of frequency analysis of the resting awake EEG in mild probable Alzheimer's disease. Electroencephalogr Clin Neurophysiol 75:148–154, 1990.)

patients than did standard EEG. Some investigators feel that attention to the duration of what has been termed "EEG microstates" may be helpful in distinguishing normal aging from dementia. A microstate is a transient period of time during which distinct, stable topographic voltage patterns occur. Stevens and Kircher (1998) showed that cognitively impaired elderly subjects had significantly shorter microstate durations than normal controls, suggesting that fragmentation of these electrophysiologic processes may underlie the cognitive impairment seen in these patients.

TBM may be able to differentiate subgroups of AD patients based on predominant clinical features. Albert and colleagues (1990) showed that AD patients with predominant memory impairment could be differentiated from those with signs of disturbed spatial orientation based on TBM. In their study, a reduction in parietal beta activity was seen in those patients with impairment of spatial orientation relative to those without this clinical feature. TBM may also distinguish senile- from presenile-onset AD. Duffey and colleagues

(1984) found that patients younger than 65 years tended to have increased theta and decreased beta activities in parietal and temporal areas, whereas older patients showed an increase in both theta and delta activities accompanied by decreased beta activity in the frontal area. Although a variety of patterns have been seen in AD, increased slow activity in the left temporal region may be the most characteristic finding in these patients (Breslau et al., 1989; Rice et al., 1990).

HIV-1 Dementia

There have been a limited number of studies utilizing QEEG techniques in patients with HIV. However, CSA has been shown by at least one group to demonstrate a shift to slower frequencies in some asymptomatic HIV seropositive patients (Parisi et al., 1989). In addition, this group demonstrated that those patients with an abnormal CSA at entry into the study tended to progress to dementia over a period of 11 months, and the rate of progression correlated with the severity of abnormalities on CSA. This suggests that CSA may be a useful technique for predicting neurologic outcome in these patients. However, QEEG changes should not be attributed to serostatus alone because they are more likely to be caused by other associated diseases (Nuwer et al., 1992).

Other Dementias

It is unclear if multi-infarct dementia (MID) can be differentiated from AD by QEEG techniques. Using CSA, Erkinjunttiet and associates (1988) found little difference between these two patient groups; both had a pattern consisting of increased theta and delta power. However, Leuchter and Walter (1989) showed that AD patients had characteristic deficits in left temporoparietal activity, whereas those patients with MID did not. D'Onofrio and co-investigators (1996) found that patients with MID had increased delta activity in occipital regions and a widespread increase of theta, and decrease of alpha activities, whereas AD patients had widespread increased delta and theta, and decreased alpha activities. CSA frequency and coherence analysis (evaluating frequency similarities between different brain regions in one hemisphere or homologous regions in both) may correctly differentiate MID from AD in more than 90% of patients (Leuchter et al., 1987). Sloan and coworkers (1995) found that the predictive power of CSA to differentiate these two causes of dementia was 90%, whereas that of single photon emission computed tomography (SPECT) was 83%. In this study, approximately 75% of AD and MID patients had appropriate abnormalities on EEG and SPECT, and only 1 of the 68 demented patients they studied had normal results on both tests. Areas of increased delta activity seen in MID have been shown to correlate with regions of reduced glucose metabolism on fluodeoxyglucose positron emission tomography (PET) scans (Szelies et al., 1999).

Patients with FTD tend to have fewer abnormalities on CSA than do those with AD (Yener et al., 1996). The abnormalities that are seen include decreased beta power anteriorly with increased theta and delta activities in frontal and anterior temporal locations. Alpha activity is usually well preserved. DLBD has been reported to be associated with increased fluctuation in the mean EEG frequency recorded in 90-second epochs (Walker et al., 2000) and may be distinguishable from AD due to more marked slowing of the posterior dominant rhythm and presence of temporal slow activity in these patients (Briel et al., 1999).

Head Trauma

A number of investigators have reported that CSA is useful in determining prognosis in patients with acute head injury. Bricolo and colleagues (1979) showed that if the CSA was characterized by a predominance of monotonous slow activity with a fixed frequency, mortality was 86%. In contrast, if there was a fluctuating, changeable pattern or if a sleeplike pattern was recorded, death occurred in 41.3% and 13.3%, respectively. Similar findings have been noted by Strnad and Strnadova (1987). CSA has also been shown to be superior to the routine EEG in accurately predicting outcome in the acute setting by at least one group (Bricolo et al., 1979). Thatcher and colleagues (1998) showed that increased amplitude of delta and decreased amplitude of alpha and beta correlated with the presence of increased T2 white matter lesions on MRI. Also, both the MRI and QEEG results they obtained correlated with decreased cognitive function on neuropsychological assessments at follow-up. They concluded that these findings implied the presence of a biophysical linkage between post-traumatic structural changes and functional impairment. However, Kane and associates (1998) found limited correlations between QEEG measures of alpha and beta power, interhemispheric coherence, and outcome at 6 months and 1 year after injury. Also, the brains of 10 fatal cases in their series were examined for histopathologic evidence of diffuse oxonal injury (DAI). They were unable to find evidence of either a significant correlation between interhemispheric coherence and outcome or a consistent relationship between this QEEG measure and severity of DAI.

In patients with the postconcussive syndrome, CSA has been reported to show a shift of both alpha and beta activity to lower frequencies regardless of whether or not the patient actually suffered loss of consciousness (Tebano et al., 1988). The routine EEG was shown to be less able to detect these subtle frequency changes but was superior to CSA in identifying paroxysmal theta bursts. Using an analysis of coherence and phase, Thatcher and colleagues (1989) found an increase in coherence and a decrease in phase in the frontal and frontotemporal regions, a decrease in power differences between anterior and posterior regions, and a decrease in posterior alpha power. These abnormalities were noted within a few hours or days and showed very little decline over an extended period of observation. They speculated that these findings correlated with shear-strain and rotational white matter damage and localized gray matter contusions, although no imaging or pathologic information was reported. Thatcher and colleagues also believed that the 80% to 95% discriminant accuracy of these techniques compared favorably with the reported accuracy of neuropsychological studies.

Brain mapping has been reported by Jerrett and Corsak (1988) to be superior to routine EEG in head-injured patients. In 8 head-injured patients they studied, 4 had abnormal brain maps, only 2 of whom also showed abnormalities on routine EEG. The EEG most frequently missed low-amplitude slow activity. Another study of 135 patients who were evaluated by brain mapping several years after head injury showed abnormalities, mostly in the temporo-occipital regions, in 56%. In contrast, the routine EEG was abnormal in only 30% and consisted mostly of nonspecific, diffuse slowing (Hooshmand et al., 1989). Watson and colleagues (1995) found a strong correlation between delay in left temporal recovery and residual psychiatric symptoms 12 months after head injury in the 26 patients they studied. However, Haglund and Persson (1990) found no additional benefit of CSA and brain mapping over routine EEG in their cohort of head-injured boxers.

EVOKED POTENTIALS

Evoked potentials (EPs) are generated in response to a repetitive sensory stimulus; with computer-assisted averaging, the desired signal is enhanced while unwanted background EEG signals and artifacts are suppressed. Visual, auditory, and somatosensory stimuli are the sensory modalities typically used. They are divided into short-, middle-, and long-latency responses, depending on the time period following the stimulus at which the potentials are recorded. Visual EP (VEP), middle- and long-latency auditory EP (AEP), and somatosensory EP (SEP) peaks are usually named according to the polarity of the response (expressed as "P" for positive and "N" for negative), followed by the mean latency of that response (in milliseconds) recorded from normal controls (e.g., P100 for the VEP). The nomenclature used for the short-latency AEPs, which are commonly referred to as brainstem auditory evoked potentials (BAEPs), is different; peaks are simply designated I through V. Although some controversy still remains, the neural generators for the short-latency AEPs are known with a fair degree of certainty. The striate and peristriate occipital cortices appear to generate the P100 potential of the VEP when a pattern reversal stimulus is used. However, a more complex waveform is produced that may be generated by a variety of cortical and subcortical projection systems when a flash is used to stimulate visual pathways, as is sometimes done in studies of inattentive patients (Allison et al., 1977). The exact generators of all of the BAEP peaks are unknown, but there is general consensus that wave I corresponds to the distal auditory nerve, waves II and III are generated at the pontomedullary region, whereas the rostral pons and mesencephalon are the sites of origin of waves IV and V. Short-latency SEP responses recorded after median nerve stimulation at the wrist originate in structures following primary somatosensory pathways in the brachial plexus, cervical spinal cord, brainstem, thalamus, thalamocortical projections, and cortex. The generators of the middle- and late-latency SEPs are more controversial but may include thalamocortical projections and primary and secondary cortical association areas (Yamada et al., 1984).

Another EP technique that has been developed specifically with the intent of physiologically assessing cognitive function is what has been commonly referred to as the event-related potential (ERP). In contrast to the stimulus-specific EPs described previously, ERPs are recorded independently of the type of sensory stimulus used and are felt to represent the electrophysiologic equivalent of the patient's psychological response to a novel stimulus (Oken, 1997). The precise nature of the psychological processes being evaluated is not known with certainty but may include memory and attention (Papanicolaou et al., 1984; Olbrich et al., 1986). The two ERPs that have been studied most frequently in cognitively impaired patients are the P300 (or "P3") response and contingent negative variation (CNV). The P300 is elicited by an anticipated stimulus (usually auditory) that occurs randomly in an "odd ball" pattern among frequent stimuli that the patient has been instructed to ignore. It is a large-amplitude positive potential with maximal distribution over the midline central and parietal regions, as demonstrated in Figure 8-9 (Goodin et al., 1978). The CNV is a slow, negative potential recorded between paired stimuli, of which the first acts as a warning and the second as an imperative stimulus to which the patient is instructed to make a response. The neural generators for these potentials are unknown. However, depth electrode studies have shown that mesial temporal lobe structures, including the hippocampus, may be important in generating the scalp-recorded P300 (Smith et al., 1990). In part because of this, some authors have speculated that ERPs are generated by tasks that require maintenance of working memory (Donchin et al., 1986). Indeed, experimental evidence indicates that the amplitude of P300 is directly correlated to performance on tests of memory (Fabiani et al., 1990). The latency of P300 appears to be related to the speed by which subjects are able to differentiate previously detected and recalled stimuli from novel and different "odd" stimuli (Magliero et al., 1984; Emmerson et al., 1990). Some subjects have a bifid P300 response, the earlier peak sometimes labeled P3a and the later P3b. P3a is seen more anteriorly over the scalp and has been felt to represent an early alerting response (Knight, 1984), whereas P3b is somewhat more posteriorly distributed and may reflect memory-updating and attentional processes (Donchin et al., 1986).

Despite numerous studies in a variety of disease states, the sensitivity and specificity of these responses has not proved to be great (Oken, 1997). This may be in part explained by the fact that a variety of nonpathologic factors appear to affect the amplitude and latency of P300 and, if not adequately controlled for, lead to considerable intrapatient and interpatient variability. Perhaps most important of these variables is the effect of

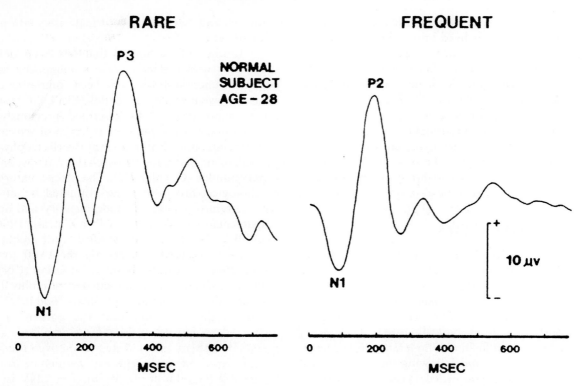

FIGURE 8-9. Event-related potentials recorded from the vertex in a normal subject using an "oddball" paradigm. Averaged responses on the left were obtained following infrequently presented target stimuli. Note that P3 (labeled P300 in the text) appears only with the target stimuli. (Reproduced with permission from Goodin DS, Squires KC, Starr A: Long latency event-related components of the auditory evoked potential in dementia. Brain 101:635–648, 1978.)

age; advancing age in adults leads to a prolongation of the P300 latency by about 1.4 msec/yr (Goodin et al., 1978). The reduction in P300 amplitude is somewhat less predictable but tends to reduce as one ages (Picton et al., 1984). This is particularly important in the evaluation of patients with dementia, which will be discussed later. Other factors include recent food ingestion, body temperature, and degree of effort required to sustain attention (Geisler & Polich, 1990; Ford et al., 1997). Rather curiously, such factors as season of the year, subject personality traits (introverted versus extroverted), and diurnal preference times have been reported by some authors to affect the results of these studies (Daruna et al., 1985; Polich & Geisler, 1991; Geisler & Polich, 1992). Differences in these factors may explain, at least in part, the rather high degree of intersubject ERP variability. These factors should be considered when performing and interpreting these studies.

Alzheimer Disease

As mentioned previously, the latency and to a lesser degree amplitude of the P300 are affected by advancing age in normal control subjects. However, ERPs have been reported to be capable of differentiating normal,

age-related changes from those seen in patients with early AD (Polich et al., 1990). In dementing illnesses, the latency of P300 is prolonged relative to age-matched controls (Fig. 8-10). Squires and colleagues (1980) found that 80% of their demented patients had a P300 latency that exceeded the upper limit of normal (mean + 2 SD) at a given age. Longitudinal studies of patients with dementia have shown that there is a progressive latency prolongation as the disease progresses (Ball et al., 1989; Polich et al., 1986). Reisberg and co-investigators (1982) showed that ERPs correlated well with the severity of the dementia as indexed by the Global Deterioration Scale; at lower levels of disability there is a gradual prolongation of latency prolongation, but at the higher extreme of the scale, P300 latency prolongs dramatically. In addition, evidence suggests that ERPs may be able to differentiate cortical dementias, such as AD from the subcortical dementias of HD and PD (Goodin & Aminoff, 1986). Attention to changes in scalp topography of P300 and CNV may aid in differentiating AD from MID (Yokoyama et al., 1995; Oishi & Mochizuki, 1998). Pattern reversal and flash VEPs have also been found to be abnormal in demented patients with PD (Okuda et al., 1995).

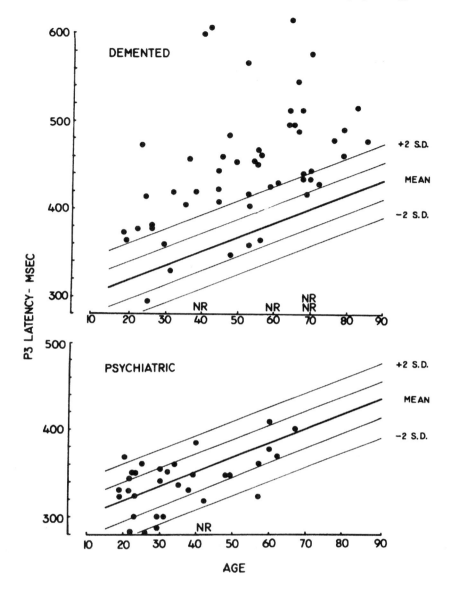

FIGURE 8-10. Plot of values obtained from 52 demented patients compared to age-matched nondemented subjects (labeled "psychiatric"). Normal limits reflect mean plus 1 and 2 SDs. NR, no response. (Modified from Squires KC, Chippendale TJ, Wrege KS, et al: Electrophysiological assessment of mental function in aging and dementia, in Poon LW [ed]: Aging in the 1980's: Selected Contemporary Issues in the Psychology of Aging. Washington, DC: American Psychological Association, 1980, pp. 125–134.)

What information might ERPs add in the evaluation of demented patients that cannot be obtained by other means, such as conventional neuropsychological batteries? A significant correlation has been reported between P300 latency and scores on tests of cognitive function, such as the Global Deterioration Scale and Weschler Adult Intelligence Scale in some studies (Reisberg, et al., 1982; Polich et al., 1986; Neshige et al., 1988), but not in others (Canter et al., 1982). However, the sensitivity of psychometric tests is probably superior to that of P300 latency prolongation in correctly identifying the presence of a dementia (Kraiuhin et al., 1986). Cohen and coworkers (1995) followed 29 demented patients for 4 years after initial diagnosis with neuropsychologoical assessments and ERP's. Functional outcome in terms of incontinence, institutionalization, activities of daily living (ADL) dependence, verbal responsiveness, recognition of family members, and capacity for social interaction were better predicted by neuropsychological measures. Only mortality was predicted more accurately by prolongation of the P300 latency. Hence, the role of ERP is probably limited in this setting. On the other hand, a fairly common clinical problem that may be clarified by ERPs is the situation in which differentiation of a genuine dementia from a depressive pseudodementia is clinically difficult. Because ERPs have been found to be normal in depressed patients, this technique may be useful in identifying this potentially treatable group of patients (Squires et al., 1980). However, a normal result would certainly not exclude the presence of an organic dementia.

HIV-1 Dementia

Short-latency EPs, especially BAEPs and SEPs, may be abnormal in both asymptomatic seropositive patients and those with AIDS. Pierelli and colleagues (1996) found abnormal EPs in 43.6% of their asymptomatic patients, whereas abnormalities were found in 76.5% of those with AIDS. The most striking finding was the high incidence of subclinical involvement of BAEP interpeak intervals and SEP conduction times. Goodin and coworkers (1990) have reported that ERPs are frequently abnormal in patients with HIV-1 dementia and not uncommonly affected in asymptomatic seropositive patients (Fig. 8-11). In their study, latencies were prolonged in 78% of the demented patients and 28% of those that were asymptomatic at the time of their evaluation. Others have found abnormal ERPs in most, if not all, seropositive patients, and the degree of severity correlates inversely with CD4 counts (Arendt et al., 1993; Schroeder et al., 1994). ERPs may also be useful in monitoring the response to antiretroviral therapy. Evers and colleagues (1998) followed 154 seropositive patients without evidence of central nervous system involvement that had been randomized to either zidovudine or placebo over a period of 2 years. They found a significant inverse correlation between P300 latency and CD4 count at any time during the course of the study, and treatment with zidovudine prevented the latency prolongation seen in the placebo group.

Head Trauma

EPs have been used in the acute period after head injury to determine long-term prognosis. SEPs have been shown to be superior in predicting outcome to VEPs and AEPs, intracranial pressure (ICP) monitoring, CT, and clinical examination by several investigators (Greenberg et al., 1982; Anderson et al., 1984; Cant et al., 1986; Firsching & Frowein, 1990; Cusumano et al., 1992). Short-latency EPs have been shown to be superior to EEG in predicting outcome in large part owing to their stability in the face of sedative medications and other confounding variables (Hutchinson et al., 1991; Moulton et al., 1998). Gutling and coworkers (1995) found that SEPs correctly predicted long-term outcome in 82% of their patients, whereas the presence or

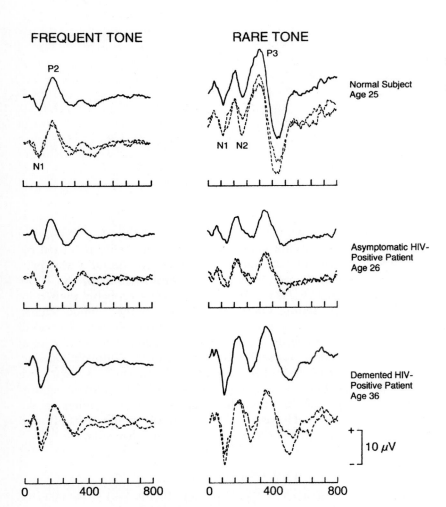

FIGURE 8-11. ERPs from a normal control, an asymptomatic HIV-1 seropositive patient, and a patient with AIDS-associated dementia. Note prolongation of latencies in the patients relative to the control. (Reproduced with permission from Goodin DS, Aminoff MJ, Chernoff DN, et al: Long latency event-related potentials in patients infected with human immunodeficiency virus. Ann Neurol 27:414–419, 1990.)

absence of EEG reactivity was correct in 92%. By combining both SEPs and EEG reactivity, they were able to correctly classify 98% of their patients.

EPs in the chronic phase of head injury have been suggested as being helpful in assessing the extent of cognitive impairment and predicting the potential for additional recovery. VEPs have been shown in one study (Gupta et al., 1986) to correlate with the extent of cognitive impairment. In this study, 50% of those with severe cognitive impairment had abnormal VEPs, whereas those with moderate or mild impairment had VEP abnormalities in 38% and 11% of cases, respectively. Prolongation of BAEP interpeak intervals may be seen in more than 25% of patients with the postconcussive syndrome (Benna et al., 1982). One group of investigators has shown that those patients with persistently abnormal or deteriorating EPs 1 year after trauma typically had a poor outcome, whereas those with normal or improving EPs did well (Newlon et al., 1982). Of particular interest is the fact that an improvement in EP abnormalities was seen in some but not all patients before clinical improvement was apparent.

Not all studies have found EPs to be helpful in this setting, however. Rappaport and coworkers (1977) noted positive correlations with a disability rating scale only when long-latency SEPs and AEPs were recorded. Even still, EPs were able to differentiate only those patients with very severe impairments from those with none; milder cases, in which the distinction is more critical, could not be differentiated from the more severely impaired. Shin and colleagues (1989) found no correlation between BAEPs and SEPs and a clinical evaluation of cognitive abilities. These EPs had only a 15% predictive power in assessing ultimate functional ability at the end of rehabilitation; the initial clinical evaluation and age of the patient were superior to EPs in this regard. EPs are particularly insensitive in comparison with such clinical features as age and duration of unconsciousness and amnesia in patients who have suffered mild head injuries (Werner & Vanderzant, 1991). The lack of predictive value in these later studies probably reflects the fact that EPs, like the routine EEG and QEEG, assess function indirectly; when the patient can be assessed directly by clinical evaluations and neuropsychological batteries, their value diminishes.

Despite the uncertainty concerning their role in assessing cognitive function, several investigators have attempted to use ERPs to evaluate patients with head injuries. The P300 has been reported to be absent in patients who have suffered severe head injuries (Curry, 1980), whereas no significant abnormalities have been reported in milder cases (Werner & Vanderzant, 1991). Curry (1980) showed that P300 abnormalities correlated well with the severity of head injury and were able to differentiate severely injured patients from those with milder degrees of trauma. Olbrich and coworkers

(1986) studied 18 severely head-injured patients acutely and, 3 to 6 months later, found that the latency of P300 significantly correlated with impairments on initial neuropsychological testing. At follow-up, however, neuropsychological deficits improved, whereas the P300 remained abnormal in many patients. Hence, they concluded that ERPs were more sensitive in identifying residual cognitive dysfunction than neuropsychological testing in some patients.

If it is true that persistently abnormal ERPs occur in some head-injured patients, what significance does this have in terms of the behavioral or cognitive state of the patient? An interesting approach to answering this question was taken by Granovsky and colleagues (1998) who used visually presented words rather than auditory tones as the stimuli. Target stimuli consisted of words that were emotionally charged and accident related, such as "crashed car" and "ambulance," whereas nontarget words were accident neutral (e.g., "pigeon," "joke"). The head-injured patients showed a significantly larger P300 response to target words, whereas controls did not. Also, the change in amplitude correlated with results on the Zung state anxiety score. Their interpretation of these findings was that ERPs were capable of providing an objective assessment of the emotional state of patients with head injuries. Some investigators have felt that P300 abnormalities represent the electrophysiologic correlate of post-traumatic amnesia (Papanicolaou et al., 1984; Onofri, 1991) or impaired orientation and memory (Olbrich et al., 1986). Others have considered the P300 as simply a nonspecific alerting response in severely injured patients (Rappaport et al., 1991).

CNV abnormalities in head-injured patients have included absence, attenuation, and asymmetry of responses, as well as an abnormal topographic distribution of the maximal negativity (Curry, 1980). The latter finding has been seen in patients suffering diffuse frontal injury with maximal negativity seen more anteriorly than usual, suggesting that this shift in distribution represents a "release" phenomenon of normally suppressed processes originating in the frontal lobes (Curry, 1980). Despite the suggestion that CNV is able to identify specific areas of cerebral trauma, another study (Low, 1979) was unable to demonstrate any correlation between CNV abnormalities and proven brain lesions. What is more, this technique was found to be even less reliable than the routine EEG in identifying cerebral pathology.

Anoxia

Prediction of outcome following an anoxic insult may be aided by combing results of routine EEG (see previous section) and short-latency SEPs. Chen and coworkers (1996) found both the EEG and SEPs to be strongly associated with outcome; the predictive power of EEG was 90% and SEPs 100%. They concluded that results of the clinical examination, EEG, and SEP performed on the third day after the event were able to provide a definitive prognosis in the majority of patients. Similar conclusions have been published by some authors (Berkhoff et al., 2000), whereas others feel that SEPs alone are sufficient for determining prognosis (Zandbergen et al., 1998). In contrast, Rothstein and colleagues (1991) reported that SEPs were useful only when cortical responses were absent bilaterally, in which case they correctly predicted an unfavorable outcome in 81%. However, SEPs were unable to differentiate those patients who made a good outcome from those left in a PVS when they were normal or only showed a delay in central conduction time.

EPs have also been used to evaluate patients in the later stages following an anoxic event. Using multimodality EPs, Guerit (1994) found that patients in a PVS due to anoxic-ischemic encephalopathy typically showed absent cortical VEP and SEP responses, whereas subcortical SEP and BAEP responses were preserved. These findings were distinguishable from those seen following head trauma where abnormal conduction to the midbrain level was noted. Prognosis for recovery from PVS was better in those patients who had improvement in brainstem-localized abnormalities on serial studies, and residual cognitive abilities were more likely to be present in patients with preserved cortical responses and ERPs. Mecklinger and associates (1998), based on results of ERPs, argued that postanoxic memory disorders are characterized by degradation of explicit memory functions, whereas implicit functions such as cognitive skill learning are unaffected. In this study, eight patients who had previously suffered an anoxic episode due to a cardiac arrest were compared to matched controls in a visual recognition memory task that required subjects to make a judgment for either object forms or spatial locations and a visual classification task that required little memory function. In the memory task, P300 amplitudes were larger for previously studied items compared to unstudied ones in the controls, whereas patients showed either no amplitude differences or an inversion of response polarity. However, the patients had relatively preserved recognition performance. Their interpretation of these findings was that retrieval memory is degraded in patients who have suffered an episode of cerebral anoxia-ischemia. In experimentally induced acute hypoxia, P300 latency and behaviorly determined reaction time prolong at oxygen saturation values less than 82%, suggesting similar cognitive processes are being assessed by these two techniques (Fowler & Prlic, 1995).

CONCLUSIONS

The potential usefulness of the techniques described in this chapter for evaluating cognitively impaired patients rests on the fact that they are tests of central nervous system function. The EEG records electrical potentials generated by the cortex that are influenced by input from the thalamus, as well as other parts of the cortex. Short-latency EPs assess function in various sensory pathways, and ERPs provide a means of quantitatively evaluating some aspects of memory and attention. In addition, these techniques are relatively inexpensive and readily available in most medical centers. However, other testing methods, from imaging studies to neuropsychological batteries, are also readily available and probably provide more complete information. CT and MRI are unquestionably superior to any of the electrophysiologic techniques for assessing structural changes, and the wealth of information that can be learned by a neuropsychological evaluation cannot be duplicated by any of them. So, what role do electrophysiologic studies play in the evaluation of patients with disordered cognition? The routine EEG is probably best suited to identifying potentially treatable conditions, such as nonconvulsive status epilepticus, toxic-metabolic encephalopathies, and depressive pseudodementia. Supportive information may also be learned about other causes of dementia, such as CJD. The EEG is also useful in assessing patients in the acute phase of an anoxic-ischemic or traumatic insult but likely has little or no place later on when more direct means of evaluating cognition are possible. The role for QEEG techniques remains to be defined and, as yet, is probably quite limited. EPs appear to be useful in determining prognosis in patients after anoxia-ischemia or trauma but seem to have a very limited place in the chronic setting. On the other hand, ERPs may be helpful in this chronic setting, perhaps by differentiating depression from an organic cause of cognitive decline or in documenting the development of dementia in patients with AIDS. Whenever the electrophysiologic techniques of EEG, QEEG, and EPs are used to evaluate patients with disorders of cognition, one must bear in mind that negative results cannot exclude the presence of significant nervous system dysfunction. This is particularly pertinent in those with milder degrees of cognitive involvement. When abnormal, the findings on these tests are usually nonspecific and are rarely capable of making a definitive etiologic diagnosis. Despite this these techniques may provide unique, useful information in the specific situations described above. This is particularly true if they are interpreted by an experienced electrophysiologist and especially when the results are considered in light of the entire clinical picture.

■ KEY POINTS

☐   The potential usefulness of EEG and EPs is based on the fact that they are tests of central nervous system function.

☐   EEG and EP findings are often nonspecific, and normal results do not exclude the presence of significant neurologic dysfunction. The clinical value of these techniques is highly dependent on accurate interpretation and correlation of the results with the patient's history and clinical examination, as well as other diagnostic studies.

☐   The role of the EEG in evaluating cognitively impaired patients is best limited to identification of potentially reversible conditions (e.g., nonconvulsive status epilepticus).

☐   The EEG and short-latency EPs may be useful in determining prognosis in acute head trauma and anoxic encephalopathy but probably add little to the evaluation of these patients in later stages.

☐   ERPs may be useful in differentiating depressive pseudodementia from organic cognitive decline and documenting the development of dementia in patients with AIDS.

KEY READINGS

Coben LA, Chi D, Snyder AZ, et al: Replication of a study of frequency analysis of the resting awake EEG in mild probable Alzheimer's disease. Electroencephalogr Clin Neurophysiol 75:148–154, 1990.

Goodin DS, Aminoff MJ: Electrophysiological differences between subtypes of dementia. Brain 109:1103–1113, 1986.

Polich J, Ladish C, Bloom FE: P300 Assessment of early Alzheimer's disease. Electroencephalogr Clin Neuorophysiol 77:179–189, 1990.

Rae-Grant A, Blume W, Lau C, et al: The electroencephalogram in Alzheimer's-type dementia: A sequential study correlating the electroencephalogram with psychometric and quantitative pathologic data. Arch Neurol 44:50–54, 1987.

Soininen H, Partanen VJ, Heilkala EL, et al: EEG findings in senile dementia and normal aging. Acta Neurol Scand 65:59–70, 1982.

REFERENCES

Abraham K, Ajmone-Marsan C: Patterns of cortical discharge and their relation to routine scalp electroencephalography. Electroencephalogr Clin Neurophysiol 10:447–461, 1958.

Albert MS, Duffy FH, McAnulty GB: Electrophysiologic comparisons between two groups of patients with Alzheimer's disease. Arch Neurol 47:857–863, 1990.

Allison T, Matsumiya Y, Goff GD, et al: The scalp topography of human visual evoked potentials. Electroencephalogr Clin Neurophysiol 42:185–197, 1997.

Anderson DC, Bundlie S, Rockswold GL: Multimodality evoked potentials in closed head trauma. Arch Neurol 41:369–374, 1984.

Arendt G, Hefter H, Jablonowski H: Acoustically evoked event-related potentials in HIV-associated dementia. Electroencephalogr Clin Neurophysiol 86:152–160, 1993.

Au WJ, Gabor AJ, Viyan N, et al: Periodic lateralized epileptiform complexes (PLEDs) in Creutzfeldt-Jakob disease. Neurology 30:611–617, 1980.

Ball SS, Marsh JT, Schubarth G, et al: Longitudinal P300 latency changes in Alzheimer's disease. J Gerontol 44:M195–200, 1989.

Benna P, Bergamasco B, Bianco C, et al: Brainstem auditory evoked potentials in postconcussion syndrome. Ital J Neurol Sci 3:281–287, 1982.

Benson DF: Subcortical dementia: A clinical approach, in Mayeux R, Rosen WG (eds): Advances in Neurology: The Dementias. New York: Raven Press, 1983, Vol. 38, pp. 185–194.

Berkhoff M, Donati F, Bassetti C: Postanoxic alpha (theta) coma: A reappraisal of its prognostic significance. Clin Neurophysiol 111:297–304, 2000.

Berger H: Über das Elektroenkephalogramm des Menschen: 1st report. Arch Psychiatr Nervenkr 87:527–570, 1929.

Bickford RG, Butt HR: Hepatic coma: The electroencephalographic pattern. J Clin Invest 34:790–799, 1955.

Binder LM: Persisting symptoms after mild head injury: A review of the postconcussive syndrome. J Clin Exp Neuropsychol 8:323–346, 1986.

Binetti G, Locascio JJ, Corkin S, et al: Differences between Pick disease and Alzheimer disease in clinical appearance and rate of cognitive decline. Arch Neurol 57:225–232, 2000.

Blatt I, Brenner RP: Triphasic waves in a psychiatric population: A retrospective study. J Clin Neurophysiol 13:324–329, 1996.

Brenner RP, Reynolds CF, Ulrich RF: Diagnostic efficacy of computerized spectral versus visual EEG analysis in elderly normal, demented and depressed subjects. Electroencephalogr Clin Neurophysiol 69:110–117, 1988.

Brenner RP, Schaul N: Periodic EEG patterns: Classification, clinical correlation and pathophysiology. J Clin Neurophysiol 7:249–267, 1990.

Brenner RP, Ulrich RF, Spiker DG, et al: Computerized EEG spectral analysis in elderly normal, demented and depressed subjects. Electroencephalogr Clin Neurophysiol 64:483–492, 1986.

Breslau J, Starr A, Sicotte N, et al: Topographic EEG changes with normal aging and SDAT. Electroencephalogr Clin Neurophysiol 72:281–289, 1989.

Bricolo A, Turazzi S, Faccioli F: Combined clinical and EEG examinations for assessment of severity of acute head injuries. Acta Neurosurg 28 (Suppl. 1):35–39, 1979.

Briel RC, McKeith IG, Barker WA, et al: EEG findings in dementia with Lewy bodies and Alzheimer's disease. J Neurol Neurosurg Psychiatry 66:401–403, 1999.

Brown DG, Goldensohn ES: The electroencephalogram in normal pressure hydrocephalus. Arch Neurol 29:70–71, 1973.

Bucht G, Adolfsson R, Winblad B: Dementia of the Alzheimer type and multi-infarct dementia: A clinical description and diagnostic problems. J Am Geriatr Soc 32:491–498, 1984.

Cant BR, Hume AL, Judson JA, et al: The assessment of severe head trauma by short-latency somatosensory and brain stem auditory evoked potentials. Electroencephalogr Clin Neurophysiol 65:188–195, 1986.

Canter NL, Hallett M, Growdon JH: Lecithin does not affect EEG spectral analysis or P300 in Alzheimer's disease. Neurology 32:1260–1266, 1982.

Celesia GG, Grigg MM, Ross E: Generalized status myoclonicus in acute anoxic and toxic-metabolic encephalopathies. Arch Neurol 45:781–784, 1988.

Chen R, Bolton CF, Young B: Prediction of outcome in patients with anoxic coma: A clinical and electrophysiologic study. Crit Care Med 24:672–678, 1996.

Chiofalo N, Fuentes A, Galvez S: Serial EEG findings in 27 cases of Creutzfeldt-Jakob disease. Arch Neurol 37:143–145, 1980.

Coben LA, Danziger W, Berg L: Frequency analysis of the resting awake EEG in mild senile dementia of Alzheimer type. Electroencephalogr Clin Neurophysiol 55:372–380, 1983.

Coben LA, Danziger W, Storandt M: A longitudinal EEG study of mild senile dementia of Alzheimer type: Changes at 1 year and at 2.5 years. Electroencephalogr Clin Neurophysiol 61:101–112, 1985.

Coben LA, Chi D, Snyder AZ, et al: Replication of a study of frequency analysis of the resting awake EEG in mild probable Alzheimer's disease. Electroencephalogr Clin Neurophysiol 75:148–154, 1990.

Cohen RA, O'Donnell BF, Meadows ME, et al: ERP indices and neuropsychological performance as predictors of functional outcome in dementia. J Geriatr Psychiatry Neurology 8:217–225, 1995.

Courjon J, Scherzer E: Traumatic disorders, in Remond A, Magnus O, Courjon J (eds): Handbook of Electroencephalography and Clinical Neurophysiology. Clinical EEG (IV). Amsterdam: Elsevier, 1972, Vol. 14, Part B, pp. 8–104.

Creutzfeldt O, Houchin J: Neuronal basis for EEG waves, in Remond A (ed): Handbook of Eelectroencephalography and Clinical Neurophsyiology Amsterdam: Elsevier, 1974, Vol. 2, Part C, pp. 5–55.

Crystal HA, Dickson DW, Lizardi JE, et al: Antemortem diagnosis of diffuse Lewy body disease. Neurology 40:1523–1528, 1990.

Curry SH: Event-related potentials as indicants of structural and functional damage in closed head injury. Prog Brain Res 54:507–515, 1980.

Cusumano S, Paolin A, Di Paolo F, et al: Assessing brain function in post-traumatic coma by means of bit-mapped SEPs, BAEPs, CT, SPET and clinical scores. Prognostic implications. Electroencephalogr Clin Neurophysiol 84:499–514, 1992.

Daruna JH, Karrer R, Rosen AJ: Introversion, attention and the late positive component of event-related potentials. Biol Psychol 20:249–259, 1985.

De Armond SJ, Prusiner SB: Prion diseases, in Lantos P, Graham D (eds): Greenfield's Neuropathology, ed 6. London: Edward Arnold, 1997, pp. 235–280.

Denker PG, Perry GF: Postconcussion syndrome in compensation and litigation: Analysis of 95 cases with electroencephalographic correlations. Neurology 4:912–918, 1954.

Donchin E, Karis D, Bashore TR, et al: Cognitive psychophysiology and human information processing, in Coles MGH, Donchin E, Porges SW (eds): Psychophysiology: Systems, Processes, and Applications. New York: Guilford Press, 1986, pp. 244–267.

D'onofrio F, Salvia S, Petretta V, et al: Quantified-EEG in normal aging and dementia. Acta Neurol Scand 93:336–345, 1996.

Dow RS, Ulett G, Raaf J: Electroencephalographic studies immediately following head injury. Am J Psychiatry 101:174–183, 1944.

Duffy FH, Albert MS, McAnulty G: Brain electrical activity in patients with presenile and senile dementia of the Alzheimer type. Ann Neurol 16:439–448, 1984.

Dusser A, Navelet Y, Devictor D, et al: Short- and long-term prognostic value of the electroencephalogram in children with severe head injury. Electroencephalogr Clin Neurophysiol 73:85–93, 1989.

Ebert U, Kirch W: Scopolamine model of dementia: Electroencephalogram findings and cognitive performance. Eur J Clin Invest 28:944–949, 1998.

Emmerson R, Dustman R, Shearer D, et al: P3 latency and symbol digit performance correlations in aging. Exp Aging Res 15:151–159, 1990.

Epstein CM: Computerized EEG in the courtroom. Neurology 44:1566–1569, 1994.

Erkinjuntti T, Larsen T, Sulkava R, et al: EEG in the differential diagnosis between Alzheimer's disease and vascular dementia. Acta Neurol Scand 77:36–43, 1988.

Evers S, Grotemeyer KH, Reichelt D, et al: Impact of antiretroviral treatment on AIDS dementia: A longitudinal prospective event-related potential study. J AIDS 17:143–148, 1988.

Fabiani M, Karis D, Donchin E: Effects of mnemonic strategy manipulation in a Von Restorff paradigm. Electroencephalogr Clin Neurophysiol 75:22–35, 1990.

Firsching R, Frowein RA: Multimodality evoked potentials and early prognosis in comatose patients. Neurosurg Rev 13:141–146, 1990.

Ford JM, Roth WT, Isaaks BG, et al: Automatic and effortful processing in aging and dementia: Event-related brain potentials. Neurobiol Aging 18:169–180, 1997.

Fowler CJ, Harrison MJG: EEG changes in subcortical dementia: A study of 22 patients with Steel-Richardson-Olszewski (SRO) syndrome. Electroencephalogr Clin Neurophysiol 64:301–303, 1986.

Fowler B, Prlic H: A comparison of visual and auditory reaction time and P300 latency thresholds to acute hypoxia. Aviat Space Environ Med 66:645–650, 1995.

Freeman MJ: Mass Action in the Nervous System. New York: Academic Press, 1975.

Gabuzda DH, Hirsh MS: Neurological manifestations of infection with human immunodeficiency virus. Ann Intern Med 107:383–391, 1987.

Geisler MW, Polich J: P300 and time-of-the day: Circadian rhythms, food intake, and body temperature. Biol Psychol 31:1–20, 1990.

Geisler MW, Polich J: P300, food and morning/evening activity cycle preference. Psychophysiology 29:86–94, 1992.

Gennarelli TA, Thibault LH, Adams JH, et al: Diffuse axonal injury and traumatic coma in the primate. Ann Neurol 12:564–574, 1982.

Goodin DS, Aminoff MJ: Electrophysiological differences between subtypes of dementia. Brain 109:1103–1113, 1986.

Goodin DS, Aminoff MJ, Chernoff DN, et al: Long latency event-related potentials in patients infected with human immunodeficiency virus. Ann Neurol 27:414–419, 1990.

Goodin DS, Squires KC, Starr A: Long latency event-related components of the auditory evoked potential in dementia. Brain 101:635–648, 1978.

Granner MA, Lee SI: Nonconvulsive status epilepticus: EEG analysis in a large series. Epilepsia 35:42–47, 1994.

Granovsky Y, Sprecher E, Hemli J, et al: P300 and stress in mild head injuries. Electroencephalogr Clin Neurophysiol 108:554–559, 1998.

Grass AM: The electroencephalographic heritage. Am J EEG Technol 24:133–173, 1984.

Greenberg RP, Newlon PG, Becker DP: The somatosensory evoked potential in patients with severe head injury: Outcome prediction and monitoring of brain function. Ann N Y Acad Sci 388:683–688, 1982.

Guerit JM: The interest of multimodality evoked potentials in the evaluation of chronic coma. Acta Neurol Belg 94:174–182, 1994.

Gupta NK, Verma NP, Guidice MA, et al: Visual evoked response in head trauma: Pattern-shift stimulus. Neurology 36:578–581, 1986.

Gurvitch AM, Ginsberg DA: Types of hypoxic and posthypoxic delta activity in animals and man. Electroencephalogr Clin Neurophysiol 42:297–308, 1977.

Gutling E, Gosner A, Imnof H-S, et al: EEG reactivity in the prognosis of severe head injury. Neurology 45:915–918, 1985.

Haglund Y, Persson HE: Does Swedish amateur boxing lead to chronic brain damage: 3. A retrospective clinical neurophysiology study. Acta Neurol Scand 82:353–360, 1990.

Harner RN: EEG evaluation of the patient with dementia, in Benson FD, Blummer D (eds): Psychiatric Aspects of Neurological Diseases. New York: Grune & Stratton, 1975, pp. 63–82.

Harrison MJ, Newman SP, Hall-Craggs MA, et al: Evidence of CNS impairment in HIV infection: Clinical, neuropsychological, EEG, and MRI/MRS study. J Neurol Neurosurg Psychiatry 65:301–307, 1998.

Helkala EL, Laulumaa V, Soininen H, et al: Different patterns of cognitive decline related to normal or deteriorating EEG in a four year follow-up study with patients of Alzheimer's disease. Neurology 41:528–532, 1991.

Hockaday JM, Potts F, Bonazzi A, et al: Electroencephalographic changes in acute cerebral anoxia from cardiac or respiratory arrest. Electroencephalogr Clin Neurophysiol 18:575–586, 1965.

Hooshmand H, Beckner E, Radfor F: Technical and clinical aspects of topographic brain mapping. Clin Electroencephalogr 20:235–247, 1989.

Hubbard O, Sunde D, Goldensohn ES: The EEG in centenarians. Electroencephalogr Clin Neurophysiol 40:407–417, 1976.

Hutchinson DO, Frith RW, Shaw NA, et al: A comparison between electroencephalography and somatosensory evoked potentials for outcome prediction following severe head injury. Electroencephalogr Clin Neurophysiol 78:228–233, 1991.

Jacome DE, Risko M: EEG features in post-traumatic syndrome. Clin Electroencephalogr 15:214–221, 1984.

Janati A, Archer RL, Osteen PK: Coexistence of ectopic rhythms and periodic EEG patterns in anoxic encephalopathy. Clin Electroencephalogr 17:187–194, 1986.

Jerrett SA, Corsak J: Clinical utility of topographic EEG brain mapping. Clin Electroencephalogr 19:134–143, 1988.

Jordan SE, Nowacki R, Nuwer M: Computerized electroencephalography in the evaluation of early dementia. Brain Topogr 1:271–282, 1989.

Jorgensen EO, Malchow-Moller A: Natural history of global and critical brain ischemia. Resuscitation 9:133–188, 1981.

Kane NM, Moss TH, Curry SH, et al: Quantitative electroencephalographic evaluation of non-fatal and fatal traumatic coma. Electroencephalogr Clin Neurophysiol 106:244–250, 1998.

Karnaze DS, Marshall LF, Bickford RG: EEG monitoring of clinical coma: The compressed spectral array. Neurology 32:289–292, 1982.

Kazis A, Karlovasitou A, Xafenias D: Temporal slow activity of the EEG in old age. Arch Psychiatr Nervenkr 231:547–554, 1982.

Knight RT: Decreased response to the novel stimuli after prefrontal lesions in man. Electroencephalogr Clin Neurophysiol 59:9–20, 1984.

Koralnik IJ, Beaumanor A, Hausler R, et al: A controlled study of early neurologic abnormalities in men with asymptomatic human immunodeficiency virus infection. N Engl J Med 323:864–870, 1990.

Kraiuhin C, Gordon D, Meares R, et al: Psychometrics and event-related potentials in the diagnosis of dementia. J Gerontol 41:154–162, 1986.

Lee RG, Blair RDG: Evolution of EEG and visual evoked response changes in Creutzfeldt-Jacob disease. Electroencephalogr Clin Neurophysiol 35:133–142, 1973.

Leuchter AF, Walter DO: Diagnosis and assessment of dementia using functional brain imaging. Int Psychogeriatr 1:63–71, 1989.

Leuchter AF, Spar JE, Walter DO, et al: Electroencephalographic spectra and coherence in the diagnosis of Alzheimer's type and multi-infarct dementia. Arch Gen Psychiatry 44:993–998, 1987.

Levy SR, Chiappa KH, Burke CJ, et al: Early evolution and incidence of electroencephalographic abnormalities in Creutzfeldt-Jakob disease. J Clin Neurophysiol 3:1–21, 1986.

Lopez OL, Becker JT, Brenner RP, et al: Alzheimer's disease with delusions and hallucinations: Neuropsychological and electroencephalographic correlates. Neurology 41:906–912, 1991.

Low MD: Event-related potentials and the electroencephalogram in patients with proven brain lesions, in Desmedt JE (ed): Progress in Clinical Neurophysiology: Cognitive Components in Cerebral Event Related Potentials and Selective Attention. Basel: Karger, 1979, Vol. 6, pp. 258–264.

Macdonell RA, Donnan GA, Bladin PF, et al: The electroencephalogram and acute ischemic stroke: Distinguishing cortical from lacunar infarction. Arch Neurol 45:520–524, 1988.

Magliero A, Bashore T, Coles MGH, et al: On the dependence of P300 latency on stimulus evaluation processes. Psychophysiology 21:171–186, 1984.

Malone M, Prior P, Scholtz CL: Brain damage after cardiopulmonary by-pass: Correlations between neurophysiological and neuropathological findings. J Neurol Neurosurg Psychiatry 44:924–931, 1981.

Markland ON: Organic brain syndromes and dementias, in Daley DD, Pedley TA (eds): Current Practice of Clinical Electroencephalography, ed 2. New York: Raven Press, 1990, pp. 401–423.

Matsuo F: EEG features of the apallic syndrome resulting from cerebral anoxia. Electroencephalogr Clin Neurophysiol 61:113–122, 1985.

Mecklinger A, von Cramon DY, Matthes-von Cramon G: Event-related potential evidence for a specific recognition memory deficit in adult survivors of cerebral hypoxia. Brain 121:1919–1935, 1988.

Miyauchi T, Hagimoto H, Ishii M, et al: Quantitative EEG in patients with presenile and senile dementia of the Alzheimer's type. Acta Neurol Scand 89:56–64, 1994.

Moulton RJ, Brown JI, Konasiewicz SJ: Monitoring severe head injury: A comparison of EEG and somatosensory evoked potentials. Can J Neurol Sci 25:S7–11, 1998.

Neshige R, Barrett G, Shibasaki H: Auditory long latency event-related potentials in Alzheimer's disease and multi-infarct dementia. J Neurol Neurosurg Psychiatry 51:1120–1125, 1988.

Newlon PG, Greenberg RP, Hyatt MS, et al: The dynamics of neuronal dysfunction and recovery following severe head injury assessed with serial multimodality evoked potentials. J Neurosurg 57:168–177, 1982.

Niedermeyer E: Historical aspects, in Niedermeyer E, Da Silva FL (eds): Electroencephalography: Basic Principals, Clinical Applications, and Related Fields, ed 3. Baltimore, MD: Williams & Wilkins, 1993, pp. 1–14.

Nuwer MR: The development of EEG brain mapping. J Clin Neurophysiol 7:459–471, 1990.

Nuwer MR, Miller RN, Visscher, BR, et al: Asymptomatic HIV does not cause EEG abnormalities: Results from the Multicenter AIDS Cohort Study (MACS). Neurology 42:1214–1219, 1992.

Obrist WD: Problems of aging, in Remond A (ed): Handbook of Electroencephalography and Clinical Neurophysiology. Amsterdam, NL: Elsevier, 1976, pp. 275–292.

Oishi M, Mochizuki Y: Correlation between contingent negative variation and regional cerebral blood flow. Clin Electroencephalogr 29:124–127, 1998.

Oken BS: Endogenous event-related potentials, in Chiappa KH (ed): Evoked Potentials in Clinical Medicine, ed 3. New York: Raven Press, 1997, pp. 539–563.

Okuda B, Tachibana H, Kawabata K, et al: Visual evoked potentials (VEPs) in Parkinson's disease: Correlation of pattern VEPs abnormality with dementia. Alzheimer Dis Assoc Disord 9:68–72, 1995.

Olbrich HM, Nau HE, Lodemann E, et al: Evoked potential assessment of mental function during recovery from severe head injury. Surg Neurol 26:112–118, 1986.

Onofri M, Curatola L, Malatesta P, et al: Reduction of P3 latency during outcome from post-traumatic amnesia. Acta Neurol Scand 83:273–279, 1991.

Papanicolaou AC, Levin HS, Eisenberg HM, et al: Evoked potential correlates of post-traumatic amnesia after closed head injury. Neurosurgery 14:676–678, 1984.

Parisi A, DiPerri G, Stosselli M, et al: Usefulness of computerized electroencephalography in diagnosing, staging and monitoring AIDS-dementia complex. AIDS 3:209–223, 1989.

Pedley TA, Miller JA: Clinical neurophysiology of aging and dementia, in Mayeux R, Rosen WG (eds): Advances in Neurology: The Dementias. New York: Raven Press, 1983, pp. 31–49.

Picton TW, Stuss DT, Champagne SC, et al: The effects of age on human event-related potentials. Psychophysiology 21:312–324, 1984.

Pierelli F, Garrubba C, Tilia G, et al: Multimodality evoked potentials in HIV-1 seropositive patients: Relationship between the immune impairment and the neurophysiological function. Acta Neurol Scand 93:266–271, 1996.

Polich J, Ehlers CL, Otis S, et al: P300 latency reflects the degree of cognitive decline in dementing illness. Electroencephalogr Clin Neurophysiol 63:138–144, 1986.

Polich J, Geisler MW: P300 seasonal variation. Biol Psychol 32:173–179, 1991.

Polich J, Ladish C, Bloom FE: P300 assessment of early Alzheimer's disease. Electroencephalogr Clin Neurophysiol 77:179–189, 1990.

Poser S, Mollenhauer B, Kraubeta A, et al: How to improve the clinical diagnosis of Creutzfeldt-Jakob disease. Brain 122:2345–2351, 1999.

Rae-Grant A, Blume W, Lau C, et al: The electroencephalogram in Alzheimer-type dementia: A sequential study correlating the electroencephalogram with psychometric and quantitative pathologic data. Arch Neurol 44:50–54, 1987.

Rae-Grant AD, Barbour PJ, Reed J: Development of a novel EEG rating scale for head injury using dichotomous variables. Electroencephalogr Clin Neurophysiol 79:349–357, 1991.

Rappaport M, Hall K, Hopkins K, et al: Evoked brain potentials and disability in brain-damaged patients. Arch Phys Med Rehabil 58:333–338, 1977.

Rappaport M, McCandless KL, Pond W, et al: Passive P300 response in traumatic brain injury patients. J Neuropsychiatry Clin Neurosci 3:180–185, 1991.

Reisberg B, Ferris SH, De Leon MJ: Global deterioration scale for age-associated cognitive decline and Alzheimer's disease. Am J Psychiatry 139:1136–1139, 1982.

Rice DM, Buchsbaum MS, Starr A, et al: Abnormal EEG slow activity in left temporal areas in senile dementia of the Alzheimer type. J Gerontol A Biol Sci Med Sci 45:M145–151, 1990.

Rothstein TL, Thomas EM, Sumi SM: Predicting outcome in hypoxic-ischemic coma. A prospective clinical and electrophysiologic study. Electroencephalogr Clin Neurophysiol 79:101–107, 1991.

Rumpl E, Lorenzi E, Hackl JM, et al: The EEG at different stages of acute secondary traumatic midbrain and bulbar brain syndromes. Electroencephalogr Clin Neurophysiol 46:487–497, 1979.

Rumpl E, Prugger M, Bauer G, et al: Incidence and prognostic value of spindles in post-traumatic coma. Electroencephalogr Clin Neurophysiol 56:420–429, 1983.

Sannita WG, Maggi L, Rosadini G: Effects of scopolamine (0.25-0.75 mg im.) on the quantitative EEG and the neuropsychological status of healthy volunteers. Neuropsychobiology 17:199–205, 1987.

Schroeder MM, Handelsman L, Torres L, et al: Early and late cognitive event-related potentials mark stages of HIV-1 infection in the drug-user risk group. Biol Psychiatry 35:54–69, 1994.

Shaw GM, Harper ME, Hann BH, et al: HTLV-III infection in brains of children and adults with AIDS encephalopathy. Science 227:177–181, 1985.

Shin DY, Ehrenberg B, Whyte J, et al: Evoked potential assessment: Utility in prognosis of chronic head injury. Arch Phys Med Rehabil 70:189–193, 1989.

Simard M, van Reekum R, Cohen T: A review of the cognitive and behavioral symptoms in dementia with Lewy bodies. J Neuropsychiatry Clin Neurosci 12:425–450, 2000.

Sloan EP, Fenton GW, Kennedy NS, et al: Electroencephalography and single photon emission computed tomography in dementia: A comparative study. Psychol Med 25:631–638, 1995.

Smith ME, Halgren E, Sokolik M, et al: The intracranial topography of the P3 event-related potential elicited during auditory oddball. Electroencephalogr Clin Neurophysiol 76:235–248, 1990.

Smith SJM, Kocen RS: A Creutzfeldt-Jakob like syndrome due to lithium toxicity. J Neurol Neurosurg Psychiatry 51:120–123, 1988.

Soikkeli R, Partanen J, Soininen H, et al: Slowing of EEG in Parkinson's disease. Electroencephalogr Clin Neurophysiol 79:159–165, 1991.

Speckmann E-J, Caspers H, Elger CE: Neuronal mechanisms underlying the generation of field potentials, in Elbert T, Rockstroh B, Lutzenberger W, et al (eds): Self-regulation of the Brain and Behavior. New York: Springer, 1984, pp. 9–25.

Sperfeld AD, Collatz MB, Baier H, et al: FTDP-17: An early-onset phenotype with parkinsonism and epileptic seizures caused by a novel mutation. Ann Neurol 46:708–715, 1999.

Squires KC, Chippendale TJ, Wrege KS, et al: Electrophysiological assessment of mental function in aging and dementia, in Poon LW (ed): Aging in the 1980's: Selected Contemporary Issues in the Psychology of Aging. Washington, DC: American Psychological Association, 1980, pp. 125–134.

Stevens A, Kircher T: Cognitive decline unlike normal aging is associated with alterations of EEG temporo-spatial characteristics. Eur Arch Psychiatry Clin Neurosci 248:259–266, 1998.

Stigsby B, Johannesson G, Ingvar DH: Regional EEG analysis and regional cerebral blood flow in Alzheimer's and Pick's diseases. Electroencephalogr Clin Neurophysiol 51:537–547, 1981.

Stockard JJ, Bickford RG, Aung MH: The electroencephalogram in traumatic brain injury, in Vinken PJ, Bruyn GW (eds): Handbook of Neurology: Injuries of the Brain and Skull. Amsterdam, NL: North-Holland, 1975, Vol. 23, Part 1, pp. 317–367.

Striade M, Deschenes M: Intrathalamic and brainstem-thalamic networks involved in resting and alert states, in Bentivoglio M, Spreafico R (eds): Cellular Thalamic Mechanisms. Amsterdam, NL: Elsevier, 1988, pp. 37–62.

Strnad P, Strnadova V: Long-term follow-up EEG studies in patients with traumatic apallic syndrome. Eur Neurol 26:84–89, 1987.

Sulg IA, Dencker SJ: Electroencephalographic findings in MZ twin pairs, discordant for closed head injury. Acta Genet Med Gemellol 17:389–401, 1968.

Synek VM: Value of a revised EEG coma scale for prognosis after cerebral anoxia and diffuse head injury. Clin Electroencephalogr 21:25–30, 1990.

Szelies B, Mielke R, Kessler J, et al: EEG power changes are related to regional cerebral glucose metabolism in vascular dementia. Clin Neurophysiol 110:615–620, 1999.

Tebano MT, Cameroni M, Gallozzi G, et al: EEG spectral analysis after minor head injury in man. Electroencephalogr Clin Neurophysiol 70:185–189, 1988.

Thatcher RW, Biver C, McAlaster R, et al: Biophysical linkage between MRI and EEG amplitude in closed head injury. Neuroimage 7:352–367, 1998.

Thatcher RW, Walker RA, Gerson I, et al: EEG discriminant analysis of mild head trauma. Electroencephalogr Clin Neurophysiol 73:94–106, 1989.

Torres F, Faoro A, Loewenson R, et al: The electroencephalogram of elderly subjects revisited. Electroencphalogr Clin Neurophysiol 56:391–398, 1983.

Torres F, Shapiro SK: Electroencephalograms in whiplash injury. Arch Neurol 5:28–35, 1961.

Tyner FS, Knott JR, Mayer WB: Artifacts, in Fundamentals of EEG Technology: Basic Concepts and Methods. Philadelphia: Lippincott Williams & Wilkins, 1983, Vol. 1, pp. 280–311.

Walker MP, Ayre GA, Cummings JL, et al: Quantifying fluctuation in dementia with Lewy bodies, Alzheimer's disease, and vascular dementia. Neurology 54:1616–1625, 2000.

Walter WG: The location of brain tumors by electroencephalogram. Proc R Soc Med 30:579–598, 1936.

Wang HS, Busse EW: EEG of healthy old persons—a longitudinal study: I. Dominant background activity and occipital rhythm. J Gerontol 24:419–426, 1969.

Watson MR, Fenton GW, McClelland RJ, et al: The post-concussional state: Neurophysiological aspects. Br J Psychiatry 167:514–521, 1995.

Werner RA, Vanderzant CW: Multimodality evoked potentials testing in acute mild closed head injury. Arch Phys Med Rehabil 72:31–34, 1991.

Williams GW, Luders HO, Brickner A, et al: Interobserver variability in EEG interpretation. Neurology 35:1714–1719, 1985.

Yamada T, Kayamori R, Kimura J, et al: Topography of somatosensory evoked potentials after stimulation of the median nerve. Electroencephalogr Clin Neurophysiol 59:29–43, 1984.

Yener GG, Leuchter AF, Jenden D, et al: Quantitative EEG in frontotemporal dementia. Clin Electroencephalogr 27:61–68, 1996.

Yokoyama Y, Nakashima K, Shimoyama R, et al: Distribution of event-related potentials in patients with dementia. Electromyogr Clin Neurophysiol 35:431–437, 1995.

Yoshii N, Matsumoto K, Oshida K, et al: Clinico-electroencephalographic study of 3200 head injury cases: A comparative work between aged adults and children. Keio J Med 19:31–46, 1970.

Zandbergen EG, de Haan RJ, Stoutenbeck CP, et al: Systematic review of early prediction of poor outcome in anoxic-ischemic coma. Lancet 352:1808–1812, 1998.

CHAPTER 9

Safe and Unsafe Driving

Matthew Rizzo

Aging

Alzheimer disease (AD)

Attention

Car crash

Heinrich's Triangle

Instrumented vehicle

Neuroergonomics

Road Rage

Simulator adaptation syndrome

Stroke

Useful field of view (UFOV)

Working memory

INTRODUCTION

Automobile driving is a crucial aspect of everyday life, yet vehicular crashes represent a serious public health problem. Vehicular crashes are an ancient problem. During the Pax Romana, the Mediterranean was safe to travel and voyagers jockeyed for position on crowded roads (Perrottet, 2002). There was no consensus on left- or right-lane driving, conical stones were positioned to keep chariots from careening onto the sidewalk, mule drivers raced the roads, and crashes were a source of incessant litigation. The advent of automobiles has amplified this ancient problem.

The automobile claimed its first U.S. fatality, Mr. Henry H. Bliss, a deaf sexagenarian widower whose skull was crushed on September 13, 1899, by the tires of a car that ran over him as he and a lady alighted from a streetcar at 74th Street and Central Park West (Fig. 9-1). Mr. Bliss died the next day, and about 30 million people worldwide have perished in car crashes since. There are about 6.2 million reported crashes in the United States each year that regularly claim about 40,000 lives and cause millions more injuries at a cost of about $150 billion dollars (NHTSA, 2001). Millions more crashes and even greater numbers of driver error safety are not reported.

Drivers with neurobehavioral disorders are at risk for a crash resulting from cognitive impairment. Some are unaware of their impairment and are liable to keep driving despite being at greater risk. This review addresses cognitive errors in the driving task in patients with neurobehavioral impairments and potential tools for discriminating between safe and unsafe drivers,

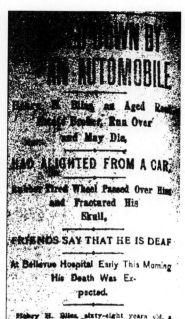

A

AUTOMOBILE VICTIM DEAD.

M. H. Bliss Mortally Injured by a Horseless Cab.

H. H. Bliss, a real-estate dealer, of No. 235 West Seventy-fifth Street, who was injured by an automobile last night at Seventy-fourth Street and Central Park West, died at 6:45 o'clock this morning in Roosevelt Hospital as a result of his injuries.

Mr. Bliss and a woman were alighting from a south-bound Eighth Avenue electric-car, when Mr. Bliss was knocked down by an automobile, operated by Arthur Smith of No. 151 West Sixty-second Street. His skull and chest were crushed, two wheels passing over him.

Dr. David Orr Edson of No. 38 West Seventy-fifth Street was the occupant of the cab. He rendered what aid he could until the injured man was taken to Roosevelt Hospital. Smith was locked up in the West Sixty-eighth Street police station.

Later Smith was arraigned in the West Side Court on a charge of homicide. Magistrate Flammer held him without bail until the afternoon session, to enable the police to get the witnesses of the accident to court.

Mr. Bliss was born sixty-one years ago in Maine, and has for many years had a real-estate office at No. 41 Wall Street. A daughter and a son survive him, Miss Florence Bliss and Collins P. Bliss, a professor in

B

FIGURE 9-1. Reproduction of *New York Herald* (A) and *New York Evening Post* (B) accounts of the first fatal car crash.

including neuropsychological tests, driving simulators, and instrumented vehicles. It also points to the conclusion that studying normal and cognitively impaired operators in controlled circumstances, as in a driving simulator, and in field studies using instrumented vehicles, can uncover rich information about coordinated activities of neural systems (such as attentional, visuo-motor, and decision making) in complex real-world activities that cannot be measured in any other way.

Note that we avoid the use of the term "accident" throughout because many crashes could be avoided through scientifically targeted interventions aimed at better roadway and vehicle design, including safety devices, and improved driver screening and training.

CONCEPTUAL FRAMEWORK

Safe driving requires the coordination of several ongoing cognitive processes, including attention, perception, memory (declarative, procedural, and working memory), and executive functions (decision making and implementation) (Rizzo & Dingus, 1996). These processes are impaired, increasing the risk of driver error and a motor vehicle crash, in different populations of drivers with neurologic or psychiatric diagnoses (Nouri et al., 1987; Van Zomeren et al., 1987; Reuben et al., 1988; Galski et al., 1990, 1992; Korteling, 1990; Madeley et al., 1990; Ball & Owsley, 1991; Kumar et al., 1991; Dubinsky et al., 1991, 1992; Waller, 1991; Lings & Dupont, 1992; Underwood, 1992; Guerrier et al., 1995) (Tables 9-1 and 9-2).

Empirically derived models and theories of traffic psychology provide frameworks for organizing and interpreting data on driver error (Wilde, 1982; Grayson, 1997; Huguenin, 1997). Relationships between driver performance factors and safety errors can be represented by an imaginary triangle (Fig. 9-2) (Heinrich et al., 1980) or "iceberg" (Maycock, 1997). Visible safety errors (above the "water line") include car crashes resulting in fatality, serious injury, mild injury, or, most commonly, property damage only. Crash events are relatively infrequent and tend to follow a Poisson distribution (e.g., Siskind, 1996; Thomas, 1996). Submerged (below the "water line") are several behavioral variables that are theoretically related to crashes and occur more frequently. As the frequency of events increases, the relevance to serious driver safety errors and crashes decreases.

Figure 9-3 depicts a simple information-processing model for understanding driver error. The driver:

1. Perceives and attends to stimulus evidence (e.g., through vision, audition, vestibular and proprioceptive inputs) and interprets the situation on the road.
2. Formulates a plan based on the particular driving situation and relevant previous experience or memory.
3. Executes an action (e.g., by applying the accelerator, brake, or steering controls). The

TABLE 9-1. Neurologic Conditions and Cognitive-Behavioral Impairments That May Pose Increased Driving Risk

Conditions/impairments	Driving-related cognitive and behavioral problems
Amnesia	Failure to remember the rules of the road, vehicle operations, or the location of nearby vehicles
Aphasia	Trouble deciphering road maps or signs
"Executive dysfunction"	Strategic and tactical errors, e.g., driving in bad weather or in an unsafe vehicle; failure to formulate and implement plans for evasive maneuvers in emergency situations
Visual field loss, i.e., hemianopia	Failure to detect objects in one visual field
Hemineglect syndrome: UFOV constriction; tunnel vision	Failure to orient to objects on one side, often accompanied by other visuospatial disorders
Sleep and arousal disorders and fatigue	Falling asleep at the wheel
Topographic disorientation	Getting lost
Epilepsy	Loss of contact or consciousness
Transient ischemic attacks	Loss of control, contact, or consciousness during an attack
Visuospatial disorders	Failure to perceive the location, speed and direction of one's own vehicle, the structure of the roadway, the changing distance from other road objects, and the time to collision
Motor dysfunction: weakness; incoordination; bradykinesia; ataxia	Inability to operate the steering, accelerator pedal, brake pedal, or other controls
Loss of limb sensation, e.g., due to neuropathy, spinal cord or cerebral lesion, etc.	Inability to operate the steering, accelerator pedal, brake pedal, or other controls

TABLE 9-2. Medical Factors that May Pose Increased Road Risk

Condition	Problem/s
Cardiac disease	Syncope; distraction by cardiac sensations
Cervical arthritis	Trouble checking the mirrors; distraction by pain
Deafness	Lack of response to hazard cues in the auditory panorama
Medications, alcohol, illegal drugs, metabolic disease	Sedation; psychosis on the road
Psychiatric disease	Hostile or paranoid driving; response to hallucinations or delusions; suicidal intent
Syncope	Loss of vehicular control
Vestibular disease	Vertigo on the road
Visual dysfunction	Failure to resolve roadway objects or signs; failure to cope with glare or low ambient light conditions

driver's behavioral response is either safe or unsafe as a result of errors at one or more stages in the driving task. The outcome of the behavior provides a source of potential feedback for the driver to take subsequent action.

The risk of human errors in complex systems, such as a driver operating a motor vehicle, increases with deficits of attention, perception, response selection (which depends on memory and decision making) and response implementation (a.k.a., executive functions). Psychomotor factors and general mobility are also relevant (e.g., Marottoli et al., 1994). Individuals with deficits in these abilities are more likely than normal drivers to commit errors that cause motor vehicle crashes. Some errors can be detected because drivers normally monitor their performance (Wickens, 1992). When feedback on driving fails to match expectations based on correctly formulated intentions, the discrepancy is often detected "on line." Drivers with cognitive impairment are less likely to realize their errors. In short, cognitive abilities and impairments determine specific driver behaviors and safety errors, which in turn predict crashes.

PERCEPTION

Automobile driving is a highly visual task (e.g., Hills, 1980). Crashes and traffic violations (3-year records) in 17,500 California driver's license applicants increased with impairments of static visual acuity, dynamic visual acuity (i.e., acuity for moving letter shapes), glare recovery, and visual fields (Burg, 1968). The binocular visual fields normally span more than 180 degrees. The need to search for critical information in the areas of impaired vision may create an extra cognitive load, tantamount to the burden of multitasking. The many possible patterns of visual field loss correspond to different lesions in visual pathways and create different risks for drivers. Macular degeneration affects areas of high detail vision around fixation. The fovea has the highest acuity and spans about 3 degrees around fixation; the macula spans about 10 degrees and participates in detail-oriented tasks such as map reading. The peripheral visual fields have low visual acuity, but good temporal resolution and movement detection. Retinitis

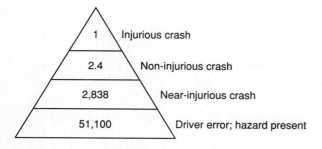

FIGURE 9-2. Heinrich's Triangle. Each injurious crash is theoretically related to many more non-injurious events. Mock counts are shown.

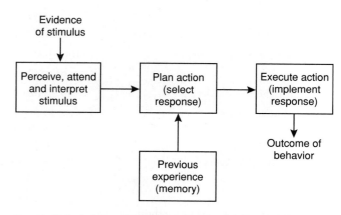

FIGURE 9-3. Information-processing model for understanding driver error.

pigmentosa produces marked constriction of the peripheral visual fields, causing drivers to be unable to detect objects approaching from the side.

Drivers with lesions in visual areas of the occipital lobe and adjacent temporal and parietal lobes have various visual field defects (such as homonymous hemianopia or quadrantanopia) and likewise may fail to register critical objects or events on one side of their vehicle (Rizzo & Kellison, 2004). These drivers may also have a variety of visual perceptual impairments, depending on the location of the lesion (see Chapters 10 and 12).

Damage to ventral areas in the occipital lobe and temporal lobe (along a "What" pathway) can cause (1) impairments of object recognition (visual agnosia) affecting interpretation of roadway targets; (2) reading (pure alexia), affecting roadway sign and map reading; and (3) color perception (cerebral achromatopsia), impeding use of color cues in traffic signals and road signs and detection of roadway boundaries and objects defined by hue contrast (Fig. 9-4).

Damage in dorsal structures in the occipital and parietal lobes (in the "Where" pathway) can impair processing of movement cues as in cerebral akinetopsia, and reduce visuospatial processing and attention abilities, as in Balint syndrome (simultanagnosia/spatial disorientation, optic ataxia, and ocular apraxia) and hemineglect syndrome (most often a failure to orient to targets in the left visual hemifields in patients with right parietal lobe lesions).

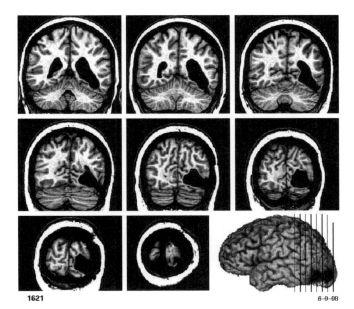

FIGURE 9-4. 3D MRI surface reconstruction of the brain of a patient who had a stroke while driving that resulted in right homonymous hemianopia, achromatopsia, and pure alexia. She could not tell the color of the traffic lights. The defects persisted and she never drove again. (Image courtesy of H. Damasio.)

Patients with cerebral lesions may have various deficits that affect perception of structure and depth that are not measured by standard clinical tests. Information on object structure and depth is so critical for interacting with and moving around objects and obstacles that the brain employs multiple cues (see Rizzo & Vecera, 2002). Motion and attention are thought to be particularly important for safe driving.

Perception of structure-from-motion (SFM) or kinetic depth is a likely real-world use of motion cues that may fail in drivers with cerebral lesions. Models of SFM extract discontinuity boundaries in a field of local motion vectors, with grouping based on common direction or speed (see Chapter 12). To measure SFM, we developed a task in which accurate performance depends on the subject's perception of the figure's shape from moving random dot elements. Varying amounts of random dot noise are added to a background region surrounding the target to prevent shape identification from non-motion cues (such as edges or dot density) and to index the difficulty of the task. The perception of SFM was impaired in early Alzheimer disease (AD) and "motion blindness" (a.k.a., cerebral akinetopsia) (Rizzo et al., 1995; Rizzo & Nawrot, 1998). SFM deficits in drivers with brain lesions are associated with increased relative risk for safety errors and car crashes in high-fidelity driving simulation scenarios (Rizzo et al., 1997b, 2001a).

Motion parallax (like binocular stereopsis) provides unambiguous cue to relative depth. There is an orderly geometric relationship between relative velocities of images across the retina and relative distances of objects in the scene. For motion parallax, relative movement of objects is produced by moving the head along the inter-aural axis. Impairments of motion parallax may be a factor in vehicle crashes in drivers with cerebral impairments, when drivers must make quick judgments with inaccurate or missing perceptual information on the location of surrounding obstacles (Nawrot, 2001).

Displacement of images across the retina during travel produces optic flow patterns (Gibson, 1979). Optic flow can specify the trajectory of self-motion (egomotion) with up to 1 degree of accuracy (Warren & Hannon, 1988; Warren et al., 1991), depending where a driver looks. Perception of heading from optical flow patterns is optimal in a limited part of the flow field surrounding the future direction of travel (Mestre, 2001; Fig. 9-5). On curved roads, drivers will fixate the inside edge of the road where the curve changes direction (Land & Lee, 1994). The findings may be construed in terms of a dynamic useful field of view (cf., the work of Ball et al., 1993, discussed in the following section) and are relevant to detection of collisions, design of roads and positioning of traffic warnings within a driver's dynamic visual environment.

Detecting impending collisions requires information on approaching objects and the driver's vehicle. Objects

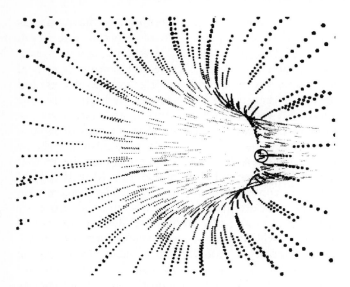

FIGURE 9-5. Perception of heading from optical flow. Drivers tend to fixate the focus of greatest expansion of motion vectors. On a straight road this is a point straight ahead of the driver around the junction between earth and sky. On a curve or in a tunnel, drivers fixate a tangent point where the inner curve changes direction (the small circle) and optical velocity is zero. When driver trajectory is aligned with this point, the driver is on course. (Courtesy of Mestre; Mestre DH: Dynamic evaluation of the useful field of view in driving. Proceedings of the First International Driving Symposium on Human Factors in Driving Assessment, Training, and Vehicle Design. Iowa City, IA: University of Iowa, 2001, p. 237.)

on collision course with the driver will maintain a fixed location in the driver's field of view, whereas "safe" objects will translate to the left or right side. Time to contact (TTC) is estimated from the expanding retinal image of the approaching object. Older drivers are less accurate than younger drivers at detecting an impending collision during braking (Andersen et al., 1999, 2000) and at judging if an approaching object in a driving scene will crash into them (Andersen et al., 2001). Performance is worse for longer TTC conditions, possibly as a result of a greater difficulty in detecting the motion of small objects in the driver's field of view (Andersen et al., 2000).

Visibility of pedestrians is another key traffic safety issue. On August 17, 1896, Bridget Driscoll of Croydon, Surrey, was knocked down by a car as she stepped off the curb, becoming the first pedestrian in the United Kingdom to be killed by a car (antedating the 1899 New York death of Mr. Bliss). About 80,000 pedestrians are struck by cars each year in the United States, and of these about 5000 are killed, especially at night (NHTSA, 2001). Use of reflectors on clothing around the joints (wrists, elbows, knees, ankles) produces biologic motion cues and provides a more effective means of protecting nocturnal pedestrians than a reflective vest or white clothing (Wood et al., 2002).

ATTENTION AND WORKING MEMORY

James (1890) underscored that we remember and act upon attended items, not unattended items. Defects of attention clearly impair driving performance (e.g., Owsley et al., 1991; Parasuraman & Nestor, 1991; Ball et al., 1993; Rizzo et al., 1997b, 2001b). The effects of attention defects on driving are complex, as there are several varieties of attention (Parasuraman, 1984) (e.g., ability to switch, sustain, or divide attention) that draw, theoretically, on "automatic" and "controlled" processes (see Chapter 10). Automatic processes are fast and involuntary and should contribute to subconscious corrections during driving, including reversals of steering wheel or accelerator pedal position during uneventful driving on mundane highway segments. These corrections help maintain the lateral and longitudinal control of the vehicle and ensure that drivers follow the rules of the road despite minimal conscious effort and can be measured in a driving simulator or instrumented vehicle. Defects of automatic control processes in drivers with cerebral lesions may resemble patterns observed in rested individuals under the demands of increased mental workload or divided attention. This includes an overall reduction in the number of steering wheel and accelerator pedal adjustments. When corrections do occur, they must be larger to keep the vehicle tracking within the lane and within legal speed limits. For example, under normal attention circumstances, the amplitude of steering wheel rotations tends to stay between 2 and 6 degrees. However, under attention load, steering wheel rotations of 6 degrees or larger tend to increase (Dingus et al., 1989). This may correlate with increased excursions over the center line or shoulder line of the road. Due to reduced acceleration corrections there may be increased velocity variance and failure to maintain the legal speed. Drivers who find the attention workload to be high may drive substantially below the legal limit.

Controlled attention processes are slow and operate during capacity-demanding tasks and conscious decision making. Examples include glancing between the road and rear-view mirror while maneuvering in and out of a traffic convoy, and the deliberate surveillance of a busy intersection, changing traffic signals, using eye and head movements. This is a "dilemma zone" where critical Go/No-Go decisions must be made (Mahelel et al., 1985. The decision to accelerate or brake depends on driving speed and the time for which green or yellow signals are visible (Allsop et al., 1991).

Owsley and colleagues (1991) and Ball and colleagues (1993) linked driving impairment with reduction in the useful field of view (UFOV), the visual area from which information can be acquired without moving the eyes or head (Ball et al., 1988; 1990; Fig. 9-6). They studied a large number of older drivers to determine what measures of visual perception and cognition correlated best with driving performance.

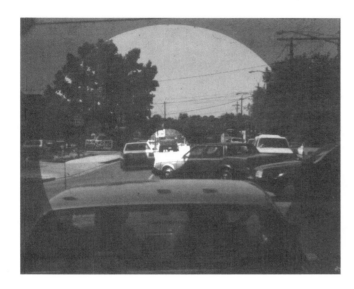

FIGURE 9-6. UFOV loss. Attention impairment (divided and selective attention) and reduced speed of processing may effectively reduce a driver's useful field of view. A driver may perform as if he or she has tunnel vision, yet show no abnormality on standard perimetry—which minimizes effects of attention to gain maximal estimates of sensory function.

Older drivers who had a reduced attentional field as determined on a UFOV task (40% or greater loss), or who had poor scores on the Mattis Organic Mental Status Syndrome Examination (MOMSSE), a shortened version of the Dementia Rating Scale (DRS) (see Chapter 1), had 3–4 times more crashes of any type, and 15 times more intersection crashes than did unaffected drivers. The UFOV task depends on speed of processing, divided attention, and selective attention, and is likely to tap abilities that contribute to the driving task at attentive and preattentive levels. UFOV begins to deteriorate by age 20 and may be construed as shrinking of the field of view or decrease in efficiency with which drivers extract information from a cluttered scene (Sekuler et al., 2000) when the focus of attention is divided between central and peripheral visual tasks. Driving behavior may also change when attention is divided between the road and an onboard task. The number, duration, and location of glances change (Wierwille et al., 1988) and gaps of >2 seconds may interrupt scanning of the road.

Many sources of information compete for driver attention in modern vehicles. Modern cars may include multiple dials, gauges, and displays, including windshield projected "heads-up" information that may distract drivers' focus of attention away from the driving task. Streams of distracting information come from wireless internet, communications devices such as cell phones (hand-held and hands-free), navigation equipment (using global positioning system [GPS] and map display software), "infotainment" devices (including CD/DVD, MP3, and complicated radios), weather gauges, temperature control devices, thermal seats, safety and security devices such as night vision (to extend the view beyond the highbeams), rear-end collision detection devices, and a host of warning signals, including auditory, visual, and haptic devices (e.g., vibrating seats).

Executive functions control our focus of attention (Vecera & Luck, 2002). Focused attention is thought to permit consolidation of information temporarily stored in visual working memory. Without focused attention, we can be unaware of marked changes in an object or a scene, made during a saccade, flicker, blink, or movie cut (change blindness) (Rensink et al., 1997; Simons & Levin, 1997; O'Regan et al., 1999; Rensink et al., 2000), and traces of retinal images in visual working memory will fade without being consciously perceived or remembered ("inattentional amnesia"). The very act of perceiving one item in a rapid series of images briefly inhibits ability to perceive another image, the "attentional blink" (Rizzo et al., 2001a). These perceptual errors depend on interactions between attention and working memory. Perceptual errors are likely if working memory is still occupied by one item when another item arrives, due to interference or to capacity limitations (at a bottleneck stage that admits only one item at a time) (Fig. 9-7).

Driver errors occur when attention is focused away from a critical roadway event in which vehicles, traffic signals, and signs are seen but not acted upon, or are missed altogether (Treat, 1980). Failure to detect roadway events increases when information load is high, as at complex traffic intersections with high traffic and visual clutter (Caird et al., 2001). Sometimes eye gaze is captured by irrelevant distracters (Theeuwes et al., 1999; Kramer et al., 2001), such as "mudsplashes" on a windscreen, that prevent a driver from seeing a critical event (O'Regan et al., 1999) such as an incurring vehicle or a child chasing a ball. Drivers with cerebral visual impairments are liable to be "looking but not seeing" despite low information load (Rizzo et al., 1997b), resembling the effects in neurologically normal operators under conditions of extreme fatigue, such as air-traffic controllers during prolonged intensive monitoring of radar displays or aircraft pilots who are sleep deprived (Russo et al., 1999) (Fig. 9-8).

Safe driving also requires executive control to switch the focus of attention between critical tasks such as tracking the road terrain, monitoring the changing locations of neighboring vehicles, reading signs, maps, traffic signal, and dashboard displays, and checking the mirrors (Owsley et al., 1991). This requires switching attention between disparate spatial locations, local and global object details, different visual tasks, and also between sensory modalities. Drivers must also switch attention between modalities when they drive while conversing with other vehicle occupants, listening to the radio or tapes, using a cell phone, and interacting with

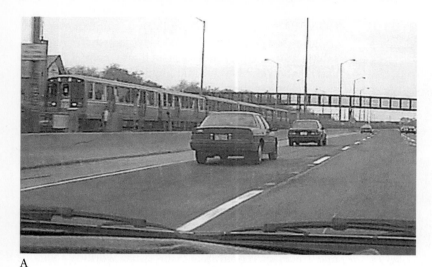

A

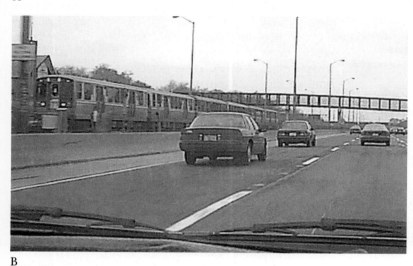

B

FIGURE 9-7. Change blindness. A driver whose focus of attention is distracted by another object or task may fail to appreciate a critical change, such as the unexpected appearance of another vehicle into the lane ahead of the driver. (Courtesy of Dr. Art Kramer.)

in-vehicle devices (Kantowitz, 2000, 2001). The attention abilities can fail in drivers with cerebral lesions (see Chapter 10).

Functional neuroimaging studies suggest that engaging in conversation distracts the brain from processing information in a visually demanding task such as driving, and vice versa (Just et al., 2001). Cell phone conversation disrupts driving performance by diverting attention to an engaging cognitive context other than the one immediately associated with driving (Strayer & Johnston, 2001). A host of other modern infotronic devices also distract cognitive resources away from the driving task (Kantowitz, 2000; Ehret et al., 2000; Stutts et al., 2003). The interference occurs at the level of central attentional processes that can be disrupted by cerebral lesions. Relevant interactions in aging and brain injury can be measured by administering a controlled auditory verbal processing load (such as the Paced Auditory Serial-Addition Task [PASAT]; Gronwall, 1977) during driving tasks (Rizzo et al., 2000c; Boer, 2001; Kantowitz, 2001).

EXECUTIVE FUNCTIONS

Decision-making requires the evaluation of immediate and long-term consequences of planned actions, and is often included with impulse control, insight, judgment, and planning under the rubric of executive functions (e.g., Benton, 1991; Damasio & Anderson, 1993; Tranel et al., 1994; Damasio, 1996, 1999; Rolls, 1999, 2000). Impaired decision-making is a critical factor in driver errors that lead to vehicle crashes (Van Zomeren et al., 1987). Pathologic causes include acquired brain lesions (due to stroke, trauma, or neurodegenerative impairment) affecting prefrontal areas, antisocial personality disorder, and effects of drugs and alcohol (Stuss et al., 1992; Rolls et al., 1994; Bechara et al., 1996; Fuster, 1996). Executive functions strongly interact with working memory (the process of brief storage of information until it is available for use) and attention (operating on contents of working memory) (Baddeley, 1992; Dias et al., 1996; Norman & Shallice, 1996), and are a key determinant of driver strategies and tactics.

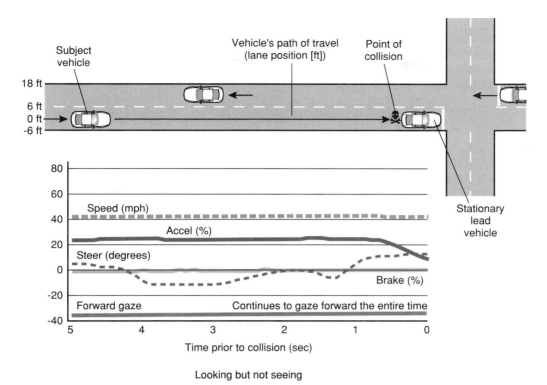

FIGURE 9-8. Looking but not seeing (Rizzo et al., 1997b). Driver behavior is shown moments before a simulated crash. The abscissa shows time in seconds. The ordinate scale shows vehicle speed in mph, percent pedal application for the accelerator and brake, and steering wheel rotations in degrees (upward deflections are counterclockwise rotations). The path (and lane position in feet from the center of the lane) of the driver and other vehicles is depicted to scale at the top of the panel. A subject with AD drives at 40 mph into the back of a stopped vehicle; in the final second he makes small and ineffective brake pedal and steering adjustments that may or may not be in response to the impending crash. Eye gaze was directed forward, suggesting he should have seen the danger ahead. Such a rear-end collision could have killed the elderly driver or other occupants of both cars.

Driver strategies include sequence of trips or stops (for gas, food, directions or naps), evaluation of traffic and weather risks, and making go/no-go decisions whether to take a trip. Tactics include adapting to speed changes near a school, choosing to switch on the headlights at twilight or in rain, changing gears on a hill, and making go/no-go decisions on whether and when to overtake another vehicle, change lanes in traffic, or pass through intersections and traffic signals. Drivers with impaired decision making may also show impairments of impulse control.

Impulse control is related to decision making but it does not require evaluation of immediate and long-term consequences (Barratt, 1994; Evenden, 1999). "Impulsiveness" can be perceptual, cognitive, or motor. Motor impulsiveness may be "nonaffective" as on the Stroop (1935) test, in which subjects must identify the color ink used to print a conflicting color name by inhibiting the compulsion to read the color name. Affective motor impulsiveness occurs when a person cannot inhibit a habit of responding to a stimulus that predicts a reward with affective value (Zuckerman, 1996), for example, a driver impulsively speeding up to prevent another car from merging ahead of the driver. In

perceptual impulsiveness, failure of inhibition occurs at the level of working memory, before a response can be readied and executed. Observers may have more trouble identifying a visual target among distracters if the distracters are familiar. For instance, a driver traveling in a stable convoy of vehicles may follow the convoy through an intersection without noticing that the signal has turned red. Cognitive impulsiveness reflects inability to evaluate the outcome of a planned action and may give the appearance of failure to perceive or evaluate risk. For example, a driver may embark on a long road trip despite poor weather conditions or an unsound vehicle.

Perceptual impulsiveness resembles "lapses" in the Reason (1984) taxonomy of error. Lapses represent failure to carry out an action rather than commission of an incorrect action. Lapses may be caused by interruption of an ongoing sequence by another task and give the appearance of forgetfulness. For example, a driver returning home from work may begin talking on a cell phone and miss ("forget") to take a highway exit. A driver approaching a tollbooth may be distracted by an on-board warning light, fail to decelerate, and strike a slower lead car. Response inhibition failures in executive dysfunction may contribute to "slips," errors in which an intention is incorrectly executed because the intended action sequence departs slightly from routine, resembles an inappropriate but more frequent action, or is relatively automated (Norman, 1981). The "reins of action" or perception are captured by a contextually appropriate strong habit due to lack of close monitoring by attention. A driver whose destination requires deviation from a familiar route may make a wrong turn toward a more habitual destination.

Drivers with executive dysfunction may commit rule-based errors when they believe they understand a situation and formulate a plan by "if-then" rules, but the "if" conditions are not met, a "bad" rule is applied, or the "then" part of the rule is poorly chosen. For instance, a driver may dismiss an engine temperature warning light, fail to service the vehicle, and suffer a vehicle breakdown in traffic.

Decision-making impairment can occur independently of memory impairment, yet memory impairment tends to compromise a driver's decision making because the driver cannot learn or recall all the situational contingencies required to make optimal decisions (Skaar et al., 2003a). Knowledge-based errors signify inappropriate decision making and planning due to failure to comprehend. In this case a driver may be overwhelmed by the complexity of a traffic situation and lack information to interpret it correctly. It may be difficult to unambiguously classify real-world data on driver performance into the above theoretic categories. This difficulty has motivated development of pragmatic, data-driven taxonomies to classify driver behavior (see the section on instrumented vehicles).

Awareness

Further, drivers with impaired decision making may be unaware of their incapacity. Lack of awareness of acquired impairments, known as anosognosia, may exacerbate the functional consequences of impairments in other aspects of cognition (Anderson & Tranel, 1989). Drivers with anosognosia have impaired awareness of their compromised cognitive condition and are liable to place themselves in harm's way while driving because they fail to take steps that might compensate for their impairments, as a result of acquired brain damage (especially in prefrontal areas), as well as with alcohol and drug intoxication, fatigue, and sleep deprivation.

MEMORY AND LANGUAGE

Disordered memory is a common sequela of many diseases including stroke, AD, traumatic brain injury, herpes simplex encephalitis, HIV dementia, and chronic alcoholism, and has several potentially undesirable effects on the driving task. Affected persons may forget the rules of the road, the location of the controls, or the location of vehicles surrounding their own; they may forget to fasten

their seat belts, check the mirrors and gauges, and fuel or service the car, as well as where they are going. Patients with "topographic disorientation" have trouble finding their way as a result of impaired visuospatial perception or visual agnosia, a condition in which visual objects are "stripped" of their meaning. Previously known routes and driving patterns may become unfamiliar. These drivers may fail to recognize important landmarks and may misinterpret previously familiar road signs or symbols (Uc et al., 2003). Aphasics or alexics (see Chapters 12 and 17) may experience similar difficulties interpreting information from glimpses of maps or roadway signs. These individuals are at high risk of getting lost. As a result of memory impairments, cognitive resources may also be diverted from critical driving tasks. For example, heightened anxiety in drivers due to uncertainty of location, extended searching for landmarks, or attempts to read maps or signs can divert key resources.

In a different vein, a morphometric study of London taxi drivers suggested the gray matter volume in the posterior hippocampus is greater than that of age-matched controls, and the amount of increase correlates with time spent taxi driving (Maguire et al., 2000). Whether this anatomophysiologic link between brain morphology and the overlearned real-world task of driving is replicable remains to be seen.

AROUSAL, ALERTNESS, AND FATIGUE

Ongoing cognitive processes, including attention, perception, memory, and executive functions that are critical to the driving task are critically affected by drugs and fatigue (See Chapter 31). A significant proportion of motor vehicle crashes are caused by sleepy drivers (Leger, 1994; Horne & Reyner, 1995, 1996 Laube et al., 1998; Lyznicki et al., 1998). Neurologically normal, high-performing young adult aircraft pilots may perform as if they have visual constriction or simultanagnosia, as in Balint syndrome (Russo et al., 1999; Throne et al., 1999).

At particular risk for a crash are drivers with sleep disorders such as obstructive sleep apnea syndrome (OSAS), which affects 4% to 5% of the general population (Young et al., 1993). Drivers with severe OSAS may have as much as a 15-fold increase in the risk of motor vehicle crashes compared with the general population (George & Smiley, 1999; Horstmann et al., 2000). Some patients with OSAS minimize the degree to which they are sleepy, as in classical descriptions of the syndrome (Dement et al., 1978). Engleman and colleagues (1997) found that 62% of the OSAS patients they studied minimized the degree of sleepiness before treatment with continuous positive airway pressure (CPAP) and that 25% of those still driving acknowledged only later that they had had trouble driving. Some drivers in sleep-related crashes deny having felt tired beforehand (Jones et al., 1979), and sleep-deprived truck drivers often underestimate their fatigue (Arnold et al., 1997). Symptom minimization may be intentional or a result of unawareness of sleepiness (Stutts et al., 1999), possibly caused by an altered frame of reference for fatigue. Also, the border between wakefulness and sleep is indistinct.

Gastaut and Broughton (1965) found that 2 to 4 minutes of electroencephalogram (EEG)-defined sleep must elapse before more than 50% of subjects recognize that they had actually been sleeping. Rather than a discrete occurrence, sleep onset can be conceived of as an evolving process characterized by steadily decreasing arousal, lengthening response time, and intermittent response failure (Ogilvie et al., 1989). The EEG may show progression from wakefulness to stages I and II sleep, or be preceded by "microsleeps" in which the EEG shows 5 or more seconds of alpha drop-out and an increase in theta activity (Harrison & Horne, 1996). These periods of approaching sleep onset have been correlated with subjective sleepiness among long-haul truck drivers (Kecklund & Akerstedt, 1993) and healthy, sleep-deprived drivers (Horne & Reyner, 1996; Reyner & Horne, 1998), and with deteriorating driving simulator performance in healthy, sleep-deprived drivers (Horne & Reyner, 1996; Reyner & Horne, 1998) and OSAS patients (Risser et al., 2000).

Drivers with OSAS have cognitive dysfunction due to acute and chronic sleep deprivation. Further research is needed to address how the magnitude of these impairments is related to the magnitude of sleep apnea, measured by polysonography (PSG) and the Multiple Sleep Latency Test (MSLT). There may be a critical threshold of sleep apnea that puts patients at substantial risk of cognitive impairments. The likelihood of driving safety errors in OSAS should increase as a function of severity of sleep apnea. Because drivers with OSAS may be unaware of their increasing drowsiness and deteriorating driving performance, they are more likely to continue to drive despite being at increased risk for a crash, as are some patients with Alzheimer disease. Some drivers with OSAS have anosognosia and are unaware of their cognitive impairment, of having fallen asleep at the wheel, and of committing driving safety errors. Observed drowsiness can be quantified through physiologic and cognitive performance measures. Self-reported estimates of acute drowsiness can be obtained using the Stanford Sleepiness Scale (Hoddes et al., 1973) and of chronic drowsiness using the Epworth Sleepiness Scale (Johns, 1991). CPAP therapy in drivers with OSAS should lead to improvement in cognitive function, driving performance, and awareness of impairment, and is an area for further research.

Issues of sleep-related cognitive decline and sudden sleep have also raised concerns of falling asleep at the wheel in drivers with Parkinson disease (PD). In addition to the hallmark motor disorder, cognitive, psychiatric, autonomic, and sleep disturbances can occur in patients with PD as a result of varied involvement of noradrener-

gic, cholinergic, and serotoninergic systems, as well as side effects of antiparkinsonian medications (Lang & Lozano, 1998a,b). Frucht and colleagues (1999, 2000) observed that patients with PD taking the newer dopamine agonists ropinirole and pramipexole may experience "sleep attacks" leading to car crashes. Excessive daytime sleepiness (EDS) or "sleep attacks" have been reported with all dopaminergic medications used to treat PD (Ferreira et al., 2000a–d; Hauser et al., 2000; Homan et al., 2000; Montastruc et al., 2000; Paladini et al., 2000; Ryan et al., 2000; Schapira, 2000). Olanow and colleagues (2000) criticized the term *sleep attack* and attributed the reported lack of warning before falling asleep to amnesia or lack of awareness for the prodrome of sleepiness. Passive movement in normal rested individuals may cause drowsiness or nausea, and even lull a driver to sleep, as in "sopite syndrome" (Graybiel & Knepton, 1976).

Physiologic indices of impending sleep include electroencephalogram (EEG) (patterns of drowsiness or microsleeps), decreased galvanic skin response (GSR), decreased respiratory rate, increased heart rate variability, reduced electromyogram (EMG) activity (e.g., in cervical paraspinous muscles), and increased percent lid closure (PERCLOS). PERCLOS scores of 80% or greater are highly correlated with falling asleep (Dinges, 2000) and can be measured in a vehicle, using a variety of techniques. These physiologic indices might be used to trigger an auditory or haptic warning (e.g., vibrating seats in a long haul-truck) in attempts to reduce injuries caused by sleep- or drowsiness-related crashes.

EMOTIONS

Driving a motor vehicle can be a pleasure; understanding the reasons why, and learning how to make driving even more fun, are major efforts of automobile designers and manufacturers, who want to increase sales. Driving can also be a major annoyance, an anxiety-provoking, maddening chore, especially to aggressive drivers (Sivak, 1983). Furthermore, aggressive driving and emotional disturbances are risk factors for car crashes.

Aggressive drivers may curse, shout, gesticulate obscenely, and drive illegally and dangerously. They may speed, fail to signal, flash their lights, ignore traffic signals, drive under the influence of drugs and alcohol, demonstrate territoriality, deliberately tailgate, or even use their car as a weapon to block or strike another car or a pedestrian. Such behaviors are known colloquially as "road rage" (Brewer, 2000), a media term used to describe extremely aggressive, and generally criminal events. A jehu (JAY hoo) is a reckless driver, named after the maniacal charioteer and Israeli king Jehu, who killed the pagan king Ahab and slew the harlot Jezebel. Today, we might say he had "road rage" and try to revoke his driver's license.

Aggressive drivers are more likely to be young, male, and single and use alcohol or drugs and have a premorbid personality disorder and increased stress at home, at work, and in a car (DiFranza et al., 1986; Holzapfel, 1995; Deery & Fildes, 1999). Stresses in a car can include high ambient temperature, crowded roadways, vehicle breakdowns, getting lost, and slow drivers ahead. Having a gun in the car is a marker for dangerous and aggressive driving behavior (Miller et al., 2002). The Dula Dangerous Driver Index (DDDI) was designed to measure a driver's likelihood to drive dangerously. Each DDDI scale (i.e., DDDI Total, Aggressive Driving, Negative Emotional Driving, and Risk Driving) has been shown to have strong internal reliability (Dula & Ballard, 2003).

Personality factors associated with aggressive driver crash involvement are thrill-seeking, impulsiveness, hostility/aggression, emotional instability, and depression (Beirness, 1993; Jonah, 1997). Crash-prone drivers have been described as emotionally immature, irresponsible, antisocial, and poorly adjusted, with a history of a traumatic childhood, delinquency, family disruption, and poor work records (Suchman, 1970). Psychiatric factors related to impaired driving ability include alcoholism, antisocial personality disorder, and depression (Noyes, 1985; Tsuang et al., 1985).

Some car crashes are preceded by stressful life events, such as disruption of key relationships. In rare instances, crashes are methods of committing suicide, like the death of Arthur Miller's salesman, Willy Loman. A depressed driver may fail to focus attention adequately on the road. Antipsychotic, antidepressant, and anxiolytic medications may decrease arousal and slow driver reactions times. A schizophrenic driver may be distracted by pathologic thoughts or hallucinations.

The New York State Department of Motor Vehicles Governor's Traffic Safety Committee has a website with excellent advice for avoiding the fallout of aggressive driving (*http://www.nysgtsc.state.ny.us/aggr-ndx.htm*; 11/20/02). The roles of personality and personality disorders, aggression, risk taking, and psychiatric disorders and drugs on driver safety and crash risk all require further study.

DRUG EFFECTS

Certain medications have been associated with greater relative risk of automobile crashes in the epidemiologic record (e.g., Ray et al., 1993). Antidepressants, pain medications, antihistamines, anticonvulsants, antihypertensives, antilipemics, hypoglycemic agents, sedatives, and hypnotics have all been implicated. Specific mechanisms besides general drowsiness, whereby these medications impair driving performance, remain unclear. Alcohol and illicit drugs also pose serious driving safety risks (e.g., Lamers & Ramaekers, 2001). Driving performance is often impaired at legally defined cutoffs for sobriety (usually 0.8–1.0 mg/dL of ethanol), but may be impaired at levels as low as 0.5 mg/dL (Borkenstein et al., 1964)(Fig. 9-9).

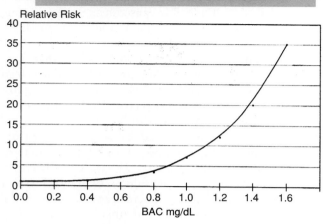

FIGURE 9-9. The Borkenstein curve shows that the risk of accidents for drivers with blood alcohol concentrations (BAC) as low as 0.5 mg/dL is greater than the risk in drivers who do not consume acohol, but still lower than the risk at 0.8 mg/dL (a common legal cut-off for drunk driving in the United States.) (Adapted from Borkenstein et al., 1974).

Deleterious effects of drugs on driving seem likely to depend in part on neurotransmitter systems involved in "executive functions" that are known to be critical for driving: decision making and working memory. According to a "somatic marker hypothesis" (Damasio, 1994; Damasio & Tranel, 1996), decision making is guided by somatic (emotional) signals linked to prior experiences with reward and punishment. The generation of somatic states is linked to a neural system that includes ventromedial (VM) prefrontal cortex, amygdala, and somatosensory cortices (SI, SII, and insula). Working memory defects result from dysfunction in a neural system in which the dorsolateral prefrontal cortex is a critical region (see earlier discussion and also Chapter 10). Elucidation of the chemical substrates (e.g., serotonin, dopamine, and acetylcholine) that modulate frontal lobe functions in at-risk older drivers may help guide development of pharmacologic interventions that improve cognitive performance in the driving task.

Studies of the effects of pharmacologic agents on driving performance can be studied most safely in a driving simulator (see discussion in following section), as in our ongoing studies of driving performance in users of Ecstasy (MDMA) and marijuana, in collaboration with C. Lamers and J. Ramaekers of the University of Maastricht (Rizzo et al., 2003a). A drug company–sponsored driving simulator study (Weiler et al., 2000) that failed to show differences between individuals taking the antihistamine fexofenadine (Allegra) and a placebo group was criticized for its methodology (Angello & Druce, 2000; de Waard & Brookhuis, 2000) and funding source (Lee & Dudley, 2000), yet the manufacturer (Aventis Pharmaceuticals, Bridgewater, NJ) continued to cite the study to market its drug in full-page ads (e.g., "Nonimpairing while Driving!", *American Medical News*, November 11, 2002).

ASSESSMENT OF DRIVING PERFORMANCE

Road Tests

States generally consider a road test, conducted under the direct observation of a trained expert, to be the "gold standard" of driver fitness. The expert grades driver performance on several standard driving tasks to calculate a cutoff score that is used to designate a driver as safe or unsafe for licensure. Several disadvantages are: (1) road tests were developed to ensure that novice drivers know and can apply the rules of the road, not to test experienced drivers who may be impaired; (2) few data exist that show that road tests are correlated with crash involvement; (3) road testing carries the risk inherent in the real-world road environment; (4) road test conditions can vary depending on the weather, daylight, traffic, and driving course; and (5) driving experts may have different biases and grading criteria.

Use of an Instrumented Vehicle

Instrumented vehicles permit quantitative assessments of driver performance in the field, under actual road conditions. These quantitative performance measurements are not subject to the type of human bias that can affect inter-rater reliability on a standard road test. For these reasons, we developed a multipurpose field research vehicle known as ARGOS (the Automobile for Research in eRGonomics and Safety) (Fig. 9-10), a mid-sized vehicle with extensive instrumentation and sensors hidden within its infrastructure (Rizzo et al., 1997a). The driving assessment in ARGOS can incorporate several standard maneuvers deemed essential to the driving task such as turns, observance of traffic signs and signals, and maintenance of vehicle control. Also, standardized challenges can be introduced that stress critical cognition abilities during the driving task. These include route finding, sign identification, multitasking (e.g., driving while performing an auditory verbal distracter task, as in holding a conversation, performing mental arithmetic, or using modern in-vehicle telematics devices such as cell phones and navigation devices), and even response to a simulated "emergency" (e.g, a low fuel light coming on).

Using an on-board radar device (LIDAR, Applied Concepts, Inc., Plano, TX) we can test whether drivers parked by the roadside in ARGOS can judge speed and distance of approaching vehicles to decide safely whether to enter traffic (Fig. 9-11). Results in 18 neurologically normal drivers show that drivers over 65 years of age

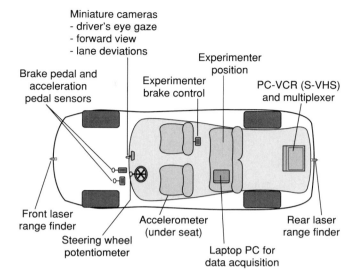

FIGURE 9-10. Schematic of Automobile for Research in eRGonomics and Safety (ARGOS).

allow a longer time cushion between themselves and an approaching vehicle in judging when to enter traffic to compensate for their greater time to maneuver (e.g., into and across traffic), compared to drivers under 65 years of age (Skaar et al., 2003b). This pattern of results could be due to perceptual and decision-making differences between the older and younger drivers. An instrumented vehicle (IV) can also be used to assess excessive risk taking in younger drivers (Rizzo et al., 2002) (Fig. 9-12).

Of note, the internal network of modern vehicles makes it possible to obtain information from the driver's own car. Modern vehicles are mandated to report certain variables pertaining to speed, emissions controls, and vehicle performance, and some allow more detailed reporting options on seatbelt and headlight use, climate and traction control, wheel speed, and antilock brake (ABS) activation. Global positioning systems can show where and when a driver drives, takes risks, and commits safety errors. Radar and video systems installed in the vehicle can gather information on the proximity, lane-keeping, merging, and following behavior of the driver and other vehicles on the road. Accelerometers can detect *g* forces associated with hazardous events such as abrupt braking, swerving, or loss of vehicle control. Wireless systems can check the instrumentation and send performance data to remote locations. Together, these developments can provide direct real-time information on driver strategy, vehicle usage, upkeep, drive lengths, route choices, and decisions to drive during inclement weather and high traffic. The unprecedented new electronic window on driver behavior offers great advantages over current insights on vehicle usage (that rely on questionnaires completed by drivers who may have

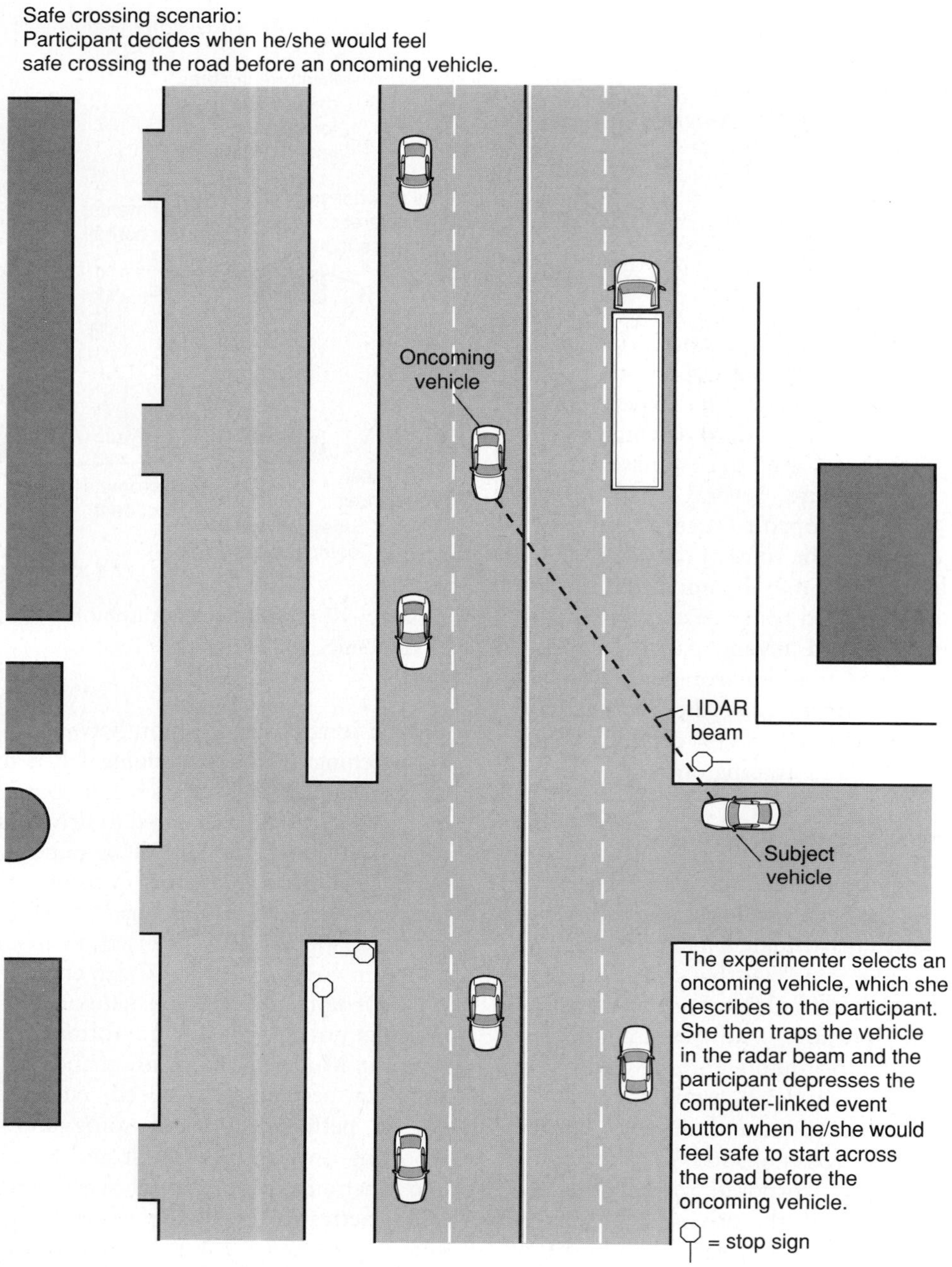

Safe crossing scenario:
Participant decides when he/she would feel
safe crossing the road before an oncoming vehicle.

Oncoming
vehicle

LIDAR
beam

Subject
vehicle

The experimenter selects an
oncoming vehicle, which she
describes to the participant.
She then traps the vehicle
in the radar beam and the
participant depresses the
computer-linked event
button when he/she would
feel safe to start across
the road before the
oncoming vehicle.

= stop sign

FIGURE 9-11. Using a radar device (LIDAR, Applied Concepts, Inc., Plano, TX) we can test whether drivers parked by the roadside in the Automobile for Research in eRGonomics and Safety (ARGOS) can judge speed and distance of approaching vehicles to decide safely whether to enter traffic.

defective memory and cognition). These advantages must be balanced against issues of privacy for the driver, others who may drive the driver's car (generally family members), and passengers.

Another issue is how to manage and analyze the huge amount of data from continuous driver monitoring and how to classify driver performance errors. In practice it is often difficult to determine unambiguously whether an error leading to a critical incident was the result of a driver lapse, slip, or rule-based or knowledge-based error (discussed previously, in

section on Executive Functions). Practical solutions can employ a set of specific operational definitions for detecting critical incidents and empirically derived "decision tree" tools for classifying these unsafe incidents and identifying their likely causes. Such empirically derived tools and models provide taxonomic frameworks for organizing and interpreting data on driver error and identifying common causes and mitigation strategies from seemingly unrelated instances (Wilde, 1982; Grayson, 1997; Huguenin, 1997; Dingus et al., 1999; Rizzo et al., 2001b).

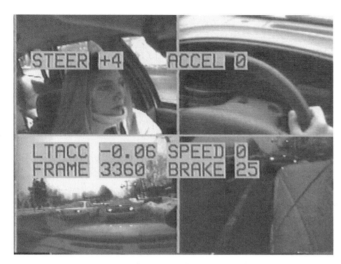

FIGURE 9-12. Younger driver in the Automobile for Research in eRGonomics and Safety (ARGOS) with neck brace restricting visual search of road and mirrors.

In particular, raw data obtained from an IV can be filtered using specific criteria to flag where a critical incident may have occurred in the IV data stream. For example, longitudinal accelerometers or lateral accelerometers measure *g* forces as drivers apply their brakes or swerve to miss an obstacle, and are used to flag critical driving situations in the data stream. The specific value of *g*-force values used to identify critical driving situations (e.g., 0.4 *g* indicating abrupt deceleration) can be systematically determined in large-scale studies using IVs such as the "100 Car Study" being conducted by our collaborators at Virginia Tech Transportation Institute (VTTI) under sponsorship of the National Highway Transportation Safety Administration (NHTSA).

Driving Simulator

Driving simulators have been applied to quantify driver performance in cognitively impaired drivers, study basic aspects of cognition in drivers with brain lesions, probe the effects of information processing overload on driver safety, and optimize the ergonomics of vehicle design. Whereas some simulators are relatively crude "video game" devices, others are sophisticated instruments that incorporate divided attention tasks and record lane tracking, speed and steering rate variation, and number of crashes.

Driving simulation offers several advantages over the use of road tests or driving records in assessments of driver fitness. Simulator studies provide the only means to replicate exactly the experimental road conditions under which driving comparisons are made and simulations are safe, with none of the risk of the road or test track. Simulation has been successfully applied to assess performance profiles in drivers who are at risk for a crash due to a variety of different conditions such as

sleep apnea, drowsiness, alcohol and other drug effects, old age, AD, PD, or traumatic brain injury (Dingus et al., 1987; McMillen & Wells-Parker, 1987; Brouwer et al., 1989; Haraldsson et al., 1990; Katz et al., 1990; Madeley et al., 1990; Guerrier et al., 1995; Rizzo et al., 1997b, 2000a).

Special concerns are often raised about fitness to drive in AD, the most common cause of abnormal cognitive decline in older adults (Cummings & Cole, 2002; see Chapter 22). Johansson and colleagues (1997) analyzed brain autopsies in 98 older drivers who perished in single and multi-vehicle crashes. Fifty-two of 98 (53%) had sufficient neuritic plaques to fulfill Consortium to Establish a Registry for Alzheimer's Disease (CERAD) neuropathologic criteria, suggesting (20%) or indicating (33%) AD. None of these drivers had a diagnosis of AD, and family members were often unaware of a problem (Lundberg et al., 1998), raising the concern that the first manifestation of AD may sometimes be a fatal crash. In deceased drivers over age 76, apolipoprotein E epsilon 4 allele (a risk factor for AD) was found more often than in age- and gender-matched paired controls. Further analyses indicated that preclinical AD increases the relative risk of fatal crashes in older drivers more than tenfold. Similar concerns of driver safety arise in PD, a significant risk factor for dementia that increases with age, severity of parkinsonism, or low score on cognitive screening at baseline (Dubois & Pillon, 1997; Aarsland et al., 2001) (Fig. 9-13).

These safety concerns can be addressed using high-fidelity driving simulation and collision avoidance scenarios. To create an immersive real-time virtual environment for assessing at-risk drivers in a medical setting we developed SIREN, the Simulator for Interdisciplinary Research in Ergonomics and Neuroscience (Rizzo et al., 2000b). We removed all running gear of a 1994 GM Saturn, cut the vehicle in half at the doorposts and installed a steel frame and instrumentation. We moved each half through our university hospital

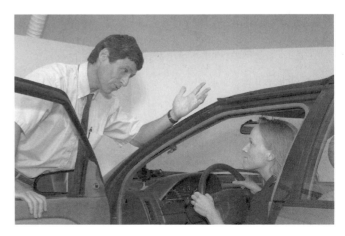

FIGURE 9-13. The Simulator for Interdisciplinary Research in Ergonomics and Neuroscience (SIREN).

and a temporary 10-foot gap in our laboratory wall. SIREN comprises the reassembled car, embedded electronic sensors, and pinhole video cameras for recording driver performance. SIREN also includes a sound system and surrounding screens (150° forward field of view [FOV], 50° rear FOV), four LCD projectors with image generators and an integrated host computer, and another computer for scenario design, control, and data collection. A tile-based scenario development tool (DriveSafety, Fort Collins, CO) allows us to select from multiple road types and populate roadways with different vehicles that interact with the driver and each other according to experimental needs.

We are applying SIREN to study the driving performance of motorists with medical disorders that can impair cognitive abilities that are crucial to the driving task. The motorists drive on simulated rural highways with interactive traffic, resembling a drive around Iowa City on roads that most drivers would travel regularly. The simulation consists of multiple "events" associated with potential crashes interspersed with uneventful highway segments (Fig. 9-14).

Participants in one such study of drivers with mild-to-moderate cognitive impairment AD drove on a virtual highway in a simulator scenario where the approach to within a few seconds of an intersection triggered an illegal incursion by another vehicle (see Fig. 9-14; Rizzo et al., 2001a). To avoid collision with the incurring vehicle, the driver had to perceive, attend to, and interpret the roadway situation; formulate an evasive plan; and then exert appropriate action upon the accelerator, brake, or steering controls, all under

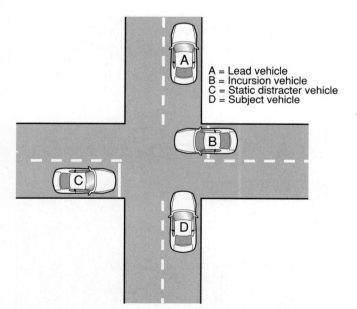

FIGURE 9-14. Schematic depiction of intersection incursion scenario to test collision avoidance behavior in the Simulator for Interdisciplinary Research in Ergonomics and Neuroscience (SIREN). (From Rizzo et al., 2001b.)

pressure of time. The drivers with AD showed a significantly increased risk of a crash compared with nondemented drivers of similar age, similar to findings in an earlier study of drivers with AD that focused on avoidance of potential rear-end collisions (Rizzo et al., 1997b). Predictors of crashes in the combined studies included visuospatial impairment, disordered attention, reduced processing of visual motion cues, and overall cognitive decline (Table 9-3).

Use of a visual tool that plots control over steering wheel position, brake and accelerator pedals, vehicle speed, and vehicle position during the five seconds preceding a crash event in these studies showed driver inattention and control responses that were inappropriate or too slow. In one type of crash, a driver was looking directly out the front windshield but took no action (as in Fig. 9-8). Such "looking without seeing" has been reported in patients with lesions of the dorsolateral visual association cortex (Rizzo & Hurtig, 1987). Other drivers reacted too late or evaded a primary hazard, only to experience a secondary collision. Another crash type occurred on a straight-away segment, possibly because the driver lost control of the car while distracted. Analysis of crash circumstances taking vehicle speed into account (using the NHTSA General Estimates System) showed that several of the crashes in these studies would likely have been fatal.

A relative drawback to simulation research is simulator adaptation syndrome (SAS), characterized by autonomic symptoms including nausea and sweating (Stanney et al., 2002). The discomfort is thought to be due to a mismatch between visual cues of movement, which are plentiful, and inertial cues, which are lacking or imperfect, even in simulators with a motion base. Similar cue conflicts are encountered in IMAX theaters. The likelihood of SAS appears to increase with peripheral visual field stimulation, as with large field of view displays or with turns (especially left turns) in which movement cues sweep across the peripheral fields, and with abrupt braking actions (Rizzo et al., 2003c). In contrast to SAS, motion sickness is associated with cue conflicts in places where inertial cues of movement are high and corresponding visual movement cues are lacking, such as below deck in boats or in elevators. In our experience SAS is also more likely with crowded displays (as in simulated urban traffic), advanced age, female gender, and history of migraine or motion sickness. SAS may also result from conflicts between visual cues that are represented with differing success in modern computer displays.

Another issue in simulator-based research is the need to test the validity of the simulation. This may involve detailed comparisons of driver performance in a simulator with performance in an instrumented vehicle and with state records of crashes and moving violations in each population of drivers being studied. The apparent face validity of the simulation (i.e. that the driver

TABLE 9-3. Predictors of Crashes in Simulated Collision Avoidance Scenarios

Predictor variable	Odds ratio estimates (95% CI)/P values		
Temporal orientation < 0	13.26	(2.39, 140.67)	/ <0.001
WAIS-R information < 10	10.21	(2.15, 67.23)	/ 0.002
COWA < 30	32.05	(5.40, 361.44)	/ <0.001
WAIS-R Digit Span < 10	14.36	(1.88, 656.13)	/ 0.004
Rey-Osterrieth CFT-Copy < 20	32.85	(5.41, 370.03)	/ <0.001
FRT < 40	7.15	(1.55, 36.42)	/ 0.009
WAIS-R Block Design < 6	19.28	(3.65, 138.28)	/ <0.001
VRT Correct < 4	5.28	(1.05, 35.52)	/ 0.042
Trail-Making Test (Part B) < 3	35.90	(4.57, 1663.21)	/ <0.001
UFOV Total Loss > 50%	9.76	(1.84, 99.66)	/ 0.003
Starry Night (d') < 1	10.34	(2.13, 70.10)	/ 0.002
3-D SFM > 15	16.88	(3.37, 118.26)	/ <0.001
MDD > 30	7.75	(1.69, 43.51)	/ 0.006
Alzheimer disease	16.91	(2.61, 8)	/ 0.001
Age > 70 y	0.62	(0.15, 2.63)	/ 0.652
Gender, M	1.63	(0.38, 8.37)	/ 0.682

CI, confidence interval; COWA, Controlled Oral Word Association; CFT, Complex Figure Test; FRT, Facial Recognition Test; MDD, Motion Direction Discrimination; SFM, structure-from-motion; UFOV, useful field of view; WAIS-R, Wechsler Adult Intelligence Scale–Revised.

appears to be driving a car and is immersed in the task) does not guarantee a lifelike performance. Drivers may behave differently in a simulator where no injury can occur, compared with real-life driving situations in which life, limb, and licensure are at stake.

Efforts to improve driving simulators have often focused on making the simulations more "lifelike," yet the added cost (e.g., of a mechanical motion base) might not translate to better assessments of driver safety. Abstract versions of reality that enhance some critical environmental cues (say, dynamic texture or shading) and minimize others might provide more effective tests (of "functional reality") that correlate even better with actual driver performance. Advances in understanding the role and representations of key visual cues from the environment in dynamic graphic displays should improve the acceptance and measurement characteristics of driving simulator tools.

We recently designed an abstract virtual environment tool to assess go/no-go decision-making by cognitively impaired drivers (Rizzo et al., 2003b). This design was motivated by modern aviation information display systems research that uses enhanced visual cues to represent the external environment within a small field of view (allowing pilots of sophisticated aircraft to maintain high situation awareness and make safe flight decisions). The environment comprised a straight, flat, two-lane road intersected by 100 crossroads (Fig. 9-15). The task was run on a PC and presented on a standard 21-inch video monitor.

In this surreal environment, each subject drove through a series of intersections having gates that opened and closed as the driver approached. Half the gates closed fully and the rest only partially, without blocking the subject's route ("open gates"). Traffic signals correctly

predicted impending gate closure state at ~80% of the gates, displaying red (Stop) for fully closed and green (Go) for open gate intersections. Traffic signals were incorrect (misleading) for the remaining (~20%) gates (displaying Go for closed and Stop for open gate intersections). Misleading and accurate traffic signals were randomly interspersed, so that while the traffic signals

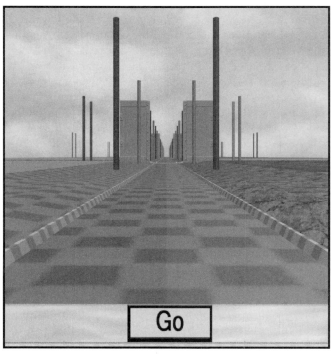

FIGURE 9-15. The Go/No-Go scenario tool—a static image from a single frame is shown.

were usually accurate, the truthfulness of each specific signal was not known to the driver.

Thirty-two licensed drivers participated in a study using the Go/No-Go scenario tool. Fourteen were recruited from the Iowa Patient Registry of patients with behavioral impairments due to chronic focal brain lesions (Palca, 1990), two had early AD, and the rest were neurologically normal. Each driver was instructed to drive through the intersections as quickly as possible without hitting the gates, using the traffic signals to help. Driver inputs were recorded from steering wheel and accelerator/brake hardware peripherals. Dependent measures included time to completion, number of crashes into closed gates, number of stops at open gates, and number of successes (i.e., stopping at closed gates and going at open gates).

Results showed that the neurologically impaired drivers took longer to complete the task and had more errors at the gates, as hypothesized. Three drivers with frontal lobe lesions, including the well-known subject E.V.R. with bilateral frontal lobe amputations after resection of a meningioma (e.g., Damasio et al., 1985; Eslinger & Damasio, 1985), had special difficulty. Among the drivers with lesions, the two fastest had very high incidences of Go failures (crashing into closed gates). Also, cognitively impaired drivers who had crashes at gates or took longer to get through the task continued to show good control of the vehicle and did not exceed the lane boundaries, indicating that visuomotor control can be intact in drivers with decision-making impairment, and that measures of visuomotor control in the driving task (such as steering and lane position variability) alone are not sensitive predictors of critical incidents caused by decision-making-impaired drivers. There were no complaints of simulator adaptation syndrome with the small field display.

Future application of driving simulation to study drivers with medical impairments will benefit from a standardized approach to scenario design, certification standards for ecological validity of simulator graphics and vehicle dynamics, uniform definitions of measures of system performance, and cost-effective methods for geo-specific visual database development.

PRACTICAL CONSIDERATIONS

Demographic and health factors may impact driving ability. Relevant factors are age, education, gender, general health, vision status, mobility, and driving frequency. Frequency of driving can be assessed using a questionnaire tool (e.g., the University of Alabama at Birmingham [UAB] Driving Habits Questionnaire [DHQ]; Ball et al., 1998; Stalvey et al., 1999). Health status information can be obtained using a checklist of medical conditions (e.g., heart disease, cancer) and when they occurred. Certain medical factors may pose increased risk of driving errors (see Table 9-2). Psycho-

logical state of the drivers can be collected using the General Health Questionnaire (GHQ) (Goldberg, 1972). Medication use can be assessed by asking drivers to bring all prescription and over-the-counter medication to the clinic. A driver's chronic sleep disturbance can be assessed from the driver's self-report on the Epworth Sleepiness Scale.

According to recent American Academy of Ophthalmology guidelines (available at URL http://www.aao.org/aao/member/policy/driving.cfm), relevant visual assessment can include tests of letter acuity, for example, the Early Treatment Diabetic Retinopathy Study (ETDRS) chart (Ferris et al., 1982), contrast sensitivity (Pelli et al., 1988), and visual field sensitivity, often assessed using automated perimetry (Trick, 2003). UFOV reduction in patients who have normal visual fields can be demonstrated using visual tasks under differing attention loads (Ball et al., 1993). Overall visual health can be assessed with the National Eye Institute (NEI) Visual Functioning Questionnaire–25 (Mangione et al., 2001).

"Bioptic lenses" are sometimes prescribed to allow drivers with low vision to see magnified images of traffic signals and signs through telescopes mounted on glasses (Peli and Peli, 2002). UFOV reduction can be partially reversed for at least one year by training (Ball et al., 2002); transfer of these training effects to driving performance is under investigation. Related research concerns rehabilitation strategies in patients with homonymous hemianopia (Tant, 2002), including prisms to shift undetected images toward the seeing fields. Enlarged side- and rear-view mirrors may mitigate effects of peripheral visual field defects in some drivers.

Table 9-4 lists several standard neuropsychological tasks of cognitive function that are essential to the driving task. Impaired performance on some of these tasks (e.g., Complex Figure Test [CFT], Trailmaking Test Part B) may be especially predictive of driving safety risk (see Table 9-3). The Swedish Road Administration (Vägverket) has proposed a set of operational guidelines for assessing fitness to drive in motorists with dementia, based on screening measures such as the Clinical Dementia Rating scale (CDR) and Mini-Mental State Examination (MMSE) (Fig. 9-16; see also Chapter 1). Reger and colleagues (2003) recently analyzed the literature on the relationship between neuropsychological test scores and driving ability in 27 studies of drivers with dementia. The American Medical Association (AMA) is recently formulating its own guidelines (American Medical Association NHTSA, 2003). Patients with moderate to severe dementia (e.g., cutoffs: MMSE ≤ 17; CDR ≥ 2) can be assessed individually but should generally not drive. However, no single test is sufficiently reliable to base judgments on fitness to drive, and a variety of sources and approaches are needed.

We note that neuropsychological test scores are often corrected (e.g., scaled for age and education) to improve the ability to detect deviations from normality;

TABLE 9-4. A Battery for the Assessment of Cognitively Impaired Drivers

Temporal Orientation	This is a quick but sensitive measure of orientation to time, which requires the subject to provide information about the date, day of week, and time of day.
Information and block design	The *Information* subtest from the WAIS-R measures general fund of information. It provides a very reliable index of verbal intellect, and has a high correlation with Verbal IQ. The Block Design subtest from the WAIS-R provides a very reliable measure of nonverbal intellectual capacity. It is highly correlated with Performance IQ.
Benton Visual Retention Test (BVRT)	The BVRT is sensitive to early mental decline in several different populations. It is well standardized and easy to administer.
Controlled Oral Word Association (COWA)	The COWA test requires subjects to generate as many words as possible that begin with a certain letter of the alphabet, within a 1-minute time limit. The test is a good detector of early abnormal decline, and it is also sensitive to language "executive functions" defects.
Facial Recognition Test	This test measures visuoperceptual capacity. The subject is asked to match unfamiliar faces presented under different lighting conditions and different viewing angles.
Rey-Osterrieth Complex Figure Test Copy	This test requires subjects to copy a complex geometric figure and provides a reliable index of visuoconstructional ability, independent of memory function.
Trail Making Test, Parts A and B	This is a reliable and sensitive measure of "executive functions." The patient must learn to track simultaneously two different types of information that require cognitive flexibility and planning.
Digit Span, Forward and Backward	The subject is required to repeat a sequence of digits forward and backward, which becomes progressively longer across trials. Both of these tasks make significant demands on "immediate" memory. The digit span backward task, in particular, makes demands on "working memory," as the subject must hold the information in a working buffer and then operate on it.

however, what matters on the road is pure ability, regardless of demographic characteristics. Consequently, studies that aim to correlate neuropsychological performance with driving performance and to generate predictions of safety in individual drivers should use raw (i.e., not corrected for age, education, or gender) neuropsychological test scores.

CONCLUSION

Safe driving requires the coordination of attention, perception, memory, executive functions (decision making and implementation) and motor functions. These abilities are impaired in some populations of drivers with neurologic disorders, increasing the risk of driver performance

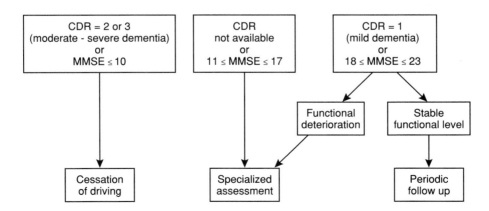

FIGURE 9-16. Algorithm for assessment of demented drivers. The specialized assessment can use a variety of techniques, including neuropsychological tests, on-road tests, and driver simulators. CDR, Clinical Dementia Rating; MMSE, Mini-Mental State Examination. (Lundber C, Johannson K, Rizzo M, et al: Dementia in driving: An attempt at consensus. Alzheim Dis Assoc Disord 11:28–37, 1997. Used with permission.)

impairments, safety errors, car crashes, and injuries. Decisions on the fitness to drive of "at-risk" drivers should be based on empirical observations of performance because age or medical diagnosis alone is often an unreliable criterion. It is desirable to observe driver errors in an environment that is challenging yet safe for the driver and tester, under conditions of optimal stimulus and response control. State road tests are designed to ensure that novice drivers know and can apply the rules of the road, not to predict crash involvement in skilled drivers who may have become impaired. Real-life crashes are sporadic, uncontrolled events during which few objective observations can be made. Personal accounts and even state crash records may be incomplete, and crashes are under-reported. The use of modern instrumented vehicles and driving simulators is helping to specify the linkage between decline in certain cognitive domains, measured by scores on neuropsychological tasks, and increased crash risk in neurologic disorders, in efforts to standardize the assessment of fitness-to-drive in persons with medical impairments. By understanding the patterns of driver safety errors that cause crashes, it may be possible to design interventions (including driver performance monitoring devices, collision warning systems, and graded licensure strategies) that will reduce these errors.

Acknowledgments

Research supported by NIA AG 15071 and NIA AG 17707.

■ KEY POINTS

☐ About 35 million crashes in the United States each year claim about 40,000 lives and cause millions more injuries at a cost of about $150 billion.

☐ Decisions on the fitness to drive of "at-risk" drivers should be based on empirical observations of performance because age or medical diagnosis alone is often an unreliable criterion.

☐ Safe driving requires coordination of several cognitive processes, including attention, perception, memory, motor functions, and executive functions (including decision making, planning, and self-awareness).

☐ Cognitive abilities and impairments determine specific driver behaviors and safety errors, which in turn predict crashes.

☐ Some errors can be detected because drivers normally monitor their performance. When feedback on driving fails to match expectations based on correctly formulated intentions, the discrepancy is often detected "on line." Drivers with cognitive impairment are less likely to realize their errors.

☐ There are few data to show that standard road tests are correlated with crash involvement.

KEY READINGS

Ball K, Owsley C, Sloane ME, et al: Visual attention problems as a predictor of vehicle crashes in older drivers. Investig Ophthalmol Visual Sci 34:3110–3123, 1993.

Reason J: Human Error. Cambridge, UK: Cambridge UP, 1990.

Rizzo M, McGehee D, Dawson J, Anderson S: Simulated car crashes at intersections in drivers with Alzheimer's disease. Alz Dis Assoc Disord 15:10–20, 2001.

Rothengatter J, Carbonell-Vaya E, eds: Traffic and transport psychology: Theory and application. Oxford: Pergamon, 1997.

REFERENCES

Aarsland D, Andersen K, Larsen JP, et al: Risk of dementia in Parkinson's disease: A community-based, prospective study. Neurology 56:730–736, 2001.

Allsop RE, Brown ID, Groeger JA, Robertson SA: Approaches to modeling driver behaviour at actual and simulated traffic light signals (Contractor report 264). Crowthorne, UK: Transport and Road Research Library, 1991.

American Academy of Ophthalmology. Policy Statement: Vision Requirements for Driving. Approved October, 2001. http://www.aao.org/aao/member/policy/driving.cfm (accessed 8/25/03).

American Medical Association. Physician's Guide to Assessing and Counseling Older Drivers. http://www.ama-assn.org/ama/pub/category/10791.html (accessed 8/18/03).

Andersen GJ, Cisneros J, Atchley P, Saidpour A: Speed, size, and edge-rate information for the detection of collision events. J Exp Psychol Hum Percept Perform 25:256–269, 1999.

Andersen GJ, Cisneros J, Saidpour A, Atchley P: Age-related differences in collision detection during deceleration. Psychol Aging 15:241–252, 2000.

Anderson SW, Tranel D: Awareness of disease states following cerebral infarction, dementia, and head trauma: Standardized assessment. Clin Neuropsychol 3:327–339, 1989.

Angello JT, Druce HM: Drug effects on driving performance [letter]. Ann Intern Med 113:657, 2000.

Arnold PK, Hartley LR, Corry A, et al: Hours of work, and perceptions of fatigue among truck drivers. Accid Anal Preven 29:471–477, 1997.

Baddeley A: Working memory. Science 255:556–559, 1992.

Ball K, Berch DB, Helmers KF, et al: Effects of cognitive training interventions with older adults: A randomized controlled trial. JAMA 288:2271–2281, 2002.

Ball K, Owsley C: Identifying correlates of accident involvement for the older driver. Hum Factors 33:583–595, 1991.

Ball K, Owsley C, Beard B: Clinical visual perimetry underestimates peripheral field problems in older adults. Clin Vision Sci 5:113–125, 1990.

Ball K, Owsley C, Sloane ME, et al: Visual attention problems as a predictor of vehicle crashes in older drivers. Investig Ophthalmol Vis Sci 34:3110–3123, 1993.

Ball K, Owsley C, Stalvey B, et al: Driving avoidance and functional impairment in older drivers. Accid Anal Preven 30:313–323, 1998.

Ball KK, Beard BL, Roenker DL, et al: Age and visual search: Expanding the useful field of view. J Optical Soc Am A 5:2210–2219, 1988.

Barratt ES: Impulsiveness and aggression, in Monahan J, Steadman HJ (eds): Violence and Mental Disorder: Developments in Risk Assessment. Chicago: University of Chicago Press, 1994, pp. 61–79.

Bechara A, Tranel D, Damasio H, Damasio AR: Failure to respond autonomically to anticipated future outcomes following damage to prefrontal cortex. Cereb Cortex 6:215–225, 1996.

Beirness DJ: Do we really drive as we live? The role of personality factors in road crashes. Alcohol, Drugs and Driving 9:129–143, 1993.

Benton AL: The prefrontal region: Its early history, in Levin H, Esenberg H, Benton A (eds): Frontal Lobe Function and Dysfunction. New York: Oxford University Press, 1991, pp. 3–12.

Boer ER: Behavioral entropy as a measure of driving performance. Proceedings of the First International Driving Symposium on Human Factors in Driver Assessment, Training and Vehicle Design. Aspen, CO. Iowa City, IA: The University of Iowa, 2001, pp. 225–229.

Borkenstein RF, Crowther RF, Shumate RP, et al: The role of the drinking driver in traffic accidents (The Grand Rapids Study), ed 2. Blutalkohol 11 (Suppl. 1):1–131, 1974.

Brewer AM: Road rage: What, who, when, where and how. Transport Reviews 20:49–64, 2000.

Brouwer WH, Ponds RWHM, Van Wolffelaar PC, et al: Divided attention 5 to 10 years after severe closed head injury. Cortex 25:219–230, 1989.

Burg A: Vision and driving: A summary of research findings. Highway Research Record 216:1–12, 1968.

Caird JK, Edwards CJ, Creaser J: The effect of time constraints on older and younger driver decisions to turn at intersections using a modified change blindness paradigm. Proceedings of the First International Driving Symposium on Human Factors in Driver Assessment, Training and Vehicle Design. Aspen, CO. Iowa City, IA: University of Iowa, 2001, p. 196.

Cummings JL Cole G: Alzheimer disease. JAMA 287:2335–2358, 2002.

Damasio A: Descartes' Error: Emotion, Reason, and the Human Brain. New York: Grosset/Putnam, 1994.

Damasio AR: The Feeling of What Happens: Body and Emotion in the Making of Consciousness. New York: Harcourt Brace & Co., 1999.

Damasio AR: The somatic marker hypothesis and the possible functions of the prefrontal cortex. Philos Trans R Soc Lond Biol Sci 351:1413–1420, 1996.

Damasio AR, Anderson SW: The frontal lobes, in Heilman KM, Valenstein E (eds): Clinical Neuropsychology, ed 3. New York: Oxford University Press, 1993.

Damasio AR, Eslinger PJ, Damasio H, et al: Multimodal amnesic syndrome following bilateral temporal and basal forebrain damage. Arch Neurol 42:252–259, 1985.

Damasio AR, Tranel D: Towards a neurobiology of the emotions. Int J Psychol 31:323, 1996.

Deery HA, Fildes BN: Young novice driver subtypes: Relationship to high-risk behavior, traffic accident record, and simulator driving performance. Hum Factors 41 628–643:1999.

Dement WC, Carskadon MA, Richardson G: Excessive daytime sleepiness in the sleep apnea syndrome, in Guilleminault C, Dement WC (eds): Sleep Apnea Syndromes. New York: Alan R. Liss, 1978, pp. 23–46.

De Waard D, Brookhuis KA: Drug effects on driving performance [letter]. Ann Int Med 133:656, 2000.

Dias R, Robbins TW, Roberts AC: Dissociation in prefrontal cortex of affective and attentional shifts. Nature 380:69–72, 1996.

DiFranza JA, Winters TH, Goldberg RJ, et al: The relationship of smoking to motor vehicle accidents and traffic violations. New York State J Med 86:464–467, 1986.

Dinges D: Accidents and fatigue. Proceedings of the International Conference: The Sleepy Driver and Pilot. National Institute for Psychosocial Factors and Health, Stockholm, May 28–31, 2000.

Dingus TA, Antin JF, Hulse MC, et al: Attentional demand requirements of an automobile moving-map navigation system. Transportation Res 4:301–315, 1989.

Dingus TA, Hardee HL, Wierwille WW: Development of models for on-board detection of driver impairment. Accid Anal Preven 19:271–283, 1987

Dingus TA, Hetrick S, Mollenhauer M: Empirical methods in support of crash avoidance model building and benefits estimation. ITS J 5:93–125, 1999.

Dubinsky RM, Gray C, Husted D, et al: Driving in Parkinson's disease. Neurology 41:517–520, 1991.

Dubinsky RM, Williamson A, Gray CS, et al: Driving in Alzheimer's disease. J Am Geriatr Soc 40:1112–1116, 1992.

Dubois B, Pillon B: Cognitive deficits in Parkinson's disease. J Neurol 244:2–8, 1997.

Ehret BD, Gray WD, Kirschbaum SS: Contending with complexity: Developing and using a scaled world in applied cognitive research. Hum Factors 42:8–23, 2000.

Engleman HM, Hirst WSJ, Douglas NJ: Under reporting of sleepiness and driving impairment in patients with sleep apnea/hypopnea syndrome. J Sleep Res 6:272–275, 1997.

Eslinger PJ, Damasio AR: Severe disturbance of higher cognition after bilateral frontal lobe ablation: Patient EVR. Neurology 35:1731–1741, 1985.

Evenden J: Impulsivity: A discussion of clinical and experimental findings. J Psychopharmacol 13:180–192, 1999.

Ferreira JJ, Galitzky M, Brefel-Courbon C, et al: "Sleep attacks" as an adverse drug reaction of levodopa monotherapy. Mov Disord 15 (Suppl. 3):129, 2000a.

Ferreira JJ, Galitzky M, Montastruc JL, Rascol O: Sleep attacks in Parkinson's disease. Lancet 355:1333–1334, 2000b.

Ferreira JJ, Pona N, Costa J, et al: Somnolence as an adverse drug reaction of antiparkinson drugs: A meta-analysis of published randomized placebo-controlled trails. Mov Disord 15 (Suppl. 3):128, 2000c.

Ferreira JJ, Thalamas C, Galitzky M, et al: "Sleep attacks" and Parkinson's disease: results of a questionnaire survey in a Mov Disord outpatient clinic. Mov Disord 15 (Suppl. 3):187, 2000d.

Ferris, FL III, Kassoff A, Bresnick GH, et al: New visual acuity charts for clinical research. Am J Ophthalmol 94:91–96, 1982.

Frucht S, Rogers JD, Green PE, et al: Falling asleep at the wheel: Motor vehicle mishaps in persons taking pramipexole and ropinirole. Neurology 52:1908–1910, 1999.

Frucht SJ, Greene PE, Fahn S: Sleep episodes in Parkinson's disease: A wake-up call. Mov Disord 15:601–603, 2000.

Fuster JM: The prefrontal cortex: Anatomy, physiology, and neuropsychology of the frontal lobe, ed 3. New York: Raven Press, 1996.

Galski T, Bruno RL, Ehle HT: Driving after cerebral damage: A model with implications for evaluation. Am J Occup Ther 46:324–332, 1992.

Galski T, Ehle HT, Bruno R: An assessment of measures to predict the outcome of driving evaluations in patients with cerebral damage. Am J Occup Ther 44:709–713, 1990.

Gastaut H, Broughton R: A clinical and polygraphic study of episodic phenomena during sleep, in Wortis J (ed). Recent

Advances in Biological Psychology. New York: Plenum Press, 1965, pp. 197–223.

George CFP, Smiley A: Sleep apnea and automobile crashes. Sleep 22:790–795, 1999.

Gibson JJ: The Ecological Approach to Visual Perception. Boston: Houghton Mifflin, 1979.

Goldberg D. GHQ: The Selection of Psychiatric Illness by Questionnaire. London: Oxford University Press, 1972.

Graybiel A, Knepton J: Sopite syndrome: A sometimes sole manifestation of motion sickness. Aviat Space Environ Med 47:873–882, 1976.

Grayson GB: Theories and models in traffic psychology: A contrary view, in Rothengatter T, Carbonnell Vaya E (eds): Traffic and Transport Psychology: Theory and Application. Amsterdam/New York: Elsevier, 1997, pp. 93–96.

Gronwall DMA: Paced Auditory Serial-Addition Task: A measure of recovery from concussion. Percept Mot Skills 44:367–373, 1977.

Guerrier JH, Manivannan P, Pacheco A, et al: The relationship of age and cognitive characteristics of drivers to performance of driving tasks on an interactive driving simulator. Proceedings of the 39th Annual Meeting of the Human Factors and Ergonomics Society. San Diego: Human Factors and Ergonomics Society, 1995, pp. 172–176.

Haraldsson P-O, Carenfelt C, Diderichsen F, et al: Clinical symptoms of sleep apnea syndrome and automobile accidents. J Oto-Rhino-Laryngol Related Specialties 52:57–62, 1990.

Harrison Y, Horne JA: Occurrence of "microsleeps" during daytime sleep onset in normal subjects. Electro-encephalogr Clin Neurophysiol 98:411–416, 1996.

Hauser RA, Gauger L, Anderson WM, Zesiewicz TA: Pramipexole-induced somnolence and episodes of daytime sleep. Mov Disord 15:658–663, 2000.

Heinrich HW, Petersen D, Roos N: Industrial Accident Prevention. New York: McGraw-Hill, 1980.

Hills BL: Vision, visibility and driving. Perception 9:183–216, 1980.

Hoddes E, Zarcone V, Smythe H, et al: Quantification of sleepiness: A new approach. Psychophysiology 10:431–436, 1973.

Holzapfel H: Violence and the car. World Transport Policy and Practice 1:57–65, 1995.

Homan, CN, Wenzyl K, Suppan M, et al: Sleep attacks after acute administration of apomorphine. Mov Disord 15 (Suppl. 3): 108, 2000.

Horne JA, Reyner LA: Counteracting driver sleepiness: Defects of napping, caffeine, and placebo. Psychophysiology 33:306–309, 1996.

Horne JA, Reyner LA: Sleep related vehicle accidents. BMJ 310:565–567, 1995.

Horstmann S, Hess CW, Bassetti C, et al: Sleepiness-related accidents in sleep apnea patients. Sleep 23:383–389, 2000.

Huguenin RD: Do we need traffic psychology models?, in Rothengatter T, Carbonell-Vaya E (eds): Traffic and Transport Psychology: Theory and Application. Amsterdam/New York: Elsevier, 1997, pp. 31–52.

James W: The Principles of Psychology, Vol. I. New York: Holt, 1890, pp. 403–404.

Johansson K, Bogdanovic N, Kalimo H, et al: Alzheimer's disease and apolipoprotein E epsilon 4 allele in older drivers who died in automobile accidents. Lancet 349:1143–1144, 1997.

Johns MW. A new method for measuring daytime sleepiness: The Epworth Sleepiness Scale. Sleep 14:540–545, 1991.

Jonah BA. Sensation seeking and risky driving: A review and synthesis of the literature. Accid Anal Preven 29:651–665, 1997.

Jones TO, Kelly AH, Johnson DR. Half a century and a billion kilometres safely. Trans Soc Automotive Engineering 87:2271–2302, 1979.

Just MA, Carpenter PA, Keller TA, et al: Interdependence of nonoverlapping cortical systems in dual cognitive tasks. NeuroImage 14:417–428, 2001.

Kantowitz BH: Effective utilization of the in-vehicle information: Integrating attractions and distractions. Proceedings of Convergence 2000 International Congress on Transportation Electronics. Detroit, MI: Society of Automotive Engineers, 2000, pp. 43–49.

Kantowitz BH: Using microworlds to design intelligent interfaces that minimize driver distraction. Proceedings of the First International Driving Symposium on Human Factors in Driver Assessment, Training and Vehicle Design. Aspen, CO. Iowa City, IA: The University of Iowa, 2001, pp. 42–57.

Katz RT, Golden RS, Butter J, et al: Driving safely after brain damage: Follow up of twenty-two patients with matched controls. Arch Physical Med Rehab 71:133–137, 1990.

Kecklund G, Akerstedt T: Sleepiness in long distance truck driving: An ambulatory EEG study of night driving. Ergonomics 36:1007–1017, 1993.

Korteling JE: Perception-response speed and driving capabilities in brain-damaged and older drivers. Hum Factors 32:95–108, 1990.

Kramer AF, Cassavaugh ND, Irwin DE, Peterson MS: Influence of single and multiple onset distractors on visual search for singleton targets. Percep Psychophysics 63:952–968, 2001.

Kumar R, Powell B, Tani N, et al: Perceptual dysfunction in hemiplegia and automobile driving. Gerontologist 31:807–810, 1991.

Lamers CTJ, Ramaekers JG: Visual search and urban city driving under the influence of marijuana and alcohol. Hum Psychopharmacol Clin Exp 16:393–401, 2001.

Land M, Lee DN: Where we look when we steer. Nature 369:742–744, 1994.

Lang AE, Lozano AM: Parkinson's disease. First of two parts. N Engl J Med 339:1044–1053, 1998a.

Lang AE, Lozano AM: Parkinson's disease. Second of two parts. N Engl J Med 339:1130–1143, 1998b.

Laube I, Seeger R, Russi EW, et al: Accidents related to sleepiness: Review of medical causes and prevention with special reference to Switzerland. Schweizerische medizinische Wochenschrift. J Suisse de Medecine 128:1487–1499, 1998.

Leger D: The cost of sleep-related accidents: A report for the National Commission on Sleep Disorders Research. Sleep 17:84–93, 1994.

Lee TH, Dudley J: Drug effects on driving performance [letter]. Ann Intern Med 133:656–657, 2000.

Lings S, Dupont E: Driving with Parkinson's disease: A controlled laboratory investigation. Acta Neurolog Scand 86:33–39, 1992.

Lundberg C, Hakamies-Blomqvist L, Almkvist O, Johansson K: Impairments of some cognitive functions are common in crash-involved older drivers. Accid Anal Preven 30:371–377, 1998.

Lundberg C, Johannson K, Rizzo M, et al: Dementia in driving: An attempt at consensus. Alzheimer Dis Assoc Disord 11:28–37, 1997.

Lyznicki JM, Doege TC, Davis RM, et al: Sleepiness, driving, and motor vehicle crashes. Council on Scientific Affairs, American Medical Association. JAMA 279:1908–1913, 1998.

Madeley P, Hully JL, Wildgust H, Mindham, RH: Parkinson's disease and driving ability. J Neurol Neurosurg Psychiatr 53:580–582, 1990.

Maguire EA, Gadian DG, Johnsrude IS, et al: Navigation-related structural change in the hippocampi of taxi drivers. PNAS 97:4398–4403, 2000.

Mahelel D, Zaidel DM, Klein T: Drivers' decision process on termination of the green light. Accid Anal Preven 17:373–380, 1985.

Mangione CM, Lee PP, Gutierrez PR, et al: Development of the 25-item National Eye Institute Visual Function Questionnaire. Arch Ophthalmol 119:1050–1058, 2001.

Marottoli RA, Cooney LM, Wagner DR et al: Predictors of automobile crashes and moving violations among elderly drivers. Ann Intern Med 121:842–846, 1994.

Maycock G. Accident liability-the human perspective, in Rothengatter T, Carbonell-Vaya E (eds): Traffic and Transport Psychology: Theory and Application. Amsterdam/New York: Elsevier, 1997, pp. 65–76.

McMillen DL, Wells-Parker E: The effect of alcohol consumption on risk-taking while driving. Addict Behav 12:241–247, 1987.

Mestre DR: Dynamic evaluation of the useful field of view in driving. Proceedings of the First International Driving Symposium on Human Factors in Driving Assessment, Training, and Vehicle Design. Iowa City, IA: University of Iowa, 2001, pp. 234–239.

Miller M, Azrael D, Hemenway D, et al: "Road rage" in Arizona: Armed and dangerous. Accid Anal Preven 34:807–814, 2002.

Montastruc JL, Brefel-Courbon C, Senard JM, et al: Sudden sleep attacks and antiparkinsonian drugs: A pilot prospective pharmacoepidemiological study. Mov Disord 15 (Suppl. 3):130, 2000.

Nawrot M: Depth perception in driving: Alcohol intoxication, eye movement changes, and the disruption of motion parallax. Proceedings of the First International Driving Symposium on Human Factors in Driving Assessment, Training, and Vehicle Design. Iowa City, IA: University of Iowa, 2001, pp. 76–80.

NHTSA: National Highway Traffic Safety Administration Highway Safety Facts 2000. U.S. DOT, 2001.

Norman DA: Categorization of action slips. Psycholog Rev 88:1–15, 1981.

Norman DA, Shallice T: Attention to action: Willed and automatic control of behavior, in Davidson RJ, Schwartz GE, Shapiro D (eds): Consciousness and Self-regulation. New York: Plenum, Vol. 4, 1996, pp. 1–18.

Nouri FM, Tinson DJ, Lincoln NB: Cognitive ability and driving after stroke. Int Disabil Studies 9:110–115, 1987.

Noyes R: Motor vehicle accidents related to psychiatric impairment. Psychosomatics 26:569–580, 1985.

Ogilvie RD, Wilkinson RT, Allison S: The detection of sleep onset: Behavioral, physiological, and subjective convergence. Sleep 21:458–474, 1989.

Olanow CW, Schapira AH, Roth T: Waking up to sleep episodes in Parkinson's disease. Mov Disord 15:212–215, 2000.

O'Regan, JK, Rensink RA, Clark JJ: Change–blindness as a result of "mudsplashes." Nature 398:34, 1999.

Owsley C, Ball K, Sloane ME, et al: Visual/cognitive correlates of vehicle accidents in older drivers. Psychol Aging 6:403–415, 1991.

Paladini D: Sleep attacks in two Parkinson's disease patients taking ropinirole. Mov Disord 15 (Suppl. 3):130–131, 2000.

Palca J: Insights from broken brains. Science 248:812–814, 1990.

Parasuraman R: Varieties of Attention. Orlando, FL: Academic Press, 1984.

Parasuraman R, Nestor PG: Attention and driving skills in aging and Alzheimer's disease. Hum Factors 33:539–557, 1991.

Peli E, Peli D: Driving with confidence: A practical guide to driving with low vision. World Scientific Company, 2002.

Pelli DG, Robson JG, Wilkins AJ: The design of a new letter chart for measuring contrast sensitivity. Clin Vision Sci 2:187–199, 1988.

Perrottet T: Route 66 AD. New York: Random House, 2002, p. 141.

Ray WA, Thapa PB, Shorr RI: Medications and the older driver. Clin Geriatr Med 9:413–438, 1993.

Reason JT: Lapses of attention, in Parasuraman R, Davies R (eds): Varieties of Attention. New York: Academic Press, 1984, pp. 515–549.

Reger MA, Welsh RK, Watson GS, et al: The relationship between neuropsychological functioning and driving ability in dementia: A meta-analysis. Neuropsychology, 2003, in press.

Rensink RA, O'Regan JK, Clark JJ: To see or not to see: The need for attention to perceive changes in scenes. Psycholog Sci 8:368–373, 1997.

Rensink RA, O'Regan JK, Clark JJ: On the failure to detect changes in scenes across brief interruptions. Vis Cogn 7:127–145, 2000.

Reuben DB, Silliman RA, Traines M: The aging driver: Medicine, policy and ethics. J Am Geriatr Soc 36:1135–1142, 1988.

Reyner LA, Horne JA: Falling asleep whilst driving: Are drivers aware of prior sleepiness? Int J Legal Med 111:120–123, 1998.

Risser MR, Ware JC, Freeman FG: Driving simulation with EEG monitoring in normal and obstructive sleep apnea patients. Sleep 23:393–398, 2000.

Rizzo M, Dingus T: Driving in neurological disease. Neurologist 2:140–160, 1996.

Rizzo M, Hurtig R: Looking but not seeing: Attention, perception, and eye movements in simultanagnosia. Neurology 37:1642–1648, 1987.

Rizzo M, Nawrot M: Perception of movement and shape in Alzheimer's disease. Brain 121:2259–2270, 1998.

Rizzo M, Vecera SP: Psychoanatomical substrates of Bálint's syndrome. J Neurol Neurosurg Psychiatr 72:162–178, 2002.

Rizzo M, Akutsu H, Dawson J: Increased attentional blink after focal cerebral lesions. Neurology 57:795–800, 2001a.

Rizzo M, Anderson SW, Dawson J, et al: Visual attention impairments in Alzheimer's disease. Neurology 54:1954–1959, 2000a.

Rizzo M, Jermeland J, Stevenson J: Instrumented vehicles and driving simulators. Gerontechnology [Special Issue. Driving in Old Age: Use of Technology to Promote Independence] 2:291–296, 2002.

Rizzo M, Kellison IL: Eyes, brains, and autos. Blodi B, Ferris F (eds). Special Issue. Archives of Ophthalmology, in press.

Rizzo M, Lamers CTJ, Skaar N, et al: Perception of heading in abstinent MDMA and THC users. Vision Sciences Society. 3rd Annual Meeting, Sarasota, FL, May 10, 2003a.

Rizzo M, McGehee D, Dawson J, Anderson S: Simulated car crashes at intersections in drivers with Alzheimer's disease. Alzheimer Dis Assoc Disord 15:10–20, 2001b.

Rizzo M, McGehee DV, Dingus TA, Petersen AD: Development of an unobtrusively instrumented field research vehicle for objective assessments of driving performance, in Rothengatter J, Carbonell-Vaya E (eds): Traffic and Transport Psychology: Theory and Application. Oxford: Pergamon, 1997a, pp. 203–208.

Rizzo M, McGehee D, Jermeland J: Design and installation of a driving simulator in a hospital environment, in Brookhuis KA, DeWaard D, Weikert CM (eds): Human System Interaction: Education, Research and Application in the 21st Century. Maastricht, The Netherlands: Shaker Publishing, 2000b, pp. 69–77.

Rizzo M, Nawrot M, Zihl J: Motion and shape perception in cerebral akinetopsia. Brain 118:1105–1128, 1995.

Rizzo M, Raby M, McGehee DV, et al: Quantification of driving performance during an auditory-verbal mental processing load. Paper presented at the International Conference on Traffic and Transport Psychology (ICTTP), Berne, Switzerland, September 4–7, 2000c. (Also available on CD-ROM.)

Rizzo M, Reinach S, McGehee D, Dawson J: Simulated car crashes and crash predictors in drivers with Alzheimer disease. Arch Neurol 54:545–551, 1997b.

Rizzo M, Severson J, Cremer J, Price K: An abstract virtual environment tool to assess decision-making in impaired drivers. 2nd International Driving Symposium on Human Factors in Driving Assessment, Training, and Vehicle Design, Park City, UT, July 21–24, 2003b.

Rizzo M, Sheffield R, Stierman L: Demographic and driving performance factors in simulator adaptation syndrome. 2nd International Driving Symposium on Human Factors in Driver Assessment, Training, and Vehicle Design, Park City, UT, July 21–24, 2003c.

Rolls ET: The brain and emotion. Oxford, UK: Oxford University Press, 1999.

Rolls ET: The orbitofrontal cortex and reward. Cereb Cortex 10:284–294, 2000.

Rolls ET, Hornak J, Wade D, McGrath J: Emotion-related learning in patients with social and emotional changes associated with frontal lobe damage. J Neurol Neurosurg Psychiatr 57:1518–1524, 1994.

Russo M, Thorne D, Thomas M, et al: Sleep deprivation induced Bálint's syndrome (peripheral visual field neglect): A hypothesis for explaining driving simulator accidents in awake but sleepy drivers. Sleep 22 (Suppl. 1):327, 1999.

Ryan M, Slevin JT, Wells A: Non-ergot dopamine agonist-induced sleep attacks. Pharmacotherapy 20:724–726, 2000.

Schapira AH: Sleep attacks (sleep episodes) with pergolide. Lancet 355:1332–1333, 2000

Sekuler AB, Bennett PJ, Mamelak M: Effects of aging on the useful field of view. Exp Aging Res 26:103–20, 2000.

Simons DJ, Levin DT: Change blindness. Trends Cognitive Sci 1:261–267, 1997.

Siskind V. Does license disqualification reduce reoffence rates? Accid Anal Preven 28:519–524, 1996.

Sivak M: Society's aggression level as a predictor of traffic fatality rate. J Safety Res 14:93–99, 1983.

Skaar N, Anderson SW, Dawson J, Rizzo M: Automobile driving with severe amnesia. [abstract] Second International Driving Symposium on Human Factors in Driver Assessment, Training, and Vehicle Design, Park City, UT, July 21–24, 2003a.

Skaar N, Rizzo M, Stierman L: Traffic entry judgments by aging drivers. Proceedings of Driving Assessment 2003. Second International Driving Symposium on Human Factors in Driver Assessment, Training, and Vehicle Design, Park City, UT, July 21–24, 2003b.

Stalvey B, Owsley C, Sloane ME, Ball K: The Life Span Questionnaires: A measurement of the extent of mobility of older adults. J Appl Gerontol 18:479–498, 1999.

Stanney KM (ed): Handbook of Virtual Environments: Design, Implementation, and Applications. Mahwah, NJ: Lawrence Erlbaum Associates, 2002.

Strayer DL, Johnston WA: Driven to distraction: Dual-task studies of simulated driving and conversing on a cellular phone. Psycholog Sci 12:462–466, 2001.

Stroop JR: Studies of interference in serial verbal reaction. J Exp Psychol 18:643–662, 1935.

Stuss DT, Gow CA, Hetherington CR: "No longer Gage": Frontal lobe dysfunction and emotional changes. J Consult Clin Psychol 60:349–359, 1992.

Stutts J, Feaganes J, Rodgman E, et al: Distractions in everyday driving. June, 2003. [University of North Carolina/Chapel Hill Highway Safety Research Center]. Prepared for AAA Foundation for Traffic Safety, Washington DC, June 2003.

Stutts JC, Wilkins JW, Vaughn BV: Why do people have drowsy driving crashes? Input from drivers who just did. Washington, DC: AAA Foundation for Traffic Safety. http://www.aaafts.org/text/research/rsrchcat.htm (accessed October 9, 1999).

Suchman EA: Accidents and social deviance. J Health Soc Behav 11:4–15, 1970.

Tant MLM, Brouwer WH, Cornelissen FW, Kooijman AC: Driving and visuospatial performance in people with hemianopia. Neuropyschol Rehab 12:419–437, 2002.

Theeuwes J, Kramer A, Hahn S, et al: Influence of attentional capture on eye movement control. J Exp Psychol Hum Percept Perform 25:1595–1608, 1999.

Thomas I: Spatial data aggregation: Exploratory analysis of road accidents. Accid Anal Preven 28:251–264, 1996.

Throne D, Thomas M, Russo M, et al: Performance on a driving-simulator divided attention task during one week of restricted nightly sleep. Sleep 22 (Suppl. 1): 301, 1999.

Tranel D, Anderson SW, Benton AL: Development of the concept of executive functions and its relationship to the frontal lobes, in Boller F, Grafman J (eds): Handbook of Neuropsychology, Vol. 9. New York: Elsevier, 1994, pp. 125–148.

Treat JR: A study of precrash factors involved in traffic accidents. HRSI Res Rev 10:1–35, 1980.

Trick G: Beyond visual acuity: New and complementary tests of visual function, in Barton JJS, Rizzo M (eds): Neuro-ophthalmology: Vision and Brain. Neurologic Clinics of North America series. Philadelphia: Saunders, 2003.

Tsuang MT, Boor M, Fleming AA: Psychiatric aspects of traffic accidents. Am J Psychiatr 142:538–546, 1985.

Uc EY, Smothers JL, Shi Q, Rizzo M: Driver navigation and safety errors in Alzheimer's disease and stroke. [abstract] Second International Driving Symposium on Human Factors in Driver Assessment, Training, and Vehicle Design, Park City UT, July 21–24, 2003.

Underwood M: The older driver: Clinical assessment and injury prevention. Arch Intern Med 152:735–740, 1992.

Van Zomeren AH, Brouwer WH, Minderhoud JM: Acquired brain damage and driving: A review. Arch Phys Med Rehab 68:697–705, 1987.

Vecera SP, Luck SJ: Attention, in Ramachandran VS (ed): Encyclopedia of the Human Brain, Vol. 1. San Diego: Academic Press, 2002, pp. 269–284.

Waller PF: The older driver. Hum Factors 33:499–505, 1991.

Warren WH, Hannon DJ: Direction of self-motion is perceived from optical flow. Nature 336:162–163, 1988.

Warren WH, Mestre DR, Blackwell AW, et al: Perception of circular heading from optical flow. J Exp Psychol Hum Percept Perform 17:28–43, 1991.

Weiler JM, Bloomfield JR, Woodworth GG, et al: Effects of fexofenadine, diphenhydramine, and alcohol on driving performance. Ann Intern Med 132:354–363, 2000.

Wickens CD: Engineering, psychology and human performance, ed 2. New York: HarperCollins, 1992, pp. 412–444.

Wierwille WW, Hulse MC, Fischer TJ, et al: Effects of variation in driving task attentional demand on in-car navigation system usage. Contract Report. Virginia Polytechnic Institute and State University. Warren, MI: General Motors Research Laboratories, 1988.

Wilde GJS: The theory of risk homeostasis: Implications for safety and health. Risk Analysis 2:249–258, 1982.

Wood JM, Owens D, Woolf MI, Owens J: Predicting night-time visibility while driving. [abstract]. J Vis 2:331a, 2002.

Young T, Palta M, Dempsey J, et al: The occurrence of sleep-disordered breathing among middle-aged adults. N Engl J Med 328:1230–1235, 1993.

Zuckerman M: The psychobiological model for impulsive unsocialized sensation seeking: A comparative approach. Neuropsychobiology 34:125–129, 1996.

III

Disorders of Higher Brain Functions

Attention: Normal and Disordered Processes

Shaun P. Vecera

Matthew Rizzo

Attention

Biased competition model

Executive control

Extinction

Frontal lobe

Neglect

Object-based attention

Parietal lobe

INTRODUCTION

The brain receives thousands of sensory inputs from the environment at every moment and only some are relevant to current behavior. For example, the location and speed of an approaching automobile are relevant inputs for the task of safe driving, but the song on the radio is not. Because the brain does not have the capacity to process all inputs simultaneously, processes exist that select relevant inputs (the approaching car) and filter out others (the song on the radio). These processes collectively are referred to as "attention."

Attentional selection has been studied intensively by both the cognitive and brain sciences (see Pashler, 1998, and Luck & Vecera, 2002, for recent reviews; also see Vecera & Luck, 2002). Early research assumed that attention is a unitary process, but current evidence suggests that there are multiple forms of attentional selection (Allport, 1993). This chapter addresses major neuropsychological syndromes and reviews several etiologies for these impairments, consistent with the view of multiple attentional processes. We begin with a brief overview of normal attentional processes.

NORMAL ATTENTIONAL PROCESSES: A BRIEF REVIEW AND FRAMEWORK

Behavioral neurologists and neuropsychologists should understand the normal operation of attentional selection. Appreciating how different attention processes are studied can help guide assessments in patients with brain damage. Knowing which attentional process or subprocess is disrupted may be useful for developing caregiving strategies and rehabilitation. In reviewing the cognitive psychology of attention, we focus on four major types of attentional selection: spatial attention, object-based attention, working memory-level attention, and executive attention. For each process, we review the methods for studying attention and discuss key results from behavioral studies of normal populations. Before discussing the types of attentional selection, we must address two fundamental questions: How is "attention" defined? and under what circumstances is attention required?

Task-Defined and Process-Defined Attention

We often speak of "paying attention" to something or someone, yet the term attention is difficult to define because it has many intuitive, folk-psychological definitions. In the psychological literature, "attention" often is used in reference to *tasks* that require attention (Luck & Vecera, 2002). Suppose an observer views a blue square and a red circle and must report the shape of the red item (i.e., report "circle"). This task requires attention; the observer must select one item (the red stimulus) over another (the blue stimulus). Task-defined attention, however, tells nothing about mechanisms or processes that permit the selection to occur. We can develop a more precise mechanistic, or *process-oriented,* definition of attention, in line with William James (1890), who defined attention as "the taking possession by the mind, in clear and vivid form, of one out of what seem several simultaneously possible objects or trains of thought.... It implies withdrawal from some things in order to deal effectively with others...." (pp. 381–382). This definition underscores that attention operates by restricting processing to some items over others and makes an attended item mentally more salient than unattended items. Because we are interested in the neural mechanisms of attentional selection, we rely on a process-oriented definition of attention and consider mechanisms that allow observers to select one stimulus over others.

When is attention necessary? Consider the two displays shown in Figure 10-1 in which observers are asked to search for a black vertical bar. In Figure 10-1*A*, this search is efficient—observers readily report there is a black bar present: Search time is independent of the number of items in the display ("set size"), and reaction time (RT) does not increase as more white bars ("distractors") are added. However, in Figure 10-1*B*, the search for a black vertical bar is inefficient: RTs increase linearly as the set size increases (i.e., distractors are added to the display). Some visual searches are efficient and rely on attention little, if at all, whereas other visual searches are inefficient and rely on attention to examine each stimulus (see Wolfe, 1998, for a review of visual search). Current evidence (see Luck & Vecera, 2002, for a detailed discussion) indicates that several factors determine when attention is necessary in such situations.

1. Attention may be required when an observer's cognitive resources are insufficient for processing stimuli. Under this *resource-allocation view* (Kahneman, 1973), attention restricts processing to allow limited cognitive resources to be allocated to the attended item. The inefficient search in Figure 10-1*B* requires greater cognitive resources than the efficient search in Figure 10-1*A*, making the inefficient search depend on attention. Attention may also be needed to regulate the inputs to a limited working memory system. When stimuli exceed the capacity of working memory, attention may exclude some items from the working memory system.

2. Attention may reduce an observer's uncertainty in making judgments about a stimulus. Under this *decision-noise account* (Pashler, 1998), optimal performance decreases as the number of stimuli increases because each stimulus contains some uncertainty (or noise). Attention reduces the noise associated with an attended stimulus. Attention may also reduce noise at a perceptual level by enhancing the signal-to-noise ratio of attended items. This *sensory-gain account* hypothesizes that attention enhances the perception of attended items compared to unattended items.

3. Attention may be needed to bind together the features of an object (Treisman, 1996). Consider again a display that contains a red circle and a blue square. How does the visual system bind the features "red" and "circle" and avoid the error of binding "red" to "square"? One solution to this *binding problem* is to focus attention on a single stimulus, thereby gluing or binding the features together.

The situations that require attention remain a topic of active research. Assuming that there are multiple attention systems, certain forms of attention may be necessary in some situations but not others.

Major Forms of Attention

Having considered the term attention and circumstances when attention operates, we now discuss the

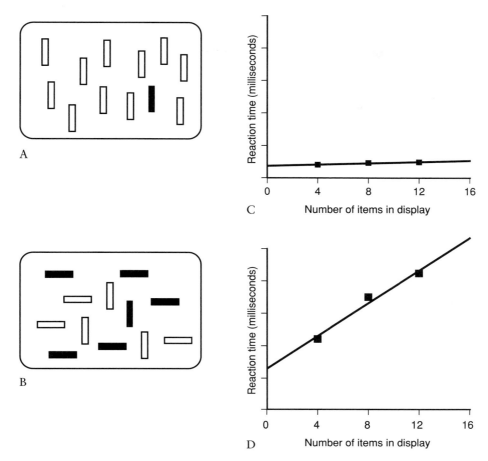

FIGURE 10-1. (*A* and *B*) Visual search displays and (*C* and *D*) typical results from a visual search task. Panel *C* shows an efficient search for a target that differs from distractors on a single feature dimension, such as color (see panel *A*). Panel *D* shows an inefficient search for a target that differs from distractors on two feature dimensions (see panel *B*).

main forms of attention and procedures for studying them. We consider (1) spatial attention, in which stimuli are selected based on their position in space; (2) object-based attention, in which stimuli are selected based on their identity; (3) attentional selection in visual working memory, in which attention selects items that will be remembered; and (4) executive attention, in which attention is involved in choosing the task or behavior that an observer will perform.

Spatial Attention

Perhaps the most complete understanding of attention comes from the visuospatial domain, in which visual stimuli at specific locations are selected for further processing. Spatial attention is closely associated with early processing, before stimulus identity is known. Attention is directed to a location in visual space and an item there is identified, possibly by enhancing the perception or binding the features of that item.

Spatial attention has mainly been studied with visual search paradigms and cueing paradigms. In typical cueing paradigms, a stimulus or instruction precedes a target stimulus. In Posner's (1980) widely used task (Fig. 10-2) each trial begins with a cue intended to orient an observer's attention to one of several locations. The cue can be a peripheral flicker (Fig. 10-2*A*) at the peripheral location where a target may appear or a centrally presented symbol such as an arrow (Fig. 10-2*B*) that points to the location where a target may appear. After a delay, a target is presented and the observer indicates that he or she detects the target (e.g., by pressing a button as soon as the target appears) or discriminates among several targets (e.g., reporting whether the target was a T or an L). On "valid" trials the cue correctly predicts the target's location; on "invalid" trials the cue is misleading. Some experiments also include neutral trials (in which all locations or no locations are cued), providing no information about the target's location. Observers typically respond fastest to valid trials,

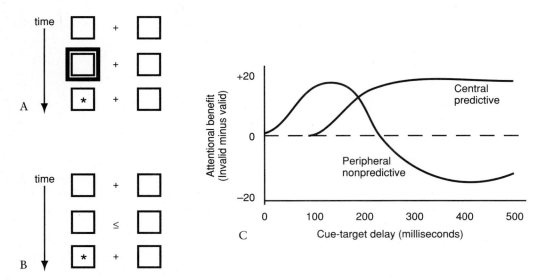

FIGURE 10-2. The order of events in the spatial cuing task. Observers are asked to detect the appearance of a target that has been validly or invalidly precued. (*A*) Peripheral precue that automatically summons spatial attention to the cued region. (*B*) Central, symbolic precue that can be used to voluntarily shift spatial attention to the cued region. (*C*) Typical results from spatial cuing studies. The graph plots the difference between response times to invalid and valid trials. Nonpredictive peripheral precues, in which valid and invalid trials are equally likely, result in attentional benefits initially, followed by a period of inhibition termed "inhibition of return." Predictive central precues require more time to produce an attentional benefit, and these cues may not produce inhibition of return in some circumstances.

slowest to invalid trials, and at some intermediate level to neutral trials (Fig. 10-2C).

To ensure they are studying effects of spatial attention shifts and not eye fixation position changes, many researchers use combined cue and target durations of less than 200 msec. This minimizes the chance of making eye movements to a cued location because it takes at least 200 msec to program and execute a saccadic eye movement to a cued location.

Peripheral and central cues control attention differently (Jonides, 1981). Observers cannot ignore peripheral cues, which appear to attract attention to the cued location automatically, but they can ignore these central cues if instructed to do so. Peripheral cues also operate faster than central cues; the difference between valid and invalid trials emerges sooner with peripheral cues than with central cues. Studies that use central, symbolic cues tend to present more valid trials than invalid trials to encourage observers to attend to the cued location. For example, 75% of the trials may be valid and 25% invalid. In contrast, peripheral cues will summon attention to the cued location even if valid and invalid trials occur equally (50% valid trials and 50% invalid trials).

Subjects usually respond faster to valid trials than invalid trials, but this pattern is sometimes reversed. In studies using unpredictive peripheral cues (50% valid and 50% invalid), observers respond faster to valid trials than invalid trials when the interval between the cue and target is less than 200 msec. As the interval exceeds 200 msec, observers respond faster to targets at the uncued location (invalid trials). This effect is called inhibition of return (Posner & Cohen, 1984), and one hypothesis is that inhibition of return prevents attention from returning to a recently attended location.

A second paradigm used to investigate spatial selection is the visual search paradigm (see Fig. 10-1). Visual search is the act of looking for a visual target among distractors (e.g., finding a friend's face in a crowd). In a typical visual search task, observers are asked to search for a particular target amid a field of distractors. The number of distractors—the set size—is varied across trials, and the RT is measured as a function of the set size. As noted earlier, efficient visual search is characterized by search functions with shallow slopes (see Fig. 10-1A) and inefficient search with steep slopes (see Fig. 10-1B). Although early studies on visual search equated shallow search functions with parallel processing and steep search functions with serial, attentive processing (Treisman & Gelade, 1980), this parallel/serial distinction has fallen out of favor because some serial-looking results can arise from parallel processing mechanisms. For example, serial-looking search, in which responses become slower as more items are added to a display, can be produced from a limited-capacity parallel search mechanism. In a limited-capacity parallel search, multiple items can be processed in parallel, but because this search has a limited capacity, searching through multiple items will take longer than searching through fewer items. For this reason, most theorists discuss efficiency of visual search, with efficient searches being characterized by shallow search functions (slopes <10 msec/item) and inefficient searches being characterized by steep search functions (slopes >20 msec/item; Wolfe, 1998).

Several studies suggest that visual search involves spatial attention. Prinzmetal and colleagues (1986) showed that adding cues to a visual search task could improve target identification on valid trials compared to invalid trials. Thus, knowing the spatial region of a target helps observers correctly identify a target. A more recent study showed that a visual search display can influence how quickly an observer responds to a spatial probe (Kim & Cave, 1995). In this task, observers performed a visual search task and determined if a target was present or absent from a display. After some of the visual search displays, a small dot appeared and observers had to press a button as soon as they detected this dot. Observers were fastest to detect the dot when it appeared in the same location as the target in the visual search task, suggesting that spatial attention had

been directed to the target location, which then allowed the subsequent dot to be detected rapidly.

Object-Based Attention

Visual attention also can select entire objects. In some situations, object selection can occur irrespective of where the object appears, suggesting that object and spatial attention involve separate processes (see Vecera, 2000, for an overview). Studies of object-based attention must be cautious to rule out selection by spatial attention, because objects necessarily occupy locations. Consequently, most studies of object attention have minimized or held constant the spatial separation between objects.

Several object-based attention paradigms have been developed; we discuss two of the most widely used tasks. In the object attribute task developed by Duncan (1984; Vecera & Farah, 1994), observers see two overlapping objects, a box and a line (Fig. 10-3A). Each object has two features: The box is short or tall and has a gap on the left or right side, and the line is dotted or dashed and tilted to the left or right. A box/line stimulus is presented very briefly (<100 msec) and followed by a pattern mask that disrupts perception. Observers are

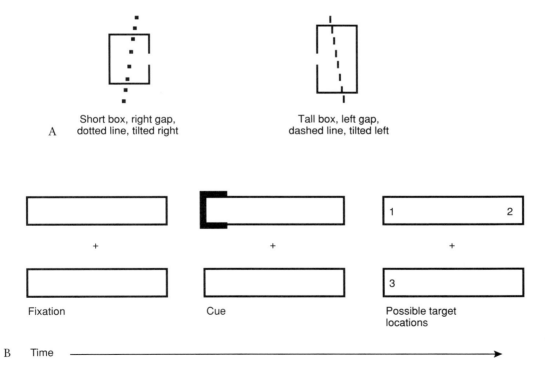

FIGURE 10-3. Stimuli used to study object-based attention. (*A*) Box and line stimuli developed by Duncan (1984). Participants report features from the same object (e.g., box height and side of gap) or from different objects (e.g., box height and line tilt). (*B*) Object cuing procedure developed by Egly and colleagues (1994). Following a precue, a target appears at the cued location (1), at an uncued location in the cued object (2), or at an uncued location in the uncued object (3). Response times are faster to targets that appear in the cued object (location 2) than in the uncued object (location 3), although these two locations are the same spatial distance from the cued region.

instructed to report two of four features, and the features can come from the same object (e.g., box height and side of gap) or from different objects (e.g., box height and tilt of line). Typically, observers are more accurate reporting features when they come from the same object than when they come from different objects.

A second paradigm for studying object-based attention resembles Posner's cueing task discussed earlier (Egly et al., 1994). In the object cueing task, attention is directed within an object or across objects. Observers view two rectangles, as depicted in Figure 10-3B. An end of one of the rectangles is cued with a brief flash, followed by a target that requires a response. The target usually appears at the cued location (a valid trial), but sometimes it appears at an uncued location within either the cued object or uncued object. Both uncued locations are the same spatial distance from the cued region and the target is equally unlikely to appear at either of them, yet observers are faster to respond to targets appearing in the uncued end of the cued rectangle than in the uncued rectangle. Thus, attention appears to cover the entire cued rectangle even though only one end was cued.

Although object attention may rely on mechanisms separate from spatial attention, some forms of object selection may involve a modified form of spatial attention. Some object selection appears to involve attending to perceptual objects that are defined in a spatial reference frame—a "grouped array" (Vecera & Farah, 1994). The grouped array is a spatial map in which locations and features are grouped according to Gestalt principles such as similarity (e.g., features that are the same color grouped together) or closure (e.g., features that form closed shapes grouped together). Selection from a grouped array representation involves attending to the *locations* of items that are grouped together, not the objects that occupy those locations. Some studies have demonstrated selection from a "grouped array" by manipulating both grouping principles and spatial position in the object cueing task discussed above (Vecera, 1994). Both grouping principles and spatial position influence attentional selection; specifically, moving the rectangles (Fig. 10-3B) closer to one another reduces the cost of switching attention from the cued rectangle to the uncued rectangle. Thus, some forms of "object-based attention" may occur within a spatially formatted representation. Other findings, however, suggest that objects can be selected irrespective of spatial position (Vecera & Farah, 1994).

Attention and Visual Working Memory

Both spatial and object attention appear to involve selection of perceptual characteristics that do not persist. Visual working memory provides a storage mechanism for holding three to four objects in a more durable form over longer time periods (Vogel et al., 2001). Recent research suggests that attention helps information enter into visual working memory, acting as a protective gate that prevents visual working memory from becoming overloaded with more information than can be remembered.

The effect of attention on visual working memory is apparent in a phenomenon known as the "attentional blink." In the attentional blink task, shown in Figure 10-4A, observers view a stream of approximately 20 stimuli presented one at a time at a rate of about 10 stimuli per second; observers are asked to detect two targets from this stream (Raymond et al., 1992). For example, the first target (T1) may be a number that observers must classify as even or odd, and the second target (T2) could be a letter that observers must classify as a consonant or vowel. Observers make both responses at the end of the stimulus stream. Observers often fail to identify T2 if it appears as the third or fourth item after T1; if T2 appears somewhat later (as the fifth or sixth item after T1), observers are more accurate at reporting its identity. The temporary impairment in identifying T2 is referred to as the "attentional blink," because, as in an eyeblink, there is a brief period during which targets cannot be detected. Typical results from an attentional blink task are shown in Figure 10-4B. Note that the recognition of T2 depends on occurrence of T1; if no T1 target appears, observers are accurate at reporting T2, and there is no attentional blink.

The attentional blink appears to be caused by a failure to store T2 in visual working memory. Attention selects T1 so that it can be reported at the end of the stream, and T1 is entered into visual memory. When there are a large number of items (i.e., 5 or 6) between T1 and T2, T1 has been attended completely and stored into memory, leaving attention ready to select T2 and assist this item into memory. Both T1 and T2 can be reported accurately because both were stored in visual working memory. However, when there are fewer items (i.e., 2 or 3) between T1 and T2, the T2 item appears before the processing of T1 is complete. Consequently, T2 receives little attention and is not entered into memory as durably as T1, which results in poor accuracy of the T2 item.

Executive Attention and Task Set

The last form of attentional selection that we discuss is the selection of one task from among many possible tasks that can be performed (Allport et al., 1994; Rogers & Monsell, 1995). In the procedures discussed above, observers perform the same attention task throughout, yet in real life we often perform different tasks concurrently or in series, such as rehearsing a phone number that was looked up, dialing the phone number, and conversing with the person we have just

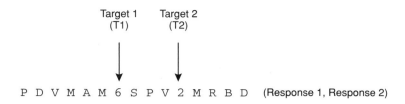

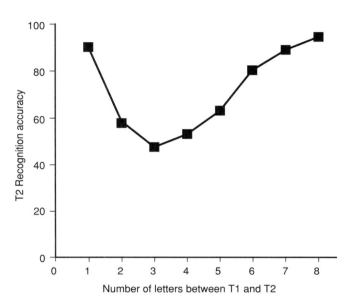

FIGURE 10-4. Attentional blink paradigm and typical results from this paradigm. The top panel shows a rapid serial visual presentation (RSVP) stream of letters and numbers. Observers are asked to identify the numbers and to report them at the end of the stream. The bottom panel shows a typical attentional blink result. After identifying the first target digit (T1), observers fail to correctly identify the second target digit (T2) when it appears shortly after T1.

called. Recent studies have examined the ability to voluntarily switch the *task set*, the task that an observer is prepared to perform.

The general finding from different task-set paradigms is that performance is impaired dramatically when multiple tasks are performed concurrently or alternated in succession. These attentional costs occur even when the individual tasks are highly practiced. Attentional processes may be involved in selecting an individual task for current behavior, with a cost in performance arising when attention is divided or switched between different tasks. One task that demonstrates the influence of one task on another is the Stroop task, in which two different tasks are performed in different blocks of trials. In this task, observers view color words (e.g., the words RED or BLUE) printed in different ink colors. The words are written either in a compatible ink color (RED printed in red ink) or in incompatible colors (RED printed in blue ink). Observers are asked to read the color name or name its ink color. Observers read words with little effect of ink color, perhaps because reading words is more practiced than naming colors. They are just as fast to read color words printed in a compatible as in an incompatible ink color. In contrast, naming the color ink is highly influenced by the color word, that is, observers are slower to name ink colors used to print an incompatible word (RED printed in blue ink) than ink colors used to print a compatible word (RED printed in red ink).

A difficulty in using the Stroop task to study task-based attention is that the word-reading task is much easier than the color-naming task. Also, the Stroop task may involve more than task-based attention. Word information influences the color-naming task, yet this is not due to alternating between the two tasks because observers perform only one task at a time. Rogers and Monsell (1995) developed a task-switching paradigm to investigate time required to switch from one task to another. They asked subjects to report whether (1) a digit was even or odd and (2) a letter was a consonant or vowel. Subjects performed each task on two consecutive trials, then switched between tasks, in a predictable alternating sequence. Comparison of RTs between trials in the same-task condition and between different tasks showed a cost of task-switching that persisted even when the time lag between the two different tasks was as much as 1200 msec. Evidently task set-switching does not occur automatically and requires time, effort, and higher cognitive control, even for simple tasks.

Putting the Pieces Together: A General Framework for Attentional Selection

Although the various forms of attentional selection reviewed above have not been integrated into a single theory of attention, they can be fit into a coherent framework for explaining different attentional phenomena. This general approach involves multiple constraint satisfaction performed by artificial neural network models. There are several specific network models of attention (Mozer & Sitton, 1998), and although each model simulates different attentional phenomena, the models all use similar computational processes.

Computational models can help explain different attentional phenomena, including spatial attention and object-based attention (Mozer & Sitton, 1998; Mozer, 2002). Attentional phenomena may be construed as arising from bottom-up (data-driven) information from the external world and top-down (goal-driven) information within an observer. Bottom-up information would involve spatial cues or the presence of a stimulus array in a visual search task. Top-down information would involve an observer's knowledge of a cue's usefulness or the target that an observer is searching for in a visual search task. In computational models, the control parameters of attention (bottom up or top down) can be specified formally and explicitly. These two sources of information each can control attentional selection.

A similar view of attention also has been presented by theories that do not involve computational models, such as "biased competition" accounts of visual search (Desimone & Duncan, 1995) and object-based attention (Vecera, 2000). In a biased competition account, visual stimuli provide bottom-up inputs that compete with each other for attention. An observer's goals—such as the target that is being searched for—provide the top-down control of attention. The top-down inputs can bias processing to favor one of the bottom-up inputs over the others. The competition among items is biased by a top-down signal, hence the name "biased competition."

A biased competition account of attention may help explain how attentional selection occurs, such as knowing if an item is selected based on bottom-up or top-down information. The biased competition framework also may explain effects of brain damage on attentional processes; that is, does the damage disrupt bottom-up or top-down control of attention, or both? This general view guides the discussion and interpretation of different disorders of attention.

DISORDERS OF SPATIAL ATTENTION

As in neurologically normal participants, most studies of attention in individuals with brain damage have focused on spatial attention. Because behavioral neurology and neuropsychology have benefited from theoretical analyses of attention and vice versa, our discussion of behavioral disturbances will emphasize what neuropsychology can contribute to cognitive

theory and how cognitive theory can assist clinical practice.

The Parietal Lobes, Neglect, and Extinction

Multiple cortical and subcortical areas process spatial attention, and, of these, the posterior parietal region may have been studied most extensively. Unilateral damage to the human parietal lobe results in a profound syndrome referred to as neglect or hemineglect (e.g., Bisiach & Vallar, 1988; Heilman et al., 1993; Rafal & Robertson, 1995; Heilman et al., 2000; Rafal, 2000). Because neglect and extinction most often follow right parietal damage, clinical symptoms are most evident for the left side of extrapersonal space or the left side of the patient (also known as left hemineglect). Patients fail to attend to stimuli falling on the hemispace opposite to the lesion (the contralesional side) and may fail to acknowledge a person sitting on the left, eat food on the left half of the plate, read words on the left half of a page, and make head or eye movements to the left. In hemineglect, failure to respond to stimuli in the fields opposite the lesion is not due to sensory deficits (e.g., a visual scotoma or hemianopia). A left-sided hemiparesis may be present, but this needs to be distinguished from motor inattention associated with hemineglect syndrome. Neglect patients can be contrasted with patients who have sensory-level impairments. Patients with sensory disturbances alone are aware of their defects and will orient to a contralesional hemifield stimulus to compensate for their impairment. However, patients with hemineglect are generally unaware of their deficit and if confronted with a defect on the impaired side (such as a hemiparesis) may even deny it, a phenomenon known as anosognosia.

Auditory testing can sometimes distinguish neglect from sensory deficits (Heilman et al., 2000). A patient with neglect may not notice sounds from the contralesional side of space, even though localized sounds reach both ears and afferent projections in the auditory system are bilateral (i.e., each ear projects to both hemispheres). In a neglect patient, failure to notice a contralesional sound would not be produced by a peripheral sensory impairment. A patient with a peripheral auditory sensory deficit would remain able to detect sounds localized to either side of space because the sound could be carried to both hemispheres by the intact ear's projections.

In addition to the attentional deficits observed in neglect and extinction patients, these patients can also present with motor neglect. In motor neglect, the patient might not move a contralesional limb, although the patient has normal strength in this limb (Heilman et al., 2000). Because motor neglect could be produced by damage to lower-level motor pathways, it can be difficult to distinguish motor neglect from a general hemiparesis. Motor extinction is more easily distinguished from lower-level impairments. In motor extinction, the patient can move a contralesional limb when the ipsilesional limb is stationary, but the contralesional limb is not moved when the ipsilesional limb is moved (Heilman et al., 2000). The co-occurrence of attentional neglect and extinction with motor neglect and extinction suggests that attentional and motoric processes may share neural mechanisms.

Neglect typically occurs immediately after damage to the parietal region, although attentional impairments can arise after damage to primary visual cortex (Rizzo & Robin, 1996). As a patient recovers and the neglect becomes less severe, patients can process a single stimulus presented in the contralesional visual field. However, they may show another disorder, extinction, in which they extinguish or fail to notice the stimulus in the contralesional field when two stimuli are presented simultaneously in both visual fields. In other words, patients with extinction exhibit neglect of contralesional stimuli only in the presence of ipsilateral stimuli. Of course, damage to the parietal cortices may produce a variety of visual perceptual disturbances (such as akinetopsia and Bálint syndrome; see Chapter 12) and cognitive disturbances (such as aphasia with damage to the left hemisphere; see Chapter 17), but we focus here only on the attentional impairments of neglect and extinction.

Neglect and extinction can be easily diagnosed at the bedside or clinic. The patient is asked to fixate the examiner's nose and to indicate (verbally or by pointing) which field contains the examiner's wiggling fingers. Patients with neglect fail to report on single stimuli in the aberrant field, whereas those with extinction fail to detect targets in the aberrant field with double simultaneous stimulation (finger wiggling) in both hemifields. However, even a patient with extinction may have difficulty detecting multiple stimuli presented in the aberrant field, resembling the perceptual defect in simultanagnosia, a full field defect of simultaneous perception often associated with bilateral parietal lobe lesions (see Chapter 12).

Neglect and extinction are also diagnosed using a variety of widely used paper-and-pencil tasks (Rafal & Robertson, 1995; Heilman et al., 2000; Rafal, 2000). Simple copying tasks (Fig. 10-5) show that these patients neglect features on the contralesional side of space (and on the contralesional side of objects). In line bisection, patients are asked to divide a horizontal line in half. Patients with hemispatial neglect often bisect the line to the right of center, presumably because they do not attend to the left-most portion of the line. In object cancellation, patients view a cluttered display containing several objects (e.g., lines, letters, geometric shapes, etc.) and are asked to cross out (i.e., cancel) all the

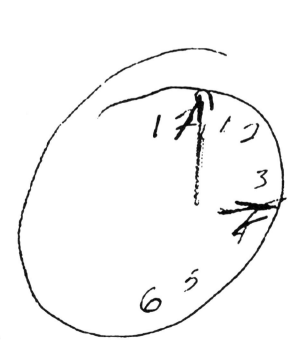

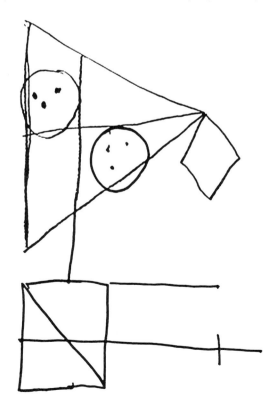

A

B

FIGURE 10-5. Sample results from patients with parietal damage that demonstrate the contralesional impairment in copying geometric stimuli or drawing objects from memory. (*A*) Defective drawing from memory of a clock omits numbers on the left. (*B*) Failure to copy the left half of the Rey Complex Figure.

objects in the display. Again, patients with damage to the right parietal area will fail to detect objects in the left visual field, and the objects are not cancelled by the patient. Severely affected patients may fail to detect their errors on visual inspection. Patients with visual loss alone (e.g., homonymous hemianopia) do not make these types of errors as long as gaze and head movements are not restricted and viewing time is longer than a few seconds.

Insights into the attentional impairments in neglect have come from studies using attentional paradigms discussed above. Posner and colleagues (1984) were among the first to study patients with damage to the parietal lobe using the guidance of an explicit cognitive theory of attention. Using Posner's spatial cueing task, Posner and coworkers (1984) found asymmetry in attentional orienting in parietal-damaged patients, who were slower to detect invalidly cued targets presented in the contralesional field. That is, a patient with right parietal damage was slower to detect a target in the left field following a cue in the right field, than to detect a target in the right field following a cue in the left field. (These patients could detect validly cued targets appearing in each visual hemifield, although RTs may be longer to targets in the contralesional field.)

Based on this response asymmetry, Posner and colleagues (1984) suggested that the parietal lobes allow disengagement of attention and that right parietal lesions cause a "disengage deficit," which hinders disengagement from the ipsilesional visual field. Thus, when a cue appears in the ipsilesional field and a target follows in the contralesional field, a right parietal patient would have difficulties detecting the target.

An odd aspect of the disengage deficit hypothesis is that each parietal lobe must mediate disengagement of attention from the ipsilesional field; that is, the right parietal lobe is needed for disengaging from the right visual field, a counterintuitive mechanism given the crossed visual pathways and the predominant left-sided deficit following right parietal damage. Cohen and colleagues (1994) presented a neural network model as an alternative explanation of the disengage deficit. In their model, neural representations of the visual hemifields compete with each other for attentional selection. If the representation of the left field was damaged, it competed less effectively with the representation of the right field. As a consequence, when attention is directed to the right (good) field, a target appearing in the left (damaged) field is at a competitive disadvantage. Thus, detecting the invalidly cued target that appeared in the left field was difficult. In contrast, when attention is directed to the disordered left field, a target appearing in the intact right field could compete effectively for attention, allowing this target to be detected relatively quickly. Under this account, no mention of "attentional disengaging" is required. Patients' behavior appears as

though there is a disengagement of attention, but the mechanism underlying the patients' behavior is based on competition between damaged and intact representations of space, not on an "attentional disengager."

Effects of right parietal damage on visual search are consistent with results from spatial cueing paradigms. Eglin and colleagues (1989) asked patients with parietal damage to search for conjunctions between features (e.g., color and shape) amid varying numbers of distractors (refer to Fig. 10-1B). The patients were dramatically slowed when the distractors appeared in the ipsilesional field compared to the contralesional field. The presence of ipsilesional distractors prevented the contralesional representation of the target from competing effectively for attention, consistent with Cohen and colleagues' (1994) account of the disengage deficit associated with parietal lobe damage.

Frames of Reference for Neglect

The phenomena of spatial neglect and extinction can be interpreted with respect to several coordinate frames. A coordinate frame determines the reference point (origin) from which space is measured. Visual locations can be represented with respect to the environment (e.g., the left or right side of a room—an environmental reference frame), observer (e.g., on the observer's left or right side—a viewer-centered reference frame), or an object (e.g., the left or right side of the letter "B"—an object-centered reference frame).

Attempts to define effects of hemineglect in different coordinate systems must consider issues of overlap and alignment; for example, a ceiling is "up" in both environmental coordinates and in viewer-centered coordinates (i.e., it appears above the viewer's head). Calvanio and associates (1987) found different effects in patients who viewed objects in a cluttered field while sitting upright versus lying on one side (in which case the viewer's left side is no longer aligned with the left side of the environment). Upright patients reported fewer objects from the left side of space. Patients lying on a side reported few objects from body-centered left and environmental left, suggesting that hemineglect disrupted both viewer-centered (or body-centered) and environmental-centered reference frames. Ladavas (1987) reported similar results, suggesting that neglect occurs in both head-centered coordinates (i.e., worse performance on stimuli to the left of the head) and either environmental- or body-centered coordinates (i.e., worse performance on stimuli on the left of the patient's body or left of the room).

Neglect may occur with respect to object-centered coordinates. Some patients with right parietal damage are less likely to report items from the left side of an object than from the right side of an object, even when the left side of the object appears in the right (ipsilesional) visual field (Driver & Halligan, 1991; also see Rafal, 2000, for a review). Failure to find object-centered neglect (Farah et al., 1990) may occur when the objects are secondary to the task that patients are asked to perform.

Also, neglect occurs across different sensory modalities. Neglect patients have difficulty attending to both visual and auditory stimuli in contralesional space, suggesting that parietal lobe attentional processes operate on a representation of space that codes both visual and auditory stimuli. Farah and coworkers (1989) found evidence for cross-modal neglect in parietal-damaged patients who were asked to detect a lateralized visual stimulus on a multimodal version of Posner's spatial cueing task. This visual target was preceded by a cue presented in either the visual or auditory modality. Parietal-damaged patients oriented similarly to both types of cues; they had difficulty "disengaging" attention from cues presented on the ipsilesional side of peripheral space regardless of cue modality. These results suggest that parietal lobe attention mechanisms are supramodal.

Control Parameters and Effects of Spatial Attention

As discussed earlier, attention can be deployed—or controlled—by a number of factors. Some are environmental (bottom-up, exogenous) factors, such as the appearance of a new object or event. Others are endogenous (top-down) factors that arise from within the observer based on goals or expectations.

The disorder of attention in parietal-damaged patients appears to involve bottom-up control parameters. This is not meant to imply that neglect is a sensory-level impairment. Perceptual processing is largely intact in neglect patients, but attention is not effectively captured by stimuli on the contralesional side of space. Although these stimuli have intact perceptual representations, they do not fully capture or drive the damaged attentional processes.

Evidence for poor bottom-up control comes from simulating aspect of neglect in neurologically normal observers by degrading one side of a visual scene (Farah et al., 1991). These observers show the "disengage deficit" if half of a computer monitor is degraded with translucent tracing paper (Vecera et al., unpublished data). Targets on the degraded side of the display are more difficult to detect following a cue on the non-degraded side than targets that appear on the non-degraded side following a cue to the degraded side.

Studies using the Posner cueing paradigm suggest that some forms of top-down attentional control are intact after parietal damage. Use of a central arrow cue (considered an endogenous cue) pointing to the left (contralesional) side can reduce the number of

targets missed by right parietal patients; the same reduction in misses does not occur for exogenous peripheral cues (Làdavas et al., 1994). As central arrows and peripheral cues are physically unalike, these differences could be due to perceptual not attentional processes. Bartolomeo and coworkers (2001) addressed this issue using peripheral cues only; to manipulate exogenous and endogenous attention, the cue's informativeness was manipulated by making the cue informative. Informative peripheral cues, which indicate the likely location of the target, tap endogenous attentional processes, whereas uninformative cues tap exogenous processes. Bartolomeo and colleagues (2001) reported that parietal-damaged patients could reduce their response times to contralesional stimuli if most of the invalidly cued targets appeared in the contralesional field. The patients correctly anticipated the target's expected location in the contralesional field and directed attention accordingly. Finally, parietal patients can make use of top-down expectancies or task-relevant goals. A contralesional stimulus may not be extinguished if the ipsilesional stimulus is task irrelevant and the patient is asked to ignore it (Baylis et al., 1993). For example, a right parietal patient, who is asked to name the color of each of two stimuli, one in each visual field, is more likely to extinguish the contralesional stimulus if the two stimuli are the same color. However, if the two stimuli are the same shape (e.g., both circles) or different shapes (e.g., one circle and one square), only the task-relevant attribute of color influences extinction. The task-irrelevant shape dimension does not influence extinction.

Having discussed the attentional control processes that appear disrupted following parietal damage, we now turn to the effects produced by parietal damage. Recall that attention has many hypothesized effects: (1) Attentional selection may provide attended stimuli with greater resources than unattended stimuli; (2) either the sensory-level or decision-level representations may be enhanced for attended items compared to unattended items; and (3) attention may bind together the features of an object. The attentional impairments following parietal damage appear to disrupt some of these attentional effects.

Little is known about attentional resources following parietal damage. However, some results from these patients support the sensory enhancement effect of spatial attention in which attention may "amplify" sensory information transmission (Hillyard et al., 1998). The results that suggest that bottom-up control is impaired in parietal patients (Làdavas, et al., 1994; Bartolomeo, et al., 2001) also suggest that sensory amplification effects may be diminished in these patients. One reason that attention may not be captured effectively by events in the contralesional field is because the damaged attentional processes do not amplify signals coming from contralesional space. More direct evidence is needed for the effect of sensory amplification following parietal damage. Future research could address sensory amplification by examining early visual evoked potentials following parietal damage or could use rigorous psychophysical techniques that have been used to investigate amplification effects (Lu & Dosher, 1998).

As with both resource allocation and sensory amplification, little is known about the role of parietal cortex in reducing decision noise, one of the hypothesized effects of spatial attention. Spatial cues appear to reduce the uncertainty of observer's decisions (Pashler, 1998), and the disrupted spatial orienting observed suggests that parietal patients may have difficulties making decisions about targets in the contralesional field. We have preliminary data from a study that investigates decision noise effects following right parietal lobe damage (Vecera & Rizzo, unpublished data). Consistent with a decision-noise deficit, our patient showed a larger difference between validly and invalidly cued targets in her contralesional field than in her ipsilesional field. These observations need to be replicated in this patient and others, but our results suggest that parietal damage may influence a host of attentional effects, including the reduction of decision noise.

Perhaps the most-studied effect with parietal patients is the role of spatial attention in solving the binding problem. When neurologically intact observers are distracted by asking them to perform a secondary task, features of different objects can become miscombined, resulting in *illusory conjunctions* of features (Treisman & Schmidt, 1982). Results from parietal patients also suggest that spatial attention is involved in binding or conjoining the features of objects because these patients mis-conjoin features and show high rates of illusory conjunctions. Cohen and Rafal (1991) asked a parietal-damaged patient to perform two tasks concurrently. The first task was a digit identification task; two digits, one large and one small, were presented at fixation, and the patient was instructed to identify the large digit. The second task was a letter identification task. One of the letters was a target (F or X) and the other was a distractor (O). The letters were colored, and the patient was instructed to name both the color and the identity of the target letter (i.e., was it F or X and what color was it?). In the second task, there are two types of errors. The first is a feature error, in which either letter name or color is reported incorrectly. For example, if the patient was presented with a blue F and a red O, reporting a yellow F would be a feature error. The second type of error is a conjunction error, in which a feature of the distractor letter O "migrates" to the target letter, forming an illusory conjunction. For example, if the patient was presented a blue F and a red O and reported a red F, the color of the red O was misconjoined with the target letter F. Cohen and Rafal's patient showed a larger number of conjunction errors in the contralesional field than in the ipsilesional field. Similar numbers of feature errors were made in the contralesional and ipsilesional fields, indicating that feature perception was similar in both fields. Presumably, the damaged parietal-based spatial attention system impaired feature integration, although the individual features are represented, allowing for accurate perception of individual features.

Even more direct evidence for the role of parietal attention areas in solving the binding problem comes from Robertson and colleagues (1997); also see Friedman-Hill and coworkers (1995), who investigated illusory conjunctions in a patient with bilateral parietal damage and Balint syndrome (also called "dorsal simultanagnosia"; see Farah, 1990). Patients with Balint syndrome typically have deficits in visually guided reaching (optic ataxia), spatial confusion (e.g., inability to judge the relative depths of objects as in "visual discrimination"), and an extreme inability to perceive more than one object or shape at a time (simultanagnosia). The patient of Robertson and coworkers could search effectively for a target defined by a single feature (e.g., search for a red target or search for an X). However, the patient was dramatically impaired at searching for conjunctions (e.g., finding a red X) and integrating the features of objects. This same patient showed illusory conjunction errors even when the visual display was present for 10 seconds, an exposure duration at which neurologically intact observers should make no illusory conjunctions. Presumably, this patient's spatial confusion and simultanagnosia prevented him from having an accurate representation of spatial location, which is necessary for conjoining the features of an object.

Summary

Patients with damage to parietal lobe areas have a variety of attentional impairments. These impairments extend across different visual reference frames and across different modalities, and many of the typical effects of attention, such as the ability to bind features of an object, appear to be defective. The bottom-up capture of attention appears to be disrupted in association with a failure of sensory amplification. The lack of capture also may prevent the damaged hemisphere from competing with the intact hemisphere for attention, resulting in an attentional imbalance that appears to favor the ipsilesional field (and may appear as a "disengage deficit").

Understanding the control and effects of spatial attention following parietal damage may offer insights for rehabilitation. If parietal damage disrupts bottom-up capture of spatial attention and involves an attentional imbalance between the cerebral hemispheres, then rehabilitation that increases the input to the disrupted hemisphere may reduce the attentional imbalance and the associated neglect or extinction. Indeed, neglect symptoms can be reduced by patching the ipsilesional eye, which (1) reduces some of the ipsilesional visual input and (2) reduces the activation of the ipsilateral colliculus (see Heilman et al., 2000, for a brief discussion of treatments for neglect). Unfortunately, most treatments that have been investigated only provide temporary relief from neglect (Heilman et al., 2000).

The Frontal Lobes and Overt Attention to Locations

Although deficits in spatial attention have been studied most extensively in patients with parietal lobe damage, spatial neglect and other spatial deficits can occur following lesions to frontal cortices (Heilman et al., 2000). However, because the frontal lobes participate in the operation of multiple cognitive processes, including language, motor control, working memory, and attention, less is known about the particular attentional processes associated with frontal areas. For example, little is known about the neuropsychology of visual search in patients with frontal lobe damage; this lack of knowledge may occur because studies of neglect sometimes include patients with frontal damage/parietal damage and patients with parietal damage, thereby obscuring possible differences between these groups. Patients with frontal damage have attentional impairments that typically are not associated with parietal damage (see Swick & Knight, 1998, for an overview).

One area of spatial attention that has been studied in patients with frontal lobe damage is the control of overt attention—the production of eye movements. Typically, directing the eyes to a region of space is preceded by directing covert spatial attention to the target region (Colby & Goldberg, 1999). Lesions of superior frontal lobe areas that include the frontal eye fields (FEFs) appear to disrupt some types of overt eye movements. Guitton and coworkers (1985) demonstrated that eye movements to an abruptly appearing visual target (a "prosaccade" in which the eyes move to the target) do not differ between frontal patients with FEF damage and control patients with temporal lobe damage. However, eye movements in a direction opposite an abruptly appearing target ("antisaccades") are dramatically impaired in frontal patients. In the antisaccade task, the FEF patients often made reflexive eye movements to the target location instead of moving in the opposite direction. When the FEF patients did make antisaccades, the latency of their eye movements was longer than those of control patients. FEF appears to play an inhibitory role in overt attention by preventing unwanted reflexive eye movements.

Although the study by Guitton and colleagues (1985) is important for demonstrating the role of frontal lobe areas in overt attention, this study does not speak to the different types of spatial cues that can control covert and overt attention. To address the role of different spatial cues (peripheral versus central/symbolic), Henik and colleagues (1994) studied patients with frontal lobe lesions that included superior dorsolateral prefrontal cortex, which included the FEF, and patients with frontal damage that excluded FEF. The patients performed two tasks. One task was a saccade task, in which eye movements were made to a peripheral location that was cued with either a central arrow cue or a peripheral cue. The other task was a detection task in which the patients pressed a key that corresponded to a target signal; this target signal was preceded by either a central arrow cue or a peripheral cue. In both tasks, half the cues (central and peripheral) were valid and half were neutral; there were no invalid cues.

Henik and coworkers (1994) found that FEF lesions disrupted eye movements to peripheral locations, but not all eye movements were disrupted equally. The FEF patients were slower to make eye movements into the contralesional field than into the ipsilesional field following central cues. Also, following peripheral cues, the FEF patients made faster eye movements into the contralesional field than into the ipsilesional field. Patients with intact FEF made eye movements into the contralesional and ipsilesional field approximately equally following both central and peripheral cues. The results from the FEF patients indicate that voluntary overt orienting is impaired in this group—these patients are only slowed in directing eye movements to the contralesional field following the symbolic arrow cue. The authors hypothesize that the FEF patients may be speeded in directing overt attention into contralesional space following a peripheral cue because the FEF lesion may disinhibit ipsilesional midbrain areas; this disinhibition has the effect of inhibiting the opposite colliculus and delaying reflexive eye movements into the ipsilesional field. Finally, the FEF group did not show any impairment in the detection task, suggesting that the attentional impairments were confined to overt attention (eye movements); covert attention could be directed to cued locations and facilitate responses that did not involve an eye movement.

Superior Colliculus and Pulvinar: Subcortical Influences on Spatial Attention

In addition to the cortical control of spatial attention, there are at least two subcortical regions that appear critical for spatial selection: the superior colliculus and the pulvinar nucleus of the thalamus. Most studies investigating the role of these subcortical regions have used Posner's spatial cueing task to investigate covert spatial attention.

Progressive supranuclear palsy (PSP) is a neurodegenerative disorder that resembles Parkinson disease and also affects the basal ganglia. One difference between these two degenerative disorders is that PSP produces a marked impairment of voluntary gaze control, likely due to degeneration of dorsal midbrain structures, especially the superior colliculus (Rafal & Grimm, 1981). PSP patients have an inability to make voluntary saccadic eye movements, especially vertical eye movements. For example, PSP patients often do not look up at a person who is speaking to them and cannot make saccades to move their eyes upward if given a command to do so. However, if the PSP patient is asked to continue to fixate a target while the head is being tilted downward, the eyes are able to maintain fixation by moving upward slowly using vestibulo-ocular mechanisms more closely related to smooth pursuit movements.

In a series of studies, Posner, Rafal, and colleagues investigated spatial orienting in PSP patients (Posner et al., 1982; Rafal et al., 1988). Patients with PSP were cued to locations that appeared in one of four locations: above, below, left, or right of fixation. Following the cue, a target appeared at the validly cued location or at an invalidly cued location, and patients were instructed to press a button as soon as they detected the target. There were two cue conditions in these studies. In the exogenous condition, the cue was a peripheral flicker that was equally valid and invalid (valid on 50% of trials and 50% of invalid trials); in the endogenous condition, the cue was a central arrow that was predictive (valid on 80% of the trials and invalid on 20% of the trials). The patients were faster at the validly cued location than at the invalidly cued location in the horizontal direction but not in the vertical direction; control patients with Parkinson disease showed no differences between orienting horizontally or vertically (Rafal et al., 1988). Also, the movement of attention in PSP patients was slower in the vertical direction than in the horizontal direction. Finally, there was a slight, but nonsignificant trend for a greater impairment in the exogenous cue condition than in the endogenous cue condition. One might predict less impairment in orienting to endogenous cues because they involve cortical processing.

Based on their results, Posner, Rafal, and colleagues suggested that the superior colliculus might be involved with one specific component of spatial attention. Spatial attention may involve several component operations for normal performance, including disengaging from an attended location, moving attention to a new location, and engaging attention at the new location. Because PSP patients orient slower vertically than horizontally, the superior colliculus may be involved with the movement of spatial attention.

Another component of spatial attention that appears to involve midbrain mechanisms is inhibition of return (described above in studies of neurologically normal subjects performing Posner's task). Inhibition of return (IoR) is the decreased tendency to re-orient attention to a previously attended location. In spatial cueing tasks, IoR typically is observed at longer delays between the cue and target. PSP patients also show reduced IoR effects in the vertical direction than in the horizontal direction. Other patient populations, including patients with frontal lesions and parietal lesions, do exhibit IoR, suggesting that IoR is linked to the eye movement system controlled by the superior colliculus and not linked to neural systems that mediate other attentional operations.

In addition to the superior colliculus, the pulvinar nucleus of the thalamus appears involved in the subcortical control of spatial attention. Pulvinar lesions can cause neglect (Rafal & Posner, 1987), and following the initial recovery, these patients exhibit attentional impairments. Rafal and Posner (1987) had pulvinar patients perform a spatial cueing task with a highly predictive (80% valid and 20% invalid) peripheral cues. Not surprisingly, the patients were slower to detect targets in the contralesional field than in the ipsilesional field. However, this visual field difference persisted across very long cue-target intervals; even when there was almost a full second between the cue and target, the pulvinar patients responded faster in the ipsilesional field than in the contralesional field. Consideration of these findings led Rafal and Posner to conclude that the pulvinar may be responsible for engaging spatial attention at a cued location. Across both the contra- and ipsilesional fields, the pulvinar patients showed a decrease in RT to validly cued targets as the time between the cue and target increased. Thus, these patients appear to deploy (move) spatial attention similarly in both visual fields, unlike PSP patients. In addition, the pulvinar patients showed a "disengage deficit" similar to that shown by parietal patients. However, the pulvinar patients only showed this pattern for short cue-target intervals, unlike parietal patients, suggesting that pulvinar patients may not have the same type of disengage deficit. The results from pulvinar patients suggest that attention can be disengaged (eventually) from an attended location and moved to a new location but that attention is ineffectively engaged at the new location. Although there are very few studies with pulvinar patients, the role of the pulvinar in visual attention is supported by neuroimaging studies with normal observers, which suggest that the pulvinar may be involved with filtering irrelevant stimuli (LaBerge & Buchsbaum, 1990).

Spatial Attention: Summary

Spatial attention is the variety of attention most widely studied in neuropsychological populations. However, gaps remain in our knowledge of the neuropsychological mechanisms involved in attending to space. For example, most studies have used a very simple spatial cueing paradigm with highly predictive cues. Although this task yields robust results and can be adapted for use with many different patient groups, spatial cueing effects have multiple interpretations (e.g., allocation of resources, reduction of decision noise, perceptual enhancement, response bias; see Luck & Vecera, 2002, for a discussion of these effects).

Application of cognitive theory and tasks in studies of patients with brain damage has provided important clues to the neuropsychology of spatial attention. Spatial attention is composed of several component processes, and different neuropsychological syndromes may involve different components. However, we should be cautious in interpreting deficits in terms of simple components, such as a "disengage" or "move" component. These components typically have not been described in sufficient detail to provide an understanding of the attentional processes involved. Labeling an attentional component or process is not the same as understanding the operation of that process. Supplementing neuropsychological observations with computational models (e.g., Cohen et al., 1994) may provide a way to understand the attentional processes that are disrupted in a neuropsychological population.

As we noted in the introduction, there are many forms of attentional selection. There have been neuropsychological investigations of other forms of attentional selection, and we now turn to a review of these other attentional processes.

NEUROPSYCHOLOGY OF OTHER ATTENTIONAL PROCESSES

In this section, we focus on three broad classes of nonspatial attentional selection that have been studied in neuropsychological populations: object-based attention, working memory–level attention, and executive attention. As with our discussion of spatial attention, we will focus on how cognitive theory can inform neuropsychological observations and vice versa.

Object-Based Attention

Object-based attention is the visual process that selects one shape from among several shapes (for reviews, see Vecera, 2000, and Vecera & Behrmann, 2001). Typical studies of object-based attention investigate either the time to switch attention within an object or between objects (Egly et al., 1994) or the effect of focusing attention on one object or dividing attention across objects (Duncan, 1984; Vecera & Farah, 1994). Typically, observers are faster and more accurate in switching attention within an object rather than between objects or are faster and more accurate attending to a single object than attending to multiple objects.

There have been two neuropsychological populations that have been studied using object attention tasks. We have already discussed one of these groups—neglect patients who have damage to parietal areas. These patients can exhibit object-based neglect, in which the left side of an object is ignored, suggesting that object-centered neglect may arise from a spatial gradient of damage (Mozer, 1999) and that some forms of object-based attention may be due to spatial attention being influenced by early perceptual organization processes (Vecera, 1994; Vecera, 2000; Vecera & Behrmann, 2001).

Egly and coworkers (1994) directly investigated object-based selection in parietal patients using a cued detection task (see Fig. 10-3). Recall that in this task a cue appears in the end of one of two objects, followed by a target. The target can be validly cued or invalidly cued, and a comparison of these two trial types provides a measure of spatial attention. Further, there are two types of invalidly cued targets, those that appear in the cued object and those that appear in the uncued object. Neurologically intact observers typically are faster to detect invalid targets appearing in the cued object than those appearing in the uncued object. This latter result demonstrates object-based attention because the locations of the two invalid trial types are equidistant from the cued location.

Egly and coworkers tested patients with lesions to either the left or right parietal lobe and found that these groups exhibited different attentional impairments. Both patient groups showed a spatial selection impairment characteristic of the "disengage deficit": The patients showed a larger difference between valid and invalid targets when the targets appeared in the contralesional visual field than in the ipsilesional visual field. However, the two groups differed in object-based selection. The patients with right parietal lesions showed a normal-looking object effect; they were faster to detect invalid targets that appeared in the cued object than those that appeared in the uncued object, regardless of the target field. The patients with left parietal lesions, in contrast, showed a larger object effect in their contralesional field than in their ipsilesional field, suggesting that it was difficult to switch attention between the objects appearing in the contralesional field. Based on these results, Egly and associates suggested that object-based attention may involve left parietal lobe processes and spatial attention may involve right parietal lobe processes.

In addition to the object attention impairments observed in parietal patients, there are patients with damage to the ventral visual pathway who have impairments in shape perception (see Vecera & Behrmann, 2001, for recent reviews), and these shape perception impairments result in disrupted object-based attention. Patients with visual agnosia have a profound inability to recognize common objects presented visually, although an agnosic patient typically has preserved recognition through other modalities. Semantic information (i.e., what an object is used for or the category of an object) typically is preserved, suggesting that the recognition impairment is due to a visual disturbance (Farah, 1990). The object recognition impairments in visual agnosia can arise from a range of neural damage, suggesting that visual agnosia is not a unitary neuropsychological syndrome. Object recognition can be disrupted by (1) a low-level deficit such as the inability to extract the features (e.g., edges) from a scene, (2) a mid-level deficit such as the inability to organize or group the features in a scene, or (3) a high-level deficit such as the failure to assign meaning to an object despite the derivation of an intact percept. Neuropsychological studies of object-based attention have studied agnosic patients who are unable to group or organize the elementary visual features in a scene. These patients have problems with processes involved in perceptual organization, including figure-ground segregation, binding shapes from featural forms, and binding surface properties to shapes. The consequence of the failure to segregate (or isolate) an object from other objects prevents attention from knowing what collection of features to select. The typical behavioral effects associated with object-based attention, such as faster or more accurate responses to a single object, typically are not obtained with these patients. Interestingly, some patients with visual-form agnosia also appear to exhibit impairments in object-based attention. One straightforward interpretation of this impairment is that these patients cannot use perceptual grouping processes to define the relevant surfaces and objects in a visual scene, thereby preventing attention from knowing what to be directed toward.

The inability to organize an image perceptually is also observed in patients with integrative agnosia (Riddoch & Humphreys, 1987), who can perceive features and edges but fail to integrate (i.e., organize) the features appropriately. As with J.W. (see the accompanying box), patients with integrative agnosia do not exhibit object-based attention effects because they cannot organize images or organize them inappropriately. However, the perceptual performance of patients with integrative agnosia tends to be better than J.W.'s perceptual performance, which is severely impaired and may be due in part to impaired feature perception. Those with integrative agnosia, such as Riddoch and Humphreys' patient, are able to perceive individual features, as indicated by efficient visual search on "pop out" displays (e.g., Fig. 10-1A).

Behrmann and colleagues recently have studied patient C.K., who has integrative agnosia. This patient is impaired at segregating foreground figures from backgrounds, and his performance is poor when objects

PATIENT JW: ILLUSTRATION OF OBJECT-BASED ATTENTION DEFICITS IN VISUAL-FORM AGNOSIA

The absence of these object-based attention effects is exemplified in the performance of a patient with visual-form agnosia (or apperceptive agnosia), patient J.W. (Vecera & Behrmann, 1997). J.W. was in his late 30s when he suffered a severe cardiac event that deprived his brain of oxygen. Although J.W. has no obvious focal lesion, he does present with multiple hypodensities in both occipital lobes, as well as more minor hypodensities in his right parietal lobe. J.W. has a mild upper left visual field, although this has no adverse effect on his perceptual performance. Consistent with the diagnosis of visual-form agnosia, J.W. is unable to group the contours and edges in a visual scene, indicated by his inability to trace around the edges of two overlapping rectangles (Fig. 10-6). He also performs at chance on the Efron (1968) shape matching task in which he is asked to determine if two rectangles of equal area are the same or different. Although J.W. is able to group image elements using the Gestalt properties such as similarity of color or proximity, he is unable to organize an image based on good continuation, closure, or symmetry (Vecera & Behrmann, 1997).

In addition to his impairments in object recognition, J.W. also exhibits difficulties with object-based attention. Specifically, J.W. is no faster to shift or divide attention within a single object than across objects (Vecera & Behrmann, 1997). When J.W. performed Egly's object attention task (see Fig. 10-3B), he demonstrated a normal spatial cueing effect: J.W. was faster to detect targets appearing at a validly cued location than at an invalidly cued location. However, J.W. was just as fast to detect targets appearing in the uncued object as targets appearing in the cued object. Neurologically normal observers are faster to detect targets that appear in the cued object than in the uncued object. J.W.'s inability to organize the edges in the image may prevent him from determining the boundaries of the objects and knowing where one object ends and the other begins. If the objects are not defined by mid-level grouping processes, then attention only can select locations in the image; the objects are nonexistent and, therefore, cannot control the allocation of attention. Importantly, spatial attention does not depend on perceptual grouping and operates independently and apparently normally in visual-form agnosia.

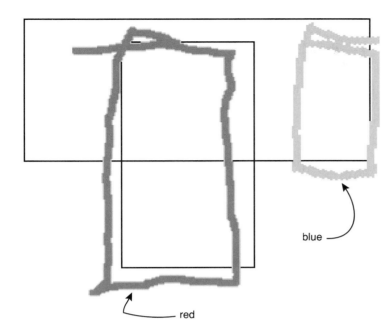

blue

red

FIGURE 10-6. Results from a patient with visual-form agnosia, patient JW. JW was unable to segregate overlapping objects from one another, indicating a difficulty with perceptual grouping processes. Patient JW also exhibits impairments on object-based attentional selection, although his spatial selection is intact.

overlap one another (Behrmann, et al., 1994). In an object-based attention task, C.K. is no faster to attend to a single object than to multiple objects. For example, when tested on a task in which observers are required to determine if two features are the same or different (Behrmann, et al., 1998), C.K. performs just as well when the features are on one object as when the features are on two different objects. Additional results from C.K. suggest that he does not perform perceptual completion; when an object is occluded by another object, C.K. is slower to attend to the occluded object than to the occluding object.

There are relatively few neuropsychological studies of object-based attention. The few studies that we reviewed, however, suggest object attention may involve a complex network of cortical visual areas to support normal performance. Additional research in this area, particularly studies of visual agnosia, may provide an understanding of the shape representation processes involved in object attention.

Visual Working Memory and the Attentional Blink

As mentioned above, the effect of attention on visual working memory is apparent in the "attentional blink" phenomenon. The attentional blink can increase pathologically after cerebral lesions, making it more difficult to perceive successive visual targets. Husain and co-workers (1997) suggested that an increased attentional blink represents a temporal form of visual neglect. Eight older subjects were studied 1 month (on average) after a right hemisphere stroke affecting inferior parietal lobe,

inferior frontal lobe, or basal ganglia. These subjects had visual neglect defined clinically on a shape cancellation task and could not identify the second target in a dual-target task until 1440 msec had elapsed after they had identified the first target. The performance of these subjects with right hemisphere lesions (in superior parietal lobe, temporal lobe, medial frontal lobe, or subcortical regions) and no neglect was similar to that of normal subjects without brain damage. The study concluded that visual neglect is a disorder that affects the patient's ability to direct attention in time as well as space, suggesting a need to reformulate prevailing spatial accounts of visual neglect. However, Rizzo and colleagues (2001) found that an abnormal attentional blink (1) could occur with lesions in either hemisphere; (2) does not require a lesion in the parietal lobe, frontal lobe, or basal ganglia; (3) could occur independently of spatial neglect; and (4) can persist after spatial neglect has resolved. They concluded that an increased attentional blink has no special status in neglect and that the mechanisms of spatial attention that are disrupted in visual hemineglect syndrome differ from the mechanisms that underlie attentional blink. The findings of Rizzo and coworkers highlight the complexity of the attentional blink and suggest that multiple mechanisms might be involved in producing this phenomenon.

Executive Control, Distraction, and Inhibition

The final aspects of attentional selection that we discuss involve a constellation of deficits that are reported in patients with frontal lobe lesions. We must acknowledge that attentional impairments following frontal damage are heterogeneous. It is clear that there are functional subdivisions of the frontal lobes, and each of these subdivisions may participate in different aspects of cognitive control. For example, patients with damage to ventromedial prefrontal cortex do not appear to be impaired in basic forms of attention or working memory, although the same patients show dramatic impairments in decision making (Damasio, 1999). In contrast, patients with damage to dorsolateral prefrontal cortex may show impairments in some forms of attention, working memory, or "executive control" (Tranel et al., 1994), although this group of patients may not show homogeneous deficits (Baddeley et al., 1997). Because of the relevance for attentional and cognitive control, we will focus on patients with impairments in executive control or executive attention.

Several views of cognitive control have emerged from cognitive psychology. Shallice (Shallice, 1982, 1988; Shallice & Burgess, 1996) suggested that frontal areas form a supervisory attention system that plays a role in *contention scheduling*, which involves control of nonautomatic behaviors and actions including (1) resolving competition between two responses, (2) preventing or inhibiting a highly practiced or frequently used action or cognitive process, and (3) coordinating the sharing of processes or resources used by several cognitive operations (Norman & Shallice, 1986). Another widespread view of cognitive control is Baddeley's "central executive" (Baddeley & Della Sala, 1996; Baddeley, 1986). Under this account, a central executive is part of a larger cognitive system that also involves working memory "slave" systems, one for verbal working memory and another for visuospatial memory. The central executive controls the two working memory slave systems and coordinates the concurrent operation of these two systems, as when someone performs two tasks at once (a dual-task situation).

Patients with frontal lobe damage can exhibit a constellation of impairments that includes distractibility, working memory impairments, difficulty learning new tasks, and inhibiting well-learned responses (see Kimberg et al., 2000, for an overview). These impairments appear in a variety of neuropsychological tests and cognitive paradigms. The one task perhaps most closely associated with frontal lobe impairments is the Wisconsin Card Sorting Task. In this task, patients are given a set of cards that contain colored shapes; the number of shapes appearing on a card differs (e.g., between one and four red stars). The patients are instructed to sort the cards by placing a card into one of four piles, and the pile a card is placed in depends on the sorting strategy the patient is using. For example, if the patient is grouping cards by color, the red cards are placed in one pile, the blue cards in another, and so on. The experimenter provides feedback after each card is placed in a pile; the patient is told either that the sort was correct or incorrect. The patient must determine how to sort the cards correctly—is the correct sorting based on color, shape, or number? Patients with damage to dorsolateral prefrontal cortex exhibit a large number of errors on this sorting task. In particular, these patients are impaired in switching sorting strategies; when the experimenter changes the correct sorting from color to shape, for example, frontal patients often will continue to sort by color, although they know that this is the incorrect sorting scheme.

Although the Wisconsin Card Sorting Task is a widely used neuropsychological tool, many component cognitive processes are necessary for correct performance in this task. For example, switching sorting strategies may involve a shift of task-based attention, but it also might involve inhibiting a previous sorting strategy. Using more restricted cognitive paradigms, several studies have attempted to focus on the processes that are impaired following frontal lobe damage. The cognitive neuropsychological picture of these patients is far from simple, although they do appear to have several impairments relevant to higher-level, or executive, attentional control.

The attentional impairments associated with frontal lobe damage are specific, and some attention tasks do not appear to be disrupted by frontal damage. Lee and colleagues (1999) demonstrated that frontal patients are not impaired on a flanker task, in which observers must respond to the central item in an array. The attended item is surrounded by (i.e., flanked by) items that are either consistent with the correct response or inconsistent with the correct response. Neurologically normal observers are slowed by the presence of incompatible flankers (Eriksen & Hoffman, 1973; Eriksen & Eriksen, 1974). Patients with frontal lobe damage also showed slower responses to incompatible flankers compared to compatible flankers, although the patients responded more slowly than control subjects (Lee, et al., 1999).

The results from the flanker task suggest that frontal patients do not appear to be disproportionately influenced by information that is incompatible with an attended stimulus. In other situations, however, frontal patients are affected more by incompatible information than control groups. Another widely studied cognitive paradigm that manipulates the consistency of information is the Stroop task, discussed earlier. Patients with damage to the right frontal lobe, but not the left, show more errors on the Stroop task than other patient groups (Vendrell et al., 1995). For example, when the word BLUE was written in red ink, patients with damage to the right frontal lobe made many errors in correctly naming the ink color.

How can the results from the flankers task be reconciled with the results from the Stroop task? Although both tasks present observers with incompatible information, there is an important difference between these tasks. The flankers task creates compatible and incompatible conditions by assigning letters to arbitrary response categories. For example, the letter "X" may indicate a left button response and the letter "P" a right button response. There is no previously learned association between these letters and their responses. In contrast, the Stroop task relies on highly learned stimuli (words) that have a direct correspondence with a response. That is, the word BLUE is associated with a specific response—saying the word "blue." Thus, some frontal patients are impaired on the Stroop task because word reading is highly practiced and automatic and the stimulus-response mapping is nonarbitrary. Frontal patients may have difficulties in inhibiting a well-learned response, such as reading a word. Impairments of patients with frontal lesions on a variety of tasks, including "go-no-go" tasks in which the patient must withhold a response (no-go) on some trials, suggest impairment in inhibiting responses (e.g., Drewe, 1975). The poor performance of patients with frontal lesions on the Wisconsin Card Sorting Task could be influenced by an inability to inhibit the current sorting procedure.

Patients with frontal lesions also appear impaired on other executive processes, such as the ability to switch between tasks. Owen and coworkers (1991) asked several patient groups to learn to choose a correct stimulus from a pair of shapes. During learning, correct performance was determined by focusing on one dimension (e.g., white shapes) and ignoring an irrelevant dimension (e.g., irregular purple shapes). That is, by focusing on the white shapes, an observer could know which of the two stimuli would be the correct choice. There were two important conditions in this study. First, after patients had performed simple discrimination learning, a new set of stimuli was introduced. The patient continued to choose one of two shapes; the correct choice was determined by the previously used dimension (white shapes, in this case). This condition involved an intradimensional shift of attention or learning. Next, after the intradimensional shift condition, another new set of shapes were introduced, but now patients had to focus on the other, ignored dimension (the irregular purple shapes) to learn which shape to choose correctly. This condition involved an extradimensional shift of attention or learning. Although extradimensional shifts were difficult for all of the patient groups studied, patients with frontal lobe damage performed the most poorly in this condition. These findings suggest that switching attention across categories, dimensions, or tasks may be impaired by frontal damage. However, because a learning paradigm was used, the impairment shown by patients with frontal damage could have been influenced by working memory impairments. Although a working memory

impairment might not account for all of the performance of patients with frontal damage, the involvement of working memory could have made frontal patients disproportionately impaired relative to the other patient groups. Future research should examine task switching in a cognitive paradigm that does not involve extensive learning (see Rogers & Monsell, 1995, for such a task).

Consistent with the hypothesis that patients with frontal damage have difficulty alternating between tasks, recent research has studied frontal patients in dual-task situations. In the dual-task approach to investigating attentional phenomena, observers are asked to perform two tasks. The tasks are performed alone (single-task condition) or concurrently (dual-task condition). If two tasks rely on the same attentional resources, the dual-task condition should be performed more poorly than the single-task condition. According to Baddeley's model of cognitive control, the central executive should be involved in coordinating performance between tasks that are performed simultaneously. To test this hypothesis, Baddeley and associates (1997) investigated dual-task performance in two groups of frontal patients, one with dysexecutive syndrome and one without. Assessment of dysexecutive syndrome was made through interviews with the patients' families and from existing clinical records; dysexecutive patients were those who exhibited perseveration, confabulation, and distractibility, among other criteria. The frontal patients characterized as having dysexecutive syndrome were more impaired in the dual-task condition than in the single-task condition compared to a group of frontal patients who did not have dysexecutive syndrome. Interestingly, standard clinical measures, such as the Wisconsin Card Sorting Task, were not reliable predictors of which patients had dysexecutive syndrome and which did not.

Finally, in addition to the many impairments we have just reviewed, patients with frontal damage also exhibit impairments in sustaining processing over time. Patients with lesions to right frontal areas have a difficult time counting digits in a list presented at a rate of one item per second; these patients are impaired little, if at all, when the list is presented at a rate of seven items per second (Wilkins et al., 1987). These results suggest that right frontal patients have difficulty sustaining their attention during the slower presentation rate. Presumably, the patients' deficit is not due to memory because memory impairment would disrupt performance at both presentation rates. However, if the faster presentation rate allows pairs of digits to be "chunked" or grouped with one another because of temporal proximity, performance could differ between the slow and fast presentation rates, and the impairment might be influenced by working memory. Similarly, a recent study by Chao and Knight (1995) demonstrated that frontal patients cannot sustain processing in the face of distractor items. Patient groups were asked to listen to an auditory stimulus and to determine if a sound played between 4 and 12.6 seconds later were the same or different. In a no-distractor condition, the delay period contained silence; in a distractor condition, the delay period contained between 3 and 18 irrelevant tones, depending on the duration of the interval. Frontal patients were more impaired by the distractors than the other patient groups. However, the frontal patients performed similarly to the other groups in the no-distractor condition, suggesting that their impaired performance was not caused by elementary perceptual or memory problems. However, this study confounded the delay period interval with the number of distractors, making the distractor condition difficult to interpret.

The results from patients with frontal lobe damage suggest that a complex set of cognitive processes are involved in "executive attention." Some of the cognitive processes controlled by frontal areas may be dissociable, as suggested by differences between patients with and without dysexecutive syndrome and between patients with lesions to left versus right frontal areas. As with the other patient groups we have reviewed, the evidence from frontal patients suggests that there are multiple forms of attentional selection, and that these forms of selection appear to be associated with different neural areas and processes.

TREATMENT OF ATTENTIONAL IMPAIRMENTS

Before concluding, it is important to address the poorly understood topic of treatment of attentional disorders. Although study of this topic is still in its infancy, some relevant clinical observations need to be discussed. Most treatment attempts have focused on the neglect syndrome, probably because this is the most frequently studied attentional impairment following focal brain damage. There have been several approaches to treating attentional impairments in neglect, including behavioral approaches and pharmacologic therapies (Bisiach & Vallar, 1988; Heilman et al., 1993; Rafal & Robertson, 1995; Heilman et al., 2000; Rafal, 2000).

Unilateral caloric stimulation of the vestibular system by placing ice water in the left ear temporarily reduces neglect (Rubens, 1985). Stimulation of the neck muscles also reduces symptoms of neglect (Karnath et al., 1993; Karnath, 1997). The latter intervention was developed from experimental observations of neglect, which suggested that neglect might occur in body-centered coordinates (see the above section on the coordinate system of neglect, also see Bisiach et al., 1985). Interestingly, neither caloric stimulation nor neck muscle vibration influences the allocation of spatial attention in neurologically normal observers, which rules out some explanations of the neglect syndrome

(Rorden et al., 2001). Unfortunately, both caloric stimulation and neck muscle vibration only reduce neglect temporarily.

Pharmacologic treatments have shown some promise for the treatment of neglect. Based on animal research that demonstrated that unilateral damage to the dopaminergic system could produce neglect, Fleet and colleagues (1987) showed an improvement in two neglect patients following the administration of a dopamine agonist. Other studies have investigated pharmacologic treatments in less-specific attentional impairments, such as those observed after traumatic brain injury (Whyte et al., 1997). Although some treatments appear to reduce the effects of neglect and other attentional impairments, a complete understanding of attentional impairments and the treatment of these impairments will require additional research, including an understanding of the neurochemistry of attention in individuals without brain damage (see Marrocco & Davidson, 1998, for a review of the neurochemistry of attention).

SUMMARY

Although attention can be a very general term in everyday use, using research in cognitive psychology to focus on the processes associated with attention can make "attention" a concept that can be studied rigorously. Attention is necessary for eliminating unwanted sensory inputs or irrelevant behavioral tasks. In general, attentional processes will be useful when some cognitive system or process receives too many inputs; attention can act to restrict the number of inputs and allow processing to continue in an effective manner.

Many different cognitive processes can receive unwanted or irrelevant inputs, ranging from perceptual processes to more executive processes. Because a wide range of systems can receive such irrelevant inputs, we might expect attention to operate on different processes depending on someone's ongoing behavior. We have tried to argue that attention is not a single process or a single "bottleneck" or selection mechanism. Many attentional processes and effects are possible.

It is relatively easy to speculate that there are multiple forms of attention. Future research needs to test this hypothesis. In addition to behavioral studies performed by cognitive psychologists, neuropsychological investigations of attention can and should play a central role in determining if there are multiple forms of attention. As was evident from our review, different neuropsychological syndromes can be characterized by the types of attention or attentional processes that are spared or damaged. Different neural sites appear to be responsible for different forms of attentional control. Understanding the integration of these neural sites and their relationship to cognitive processes and, ultimately, behavior will increase our understanding of both normal and disordered attentional selection.

■ KEY POINTS

☐ Attention is a set of mechanisms that allow processing to be restricted to some stimuli, events, or goals over others.

☐ There are multiple forms of attention, and some of these attentional processes are separate from each other.

☐ Attentional deficits can arise from damage to different areas of the brain, but the parietal lobes and frontal lobes appear to control specific and important attentional parameters. The parietal attention system appears to involve the bottom-up control of attention, whereas the frontal attention system appears to involve top-down, or goal-driven, control of attention.

☐ A general framework, the biased competition account, provides a useful theoretical tool for studying attention in both normal populations and patient populations.

Acknowledgments. This chapter was prepared with partial support from grants from the National Science Foundation (BCS 99-10727), the National Institute of Mental Health (MH60636), and the National Institute of Neurological Disease and Stroke (P01 NS19632) and the National Institute on Aging (AG15071; AG17717). Correspondence can be addressed to the first author at the Department of Psychology, E11 Seashore Hall, University of Iowa, Iowa City, IA, 52242-1407. Electronic mail can be sent to shaun-vecera@uiowa.edu.

KEY READINGS

Desimone R, Duncan J: Neural mechanisms of selective visual attention. Ann Rev Neurosci 18:193–222, 1995.

Luck SJ, Vecera SP: Attention: From tasks to mechanisms, in Yantis S (ed): Stevens' Handbook of Experimental Psychology, Vol 1. Sensation and Perception. New York: John Wiley & Sons, 2002, pp. 235–286.

Pashler H: The Psychology of Attention. Cambridge, MA: MIT Press.

Rafal RD: Neglect II: Cognitive neuropsychological issues, in Farah MJ, Feinberg TE (eds): Patient-Based Approaches to Cognitive Neuroscience. Cambridge, MA: MIT Press, 2000, pp. 125–141.

Vecera SP, Luck SJ: Attention, in Ramachandran VS (ed): Encyclopedia of the Human Brain. San Diego, CA: Academic Press, 2002, Vol. 1, pp. 269–284.

REFERENCES

Allport A: Attention and control. Have we been asking the wrong questions? A critical review of twenty-five years, in Meyer DE, Kornblum S (eds): Attention and Performance. Cambridge, MA: MIT Press, 1993, Vol. XIV, pp. 183–218.

Allport DA, Styles EA, Hsieh S: Shifting intentional set: Exploring the dynamic control of tasks, in Umiltá C, Moscovitch M (eds): Attention and Performance XV: Conscious and Nonconscious Information Processing. Cambridge, MA: MIT Press, 1994, pp. 421–452.

Baddeley A, Della Sala S: Working memory and executive control. Philos Trans R Soc Lond 351:1397–1404, 1996.

Baddeley A, Della Sala S, Papagno C, et al: Dual-task performance in dysexecutive and nondysexecutive patients with a frontal lesion. Neuropsychology 11:187–194, 1997.

Baddeley AD: Working Memory. Oxford, England: Clarendon, 1986.

Bartolomeo P, Siéroff E, Decaix C, et al: Modulating the attentional bias in unilateral neglect: The effects of the strategic set. Exp Brain Res 137:432–444, 2001.

Baylis GC, Driver J, Rafal RD: Visual extinction and stimulus repetition. J Cogn Neurosci 5:453–466, 1993.

Behrmann M, Moscovitch M, Winocur G: Intact visual imagery and impaired visual perception in a patient with visual agnosia. J Exp Psychol Hum Percept Perform 20:1068–1087, 1994.

Behrmann M, Zemel RS, Mozer MC: Object-based attention and occlusion: Evidence from normal participants and a computational model. J Exp Psychol Hum Percept Perform 24:1011–1036, 1998.

Bisiach E, Capitani E, Porta E: Two basic properties of space representation in the brain: Evidence from unilateral neglect. J Neurol Neurosurg Psychiatry 48:141–144, 1985.

Bisiach E, Vallar G: Hemineglect in humans, in Boller F, Grafman J (eds): Handbook of Neuropsychology. New York: Elsevier, 1988, Vol. 1, pp. 195–222.

Calvanio R, Petrone PN, Levine DN: Left visual spatial neglect is both environment-centered and body-centered. Neurology 37:1179–1183, 1987.

Chao LL, Knight RT: Human prefrontal lesions increase distractability to irrelevant sensory inputs. Neuroreport 6:1605–1610, 1995.

Cohen A, Rafal RD: Attention and feature integration: Illusory conjunctions in a patient with a parietal lobe lesion. Psychol Sci 2:106–110, 1991.

Cohen JD, Romero RD, Servan-Schreiber D, et al: Mechanisms of spatial attention: The relation of macrostructure to microstructure in parietal neglect. J Cogn Neurosci 6:377–387, 1994.

Colby CL, Goldberg ME: Space and attention in parietal cortex. Annu Rev Neurosci 22:319–349, 1999.

Damasio AR: The somatic marker hypothesis and the possible functions of prefrontal cortex. Philos Trans R Soc Lond B351:1413–1420, 1999.

Desimone R, Duncan J: Neural mechanisms of selective visual attention. Annu Rev Neurosci 18:193–222, 1995.

Drewe EA: Go-no-go learning after frontal lobe lesions in humans. Cortex 11:8–16, 1975.

Driver J, Halligan PW: Can visual neglect operate in object-centered co-ordinates? An affirmative single-case study. Cogn Neuropsychol 8:475–496, 1991.

Duncan J: Selective attention and the organization of visual information. J Exp Psychol Gen 113:501–517, 1984.

Efron R: What is perception? in Cohen RS, Wartofsky M (eds): Boston Studies in the Philosophy of Science. New York: Humanities Press, 1968, Vol. IV, pp. 137–173.

Eglin M, Robertson LC, Knight RT: Visual search performance in the neglect syndrome. J Cogn Neurosci 1:372–385, 1989.

Egly R, Driver J, Rafal RD: Shifting visual attention between objects and locations: Evidence from normal and parietal lesion subjects. J Exp Psychol Gen 123:161–177, 1994.

Eriksen BA, Eriksen CW: Effects of noise letters upon the identification of a target letter in a nonsearch task. Percept Psychophys 16:143–149, 1974.

Eriksen CW, Hoffman JE: The extent of processing of noise elements during selective encoding from visual displays. Percept Psychophys 14:155–160, 1973.

Farah MJ: Visual agnosia. Cambridge, MA: MIT Press, 1990.

Farah MJ, Brunn JL, Wong AB, et al: Frames of reference for allocation of spatial attention: Evidence from the neglect syndrome. Neuropsychologia 28:335–347, 1990.

Farah MJ, Monheit MA, Wallace MA: Unconscious perception of "extinguished" visual stimuli: Reassessing the evidence. Neuropsychologia 29:949–958, 1991.

Farah MJ, Wong AB, Monheit MA, et al: Parietal lobe mechanisms of spatial attention: Modality-specific or supramodal? Neuropsychologia 27:461–470, 1989.

Fleet WS, Valentstein E, Watson RT, et al: Dopamine agonist therapy for neglect in humans. Neurology 37:1765–1771, 1987.

Friedman-Hill SR, Robertson LC, Treisman A: Parietal contributions to visual feature binding: Evidence from a patient with bilateral lesions. Science 269:853–855, 1995.

Guitton D, Buchtel HA, Douglas RM: Frontal lobe lesions in man cause difficulties in suppressing reflexive glances and in generating goal-directed saccades. Exp Brain Res 58:455–472, 1985.

Heilman KM, Watson RT, Valenstein E: Neglect and related disorders, in Heilman KM, Valenstein E (eds): Clinical Neuropsychology, ed 3. New York: Oxford University Press, 1993, pp. 279–336.

Heilman KM, Watson RT, Valenstein E: Neglect I: Clinical and anatomic issues, in Farah MJ, Feinberg TE (eds): Patient-Based Approaches to Cognitive Neuroscience. Cambridge, MA: MIT Press, 2000, pp. 115–123.

Henik A, Rafal R, Rhodes D: Endogenously generated and visually guided saccades after lesions of the human frontal eye fields. J Cogn Neurosci 6:400–411, 1994.

Hillyard SA, Vogel EK, Luck SJ: Sensory gain control (amplification) as a mechanism of selective attention: Electrophysiological and neuroimaging evidence. Philos Trans R Soc Lond Biol Sci 353:1257–1270, 1998.

Husain M, Shapiro K, Martin J, et al: Abnormal temporal dynamics of visual attention in spatial neglect patients. Nature 385:154–156, 1997.

James W: Principles of Psychology. New York: Holt, 1890.

Jonides J: Voluntary versus automatic control over the mind's eye's movement, in Long JB, Baddeley AD (eds): Attention and Performance IX. Hillsdale, NJ: Erlbaum, 1981, pp. 187–203.

Kahneman D: Attention and Effort. Englewood Cliffs, NJ: Prentice Hall, 1973.

Karnath H-O: Neural encoding of space in egocentric coordinates?, in Thier P, Karnath H-O (eds): Parietal Lobe Contributions to Orientation in 3D-Space. Heidelberg: Springer-Verlag, 1997, pp. 497–520.

Karnath H-O, Christ K, Hartje W: Decrease of contralateral neglect by neck muscle vibration and spatial orientation of trunk midline. Brain 116:383–395, 1993.

Kim M-S, Cave KR: Spatial attention in visual search for features and feature conjunctions. Psychol Sci 6:376–380, 1995.

Kimberg DY, D'Esposito M, Farah MJ: Frontal lobes II: Cognitive issues, in Farah MJ, Feinberg TE (eds): Patient-Based Approaches to Cognitive Neuroscience. Cambridge, MA: MIT Press, 2000, pp. 317–326.

LaBerge D, Buchsbaum MS: Positron emission tomographic measurements of pulvinar activity during an attention task. J Neurosci 10:613–619, 1990.

Ladavas E: Is the hemispatial deficit produced by right parietal lobe damage associated with retinal or gravitational coordinates? Brain 110:167–180, 1987.

Làdavas E, Carletti M, Gori G: Automatic and voluntary orienting of attention in patients with visual neglect: Horizonal and vertical dimensions. Neuropsychologia 32:1195–1208, 1994.

Lee SS, Wild K, Hollnagel C, et al: Selective visual attention in patients with frontal lobe lesions or Parkinson's disease. Neuropsychologia 37:595–604, 1999.

Lu Z, Dosher BA: External noise distinguishes attention mechanisms. Vision Res 38:1183–1198, 1998.

Luck SJ, Vecera SP: Attention: From tasks to mechanisms, in Yantis S (ed): Stevens' Handbook of Experimental Psychology. Sensation and Perception. New York: John Wiley & Sons, 2002, Vol. 1, pp. 235–286.

Marrocco RT, Davidson MC: Neurochemistry of attention, in Parasuraman R (ed): The Attentive Brain. Cambridge, MA: MIT Press, 1998, pp. 35–50.

Mozer MC: Explaining object-based deficits in unilateral neglect without object-based frames of reference, in Reggia JA, Ruppin E, Glanzman D (eds): Disorders of Brain, Behavior, and Cognition: The Neurocomputational Perspective. Amsterdam: Elsevier, 1999, pp. 99–119.

Mozer MC: Frames of reference in unilateral neglect and visual perception: A computational perspective. Psychol Rev 109:156–185, 2002.

Mozer MC, Sitton M: Computational modeling of spatial attention, in Pashler H (ed): Attention. Hove, England: Psychology Press/Erlbaum (UK) Taylor & Francis, 1998, pp. 341–393.

Norman DA, Shallice T: Attention to action: Willed and automatic control of behavior, in Davidson RJ, Schwartz GE, Shapiro D (eds): Consciousness and Self-Regulation. New York: Plenum Press, 1986, Vol. 4, pp. 1–18.

Owen AM, Robert AC, Polkey CE, et al: Extra-dimensional versus intra-dimensional set shifting performance following frontal lobe excisions, temporal lobe excisions, or amygdalohippocampectomy in man. Neuropsychologia 29:993–1006, 1991.

Pashler HE: The Psychology of Attention. Cambridge, MA: MIT Press, 1998.

Posner MI: Orienting of attention. Q J Exp Psychol 32:3–25, 1980.

Posner MI, Cohen Y: Components of visual orienting, in Bouma H, Bouwhuis DG (eds): Attention and Performance X. Hillsdale, NJ: Erlbaum, 1984, pp. 531–556.

Posner MI, Cohen Y, Rafal RD: Neural systems control of spatial orienting. Philos Trans R Soc Lond B298:187–198, 1982.

Posner MI, Walker JA, Friedrich FJ, et al: Effects of parietal lobe injury on covert orienting of visual attention. J Neurosci 4:1863–1874, 1984.

Prinzmetal W, Presti DE, Posner MI: Does attention affect visual feature integration? J Exp Psychol Hum Percept Perform 12:361–369, 1986.

Rafal R, Grimm RJ: Progressive supranuclear palsy: Functional analysis of the response to methysergide and antiparkinsonian agents. Neurology 31:1507–1518, 1981.

Rafal R, Robertson L: The neurology of visual attention, in Gazzaniga MS (ed): The Cognitive Neurosciences. Cambridge, MA: MIT Press, 1995 pp. 625–648.

Rafal RD: Neglect II: Cognitive neuropsychological issues, in Farah MJ, Feinberg TE (eds): Patient-Based Approaches to Cognitive Neuroscience. Cambridge, MA: MIT Press, 2000, pp. 125–141.

Rafal RD, Posner MI: Deficits in human visual spatial attention following thalamic lesions. Proc Natl Acad Sci U S A 84:7349–7353, 1987.

Rafal RD, Posner MI, Friedman JH, et al: Orienting of attention in progressive supranuclear palsy. Brain 111:267–280, 1988.

Raymond JE, Shapiro KL, Arnell KM: Temporary suppression of visual processing in an RSVP task: An attentional blink? J Exp Psychol Hum Percept Perform 18:849–860, 1992.

Riddoch MJ, Humphreys GW: A case of integrative visual agnosia. Brain 110:1431–1462, 1987.

Rizzo M, Akutsu H, Dawson J: Increased attentional blink after focal cerebral lesions. Neurology 57:795–800, 2001.

Rizzo M, Robin DA: Bilateral effects of unilateral visual cortex lesions in human. Brain 119:951–963, 1996.

Robertson L, Treisman A, Friedman-Hill S, et al: The interaction of spatial and object pathways: Evidence from Balint's syndrome. J Cogn Neurosci 9:295–317, 1997.

Rogers RD, Monsell S: Costs of a predictable switch between simple cognitive tasks. J Exp Psychol Gen 124:207–231, 1995.

Rorden C, Karnath H-O, Driver J: Do neck-proprioceptive and caloric-vestibular stimulation influence covert visual attention in normals, as they influence visual neglect? Neuropsychologia 39:364–375, 2001.

Rubens AB: Caloric stimulation and unilateral visual neglect. Neurology 35:1019–1024, 1985.

Shallice T: From Neuropsychology to Mental Structure. New York: Cambridge, 1988.

Shallice T: Specific impairments of planning. Philos Trans R Soc Lond B298:199–209, 1982.

Shallice T, Burgess P: The domain of supervisory processes and temporal organization of behaviour. Philos Trans R Soc Lond 351:1405–1412, 1996.

Swick D, Knight RT: Cortical lesions and attention, in Parasuraman R (ed): The Attentive Brain. Cambridge, MA: MIT Press, 1998, pp. 143–162.

Tranel D, Anderson SW, Benton AL: Development of the concept of "executive function" and its relationship to the frontal lobes, in Boller F, Spinnler H (eds): Handbook of Neuropsychology. Amsterdam: Elsevier, 1994, Vol. 9, pp. 125–148.

Treisman A: The binding problem. Curr Opin Neurobiol 6:171–178, 1996.

Treisman A, Schmidt H: Illusory conjunctions in the perception of objects. Cogn Psychol 14:107–141, 1982.

Treisman AM, Gelade G: A feature-integration theory of attention. Cogn Psychol 12:97–136, 1980.

Vecera SP: Grouped locations and object-based attention: Comment on Egly, Driver, and Rafal (1994). J Exp Psych Gen 123:316–320, 1994.

Vecera SP: Toward a biased competition account of object-based segregation and attention. Brain Mind 1:353–384, 2000.

Vecera SP, Behrmann M: Attention and unit formation: A biased competition account of object-based attention, in Shipley TF, Kellman P (eds): From Fragments to Objects: Segmentation and Grouping in Vision. Amsterdam: Elsevier, 2001, pp. 145–180.

Vecera SP, Behrmann M: Spatial attention does not require preattentive grouping. Neuropsychology 11:30–43, 1997.

Vecera SP, Farah MJ: Does visual attention select objects or locations? J Exp Psychol Gen 123:146–160, 1994.

Vecera SP, Luck SJ: Attention, in Ramachandran VS (ed): Encyclopedia of the Human Brain. San Diego, CA: Academic Press, 2002, Vol. 1, pp. 269–284.

Vendrell P, Junqué C, Pujol J, et al: The role of prefrontal regions in the Stroop task. Neuropsychologia 33:341–352, 1995.

Vogel EK, Woodman GF, Luck SJ: Storage of features, conjunctions, and objects in visual working memory. J Exp Psychol Hum Percept Perform 27:92–114, 2001.

Whyte J, Hart T, Schuster K, et al: Effects of methylphenidate on attentional function after traumatic brain injury. Am J Phys Med Rehabil 76:440–450, 1997.

Wilkins AJ, Shallice T, McCarthy R: Frontal lesions and sustained attention. Neuropsychologia 25:359–365, 1987.

Wolfe JM: Visual search, in Pashler H (ed): Attention. Hove, England: Psychology Press/Erlbaum (UK) Taylor & Francis, 1998, pp. 13–73.

Memory and Learning

John DeLuca

Jean Lengenfelder

Paul J. Eslinger

Amnesia

Anterograde amnesia

Consolidation

Declarative memory

Hippocampus

Learning

Procedural memory

Retrograde amnesia

Working memory

INTRODUCTION

The aims of this chapter are to outline how memory is organized in the brain and to summarize the most common forms of memory and learning impairments associated with neurologic disease. Evaluation of memory disorders is reviewed together with intervention and management approaches.

Memory can be defined as the ability to retain information and experiences and represents a fundamental adaptive capacity of the brain. Memory underlies children's achievement of developmental milestones, such as walking and talking, academic progress, social maturation, and other major activities and achievements throughout adolescence and adulthood, including education, vocation, family life, automobile driving, and most aspects of everyday life. Patients who acquire amnesia, the most profound form of memory impairment, accomplish little on a day-to-day basis. In describing the well-known case of H.M. (Scoville & Milner, 1957), who developed amnesia after bilateral medial temporal resections for intractable epilepsy, Scoville (1968) noted the following characteristics several years after his surgery:

> He reads magazines and newspapers but totally forgets the contents after 15 minutes; similarly, he solves difficult crossword puzzles and forgets them thereafter. He is unable to find his way home from a nearby store and is therefore not encouraged to go out of the house unaccompanied. . . . Of special interest is a slight but definite improvement in memory function, noted recently, more than 14 years after operation. H.M. now has a vague notion of some present-day occurrences, with recognition of the name of our President and of past wars, though still cannot spontaneously remember them. (p. 212)

Stefanacci and colleagues (2000) recently described the daily routine of case E.P., who suffered profound amnesia after a bout of herpes simplex encephalitis, as follows:

> On a typical day, E.P. has a light breakfast when he wakes up, and then he returns to bed where he listens to the radio. His wife reports that when he arises a second time, he will often return to the kitchen and have breakfast again, and sometimes he again returns to bed. He has had breakfast as many as three times in one morning before staying up for the day. E.P. chooses his own clothes and dresses himself. He needs no assistance in bathing or shaving, although he often needs reminders about those activities from his wife. In the morning, he alternates between taking short walks around his neighborhood and sitting in the backyard or in the living room. After lunch, he watches television or reads the newspaper or a magazine. Often, he will suggest that he and his wife go out, but once they leave the house (to go shopping, for example), he will become confused and ask to return home. He watches television after dinner, and retires early (7:00 P.M. or 8:00 P.M.). (p. 7024)

These brief vignettes underscore that amnesias are disabling conditions that severely limit a person's ability to function independently. A heavy burden of providing daily care often falls on family members who must steadfastly manage these patients' everyday activities and safety.

Memory impairments occur in many clinical forms and degrees, the most severe being amnesia. It is important to distinguish isolated memory loss (also called focal or selective memory loss) from memory loss in the context of more widespread or global cognitive impairments, as in dementia. Selective amnesia implies intact intellectual, attentional, perceptual, and communicative abilities. In many behavioral neurology and neuropsychology settings, memory complaints are common. Although strongly associated with advancing age, memory disorders can also be observed in young children (Vargha-Khadem et al., 1997). Amnesia may follow traumatic brain injury (TBI), which is a special risk in adolescent and young adult men (see Chapter 27). Although there are few systematic survey data, memory disorders are known to occur in neurodevelopmental (e.g., learning disabilities, autism, retardation), neurologic (e.g., Alzheimer disease [AD], stroke, epilepsy, head trauma), and psychiatric (e.g., schizophrenia, depression) populations.

APPROACH TO EVALUATION OF MEMORY DISORDERS

Memory Disorders Clinic

Specialized "memory disorders clinics" have been established at many university hospitals to provide multidisciplinary evaluation, treatment, patient education, and opportunities to participate in drug trials and other research protocols. These clinics are often organized through neurology departments and clinical neuroscience and neurorehabilitation programs with physician, psychologist, nursing, and social service support staff.

Hogh and colleagues (1999) reported their experiences with 400 consecutive patients referred to the Copenhagen University Hospital memory clinic over approximately a 2-year period. The results illustrate a working model of a memory disorders clinic. Referrals were received from general practitioners and specialists. Patients requiring immediate hospitalization (such as those with acute confusion, severe dementia, behavioral problems, and normal pressure hydrocephalus) were referred to emergency services and excluded from the sample. Medical evaluation typically included:

- A mailed questionnaire about health problems, medications, automobile driving, and other background information (often completed by a caregiver who accompanied the patient to the clinic visit)

- Interview, history, neurologic, and physical examinations with Mini-Mental State Examination screening test (see Chapter 1 on Mental Status Screening for further details on this and other mental status screening tests), laboratory (blood) screening tests, and electrocardiography.

- Further laboratory and clinical assessments as needed for each case, such as neuropsychological testing (see Chapter 2 on Neuropsychological Assessment for rationale and methods in neuropsychological testing), psychiatric evaluation (see Chapter 3 for details of neuropsychiatric examination), brain computed tomography (CT) or magnetic resonance imaging (MRI), and single photon emission computed tomography (SPECT). Neuropsychological testing typically encompassed six major cognitive domains with identification of scores that were more than two standard deviations below the mean (see end of this section for more details on brief mental status screening and comprehensive neuropsychological testing in memory disorders).

- Additional evaluation options included cerebrospinal fluid examination (spinal tap), intracranial pressure monitoring, and ventricular infusion study, positron emission tomography (PET), electroencephalography (EEG), quantitative EEG, and blood tests for rare conditions.

Following the evaluation phase, a multidisciplinary conference was convened to gather consensus on diagnosis, treatment, and further evaluation for each patient. Patients were classified into one of four categories: (1) dementia, (2) selective (isolated) amnesia, (3) other selective cognitive impairments, and (4) no cognitive impairments. Underlying diagnostic etiology was also established based on reference criteria such as DSM-IV (American Psychiatric Association, 1994), NINCDS-ADRDA (McKhann et al., 1984), and ICD-10 (World Health Organization, 1994) classification. Concomitant diseases and risk factors were also noted. Concerns pertinent to caregiver, treatment, and social, occupational, economic, automobile driving, and other real-life issues for each patient were identified and discussed. The patient and caregiver were given feedback on the diagnosis and proposed treatment plan. A written summary was sent to the referral source and follow-up was scheduled as needed.

Characteristics of the Copenhagen memory disorders clinic are outlined in Table 11-1. The structure and pattern of evaluation reported by these authors describe a successful prototype for divising other

memory disorder clinics. Frequency of diagnoses will vary among such clinics depending on patient referral patterns and clinic settings. A neurologist often leads the multidisciplinary evaluation team that works together to accomplish the following: (1) identify and treat reversible causes of memory loss, (2) understand disease prognosis, (3) develop management plans for untreatable memory and cognitive conditions, and (4) treat secondary conditions to improve the overall health of the patient. It is also vital to (5) educate caregivers, patients, and other involved persons to aid them in coping and planning, and (6) identify local services within patients' communities (e.g., support groups, adult day care, "meals-on-wheels" programs, respite care, long-term care facilities, etc.). Finally, (7) inviting patients with memory impairment and their caregivers to participate in treatment trials and research protocols can offer them a sense of hope and the chance to make a positive contribution toward conquering these often devastating diseases.

Brief Mental Status Screening Versus Neuropsychological Testing

The clinical assessment of memory can range from a brief office or bedside screening exam (e.g., mental status evaluation) to comprehensive neuropsychological assessment of the major features of learning and memory and other processes that contribute to memory functions (further details about mental status tests and neuropsychological testing are described in Chapters 1 and 2).

The assessment of memory is an important part of the mental status evaluation. Typically, examiners assess attention and simple working memory with digit span tasks and short-term verbal memory through orientation questions and patient recall of three or four words after a 5-minute delay. More elaborate mental status assessments will attempt to add a visuospatial memory component (e.g., recall four objects hidden in a room) in addition to assessing other aspects of cognition such as language and spatial cognition.

Although screening tests have the benefit of being brief, they also have limited sensitivity and specificity. They are likely to detect severe memory impairment (as in amnesia and dementia) but may miss or underestimate less severe forms of impaired memory (e.g., in multiple sclerosis [MS] or traumatic brain injury [TBI]). Mild to moderate memory disorders may limit everyday independent functioning (Rosenthal & Ricker, 2000). Consequently, referral for more in-depth neuropsychological evaluation should take into account information from the history (complaints of decreased work efficiency; family subjective reports) or other medical factors (lesions on CT or MRI), and not just results of a

TABLE 11-1. Characteristics of the Copenhagen University Hospital Prototypical Memory Disorders Clinic over a 2-year Period (Hogh et al., 1999)

400 consecutive patients: 190 women, 210 men	
Mean age 63.6 yr (range, 19–97 yr)	
Mean Mini-Mental State Exam score 23.2/30 (range 0–30)	
Referral from general practitioners 191; from specialists and hospital departments 183	
Neuropsychological testing completed in 241 patients (60%)	
Psychiatric evaluation completed in 150 patients (37%)	
Cerebrospinal fluid exam completed in 77 patients (19%)	
Final behavioral diagnoses:	
Dementia	46%
Selective amnesia	5%
Selective other cognitive impairment	14%
No cognitive deficits	31%
Ten most frequent medical diagnoses (comprising 72% of all patients):	
Alzheimer disease	18.50%
No neuropsychiatric diagnosis	11.25%
Depression	8.50%
Vascular dementia	7.00%
Sequelae of stroke	6.50%
Unspecified dementia	5.75%
Normal pressure hydrocephalus	4.75%
Organic amnesia	3.25%
Alcohol dependence	3.25%
Mixed Alzheimer dementia	3.00%
Alzheimer potentially treatable conditions	26.00%
Potentially reversible underlying disease in patients 65 yr and older (37/214)	17.00%

mental status screening test score. In the study by Hogh and colleagues (1999), two thirds of the patients with normal screening mental status scores were referred for neuropsychological testing, principally to rule out memory and other cognitive impairments suspected on the basis of history, interview, and clinical exam.

Referrals for neuropsychological examination have increased substantially over the last few decades (Lezak, 1995). The neurologic community recognizes this examination as an established and clinically informative service (Subcommittee of American Academy of Neurology, 1996). The practice of clinical neuropsychology implies specialized training, often at the postdoctoral level, in the assessment of brain-behavior relationships. Appropriately, referral for neuropsychological services should be made to specialists who are qualified to conduct a comprehensive neuropsychological evaluation.

Why is a comprehensive evaluation often needed rather than a simplified assessment of memory? What may appear to be a memory problem may actually be a problem that lies outside the domain of memory. For instance, most persons who complain of impaired cognition will usually point to memory as the primary difficulty. Rarely do individuals self-refer for impairments in attention, information processing, and executive functions. Many persons who report subjective memory impairment, such as persons with TBI or MS, may have difficulties primarily in areas of speed of processing, attention, or executive functions (EF), rather than declarative memory (Demaree et al., 1999). The comprehensive neuropsychological evaluation can identify and quantify these distinctions.

Comprehensive neuropsychological testing can also identify which specific memory processes are defective, which can be helpful for differential diagnosis. For instance, persons with TBI, MS, Huntington chorea, and other neurologic diseases are more likely to have difficulties in the initial acquisition or learning of information rather than in consolidation (i.e., rate of forgetting) or in memory retrieval (DeLuca et al., 1998, 2000). Learning impairments may be due to difficulties in speed of processing, attention, or EF. In contrast, persons in early stages of AD and other forms of medial temporal lobe pathology are more likely to show comparatively preserved immediate recall but rapid rates of forgetting that affect memory retention.

Neuropsychological assessment can delineate the severity of memory impairment and provide recommendations for treatment, modifications to home and work settings, and compensatory approaches. Neuropsychological evaluation can identify potential non-neurologic explanations for memory complaints. These include issues of patient effort in testing, malingering, depression, anxiety, stress, pain, medication effects, remote head trauma, and normal aging changes.

A MODEL OF MEMORY ORGANIZATION IN THE BRAIN

Multiple Memory Systems

Historically, memory was thought to be part of the "intellectual faculties" in humans (e.g., Markowitsch, 2000). By the mid-1800s, human intelligence was associated with the functions of the frontal lobes; as such, memory processing was also linked to frontal lobe structures. By the turn of the 20th century, a clinical amnestic syndrome became recognized and was most notably associated with Wernicke-Korsakoff syndrome as a result of chronic alcoholism. Neuropathologic studies of patients with Wernicke-Korsakoff syndrome subsequently identified degenerative changes in the dorsomedial thalamic nuclei and the mammillary bodies, which then became a primary anatomic focus for memory-related function and impairment. Despite scattered reports, the role of mesial temporal lobe structures (primarily the hippocampus) was not recognized as a critical memory structure until the middle of the 20th century. The role of the basal forebrain in memory processes has been gaining increased attention as well. The frontal lobes have also reemerged as important for memory, particularly encoding and retrieval processes.

Memory is often referred to as a singular concept (e.g., "How is the patient's memory?"). In fact, memory is a complex and complicated construct. Is recalling the name of a second grade teacher the same as recalling what one ate for breakfast or remembering how to ride a bicycle or memorizing the number from a phone book to call for pizza? The answer is no. From cognitive and anatomic perspectives, each of these functional activities depends on different memory systems in the brain that are specialized for learning, storage and retrieval of knowledge, experiences, events, and skills.

Importantly, there can be no memory without learning. Learning refers to "the process of acquiring new information," whereas memory refers to "the per-

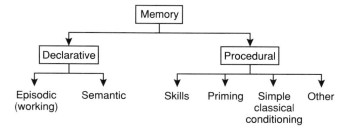

FIGURE 11-1. Proposed classification of memory systems in the brain. (Adapted from Squire LR: *Memory and Brain*. New York: Oxford University Press, 1987.)

sistence of learning in a state that can be revealed at a later time" (Squire, 1987). The integrity of memory systems cannot be assessed adequately without reference to the quality and quantity of learning-related processes.

Learning and memory can be divided into two general constructs: declarative and procedural (Fig. 11-1). Declarative memory refers to the conscious recollection of facts, knowledge, experiences, and events (e.g., Where did you spend your last holiday? Who is the president? What day of the week is it?). This system mediates the general, specific, and personal aspects of declarative knowledge that are acquired through learning and is highly sensitive to acquired brain damage. The neural substrate of the declarative memory system consists of complex interactions among medial temporal lobe (especially parahippocampal gyrus, entorhinal cortex, and hippocampus), diencephalic (primarily medial nuclear structures), basal forebrain, and diverse cortical association structures dedicated to sensory-perceptual processing and executive functions (see following section for more details). In contrast, procedural memory refers to sensory-motor and skill-based learning (e.g., knowledge of how to ride a bike, play the piano) and is generally viewed as memory that is not necessarily accessible to conscious experience (e.g., Cohen & Eichenbaum, 1994). Specifically, procedural memory does not require explicit recollection of past experiences to access and implement related aspects of those memories.

One can view the declarative memory system as consciously knowing *that* something was learned (e.g., learning to swim) and the procedural memory system as knowing *how* to perform the learned skill in the absence of conscious awareness of the learning experiences (Eslinger & Damasio, 1986; Baur et al., 1993). Procedural memory is typically spared following brain damage and is thought to be mediated by a network of structures that includes the basal ganglia and the cerebellum along with cortical sensory-perceptual areas. Although controversial, some have used the terms *explicit* and *implicit memory* as synonymous with declarative and procedural memory, respectively.

Declarative Memory

Declarative memory can be subdivided into a variety of different memory constructs. These divisions are usually based on differences in how declarative memory defects are manifested, often following brain damage. The oldest and most common division is between short-term memory (increasingly referred to as working memory in contemporary discussions) and long-term memory.

Working Memory

Working memory (WM) encompasses the representational processes that allow us to keep information active or "in mind" for various periods of time. It involves both temporary storage and processing operations that are critical to learning. Baddeley (1992) proposed that WM consists of two main components: a central executive and sensory-perceptual slave systems. The slave systems are purported to be limited capacity, temporary storage sites for rapidly changing information. At least two slave systems are proposed: (1) a phonological loop that temporarily stores auditory information and (2) a visuospatial sketchpad that temporarily stores visual information. These slave systems are functionally equivalent to what has been termed *short-term memory*. If unrehearsed or otherwise not used, such information will decay rapidly. The central executive component of WM refers to the limited-capacity attentional system that catalyzes the active manipulation and processing of information stored in the slave systems (see Chapter 10). That is, the central executive serves as the overall organizer, controller, planner, and resource allocation system for the active manipulation of representational information in WM. Importantly, WM is one of the most sensitive cognitive constructs to brain damage, imposing rate-limiting constraints on speed, complexity, and extent of new information processing. WM has been conceptualized as the "encoding stage" in information processing that sets in motion beginning mechanisms of consolidation for eventual long-term memory storage (Johnson, 1992).

Long-Term Memory

Long-term memory (LTM) refers to information that has been encoded and consolidated to a degree sufficient to permit stable representations in the brain. Such memory is rarely, if ever, processed in isolation and is often repeatedly elaborated and associated in relationship to existing and subsequently acquired memory. These inter-related perceptual, cognitive, and memory processes yield not only specific memory traces but also their accumulation into diverse knowledge structures that underlie semantic memory systems such as language and object recognition, episodic memory systems including autobiographical memory, and higher-level conceptual and categorical knowledge.

LTM can be divided into many different compartments. One useful distinction for diagnostic and rehabilitative purposes is *anterograde* and *retrograde* memory. Anterograde memory refers to learning and memory that occurs after damage to the brain. Hence, anterograde amnesia refers to impairment of new learning and memory capabilities, which is the most common presentation. Retrograde memory refers to information and experiences acquired before the onset of brain damage. Retrograde amnesia, therefore, indicates that the individual is unable to retrieve or access past memory stores. In most amnestic disorders, a temporal gradient in retrograde memory can be observed, indicating that patients have better recall the farther back in time events were initially acquired (Ribot, 1881). Although rare, there are cases of focal retrograde amnesia with normal or near-normal anterograde memory (Kapur, 1993).

Another useful distinction uncovered through neuropsychological research is the difference between *episodic* and *semantic* memory. Episodic memory refers to events, facts, and experiences that have occurred within specific spatial-temporal contexts (e.g., what you ate for breakfast today, what you remember about your 21st birthday, accomplishments during your college years, etc.). Episodic memory is a highly autobiographical form of memory that is critical for adaptive social functioning, relationships, judgment, goal-directed behavior, and the continuous sense of "self" across time (Levine et al., 1998). In contrast, semantic memory reflects general knowledge, recognition, and meaning of words, objects, actions, and facts that are not tied to specific time and place of learning. Neuropsychological studies have documented that amnesic individuals can retain intellectual, linguistic, perceptual, and semantic knowledge and skills but show profound deficits in the ability to recall specific details and episodes of learned information. The following case demonstrates this remarkable dissociation.

CASE STUDY

The patient, a 40-year-old man, working as a physician, suffered a bout of status epilepticus related to deficient compliance with longstanding treatment for seizure disorder. Brain MRI scan showed abnormal signal confined to the medial temporal regions bilaterally, involving the hippocampus (Fig. 11-2). The patient presented clinically as densely amnesic but without other neurologic and neuropsychological impairments. He was fully conversant and handled his daily needs without difficulty though he needed frequent cueing. He could recall bits of new information and experiences for only 3 to 4 minutes (i.e., rapid forgetting). General intelligence measured on the WAIS-R yielded a full-scale IQ of 117 (above average). In contrast, memory index scores from the WMS-R were as follows:

Verbal   = 57 (very impaired)
Visual   = 78 (borderline)
General = 56 (very impaired)
Delayed = 50 (very impaired)

These scores indicated severely impaired immediate recollection and virtually no delayed recollection of both verbal and visual information, even when examined 2 weeks after onset of his illness when he had stabilized and been seizure free for 12 days. This pattern has remained stable for 2 years and disabled him from independent employment. He is independent in certain daily activities around his home and community but these are highly routine. He has been able to use limited self-cueing strategies to accomplish local shopping and driving. It is important to note that despite his longstanding seizure disorder, The patient was above average in his academic achievement and general adaptation. He had completed college, medical school, and residency training and had been working as a physician for 14 years prior to his acute-onset illness. His bilateral medial temporal damage was likely related to anoxic-ischemic effects of a bout of status epilepticus (Eslinger, 1998).

Procedural Memory

Procedural memory can take many forms (see Fig. 11-1) that can include skill learning and memory, priming, and classical conditioning.

Skill Learning and Memory

Learning sensory-motor skills such as typing, playing musical instruments, riding a bike, and swimming is mediated by the procedural memory system and its interactions with diverse sensory-perceptual and motor system structures. Patients with dense amnesias can acquire new perceptual, cognitive, and motor skills despite their lack of awareness of and inability to recall the learning experience. For example, amnesic individuals have been taught to play a melody on the piano (Gardner, 1975), show normal learning and recall of visual motor skills (Damasio et al., 1985), and learn to use word processing on a computer (Glisky, 1995) despite the failure to recall the learning sessions or demonstrate any awareness of them. An important role for the basal ganglia in skill learning has been supported through studies of individuals with damage to these structures (e.g., Huntington disease, Parkinson disease), who demonstrate specific deficits in motor skill learning but not in declarative memory.

Priming

Priming refers to biased processing of information because of preceding exposure to the specific stimulus materials. In such situations, there need not be conscious awareness of the prior exposure when subjects are asked to respond to similar information. For instance, in a priming experiment, subjects can be shown a series of words and instructed to make some decision about each (e.g., "Is this a type of animal?"). They are not instructed to remember the words. At a later time, they are asked to fill in a series of word stems with any word they wish (e.g., the word stem "cel" or "sto"). Results typically demonstrate that amnesics will fill in the word stems with words previously shown to them at a rate that is well above chance (e.g., the words "celery" and "stone" from the previous examples). In another priming experiment, subjects will show much faster and more accurate reading of previously exposed words than novel items, even though they cannot recall those words in any demonstrable way. Importantly, these priming effects are similar for both amnesic patients and healthy controls.

Classical Conditioning

In classical conditioning, a stimulus that does not produce an unconditioned response (conditioned stimulus) is paired with one that does (unconditioned stimulus) until the conditioned stimulus also begins to elicit the same response. Delay eye-blink conditioning

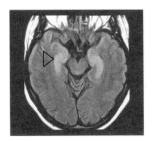 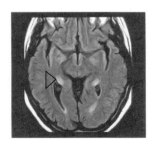

FIGURE 11-2. Brain MRI scan of the patient, who developed profound amnesia and abnormal signal in the bilateral medial temporal lobe after a bout of status epilepticus.

involves learning to blink in anticipation of an airpuff to the eye by the advanced presentation of a previously neutral cue such as a tone. Eye-blink conditioning is known to be critically dependent on the cerebellum in both humans and animals. Furthermore, it has been shown in both humans and animals that damage to the hippocampus and surrounding areas does *not* disrupt the acquisition of delay eye-blink conditioning. Conversely, cerebellar damage in humans and animals impairs or abolishes delay eye-blink conditioning (Myers et al., 2001). Taken together, these data strongly suggest that classical conditioning is not dependent on the medial temporal lobe and declarative memory system and can be preserved in amnesia.

Information Processing Approach to Memory

An important approach to examining memory dysfunction is to examine the "process" by which memory becomes impaired. That is, an information processing approach examines where in the process of memory formation that performance becomes deficient. In this model, memory formation can be divided into "acquisition" and "retrieval" phases. *Acquisition* refers to "the sensory uptake of information, its initial encoding, and further consolidation" (Markowitsch, 2000). *Retrieval* refers to "the process of recovering previously encoded (and stored) information" (Brown & Craik, 2000). Some authors further differentiate memory acquisition into encoding and consolidation phases, whereas others completely separate encoding from consolidation processes.

Dichotomizing the memory process into acquisition versus retrieval mechanisms allows for the examination of where in the learning and memory process a patient is experiencing difficulty. Is the patient having difficulty in the initial learning of information or is the difficulty in the retrieval of information from long-term storage? Recent work in persons with TBI and MS illustrates how an information processing approach can help clarify the nature of impaired learning and memory.

Numerous studies have concluded that impaired memory in TBI and MS is due to difficulties in the retrieval of information from long-term storage (DeLuca et al., 1998, 2000). However, close examination of many of these studies reveals that investigators have typically failed to control for the amount of information initially acquired (or learned). If subjects acquire less information during learning, it cannot be distinguished whether impaired recall is due to lower initial learning or retrieval failure.

The need to control for the amount of information initially acquired is well documented (Huppert & Piercy, 1979; Baur et al., 1993; Hart & O'Shanick, 1993; Hart, 1994). In fact, Hart (1994) argued that only paradigms that "attempt to minimize the confounding effects of deficient encoding by matching samples on initial learning" (p. 331) can appropriately be used to disentangle the complex issues of encoding, storage, and retrieval.

To address this issue, DeLuca and colleagues (1998, 2000) designed studies to control the amount of information initially learned by equating TBI and MS samples on acquisition. This was accomplished by training the clinical groups and healthy controls to a learning criterion (e.g., recitation of 10 of 10 words on two consecutive trials of a list learning task). Once equated for level of acquisition, retrieval capacities can then be more clearly examined through recall and recognition paradigms. It was reasoned that if impaired learning was occurring in the clinical samples, then equating their learning levels should lead to no differences in recall or recognition between groups. In contrast, a retrieval-failure hypothesis would suggest that, even after being equated for initial acquisition, the clinical groups should still show impaired recall but intact recognition.

The results of these two studies were clear. Both the TBI and MS groups took significantly more trials to reach the learning criterion. However, the two clinical groups did not differ from healthy controls in both recall and recognition. In fact, no group differences were noted in recall and recognition up to 1 week after learning in MS (TBI subjects were not examined 1 week later). These results show that the major deficit experienced by persons with TBI and MS is in the initial acquisition of information, not retrieval from long-term storage. Since this initial work, other investigators have replicated and extended these findings (Demaree et al., 2000; Vanderploeg et al., 2001). A similiar approach has also been used in other clinical populations (Weingartner et al., 1979; Ryan & Butters, 1983).

The advantage of an information processing approach to the study of impaired memory is that the findings have significant implications for rehabilitation and treatment. Treatment for acquisition difficulties should focus on techniques to improve learning, whereas treatment for retrieval failure would rely more on techniques to aid in the search of stored memories.

Neural Structures Critical to Learning and Memory

Learning and memory capacities are mediated by multiple neural systems. During the first half of the 20th century, the neural basis of memory was considered to be an emergent property of the central nervous system and not "localizable" in any clear fashion (Lashley, 1950). Concepts of mass action and equipotentiality prevailed and suggested that the search for the engram or neural equivalent of memory traces was largely futile because memory traces were equally embedded throughout numerous brain structures and were disrupted in proportion to the size of a brain lesion, regardless of its specific location. These concepts changed dramatically with the description of case of H.M. by Scoville and Milner (1957) and subsequent cases that confirmed their findings. Because of intractable epilepsy related to medial temporal lobe irritative lesions, H.M. underwent bilateral resection of the anterior and medial temporal lobes (Corkin et al., 1997). This surgical treatment was actually quite effective in controlling his epilepsy but had the unintended effect of causing a profound anterograde amnesia that has changed little over the past 50 years. H.M. has been able to learn certain daily routines and has retained his intellectual, sensorimotor, perceptual, and communicative abilities. However, he has been unable to retain new information and experiences with few exceptions (e.g., he has been able to learn a very limited amount of new vocabulary words and factual information). H.M. shows full preservation of sensory and motor learning (i.e., procedural memory), which is a characteristic finding with medial temporal lobe amnesia as well as in AD (Milner, 1965; Corkin, 1968; Damasio et al., 1985; Eslinger & Damasio, 1986). However, he has required daily supervision and has been a resident of a long-term care facility since his parents died.

The anatomic structures damaged in H.M. and in other cases confirming medial temporal lobe amnesia include the hippocampus most prominently but other nearby structures as well including the amygdala, entorhinal cortex, parahippocampal gyrus, subiculum, and in some cases part of the temporal polar cortex. Subsequent anatomic studies, using radioactive tracers that are transported in retrograde and anterograde fashion within neurons, have been able to decipher the pattern of projections both within the medial temporal region as well as between the medial temporal lobe and various associational cortices (Van Hoesen et al., 1972; Seltzer & Pandya, 1976; Van Hoesen, 1982). These studies have indicated that projections from primary sensory cortices (i.e., for vision, audition, and somatosensory functions) are directed to their modality-specific association cortices. These association cortices, in turn, project into multimodal association areas, including the inferior parietal lobule and dorsolateral prefrontal cortex. Most importantly, these modality-specific and multimodal association areas send converging projections to the parahippocampal gyrus in the medial temporal lobe region. This convergence zone is the primary staging area for input to the hippocampus, which occurs via the entorhinal cortex and perforant pathway. Processing within the hippocampus involves its various CA 1–4 zones with output directed via the subiculum and fimbria-fornix system back to sensory association cortices, largely reciprocating the pattern of afferent projections to the medial temporal region. In addition to these reciprocal projection systems between various sensory association cortices and the medial temporal lobe, there are extensive interconnections between the medial temporal lobe and other limbic system structures including the basal forebrain, medial diencephalon (particularly the dorsomedial thalamic nucleus and mammillary bodies), amygdala, and retrosplenial cortex via many important pathways.

Clinical and behavioral validation of the functional significance of these various structures and pathways has been possible through the study of patients who present with cerebral lesions and behavioral changes (Damasio et al., 1985; von Cromen et al., 1985; Valenstein et al, 1987; van Squire, 1987; Rempel-Clower et al., 1996; Graham & Hodges, 1997). The neural substrate of declarative memory and associated memory-related impairments are summarized in Figure 11-3.

Lesions to the primary cortical sensory areas cause pure cortical sensory syndromes (e.g., cortical blindness, cortical deafness), whereas lesions to modality-specific cortical association areas result in agnosias (or loss of modality-specific knowledge leading to perception and recognition deficits, such as visual agnosia or auditory agnosia). Associative processing in these modality-specific cortical regions is essential if adequate learning is to occur, because they mediate basic sensory-perceptual, WM, and long-term recognition memory capacities. Hence, cortical sensory and agnosic syndromes are associated with impaired learning within specific modalities. Lesions to multimodal association areas will cause diverse cognitive and memory impairments, such as fluent aphasias with impaired comprehension, hemispatial neglect and spatial cognitive impairments, dysexecutive syndromes, and other losses of semantic knowledge that significantly interfere with specific types of learning and memory capacities. These can include verbal and visuospatial WM, encoding, and retrieval processes.

Medial temporal lobe functions depend on numerous cortical regions for accurate, coordinated, detailed, and timely modality-specific and multimodal sensory-perceptual processing. Damage to the medial temporal region and its limbic system counterparts lead to amnesias that are multimodal in nature. As is characteristic of medial temporal lobe amnesia, the most profound deficit is in retention of new information and experiences, with much less loss of previously acquired memory or long-term knowledge. The role of the medial temporal lobe, and particularly the hippocampus, has been linked to registering inter-related, multimodal information and experiences and setting up physiologic connections among the respective modality-specific and multimodal areas that underlie that new information processing. These physiologic connections are thought to involve the formation of new synapses and other

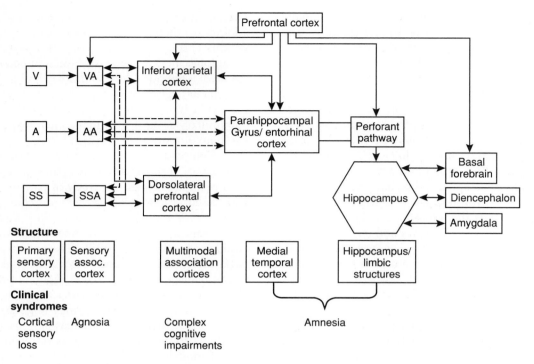

FIGURE 11-3. Schematic illustration of structures and pathways involved in declarative learning and memory. (V, visual cortex; VA, visual association cortex; A, auditory cortex; AA, auditory association cortex; SS, somatosensory cortex; SSA, somatosensory association cortex.)

physiologic events that become established through processes of memory consolidation. Consolidation occurs over a period of time from minutes to months and can be influenced by numerous neurobiologic, cognitive, emotional, and environmental factors. Impaired consolidation leads to rapid forgetting (or physiologic decay of temporary memory representations). Hence, patients with medial temporal lobe amnesia will show relatively preserved immediate recall of limited amounts of new information and experiences, but these traces will decay rapidly due to lack of consolidation.

The hippocampus and amygdala have strong interconnections. The role of the amygdala, which lies just rostral to the hippocampus, has become clearer through recent research. Though severe memory disorder has not been characteristic of amygdala damage, these patients develop memory difficulties, particularly in cross-modal learning and emotion-based learning.

CLINICAL DISORDERS OF MEMORY

Alcoholic Korsakoff Syndrome

Wernicke-Korsakoff syndrome (Korsakoff psychosis) is most often due to chronic alcohol abuse but may also be caused by other metabolic and nutritional disorders that deplete thiamine. In the acute presentation phase, patients develop gait ataxia, confusion, and ophthalmo-

plegia. With thiamine and folate loading, about 25% of patients recover adequately, but most develop amnesia in the chronic phase (Victor et al., 1989). Sensory-motor, intellectual, language, and perceptual abilities are otherwise well preserved. The pattern of memory impairment is typically profound anterograde amnesia with a temporally graded retrograde amnesia (i.e., preserved remote memory but impaired recent memory) and strong tendencies toward confabulation (Butters & Cermak, 1980). Chronic alcoholism itself may be associated with gradual progression of memory loss that dramatically escalates with development of Wernicke-Korsakoff disease (Ryan & Butters, 1983).

One of the difficulties in delineating the neuropathologic bases of Wernicke-Korsakoff syndrome is the complicating effect of chronic alcohol abuse including direct alcohol toxicity, nutritional deficiencies, and head traumas. Postmortem studies have emphasized degeneration of the dorsomedial nucleus of the thalamus and mammillary bodies as the key lesions. In a recent neuropathologic study of amnesic and nonamnesic alcoholics, Harding and colleagues (2000) reported that the most decisive difference occurred in the anterior thalamic nucleus, where neuronal loss was observed only in the alcoholic Korsakoff amnesic patients.

Personality, motivational, and EF impairments have also been reported in alcoholic Wernicke-Korsakoff syndrome but it remains unclear whether these represent specific, acute-onset changes or gradual and progressive changes due to complications of chronic alcoholism.

Herpes Simplex Encephalitis

Infection with the herpes simplex virus can cause a rare neurologic disorder known as herpes simplex encephalitis (HSE). Acute symptoms include fever, headache, vomiting, and seizures. Untreated, infection can result in severe brain damage within 24 hours of exposure (Schlitt et al., 1986). Predilection for the anterior and medial temporal lobe is typical with progression of necrotizing lesions into orbital and medial frontal lobes (Damasio et al., 1985; Eslinger et al., 1993). Early neurobehavioral defects include severe amnesia, confusion, fluent dysphasia, and symptoms associated with Klüver-Bucy syndrome (hyperphagia [indiscriminant ingestion, including nonfood items], aggressive behavior, hypersexuality, and emotional flaccidity). Acute symptoms tend to ameliorate with time, but social-emotional defects and severe amnesia often remain. Treatment with acyclovir is recommended but it remains uncertain just how effective this regimen is.

In chronic cases, many aspects of short-term or working memory are intact; however, memory retention is frequently profoundly impaired. Patients experience a rapid rate of forgetting, thought to be more severe than that observed in diencephalic amnesia (Squire, 1987). There is usually a retrograde amnesia, which varies across subjects in severity and extent of temporal gradient. Retrograde amnesia affects both general learned facts (e.g., well-known public events, famous persons) as well as autobiographical information. Procedural memory is typically intact on a variety of tasks including eye-blink conditioning and pursuit rotor learning (Damasio et al., 1985; Parkin & Lang, 1993). Integrity of frontal lobe–related tasks such as abstraction, set shifting, associative fluency, and cognitive estimation is variable and depends on encroachment of the necrotic lesions into prefrontal structures. Spontaneous confabulations, which are associated with frontal lobe pathology (DeLuca et al., 2000), can occur but are rare. When documented, they are often associated with a confusional state.

HSE can result in bilateral symmetrical or asymmetrical lesions as well as unilateral lesions in temporal lobe structures, with similar variations in encroachment of lesions into mesial and orbital frontal cortices. For example, Eslinger and colleagues (1996) compared and contrasted two patients with HSE with highly asymmetrical temporal lobe lesions (Figs. 11-4 and 11-5). Results demonstrated that profound loss of verbal learning and memory occurred in patient 061, who suffered predominant left temporal lobe damage.

Her visual learning and memory, in contrast, remained exceptional. She easily navigated routes around her town and throughout neighboring states and recognized famous faces though she could name virtually none of them. Patient 075, with unilateral right temporal lobe damage after HSE, was less severely impaired overall, but unable to return to work installing large kitchen appliances because of difficulties in spatial memory and imagery. He showed relative difficulties in certain face processing tasks but was not prosopagnosic. Another case with more extensive damage to right hemisphere temporal and parietal structures after HSE was able to navigate spatial routes only via specific verbal instructions (she was lost if this route was changed because of detours or other spatial variations), could not track where she parked her car, or even recognize her car except by license plate (Eslinger et al., 1993). Hence, the presentation of amnesia in HSE can be quite variable but strongly linked to location and extent of necrotic lesions within temporal lobe and related structures.

Cerebrovascular Diseases

Memory impairments can result from cerebrovascular lesions that affect the diverse memory systems described above. The most striking presentations of profound amnesia result from ischemic stroke in the lateral branch of the posterior cerebral artery (PCA) and in the interpeduncular profundus artery. The PCA stroke can extend from the occipital pole forward to the medial temporal lobe (Fig. 11-6), damaging the parahippocampal gyrus and the hippocampus. This frequently occurs in unilateral fashion and can give rise to material-specific types of memory impairments. With such left hemisphere strokes, the memory impairments are usually related to processing of verbal materials as well as temporal orientation and can be accompanied by alexia and right visual field cuts. This partial amnesia is generally confined to the anterograde sphere, without significant retrograde amnesia beyond the recent 1 to 2 years. When the PCA stroke occurs in the right hemisphere, the memory impairment is not as profound but does compromise learning and retention of faces, designs, and other visuospatial types of materials.

Stroke in the interpeduncular profundus artery affects the medial thalamus including the dorsomedial nucleus. Ischemic damage can be unilateral and cause similar material-specific memory impairments as PCA strokes or bilateral and cause a profound anterograde and retrograde amnesia, or so-called diencephalic amnesia (Graff-Radford et al., 1985). The bilateral lesions usually arise from an anatomic variant of this artery whereby a single artery bifurcates to supply both medial thalamic regions. Hence, occlusion in a single artery can cause bilateral ischemic lesions.

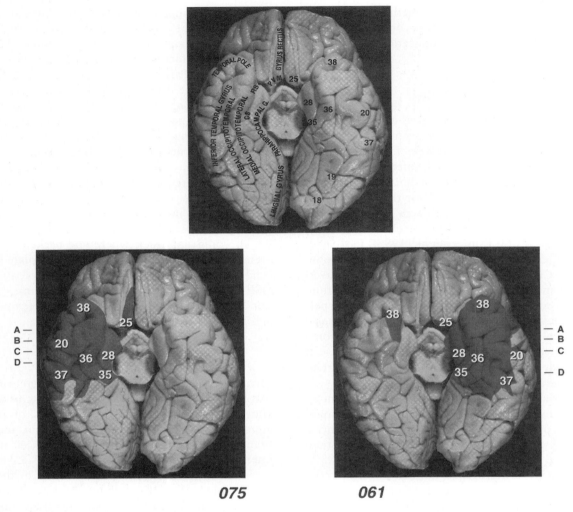

FIGURE 11-4. Comparison of cases with asymmetrical lesions after HSE with reference to inferior surface of the temporal lobes.

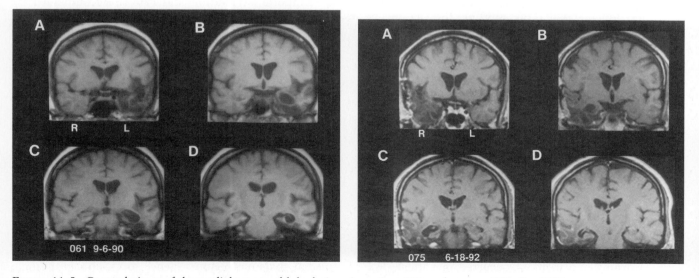

FIGURE 11-5. Coronal views of the medial temporal lobe lesions in patient 061 and patient 075 after HSE.

R L

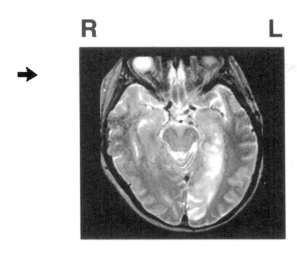

FIGURE 11-6. Axial view of left posterior cerebral artery stroke affecting medial temporal lobe structures in addition to the occipital lobe.

Aneurysmal subarachnoid hemorrhage (SAH) often results in impaired memory. Aneurysm of the anterior communicating artery (ACoA) commonly leads to significant memory impairment (DeLuca & Diamond, 1995). This is thought to be due to damage to the basal forebrain, an area perfused by perforating branches of the ACoA. The observed memory impairment may result from impaired modulation of hippocampal activity by a damaged basal forebrain (DeLuca & Chiravalloti, 2002). Among ACoA patients, impaired declarative memory is the primary problem, with intact procedural memory. Although immediate memory is generally intact, severe deficits in delayed recall are often observed. There is little evidence for severe and persistent retrograde memory impairment, but when it occurs, it is usually during the acute epoch.

It is important to recognize that aneurysmal SAH (not just from ACoA) can also result in significant memory and other cognitive impairments even in individuals with little or no other neurologic dysfunction (Ljunggren et al., 1985; Bornstein et al., 1987; Sonesson et al., 1987).

Confabulation, distortions in memory that frequently consist of temporally misplaced recollections of actual events as well as intrusions of often bizarre fabrications, is frequently observed following ACoA (DeLuca et al., 2000). Confabulation is always associated with an amnesic condition. Confabulation following ACoA has been shown to require both ventromedial frontal pathology and basal forebrain damage (DeLuca & Chairavalloti, 2002).

Epilepsy

Both temporal lobe epilepsy and lobectomy for the surgical treatment of intractable epilepsy have been associ-

ated with memory impairments. The hippocampal complex is the most epileptic-prone structure in the brain, leading to irritative lesions (e.g., hippocampal sclerosis) that have significant disruptive effects on normal functioning. Studies have established consistent "material-specific" deficits in memory after left and right temporal lobe epilepsy. That is, left temporal lobe pathology has been associated with predominantly verbal memory deficits, whereas right temporal lobe pathology has been associated with nonverbal, visual-spatial and face-processing memory impairments (Barr et al., 1990; Barr, 1997; Crane & Milner, 2002; Viskontas et al., 2002). Such deficits have been delineated primarily in the anterograde sphere but can also occur in the retrograde sphere.

Head Trauma

TBI has been associated with anterior temporal and orbitofrontal lobe contusions as well as shear injury that can affect multiple pathways in the brain, typically in frontal regions. Post-traumatic amnesia (PTA) refers to the anterograde amnesia that occurs after significant head trauma, often accompanied by a varied degree of retrograde amnesia as well. In mild and moderate cases of TBI, a substantial recovery of function can be expected, with resolution of most memory impairments, though residual alterations in attention, speed of processing, and WM can be observed (see Chapter 27 for more details).

Alzheimer Disease and Related Disorders

Alzheimer disease (AD) is a progressive neurodegenerative condition characterized by cognitive deterioration in multiple areas of cognition. AD is associated with an insidious onset and gradual course. It is the most common cause of dementia with prevalence rates of 5% to 10% in the population ages 65 and older and 25% to 50% in individuals 85 and older (see Chapter 22).

Memory impairment is a major feature of AD and is usually the presenting symptom. As the disease progresses, more widespread cognitive deficits progressively emerge (Flicker et al., 1991; Rossor, 1993). Symptoms of memory impairment in AD include rapid forgetting of new information, recall and recognition deficits, consolidation deficits, and impaired incidental learning. Some examples of memory difficulties apparent in daily life include misplacing items, trouble recalling details of conversations and recent events, forgetting names, and repeating questions and conversations (Morris, 1994; Morris et al., 1996). In contrast to impaired declarative memory processing, there is preservation of motor skill learning (Eslinger & Damasio, 1986).

Initially, memory deficits are most prominent in recalling recent events, whereas remote events and recent events with high emotional significance remain preserved (Price et al., 1993, Feinberg & Farah, 1997). For a period of time, memory prompts may aid in retrieving information but as the disease progresses retrieval becomes more impaired. Studies attempting to minimize the demands on retrieval by using various cueing and recognition paradigms have identified that memory performance improves only minimally. Incidental recall has also been shown to be impaired in individuals with AD but not in age-matched healthy individuals (Weintraub et al., 2000). There is a reduced ability to learn new information. Individuals with AD are also susceptible to retroactive interference effects, such that retention of previously learned information becomes disrupted by learning of new information (Wilson et al., 1983). For example, in a list-learning task such as the California Verbal Learning Test (Delis et al., 1987), learning the second list of words can interfere with recall of the first list of words presented.

As the disease progresses, recognition memory becomes impaired and individuals with AD are not able to retain new information for longer than a few minutes. In end-stage AD, individuals are often unable to even recognize well-known family members (Mesulam, 2000).

Vascular Dementia

Vascular dementia (VD) is the most common cause of dementia after AD and is characterized by cognitive impairment due to cerebrovascular lesions/disease. VD is generally associated with an abrupt onset and stepwise deterioration or fluctuating course. Additionally, other features may be present such as a history of stroke, more focal neurologic and neuropsychological deficits, and vascular risk factors such as hypertension. Two types of dementia are often distinguished in the literature. *Multi-infarct dementia (MID)* occurs after multiple strokes involving both cortical and subcortical regions. *Binswanger disease* occurs following strokes that primarily involve subcortical white matter.

Studies comparing memory impairments in VD and AD have not clearly identified consistent differences. Some report that certain aspects of memory are more severely impaired in AD (Carlesimo et al., 1993; Villardita, 1993; Kertesz & Clydesdale, 1994), whereas others have found no differences in memory impairments between the two groups (Almkvist et al., 1993; Erkinjuntti, 1987; Fischer et al., 1990). The pattern of memory deficits in VD tends to be more variable, depending on the nature, location, and extent of vascular disease.

Frontotemporal Dementia

Three clinical subtypes of frontotemporal dementia (FTD) have been identified: progressive nonfluent aphasia (PNFA), semantic dementia (SD), and frontal variant or behavior disorder-dysexecutive (BDD; Neary et al., 1998; Grossman, 2002). Common to all three subtypes is an insidious onset of symptoms with a slow gradual progression.

Changes in personality and behavior often emerge prior to the onset of memory deficits and these behavioral changes can include disinhibition, irritability, apathy, lack of insight, emotional lability, and paranoia (Neary et al., 1988; Knopman et al., 1990; Miller et al., 1991; Hodges et al., 1999). Impairment in executive abilities in the BDD subgroup is disproportionate to memory abilities, but nonetheless contributes to impairments in learning, utilization, and retrieval of information (Neary & Snowden, 1996). This pattern is opposite to that in AD where memory is often more impaired than executive abilities in the earlier stages of the disease (Neary et al., 1986; Jagust et al., 1989; Johansen & Hagberg, 1989; Pachana et al., 1996). Among the language-impaired subgroups (PNFA and SD), memory impairments develop as secondary effects of primary language-based deficits.

Lewy Body Disease

Lewy body disease (LBD) is characterized by visual hallucinations, parkinsonism, and fluctuating cognition with variations in alertness or attention. Pathologic Lewy bodies are present at autopsy and are found in the brainstem, limbic structures, and neocortex (McKeith et al., 1996).

Prominent or persistent memory impairment may not necessarily occur in the early stages of the disease but is usually evident with progression. AD patients typically perform worse on episodic memory and rate of forgetting measures, whereas LBD patients perform worse on measures of praxis, visuospatial ability, and attention (Sahgal et al., 1992; Connor et al., 1998; Ballard et al., 1999).

Frontal Lobe Syndromes

The frontal lobe contribution to memory and learning processes is quite different from those of the medial temporal lobe and other association cortices. As an important substrate for executive functions, prefrontal cortex has been linked to diverse attention, WM, and cognitive processes that influence how we process information as well as how we manipulate and retrieve it. In addition, the prefrontal cortex has been associated with metacognition, which encompasses our awareness of how we learn and why we learn (e.g., motivation, goal-directed behavior).

Clinically, patients with frontal lobe damage have been described with memory deficits, such as "forgetting to remember," which implies a metacognitive type of deficit. That is, rather than dysfunction in the memory system per se, this kind of impairment is manifested in the impaired use of memory in daily activities and tasks (see Chapter 20). Frontal lobe damage has also been linked to impaired source memory, that is, remembering the original spatial-temporal context of specific memories. Learning capacities of patients with frontal lobe damage have been described as more disorganized, shallower in level of processing, and atypical in learning curve characteristics. Impairments of temporal order and frequency processing have also been linked to frontal lobe damage. Shimamura (2000) has conceptualized the role of the frontal lobe in memory as a dynamic filtering system that selects, maintains, updates, and reroutes information processing and retrieval in association with other cortical regions.

Age-Associated Memory Changes

In the process of standardization, tests of memory are applied to samples of normal volunteers to gauge and establish the range, mean score, and other statistical properties of typical performance. In addition, effects of variables, such as age, education attainment, gender, processing speed, and general intellectual level, are often analyzed. Hence, the influence of such variables can be considered and their specific interactive effects with memory identified. An illustrative case is the recent renorming of the Wechsler Memory Scale (WMS-III), which identified clear effects of advancing age on diverse WM, verbal, and visual memory retention tasks. These tests provide normative observations for interpretation of test scores relative to the patient's age group. Hence, the mean number of items recalled or recognized on a verbal list-learning task will decrease with age but may remain at the average level (e.g., 50th percentile) because the overall performance of the older age group declines as well.

Age-associated memory changes are also referred to as "benign senescent forgetfulness" and refer to inefficiencies in learning, retention, and memory retrieval that are not associated with any known disease, trauma, or illness. These are annoying and frustrating to most people but neither disabling nor problematic if compensatory measures are taken. Adaptive strategies can be applied to people's occupational settings, daily and domestic affairs as well as leisure and recreational activities. An interesting trade-off, as it were, occurs in memory processing with age. That is, young adults are able to freely recall more items from most memorization-type tasks, but older adults generate comparatively more cohesive and integrated recall of information.

Neuropsychological testing of older persons with subjective complaints of memory changes can identify mild changes that bear watching and follow-up check for any progression (i.e., possible "mild cognitive impairment"), affective changes (e.g., depression, grief and adjustment reactions) that are disrupting normal memory abilities and require primary treatment, as well as an entirely normal range of results that are reassuring to patients and their families (see discussion on impairments in cognitive function with age in Chapter 36).

Psychiatric Disorders

Memory impairments have been reported in both schizophrenia and major depression. In schizophrenia, the deficits have been observed for verbal and visuospatial memory in the encoding and retrieval phases of memory processing rather than consolidation per se (Saykin et al., 1991; Paulsen et al., 1995). For treatment of intractable major depression, electroconvulsive therapy can be an effective option, with an estimated 100,000 people per year receiving treatment in the United States. Despite effectiveness, memory impairments have been a steadfast complication. These include deficits in declarative memory with relatively preserved immediate recall capacities (Lisanby et al., 2000; Rami-Gonzalez et al., 2001). The anterograde amnesia tends to resolve over weeks but retrograde amnesia has been reported to persist. Both are more common after bilateral than unilateral treatments (see Datto, 2000, for a recent review).

Other Medical Conditions

A number of other neurologic diseases, generally of a degenerative nature, are associated with impairments of memory and learning though not necessarily as the primary or most prominent symptom. These include Parkinson disease, Huntington chorea, MS, progressive supranuclear palsy (PSP), and corticobasal degeneration (CBD). (See Chapters 24 and 35 for detailed descriptions of associated memory and cognitive impairments in these conditions.) Two main points need to be made about these other neurodegenerative conditions and associated memory functions in comparison to the profound amnesias related to medial temporal lobe and diencephalic pathology. First, none show the prominent consolidation deficit with otherwise normal registration of new information. Their pattern of memory and learning deficit commonly revolves around a mix of attentional, cognitive, memory, and other disease-related deficits (e.g., slowed processing), sometimes exacerbated by side effects of medication. Second, the study of basal ganglia-related diseases has shown profound deficits in procedural memory as compared to declarative memory processing. This is the opposite of the medial temporal/diencephalic amnesia pattern in which procedural memory is normal.

Functional Memory Disorders

The accurate assessment of memory must occur with the confidence that the patient is providing full effort or motivation. "Functional" contributions to impaired memory range from "unconscious" (or thought to be psychogenic or "pseudoneurologic" in nature) to the active attempt to feign a memory disorder (malingering). Despite the development of numerous methodological procedures, it is not always easy to differentiate between the so-called psychogenic conditions (e.g., somatoform and factitious disorders, dissociative amnesia) versus malingering. DSM-IV requires that external incentives for the memory problem must be absent for factitious disorders, whereas they are often present for malingering. A number of specific tests have been developed to specifically address malingering of memory disorders. Among the most sensitive are the forced choice paradigms where patients are asked to examine simple pictures or words, or are presented with a string of digits to keep in mind. After a short delay or mild distraction, the patient is presented with two alternatives: a previously presented item and a novel item. The patient is asked to indicate which was presented earlier. The strength in such procedures is the normative finding that persons with severe brain damage (e.g., dementia) do as well as healthy controls on such tests. As such, poor performance on these measures strongly suggests poor effort or compromised motivation.

Additionally, given our knowledge of how declarative memory works, a number of observations can raise the suspicion of problems with effort or motivation. These include recognition memory worse than recall performance, complaints of impaired procedural memory (e.g., "I forgot how to play the piano."), and complaints of impaired very remote recall (e.g., "I can't recall the name of my high school.").

Certain contextual factors have also been associated with decreased effort or motivation. These include compensation seeking, disability and forensic evaluations, need to maintain a "sick role," and workers' compensation-related evaluations. It should be emphasized that the presence of such variables alone is not an indication of reduced effort or motivation and should never be used to support such hypotheses in isolation. For a more in-depth discussion on functional memory disorders, see Lezak (1995) and Chapter 53.

INTERVENTION AND MANAGEMENT APPROACHES

Behavioral Compensatory Approaches

Depending on the degree and type of memory impairment, cognitive and behavioral interventions can be helpful toward restoring a greater range of independent functioning in patients (see Glisky & Glisky, 2002, for a recent review; see Chapter 48 in this volume). Potential approaches include the following:

- Practice and rehearsal—can be helpful in learning/relearning limited and specific types of information, usually for daily living needs
- Mnemonic strategies—teaching and implementation of cognitively based strategies to improve learning of association, action sequences, and text; uses such strategies as visual imagery, verbally based organization and rules, and associative strategies
- Environmental supports and external aids— encourages the use of adaptive external memory devices to aid self-cueing, such as labels, instructions, notebooks and pads, calendars, alarm watches, timers, pagers, and electronic organizers specifically geared to the functional tasks and activities of individual patients
- Domain-specific learning—teaches very specific tasks and activities to patients with severe memory impairments. This is a slow and gradual process that capitalizes on the preserved abilities of patients to acquire skills through procedural memory mechanisms.

An integrated approach that uses several of these methods can be beneficial to patients with significant memory impairments (Glisky & Glisky, 2002). The most successful outcomes are those focused on well-defined and specific behavioral goals rather than on attempts to remediate the basic mechanisms of memory processing. The proliferation of handheld electronic organizers has tremendous potential for furthering the adaptive functioning of individuals with mild and moderate memory loss and otherwise intact cognitive capacities. Not only are they socially acceptable in most circumstances, but they also offer the benefits of low cost, application to many functional goals and circumstances, portability, and ease of use (Eslinger, 2002). Consultation with a rehabilitative neuropsychologist, speech pathologist, occupational therapist, and vocational counselor can help identify potential approaches and their implementation.

Medication Approaches

Prescription medications that have specific and proven beneficial effects on memory impairments are extremely limited. The only compounds that have undergone phase 3 trials are those approved for treatment of cognitive deficits in AD. These act as acetylcholinesterase inhibitors, blocking the reuptake of acetylcholine in the synaptic cleft, essentially prolonging its potential neurotransmitter effects (i.e., donepezil [Aricept], rivastigmine tartrate [Exelon], and galantamine hydrobromide [Reminyl]). The beneficial effects are modest but often noticeable on mental status screening tests and by patient and family reports. These medicines act to slow the rate of cognitive and memory loss characteristic of AD. There have been reported off-label uses for memory impairments in TBI, VD, and stroke, with some beneficial effects noticed (e.g., Taverni et al., 1998). An important avenue of research at this time is the exploration of potential effective combinations of medications and behavioral-cognitive remediation approaches.

Reports in the literature suggest a modest beneficial effect of ginkgo biloba for the memory impairment in early AD. Dosage varied within the 120- to 240-mg/d range, with about a 5% improvement in mental status screening test scores. Other drug intervention possibilities that have not been adequately tested include low-dose stimulants and dopamine agonists.

Patient and Family Adjustments

An important part of living with memory impairment is the recognition of the practical limitations that it imposes on people's lives and those of their family members. Cognitive and behavioral therapy with a clinical neuropsychologist can be geared toward defining and managing these limitations. In our experience, some of the major issues that must be addressed include ways to reduce the memory load in patients, how to modify the memory demands of their daily activities, occupational pursuits, and community interactions, and adjusting to supervised care or extended-care settings.

SUMMARY

Memory disorders are common complications of neurologic disease and trauma. The frequency of memory impairments is attributed to the many interactions among many brain structures that are necessary for encoding, consolidation, and retrieval aspects of memory. Significant memory impairments are quite disabling and can leave individuals in need of long-term supervised care. Focal or isolated amnesias most commonly result from lesions to the medial temporal lobe regions, including the hippocampus, entorhinal cortex, and parahippocampal gyrus together with related limbic system structures particularly the medial diencephalon, basal forebrain, and retrosplenial cortex. Diagnosis of memory disorders through routine office and comprehensive evaluations with specialists can lead to identification of potentially reversible causes. After evaluation for treatable causes, perhaps the most important distinction to be made is between isolated or focal memory impairments and memory impairments that are part of more widespread cognitive disorders. Aspects of memory impairment can be managed through medication (particularly procholinergics), cognitive remediation, and environmental modifications that reduce demands on memory systems and provide self-cueing strategies.

■ KEY POINTS

☐ Memory can be defined as the ability to retain information and experiences. It is perhaps the most fundamental adaptive capacity of the brain. Memory underlies children's achievement of developmental milestones, such as walking and talking, their academic progress and social maturation, as well as most major tasks and accomplishments throughout adolescence and adulthood. The latter include the demands of education, vocational productivity, family life, driving, and most aspects of everyday, independent functioning within the world.

☐ Memory impairments can occur in many clinical forms and degrees of severity. The most profound form of memory impairment is amnesia. It is important to distinguish between isolated memory loss (also called focal or selective memory loss) and memory loss due to global cognitive impairments in patients with dementia. Selective amnesia implies intact intellectual, attentional, perceptual, and communicative abilities.

☐ Memory can be divided into two general constructs: declarative and procedural. Declarative memory refers to the conscious recollection of facts, knowledge, experiences, and events. This system is highly sensitive to acquired brain damage. The neural substrate of declarative memory consists of complex interactions among medial temporal lobe (especially parahippocampal gyrus, entorhinal cortex, and hippocampus), diencephalic (primarily medial nuclear structures), basal forebrain, and diverse cortical association structures. Procedural memory refers to sensory-motor and skill-based learning that is not necessarily accessible to conscious experience. Procedural memory does not require explicit recollection of past experiences to access and implement related aspects of those memories. It is mediated by a network of structures that includes the basal ganglia and cerebellum along with cortical sensory-perceptual areas.

☐ An increasing variety of cognitive, behavioral and medical interventions can help restore a greater range of independent functioning in patients with memory disorders.

KEY READINGS

Baddeley A: Working memory. Science 255:556–559, 1992.

Squire LR: Memory and Brain. New York: Oxford University Press, 1987.

Tulving E, Craik FIM (eds): The Oxford Handbook of Memory. New York: Oxford University Press, 2000.

REFERENCES

Almkvist O, Backman L, Basun H, et al: Patterns of neuropsychological performance in Alzheimer's disease and vascular dementia. Cortex 29:661–673, 1993.

American Psychiatric Association: Diagnostic and Statistical Manual of Mental Disorders-DSM-IV. Washington, DC: Author, 1994.

Baddeley A: Working memory. Science 255:556–559, 1992.

Ballard CG, Ayre G, O'Brien J, et al: Simple standardized neuropsychological assessments aid in the differential diagnosis of dementia with Lewy bodies from Alzheimer's disease and vascular dementia. Dement Geriatr Cogn Disord 10:104–108, 1999.

Barr WB: Examining the right temporal lobe's role in nonverbal memory. Brain Cogn 35:26–41, 1997.

Barr WB, Goldberg E, Wasserstein J, et al: Retrograde amnesia following unilateral temporal lobectomy. Neuropsychologia 28:243–255, 1990.

Baur RM, Tobias B, Valenstein E: Amnesic disorders, in Heilman KM, Valenstein E (eds): Clinical Neuropsychology, ed 3. New York: Oxford University Press, 1993, pp. 523–602.

Bornstein RA, Weir BK, Petruk KC, et al: Neuropsychological function in patients after subarachnoid hemorrhage. Neurosurgery 21:651–654, 1987.

Brown SC, Craik FIM: Encoding and retrieval of information, in Tulving E, Craik FIM (eds): The Oxford Handbook of Memory. New York: Oxford University Press, 2000, pp. 93–107.

Butters N, Cermak L: Alcoholic Korsakoff's Syndrome. An Information Processing Approach to Amnesia. New York: Academic, 1980.

Carlesimo GA, Fadda L, Bonci A, et al: Differential rates of forgetting from long-term memory in Alzheimer's and multi-infarct dementia. Intl J Neurosci 73:1–11, 1993.

Cohen NJ, Eichenbaum H: Memory, Amnesia, and the Hippocampal System. Cambridge, MA: MIT Press, 1994.

Connor DJ, Salmon DP, Sandy TJ, et al: Cognitive profiles of autopsy-confirmed Lewy body variant vs pure Alzheimer disease. Arch Neurol 55:994–1000, 1998.

Corkin S: Acquisition of motor skill after bilateral medial temporal-lobe excision. Neuropsychologia 6:255–265, 1968.

Corkin S, Amaral DG, Gonzalez RG, et al: H. M.'s medial temporal lobe lesion: Findings from magnetic resonance imaging. J Neurosci 17:3964–3979, 1997.

Crane J, Milner B: Do I know you? Face perception and memory in patients with selective amygdalo-hippocampectomy. Neuropsychologia 40:530–538, 2002.

Damasio AR, Eslinger PJ, Damasio H, et al: Multimodal amnesic syndrome following bilateral temporal and basal forebrain damage. Arch Neurol 42:252–259, 1985.

Datto CJ: Side effects of electroconvulsive therapy. Depress Anxiety 12:130–134, 2000.

Delis DC, Kramer JH, Kaplan E, et al: California Verbal Learning Test. San Antonio, TX: Psychological Corporation, 1987.

DeLuca J, Chiaravalloti ND: Neuropsychological consequences of ruptured aneurysms of the anterior communicating artery, in Harrison JE, Owen AM (eds): Cognitive Deficits in Brain Disorders. London: Martin Duntz, 2000, pp. 17–36.

DeLuca J, Diamond BJ: Aneurysm of the anterior communicating artery: A review of neuroanatomical and neuropsychological sequelae. J Clin Exp Neuropsychol 17:100–121, 1995.

DeLuca J, Gaudino EA, Diamond BJ, et al: Acquisition and storage deficits in multiple sclerosis. J Clin Exp Neuropsychol 20:376–390, 1998.

DeLuca J, Schultheis MT, Madigan NK, et al: Acquisition vs. retrieval deficits in brain injury: Implications for memory rehabilitation. Arch Phys Med Rehabil 81:1327–1333, 2000.

Demaree HA, DeLuca J, Guadino EA, et al: Speed of information processing as a key deficit in multiple sclerosis: Implications for rehabilitation. J Neurol Neurosurg Psychiatry 67:661–663, 1999.

Demaree HA, Gaudino EA, DeLuca J, et al: Learning impairment is associated with recall ability in multiple sclerosis. J Clin Exp Neuropsychol 22:865–873, 2000.

Erkinjuntti T: Differential diagnosis between Alzheimer's disease and vascular dementia: evaluation of common clinical methods. Acta Neurol Scand 76:433–442, 1987.

Eslinger PJ: Autobiographical memory after temporal lobe lesions. Neurocase 4:481–495, 1998.

Eslinger PJ: Summary and analysis of emerging interventions models, in Eslinger PJ (ed): Neuropsychological Interventions. New York: Guilford Press, 2002, pp. 339–354.

Eslinger PJ, Damasio AR: Preserved motor learning in Alzheimer's disease: Implications for anatomy and behavior. J Neurosci 6:3006–3009, 1986.

Eslinger PJ, Damasio H, Damasio AR, et al: Nonverbal amnesia and asymmetric cerebral lesions following encephalitis. Brain Cogn 21:140–152, 1993.

Eslinger PJ, Easton A, Grattan LM, et al: Distinctive forms of partial retrograde amnesia after asymmetric temporal lobe lesions: Possible role of the occipitotemporal gyri in memory. Cereb Cortex 6:530–539, 1996.

Feinberg TE, Farah MJ: Behavioral Neurology and Neuropsychology. New York: McGraw-Hill, 1997.

Fischer P, Gatterer G, Marterer A, et al: Course characteristics in the differentiation of dementia of the Alzheimer type and multi-infarct dementia. Acta Psychiatr Scand 81:551–553, 1990.

Flicker C, Ferris SH, Reisberg B: Mild cognitive impairment in the elderly: Predictors of dementia. Neurology 41:1006–1009, 1991.

Gardner H: The Shattered Mind. New York: Knopf, 1975.

Glisky E: Acquisition and transfer of word processing skill by an amnesic patient. Neurorehabilitation 5:299–318, 1995.

Glisky EL, Glisky ML: Learning and memory impairments, in Eslinger PJ (ed): Neuropsychological Interventions. New York: Guilford Press, 2002, pp. 137–162.

Graff-Radford NR, Damasio H, Yamada T, et al: Nonhaemorrhagic thalamic infarction. Clinical, neuropsychological and electrophysiological findings in four anatomical groups defined by computerized tomography. Brain 108:485–516, 1985.

Graham KS, Hodges JR: Differentiating the role of the hippocampal complex and the neocortex in long-term memory storage: Evidence from the study of semantic dementia and Alzheimer's disease. Neuropsychology 11:77–89, 1997.

Grossman M: Frontotemporal dementia: A review. JINS 8:566–583, 2002.

Harding A, Halliday G, Caine D, et al: Degeneration of anterior thalamic nuclei differentiates alcoholics with amnesia. Brain 123:141–154, 2000.

Hart RP: Forgetting in traumatic brain-injured patients with persistent memory impairment. Neuropsychology 8: 325–332, 1994.

Hart RP, O'Shanick GJ: Forgetting rates for verbal, pictorial, and figural stimuli. J Clin Exp Neuropsychol 15:245–265, 1993.

Hodges JR, Patterson K, Ward R, et al: The differentiation of semantic dementia and frontal lobe dementia (temporal and frontal variants of frontotemporal dementia) from early Alzheimer's disease: A comparative neuropsychological study. Neuropsychology 13:31–40, 1999.

Hogh P, Waldemar G, Knudseu GM, et al: A multidisciplinary memory clinic in a neurological setting: Diagnostic evaluation of 400 consecutive patients. Eur J Neurol 6:279–288, 1999.

Huppert FA, Piercy M: Normal and abnormal forgetting in organic amnesia: Effect of locus of lesion. Cortex 15:385–390, 1979.

Jagust WJ, Reed BR, Seab JP, et al: Clinical-physiologic correlates of Alzheimer's disease and frontal lobe dementia. Am J Physiol Imaging 4:89–96, 1989.

Johanson A, Hagberg B: Psychometric characteristics in patients with frontal lobe degeneration of non-Alzheimer type. Arch Gerontol Geriatr 8:129–137, 1989.

Johnson MK: MEM: Mechanisms of recollection. J Cogn Neurosci 4:268–280, 1992.

Kapur N: Focal retrograde amnesia in neurological disease: A critical review. Cortex 29:217–234, 1993.

Kertesz A, Clydesdale S: Neuropsychological deficits in vascular dementia vs Alzheimer's disease. Frontal lobe deficits prominent in vascular dementia. Arch Neurol 51:1226–1231, 1994.

Knopman DS, Mastri AR, Frey WH, et al: Dementia lacking distinctive histologic features: a common non-Alzheimer degenerative dementia. Neurology 40:251–256, 1990.

Lashley KS: In search of the engram. Soc Exp Biol Symp 4:454–482, 1950.

Levine B, Black SE, Cabeza R et al: Episodic memory and the self in a case of isolated retrograde amnesia. Brain 121:1951–1973, 1998.

Lezak MD: Neuropsychological Assessment, ed 3. New York: Oxford University Press, 1995.

Lisanby SH, Maddox JH, Prudic J, et al: The effects of electroconvulsive therapy on memory of autobiographical and public events. Arch Gen Psychiatry 57:581–590, 2000.

Ljunggren B, Sonesson B, Saveland H, et al: Cognitive impairment and adjustment in patients without neurological deficits after aneurysmal SAH and early operation. J Neurosurg 62:673–679, 1985.

Markowitsch HJ: Memory and amnesia, in Mesulam MM (ed): Principles of Behavioral and Cognitive Neurology. New York: Oxford University Press, 2000, pp. 257–293.

McKhann G, Drachman D, Folstein M, et al: Clinical diagnosis of Alzhimer's disease: Report of the BUBCDS-ADRDA work group under the auspices of Department of Health and Human Service Task Force on Alzheimer Disease. Neurology 34:939–944, 1984.

McKeith IG, Galasko D, Kosaka K, et al: Consensus guidelines for the clinical and pathologic diagnosis of dementia with Lewy bodies (DLB): Report of the consortium on DLB international workshop. Neurology 47:1113–1124, 1996.

Mesulam MM: Principles of Behavioral and Cognitive Neurology. New York: Oxford University Press, 2000.

Miller BL, Cummings JL, Villanueva-Meyer J, et al: Frontal lobe degeneration: Clinical, neuropsychological, and SPECT characteristics. Neurology 41:1374–1382, 1991.

Milner B: Visually-guided maze learning in man: Effects of bilateral hippocampal, bilateral frontal and unilateral cerebral lesions. Neuropsychologia 3:317–338, 1965.

Morris JC: Differential diagnosis of Alzheimer's disease. Clin Geriatr Med 10:257–276, 1994.

Morris JC: Classification of dementia and Alzheimer's disease. Acta Neurol Scand Suppl 165:41–50, 1996.

Myers CE, DeLuca J, Schultheis MT, et al: Impaired eyeblink classical conditioning in individuals with anterograde amnesia resulting from anterior communicating artery aneurysm. Behav Neurosci 11:560–570, 2001.

Neary D, Snowden J: Fronto-temporal dementia: Nosology, neuropsychology, and neuropathology. Brain Cogn 31:176–187, 1996.

Neary D, Snowden JS, Bowen DM, et al: Neuropsychological syndromes in presenile dementia due to cerebral atrophy. J Neurol Neurosurg Psychiatry 49:163–174, 1986.

Neary D, Snowden JS, Gustafson L, et al: Frontotemporal lobar degeneration: A consensus on clinical diagnostic criteria. Neurology 51:1546–1554, 1998.

Neary D, Snowden JS, Northen B, et al: Dementia of frontal lobe type. J Neurol Neurosurg Psychiatry 51:353–361, 1988.

Pachana NA, Boone KB, Miller BL, et al: Comparison of neuropsychological functioning in Alzheimer's disease and frontotemporal dementia. J Intl Neuropsychol Soc 2:505–510, 1996.

Parkin AJ, Leng NRC: Neuropsychology of the Amnesic Syndrome. Hillsdale, NJ: Lawrence Erlbaum Associates, 1993.

Paulsen JS, Heaton RK, Sadek JR, et al: The nature of learning and memory impairments in schizophrenia. J Intl Neuropsychol Soc 1:88–99, 1995.

Price BH, Gurvit H, Weintraub S, et al: Neuropsychological patterns and language deficits in 20 consecutive cases of autopsy-confirmed Alzheimer's disease. Arch Neurol 50:931–937, 1993.

Rami-Gonzalez L, Bernardo M, Boget T, et al: Subtypes of memory dysfunction associated with ECT: Characteristics and neurobiological cases J ECT 17:129–135, 2001.

Rempel-Clower NL, Zola SM, Squire LR, et al: Three cases of enduring memory impairment after bilateral damage limited to the hippocampal formation. J Neurosci 16:5233–5255, 1996.

Ribot T: Les maladies de la memoire [Diseases of memory]. New York: Appleton-Century-Crofts, 1881.

Rosenthal M, Ricker JH: Traumatic brain injury, in Frank R, Eliott T (eds): Handbook of Rehabilitation Psychology. Washington, DC: American Psychological Association, 2000, pp. 49–74.

Rossor M: Alzheimer's disease. BMJ 307:779–782, 1993.

Ryan C, Butters N: Cognitive deficits in alcoholics, in Kissin, Begleiter (eds): The Pathogenesis of Alcoholism. New York: Plenum Press, 1983, pp. 485–538.

Sahgal A, Galloway PH, McKeith IG, et al: Matching-to-sample deficits in patients with senile dementias of the Alzheimer and Lewy body types. Arch Neurol 49:1043–1046, 1992.

Saykin AJ, Gur RC, Gur RE: Neuropsychological function in schizophrenia: Selective impairment in memory and learning. Arch Gen Psychiatry 48:618–624, 1991.

Schlitt MJ, Morawertz RB, Bonnin JM, et al: Brain biopsy for enchephalitis. Clin Neurosurg 33:591–602, 1986.

Scoville WB: Amnesia after bilateral mesial temporal-lobe excision: Introduction to case H.M. Neuropsychologia 6:211–213, 1968.

Scoville WB, Milner B: Loss of recent memory after bilateral hippocampal lesions. J Neurol Neurosurg Psychiatry 20:11–21, 1957.

Seltzer B, Pandya DN: Some cortical projections to the parahippocampal area in the rhesus monkey. Exp Neurol 50:146–160, 1976.

Shimamura AP: The role of the prefrontal cortex in dynamic filtering. Psychobiology 28:207–218, 2000.

Sonesson B, Ljunggren B, Saveland H, et al: Cognition and adjustment after late and early operation for ruptured aneurysm. Neurosurgery 21:279–287, 1987.

Squire LR: Memory and Brain. New York: Oxford University Press, 1987.

Stefanacci L, Buffalo EA, Schmolck H, et al: Profound amnesia after damage to the medial temporal lobe: A neuroanatomical and neuropsychological profile of patient E. P. J Neurosci 20:7024–7036, 2000.

Subcommittee of American Academy of Neurology: Report of the therapeutics and technology assessments. Assessment: Neuropsychological assessment of adults. Consideration for neurologists. Neurology 47:592–599, 1996.

Taverni JP, Seliger G, Lichtman SW: Donepezil mediated memory improvement in traumatic brain injury during post acute rehabilitation. Brain Injury 12:77–80, 1998.

Valenstein E, Bowers D, Verfaellie M, et al: Retrosplenial amnesia. Brain 16:1631–1646, 1987.

Vanderploeg RD, Crowell TA, Curtiss G: Verbal learning and memory deficits in traumatic brain injury: encoding, consolidation, and retrieval. J Clin Exp Neuropsychol 23:185–195, 2001.

Van Hoesen GW: The parahippocampal gyrus. New observations regarding its cortical connections in the monkey. Trends Neurosci 5:345–350, 1982.

Van Hoesen GW, Pandya DN, Butters N: Cortical afferents to the entorhinal cortex of the rhesus monkey. Science 175:1471–1473, 1972.

Vargha-Khadem F, Gadian DG, Watkins KE, et al: Differential effects of early hippocampal pathology on episodic and semantic memory. Science 277 :376–380, 1997.

Victor M, Adams R, Collins G: The Wernicke-Korsakoff Syndrome and Related Neurological Disorders due to Alcoholism and Malnutrition. Philadelphia, PA: Davis, 1989.

Villardita C:. Alzheimer's disease compared with cerebrovascular dementia. Neuropsychological similarities and differences. Acta Neurol Scand 87:299–308, 1993.

Viskontas IV, McAndrew MP, Moscovitch M: Memory for famous people in patients with unilateral temporal epilepsy and excision. Neuropsychology 16:472–480, 2002.

von Cromen D, Hebel N, Schuri U: A contribution to the anatomical basis of thalamic amnesia. Brain 108:993–1008, 1985.

Weingartner H, Caine ED, Ebert MH: Imagery, encoding, and retrieval of information from memory: Some specific encoding-retrieval changes in Huntington's disease. J Abnorm Psychol 88:52–58, 1979.

Weintraub S, Peavy GM, O'Connor M, et al: Three words three shapes: A clinical test of memory. J Clin Exp Neuropsychol 22:267–278, 2000.

Wilson RS, Bacon LD, Fox JH, et al: Primary memory and secondary memory in dementia of the Alzheimer type. J Clin Neuropsychol 5:337–344, 1983.

World Health Organization: The ICD-10 Classification of Mental and Behavioral Disorders. Geneva, Switzerland, 1994.

Visual Dysfunction

Jason J. S. Barton

Acquired alexia
Akinetopsia
Balint syndrome
Blindsight
Color anomia
Hemianopia
Optic ataxia
Simultanagnosia
Topographagnosia

INTRODUCTION

The cerebral organization of visual processing involves two distinct components. First is serial relay of information from the retina to the lateral geniculate nucleus and then to striate cortex (area V1). Striate cortex and the optic radiations projecting to it have a precise topographic distribution, which is limited to the contralateral visual hemifield. After the striate cortex, visual information fans out in multiple projections to various areas in an interconnected hierarchical network of extrastriate cortical areas. In the monkey, over 40 areas have been identified (Felleman & van Essen, 1991) (Fig. 12-1). As information proceeds through this hierarchy, the visual areas become increasingly specialized for specific types of visual analysis, and topographic representation becomes coarser, with many neurons in high-level areas responding to stimuli from a wide expanse of both ipsilateral and contralateral visual fields.

Cerebral lesions affect vision in one of two ways. First, homonymous field defects result from lesions of the striate cortex or the optic radiations. These are localized to regions of the contralateral visual field and impair all aspects of vision in the affected region. Thus, they are specific for location but not for modality. In contrast, lesions of the extrastriate cortex disturb some visual modalities but not others, and the defects are much less specific for location in the visual field.

There is evidence that these extrastriate regions are grouped into two distinct processing streams, a ventral and a dorsal one. One hypothesis is that these subserve object recognition and spatial processing, respectively, the so-called What and Where pathways (Ungerleider & Mishkin, 1982). Another hypothesis proposes that the distinction is between processing for recognition and processing for action, the guidance of responses to stimuli (Milner & Goodale, 1995). The ventral or temporal stream extends below the calcarine fissure into the medial temporal lobe. Damage to these regions causes problems such as agnosia, alexia, and achromatopsia. The dorsal or parietal pathway extends superiorly and laterally from striate cortex and includes the occipitoparietal and temporoparieto-occipital areas. Damage causes defects such as akinetopsia, Balint syndrome, and hemispatial neglect.

Like all theoretical constructs, this view of extrastriate function is simplified. For one, the many extrastriate areas are highly interconnected, including lateral, feed-forward, and feedback projections. Lesions in one area may therefore have secondary effects in others. Also, many visual processes are complex, involving both dorsal and ventral functions. Consider reading, which can be impaired not only by a type of visual agnosia that affects identification of letters and words, but also by simultanagnosia, hemineglect, and even hemianopia.

Another factor to consider is the normal variation in human neuroanatomy and vascular anatomy. The exact location of different extrastriate cortical areas varies between subjects; for instance, the V5 motion area varies by up to 3 cm in location (Watson et al., 1993). The exact juncture between middle and posterior cerebral arterial territories also differs, affecting the pattern of deficit in patients with stroke. The net result is considerable intersubject variation in patterns of damage, which often cross the boundaries between areas and streams, affecting both segments of the geniculostriate relay and extrastriate hierarchy, and cre-

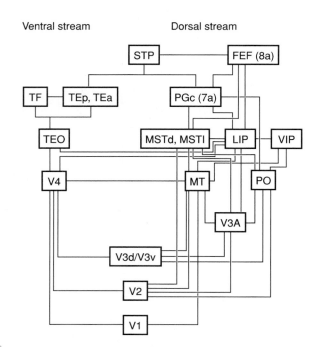

FIGURE 12-1. One version of the cortical processing stream for vision.

ating unique combinations of high-level and low-level deficits in vision.

HOMONYMOUS FIELD DEFECTS

Lesions of the retinogeniculostriate relay after the decussation at the optic chiasm cause homonymous defects in the contralateral hemifield (Fig. 12-2). The *optic tract*, the portion of the relay between the optic chiasm and the lateral geniculate nucleus, lies inferior to the hypothalamus and adjacent to the medial temporal lobe. Hence, though an extracerebral structure, it can be affected by cerebral masses or procedures such as temporal lobectomy (Anderson et al., 1989). Infarction of the optic tract is also one manifestation of anterior choroidal arterial ischemia. The homonymous field defects of a tract lesion are often *incongruous* when partial (Newman & Miller, 1983), reflecting poor alignment of binocular retinotopy at this point in the relay. Two other signs indicate a tract lesion. First, because the axons in the tract originate from retinal ganglion cells, a lesion of more than a few months' duration will have associated partial *optic atrophy* in both eyes. Second, because the tract also contains fibers projecting to the pretectal nuclei, the pupil light responses are affected, most commonly with a *relative afferent pupillary defect* in the eye with temporal field loss (Newman & Miller, 1983).

Lesions of the *lateral geniculate nucleus* cause hemianopia with partial bilateral optic atrophy also. However, the pupil responses are not affected because these fibers have already left for the pretectal nuclei.

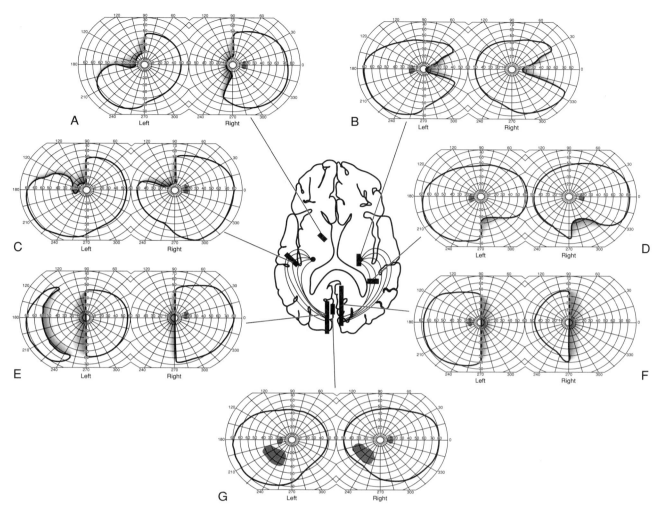

FIGURE 12-2. Homonymous visual field defects from lesions of the postchiasmal pathway. *A,* Right optic tract lesion causing incongruous left hemianopia. *B,* Lateral geniculate nucleus infarct from posterior choroidal arterial ischemia, causing right sectoranopia. *C,* Partial left superior quadrantanopia, mildly incongruous, from damage to right temporal optic radiations (Meyer's loop). *D,* Partial right inferior quadrantanopia from a left parietal lesion of the optic radiations. *E,* Sparing of the monocular temporal crescent, with a right striate lesion sparing the retrosplenial region. *F,* Macular-sparing left hemianopia, from a right striate lesion sparing the occipital pole. *G,* Homonymous scotoma from a lesion of the mid-portion of the striate cortex.

This nucleus has two blood supplies. An infarct in the territory of the lateral posterior choroidal artery causes a *sectoranopia,* a wedge-shaped defect straddling the horizontal meridian (Frisèn et al., 1978). Geniculate infarction in the territory of the anterior choroidal artery produces the mirror image: a hemianopia sparing the zone around the horizontal meridian (Helgason et al., 1986). Complete hemianopias occur with larger lesions.

Complete hemianopia with *optic radiation* infarction usually occurs with large lesions, often middle cerebral arterial ischemia, invariably with other major dysfunction such as hemiparesis, hemisensory loss, aphasia, or hemineglect. Complete hemianopia with few other signs indicates damage in the retrolenticular internal capsule proximally or in the distal radiations occipitally, with or without striate damage. More typically optic radiation damage causes partial defects with mild *incongruity*. Lesions of the temporal optic radiations in Meyer's loop cause a *superior quadrantanopia.* Damage to the parietal optic radiations causes *inferior quadrantanopia.* Quadrantic defects usually abut the vertical meridian and extend variably toward the remaining field on the same side, seldom aligning on the horizontal meridian (Jacobson, 1997). Damage to the radiation midzone causes a *sectoranopia* that mimics a geniculate lesion, but without optic atrophy (Carter et al., 1985).

Lesions of *striate cortex* are most frequently caused by posterior cerebral arterial ischemia. In about half the patients the field defect is the sole finding. Others have amnesia, prosopagnosia, and color perception defects, too (Pessin et al., 1987). Lesions extending to the parahippocampus and hippocampus cause a syndrome of *agitated delirium with hemianopia* (Medina et al., 1977). Striate damage causes highly *congruent* homonymous hemifield defects; that is, the shapes and location of the visual field defects in the two eyes appear the same when superimposed. Hemianopia can be complete or spare the central 5 degrees, known as *macula-sparing* (Gray et al., 1997). Whether or not macular vision is spared by posterior cerebral arterial infarcts depends on whether the occipital pole, which represents this region of the field, is supplied by the posterior or the middle cerebral artery. Macula-sparing is pathognomonic of striate lesions. Partial lesions of the striate cortex are also common. A lesion that involves all but the most anterior portion of striate cortex causes a hemianopia with *sparing of the monocular temporal crescent.* This too is pathognomonic of striate lesions (Benton et al., 1980). Infarction of the lower bank of the calcarine fissure causes *superior quadrantanopia* and infarction of the upper bank causes *inferior quadrantanopia.* As with radiation lesions, the horizontal boundary varies. Striate quadrantanopia is more frequently an isolated sign, sometimes with other visual dysfunction such as alexia or hemiachromatopsia, but there is usually hemiparesis, dysphasia, or amnesia with optic radiation quadrantanopia (Jacobson, 1997). Small lesions can cause *homonymous scotomas* (Gray et al., 1997) and are best detected by coronal magnetic resonance (MR) images.

Defects of both visual fields are most common with occipital lesions because the striate cortices are adjacent to each other and the two posterior cerebral arteries have a shared origin from the basilar artery tip. Bilateral large lesions cause complete *cerebral blindness* (Aldrich et al., 1987), distinguished from bilateral ocular disease by normal pupillary light reflexes. Incomplete bilateral hemianopia is distinguished from bilateral ocular disease by the congruity of the defects and a step defect along the vertical meridian, which reveals an asymmetry between the hemifields. The prognosis for cerebral blindness varies with cause. It is permanent in 25% of ischemic cases and residual partial field defects are common. Bioccipital lucencies on computed tomography (CT) scans carry a poor prognosis for recovery, but the status of visual evoked potentials is not informative (Aldrich et al., 1987).

Behavioral Issues in Hemianopia

Homonymous field defects impairing the central 5 degrees cause *hemianopic dyslexia* (Zihl, 1995;

Trauzettel-Klosinski & Brendler, 1998). Overall reading speed is more prolonged with right hemianopia than with left hemianopia. With languages written left to right, left hemianopia causes trouble finding the beginning of lines, because the left margin disappears when they scan rightward. Marking the line onset with an L-shaped ruler helps. Right hemianopia prolongs reading times, with increased fixations and reduced amplitude of reading saccades to the right. Smaller type and reading with the page turned nearly 90 degrees may help. Reading performance improves with time as patients learn adaptive strategies.

Differentiating hemianopia from *hemineglect* is important, particularly with right-sided lesions. Both conditions cause the patient to be unaware of stimuli on the contralateral side. There are two key features to note: the spatial distribution of unawareness and the pattern of exploration of space with eye movements. In retinal coordinates, hemianopia is sharply demarcated at the vertical meridian. Thus, as long as patients maintain stable fixation, they will have a reproducible moment of sudden awareness of a moving stimuli when it crosses over from the blind to the seeing hemifield. In contrast, there is no sharp demarcation at the midline in hemineglect. Rather, there is a gradient of inattention in this condition (Behrmann et al., 1997), and the moment at which a patient notices a stimulus moving toward the side of the lesion will vary from moment to moment and with stimulus intensity. Furthermore, the hemineglect in some cases is referenced to body rather than retinal coordinates, so that turning the head (and retina) toward the side of the lesion will lessen the neglect. This maneuver does not improve hemianopia.

Studies of eye movements in hemianopia and hemineglect reveal differences that can be detected at the bedside (Fig. 12-3). Patients with established hemianopia and awareness of their deficit compensate by making more saccades toward their blind side, thus increasing the likelihood of detecting stimuli with their intact hemifield. Studies with line bisection or letter arrays show that this forms an adaptive gradient of eye movements increasing toward the contralateral blind side (Behrmann, et al., 1997; Barton et al., 1998). In contrast, patients with hemineglect make fewer eye movements into contralateral hemispace than normal and have a pathologic gradient increasing toward the ipsilateral side.

RESIDUAL VISION AND BLINDSIGHT

Patients with visual loss due to lesions of the striate cortex or optic radiations may have a remnant of visual function in their supposedly blind fields. Some of these patients still have some awareness of visual stimuli, or *residual vision,* implying a relative rather than absolute field defect. Others deny awareness even though they

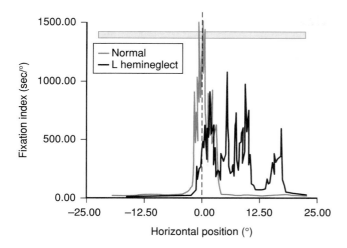

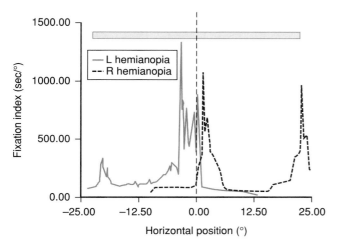

FIGURE 12-3. Eye movements during line bisection. Fixation index measures the number and duration of fixations spent near a given point. The line is represented as the gray horizontal bars. In the top graph, normal subjects concentrate their fixations near line center, whereas patients with left hemineglect scatter their fixation in the right half of the line. In the bottom graph, hemianopic patients explore to the contralateral line end and have a central peak biased into the contralateral hemifield. (Adapted from Barton J, Behrmann M, Black S: Ocular search during line bisection. The effects of hemi-neglect and hemianopia. Brain 121:1117–1131, 1998.)

perform above chance when asked to indicate some property of the stimulus, such as location, motion, color, or form; these have blindsight. Unwieldy terms of "blindsight type I" or "agnosopsia" for blindsight and "blindsight type II" or "gnosanopsia" for residual vision have been proposed (Weiskrantz, 1998; Zeki & ffytche, 1998). Whether residual vision and blindsight have different or shared pathophysiologies is not clear. The phenomenological distinction between the two is not sharp. Perceptual awareness varies along a spec-

trum; with a very brief stimulus, patients may retain a vague awareness of its presence but not of particular features, which they can nonetheless discriminate or act on (Marcel, 1998). Stimulus parameters can be manipulated so that a patient shows residual vision with awareness under some conditions and blindsight without awareness under others (Weiskrantz, et al., 1995; Sahraie et al., 1997). Similar stimulus manipulations can degrade awareness and generate blindsight-like performance in normal subjects (Meeres & Graves, 1990; Kolb & Braun, 1995; Morgan et al., 1997).

Varieties of Blindsight Phenomena

Localization

Some blindsight studies show a weak correlation of saccadic size and target position (Sanders et al., 1974, Weiskrantz et al., 1974; Perenin & Jeannerod, 1975). Studies of manual reaching and pointing generally find weak and variable results (Perenin et al., 1980; Blythe et al., 1987; Corbetta et al., 1990), but a few claim nearly normal localization (Weiskrantz et al., 1974; Marcel, 1998). However, other results cast doubts on the existence of blindsight localization. In at least one prominent blindsight patient (D.B.) the validity of the data can be questioned, because the localization ability was restricted to a zone that recovered on later perimetry (Weiskrantz, 1987). Other studies have failed to find saccadic localization without awareness (Meienberg et al., 1981; Blythe et al., 1986; Barton & Sharpe, 1997b).

Motion

Some studies report that localization is easier with moving or oscillating targets, others do not. Patient G.Y. has some residual speed and direction discrimination (Blythe et al., 1987; Morland et al., 1999), as do some other patients (Perenin, 1991). Some experience self-motion with large optokinetic gratings (Heide et al., 1990). A larger study using random dot stimuli found no blindsight motion perception (Barton & Sharpe, 1997b). Eye movements could reveal blindsight motion perception. Although residual optokinetic responses were found in one patient with cortical blindness (ter Braak et al., 1971), it has not been found in others with cortical blindness or hemianopic fields (Perenin, 1991; Barton & Sharpe, 1997a; Verhagen et al., 1997).

Form

Although patient D.B. was reported to use line orientation to discriminate large Xs from Os (Weiskrantz, 1987), form and orientation discrimination has not been found in other patients (Morland et al., 1996; Perenin & Rossetti, 1996). However, a few patients appear to alter their grasp correctly as they reach for objects in their blind field (Perenin & Rossetti, 1996; Marcel, 1998). This is consistent with a dissociation between pathways for object recognition and action (Milner, & Goodale, 1995).

Color

Some studies report color detection and color-opponent interactions in spectral sensitivity curves (Stoerig, 1987; Stoerig & Cowey, 1991). Patient G.Y. can discriminate the motion of equiluminant colored spots (Guo et al., 1998) and is aware of hue, based on averaged responses across areas of differing sensitivity in the entire blind hemifield (Morland & Ruddock, 1997). G.Y. can match and discriminate the color and motion of stimuli, but cannot compare the brightness of stimuli between his blind and seeing fields (Morland et al., 1999).

Interactions between Blind and Normal Hemifields

Traditional blindsight methods ask patients to respond to targets they cannot see. However, some studies have examined whether responses to visible stimuli are modified by stimuli in the blind field.

Spatial summation of two simultaneously presented stimuli generates faster responses than a single stimulus. Likewise, *temporal summation* of a preceding prompt with a target stimulus will reduce the reaction time to the target. Evidence for spatial or temporal summation between the seeing and blind fields has been inconsistent (Marzi et al., 1986; Corbetta et al., 1990). A *distraction effect*, in which targets in the blind field slow down response times to stimuli in the seeing field, has been shown for saccades (Rafal et al., 1990). A stimulus delays the detection of a target appearing in the same location a short time later, in *inhibition of return* (see Chapter. 10). Because this effect is coded for position in external space rather than retinal position, a study showed in one patient that a light flashed in the hemianopic field delayed responses to a target that appeared at the same spot after a saccade had placed the spot in the seeing field (Danziger et al., 1997). From monkey physiology, they argued that this was mediated by the superior colliculus.

Evidence for form and letter perception using traditional methods has been mixed. In two patients blindsight word perception emerged only with an indirect strategy in which the choice of meaning of an ambiguous word (i.e., LIGHT) in the seeing field was influenced by another word in the blind field (i.e., DARK versus HEAVY) (Marcel, 1998). *Completion effects* with stimuli that lie partly in the blind field have been reported. Three patients could discriminate circles from semicircles even when the critical half lay in the hemianopic field (Torjussen, 1978), but the macular sparing of their deficit complicates the results. Two patients had completion effects for afterimages or illusory contours that depended on a component in the blind field (Marcel, 1998). Another study of a patient with an occipital lesion used an interference task that flanked a stimulus with distractors that were either the same as or different from the stimulus. Reaction times to seen letters and colors were prolonged when flankers in the blind field differed from the stimulus (Danckert et al., 1998).

Pupillary Responses

There are pupillary responses to changes in gratings and colors that do not alter luminance. Although such pupillary responses may be modulated by cortical activity, it is unclear whether cortex is critical for responses to isoluminant stimuli (Barbur et al., 1999). Pupillary responses to such stimuli in the blind hemifield have been shown in G.Y., with or without awareness (Weiskrantz et al., 1999).

Blindsight and Hemidecortication

Studies of patients lacking a cerebral hemisphere are of obvious interest in the debate over the role of extrastriate cortex in blindsight functions, because they may help clarify the role of ipsilateral cortex in blindsight. Findings of blindsight abilities in hemidecorticate patients in some studies (Perenin & Jeannerod, 1978; Ptito et al., 1991; Braddick et al., 1992; Tomaiuolo et al., 1997) have been attributed to light scatter in others (King et al., 1996; Stoerig et al., 1996; Faubert et al., 1999). A functional magnetic resonance imaging (fMRI) study claimed that moving stimuli activated V5 and V3A but not V1 in the remaining hemisphere of one of three patients with hemispherectomies (Bittar et al., 1999); V1 should have been activated as well if scatter had been responsible.

Artifact and Blindsight

There are many pitfalls in studying blindsight. Detailed perimetry may reveal surviving islands of vision that explain remnant perception (Fendrich et al., 1992, Kasten et al., 1998, Scharli et al., 1999). Some studies claim to exclude this possibility based on lack of visual activation of striate cortex on fMRI (Stoerig et al., 1998), but this imaging technique is probably not sensitive enough to exclude low-level activity in area V1. Poor fixation is a problem if stimulus location is predictable or duration is more than 150 msec; electro-oculographic or infrared eye-movement monitors detect eye-in-head shifts but not gaze shifts accomplished by head motion (Balliet et al., 1985). Rigid head immobilization is thus essential though seldom implemented. Many studies show that light scatter can mimic blindsight (Campion et al., 1983; King et al., 1996; Stoerig et al., 1996; Barton & Sharpe, 1997a; Faubert et al., 1999). Because the eye is more sensitive than electronic equipment to light scatter, negative readings on electronic equipment cannot exclude this possible mechanism (Barton & Sharpe., 1997a). Physiologic controls in studies of blindsight include comparison with the normal blind spot (Weiskrantz, 1987), patients with pregeniculate lesions (Pöppel et al., 1973; Perenin & Jeannerod, 1975, 1978), or controls with simulated hemianopia (Barton & Sharpe, 1997a). Claims that scatter accounts for residual responses in hemispherectomy patients (King et al., 1996) raise questions about the scatter in other cases. Note that flooding the seeing field with light can minimize effects of scatter.

It has also been argued that blindsight may represent a simple *criterion shift*. That is, subjects reply more conservatively in detection tasks than when discriminating between alternatives (Campion et al., 1983). Indeed, normal subjects show criterion shift with very brief stimuli (Campion et al., 1983; Meeres & Graves, 1990; Kolb & Braun, 1995). Signal detection analysis has been used to answer this criticism by calculating a measure of sensitivity independent of the response criterion (Azzopardi & Cowey, 1997; Stoerig, 1987).

Explanations of Blindsight

Blindsight is usually attributed to pathways alternative to the retinogeniculostriate relay. The retinotectal system alone may serve some functions such as spatial localization (Wessinger et al., 1996). Others like pattern or motion detection may require a relay from the tectum, through the pulvinar, to extrastriate cortex. Chromatic blindsight may require direct projections to extrastriate cortex from the lateral geniculate nucleus (Cowey & Stoerig, 1995).

The evidence from monkeys most strongly supports the retinotectopulvinar relay to extrastriate regions, particularly those involved in motion perception; lesions of V1 do not abolish responses in V5 or V3A unless accompanied by lesions of the superior colliculus (Rodman et al., 1989; Girard et al., 1992). On the other hand, there is no neuronal evidence yet of remnant responses in regions of the monkey's ventral stream (Girard & Bullier, 1989; Girard et al., 1991; Gross, 1991), at odds with the demonstrations of residual color and form perception in humans and recently in monkeys (Cowey & Stoerig, 1999).

Not all hemianopic patients have blindsight or residual vision. In fact, recent series representing 46 patients in total suggest that blindsight is quite rare (Barton & Sharpe, 1997a,b; Kasten et al., 1998, Scharli et al., 1999). Several factors may be critical. One is the variable sparing of optic radiations and extrastriate

cortex by natural lesions. If extrastriate cortical function is responsible for blindsight, then which extrastriate regions survive will determine if a given patient will have blindsight and for what type of visual ability. However, correlations between abilities and lesion anatomy have proven elusive (Blythe et al., 1986; Magnussen & Mathiesen, 1989; Barton & Sharpe, 1997a). If blindsight requires neural plasticity, age at onset, lesion duration, and even training may be important. Of note, G.Y. sustained his lesion at age 8 and has had extensive practice over many years. Infants or children may be more likely to develop blindsight or residual vision in both nonhuman primates and man (Moore et al., 1996; Payne et al., 1996). However, not all studies find that age matters (Ptito et al., 1987).

At present, a major problem in blindsight research is the dominance of reports involving one patient, G.Y. While these studies show what is possible in a subject extensively trained after the loss of striate cortex at a young age, the generalizability of the findings and the validity of the anatomic conclusions are suspect without corroboration in other hemianopic patients. It is disturbing that recent large series have concluded that remnant perception in their subjects was due to spared striate cortex and not blindsight (Kasten et al., 1998; Scharli et al., 1999), and that the results in studies of hemispherectomized patients were due to light scatter (King et al., 1996). Although one can always argue that stimulus parameters were suboptimal in negative studies (Weiskrantz et al., 1995), at some point one must question whether G.Y. and other unusual subjects with blindsight differ from other hemianopic patients in some anomalous way.

DISORDERS OF COLOR
Cerebral Dyschromatopsia

Patients with cerebral achromatopsia see the world in shades of gray. Those with dyschromatopsia have some residual color perception, with faded or reduced range of hues (Heywood et al., 1991). A few see the world as through a colored filter or find that colors spread beyond object boundaries. Hemiachromatopsia, with impaired color perception restricted to the contralateral hemifield, is under-recognized because it is asymptomatic and few clinicians test for it (Paulson et al., 1994).

Testing color perception requires care. Asking patients to name colors is not sufficient. This confuses color anomia with achromatopsia. Also, some patients with partial defects in color perception can still make the coarse categorizations needed to name colors. Pseudo-isochromatic plates such as the AO-14 and Ishihara tests were designed for congenital red-green defects; some patients with cerebral achromatopsia achieve normal scores on these tests if the plates are far enough away to obscure the perception of the individual dots on the plates (Victor et al., 1989; Heywood et al., 1991). This is attributed to the detection of chromatic boundaries by intact color-opponent mechanisms in striate cortex, even though the colors cannot be identified. Color-sorting tests provide the best evidence of impaired color perception. The Farnsworth-Munsell 100 Hue Test is the gold standard for hue perception. Shorter hue tests include the Farnsworth D-15 and the Lanthony New Color Test. The Sahlgren Saturation Test measures saturation discrimination. Cerebral achromatopsia impairs perception of hue and saturation, and along both red-green and blue-yellow axes, though they may be asymmetrically affected (Victor, et al., 1989; Heywood et al., 1991; Rizzo et al., 1993). Patients with hemiachromatopsia use their normal field to score normally on these tests; they are usually diagnosed by poor matching or naming of colors in one hemifield but not the other, despite otherwise normal visual fields. Clinical color-matching tasks can be used in the peripheral field but are less well calibrated.

Some color function is preserved. Photopic spectral sensitivity curves (Kennard et al., 1995; Heywood et al., 1996), anomaloscope tests (Pearlman et al., 1979), and chromatic contrast sensitivity measured by evoked potentials or psychophysical tests (Heywood et al., 1996) show preserved trichromacy and color opponency. However, this is not true of all patients; abnormal spectral sensitivity curves in three patients suggest that some extrastriate processing is required for color opponency (Cavanagh et al., 1998). Motion perception for chromatic stimuli is present (Heywood et al., 1998) and can be normal at suprathreshold chromatic contrast (Cavanagh et al., 1998), implying processing by a pathway alternate to the regions damaged in achromatopsia, possibly a dorsal V4 analogue.

Color constancy is an important issue. The spectral composition of light reflected from an object depends on both the light-absorption characteristics of the object and the ambient lighting. Yet, for natural ranges of illumination we see colors as stable properties of objects; somehow we must "discount the illuminant." The spectral output of the illuminant must be deduced indirectly, from considering the color profile of the environment surrounding the object. Thus color constancy requires color data over large portions of the visual scene (Land, 1986), and in monkeys emerges only in area V4 (Zeki, 1983a,b). Although achromatopsia is a more severe deficit than impaired color constancy, in that color perception is not just unstable but absent, there are reports of poor color constancy in some patients with partial dyschromatopsia or after achromatopsia resolved (Kennard, et al., 1995; Clarke et al., 1998; D'Zmura et al., 1998; Hurlbert et al., 1998). Another report asserted that impaired color constancy without any dyschromatopsia could occur with lateral

parietotemporal lesions (Rüttiger et al., 1999), implicating a larger network of cortical regions in color perception than traditionally thought.

Can achromatopsic patients accurately imagine colors? This requires careful study because stereotyped color associations can be derived from verbal associations (i.e., yellow banana) without visual imagery. Good evidence indicates that at least two patients with complete achromatopsia have normal imagery for colors (Shuren et al., 1996; Bartolomeo et al., 1997; Bartolomeo et al., 1998). Other patients can match hues but cannot imagine them or associate colors correctly with objects (de Vreese, 1991). This double dissociation may be explained by a separate color "image buffer," which can be disconnected from either perceptual input about color or color memories (Shuren et al., 1996).

Other clinical signs are frequent. Usually there is superior quadrantanopia in both hemifields, sometimes with complete hemianopia on one side. Associated agnosias include prosopagnosia, topographagnosia, and pure alexia in those with right hemianopia. More anterior temporal lobe impairment may produce memory deficits. Problems with directing attention to less salient stimuli are evident experimentally (Mendola & Corkin, 1999), replicating a defect in attentional allocation during form processing that was described in monkeys with V4 lesions.

Lesions of the lingual and fusiform gyri cause achromatopsia (Zeki, 1990). Lesions of the middle third of the lingual gyrus or the white matter behind the posterior tip of the lateral ventricle may be critical (Rizzo et al., 1993). fMRI has confirmed the participation of this region in normal color perception (Merigan et al., 1997). Unilateral lesions cause a contralateral hemiachromatopsia. Complete achromatopsia requires bilateral lesions. These are most commonly posterior cerebral arterial strokes, either simultaneous or sequential, sometimes as the residue of a more severe cerebral blindness. Other causes include lobar hemorrhage from amyloidosis or coagulopathy, focal encephalitis such as herpes simplex, metastatic disease, posterior cortical dementia, or repeated focal seizures. A transient form can occur with migraine. Subcortical temporo-occipital white matter damage caused reversible dyschromatopsia in one patient with carbon monoxide poisoning (Fine & Parker, 1996), a condition that more often causes an apperceptive agnosia with relative sparing of color perception (Zeki, 1990).

A controversial issue is whether the region damaged in cerebral achromatopsia is homologous to monkey area V4. Area V4 has color-specific responses and is implicated in color constancy (Zeki, 1983b). However, severe deficits in hue discrimination occur not with lesions of monkey V4 but with more anterior temporal lesions (Heywood et al., 1995). In humans, fMRI has identified a more anterior area, named V8, which is involved in conscious color perception and the perception of color afterimages, and this may be the region critically damaged in achromatopsia (Hadjikhani et al., 1998).

Achromatopsia may resolve with time, leaving more subtle deficits in color constancy, discrimination, imagery, or color-object association. More often it is permanent. Rehabilitation cannot restore color perception, but can foster substitutive strategies using texture and contrast cues in tasks that traditionally emphasize color.

Color Anomia and Agnosia

Whereas patients with achromatopsia cannot discriminate hue and saturation (though some can name colors correctly), those with color anomia or agnosia can discriminate colors but not name or recognize them. Such patients may not be aware of their deficits. Positron emission tomography (PET) studies show that color words activate the posterior inferior ventral temporal lobe just anterior to the zone activated by color perception, the parieto-occipital junction, and left lingual gyrus (Martin et al., 1995; Paulesu et al., 1995).

Color anomia can occur without other linguistic dysfunction. When it accompanies pure alexia and right homonymous hemianopia, it may be due to an *interhemispheric visual-verbal disconnection* (de Vreese, 1991). Though colors are perceived normally in the remaining left hemifield, disruption of splenial connections between the right striate cortex and the left angular gyrus blocks the transfer of color information to language processors. Naming for visual objects may be spared. This is attributed to coactivation of right-sided somatosensory representations of objects, which may be transferred to the left hemisphere by more anterior callosal connections.

In *color dysphasia*, patients cannot name the colors they see or name the colors that belong to familiar objects they see or imagine (Oxbury et al., 1969). These patients may have lost their color lexicon, and often have left angular gyrus lesions, with associated alexia and agraphia, right hemifield defects, and Gerstmann syndrome.

Color agnosia is rare. Patients are similar to those with color anomia, but also cannot color line drawings correctly or learn associations between objects and colors (Kinsbourne & Warrington, 1964).

VISUAL AGNOSIA

Patients with visual agnosia cannot recognize objects they have seen before. They cannot name a previously familiar but unrecognized object and show no knowledge of its use, context, or history. Patients with anomia cannot name the objects but do possess such knowledge. With purely visual agnosia, recognition is possible through other modalities such as hearing or touch.

Agnosia is traditionally divided into two broad categories, apperceptive and associative. Apperception implies that recognition is impaired because the patient does not perceive the object properly, despite intact low-level visual functions. In associative agnosia, the percept is adequate but the patient cannot match this to representations from past experience. It is probable that this apperceptive/associative distinction forms a spectrum rather than an absolute dichotomy.

A severe generalized (apperceptive) agnosia is caused by diffuse anoxia, as with carbon monoxide poisoning (Sparr et al., 1991). This affects the perception of many visual objects. More selective agnosias affect the recognition of only certain types of objects. The most characteristic of these are alexia and prosopagnosia. Farah (1990) proposed that these two disorders are the most prominent manifestations of impaired higher level visual processing, with alexia reflecting mainly left and prosopagnosia mainly right extrastriate cortical dysfunction. According to this proposal visual agnosia without either alexia or prosopagnosia, or prosopagnosia and alexia without general agnosia, should not occur. However, two patients who possess the latter syndrome have been described (de Renzi & di Pellegrino, 1998; Buxbaum et al., 1999), challenging this hypothesis. It appears selective agnosias may be caused by a variety of perceptual and memory deficits and other mechanisms such as interhemispheric dissociations (see below).

DISORDERS OF READING

Acquired alexia is loss of reading fluency. Reading is a highly complex task. It requires intact foveal visual acuity and paracentral fields, form perception, visuospatial attention, and ocular motor skills to generate the series of alternating fixations and saccades in scanning lines of text, and linguistic functions such as grapheme-to-phoneme conversion and lexicon access. Consequently, many different lesions and dysfunctions can impair reading.

Pure alexia, or alexia without agraphia is discussed in Chapter 17. That chapter also discusses central dyslexias, such as surface dyslexia, phonological dyslexia, and deep dyslexia, which are not so much related to visual dysfunction as to failures in linguistic processes. Here we describe briefly a few of the dyslexias that can occur secondary to other visual factors.

Acquired Alexias Secondary to Visual, Attentional, or Ocular Motor Dysfunction

Any disorder that reduces acuity in both eyes impairs reading, ranging from cataracts to bilateral occipital pole infarcts. Visual field loss in the central 5 degrees impairs reading also, even if central acuity is normal (see hemianopic dyslexia). Bitemporal hemianopia causes *hemifield slide*, in which the loss of overlap between one eye's visual field and that of the other leads to unstable binocular alignment. Words or letters transiently duplicate or disappear during reading when the eyes lose horizontal alignment (Kirkham, 1972). When vertical conjugacy is lost, a vertical step develops in the line of text, sometimes causing the left side of one line to merge with the right side of another.

Patients with left hemineglect can have *neglect dyslexia* (Behrmann et al., 1990). They omit reading the left side of lines or pages. With words, they make left-sided omissions, additions, or substitutions. Vertically printed text is not affected. Rarely, it may occur without other signs of hemineglect (Patterson & Wilson, 1990).

Abnormal fixation and saccades impair reading. Most unilateral cortical lesions cause only minor eye movement problems, but the acquired ocular motor apraxia from bilateral frontal or parietal lesions impairs reading severely (Baylis et al., 1994). Saccadic intrusions such as square wave jerks or opsoclonus, which disrupt fixation, impair line scanning, as in patients with progressive supranuclear palsy (Friedman et al., 1992).

DISORDERS OF FACE PERCEPTION

Prosopagnosia

Patients with prosopagnosia cannot recognize the faces of familiar people or learn new faces. They are usually aware of their social difficulty, though some with childhood onset may not be aware of their difference from others. They recognize some faces by odd features, such as glasses, hairstyle, or scars, or else rely on voice, gait, or mannerisms to identify people. The context of the encounter can aid their recognition.

Testing face recognition usually involves a battery of photographs of public persons, sometimes with unfamiliar faces as distractors. The patient indicates which faces are familiar and provides names or other information about the faces. Ideally, failure should be contrasted with intact recognition of famous voices. Interpretation of results must take into account the cultural and social background of the patient. It should be verified that the subject knows the public persons whose faces are used, by presenting their names and asking the patient to provide some information about them. Photographs of friends or relatives can be used instead for patients with limited public knowledge.

Other face tests include the Benton Face Recognition Test (Benton & van Allen, 1972), which shows subjects anonymous faces and asks them to find the matching face in an array, which can differ in lighting or viewpoint. This test probes the adequacy of face perception (not recognition). The Warrington Recognition Test (Warrington, 1984) presents 50 unknown faces briefly and then, after a short interval, presents them again mixed with other unfamiliar faces. The subject is asked which faces were the ones previously shown. Thus this tests short-term memory for faces. A second part of the Warrington test uses words instead of faces, providing a useful index of the selectivity of the defect for faces.

The pathophysiology of prosopagnosia is quite variable, reflecting the complexity of normal face processing. Face recognition involves a series of stages (Bruce & Young, 1986). Visual processing generates a facial percept, which is matched to a store of templates or facial memories ("face recognition units"). A match activates person-identity nodes containing name and biographical information. Impaired visual processing would constitute an apperceptive type of prosopagnosia (de Renzi et al., 1991). The nature of this perceptual impairment is still unclear. Many investigators believe that it is a "configural" or holistic mode of processing that is lost. Thus patients see individual facial features but not the whole facial structure (Levine & Calvanio, 1989; Sergent & Villemure, 1989). This may explain why some patients resort to a feature-by-feature strategy in processing faces. Other indirect evidence for this includes impaired perception of objects in overlapping figures, silhouettes, Gestalt completion tests, and global texture or Moiré patterns (Levine & Calvanio., 1989; Rentschler et al., 1994).

Dysfunction of face recognition units is often claimed too (de Renzi et al., 1991); these patients should neither recognize familiar faces nor imagine them (Takahashi et al., 1995). Disconnection between intact perceptual encoding and intact face recognition units was hypothesized in a patient who could both match unknown faces and recall images of familiar faces (Takahashi, et al., 1995). A disconnection between face recognition units and person-identity nodes may impair the ability to provide name or biographical information about a face that is nevertheless recognized as familiar (Verstichel & Chia, 1999). Dysfunction of person-identity nodes causes a people-specific amnesia rather than prosopagnosia. These patients cannot identify people by faces or other nonfacial cues and are described with right temporal pole lesions (Ellis et al., 1989; Hanley et al., 1989; Evans et al., 1995).

Faces can also yield other social information. Some prosopagnosic patients are also impaired in using faces to judge age, sex, expression, and the direction of gaze, an important social signal (Young & Ellis, 1989; Campbell et al., 1990; de Haan & Campbell, 1991) but others are not (Sergent & Poncet, 1990; Evans et al., 1995). Although deficiencies in these other face-related skills are often taken to indicate that prosopagnosia is apperceptive, this may be incorrect. These defects can exist as isolated entities without prosopagnosia (see below), and fMRI shows that the processing of gaze and

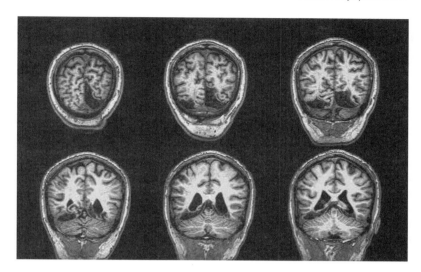

FIGURE 12-4. Coronal MR images of a prosopagnosic patient with bilateral occipitotemporal lesions.

expression involves lateral temporal sites distinct from the areas implicated in the recognition of facial identity (Haxby et al., 2000).

Patients with prosopagnosia can recognize that a face is a face, just not whose face it is. This normal basic-level object recognition distinguishes them from patients with severe generalized visual agnosia. Whether their dysfunction in identifying specific faces ("exemplar-level processing") affects other classes of objects is controversial. Certainly some patients cannot identify their own car or makes of cars, types of food, coins, or unique items such as buildings, handwriting, and personal clothing. However, many others can, at least for some classes (Farah et al., 1995; Henke et al., 1998). Part of the difficulty with the question of selectivity lies in finding other subordinate-level distinctions that are as difficult as individuating faces, so that the issue of selectivity does not degenerate into one of severity. Another complication is that the ability of a subject to individuate members of an object class depends on prior experience and interest in making that identification (Diamond & Carey, 1986). Although experience with faces is universal, expertise in flowers, dogs, and cars, for example, is not. Nevertheless, a recent review with measures of reaction time and signal detection parameters in two prosopagnosic patients has argued that deficits with nonface objects are present, even when accuracy rates suggest otherwise (Gauthier et al., 1999). Thus face recognition may be merely the most dramatic example of a type of perception that requires distinction of subtle differences in a basic configuration shared by all objects in that class.

Prosopagnosia is caused by lesions in either the lingual and fusiform gyri (Meadows, 1974) or the more anterior temporal cortex (Evans et al., 1995). fMRI has confirmed face identity-related activity in the right fusiform gyrus (Kanwisher, et al., 1997; Haxby et al., 2000). Bilateral lesions have been reported in many cases on autopsy (Meadows, 1974) and neuroimaging

(Fig. 12-4). Indeed, prosopagnosia may only emerge after a second left-sided stroke in patients with a prior right-sided lesion (Ettlin et al., 1992). However, increasing evidence from pathology (Landis et al., 1988) and imaging indicates that a right-sided lesion alone can cause prosopagnosia (Fig. 12-5). Variations in laterality and location of damage in prosopagnosia may relate ultimately to the various functional defects that can impair recognition. One hypothesis is that unilateral right occipitotemporal lesions cause an apperceptive defect, whereas bilateral, more anterior temporal lesions cause an associative one (Damasio et al., 1990). However, one study of two patients found that perceptual status as indexed by face-matching ability did not correlate in the expected fashion with the anterior/posterior location of lesions (Clarke et al., 1997). Whether this speaks to the inadequacy of the hypothesis or of the use of face matching to index perception is not settled. Some bilateral cases with left hemianopia may even represent a disconnection like that in pure alexia, with the left-sided lesions disconnecting the remaining right field visual input from the right hemispheric regions involved in facial recognition (Kay & Levin, 1982; de Renzi, 1986).

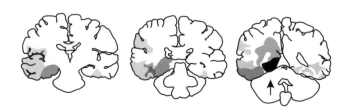

FIGURE 12-5. Template of lesions of four patients with prosopagnosia with predominantly right-sided lesions. Two had no evidence of left-sided damage. The area of overlap (*black region*) included the location of the fusiform face area identified from functional MRI experiments in normal subjects.

Covert processing of faces has also been reported in prosopagnosia (Bruyer, 1991). Physiologic techniques include galvanic skin response and visual evoked potentials (Bauer & Verfaellie, 1988; Renault et al., 1989). Psychological techniques include eye scan patterns, forced-choice responses, and the speed of learning to pair correct versus incorrect names with faces (Rizzo et al., 1987; Sergent et al., 1990; McNeil & Warrington, 1991). These can show either a retained sense of familiarity or retained semantic information about known faces, such as names and occupations (Fig. 12-6). The pathophysiologic implications of covert processing are not yet clear. Some argue that covert processing requires normal perceptual stages and indicates that prosopagnosia is associative in individuals who possess it. Some hypothesize that covert abilities are mediated by activity in a dorsal pathway involving the superior temporal cortex (Bauer, 1986), whereas others believe it can be generated in the surviving portions of the ventral face-recognition network (Farah et al., 1993).

Prosopagnosia is frequently associated with upper quadrantanopia, either left or bilateral, or with left homonymous hemianopia. Achromatopsia is frequent but not always present. Some patients have topographagnosia and those with anteromedial temporal damage have impaired visual or verbal memory. The most common causes are posterior cerebral arterial infarctions, head trauma, and viral encephalitis. Tumors, hematomas, abscesses, and surgical resections are less frequent. Progressive forms occur with Alzheimer dementia or focal temporal atrophy.

There is no known treatment for prosopagnosia. Patients may benefit socially from learning to use nonfacial and nonvisual cues more effectively to identify people. One report claimed that a patient learned new faces more effectively with "deep" encoding instruc-

tions to rate the personality trait or remember semantic data about a presented face, than with instructions to focus on features (Polster & Rapcsak, 1996). However, this benefit did not translate to recognition of other views of the same faces.

Other Disorders of Face Perception

A rare group of patients recognize long-known faces but cannot learn new ones since their lesion (Young et al., 1995). This *anterograde prosopagnosia* occurs with bilateral damage to the amygdala, usually from epileptic surgery (Young et al., 1995). There is associated dysnomia, and patients cannot judge facial expressions or the direction of gaze, consistent with the role of the amygdala in social behavior.

A rare *developmental prosopagnosia* exists (de Haan & Campbell, 1991; Kracke, 1994). These patients may not be aware of their problem but come to attention because of consequent social difficulties, which can resemble Asperger syndrome, or their parents may realize that their vision is not normal in some way. Most have other problems in face perception, with difficulty judging facial age, sex, and expressions, and slow performance of facial matching tasks. As with acquired prosopagnosia, other general perceptual skills may be relatively spared or also affected. Developmental prosopagnosia can be familial, possibly an autosomal dominant trait. Imaging may not show a lesion.

Some patients with right hemispheric lesions but without prosopagnosia have trouble matching unfamiliar faces or determining age from faces (de Renzi et al., 1989). Left hemisphere lesions can selectively impair perception of facial expressions (Young et al., 1993). These deficits are asymptomatic and found only with detailed psychological tests.

On occasion, one encounters patients who have a *false sense of familiarity* with unknown faces. They mistake strangers for people known to them (Young et al., 1993) and can persist in the delusion despite evidence to the contrary. Most have large middle cerebral arterial strokes, affecting lateral frontal, temporal, and parietal cortex. Some have prosopagnosia on testing, though they deny problems recognizing faces; others do not (Young et al., 1993; Rapcsak et al., 1996). Right prefrontal damage appears to be critical in both groups. This may cause dysfunction in self-monitoring and decision making, leading to fragmentary judgments of facial similarity with failure to reject incorrect matches (Rapcsak et al., 1996). This likely accounts also for failure to recognize associated prosopagnosia and persistence in mistaken delusions.

Somewhat related is *Capgras syndrome*, in which a patient believes that familiar people have been replaced by impostors. Although this can be associated with psychiatric syndromes, there are also cases with

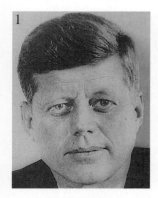

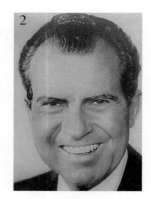

John F Kennedy   Lyndon B Johnson

FIGURE 12-6. Example of a covert face perception task. The patient has to learn to pair a name with a face. Fewer repetitions are required for the patient to learn this if the name truly belongs to the face (*1*), than when it does not (*2*).

neurologic origins. Frontal lesions are common, often bilateral, and sometimes are combined with right posterior hemispheric lesions. Many of these patients are said to be impaired on tests of face matching, but the evidence for associated prosopagnosia is more sparse and variable.

DISORDERS OF MOTION PERCEPTION (AKINETOPSIA)

Compared to achromatopsia, selective deficits in motion perception have a much more recent history, only emerging after the delineation of motion-selective extrastriate regions in monkeys. Only two cases of akinetopsia from bilateral lesions have been well described, L.M. and A.F. L.M., in particular, has been the subject of many reports. Symptomatically, L.M. had no impression of motion in depth or of rapid motion (Zihl et al., 1983), with fast targets appearing to "jump" rather than move (Zihl et al., 1991). Patients with motion deficits from unilateral lesions are either asymptomatic or have more subtle complaints, such as "feeling disturbed by visually cluttered moving scenes" (Vaina & Cowey, 1996), and trouble judging the speed and direction of cars (Vaina et al., 1998).

Tests for motion perception require animated computer displays, currently available only in research laboratories. Inferring perceptual deficits from impaired motor responses to moving stimuli, such as smooth pursuit eye movements or manual reaching, is not possible because these are dissociable deficits (Barton et al., 1996a).

Experimentally, many different aspects of motion perception can be tested. These show that, even with extensive bilateral lesions, not all motion perception is lost. Distinguishing moving from stationary stimuli is still possible (Zihl et al., 1983), and the contrast sensitivity for moving striped patterns is almost normal (Hess et al., 1989). L.M. could discriminate the direction of small spots (Zihl et al., 1991) and random dot patterns in which all dots were moving in the same direction (Baker et al., 1991; Rizzo et al., 1995). However, L.M. and A.F. had trouble discriminating differences in speed, and their discrimination of direction was severely affected when even small amounts of random motion or even stationary noise was added to displays (Baker et al., 1991; Vaina, 1994; Rizzo et al., 1995).

These deficits are reflected in a number of perceptual tasks involving motion cues. When searching among multiple objects for a target, L.M. could restrict her attention to objects with specific shapes or colors if required, but could not do so to moving ones, implying lack of a "motion filter" (McLeod et al., 1989). L.M. and A.F. could not identify two-dimensional shapes encoded by differences in motion between object and background, especially with added noise; L.M. was also impaired for three-dimensional shapes defined by motion but A.F. was not (Vaina, 1994; Rizzo et al., 1995). When lip-reading, L.M. has trouble with polysyllables uttered rapidly, and her judgment of sound is biased by auditory rather than visual cues when there are discrepancies (Campbell et al., 1997). On the other hand, L.M. can easily see "biologic motion" (e.g., identifying body movements of a person).

L.M. suffered sagittal sinus thrombosis with bilateral cerebral infarction of lateral aspects of Brodmann areas 18, 19, and 39 (Zihl et al., 1991) and a PET study (Shipp et al., 1994) showed that visual motion induced activity in probable homologues of V3 and the superior temporal lobe but not in the human V5 region. A.F. had acute hypertensive hemorrhage with similar bilateral lateral occipitotemporal lesions (Vaina, 1994). The likelihood that this lateral occipitotemporal area in humans corresponds to monkey V5 was strengthened by a study showing that similar patterns of deficits and spared abilities were shared by L.M. and monkeys with V5 ablations (Marcar et al., 1997).

Unilateral lesions of extrastriate cortex cause more subtle abnormalities of motion perception (Fig. 12-7). Some small series of patients report that in the contralateral peripheral there are hemifield defects in speed discrimination (Plant, et al., 1993; Greenlee et al., 1995), detecting boundaries between regions with different motion and discriminating direction amidst motion noise (Barton et al., 1995). As in L.M. and A.F., motion detection and contrast thresholds for motion direction were normal (Plant et al., 1993; Greenlee et al., 1995). In the central visual field, there are similar defects in discerning direction in noisy displays (Barton et al., 1995) and in the perception of motion-defined form (Vaina, 1989; Regan et al., 1992).

In most of these studies of unilateral lesions, the areas damaged were located in lateral occipitotemporal cortex or the inferior parietal lobule. The lateral occipitotemporal area has been identified from histologic markers (Clarke & Miklossy, 1990, Tootell & Taylor, 1995) and functional imaging as homologous to monkey area V5 (or MT, the middle temporal area; Fig. 12-8). At present, there are few data on hemispheric differences; although an earlier study found a predominance of right-sided lesions (Vaina, 1989), similar defects have been identified subsequently with damage to either side (Regan et al., 1992; Barton et al., 1995).

Are different types of motion perception affected by different lesions? First-order (Fourier) motion refers to stimuli from which motion can be computed by correlating the spatial distribution of luminance in the visual scene over time. However, we can also discern the motion of other types of stimulus attributes besides luminance, such as contrast, texture, stereopsis, and flicker, which do not generate a motion signal in the Fourier domain—these are known as second-order

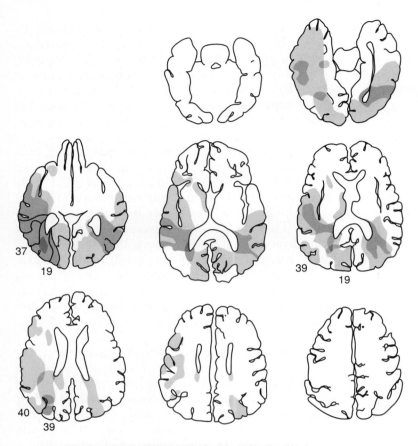

FIGURE 12-7. Lesions of six patients with unilateral lesions (two left-sided, four right-sided) and impaired motion direction discrimination. The darkest area represents the maximum overlap, which occurs at the junction of Brodmann areas 19 and 37, in lateral occipitotemporal cortex. (Reproduced with permission from Barton J, Sharpe J, Raymond J: Retinotopic and directional defects in motion discrimination in humans with cerebral lesions. Ann Neurol 37:665–675, 1995.)

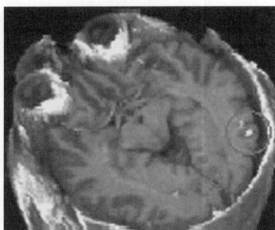

FIGURE 12-8. Functional MRI of a normal subject. Control stimulus was a stationary dot pattern; experimental conditions were random dot motion and an optic flow pattern of visual motion. Bright pixels superimposed on axial slice show activations by optic flow, random dot motion, or both. Note the cluster of activity in the lateral occipitotemporal area (circle).

(non-Fourier) motion. Initial case studies suggested that first- and second-order motion may have separate loci, with a lesion near the V5 region impairing the latter (Vaina & Cowey, 1996; Vaina et al., 1999) and a medial occipital lesion thought to affect homologues of V2 and

V3 impairing the former (Vaina et al., 1998). However, recent group studies have found that deficits of first- and second-order motion perception in the contralateral hemifield colocalize to the V5 region or the inferior parieto-occipital region (Greenlee & Smith, 1997; Braun et al., 1998). Some segregated processing of these is still possible though as dissociations between impaired first-order and preserved second-order motion perception were occasionally encountered in patients with smaller peri-V5 lesions (Greenlee & Smith, 1997). An fMRI study (Smith et al., 1998) suggested that signals from second-order motion first emerge in areas V3 and VP and may be later integrated with first-order motion signals in area MT.

The relation of pursuit eye movements to motion perception is interesting. During pursuit, the fMRI signal related to motion perception is enhanced in V5 and a dorsal parieto-occipital location (Barton et al., 1996b; Freitag et al., 1998). Some of the neuronal activity in the middle superior temporal (MST) area during pursuit may be information about the eye movement itself ("efference copy"). Because movement of images on the retina can be generated either by moving objects while the eye remains still, or by eye movement while the world remains still, efference copy may serve to disambiguate the two. A patient with vertigo induced by moving objects could not take his own eye movements into account when estimating object motion (Haarmeier et al., 1997). He had bilateral occipitoparietal lesions, possibly of MST homologues.

The pattern of deficits associated with damage to the V5 region requires further delineation. The proximity of the optic radiations means that hemianopic defects are frequent and may obscure motion perception defects in the contralateral hemifield. The two akinetopsic patients had large lesions and, not surprisingly, defects on other nonmotion perceptual tasks. A.F. was poor at recognizing objects seen from unusual angles and in incomplete line drawings, and on spatial tests such as hyperacuity, line orientation, line bisection, and spatial location, and stereopsis. L.M. also had poor perception of forms constructed from cues of texture, stereopsis, or density (Rizzo et al., 1995).

The prognosis of motion perceptual deficits is still unclear. At least two cases have been studied sequentially (Barton & Sharpe, 1998; Braun et al., 1998), showing significant improvement over the first 6 to 12 months. In monkeys the pace and degree of recovery correlates with the extent of damage to both V5 and V5a (Yamasaki & Wurtz, 1991). Recovery with larger lesions presumably reflects adaptation within other surviving motion-responsive regions of cortex.

DISORDERS OF SPATIAL PERCEPTION (BALINT SYNDROME)

Balint syndrome consists of a loosely associated triad of visuospatial dysfunctions, which are traditionally considered to be simultanagnosia, optic ataxia, and ocular motor apraxia.

Patients have a deficit in *distributing spatial attention*, in which they cannot pay attention to more than a few objects at a time. Thus these patients have trouble with attentionally demanding visual search tasks (Coslett & Saffran, 1991) and in maintaining attentional surveillance consistently over large regions of space (Rizzo & Robin, 1990). This defect may be equated to *simultanagnosia*, the inability to interpret a complex scene with multiple inter-related elements, despite being able to perceive those individual elements. What constitutes an element or object is a complex matter, depending not only on visual properties but cognitive factors. For example, such patients can identify single letters but have difficulty identifying multiple letters in a random string. However, if that string is a word or even a pronounceable nonword, performance is better, indicating that the letters have been grouped into a single linguistic element (Baylis et al., 1994). Similarly, the detection of multiple objects improves if they are semantically related (Coslett & Saffran, 1991).

An additional spatial problem is *visual disorientation*, a defect in judging the spatial position and distance of objects. This deficit may contribute to *optic ataxia*, defective hand movements under visual guidance despite normal limb strength and position sense. Misreaching may represent more than just visuospatial misperception because it can affect one arm more than the other or impair reaching to somatosensory targets, such as the patient's own body parts. Thus, a multimodal spatial targeting for hand guidance may be at fault. Laboratory measures of reaching, pointing, and grasping have shown increased latency, abnormal hand trajectories, increased variability of the end of the reach, tendency to reach to one side, and dissociations of distance and direction control (Jakobson et al., 1991; Rizzo et al., 1992).

The ocular motor abnormalities of Balint syndrome are not well characterized. There are probably several potentially dissociable components. Difficulty initiating saccades to visual targets is variably known as *psychic paralysis of gaze* or *acquired ocular motor apraxia*. Saccades to targets prompted by a verbal command are difficult if not impossible, whereas "reflexive" saccades to suddenly appearing visual objects or noises, or even random spontaneous saccades are normal. A related problem is *spasm of fixation*, which is more narrowly defined now as a problem in initiating saccades away from a fixation point that remains visible (Johnston et al., 1992). Once saccades are generated, there may be gross *inaccuracies in saccadic targeting*, which causes the eyes to wander in a series of saccades searching for targets. Furthermore, once on the target, patients can have trouble maintaining the fixation.

Diagnosis of Balint syndrome requires careful exclusion of more general cognitive dysfunction, hemineglect, and elementary visual defects in acuity and peripheral fields. Perimetry can be difficult, due to inattention, fatigue, and difficulty maintaining fixation. Many reports of Balint are marred by inadequate documentation of visual fields. Extensive peripheral scotomata leaving only "keyhole vision" can create signs that mimic all components of the Balint triad. Simultanagnosia is usually tested by asking the patient to report all items and describe the events depicted in a complex visual display with a balance of information in all quadrants, such as the Cookie Theft Picture from the Boston Diagnostic Aphasia Examination (Goodglass & Kaplan, 1983). Patients will omit elements and fail to realize the story being shown. At the bedside, patients can be asked to pick up a number of coins scattered on a table. To test for optic ataxia, easily seen items are placed at different locations within arm's reach of the patient, who is asked to touch or grasp them, with each hand tested separately for each side of hemispace (Castaigne et al., 1975). With unilateral lesions, the problem tends to be worse for reaches initiated with the contralateral hand and hemispace. Misreaching for visual targets is contrasted with reaching to parts of their own bodies, though more diffuse disturbances in parietal spatial representation may impair both. Such generalized misreaching can be confused with cerebellar dysmetria, but the latter is usually accompanied by intention tremor and dysdiadocokinesia also. Ocular motor apraxia is confirmed by comparing the patient's difficulty in making saccades to command with ease in making reflexive saccades to sudden targets in the natural environment, such an unexpected noise or a person walking by in the hall. Spasm of fixation can only be diagnosed with eye movement recordings (Johnston et al., 1992).

Although optic ataxia and ocular motor apraxia have at times been blamed on simultanagnosia, and optic ataxia on inadequate saccadic targeting (Vighetto & Perenin, 1981), each of the elements of Balint syndrome are dissociable (Cummings et al., 1986), and therefore can have different pathophysiologic origins, even if they can also contribute to each other's manifestations. The incapacity to combine elements into a whole seen in simultanagnosia was thought to reflect an inhibitory action of a focus of attention on surrounding regions. Failure of long-range spatiotemporal processes to sustain and distribute attention is likely, though the ability to direct attention serially and with cueing is better preserved (Rizzo & Robin, 1990; Coslett & Saffran 1991). Reaching under visual guidance may be mediated by recursive processes involving intercommunication among a cerebral network (Battaglia Mayer et al., 1998), which can be disrupted at a number of key points, including parietal and frontal cortex (Nagaratnam et al., 1998). Inaccurate saccades and difficulty initiating saccades reflect damage to specific structures involved in saccadic control, likely homologues of the lateral intraparietal area or the frontal eye field.

There are often other disturbances. These include a variety of bilateral visual field defects, usually affecting the lower quadrants more severely, and other visuospatial defects such as left hemineglect, akinetopsia, and astereopsis (Rizzo, 1993; Rizzo & Vecera, 2002). Smooth pursuit is often impaired. Patients may complain of distortions of perception such as metamorphopsia, micropsia and macropsia, or visual perseverations such as palinopsia and monocular polyopia. Visual agnosias may be present with even more extensive lesions. Visual evoked potentials may be normal (Onofrj et al., 1995) or abnormal (Jarry et al., 1999), probably depending on the extent of associated damage.

Balint syndrome results from bilateral occipitoparietal damage, though at least optic ataxia has been described with unilateral right or left parietal lesions alone (Ando & Moritake, 1990; Nagaratnam et al., 1998, Perenin & Vighetto, 1988). The early reports emphasized the role of the angular gyri in particular, though the lesions clearly were more extensive, involving the splenium, white matter, and pulvinar. Modern imaging associates simultanagnosia with lesions of the dorsal occipital lobes in Brodmann areas 18 and 19 (Rizzo & Robin, 1990). The lesions of optic ataxia are more variably localized, including premotor cortex, occipitoparietal regions, cortex inferomedial to the angular gyri (Rizzo et al., 1992), and occipital-frontal white matter connections (Auerbach & Alexander, 1981; Nagaratnam et al., 1998), and can be unilateral. Acquired ocular motor apraxia in its dramatic form requires bilateral lesions of the frontal eye fields, inferior parietal lobes, or both (Pierrot-Deseilligny et al., 1986); it has even been described in one patient after unilateral pulvinar resection (Ogren et al., 1984).

The most common causes of Balint syndrome are ischemia, particularly watershed infarctions, and degenerative disorders such as Alzheimer disease and posterior cortical atrophy, in which it can be an early sign. Other causes include tumors, abscesses, trauma, leukoencephalopathies, Marchiafava-Bignami disease, prion disorders, and, in patients with AIDS, progressive multifocal leukoencephalopathy and HIV encephalitis. Recurrent transient episodes of the Blint triad can occur rarely with migraine.

The prognosis for Balint syndrome varies with etiology. Patients with acute infarction can recover significantly with time, whereas those with posterior cortical atrophy deteriorate. Little is known about treatment. Cognitive and perceptual rehabilitative approaches involving verbal cues and organizational search strategies have been reported to improve visual function and reaching in three patients (Perez et al., 1996).

TOPOGRAPHAGNOSIA

Patients with topographagnosia get lost in familiar surroundings. This can be due to a problem in either the ventral or dorsal visual association cortices. Ventral lesions are associated with prosopagnosia and achromatopsia and reflect agnosia for familiar landmarks and buildings. This occurs with right medial temporo-occipital lesions (McCarthy et al., 1996; Pai, 1997), sometimes without prosopagnosia, and may reflect more of a selective multimodal memory disturbance than a strictly visual problem (McCarthy et al., 1996). In the dorsal form of topographagnosia, the spatial processing needed to describe, follow, or memorize routes is disrupted, usually by right parietotemporal lesions (Pai, 1997).

TESTING VISION

Familiarity with the features of the above syndromes is key to obtaining an accurate history of symptoms and performing a useful examination of the patient with visual dysfunction. Not all of these syndromes have readily available clinical tests (i.e., motion perception defects), and some are diagnosed primarily on history (i.e., topographagnosia). Of the tests that are currently used, these can be divided into two main groups: those used by physicians and those traditionally administered by neuropsychologists (Lanca et al., 2003). Most of the relevant neuropsychological tests that are commercially available have been discussed above with each disorder. Here we describe briefly a few tools that we find useful in the clinic, as well as an approach to perimetry.

Clinic Tests

In the clinic, most visual examination is directed toward uncovering low-level visual deficits. A standard battery includes visual acuity (best corrected or with pinhole) and confrontation visual fields, as well as an assessment of pupil light reactions and fundoscopy, all done on each eye separately. Significant asymmetries between the two eyes indicate an element of ocular dysfunction, rather than cerebral visual loss. Low-level factors such as cataracts need to be taken into account when assessing cerebral visual function. The blur, reduced acuity, decreased illumination, and altered spectral transmission from these factors may impair performance on a wide range of tests of high-level visual function, including face perception, color discrimination, and reading, among others.

Beyond these, it is useful to have several simple objects in the clinic to serve as quick but coarse tests of high-level function. A handful of colored caps can be presented to a patient, asking the patient to point to one of a named hue. This may not detect subtle color deficits, but patients with severe achromatopsia will fail. Colored targets can also be presented in the peripheral fields, comparing the ipsilateral and contralateral hemifields. A handful of line drawings from the Boston Naming Test, or photographs of common objects (both man-made and living things) are useful in assessing object agnosia. A few large, clearly printed sentences on a card are helpful in assessing reading. These sentences should contain a variety of words of different length, so that word length effects can be discerned, and should cover several lines, so that defects in returning to the start of the next line in hemianopic dyslexia are revealed. Screening tests of face recognition can use a variety of magazine pictures of famous faces as long as the patient is familiar with the celebrity in question and there are no "give-away" cues that can circumvent the need to recognize the face (e.g., Elton John's glasses, Abraham Lincoln's beard). Formal assessment requires standardized neuropsychological procedures (see Chapter 2), detailed analysis of visuoperception and cognitive abilities such as visuoconstructive, visual memory, reading, and visual problem solving.

Perimetry

In addition to confrontation visual fields, formal perimetry can be very useful in detecting subtle relative scotomata. To do automated perimetry, a patient must be alert, cooperative, and attentive. This method, when measuring thresholds rather than just performing a general screen, is the best at detecting subtle paracentral depressions of luminance sensitivity. It can be adjusted to test various regions of interest, such as the central 30 degrees, the central 10 degrees, or even just the macular region. Careful examination of the central-most zone of vision is useful in excluding a paracentral scotoma as a cause of impaired reading, for example.

For a wider view of the entire visual field, though, manual kinetic perimetry (Goldmann) is still the best compromise between speed and accuracy. Careful exploration of the wider perimetry is important in excluding peripheral field defects in patients who complain of problems navigating their environment. For example, a patient who notes tripping over objects and hesitancy going down stairs may have an inferior field defect. A patient who bumps into objects on the right likely has a right hemianopic defect.

Goldmann perimetry is also the method of choice in a patient suspected of having simultanagnosia. The attentional deficits of these patients lead them to perform miserably on automated perimetry. A patient interaction between the perimetrist and the subject is key to determining if multiple scotomata are present in the visual field of the patient. It is not easy to determine if patients fail to see a target because they have a field defect or if it is because they have a variable and limited attentional capacity. Repeated testing under conditions with limited distractions is needed to determine if any failures to detect a target are consistent within a given region and whether a zone of failure has a consistent clear demarcation from normal visual field. Attentional deficits tend to give more spatially variable performance than low-level loss of peripheral visual sensitivity.

Reduced visual attention and processing speed can effectively reduce the useful field of view in the absence of true visual field defects (Ball et al., 1993).

The key point to be made in a discussion of perimetry, then, is that when requesting this from an ophthalmology clinic, it is important to describe the type of problem the patient has, what confrontation testing has already shown, and what type of field defect one wishes to exclude or confirm. These patients are not routine to the eye clinic, and an experienced perimetrist who has been informed about the nature of the patient's problem is needed to produce a meaningful result.

CONCLUSION

This chapter can provide only a broad overview of some of the more important disorders of higher cortical visual function. Hemianopic field defects are common and can provide useful localizing information. It is important also to consider the impact of these low-level deficits on high-level visual performance and behavior, because they can interfere with tasks such as visual search and reading. True deficits of high-level vision can lead to a variety of selective visual disturbances that perplex clinicians. Failures in recognizing the properties of objects, such as color, face and object recognition, or the spatial distribution of visual scenes, such as motion and location, can occur in isolation or as loosely bound syndromes, corresponding to divisions of extrastriate processing into a ventral occipitotemporal "where" and occipitoparietal "what" stream. Knowledge of these entities, the manner in which they present, and simple ways to test for their existence is important to diagnosing and understanding the difficulties these patients have. Whether they can be successfully treated remains a topic for future research.

■ KEY POINTS

☐   Cerebral visual disorders that affect the terminal portion of the relay from retina to striate cortex cause hemifield defects that impair processing of all visual cues. Those that affect extrastriate cortex cause defects that are selective for the type of information processed but not its location in the visual field. Hemianopic defects are common and contain useful localizing information.

☐   Extrastriate cortical defects can be loosely grouped into those that affect a ventral occipitotemporal stream involved in object identification and those that affect a dorsal occipitoparietal stream involved in visuospatial analysis. Ventral stream defects include achromatopsia, object agnosia, alexia, and prosopagnosia. Dorsal stream defects include akinetopsia and the various components of Balint syndrome. Topographagnosia, loss of orientation in familiar surroundings, can occur from either dorsal or ventral deficits.

☐   The congruity of hemifield defects is greatest with striate lesions and least with optic tract lesions.

☐   Hemianopia can impair high-level tasks such as reading and visual search. However, the pattern of the impairments differ from those of alexia and neglect.

☐   Cerebral achromatopsia is most often associated with lesions of the fusiform gyri.

☐   Blindsight is an uncommonly reported finding in patients with cerebral visual loss. Its anatomic basis and whether it confers any functional benefit to patients is unclear.

☐   Artifacts such as light scatter into the seeing fields must be excluded. Although hemianopic defects are usually severe, recent studies suggest that some patients with striate damage may yet have some residual or unconscious visual experience, a phenomenon known as "blindsight."

☐   Patients with color anomia and agnosia can still discriminate hues correctly, in contrast to patients with achromatopsia.

☐   Before diagnosing acquired alexia, consider other causes of a secondary alexia, from disorders of eye movements, neglect, and field loss.

☐   Akinetopsia is rare and requires bilateral lesions of the lateral occipitotemporal area.

☐   Prosopagnosia is a family of disorders affecting various stages of perceptual and memory processing for faces in the ventral occipitotemporal stream, predominantly in the right hemisphere.

☐   Balint syndrome is a loose triad of simultanagnosia, optic ataxia, and defects in initiating and targeting saccades. These impairments may occur in isolation.

☐   Topographagnosia can result from either failure to recognize landmarks or inability to find correct routes.

KEY READINGS

Aldrich M, Alessi A, Beck R, et al: Cortical blindness: Etiology, diagnosis and prognosis. Ann Neurol 21:149–158, 1987.

Barton JJS, Rizzo M (eds): Vision and the Brain I and II. Neurologic Clinics, Vol. 21. Philadelphia: Saunders, 2003.

Cowey A, Stoerig P: The neurobiology of blindsight. Trends Neurosci 14:140–145, 1995.

Damasio A, Tranel D, Damasio H: Face agnosia and the neural substrates of memory. Ann Rev Neurosci 13:89–109, 1990.

Rizzo M, Vecera SP: Psychoanatomical substrates of Bálint's syndrome. J Neurol Neurosurg Psychiatry 72:162–178, 2002.

Zeki, SM: A century of cerebral achromatopsia. Brain 113:1721–1777, 1990.

REFERENCES

Aldric, M, Alessi A, Beck R, et al: Cortical blindness: Etiology, diagnosis and prognosis. Ann Neurol 21:149–158, 1987.

Anderson D, Trobe J, Hood T, et al: Optic tract injury after anterior temporal lobectomy. Ophthalmology 96:1065–1070, 1989.

Ando S, Moritake K: Pure optic ataxia associated with a right parieto-occipital tumour. J Neurol Neurosurg Psychiatry 53:805–806, 1990.

Auerbach S, Alexander M: Pure agraphia and unilateral optic ataxia associated with a left superior parietal lobule lesion. J Neurol Neurosurg Psychiatry 44:430–402, 1981.

Azzopardi P, Cowey A: Is blindsight like normal, near-threshold vision? Proc Natl Acad Sci U S A 94:14190–14194, 1997.

Baker CJ, Hess R, Zihl J: Residual motion perception in a "motion-blind" patient, assessed with limited-lifetime random dot stimuli. J Neurosci 11:454–461, 1991.

Ball K, Owsley C, Sloane ME, et al: Visual attention problems as a predictor of vehicle crashes in older drivers. Invest Ophthalmol Vis Sci 34:3110–3123, 1993.

Ballie, R, Blood KM, Bach-y-Rita P: Visual field rehabilitation in the cortically blind? J Neurol. Neurosurg Psychiatry 48:1113–1124, 1985.

Barbur JL, Weiskrantz L, Harlow JA: The unseen color aftereffect of an unseen stimulus: Insight from blindsight into mechanisms of color afterimages. Proc Natl Acad Sci U S A 96:11637–11641, 1999.

Bartolomeo P, Bachoud-Lévi A-C, De Gelder B, et al: Multiple-domain dissociation between impaired visual perception and preserved mental imagery in a patient with bilateral extrastriate lesions. Neuropsychologia 36:239–249, 1998.

Bartolomeo P, Bachoud-Levi AC, Denes G: Preserved imagery for colours in a patient with cerebral achromatopsia. Cortex 33:369–378, 1997.

Barton J, Behrmann M, Black S: Ocular search during line bisection. The effects of hemi-neglect and hemianopia. Brain 121:1117–1131, 1998.

Barton J, Sharpe J: Smooth pursuit and saccades to moving targets in blind hemifields. A comparison of medial occipital, lateral occipital, and optic radiation lesions. Brain 120:681–699, 1997a.

Barton J, Sharpe J: Ocular tracking of step-ramp targets by patients with unilateral cerebral lesions. Brain 121:1165–1183, 1998.

Barton J, Sharpe J, Raymond J: Retinotopic and directional defects in motion discrimination in humans with cerebral lesions. Ann Neurol 37: 665–675, 1995.

Barton J, Sharpe J, Raymond J: Directional defects in pursuit and motion perception in humans with unilateral cerebral lesions. Brain 119:1535–1550, 1996a.

Barton J, Simpson T, Kiriakopoulos E, et al: Functional magnetic resonance imaging of lateral occipitotemporal cortex during pursuit and motion perception. Ann Neurol 40:387–398, 1996b.

Barton JJS, Sharpe JA: Motion direction discrimination in blind hemifields. Ann Neurol 41:255–264, 1997b.

Battaglia Mayer A, Ferraina S, Marconi B, et al: Early motor influences on visuomotor transformations for reaching: A positive image of optic ataxia. Exp Brain Res 123:172–189, 1998.

Bauer R: The cognitive psychophysiology of prosopagnosia, in Ellis H, Jeeves M, Newcombe F, et al (eds): Aspects of Face Processing. Dordecht, The Netherlands: Martinus-Nijhoff, 1986, pp. 253–267.

Bauer R, Verfaellie M: Electrodermal discrimination of familiar but not unfamiliar faces in prosopagnosia. Brain Cogn 8:240–252, 1988.

Baylis G, Driver J, Baylis L, et al: Reading of letters and words in a patient with Balint's syndrome. Neuropsychologia 32:1273–1286, 1994.

Behrmann M, Moscovitch M, Black S, et al: Perceptual and conceptual factors in neglect dyslexia: Two contrasting case studies. Brain 113:1163–1183, 1990.

Behrmann M, Watt S, Black S, et al: Impaired visual search in patients with unilateral neglect: An oculographic analysis. Neuropsychologia 35:1445–1458, 1997.

Benton A, van Allen M: Prosopagnosia and facial discrimination. J Neurol Sci 15:167–172, 1972.

Benton S, Levy I, Swash M: Vision in the temporal crescent in occipital infarction. Brain 103:83–97, 1980.

Bittar RG, Ptito M, Faubert J, et al: Activation of the remaining hemisphere following stimulation of the blind hemifield in hemispherectomized subjects. Neuroimage 10:339–346, 1999.

Blythe I, Kennard C, Ruddock K: Residual vision in patients with retrogeniculate lesions of the visual pathways. Brain 110:887–905, 1987.

Blythe IM, Bromley JM, Kennard C, et al: Visual discrimination of target displacement remains after damage to the striate cortex in humans. Nature 320:619–621, 1986.

Braddick O, Atkinson J, Hood B, Harkness W, et al: Possible blindsight in infants lacking one cerebral hemisphere. Nature 360:461–463, 1992.

Braun D, Petersen D, Schonle P, et al: Deficits and recovery of first- and second-order motion perception in patients with unilateral cortical lesions. Eur J Neurosci 10:2117–2128, 1998.

Bruce V, Young A: Understanding face recognition. Br J Psychol 77:305–327, 1986.

Bruyer R: Covert facial recognition in prosopagnosia: A review. Brain Cogn 15:223–235, 1991.

Buxbaum L, Glosser G, Coslett H: Impaired face and word recognition without object agnosia. Neuropsychologia 37:41–50, 1999.

Campbell R, Heywood C, Cowey A, et al: Sensitivity to eye gaze in prosopagnosic patients and monkeys with superior temporal sulcus ablation. Neuropsychologia 28:1123–1142, 1990.

Campbell R, Zihl J, Massaro D, et al: Speechreading in the akinetopsic patient, L.M. Brain 120:1793–1803, 1997.

Campion J, Latto R, Smith YM: Is blindsight an effect of scattered light, spared cortex, and near-threshold vision? Behav Brain Sci 6:423–486, 1983.

Carter J, O'Connor, P, Shacklett D, et al: Lesions of the optic radiations mimicking lateral geniculate nucleus visual field defects. J Neurol Neurosurg Psychiatry 48:982–928, 1985.

Castaigne P, Rondot P, Dumas J, et al: Ataxie optique localisee au cote gauche dans les deux hemichamps visuels homonymes gauches. Rev Neurol (Paris) 131:23–28, 1975.

Cavanagh P, Hénaff M-A, Michel F, et al: Complete sparing of high-contrast color input to motion perception in cortical color blindness. Nat Neurosci 1:242–247, 1998.

Clarke S, Lindemann A, Maede, P, et al: Face recognition and postero-inferior hemispheric lesions. Neuropsychologia 35:1555–1563, 1997.

Clarke S, Miklossy J: Occipital cortex in man: Organization of callosal connections, related myelo- and cytoarchitecture, and putative boundaries of functional visual areas. J Comp Neurol 298:188–214, 1990.

Clarke S, Walsh V, Schoppig A, et al: Colour constancy impairments in patients with lesions of the prestriate cortex. Exp Brain Res 123:154–158, 1998.

Corbetta M, Marzi C, Tassinari G, et al: Effectiveness of different task paradigms in revealing blindsight. Brain 113:603–616, 1990.

Coslett H, Saffran E: Simultanagnosia. To see but not two see. Brain 114:1523–1545, 1991.

Cowey A, Stoerig P: The neurobiology of blindsight. Trends Neurosci 14:140–145, 1995.

Cowey A, Stoerig P: Spectral sensitivity in hemianopic macaque monkeys. Eur J Neurosci 11:2114–2120, 1999.

Cummings J, Houlihan J, Hill M: The pattern of reading deterioration in dementia of the Alzheimer type. Brain Lang 29:315–323, 1986.

Damasio A, Tranel D, Damasio H: Face agnosia and the neural substrates of memory. Ann Rev Neurosci 13:89–109, 1990.

Danckert J, Maruff P, Kinsella G, et al: Investigating form and colour perception in blindsight using an interference task. Neuroreport 9:2919–2925, 1998.

Danziger S, Fendrich R, Rafal RD: Inhibitory tagging of locations in the blind field of hemianopic patients. Conscious Cogn 6:291–307, 1997.

de Haan E, Campbell R: A fifteen year follow-up of a case of developmental prosopagnosia. Cortex 27:489–509, 1991.

de Renzi E: Current issues in prosopagnosia, in Ellis H, Jeeves M, Newcome F, et al. (eds): Aspects of Face Processing. Dordecht, The Netherlands: Martinus Nijhoff, 1986, pp. 243–252.

de Renzi E, Bonacini M, Faglioni P: Right posterior brain-damaged patients are poor at assessing the age of a face. Neuropsychologia 27:839–848, 1989.

de Renzi E, di Pellegrino G: Prosopagnosia and alexia without object agnosia. Cortex 34:403–415, 1998.

de Renzi E, Faglioni P, Grossi D, et al: Apperceptive and associative forms of prosopagnosia. Cortex 27:213–321, 1991.

de Vreese LP: Two systems for color-naming defects: Verbal disconnection versus colour imagery disorder. Neuropsychologia 29:1, 1991, pp. 1–18.

Diamond R, Carey S: Why faces are and are not special: An effect of expertise. J Exp Psychol Gen 115:107–117, 1986.

D'Zmura MD, Knoblauch K, Henaff M-A, et al: Dependence of color on context in a case of cortical color vision deficiency. Vision Res 38:3455–3459, 1998.

Ellis A, Young A, Critchley E: Loss of memory for people following temporal lobe damage. Brain 112:1469–1483, 1989.

Ettlin T, Beckson M, Benson D, et al: Prosopagnosia: A bihemispheric disorder. Cortex 28:129–134, 1992.

Evans J, Heggs A, Antoun N, et al: Progressive prosopagnosia associated with selective right temporal lobe atrophy. Brain 118:1–13, 1995.

Farah M: Visual Agnosia. Cambridge, MA: MIT Press, 1990.

Farah M, Levinson K, Klein K: Face perception and within-category discrimination in prosopagnosia. Neuropsychologia 33:661–674, 1995.

Farah M, O'Reilly R, Vecera S: Dissociated overt and covert recognition as an emergent property of a lesioned neural network. Psychol Rev 100:571–588, 1993.

Faubert J, Diaconu V, Ptito M, et al: Residual vision in the blind field of hemidecorticated humans predicted by a diffusion scatter model and selective spectral absorption of the human eye. Vision Res 39:149–157, 1999.

Felleman D, van Essen D: Distributed hierarchical processing in the primate cerebral cortex. Cereb Cortex 1:1–47, 1991.

Fendrich R, Wessinger CM, Gazzaniga MS: Residual vision in a scotoma: Implications for blindsight. Science 258:1489–1491, 1992.

Fine R, Parker G: Disturbance of central vision after carbon monoxide poisoning. Aust N Z J Ophthalmol 24:137–141, 1996.

Freitag P, Greenlee M, Lacina T, et al: Effect of eye movements on the magnitude of functional magnetic resonance imaging responses in extrastriate cortex during visual motion perception. Exp Brain Res 119:409–414, 1998.

Friedman D, Jankovic J, McCrary J: Neuro-ophthalmic findings in progressive supranuclear palsy. J Clin Neurophthalmol 12:104–109, 1992.

Frisèn L, Holmegaard L, Rosenkrantz M: Sectoral optic atrophy and homonymous horizontal sectoranopia: A lateral choroidal artery syndrome? J Neurol Neurosurg Psychiatry 41:374–380, 1978.

Gauthier I, Behrmann M, Tarr M: Can face recognition really be dissociated from object recognition? J Cogn Neurosci 11:3 49–370, 1999.

Girard P, Bullier J: Visual activity in area V2 during reversible inactivation of area 17 in the macaque monkey. J Neurophysiol 62:1989, pp. 1287–1302.

Girard P, Salin P, Bullier J: Visual activity in areas V3a and V3 during reversible inactivation of area V1 in the macaque monkey. J Neurophysiol 66:1493–1503, 1991.

Girard, P, Salin, P and Bullier, J. Response selectivity of neurons in area MT of the macaque monkey during reversible inactivation of area V1. J Neurophysiol 67: 1437–1446, 1992.

Goodglass H, Kaplan E: The Assessment of Aphasia and Related Disorders. Philadelphia: Lea & Febiger, 1983.

Gray L, Galetta S, Siegal T, et al: The central visual field in homonymous hemianopia. Evidence for unilateral foveal representation. Arch Neurol 54:312–317, 1997.

Greenlee M, Lang H, Mergner T, et al: Visual short-term memory of stimulus velocity in patients with unilateral posterior brain damage. J Neurosci 15:2287–3000, 1995.

Greenlee M, Smith A: Detection and discrimination of first- and second-order motion in patients with unilateral brain damage. J Neurosci 17:804–818, 1997.

Gross C: Contributions of striate cortex and the superior colliculus to visual functions in area MT, the superior temporal polysensory area and inferior temporal cortex. Neuropsychologia 29:497–515, 1991.

Guo K, Benson PJ, Blakemore C: Residual motion discrimination using colour information without primary visual cortex. Neuroreport 9:2103–2107, 1998.

Haarmeier T, Thier P, Repnow M, et al: False perception of motion in a patient who cannot compensate for eye movements. Nature 389:849–852, 1997.

Hadjikhani N, Liu AK, Dale AM, et al: Retinotopy and color sensitivity in human visual cortical area V8. Nat Neurosci 1:235–241, 1998.

Hanley J, Young A, Pearson N: Defective recognition of familiar people. Cogn Neuropsychol 6:179–210, 1989.

Haxby J, Hoffman E, Gobbini M: The distributed human neural system for face perception. Trends Cogn Sci 4:223–233, 2000.

Heide W, Koenig E, Dichgans J: Optokinetic nystagmus, self-motion sensation and their aftereffects in patients with occipit-parietal lesions. Clin Vision Sci 5:145–156, 1990.

Helgason C, Caplan L, Goodwin J, et al: Anterior choroidal artery-territory infarction. Report of cases and review. Arch Neurol 43:681–686, 1986.

Henke K, Schweinberger S, Grigo A, et al: Specificity of face recognition: Recognition of exemplars of non-face objects in prosopagnosia. Cortex 34:289–296, 1998.

Hess R, Baker CJ, Zihl J: The "motion-blind" patient: Low-level spatial and temporal filters. J Neurosci 9:1628–1640, 1989.

Heywood C, Gaffan D, Cowey A: Cerebral achromatopsia in monkeys. Eur J Neurosci 7:1064–1073, 1995.

Heywood CA, Cowey A, Newcombe F: Chromatic discrimination in a cortically colour blind observer. Eur J Neurosci 3:802–812, 1991.

Heywood CA, Kentridge RW, Cowey A: Form and motion from colour in cerebral achromatopsia. Exp Brain Res 123:145–153, 1998.

Heywood CA, Nicholas JJ, Cowey A: Behavioural and electrophysiological chromatic and achromatic contrast sensitivity in an achromatopsic patient. J Neurol Neurosurg Psychiatry 61:638–643, 1996.

Hurlbert AC, Bramwell DI, Heywood C, et al: Discrimination of cone contrast changes as evidence for colour constancy in cerebral achromatopsia. Exp Brain Res 123:136–144, 1998.

Jacobson D: The localizing value of a quadrantanopia. Arch Neurol 54:401–404, 1997.

Jakobson L, Archibald Y, Carey D, et al: A kinematic analysis of reaching and grasping movements in a patient recovering from optic ataxia. Neuropsychologia 29:803–809, 1991.

Jarry D, Rigolet M-H, Rivaud S, et al: Diagnostic électrophysi-ologique de deux syndromes psycho-visuels: Syndrome de Balint et cécité corticale. J Fr Ophtalmol 22:876–880, 1999.

Johnston JL, Sharpe JA, Morrow MJ: Spasm of fixation: A quantitative study. J Neurol Sci 107:166, 1992, pp. 166–171.

Kanwisher N, McDermott J, Chun M: The fusiform face area: A module in human extrastriate cortex specialized for face perception. J Neurosci 17:4302–4311, 1997.

Kasten E, Wuest S, Sabel B: Residual vision in transition zones in patients with cerebral blindness. J Clin Exp Neuropsychol 20:581–598, 1998.

Ka, M, Levin H: Prosopagnosia. Am J Ophthalmol 94:75–80, 1982.

Kennard C, Lawden M, Morland AB, et al: Colour identification and colour constancy are impaired in a patient with incomplete achromatopsia associated with prestriate lesions. Proc Roy Soc Lond B 260:169–175, 1995.

King S, Azzopardi P, Cowey A, et al: The role of light scatter in the residual visual sensitivity of patients with complete cerebral hemispherectomy. Visual Neurosci 13:1–13, 1996.

Kinsbourne M, Warrington EK: Observations on colour agnosia. J Neurol Neurosurg Psychiatry 27:296, 1964, pp. 296–299.

Kirkham T: The ocular symptomology of pituitary tumors. Proc Roy Soc Med 65:517–518, 1972.

Kolb FC, Braun J: Blindsight in normal observers. Nature 377:336–338, 1995.

Kracke I: Developmental prosopagnosia in Asperger syndrome: Presentation and discussion of an individual case. Dev Med Child Neurol 36:873–886, 1994.

Lanca M, Jerskey BA, O'Connor MG: Neuropsychologic assessment of visual disorders, in Barton JJS, Rizzo M (eds): Vision and the Brain I. Neurologic Clinics, Vol. 21. Philadelphia: Saunders, pp. 387–416, 2003.

Land E: Recent advances in retinex theory. Vision Res 26:7–21, 1986.

Landis T, Regard M, Blieste A, et al: Prosopagnosia and agnosia for noncanonical views. Brain 111:1287–1297, 1988.

Levine D, Calvanio R: Prosopagnosia: A defect in visual configural processing. Brain Cogn 10:149–170, 1989.

Magnussen S, Mathiesen T: Detection of moving and stationary gratings in the absence of striate cortex. Neuropsychologia 27:725–728, 1989.

Marcar V, Zihl J, Cowey A: Comparing the visual deficits of a motion blind patient with the visual deficits of monkeys with area MT removed. Neuropsychologia 35:1459–1465, 1997.

Marcel A: Blindsight and shape perception: Deficit of visual consciousness or of visual function? Brain 121:1565–1588, 1998.

Martin A, Haxby JV, Lalonde FM, et al: Discrete cortical regions associated with knowledge of color and knowledge of action. Science 270:102–105, 1995.

Marzi C, Tassinari G, Agliotti S, et al: Spatial summation across the vertical meridian in hemianopics: A test of blindsight. Neuropsychologia 24:749–758, 1986.

McCarthy R, Evans J, Hodges J: Topographic amnesia: Spatial memory disorder, perceptual dysfunction, or category specific semantic memory impairment? J Neurol Neurosurg Psychiatry 60:318–325, 1996.

McLeod P, Heywood C, Driver J, et al: Selective deficit of visual search in moving displays after extrastriate damage. Nature 339:466–467, 1989.

McNeil J, Warrington E: Prosopagnosia: A reclassification. Q J Exp Psychol 43A:267–287, 1991.

Meadows J: The anatomical basis of prosopagnosia. J Neurol Neurosurg Psychiatr 37:489–501, 1974.

Medina J, Chokroverty S, Rubino F: Syndrome of agitated delirium and visual impairment: A manifestation of medial temporo-occipital infarction. J Neurol Neurosurg Psychiatry 40:861–864, 1977.

Meeres SL, Graves RE: Localization of unseen stimuli by humans with normal vision. Neuropsychologia 28:1231–1237, 1990.

Meienberg O, Zangemeister WH, Rosenberg M, et al: Saccadic eye movement strategies in patients with homonymous hemianopia. Ann Neurol 9:537–544, 1981.

Mendola J, Corkin S: Visual discrimination and attention after bilateral temporal-lobe lesions: A case study. Neuropsychologia 37:91–102, 1999.

Merigan W, Freeman A, Meyers SP: Parallel processing streams in human visual cortex. Neuroreport 8:3985–3991, 1997.

Milner A, Goodale M: The visual brain in action. Oxford: Oxford University Press, 1995.

Moore T, Rodman H, Repp A, et al: Greater residual vision in monkeys after striate damage in infancy. J Neurophysiol 76:3928–3933, 1996.

Morgan MJ, Mason AJS, Solomon JA: Blindsight in normal subjects? Nature 385:401–402, 1997.

Morland A, Ogilvie J, Ruddock K, et al: Orientation discrimination is impaired in the absence of the striate cortical contribution to human vision. Proc Roy Soc Lond B Biol Sci 263:633–640, 1996.

Morland AB, Jones SR, Finlay AL, et al: Visual perception of motion, luminance and colour in a human hemianope. Brain 122:1183–1198, 1999.

Morland AB, Ruddock KH: Retinotopic organisation of cortical mechanisms responsive to colour: Evidence from patient studies. Acta Psychol 97:7–24, 1997.

Nagaratnam N, Grice D, Kalouche H: Optic ataxia following unilateral stroke. J Neurol Sci 155:204–207, 1998.

Newman S, Miller N: Optic tract syndrome. Neuro-ophthalmologic considerations. Arch Ophthalmol 101:1241–1250, 1983.

Ogren MP, Mateer CA, Wyler AR: Alterations in visually related eye movements following left pulvinar damage in man. Neuropsychologia 22:187–196, 1984.

Onofrj M, Fulgente T, Thomas A: Event related potentials recorded in dorsal simultanagnosia. Brain Res Cogn Brain Res 3:25–32, 1995.

Oxbury JM, Oxbury SM, Humphrey NK: Varieties of colour anomia. Brain 92:847–860, 1969.

Pai M: Topographic disorientation: Two cases. J Formos Med Assoc 96:660–663, 1997.

Patterson K, Wilson B: A rose is a nose: A deficit in initial letter identification. Cogn Neuropsychol 13:447–478, 1990.

Paulesu E, Harrison J, Baron-Cohen S, et al: The physiology of coloured hearing: A PET activation study of colour-word synaesthesia. Brain 118:661–676, 1995.

Paulson HL, Galetta SL, Grossman M, et al: Hemiachromatopsia of unilateral occipitotemporal infarcts. Am J Ophthalmol 118:518–523, 1994.

Payne B, Lomber S, Macneil M, et al: Evidence for greater sight in blindsight following damage of primary visual cortex early in life. Neuropsychologia 34:741–774, 1996.

Pearlman AL, Birch J, Meadows JC: Cerebral color blindness: An acquired defect in hue discrimination. Ann Neurol 5:253–261, 1979.

Perenin M, Vighetto A: Optic ataxia: A specific disruption in visuo-motor mechanisms. I. Different aspects of the deficit in reaching for objects. Brain 111:643–674, 1988.

Perenin M-T: Discrimination of motion direction in perimetrically blind fields. Neuroreport 2:397–400, 1991.

Perenin M-T, Jeannerod M: Residual vision in cortically blind hemifields. Neuropsychologia 13:1–7, 1975.

Perenin M-T, Jeannerod M: Visual functions within the hemianopic field following early cerebral hemidecortication in man—I. Spatial localization. Neuropsychologia 16:1–13, 1978.

Perenin M-T, Rossetti Y: Grasping without form discrimination in a hemianopia field. Neuroreport 7:793–797, 1996.

Perenin M-T, Ruel J, Hécaen H: Residual visual capacities in a case of cortical blindness. Cortex 6:605–612, 1980.

Perez FM, Tunkel RS, Lachman EA et al: Balint's syndrome arising from bilateral posterior cortical atrophy or infarction: Rehabilitation strategies and their limitation. Disabil Rehabil 18:300–304, 1996.

Pessin M, Lathi E, Cohen M, et al: Clinical feature and mechanism of occipital lobe infarction. Ann Neurol 21:290–299, 1987.

Pierrot-Deseilligny C, Gray F, Brunet P: Infarcts of both inferior parietal lobules with impairment of visually guided eye movements, peripheral inattention and optic ataxia. Brain 109:81–97, 1986.

Plant G, Laxer K, Barbaro N, et al: Impaired visual motion perception in the contralateral hemifield following unilateral posterior cerebral lesions in humans. Brain 116:1303–1335, 1993.

Polster M, Rapcsak S: Representations in learning new faces: Evidence from prosopagnosia. J Int Neuropsychol Soc 2:240–248, 1996.

Pöppel E, Held R, Frost D: Residual visual function after brain wounds involving the central visual pathways in man. Nature 243:295–296, 1973.

Ptito A, Lassonde M, Lepore F, et al: Visual discrimination in hemispherectomized patients. Neuropsychologia 25:869–879, 1987.

Ptito A, Lepore F, Ptiito M, et al: Target detection and movement discrimination in the blind field of hemispherectomized patients. Brain 114:497–512, 1991.

Rafal R, Smith J, Krantz J, et al: Extrageniculate vision in hemianopic humans: Saccade inhibition by signals in the blind field. Science 250:118–121, 1990.

Rapcsak S, Polster M, Glisky M, et al: False recognition of unfamiliar faces following right hemisphere damage: Neuropsychological and anatomical observations. Cortex 32:593–611, 1996.

Regan D, Giaschi D, Sharpe J, et al: Visual processing of motion-defined form: Selective failure in patients with parietotemporal lesions. J Neurosci 12:2198–2210, 1992.

Renault B, Signoret J-L, DeBruille B, et al: Brain potentials reveal covert facial recognition in prosopagnosia. Neuropsychologia 27:905–912, 1989.

Rentschler I, Treutwein B, Landis T. Dissociation of local and global processing in visual agnosia. Vision Res 34:963–971, 1994.

Rizzo M: Bálint's syndrome and associated visuospatial disorders, in Kennard C (eds):Bailliere's International Practice and Research. Philadelphia: Saunders, 1993, pp. 415–437.

Rizzo M, Hurtig R, Damasio A: The role of scanpaths in facial recognition and learning. Ann Neurol 22:41–45, 1987.

Rizzo M, Nawrot M, Zihl J: Motion and shape perception in cerebral akinetopsia. Brain 118:1105–1127, 1995.

Rizzo M, Robin DA: Simultanagnosia: A defect of sustained attention yields insights on visual information processing. Neurology 40:447–455, 1990.

Rizzo M, Rotella D, Darling W: Troubled reaching after right occipito-temporal damage. Neuropsychologia 30:711–722, 1992.

Rizzo M, Smith V, Pokorny J, et al: Color perception profiles in central achromatopsia. Neurology 43:995–1001, 1993.

Rizzo M, Vecera SP: Psychoanatomical substrates of Bálint's syndrome. J Neurol Neurosurg Psychiatry 72:162–178, 2002.

Rodman H, Gross C, Albright T: Afferent basis of visual response properties in area MT of the macaque. I. Effects of striate cortex removal. J Neurosci 9:2033–2050, 1989.

Rüttiger L, Braun DI, Gegenfurtner KR, et al: Selective color constancy deficits after circumscribed unilateral brain lesions. J Neurosci 19:3094–3106, 1999.

Sahraie A, Weiskrantz L, Barbur J, et al: Pattern of neuronal activity associated with conscious and unconscious processing of visual signals. Proc Natl Acad Sci U S A 94:9406–9411, 1997.

Sanders MD, Warrington E, Marshall J, et al: Blindsight: Vision in a field defect. Lancet, April 20, 1974, pp. 707–708.

Scharli H, Harman A, Hogben J: Blindsight in subjects with homonymous visual field defects. J Cogn Neurosci 11:52–66, 1999.

Sergent J, Poncet M: From covert to overt recognition of faces in a prosopagnosic patient. Brain 113:989–1004, 1990.

Sergent J, Villemure J-G: Prosopagnosia in a right hemispherectomized patient. Brain 112:975–995, 1989.

Shipp S, de Jong B, Zihl J, et al: The brain activity related to residual motion vision in a patient with bilateral lesions of V5. Brain 117:1023–1038, 1994.

Shuren J, Brott T, Shefft B, et al: Preserved color imagery in an achromatopsic. Neuropsychologia 34:485–489, 1996.

Smith A, Greenlee M, Singh K, et al: The processing of first- and second-order motion in human visual cortex assessed by functional magnetic resonance imaging. J Neurosci 18:3816–3830, 1998.

Sparr S, Jay M, Drislane F, et al: A historic case of visual agnosia revisited after 40 years. Brain 114:789–800, 1991.

Stoerig P: Chromaticity and achromaticity. Evidence for a functional differentiation in visual field defects. Brain 110:869–886, 1987.

Stoerig P, Cowey A: Increment-threshold spectral sensitivity in blindsight. Evidence for colour opponency. Brain 114:1487–1512, 1991.

Stoerig P, Faubert J, Ptito M, et al: No blindsight following hemidecortication in human subjects? Neuroreport 7:1990–1994, 1996.

Stoerig P, Kleinschmidt A, Frahm J: No visual responses in denervated V1: High-resolution functional magnetic resonance imaging of a blindsight patient. Neuroreport 9:21–25, 1998.

Takahashi N, Kawamura M, Hirayama K, et al: Prosopagnosia: A clinical and anatomic study of four patients. Cortex 31:317–329, 1995.

ter Braak J, Schenk V, van Vliet A: Visual reactions in a case of long-lasting cortical blindness. J Neurol Neurosurg Psychiatry 34:140–147, 1971.

Tomaiuolo F, Ptito M, Marzi C, et al: Blindsight in hemispherectomized patients as revealed by spatial summation across the vertical meridian. Brain 120:795–803, 1997.

Tootell R, Taylor J: Anatomical evidence for MT and additional cortical visual areas in humans. Cereb Cortex 5:39–55, 1995.

Torjussen T: Visual processing in cortically blind hemifields. Neuropsychologia 16:15–21, 1978.

Trauzettel-Klosinski S, Brendler K: Eye movements in reading with hemianopic field defects: The significance of clinical parameters. Graefes Arch Clin Exp Ophthalmol 236:91–102, 1998.

Ungerleider L, Mishkin M: Two cortical visual systems, in Ingle DJ, Mansfield RJW, Goodale MS (eds): The Analysis of Visual Behaviour. Cambridge, MA: MIT Press, 1982, pp. 549–586.

Vaina L: Selective impairment of visual motion interpretation following lesions of the right occipito-parietal area in humans. Biol Cybern 61:347–359, 1989.

Vaina L: Functional segregation of color and motion processing in the human visual cortex: Clinical evidence. Cereb Cortex 5:555–572, 1994.

Vaina L, Cowey A: Impairment of the perception of second order motion but not first order motion in a patient with unilateral ocal brain damage. Proc R Soc Lond B Biol Sci 263:1225–1232, 1996.

Vaina L, Cowey A, Kennedy D: Perception of first- and second-order motion: Separable neurological mechanisms? Hum Brain Mapp 7:67–77, 1999.

Vaina L, Makris N, Kennedy D, et al: The selective impairment of the perception of first-order motion by unilateral cortical brain damage. Vis Neurosci 15:333–348, 1998.

Verhagen W, Huygen P, Mulleners W: Lack of optokinetic nystagmus and visual motion perception in acquired cortical blindness. Neurophthalmology 17:211–218, 1997.

Verstichel P, Chia L : Trouble d'identification des visages apres lesion hemispherique gauche. Rev Neurol 155:937–943, 1999.

Victor JD, Maiese K, Shapley R, et al: Acquired central dyschromatopsia: Analysis of a case with preservation of color discrimination. Clin Vis Sci 4:183–196, 1989.

Vighetto A, Perenin M : Ataxie optique: Analyse des reponses oculaires et manuelles dans une tache de pointage vers une cible visuelle. Rev Neurol (Paris) 137:357–372, 1981.

Warrington E: Warrington Recognition Memory Test. Los Angeles: Western Psychological Services, 1984.

Watson J, Myers R, Frackowiak R, et al: Area V5 of the human brain: Evidence from a combined study using positron emission tomography and magnetic resonance imaging. Cereb Cortex 3:79–94, 1993.

Weiskrantz L: Residual vision in a scotoma: A follow-up study of "form" discrimination. Brain 110:77–92, 1987.

Weiskrantz L: Blindsight: A Case Study and Implications. Oxford: Oxford University Press, 1998.

Weiskrantz L, Barbur J, Sahraie A: Parameters affecting conscious versus unconscious discrimination with damage to the visual cortex (V1). Proc Natl Acad Sci U S A 92:6122–6126, 1995.

Weiskrantz L, Cowey A, Barbur JL: Differential pupillary constriction and awareness in the absence of striate cortex. Brain 122:1533–1538, 1999.

Weiskrantz L, Warrington E, Sanders M, et al: Visual capacity in the hemianopic field following a restricted occipital ablation. Brain 97:709–728, 1974.

Wessinger CM, Fendrich R, Gazzaniga MS, et al: Extrageniculostriate vision in humans: Investigations with hemispherectomy patients. Prog Brain Res 112: 405–413, 1996.

Yamasaki D, Wurtz R: Recovery of function after lesions in the superior temporal sulcus in the monkey. J Neurophysiol 66: 651–673, 1991.

Young A, Aggleton J, Hellawell D, et al: Face processing impairments after amygdalotomy. Brain 118:15–24, 1995.

Young A, Ellis H: Childhood prosopagnosia. Brain Cogn 9:16-47, 1989.

Young A, Flude B, Hay D, et al: Impaired discrimination of familiar from unfamiliar faces. Cortex 29:65–75, 1993.

Young A, Newcombe F, de Haan E, et al: Face perception after brain injury. Brain 116:941–959, 1993.

Zeki S, ffytche DH: The Riddoch syndrome: Insights into the neurobiology of conscious vision. Brain 121:25–45, 1998.

Zeki SM: Colour coding in the cerebral cortex: The reaction of cells in monkey visual cortex to wavelengths and colours. Neuroscience 9:741–765, 1983a.

Zeki SM: Colour coding in the cerebral cortex: The responses of wavelength-selective and colour-coded cells in monkey visual cortex to changes in wavelength composition. Neuroscience 9:767-781, 1983b.

Zeki SM: A century of cerebral achromatopsia. Brain 113:1721-1777, 1990.

Zihl J: Eye movement patterns in hemianopic dyslexia. Brain 118:891-912, 1995.

Zihl J, von Cramon D, Mai N: Selective disturbance of movement vision after bilateral brain damage. Brain 106:313-340, 1983.

Zihl J, von Cramon D, Mai N, et al: Disturbance of movement vision after bilateral posterior brain damage. Further evidence and follow-up observations. Brain 114:2235-2252, 1991.

Functional Organization of the Auditory System

Sylvie Hébert

Isabelle Peretz

Amusia
Auditory agnosia
Auditory phantom phenomena.
Auditory system
Brain specialization for music
Brain specialization for speech
Functional organization
High-level audition
Low-level audition

INTRODUCTION

Over a life span, the auditory system is highly vulnerable to damage from the peripheral organ up to its most central structures. Hearing functions start to decline as early as the fourth decade of life and decrease with age, such that hearing abilities at midlife may already be compromised in comparison to those of young adults. Presently, the impact that a deficit in basic sound analysis has on higher auditory processing is not fully understood. It is probable that such a deficit impedes the ability to adequately process the sound signal from its early to its latest stages. For example, one study (Griffiths et al., 1997) has shown that a deficit in higher-level auditory function, namely, an impairment in recognizing familiar music, may result from more basic impairments in sound analysis. HV, a patient with brain damage, showed a deficit in the analysis of rapid temporal sequences of notes and also in apparent sound-source movement that was associated with difficulty in music processing. High-level auditory functions are particularly liable to cerebral damage because the auditory cortical structures are irrigated by the middle cerebral arteries, which are the most likely loci for aneurysm ruptures and ischemia. Depending on the cortical areas (primary or associative) involved, such changes may affect different levels and domains of auditory processing. For instance, we have documented that a ruptured aneurysm on the middle cerebral artery is very likely to result in impaired auditory processing of music (Ayotte et al., 2000). However, because there is not as yet any comprehensive model that accounts for how the sound signal is processed from the periphery to the brain, the role of subtle, lower-level impairments on higher-level functions remains to be disclosed. This chapter presents an overview of the functional organization of the auditory system through an examination of specific deficits resulting from damage along various stages of the auditory pathways. Particular attention is paid to aspects of music processing.

FUNCTIONAL DEFICITS DUE TO PERIPHERAL ASPECTS OF AUDITION

It is the auditory system as a whole that enables one to process sound information coming from the environment. Classically, it is divided into four anatomic parts: the outer ear, the middle ear, the inner ear, and the central auditory system. The latter encompasses all the complex interconnections between the auditory nerve, located at the output of the inner ear, and the auditory cortex, which is the part of the brain responsible for auditory information processing (Fig. 13-1).

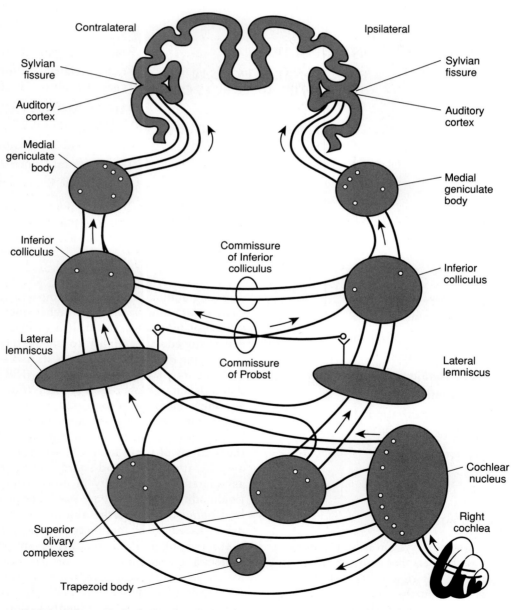

FIGURE 13-1. Schematic diagram of the ascending pathways of the central auditory system from the right cochlea to the auditory cortex. (From Yost WA: Fundamentals of Hearing: An Introduction. San Diego, CA: Academic Press, 2000, p. 228, Fig 15.1, with permission.)

The outer ear is composed of the pinna and the external auditory canal ending extending to the eardrum. Due to their particular shape, the pinnae capture sound in a specific way, depending on the direction of the sound, and play a role in sound localization. The physical separation between the two ears is a determining factor for the encoding of sound localization information along the horizontal plane. This phenomenon is explained by the fact that sound from one side of the head will arrive to the ear closer to the sound source with a different time/phase and intensity as compared to the opposite ear (i.e., the ear farthest from the sound source). The sound vibration is then transmitted from the eardrum to the middle ear, which is composed of three tiny ossicles (the smallest bones of the human body, about 1 cm³ in total volume) referred to as incus, malleus, and stapes. The middle ear principally serves to amplify the vibration an aerial environment in the outer ear, to a liquid, denser environment, in the inner ear.

The inner ear, more specifically the organ of Corti located in the cochlea, contains both inner and outer hair cells. The inner hair cells are the true sound receptors, whereas the outer hair cells are mainly innervated by efferent fibers, which are inhibitory in nature. Indeed, considerable outer hair cell damage (up to 30%) may exist and remain imperceptible on the audiogram (a device used to measure an auditory threshold at various pure tone frequencies). The inner ear translates the sound vibration into nerve pulses, which are transmitted to the cortex and subsequently analyzed.

At the functional level, the peripheral auditory system has encoded frequency, amplitude (intensity), and temporal/phase characteristics of the acoustic waveform. Before it is translated into a neural impulse, the sound wave causes the basilar membrane of the inner ear to oscillate at maximum amplitude at a location that depends on the frequency of the stimulation. Such selectivity may be explained by the basic mechanical properties of the membrane, which is stiff and narrow at the base, and supple and wide at the apex. If the sound wave is a complex one, that is, when it is composed of several frequencies, each frequency will cause the basilar membrane to vibrate maximally at a particular point. High frequencies will reach maximal vibration at the basal end of the membrane, whereas low frequencies will reach maximal vibration at the apical end. Hair cells placed along the basilar membrane also follow this frequency-dependent arrangement. The information about frequency is encoded via the periodicity of the neural discharge rate because neurons tend to fire at a fixed point of the sound wave cycle. Therefore, discharges are locked to specific sound periods and hence, to its frequency, where the period refers to the time required for the sound wave to complete one cycle. Increases in sound wave intensity are assumed to be encoded via an increase in the discharge rate within the auditory system. Because each individual neuron will increase its discharge over a relatively small range of level changes, intensity is likely determined by an increase in discharge rate of a large number of fibers (see Yost, 2000, for a summary).

With the exception of a blockage of the ear canal or a disease affecting the middle ear, the outer and middle ear structures do not produce significant hearing loss or distortions in sound perception. Essentially, it is the inner ear structures and functions that lead to such impairments. The tonotopic arrangement of inner hair cells along the basilar membrane in the cochlea (tonotopy that is preserved up to the auditory cortex) explains why high-frequency hearing loss appears sooner with age than a low-frequency one. The inner hair cells, concentrated on the basal end, carry information about high-frequency sounds and those at the apex carry information about low-frequency sounds. Sounds of all frequencies cause the bending of all hair cells, from the base to the apex, whereas sounds of low frequencies cause the bending of hair cells at the apex only. Hair cells at the base therefore wear out before those at the apex. Accordingly, a selective high-frequency hearing loss is typical of damage to the cochlea.

Damage to the cochlea, by virtue of age or an acoustic trauma, may lead to a host of perceptual deficits, present to variable degrees depending on the individual. These include loudness recruitment, which is a narrowing of the dynamic range; absolute thresholds are higher than normal, whereas pain thresholds remain normal. This causes the loudness of sounds to grow more rapidly than normal with the increase in sound level. Filter broadening also results from cochlear damage and impedes the frequency-resolving power of the inner ear. Sound is more susceptible to interference and masking, and perceptually, this may lead to a decreased ability to follow a conversation in noisy backgrounds (see Moore, 1995, for an in-depth account of perceptual deficits due to cochlear damage).

In addition to such deficits, other abnormal percepts may occur following cochlear damage. One of the most common hearing problems following cochlear damage is *tinnitus*, which is the illusory perception of a sound (often permanent) in the head or the ears. Tinnitus is usually described as a buzzing, whistling, or ringing sound and is conservatively estimated to occur in 10% to 15% of the adult population (Davis & Rafaie, 2000). Presently, there is not a unanimous explanation for tinnitus. One possible cause is articulated in terms of an interaction between peripheral and central factors. In time, resultant peripheral damage (hearing loss) would lead to more central changes. Brain regions devoted to the analysis of frequencies that are lost (usually high frequencies) would be invaded by other regions responsible for the analysis of adjacent frequencies. These brain changes would probably be implemented by a breakdown in the balance of efferent and afferent pathways. Tinnitus, corresponding to the frequencies in the region of the hearing loss, would therefore be the perceptual correlate of brain plasticity (Mühnickel et al., 1998).

Central subcortical structures are located in the brainstem and consist of many nuclei and connections that are intricate and complex (see Fig. 13-1). There are both ascending and descending auditory pathways, the latter being mainly (but not exclusively) inhibitory. The ascending pathways receive and send input from both ears at and above the superior olivary complex. Due to the fact that these nuclei are relatively intricate and inaccessible, much is still unknown about their functioning and exact role in audition. Their functioning is observed indirectly in humans by several methods, such as evoked potentials. For instance, brainstem evoked potentials are used to assess the speed of transmission of the auditory input up to this structure and above, and more generally to detect possible deficiencies in the auditory pathways of the brainstem. The main nuclei in the brainstem function to refine the code for sound by performing neural comparisons, to combine information coming from both ears and make binaural comparisons, and to refine the processing of sound source locations. Damage to brainstem structures of nuclei may disrupt the transmission of the sound characteristics to higher structures, that is, at the cortex level (Musiek et al., 1994; Popper & Fay, 1991).

FUNCTIONAL DEFICITS DUE TO CENTRAL ASPECTS OF AUDITION

In everyday situations, the acoustic environment is composed of several different sound sources, themselves consisting of complex sounds, of which acoustic characteristics may be similar or even overlap to a great extent. Sound vibrations created by these different sound sources arrive at the eardrum under the form of a complex, but unique, vibratory pattern. One of the most important tasks of higher auditory functions is to disentangle elements belonging to various sound sources in order that they may be correctly identified and localized in space. There is no a priori argument to postulate that the auditory system possesses specific "channels" for a certain type of sound source, for instance a channel for "speech," another for "music," still another for "human voices," and so forth (see Mann & Liberman, 1983, for the proposition of the existence of such a specific channel for speech). Rather, all sound patterns produced by different sources must be decoded according to their basic acoustic properties, recoded into some coherent "stream" or "group" according to several physical variables (such as spectral separation, spectral profile, spatial separation, etc.), and

further compared with mental representations or "auditory objects" of sound sources previously encoded in memory, so that a correct recognition and identification can occur (see Bregman, 1990, for an extensive account of the auditory scene analysis problem).

However, evidence suggests that once the basic acoustic properties of the sound have been decoded, there is a specialization in the analysis of the auditory input that occurs (at what stage exactly is as of yet unknown), such that sound sources of differing natures are processed by particular anatomic brain regions and are subserved by specific neural networks. In this respect, studies on brain lesions have provided a richness of information, because the specific patterns of selective breakdowns and preservation of abilities displayed by patients with cerebral lesions are indicative of the highest levels of organization of auditory functions.

Neurologists were the first to observe patients with specific brain lesions that could selectively impair speech (Broca, 1861; Wernicke, 1874). Other selective impairments of auditory functions, such as music, were reported soon after (Bouillaud, 1865, in Dorgeuille, 1966). Specific terminology already reflected the will to classify cerebral damages in functional terms: agnosias, aphasias, amusias were put forth to designate specific types of auditory deficits, depending on the impaired domain. One line of research in neuropsychology (the study of the relationship between cerebral organization and mental functioning) is the study of higher auditory functions. The next section will review neuropsychological evidence in favor of the idea that different subdivisions of these higher auditory functions may result from brain specialization for particular domains.

One classical and powerful method used in neuropsychology to determine whether auditory functions are distinct, that is, subserved by different neural networks, is a *double dissociation* paradigm. (Teuber, 1955; Shallice, 1988). The dissociations are of two basic types: selective loss and selective sparing. The rational of the dissociation is the following. If a patient can no longer accomplish operation X (selective loss) but is able to perform operation Y (selective sparing) then the dissociation of X from Y suggests that the two operations are performed by different mechanisms. There are, however, alternative explanations, such as a continuum of difficulty between operation X and Y. Poor performance on operation X may merely reflect that it is more difficult than operation Y. The inference is therefore much stronger if another patient is found to display the inverse dissociation, that is, the loss of Y and the sparing of X. These two patients then form an instance of a double dissociation. Simple and double dissociations between patterns of losses and sparings are used to document which auditory domains are independent from one another.

Cortical Deafness

The term "cortical deafness" refers to a deficit involving damage to the auditory cortical areas that leads to a global deficit in auditory recognition of sound events. Peripheral hearing (pure-tone audiogram, tympanogram, stapedius reflex, etc.) is typically normal. Michel and colleagues (1980) described the case of a patient who could speak, read, and write normally, but who could not understand what was said to him. He also could not recognize environmental sounds and simple musical tunes, though sound localization was very inaccurate. Although his peripheral hearing was functionally intact, he did not show any response to late auditory evoked potentials (known in audiology as auditory late response, or ALR). The latter have a cortical origin, although the specific site of generation is still unknown. Thus, the absence of neurophysiological responses indicated that auditory cortices were dysfunctional. In this case, then, the sensory deficit (i.e., the absence of ALR) was sufficient to explain the lack of recognition of sound events.

Although diagnosis can point to clinical and electrophysiological data, the concept of cortical deafness still invites controversy. Despite the fact that correlation can occur between clinical and elctrophysiological data, pure clinical cases are rare, recording techniques are diverse, and ALRs are not that well known. Moreover, there may be residual auditory functions (e.g., some understanding of speech under certain conditions) involving related auditory-processing structures (i.e., auditory associative cortices, medial geniculate nucleus of the thalamus) that are not fully understood (Michel et al., 1980). However, cortical deafness should be considered within a differential diagnosis of aphasia, auditory agnosia, and related auditory processing disorders. Its occurrence would be similar to cortical blindness (Anton syndrome) and cortical anesthesia/somatosensory loss.

Auditory Agnosia

An auditory disorder following a brain lesion is usually general or global, in the sense that it applies to all types of auditory events. The typical patient complains of hearing all sounds as unintelligible or as noise. The patients behave as deaf people who retain the ability to speak, read, and write; however, they are not completely deaf because they can usually perceive basic characteristics of the sounds, such as changes in frequency, intensity, and duration. By way of example, a patient studied by Klein and Harper (1956, p. 114) made the following remarks: ". . . I know exactly what I want to say but I don't know whether it is right or wrong. . . . I know I am speaking but I can't hear the words right, not the actual words, I can hear the voice." Such a disorder involves a problem of recognition and identification that cannot be explained by deafness as such nor by a difficulty in verbal expression. This condition is referred to as *auditory agnosia.*

Brain Specialization for Speech

Most early descriptions of auditory agnosia are limited to this general characterization. However, since the 1970s, further subdivisions have been drawn (see Polster & Rose, 1998, for a recent historical review). A major line of division lies between verbal agnosia (involving comprehension of speech) and nonverbal agnosia (involving recognition of sounds other than speech). This differentiation echoes the claim of Liberman and his colleagues (1967) that speech perception involves special mechanisms. They argue that there are essentially two modes of auditory perception. One is dedicated to speech—the phonetic or speech mode; and the other—the auditory mode—is a general-purpose system handling all the nonspeech sounds. Thus, it is suggested that there are two types of dissociable systems depending on whether the information to be processed is speech or nonspeech.

There is much empirical evidence in support of this claim. Table 13-1 shows several reports of agnosia for speech, sparing either music or environmental sounds. Conversely, there are cases of impaired processing for both musical patterns and common environmental sounds (such as animal cries, traffic noises, etc.), with no speech impairment. This set of studies therefore constitutes evidence of a double dissociation between the recognition of speech and nonspeech sounds.

Several models of speech recognition have been proposed. Although there is not as yet a full understanding as to what acoustic units of spoken language are processed, and how (but see Philipps, 1998), all models involve a specialization for the processing of perceptual linguistic units, specific to each language. For example, the perceptual unit would be the stressed syllable in English, the syllable in French, and the mora in Japanese (Otake & Cutler, 1996). Because models of speech recognition have been detailed elsewhere, they will not be described here (McClelland & Elman, 1986; Schouten, 1992).

Brain Specialization for Music

A single system does not, however, govern all nonspeech sounds. Indeed, an overall distinction such as verbal/nonverbal is deemed too coarse to account for the specificity of patients' disorders. Within the nonverbal auditory domain, some specialization exists as well, specifically in the musical domain. We have observed that patients with brain damage who have lost the ability to recognize well-known tunes may retain the

TABLE 13-1. Case Reports of Selective Impairment in the Recognition of Speech Sounds, Music, and Environmental Sounds

Reports	Domain		
	Speech	Music	Environmental sounds
Metz-Lutz & Dahl, 1984	−	+	+
Yaqub et al., 1988	−	+	+
Takahashi et al., 1992	−	+	+
Spreen et al., 1965	+	−	−
Habib et al., 1995	+	−	−
Peretz et al., 1994, CN and GL	+	−	+
Peretz et al., 1997, IR	+	−	+
Griffiths et al., 1997	+	−	+
Piccirilli et al., 2000	+	−	+
Laignel-Lavastine & Alajouanine, 1921	−	+	−
Godefroy et al., 1995*	−	−	+
Mendez, 2001	+	−	−
Tanaka et al., 1987	−	−	+
Eustache et al., 1990, case I	−	−	+
Mendez & Geehan, 1988,* case II	−	−	+
Motomura et al., 1986*	+	+	−

*During recovery.

+ = normal recognition;− = impaired recognition

ability to recognize song lyrics, familiar voices, intonation, animal cries, and other environmental sounds (Dalla Bella & Peretz, 1999, summarize three such cases). Such a selective loss for music has also been observed in other laboratories (Griffiths et al., 1997; Piccirilli et al., 2000). Moreover, a few cases have been described where both speech and environmental sounds are impaired and music is spared (Laignel-Lavastine & Alajouanine, 1921; Godefroy et al., 1995; Mendez, 2001). Therefore, a double dissociation exists between music and other domains, such as speech and environmental sounds.

The idea of brain specialization for music stems not only from these lesion studies but also from converging evidence from alternative approaches and methodologies. For instance, some brain areas seem to respond exclusively to music, as was observed by Penfield and Perot (1963), who found that electrical stimulation of certain cortical areas in patients evoked the auditory experience of hearing songs or tunes. The very existence of musicogenic epilepsy, that is, epilepsy triggered exclusively by music (Wieser et al., 1997; Nakano et al., 1998), or lessened by it (Hughes et al., 1998), renders it very unlikely that these neural circuits would respond to other types of acoustic stimuli.

Furthermore, the observation that musical talent can exist despite very low-level general cognitive functioning, for example, as in autism (Mottron et al., 1999, 2000) and in Williams syndrome (Don et al., 1999), is consistent with the idea that music abilities are dissociable from other general cognitive abilities (Steinke et al, 1997).

Another intriguing phenomenon that suggests that there exists a brain specialization for music is *musical hallucination*. Musical hallucinations are, in a sense, the "opposite of deficits" because they refer to an illusory perception of music in the absence of any external sound source. Musical hallucinations are the " formed, "or complex version, of the more common tinnitus as detailed above.

A typical sufferer of musical hallucinations has been illustrated by Oliver Sacks (1985) in his popular book *The Man Who Mistook His Wife for a Hat*, in the character of Mrs O'C. Mrs O'C is an old lady who has a long history of deafness but who is psychologically sane. She would wake up in the morning hearing loud music from her childhood and would believe that her radio station had been on throughout the night, or that her neighbors were simply being noisy. She would search for a sound source, and eventually realize that the sound was coming from inside her head. If fortunate, she may meet a clinician who will provide a correct diagnosis and will reassure her that she is not insane (Sacks, pp. 125–126).

There are four major etiologies for musical hallucinations, namely, ear pathology, brain disease, psychopathology, and toxic states (Table 13-2). Ear pathology is by far the major cause for musical hallucinations, followed by brain disease. It appears that some degree of sensorineural hearing loss (i.e., involving the inner ear), most often bilateral, is a very prominent clinical characteristic of patients experiencing musical hallucinations (for reviews, see Keshavan et al., 1992; Pasquini & Cole, 1997). This type of hallucination associated with sensory deprivation represents an auditory form of the Charles-Bonnet syndrome, reported in patients with long-standing visual deficits. The profiles of patients for each type of deficit are remarkably similar, suggesting similar mechanisms but in differing modalities. In patients where both auditory and visual deficits occur, both types of hallucinations may be present (Fenelon et al., 2000).

Another major etiology for musical hallucinations is brain disease. This can take several forms, such as focal tumors, brain lesions due to cerebrovascular disease, lobectomies, temporal lobe abnormality (e.g., epilepsy), or even brainstem abnormality and lesions (e.g., Douen & Bourque, 1997). The relationship between lesion site and hallucination type is not clear. The content of hallucinations is of interest to clinicians because they may have important diagnostic implications. However, the fact that hallucinations are not a unitary phenomenon explains why they do not bear a regular relationship with one side of the brain of the other. Several recent cases of hallucinations associated with degenerative brain diseases, and therefore involving the whole cortex (e.g., Parkinson and Alzheimer diseases) have been reported (Bassionny et al., 2000; Fenelon et al., 2000).

Finally, psychopathology and toxic states may also be etiologies for auditory hallucinations. In the reported cases, about one third of the patients suffered from some form of psychopathology, mainly depression, a prevalent problem among the aged. Toxic states such as intoxication by alcohol, or by common medication such as salicylates, benzodiazepines, or propranolol, are also often reported as an etiology. In contrast to other etiologies in these cases, hallucinations usually stop when medication is withdrawn. These etiologies suggest that some chemical mechanisms involving neurotransmitters are potentially active in the onset of hallucinations.

It is generally acknowledged that some combination of peripheral and central factors is required to produce hallucinations. Because hallucinations arise in the elderly where there is both some degree of hearing loss and brain changes (such as diffuse cortical atrophy, plastic changes, etc.), it is almost impossible to exclude one factor or the other in the onset of hallucinations. Given the scarcity of the data on the phenomenon (*bl1% according to the only study that assessed prevalence rate of musical hallucinations; Fukunishi et al., 1998), it is likely that multiple factors are involved.

As is the case for simple tinnitus, we suggest that cortical reorganization is of paramount importance in musical hallucinations, most probably via disinhibition, that is, the unmasking of previously hidden brain connections. Besides tinnitus, cortical plasticity has been shown to be involved in complex phenomena involving "missing" body parts or abilities such as phantom limb pain (Flor et al., 1995) and spatial localization in the blind (Lessard et al., 1998). For instance, if an upper limb is amputated, the cortical area originally corresponding to the hand will be taken over by sensory input from adjacent areas, such as the cortical area responsible for sensation in the face. When a stroke occurs, the facial area creates an additional sensation of pain in the missing limb; the pain in the phantom limb would therefore be the perceptual correlate of this brain reorganization. The cortical representation of the hand is "invaded." In the case of musical hallucinations, because of the hearing loss, some adjacent brain regions would take over the neural networks devoted to music processing, so that musical hallucinations would be the perceptual correlate of brain plasticity. Why music in

Table 13-2. Main Etiologies and General Characteristics of Musical Hallucinations

Etiology	Pathology	General Characteristics
Ear pathology	Deafness (usually bilateral, moderate or severe)	Songs from childhood, carols, popular songs, folk songs, unfamiliar music, vocal and instrumental music, choirs, religious songs, etc.
Brain disease	Cerebrovascular accident, epilepsy, space-occupying tumor	
Psychopathology	Depression, psychosis	
Toxic states	Intoxication by alcohol or medication	

particular may be the privileged perceptual correlate to brain plasticity is still a matter of speculation. More case descriptions of other types of auditory hallucinations, such as verbal hallucinations, best known in relation to schizophrenia, and vocal hallucinations, that is, voices heard without a specific verbal content (i.e., murmurs, whispers, blurred conversations, etc.) are required to cement a clearer picture. This last category of hallucinations has been generally overlooked.

Whatever the exact mechanisms of musical hallucinations are, the important prerequisite is that the music hallucinated has already been stored in memory. Moreover, as for musicogenic epilepsy, it is difficult to imagine that "disinhibited" networks that can produce a highly organized percept such as music of one's childhood would also respond to other forms of auditory sources. In addition, the majority of patients with musical hallucinations have no particular musical training, suggesting that specialization for music exist in the brain of the majority (Peretz, 2000; Peretz & Hébert, 2000). A model of music perception derived from studies of patients with brain damage patients is presented below.

Brain Specialization for Other Types of Auditory Sources

To date there have been no reported cases of patients with selective impairment involving only environmental sounds (i.e., while sparing speech and music), except those cases occurring during recovery (see Table 13-1). The fact that this domain can be selectively spared suggests, however, that environmental sounds may constitute a category distinct from speech and music. Brain damage causing selective impairments in processing of speech, music, and the recognition of environmental sounds strongly suggests at least three distinct systems for auditory recognition. These domain divisions seem to correspond to differences in kind and not in degree. Indeed, if the three domains under consideration were differentially vulnerable to brain damage, while being mediated by a single system, observations of double dissociations should never occur. Only single dissociations should be observed in a constant direction. Moreover, if a single system were involved, recovery of auditory functions should proceed in a consistent order, that is, in the order of increasing difficulty. Yet, two case studies present diametrically opposed sequences of recovery. In the first (Mendez & Geehan, 1988), environmental sounds were recovered first, followed by music and finally speech, whereas, in the second (Motomura et al., 1986), the order was reversed. Yet, both cases were similar because they suffered primarily from perceptual deficits.

There is also another important class of recognizable sounds that is generally neglected: that of human *voices*. Both the existence of phonagnosia (i.e., the inability to recognize human voices; Van Lancker & Canter, 1982) and evidence from recent functional imagery studies (Belin et al., 2000) suggest that voice recognition appears mediated by a further specialized auditory system. Phonagnosia seems to occur without accompanying an auditory speech comprehension disorder (Van Lancker & Kreiman, 1987). However, the reverse condition, that of a speech comprehension deficit with the retention of voice recognition abilities has, to our knowledge, never been reported. The recent discovery of specialized areas in the superior temporal gyri for voices, as measured by functional magnetic resonance imagery (fMRI) in neurologically intact subjects by Belin and collaborators (2000), suggests that selective cases of phonagnosia should be observed.

The most prominent obstacle to the study of voice and common sounds recognition, in both the clinical assessment and research environments, is the lack of theoretical models. To overcome this lack, future studies should aim to develop such models. In summary, the general label of auditory agnosia covers a wide range of deficits involving different types of auditory events. There are at least two types of auditory events, and most probably four (speech, music, environmental sounds, and voices) for which there is known brain specialization. However, the relationships among these domain-specific disorders of auditory recognition remain poorly understood. Yet the selectivity of the cases suggests that recognition of words, music, and other familiar sounds differ in several important ways. Understanding the nature of each type of disorder in such selective cases will serve to delineate at what level of auditory processing each type of auditory stimulus differs from other classes of auditory patterns. What is necessary at this stage is a grid for decomposing the whole system into its relevant components and to compare them across domains. For example, next we present the case of music recognition, for which a high degree of brain specialization exists.

THE MUSIC RECOGNITION SYSTEM: AN OVERVIEW

Recognition of familiar music is immediate and easy for all humans. Despite its apparent effortlessness, music recognition is a complex procedure that requires multiple processing components. At the very least, the perceptual input must be processed along the *melodic dimension* (defined by sequential variations in pitch) and the *temporal dimension* (defined by sequential variations in duration) and then mapped onto a stored long-term representation that represents some of the invariant properties of the musical selection. This outline is shown in Figure 13-2.

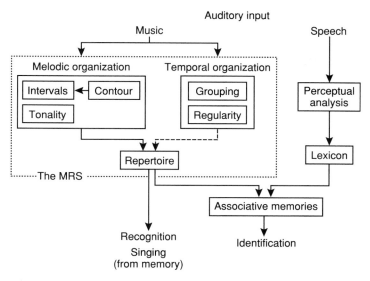

Auditory input

FIGURE 13-2. Functional model of the music recognition system.

—— Primary access
--- Secondary access

Figure 13-2 represents a plausible functional architecture of the music recognition system (MRS), and is based, to a large degree, on studies with brain-damaged patients (Peretz, 2000, offers a more detailed account). The musical input is analyzed by two parallel and largely independent subsystems whose functions are to specify, respectively, the melodic content, that is, representing the melodic contour and the tonal functions of the successive pitches, and the temporal content, that is, representing the metrical organization as well as the grouping of the successive durations. To simplify, the melodic route represents the *what* and the temporal route represents *when* events occur in the auditory musical input. Both routes, defining the musical analysis components, send their respective outputs—or perhaps a combination of the two—to the *repertoire*. The *repertoire* is conceived as a perceptual representation system, available to all listeners, which contains all the representations of the specific musical pieces to which one has been exposed during one's lifetime. In turn, the repertoire output can activate stored representations in other systems, such as the lexicon for the retrieval of the accompanying lyrics, if any, or the associative memories for retrieving and pronouncing the title (i.e., identification) of the musical excerpt and for retrieval of all sorts of nonmusical information (such as an episode related to the first hearing of the music concerned). Naming a musical excerpt via associative memories is, however, not necessary for recognition. Successful activation (or selection) of one particular musical candidate in the *repertoire* will evoke a sense of familiarity and, hence, lead to recognition.

The Melodic Dimension

As posited in Figure 13-2, the musical input is conceived as undergoing transformations along two parallel perceptual routes: the melodic and temporal routes. This is a controversial issue in the literature on neurologically intact listeners, in that some authors (e.g., Jones, 1987; Bigand, 1997) argue that melody and rhythm are not perceptually independent, but rather treated along a unified dimension.

However, the neuropsychological evidence is rather consistent in showing a separation of these two organization principles in the music domain. We have documented dissociation between melodic and temporal processing several times in various experimental settings. The task usually involves a "same-different" classification of successive musical sequences. In the melodic conditions, the comparison stimuli are altered by changing the pitch structure but retaining the original temporal structure. In the rhythmic conditions, the stimuli are the same, but this time, the temporal structure is modified in the comparison sequence and the pitch structure is left constant. A comparison of results obtained with unilaterally brain-damaged patients with those of neurologically healthy subjects (matched in terms of age and education) reveals dissociations that are very robust. Some patients score well below the normal range (established by control subjects) in the deficient dimension, but within the normal range in the unaffected dimension. In each study, involving different populations of brain-damaged patients (Peretz, 1990; Liégeois-Chauvel et al., 1998; Ayotte et al., 2000; Piccirilli et al., 2000), there were patients who could no longer discriminate the musical stimuli when the discrimination cue was melodic and who performed normally when the distinguishing cue was rhythmic, and vice versa. In a further case, CN (Peretz & Kolinsky, 1993), we were able to show that such a dissociation between melody and rhythm could be still observed in situations that promote integration of the melodic and rhythmic dimensions in an intact brain. A Stroop-like situation was created with sequences varying in both melody and rhythm, while maintaining the "same-different" classification requirements. Subjects (CN and her matched controls) were asked to pay selective attention to rhythm despite any potential changes in melody. Control subjects failed to ignore the irrelevant melodic variations, thus showing Stroop interference effects (with an average performance of 67%). CN did not (with an average performance of 83%). For her, melody and rhythm were entirely separable. Thus, brain damage can produce a selective loss for either melody or rhythm. The evidence strongly supports the claim that these two dimensions involve the operation of separable perceptual subsystems (for melodic/rhythm dissociations in other modalities see also Mann, 1898, and Josmann, 1926, reported in Dorgeuille, 1966; Brust, 1980; Mavlov, 1980).

Recognition of a single melodic line relies on essentially three kinds of features: contour, intervals, and scale degree. Pitch directions contribute to the *contour* of the melody. Pitch distance between consecutive notes defines the melodic *intervals*. The exact pitch level is not important for music recognition. A familiar tune can be easily recognized whether sung by a man or a woman, for example. Contour, however, plays a crucial role in melodic discrimination, whereas intervals provide critical information as well. Intervals typically evoke a particular *scale*, which refers to a particular subset of pitch intervals. These intervals, or scale degrees, confer in turn a particular structure to the melodic line. In our Western musical system, this structure reflects a set of tonal constraints by which each tone receives a varying degree of stability. For instance, a tonal piece usually begins and ends on the most stable pitch (called the tonic or the first degree). The second in order of importance is the fifth degree and often replaces the tonic. The contribution of contour, intervals, and scale to melodic perception has been relatively well documented in both neurologically intact subjects and in brain-damaged patients. In brain-damaged patients, a lesion in the left hemisphere was found to spare the ability of representing melodies in terms of their contour but to interfere with an interval-based procedure, whereas a lesion in the right hemisphere was found to disrupt both procedures (Peretz, 1990; Liégeois-Chauvel et al., 1998; Ayotte et al., 2000).

The tonal encoding of pitch is presumably mediated by several cognitive operations. Because these operations have not yet been distinguished, they are grouped in a single component in Figure 13-2 under the term "tonality." There is substantial empirical evidence that listeners use these tonal regularities in perception, albeit in an implicit manner (Tillmann et al., 2000). Tonal encoding of pitch can also be selectively impaired by brain damage (Peretz, 1993).

The Temporal Dimension

Two types of temporal organization appear fundamental to the perception of musical "rhythm": the segmentation of an ongoing sequence into temporal groups of events on the basis of their durational values and the extraction of an underlying temporal regularity or beat. The first type of temporal organization corresponds to the tendency to group events according to temporal proximity, without regard to periodicity. The second type of fundamental temporal organization is regularity and refers to the tendency to perceive events that occur at regular intervals in time, in the form of an underlying beat. Beat perception leads to the perception of a metrical organization corresponding to periodic alternation between strong and weak beats (the strong beats generally correspond to the spontaneous tapping of the foot). In Western music, metrical patterns contain either binary or ternary beats, by inducing a major accent on the first beat of two or three beats (as in a waltz: ONE, two, three, ONE, two, three,...).

Temporal grouping and metric interpretation of music have rarely been distinguished in neuropsychological studies. The three studies that have addressed this question (not intentionally in all cases) have showed neuropsychological dissociations, thus validating the independence view. For example, Ibbotson and Morton (1981) were the first to show that subjects tapped a rhythmic pattern far more easily with their right hand and the beat with their left hand, than the other way around. These findings suggest that the beat is better handled by the right hemisphere, whereas grouping would rely essentially on the left hemisphere. Such hemispheric separation for the two types of organization mediating temporal pattern processing is consistent with the claim that these two aspects are mediated by distinct mechanisms. Further support has been provided by the study of a patient with a right-hemispheric lesion (but in a left-hander) who could no longer tap the beat but who was still able to reproduce temporal patterns (Fries & Swihart, 1990). In both studies, however, it can be argued that the outcome is more related to the programming and coordination of fine motor skills than to temporal processing per se. Nevertheless, in our studies in which more perceptual aspects of temporal processing were assessed, convergent evidence for dissociating meter from grouping was also found (Peretz, 1990; Liégeois-Chauvel et al., 1998; Sakai et al., 1999).

Access to the Repertoire

Melodic cues play a prominent role in accessing the music representations within the repertoire. This hypothesis comes from our neuropsychological investigations of CN and GL (Peretz et al., 1994). Both patients were no longer able to recognize highly familiar music such as "Happy Birthday." Yet, neither CN nor GL had any impairment in discriminating and retaining rhythmic patterns. In theory, both patients could have used rhythm as a basis to recognize music. The fact that they did not raises the possibility that the melodic route, which was disrupted in both patients, is the most diagnostic of music identity. In support of this idea is the reputable study of White (1960), who found that neurologically intact listeners correctly identified 88% of familiar melodic lines of which temporal variations were removed, whereas they were only 33% correct when presented with the rhythmic pattern deprived from its pitch variations. We have replicated and extended this result with unanticipated musical excerpts in university students (Hébert & Peretz, 1997). In the first experiment, we used both identification (i.e., title identification) and familiarity ratings as response measures. Subjects were found to be able to name only 1 of 25 excerpts from their rhythmic patterns, whereas the subjects successfully identified half of the excerpts from hearing the melodic variations alone. The same pattern of results emerged on the familiarity ratings and in subsequent experiments. Altogether the results consistently showed that the melodic pattern is more diagnostic for music identification than the rhythmic pattern and that this advantage is basically perceptual.

The implication of this finding is that patients, like CN and GL, who are impaired along the melodic route should systematically experience difficulties in recognizing familiar music. These patients would thus be music agnosic because of a perceptual defect. In contrast, patients who are selectively impaired along the temporal route should not be agnosic, unless their repertoire is damaged as well. These predictions remain to be verified.

Songs

The idea that music and speech are intrinsically related through song challenges the existence of a brain specialization for music. However, substantial evidence now indicates that, in songs, melody and text are perceptually separable. Neurologically intact listeners can monitor opera excerpts for incongruities in speech and in music independently and, in doing so, elicit distinctive brain potentials (Besson et al., 1998). When presented with sung digits, musicians engage opposite cerebral hemispheres for the recall of the pitch patterns and of the digits (Goodglass & Calderon, 1977).

Finally, brain-damaged patients can recognize lyrics normally while failing to recognize the melody (Peretz et al., 1994) even when lyrics and melody are sung together in their original pairing or in a false pairing (Hébert & Peretz, 2001). Melody and text that are integrated in songs appear nevertheless separable for the brain.

There is, however, a paradox. It has been repeatedly shown that, in a memory recognition task, neurologically intact listeners behave as though they cannot access the melody without having access to the text of the studied song. The task consists of a forced-choice memory task in which subjects are required to recognize the tune, the lyrics, or both, of *novel songs* that they had previously heard; among the alternatives are excerpts in which the tune of one song and the lyrics of another song are combined (mismatch songs). The integration effects are revealed by the systematic superiority of recognition scores for match songs over mismatch songs. This recurrent finding, which is taken as evidence for lyrics and tune integration in song memory, has been documented in adults (Crowder et al., 1990; Serafine et al., 1984, 1986), in preschool children (Morrongiello & Roes, 1990), and in patients with epilepsy after unilateral temporal lobe resections (Samson & Zatorre, 1991). However, all these studies were derived from the use of the same paradigm that does not allow us to distinguish between an integrated stored representation, where the musical and the linguistic component would be represented in some combined or common code, from an associative organization, where the musical and linguistic components would be represented as distinct entities related by associative links (but see Crowder et al., 1990, Experiment 3, for providing support to the latter option). Thus, there is a particular need here for both diversity in experimental tasks and systematic neuropsychological investigations before we can draw any firm conclusions about the relation between music and language in song memory.

Similarly, singing performance should be more systematically explored. For example, it is known that subjects with nonfluent aphasia can sing words that they cannot pronounce (as initially reported by Broca, 1861). However, the significance of this behavior to the relation of melody and text representation is not yet clear because studies of aphasic singing have been anecdotal (e.g., Yamadori et al., 1977). We (Gagnon et al., 1998; Hébert et al., 2001) have documented the case of an aphasic patient who had great difficulties in spontaneous speech but whose singing performance was not different from his spoken performance (in terms of number of words correctly pronounced). Further studies are needed to provide convergent evidence.

Therefore, in the current state of knowledge, strong evidence suggests that music and speech are treated independently up to the repertoire and the phonological input lexicon. This position may, however, be too extreme because, as we have seen here, some processing components may be shared by music and speech.

CONCLUSION

We have overviewed functional auditory deficits that can result from damage at several levels of the auditory system, from the periphery up to the most central levels. A particularly important aspect underlined in this overview is that an assessment of auditory functions demands the involvement of several disciplines of audition, such as otology, neurology, and neuropsychology, to provide a thorough understanding of the deficits.

Acknowledgments

This chapter was prepared thanks to the financial support and grant from Fonds de la recherche en santé du Québec to S.H., and to a grant from Canadian Institute of Health Research of Canada to I.P.

KEY POINTS

☐   Peripheral audition, is, basically, damage to the inner ear and central auditory structures that leads to significant hearing loss or distortions in sound perception. These include sensorineural hearing loss, loudness recruitment, tinnitus, difficulty in sound localization, difficulty in detecting a signal in background noise, and so forth.

☐   Central audition is concerned by the allocation of the correct attributes to the incoming sound sources that arrive at the eardrum under the form of a complex, but unique, vibratory pattern. Central audition involves higher subcortical and cortical structures and plays a key role in disentangling elements belonging to various sound sources in order that they may be correctly identified and localized in space.

☐   Auditory agnosia is a general term that designates a deficit in recognizing auditory events after brain damage and that cannot be explained by deafness or by a difficulty of verbal expression. Auditory agnosia may selectively impair the domains of language (aphasia), or music (amusia). It is also likely that patients with selective disorders in perception and recognition of environmental sounds (no specific term has been as yet coined, but we would suggest the term "ecoagnosia," in which eco stands for habitat, environment), and human voice (phonagnosia) will be reported in the future. All these selective deficits may be decomposed in fine-grained impairments of subcomponents.

☐   In the music recognition system, the musical perceptual input must be at the very least processed along the melodic and the temporal dimensions. A melodic line is decomposable in key features, that is, contour, intervals, and tonality. The temporal dimension is decomposable in meter and grouping. There is also evidence that in songs, music and speech are treated independently up to the repertoire, which contains all the representations of musical (experiences) to which one has been exposed.

☐   Auditory phantom phenomena appear following damage to some auditory structures. They are different from other deficits, in that they refer to an illusory auditory perception in the absence of any external sound source. Depending on the brain structure involved, auditory phantom phenomena may be simple (e.g., tinnitus, a buzzing or ringing in the ear) or complex (e.g., musical or voice hallucinations), and they can exist without any other psychiatric disease.

KEY READINGS

Moore BCJ: Perceptual Consequences of Cochlear Damage. Oxford, England: Oxford Medical Publications, 1995.

Caplan D: Language: Structure, Processing, and Disorders. Cambridge, MA: MIT Press, 1992.

Zatorre RJ, Binder JR: (2000). Functional and structural imaging of the human auditory system, in Toga AW, Mazziotta JC (eds): Brain Mapping: The Systems. San Diego, CA: Academic Press, 2000, pp. 365–402.

REFERENCES

Ayotte J, Peretz I, Rousseau I, et al: Patterns of music agnosia associated with middle cerebral artery infarcts. Brain 123:1926–1938, 2000.

Bassionny MM, Steinberg MS, Warren A, et al: Delusions and hallucinations in Alzheimer's disease: Prevalence and clinical correlates. Int J Geriatr Psychiatry 15:99–107, 2000.

Belin P, Zatorre R, Lafaille P, et al: Voice-selective areas in human auditory cortex. Nature 403:309–331, 2000.

Besson M, Faïta F, Peretz I, et al: Singing in the brain: Independence of lyrics and tunes. Psychol Sci 9:494–498, 1998.

Bigand E: Perceiving musical stability: The effects of tonal structure, rhythm, and musical expertise. J Exp Psychol Hum Percept Perform 23:808–822, 1997.

Bregman AS: Auditory Scene Analysis: The Perceptual Analysis of Sound. Cambridge, MA: MIT Press, 1990.

Broca P: Remarques sur le siège de la faculté du langage articulé, suivies d'une observation d'aphémie. Bull Soc Anat Paris 36:330–357, 1861.

Brust J: Music and language: Musical alexia and agraphia. Brain 103:367–392, 1980.

Crowder R, Serafine ML, Repp B: Physical interaction and association by contiguity in memory for the words and melodies of songs. Mem Cognit 18:469–476, 1990.

Dalla Bella S, Peretz I: Music agnosias: Selective impairments of music recognition after brain damage. J New Music Res 28:209–216, 1999.

Davis A, Rafaie EA: Epidemiology of tinnitus, in Tyler R (ed): Tinnitus Handbook. San Diego, CA: Singular Publishing Group, 2000, pp. 1–23.

Don AJ, Schellenberg EG, Rourke BP: Music and language skills of children with Williams syndrome. Child Neuropsychol 5:154–170, 1999.

Dorgeuille C: Introduction à l'étude des amusies. Unpublished doctoral dissertation. Paris, 1966.

Douen AG, Bourque PR: Musical auditory hallucinosis from listeria rhombencephalitis. Can J Neurol Sci 24:70–72, 1997.

Eustache F, Lechevalier B, Viader F, Lambert J: Identification and discrimination disorders in auditory perception: A report of two cases. Neuropsychologia 28:257–270, 1990.

Fenelon G, Mahieux F, Huon R, Ziegler M: Hallucinations in Parkinson's disease: Prevalence, phenomenology and risk factors. Brain 123:733–745, 2000.

Flor H, Elbert T, Knecht S, et al: Phantom-limb pain as a perceptual correlate of cortical reorganization following arm amputation. Nature 375:482–484, 1995.

Fries W, Swihart A: Disturbance of rhythm sense following right hemisphere damage. Neuropsychologia 28:1317–1323, 1990.

Fukunishi I, Horikawa N, Onai H: Prevalence rate of musical hallucinations in a general hospital setting. Psychosomatics 39:175, 1998.{AU: Please add inclusive page number.}

Gagnon L, Macoir J, Peretz I:. Indépendance de la production du langage et de la musique: étude d'un cas d'aphasie primaire progressive. VIe Congrès International Francophone de Gérontologie. Palexpo, Genève, Switzerland, 1998.

Godefroy O, Leys D, Furby A, et al: Psychoacoustical deficits related to bilateral subcortical hemorrhages. A case with apperceptive auditory agnosia. Cortex 31:149–159, 1995.

Goodglass H, Calderon M: Parallel processing of verbal and musical stimuli in right and left hemisphere. Neuropsychologia 15:397–407, 1977.

Griffiths T, Rees A, Witton C, et al: Spatial and temporal auditory processing deficits following right hemisphere infarction: A psychophysical study. Brain 120:785–794, 1997.

Habib M, Daquin G, Milandre L, et al: Mutism and auditory agnosia due to bilateral insular damage—role of the insula in human communication. Neuropsychologia 33:327–339, 1995.

Hébert S, Peretz I: Recognition of music in long term memory: Are melodic and temporal patterns equal partners? Mem Cognit 25:518–533, 1997.

Hébert S, Peretz I. Are text and tune of familiar songs separable by brain damage? Brain Cognit 46:169–175, 2001.

Hébert S, Racette A, Gagnon L, et al: Production of speech and songs in aphasic patients: A case study. Paper submitted for publication.

Hughes JR, Daaboul Y, Fino JJ, et al: The "Mozart effect" on epileptiform activity. Clin Electroencephalogr 29:109–119, 1998.

Ibbotson N, Morton J: Rhythm and dominance. Cognition 9:125–138, 1981.

Jones MR: Dynamic pattern structure in music: Recent theory and research. Percept Psychophys 41:621–634, 1987.

Keshavan MS, David AS, Steingard S, et al: Musical hallucinations: A review and synthesis. Neuropsychiatry Neuropsychol Behav Neurol 5:211–223, 1992.

Klein R, Harper J: The problem of agnosia in the light of a case of pure word deafness. J Ment Sci 102:112–120, 1956.

Laignel-Lavastine M, Alajouanine T: Un cas d'agnosie auditive. Rev Neurol 37:194–198, 1921.

Lessard N, Pare M, Lepore F, et al: Early-blind human subjects localize sound sources better than sighted subjects. Nature 395:278–280, 1998.

Liberman A, Cooper F, Shankweiler D, et al: Perception of the speech code. Psychol Rev 74:431–461, 1967.

Liégeois-Chauvel C, Peretz I, Babaï M, et al: Contribution of different cortical areas in the temporal lobes to music processing. Brain 121:1853–1867, 1998.

Mann V, Liberman P: Some differences between phonetic and auditory modes of perception. Cognition 14:211–235, 1983.

Mavlov L: Amusia due to rhythm agnosia in a musician with left hemisphere damage: A non auditory supramodal defect. Cortex 16:321–338, 1980.

McClelland JL, Elman J: The trace model of speech perception. Cogn Psychol 18:1–86, 1986.

Mendez MF: Generalized auditory agnosia with spared music recognition in a left-hander. Analysis of a case with a right temporal stroke. Cortex 37:139–150, 2001.

Mendez MF, Geehan GR: Cortical auditory disorders: Clinical and psychoacoustic features. J Neurol Neurosurg Psychiatry 51:1–9, 1988.

Metz-Lutz MN, Dahl E: Analysis of word comprehension in a case of pure word-deafness. Brain Lang 23:13–25, 1984.

Moore BCJ: Perceptual Consequences of Cochlear Damage. New York: Oxford University Press, 1995.

Morrongiello B, Roes C: Children's memory for new songs: Integration or independent storage of words and tunes? J Exp Child Psychol 50:25–38, 1990.

Motomura N, Yamadori A, Mori E, et al: Auditory agnosia: Analysis of a case with bilateral subcortical lesions. Brain 109:379–391, 1986.

Mottron L, Peretz I, Belleville S, et al: Absolute pitch in autism: A case study. Neurocase 3:485–501, 1999.

Mottron L, Peretz I, Ménard E: Local and global processing of music in high-functioning persons with autism: Beyond cerebral coherence? J Child Psychol Psychiatry 41:1057–1065, 2000.

Mühnickel W, Elbert T, Taub E, et al: Reorganization of auditory cortex in tinnitus. Proc Natl Acad Sci U S A 95:10340–10343, 1998.

Musiek FE, Baran JA, Pinheiro ML (eds): Neuroaudiology: Case Studies. San Diego, CA: Singular, 1994.

Nakano M, Takase Y, Tatsumi C: A case of musicogenic epilepsy induced by listening to an American pop music. Clin Neurol 38:1067–1069, 1998.

Otake T, Cutler A (eds): Phonological Structure and Language Processing: Cross-Linguistic Studies. van Heuve VJ, Pols LCW (General Series Editors), Speech Research 12. New York: Mouton de Gruyter, 1996.

Pasquini F, Cole MG: Idiopathic musical hallucinations in the elderly. J Geriatr Psychiatry Neurol 10:11–14, 1997.

Penfield W, Perot P: The brain's record of auditory and visual experience. Brain 94:595–694, 1963.

Peretz I: Processing of local and global musical information in unilateral brain damaged patients. Brain 113:1185–1205, 1990.

Peretz I: Auditory atonalia for melodies. Cogn Neuropsychol 10:21–56, 1993.

Peretz I: Music perception and recognition, in Rapp B (ed): The Handbook of Cognitive Neuropsychology: What Deficits Reveal About the Human Mind. Philadelphia, PA: Taylor & Francis, 2000, pp. 519–542.

Peretz I, Belleville S, Fontaine FS: Dissociations entre musique et langage après atteinte cérébrale: un nouveau cas d'amusie sans aphasie. Rev Can Psychol Exp 51:354–367, 1997.

Peretz I, Hébert S: Toward a biological account of musical experience. Brain Cognit 42:131–134, 2000.

Peretz I, Kolinsky R: Boundaries of separability between melody and rhythm in music discrimination: A neuropsychological perspective. Q J Exp Psychol 46A:301–325, 1993.

Peretz I, Kolinsky R, Tramo M, et al: Functional dissociations following bilateral lesions of auditory cortex. Brain 117:1283–1301, 1994.

Philipps DP: Sensory representations, the auditory cortex, and speech perception. Semin Hearing 19:319–332, 1998.

Piccirilli M, Sciarma T, Luzzi S: Modularity of music: Evidence from a case of pure amusia. J Neurol Neurosurg Psychiatry 69:541–545, 2000.

Polster M, Rose S: Disorders of auditory processing: Evidence for modularity in audition. Cortex 34:47–65, 1998.

Popper AN, Fay RR (eds): The Mammalian Auditory Pathway: Neurophysiology. New York: Springer-Verlag, 1991.

Sacks O: The Man Who Mistook His Wife for a Hat. London: Duckworth, 1985.

Sakai K, Hikosaka O, Miyauchi S, et al: Neural representation of a rhythm depends on its interval ratio. J Neurosci 19:10074–10081, 1999.

Samson S, Zatorre RJ: Recognition for text and melody of songs after unilateral temporal lobe lesion: Evidence for dual encoding. J Exp Psychol Learn Mem Cogn 17:793–804, 1991.

Schouten M (ed): The Auditory Processing of Speech: From Sounds to Words. Berlin: Mouton de Gruyter, 1992.

Serafine ML, Crowder RG, Repp B: Integration of melody and text in memory for song. Cognition 16:285–303, 1984.

Serafine ML, Davidson J, Crowder RG, et al: On the nature of melody-text integration in memory for songs. J Mem Lang 25:123–135, 1986.

Shallice T: From Neuropsychology to Mental Structure. Cambridge: Cambridge University Press, 1988.

Spreen O, Benton A, Fincham R: Auditory agnosia without aphasia. Arch Neurol 13:84–92, 1965.

Steinke W, Cuddy L, Holden R: Dissociation of musical tonality and pitch memory from nonmusical cognitive abilities. Can J Exp Psychol 51:316–335, 1997.

Takahashi N, Kawamura M, Shinotou H, et al: Pure word deafness following bilateral lesions. A psychophysical analysis. Brain 110:381–403, 1992.

Tanaka Y, Yamadori A, Mori E: Pure word deafness following bilateral lesions. A psychophysical analysis. Brain 110:381–403, 1987.

Teuber H: Psychophysiological psychology. Annu Rev Psychol 9:267–296, 1955.

Tillmann B, Bharucha JJ, Bigand E: Implicit learning of tonality: A self-organizing approach. Psychol Rev 107:885–913, 2000.

Van Lancker D, Canter D: Impairments of voice and face recognition in patients with hemispheric damage. Brain Cogn 1:185–192, 1982.

Van Lancker D, Kreiman J: Voice discrimination and recognition are separate abilities. Neuropsychologia 25 829–834, 1987.

Wernicke C: The symptom complex of aphasia. Boston Studies in the Philosophy of Sciences 4:34–97, 1874.

White B: Recognition of distorted melodies. Am J Psychology 73:100–107, 1960.

Wieser HG, Hungerbuhler H, Siegel AM, et al: Musicogenic epilepsy: Review of the literature and case report with ictal single photon emission computed tomography. Epilepsia 38:200–207, 1997.

Yamadori A, Osumi Y, Masuhara S, et al: Preservation of singing in Broca's aphasia. J Neurol Neurosurg Psychiatry 40:221–224, 1977.

Yaqub BA, Gascon GG, Al-Nosha M, et al: Pure word deafness (acquired verbal auditory agnosia) in an Arabic speaking patient. Brain 111:457–466, 1988.

Yost WA: Fundamentals of Hearing: An Introduction. San Diego, CA: Academic Press, 2000.

Somatosensory System

Mehrdad Razavi

Somatosensory processing

Astereognosis

Tactile agnosia

Tactile anomia

Tactile apraxia

Tactile hallucinations

Tactile neglect

INTRODUCTION

To perceive how the world impinges on the body and to read the body's own internal state, the brain processes streams of information from receptor organs located in the skin, limbs, joints, and viscera. Information from this somatosensory system must be integrated with other sensory, motor, and cognitive system functions to generate actions for human survival. This chapter reviews the functional organization of the somatosensory system and the behavioral disorders associated with its dysfunction and provides examples of how this knowledge can be used to plan effective treatment for patients with somatosensory disorders.

SOMATOSENSORY SYSTEM: CODING, ORGANIZATION, AND PATHWAYS

The study of the relationship between the somatosensory stimuli and conscious experience began in the 19th century with the pioneering work in sensory psychophysics of Weber (1846) and Fechner (1860), who emphasized that all sensory systems convey information on stimulus modality, location, timing, and intensity (Gescheider, 1997).

Along with Helmholz and von Frey, they developed experiments to compare how stimuli of different intensities are distinguished. We easily perceive that 1 kg is different from 2 kg; why is it difficult to distinguish 50 kg from 51 kg? Weber demonstrated that the ability to detect a difference between a target and reference stimulus depends on the difference in strength of the two stimuli divided by the strength of the reference stimulus. Fechner (1860) discovered that the intensity of (stimulus) perception depends on the logarithm of the ratio: the strength of the target stimulus/strength of the stimulus that can be detected at threshold. Stevens (1953) later noted that this intensity is better described by a power function, rather than a logarithmic function. This logarithmic relationship between somatosensory stimuli and conscious experience may have implications for treatment strategies for behavioral disorders of the somatosensory system.

The four major modalities in the somatosensory system are: (1) discriminative touch (the sense of texture and shape of objects and their movement across the skin); (2) proprioception (the sense of static position and movement of the limbs and body); (3) nociception (the signaling of tissue damage or chemical irritation, typically perceived as pain or itch); and (4) temperature sense (warmth and cold).

Each modality is mediated by a distinct system of peripheral and central pathways to the brain (Parent, 1996; Afifi & Bergmann, 1998; Kandel et al., 2000), reminiscent of the parallel pathways identified in vision and audition (see Chapters 12 and 13). This chapter focuses on touch and proprioception. Pain and temperature sensation are reviewed in Chapter 33.

Peripheral Somatosensory System and Pathways to Cortex

The peripheral somatosensory system consists of receptors and dorsal root ganglion neurons. Receptors are the distal terminals of the peripheral branches of dorsal root ganglion neurons. Morphologic and molecular spe-

cializations determine receptor sensory function modality (Table 14-1; Fig. 14-1; Johnson et al., 2000; Kandel et al., 2000; Johnson, 2001).

Information from sensory receptors is conveyed by dorsal root ganglion neurons. The neuron cell body lies in a ganglion on the dorsal root of a spinal nerve. The axon has two branches. The terminals of the peripheral branch meet the receptors, and the central branch transmits the encoded stimulus information to the central pathways.

The sensory specialization of the receptors and the dorsal root ganglion neurons is preserved in the central nervous system (CNS) through distinct pathways for the various somatosensory modalities. These pathways ascend through the spinal cord, brainstem, and thalamus to reach the somatosensory cortices (Fig. 14-1) as follows (Parent, 1996; Afifi & Bergmann, 1998; Kandel et al., 2000):

- Axons of dorsal root ganglion neurons for discriminative touch and proprioception travel in the spinal cord ipsilaterally as the posterior or dorsal column, decussate in the tegmentum of the medulla oblongata, and then ascend as the medial lemniscus to synapse in the neurons of the contralateral ventral posterolateral nucleus (VPL) of the thalamus.
- Axons of dorsal root neurons for conveying information on pain and temperature decussate in the spinal cord and travel as the anterolateral spinothalamic tract to synapse in the neurons of contralateral VPL of the thalamus.
- The trigeminal pathway mediates all four somatosensory modalities (touch, proprioception, pain, and temperature) of sensation for the face. The peripheral pathway includes ophthalmic, maxillary, and mandibular branches of the trigeminal nerve, whose neurons are located in the gasserian ganglion. The central processes of these unipolar neurons of the gasserian ganglion enter the lateral aspect of the pons and ascend to synapse in the neurons of the contralateral ventral posteromedial nucleus (VPM) of the thalamus.
- Axons of neurons in the contralateral VPM and VPL project on the terminal station of all these pathways in the primary somatosensory cortex (also called S-I) of the contralateral parietal lobe.

Primary Somatosensory Cortex

Maps of the body are created in the CNS by the topographic arrangement of afferent inputs from dorsal root

TABLE 14-1. Somatosensory Receptors

Receptor type	Location	Terminology	Function
Mechanoreceptors	Superficial skin	Merkel disk	Slowly adapting receptors that signal the texture and shape of objects
		Meissner corpuscle	Rapidly adapting receptors that signal the motion of objects on the skin
	Deep skin	Ruffini ending	Same as Merkel disk receptor; also signal skin stretch and motion direction
		Pacinian corpuscle	Same as Meissner corpuscle; also signal vibration
Proprioceptors	Muscle	Muscle spindle	Signal changes in muscle length
	Muscle/tendon junction	Golgi tendon organs	Signal changes in muscle tension
	Joint	Joint capsule	Signal flexion or extension of the joint and provide information about joint movements
Pain and temperature receptors	Superficial skin	Pain receptors	Signal pain or temperature

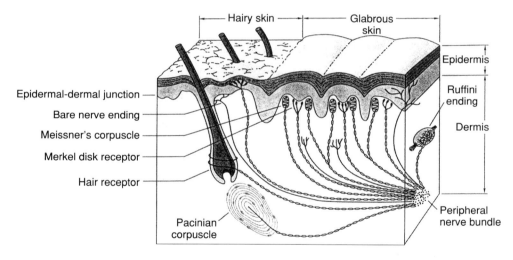

FIGURE 14-1. The location and morphology of mechanoreceptors in the skin of the human hand. The mechanoreceptors are located in the superficial skin, at the junction of the dermis and epidermis, and more deeply in the dermis and subcutaneous tissue. The structure of the receptor organ determines its physiologic function. (From Gardner EP, Martin JH, Jessel TM: The bodily senses, in Kandel ER, Schwartz JH, Jessel TM [eds]: Principles of Neural Science, ed 4. New York: McGraw-Hill, 2000, p. 433.)

ganglion cells. This somatotopic organization of axons relaying sensory input from the receptors in the skin and joints is maintained throughout the entire ascending somatosensory pathway. The contralateral half of the body is represented in a precise but disproportionate manner as a sensory homunculus in the S-I (Fig. 14-2; Penfield & Jasper, 1954). The pharynx, tongue, and jaw are represented in the most ventral portion of the lateral S-I, followed in ascending order by the face, hand, arm, trunk, and thigh. The leg and foot are represented on the medial surface of the cerebral hemisphere. The anal and genital regions (see Chapter 32) are represented in the most ventral portion of the medial surface just above the cingulate gyrus. The face and tongue are represented bilaterally; the representation of the face, lips, hand, thumb, and index fingers is disproportionately large in comparison with their relative size in the body. This disproportionate representation of the body surface in the S-I is thought to reflect the density of the peripheral innervation. Those regions of the body with higher densities of somatosensory receptors have more extensive cortical representations, whereas those

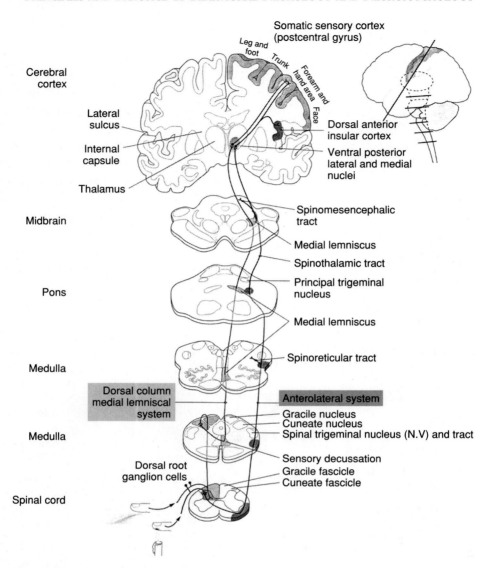

FIGURE 14-2. Distinct pathways mediate different somatosensory modalities from periphery to the somatosensory cortices. The dorsal (or posterior) column mediates touch and proprioception, whereas the anterolateral spinothalamic tract mediates pain and temperature. (From Gardner EP, Martin JH, Jessel TM: The bodily senses, in Kandel ER, Schwartz JH, Jessel TM [eds]: Principles of Neural Science, ed. 4. New York: McGraw-Hill, 2000, p. 447.)

regions with relatively few receptors have less extensive representation. This reflects the functional importance of these parts in somatosensory function (and recalls the cortical magnification factor in the visual system, whereby the central 10 degrees of vision subtends about half the volume of primary visual cortex).

The S-I is located in the postcentral gyrus of the parietal lobe (areas 1, 2, and 3 of Brodmann) and the posterior part of the paracentral lobule (Figs. 14-3 and 14-4; Penfield & Jasper, 1954; Geyer et al., 1999, 2001). Area 3 is divided into two parts, 3a in the depths (fundus) of the central sulcus and 3b on the posterior wall of the central sulcus. Areas 1 and 2 form, respectively, the crown and posterior (caudal) wall of the postcentral gyrus. The afferents to these areas convey touch, position, vibration, pain, and temperature. Each area has its own homunculus-like organization based on projections from different populations of thalamic neurons. As a result, each area is responsible for a different aspect of somatosensory perception and function (Fig. 14-5; Mima et al., 1997; Moore et al., 2000; Bodegård et al., 2000; 2001; Geyer et al., 2001), as follows:

- Area 3b receives input from cutaneous receptors.
- Area 3a receives input from muscle stretch receptors.
- Area 2 receives input from both cutaneous and deep receptors.

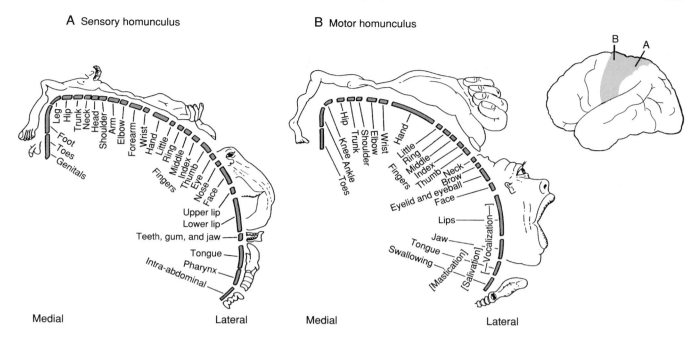

FIGURE 14-3. The entire body surface is represented in the primary somatosensory cortex (S-I) as a homunculus. The area of cortex dedicated to a particular part of the body is not proportional to the size of the body part but, instead, reflects the degree of innervation, and therefore the functional importance of that part. (From Amaral DG: The functional organization of perception and movement, in Kandel ER, Schwartz JH, Jessel TM [eds]: Principles of Neural Science, ed 4. New York: McGraw-Hill, 2000, p. 344.)

- Neurons in areas 3b and 1 predominantly mediate the sense of touch.
- Neurons in area 3a predominantly mediate the sense of position.
- Neurons in area 2 mediate both touch and position sense.

Area 3b has neurons with small receptive fields and therefore contains the greatest spatial fidelity, whereas neurons in areas 1 and 2 have large receptive fields (Geyer et al., 2001). Although area 3b contains some neurons that respond to different tactile submodalities, these occur in increasing numbers in area 1 and beyond, suggesting progressively increasing degrees of abstraction as the neuronal activity moves away from area 3b to areas 1 and 2 (see Fig. 14-4; Mima et al., 1997; Bodegård et al., 2000; Geyer et al., 2001).

Different material features are processed in parallel pathways in S-I (Fig. 14-6; see also Fig. 14-5; Roland et al., 1998; Saetti et al., 1999; Moore et al., 2000; Bodegård et al., 2000, 2001; Geyer et al., 2001). Area 3b projects to both areas 1 and 2. The projection to area 1 is concerned primarily with texture (roughness, softness) perception (a.k.a. hylognosis), whereas the projection to area 2 is concerned with shape (size, length, geometry) perception (aka morphognosis). Both these systems contribute to stereognosis (tactile perception of shape and texture of objects). In monkeys, selective lesion of area 3b results in impairment of all

aspects of tactile discrimination learning. Selective lesions of area 1 produce loss of texture, but spares shape discriminations. The opposite pattern is seen with area 2 lesions (Randolph & Semmes, 1974; Carlson, 1981).

Besides stereognosis, S-I mediates touch localization, two-point discrimination, position sense, and graphesthesia (the ability to recognize from tactile sensation, numbers or letters written on the skin). Electrophysiologic, functional neuroimaging, along with lesion studies have helped in determining the localization of these different cortical somatosensory functions. Experiments using somatosensory evoked potentials (SEP) suggest that touch threshold, vibration sense, thermesthesia, and nociception are mediated mainly by subcortical structures (Knecht et al., 1996). Two-point discrimination tasks involve SI, whereas graphesthesia and stereognosis involve more posterior regions, possibly areas 2 to 5. It has been postulated that the serial processing of information from S-I to posterior parietal association cortex is a precondition for stereognosis (Knecht et al., 1996). Sensory input from S-I to posterior parietal cortex and their connections to motor cortex can update or reinforce existing motor programs, and further strengthen the feed-forward model of sensory-motor learning.

Acute S-I lesions impair the perception of all somatosensory cue types. Appreciation of pain and temperature sensations is probably mediated at the

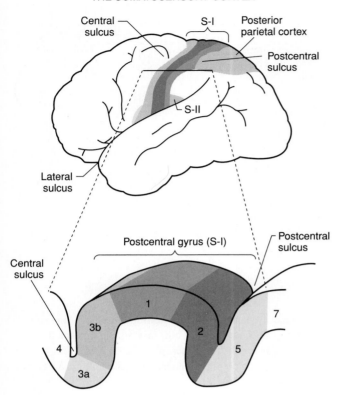

THE SOMATOSENSORY CORTEX

FIGURE 14-4. The somatosensory cortices are divided in the primary somatosensory cortex (S-I) and the association somatosensory cortices. These association cortices include the secondary somatosensory cortex (S-II) and the posterior parietal cortex (areas 5 and 7). The four distinct cytoarchitectonic regions of S-I (Brodmann areas 3a, 3b, 1, and 2) and their relationship to S-II, and to areas 5 and 7 of the posterior parietal cortex, are shown. (From Kandel ER: From nerve cells to cognition: The internal cellular representation required for perception and action, in Kandel ER, Schwartz JH, Jessel TM [eds]: Principles of Neural Science, ed 4. New York: McGraw-Hill, 2000, p. 384.)

thalamic level and generally recovers after acute S-I lesion. However, appreciation of the source, severity, and quality of pain and temperature sensation depends on the integrity of S-I and does not recover after acute S-I lesions. Chronic effects of S-I lesions include reduced appreciation of source, severity, and quality of pain and temperature sensation, and loss of touch localization, two-point discrimination, position sense, graphesthesia, and stereognosis. There is also impaired ability to learn new motor skills, but execution of previously acquired motor skills generally remains intact (Debowy et al., 2001).

Somatosensory Association Cortices

Association areas for the somatosensory system are diverse and include unimodal regions (S-II [Brodmann area 43] and area 5), heteromodal regions (area 7), and multimodal regions (areas 39 and 40, and cortices in the superior temporal sulcus; see Figs. 14-4 and 14-5; Afifi & Bergmann, 1998; Mesulam 2000; Bodegård et al., 2001; Harris et al., 2001; Ruben et al., 2001). Areas 5 and S-II are the only areas that receive direct afferent projections from S-I. They also allow interhemispheric transfer of somatosensory information via posterior corpus callosum (Iwamura et al., 1994; Fabri et al., 2001).

Physiologic and lesion studies have suggested a strong functional distinction between two systems of somatosensory association cortices: a ventral and a dorsal system (Caselli, 1993; Reed & Caselli, 1994; Reed et al., 1996). These systems represent dual streams of somatosensory information processing (see Fig. 14-6). The ventral stream mediates tactile object perception, recognition, learning, and memory ("what" pathway). The dorsal stream mediates tactile localization, spatiotemporal functions, body representation, and sensorimotor transformation ("where" pathway). These "what" and "where" pathways work together to produce necessary somatosensory information for purposeful motor behavior. Lesions in these tactile processing streams could lead to a variety of cortical or behavioral somatosensory disorders (discussed below). Examples of disorders of the "what" pathway include astereognosis, tactile agnosia, tactile anomia, and graphesthesia. Examples of disorders of the "where" pathway include tactile apraxia and optic ataxia. (See Chapter 12 for a discussion of ventral "what" and dorsal "where" pathways in visual systems.)

Ventral Streams (S-II; "What" Pathway)

In humans, S-I is bounded ventrolaterally by S-II, located on the most inferior aspect of the postcentral gyrus and in the superior bank and depth of the lateral sulcus (parietal operculum) (see Figs. 14-4, 14-5, 14-7; Caselli, 1993; Afifi & Bergmann, 1998; Ruben et al., 2001). In monkeys S-I is bounded by S-III (inferior parietal cortex) and S-IV (posterior insula and retroinsular cortex). Whereas S-II responds to low threshold somatosensory stimuli, S-IV responds to nociceptive stimuli. Body representation in the S-II area is bilateral with contralateral predominance (Iwamura et al., 1994; Fabri et al., 2001; Ruben et al., 2001), and is the reverse of that in S-I, so that the two face areas are adjacent to each other. S-II contains neurons with receptive fields that are large, poorly demarcated, and overlap extensively (Caselli, 1993; Reed & Caselli, 1994; Roland et al., 1998; Harris et al., 2001; Valenza et al., 2001).

Within the "what" pathway there are dual streams for processing different somatosensory cues (see Fig. 14-6). Appreciation of texture depends on S-I (most

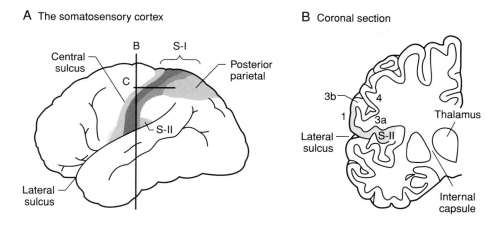

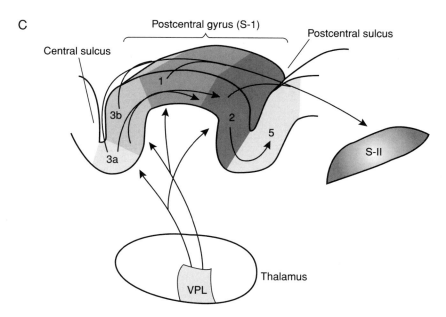

FIGURE 14-5. The somatosensory information processing in the primary and association somatosensory cortices. The inputs to the somatosensory cortices originate from thalamic nuclei, which project to S-I, mainly to Brodmann areas 3a and 3b. These two areas project to areas 1 and 2, which, in turn, project to the somatosensory association cortices, S-II, and posterior parietal cortex. (From Gardner EP, Kandel ER: Touch, in Kandel ER, Schwartz JH, Jessel TM [eds]: Principles of Neural Science, ed 4. New York: McGraw-Hill, 2000, pp. 453-459.)

likely area 3b and area 1; Caselli, 1993; Saetti et al., 1999; Bodegård et al., 2001), whereas processing of shape depends on S-I (mainly area 2), and area 5 (Roland et al., 1998; Saetti et al., 1999; Bodegård et al., 2000, 2001). Appreciation of shape is achieved through either active tactile exploration or passive touch guided by the examiner (Vega-Bermudez et al., 1991; Roland et al., 1998; Valenza et al., 2001). Both streams (texture and shape) converge and integrate in S-II, contributing to tactile perception ("what" pathway). The connection of S-II to semantic memory areas, in the inferior temporal lobe (Pandya et al., 1981), mediates more extended associative processing tactually for perceived objects, that is, tactile recognition and memory (Nakamura et al., 1998; Valenza et al., 2001). Finally, naming of pal-

pated objects is mediated through the connection of S-II to the language areas ipsilaterally or through corpus callosum (Yamadori et al., 1980; Endo et al., 1992, 1996; Fukatsu et al., 1998; Nakamura et al., 1998). Lesions in these areas can result in astereognosis, tactile agnosia, or tactile anomia.

Dorsal Stream (Areas 5 and 7, Supplementary Sensory Area; "Where" Pathway)

The dorsal somatosensory association cortices are thought to contribute to a somatosensory "where" pathway. This pathway is divided anatomically and functionally into two systems: the dorsomedial system

Figure 14-6. Localization of disorders in processing pathways.

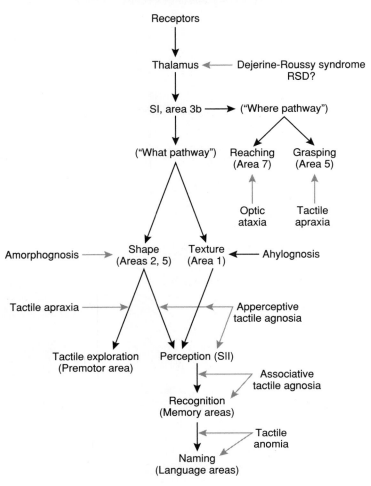

PROCESSING OF SOMATOSENSORY INFORMATION

(mesial areas 5 and 7) and the dorsolateral system (nonmesial areas 5 and 7).

Dorsomedial Somatosensory Association Cortices (Mesial Areas 5 and 7, SSA). S-I is bounded dorsomedially by another somatosensory association area, originally defined by Penfield during inoperative stimulation studies in humans. He labeled this region the supplementary sensory area (SSA) (Penfield & Rasmussen, 1950; Penfield et al., 1954; Caselli, 1993; Allison et al., 1996; Afifi & Bergmann, 1998; Kandel et al., 2000). Anatomic studies in monkeys suggest that SSA encompasses the mesial portion of Brodmann areas 5 and 7. SSA neurons have much larger receptive fields than do neurons in S-I and S-II. They receive afferent projections from medial thalamic nuclei that receive nociceptive input and are involved in pain processing (Dowman & Schell, 1999). They also receive afferent projections from SI and have efferent projections to premotor and SMA. Their pattern of connections is very similar to the supplementary motor area (SMA) (Murray & Coulter, 1982), and the two areas are strongly interconnected, suggesting that SSA is a somatosensory analog of SMA

(Golberg, 1985). SSA has been implicated in movement sense generation and maintenance and in somatosensory spatiotemporal functions, for example, touch localization (Caselli, 1993; Radovanovic, 2002).

Dorsolateral Somatosensory Association Cortices (Nonmesial Area 5 and 7). The nonmesial parts of areas 5 (unimodal) and 7 (heteromodal) are located in the anterior and posterior portion of the superior parietal lobe, respectively (see Fig. 14-4; Afifi & Bergmann, 1998; Mesulam, 2000). Unlike S-I and S-II, there are less distinct somatotopic representations in these areas (Gelnar et al., 1997). Their neuronal responses are complex and involve integration of a number of cortical and thalamic inputs. Inputs derive mainly from S-I, but they also have reciprocal connections with the pulvinar nucleus of the thalamus and are connected bilaterally through the corpus callosum. Areas 5 and 7 both project to S-II (important for shape perception), to the dorsolateral portion of the frontal lobe (important for sensorimotor transformation), and to multimodal association areas in the inferior parietal lobe, the supramarginal, and angular gyri

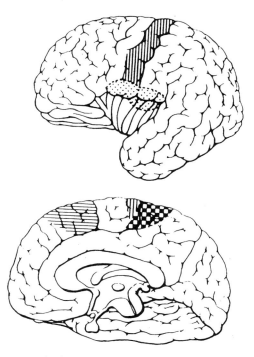

FIGURE 14-7. The human somatosensory cortices are shown. The vertical lines delineate S-I, small dots delineate S-II and posterior insula, checkerboard delineates the supplementary somatosensory area (SSA; mesial areas 5 and 7), and horizontal lines delineate the supplementary motor cortex (SMA). The dorsolateral somatosensory association cortices in the nonmesial areas 5 and 7 are not delineated here. (From Caselli RJ: Ventrolateral and dorsomedial somatosensory association cortex damage produces distinct somesthetic syndromes in humans. Neurology 43:762, 1993.)

(areas 39 and 40) (important for intermodal integration and multisensory perceptions).

Sensorimotor Transformation. The projections of non-mesial areas 5 and 7 to the dorsolateral portion of the frontal lobe allow sensory stimuli to be converted into motor commands, a process referred to as "sensorimotor transformation" (Figs. 14-8 and 14-9; Soechting & Flanders, 1992; Jeannerod et al., 1995; Rizzo & Darling, 1997; Blakemore et al., 1998; Wolpert et al., 1998; Pouget & Snyder, 2000; Darling et al., 2001; Freund, 2001; Rizzo & Vecera, 2002). The integration of sensory and motor function requires interconnection of several cortical areas, including the above-mentioned primary sensory, unimodal sensory association, multimodal sensory association, multimodal motor association, unimodal motor association, and primary motor cortices (see Fig. 14-9). Each primary sensory cortex (e.g., S-I) projects to nearby higher order sensory cortex, a unimodal association area, for example, area 5 that integrates afferent information for a single sensory modality. The unimodal association areas in turn converge in multimodal sensory association areas (e.g., area 7 and angular gyrus) that project to premotor and prefrontal cortex. The higher-order motor areas transform sensory information into planned movement and compute the programs for these movements, which are then conveyed to the premotor and primary motor cortex for implementation. The sequence of information processing in the motor system is essentially the reverse of that in the sensory systems. Thus, the primary sensory areas are the initial sites of cortical processing of sensory information, whereas the primary motor areas are the final sites for the cortical processing of motor commands.

Mechanisms of sensorimotor transformation enable us to act efficiently in environments where spatial relations are defined with respect to coordinates external to the organism. For example, reaching and grasping of targets under visual guidance require specification of target location in a visual coordinate system and a series of transformations into motor commands that move the hand to a position to acquire the

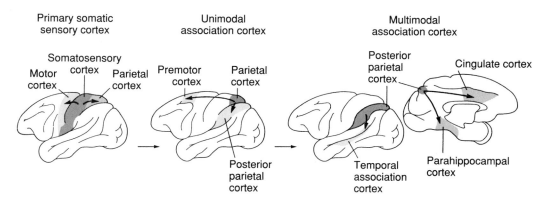

FIGURE 14-8. The processing of sensory information in the cerebral cortex begins with primary sensory cortices, continues in unimodal association cortices, and multimodal association cortices, all of which then project to premotor and motor cortices. These cortices provide the network necessary for sensorimotor transformation. (From Amaral DG: The functional organization of perception and movement, in Kandel ER, Schwartz JH, Jessel TM [eds]: Principles of Neural Science, ed 4. New York: McGraw-Hill, 2000, p. 345.)

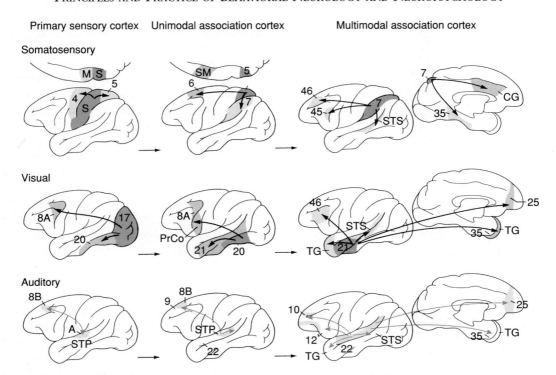

FIGURE 14-9. Cortices involved in sensorimotor transformation in different sensory modalities, for example, somatosensory, visual, and auditory domains. (From Saper CB, Iversen S, Frackowiak R: Integration of sensory and motor function: The association areas of the cerebral cortex and the cognitive capabilities of the brain, in Kandel ER, Schwartz JH, Jessel TM [eds]: Principles of Neural Science, ed 4. New York: McGraw-Hill, 2000, p. 354.)

target (Jeannerod et al., 1995; Rizzo & Darling, 1997; Darling et al., 2001; Rizzo & Vecera, 2002). To determine how sensory information is used to coordinate these movements we must understand how spatial parameters are encoded in brain.

Frames of Reference. Various senses sample space in different coordinates: for example, vision is retinotopic, tactile is somatotopic, and audition and vestibular sense are head-centered (Driver & Spence, 1998). Sensorimotor transformation requires that information from these different senses be represented in a common space, spatial coordinates, or frames of reference. An important role for the nonmesial areas 5 and 7 is to construct and transform the three successive frames of reference: retinotopic, head-centered, and body-centered frames of reference (Soechting et al., 1992; Andersen, 1997; Berlucchi & Aglioti, 1997; Goldenberg, 1997; Snyder et al., 1998). Visual information leaving the retina is organized into a two-dimensional map of the visual field. We refer to this map as a retinotopic map or a retinotopic frame of reference that is fixed to the eyes. Each time the eye moves, the retinotopic frame of reference moves as well. A head-centered frame of reference is constructed by combining the retinotopic frame of reference with information about the eye position. Likewise, a body-centered frame of reference is constructed by combining the head-centered frame of refer-

ence with information about posture and position of the head in relation to the body in space (see Chapter 16). Thus, one frame of reference is built on another.

These frames of reference depend on neurons in the parietal cortex to mediate multimodal mapping of salient body-related events in multiple frames of reference. According to Mountcastle and colleagues (1980, p. 522), "the parietal lobe, together with the distributed system of which it is a central node, generates an internal neural construction of the immediately surrounding space, of the location and movements of objects within it in relation to body position, and of the position and movement of the body in relation to that immediately surrounding space. The region appears in general to be concerned with continually updating information regarding the relation between internal and external coordinate systems."

These three constantly changing, dynamic frames of reference provide the necessary information for sensorimotor transformation that is used for organization of posture, and planning and execution of movements directed at external targets (Jeannerod et al., 1995; Rizzo & Darling, 1997; Darling et al., 2001; Debowy et al., 2001; Rizzo & Vecera, 2002). There may be a segregation of neurons encoding different frames of reference (see Fig. 14-6; Bonda et al., 1995; Snyder et al., 1998). For example, area 5 (intraparietal sulcus) is involved in constructing a body-centered frame of reference based on somatosensory input, which is important for tactile-guided movements such as grasping or tactile exploration. In contrast, area 7 is more closely involved in constructing a world-centered frame of reference based on vestibular and visual input, important for visually guided movement such as reaching. These two examples, grasping and reaching, will be discussed in more detail below (see Fig. 14-6).

Tactile-Guided Movement and Tactile Exploration. Neurons in nonmesial area 5 have bilateral hand representation and integrate information necessary for the cooperative actions of the two hands. They also ascertain the information on the spatial relationship between the body and the limbs at rest and in motion, which can be used in tests such as grasping and reaching in the dark (Jeannerod et al., 1995; Rushworth et al., 1997; Binkofski et al., 1998). These neurons integrate tactile inputs from mechanoreceptors in the skin with proprioceptive input from the fingers to encode the shape of objects (morphognosis) grasped and explored by both hands. When an object is palpated, these neurons process these sensory and proprioceptive cues and interact with premotor and motor regions to direct a series of coordinated movements necessary to construct a "tactile image" of the object. Although morphognosis usually depends on active tactile palpation/exploration, it can also be based on passive touching guided by the examiner (Vega-Bermudez et al., 1991; Valenza et al., 2001). The projection of area 5 to premotor cortex is believed to be important for tactile exploration. A lesion in this area may result in defective shape perception seen in tactile amorphognosis or in abnormal sensorimotor transformation seen in tactile apraxia (Binkofski et al., 2001; Valenza et al., 2001).

Visually Guided Movements. Reaching for objects under visual guidance requires that the retinotopic coordinates of the perceived object be transformed into body-centered coordinates (Jeannerod et al., 1995; Rizzo & Darling, 1997; Darling et al., 2001; Rizzo & Vecera, 2002). This transformation has to take into account the current position of the eyes relative to the head and of the head relative to the trunk. In addition to the representation of the target in body-centered coordinates, the brain must also represent the initial arm configuration to plan the trajectory. Single-cell recordings in monkeys have provided evidence that cells in areas 7 in the posterior parietal lobe receive both tactile and visual input about the current position and configuration of the eyes, head, body, and limbs, and perform the computations necessary for transforming visually perceived locations (i.e., retinotopic frame of reference) into body-centered coordinates. These cells not only receive information about body part interrelationships (such as are maintained by area 5), but also about the interaction of the body with external objects and events. Indeed, many cells in this vicinity become highly active when the hand is moved toward an object or while reaching for and manipulating objects. Similarly, using fMRI, activation of area 7 has been found with reaching tasks. Lesions in these areas may result in abnormal sensorimotor transformations, seen in optic ataxia and Balint syndrome (see Chapters 10 and 12).

Body Schema (Awareness) and Body Knowledge. In addition to their involvement in building frames of reference necessary for sensorimotor transformations, nonmesial area 5 and area 7 are also involved in awareness and knowledge about the body (Bonda et al., 1995; Iriki et al., 1996; Berlucchi & Aglioti, 1997; Goldenberg, 1997).

Assessment of the body target location in terms of body-centered coordinates does not require conscious awareness of one's body. That is, while somatosensory, vestibular, and visual afferents provide information about the actual position and configuration of one's body, one has a basic feeling of where one's body parts are, even without these inputs. The basic awareness of one's own body has been conceptualized as a mental body schema; moreover, there is a general (conscious) knowledge about the functions, locations, and names of human body parts (Sirigu et al., 1991). Examples of disorders with impaired awareness of the mental body schema, but preserved knowledge of the human body, are phantom limb syndrome and hemineglect syndrome. In contrast, patients with autotopagnosia have preserved awareness of the mental body schema, but impaired knowledge of the human body. These disorders will be discussed in the next section.

Multimodal Association Cortices (Areas 39 and 40 and Superior Temporal Sulcus)

The supramarginal and angular gyri in the inferior parietal lobule (areas 39 and 40) are multimodal association areas that receive inputs from several modalities (visual, auditory, tactile) and serve intermodal integration and multisensory perceptions. Lesions in these areas can result in Gerstmann syndrome (discussed later). Cortical areas in the superior temporal sulcus (STS) also belong to multimodal association areas that send feedback connections to unimodal sensory cortices and contain neurons responsive to feature-level aspects of stimuli in multiple sensory modalities (Seltzer & Pandya, 1978; Schlitz et al., 1999). This area may be involved in synesthesia (discussed later).

BEHAVIORAL DISORDERS OF THE SOMATOSENSORY SYSTEM

Symptoms and Signs

Like any other sensory modality, there are positive as well as negative symptoms and signs in the somatosensory system (Asbury, 1998; Campero et al., 1998).

TABLE 14-2. Positive Symptoms

Dysesthesia		Abnormal sensation described as unpleasant. It may be spontaneous or provoked by maneuvers on physical examination
Paresthesia		Abnormal but not unpleasant or painful sensation that may be spontaneous or evoked
Allodynia	Mechanical	Abnormal perception of pain from usually nonpainful mechanical stimulation; e.g., pain that is caused by contact with clothing, bed sheets, or wind. It can be one of the most disabling physical symptoms
	Thermal	Abnormal sensation of pain from what is normally nonpainful thermal stimulation, such as cold or warmth; patients may experience a delay in response to thermal stimuli followed by a stronger or irritating sensory experience that continues for longer than normal
Hyperalgesia		Exaggerated pain response from a usually painful stimulation; does not have a symptom analogue and can only be determined by physical examination; may be mechanical or thermal, depending on the type of stimulus
Hyperpathia		Complex abnormal sensation that refers to an abnormally painful and exaggerated reaction to a stimulus

Data from Merskey H, Bogduk N: Classification of Chronic Pain. Seattle, WA: IASP Press, 1994.

Positive somatosensory phenomena (Table 14-2) include spontaneous somatosensory perceptual experiences that occur in the absence of an appropriate stimulus (paresthesia), altered sensation or unpleasant distortions of actual sensory stimuli (dysesthesia), exaggerated sensations (hyperesthesia), exaggerated painful sensation to mildly painful stimuli (hyperalgesia), and painful sensation to nonpainful stimuli (allodynia) (Merskey & Bogduk, 1994; McKnight & Adcock, 1997; Asbury, 1998). Despite their common occurrence, these simple positive sensory phenomena are poorly understood with respect to their pathophysiology (Rizzo et al., 1996). Positive somatosensory phenomena can also be complex (Table 14-3).

Negative somatosensory phenomena refer to diminished (anesthesia) or decreased (hypoesthesia) somatosensation, or deficits in higher order somatosensory functions (Table 14-4; McKnight & Adcock, 1997; Asbury, 1998).

Both positive and negative somatosensory symptoms and signs can result from lesions at any level of the somatosensory system. The distribution and nature of these sensory symptoms and signs can help localize their source (Haerer, 1992; Asbury, 1998). In the next section, we review the positive as well as negative behavioral disorders of the somatosensory system, and later we address various treatment options available for these disorders.

Reflex Sympathetic Dystrophy

As early as 1864, Silas Weir Mitchel, the founding father of American neurology, described the clinical condition of causalgia in soldiers injured in the American Civil War (Schott, 2001). This term was used to describe a partic-ular burning pain condition, which followed a partial nerve injury, usually affecting a limb. The burning pain was often accompanied by additional features including various sensory disturbances; temperature and sweating changes; changes of skin, subcutaneous tissues, muscle, and joints; paralysis; and involuntary movement (Gordon, 1996; Schott, 2001). Earlier this century, others noted that there were patients with a similar but less severe condition that again followed trauma but without major nerve injury. This condition was referred to as reflex sympathetic dystrophy (RSD) and was introduced first by Evans in 1946.

In 1994, the International Association for the Study of Pain (IASP) introduced the term *complex regional pain syndrome* (CRPS) (Merskey & Bogduk, 1994). Type I CRPS is synonymous with RSD, defined as a syndrome that usually develops after an initiating noxious event, is not limited to the distribution of a single peripheral nerve, and is apparently disproportionate to the inciting event (see Chapter 33). It is associated at some points with evidence of edema, changes in skin blood flow, abnormal sudomotor activity, allodynia, or hyperalgesia. Type II CRPS is the term used when this condition is associated with clear nerve injury (i.e., causalgia) (Schott, 2001).

To describe the clinical features of RSD, we will use an example of wrist fracture described previously (Schott, 2001). The affected part may become warm, red, puffy, sweaty, and painful. After some weeks or months the area becomes cold, blue, and dry and remains painful. Atrophy of the affected limb (including the skin, muscle, and bone) follows. The warm stage has been attributed to the loss of cutaneous vasoconstrictor activity at the spinal level, leading to disturbances of the skin microvasculature. This sympathetic inhibition

TABLE 14-3. Positive Somatosensory Syndromes and Localization

Syndrome		Lesion	Definition
Reflex sympathetic dystrophy (RSD)		Probable supersensitivity of CNS, particularly thalamus, to sympathetic neurotransmitters	A particular burning pain condition, which follows a partial nerve injury, typically affecting a limb, and often accompanied by temperature and sweating changes, edema, abnormal sudomotor activity, allodynia, or hyperalgesia
Déjérine-Roussy syndrome		Nucleus ventrocaudalis of the thalamus	Spontaneous paroxysmal burning pain over the contralesional half of the body
Tactile hallucination	Simple	Peripheral somatosensory system up to thalamus	Perceptual somatosensory experience in the absence of stimuli as described in Table 14-2, RSD, and Déjérine-Roussy syndrome
	Complex	S-I and area 5	Perceptual somatosensory experience of being touched or having object put in one's hands, in the absence of stimuli
Phantom limb phenomena	**Phantom limb pain**	S-I and thalamus	Perceptual experience of pain in an amputated limb
	Phantom limb perception	S-II and area 5	Perceptual experience that an amputated limb is present
Synesthesia	**Synesthetic perception**	Association cortices, right prefrontal cortex, insula, and superior temporal gyrus	Perceptual experience in a modality by a stimulus in another modality, so that the individual has multimodal perceptual experience from a unimodal sensory event
	Synesthetic conception	Association cortices, right prefrontal cortex, insula, and superior temporal gyrus	Perception in a modality by just thinking about a particular concept in another modality

resolves after the early stages of RSD. However, these vascular changes may be nonspecific because they are normally seen after most injuries. There are also changes in bone, which can be assessed by isotropic bone scanning and magnetic resonance imaging (MRI).

The etiology of RSD could be peripheral or central, including stroke, multiple sclerosis, spinal trauma, shingles, systemic diseases such as myocardial infarction, cardiac surgery, drugs such as phenobarbital, and pregnancy (Gordon, 1996; Schott, 2001). By far the most common cause (50%) of RSD is peripheral trauma, both accidental and surgical. Although the changes in RSD may resemble sympathetically mediated ones, and the pain in RSD is sometimes relieved by interrupting the sympathetic outflow to the limb, RSD may occur in a sympathectomized limb and its features do not resemble those usually associated with diseases of the central and peripheral autonomic systems. Moreover, microneurographic studies of sympathetic nerve fibers of these or concentration of adrenalin and noradrenalin in their affected limbs are normal. This profile of findings argues against a disease of the sympathetic nervous system and favors supersensitivity to sympathetic neurotransmitters as being the pathophysiologic basis for RSD.

Whereas the changes in RSD suggest a peripheral cause, the presence of hyperhidrosis, urinary dysfunction, and abnormal thalamic perfusion on the contralateral side shown by single photon emission computed tomography (SPECT; Fig. 14-10) suggests a central etiology (Fukumoto et al., 1999; Schott, 2001).

TABLE 14-4. Negative Somatosensory Syndromes and Localization

Syndrome		Lesion	Definition
Astereognosis	Ahylognosis	Area 1	Inability to tactually perceive texture (e.g., roughness, density, weight, etc.)
	Amorphognosis	Areas 2 to 5	Inability to tactually perceive shape (e.g., size, length, etc.)
Tactile agnosia	Apperceptive	Connections of areas 1, 2, and 5 to area S-II, or area S-II	Inability to tactually recognize objects despite intact tactile texture and shape perception
	Associative	Connections of area S-II to the semantic memory areas in the inferior temporal lobe	Inability to attribute meaning to tactually correctly explored and perceived objects
Tactile anomia		Connections of area S-II to the language areas in the left temporal lobe	Inability to name tactually recognized objects
Graphesthesia		Left intraparietal sulcus	Inability to recognize and name, from tactile stimulation, numbers written on the hand skin
Tactile neglect		Right-sided areas 5 and 7 in the inferior part of the superior parietal lobe	Failure to detect a tactile stimuli contralateral to the lesion, under conditions of simultaneous bilateral tactile stimulation of the body
Tactile apraxia		Area 5, particularly the anterior intraparietal sulcus, and their projections to premotor and supplementary motor areas	Impairment in tactile exploration, exploitable for tactile object recognition
Optic ataxia		Area 7 and its projections to premotor and supplementary motor areas	Inability to reach under visual guidance despite normal proprioception and normal limb strength
Autotopagnosia		Left posterior parietal lobe	Inability to localize body parts on one's own or on someone else's body, on verbal or nonverbal command, despite preserved knowledge of location and names of the body parts
Gerstmann syndrome		Left angular gyrus	Acalculia, agraphia, finger agnosia, and left-right disorientation
Hysteria (psychogenic somatosensory symptoms and signs)		Orbitofrontal, anterior cingulate, and prefrontal cortices	Somatosensory symptoms and signs that cannot be attributed to organic pathology, but suggest a neurologic cause

Furthermore, thalamic perfusion changes over time, initially increasing (in acute pain) and then decreasing (in chronic pain), which may reflect the evolution of the clinical picture (Fukumoto et al., 1999).

In summary, RSD may be due to supersensitivity of CNS to sympathetic (possibly thalamic) neurotransmitters. This may have implications for designing drugs for treatment (e.g., capable of passing the blood-brain barrier), and also emphasizes the behavioral and cognitive approach, currently under research to treat this central/behavioral somatosensory disorder (Gordon, 1996; Schott, 2001).

Déjérine-Roussy Syndrome

In 1903, Déjérine and Egger described a clinical syndrome caused by a thalamic lesion, more fully described in the 1906 report of Déjérine and Roussy (Schott, 1995; Nasreddine & Saver, 1997). The cardinal symptom in this case was pain. There is usually no rela-

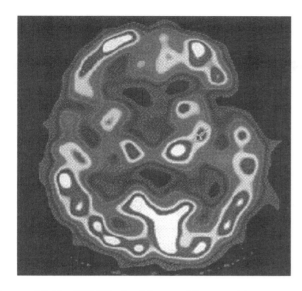

FIGURE 14-10. SPECT of a 56-year-old man with symptoms of RSD in his right arm for 5 months shows an increase in contralateral (left) thalamic perfusion.

tionship between the degree of sensory deficiency and appearance of pain. Patients have minimal signs at time of onset, but over a period of a few weeks, severe spontaneous paroxysmal burning pain appears over the contralesional half of the body (Gonzales et al., 2001).

Recent observations suggest that the key lesions in Déjérine-Roussy syndrome affect the nucleus ventrocaudalis of the thalamus, often due to occlusion of the geniculothalamic artery, a branch of the posterior cerebral artery (PCA) (Graff-Radford, 1997; Paciaroni & Bogousslavsky, 1998). The frequency of pain after geniculothalamic stroke is estimated to be 24%, and more common with right than left thalamic lesions. This specificity suggests a particular vulnerability of pain processing to right thalamic lesion, consistent with right hemispheric dominance for processing of somatic representation and monitoring somatic states (Nasreddine & Saver, 1997). This was recently postulated by the theories of somatic markers in the guidance of behavior (Damasio, et al., 1991; Bechara, et al., 1994) and supported by findings of right hemispheric specialization for processing of pain, because pain signals are critically important for acquisition of somatic knowledge and avoidance behavior.

Tactile Hallucinations

Hallucinations are (positive) perceptual experiences in the absence of external sensory stimuli. They can occur in any sensory modality, including visual, auditory, and the tactile domain. They are generally divided into simple and complex hallucinations. The positive somatosensory phenomena described so far, that is, symptoms due to peripheral somatosensory disorders

(see Table 14-3), RSD, and Déjérine-Roussy syndrome, are examples of simple tactile hallucinations. They stand in sharp contrast to complex tactile hallucinations, also called spontaneous stereognostic sensations (Stacy, 1987; Shergill et al., 2001). The following two examples illustrate complex hallucinations: (1) An 80-year-old woman with biparietal lesions who had normal reaching but difficulty with grasping (intact area 7; but abnormal area 5) had episodes of feeling that an object was being placed into her hand (Stacy, 1987); and (2) a 36-year-old man with schizophrenia who reported the perception of being touched. Using functional MRI (fMRI), it was demonstrated that his complex tactile hallucinations were associated with activity in the thalamus, S-I, and posterior parietal cortex (Shergill et al., 2001). These findings suggest that simple tactile hallucinations involve subcortical structures from the periphery to the thalamus, whereas complex tactile hallucinations involve cortical structures such as S-I and areas 5 and 7.

Astereognosis

According to an early classification by Delay (Delay et al., 1935; Endo et al., 1992), astereognosis was defined as a complex somatosensory disorder that has three main parts: (1) ahylognosis, the inability to discriminate texture, mediated by area 1; (2) amorphognosis (Saetti et al., 1999), the inability to perceive shape, mediated by areas 2 and 5; and (3) tactile asymboly (tactile agnosia), the inability to identify an object by touch in the absence of amorphognosis and ahylognosis, mediated by area S-II (see Fig. 14-6; Caselli, 1991, 1993). However, the term *astereognosis* should be restricted to impaired tactile perception that is due to severely impaired basic somatosensory functions (i.e., due to ahylognosis and amorphognosis). That is, patients with astereognosis are not able to tactually recognize objects *because of* their inability to perceive texture or shape. In contrast, tactile agnosia is a selective disturbance of tactile object recognition that occurs in the absence of any impairment of basic somatosensory functions (texture and shape perception) (Caselli, 1991, 1993; Reed & Caselli, 1994; Reed et al., 1996; Valenza et al., 2001). That is, patients with tactile agnosia are unable to tactually recognize objects *despite* intact ability to perceive texture and shape (see Fig. 14-6). Astereognosis can result from cortical deafferentation arising from damage to any level of the somatosensory system including the peripheral nerves (particularly severe large-fiber peripheral neuropathies, such as Guillain-Barré syndrome), spinal cord (especially posterior column pathways), brainstem (interruption of the medial lemniscus), thalamus (VPL) nucleus, S-I, or area 5. Astereognosis is generally more severe when caused by a cortical lesion than by a peripheral nerve, spinal cord, brainstem, or thalamic lesion.

Tactile Agnosia

Tactile agnosia is the selective impairment of tactile object recognition despite intact basic somatosensory functions such as texture perception and shape perception (see Fig. 14-6). If the selective impairment occurs before or at the integration of texture and shape perception, such as with S-II lesions, it leads to the syndrome of apperceptive tactile agnosia (see Fig. 14-6; Caselli, 1991, 1993; Reed & Caselli, 1994; Reed et al., 1996; Valenza et al., 2001). If this selective impairment occurs after intact integration of intact texture and shape perception in S-II, it leads to the syndrome of associative tactile agnosia (see Fig. 14-6; Endo et al., 1992; Nakamura et al., 1998; Valenza et al., 2001).

Apperceptive tactile agnosia is a modality-specific deficit in somatosensory integration that combines the preserved submodal features into a coherent somesthetic image and permits recognition; that is, these patients have difficulty accurately integrating decoded object parts into cohesive tactile representation sufficient to permit recognition. In contrast to patients with astereognosis, patients with apperceptive tactile agnosia can draw the object they are touching, demonstrating their preserved ability to decipher the salient somatosensory characteristics of the object they fail to recognize. Apperceptive tactile agnosia is a unilateral disorder affecting the left or right hand that results from unilateral contralateral lesion. The generally unilateral nature of tactile apperceptive agnosia implies a perceptual, as opposed to semantic or mnemonic, impairment because if memory representations were destroyed, then it should not matter which hand is used to access those representations. Furthermore, the normal tactile imagery ability in these patients indicates intact memory representation. In these patients, tactile exploration strategies are normal, suggesting that these strategies are not critical for tactile object recognition. Apperceptive tactile agnosia is seldom disabling because patients can compensate in several ways. For example, an object may be described in approximate terms, "safety pin" for a paper clip, or in a more generic way, "a tool" for a wrench.

In contrast to patients with apperceptive tactile agnosia, patients with associative tactile agnosia have intact tactile perception (Endo et al., 1992; Nakamura et al., 1998; Valenza et al., 2001). However, they are unable to attribute meaning to the correctly explored and perceived objects, as evidenced by patients' inability to classify objects according to their function out of vision. This can be caused by a lesion in the connection of S-II to the semantic memory areas in the inferior temporal lobe, for example, damage in arcuate fasciculus, or inferior longitudinal fasciculus in the subcortical regions of angular gyrus (see Fig. 14-6).

Tactile Anomia

Tactile anomia is the inability to name tactually recognized objects in the absence of aphasic anomia (Yamadori et al., 1980; Endo et al., 1992, 1996; Fukatsu et al., 1998; Nakamura et al., 1998). These patients demonstrate intact tactile object recognition, as evidenced by correct classification, but they are unable to name the objects correctly. This is due to disconnection of the tactile recognition system from language areas (see Fig. 14-6). Lesions of the corpus callosum (cerebral commissurotomy) in patients with complete separation of the cerebral hemispheres can result in a clinical picture in which objects presented to the left hand are well recognized, but cannot be named by the linguistically deprived right hemisphere.

Graphesthesia

Graphesthesia refers to the inability to recognize and name, from tactile sensation, letters or numbers written on the skin and is usually associated with lesions of left intraparietal sulcus. Consistent with this is the recently reported functional imaging experiment showing activation of the intraparietal sulcus in the tactile reading phonograms in Japanese patients (Takeda et al., 1999). The proposed mechanism is that such a lesion disconnects tactile letter representation in somatosensory associative cortex from language-related and memory areas (Fukatsu et al., 1998). In these patients, the nonlexical as well as lexical (visual-verbal, auditory-visual) routes are preserved.

Tactile Apraxia

Extraction of sensory information relies on the adequacy of purposeful motion, motor-sensory transformation. The inability to integrate this tactile feedback with stored tactile shape information to generate the exploratory hand movement exploitable for tactile object recognition is known as tactile apraxia (see Fig. 14-6) (Binkofski et al., 2001; Valenza et al., 2001). It is a unimodal disorder of tactile exploration that can result in impaired tactile object recognition. In patients with tactile apraxia, tactile recognition based on passive touch (e.g., guided by the examiner) may remain intact (Valenza et al., 2001). Tactile apraxia is usually caused by lesion of the projections from area 5, particularly from the anterior intraparietal sulcus to premotor and supplementary motor areas.

Tactile apraxia can be tested quantitatively by kinematic recording of exploratory finger movements (transitive movements) and rapid alternating finger movements (intransitive movements; Binkofski et al., 2001). Infrared light-emitting diodes are fixed to the fingers, and their movements are monitored with a two-camera opto-electronic recording system. Subjects are asked to perform exploratory finger movements and rapid alternating forefinger-thumb opposition movements. Another method of testing exploratory movements is by videotaping and tracking a small colored point at the center of the nails of fingers, used as reference points (Valenza et al., 2001).

Optic Ataxia

Optic ataxia is a defect of reaching under visual guidance, despite normal proprioception and limb strength (Rizzo, 1993; Rizzo & Vecera, 2002). Usually it is caused by lesions in the posterior parietal and parieto-occipital areas (such as 5, 7, 39, 39, and 37). These patients may have defective sensorimotor transformation, that is, an inability to transform object coordinates in retinotopic frame of reference into a body-centered frame of reference. However, these patients can actively reach for parts of their own bodies because body parts are a-priori coded in a body-centered frame of reference. The difficulty reaching is generally worse with the contralesional hand (to both hemifields) and with both hands (to the contralesional hemifield). Such patients may be unable to pour water from a bottle into a glass without spilling yet can accurately reach targets on their own bodies. It is important in screening for optic ataxia that the patient accurately detects and perceives the target for a reach before reaching for it.

Tactile Neglect and Extinction

Tactile neglect and extinction are disorders of impaired awareness of the mental body schema, but with preserved knowledge of the human body, and are attributed to disorders of attention (see Chapter 10 for a discussion of their occurrence in the visual domain).

Tactile attention, mediated by synchronous activity of neurons in the right posterior parietal lobe, modulates activity of both S-I and S-II (Mima et al., 1998; Hämäläinen et al., 2000; Johansen-Berg et al., 2000). The finding that tactile extinction may affect only complex stimuli may only reflect the higher attentional demand required for perception of more complex stimuli (Ito et al., 1989).

Both visual and tactile extinction seem to be related mainly to lesions of right posterior inferior parietal lobe, which is involved in control of attention, and representation of personal, peripersonal, and extrapersonal space. However, they can be double-dissociated, both functionally and anatomically (Vallar et al., 1994; Smania & Aglioti, 1995).

Functionally, extinction may be considered in the three frames of references described above (Smania & Aglioti, 1995; Berti et al., 1999). Smania and Aglioti (1995) studied patients with right brain damage and somatosensory extinction, visual extinction, or both. Patients verbally reported light touches delivered to each hand, or simultaneously to both hands, in two experimental situations. In the "anatomic" situation, each hand was in its homonymous hemispace. In the "crossed situation," each hand was held across the midline. Under both single- and double-stimulated conditions, the stimuli delivered to the contralateral hand were detected with lower accuracy. The accuracy was lower for the anatomic than for the crossed position. Processing sensory information in S-I should not be influenced by the hemispatial position of the stimulated body parts. This suggests that the somatosensory extinction is due mainly to sensory factors, but also to attentional factors. The attentional impairment in the somatosensory domain is not related to the defective coding in extrapersonal space, but in the somatotopic (or personal) coordinates. Thus, whereas visual stimuli are coded mainly in terms of extrapersonal space, tactile stimuli are coded mainly in the personal space. The interaction between the visual and tactile system occurs between extrapersonal and personal (somatotopic) space, respectively, namely, in the peripersonal space, at the level of neurons in area 7 that receive both tactile and visual inputs (Moscovitch & Behrmann, 1994; Làdavas et al., 1998). This interaction is relevant to treatment and rehabilitation strategies in patients with tactile extinction and neglect (Làdavas et al., 1994, 1998).

The anatomic correlates of tactile and visual extinction are also different (Vallar et al., 1994). In visual extinction, internal representation of extrapersonal space is disrupted by lesions in the posterior inferior parietal cortex and the posterior thalamus. The anatomic correlates of tactile extinction are not confined to cortical lesions involving the parietal cortex (area 5), as traditionally maintained, but also involve the dorsolateral frontal cortex and subcortical structures such as paraventricular occipital white matter. The subcortical structures involving ascending pathways may be a neural correlate of a sensory component of tactile extinction.

Phantom Limb Perception and Phantom Pain

Other examples of disorders with impaired awareness of the mental body schema, but preserved knowledge of the human body, are phantom limb perception and phantom limb pain. In tactile neglect there is lack of awareness of one's own body parts; in phantom phenomena there is perception of body parts that are not really present.

Visual, auditory, and olfactory phantom perceptions or sensations have been reported after deafferentation of the corresponding sense organs, but the most recently studied phantom phenomena are somatosensory in nature, including all submodalities from touch perception to pain.

The term phantom limb was introduced by Silas Weir Mitchell in 1871, in reference to a condition in which patients experience that an amputated extremity is still present, and in some cases also experience pain in the missing limb (Ramachandran, 1998; Ramachandran & Hirstein, 1998). Phantom phenomena occur not only after amputation but can also be caused by lesions that interrupt all afferents from the affected body part. This may be the case with lesions of the peripheral nerves, the plexus, and the spinal cord or with subcortical cerebral lesions. If the deafferented limb is still present and visible, the phantom phenomena may involve a supernumerary limb. Patients recognize that the perceptions or sensations are not real; that is, what they experience is an illusion, not a delusion.

The occurrence of phantom limb sensations suggests that the brain houses a mental body schema that continues to exist even if it has lost its correlate in the real body (Ramachandran, 1998; Ramachandran & Hirstein, 1998). The phenomena are less common in children, suggesting that there may not have been enough time for the body schema image to "consolidate." Until recently it was assumed that cortical maps of the body surface were "hard wired" and the pathways from receptors in the skin to the cortex were fixed early in development, but recent reports indicate that this may not be the case, particularly during childhood and after amputation in adults.

Using microelectrode recording and tracer injections in monkeys with limb amputation, it was shown that cortical areas 3b and 1 contralateral to the amputated limb have expanded lateral connections (Faggin et al., 1997; Florence et al., 1998; Wall et al., 2002). This reorganization of neuronal connections not only occurs at the cortical level, but also at the thalamic and brainstem levels. Although some changes occur immediately, the full spectrum of these changes takes months to years to develop. Multiple mechanisms of reorganization have been identified:

1. The immediate reorganization is due to the disinhibition of existing, previously silent input, probably mediated through γ-aminobutyric acid (GABA) receptors.
2. The more slowly developing changes are due to potentiation of weak connections, probably mediated through N-methyl-D-aspartate (NMDA) receptors.
3. The long-term changes are due to growth of new connections, probably mediated through growth factors (e.g., growth-associated protein-43 [GAP-43]).

One frequently encountered feature of this somatosensory reorganization is that it involves shift of representations among neighboring regions in the somatosensory maps. This leads to reactivation of the region deprived of its dominant input by other inputs physically adjacent to the deprived region. Several findings described below indicate that following amputation similar mechanisms might operate in humans.

Stimulation of the face area of these patients can lead to referred sensation in the phantom limb (Ramachandran, 1998; Ramachandran & Hirstein, 1998). This may be a perceptual correlate of the cortical reorganization. The finding that referred sensations could be elicited from both the intact and the amputation side as well as from distal areas, such as the legs, suggests an involvement of S-II where the leg and arm representations are adjacent (Grüsser et al., 2001).

Magnetic source imaging studies in humans have supported the hypothesis that phantom pain is related to and may be a consequence of somatosensory cortical reorganization (Flor et al., 1995, 2001). In patients with phantom limb pain but not perception, imagined movement of phantom hand activated the neighboring face area (Lotze et al., 2001). Positron emission tomography (PET) and transcranial magnetic stimulation (TMS) studies have demonstrated increased excitability of the somatosensory cortex and posterior parietal cortex contralesional to the amputated limb (Kew et al., 1994; Schwenkres et al., 2000). These data suggest that phantom limb perception is produced by the same processes that represent body schema, whereas phantom limb pain is mediated through hyperactivity of thalamus, anterior cingulate, and lateral prefrontal cortex (Willoch et al., 2000). It is postulated that reorganization in the thalamus and S-I underlie the phenomenon of phantom limb pain, whereas the reorganization in S-II and posterior parietal cortex may underlie the phantom limb perception (Grüsser et al., 2001). Consistent with this hypothesis is the finding that a lesion in the posterior parietal cortex could result in disappearance of the phantom limb perception (Appenzeller & Bicknell, 1969).

Finally, it has been suggested that the phantom limb perception and phantom limb pain are not advantageous (Moore et al., 2000), and therefore are referred to as "maladaptive" plasticity (Karl et al., 2001). Study of phantom limb phenomena may shed light on plasticity and the neural basis of conscious experience.

Autotopagnosia

Autotopagnosia is a disorder of impaired knowledge about the human body, with preserved awareness of the mental body schema (Sirigu et al., 1991; Goldenberg, 1997; Denes et al., 2000; Guariglia et al., 2002). It is the inability to localize body parts on one's own or on someone else's body, on verbal or nonverbal command, despite preserved knowledge of their location and the ability to name them. When asked to give verbal descriptions of body parts, some patients describe the function and the individual visual appearance of body parts, but when asked to describe their location, could not. The reverse finding was reported by Dennis (1976) in a patient who could localize body parts (with nonverbal instructions) but could not define or understand names of body parts. This suggests a double dissociation of the processing systems involved in these two systems (lexical and visuospatial representations of body). In patients with autotopagnosia both systems seem to be intact. These patients have an intact lexical representation and are able to name the body parts pointed at by someone else or shown in pictures. They can locate their own body parts to which small objects are attached, suggesting intact visuospatial representation of their bodies. However, they seem to suffer from an inability to link these two preserved systems, i.e., visuospatial representation of one's own body with lexical (semantic) knowledge about the body. Autotopagnosia is usually associated with lesions of the left posterior parietal lobe.

Gerstmann Syndrome

Lesions involving the heteromodal regions of the angular gyrus in the language-dominant hemisphere give rise to complex combinations of anomia, alexia, acalculia, agraphia, finger agnosia, and left-right disorientation in the absence of additional language deficits (Benton 1992; see Chapter 17). This collection of impairments is collectively known as the left angular gyrus (or left parietal) syndrome. The term *Gerstmann syndrome* is used to identify the clinical picture when only the last four of these deficits emerge in isolation (Benton et al., 1992). The four components of Gerstmann syndrome are discussed below.

Finger agnosia is an impairment in recognizing, identifying, differentiating, naming, selecting, indicating, and orienting individual fingers from either one's own hands or those of another person. It includes pointing to fingers named by the examiner or moving or indicating a particular finger on one hand when the same finger is stimulated on the opposite hand. In its classic form, the fingers of both hands are affected. It is often a partial defect, with the patient identifying fingers inconsistently. For example, the patient may correctly recognize his thumb and little finger but not identify the index, middle, or ring fingers, or any of the examiner's fingers. In general, the middle three fingers are hardest to recognize.

Comprehension deficit and loss of visual or somatosensory input may interfere with finger recognition and must be excluded before finger agnosia is diagnosed. The value of verbal tasks of finger identification has been called into question because they may be more sensitive to language disorders than to defective orientation on the body. However, a considerable number of patients with brain damage fail on nonverbal tasks of finger localization. To exclude a language disturbance, the patient may be asked to point to the correct finger, touched on the patient's own hand, on a hand model, or on a drawing. Formal tests are available and explained in the next section.

Right-left disorientation is the inability to name or point to the right and left sides of objects, including body parts of the patient or examiner. It can represent an aphasic disturbance (i.e., incorrect verbal labeling or understanding of the words "right" and "left") or a true disturbance of egocentric spatial orientation. To assess verbally mediated right-left discrimination, the patient is asked to indicate and label right and left on his or her own body and on the examiner's. Complexity is increased with commands such as "Put your left hand on your right eye" or "Point with your left hand to my right ear." Even though these tests are used to assess right-left disorientation, they really test verbal labeling for right and left. In order to assess spatially mediated right-left discrimination, the patient can be asked, nonverbally, to touch locations on his or her own limbs corresponding to those on the examiner's body. More formal tests such as the Culver test and the standardized road map test are available (Table 14-5).

Patients with the right-left disorientation of Gerstmann syndrome are not impaired in their route-finding ability, suggesting that this is a lexical deficit rather than a manifestation of spatial disorientation. However, right-left disorientation of the type seen in Gerstmann syndrome is diagnosed only if it occurs either in the absence of aphasia or when its severity is out of proportion to the aphasia.

Acalculia (or anarithmetria) is an acquired loss of arithmetic skills (Grafman et al., 1997; Dehaene, 2003; Denburg & Tranel, 2003). Arithmetic skills include numerical facts and knowledge about execution of basic mathematical operations (i.e., addition, subtraction, multiplication, and division), each of which can be selectively disrupted by brain damage. Acalculia is a significant burden for patients because it may restrict their ability to use a checkbook, pay a bill, or exchange money.

Performance on calculation can be impeded by several factors. Poor concentration interferes with mental calculation and can also result in careless errors in written calculation (e.g., failure to notice the sign). Aphasia and alexia may interfere with number reading and writing. Hemispatial neglect interferes with perception of digits in the leftmost position while calculating. Frontal lesions may interfere with maintaining order and correctly planning in sequence, resulting in impairment of calculation skill. Primary acalculia (anarithmetria) should not be diagnosed if calculation failure is secondary to any of these factors. It has been suggested that the left hemisphere is important for precise calculations, whereas the right hemisphere is important for approximate calculations (Dehaene, 2003). It comprises up to 6% of acalculic patients with right-hemispheric lesions and 23% of acalculic patients

TABLE 14-5. Standardized Neuropsychological Tests

Tactile acuity		• von Frey's Hair Test
Tactile attention		• Face-hand test
		• Single and Double Simultaneous Stimulation Test
		• Quality Extinction Test
Body orientation	**Body part orientation**	• Orientation Test to Body Part
	Finger recognition	• Boston Diagnostic Aphasia Examination (BDAE)
		• Benton Finger Agnosia Test
	Right-left orientation	• Laterality Discrimination Test (Culver Test)
		• Standardized Road Map Test
		• Right-Left Orientation Test (RLOT)
Graphesthesia		• Ray Skin Writing Test
Acalculia		• Boston Diagnostic Aphasia Examination (BDAE)
		• Wechsler Adult Intelligence Scale III (WAIS III) (arithmetic subset)
		• Wide Range Achievement Test–3rd Edition (WRAT3)
		• Key Math Diagnostic Arithmetic Test–Revised (Key Math–R)
		• Woodcock-Johnson Tests for Achievement–Revised (WJ-R)

with left-hemispheric lesions. Different arithmetic skills (i.e., subtraction, addition) can be selectively affected.

To test basic mathematical operations, paper-and-pencil arithmetic examples can be used at bedside. Standardized tests are available (see Table 14-5).

Agraphia is the acquired loss of writing skills and is discussed in Chapter 17.

There has been considerable controversy surrounding the specificity and even the existence of Gerstmann syndrome. Skeptics have argued that the degree of intercorrelation among the four components is low, questioning the existence of a syndrome. However, it is of no importance whether the intercorrelation is low or whether it is no higher than the correlation of any component with other deficits. What is important is the predictive ability of the entire complex of components (i.e., Gerstmann syndrome). When all four components are present, it predicts with a high degree of accuracy the presence of a left angular gyrus lesion. Because counting relies on fingers, it is not surprising that calculation, finger recognition, left-right discrimination, and writing ability could all be impaired following a single lesion in the left angular gyrus.

Synesthesia

Integration of information from multiple sensory channels is a necessary prerequisite for many tasks (Schlitz et al., 1999). Besides the physiologic intersensory integration, nonphysiologic integration of sensory experiences from different modalities might rarely occur in otherwise neurologically and psychologically healthy individuals, so that a modality-specific stimulus can rarely produce perception in another modality (synesthetic perception; Rizzo & Eslinger, 1989; Grossenbacher & Lovelace, 2001). Thus, the individual has multimodal perceptual experiences from a unimodal sensory event (Rizzo & Eslinger, 1989; Palmeri et al., 2002). For example, the individual might experience the intense feeling of touching shapes on tasting something (taste-shape synesthesia). Synesthesia can also be induced by only thinking about a particular concept (synesthetic conception). For example, in number-location synesthesia, each counting number has a location in space relative to its neighbors.

Synesthesia may be developmental or acquired, and many cases have a clear neural basis (Schlitz et al., 1999). Acquired cases may follow brain lesion, sensory deafferentation or drug effects (e.g., LSD or mescaline) (Grossenbacher & Lovelace, 2001).

In synesthesia there is a remarkable consistency of association over time. Although there is inter-individual variability, a given individual's synesthesia is specific and consistent. There also appears to be a strong familial clustering of synesthesia, with a female-to-male ratio of 6:1, suggesting a genetic basis (Schlitz et al., 1999).

Cerebral blood flow changes that have been reported during synesthesia include areas in the association cortices, right prefrontal cortex, insula, and superior temporal gyrus, but not in the primary sensory areas (Nunn et al., 2002).

Several studies suggest that synesthesia arises from cross-modal associative ability of the limbic systems, which have multiple sensory inputs essential for multimodal associations (Rizzo & Eslinger, 1989; Grossenbacher et al., 2001). In particular, the cortical areas in the STS, which are connected to unimodal sensory cortices and contain neurons responsive to stimuli in multiple sense modalities, may mediate pathway convergence necessary for synesthesia. If synesthesia involves normal neural connections, then the study of synesthesia might improve our understanding of multisensory issues in normal, the nonsynesthetic perception.

Psychogenic (Hysteric) Somatosensory Symptoms and Signs

Somatic symptoms and signs that cannot be attributed to organic pathology constitute a broad spectrum of disorders, referred to as the somatoform disorders (Ron, 1994). As one of these disorders, hysteria refers to those unexplained symptoms and signs that suggest a neurologic cause, for example, somatosensory deficits or paralysis (Marsden, 1986; Vuilleumier et al., 2001). Its incidence is about 1% of all neurologic patients (Marsden, 1986). Interestingly, most of these patients have an underlying organic disease (Slater et al., 1965; Whitlock et al., 1967), and psychological factors are evident in only 20% of the cases (Marsden, 1986). One study demonstrated that 13% of patients with neurologic disease were originally thought to have a psychiatric disorder (Tissenbaum et al., 1951). Patients attempt to convince the doctor to determine the real cause of the problem. Their anxiety leads to elaboration and exaggeration of their symptoms.

In the *Diagnostic and Statistical Manual of Mental Disorders IV-R*, the American Psychiatric Association adopts the term conversion disorder (American Psychiatric Association, 2000). Conversion was an idea, introduced by Freud, to explain hysterical symptoms as the result of transformation of inner subconscious conflict into physical complaints. The resolution of this unconscious conflict is the primary gain, and the advantage resulting from the assumption of the sick role is the secondary gain (Ron, 1994). It has to be differentiated from malingering (for secondary gain, see Chapter 53) or factitious disorder (primary gain: being the center of attention) (American Psychiatric Association, 2000).

The most common symptom in conversion disorder is gait disturbances, followed by tremor and paralysis (Marsden, 1986). However, somatosensory complaints are not uncommon. The somatosensory evoked potential and the response of primary motor cortex to stimulation are normal in these patients (Kaplan et al., 1985; Morota et al., 1994), but the normal arrival of sensory signal to somatosensory cortex does not lead to a conscious perception (Marsden, 1986). It seems that the brain dissociates conscious awareness from mechanism of somatosensory perception.

PET experiments in patients with conversion disorder showed that the attempt to move the paralyzed leg failed to activate the corresponding motor cortex, but instead activated the right orbitofrontal and anterior cingulate cortex, which inhibited the prefrontal (willed) effects on the right primary motor cortex (Marshall et al., 1997). This finding is also consistent with the previous report that psychogenic paresthesia was associated with simultaneous activation of frontal inhibitory areas and inhibition of the somatosensory cortex (Tiihonen et al., 1995). Several studies demonstrate hypoactivity of contralateral thalamus and basal ganglia circuits during bilateral hand vibration, despite normal activity in the primary somatosensory and premotor cortices (Vuilleumier et al., 2001). It has been suggested that abnormal striatal and thalamic activity represent only downstream effects due to primary dysfunction in orbitofrontal, cingulate, or prefrontal cortex. Anterior cingulate has been implicated in both cognitive and motivational processes. In short, conversion disorder may depend on pathologic interactions between limbic structures and striatothalamocortical circuits.

Because conversion and neglect symptoms are more common on the left side, similar pathophysiology has been postulated (Marshall et al., 1997; Vuilleumier et al., 2001). Indeed, both phenomena involve the striatothalamocortical loop, and in both cases there is a discrepancy between awareness in the patients and objective neurologic functions. Whereas in neglect, patients have deficits due to physical damage but have no awareness, in conversion disorder, patients experience deficit in the absence of physical damage. It is postulated that the selective impairment of attentional or motivational mechanisms, operating at the level of thalamus or basal ganglia to influence cortical sensorimotor processes, can lead to neglect and conversion disorder, respectively. This attentional or motivational modulation may be triggered outside conscious will by various emotional stressors. Interestingly, altered activity in these areas have been shown in patients with fibromyalgia (Mountz et al., 1995), and in individuals undergoing acupuncture treatment (Hui et al., 2000), two conditions where, presumably, both physiologic and motivational factors are involved.

AGING OF SOMATOSENSORY SYSTEM

The effects of lesions in the somatosensory system are compounded by the effects of aging. During normal aging, tactile sensitivity declines in a variety of domains, such as von Frey thresholds (described below), spatial acuity, and discrimination of vibratory frequency, especially in the high-frequency range (Sathian et al., 1997). Tactile spatial threshold and its inter-individual variation increase significantly (25%) with age. The loss in tactile spatial acuity was found on a variety of tests, which included discrimination of length and orientation, accurate tactile localization, and two-point discrimination (Sathian et al., 1997). This loss may be due to age-related biologic changes, such as thinning of the epidermis and a decrease in collagen, in elastin, or in the density of Meissner corpuscles (Thornbury & Mistretta, 1981). Stevens and Choo (1996) measured spatial acuity at 13 different body sites and found that sensitivity declined with age at some sites more than at others. The feet and hands showed the greatest drop in sensitivity, a result that may be due to reduced circulation (Craig & Rollman, 1999).

APPROACH TO DIAGNOSIS OF SOMATOSENSORY DISORDERS

Assessment Tools

Clinical Neurologic Evaluation

Somatosensory disorders have been diagnosed mainly with "bedside" screening techniques that vary between examiners and are rarely standardized. Nevertheless, neurologists have used these techniques successfully over many years (Haerer et al., 1992).

The clinical sensory examination is performed to determine the quality, severity, and localization of somatosensory change. There may be any of the following: loss, decrease, or increase of sensation; dissociation of sensation with loss of one type but not of others; and abnormal sensation (discussed earlier). More than one of these may occur simultaneously.

Before starting the examination, the examiner should determine whether the patient is aware of subjective change in sensation or is experiencing spontaneous sensations of an abnormal type. If such symptoms are present, the examiner should attempt to determine their type and character, intensity, exact distribution, duration, and periodicity, as well as factors that trigger, increase, and decrease them. Psychogenic symptoms and signs are often associated with inappropriate affect (either excessive emotion or indifference) and are vague in character or location, and reactions to them are not consistent with the degree of disability.

The main principle of somatosensory examination is that it relies on a patient's subjective responses and her or his full cooperation. Although negative somatosensory phenomena should be verified through physical examination, positive somatosensory phenomena may not be associated with any physical findings. It is advisable to perform the investigation of the sensory system early in the course of the neurologic examination. It is most accurate if the patient is alert. Fatigue makes the findings less reliable. During the examination the patient should be warm and comfortable. The proximal sensory examination should be compared with the distal as well as the contralateral area. The patient's eyes must remain closed during the entire examination.

The clinical sensory examination includes the sense of pain, temperature, touch, vibration, position, and cortical sensory testing.

Pain sensation is generally tested by holding the sharp end of a safety pin between the thumb and index finger with sufficient pressure so that it slides slightly to contact the patient. The patient should not be asked "Do you feel this?" or "Is this sharp?" but instead should be instructed to reply "sharp" or "dull." The pin or safety pin should be sterile and must be discarded after use on a single patient to avoid the risk of transmitting disease from accidental puncturing of the patient's skin.

Temperature sense is tested by touching the skin in the area with cold metal such as a tuning fork. Areas of temperature loss often overlap with areas of loss of sensitivity to pain.

Light touch is adequately tested with a wisp of cotton.

Vibration sense is tested by placing a tuning fork in vibration and holding it on the great toe or over the lateral or medial malleolus until the patient no longer feels it vibrate. The fork is then quickly moved to the corresponding point on the opposite limb. A tuning fork of 128 Hz is most frequently used, although some experts believe that a fork of 256 Hz may detect finer changes in the vibratory threshold. Many examiners consider vibration sense to be "normal" when the patient perceives maximum vibration; a much more sensitive criterion, however, is the ability to feel the fork when it has almost stopped vibrating. An asymmetry or difference between the two sides usually indicates a structural lesion.

Position sense is tested by grasping the side of the finger or the great toe and asking the patient, with his eyes closed, to indicate whether the digit is moved into an up or down position. Thus, passive movement of the joint is being tested. The digit should be grasped proximally and laterally to eliminate pressure cues. The digit should also be separated from adjoining ones so that no clues from contact are provided. The patient should be instructed not to attempt active movement of the digit, which may help to judge its position. If there is distal position sense loss, the proximal joint should be assessed. Position sense can also be examined by observation of the station and gait. A patient with significantly diminished sensations of movement and of position in the lower extremities is not aware of the position of his feet or of the posture of his body. The patient can assume a stable, erect posture when standing with eyes open, but sways and falls with eyes closed (positive Romberg sign). The patient can walk fairly well with eyes open, but with eyes closed, staggers and may fall (sensory ataxia).

Testing of higher-level somatosensory functions includes two-point discrimination: touch localization, tactile attention, graphesthesia, stereognosis, tactile perception, tactile recognition, tactile memory, and tactile naming.

Two-point discrimination is usually tested by a compass or a calibrated two-point esthesiometer. Bending a paper clip to different distances between its two points is less quantitative but available for quick evaluation. The patient is stimulated randomly by a single point and by two points. Stimuli that are about 1 mm apart can be detected on the normal fingertips, whereas they may have to be as far as 7 cm apart in areas of the back.

Topesthesia, or topognosia, is the ability to localize a tactile sensation. It is usually tested by light pressure of the examiner's fingertip, asking the patient, whose eyes are closed, to localize the site of touch. Neurologically normal individuals will immediately identify each finger touched, although they may make an error in distinguishing the third and fourth fingers. Note that a defective performance does not imply the presence of "finger agnosia," which affects both hands and is tested with eyes open.

Tactile attention is usually tested by bilateral simultaneous stimulation at analogous sites, for example, dorsa of both hands, to determine if the patient's perception of touch is extinguished on one side of the body. Cotton or touch with the fingertip can be used as stimuli.

Graphesthesia is tested by the ability to recognize numbers or letters drawn on the patient's palm by the examiner's fingertip or by a pencil or a dull pen. The patient is then asked to identify them. Easily identifiable, dissimilar numbers should be used, for example, 3 and 4 rather than 3 and 8.

Stereognosis includes perception of texture (roughness, softness) and shape (size, length, geometry, etc.). Texture perception can be examined by the use of solid objects, such as sandpaper or a plastic or wooden ball. Shape perception may be tested by the use of objects of the same size but different shapes, such as a circle, a square, or a triangle cut out of paper or plastic.

Tactile perception, recognition, and *naming* are evaluated by placing simple objects such as a key, button, comb, pencil, or safety pin in the hand of the blindfolded patient and asking her to identify them, through verbal, pointing, and matching tasks. Cross-modal matching (tactile-verbal, tactile-visual) is also important in evaluating the scope of the recognition defect, by asking the patient to draw misidentified objects or to tactually select them from a group. Tactile exploratory behavior should also be carefully observed. Organically intact adults are able to perform tactile recognition and discrimination tests with virtually complete accuracy. A single erroneous response or even evidence of hesitancy suggests that this function may be impaired. However, if not, the other hand needs to be tested, and used as a control.

Neuropsychological Evaluation

Although neurologic "bedside" techniques are rarely standardized, there are standardized neuropsychological tests for the somatosensory system (Lezak, 1995), as follows.

Tests of Tactile Sensation, Acuity, or Threshold. Before examining higher-order or cortical tactile-perceptual functions, the integrity of the somatosensory system in the area of neuropsychological interest—usually the hands—should be evaluated (see discussion of the neurologic examination in the previous section). A more quantitative method to test the tactile threshold or tactile acuity is to use the von Frey's hair set (Von Frey & Kiesow, 1899; Thornbury & Mistretta, 1981; Pitcher et al., 1999). A set contains a certain number of nylon monofilaments of equal length but different diameter in millimeters. The force (gm) required to bend each monofilament is precalibrated and measured in gm. A see-through and irregular surface such as wire mesh or a smooth opaque surface is a commonly used apparatus to allow their application. Mechanical force is exerted via application of a particular hair to the cutaneous receptor field until buckling of the hair occurs. The bending force necessary to induce touch sensation is a measure for touch threshold.

Higher-Order Somatosensory Tests. Tests for astereognosis, tactile perception, recognition, and naming are commonly performed in neurologic examinations and were discussed earlier. Other standardized neuropsychological tests that assess for graphesthesia, tactile attention, body orientation, and acalculia are available (Lezak, 1995; see Table 14-5).

Electrophysiologic Evaluation

In the clinical setting, nerve conduction study and electromyography (NCS/EMG) are used to evaluate peripheral nerve function, and SEPs are used to evaluate central somatosensory conduction pathways (Nuwer, 1998).

SEPs are event-related potentials attributed mainly to synchronized extracellular currents from summated postsynaptic potentials or pyramidal cells in S-I (Knecht et al., 1996; Mima et al., 1997; Nuwer, 1998) (see Chapter 8). It is performed by stimulating the median nerve in the upper extremity or posterior tibial nerve in the lower extremity with a transcutaneous delivery of an electrical stimulus. The transmission of the nerve action potential can be recorded at several points, including somatosensory cortices using a scalp needle electrode. It can be used clinically to detect, localize, and quantify a focal interruption or lesions along these pathways.

The early component of the somatosensory evoked potential, the N20 component, can be used as an indicator for the integrity of S-I (Knecht et al., 1996).

Touch threshold, vibration sense, thermesthesia, and nociception are not correlated with N20, suggesting that these functions are mediated mainly by subcortical structures. Two-point discrimination, graphesthesia, and stereognosis are correlated with N20, suggesting that they are primarily mediated by cortical structures. Using SEPs, localizations of these cortical sensory functions were determined as located anterior to posterior (S-I to area 5): two-point discrimination, position sense, and stereognosis.

Somatosensory evoked magnetic fields (SEFs) can be recorded using magnetoencephalography (MEG) (Hari & Forss, 1999; Korvenoja et al., 1999). In MEG studies, weak magnetic fields generated by cerebral currents are detected outside the head with superconducting sensors. The magnetic field pattern is then mapped and the most probable source current distribution within the brain is calculated. It has been used to confirm noninvasively the well-known somatotopic representation of S-I, detected during cortical stimulation and by intracranial recording. Using simple tactile stimulation, activity within areas S-I, S-II, 5, 7, SSA, and SMA were recorded. The serial versus parallel processing in the somatosensory network can be studied with MEG. The excellent temporal resolution of MEG nicely complements anatomically accurate fMRI and PET and allows detailed investigations of somatosensory processing. They measure not only simple primary sensory pathways, but also higher-order somatosensory functions.

Neuroimaging

The structure of the human somatosensory system can be studied using detailed structural neuroimaging techniques such as CT and MRI. The organization and function of human somatosensory systems can be studied noninvasively, using functional neuroimaging such as PET (Bonda et al., 1995; Roland et al., 1998; Banati et al., 2000; Bodegård et al., 2000; Coghill et al., 2001; see Chapter 6) and fMRI (Gelnar et al., 1998; Gordon et al., 1998; Maldjian et al., 1999; Polonara et al., 1999; Takeda et al., 1999; Moore et al., 2000; Fabri et al., 2001; Ruben et al., 2001; Deuchert et al., 2002; see Chapter 7). Their clinical applications are areas for future research.

Localization

Sensory symptoms and signs can result from lesions at any level of the nervous system. It is important to emphasize that patients with central behavioral somatosensory disorders may also have peripheral disease of the somatosensory system (e.g., head injury associated with spinal injury or stroke in a patient with alcoholic polyneuropathy). There may be diminished sensation (hypoesthesia) or loss of sensation (anesthesia) in one or more modalities, or abnormal sensation (paresthesia, pain) that can be either constant on intermittent. The distribution and nature of sensory symptoms and signs can help localize the lesion (Haerer, 1992; Asbury, 1998).

With peripheral nerve lesions, the distribution of symptoms and signs follows the areas innervated by those specific nerves. In mononeuropathy (e.g., carpal tunnel syndrome), the distribution follows the territory innervated by the specific nerve. In cases of radiculopathy (nerve root), the distribution is segmental and follows the corresponding dermatome. The distribution in polyneuropathy follows a stocking-glove pattern.

With spinal cord or brainstem lesions, the sensory loss is usually dissociated, with impairment of certain modalities and sparing of others. In diseases of the spinal cord there is usually a dissociation of proprioception from pain and temperature sensation. In hemisection of the spinal cord (the Brown-Sequard syndrome) there is contralesional loss of pain and temperature sensation and ipsilesional loss of proprioception and motor strength. There may be bowel and bladder incontinence and hyperreflexia. The Lhermitte sign, which consists of sudden electric-like or painful sensations, spreading down the body or into the back or extremities on flexion of the neck, can be seen in diseases of the posterior columns, particularly of the cervical cord (e.g., multiple sclerosis). There may be sensory loss with brainstem lesions, ipsilateral on the face and contralateral on the body (paradoxical dissociation). With thalamic lesion one can see a hemisensory loss that may be associated with pain (see Déjérine-Roussy syndrome).

Cortical lesions may show cortical sensory loss, such as diminished two-point discrimination or touch localization, astereognosis, agraphesthesia, tactile agnosia, tactile anomia, tactile extinction or neglect, autotopagnosia, finger agnosia, tactile hallucinations, or synesthesia (see Table 14-3 through 14-5).

In hysteria (conversion disorder), changes in sensory perception do not correspond to known physiologic distribution. The borders of the anesthetic area may be sharply defined (e.g., exactly in the midline). There may be a midline change for the sense of vibration over the bony areas, such as the skull or sternum, anatomically impossible because of the continuity of the bone stimulated. Despite complaints of marked anesthesia, some of these individuals may identify objects by touch and perform skilled movements and fine acts for which cutaneous sensations are indispensable and retain postural sensation even though all other sensations are lost. These patients are influenced by suggestion and may vary their report from examination to examination. Hysterical changes and malingering can often be demonstrated by asking the patient to say "yes" when he is stimulated and "no" when he is not stimulated; he will often say "no" every time the pseudoanesthetic area is touched. In conclusion, it should be emphasized that all so-called hysterical somatosensory symptoms and signs require thorough investigation.

Common Etiologies

By far the most common causes for somatosensory symptoms and signs are diseases of the peripheral nervous system, such as compressive mononeuropathy (e.g., carpal tunnel syndrome), polyneuropathy (e.g., due to diabetes or alcohol use), and radiculopathy (e.g., due to a herniated disk). However, they may also result from diseases of the CNS. Although migraine and epilepsy cause episodic positive sensations at all ages, other diseases have predilections for certain ages; for example, multiple sclerosis in young to middle-aged patients, brain tumor in middle-aged to elderly patients, and stroke and degenerative diseases in elderly patients. Degeneration of primary and association somatosensory cortices can cause gradually progressive astereognosis. Tactile object recognition occasionally is more severely affected than more basic somatosensory functions, though it is rarely pure when it occurs in a degenerative context. Although a tumor or other structural lesion should be sought, severe somatosensory impairment evolving over a few years in an elderly patient is commonly degenerative. Several pathologic patterns have been described, including corticobasal degeneration, Alzheimer disease, and Pick disease.

TREATMENT OF SOMATOSENSORY DISORDERS

Whereas positive syndromes (see Table 14-3) are treated mainly with medication, negative syndromes (see Table 14-4), including many of the behavioral somatosensory disorders discussed above, benefit primarily from cognitive rehabilitation. Several examples follow.

Medical Therapy for Positive Symptoms and Signs

Déjérine-Roussy Syndrome

Treatments include pharmacologic, physical, and stimulation therapy (Schott, 1995; Berić et al., 1998). Pharmacotherapies include tricyclic antidepressants such as nortriptyline; anticonvulsants such as carbamazepine, gabapentin, or lamotrigine; lidocaine patches; and clonidine. Narcotics such as morphine can be used as adjuvant therapy. For more intractable pain, stimulation techniques range from simple noninvasive transcutaneous electrical nerve stimulation (TENS) units to spinal cord and possibly deep brain stimulation. There are also recent reports that motor cortex stimulation may be helpful. The rationale behind this approach is that it may stimulate the descending inhibitory nonnociceptive sensory pathways present in the motor cortex.

Reflex Sympathetic Dystrophy

For RSD, a specific treatment plan is necessary (Gordon, 1996; Nikolajsen & Jensen, 2001; Schott, 2001). The most effective preventive measure is the efficient control of pain as soon as possible and early mobilization (Gordon, 1996; Schott, 2001). Apart from sympathetic blocking procedures (paravertebral and epidural injection with local anesthetics), there are pharmacologic, physical, and psychological treatments. Pharmacologic treatments include tricyclic antidepressants, sodium channel blocking drugs such as carbamazepine, GABA agonist agents such as gabapentin, calcitonin (100–160 IU/d by intramuscular injections), and steroids (prednisone 60 mg/d and a slow taper over a month). Stimulation procedures include acupuncture, TENS unit, and spinal cord and deep brain stimulation. Physical therapy is very important and consists of resting and elevating the affected joints to prevent vascular stasis. The joints should be gently mobilized several times a day. If the patient does not respond to these treatments, surgical sympathectomy may be considered. New developments include the use of neurotrophic factors to reverse the phenotypic changes that occur in the dorsal horn and the use of pharmacologic agents to block the activity-dependent NMDA channels that appear to be instrumental in maintaining central sensitization. In view of the difficulties of treatments for RSD, cognitive behavioral and other psychological techniques that aim to help patients deal with their pain rather than to cure it are becoming more important.

Phantom Limb Perception and Pain

Pharmacologic, neurosurgical, physical, environmental, and psychological treatments are available (Finnoff, 2001; Nikolajsen & Jensen, 2001). Pharmacologic treatments include β-blockers, anticonvulsants, tricyclic antidepressants, baclofen, tizanadine, neuroleptics, calcitonin, ketamine, and epidural and regional anesthesia. Neurosurgical treatment includes deep brain stimulation of thalamus or periaqueductal gray. For further information on pain, see Chapter 33. Physical treatments include acupuncture, ultrasound, massage, TENS, and rigid postoperative dressing for edema control, with TENS being the most effective. Environmental treatments include avoidance of food and physical behavior that exacerbate the pain. Psychological treatments include preamputation counseling regarding body image, limb loss, relaxation, and biofeedback.

Cognitive Rehabilitation for Negative Symptoms and Signs

Whereas neuronal regeneration is almost nonexistent in the human CNS, neuronal plasticity does exist. The focus of rehabilitation is to use this plasticity to reorganize the sensorimotor representation in brain (Carel et al., 2000). Patients may adapt better to an existing strategy than learning new strategies (Swinnen et al., 2000).

This can be achieved through passive training with repeated proprioceptive stimulation (Loubinoux et al., 2000), a multicontext approach with intense verbal cueing and organizational strategies, or computer-assisted training (Perez et al., 1996).

One such example is the recent report of successful treatment of patients with phantom limb pain. Because in these patients the cortical representation of the mouth area expands to the area that formerly represented the amputated limb, sensory discrimination training, that is, synchronous or asynchronous tactile stimulation of the lip and residual limb, has been used to segregate both regions, and could provide an effective intervention for phantom limb pain (Flor et al., 2001; Huse et al., 2001). Furthermore, chronic motor cortex stimulation, through virtual movement of the amputated limb, led to inhibition of somatosensory cortex and reduction of phantom limb phenomena (Roux et al., 2001). Finally, visual feedback via a mirror has been used successfully to simulate virtual movement of the phantom limb, unclenching the spasms, and successful pain relief (Ramachandran & Rogers-Ramachandran, 2000).

Another example of behavioral training as treatment for a behavioral somatosensory disorder has been described for patients with neglect phenomenon (Làdavas et al., 1994). The interaction between the visual and tactile system has been used to treat and rehabilitate patients with extinction and neglect. Stimulation of one side in one modality may reduce extinction of another modality.

SUMMARY

The somatosensory stimuli we encounter in everyday life are complex. Different properties of these stimuli selectively activate different receptor organs. This information is then transmitted by a population of different types of sensory neurons and conveyed in parallel pathways to the somatosensory cortices, where it all is combined into a unified somatosensory percept. Different areas of the brain are involved in different aspects of tactile perception, recognition, memory, and naming. Information processing can be disrupted at any of these different levels, resulting in different but specific and recognizable clinical entities, both positive and negative behavioral somatosensory disorders. Knowledge about the somatosensory system, combined with comprehensive neurologic, neuropsychological, electrophysiologic, and recently functional imaging examinations provide the necessary tools for accurate diagnosis and effective treatment of patients with behavioral somatosensory disorders.

Acknowledgments

I would like to dedicate this chapter first and foremost to my dear parents: Masoumeh and Mahmood Razavi; my dear sister and her family: Marjan, Johann, David, and Daniel Kreuter; my dear brother and his family: Behzad, Lida, and Nasim Razavi; my dear extended family: Jamileh, Faramarz, Farzin, Farshad, Fariborz, Majid, Masoud, and Manootchehr Razavi, Hosein Esfandiari, and Ali Sadeghi; and my dear mentors: Arezou and Saeed Tofighi, Amir Arsham Amini, Mehrdad Baghestanian, Richard Marz, and the late Werner Resch. You all inspired and supported me, and I owe you my deepest gratitude.

■ KEY POINTS

☐   Somatosensory information is processed in both hierarchical and parallel pathways from receptor organs in the periphery to somatosensory cortices. This information is processed in dual streams by the somatosensory cortices.

☐   The ventral stream mediates tactile object perception, recognition, learning, and memory ("what" pathway). Lesion in this pathway can result in astereognosis (ahylognosis, amorphognosis), apperceptive tactile agnosia, associative tactile agnosia, or tactile anomia.

☐   The dorsal stream mediates tactile object localization, spatiotemporal functions, body representation, and sensorimotor integration ("where" pathway). Lesions in this pathway can result in tactile apraxia or optic ataxia.

☐   The basic awareness of one's own body has been conceptualized as a mental body schema. One also has a general knowledge about the functions, locations, and names of body parts. Examples of disorders with impaired awareness of the mental body schema, but preserved knowledge of the human body, are phantom limb syndrome and hemineglect syndrome. In contrast, patients with autotopagnosia have preserved awareness of the mental body schema, but impaired knowledge of the human body.

☐   Positive somatosensory syndromes include reflex sympathetic dystrophy (RSD), Déjérine-Roussy syndrome, tactile hallucination (simple and complex), phantom limb phenomena (perception and pain), and synesthesia.

☐   Whereas positive syndromes are treated mainly with medication, negative syndromes, including many of the behavioral somatosensory disorders, benefit primarily from cognitive rehabilitation.

KEY READINGS

Bodegård A, Geyer S, Grefkes C, et al: Hierarchical processing of tactile shape in the human brain. Neuron 31:317–328, 2001.

Caselli RJ: Ventrolateral and dorsomedial somatosensory association cortex damage produces distinct somesthetic syndromes in humans. Neurology 43:762–771, 1993.

Saetti MC, De Renzi E, Comper M: Tactile morphagnosia secondary to spatial deficits. Neuropsychologia 37:1087–1100, 1999.

Valenza N, Ptak R, Zimine I, et al: Dissociated active and passive tactile shape recognition. A case study of pure tactile apraxia. Brain 124:2287–2298, 2001.

REFERENCES

Afifi A, Bergmann RA: Functional Neuroanatomy. New York: McGraw-Hill, 1998.

Allison T, McCarthy G, Luby M, et al: Localization of functional regions of human mesial cortex by somatosensory evoked potential recording and by cortical stimulation. Electroencephalogr Neurophysiol 100:126–140, 1996.

American Psychiatric Association: Diagnostic and Statistical Manual of Mental Disorders, ed 4, revised. Washington, DC: Author, 2000.

Andersen RA: Multimodal integration for the representation of space in the posterior parietal cortex. Phil Trans R Soc Lond B Biol Sci 352:1421–1428, 1997.

Appenzeller O, Bicknell JM: Effects of nervous system lesions on phantom experience in amputees. Neurology 19:141–146, 1969.

Asbury AK: Numbness, tingling, and sensory loss, in Isselbacher KJ, Braunwald E, Wilson JD, et al (eds): Harrison's Principles of Internal Medicine, ed 14. New York, NY: McGraw-Hill, 1998, pp. 128–132.

Banati RB, Goeres GW, Tjoa C, et al: The functional anatomy of visual-tactile intergration in man: A study using positron emission tomogrpahy. Neuropsychologia 38:115–124, 2000.

Bechara A, Damasio AR, Damasio H, et al: Insensitivity to future consequences following damage to human prefrontal cortex. Cognition 50:7–15, 1994.

Benton AL: Gerstmann's syndrome. Arch Neurol 49:445–447, 1992.

Berić A: Central pain and dysesthesia syndrome. Neuropathic Pain Syndr 16:899–918, 1998.

Berlucchi G, Aglioti S: The body in the brain. Neural bases of corporeal awareness. Trends Neurosci 20:560–564, 1997.

Berti A, Oxbury S, Oxbury J, et al: Somatosensory extinction for meaningful objects in a patient with right hemispheric stroke. Neuropsychologia 37:333–343, 1999.

Binkofski F, Dohle C, Posse S, et al: Human anterior intraparietal area subserves prehension: A combined lesions and functional MRI activation study. Neurology 50:1253–1259, 1998.

Binkofski F, Kunesch E, Classen J, et al: Tactile apraxia unimodal apractic disorder of tactile object exploration associated with parietal lobe lesions. Brain 124:132–144, 2001.

Blakemore SJ, Goodbody SJ, Wolpert DM: Predicting the consequences of our own actions: The role of sensorimotor context estimation. J Neurosci 18:7511–7518, 1998.

Bodegård A, Geyer S, Grefkes C, et al: Hierarchical processing of tactile shape in the human brain. Neuron 31:317–328, 2001.

Bodegård A, Ledberg A, Geyer S, et al: Object shape differences reflected by somatosensory cortical activation in human. J Neurosci 20:RC51(1–5), 2000.

Bonda E, Petrides M, Frey S, et al: Neural correlates of mental transformations of the body-in-space. Proc Natl Acad Sci U S A 92:11180–11184, 1995.

Campero M, Serra J, Marchettini P, et al: Ectopic impulse generation and autoexcitation in single myelinated afferent fibers in patients with peripheral neuropathy and positive sensory symptoms. Muscle Nerve 21:1661–1667, 1998.

Carel C, Loubinoux I, Boulanouar K, et al: Neural substrate for the effects of passive training on sensorimotor cortical representation: A study on the functional magnetic resonance imaging in healthy subjects. J Cereb Blood Flow Metab 20:478–484, 2000.

Carlson M: Characteristics of sensory deficits following lesions of Brodmann's areas 1 and 2 in the postcentral gyrus of *Macaca mulatta*. Brain Res 204:424–430, 1981.

Caselli RJ: Rediscovering tactile agnosia. Mayo Clin Proc 66:129–142, 1991.

Caselli RJ: Ventrolateral and dorsomedial somatosensory association cortex damage produces distinct somesthetic syndromes in humans. Neurology 43:762–771, 1993.

Coghill RC, Gildron I, Iadarola J: Hemispheric lateralization of somatosensory processing. J Neurophysiol 85:2602–2612, 2001.

Craig JC, Rollman GB: Somesthesis. Annu Rev Psychol 50:305–331, 1999.

Damasio AR, Tranel D. Damasio H: Somatic markers and the guidance of behavior: Theory and preliminary testing, in Levin H, Eisenberg H, Benton A (eds): Frontal Lobe Function and Injury. New York: Oxford University Press, 1991, pp. 217–229.

Darling WG, Rizzo M, Butler AJ: Disordered sensorimotor transformations for reaching following posterior cortical lesions. Neuropsychologia 39:237–254, 2001.

Debowy DJ, Ghosh S, Ro JY, et al: Comparison of neuronal firing rates in somatosensory and posterior parietal cortex during prehension. Exp Brain Res 137:269–291, 2001.

Dehaene S: Acalculia and number processing disorders, in Feinberg TE, Farah MJ (eds): Behavioral Neurology and Neuropsychology. New York: McGraw-Hill, 2003, pp. 207–215.

Delay JPL: Les astéréognosies: Pathologie du toucher, clinique, physiologie, topographie. Paris, France: Masion, 1935.

Denburg N, Tranel D: Acalculia and disturbances of the body schema, in Heilman KM, Valenstein E (eds): Clinical Neuropsychology, ed 4. New York: Oxford University Press, pp. 161–184.

Denes G, Cappelletti JY, Zilli T, et al: A category-specific deficit of spatial representation: The case of autotopagnosia. Neuropsychologia 38:345–350, 2000.

Dennis M: Dissociated naming and locating of body parts after left anterior temporal lobe resection: An experimental case study. Brain Lang 3:147–163, 1976.

Deuchert M, Ruben J, Schwiemann J, et al: Event-related fMRI of the somatosensory system using electrical finger stimulation. Neuroreport 13:365–369, 2002.

Dowman R, Schell S: Evidence that the anterior cingulate and supplementary somatosensory cortices generate the pain-related negative difference potential. Clin Neurophysiol 111:2117–2126, 1999.

Driver J, Spence C: Attention and the crossmodal construction of space. Trends Cogn Sci 2:254–262, 1998.

Endo K, Makishita H, Yanagisawa N, et al: Modality specific naming and gesture disturbances: A case with optic aphasia, bilateral tactile aphasia, optic apraxia and tactile apraxia. Cortex 32:3–28, 1996.

Endo K, Miyasaka M, Makishita H, et al: Tactile agnosia and tactile aphasia. Symptomatological and anatomical differences. Cortex 28:445–469, 1992.

Evans JA: Reflex sympathetic dystrophy. Surg Clin North Am 26:780–790, 1946.

Fabri M, Polonara G, Del Pesce M, et al: Posterior corpus callosum and interhemispheric transfer of somatosensory information. An fMRI and neuropsychological study of a partially callosotomized patient. J Cogn Neurosci 13:1071–1079, 2001.

Faggin BM, Nguyen Kt, Nicolelis MA: Immediate and simultaneous sensory reorganization at cortical and subcortical levels of the somatosensory system. Proc Nat Acad Sci U S A 94:9428–9433, 1997.

Fechner G: Elements of psychophysics, in Howes DH, Boring EG (eds): Elemente der Psychophysik [Elements of Psychophysics]. Adler HE (translator). New York: Holt, Rinehart and Wilson, Vol. 1, 1968.

Finnoff J: Differentiation and treatment of phantom sensation, phantom pain, and residual-limb pain. J Am Podiatr Med Assoc 91:23–33, 2001.

Flor H, Elbert T, Knecht S: Phantom-limb pain as a perceptual correlate of cortical reorganization following arm amputation. Nature 375:482–484, 1995.

Flor H, Denke C, Schaefer M, et al: Effect of sensory discrimination training on cortical reorganization and phantom limb pain. Lancet 357:1763–1764, 2001.

Flor H, Mühlnickel W, Karl A, et al: A neural substrate of nonpainful phantom limb phenomena. Neuroreport 11:1407–1411, 2000.

Florence SH, Taub HB, Kaas JH: Large-scale sprouting of cortical connections after peripheral injury in adult macaque monkeys. Science 282:1117–1121, 1998.

Freund H-J: The parietal lobe as a sensorimotor interface: A perspective from clinical and neuroimaging data. Neuroimage 14:S142–S146, 2001.

Fukatsu R, Fujii T, Yamadori A: Pure somaesthetic alexia: Somaesthetic-verbal disconnection for letters. Brain 121:843–850, 1998.

Fukumoto M, Ushida T, Zinchuk VS, et al: Contralateral thalamic perfusion in patients with reflex sympathetic dystrophy syndrome. Lancet 354:1790–1791, 1999.

Gelnar PA, Krauss BR, Szeverenyi NM, et al: Fingertip representation in the human somatosensory cortex. An fMRI study. Neuroimage 7:261–283, 1998.

Gescheider GA: Psychophysics: The Fundamentals. Mahwah, NJ: Lawrence Erlbaum, 1997.

Geyer S, Schleicher A, Schormann T, et al: Integration of microstructural and functional aspects of human somatosensory areas 3a, 3b, and 1 on the basis of a computerized brain atlas. Anat Embryol 204:351–366, 2001.

Geyer S, Schleicher A, Zilles K: Areas 3a, 3b, and 1 of human primary somatosensory cortex. Neuroimage 10:63–83, 1999.

Goldberg G: Supplementary motor area structure and function: Review and hypothesis. Behav Brian Sci 8:567–616, 1985.

Goldenberg G: Disorders of body perception, in Feinberg TE, Farah M (eds): Behavioral Neurology and Neuropsychology, ed 2. New York: McGraw-Hill, 2003, pp. 285–300.

Gonzales GR, Lewis SA, Weaver AL: Tactile illusion perception in patients with central pain. Mayo Clin Proc 76:267–274, 2001.

Gordon AM, Lee J-H, Flament D, et al: Functional magnetic resonance imaging of motor, sensory, and posterior parietal cortical areas during performance of sequential typing movements. Exp Brain Res 121:153–166, 1998.

Gordon N: Reflex sympathetic dystrophy. Brain Dev 18:257–262, 1996.

Graff-Radford NR: Syndromes due to acquired thalamic damage, in Feinberg TE, Farah M (eds): Behavioral Neurology and Neuropsychology. New York: McGraw-Hill, 1997, pp. 433–443.

Grafman J, Rickard T: Acalculia, in Feinberg TE, Farah M (eds): Behavioral Neurology and Neuropsychology. New York: McGraw-Hill, 1997, pp. 219–225.

Grossenbacher PG, Lovelace CT: Mechanisms of synesthesia. Cognitive and physiological constraints. Trends Cogn Sci 5:36–41, 2001.

Grüsser SM, Winter C, Mühlnickel W, et al: The relationship of perceptual phenomena and cortical reorganization in upper extremity amputees. Neuroscience 102:263–272, 2001.

Guariglia C, Piccardi L, Puglisi Allegra MC, et al : Is autotopagnosia real? EC says yes. A case study. Neuropsychologia 40:1744–1749, 2002.

Haerer AF: Dejong's The Neurologic Examination, ed 5. Philadelphia: JB Lippincott, 1992.

Hämäläinen H, Hiltunen J, Titievskaja I: FMRI activations of the SI and SII cortices during tactile stimulation depend on attention. Neuroreport 11:1673–1676, 2000.

Hari R, Forss N: Magnetoencephalography in the study of human somatosensory cortical processing. Philos Trans R Soc Lond B Biol Sci 354:1145–1154, 1999.

Harris JA, Harris IM, Diamond ME: The topography of tactile learning in humans. J Neurosci 21:1056–1061, 2001.

Hui KK, Liu J, Makris N, et al: Acupuncture modulates the limbic system and subcortical gray structures of the human brain: Evidence from fMRI studies in normal subjects. Hum Brain Map 9:13–25, 2000.

Huse E, Preissl, H, Larbig W, et al: Phantom limb pain. Lancet 358:1015, 2001 (Letter).

Iriki A, Tanaka M, Iwamura Y: Coding of modified body schema during tool use by macaque postcentral neurones. Neuroreport 7:2325–2330, 1996.

Ito K, Tanabe H, Ikejiri Y, et al: Tactile extinction to simple (elementary) and complex stimuli. Acta Neurol Scand 80:68–77, 1989.

Iwamura Y, Iriki A, Tanaka M: Bilateral hand representation in the postcentral somatosensory cortex. Nature 369:554–556, 1994.

Jeannerod M, Arbib MA Rizzolatti G, et al: Grasping objects: The cortical mechanisms of visuomotor transformation. Trends Neurosci 18:314–320, 1995.

Johansen-Berg H, Christensen V, Woolrich M, et al: Attention to touch modulates activity in both primary and secondary somatosensory areas. Neuroreport 11:1237–1241, 2000.

Johnson KO: The roles and functions of cutaneous mechanoreceptors. Curr Opin Neurobiol 11:455–461, 2001.

Johnson KO, Yoskioka T, Vega-Bermudez F: Tactile functions of mechanoreceptive afferents innervating the hand. J Clin Neurophysiol 17:539–558, 2000.

Kandel E, Schwartz JH, Jessell TM: Principles of Neural Science, ed 4. New York: McGraw-Hill, 2000.

Kaplan BJ, Friedman WA, Gravenstein D: Somatosensory evoked potentials in hysterical paraplegia. Surg Neurol 23:502–506.

Karl A, Birbaumer N, Lutzenberger W, et al: Reorganization of motor and somatosensory cortex in upper extremity amputees with phantom limb pain. J Neurosci 21:3609–3618, 2001.

Kew JM, Ridding MC, Rothwell JC, et al: Reorganization of cortical blood flow and 12 transcranial magnetic stimulation maps in human subjects after upper limb amputation. J Neurophysiol 72:2517–2524, 1994.

Knecht S, Kunesch E, Schnitzler A: Parallel and serial processing of haptic information in man. Effects of parietal lesions on sensorimotor hand function. Neuropsychologia 34:669–687, 1996.

Korvenoja A, Huttunen J, Salli E, et al: Activation of multiple cortical areas in response to somatosensory stimulation. Combined magnetoencephalographic and functional magnetic resonance imaging. Hum Brain Map 8:13–27, 1999.

Làdavas E, Menghini G, Umiltá C: A rehabilitation study of hemispatial neglect. Cogn Neuropsychol 11:75–95, 1994.

Làdavas E, di Pellegrino G, Farnè, et al: Neuropsychological evidence of an integrated visuotactile representation of peripersonal space in humans. J Cogn Neurosci 10:581–589, 1998.

Lezak MD: Neuropsychological Assessment, ed 3. New York: Oxford University Press, 1995.

Lotze M, Flor H, Grodd W: Phantom movements and pain an fMRI study in upper limb amputees. Brain 124:2268–2277, 2001.

Maldjian JA, Gottschalk A, Patel RS, et al: Mapping of secondary somatosensory cortex activation induced by vibrational stimulation. An fMRI study. Brain Res 824:291–295, 1999.

Marsden CD: Hysteria—A neurologist's view. Psychol Med 16:277–288, 1986.

Marshall JC, Halligan PW, Fink GR, et al: The functional anatomy of a hysterical paralysis. Cognition 64:B1–B8, 1997.

Mcknight JT, Adcock BB: Paresthesia. A practical approach. Am Fam Physician 56:2253–2260, 1997.

Merskey H, Bogduk N: International Association for the Study of Pain (IASP): Classification of Chronic Pain, ed 2. Seattle, WA: IASP Press, 1994.

Mesulam MM: Principles of Behavioral and Cognitive Neurology, ed 2. New York: Oxford University Press, 2000.

Mima T, Ikeda A, Terada K, et al: Modality-specific organization for cutaneous and proprioceptive sense in human primary sensory cortex studied by chronic epicortical recording. Electroencephalogr Clin Neurophysiol 104:103–107, 1997.

Mima T, Nagamine T, Nakamura K, et al: Attentiona modulates both primary and second somatosensory cortical activities in humans: A magnetoencephalographic study. J Neurophysiol 80:2215–2221, 1998.

Moore CI, Stern CE, Corkin S, et al: Segregation of somatosensory activation in the human Rolandic cortex using fMRI. Am Physiol Soc 84:558–569, 2000.

Morota N, Deletis V, Kiprovski K, et al: The use of motor evoked potentials in the diagnosis of psychogenic quadriplegics: A case study. Pediatr Neurosurg 20:203–206.

Moscovitch M, Behrmann M: Coding of spatial information in the somatosensory system: Evidence from patients with neglect following parietal lobe damage. J Cogn Neurosci 6:151–155, 1994.

Mountcastle VB, Motter BC, Andersen RA: Some further observations on the functional properties of neurons in the parietal lobe of waking monkey. Behav Brain Sci 1980:520–529, 1980.

Mountz JM, Bradley LA, Modell JG, et al: Fibromyalgia in women: Abnormalities of regional cerebral blood flow in the thalamus and the caudate nucleus are associated with low pain threshold levels. Arthritis Rheum 38:926–938, 1995.

Murry EA, Coulter JD: Supplementary sensory cortex: The medial parietal cortex in the monkey, in Woolsey CN (ed): Cortical Sensory Organization. Vol. 1. Multiple Somatic Areas. Clifton, NJ: Humana Press, 1982, pp. 167–195.

Nakamura J, Endo K, Sumida T, et al: Bilateral tactile agnosia: A case report. Cortex 34:375–388, 1998.

Nasreddine ZS, Saver JL: Pain after thalamic stroke. Right diencephalic predominance and clinical features in 180 patients. Neurology 48:1196–1199, 1997.

Nikolajsen L, Jensen TS: Phantom limb pain. Br J Anaesth 87:107–116, 2001.

Nunn JA, Gregory LJ, Brammer M, et al: Functional magnetic resonance imaging of synesthesia. Activation of V4/V8 by spoken words. Nat Neurosci 5:371–375, 2002.

Nuwer MR: Fundamentals of evoked potentials and common clinical applications today. Electroencephalogr Clin Neurophysiol 106:142–148, 1998.

Paciaroni M, Bogousslavsky J: Pure sensory syndromes in thalamic stroke. Eur Neurol 39:211–217, 1998.

Palmeri TJ, Blake R, Marois R, et al: The perceptual reality of synesthetic colors. Proc Natl Acad Sci U S A 99:4127–4131, 2002.

Pandya DN, Van Hoesen GW, Mesulam MM: Efferent connections of the cingulate gyrus in the rhesus monkey. Exp Brain Res 42:319–330, 1981.

Parent A: Carpenter's Human Neuroanatomy, ed 9. Baltimore: William & Wilkins, 1996.

Penfield W, Jasper H: Epilepsy and the Functional Anatomy of Human Brain. Boston: Little, Brown, 1954.

Penfield W, Rasmussen T: Secondary Sensory and Motor Representation. New York: MacMillan, 1950.

Perez FM, Tunkel RS, Lachmann EA, et al: Balint's syndrome arising from bilateral posterior cortical atrophy or infarction. Rehabilitation strategies and their limitation. Disabil Rehabil 18:300–304, 1996.

Pitcher GM, Ritchie J, Henry JL: Paw withdrawal threshold on the von Frey hair test is influenced by the surface on which the rat stands. J Neurosci Methods 87:185–193, 1999.

Polonara G, Fabri M, Manzoni T, et al: Localization of the first and second somatosensory areas in the human cerebral cortex with functional MR imaging. Am J Neuroradiol 20:199–205, 1999.

Pouget A, Snyder LH: Review. Computational approaches to sensorimotor transformations. Nata Neurosci Suppl 3:1192–1198, 2000.

Radovanovic S, Korotkov A, Ljubisavljevi M, et al: Comparison of brain activity during different types of proprioceptive inputs: A positron emission tomography study. Exp Brain Res 143:276–285, 2002.

Ramachandran VS : Consciousness and body image: Lessons from phantom limbs, Capgras syndrome and pain asymbolia. Philos Trans R Soc Lond B Biol Sci 353:1851–1859, 1998.

Ramachandran VS, Hirstein W: The perception of phantom limbs. The D.O. Hebb Lecture. Brain 121:1603–1630, 1998.

Ramachandran VS, Rogers-Ramachandran D: Phantom limbs and neural plasticity. Arch Neurol 57:317–320, 2000.

Randolph M, Semmes J: Behavioral consequences of selective subtotal ablations in the postcentral postcentral gyrus of *Macaca mulatta*. Brain Res 70:55–70, 1974.

Reed CL, Caselli RJ: The nature of tactile agnosia. A case study. Neuropsychologia 32:527–539, 1994.

Reed CL, Caselli RJ, Farah MJ: Tactile agnosia underlying impairment and implications for normal tactile object recognition. Brain 119:875–888, 1996.

Rizzo M: "Bálint's syndrome" and associated visuospatial disorders, in Kendall C (ed): Bailliére's Clinical Neurology. London: Harcourt Brace Jovanovich, 1993, Vol. 2, pp. 415–437.

Rizzo M, Darling W: Reaching with cerebral tunnel vision. Neuropsychologia 35:53–63, 1997.

Rizzo M, Eslinger PJ: Colored hearing synesthesia: An investigation of neural factors. Neurology 39:781–784, 1989.

Rizzo M, Vecera SP: Psychoanatomical substrates of Bálint's syndrome. J Neuro Neurosurg Psychiatry 72:162–178, 2002.

Rizzo MA, Kocsis JD, Wavman SG: Mechanisms of paresthesiae, dysesthesiae, and hyperesthesiae: Role of Na channel heterogeneity. Eur Neurol 36:3–12, 1996.

Roland PE, O'Sullivan B, Kawashima R: Shape and roughness activate different somatosensory areas in the human brain. Proc Natl Acad Sci U S A 95:3295–3300, 1998.

Ron MA: Somatisation in neurological practice. J Neurol Neurosurg Psychiatry 57:1161–1164, 1994 (Editorial).

Roux F-E, Ibarrola D, Lazorthes Y, et al: Chronic motor cortex stimulation for phantom limb pain: A functional magnetic resonance imaging study: Technical case report. Neurosurgery 48:681–688, 2001.

Ruben J, Schwiemann J, Deuchert M, et al: Somatotopic organization of human secondary somatosensory cortex. Cereb Cortex 11:463–473, 2001.

Rushworth MFS, Nixon PD, Passingham RE: Parietal cortex and movement. 1. Movement selection and reaching. Exp Brain Res 117:292–310, 1997.

Saetti MC, De Renzi E, Comper M: Tactile morphagnosia secondary to spatial deficits. Neuropsychologia 37:1087–1100, 1999.

Sathian K, Zangaladze A, Green J, et al: Tactile spatial acuity and roughness discrimination. Impairments due to aging and Parkinson's disease. Neurology 49:168–177, 1997.

Schiltz K, Trocha K, Wieringa BM: Neurophysiological aspects of synesthetic experience. J Neuropsychiatry Clin Neurosci 11:58–65, 1999.

Schott GD: From thalamic syndrome to central poststroke pain. J Neurol Neurosurg Psychiatry 61:560–564, 1995 (Editorial).

Schott GD: Reflex sympathetic dystrophy. J Neurol Neurosurg Psychiatry 71:291–295, 2001.

Schwartzman RJ, Popescu A: Reflex sympathetic dystrophy. Curr Rheumatol Rep 4:165–169, 2002.

Schwenkreis P, Witscher K, Janssen F, et al. Changes of cortical excitability in patients with upper limb amputation. Neurosci Lett 293:143–146, 2000.

Seltzer B, Pandya DN: Afferent cortical connections and architectonics of the superior temporal sulcus and surrounding cortex in the rhesus monkey. Brain Res 149:1–24, 1978.

Shergill SS, Cameron LA, Brammer MJ, et al: Modality specific neural correlates of auditory and somatic hallucinations. J Neurol Neurosurg Psychiatry 71:688–690, 2001.

Sirigu A, Grafman J, Bressler K, et al: Multiple representations contribute to body knowledge processing. Brain 114:629–642, 1991.

Slater E: Diagnosis of "hysteria." BMJ 1:1395–1399, 1965.

Smania N, Aglioti S: Sensory and spatial components of somaesthetic deficits following right brain damage. Neurology 45:1725–1730, 1995.

Snyder LH, Grieve KL, Brotchie P, et al: Separate body- and world-referenced representations of visual space in parietal cortex. Nature 394:887–893, 1998.

Soechting JF, Flanders M: Moving in three-dimensional space: Frames of reference, vectors, and coordinate systems. Annu Rev Neurosci 15:167–191, 1992.

Stacy CB: Complex haptic hallucinations and palinaptia. Cortex 23:337–340, 1987.

Stevens JC, Choo KK: Spatial acuity of the body surface over the life span. Somatosens Mot Res 13:153–166, 1996.

Stevens SS: On the brightness of lights and the loudness of sounds. Science 118:576, 1953.

Swinnen SP, Steyvers M, Van Den Bergh L, et al: Motor learning and Parkinson's disease. Refinement of within-limb and between-limb coordination as a result of practice. Behav Brain Res 111:45–49, 2000.

Takeda K, Kaminaga T, Furui S, et al: Functional magnetic resonance imaging localization of tactile reading phonograms in Japanese subjects. Neurosci Lett 259:87–90, 1999.

Thornbury JM, Mistretta CM: Tactile sensitivity as a function of age. J Gerontol 36:34–39, 1981.

Tiihonen J, Kuikka J, Viinamäki H, et al: Altered cerebral blood flow during hysterical paresthesia. Biol Psychiatry 37:134–135, 1995 (Letter).

Tissenbaum MJ, Harter HM, Friedman AP: Organic neurological syndromes diagnosed as functional disorders. JAMA 147:1519–1521, 1951.

Valenza N, Ptak R, Zimine I, et al: Dissociated active and passive tactile shape recognition. A case study of pure tactile apraxia. Brain 124:2287–2298, 2001.

Vallar G, Rusconi ML, Bignamini L: Anatomical correlates of visual and tactile extinction in humans. A clinical CT scan study. J Neurol Neurosurg Psychiatry 57:464–470, 1994.

Vega-Bermudez F, Johnson KO, Hsiao SS: Human tactile pattern recognition: Active versus passive touch, velocity effects, and patterns of confusion. J Neurophysiol 65:531–546, 1991.

Von Frey M, Kiesow F: Ueber die Function der Tastkoerperchen. Z Psychol 20:126–163, 1899.

Vuilleumier P, Chicherio C, Assal F, et al: Functional neuroanatomical correlates of hysterical sensorimotor loss. Brain 124:1077–1090, 2001.

Wall JT, Xu J, Wang X: Human brain plasticity: An emerging view of the multiple substrates and mechanisms that cause cortical and related sensory dysfunctions after injuries of sensory inputs from the body. Brain Res Brain Res Rev 39:181–215, 2002.

Weber EH: Der Tastsinn und das Gemeingefühl, in Ross HE, Murray DJ (eds): E.H. Weber on the Tactile Senses. Hove, UK: Erlbaum (UK), 1995. [Originally published in Wagner R (ed): Handwörterbuch der Physiologie. Braunschweig, 1846, Vol. 3, Pt 2, pp. 481–588, 709–728].

Whitlock FA: The aetiology of hysteria. Acta Psychiatr Scand 43:144–162, 1967.

Willoch F, Rosen G, Tölle TR, et al: Phantom limb pain in the human brain: Unraveling neural circuitries of phantom limb sensations using positron emission tomography. Ann Neurol 48:842–849, 2000.

Wolpert DM, Goodbody SJ, Husain M: Maintaining internal representations: The role of the human superior parietal lobe. Nat Neurosci 1:529–533, 1998

Yamadori A, Osumi Y, Ikeda H, et al: Left unilateral agraphia and tactile anomia. Arch Neurol 37:88–91, 1980.

Smell and Taste Disorders

Thomas C. Pritchard

Paul J. Eslinger

JianLi Wang

Qing Yang

Ageusia

Anosmia

Chemosensory disorders

Dysosmia

Dysgeusia

Flavor

Olfaction

Psychophysical testing

Taste

INTRODUCTION

Olfactory and gustatory deficits are more common than most people believe. Each year more than 200,000 people in the United States seek medical attention for a taste or smell disorder. An estimated 2.7 million Americans report chronic olfactory impairment (Hoffman et al., 1998) and 2 million adults with chemosensory problems are not currently under a physician's care. The incidence of olfactory problems increases gradually with age until by age 65 more than one half of the populace has an olfactory deficit. The percentage of people over age 80 who report an inability to either detect or identify odors exceeds 75% (Doty et al., 1984a). With the National Institute on Aging predicting that more than 70 million people (20% of the population) in the United States will be older than 65 by the year 2030, physicians should expect a dramatic increase in the number of patients with chemosensory complaints. Most patients with chemosensory complaints report a partial or complete loss of taste or smell. Others describe various distortions of tastes and odors or gustatory/olfactory hallucinations. These deficits are more than a minor inconvenience for those afflicted. Patients experience a diminished quality of life and increased safety risk. More serious chemosensory deficits interfere with eating and drinking and undermine nutrition and metabolism (Duffy & Ferris, 1989). When patients with renal impairment, diabetes mellitus, or congestive heart failure attempt to compensate for a taste loss by adding salt or sugar to their food, there can be serious consequences. This is especially true for older persons, the segment of society with the highest incidence of chemosensory problems.

Taste and smell deficits can be caused by disease, trauma, or iatrogenic interventions that affect peripheral or central chemosensory structures. Most chemosensory alterations, however, are secondary to another disease process or treatment that does not directly involve structures typically associated with the chemical senses. For this reason gustatory and olfactory disorders need to be evaluated in the context of the patient's overall health. Gustatory and olfactory testing should be considered only after a complete patient history and a thorough medical examination have been obtained. Even after a thorough medical work-up has been completed, the origins of 17% to 26% of all chemosensory complaints are listed as idiopathic (Goodspeed et al., 1987; Seiden, 1997). The incidence of chemosensory complaints of idiopathic origin is likely to decrease as testing and differential diagnoses improve.

This chapter provides an overview of olfactory and gustatory disorders, their diagnostic evaluation, and their potential for treatment. Given the high incidence of olfactory and taste confusion that many patients experience, we first describe a combined approach to evaluation and then more specific details about each sensory system and its clinical presentations.

MEDICAL EVALUATION OF CHEMOSENSORY IMPAIRMENTS

Patient History

In addition to a detailed description of the specific chemosensory problems, a patient's medical, professional, and social histories must be obtained. Less emphasis usually is placed on the patient's professional and social histories unless they appear relevant to the etiology of complaints. For example, professional and social histories may deserve additional attention when the physician suspects that a chemosensory disorder may be related to environmental toxin exposure or the use/abuse of tobacco, alcohol, or illegal drugs. Although gustatory and olfactory functions generally attenuate with age (Schiffman, 1997; Murphy et al., 2002), it would be a mistake to ascribe a patient's chemosensory complaints to aging alone without ruling out other possibilities.

The most accurate and complete descriptions of chemosensory symptoms are obtained when the patients are permitted to tell their own story in their own way. When patients are allowed to speak freely, they not only describe their symptoms in the proper context but also provide factual information that the physician would be unlikely to elicit with direct questioning. Once the patient's story has been completed, more direct follow-up questions should be asked about points that may have been covered superficially. For example, if the patient's chief complaint is that "food no longer tastes or smells good," the physician should ask how taste or smell has changed. Open-ended questions that encourage patients to describe the symptoms are more effective than closed-ended questions that may be answered with one or two words. Under favorable circumstances, the interview should yield answers to the following questions:

- Is taste or smell absent (indicating ageusia or anosmia)?
- Is the taste or smell weak (indicating hypogeusia or hyposmia)?
- Is the taste or smell distorted (indicating dysgeusia or dysosmia/parosmia)?
- Are the symptoms always the same; if not, under what circumstances do they appear or disappear?
- Is the problem restricted to one nostril or only part of the tongue?
- Is this a recent or longstanding problem?
- Was the onset sudden, stepwise, or gradual?
- Was the onset of the chemosensory disorder coincident with any changes in the patient's medical (i.e., illness, diagnosis, medication usage, treatment), professional, community, or personal circumstances, including toxic exposure?

The answers to these questions, especially those related to the circumstances surrounding the onset of the chemosensory disorder, will help guide the selection of the appropriate tests and establish a differential diagnosis.

Despite patients' best efforts to provide complete and accurate descriptions of their symptoms, it is not uncommon to encounter erroneous, incomplete, or contradictory information during history taking. This problem is more acute when dealing with patients who have cognitive and chemosensory deficits. Confusion regarding symptoms also may arise because odors encountered during feeding are typically perceived as originating from the palate (Deems et al., 1991). Indeed, many patients with olfactory disturbances will report that they have lost their sense of taste (Gent et al., 1987). According to Gent and colleagues (1987), only a small fraction (3%–13%) of the patients who report a gustatory deficit actually have a gustatory deficit. The accuracy of history taking can be improved, however, by ensuring that patients understand the differences between taste, smell, and flavor. The distinctions between *taste*, *smell*, and *flavor* are more than a formality; each is the perceptual correlate of a separate sensory system whose unique receptors and separate peripheral/central pathways respond to different classes of stimuli.

Taste, the sensation produced by stimulation of taste buds distributed throughout the oral cavity, is typically described as salty, sweet, sour, and bitter. Taste does *not* include tactile sensations such as stickiness (e.g., peanut butter) or crunchiness (e.g., crackers), thermal sensations (e.g., hot, cold), or the burn of spicy foods (e.g., chili). Taste also does not include the bouquet of a fine wine or the aroma of coffee, even though these fluids are taken orally. The sense of *smell* is stimulated by airborne molecules that enter the nose either through the nostrils (as food enters the mouth) or retronasally through the nasopharynx (during chewing, drinking, and swallowing). Tactile and thermal sensations as well as spiciness are conveyed by receptors innervated by the trigeminal nerve and distributed throughout the oral-nasal cavities. People who report problems with hot/cold, spicy, or strong-tasting foods may have a trigeminal problem rather than a chemosensory one. Normally, sensations conveyed by the gustatory, olfactory, and trigeminal nerves fuse into a single percept called *flavor*. Patients often use the terms taste and flavor interchangeably because both are perceived as originating within the mouth. By inquiring about the specific foods and beverages that trigger the patient's symptoms, it may be possible to determine which sensory system has been affected. If necessary, patients can be asked if their symptoms appear when they encounter certain exemplars for taste (e.g., peanuts [salty], lemon juice [sour]), odor (e.g., flowers, perfume), or spicy foods (e.g., chili). Also note that people typically describe tastes by quality (e.g., salty, bitter) and smells by the origin of the odor (e.g., lemon, feces).

The information contained in the patient history will help determine the differential diagnosis for the chemosensory disorder as well as the locus and time of onset. This information will help guide the physical examination and, ultimately, the course of treatment. For these reasons, history taking should include a comprehensive list of the patient's other medical conditions, even those that the patient may feel are unrelated to the senses of smell and taste. Patients also should be asked about all previous surgeries and illnesses; those involving the head or neck should be discussed in detail. Specific inquiries should be made about traumatic head injury, which is a well-documented cause of olfactory dysfunction (Doty et al., 1997). Table 15-1 lists some of the dozens of factors known to affect the olfactory system; see Schiffman and Zervakis (2002) for a more complete listing.

Information also should be gathered about the patient's current medications, with particular attention paid to any medication changes that occurred around the time chemosensory symptoms began (Table 15-2).

The gustatory system is not as prone to damage as the olfactory system, but taste deficits do accompany or are caused by a variety of oral and dental conditions as well as certain disease processes and their treatments (Deems et al., 1991; Table 15-3). In addition, there is a high degree of comorbidity of taste and smell disorders. For example, taste perception may be affected by upper respiratory infections (Goodspeed et al., 1986), allergic rhinitis (Rydzewski et al., 2000), and head trauma (Costanzo & DiNardo, 1995), three of the leading causes of olfactory dysfunction.

Table 15-4 includes a sample of the more than 250 medications known to cause taste deficits (Ackerman & Kasbekar, 1997; Finkelstein & Schiffman, 1999; Schiffman & Zervakis, 2002). Although the list is long, for reasons that are not well understood, the number of patients who report problems with these drugs is quite small. The gustatory system also is susceptible to fluctuations in the oral environment such as changes in saliva composition caused by salivary gland damage, xerostomia, or a deterioration of oral hygiene precipitated by xerostomia (Kuten et al., 1986). Some patients with burning-mouth syndrome, a trigeminal rather than a gustatory disorder, report alterations in taste perception (Grushka & Epstein, 1997). Early research on trace metal deficiencies suggested that zinc supplements ameliorated taste deficits, but more recent studies have shown that zinc therapy is rarely effective unless the patient has a medical condition such as chronic liver disease, which predisposes patients to zinc deficiency (Price, 1986).

The chief obstacle to obtaining a complete and accurate patient history is the patient's inability to appreciate the relationship between the chemosensory disturbance and other seemingly unrelated medical conditions. It is for just this reason, however, that a broad-based approach be taken when obtaining the patient history. Questionnaires can help ensure that important areas of inquiry are not missed, but the key to successful history taking is patient cooperation.

Text continues on page 342

TABLE 15-1. Medical Conditions and Exposures that Alter Olfaction

Neurologic	Reference	Symptom
Alzheimer disease	Lehrner et al., 1997	Identification, threshold, memory
Alcoholic Korsakoff syndrome	Eslinger et al., 1982 (review)	Threshold, identification, memory
Brain tumor	Olsen & DeSanto, 1983	Anosmia
Epilepsy	Currie et al. 1971	Hallucination, dysosmia
Head trauma	Doty et al., 1997	Anosmia
Herpes simplex encephalitis	McGrath et al., 1997	Anosmia
Huntington disease	Hamilton et al, 1999	Threshold
Migraine	Wolberg & Ziegler, 1982	Hallucination
Multiple sclerosis	Pinching, 1977	Hyposmia, anosmia
Parkinson disease	Lehrner et al., 1997	Identification
Temporal lobectomy	Eskenazi et al., 1986	Identification

Nutritional and metabolic		
Renal failure	Griep et al., 1997	Threshold
Liver disease (end-stage)	Bloomfield et al., 1999	Hyposmia
Vitamin B_{12} deficiency	Rundles, 1946	Parosmia, anosmia

Developmental/Endocrine		
Adrenal cortical insufficiency	Henkin, 1975	Hyperosmia
Attention-deficit/hyperactivity disorder	Gansler et al., 1998	Identification
Cushing's syndrome	Henkin, 1975	Hyposmia
Diabetes mellitus	Jorgensen & Buch, 1961	Hyposmia, anosmia
Down syndrome	Warner et al., 1988	Identification
Gonadal dysgenesis (Turner syndrome)	Henkin, 1967	Hyposmia
Hypothyroidism	McConnell et al., 1975	Hyposmia
Kallmann syndrome (hypogonadotropic hypogonadism)	Males et al., 1973	Anosmia
Primary amenorrhea	Marshall & Henkin, 1971	Hyposmia
Pseudohypoparathyroidism	Weinstock et al., 1986	Hyposmia

Local		
Adenoid hypertrophy	Ghorbanian et al., 1978	Hyposmia
Rhinitis	Rydzewski et al., 2000	Anosmia, hyposmia
Facial hypoplasia	Henkin et al., 1966	Hyposmia
Nasal and sinus disease and neoplasms	Doty & Mishra, 2001 (review)	Identification
Sjögren syndrome	Weiffenbach & Fox, 1993	Identification

Viral infections		
Acute viral hepatitis	Henkin & Smith, 1971	Hyposmia
HIV infection	Grahm et al., 1995	Identification
Herpes simplex encephalitis	McGrath et al., 1997	Anosmia
Upper respiratory infections	Leopold et al., 1991	Hyposmia

TABLE 15-1. Medical Conditions and Exposures that Alter Olfaction—cont'd

Environmental exposure		
Cigarette smoking	Frye et al., 1990	Identification
Formaldehyde, toluene	Elsner, 2001	Threshold
Radiation (therapeutic, cranial)	Ophir et al., 1988	Threshold
Other		
Aging	Murphy et al. 2002	Identification
Alcoholism	Shear et al., 1992	Identification
Congenital	Jafek et al., 1990	Anosmia
Laryngectomy	Hilgers et al., 2002	Anosmia, hyposmia
Schizophrenia	Kopala et al., 1992	Identification

(Adapted from Schiffman SS, Zervakis J: Taste and smell perception in the elderly: Effect of medications and disease. Adv Food Nutr Res 44:247–346, 2002.)

TABLE 15-2. Medications that Alter Smell

Class of drug	*Drug*	*Source*	*Symptom*
AIDS-related therapeutic drugs	Zalcitabine	PDR (Hivid)	Parosmia
Anesthetic (topical)	Cocaine	Zilstorff, 1965	Hyposmia
Antihypertensive/antiarrhythmic	Diltiazem	Berman, 1985	Anosmia, dysosmia
	Enalapril maleate	PDR (Vasotec)	Anosmia
	Nifedipine	Levinson & Kennedy, 1985	Dysosmia
Anti-inflammatory drugs	Beclomethasone dipropionate	PDR (Beconase)	Anosmia
	Dexamethasone sodium phosphate	PDR (Decadron Turbinaire)	Anosmia
Antimicrobial drugs	Ciprofloxacin	PDR (Cipro)	Anosmia
	Streptomycin	Zilstorff & Herbild, 1979	Parosmia
Antithyroid agents	Carbimazole	Errikssen et al., 1975	Anosmia
	Propylthiouracil	Grossman, 1953	Anosmia
Bronchodilators/antiasthmatic drugs	Bitolterol mesylate	PDR (Tornalate)	Unusual smell
Opiates	Codeine	Macht & Macht, 1940	Hyposmia
	Morphine	Macht & Macht, 1940	Hyposmia
Psychopharmacologic agents	Buspirone HCl	PDR (BuSpar)	Parosmia
	Clomipramine HCl	PDR (Anafranil)	Parosmia
Sympathomimetic drugs	Amphetamines	Schiffman, 1983	Increased acuity
Other	Strychnine	Skouby & Zilstorff-Pedersen, 1954	Decreased threshold

(Adapted from Schiffman SS, Zervakis J: Taste and smell perception in the elderly: Effect of medications and disease. Adv Food Nutr Res 44:247–346, 2002.)

TABLE 15-3. Medical Conditions and Exposures that Alter Taste

Neurologic		
Alzheimer disease	Schiffman et al., 1990	Ageusia
Brain tumors	Pritchard et al., 1999	Hypogeusia
Chorda tympani damage		
Acoustic neuromas	Magliulo et al., 1998	Ageusia
Bell's palsy	Ekstrand, 1979	Ageusia
Middle ear surgery	Jeppsson & Hallen, 1971	Ageusia
Epilepsy	Hausser-Hauw & Bancard, 1987	Hallucinations
Head trauma	Schechter & Henkin, 1974	Hypogeusia, dysgeusia
Multiple sclerosis	Catalanotto et al., 1984	Hypogeusia
Endocrine		
Adrenal cortical insufficiency	Henkin, 1975	Hypergeusia
Cushing syndrome	Henkin, 1975	Hypergeusia
Diabetes mellitus	Halter et al., 1975	Glucose detection
Local		
Third molar extractions	Shafer et al., 1999	Hypogeusia, identification
Sjögren syndrome	Henkin et al., 1972	Hypogeusia
Nutritional and metabolic		
Chronic renal failure	Ciechanover et al., 1980	Threshold
Cirrhosis of the liver	Garret-Laster et al., 1984	Hypogeusia
Niacin (vitamin B_3) deficiency	Green, 1971	Hypogeusia, dysgeusia
Environmental exposure		
Chemotherapy	Dikken & Sitzia, 1998	Changes
Radiation therapy	Mossman, 1986	Threshold
Other		
Cancer (noncranial)	Panayiotou et al., 1995	Dysgeusia
Diabetes mellitus	Settle, 1991	Hypogeusia
Psychiatric disorders	Amsterdam et al., 1987	Hypogeusia
Familial dysautonomia	Henkin & Kopin, 1964	Hypogeusia
Cystic fibrosis	Desor & Maller, 1975	Hypergeusia
Laryngectomy	Kashima & Kalinowski, 1979	Hypogeusia
Depression	Amsterdam et al., 1987	Altered sensitivity to suprathreshold concentrations of sucrose

(Adapted from Schiffman SS, Zervakis J: Taste and smell perception in the elderly: Effect of medications and disease. Adv Food Nutr Res 44:247–346, 2002.)

TABLE 15-4. Medications that Alter Taste

Class of drug	Drug	Source	Symptom
AIDS and HIV therapeutic drugs—nucleosides	Zidovudine	PDR (Retrovir)	Dysgeusia
AIDS and HIV therapeutic drugs—protease inhibitors	Indinavir	PDR (Crixivan)	Dysgeusia
Anticholesteremics and antilipidemics	Pravastatin	PDR (Pravachol)	Parageusia
Anticoagulants	Phenindione	Scott, 1960	Burning sensation on tongue; local sensitivity of the taste buds
Antihistamines	Loratadine	PDR (Claritin)	Parageusia
Antimicrobial agents	Ampicillin	Jaffe, 1970	Hypogeusia
	Bleomycin	Soni & Chatterji, 1985	Ageusia
	Tetracyclines	Magnasco & Magnasco, 1985	Intense, offensive metallic taste
Antiproliferative and immunosuppressive agents	Cisplatin	Schiffman, 1991	Dysgeusia
	Doxorubicin	Duhra & Foulds, 1988	Ageusia
	Methotrexate	Duhra & Foulds, 1988	Ageusia
	Vincristine	State et al., 1977	Ageusia, dysgeusia, parageusia
Antirheumatic, antiarthritic, analgesic, and anti-inflammatory drugs	Dexamethasone	Fehm-Wolfsdorf et al., 1989	Less sensitive to taste differences
	Hydrocortisone	Fehm-Wolfsdorf et al., 1989	Less sensitive to taste differences
	Morphine	PDR (MS Contin)	Parageusia
	Salicylates	Hellekant & Gopal, 1975	Hypogeusia, ageusia
Antiseptics	Hexetidine	Plath & Otten, 1969	Salty taste, burning sensation
Antispasmodics	Phenobarbital	PDR (Donnatal)	Ageusia
Antithyroid agents	Thiouracil	Rollin, 1978	Hypogeusia, ageusia, phantogeusia
Antiulcerative drugs	Famotidine	PDR (Pepcid)	Taste disorder
Antiviral agents	Acyclovir	PDR (Zovirax)	Medication taste
Bronchodilators and antiasthmatic drugs	Albuteral	PDR (Ventolin)	Unusual tastes
Dental hygiene	Sodium fluoride	Thumfart et al., 1980	Ageusia
	Chlorhexidine	Lang et al., 1988	Salt hypogeusia
Diuretics, antiarrhythmic, antihypertensive, and antifibrillatory drugs	Amiloride	PDR (Monduretic)	Dysgeusia
	Procainamide HCl	PDR (Procan SR)	Bitter taste
	Propranolol	Griffin, 1992	Ageusia, dysgeusia, parageusia
Hypnotics and sedatives	Midazolam HCl	PDR (Versed)	Sour taste
Muscle relaxants, drugs for Parkinson disease	Levodopa	Siegfried & Zumstein, 1971	Ageusia, dysgeusia
Psychopharmacologics and antiepileptic drugs	Buspirone HCl	PDR (BuSpar)	Dysgeusia
	Clozapine	PDR (Clozaril)	Bitter taste
	Risperidone	PDR (Risperdal)	Bitter taste
	Nicotine	PDR (Nicoderm)	Dysgeusia

Continued

TABLE 15-4. Medications that Alter Taste—cont'd

Class of drug	Drug	Source	Symptom
Sympathomimetic drugs	Amphetamine	PDR (Biphetamine)	Dysgeusia
Vasodilators	Isosorbide mononitrate	PDR (Monoket)	Bitter taste
	Nitroglycerin patch	Ewing et al., 1989	Ageusia
Other drugs	Allopurinol	Rollin, 1978	Metallic phantogeusia
	Histamine	PDR (Histatrol)	Metallic taste

(Adapted from Schiffman SS, Zervakis J: Taste and smell perception in the elderly: Effect of medications and disease. Adv Food Nutr Res 44:247–346, 2002.)

When history taking is incomplete, the probability increases that the cause of a chemosensory disorder will be listed as idiopathic.

Clinical Examination

After the patient history has been completed, a physical examination of the ears, nose, mouth, and upper respiratory system should be conducted on all patients. The decision to conduct an even more complete physical examination should be dictated by the patient history and the knowledge that many chemosensory disorders are related to medical conditions not typically associated with the chemical senses. Limiting the examination to the oral cavity in patients with taste problems or the nose and upper respiratory tract in patients with complaints about smell may miss important clues about the cause of the patient's problems. The risk of a partial examination missing important information is particularly high among patients whose taste/smell confusions are not exposed during history taking. Any noteworthy findings from the neurologic examination, especially those related to the olfactory nerve, and to the facial and glossopharyngeal nerves, which innervate most of the gustatory receptors of the oral cavity, should be pursued in more detail.

Regardless of whether the presenting symptom concerns taste or smell, the single most important test to conduct is the endoscopic examination. An endoscopic examination will reveal changes in the color and texture of the nasal mucosa and the character of the mucous discharge, as well as signs of inflammation, swelling, surface erosion, atrophy, or ulceration. When the endoscopic examination yields abnormal findings, a diagnosis of sinusitis or rhinitis should be considered. When the findings of the endoscopic examination are normal, but the patient's history strongly suggests chronic sinusitis infection, computed tomography (CT) scanning of the nasal and paranasal regions should be performed to rule out anatomic and mucosal changes in the middle and superior meati, which typically cannot be visualized with endoscopy. CT scans also may provide the definitive diagnosis when nasal sinus obstruction, polyposis, or nasal and intracranial neoplasms are suspected but cannot be confirmed (Brightman, 1994). CT scanning may not be justified for anosmic patients who do not have a significant clinical history or positive endoscopic observations (Busaba, 2001). The endoscopic examination also will expose airway obstructions of inflammatory, neoplastic, traumatic, or developmental origin that may limit or prevent odors from reaching the olfactory neuroepithelium. After ruling out a conductive deficit, a sensorineural deficit should be considered. Strokes that damage or tumors that compress the ventral surface of the frontal lobe or the anterior-medial aspect of the temporal lobe can affect the sense of smell (Welge-Luessen et al., 2001). Olfactory loss seldom is found in isolation in patients with central nervous system (CNS) damage. In addition to the more common motor and sensory symptoms, several studies have shown that olfactory deficits are among the earliest symptoms of Alzheimer disease (Doty et al., 1987; Serby et al., 1991; Lehrner et al., 1997) and Parkinson disease (Doty et al., 1988; Lehrner et al., 1997).

Unlike the nasal cavity, the oral cavity is more accessible and thus easier to examine. The oral examination should begin with a general appraisal of the dental health of the patient because common and easily treatable causes of taste dysfunction include lapses in dental hygiene. Objectionable tastes may be caused or exacerbated by excessive plaque and tartar buildup on the teeth or food lodged between severely maloccluded teeth. Bad tastes also may originate from caries, poorly maintained prosthetic devices (bridges, dentures), and dental restorations (fillings, crowns) that are overdue for replacement. Because poorly fitting dentures and bridges may cause abrasions and abscesses, they should be removed so that the patient's underlying gums and hard palate can be carefully examined. Patients with periodontal disease may taste the putrid exudate that leaks from the crevicular spaces around the teeth. Patients with questionable dental hygiene should be strongly encouraged to see a dentist or a periodontist, with specific taste testing delayed until all of the dental issues have been resolved (Langen & Yearick, 1976).

The color and texture of the inner surfaces of the cheeks and gums should be noted and examined for signs of dryness, inflammation, edema, ulceration, erosion, or changes in surface texture that may be indicative of candida (thrush), lichen planus, cheek biting, thermal or chemical burns, viral infections, focal hyperkeratosis, or leukoplakia. Palpation of the cheeks and floor of the mouth may reveal inflammation, swelling, purulence, or masses associated with the parotid, sublingual, and submandibular glands. The tongue itself should be inspected for signs of excessive bacterial growth that may impede or even prevent sapid stimuli from reaching the taste receptors. Patients lacking fungiform and circumvallate taste papillae will lack taste buds and report a complete ageusia (Henkin & Kopin, 1964); testing for familial dysautonomia (Riley-Day syndrome) is then indicated.

OLFACTORY SYSTEM

Location and Innervation of Olfactory Structures

Olfaction begins when airborne molecules bind to the distal cilia of the roughly 12 million bipolar olfactory receptor neurons located along the roof and medial wall of the nasal cavity. Olfactory transduction is facilitated by odor-binding proteins that transport these molecules to the olfactory epithelium and odorant-degrading enzymes that clear the sites (Christensen & White, 2000; Doty, 2001). Following transduction, action potentials are generated in the receptor cells and transmitted to the olfactory bulb through the fila of the olfactory nerve (cranial nerve I). The olfactory bulbs are located between the ventral surface of the frontal lobes and the underlying cribriform plate of the ethmoid bone. The delicate fila of the olfactory nerve reach the olfactory bulbs by coursing through small fenestrations in the cribriform plate of ethmoid bone. Although the distance between the olfactory epithelium and the olfactory bulbs is short, the delicate fila are very susceptible to trauma caused by sudden deceleration. For this reason, head trauma is one of the leading causes anosmia (Costanzo & Becker, 1986).

The axons of the olfactory nerve enter the bulb and terminate in glomeruli, acellular ensembles that contain the dendritic endings of periglomerular, tufted, and mitral cells, which are located in the core of the bulb. The convergence of the olfactory axons onto the glomeruli of the olfactory bulb (estimated to be 25,000:1 in the rabbit) increases the sensitivity of the system by amplifying the odorant signal. The periglomerular cells that interconnect local glomeruli, and the granule cells that form local circuits between the mitral and tufted cells, permit the olfactory bulb to perform a significant amount of processing before transmission to the brain.

Indeed, the glomerulus is believed to play such an important role in olfactory discrimination that it has been referred to as the system's fundamental coding unit (Mori et al., 1999). The output neurons of the olfactory bulb are mitral and tufted cells, whose axons form the lateral olfactory tract that projects to the primary olfactory cortices located along the ventral surface of the telencephalon and the anteromedial temporal lobe. The widespread cortical distribution of olfactory information stands in sharp contrast to the convergence of sensory input that occurs between the receptor neurons and the glomeruli of the olfactory bulb.

Primary olfactory cortex consists of six areas: anterior olfactory nucleus, olfactory tubercle, piriform cortex, anterior cortical amygdaloid nucleus, periamygdaloid nucleus, and lateral entorhinal cortex (Figs. 15-1 and 15-2). Most of the olfactory cortices are three-layered paleocortex; the exception, entorhinal cortex, is classified as transitional because it shares some characteristics with traditional six-layer neocortex. Whereas the olfactory bulb is critical for preliminary analysis and detection of odors, the primary olfactory cortices are more heavily invested in integration of this information with other brain systems. The olfactory tubercle, which is closely related to the ventral striatum (e.g., nucleus accumbens), may be related to motivation. The anterior cortical amygdaloid nucleus provides input to reproduction-related areas in the anterior hypothalamus. The anterior periamygdaloid cortex projects to the deep amygdaloid nuclei, which play a key role in emotion and may explain why the link between smell and emotions (e.g., fear and arousal) is so strong. The part of the entorhinal cortex that receives olfactory inputs project to the hippocampus, which is a key structure in memory formation.

The olfactory cortices project to a number of other areas including the lateral hypothalamus, the mediodorsal thalamus, and the posterior orbitofrontal cortex. Olfactory information reaching the hypothalamus plays a role in reproduction, maternal behavioral, feeding and drinking, and aggressive behavior (Dielenberg et al., 2001; Savic et al., 2001). The posterior orbitofrontal cortex, which receives direct projections from the piriform cortex and indirect projections via the mediodorsal nucleus of the thalamus, is the target of efferent projections from parts of gustatory cortex, fueling speculation that this may be the site where flavor emerges from the convergence of taste and smell (Rolls, 1997).

Olfactory Changes Associated with Aging

Olfactory capabilities diminish with age, although the degree varies widely (see Chaves & Ship, 2000, for a review; Murphy et al., 2002). Changes with age have been established in studies of:

FIGURE 15-1. Ventral surface of the human brain showing prominent olfactory structures. (Adapted from Eslinger P, Damasio AR, Van Hoesen GW: Olfactory dysfunction in man: Anatomical and behavioral aspects. Brain Cogn 1:259–285, 1982.)

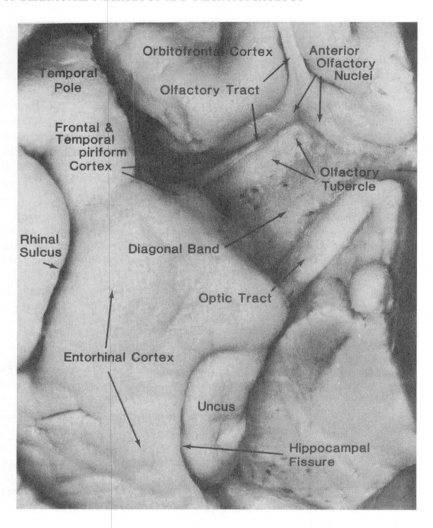

- Odor identification
- Odor discrimination
- Detection thresholds
- Intensity perception
- Adaptation to odors

Causes of age-related olfactory impairments are multifactorial and may include both peripheral and central factors. Unfortunately, the data regarding changes within the peripheral olfactory epithelium in the aged is controversial. Some studies suggest a patchy loss of olfactory epithelium, whereas others indicate that odor-responsive neurons are still vital in patients over 65 years of age (Rawson et al., 1998).

Olfactory changes with age can be a genuine threat to health and safety. For example, Cain and Stevens (1989) reported that 45% of older persons sampled failed to detect the warning odor that is added to natural gas (ethyl mercaptan). Older adults with olfactory loss also can contract oral and pharyngeal disease more easily (Ship, 1999). A recent study of 50 older persons, aged 50 to 96, in Ireland reported that prior occupational exposure to caustic fumes affected

odor thresholds and that medication usage as well as the patient's mental status was associated with odor recognition abilities (Elsner, 2001). Thus, the evaluation of olfactory abilities should include environmental exposure factors (e.g., pollutants, irritants, contaminants), as well as medications, nutritional and behavioral factors (e.g., smoking), and genetics. Management approaches revolve around minimizing risk factors within an overall health maintenance plan.

Functional Brain Imaging of Olfaction

In our nuclear magnetic resonance (NMR) imaging center, we have been using functional magnetic resonance imaging (fMRI) to map the areas of the human brain that respond to the odors peppermint and lavender. We have obtained comprehensive olfactory fMRI maps from normal young volunteers (mean age = 24 years; 6 women, 5 men) and older volunteers (mean age = 66 years; 3 women, 5 men). The imaging is done with the subjects breathing either clean air (OFF condition) or odorized air (ON condition). By subtracting the

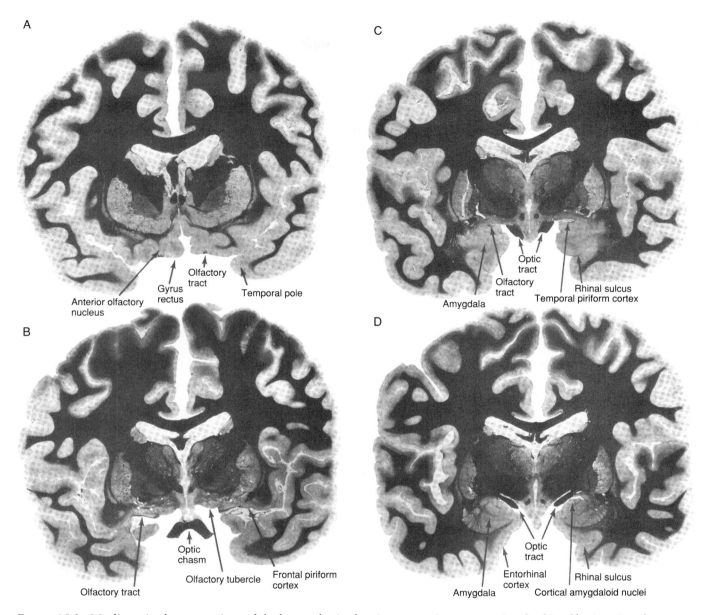

FIGURE 15-2. Myelin-stained cross-sections of the human brain showing anatomic structures involved in olfaction. Based on comparative studies, the primary olfactory cortex consists of a set of structures in the ventral forebrain and temporal lobe that receives projections from the olfactory bulb. These structures include the anterior olfactory nucleus, olfactory tubercle, piriform cortex, anterior cortical nucleus of the amygdala, part of the periamygdaloid cortex and the anterior edge of the entorhinal cortex. (Adapted from Eslinger P, Damasio AR, Van Hosen GW: Olfactory dysfunction in man: Anatomical and behavioral aspects. Brain Cogn 1:259–285, 1982.)

OFF activation from the ON activation, we have identified several areas of the brain that respond during olfactory stimulation. The olfactory stimuli produced a similar activation pattern in both the young and the old subjects. Odor-induced activation was observed in known primary olfactory cortical areas (anterior olfactory nucleus, piriform cortex, anterior cortical nucleus of the amygdala, the periamygdaloid cortex, the entorhinal cortex) as well as the hippocampus, the parahippocampal gyrus, the orbitofrontal cortex, and insula (Fig. 15-3).

Except for the insula which showed bilateral activity, there was more activation in the right hemisphere than the left. Although the overall pattern of brain activation was the same in both the younger and older subjects, the size and intensity of the active sites were significantly reduced in the latter group. The average activation volumes were 488 (±297) and 263 (±62)

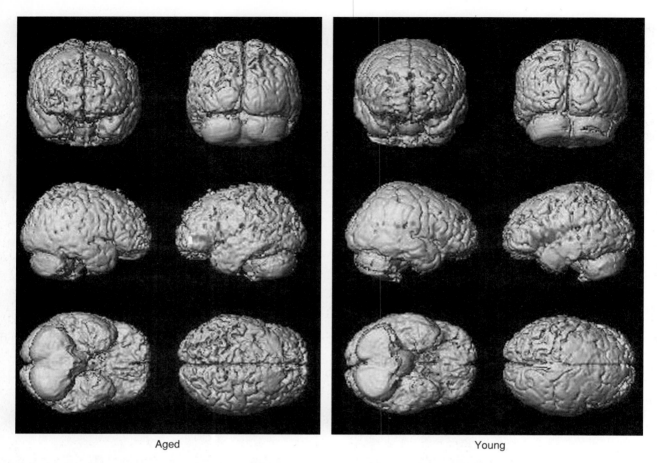

Aged

Young

FIGURE 15-3. Functional magnetic resonance image (fMRI) of aged (*left*) and young (*right*) normal volunteers showing areas of brain activation after exposure to odorants. Significant areas of activation included the primary olfactory cortex (anterior olfactory nucleus, olfactory tubercle, frontal and piriform cortex, and amygdala), the insula, and prefrontal regions. (See Color Plate 6)

pixels for the young and old subjects, respectively (*P* < 0.05; Fig. 15-4). The attenuation of olfactory activation in the older subjects accords well with age-related olfactory deficits. Further study is needed, however, to determine if the reduced activation of the brain is of peripheral or central origin. It also would be interesting and important from a therapeutic standpoint to know if the level of brain activation in older subjects is capable of increasing in response to increases in the concentration of the odorant.

Our preliminary data also showed patterns of brain activation that were specific to peppermint and lavender. For example, when subjects were tested with peppermint, an odor typically described as refreshing or arousing, brain activation was high in the areas listed above as well as several motor-related areas such as premotor cortex. Lavender, which many subjects describe as relaxing and calming, produced less overall activation but included somatosensory association cortices and the cerebellum. Further research will be needed to determine if these differences are due to peripheral or central factors and if the two patterns are related to the specific odors or to classes of similar odors.

Olfactory Dysfunction

Nordin and colleagues (1996) reported the prevalence of dysosmia in 363 patients referred to the University of California Nasal Dysfunction Clinic. Patients ranged from 19 to 90 years of age and were evenly split between women and men. Findings revealed 35% with a form of dysosmia, including 9% with parosmia, 16% with phantosmia, and 10% with combined parosmia and phantosmia. About one half of the patients with a history of head trauma or upper respiratory infection showed olfactory impairment, followed by lower percentages for patients with chronic sinusitis and allergic rhinitis. Interestingly, these rates did not change with age among this selected population of referred patients.

Olfactory Deficits in Neurological and Medical Disease

Olfactory dysfunction has been linked with a wide variety of medical and neurologic conditions (see Table 15-1). The link is particularly strong between olfactory dysfunction and epilepsy, brain tumors, cere-

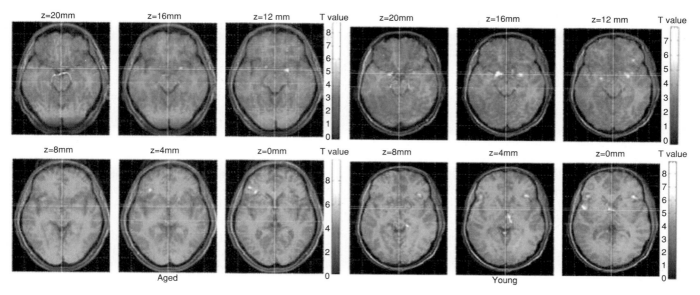

FIGURE 15-4. Olfactory fMRI maps in the axial plane from aged (*left*) and young (*right*) groups showing areas of statistically significant activation (*P* < 0.001). Stronger activation was observed in the major olfactory-related structures of the young group compared to the aged group (*P* = 0.035). (See Color Plate 7)

brovascular disease, head trauma, viral encephalitis, Korsakoff syndrome, and various neurodegenerative disorders; their impact on the olfactory perception is described below. More complete lists of the diseases and medications that affect olfaction and taste, particularly in older persons, have been published recently by Schiffman and Zervakis (2002) and Doty (2001).

Epilepsy

Olfactory auras in epilepsy provided some of the earliest observations regarding olfaction and the brain. In 1866 Hughlings-Jackson reported that the "first symptom of epileptiform seizure ... is a subjective sensation of smell, generally a disagreeable one" (p. 659). Olfactory auras or phantosmias that signal or presage a seizure are fairly accurate localizing signs that the seizure focus includes the anterior-medial temporal lobe or possibly posterior the orbitofrontal cortical region. The "uncinate group of fits" can include auras of smell, taste, epigastric sensation, mastication, and salivation, not atypical for complex partial seizures associated with medial temporal lobe gliosis. The olfactory auras are generally foul and unpleasant (e.g., burning rubber, spoiled food), but a pleasant olfactory aura will occasionally be reported. Odors can precipitate a seizure and in rare instances can avert a seizure (Efron, 1956; Passouant, 1965). Several investigators relying on clinical reports have suggested that epileptics experience hyperosmia or a heightened sense of olfactory acuity and perception (see Eslinger et al., 1982, for a summary). It is unclear how often hyperosmia occurs and what the psychophysical characteristics may be (e.g., detection threshold levels versus hedonic reactions, etc.). Such changes, however, may be related to altered zinc metabolism or neurophysiological irritability in temporal lobe epilepsy. In contrast, a recent study of patients with right temporal lobe epilepsy demonstrated a decreased ability to identify and remember odors (Carroll et al., 1993).

Surgical ablations for treatment of intractable epilepsy often involve a temporal lobectomy, a resection of anterior and medial temporal structures including the temporal pole, amygdala, hippocampus, and parahippocampal gyrus. Prior to resection, cortical mapping is often undertaken. In awake patients direct stimulation of the olfactory bulb, amygdala, and less often the uncus typically evokes unpleasant smells. Interestingly, thalamic and subthalamic stimulation also produces olfactory experiences, either of a purely sensory nature or as part of more complex experience that includes somatosensory and memory associations. Olfactory studies of patients who have undergone left or right temporal lobectomy have produced ambiguous and conflicting results regarding odor detection and recognition thresholds. Temporal lobectomy does appear to cause impairment in odor matching-to-sample, more so after right than left resections (see Eslinger et al., 1982, for further details). Because patients can detect and recognize olfactory stimuli presented to the nostril ipsilateral to the intact hemisphere (i.e., right hemisphere perception after right nostril stimulation), it is believed that both hemispheres are capable of olfactory perception. Furthermore, both hemispheres have sensory-motor integration capabilities relevant to olfaction, such as olfactory-visual, olfactory-tactile, and olfactory-motor processing.

Patients with intractable epilepsy, who are at high risk of life-threatening or repeated injuries from falls following loss of consciousness, may benefit from surgical disconnection of the cerebral hemispheres. By limiting the spread of seizures to a single hemisphere, commissurotomies allow patients to maintain consciousness and avoid injuries. Although a commissurotomy may have some impact on smell, major problems would not be expected because most olfactory information is transferred between the cerebral hemispheres through the anterior commissure (see Eslinger et al., 1982, for further details). Olfactory processing is not identical in the two hemispheres, but the scope and magnitude of these differences is not fully appreciated. We do know, however, that verbal tagging or naming of odors is more dependent on left hemisphere processing, whereas hedonic and some aspects of recognition processing reside within the right hemisphere (Homewood & Stevenson, 2001).

Head Trauma

Anosmia following head trauma was reported as early as 1870 by Ogle. Trauma-induced anosmia has been linked to all directions of blows about the head and to diverse forms of damage, including obstruction of the nasal cavity, destruction of the olfactory epithelium, shearing of the olfactory nerve as it travels through the cribriform plate, disconnection/compression of the olfactory tract, and damage to cortical olfactory areas. In addition to anosmia, olfactory distortions (i.e., dysosmia and parosmia) have been reported after head injury in as many as 52% of patients referred to smell and taste clinics (Schechter & Henkin, 1974).

The incidence of olfactory impairments after head trauma varies widely and depends on sampling and methodological procedures, which have also varied widely. Early studies suggested that smell was affected in as many as 65% of patients with head trauma (Laemmle, 1932); subsequent studies report anosmia in fewer than 10% of patients. In a recent study, olfactory impairment was reported in 14% of patients with head injury (Ogawa & Rutka, 1999). Skull fractures in the frontal, occipital, skull base, and midface were twice as likely to cause anosmia as temporal and parietal fractures.

Neurodegenerative Diseases

Significant olfactory impairments have been reported in Alzheimer disease (AD), Parkinson disease (PD), Huntington disease (HD), and motor neuron disease (Lehrner et al, 1997; Hamilton et al., 1999). AD and PD groups develop deficits in threshold detection, identification, and memory that are significantly different from age-related changes. In the case of PD, the olfactory impairments appear not to be related to cognitive impairment per se and are independent of disease

progression and treatment (Hawkes & Shephard, 1998). In AD, not only are olfactory deficits prevalent, but such deficits can be detected at an early stage. Histopathology studies show that AD patients have a disproportionate amount of degeneration in peripheral and central olfactory pathways compared to visual, auditory, motor, and other sensory systems. It has been suggested that early expression of olfactory deficits in AD (and its prodromal phase, mild cognitive impairment) may reflect the earliest pathology of the entorhinal cortex, which subsequently progresses to the hippocampus and surrounding temporal cortical olfactory regions. Olfactory impairments in the mild cognitive impairment stage, coupled with patients' lack of awareness of such changes, were predictive of progression to AD (Devanand et al., 2000). Therefore, the potential exists to use olfactory deficits as a preclinical marker of possible AD; studies investigating this possibility are currently underway.

Viral Encephalitis

Anosmia is common after herpes simplex encephalitis, a viral infection that has a particular proclivity for causing necrotizing lesions in the orbitofrontal cortex and limbic structures such as the amygdala, hippocampus, temporal pole, basal forebrain, insula, and anterior cingular cortex (Drachman & Adams, 1962; McGrath et al., 1997). Twomey and colleagues (1979) reported that the olfactory mucosa of three patients with herpes simplex encephalitis showed inflammatory changes, ulceration, and other histologic abnormalities. Hemorrhages within the perineural sheath of the olfactory nerves of these three patients and the fact that the virus could be grown from the mucosa (N = 2) or the olfactory bulb (N = 1) support the authors' assertion that the virus used the olfactory nerves as a conduit to enter the brain. The olfactory nerves appear to be the most likely route for infection, even though the authors could not completely rule out the virus traveling from the brain to the olfactory mucosa, and previous studies have shown that the herpes virus can enter the CNS through the lacrimal duct (Stroop et al., 1990).

Korsakoff Syndrome

Alcoholic Korsakoff syndrome is a neurodegenerative disorder that has been linked with prolonged alcohol abuse and olfactory deficits. After the acute neurologic phase, patients are generally left with a predominant anterograde amnesia. Anatomically, lesions have been identified in the mediodorsal nucleus of the thalamus, mammillary bodies, cerebellum, and brainstem. A series of studies in the 1970s identified specific impairments in olfactory detection threshold, intensity discrimination, identification, and memory in Korsakoff patients (see

Eslinger et al., 1982, for review). Similarities between borderline Korsakoff patients, detoxified alcoholics, and recent alcoholics suggest that these conditions lie along a continuum of olfactory impairment (and possibly neuropathology), with Korsakoff patients at the advanced end and the remaining groups at borderline to mild impairment stages (Potter & Butters, 1980).

Brain Tumors

Olfaction can be impaired by tumors that impinge on the orbitofrontal cortex and the anterior and medial temporal lobe. In fact, anosmia and dysosmia may be one of the earliest signs of such pathophysiology, which may be caused by direct structural damage or pressure/mass-mediated compression. Studies of tumor localization in the forebrain based on olfactory testing have reported accuracy rates ranging from 22% to 74% (Eslinger et al., 1982).

Cerebrovascular Disease

Although the orbitofrontal and anterior-medial temporal cortical regions are rarely affected by cerebrovascular diseases, olfactory structures can be affected by aneurysms of the anterior communicating artery (ACoA) and posterior cerebral artery strokes. Surgical clipping of leaking or ruptured ACoA aneurysms to relieve hemorrhagic mass effects may cause additional structural damage or ischemic injury due to vasospasm. Patients with aphasia from middle cerebral artery strokes are impaired in olfactory naming along with visual, auditory, and tactile naming.

Congenital Anosmia

A neurodevelopmental form of anosmia has been described and linked to the genetic defect associated with Kallmann syndrome (Rawson et al., 1995). Despite the presence of functional olfactory receptor neurons in the nasal cavity, there are no connections to the brain because the olfactory bulbs fail to develop. These individuals are also hypogonadotropic.

Olfactory Testing

Until recent developments in olfactory testing, such assessments were not standardized and typically varied widely between studies. Psychophysical methods are particularly challenging in olfaction because of rapid sensory adaptation. Rawson (2000) identified other limitations including the large number of potential stimuli, an elusive classification scheme for odors that has both biologic and perceptual bases, and technical issues that interfere with reliable control and delivery of olfactory stimuli. There are no "primary odors" and no appreci- ation for how or even if odors are differentiated by single versus multiple molecular components. Rawson (2000) offers the example of the aroma of coffee, which contains over 800 different chemicals but only 20 or 30 are linked to its aromatic quality. Despite these problems, olfactory testing can be conducted in the office and clinic as well as in research laboratories. Typically, detection thresholds are assessed along with odor identification at suprathreshold concentrations. For the latter, "scratch and sniff" blotters containing multiple choice options have become increasingly popular. For example, the University of Pennsylvania Smell Identification Test (UPSIT; Doty et al., 1984b; Doty, 2001) presents 40 odorants in "scratch and sniff" format with four choices per odor. Stimuli range from bubble gum and banana to motor oil and cinnamon. Normative values, established from over 4000 persons over a wide age range, have shown that the test has good reliability and validity. The UPSIT is available in English, Spanish, French, and German versions and a three-odor pocket version is available for screening assessment. Other tests also include the San Diego Odor Identification Test (Anderson et al., 1992), and the Scandinavian Odor Identification Test (Nordin et al., 1999). A standardized odor concentration test is also available for more detailed assessment of odor detection thresholds (The Smell Threshold Test; Doty, 2000). Tests of odor discrimination, odor memory, and odor magnitude estimation have also been implemented in research studies.

Olfactory Disorders: Recovery and Treatment

The variety of causative factors for olfactory dysfunction dilutes the effort that has been invested in follow-up study of recovery following olfactory loss. Several studies have shown that 15% to 39% of the patients who report olfactory loss following traumatic brain injury show some recovery (Zusho, 1982; Costanzo & Becker, 1986; Duncan & Seiden, 1995). In many of these patients, however, recovery was prolonged (up to 5 years), progressive (e.g., evolve from anosmia to dysosmia), and accompanied by parosmias or phantosmias. Damage to the olfactory fila generally produces a permanent olfactory deficit; "recovery of function" in these patients may reflect a local diminution of edema within the olfactory epithelium or along the cribriform plate.

Many people believe that successful treatment of conductive disorders such as allergic rhinitis, polyps, and obstructive nasal disease will restore olfactory function, but often this is not the case. Rydzewski and colleagues (2000) report that only 3 of 5 patients (60%) they treated for obstructive airway disease reported normal olfactory function afterward. Olfactory impairments caused by chronic nasal disease, asthma, rhinitis, and nasal polyps may respond to anti-inflammatory sprays and glucocorticoids (Jafek et al., 1987; Mott et al., 1997). Anosmic or hyposmic patients who have received medical or surgical treatment of sinusitis, rhinitis, or obstructive airway diseases report a transient improvement (Hosemann et al., 1993). Vitamin A therapy may also be of benefit given the important role of retinoids in the development of olfactory epithelium (Haskell et al., 2002).

Management approaches revolve around minimizing risk factors within an overall health maintenance plan. Patients with smell disorders should be strongly encouraged to regularly check that their smoke and carbon monoxide detectors at their home and workplace are in full working order. Those individuals potentially exposed to gas leaks from home heating and cooking appliances should consider purchasing a gas detector (the local gas utility will supply such information). To guard against eating food that may be spoiled, patients with olfactory impairment should regularly check expiration dates, color, and texture of foods, and when possible, ask a family member to smell the food. They also should pay particular attention to the dates stamped on most perishable foods and discard foods that are past their expiration date.

GUSTATORY SYSTEM

Distribution and Innervation of the Gustatory Receptors

Proper gustatory testing requires familiarity with both the location of the taste receptors and their neural innervation. Taste transduction occurs at the apices of taste buds scattered across the tongue, soft palate, larynx, and epiglottis. The taste buds located on the tongue are encased within fungiform, foliate, and circumvallate papillae, which can be seen with the naked eye. The fungiform papillae are located on the dorsal surface of the anterior two thirds of the tongue, primarily along the lateral edges. The highest concentration of fungiform papillae is at the anterolateral margin of the tongue; the center of the tongue has few if any taste buds. The foliate papillae are 2 to 9 vertically oriented, pinkish troughs located along the side of the tongue near the palatoglossal arch. The taste buds are buried within the trenches formed by the papillar folds. Taste buds also are buried within the trenches that surround the 7 to 10 circumvallate papillae located on the posterior tongue. Fluid access to the taste buds of the circumvallate and foliate papillae is limited unless accompanied by mechanical stimulation, which typically accompanies both drinking and chewing. The taste buds on the soft palate, epiglottis, and larynx are embedded in the surface epithelium rather than being associated with a specialized papilla.

Each of the lingual and extralingual populations of taste buds has a unique innervation pattern. The taste buds within the fungiform papillae and the rostral half of the foliate papillae are innervated by the chorda tympani nerve, a branch of the facial nerve (cranial nerve VII). The taste buds located on the soft palate are innervated by another branch of the facial nerve, the greater superficial petrosal nerves. Taste receptors within the circumvallate papillae and the posterior half of the foliate papillae are innervated by the glossopharyngeal nerve (cranial nerve IX). The remaining taste buds on the epiglottis, larynx, and esophagus are innervated by the lingual branch of the vagus nerve (cranial nerve X). Based on electrophysiological studies in animals, the vagus nerve may play a more important role in airway protection than gustatory perception (Bradley, 2000). Because gustatory information is conveyed by three different nerves, patients with damage to only one of these nerves may not notice a change in taste sensation during eating (Bartoshuk et al., 1983). However, when patient questioning and gustatory testing are guided by the different sources of innervation for the anterior and posterior tongue, it is often possible to identify patients whose taste deficits are caused by damage to only one of the gustatory nerves.

Central Gustatory Pathways

The facial, glossopharyngeal, and vagus nerves terminate in the nucleus of the solitary tract (NST) in the medulla, which, in addition to relaying taste information to the forebrain, mediates salivary, gastric, pancreatic, and intestinal reflexes related to feeding (Beckstead & Norgren, 1979). The rostral tip of the NST, which in humans is often referred to as the gustatory nucleus, receives projections from the facial nerve. The terminal area of the glossopharyngeal nerve includes the entire rostral half of the NST. Involvement of the vagus nerve in taste is probably minor and certainly dwarfed by its role as the conduit for visceral afferent information bound for the caudal NST from the thoracic and abdominal viscera.

In addition to the anterior-posterior partition on the tongue, there is an important left-right division to the gustatory system because taste information ascends from the tongue to cortex in a strictly ipsilateral fashion (Pritchard & Norgren, 2003). Thus, most taste deficits not of systemic origin are restricted to one side of the tongue (hemiageusia). When central damage is suspected, there is a strong likelihood that gustatory and somatosensory deficits will coexist given the proximity of these two systems at every level of the neuraxis (Pritchard & Norgren, 2003).

Most of what is known about the central projections of the gustatory system has been derived from studies on nonhuman primates, but it reinforces the fragmentary information available from humans

(Pritchard & Norgren, 2003). Ascending projections from the NST enter the central tegmental tract and ascend ipsilaterally to the parvicellular division of the ventroposteromedial nucleus of the thalamus (VPMpc), which lies at the medial tip of the oral somatosensory relay (Beckstead et al., 1980). Efferent projections from VPMpc terminate in the rostrodorsal insula and the adjacent inner operculum, which serve as primary taste cortex (Pritchard et al., 1986). Projections from primary taste cortex to the agranular insula and the caudal orbitofrontal cortex, which receive olfactory projections from the entorhinal cortex and the mediodorsal nucleus of the thalamus, may provide the anatomic basis for perception of flavor (Rolls, 1997).

In summary, the tongue consists of left and right halves, each of which is divisible into a large rostral portion (anterior two thirds) and a small caudal segment (posterior one third). Diagnosis and testing can be undertaken with this organization model.

Classification of Taste Deficits

Gustatory testing may focus on either quantitative or qualitative aspects of taste perception involving either specific regions of the oral cavity or the entire mouth. Given the time-consuming nature of taste testing, the types of testing to be done warrants careful consideration. Most taste tests are conducted to corroborate the patient's complaint and are especially useful when there are questions about the patient's ability to differentiate gustatory, olfactory, and somatosensory information from one another. In addition, testing the patient's sense of taste allows the physician to observe firsthand the conditions under which the chemosensory (or somatosensory) complaint emerges as well as determine the patient's degree of permanent taste impairment or disability. When the taste loss is a work-related injury, the results of gustatory testing may form the basis for a workers' compensation claim or legal action. In some cases a verifiable chemosensory loss may provide the impetus for upgrading the company's safety procedures. When pretreatment testing is done, the physician has a baseline for monitoring treatment efficacy and symptom resolution. Bearing in mind that many patients with olfactory problems complain that their sense of taste has been affected, an abbreviated taste test may be administered to patients who, based on the history, require a convincing demonstration that their deficit is, in fact, olfactory and not gustatory.

The patient history and clinical evaluation should be used to identify patients who do not require taste testing. For example, gustatory problems caused by a lapse in dental hygiene are likely to resolve after consulting a dentist. After the decision to perform gustatory testing has been made, the next step is to determine the type of taste test to perform. Ideally, each of the tests described below should be tested; in reality, taste testing is too time consuming to permit the physician that luxury. In most cases one or two taste tests should be done, and depending on how cooperative the patient is, testing may require more than one session. It is more important that gustatory testing in the clinic be efficient than comprehensive. The choice of which tests to conduct should be guided by the patient's initial taste complaint and the physician's preliminary diagnosis.

Different tests are used for patients with qualitative and quantitative taste deficits. The quantitative taste deficits are ageusias, hypogeusias, and hypergeusias. Ageusias are characterized by a complete loss of taste for one or more of the four basic taste qualities (salty, sweet, sour, bitter) included in a standard test battery. Ageusias are classified as "total" if all taste qualities are affected, "partial" if a few of the four basic taste qualities are involved, or "specific" if the deficit involves only one taste quality. A complete loss of taste sensation across the entire oral cavity is possible but rare because the gustatory receptors are both widely distributed and innervated by three different cranial nerves. Hypogeusias are characterized by a diminution of taste intensity for one or more of the gustatory stimuli and similarly may or may not involve the entire oral cavity. Total, partial, or specific hypogeusias have been reported. When either an ageusia or a hypogeusia is suspected, the goal of taste testing is to determine if the patient's perception of taste intensity lies within the normal range. Patients with hypergeusias report enhanced taste sensitivity, a rare symptom sometimes observed in association with migraine attacks (Blau & Soloman, 1985).

Qualitative taste deficits (dysgeusias or parageusias) are typically persistent and unpleasant, often being described as bitter, salty, or metallic and less often as sour or sweet. Dysgeusias described with nongustatory terms (e.g., foul, fetid, or rancid) may, in fact, be olfactory dysosmias. Sometimes spontaneously appearing dysgeusias are referred to as gustatory hallucinations, but unlike a true hallucination that occurs in the absence of sensory stimulation, many gustatory "hallucinations" have identifiable causes such as fetid secretions from intraoral cysts, abscesses, wounds, or crevicular spaces that spill onto taste receptive areas. Some dysgeusias are triggered by the presence of food or drink in the mouth; others are masked by eating. Nerve damage, toxic exposure, strokes, burning-mouth syndrome, and head trauma are known causes of dysgeusia, but in most cases the cause cannot be identified (Smith et al., 1987; Costanzo & Dinardo, 1995; Grushka & Epstein, 1997).

Stimulus Selection and General Guidelines for Gustatory Testing

It is imperative that stimulation of the gustatory system be done with as little activation of either the

TABLE 15-5. Recommended Concentrations: Focal and Whole-Mouth Taste Tests

Quality	Stimulus	Stimulus concentration	
		Focal testing	Whole mouth
Salty	Sodium chloride (NaCl)	1.0 M	0.01–1.0 M
Sweet	Sucrose	1.0 M	0.01–1.0 M
Sour	Citric acid	0.03 M	0.00032–0.032 M
Bitter	Quinine hydrochloride (QHCl)	0.001 M	0.0000032–0.001 M

(Adapted from Bartoshuk LM: Clinical evaluation of the sense of taste. Ear Nose Throat J 68:331–337, 1989.)

somatosensory or olfactory system as possible. Although a perfect method of gustatory stimulation does not exist, the use of appropriate tastants and the proper stimulation technique will ensure that the effects of concomitant tactile, thermal, and olfactory stimuli are minimized. The ideal gustatory stimulus does not have an odor and does not cool (e.g., menthol) or burn (e.g., capsaicin) the tongue. The four gustatory stimuli listed in Table 15-5 meet these criteria. Ideally, the taste stimuli should be dissolved in distilled or deionized water, but for field testing it may be necessary to use tap water. When testing suprathreshold concentrations, the use of tap water as a diluent for the sapid stimuli should have no effect provided the water does not have a distinct odor or taste.

Testing should be started at least 1 hour after the subject's last meal and several hours after the subject's last use of tobacco or alcohol. Regardless of which taste test is used, each stimulus should be thoroughly rinsed from the tongue with the same type of water used as the diluent. Testing should be done at a relaxed pace with sapid stimuli being applied 45 to 60 seconds apart; longer rest periods and additional rinses are recommended after testing sour or bitter stimuli.

Psychophysical Testing of Taste

Depending on the patient's symptoms, quantitative and qualitative testing may be conducted on selected parts or all of the oral cavity. Because whole mouth testing more closely approximates the patient's real-life experience during eating and drinking, it has some utility in a clinical setting. Whole mouth testing, however, does not allow the taste deficit to be localized within the oral cavity. The most common method of whole mouth stimulation is the "sip and spit" technique. The patient sips a small volume of the tastant, typically about 10 mL, and after swishing the fluid around the mouth, spits it into a waste container. After identifying the quality or intensity of the tastant, the patient rinses with water. A thorough rinse and the 45- to 60-second interstimulus period maximize the patient's sensitivity by limiting taste adaptation.

Focal (i.e., regional) testing, unlike whole mouth testing, enables the physician to determine the gustatory receptive field and thereby identify both the innervation and laterality of the affected area. For this reason, we recommend focal taste testing for all patients, including those who feel they can localize taste symptoms to part of the oral cavity with whole mouth stimulation. The most compelling reason for focal testing is that it may expose taste problems that escape detection with whole mouth testing (Pritchard et al., 1999). Ideally, the anterior, lateral (i.e., foliate), and posterior (i.e., circumvallate, epiglottal, and soft palate) gustatory fields should be tested, but patients with very sensitive gag reflexes may not tolerate probing of the posterior oral cavity.

Focal testing can be performed with either fluid-saturated paper disks, a pipette, or a cotton-tipped applicator soaked with the sapid stimulus. The paper disks and the cotton swabs provide excellent control of stimulus volume; their primary drawback is that stimulus application is accompanied by physical contact with the tongue, which causes unwanted somatosensory stimulation. Compared to the other techniques, cotton-tipped applicators that have long wooden shafts provide the best access to the taste buds along the side of the tongue and the posterior oral cavity. The main advantage of the paper disk technique is that it standardizes the application area, which is important because taste sensitivity increases as the stimulated area increases (Smith, 1971). Regardless of which technique is used, differences in receptor density across the tongue dictate that taste stimuli be applied to corresponding areas of the left and right sides of the tongue. For the same reason, it is imperative that the same area of the tongue/oral cavity be stimulated in all patients.

Testing for Qualitative Deficits in Taste Perception

Although the etiology of dysgeusias can be difficult to identify, it is relatively easy to verify that the patient has a problem in taste quality perception. The stimuli and concentrations of the taste stimuli used for qualitative testing are shown in Table 15-5. The concentrations of taste stimuli used for focal testing are higher than those used for whole mouth testing because the sapid stimuli are applied to restricted areas of the oral cavity.

Whether whole mouth testing or focal testing is used, the qualitative assessment simply involves asking the patient to identify that taste. The patient may describe the stimuli either verbally or by pointing to a list of descriptors; regardless of which technique is used, it should be open-ended in case the patient requires nongustatory names to describe the oral experience. It is important to bear in mind, however, that even people with normal taste perception occasionally confuse sour with either bitter or salty. When a patient appears to be confusing sour, bitter, and salty stimuli, a brief discussion with the patient after the first series of trials may enable the physician to determine if the patient is unable to distinguish the different stimuli from each other or is unable to name them correctly. This discussion may improve the patient's proficiency on the next test series. Even if some sour, bitter, salty confusion persists, patients with normal perception of taste quality will limit their descriptions of taste quality to the four basic taste qualities: salty, sweet, sour, bitter. Descriptors such as fecal, metallic, burning, caustic, and the like indicate that the patient's problem is not gustatory.

Testing of Quantitative Deficits in Taste Perception

When whole mouth stimulation is used to test patients whose chief complaint is hypogeusia, it is likely that the taste deficit will go undetected in the clinic if the problem is caused by damage to only one of the six (three per side) gustatory nerves. The probability of confirming the patient's complaint improves significantly when focal taste stimulation is used to test circumscribed areas of the tongue. Focal testing also allows the physician to locate the affected area within the oral cavity, an important step toward identifying the cause of the taste deficit. The technique we recommend is based on the one used successfully at the University of Connecticut and Yale University; see Bartoshuk (1989) for a complete description of the latter procedure.

Briefly, sapid stimuli are applied separately to the anterolateral (fungiform) and the posterior (circumvallate) gustatory fields; testing of the soft palate and epiglottal areas can be done in patients who can tolerate taste stimulation in those areas without gagging. In a departure from the Yale and Connecticut protocols, we do not recommend testing the taste buds of the lateral (foliate) field because their innervation by the facial and glossopharyngeal nerves varies significantly among patients.

Stimulation of the anterolateral field is done with the subject's tongue protruded approximately 1 inch and secured between the lips. The taste receptors of the circumvallate papillae, soft palate, and epiglottis can be accessed if a piece of gauze is used to grasp the tip of the tongue and gently deflect it to the side opposite where the sapid stimuli will be applied. The cotton-tipped applicator should be moist, but not dripping, when it is gently rolled across the target area. The affected side of the tongue, if known, should be tested first and the stimulation should be done from medial to lateral to avoid crossing the midline. Patients report the intensity of the stimulus prior to retracting the tongue to ensure that the fluid stimulus does not spread to the opposite side of the tongue or spread to a larger area than intended. Perceived taste intensity is reported with a modified magnitude estimation technique. In a departure from the traditional magnitude estimation technique, the patients rate the perceived intensity of each tastant by making a mark at the appropriate point along a 100-point scale that is marked with semantic labels such as weak, moderate, strong, and very strong (Green et al., 1993, 1996). Because the labeled magnitude scale encourages patients to use their real-life experiences to rate perceived taste intensity, interpatient variability is reduced. Parametric or nonparametric statistical tests can be used to determine if differences in taste intensity between the left and right sides of the tongue are statistically significant. When published norms for the labeled magnitude test become available, it will be possible not only to determine the percentile score of each patient but also identify malingerers.

Although some patients notice hypogeusias, in most cases the multiple innervations of the taste receptors causes focal ageusias or dysgeusias to go unnoticed.

Treatment of Gustatory Disorders and Prognosis for Recovery

The prospects and course for recovery from a gustatory deficit are as varied as the causes of the dysfunction itself. A patient's prospects for recovery are excellent when the gustatory symptoms are related to a medical or dental condition that does not directly involve the gustatory system such as allergies, upper respiratory infections, or gingivitis. In cases such as these the taste disturbance typically improves as the medical/dental condition resolves. When the problem can be traced to a specific medication or treatment, gustatory symptoms are likely to disappear shortly after their discontinuation. For example, gustatory disorders related to cancer (either the disease process itself or its treatment) often resolve within several months following a cure or termination of treatment. Persistent chemosensory deficits in cancer survivors may signal permanent damage to the oral cavity caused by the disease or the prior medical treatment. Gustatory deficits of idiopathic origin are among the most difficult to treat and the least likely to recover spontaneously.

Post-traumatic gustatory disturbances, which may account for 18% of all taste problems, typically are not amenable to treatment (Deems et al., 1991). When recovery does occur, it usually takes place without intervention, takes weeks or months to begin, and may not be uniform across the four basic taste qualities. In the trauma patients examined by Costanzo and Becker (1986), when taste recovered, sweetness returned first and bitterness last. The relationship between locus and severity of head injury and the probability and degree of recovery is not well understood and requires further study.

Chemosensory disorders that resist treatment degrade the patient's quality of life and in many instances cause both depression and anxiety. One fourth of all patients reporting a taste or smell disorder also suffered mild to severe depression, and conversely, 35% of all depressed patients complain of changes in taste or smell perception (Deems et al., 1991). When an underlying cause for the patient's chemosensory complaint cannot be identified, a psychiatric diagnosis should be considered. Regardless of whether the chemosensory or the psychiatric disorder is determined to be the causative factor, successful treatment of the patient's chemosensory disorder will require that any comorbid psychiatric problems be addressed as well.

Deems and colleagues (1996) reported that 63% of patients with dysgeusias show partial or complete spontaneous remission, typically in less than 1 year. Approximately 35% of the dysgeusias caused by upper respiratory infections resolve after treatment (Mott et al., 1993). Beyond targeting related medical or dental conditions, however, there are no established treatments that permanently improve taste acuity or abolish a dysgeusia (Mott et al., 1993). Even zinc therapy, which has been touted for years as an effective treatment for hypogeusias and dysgeusias, is of questionable value. Patients who complain of a metallic taste when eating may obtain some relief by switching to plastic eating utensils (Johnson, 2001).

Rinsing, lozenges, topical anesthetics (e.g., dyclonine), and even eating may provide temporary relief when the gustatory symptoms are of peripheral origin; obviously none of these are suitable for long-term symptomatic treatment. Patients may be able to partially reinvigorate foods by experimenting with texture (nuts, croutons, syrups, gravies), food colorings, spices (pepper, oregano), temperature, and even garnishes. Commercially available flavors (e.g., bacon, butter) have been used to augment foods for the elderly in both hospital and nursing home settings (Schiffman, 1993). Finally, the desirability of foods may be enhanced by improving the visual presentation of the meal and the table setting. All patients, but particularly those with diabetes and hypertension, should be cautioned not to augment the flavor of foods by increasing their use of table salt or sugar (Mattes et al., 1990). Professional counseling by a nutritionist may be warranted for patients who are particularly frustrated by their chemosensory loss.

SEEKING HELP FOR OLFACTORY AND GUSTATORY DISORDERS

Few general practitioners are either trained or equipped to diagnose and treat chemosensory disorders, so in most instances patients will require a referral to an otorhinolaryngologist or neuro-otolaryngologist. Even though these specialists are trained in the diagnosis and treatment of ear, nose, and throat disorders, they are unlikely to have special training in the chemical senses. Physicians who suspect that a patient will require more thorough testing than they are able to provide can still perform the preliminary tests in their office and then, if appropriate, refer the patient to a smell and taste center for more thorough testing. The staff of these chemosensory clinics includes ear, nose, and throat specialists as well as sensory physiologists and psychophysicists trained in the measurement, diagnosis, and treatment of taste and smell disorders. American taste and smell clinics listed in Table 15-6 accept self-referrals.

SUMMARY

Impairments of olfaction may accompany or be caused by many neurologic disorders, traumatic injuries, medical illnesses, and environmental toxic exposure. Olfactory problems are especially prevalent in older adults, often without an obvious cause. Upper respiratory disorders, medication side effects and behavioral habits (e.g., smoking) are also frequent contributors to olfactory alterations that are classified generally as anosmia (loss), dysosmia (reduction), parosmia (altered), or phantosmia (olfactory auras and hallucinations). Depending on the degree and type of olfactory changes, these impairments can be minor or quite bothersome and must be diagnosed, assessed, and managed for the health and safety of the patient.

Gustatory disorders may be comorbid with olfactory disorders or present in isolation. Taste perception can be affected by upper respiratory, neurologic, and medical illnesses; toxic exposures; oral and dental conditions; psychiatric disorders; nutritional deficiencies; and medication side effects. Taste disorders are classified as focal or complete ageusia (loss of salty, sweet, sour, and /or bitter), hypogeusia (reduction), and parageusia/dysgeusia. Assessment and management revolves around fairly comprehensive medical, neurologic, and oral examinations, with treatable causes sometimes being identified.

Patients with chemosensory disorders report a diminished quality of life and social isolation. After repeated unsuccessful trips to doctors' offices, considerable frustration and hopelessness may ensue. Although many taste and smell problems are difficult to treat, patients feel a sense of vindication and relief when they

TABLE 15-6. American Specialty Centers for Chemosensory Disorders

Virginia Commonwealth University/Medical College Virginia Smell and Taste Clinic
A.D. Williams Clinic Building
Suite 401
12th and Marshall Streets
Richmond, VA 23219
Director: Richard Costanzo
Tel: (804) 628-4ENT (628-4368)
Fax: (804) 828-8299
E-mail: ent@hsc.vcu.edu
Website: http://views.vcu.edu/ent/fspc.htm

State University of New York (SUNY) Smell and Taste Disorders Clinic
SUNY Health Science Center at Syracuse
750 East Adams Street
Syracuse, NY 13210
Director: Daniel Kurtz, PhD
Tel: (315) 464-5588
Fax: (315) 464-7712
E-mail: kurtzd@mail.upstate.edu
Website: www.upstate.edu/ent/smelltaste/shtml

San Diego Nasal Dysfunction Clinic
University of California, San Diego Medical Center
225 Dickinson Street
San Diego, CA 92103
Director: Terence M. Davidson, MD
Tel: (619) 543-3893 or (619) 657-8594
E-mail: tdavidson@ucsd.edu
Website: www-surgery.ucsd.edu/ent/DAVIDSON/NDC/booklet.htm#Anatomy

Chemosensory Clinical Research Center
Monell Chemical Senses Center
3500 Market Street
Philadelphia, PA 19104-3308
Director: Gary Beauchamp, PhD
Tel: (215) 898-6666
Fax: (215) 898-2084
E-mail: info@monell.org
Website: www.monell.org/contactus_h.htm

Connecticut Chemosensory Clinical Research Center
University of Connecticut Health Center
263 Farmington Avenue
Farmington, CT 06030-1718
Director: Marion Frank, PhD
Tel: (860) 679-2459
Fax: (860) 679 1382
E-mail: tasteandsmell@neuron.uchc.edu
Website: www.uchc.edu/unconntassteandsmell/index.html

The Smell and Taste Center at the University of Pennsylvania
3400 Spruce Street
5 Ravdin Pavilion
Philadelphia, PA 19104
Director: Richard L. Doty, PhD
Tel: (215) 662-6580
Fax: (215) 349-5266
E-mail: emma.barkley@uphs.med.upenn.edu
Website: www.smellandtastecenter.com

Rocky Mountain Taste and Smell Center
University of Colorado Health Science Center
4200 East Ninth Avenue, Box B-205
Denver, CO 80262
Tel: (303) 315-6600
Fax: (313) 315-8787
Website: www.uchsc.edu/rmtsc

receive an accurate description and diagnosis of their chemosensory complaint. Diagnosis of a chemosensory disorder requires a complete patient history, a thorough medical and neurological examination, appropriate chemosensory testing, and sometimes referral to a specialty center.

Acknowledgments

We would like to thank Ms. Laura Hough and Mr. Nathan Salinas for organizing the references. During the preparation of this manuscript, T.C.P.'s salary was funded, in part, by Public Health Service grants DC04436 and DK59549.

■ KEY POINTS

☐　More than 200,000 people in the United States seek medical treatment for a smell or taste disorder each year. An estimated 2.7 million Americans report chronic olfactory impairment and 2 million adults with chemosensory problems are not currently under a physician's care. The incidence of olfactory problems increases gradually with age until by age 65 more than one half of the populace has an olfactory deficit. The percentage of people over 80 who report an inability to either detect or identify odors exceeds 75%.

☐　Most patients with a chemosensory disorder report a partial or complete loss of taste or smell. Others describe various distortions of taste or odors or gustatory/olfactory hallucinations. These deficits are more than an inconvenience because affected patients experience a diminished quality of life and increased safety risk. More serious chemosensory deficits interfere with eating and drinking, and undermine nutrition and metabolism.

☐ Taste and smell alterations can be caused by disease, trauma, environmental exposures, medications, aging, psychiatric disorders, and iatrogenic interventions that affect peripheral or central chemosensory structures. Most chemosensory deficits are secondary to another disease process or treatment that does not directly involve structures typically associated with the chemical senses. For this reason, olfactory and gustatory disorders must be evaluated in the context of the patient's overall health, history, and lifestyle.

☐ Olfactory alterations include anosmia, hyposmia, parosmias, and phantosmias. Gustatory alterations include ageusias, hypogeusias, parageusias, and hypergeusias.

☐ Olfactory and taste changes can be evaluated with clinical screening tests, standardized psychophysical procedures that yield quantitative data regarding chemosensory threshold, discrimination, and identification.

☐ Treatment options for olfactory and gustatory disorders are fairly limited. Most important among them are identification and treatment of any underlying medical and oral dental conditions as well as diseases primarily affecting peripheral and central chemosensory structures. Because many medications have side effects on the chemosenses, careful evaluation of these effects is indicated. Some natural recovery of function is possible, particularly in disorders with acute onset.

KEY READINGS

Deems DA, Doty RL, Settle RG, et al: Smell and taste disorders: A study of 750 patients from the University of Pennsylvania Smell and Taste Center. Arch Otolaryngol Head Neck Surg 117:508–528, 1991.

Doty RL: Olfaction. Ann Rev Psychol 52:423–452, 2002.

Finkelstein JA, Schiffman SS: Workshop on taste and smell in the elderly. An overview. Physiol Behav 66:173–176, 1999.

Gent JF, Frank ME, Mott A: Taste testing in clinical practice, in Seiden AM (ed): Taste and Smell Disorders. New York: Thieme, 1997.

REFERENCES

Ackerman BH, Kasbekar N: Disturbances of taste and smell induced by drugs. Pharmacotherapy 17:482–496, 1997.

Amsterdam JD, Settle RG, Doty RL, et al: Taste and smell disorders in depression. Biol Psychiatry 22:1481–1485, 1987.

Anderson J, Maxwell L, Murphy C: Odorant identification testing in the young child [abstract]. Chem Senses 17: 590, 1992.

Bartoshuk LM: Clinical evaluation of the sense of taste. Ear Nose Throat J 68:331– 337, 1989.

Bartoshuk LM, Gent J, Catalanotto FA, et al: Clinical evaluation of taste. Am J Otolaryngol 4:257–260, 1983.

Beckstead RM, Morse JR, Norgren R: The nucleus of the solitary tract in the monkey: Projections to the thalamus and brain stem nuclei. J Comp Neurol 190:259–282, 1980.

Beckstead RM, Norgren R: Central distribution of the trigeminal, facial, glossopharyngeal, and vagus nerves in the monkey. J Comp Neurol 184:455–472, 1979.

Berman JL: Dysosmia, dysgeusia, and diltiazem [letter]. Ann Intern Med 102:717, 1985.

Blau JN, Solomom F: Smell and other sensory disturbances in migraine. J Neurol 232:275–276, 1985.

Bloomfeld RS, Graham BG, Schiffman SS, et al: Alterations of chemosensory function in end-stage liver disease. Physiol Behav 66:203–207, 1999.

Bradley RM: Sensory receptors of the larynx. Am J Med 108(Suppl. 4a):47S–50S, 2000.

Brightman VJ: Abnormalities of taste, in Lynch MA, Brightman VJ, Greenberg MS (eds): Burket's Oral Medicine. Philadelphia, PA: Lippincott, 1994, pp. 343–378.

Busaba NY: Is imaging necessary in the evaluation of the patient with an isolated complaint of anosmia? Ear Nose Throat J 80:892–896, 2001.

Cain WS, Stevens JC: Uniformity of olfactory loss in aging. Ann N Y Acad Sci 561:29–38, 1989.

Carroll B, Richardson JT, Thompson P: Olfactory information processing and temporal lobe epilepsy. Brain Cogn 22:230–243, 1993.

Catalanotto FA, Dore-Duffy P, Donaldson JO: Taste and smell function in multiple sclerosis, in Meiselman HL, Rivlin RS (eds): Clinical Measurement of Taste and Smell. New York: Macmillan, 1984, pp. 519–528.

Chaves EM, Ship JA: Sensory and motor deficits in the elderly: Impact on oral health. J Public Health Dent 60:279–303, 2000.

Christensen TA, White J: Representation of olfactory information in the brain, in Finger TE, Silver WL, Restrepo D (eds): The Neurobiology of Taste and Smell, ed 2. New York: Wiley-Liss, 2000, pp. 201–232.

Ciechanover M, Peresecenschi G, Aviram A, et al: Malrecognition of taste in uremia. Nephron 26:20–22, 1980.

Costanzo RM, Becker DP: Smell and taste disorders in head injury and neurosurgery patients, in Meiselman HL, Rivlin RS (eds): Clinical Measurement of Taste and Smell. New York: Macmillan, 1986, pp. 565–578.

Costanzo RM, DiNardo LJ: Head injury and taste, in Doty RL (ed): Handbook of Olfaction and Gustation. New York: Marcel Dekker, 1995, pp. 775–783.

Currie S, Heathfield KWG, Henson RA, et al: Clinical course and prognosis of temporal lobe epilepsy. A survey of 666 patients. Brain 94:173–190, 1971.

Deems DA, Doty RL, Settle RG, et al: Smell and taste disorders: A study of 750 patients from the University of Pennsylvania Smell and Taste Center. Arch Otolaryngol Head Neck Surg 117:508–528, 1991.

Deems DA, Yen DM, Kreshak A, et al: Spontaneous resolution of dysgeusia. Arch Otolaryngol Head Neck Surg 122:961–963, 1996.

Desor JA, Maller O: Taste correlates of disease states: Cystic fibrosis. J Pediatr 87:93–96, 1975.

Devenand DP, Michaels-Marston KS, Xinhua L, et al: Olfactory deficits in patients with mild cognitive impairment predict Alzheimer's disease at follow up. Am J Psychiatry 157:1399–1405, 2000.

Dielenberg RA, Hunt GE, McGregor IS: "When a rat smells a cat": The distribution of Fos immunoreactivity in rat brain following exposure to a predatory odor. Neuroscience 104:1085–1097, 2001.

Dikken C, Sitzia J : Patients' experiences of chemotherapy: Side-effects associated with 5-fluorouracil + folinic acid in the treatment of colorectal cancer. J Clin Nurs 7:371–379, 1998.

Doty RL: Odor Threshold Test Administration Manual. Haddon Heights, NJ: Sensonics, 2000.

Doty RL: Olfaction. Annu Rev Psychol 52:423–452, 2001.

Doty RL, Deems DA, Stellar S: Olfactory dysfunction in parkinsonism: A general deficit unrelated to neurologic sign, disease stage, or disease condition. Neurology 38:1237–1244, 1988.

Doty RL, Mishra A: Olfaction and its alteration by nasal obstruction, rhinitis, and rhinosinusitis. Laryngoscope 111:409–423, 2001.

Doty RL, Reyes PF, Gregor T: Presence of both odor identification and detection deficits in Alzheimer's disease. Brain Res Bull 18:597–600, 1987.

Doty RL, Shaman P, Applebaum SL, et al: Smell identification ability: Changes with age. Science 226:1441–1443, 1984a.

Doty RL, Shaman P, Dann M: Development of the University of Pennsylvania Smell Identification Test: A standardized microencapsulated test of olfactory function. Physiol Behav 32:489–502, 1984b.

Doty RL, Yousem DM, Pham L, et al: Olfactory dysfunction in patients with head trauma. Arch Neurol 57:1131–1140, 1997.

Drachman DA, Adams RD: Herpes simplex and acute inclusion body encephalitis. Arch Neurol 7:61–79, 1962.

Duffy VB, Ferris AM: Nutritional management of patients with chemosensory disturbances. Ear Nose Throat J 68:395–397, 1989.

Duhra P, Foulds IS: Methotrexate-induced impairment of taste acuity. Clin Exp Dermatol 13:126–127, 1988.

Duncan HJ, Seiden AM: Long-term follow-up of olfactory loss secondary to head trauma and upper respiratory tract infection. Arch Otolaryngol Head Neck Surg 121:1183–1187, 1995.

Efron R: The effect of olfactory stimuli in arresting uncinate fits. Brain 79:267–281, 1956.

Ekstrand T: Bell's palsy: Prognostic accuracy of case history, sialometry and taste impairment. Clin Otolaryngol 4:183–196, 1979.

Elsner RJ: Environment and medication use influence olfactory abilities of older adults. J Nutr Health Aging 5:5–10, 2001.

Erikssen J, Seegaard E, Naess K: Side-effects of thiocarbamides. Lancet 1:231–232, 1975.

Eskenazi B, Cain WS, Novelly RA, et al: Odor perception in temporal lobe epilepsy patients with and without temporal lobectomy. Neuropsychologia 24:553–562, 1986.

Eslinger P, Damasio AR, Van Hosen GW: Olfactory dysfunction in man: Anatomical and behavioral aspects. Brain Cogn 1:259–285, 1982.

Ewing RC, Janda SM, Henann NE: Ageusia associated with transdermal nitroglycerin. Clin Pharmacol 8:146–147, 1989.

Fehm-Wolfsdorf G, Scheible E, Zenz H, et al: Taste thresholds in man are differentially influenced by hydrocortisone and dexamethasone. Psychoneuroendocrinology 14:433–440, 1989.

Finkelstein JA, Schiffman SS: Workshop on taste and smell in the elderly: An overview. Physiol Behav 66:173–176, 1999.

Frye RE, Schwatz BS, Doty RL: Dose-related effects of cigarette smoking on olfactory function. JAMA 263:1233–1236, 1990.

Gansler DA, Fucetola R, Krengel M, et al: Are there cognitive subtypes in adult attention deficit/hyperactivity disorder? J Nerv Ment Dis 186:776–781, 1998.

Garrett-Laster M, Russell RM, Jacques PF: Impairment of taste and olfaction in patients with cirrhosis: The role of vitamin A. Hum Nutr Clin Nutr 38C:203–214, 1984.

Gent JF, Goodspeed RB, Zagranski RT, et al: Taste and smell problems. Validations of questions for the clinical history. Yale J Biol Med 60:27–35, 1987.

Ghorbanian SN, Paradise JL, Doty RL: Odor perception in children in relation to nasal obstruction [abstract]. Pediatr Res 12:371, 1978.

Goodspeed RB, Catalanotto FA, Gent JF, et al: Clinical characteristics of patients with taste and smell disorders, in Meiselman HL, Rivlin RS (eds): Clinical Measurement of Taste and smell. New York: Macmillan, 1988, pp. 451–466.

Goodspeed RB, Gent JF, Catalanotto FA: Chemosensory dysfunction: Clinical evaluation results from a taste and smell clinic. Postgrad Med 81:251–260, 1987.

Graham CS, Graham BG, Bartlett JA, et al: Taste and smell losses in HIV infected patients. Physiol Behav 58:287–293, 1995.

Green BG, Dalton P, Cowert B, et al: Evaluating the 'labelled magnitude scale' for measuring sensation of taste and smell. Chem Senses 21:323–334, 1996.

Green BG, Shaffer GS, Gilmore MM: Derivation and evaluation of a semantic scale of oral sensation magnitude with apparent ratio properties. Chem Senses 18:683–702, 1993.

Green RF: Subclinical pellagra and idiopathic hypogeusia. JAMA 218:1303, 1971.

Griep MI, Van der Niepen P, Sennesael JJ, et al: Odor perception in chronic renal disease. Nephrol Dial Transplant 12:2093–2098, 1997.

Griffin JP: Drug-induced disorders of taste. Adverse Drug React Toxicol Rev 11:229–239, 1992.

Grossman S: Loss of taste and smell due to propylthiouracil therapy. N Y State J Med 53:1236, 1953.

Grushka M, Epstein JB : Burning mouth syndrome, in Seiden AM (ed): Taste and Smell Disorders. New York: Thieme, 1997, pp. 159–171.

Halter J, Kulkosky P, Woods S, et al: Afferent receptors, taste perception, and pancreatic endocrine function in man [abstract]. Diabetes 24:414, 1975.

Hamilton JM, Murphy C, Paulsen JS: Odor detection, learning, and memory in Huntington's disease. J Intl Neuropsychol Soc 5:609–615, 1999.

Haskell GT, Maynard TM, Shatzmiller RA, et al: Retinoic acid signaling at sites of plasticity in the mature central nervous system. J Comp Neurol 452:228–241, 2002.

Hausser-Hauw C, Bancaud J: Gustatory hallucinations in epileptic seizures. Electrophysiological, clinical and anatomical correlates. Brain 110:339–359, 1987.

Hawkes CH, Shephard BC: Olfactory evoked responses and identification tests in neurological disease. Ann N Y Acad Sci 855:608–615, 1998.

Hellekant G, Gopal V: Depression of taste responses by local or intravascular administration of salicylates in the rat. Acta Physiol Scand 95:286–292, 1975.

Henkin RI: Abnormalities of taste and olfaction in patients with chromatin negative gonadal dysgenesis. J Clin Endocrinol Metab 27:1436–1440, 1967.

Henkin RI: The role of adrenal corticosteroids in sensory processes, in Blaschko H, Smith AD, Sayers G (eds): Handbook of Physiology Endocrinology. Baltimore: Williams & Wilkins, 1975, pp. 209–230.

Henkin RI, Christiansen RL, Bosma JF: Impairment of recognition of oral sensation and familial hyposmia in patients with facial hypoplasia and growth retardation: A new syndrome [abstract]. Clin Res 14:236, 1966.

Henkin RI, Kopin IJ: Abnormalities of taste and smell thresholds in familial dysautonomia: Improvement with methacholine. Life Sci 3:1319–1325, 1964.

Henkin RI, Smith FR: Hyposmia in acute viral hepatitis. Lancet 1:823–826, 1971.

Henkin RI, Talal N, Larson AL, et al: Abnormalities of taste and smell in Sjogren's syndrome. Ann Intern Med 76:375–383, 1972.

Hilgers FJ, Jansen HA, Van As CJ, et al: Long-term results of olfaction rehabilitation using the nasal airflow-inducing ("polite yawning") maneuver after total laryngectomy. Arch Otolaryngol Head Neck Surg 128:648–654, 2002.

Hoffman HJ, Ishii EK, MacTurk RH: Age-related changes in the prevalence of smell/taste problems among the United States adult population. Results of the 1994 disability supplement to the National Health Interview Survey (NHIS). Ann N Y Acad Sci 855:716–722, 1998.

Homewood J, Stevenson RJ: Differences in naming accuracy of odors presented to the left and right nostrils. Biol Psychiatry 58:65–73, 2001.

Hosemann W, Goertzen W, Wohlleben R, et al: Olfaction after endoscopic sinus surgery. Am J Rhinol 7:11–15, 1993.

Hughlings-Jackson JH: Clinical remarks on the occurrence of subjective sensations of smell in patients who are liable to epileptiform seizures, or who have symptoms of mental derangement, and in others. Lancet 1:659–660, 1866.

Jafek BW, Gordon AS, Moran DT, et al: Congenital anosmia. Ear Nose Throat J. 69:331–337, 1990.

Jafek BW, Moran DT, Eller PM, et al: Steroid-dependent anosmia. Arch Otolaryngol Head Neck Surg 113:547–547, 1987.

Jaffe IA: Ampicillin rashes [letter]. Lancet 1: 245, 1970.

Jeppsson PH, Hallen O: The taste after operation for otosclerosis. Pract Otorhinolaryngol (Basel) 33:215–221, 1971.

Johnson FMG: Alterations in taste sensation: A case presentation of a patient with end-stage pancreatic cancer. Cancer Nurs 24:149–155, 2001.

Jorgensen MB, Buch NH: Studies on the sense of smell and taste in diabetics. Acta Otolaryngol 53:539–545, 1961.

Kashima HK, Kalinowski B: Taste impairment following laryngectomy. Ear Nose Throat J 58:62–71, 1979.

Kopala L, Clark C, Hurwitz T: Olfactory deficits in neuroleptic naive patients with schizophrenia. Schizophr Res 12:205–211, 1992.

Kuten A, Ben-Aryeh H, Berdicevsky I, et al: Oral side effects of head and neck radiation: Correlation between clinical manifestations and laboratory data. Int J Radiat Oncol Biol Physiol 12:401–405, 1986.

Laemmle H: Uber geruchsstorungen und ihre klinische bedeutung. Arch Ohren Nasen Kehlropfheildunde 30:22–42, 1932.

Lang NP, Catalanotto FA, Knopfi RU, et al: Quality-specific taste impairment following the application of chlorhexidine digluconate mouthrinses. J Clin Periodontol 15:43–48, 1988.

Langen MJ, Yearick ES: The effects of improved oral hygiene on taste perception and nutrition in the elderly. J Gerontol 31:413–418, 1976.

Lehrner JP, Brucke T, Dal-Bianco P, et al: Olfactory functions in Parkinson's disease and Alzheimer's disease. Chem Senses 22:105–110, 1997.

Leopold DA, Hornung DE, Youngentob SL: Olfactory loss after upper respiratory infection, in Getchell TV, Doty RL, Bartoshuk LM, et al (eds): Smell and Taste in Health and Disease. New York: Raven Press, 1991, pp. 731–734.

Levinson JL, Kennedy K: Dysosmia, dysgeusia, and nifedipine [letter]. Ann Intern Med 102:135–136, 1985.

Macht DI, Macht MB: Comparison of effect of cobra venom and opiates on olfactory sense. Am J Physiol 129:P411–412, 1940.

Magliulo G, Cordeschi S, Sepe C, et al: Taste and lacrimation after acoustic neuroma surgery. Rev Laryngol Otol Rhinol (Bord) 119:167–170, 1998.

Magnasco LD, Magnasco AJ: Metallic taste associated with tetracycline therapy. Clin Pharmacol 4:455–456, 1985.

Males JL, Townsend JL, Schneider RA: Hypogonadotropic hypogonadism with anosmia-Kallman's syndrome. A disorder of olfactory and hypothalamic factors. Arch Intern Med 131:501–507, 1973.

Marshall JR, Henkin RI: Olfactory acuity, menstrual abnormalities, and oocyte status. Ann Intern Med 75:207–211, 1971.

Mattes RD, Cowert BJ Schiavo MA et al: Dietary evaluation of patients with smell and/or taste disorders. Am J Clin Nutr 51:233–240, 1990.

McConnell RJ, Menendez CE, Smith FR, et al: Defects of taste and smell in patients with hypothyroidism. Am J Med 59:354–364, 1975.

McGrath N, Anderson NE, Croxson MC, et al: Herpes simplex encephalitis treated with acyclovir: Diagnosis and long term outcome. J Neurol Neurosurg Psychiatry 63:321–326, 1997.

Mori K, Nagao H, Yoshihara Y: The olfactory bulb: Coding and processing of odor molecule information. Science 286:711–715, 1999.

Mossman KL: Gustatory tissue injury in man: Radiation dose response relationships and mechanisms of taste loss. Br J Cancer 53(Suppl. VII):9–11, 1986.

Mott AE, Cain WS, Lafreniere D, et al: Topical corticosteroid treatment of anosmia associated with nasal and sinus disease. Arch Otolaryngol Head Neck Surg 123:367–372, 1997.

Mott AE, Grushka M, Sessle BJ: Diagnosis and management of taste disorders and burning mouth syndrome. Dent Clin North Am 37:33–71, 1993.

Murphy C, Schubert CR, Cruickshanks KJ, et al: Prevalence of olfactory impairment in older adults. JAMA 288:2307–2312, 2002.

Nordin S, Bramerson A, Liden E, et al: The Scandinavian odor-Identification test: development, reliability, validity and normative data. Acta Otolaryngol 118:226–234, 1999.

Nordin S, Murphy C, Davidson TM, et al: Prevalence and assessment of qualitative olfactory dysfunction in different age groups. Laryngoscope 106:739–744, 1996.

Ogawa T, Rutka J: Olfactory dysfunction in head injured workers. Acta Otolaryngol 540:50–57, 1999.

Ogle W: Anosmia: Cases illustrating the physiology and pathology of the sense of smell. Medico-Chirurgie Transaktionen 53:263–290, 1870.

Olsen KD, Se Santo LW: Olfactory neuroblastoma: Biloogical and clinincal behavior. Acta Otolaryngol 109:797–802, 1983.

Ophir D, Guterman A, Gross-Isseroff R: Changes in smell acuity induced by radiation exposure of the olfactory mucosa. Arch Otolaryngol Head Neck Surg 114:853–855, 1988.

Panayiotou H, Small SC, Hunter JH, et al: Sweet taste (dysgeusia). The first symptom of hyponatremia in small cell carcinoma of the lung. Arch Intern Med 15:1325–1328, 1995.

Passouant P: Olfaction et epilepsie. Rev Laryngol Otol Rhinol (Bord) 86(Suppl.):935–953, 1965.

Pinching AJ: Clinical testing of olfaction reassessed. Brain 100: 377–388, 1977.

Plath P, Otten E: Untersuchungen uber die Wirksamkeit von Hexetidine bei akuten Erkrankungen des Rachens und der Mundhohle sowie nach Tonsillektomie. Therapiewocke 19:1565–1566, 1969.

Potter H, Butters N: An assessment of olfactory deficits in patients with damage to prefrontal cortex. Neuropsychology 18:621–628, 1980.

Price S: The role of zinc in taste and smell, in Meiselman HL, Rivlin RS (eds): Clinical Measurement of Taste and Smell. New York: Macmillan, 1986, pp. 443–445.

Pritchard TC, Hamilton RB, Norgen R: Projections from thalamic gustatory and lingual areas in the monkey, *Macaca facsicularis.* J Comp Neurol 244:213–228, 1986.

Pritchard TC, Macaluso DA, Eslinger PJ: Taste perception in patients with insular cortex lesions. Behav Neurosci 113:663–671, 1999.

Pritchard TC, Norgren R: Gustatory system, in Paxinos G (ed): The Human Nervous System. 2003, in press.

Rawson NE: Human olfaction, in Finger TE, Silver WL, Restrepo D (eds): The Neurobiology of Taste and Smell, ed 2. New York: Wiley-Liss, 2000, pp. 257–284.

Rawson NE, Brand JG, Cowert BJ, et al: Functionally mature olfactory neurons from two anosmic patients with Kallman's syndrome. Brain Res 681:58–64, 1995.

Rawson NE, Gomez G, Cowert B, et al: The use of olfactory receptor neurons (ORNs) from biopsies to study changes in aging and neurodegenerative diseases. Ann N Y Acad Sci 855:701–707, 1998.

Rollin H: Drug-related gustatory disorders. Ann Otol Rhinol Laryngol 87:37–42, 1978.

Rolls ET: Taste and olfactory procesing in the brain and its relation to the control of eating. Crit Rev Neurobiol 11:263–287, 1997.

Rundles RW: Prognosis in the neurologic manifestations of pernicious anemia. Blood 1:209–219, 1946.

Rydzewski B, Pruszewski A, Sulkowski WJ: Assessment of smell and taste in patients with allergic rhinitis. Acta Otolaryngol 120:323–326, 2000.

Savic I, Berglund H, Gulyas B, et al: Smelling of odorous hormone-like compounds causes sex-differentiated hypothalamic activations in humans. Neuron 31:661–668, 2001.

Schechter PJ, Henkin RI: Abnormalities of taste and smell after head trauma. J Neurol Neurosurg Psychiatry 37:802–810, 1974.

Schiffman SS: Taste and smell in disease. N Engl J Med 308: 1275–1279, 1337–1342, 1983.

Schiffman SS: Drugs influencing taste and smell perception, in Getchell TV, Doty RL, Bartoshuk LM, et al (eds): Smell and Taste in Health and Disease. New York: Raven Press, 1991, pp. 845–850.

Schiffman SS: Perception of taste and smell in elderly persons. Crit Rev Food Sci Nutr 33:17–26, 1993.

Schiffman SS: Taste and smell losses in normal aging and disease. JAMA 278:1357–1362, 1997.

Schiffman SS, Clark CM, Warwick ZS: Gustatory and olfactory dysfunction in dementia: Not specific to Alzheimer's disease. Neurobiol Aging 11:597–600, 1990.

Schiffman SS, Zervakis J: Taste and smell perception in the elderly: Effect of medications and disease. Adv Food Nutr Res 44:247–346, 2002.

Scott PJ: Glossitis with complete loss of taste sensation during Dindevan treatment: Report of a case [abstract]. N Z Med J 59:296, 1960.

Seiden AM: The initial assessment of patients with taste and smell disorders, in Seiden AM (ed): Taste and Smell Disorders. New York: Thieme, 1997, pp. 4–19.

Serby M, Larson P, Kalkstein D: The nature and course of deficits in Alzheimer's disease. Am J Psychiatry 148:367–360, 1991.

Settle RG: The chemical senses in diabetes mellitus, in Getchell TV, Doty RL, Bartoshuk LM, et al (eds): Smell and Taste in Health and Disease. New York: Raven Press, 1991, pp. 829–843.

Shafer DM, Frank ME, Gent J, et al: Gustatory function after third molar extraction. Oral Surg Oral Med Oral Pathol Oral Radiol Endod 87:419–429, 1999.

Shear PK, Butters N, Jernigan TL, et al: Olfactory loss in alcoholics: Correlations with cortical and subcortical MRI indices. Alcohol 9:247–255, 1992.

Ship JA: The influence of aging on oral health and consequences for taste and smell. Physiol Behav 66:209–215, 1999.

Siegfreid J, Zumstein H: Changes in taste under L-DOPA therapy. Z Neurol 200:345–348, 1971.

Skouby AP, Zilstorff-Pedersen K: The influence of acetylcholine-like substances, menthol and strychnine on olfactory receptors in man. Acta Physiol Scand 32:252–258, 1954.

Smith DV: Taste intensity as a function of areas and concentration: Differentiation between compounds. J Exp Psychol 87: 163–171, 1971.

Smith DV, Frank RA, Pensak ML, et al: Characteristics of chemosensory patients and a comparison of olfactory assessment procedures [abstract]. Chem Senses 12:698, 1987.

Soni NK, Chatterji P: Gustotoxicity of bleomycin. J Otorhinolaryngol Relat Spec 47:101–104, 1985.

State FA, Hamed MS, Bondok AA: Effect of vincristine on the histological structure of taste buds. Acta Anat 99:445–449, 1977.

Stroop WG, McKendall RR, Battles EK, et al: Spread of herpes simplex virus type I in the central nervous system during experimentally reactivated encephalitis. Microb Pathog 8:119–134, 1990.

Thumfart W, Plattig KH, Schlict N: Smell and taste thresholds in older people. Zeit Gerontol 13:158–188, 1980.

Twomey JA, Barker CM, Robinson G, et al: Olfactory mucosa in herpes simplex encephalitis. J Neurol Neurosurg Psychiatry 42:983–987, 1979.

Warner M, Peabody C, Berger P: Olfactory deficits and Down's syndrome. Biol Psychiatry 23:836–839, 1988.

Weiffenbach JM, Fox PC: Odor identification ability among patients with Sjogren's syndrome. Arthritis Rheum 36:1752–1754, 1993.

Weinstock RS, Wright HN, Spiegel AM, et al: Olfactory dysfunction in humans with deficient guanine nucleotide-binding protein. Nature 322:635–636, 1986.

Welge-Luessen A, Temmel A, Quint C, et al: Olfactory function in patients with olfactory groove memingioma. J Neurol Neurosurg Psychiatry 70:218–221, 2001.

Wolberg FL, Ziegler DK: Olfactory hallucination in migraine. Arch Neurol 39:382, 1982.

Zilstorff K: Sense of smell alterations by cocaine and tetracaine. Arch Otolaryngol 82:53–55, 1965.

Zilstorff K, Herbild O: Parosmia. Acta Otolaryngol 360(Suppl.): 40–41, 1979.

Zusho H: Posttraumatic anosmia. Arch Otolaryngol 108:90–92, 1982.

Vestibular System and Balance

Deema Fattal

Matthew Rizzo

Disequilibrium

Dizziness

Labyrinth

Lightheadedness

Vertigo

Vestibular

Vestibulo-ocular reflex

Dizziness is a common complaint that affects up to 20% of the general population (Yardley et al., 1998c) and one forth to one third of persons over 75 years of age (Tinetti et al., 2000). Patients may describe their dizziness in terms of spinning sensation, lightheaded-ness, giddiness, near-fainting, swimming, floating, walking on clouds, and other nonspecific language, and there may be multiple underlying conditions to diagnose and treat.

The term dizziness encompasses three main symptom types: (1) vertigo—sensations of spinning or, rarely, linear movement; (2) presyncope—sensations of near fainting or lightheadedness; and (3) disequilibrium/unsteadiness ("dizziness in the feet," as one patient put it). Vertigo is often due to vestibular dysfunction in the end-organ or its central connections in the brain (Baloh, 1999), whereas nonvertiginous dizziness has diverse causes including vestibular, cardiovascular, medication effects, metabolic, or psychological (Baloh, 1998a).

This chapter reviews symptoms and signs of peripheral and central vestibular disorders, along with approaches to the evaluation and management of patients who complain of dizziness. We begin with the anatomy and physiology of the inner ear, the vestibular nerve, and their central connections through the brainstem, cerebellum, thalamus, and the "vestibular cortex."

ANATOMY OF THE VESTIBULAR SYSTEM

Inner Ear

Anatomy and Physiology

Embryologically, the labyrinth begins with the *otic placodes*, ectodermal thickenings on each side of the rhombencephalon (Sadler, 1990). Invagination of each otic placode forms the primitive *otocyst*, which has three primary components that develop into the parts of the labyrinth: (1) the endolymphatic sac and duct, (2) the utricle and semicircular canals, and (3) the saccule and cochlear ducts. Regions in the labyrinth later differentiate into the specialized hair cells. The inner ear begins to develop at about 3 weeks of gesta-

tion. The semicircular canals are present by the end of the fourth week. The cochlear formation terminates by the eighth week (Sadler, 1990).

The basic anatomy of the inner ear is summarized in Figure 16-1 (see also Baloh, 1996, 1998a; Parent, 1996; Afifi, 1998; Brandt, 2000; Goebel, 2001). The inner ear is encased within the bony labyrinth at the apex of the petrous bone of the skull (Fig. 16-2). Within the bony labyrinth are a series of tubes and sacs called the *membranous labyrinth*. The membranous labyrinth is composed of a single cell layer and consists of the *semicircular canals*, the *otolith organs*, and the *cochlea*. It is filled with endolymphatic fluid and is surrounded by *perilymph*, which is cerebrospinal fluid, and is connected to the subarachnoid space, via the *vestibular aqueduct* (Fig. 16-3). The endolymphatic fluid is secreted by the membranous labyrinth cells and absorbed via the *endolymphatic sac*.

The three semicircular canals are the anterior (superior), posterior (inferior), and horizontal (lateral) canals. The first two are oriented vertically and perpendicular to each other. The horizontal canals are almost

FIGURE 16-1. A three-dimensional overview of the anatomy of the inner ear (see Fig. 16-3 for details). (Reprinted with permission of the Anatomical Chart Company.)

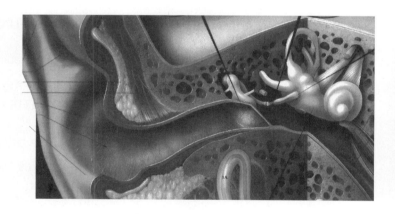

FIGURE 16-2. A bird's-eye view of the bony labyrinth embedded in the petrous bone. (Reproduced with permission from Goebel JA [ed]: Practical Management of the Dizzy Patient. Philadelphia: Lippincott Williams & Wilkins, 2001.)

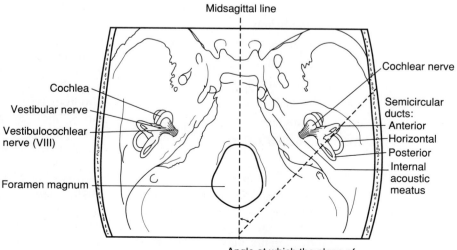

horizontal in orientation and are perpendicular to the vertical ones. The anterior canal on one side is parallel to the posterior canal on the other side.

Each canal has one enlarged ending, the ampulla (Fig. 16-4). Within each *ampulla*, the membranous labyrinth cell layer contains a patch of specialized *hair cells*. The region of the hair cells and surrounding cells supporting them is termed the *crista*. Each hair cell has cilia that are embedded in gelatinous material, the *cupula*. The cilia of each cell contain one long cilium called the *kinocilium* (Fig. 16-5). There are two types of hair cells, types I and II. The afferents on type I are flask-like and button-like terminals, whereas those on type II are only button-like. These afferents form the *vestibular division of the eighth cranial nerve*. They fire at a basal rate. With angular rotations of the head, the movement of the endolymph/ampulla causes deflection in the cilia. There is more firing if the deflection is in the direction of the kinocilia.

Each canal is stimulated by head rotation in its plane. The afferent nerve fibers of one horizontal canal increase their baseline firing rate when the head is turned ipsilateral to the canal. This causes the ampulla to deflect in the direction of kinocilia. This is also the direction toward the utricle. This is called *ampullipetal* flow. On the other hand, the nerve endings of the vertical canals increase their firing rate when the flow is away from the utricle-*ampullifugal* flow.

The otolith organs consist of the *utricle* and *saccule*. Together they are also called the *vestibule* (see Fig. 16-4). Each otolith organ has a patch of specialized hair cells called *macula*. The maculae of the utricle and saccule are perpendicular to each other (Fig. 16-6). The hair cells have cilia and kinocilia embedded in gel that is topped by calcium carbonate crystals (*otoconia*). Movement of the otoconia causes movement of the gel and deflection of the cilia (Fig. 16-7). The resultant firing in the vestibular nerve depends on the direction of the deflection of the kinocilia.

The otolith is stimulated by linear acceleration movement or by static head tilts (as the otoconia move with gravitational pull; Fig. 16-7). The otolith also provides the brain with information about position of the head with respect to gravity.

A dilemma for the brain is how to distinguish linear acceleration from simple static head tilts (Baloh, 1998a). The frequency of stimulation may provide a clue because low-frequency stimulation tends to arise with head tilt and high-frequency stimuli with linear acceleration (Leigh & Zee, 1999). Another clue is that head tilt produces asymmetrical stimulation of the vertical canals, whereas linear acceleration produces symmetrical stimulation.

Blood Supply

The *labyrinthine* artery supplies blood to the inner ear and arises usually from the anterior inferior cerebellar artery (AICA) and sometimes from the basilar artery (Fig. 16-8). The labyrinthine artery divides into the *anterior vestibular artery*, which supplies the anterior/

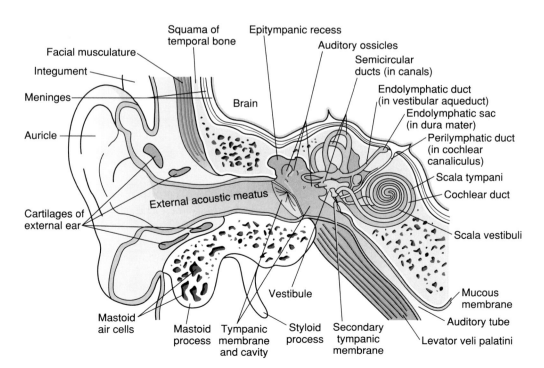

FIGURE 16-3. Coronal section of the ear. (Reproduced with permission from Tusa R, Brown S: Neuro-otologic trauma and dizziness, in Rizzo M, Tranel D [eds]: Head Injury and Postconcussive Syndrome. New York: Churchill Livingstone, 1996, pp. 177–200.)

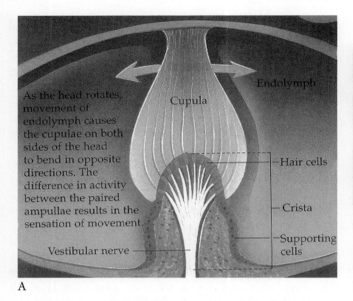

A

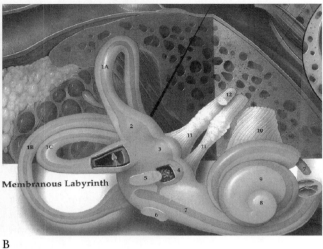

B

FIGURE 16-4. *A* is an enlargement of the ampulla of the horizontal canal of *B*. 1A, 1B, and 1C are the canals (anterior/posterior /horizontal); 2, ampulla of anterior canal; 3, utricle; 4, saccule (together 3 and 4 are called the vestibule); 4, a look into the saccule exposing the otoconia; 5, oral window; 6, round window; 7, cochlear duct; 8, cupula of cochlea; 9, cochlea; 10, cochlear division of cranial nerve VIII; 11, vestibular division of cranial nerve VIII; 12, stump of facial nerve. (Reproduced with permission from Baloh R: Dizziness, Hearing Loss, and Tinnitus: The Essentials of Neurotology. New York: Oxford University Press, 1984, p. 24.)

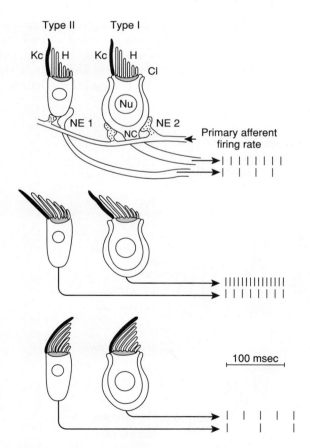

FIGURE 16-5. The hair cells have a basal firing rate (*top*) that increases with deviation of cilia in the direction of the kinocilium (Kc) (*middle*) and decreases with deviation away from Kc (*bottom*). (Reprinted with permission from the Anatomical Chart Company.)

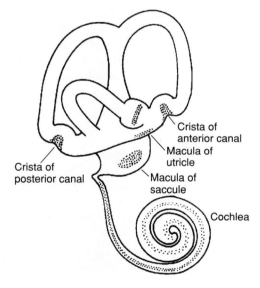

FIGURE 16-6. The areas of specialized hair cells throughout the labyrinth: the cochlea, the maculae of saccule (oriented vertically), and utricle (oriented horizontally) and the cristae of the three semicircular canals. Note that the two maculae are perpendicular to each other. (Reproduced with permission from Wersall DJ, Bagger-Sjobak D: Morphology of the vestibular sense organs, in Kornluber W [ed]: Handbook of Sensory Physiology. New York: Springer, 1974, pp. 123–170.)

horizontal canals, utricle, and the superior part of the saccule, and into the *common cochlear artery*. The common cochlear artery divides into a *posterior vestibular artery*, which supplies the posterior canal and inferior part of saccule, and the *main cochlear artery*,

Macula of Saccule *balance*

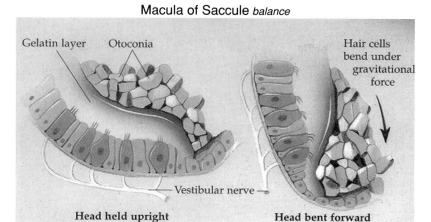

Gelatin layer   Otoconia

Hair cells bend under gravitational force

Vestibular nerve

Head held upright   Head bent forward

FIGURE 16-7. The otoconia of the maculae move with head movement depending on the pull of gravity. Their movement causes the cilia of the hair cells to bend, thus changing the firing rate of the vestibular nerve. (Reproduced with permission from the Anatomical Chart Company.)

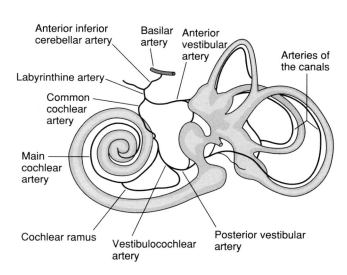

Anterior inferior cerebellar artery   Basilar artery   Anterior vestibular artery

Arteries of the canals

Labyrinthine artery

Common cochlear artery

Main cochlear artery

Cochlear ramus   Vestibulocochlear artery   Posterior vestibular artery

FIGURE 16-8. The blood supply of the inner ear. (Reproduced with permission from Schuknecht HF: Pathology of the Ear. Cambridge, MA: Harvard University Press, 1974.)

which supplies the cochlea. These are end arteries with no collaterals to protect the inner ear from infarction.

Brainstem and Cerebellum

Signals from hair cells are carried centrally via the vestibular nerve afferents to the bipolar neurons of the *Scarpa ganglion* in the internal auditory canal. From there, the central processes synapse on the *vestibular nuclei* in the upper medulla and lower pons (Fig. 16-9). A number of afferents go directly to the cerebellum (via the juxtarestiform body).

Vestibular Nuclei

The vestibular nuclei (VN) comprise four nuclei (lateral, medial, superior, and inferior). Most of their neurons receive multisensory inputs, making these nuclei "sensory integrators" (Baloh & Halmagyi, 1996). The inputs to the vestibular nuclei (see Fig. 16-9) are:

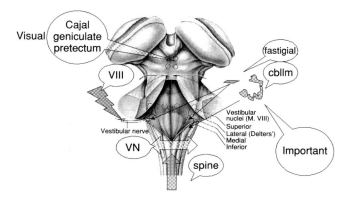

Visual   Cajal geniculate pretectum   (fastigial)   cbllm

VIII

Vestibular nerve   Vestibular nuclei (M. VIII) Superior Lateral (Delters') Medial Inferior   Important

VN   spine

FIGURE 16-9. The afferents of the vestibular nuclei (VN): (1) end-organ via cranial nerve VIII; (2) visual (interstitial nucleus of Cajal, lateral geniculate, pretectal area); (3) cerebellar input (fastigial nuclei and cortex); (4) proprioceptive input from the spine; (5) input from the contralateral VN. The cerebellar input (cbllm) has an important role. (Reproduced with permission from Kander E, Schwartz J: Principles of Neural Science. New York: Elsevier, 1985, p. 592.)

- Peripheral end-organ, the labyrinth
- The contralateral VN (inhibitory input)
- Spinovestibular input (proprioceptive)
- Cerebellar input (important and inhibitory)
- Indirect visual input (via interstitial nucleus of Cajal and superior colliculus)

- The VN output parallels the VN input (Fig. 16-10)
- Peripheral end-organ (i.e., VN modify the peripheral input)

- The contralateral VN
- Vestibulospinal tracts: lateral and medial
- Cerebellum
- Extraocular muscles nuclei—mainly via medial longitudinal fasciculus (MLF; Parent, 1996)

FIGURE 16-10. Vestibular nuclei efferents: (1) to end-organ via cranial nerve VIII; (2) to extraocular nuclei (EOM) via medial longitudinal fasciculus; (3) to cerebellum (cbllm); (4) to spine via lateral and medial vestibulospinal tracts; (5) to contralateral vestibular nuclei. All efferents are bilateral except to the cerebellum. Vestibular efferents to the cortex are via the ventroposterolateral (VPL) thalamic nuclei. (Reproduced with permission from Parent A: Carpenter's Human Neuroanatomy. Baltimore: Williams & Wilkins, 1996, p. 487.)

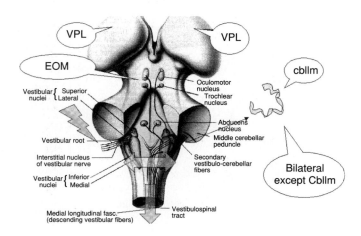

The VN also have connections with autonomic structures such as the locus ceruleus, parabrachial nucleus, nucleus solitarius and ambiguus, and the motor nucleus of the vagus nerve. VN have reciprocal connections with cerebellum, including the *flocculonodulus* (or "vestibulocerebellum"), uvula, and paraflocculus. The vestibular system remains a multisensory system at all levels rostral to the VN and up to the cortex, which may explain why a clearly demarcated unimodal primary sensory vestibular cortex has not been found (Guldin & Grusser, 1998).

Vestibular System Functions

To maintain posture and balance with ambulation, the body relies on the vestibular, visual, and proprioceptive systems. The information from these three systems is somewhat redundant, and some patients can balance with only one system functioning. On the other hand, patients with proprioceptive dysfunction who close their eyes while standing may fall straight to the floor (Adams & Victor, 1993). The cerebellum, pyramidal system, locomotor centers (mesencephalic, subthalamic, and pontine), subcortical nuclei (in the basal ganglia and thalamus), and cortical areas (frontal and, rarely, parietal) also contribute to posture, balance, and locomotion. For comprehensive reviews, see Burke (2001), Dietz (2001), and Mori and colleagues (2001).

The vestibular system maintains (1) gaze stability with head movement (e.g., during locomotion), (2) gait stability, and (3) spatial orientation, in association with three vestibular reflexes: the vestibulo-ocular reflex (VOR), the vestibulocollic reflex, and the vestibulospinal reflex (Tusa & Brown, 1996).

The *vestibulo-ocular reflex* (VOR) depends on the canal-ocular connections. The semicircular canals connect with extraocular nuclei via the MLF, which runs between the medulla, pons, and midbrain on both sides of the brainstem. Each canal is connected with the neurons controlling the muscles that move the eyes in the canal plane. For example, the horizontal canal is connected to the ipsilateral medial rectus and contralateral lateral rectus motoneurons. The horizontal canal is stimulated by turning the head ipsilaterally thus causing the eyes to deviate contralaterally.

The canal-ocular connections forming this VOR are stimulated by angular acceleration of the head. The angular VOR (aVOR) keeps visual targets in focus by preventing the slip of target images across the retina while the head moves, as during locomotion. This requires moving the eyes at the same speed and amplitude as the head movement, but in the opposite direction (180 degrees out of phase). The ratio of velocity of eyes to velocity of head is called the gain and is ideally 1 in magnitude, and is in the opposite direction. The aVOR responds to three-dimensional rotations: Yaw is rotation around a rostrocaudal axis, pitch is rotation around an interaural axis, and roll is rotation around the naso-occipital axis. Rotational head movements (especially in pitch) are normally at high frequencies (0.5–5 cycles/sec). This is commonly due to the heel strike during locomotion and is more pronounced during running. The latency of the aVOR is 7 to 15 msec (the fastest eye compensation mechanism for head movement) (Leigh & Zee, 1999).

Connections between the otolith and the extraocular muscle (EOM) motoneurons underlie the linear VOR (lVOR), which is triggered by linear movement. Otolith connections to the VN are not well mapped. The lVOR works at 2 Hz (Moore, 2000). The otolith also mediates another type of VOR called ocular counter rolling. It responds to sustained head tilt, which causes static torsional (counter rolling) of the eyes in the opposite direction to the head tilt (Leigh & Zee, 1999). The compensation is small, though, only about 10% of the tilt, and this incomplete compensation does not compromise vision because roll movements do not cause the images to slip much off the fovea.

The *vestibulocollic reflex* relies on information from the vestibular nuclei and proprioceptors in the cervical spine in the medial vestibulospinal tract to maintain orientation of head in space. The *vestibulospinal reflex* depends on the lateral vestibulospinal tract and maintains the orientation of the body in space.

The vestibular system works in conjunction with the proprioceptive and visual systems to relay information about orientation and movement of the body in space. For example, an observer on a train with a second train close by, and blocking the observer's entire field of view, may find it difficult to discern the other train as moving. In conjunction with other cues such as visual and proprioceptive cues, the vestibular function helps us to determine whether we are moving, or the environment is.

When there is conflict between cues provided by the visual, proprioceptive, and vestibular systems, a person may develop "*motion sickness.*" For example, the vestibular input of a passenger rocking in a cabin on a ship signals movement while visual inputs do not, creating a cue conflict that can trigger dizziness, nausea, sweating, tachycardia, increased swallowing, rapid breathing, and vomiting. To decrease symptoms, the passenger may rise to the deck and gaze at far objects so that the visual horizon now provides movement cues that correspond to vestibular information. Discomfort may also arise in elevators in which there are strong inertial cues without matching visual cues of movement, and in driving simulators or IMAX theaters, in which a visual scene conveys wide-field impressions of linear or angular movement that do not match the inertial cues received by the observer. Some of these effects are mitigated by learning or prolonged adaptation.

Imagine an automobile driver making a left turn at 15 miles per hour, turning the head and eyes left and right, and shifting the torso to avoid colliding with other vehicles. This offers a challenge to the vestibular system functions. Navigation through space and around obstacles depends not only on balance systems and reflexes mentioned above but also on multiple depth cues. *Motion parallax* is an important ability that allows us to discriminate depth from relative motion of objects when we are moving actively. *Motion perspective* comes into play when relative movement is produced by passive movement as when we look out the window of a moving vehicle.

Thalamus and Cortex

The vestibular nuclei connect with the cortex via the nucleus ventro-oralis intermedius (Vim), the nucleus ventrocaudalis externus (Vce), and the nucleus dorsocaudalis (Dc) of the thalamus. In animals, these correspond to nucleus ventroposterior lateralis, pars oralis (VPLo), nucleus ventroposterior lateralis, pars caudalis (VPLc), and the nucleus ventrolateralis, pars caudalis (VLc), respectively (Dieterich & Brandt, 1993). Studies of primates and nonprimates have identified several vestibular cortices (Guldin & Grusser, 1998; Fig. 16-11) These areas respond to peripheral vestibular stimulation and are connected to VN and to each other and include:

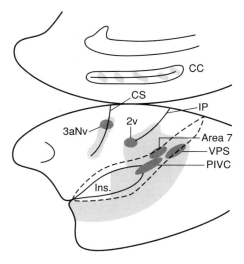

FIGURE 16-11. Monkey "vestibular" cortex. Also depicted are the insula (Ins) and the cingulate cortex (CC). The shaded areas are those that have been found to be involved in vestibular function/anatomy in primates and the black areas are those found in humans (Grusser & Guldin, 1998). PIVC, parietal insular vestibular cortex; VPS, visual posterior sylvian area; Area 7, within the lips of the sylvian fissure; 2v, at the anterior tip of the intraparietal sulcus (IP); 3aNv, neck vestibular region within the central sulcus (SC).

Frontal cortex
- Area 6v (vestibular part of area 6)
- Area VC (vestibular cingulate area)

Parietal areas
- Area 2v (intraparietal sulcus)
- Area 7 (within the lips of the sylvian fissure)

Temporal areas
- VPS (visual posterior sylvian area)
- MST (medial superior temporal)

Insular/Retroinsular region
- PIVC (parietal insular vestibular cortex)

Central sulcus
- 3aNv (3a-neck-vestibular area)
- 3aHv (3a-hand-vestibular area)

Only 30% to 50% of neurons in all the above regions respond to vestibular stimuli. These areas also receive multimodal inputs relevant to control of posture, hand movement, orientation in space, and movement of the head and neck relative to the body. The *parietal insular vestibular cortex* (PIVC) is the only area that is connected to all the above regions. Several lines of evidence indicate that the posterior insula in the vestibular system in humans plays a key role in the processing of vestibular information, as in animals. These lines of evidence are:

1. Penfield (1957) found that stimulation in the posterior superior temporal region and the posterior portion of the parietal lobe (temporoparietal bordering areas) precipitated

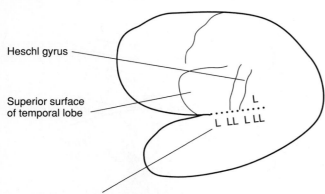

FIGURE 16-12. L refers to areas where Penfield stimulations caused sensation of dizziness or other related sensations (see text). (Reproduced with permission from Penfield W: Vestibular sensation and the cerebral cortex. Ann Otol 66:691, 1957.)

vertigo. In these experiments, application of electrical currents adjacent to Heschl gyrus caused a sensation of dizziness. Subjects also described sensations of "spinning," "swinging," "sinking," and a "full head" (Fig. 16-12). Parietal stimulation caused "bodily displacement" or "rotation," and parieto-occipital stimulation produced vertigo in one subject.

2. Tornado seizures, in which vertigo presents as an epileptic event, are thought to arise in temporal and parietal areas in and around the posterior insula (Ahmed, 1980; see also Chapter 8).

3. Patients with middle cerebral artery infarcts have perturbed sensation of the subjective vertical orientation, i.e., they cannot align a rod vertically in the dark. Anatomic analyses suggest a common key lesion in posterior insula (Fig. 16-13; Brandt et al., 1994).

4. Caloric, optokinetic, and proprioceptive stimulation (associated with parietal lesions) causes transient improvement of spatial hemineglect (Rubens, 1985; Rode et al., 1992; Karnath et al., 1993; see also Chapter 10).

5. Positron emission tomography (PET) scans involving caloric stimulation in normal individuals reveal activation of posterior insula and other areas (including temporoparietal cortex and putamen) commensurate with findings in nonhuman primates (Bottini et al., 1994; Fig. 16-14). Moreover, caloric and optokinetic stimuli and neck muscle vibration in normal individuals cause shifts in the body-fixed anterior-posterior axis that helps guide pointing movements in a "straight ahead" direction. One PET study showed involvement of the insula, retroinsular region, temporoparietal junction, and somatosensory area II (Bottini et al., 2001).

6. Functional magnetic resonance imaging (fMRI) using galvanic stimulation revealed similar findings. Galvanic stimulation involves stimulation of the vestibular nerve, bilaterally; it causes tilting in the subjective vertical orientation as well as a sensation of turning in subjects. Such studies showed involvement of the posterior insula and other areas including the temporoparietal junction, central sulcus, and intraparietal regions (Lobel et al., 1998); insula, thalamus, putamen, inferior parietal lobule, superior temporal gyrus, anterior cingulate, and others (Bense et al., 2001); and posterior insula, transverse temporal (Heschl) gyrus and thalamus (Bucher et al., 1998).

In sum, historical stimulation studies, lesions, and functional imaging studies all point to the fact that the posterior insula region plays an important role in vestibular function in humans.

VESTIBULAR DYSFUNCTION

Symptoms

Vestibular dysfunction results in dizziness, gaze and gait instability, and autonomic symptoms. First, diseases of the vestibular end-organ or its central connections cause vertigo (Latin, *vertere*, to turn) (Nagarkar et al., 2000), which is usually described as a spinning sensation and rarely as tilting or linear movement. Patients may also describe it as a merry-go-round, drunken state, world spinning, or spinning inside the head. A peripheral vestibular etiology is the most common. Second, VOR dysfunction destabilizes gaze during head movements, causing object images to de-focus and blur. When there is nystagmus, images jump back and forth causing *oscillopsia*. Unsteadiness or *disequilibrium* may arise from damage to spinal/vestibular connections that contribute to gait stability, balance, and maintenance of upright posture. Finally, autonomic symptoms (nausea, vomiting, pallor, sweating) may occur, especially with acute unilateral vestibular lesions, because of vestibular connections to autonomic centers in the brainstem.

Signs

Nystagmus

Nystagmus frequently accompanies vestibular symptoms and is characterized by rhythmic eye movements. These generally consist of slow movements in one direction and fast movements in the opposite direction. By convention, the direction of nystagmus is defined by the direction of the fast component.

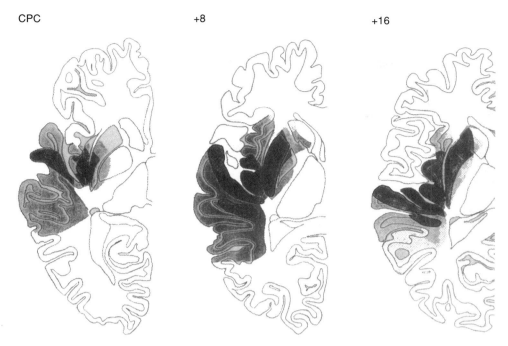

FIGURE 16-13. The areas shaded represent the overlap of lesions in patients with middle cerebral artery infarcts who also have subjective tilt of the vertical. (Reproduced with permission from Brandt T, Dieterich M, Danek A, et al: Vestibular cortex lesions affect the perception of verticality. Ann Neurol 35:403–412, 1994.)

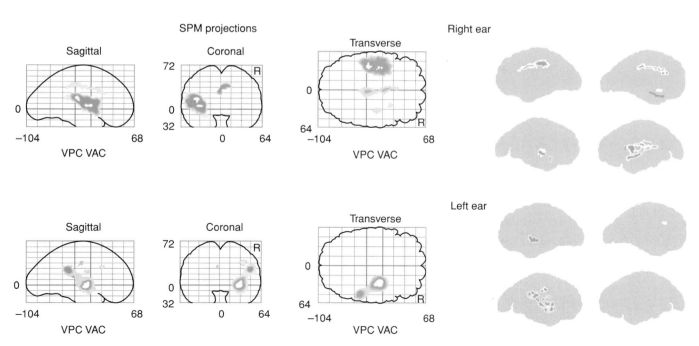

FIGURE 16-14. PET scan in normal subjects undergoing caloric stimulation. There is activation in the posterior insula. (Reproduced with permission from Bottini G, Sterzi R, Paulesu E, et al: Identification of the central vestibular projections in man. Exp Brain Res 99:164–169, 1994.)

In a peripheral vestibular lesion, the nystagmus is (1) horizontal with a torsional component, (2) unidirectional, (3) suppressed by fixation ("fixation suppression"), (4) contralateral to the lesion, and (5) obeys Alexander's law, that is, it is worse in the direction of the fast component of the nystagmus (Leigh & Zee, 1999).

Central nystagmus (1) is often pure horizontal, vertical, or torsional; (2) may change direction; and (3) is not affected by loss of fixation (Table 16-1). Examples of central nystagmus are downbeat and upbeat nystagmus (Table 16-2). Congenital nystagmus may change direction, like central nystagmus, but may be distinguished by its bizarre waveforms, early age of onset, and chronicity (Leigh & Zee, 1999).

The types of nystagmus mentioned above are forms of spontaneous nystagmus. In addition, nystagmus can be evoked by different positions. *Positional nystagmus* (also called static positional nystagmus) is present in certain positions, persists as long as the patient remains in that position, and is not often accompanied by vertigo. It may be direction-fixed or direction-changing and is mostly due to peripheral vestibular disease. If it does not suppress with fixation, the etiology is probably central.

Paroxysmal "positional" nystagmus (also called positioning nystagmus) is transient nystagmus that occurs on assuming a certain position. The most common variety, benign paroxysmal positional nystagmus (BPPN) can be elicited by Dix-Hallpike maneuver (Fig. 16-15). The presumed mechanism is debris from the otoconia of the otolith, moving within and stimulating the receptors in the semicircular canals. The debris commonly accumulates in the posterior canal, which is in a dependent position with respect to the otolith (see Fig. 16-4). The nystagmus has a brief latency of onset after movement (1–3 seconds), and usually lasts less than 30 to

TABLE 16-1. Clinical Characteristics of Peripheral vs Central Nystagmus

	Peripheral	*Central*
Orientation	Horizontal/torsional	Often pure, horizontal, vertical, or torsional
Direction	Unidirectional	May change direction
Loss of fixation	Increased	No effect
Relation to lesion site	Contralateral	Variable
Alexander's law	Obeys	Does not obey

TABLE 16-2. Clinical Downbeat and Upbeat Nystagmus

Downbeat nystagmus	*Upbeat nystagmus*
Worse with looking down and laterally	Worse with upgaze
Convergence may make it upbeat	Convergence may make it downbeat
Common locations	Common locations
Cervicomedullary junction	Pontomedullary junction
Lower cerebellum	Pontomesencephalic junction
	Medulla
	Midbrain
	Cerebellum
	Thalamus
Common causes	Common causes
Idiopathic 5–30%	Structural
Structural	Cerebellar/brainstem: stroke, tumor
Cerebellar/brainstem: stroke, tumor	Multiple sclerosis
Chiari malformation	Cerebellar degeneration
Multiple sclerosis	Thalamic arteriovenous malformation
Cerebellar degeneration	Infectious/inflammatory
Toxic/metabolic	Brainstem encephalitis
Mg/B$_{12}$ deficiency	Tobacco
Anticonvulsant/lithium toxicity	Congenital
Head injury	
Increased intracranial pressure	

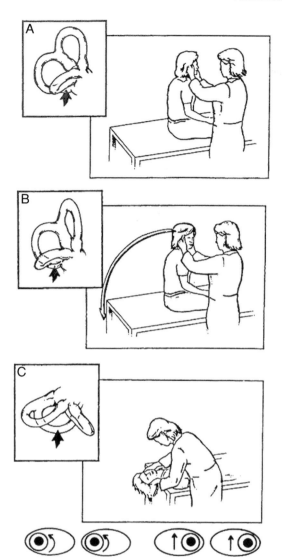

TABLE 16-3. Algorithm for Clinical Evaluation of Gait

I.   Gait evaluations

1   Romberg: check standing patient for any increased sway or falling to one side

2   Sharpened Romberg (similar to but more sensitive than Romberg): it is the same as Romberg, but even more sensitive

3   Tandem with eyes open: count how many steps the patient can walk prior to taking a side step (>10 is normal)

4   Tandem with eyes closed: administer if the above is normal, try tandem with eyes closed; this is a sensitive, but nonspecific test, of the locomotor system.

5   Check for steppage gait: ask the patient to march in place with eyes closed and observe any deviation

6   Assess for asymmetry of limb movement (hemiparetic, circumduction, asymmetrical arm swing)

7   Assess the ability of standing (without using arms) and speed of doing that

8   Assess the ability while walking to quickly stop and turn (an instability may be secondary to cerebellar disease)

9   Assess toe walking and check for any asymmetry

10   Assess heel walking and check for any asymmetry

11   Count the number of turns (normal is <2)

12   Assess for any truncal ataxia (sway back and forth as is seen with vermal disease)

13   Check for any spasticity or scissoring

14   Check for any shuffling or festination

15   Check stride length and base width

16   Check postural reflexes

FIGURE 16-15. Dix-Hallpike maneuver precipitating nystagmus in posterior canal BPPV: The eye ipsilateral to the ear down shows more torsional nystagmus and the contralateral eye shows more upbeat nystagmus. (Reproduced with permission from Herdman SJ: Vestibular Rehabilitation, ed 2. Philadelphia: FA Davis, 1999.)

60 seconds. It appears as torsional beating of the eyes toward the floor with the abnormal ear down, with a vertical component beating toward the forehead (see Fig. 16-15). If the debris is in the horizontal canal, the nystagmus is horizontal (in the plane of the canal).

Induced nystagmus is precipitated by certain maneuvers, such as hyperventilation in patients who have compression of the vestibular nerve due to a corticopontine angle (CPA) tumor, or in demyelinating disease, such as multiple sclerosis. The audiovestibular nerve is normally myelinated by oligodendrocytes even outside the brainstem and up to the point where it pierces the dura in the internal auditory canal. It is covered by oligodendrocytes for 1 to 1.5 cm of its

2.5 cm length (Jannetta, 1984). Head shaking can also trigger nystagmus in peripheral and central vestibular disease and is usually attributed to decompensation in VOR. Finally, noise can induce nystagmus (Tullio phenomenon), usually with a peripheral lesion such as a perilymph fistula.

Imbalance

Gait abnormalities are common in patients with vestibular disease (Table 16-3). Abnormal Romberg test and tandem gait are common. Romberg can be performed with the feet side by side, with more difficulty as a sharpened Romberg (standing with one foot in front of the other), or standing in Romberg position on foam. In addition, tandem gait can be done with the eyes open or closed (the more difficult version). Balance tests tend to elicit abnormalities, such as lateral sway, which is seen in acute vestibular disease, and is ipsilateral to lesions in labyrinth up to the pontomedullary region and contralesional to those in pontomesencephalic region, midbrain, or thalamus. (Brandt, 2000). In chronic states, the instability is non-localizing, because patients may fall to one side or the other due to overcompensation. For example, acute labyrinthine and vestibular nerve lesions cause ipsilateral falls. Lateral medullary infarcts cause *lateropulsion*, which is a sensation of being actively pulled to the ground ipsilaterally. This is accompanied by ocular lateropulsion, or more precisely *ipsipulsion*; when the patient closes the eyelids, the eyes drift ipsilaterally; when the patient is asked to look upward with the eyes open, the eyes drift obliquely toward the lesion side (Leigh & Zee, 1999).

Other Neurotologic Signs

"*Past-pointing*" is tested by asking the patient to elevate the arm above the head (with index finger extended) then lower it to touch the examiner's finger, first with the eyes open, then closed. Past-pointing is present if there is arm deviation to one side. As with imbalance, in acute cases the deviation is ipsilateral to lesions caudal to the pons and contralesional more rostral; chronically, it can be to either side.

Dynamic visual acuity may also fail. The patient is asked to shake the head rapidly at 2 Hz while reading the Snellen visual acuity chart. If acuity drops by more than one line, this suggests a VOR abnormality and is usually secondary to bilateral vestibular damage. This is a test of VOR suppression. In computerized versions of this test patients are asked to identify letters that move across a video monitor.

A useful clinical screen is to rotate a patient back and forth in a swivel chair while the patient fixates his or her own finger. This assesses VOR suppression. Asking the patient to fixate a spot on a far wall (without turning the head) during the rotation assesses VOR.

Head thrust is a useful maneuver for identifying unilateral vestibular end-organ disease, canal by canal (Halmagyi & Curthoys, 1988). Horizontal head thrusts test horizontal canals and up/down thrusts test the vertical canals. The patient fixates on a target 3 meters (c. 10 ft) away as the examiner thrusts the head in one quick movement; catch up saccades reflect canal paresis. Results are specific but not sensitive (Baloh & Halmagyi, 1996).

The Valsalva maneuver may occasionally precipitate nystagmus in patients with peripheral lesions such as in perilymphatic fistula. Pressure change in the external auditory canal caused by a pneumoscope (*Tragal pressure test*) may also precipitate nystagmus and aid in the diagnosis of fistula cases.

Testing for an *ocular tilt reaction* (OTR) may be useful. This reaction comprises: (1) ocular cyclorotation (ocular counter rolling); (2) head tilt; and (3) skew deviation, in which the eye ipsilateral to the head tilt is lower and the contralateral eye is higher (Baloh, 1998a,

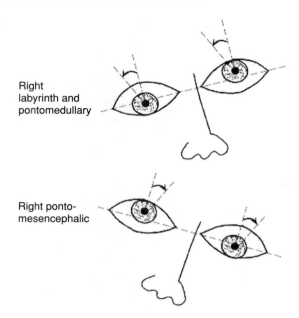

FIGURE 16-16. The ocular tilt reaction triad: head tilt; skew deviation; oculocyclotorsion. Lesions of the labyrinth/vestibular nerve/vestibular nuclei in medulla cause ipsilesional tilt, while mesencephalic lesions cause contralesional tilt. Pontine lesions cause tilts in either direction. The midbrain is the most rostral site reported to cause this triad. (Reproduced with permission from Baloh R: Dizziness, Hearing Loss, and Tinnitus: The Essentials of Neurotology. New York: Oxford University Press, 1984, p. 70.)

Fig. 16-16). This reaction occurs in peripheral and central lesions and may signify destruction of otolith-ocular connections. These connections seem to be ipsilateral below the pons and then cross in the pons to become contralateral rostrally. The head tilt is ipsilesional to damage in the labyrinth, VIII nerve, root entry zone, and with lateral medullary infarcts, and contralesional to damage in the upper pons and in mesencephalon. Pontine lesions can cause tilt to either direction (Dieterich & Brandt, 1993). Thalamic lesions, reported to cause ocular tilt reaction, have also involved the rostral midbrain. Thus, the midbrain seems to be the most rostral site to cause this triad or its components (Dietrich & Brandt, 1993; Brandt, 2000). All or some of the OTR components are present in up to 83% of brainstem lesions, making them important central signs (Dietrich & Brandt, 1993; 2000). MLF lesions may also cause an ocular tilt response (Baloh, 1998a).

Vestibular Syndromes

Damage in the vestibular system can occur at multiple points. Peripheral lesions may involve the labyrinth, vestibular nerve, or root entry zone. Central syndromes may arise with lesion of the brainstem, cerebellum, thalamus, or cortex (including superior temporal and adjacent parietal and frontal cortices). Symptoms vary depending on the locus of the lesion and whether the lesion is acute or chronic, unilateral or bilateral.

Acute vestibular syndromes generally evolve over seconds to hours or, rarely, a few days. The lesion is typically unilateral and produces acute asymmetry in signals reaching the cortex (Hotson & Baloh, 1998). An acute vestibular syndrome may also occur with asymmetrical bilateral lesions, as in head trauma.

Severe vertigo is a prominent feature of the acute vestibular syndrome. The spinning sensation is generally in the horizontal plane, that is, in the plane of the remaining healthy horizontal canal. The healthy vertical canals are perpendicular to each other and do not contribute because their effects cancel each other. Because the utricle and saccule of the healthy otolith structure are perpendicular to each other, their effects are also canceled. Thus, what is left is the healthy horizontal canal, which produces a sensation of spinning (as well as nystagmus) in its plane.

Although rare, vertigo described as either linear movement or tilting sensation may arise when signals from the otolith organ, vertical canals, or their central connections are affected differently than those from the horizontal canals.

The direction of the vertigo is a potentially misleading cue for lesion lateralization. For example, if the left ear is inflamed, signals from the functioning right horizontal canal produce the equivalent of right horizontal canal stimulation, as in turning the head to the right. The eyes (via VOR) move slowly to the left and corrective saccades move them back to the right, generating nystagmus with fast component to the right (i.e., contralesionally). If the eyes are open, the world may seem to move in the opposite direction of the slow movements of the eyes. The visual world appears to move slowly to the right, disappears suddenly, reappears on the left, and then drifts rightward again. When the eyes are closed, the patient feels unsteady and tends to fall ipsilesionally.

Strong autonomic discharges in acute vestibular syndromes, characterized by nausea, vomiting, pallor, and sweating, often accompany vertigo, blurred vision, oscillopsia, unsteadiness, and falling tendency. Patients with a peripheral lesion tend to keep their eyes open and fixate on an object. (Fixation suppression decreases peripheral nystagmus, as explained above.)

With peripheral disease, such as viral labyrinthine infection, there may also be auditory symptoms, such as unilateral hearing loss and tinnitus. With a central cause, such as brainstem stroke, central neurologic symptoms including bulbar, sensory, and others are generally present (see the section on stroke).

Patients with peripheral lesions are often much better within a few days. Although they may remain unsteady for a week and have short episodes of dizziness for 2 to 3 weeks, especially with movement, most are back to work within 1 month. Symptoms may last longer following a central lesion.

Brain Compensation and Recovery

Acute vestibular syndromes (both peripheral and central) lead to postural and oculomotor abnormalities that tend to recover over time. For example, spontaneous nystagmus with fixation following a peripheral lesion may persist a few days, and nystagmus in the absence of fixation for up to a month (Baloh & Halmagyi, 1996). The vestibular system recovers so well (due to a variety of mechanisms, often subsumed under the term "plasticity") that it is currently considered as a prototype for studying recovery from other conditions such as trauma and stroke. The mechanisms of this compensation probably depend on changing interactions between the vestibular nuclei and other brainstem nuclei (Ryu & McCabe, 1976; Vibert et al., 1999), cerebellum (Furman & Cass, 2003), and cortex, and are a topic of active research (Darlington & Smith, 2000). VOR may remain defective under dynamic conditions in the chronic phase of recovery. To compensate for this abnormal dynamic VOR, other mechanisms may be used. For example, catch-up saccades are used to complement defective VOR with head movement; patients may limit their head movement and turn only their eyes; and there is more dependence on the visual and proprioceptive systems to maintain equilibrium (Brandt, 2000). Therefore, vestibular compensation is good for static symptoms but is incomplete under dynamic conditions.

Recovery from vestibular impairments may be incomplete or delayed due to:

- Pre-existing brain disease (i.e., periventricular white matter disease, prior strokes, or lesions in brainstem/cerebellum)
- Advanced age (associated with small vessel ischemic disease)
- Prolonged use of vestibular suppressants, such as meclizine (Antivert), diazepam, or clonazepam, beyond the acute phase of several days
- Physical inactivity/slowing down (causing deconditioning)

Although vestibular suppressants decrease acute vertigo by suppressing vestibular function, their prolonged use beyond the acute phase of a vestibular syndrome (a few days) causes a cycle of further decrease in vestibular function (suppression), increased dizziness, ongoing need for medication, physical dependency, and delayed brain compensation (Baloh, 1998b). With incomplete recovery, patients may continue to experience brief episodes of lightheadedness, especially with quick head movements. This intolerance to movement has been called space and motion discomfort (SMD; Furman & Jacob, 2001) and may be due to VOR dysfunction. With quick head movements, the eyes cannot catch up, resulting in slip of retinal images, blurred vision, and dizziness. This state of movement-precipitated symptoms may contribute to more inactivity, leading to more deconditioning. SMD may depend on interplay between vestibular and psychological factors, addressed further below.

Bilateral lesions, acute or chronic, produce no vertigo if the lesions are symmetrical. Patients will have gaze and gait instability that improve over time, but may have chronic gait instability especially with loss of visual and proprioceptive inputs (e.g., in the dark and on uneven surfaces). Acutely, the gaze instability may be so severe that any head movement causes blurred vision, even the minimal movement that results from breathing. An example is vestibulotoxicity due to aminoglycosides (Table 16-4 shows other medications). Chronic unilateral vestibular lesions (such as an acoustic neuroma) cause slowly progressive unsteadiness and unilateral hearing loss, usually without vertigo.

One particular symptom seen in one inner ear disease, Meniere's disease, is *Tumarkin's otolithic crisis.* This is characterized by sudden falls without warning, altered sensorium, or other associated symptoms. Patients fall with full force, are unable to break the fall, and may even feel like they are being pushed to the ground. After the fall, patients are able to resume prior activities.

Tumarkin's crisis is in the differential diagnosis of drop attacks and occurs in 7% of patients with Meniere's disease, at any stage of disease. The pathophysiology is assumed to be secondary to otolith dys-

function. The frequency varies from a few attacks to repeated attacks throughout the disease. Treatment for patients with frequent attacks is vestibular ablation (Baloh & Halmagyi, 1996).

APPROACH TO THE DIZZY PATIENT

A systematic approach to evaluating dizziness can help delineate its cause in the majority of patients.

First, try to establish if the dizziness is:

- Vertigo (spinning or tilting/linear movement)
- Lightheadedness/near-fainting dizziness/floating/others
- Imbalance/disequilibrium without dizziness

Vertigo usually signifies an acute unilateral vestibular lesion. Fortunately, this usually lasts only a few days, and there is practically no "chronic vertigo." Whether the spinning is described in the environment or inside the head does not distinguish between vestibular and psychological causes. Duration of the vertigo, whether it is a first-time occurrence or a recurrence, and accompanying symptoms and signs will help differentiate a peripheral from a central lesion (Tables 16-5, 16-6, and 16-7).

Lightheadedness and *near-faint dizziness* occur in many settings and are described in different terms, such as giddiness, floating, dissociation from the body, swim-

TABLE 16-4. Drugs That Can Commonly Cause Dizziness

Drugs causing dizziness
Antiarrhythmics
Anticonvulsant
Antidepressants
Antihypertensives
Anti-inflammatory drugs
Antibiotics (e.g., aminoglycoside)
Chemotherapeutics
Muscle relaxants
Tranquilizers
Vestibular suppressants (e.g., benzodiazepines, antihistamine, anticholinergic, and antidopaminergic agents)

Ototoxic drugs
Antiarrhythmics
Diuretics
Aspirin
Chemotherapeutic agents (e.g., cisplatin)
Antibiotics (e.g., aminoglycoside, vancomycin, antimalarial drugs)
Heavy metals (mercury, lead)

TABLE 16-5. First Episode of Isolated Vertigo

Infection
Vestibular neuritis
Bacterial vestibulitis
Otomastoiditis
Trauma
Labyrinthine (concussion)
Infarction
Labyrinthine (artery or its branches)
Stroke/hemorrhage
Cerebellum

TABLE 16-6. First Episode of Vertigo with Associated Neurologic Symptoms/Signs

Stroke
Brainstem
Cerebellum
Hemorrhage
Brainstem
Cerebellum
Trauma
Brainstem concussion
Multiple sclerosis (could be recurrent)

TABLE 16-7. Recurrent Vertigo—by Duration

Seconds → BPPV

Minutes → Posterior circulation transient ischemic attacks

Hours → Meniere

Variable →

    Migraine (seconds-days)

    Multiple sclerosis

    Chiari malformation

    Perilymph fistula

ming, or near-fainting. Inquire if the symptoms are (1) positional (as in orthostatic hypotension, bilateral vertebral artery stenosis, or BPPV, which may not be described as spinning), (2) related to certain neck positions or pain (as in cervical spondylosis or cervicogenic dizziness), or (3) precipitated by specific factors, such as medication, postprandial hypoglycemia, congestive heart failure, pain, fear, or the sight of blood (vasovagal), standing or walking only (multisensory dizziness in elderly), palpitations or syncope (arrhythmias), or stress (psychological) (McIntosh et al., 1993a, b). Table 16-8 presents an algorithm for work-up.

On clinical examination, check the orthostatic blood pressures/pulse and consider hyperventilating the patient. Work-up will include review of medications, laboratory findings, and imaging in selected patients. Referral to cardiology is warranted when cardiac disease is suspected (arrhythmia, palpitation, syncope, heart disease). In elderly patients with unexplained dizziness, falls, or unsteadiness, search for a cardiovascular disorder is of paramount importance. Relevant tests include carotid sinus massage and event monitors.

Medications may be the cause of or a contributing factor in dizziness in over one third of the elderly (Colledge et al., 1996; Evans et al., 1997). Routine blood tests are not warranted (Davis, 1994; Colledge et al., 1996), but selective tests are recommended when suspicion is high, for example, complete blood count (looking for anemia) or glucose (looking for hypoglycemia). Lipids, thyroid function tests, and serum B12 may also provide clues to complaints of dizziness (especially if there is a concomitant large-fiber neuropathy). An MRI of the brain may show periventricular white matter disease or posterior fossa or cerebellopontine angle lesions in some patients.

For *imbalance/disequilibrium without dizziness*, if the symptoms are related to ambulation without any dizziness, then the work-up for disequilibrium is different and depends on the pattern and suspected cause of gait abnormalities (Table 16-9).

Patients may have more than one cause of dizziness, and disentangling the causes requires careful history-taking, neurovestibular examination, and diagnostic tests (Colledge et al., 1996).

EVALUATION OF DIZZINESS

Electronystagmography (ENG) relies on measuring eye movements, usually with electro-oculography (EOG) to measure movements of the corneoretinal dipole. The retina maintains a negative dipole with respect to surrounding tissue. The cornea is positive with respect to the retina, and the sclera is an insulating sheath. Using a distant electrode as a reference, an electrode close to the eye is more positive if the eyes move toward it. Clinical recordings have generally used AgCl electrodes around the eyes to detect horizontal and vertical eye movements. The EOG technique has now been supplemented by newer methods such as infrared recording. The American Academy of Neurology has published recent guidelines (Fife et al., 2000).

Caloric testing measures ocular responses after water (or air) is placed in the external ear canal. Warm water activates the ipsilateral horizontal canal and cold water deactivates it, possibly via convection currents (Baloh, 1998a; Furman & Cass, 2003). Cold stimulation results in nystagmus beating away from and warm stimulation beating to same side (COWS: cold-opposite; warm-same). Caloric testing can assess each horizontal canal and can detect unilateral canal paresis (Fig. 16-17). One limitation is patient discomfort (which often limits serial testing) and another is that calorics do not test vertical canals or otolith. Also, calorics stimulate the canals at a frequency equivalent to 0.003 Hz (Jacobson et al., 1997), which is extremely low for the vestibular system, which usually operates at a range of about 0.5–5 Hz during ambulation—and up to about 8 Hz during running (Leigh & Zee, 1999).

A rotary chair is used for bilateral horizontal canal stimulation and complements caloric testing. It is better tolerated and is used for serial follow-up assessments, as in monitoring the patient during treatment with aminoglycoside or recovery from toxicity. It uses different and higher frequencies than caloric testing and can detect residual function when the caloric responses are absent.

Eye movements are recorded with and without fixation to look for spontaneous nystagmus. The patient is then placed in various positions to assess positional or positioning nystagmus. Finally, induced nystagmus can be detected with several maneuvers (head shake, hyperventilation, Valsalva). Recordings of smooth pursuit, saccades, and optokinetic nystagmus can define eye movement abnormalities in patients with central lesions.

Posturography is a test of balance and posture that does not rely on eye movement recordings. Its use is evolving and it may be important for serial assessments of progress during balance rehabilitation; furthermore, it may play a role in assessing pseudo-astasia/imbalance.

COMMON CAUSES OF DIZZINESS

Vestibular disorders occur at the end-organ, nerve, brainstem/cerebellum, thalamus, and cortical and

TABLE 16-8. Algorithm for Suggested Diagnoses and Work-up of Lightheadedness/Near-Fainting

Symptoms/Signs	Diagnosis	Work-up
Orthostatic dizziness	Medications/dehydration/bilateral vertebral stenoses/autonomic dysfunction	Review medications Orthostatic blood pressure and pulse Autonomic function (including heart rate variability and pupil reaction) Magnetic resonance angiogram
Hyperventilation-induced dizziness	Stress Multiple sclerosis CPA lesions	Brain MRI
Sensory dysfunction in a stocking/glove distribution	Peripheral neuropathy	B_{12}, glucose, TSH, +/– serum immunofixation, EMG
Presyncope and syncope	Vasovagal (if preceded by a trigger, such as sight of blood or pain) Dehydration Anemia Cardiac arrhythmia Carotid sinus disease	Cardiac referral Cardiac holter monitor (for 1–2 days) or event monitor (for a month) Carotid massage
Dizziness of unclear cause (no obvious cause on exam)	Undiagnosed cardiac disease Undiagnosed vestibular disease Periventricular white matter or posterior fossa disease (Chiari/MS) Medication related Inactivity/deconditioned state Nonspecific dizziness of elderly Multifactorial (combination of above)	Review medications ENG Brain MRI (looking for posterior fossa/CPA/periventricular white matter disease) Cardiac evaluation Carotid sinus massage Holter or event monitor
Neck pain associated with dizziness	Cervicogenic dizziness	Cervical spine MRI
Medication related	—	Keep a diary to check temporal relationship Review/simplify medication
Headache associated with dizziness	Migraine-related	+/– brain MRI (if new headache) ENG
History of prior vestibular disease	Incomplete vestibular compensation	ENG
Otologic complaints	Meniere (occasionally causes lightheadedness without a spinning sensation) CPA lesion Perilymph fistula	Brain MRI, +/– contrast, and with thin cuts to CPA area ENG Audiogram
Dizziness associated with new eyeglasses or cataract surgery	Visual/ocular dizziness	Vestibular rehabilitation
Dizziness associated with anxiety/panic symptoms	Psychiatric dizziness Panic disorder Anxiety disorder	Psychiatric referral

CPA, cerebellopontine angle; EMG, electromyography; ENG, electronystagmography; MS, multiple sclerosis; TSH, thyroid stimulating hormone.

TABLE 16-9. Common Causes of Imbalance

Orthopedic/arthritic/pain

Motor

Sensory (proprioceptive)

Visual

Vestibular disease

Neuropathy

Myelopathy

Cerebellum

Subcortical disease (basal ganglia, thalamic)

Cortical/subcortical (normal pressure hydrocephalus, periventricular white matter disease, bifrontal subdurals/tumor/stroke)

Elderly with no other cause: multisensory loss

Symptoms with quick head movement → incomplete vestibular compensation

Deconditioned state

Psychological

subcortical areas. Table 16-10 shows the prevalence of various causes of dizziness; moreover, there may be interplay between the somatic and psychological factors explaining symptoms of dizziness.

Semicircular Canals: Benign Paroxysmal Positional Vertigo

Benign paroxysmal positional vertigo (BPPV) is the most common cause of dizziness and vertigo in the clinic and accounts for about 20% to 25% of cases. It is a rewarding condition to diagnose because it can be successfully treated in many cases. BPPV is characterized by recurrent bouts of vertigo lasting less than 1 minute and precipitated by turning in bed, getting in and out of bed, bending down then straightening up, and looking up as

in reaching for a high shelf ("shelf sign"). Patients may have a sense of unsteadiness or constant dizziness for hours or days especially after repeated bouts. The symptoms may be associated with fear, leading to avoidance behavior, and, in severe cases, significant limitations in daily activities (Nagarkar et al., 2000). In rare cases, people continue this pattern for years, even sleeping upright. Most of the time, however, the natural history is benign; 42% of the cases resolve on their own (Hausler et al., 1989). Although about half of patients will have recurrences, the symptoms tend to lessen in intensity with time; one third have symptoms for more than 1 year and 3% have symptoms that may recur for more than 10 years (Baloh et al., 1987; Nunez, 2000).

About 50% of BPPV cases are idiopathic, 15% are associated with a recent trauma (possibly within days), and 13% with viral vestibular neuritis (Baloh et al., 1987). Forty-seven percent of patients have abnormalities on ENG. BPPV is more common in patients in their sixth and seventh decades of life, although non-idiopathic forms tend to occur at a younger age. Women outnumber men by 1.6:1.

The diagnosis of BPPV is confirmed by Dix-Hallpike maneuver. The patient is swiftly moved from a sitting into a supine position with the head hanging off the table and turned to one side (ipsilateral to the symptoms). Torsional vertical nystagmus occurs after a few seconds (3–10) (Fig. 16-5). The mean latency in one study of BPPV was about 8 seconds, but the range was zero to 40 seconds (Baloh et al., 1987). Thus, zero latency does not exclude the diagnosis of BPPV and does not necessarily imply a central lesion. The duration of nystagmus in BPPV is usually 20 to 40 seconds, and always less than 1 minute. After tilting the patient up, there may be nystagmus in the reverse direction. Repeating the Dix-Hallpike maneuver causes a decrease in the nystagmus (fatigability) in 85%. About 8% or less of patients with BPPV affecting the posterior canal actually have bilateral nystagmus (Honrubia et al., 1999), but bilateral nystagmus may be seen in up to 20% of

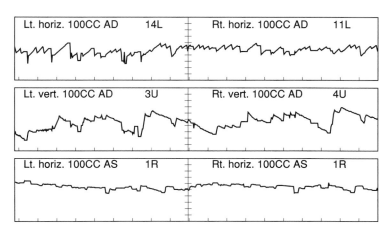

FIGURE 16-17. Nystagmus induced by calorics in a patient with acute vestibular syndrome. There is normal response with right canal stimulation (horizontal channels, *uppermost tracing*; vertical channels, *middle tracing*), but almost no nystagmus with the left-sided stimulation (*lowermost tracing*).

TABLE 16-10. Causes of Dizziness in General Population and in Elderly (in Percent)

	General*	Elderly†	Elderly‡
BPPV	31%	26%	23%
Migraine	11	—	—
Psychological	20	3	9
Vestibular neuritis	10	3	8
Unknown	7–15	14	14
Meniere	—	4	8
Stroke/central	4	10	19
Cardiac	—	5	1
Hypotension	5	3	2
Drug toxicity	—	2	2
Proprioceptive	—	7	2
Visual	—	1	2

*Neuhauser et al. (2001)
†Davis (1994)
‡Sloane and Baloh (1989)

patients with BPPV due to improper positioning during the Dix-Hallpike maneuver (Baloh et al., 1987).

Baloh and colleagues (1987) reported that only 14 of 240 patients with positional vertigo had symptoms or signs of central nervous system (CNS) involvement, all of them already known and most likely unrelated to the BPPV.

The presence of debris in the posterior canal has been documented in BPPV (Welling et al., 1997). The debris is presumed to be utricular otoconia that has degenerated and entered the posterior canal. The posterior canal is implicated because the nystagmus is in its plane, and clogging of this canal or its ampullary nerve resection results in symptom resolution.

Treatment of BPPV uses a particle repositioning maneuver. This involves putting the patient in head-hanging position and turning the patient toward the good ear in increments, then lifting the patient up (Fig. 16-18). The success rate is close to 90% (Honrubia et al., 1999). In a small percentage, patients may have a high recurrence rate thus needing other measures. For example, they may learn to perform the maneuver on themselves, although this may not always work. This is because the otoconia may move into a different canal, rendering a particular maneuver useless or potentially harmful (Baloh & Halmagyi, 1996; von Brevern et al., 2001). Alternatively, patients may be given balance exercises (Brandt, 2000). Rarely, surgical intervention such as canal plugging may be needed for severe and treatment-resistant symptoms.

If the debris is in the horizontal canal, a horizontal variant of BPPV develops. The symptoms are restricted

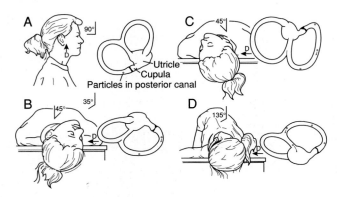

FIGURE 16-18. Particle repositioning maneuver: The patient is put in Dix-Hallpike position (from position A to B), then is turned in increments toward the good ear (from position C to D), and is then sat up. (Reproduced with permission from Furman JM, Cass SP: Balance Disorders: A Case-Study Approach. Philadelphia: FA Davis, 1996.)

to vertigo precipitated by turning in bed, or even turning side to side while seated upright. On exam, the nystagmus is horizontal (in the plane of the involved canal) and geotropic (beating to the ground). It tends to be bilateral, but worse on one side, and is treated with a different particle-repositioning maneuver, the barbeque (BBQ) maneuver. This variant accounts for only 5% of BPPV cases and is more resistant to treatment; the success rate is about 50% (Honrubia et al., 1999). Finally, there is a disputed anterior canal variant where the nystagmus is torsional to the floor but the vertical component is downward. No consensus on treatment is available.

In conclusion, BPPV is a benign, self-limited mechanical condition that rarely requires aggressive treatments such as surgery. Treatment comprises particle-repositioning maneuvers that depend on the location of canal pathology and can be repeated as needed.

Labyrinth: Vestibular Neuritis

Vestibular neuritis may be due to a viral infection (viral labyrinthitis), bacterial infection, trauma (as in labyrinthine concussion), or ischemia (as in labyrinthine infarct). All of these present as acute vestibular syndromes. Cognitive effects are limited to fatigue and to somatopsychic effects that may develop after the acute episode subsides (described below).

Vestibular Nerve: Acoustic Neuroma

The vestibular nerve may be compressed by cerebello-pontine angle tumors. Such tumors produce gradual compression of cranial nerves VII and VIII. Symptoms may evolve over months or even years and include unilateral sensorineural hearing loss, facial paresis, and a slowly progressive sense of imbalance. Vertigo is not typically a feature. In later stages the trigeminal nerve is affected, followed by cranial nerves VI, IX, and X. The brainstem and the cerebellum may also get compressed, leading to more symptoms such as dysmetria. Ninety percent of such tumors are acoustic neuromas. Other tumors in this region are meningiomas, epidermoid cysts, and facial nerve schwannomas (Baloh, 1998a).

Brainstem and Cerebellum: Stroke

Transient ischemic attacks (TIAs) are a relatively common cause of vertigo in the elderly (Baloh, 1998a). The vertigo is usually abrupt, lasts for a few minutes, and is accompanied by other symptoms including visual or somatosensory, altered mentation, imbalance, dysarthria, incoordination, weakness, headaches, diplopia, or dysphagia (Baloh et al., 1995a, 1998a). Recurrent mechanical compression of the vertebral arteries with neck extension might occur with cervical arthritic changes but has rarely been documented. Isolated vertigo that recurs over more than 6 weeks is not likely to be due to transient ischemic attacks (Caplan, 2000), although there are exceptions (Oas & Baloh, 1992).

Strokes/TIAs in the posterior circulation territory can be divided into different groups.

Extracranial Vertebral Arteries

TIAs due to extracranial vertebral arteries (EVAs) are stereotyped and frequent, but strokes are rare. The symptoms are positional dizziness/vertigo if there is bilateral disease. Thus, EVA disease is in the differential of orthostatic dizziness. The work-up includes checking brain MRI and magnetic resonance angiography (MRA).

Intracranial Vertebral Arteries: Lateral Medullary Syndrome

The lateral medullary syndrome (LMS) occurs with infarction in the lateral aspect of the rostral medulla and is often due to occlusion of the ipsilateral vertebral artery. Less frequently, occlusions of the medial branch of the posterior inferior cerebellar artery (mPICA) cause LMS.

The symptoms of such an infarct are vertigo, nausea and vomiting, ipsilateral ataxia, ipsifacial sensory loss and contralateral body sensory loss (the latter is often asymptomatic), dysphagia, hiccups, Horner syndrome, and lateropulsion (see earlier section Vestibular Dysfunction: Signs; see also Glossary). In addition, there is nystagmus, which may be ipsilesional, contralesional, or direction-changing. Moreover, there is saccadic ipsipulsion with overshooting ipsilesional saccades and undershooting contralesional saccades; there may also be an ocular tilt reaction (see Glossary). The symptoms and signs reflect damage to the vestibular nuclei, inferior cerebellar peduncle, spinal nucleus of the trigeminal nerve and its tract, spinothalamic tract, nucleus ambiguus, and sympathetic fibers.

AICA: Lateral Pontine Syndrome

Infarcts in the anterior inferior cerebellar artery (AICA) territory cause lateral pontine syndrome, which includes vertigo, ipsilateral hearing loss, ipsilateral facial weakness, ipsilateral facial and contralateral body numbness, and ipsilateral ataxia. The syndrome is distinguished from LMS by the presence of facial weakness and hearing loss.

Basilar Artery Infarcts

Basilar artery infarcts tend to affect the basis pontis causing ocular abnormalities and limb weakness. The lateral and dorsal aspects of the pons are less affected because the long circumferential arteries supplying these areas tend to have collaterals (Caplan, 2000).

Cerebellar Infarcts

Most cerebellar infarcts are "silent" and the clinically evident ones are mostly embolic in nature. Overall, cerebellar infarcts comprise 1.5% of all strokes, with posterior inferior cerebellar artery (PICA) infarcts being the most common, followed by superior cerebellar artery (SCA) and AICA infarcts (Barth, 1993; Kase et al., 1993).

An mPICA infarct typically causes gait ataxia, vertigo, nausea, vomiting and headache (Chaves, 1994). Importantly, it may mimic *acute peripheral vestibulopathies* because the mPICA supplies the nodulus and uvula of the cerebellum (Leigh & Zee, 1999). AICA infarcts are rare. They also cause vertigo, nausea and vomiting, and ipsilateral ataxia, in addition to cranial nerve abnormalities. The AICA supplies the flocculus and paraflocculus (Baloh & Halmagyi, 1996; Afifi & Bergman, 1998).

SCA infarcts cause prominent gait and limb ataxia but less prominent vertigo or headaches. Although one study reported "vertigo" in about half of patients with SCA infarcts (Erdemoglu & Duman, 1998), in general, vertigo seems infrequent and of minor importance (Kase et al., 1993). On exam, SCA infarcts cause a characteristic eye abnormality, *contrapulsion*, which is opposite to the saccadic ipsipulsion that occurs in lateral medullary infarcts. Thus, the saccades are hypermetric contralateral to the lesion and hypometric ipsilaterally. Moreover, the eyes drift obliquely contralateral to the lesion on up gaze (Leigh & Zee, 1999). The SCA supplies the superior cerebellar peduncle, near which run the fastigial output fibers to the vestibular nuclei (Parent, 1996). Cerebellar infarcts may be mistaken for a peripheral vestibular disease, and the exam is crucial because there are *central* vestibular signs present. These include impaired oculomotor responses (dysmetric saccades, impaired smooth pursuit, and optokinetic nystagmus [OKN]); central nystagmus (gaze-evoked, downbeat or upbeat); and profound ataxia (patient cannot stand). These are differentiating factors from peripheral vestibular disease (Norrving et al., 1995; Brandt, 2000). Slight dysarthria and lateropulsion may also be seen. When in doubt, the patient should be observed for 24 to 48 hours because cerebellar infarcts may swell and cause fatal brainstem compression without emergent decompressive surgery.

Thalamus

Thalamic stimulation has been reported to cause vertigo, when the ventrocaudalis (vc) nucleus is involved (Lin & Lenz, 1993; Lin & Lenz, 1994). Uncommonly, a thalamic lesion causes dizziness or imbalance (Lannuzel et al., 1994). In addition, several thalamic "syndromes" have been reported.

Thalamic astasia (Greek, loss of station) describes an inability to stand or walk after thalamic infarcts or hemorrhages, even though motor power is normal or mildly affected (Masdeu & Gorelick, 1988). Patients tend to fall ipsilaterally to the affected side (or contralesionally) and to pull themselves up using both hands to steady themselves. Underlying lesions have been reported in superoposterolateral areas of the thalamus (Masdeu & Gorelick, 1988) that receive input from the fastigial nuclei in the vestibulocerebellum and send output to Brodmann area 4. Thalamic astasia resembles the unsteadiness produced by a vermal lesion and has also been called ataxic hemiparesis (Masdeu & Gorelick, 1998) and resembles a condition known as "ease of falling" syndrome (Awerbuch & Labadie, 1989). A condition similar to thalamic astasia has also been reported in internal capsule/corona radiata and basal ganglia lesions (Awerbuch & Labadie, 1989).

Pusher syndrome is characterized by patients *actively* pushing with their normal limbs away from the lesion side, producing tilting of posture and a tendency to fall toward the symptomatic (paretic) side (Karnath, 2000). The patients resist correction of their posture by someone else. Karnath and colleagues (2000) reported 31 such patients: 80% had neglect, two thirds had right-sided and one third left-sided lesions. The lesions overlapped in the ventral posterior and lateral posterior areas of the thalamus, with a relatively frequent involvement of the posterior limb of the internal capsule and a slight part of the corpus of the caudate.

Dieterich and Brandt (1993) evaluated 35 patients in a study of thalamic infarcts and falls. Patients with medial thalamic lesions tended to show contraversive tilting of the subjective vertical. Those with posterolateral lesions had tilting to either direction of the subjective vertical and tended to fall (the direction was not specified). Patients with anterior thalamic lesions had no unsteadiness.

Despite the differing imaging techniques and nomenclature, lesions in the above syndromes affect the same general area of the posterolateral thalamus. This nuclear region receives vestibular input and vestibularly related cerebellar input into the "vestibular thalamus" (Haines, 1995).

Cortex: Insular Infarcts

Cortical infarcts do not produce dizziness as the only complaint. Brandt and colleagues (1995) reported a single case of a patient with posterior insular infarct who had nonepileptic rotational vertigo. However, an altered sensation of the gravitational vertical has been documented and may be more common than recognized. It occurs with lesions in areas thought to contain vestibular cortical areas. In one report, patients with large middle cerebral artery infarcts were unable to vertically align a light bar in a dark room, reflecting a disturbance in the perception of verticality. The area where the lesions overlapped was the posterior insula (Brandt et al., 1994).

Cortex: Epilepsy

Vertigo and epilepsy were associated together in ancient times and up until the end of the 19th century. In the 18th and 19th centuries, vertigo was believed to be a minor form of epilepsy and was used to describe mental confusion (rather than an abnormal sensation of motion). Epilepsy and vertigo were also linked with immoral/criminal behavior (Bladin, 1998). By the end of the 19th century, Jackson, then Charcot, asserted that vertigo was more likely due to vestibular or inner ear disease. In the 20th century, Cawthorne described four patients whose symptoms of epilepsy were precipitated by caloric testing. In 1969, Penfield and Jasper stimulated the posterior superior temporal and temporoparietal border areas, triggering vertigo (Bladin, 1998).

Vertigo can be an epilepsy aura, an ictal event, or postictal sensation (Kogeorgos et al., 1981) but is rare (Palmini & Gloor, 1992). Dizziness or lightheadedness may also be an aura, yet of a poor localizing value (Palmini & Gloor, 1992; Fried et al., 1995). In *tornado epilepsy* vertigo is the ictal event. This condition may be caused by trauma and may be more common in young patients and women (Ahmed, 1980).

Dizziness that is related to epilepsy may arise from the cortex or be precipitated when peripheral vestibular stimulation triggers a seizure, as in *reflex epilepsy* (Beaumanoir, 1998). Epileptic vertigo was described in one patient with left middle frontal gyrus astrocytoma (Kluge et al., 2000). There have also been about a dozen reports of epileptic nystagmus originating from frontal, temporal, or parietal regions (Furman et al., 1990).

The relationship between dizziness and epilepsy requires further study (Gordon, 1999). Certain mice have generalized epilepsy induced by tossing or spinning the mouse (vestibular stimuli, reflex epilepsy). Postnatal exposure to intense sounds induces an audiogenic seizure in otherwise seizure-resistant rats. Deaf children seem to be especially susceptible to febrile seizures, two thirds of patients with dizziness have abnormal electroencephalograms (EEGs; Hughes & Drachman, 1977), and epileptiform EEGs are seen in 70% of patients with probable cochlear hydrops.

Cortical/Subcortical: Migraine

Migraine is common, affecting 17% to 29% of women and 6% to 20% of men (Cass et al., 1997). Besides recurrent headaches, patients may have other symptoms such as visual, sensory, or motor symptoms. Up to 25% of patients with migraine have dizziness, making it as common as visual auras (Baloh, 1997). The dizziness may be prior to or during a headache, or during headache-free intervals. The headaches are temporally connected to the dizziness in about 50% of cases (Neuhauser et al., 2001).

Migraine-related complaints of dizziness range from episodes of true vertigo to imbalance, lightheadedness, motion intolerance (head movement causing dizziness), motion sickness, or susceptibility to dizziness provoked by visual stimuli (Harker & Russekh, 1988; Cass et al., 1997). Some patients actually limit their daily activities including avoiding riding in cars or elevators. Only 6% have true vertigo as an aura, and in all reports it lasted less than several hours. In general, the dizziness in its various forms may last seconds, minutes, hours, days, or even weeks and months. On average, most forms last less than a day (Neuhauser et al., 2001). Moreover, almost 90% of patients with migraine have motion sickness (versus about 10% in the general population; Cass et al., 1997).

About two thirds of migraineurs have abnormal vestibular function on calorics/rotary chair. Asymmetry in caloric response and directional preponderance on rotary chair are among the most common (Cass et al., 1997). Auditory symptoms are also common, and phonophobia may occur in two thirds of patients and fullness in the ears in one fourth. Audiometry testing is normal in 80% of patients. Fluctuating low-frequency hearing loss (as in Meniere's disease) has even been reported, especially in young women around menses. Sudden hearing loss has also been reported (Baloh, 1997).

The pathophysiology of migraine-related dizziness is not known, but relevant mechanisms may involve serotonin. Serotonin induces dilation of the cerebral vasculature, thought to be associated with the headache phase, and has a direct effect on the firing rate of the vestibular nuclei. Immunohistochemical studies have shown prominent serotonergic input to the vestibular nuclei especially in the medial vestibular nucleus, which is connected to the nucleus of tractus solitarius and the dorsal motor nucleus of vagus nerve (Cass et al., 1997). Furthermore, pain medications used to treat migraine headaches can also help improve dizziness related to migraine.

The incidence of migraine in patients with Meniere's disease (22%–76%) is about double that in the general population, and 7.5% of migraineurs have Meniere's disease (versus 0.05% in the general population; Baloh, 1997).

Basilar migraine, a term coined by Bickerstaff in 1961 (Cass et al., 1997), usually manifests as an occipital headache associated with several neurological symptoms referable to the brainstem (Cass et al., 1997; Baloh, 1998a). Symptom frequencies are vertigo 63%, gait ataxia 63%, paresthesia (usually bilateral) 61%, dysarthria 57%, weakness (usually bilateral) 55%, tinnitus 26%, impaired hearing 20%, and diplopia 16% (Baloh, 1997). There may also be altered mental states. Although basilar migraine can occur at any age, it may be more common in adolescent girls.

Benign paroxysmal vertigo of childhood is connected with migraine-like symptoms. Patients have recurrent episodes of sudden unsteadiness, sweating, pallor, and vomiting. The symptoms are worse with head movement and are occasionally accompanied by torticollis or nystagmus. Some children describe a spinning sensation, although most have difficulty describing what they feel. The episodes start suddenly and last seconds to a few minutes. The child may look afraid and refuse to move. The episodes remit suddenly and the child resumes ongoing activities and normal play. The frequency of the episodes is several times per month. They usually occur in children under 4 years of age and remit by about 7 or 8 years. Frequently these children have unilateral canal paresis on calorics (Cass et al., 1997). These children may ultimately develop migraine headaches.

Some patients have recurrent vertigo without otologic symptoms, known as recurrent vestibulopathy or "vestibular hydrops." Episodes may last hours/days and are followed by a variable period of disequilibrium. The symptoms may have common precipitants of migraine such as lack of sleep, emotional stress, or alcohol, and there is usually female preponderance and a strong positive family history of migraine. Rassekh and Harber (1992) followed 38 patients with such symptoms; 25% developed Meniere's disease and 25% had remission. Fifty percent remained unchanged; of these 80% had migraine. Other studies (comprising more than 100 total patients) have followed these patients for between 3 and 8 years.) Less than 25% of these patients developed Meniere's disease or BPPV, but about 70% had no new symptoms (Leliever & Barber, 1981; Rutka & Barber,

1986; Kentala & Pyykko, 1997). In one study of headache patients, 7 of 21 patients had vertigo, raising the possibility that migraine elicited the vertigo (Kitamura & Kudo, 1990).

Migraine patients should avoid triggers such as certain foods (chocolate, red wine, aged cheese, pickles, others). Acute treatment includes abortive medications (Baloh, 1997) and prophylactic medications to reduce the likelihood of recurrent headaches and reduce the severity of headaches, should they occur. Schedule adjustments, including regular sleep and meals, may also help. Migraine-associated dizziness responds to treatment of the migraine headaches. Vestibular suppressants such as benzodiazepines (e.g., clonazepam) or antihistamine (e.g. dimenhydrinate) are sometimes used to treat prolonged attacks.

Cortical/Subcortical: Multisensory Dizziness

Normal aging is accompanied by change in gait (see Chapter 36) and also associated with hair cell loss in cochlea and labyrinth, and decreased vision, proprioception, and processing speed (see Chapter 36; Fife & Baloh, 1993). Changes in gait seen with aging include slight anteroflexion of the torso, flexion of the arms and knees, shorter step length, and diminished arm swing. Senile, or cautious gait, is characterized by slightly wider base, slowed gait, en bloc turns, short steps, rigid arms, and careful and slow tandem gait. In advanced stages, shuffling becomes prominent, but festination is not seen. Other terms that describe similar or more severe gait abnormalities are marche à petits pas, magnetic gait, subcortical disequilibrium, frontal gait disorder, gait apraxia or ataxia, vascular or lower body parkinsonism, and frontal disequilibrium. There have been attempts to operationalize these terms (Nutt et al., 1993); however, no clear classification of cortical/subcortical gait and equilibrium disorders has yet emerged (Fattal, 2003).

Elble and colleagues (1992) reported that elderly patients with differing diagnoses (e.g., Alzheimer disease with parkinsonism features, normal pressure hydrocephalus, vascular dementia) had similar kinematic profiles and gait disturbances. These include stooping, reduced arm swing, stride (step length) and cadence (steps per minute), decreased foot floor clearance, increased time with both feet on the floor (double limb stance), and hesitancy with turning. Moreover, other studies have also noted similarities among gait disorders due to subcortical arteriosclerotic disease, hydrocephalus, frontal lobe lesions, and "senile" disorders (Thompson & Marsden, 1987). A similar "senile gait" picture is seen in young subjects who are blindfolded or are on a slippery floor, patients with bilateral subdural hematomas, Binswanger disease, parkinsonism, or high cervical myelopathy.

Baloh and colleagues assessed the gait in 100 patients aged 75 years or older who complained of insidious onset of dizziness and unsteadiness when upright that was relieved when sitting or lying down (Fife & Baloh, 1993; Baloh et al., 1995b; Kerber et al., 1998). They had objective impairments of gait on exam, with no known cause (such as cerebellar, neuropathy, CNS disease, neurodegeneration, strokes, normal pressure hydrocephalus, motor disorder, orthopedic limitations, or spinal injury). Controls were healthy older individuals with no complaint of dizziness/imbalance. All had a comprehensive evaluation including a history and exam, a questionnaire about their falls, scales of activities of daily living, gait scale, mini-mental exam, audiometry, visual acuity, visual tracking, rotational vestibular testing, and quantitative posturography. Compared to controls, patients had more falls and fear of falling, did poorer on gait exam, and swayed more on posturography. Moreover, subcortical white matter disease was moderate to severe in patients compared to mild to moderate in controls. Baloh and colleagues called this clinical picture *nonspecific disequilibrium of the elderly*.

Nonspecific disequilibrium of the elderly is seen in persons in their seventh and eighth decades. Although the prevalence is unknown (Fife & Baloh, 1993), several studies have found chronic dizziness or disequilibrium in 13% to 38% of older people (Tinetti et al., 2000). Baloh and Vinters (1995) studied the brain pathology in three such patients and found astrocytosis (as may underlie the increased T2 signal in white matter on MRI). The brain of such patients also showed more gross atrophy and severe white matter pathology (Whitman et al., 1999). A remaining research question is whether senile gait disturbances are a harbinger of neurodegenerative impairment (Kerber et al., 1998).

Psychiatry and Neurotology

Dizziness is generally a benign syndrome and patients fare well over time. In a community study of working age people with a 7-month follow-up, 60% of the dizzy individuals improved and only about 10% worsened (Yardley et al., 1998a). In another community-based study of elderly patients, dizziness did not result in increased mortality or hospitalization 1 year later (Tinetti et al., 2000).

Yet some dizzy patients report handicaps, impairments, or disabilities (for these and related classifications see Chapter 50). Patients may complain of dizziness at work and may even leave work (Yardley, 1992). Handicap levels and anxiety have been reported to increase, even when symptoms of dizziness improve (Yardley et al., 1994).

Space and motion discomfort (SMD) refers to a constellation of symptoms that may persist or even increase following vestibular dysfunction (Furman et al., 2001; Furman & Jacob, 2001). Vestibular disease causes vertigo, blurred vision, and imbalance due to VOR dysfunction. Spatial disorientation may occur because vestibular dysfunction upsets the balance between stimuli from the three systems important for balance: vestibular, somatosensory, and visual. Once the vestibular system is dysfunctional, the brain starts to rely more on the proprioceptive and the visual systems, leading to "overuse" of, and "hypersensitivity" to, visual stimuli; that is, the patient may then become dizzy and disoriented on exposure to multiple visual stimuli. Patients may complain of imbalance or dizziness with high levels of visual and kinesthetic stimulation, as when in busy malls and grocery stores. In time, even patterned wallpaper (in which different stimuli compete for visual fixation) may produce symptoms. Learned avoidance may lead to symptoms of agoraphobia (Jacob & Furman, 2001). The anxiety and fear of precipitating the symptoms may lead to panic attacks and even panic disorder (American Psychiatric Association, 2000). Of note, patients with agoraphobia without dizziness describe a symptom complex similar to SMD. In some, the symptoms of SMD may become their main focus, limiting their daily activities, leading to inactivity, and worsening central vestibular decompensation.

Individuals with combined vestibular and psychological symptoms are at increased risk for persistent difficulty. The association between somatic and psychological symptoms has been known for millennia, and Plato used terms such as "somatic" and "psychic" to describe vertigo, mental confusion, and disorientation (Furman et al., 2001). In the last half of the 19th century, agoraphobia was considered by some to be a form of vertigo, although by the end of that century, vertigo and psychiatric/psychological disorders were considered as separate entities (Furman et al., 2001).

Furman and Jacob (2001) summarized the multifaceted relation between psychiatric, psychological, and somatic factors in dizzy patients. "Psychiatric dizziness" is estimated to comprise about 10% of all dizziness cases and may be due to panic attacks, conversion disorders, or other psychiatric conditions. Psychological overlay refers to symptoms beyond those expected for a given balance disorder. For example, patients with phobic postural vertigo may have a premorbid obsessive-compulsive personality contributing to "exaggerated" symptoms (Brandt, 1996). Along similar lines, increases in body sway were found in normal subjects when they were talking loudly or after hyperventilation, an effect that correlated with reduced somatosensory potentials (Jacob & Furman, 2001). On the other hand, hyperventilation can also induce nystagmus, dizziness, or disequilibrium in patients with vestibular disorders such as acoustic neuroma (Minor et al., 1999). Similarly, nystagmus induced by calorics or rotary chair decreases with som-

nolence (Jacobson et al., 1997) and increases with mental tasks, especially in patients who report a greater level of stress and fear (Yardley et al., 1995).

In several studies, psychological or psychiatric factors were key predictors of handicap in dizzy patients. Factors included poor coping strategies and anxiety symptoms (Yardley, 1994), baseline anxiety trait (Yardley, 1992), agoraphobia, avoidance, and fainting symptoms (Yardley et al., 1998a), panic symptoms (Yardley et al., 2001), and autonomic/arousal/anxiety symptoms (Yardley et al., 1994).

Psychological or psychiatric symptoms and dizziness often coexist in a patient. In one community-based study, 10% of the patients had concurrent dizziness and psychological symptoms, twice the rate expected by chance (Yardley et al., 1998c). About one half of the patients with dizziness also had anxiety and avoidance behavior. Compared to controls, dizzy patients were three times more likely to have anxiety and four times more likely to have panic/agoraphobic symptoms (Yardley et al., 1998c). Moreover, one fourth of dizzy patients have panic disorder (Yardley et al., 2001). In a study of working-age individuals, phobic symptoms were ten times more prevalent and somatic symptoms five times more prevalent in dizzy patients than in the controls (Yardley et al., 1998c). Finally, patients with anxiety disorders are twice as likely as controls to have abnormalities on vestibular testing (Jacob et al., 1996).

"Somatopsychic" is sometimes used to refer to "organic" vestibular disease "causing" psychological symptoms. Patients with dizziness are twice as likely to seek psychiatric advice after the onset of dizziness (Yardley, 1992). Panic and agoraphobia-like symptoms are more prevalent among dizzy patients with documented vestibular dysfunction than in those without (Sullivan et al., 1993). Severe vestibular symptoms may precipitate panic because of their association with the sense of impending danger; once panic symptoms are established, they may remain after vestibular symptoms resolve. Through conditioning and stimulus generalization processes nonvestibular stimuli may then precipitate panic symptoms. For example, head movement resulted in increase in respiratory rate in dizzy patients and normal controls, but only dizzy patients reported increases in anxiety, dizziness, and autonomic symptoms (Yardley et al., 1998b). Additional risk factors for developing anxiety symptoms with vestibular diagnoses include an underlying somatization disorder (Jacob & Furman, 2001), obsessive-compulsive diagnosis (Brandt, 1996), genetic predisposition to anxiety disorders, or situational/concurrent stress (Yardley, 2000). Vestibular rehabilitation helps both vestibular and anxiety symptoms (Gurr & Moffat, 2001; Jacob & Furman, 2001; Jacob et al., 2001).

In short, the vestibular system and the systems pertaining to anxiety appear to overlap. There is monoaminergic input to the vestibular nuclei. The parabrachial nucleus network receives converging vestibular, visceral, and somatic nociceptive inputs, and connects reciprocally to sympathetic and parasympathetic systems, respiratory brainstem centers, amygdala, and other limbic cortices (Balaban & Thayer, 2001). The interactions between the psychiatric and the somatic factors in vestibular complaints are complex and should be addressed, as with a combination of vestibular rehabilitation and psychological treatment.

MANAGEMENT OF DIZZINESS

Management of dizziness is multidimensional. It is essential to treat the underlying cause, such as migraine headache in migraine-related dizziness (as discussed in previous sections). Vestibular suppressants may be used in the first few days of an acute vestibular event, but chronic use of vestibular suppressants is unwarranted, unhelpful, and commonly harmful because it leads to vestibular system suppression and delayed brain compensation (Baloh & Halmagyi, 1996; Baloh, 1998; Hotson & Baloh, 1998). Exceptions are the use of low-dose clonazepam or diazepam as needed in patients with recurrent dizziness, as in patients with Meniere's disease.

As mentioned earlier, abnormal eye movements due to CNS lesion can produce troublesome perceptual symptoms such as oscillopsia due to central nystagmus. Treatment for central nystagmus is often ineffective and may include baclofen, gabapentin, clonazepam, and retro-orbital botulinum injections into the affected extraocular muscles. If the nystagmus is present in primary gaze or if convergence dampens the nystagmus, then prisms may be useful.

A cornerstone in the treatment of dizziness is vestibular rehabilitation that uses eye, head, and body exercises to "retrain" the vestibular system. The exercises stress the deconditioned vestibular system and the VOR function and may initially trigger dizziness or nausea, but this does not mean the patient is getting worse. Patients should be encouraged to continue with the exercises, but may temporarily slow the speed of the exercises to decrease the symptoms. Typically, patients need to exercise daily at home for at least 2 months.

CONCLUSION

Dizziness is a common symptom, and many differing conditions and complaints are subsumed by this colloquial term. With a careful history and physical examination the cause of the dizziness can be identified in most patients. Most cases are benign and improve with treatment. A cornerstone of the diagnostic testing is the ENG. Brain and cervical spine MRIs are less frequently needed. "Routine" laboratory tests such as complete blood count, lipids, glucose, thyroid, vitamin B_{12}, erythrocyte sedimentation rate, or syphilis serology are not usually warranted. Elderly patients with unexplained dizziness, syncope, or falls will benefit from cardiac evaluations, including Holter or event monitors, or carotid sinus massage. The physician should (1) treat associated conditions, such as migraine, (2) avoid using chronic vestibular suppressants, (3) refer patients to vestibular therapists to learn vestibular exercises tailored to the patient's disease and symptoms, (4) appreciate that psychic and somatic factors may contribute to a patient's symptoms, and (5) refer patients to psychologists or psychiatrists as needed. Such a multidisciplinary approach can help improve symptoms more quickly, increase patient compliance (e.g., with vestibular exercises), decrease dependence on benzodiazepines or other medications, and lessen the risk of handicap and disability.

■ KEY POINTS

☐ The vestibular system is a sensory system that starts in the hair cells of the labyrinth of each ear and connects through cranial nerve VIII to the brainstem, cerebellum, thalamus, and cortical areas.

☐ The function of the vestibular system is gaze and gait stability with body and head movement, as well as orientation in space.

☐ Vestibular dysfunction leads to vertigo, oscillopsia, disequilibrium, and autonomic symptoms. A prominent sign is nystagmus. The vestibular system is capable of remarkable recovery, and plasticity.

☐ In approaching the dizzy patient, it is useful to classify the dizziness into vertigo, lightheadedness, or disequilibrium, or a combination of these.

☐ The relationship between vestibular and psychological symptoms is multifaceted.

KEY READINGS

Baloh R, Honrubia V. Clinical Neuropsychology of the Vestibular System. New York: Oxford University Press, 2001.

Brandt T: Vertigo. New York: Springer, 2000.

Fife T, Tusa R, Furman J, et al: Assessment: Vestibular testing techniques in adults and children: Report of the Therapeutics and Technology Assessment Subcommittee of the American Academy of Neurology. Neurology 55:1431–1441, 2000.

Furman J, Cass S: Vestibular Disorders: A Case Study Approach. London: Oxford University Press, 2003.

Guldin WO, Grusser OJ: Is there a vestibular cortex? Trends Neurosci 21:254–259, 1998.

REFERENCES

Adams R, Victor M: Principles of Neurology. New York: McGraw-Hill, 1993.

Afifi A, Bergman R. Functional Neuroanatomy. New York: McGraw-Hill, 1998.

Ahmed I: Epilepsia tornado. J Kans Med Soc 81:466–467, 1980.

American Psychiatric Association: Diagnostic and Statistical Manual of Mental Disorders, ed 4 rev. Washington, DC: American Psychiatric Association, 2000.

Awerbuch G, Labadie E: "Ease of falling" syndrome. Ann Neurol 25:210–211, 1989.

Balaban CD, Thayer JF: Neurological basis for balance-anxiety links. J Anxiety Disord 15:53–79, 2001.

Baloh R: The dizzy patient. Postgraduate Med 105:161–164, 167–172, 1999.

Baloh R: Dizziness, Hearing Loss and Tinnitis. Philadelphia: F.A. Davis, 1998a.

Baloh R: Neurotology of migraine. Headache 37:615–621, 1997.

Baloh R: Vertebrobasilar insufficiency and stroke. Otolaryngol Head Neck Surg 112:114–117, 1995.

Baloh R: Vertigo (seminar). Lancet 352:1841–1846, 1998b.

Baloh R, Halmagyi GM (eds): Disorders of the Vestibular System. New York: Oxford University Press, 1996.

Baloh R, Honrubia V: Clinical Neurophysiology of the Vestibular System, ed 3. London: Oxford University Press, 2001.

Baloh R, Honrubia V, Jacobson K. Benign positional vertigo: Clinical and oculographic features in 240 cases. Neurology 37:371–378, 1987.

Baloh R, Spain S, Socotch T, et al: Posturography and balance problems in older people. J Am Geriatr Soc 43:638–644, 1995a.

Baloh R, Vinters H: White matter lesions and disequilibrium in older people. II. Clinicopathologic correlation. Arch Neurol 52:975–981, 1995.

Baloh R, Yue Q, Socotch T, et al: White matter lesions and disequilibrium in older people. I. Case-control comparison. Arch Neurol 52:970–974, 1995b.

Barth A, Bogousslavsky J, Regli F: The clinical and topographic spectrum of cerebellar infarcts: A clinical-magnetic resonance imaging correlation study. Ann Neurol 33:451–456, 1996.

Beaumanoir A: History of reflex epilepsy. Adv Neurol 75:1–4, 1998.

Bense S, Stephan T, Yousry T, et al: Multisensory cortical signal increases and decreases during vestibular galvanic stimulation (fMRI). J Neurophysiol 85:886–899, 2001.

Bladin P: History of "epileptic vertigo": Its medical, social, and forensic problems. Epilepsia 39:442–447, 1998.

Bottini G, Karnath H, Vallar G, et al: Cerebral representations for egocentric space. Brain 124:1182–1196, 2001.

Bottini G, Sterzi R, Paulesu E, et al: Identification of the central vestibular projections in man. Exp Brain Res 99:164–169, 1994.

Brandt T: Phobic postural vertigo. Neurology 46:1515–1519, 1996.

Brandt T: Vertigo. New York; Berlin: Springer, 2000.

Brandt T, Botzel K, Yousry T, et al: Rotational vertigo in embolic stroke of the vestibular and auditory cortices. Neurology 45:42–44, 1995.

Brandt T, Dieterich M, Danek A, et al: Vestibular cortex lesions affect the perception of verticality. Ann Neurol 35:403–412, 1994.

Bucher S, Dieterich M, Wiesmann M, et al: Cerebral functional magnetic resonance imaging of vestibular, auditory, and nociceptive areas during galvanic stimulation. Ann Neurol 44:120–125, 1998.

Burke R: The central pattern generators for locomotion in mammals. Adv Neurol 87:11–24, 2001.

Caplan L: Caplan's Stroke, ed 3. Boston: Butterworth-Heinemann, 2000.

Cass S, Furman J, Ankerstjerne K, et al: Migraine-related vestibulopathy. Ann Otol Rhinol Laryngol 106:182–189, 1997.

Chaves C, Caplan L, Chung C, et al: Cerebellar infarcts in the New England Medical Center Posterior Circulation Stroke Registry. Neurology 44:1385–1390, 1994.

Colledge N, Barr-Hamilton R, Lewis S, et al: Evaluation of investigations to diagnose the cause of dizziness in elderly people: A community based controlled study. BMJ 313:788–792, 1996.

Darlington CL, Smith PF: Molecular mechanisms of recovery from vestibular damage in mammals: Recent advances. Prog Neurobiol 62:313–325, 2000.

Davis LE: Dizziness in elderly men. J Am Geriatr Soc 42:1184–1188, 1994.

Dieterich M, Brandt T: Thalamic infarctions: Differential effects on vestibular function in the roll plane (35 patients). Neurology 43:1732–1740, 1993.

Dietz V: Physiology of human gait: Neural processes. Adv Neurol 87:53–63, 2001.

Elble R, Hughes L, Higgins C: The syndrome of senile gait. J Neurol 239:71–75, 1992.

Erdemoglu A, Duman T: Superior cerebellar artery territory stroke. Acta Neurol Scand 98:283–287, 1998.

Evans P, Gray D, Steele R, et al: Investigations to diagnose cause of dizziness in elderly people: Algorithm should ask whether patient is taking drugs that may cause dizziness. BMJ 314:224, discussion 224–225, 1997.

Fattal D: Disequilibrium. (available by subscription at Medlink/Neurology URL: http://www.medlink.com/user/medlinklogin.asp, 2003)

Fife T, Baloh R: Disequilibrium of unknown cause in older people. Ann Neurol 34:694–702, 1993.

Fife T, Tusa R, Furman J, et al. Assessment: Vestibular testing techniques in adults and children: Report of the Therapeutics and Technology Assessment Subcommittee of the American Academy of Neurology. Neurology 55:1431–1441, 2000.

Fried I, Spencer D, Spencer S: The anatomy of epileptic auras: Focal pathology and surgical outcome. J Neurosurg 83:60–66, 1995.

Furman J, Balaban C, Jacob R: Interface between vestibular dysfunction and anxiety. Otol Neurotol 22:426–427, 2001.

Furman J, Cass S: Vestibular Disorders: A Case-study Approach. London: Oxford University Press, 2003.

Furman J, Crumrine P, Reinmuth O: Epileptic nystagmus. Ann Neurol 27:686–688, 1990.

Furman JM, Jacob RG: A clinical taxonomy of dizziness and anxiety in the otoneurological setting. J Anxiety Disord 15:9–26, 2001.

Gordon AG: Link between vertigo and epilepsy. [Comment]: Epilepsia 40:1168–1169, 1999.

Guldin WO, Grusser O-J: Is there a vestibular cortex? Trends in Neurosci 21:254–259, 1998.

Gurr B, Moffat N: Psychological consequences of vertigo and the effectiveness of vestibular rehabilitation for brain injury patients. Brain Injury 15:387–400, 2001.

Haines D: Neuroanatomy: An Atlas of Structures, Sections, and Systems, ed 4. Baltimore, MD: Williams & Wilkins, 1995.

Halmagyi GM, Curthoys IS: A clinical sign of canal paresis. Arch Neurol 45:737–739, 1988.

Harker LA, Russekh C: Migraine equivalent as a cause of episodic vertigo. Laryngoscope 98:160–164, 1988.

Hausler R, Pampurik J: Surgical and physical therapy treatment of benign paroxysmal positional vertigo. Laryngorhinootologie 68:349–354, 1989.

Honrubia V, Baloh R, Harris M, et al: Paroxysmal positional vertigo syndrome. Am J Otol 20:465–470, 1999.

Hotson J, Baloh R: Current concepts: Acute vestibular syndrome. N Engl J Med 339:680–685, 1998.

Hughes JR, Drachman DA: Dizziness, epilepsy, and the EEG. Dis Nerv Syst 38:431–435, 1977.

Jacob R, Whitney S, Detweiler-Shostak G, et al: Vestibular rehabilitation for patients with agoraphobia and vestibular dysfunction: A pilot study. J Anxiety Disord 15:131–146, 2001.

Jacob RG, Furman JM: Psychiatric consequences of vestibular dysfunction. Curr Opin Neurol 14:41–46, 2001.

Jacob RG, Furman J, Durrant J, et al: Panic, agoraphobia and vestibular dysfunction. Am J Psychiatry 153:503–512, 1996.

Jacobson G, Newman C, Kartush J: Handbook of Balance Function Testing. San Diego, CA: Singular Publishing Group, 1997.

Jannetta P, Moller M, Moller A: Disabling positional vertigo. N Engl J Med 310:1700–1705, 1984.

Karnath H-O: The origin of contraversive pushing. Neurology 55:1298–1304, 2000.

Karnath H-O, Christ K, Hartje W: Decrease of contralateral neglect by neck muscle vibration and spatial orientation of trunk midline. Brain 116:383–396, 1993.

Karnath H-O, Ferber S, Dichgans J: The neural representation of postural control in humans. Proc Natl Acad Sci U S A 97:13931–13936, 2000.

Kase C, Norrving B, Levine S, et al: Cerebellar infarction clinical and anatomic observation in 66 cases. Stroke 24:76–83, 1993.

Kentala E, Pyykko I. Benign recurrent vertigo—true or artificial diagnosis? Acta Otolaryngol Suppl 529:101–103, 1997.

Kerber K, Enrietto J, Jacobson K, et al: Disequilibrium in older people: A prospective study. Neurology 51:574–580, 1998.

Kitamura K, Kudo Y: Benign recurrent vertigo in Japanese. Auris Nasus Larynx 17:211–216, 1990.

Kluge M, Beyenburg S, Fernandez G, et al: Epileptic vertigo: Evidence for vestibular representation in human frontal cortex. Neurology 55:1906–1908, 2000.

Kogeorgos J, Scott D, Swash M: Epileptic dizziness. BMJ 282:687–689, 1981.

Lannuzel A, Moulin T, Amsallem D, et al: Vertebral–artery dissection following a judo session: A case report. Neuropediatrics 25:106–108, 1994.

Leigh RJ, Zee DS: The Neurology of Eye Movements, ed 3. New York: Oxford University Press, 1999.

Leliever WC, Barber HO: Recurrent vestibulopathy. Laryngoscope 91:1–6, 1981.

Lin YC, Lenz FA: Distribution and response evoked by microstimulation of thalamus nuclei in patients with dystonia and tremor. Chin Med J 107:265–270, 1994.

Lin YC, Lenz FA: Effective response evoked by microstimulation of thalamus nuclei in patients with tremor. Chin Med J 106:372–374, 1993.

Lobel E, Kleine J, Bihan D, et al: Functional MRI of galvanic vestibular stimulation. J Neurophysiol 80:2699–2709, 1998.

Masdeu J, Gorelick P: Thalamic astasia: Instability to stand after unilateral thalamic lesions. Ann Neurol 23:596–603, 1988.

McIntosh S, DaCosta D, Kenny R: Outcome of an integrated approach to the investigation of dizziness, falls, and syncope in elderly patients referred to a syncope clinic. Age Ageing 22:53–58, 1993a.

McIntosh S, Lawson J, Kenny R: Clinical characteristics of vasodepressor, cardioinhibitory, and mixed carotid sinus syndrome in the elderly. Am J Med 95:203–208, 1993b.

Minor L, Haslwanter T, Straumann D, et al: Hyperventilation-induced nystagmus in patients with vestibular schwannoma. Neurology 53:2158–2168, 1999.

Moore S: LVOR and AVOR during locomotion in humans. Vestibular Labyrinth in Health and Disease Symposium. November 16–18, 2000, Otolaryngology, School of Medicine, Washington University, St. Louis, MO.

Mori S, Matsuyama K, Mori F, et al: Supraspinal sites that induce locomotion in the vertebrate central nervous system, in Ruzicka E, Hallet M, Jankovic J (eds): Gait Disorders: Advances in Neurology. Philadelphia: Lippincott, Williams & Wilkins, 2001, Vol. 87, pp. 25–46.

Nagarkar A, Gupta A, Mann S: Psychological findings in benign paroxysmal positional vertigo and psychogenic vertigo. J Otolaryngol 29:154–158, 2000.

Neuhauser H, Leopold M, von Brevern M, et al: The interrelations of migraine, vertigo, and migrainous vertigo. Neurology 56:436–441, 2001.

Norrving B, Magnusson M, Holtas S: Isolated acute vertigo in the elderly: Vestibular or vascular disease? Acta Neurol Scand 91:43–48, 1995.

Nunez R: Short- and long-term outcomes of canalith repositioning for benign paroxysmal positional vertigo. Otolaryngol Head Neck Surg 122:647–652, 2000.

Nutt JG, Marsden C, Thompson P: Human walking and higher-level gait disorders, particularly in the elderly. Neurology 43:268–279, 1993.

Oas J, Baloh R: Vertigo and the anterior inferior cerebellar artery syndrome. Neurology 42:2274–2279, 1992.

Palmini A, Gloor P: The localizing value of auras in partial seizures: A prospective and retrospective study. Neurology 42:801–808, 1992.

Parent A (ed): Carpenter's Human Neuroanatomy. Baltimore, MD: Williams & Wilkins, 1996.

Penfield W: Vestibular sensation and the cerebral cortex. Ann Otol Rhinol Laryngol 66:691–698, 1957.

Rassekh CH, Harker LA: The prevalence of migraine in Meniere's disease. Laryngoscope 102:135–138, 1992.

Rode G, Charles N, Perenin M, et al: Partial remission of hemiplegia and somatoparaphrenia through vestibular stimulation in a case of unilateral neglect. Cortex 28:203–208, 1992.

Rubens A: Caloric stimulation and unilateral visual neglect. Neurology 35:1019–1024, 1985.

Rutka JA, Barber HO: Recurrent vestibulopathy: Third review. J Otolaryngol 15:105–107, 1986.

Ryu J, McCabe B: Central vestibular compensation. Arch Otolaryngol 102:71–76, 1976.

Sadler TW: Langman's Medical Embryology. Baltimore, MD: Williams & Wilkins, 1990.

Sloane P, Baloh R: Persistent dizziness in geriatric patients. J Am Geriatr Soc 37:1031–1038, 1989.

Sullivan M, Clark M, Katon W, et al: Psychiatric and otologic diagnoses in patients complaining of dizziness. Arch Intern Med 153:1479–1483, 1993.

Thompson PD, Marsden CD: Gait disorder of subcortical arteriosclerotic encephalopathy: Binswanger's disease. Mov Disord 2:1–8, 1987.

Tinetti M, Williams C, Gill T: Health, functional, and psychological outcomes among older persons with chronic dizziness. J Am Geriatr Soc 48:417–421, 2000.

Tusa RJ, Brown SB: Neuro-otologic trauma and dizziness, in Rizzo M, Tranel D (eds): Head Injury and Postconcussive Syndrome. New York: Churchill Livingstone, 1996, pp. 177–200.

Vibert N, Bantikyan A, Babalian A, et al: Post-lesional plasticity in the central nervous system of the guinea-pig: A 'top-down' adaptation process? Neuroscience 94:1–5, 1999.

von Brevern M, Clarke A, Lempert T: Continuous vertigo and spontaneous nystagmus due to canalolithiasis of the horizontal canal. Neurology 56:684–686, 2001.

Welling D, Parnes L. O'Brien B, et al: Particulate matter in the posterior semicircular canal. Laryngoscope 107:90–94, 1997.

Whitman G, DiPatre P, Lopez I, et al: Neuropathology in older people with disequilibrium of unknown cause. Neurology 35:375–382, 1999.

Yardley L: Overview of psychologic effects of chronic dizziness and balance disorders. Otolaryngol Clin North Am 33:603–616, 2000.

Yardley L. Prediction of handicap and emotional distress in patients with recurrent vertigo. Soc Sci Med 39:573–581, 1994.

Yardley L. Somatic and psychological factors contributing to handicap in people with vertigo. Br J Audiol 26:283–290, 1992.

Yardley L, Burgneay J, Nazareth I, et al: Neuro-otological and psychiatric abnormalities in a community sample of people with dizziness: A blind controlled investigation. J Neurol Neurosurg Psychiatry 65:679–684, 1998a.

Yardley L, Gresty M, Bronstein A, et al: Changes in heart rate and respiration rate in patients with vestibular dysfunction following head movements which provoke dizziness. Biol Psychol 49:95–108, 1998b.

Yardley L, Luxon L, Haacke N: A longitudinal study of symptoms, anxiety and subjective well-being in patients with vertigo. Clin Otolaryngol Allied Sci 19:109–116, 1994.

Yardley L, Owen N, Nazareth I, et al: Panic disorder with agoraphobia associated with dizziness. J Nerv Ment Dis 189:321–327, 2001.

Yardley L, Owen N, Nazareth I, et al: Prevalence and presentation of dizziness in a general practice community sample of working age people. Br J Gen Pract 48:1131–1135, 1998c.

Yardley L, Watson S, Britton J, et al: Effects of anxiety arousal and mental stress on the vestibulo–ocular reflex. Acta Otolaryngol (Stockholm) 115:597–602, 1995.

Aphasia, Alexia, Agraphia, Acalculia

Howard S. Kirshner

Acalculia

Agraphia

Alexia

Angular gyrus syndrome

Aphasia

Gerstmann syndrome

INTRODUCTION

Speech and language have a twofold claim to the interest of all students of the mind and the brain. First, language was the first "higher" function to be localized in the brain, through the pioneering work of Paul Broca and other European physicians almost a century and a half ago. Second, language is absolutely critical to our humanity, our ability to communicate with others. We define speech as the articulation of language sounds by the vocal apparatus. Language refers to the manipulation of symbols in the production and comprehension of communication. Aphasias are defined as acquired disorders of language secondary to brain disease (Alexander

& Benson, 1999). Aphasia syndromes, like more elementary neurologic syndromes, can be defined by the bedside neurologic examination, specifically the portion of the mental status examination devoted to speech and language.

Broca and other 19th century neurologists described patients with acquired language disorders, studied their brains after their death, and created the correlations of structure and function that have formed the model for behavioral neurology ever since. In recent years, such clinical observations have been greatly augmented by new technologies, especially the new brain imaging modalities. Computed tomographic (CT) and magnetic resonance imaging (MRI) have permitted precise imaging of brain lesions in the living patient. Single photon emission computed tomography (SPECT), positron emission tomography (PET), and functional MRI (fMRI), so-called functional imaging methods, have made possible the visualization of brain areas as they activate in response to specific language tasks. These technologies have advanced the study of language activity in normal individuals as well as patients with brain disorders. Another new technology is the electrophysiologic mapping of epileptic foci, which has provided an independent source of information on language localization in the brain. The analysis of language disorders has not only advanced our knowledge of brain structure and function but has also been of practical importance in the diagnosis and treatment of patients. Better treatments for many of the brain diseases that cause aphasia, including stroke, promise much more to aphasic patients.

APHASIA

Diagnosis of Aphasia

In diagnosing a patient with language difficulty, the examiner must first exclude other, confounding conditions. The definition of aphasia excludes three other causes of abnormal communication. First, we exclude developmental or congenital language disorders, which can occur either as isolated "dysphasia" or as part of a more general, retarding condition. The examiner must first ensure in the history that the deficit is acquired, that is, that premorbid speech and language skills were normally developed. Note that in the United Kingdom and Europe, the term "dysphasia" often refers to a partial, as opposed to complete, loss of language.

Second, the definition of aphasia excludes motor speech disorders, which disturb only spoken language output. In motor speech disorders, the comprehension of both spoken and written language remains intact. Muteness is especially difficult to diagnose; a patient who is mute is not always aphasic. Other causes of muteness include severe dysarthria, laryngeal disorders, frontal lobe syndromes such as "akinetic mutism," extrapyramidal disorders such as Parkinson disease, and psychogenic states such as catatonia or uncooperativeness. It is always helpful to have some language production to analyze, to diagnose aphasia with confidence. A patient who can understand language and write normally is probably not aphasic. Muteness and inability to follow commands in a patient who is seemingly alert may signify severe aphasia, especially if the patient attempts to communicate by gesturing, pointing, or making nonverbal noises. The diagnosis is made easier by "neighborhood signs" of left hemisphere injury such as right hemiparesis and right hemianopia.

Third, we must exclude disorders of language content secondary to psychiatric disorders. In psychosis, the mechanics of speech and language are normal, but the underlying thought process, or manipulation of concepts, goes awry. A psychotic patient may articulate well-constructed sentences, with normal word choice and grammar, but the content is bizarre, vague, or illogical (Docherty et al., 1996). A key difference between psychosis and aphasia is in the patient's nonlinguistic behavior. The psychotic patient manifests abnormal behavior as well as language, whereas an aphasic patient usually behaves appropriately, though unable to communicate. The presence of other focal left hemisphere signs in many aphasic patients also helps to indicate a neurologic rather than psychiatric disorder.

Bedside Aphasia Examination

Aphasias are classified by findings on the bedside language examination. We shall use the six-part outline of Benson and Geschwind, recently updated by Alexander and Benson (1999). This examination is listed in Table 17-1. Spontaneous speech is first categorized as fluent or nonfluent. Errors of speech, or paraphasic errors, are also recorded. Sound or phoneme substitutions are called literal or phonemic paraphasias; examples include "ben" for "pen" or "spork" for "fork." Substitutions of an incorrect word are called verbal or semantic paresthesias; examples include "pencil" for "pen" or "spoon" for "fork." When speech is so full of errors and neologisms (nonwords) that the meaning cannot be discerned, we speak of jargon aphasia. Naming should be tested for objects, object parts, colors, body parts, and actions. Some aphasic disorders are surprisingly selective for specific groups of items. Repetition is tested both for polysyllabic words ("Methodist Episcopal") and for grammatical phrases ("No ifs, ands, or buts"). Polysyllabic words are difficult for patients with dysarthria and apraxia of speech, whereas the grammatical phrases are difficult for aphasics. We test auditory comprehension by asking the patient to follow commands of one step ("close your eyes"), two step ("pick up your right hand and touch your nose"), or three steps ("touch your nose, then your right ear, then your left shoulder"). If the patient fails this test, it is important to be sure that the patient can hear, can understand English, is not paralyzed in the limb required for the command, and is not apraxic. Apraxia is defined as a disorder of learned movement not explained by elementary deficits in motor function or language comprehension. In case of doubt regarding apraxia, the examiner should use yes/no questions or commands to point to objects. Reading is tested both by reading aloud and reading for comprehension, using commands analogous to those used to test auditory comprehension. Writing can be tested by copying, writing to dictation, and writing spontaneous

TABLE 17-1. Bedside Aphasia Examination

Spontaneous speech

Naming: objects, object parts, colors, body parts, actions

Repetition

Auditory comprehension

Reading: aloud, for meaning

Writing: copying, writing to dictation, writing spontaneously phrases and sentences. It is important to emphasize that the alexias and agraphias, disorders of reading and writing, will be missed unless these functions are tested deliberately. The neurologist uses the results of the rest of the neurologic examination, in addition to language features, in coming to a localization of the brain disorder.

Aphasia Syndromes

Aphasias are traditionally divided into syndromes by the features of the language disorder. These behavioral aphasia syndromes have correlated to some extent with specific lesion localizations. A number of aphasia classifications have been advanced. The "Boston" classification of Benson and Geschwind, as updated by Alexander and Benson (1999), offers the most practical system for clinical neurologists, because it uses the classical syndromes described in the 19th century but incorporates new knowledge of neuroanatomy and clinical findings. In addition, this classification scheme relates directly to both the bedside language examination and to test scores obtained on the Boston Diagnostic Aphasia Examination (BDAE). A preliminary classification is made from the bedside examination, but more reliable syndrome diagnosis is obtained from either the BDAE or its shortened adaptation, the Western Aphasia Battery (WAB).

Many systems of aphasia classification begin with a dichotomous approach, such as expressive-receptive, motor-sensory, fluent-nonfluent, or anterior-posterior aphasias. The expressive-receptive and motor-sensory dichotomies are misleading, because aphasias are rarely purely expressive or receptive, motor or sensory. Nearly all aphasics have abnormal language expression. The fluent-nonfluent dichotomy has the advantage that it is merely descriptive, though there are intermediate cases. The anterior-posterior dichotomy implies an anatomic localization of the lesion, which can only be guessed from the aphasia phenomena.

The "Boston" classification divides the aphasias into eight classical syndromes: Broca, Wernicke, global, conduction, anomic, transcortical motor, transcortical sensory, and mixed transcortical aphasia, also called the syndrome of the isolation of the speech area. We shall also briefly consider the syndromes of aphemia, pure word deafness, and the subcortical aphasia syndromes, as well as the alexias, agraphias, and acalculias. Finally, we shall consider the topics of aphasia in left-handers, "crossed aphasia" associated with right hemisphere lesions in right-handers, and aphasia in bilingual or multilingual speakers.

Broca's Aphasia

Paul Broca's two original patients had a severe disorder of articulation; they could comprehend language but could produce only stereotyped utterances such as "tan tan." Broca localized the articulation of speech to the inferior left frontal region that now bears the name "Broca's area." The person with typical Broca's aphasia speaks hesitantly. The deficit can range from complete muteness, to single word utterances, to hesitant phrases and short sentences. The disorder is an aphasia, rather than just a motor speech disorder, because grammatical constructions are disturbed. Expressive speech is agrammatical or "telegraphic"; for example, a Broca's aphasic might say "go fishing son Saturday" to express his plans for the weekend. Table 17-2 shows the major clinical features of Broca's aphasia.

Naming in Broca's aphasia is usually impaired. Frequently, patients will have an idea of the name; they may be able to produce the initial letter or phoneme or correctly state the number of syllables in the word. This type of anomia is called the "tip of the tongue phenomenon." In some patients, naming of actions (verbs) is more impaired than naming of objects (nouns). Repetition in Broca's aphasia is usually only slightly better than spontaneous speech, marred by similar articulatory difficulty and hesitancy. Auditory comprehension often seems normal, but sentences with complex grammatical structure reveal deficits in syntactic decoding, just as the same types of sentences are difficult for the Broca's aphasic to speak. For example, the sentence "the present that Jane gave to Arthur was gaudy," may cause major difficulty; the patient may have difficulty answering questions regarding who received the present and who gave it. Caplan and colleagues (1997) investigated activation of the cerebral cortex by positron emission tomography during the expression and

TABLE 17-2. Features of Broca's Aphasia

Spontaneous speech	Nonfluent, hesitant, varying from mute to agrammatical, often dysarthric
Naming	Impaired ("tip-of-the-tongue")
Auditory comprehension	Intact for simple material; impaired for complex syntax
Repetition	Impaired, hesitant
Reading	Difficulty reading aloud, often poorer reading than auditory comprehension
Writing	Difficulty writing, even with left hand
Associated signs	Right hemiparesis, right hemisensory loss, apraxia of left limbs
Behavior	Frustrated, depressed, but appropriate

comprehension of sentences with embedded clauses. The left frontal "Broca's area" activated during both functions, confirming the importance of this region to syntactic processing. Reading is often more affected than auditory comprehension in Broca's aphasia. Benson (1977) referred to this reading difficulty as the "third alexia," distinguishing this alexia from the traditional syndromes of alexia with and without agraphia, to be discussed later. Writing is also deficient in Broca's aphasia. Most Broca's aphasics have partial or total paralysis of the right arm and leg, making it difficult for the right-handed patient to write with the dominant hand. Some patients refuse to attempt to write with the nondominant or left hand. Usually, however, there is nearly total inability to write. Persons with injuries to the right arm, but with normal brain function, can learn to write awkwardly but intelligibly with the left hand. The inability of patients with Broca's aphasia to write is thus not a motor disorder, but rather a part of the language disorder. Experimentally, some patients with Broca's aphasia and right hemiparesis have been able to learn to write with a device resembling a roller skate; patients with proximal arm movement can direct the skate. Many patients can write better with the paralyzed right arm in the skate device than with the nonparalyzed left arm (Whurr & Lorch, 1991).

Associated deficits with Broca's aphasia include weakness of the right face, arm, and leg, and sensory loss on the right side of the body. The visual fields are usually spared. Some studies on depression after stroke have found an association between depression and infarctions of the anterior left hemisphere (Robinson et al., 1984), though surveys with a longer time after the stroke have not found consistent differences between the hemispheres (Robinson, 2000). Patients with Broca's aphasia are generally aware of their deficits, often frustrated by them, but appropriate in their behavior. Some patients with Broca's aphasia show apraxia of the left limbs, failing to follow commands for use of the left limbs that they comprehend. It is important to recognize this apraxia and not mistake it for failure to comprehend.

The lesions that produce Broca's aphasia classically involve the posterior two thirds of the inferior frontal convolution, pars triangularis and pars opercularis, and Brodmann areas 44 and 45 (Fig. 17-1). Strokes in the territory of the frontal branches of the left middle cerebral artery are the most common cause of Broca's aphasia. Mohr and colleagues (1978) showed that lesions restricted to the cortical Broca's area allow virtually complete recovery, such that Broca's aphasia is a transitory phenomenon over several weeks. Alexander and colleagues (1990) found that patients with lesions of areas 44 and 45 had mainly a deficit in initiation of speech, not a true aphasia. Patients with lesions only of the lower motor cortex had only dysarthria and speech

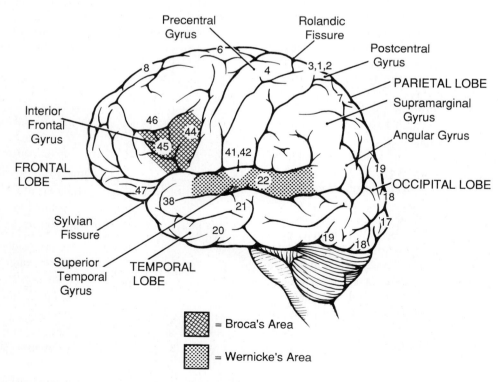

FIGURE 17-1. Drawing of the lateral surface of the left hemisphere, showing the relationship of Broca's and Wernicke's language areas to the motor and sensory cortices, the angular and supramarginal gyri, and the lobar architecture of the brain.

hesitancy. Both areas 44 and 45 and the lower motor cortex had to be damaged to produce the full picture of Broca's aphasia. Figure 17-2 shows a CT scan from a patient with Broca's aphasia and right hemiparesis. Patients with lasting Broca's aphasia usually have larger lesions, involving not only Broca's area but also much of the frontoparietal operculum. Broca's two original cases had such lesions, as have most reported cases over the ensuing century. These patients usually have global aphasia in the early days after stroke, then recover toward a deficit profile of Broca's aphasia. Mohr and colleagues (1978) referred to the transitory and permanent forms of Broca's aphasia as "Baby Broca" and "Big Broca" syndromes, respectively.

Naeser and colleagues (1989) reported that lesions associated with poor recovery of fluent speech always include two subcortical areas: (1) the subcallosal fasciculus deep to Broca's area and (2) the periventricular white matter along the body of the left lateral ventricle. The combined cortical-subcortical frontal lesion appears to be required for lasting nonfluency.

Aphemia

Broca originally used the term "aphemie" to describe the articulatory disorder of his two 1861 cases, but "aphemia" is now used to designate a more restricted syndrome of nonfluent speech, with normal comprehension and writing. Patients with aphemia are often mute initially, with hesitant speech emerging over the next few days, often with prominent phonemic errors. Patients with aphemia often have right facial weakness but no major motor deficits, and their comprehension, reading, and writing are largely normal. The lesions may involve the face area of the motor cortex (Alexander et al., 1990). In strict terms, aphemia is not a true language disorder, but a motor speech disorder.

Wernicke's Aphasia

The German physician Karl Wernicke described the second major aphasia syndrome, Wernicke's aphasia, in 1874. Wernicke's aphasia can be thought of as the opposite of Broca's aphasia. Unlike the sparse, effortful speech of Broca's aphasia, Wernicke's aphasia is characterized by fluent, effortless speech, often with normal or even increased numbers of words per unit time ("logorrhea"). The speech content, however, is empty, containing stock phrases but few meaningful nouns and verbs and many paraphasic errors of both literal (phonemic) and verbal (semantic) type. If the speech is so filled with nonwords that the meaning cannot be discerned, we speak of "jargon aphasia." In milder cases, sentences may begin appropriately, but the word order then goes awry, and the meaning becomes lost. A listener unfamiliar with the native language of a Wernicke's aphasic might not notice much amiss; the patient speaks fluently in a pattern resembling the speaker's native language, but little actual meaning is expressed. Wernicke's aphasics often comprehend little of what is said to them. Patients sometimes seem to understand family members, but extralinguistic cues such as facial expressions and gestures facilitate communication. An unbiased examiner, testing comprehension by nonrepetitive commands

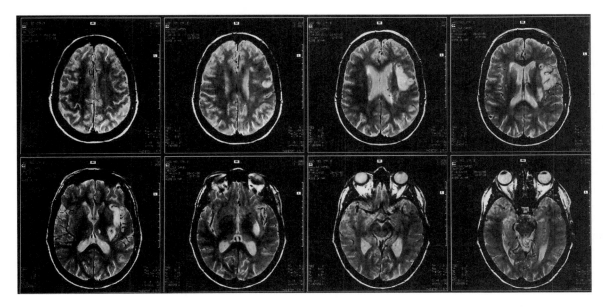

FIGURE 17-2. MRI scan from a patient with Broca's aphasia. There is a small left frontal, cortical infarct, but more extensive involvement of the subcortical white matter and insula. The patient had a hesitant speech pattern consisting of mild Broca's aphasia and apraxia of speech. Her recovery over several weeks was excellent.

TABLE 17-3. Features of Wernicke's Aphasia

Spontaneous speech	Fluent, with paraphasic errors of both phonemic and verbal type
Naming	Impaired, often paraphasic
Auditory comprehension	Impaired
Repetition	Impaired
Reading	Usually impaired
Writing	Well formed but paragraphic
Associated signs	± Right hemianopia, usually no motor or sensory deficits
Behavior	Often unaware of deficits, may be inappropriately happy, later sometimes angry, suspicious

or by yes/no questions, finds major deficits. Nonsense questions such as "Are you sitting on top of a helicopter?" rapidly establish deficits in comprehension.

The characteristics of Wernicke's aphasia are listed in Table 17-3. Naming often involves bizarre and paraphasic productions, unrelated to the target word or not a word at all. Repetition is usually impaired, with paraphasic substitutions. Reading comprehension is usually impaired, similarly to auditory comprehension. Occasionally, a patient with Wernicke's aphasia can comprehend printed better than spoken language, or the reverse (Kirshner et al., 1989). Patients can then communicate via the spared channel. Patients with Wernicke's aphasia with intact reading resemble the classical syndrome of pure word deafness (see below), whereas those with relatively spared auditory comprehension resemble the deficit of pure alexia with agraphia. The patient with Wernicke's aphasia can usually write with well-formed letters, but the writing is filled with misspellings, empty phrases, and nonwords. Abnormal spelling can be an early sign of a temporal lobe lesion with mild Wernicke's aphasia. As in the case of reading, a few atypical cases have been described in which writing is superior to spoken verbal expression.

The associated deficits of Wernicke's aphasia are often minor. Some patients have right visual field deficits, but there is usually no significant weakness or sensory loss. Because of the absence of obvious focal neurologic signs, Wernicke's aphasia may be mistaken for a psychosis or acute confusional state. Wernicke's aphasics often seem unaware of their deficits and, hence, not appropriately depressed. Lazar and colleagues (2000) recently reported data on a patient with an arteriovenous malformation who became aphasic during selective amobarbital injections into the inferior division of the left middle cerebral artery. This patient

recalled the episodes and understood the interactions better than the examiners thought.

The lesion in Wernicke's aphasia classically involves the left superior temporal gyrus. Modern brain imaging studies have confirmed this localization, though some authors include the inferior parietal lobule (supramarginal and angular gyri, Brodmann areas 39 and 40) as part of Wernicke's area. Kirshner and colleagues (1989) found differences in the deficit profile of Wernicke's aphasia; patients with temporal lesions had more severe impairment of auditory comprehension than of reading, whereas those with parietal lesions had the opposite impairment. A CT scan of a patient with Wernicke's aphasia is shown in Figure 17-3. Electrical stimulation studies have confirmed that activation of the posterior left superior temporal gyrus by surface electrodes interferes temporarily with language comprehension (Lesser et al., 1986; Boatman et al., 2000). Patients reported hearing sounds but were unable to comprehend them.

Lasting loss of auditory comprehension for single words requires complete destruction of Wernicke's area

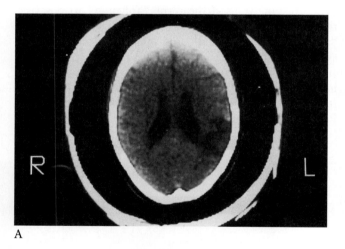

A

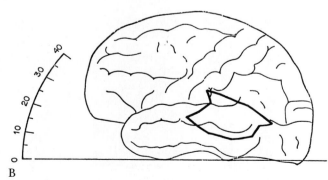

B

FIGURE 17-3. (A) CT scan from a patient with Wernicke's aphasia but spared reading ability. Note that the lesion, though very large, is predominantly temporal. (B) Lateral brain diagram, derived from the axial CT images.

(Naeser et al., 1987). Other studies, however, have indicated that lasting Wernicke's aphasia usually correlates with larger lesions, extending into the left temporal and parietal lobes (Kertesz et al., 1993). Smaller lesions of the left temporal lobe permit recovery toward the syndromes of conduction or anomic aphasia.

Pure Word Deafness

Pure word deafness is a selective deafness for auditory language. Speech, writing, naming, and reading are normal, but auditory comprehension and repetition are severely impaired. The patient is deaf only to words; normal pure tone hearing is a prerequisite for the diagnosis. The word-deaf patient can hear and interpret meaningful nonverbal sounds such as animal cries or the sound of a bell or beeper. Most patients with pure word deafness have other, mild language deficits such as paraphasic speech and impaired naming.

Geschwind explained pure word deafness neuroanatomically as a disconnection of the intact Wernicke's area from both auditory cortices. Cases of pure word deafness have been reported with bilateral, temporal lobe pathology such as herpes simplex encephalitis and bilateral strokes. Destructive lesions of both temporal lobes, involving the Heschl gyrus bilaterally, classically produce cortical deafness, comprising loss of both word comprehension and identification of other meaningful sounds. In some cases, initial cortical deafness has given way to more selective syndromes affecting language more than nonverbal auditory sounds.

Theoretically, even a unilateral, left temporal lesion could disconnect the left hemisphere Wernicke's area from both auditory cortices (Takahashi et al., 1992). This would explain the clear overlap with Wernicke's aphasia, related to unilateral lesions of the left temporal lobe.

Global Aphasia

Global aphasia can be thought of as the sum of Broca's plus Wernicke's aphasia. The aphasia profile is simply the loss of all of the elementary language functions (Table 17-4); the patient speaks like a Broca's aphasic but comprehends like a Wernicke's aphasic, the worst of both worlds. Some patients speak only a verbal stereotyped phrase or "stereotypy" such as "wawawa."

Most patients with global aphasia have severe associated deficits of right hemianopia, right hemiparesis, and right hemisensory loss. The syndrome of global aphasia without hemiparesis has been reported several times, with lesions that generally involve both Broca's and Wernicke's areas but spare the motor and sensory cortices. In general, patients with global aphasia have extensive damage involving the left frontal, temporal, and parietal lobes. The most common causes would

TABLE 17-4. Features of Global Aphasia

Spontaneous speech	Nonfluent, mute, or restricted to a stereotyped phrase
Naming	Impaired
Auditory comprehension	Impaired
Repetition	Impaired
Reading	Impaired
Writing	Impaired
Associated signs	Most have right hemianopia, right hemiparesis, right hemisensory loss, often apraxia
Behavior	Often depressed

be infarctions secondary to embolic occlusion of the middle cerebral artery or occlusion of the internal carotid artery. The syndrome also results from brain tumors, large left basal ganglia hemorrhages, and massive head trauma. The patient with global aphasia often appears depressed and withdrawn.

Global aphasia often improves over time, with the deficit evolving into another aphasia category. The evolution from global to Broca's aphasia is the most common path for these patients, as comprehension gradually improves over weeks and months (Mohr et al., 1978). In the study of Naeser and colleagues (1990), sparing of the cortical Wernicke's area in the superior temporal lobe was associated with recovery of comprehension. Occasionally patients evolve toward Wernicke's or even anomic aphasia.

Conduction Aphasia

Conduction aphasia is a relatively uncommon but important aphasia syndrome, one that was historically important in the understanding of language function in the human brain. Conduction aphasia can be thought of primarily as a disorder of repetition because this function is impaired out of proportion to other language deficits. The patient may be unable to repeat even single words or phrases. One of our patients could not repeat the word "boy" but spontaneously said, "I like girls better." Asked to repeat "hospital," he said, "Hother...my hotheral...you know, this damned place where we are." Speech in conduction aphasia is categorized as fluent, but in some cases, the speech output is so interrupted by literal paraphasic errors and attempts at self-correction that the fluency is intermittent. Some patients have more frankly paraphasic speech. Naming is variable, but auditory comprehension must be intact for conduction aphasia to be diagnosed. Reading for meaning is generally good, but reading aloud may

TABLE 17-5. Features of Conduction Aphasia

Spontaneous speech	Fluent, with literal paraphasic errors
Naming	Variably intact
Auditory comprehension	Intact
Repetition	Poor
Reading	Variable aloud, comprehension intact
Writing	Variably intact
Associated signs	Right hemiparesis, right hemisensory loss, visual field defect, apraxia
Behavior	No typical syndrome

produce errors resembling repetition. Writing is usually preserved. These features are summarized in Table 17-5.

Associated deficits in conduction aphasia are also variable. Many patients have right hemiparesis and right-sided sensory loss, and many have ideomotor apraxia. The lesion in conduction aphasia may involve the superior temporal lobe or the inferior parietal region. Conduction aphasia is an example of a "disconnection syndrome," a theory originally postulated by Wernicke and later revived by Geschwind; the lesions leave Broca's and Wernicke's areas intact but disrupt the connections between them. This theory is useful as a convenient way of remembering the syndrome, but it is likely an oversimplification. Most cases of conduction aphasia involve cortical damage in the temporal and parietal lobes; isolated cases with deep temporal lesions in the white matter are rare. The apraxia seen as part of conduction aphasia may correlate with parietal as compared to temporal lesions (Damasio & Damasio, 1980). The supramarginal gyrus, often affected in conduction aphasia, appears to be involved in phoneme selection, and lesions in this area may result in literal paraphasic errors (Demonet et al., 1992; Kirshner et al., 1999).

Another theory of conduction aphasia holds that the syndrome is caused by a failure of auditory-verbal immediate memory. Failure to keep a word string in immediate memory would result in a loss of repetition ability, as seen in conduction aphasia. In this regard, it is interesting that delayed feedback of the words to be repeated helps patients with conduction aphasia repeat better, whereas it seems to confuse normal subjects. These competing theories of conduction may both have some validity in explaining the language features of conduction aphasia.

Anomic Aphasia

Anomic aphasia, as the name implies, is a syndrome in which naming difficulty is the primary abnormality.

Spontaneous speech is fluent, with word-finding pauses and circumlocutions. Auditory comprehension, repetition, reading, and writing are all relatively intact (Table 17-6). Associated deficits are variable and often absent.

Naming is disturbed in virtually all of the aphasic syndromes. Even normal people, and especially elderly people, have occasional difficulty finding words. Anomic aphasia is often the last stage in recovery from many different types of aphasia.

Benson and Ardila (1996) divide anomia into four separate types: word production anomia, word selection anomia, semantic anomia, and disconnection anomia. *Word production anomia* is a difficulty with elicitation of words, seen particularly with left frontal lesions. Patients with word production anomia recognize the correct word and often produce it with cues. Patients with *word selection anomia* cannot produce the word or benefit from cues, but they can always point to the object if given the name. This deficit may correlate with temporal lesions, usually not involving Wernicke's area. Naming of nouns is more affected than verbs with temporal lesions; the reverse often occurs with frontal lesions. Patients with *semantic anomia* cannot elicit the name or benefit from cues, and they cannot point to the object when given the name; the patient has simply lost the meaning of the word. This third type of anomia may arise from the angular gyrus region. Semantic anomia has also been described in dementias ("semantic dementia"). *Disconnection anomia* refers to anomia for selective classes of items, in which a disconnection prevents semantic information from reaching the left hemisphere language area. Examples include category-specific anomias, such as the color anomia associated with alexia without agraphia (see below), and corpus callosum lesions, which prevent information from crossing from one hemisphere to the other. A patient with callosotomy surgery, for example, will be unable to name an object palpated with the left hand; the right hemisphere recognizes the object but cannot transfer the information to the left hemisphere for naming.

TABLE 17-6. Features of Anomic Aphasia

Spontaneous speech	Fluent, with word-finding pauses and circumlocutions
Naming	Impaired
Auditory comprehension	Intact
Repetition	Intact
Reading	Intact
Writing	Intact except for word-finding difficulty
Associated signs	Variable, often absent
Behavior	No characteristic features

The lesions of anomic aphasia are extremely variable. The sparing of repetition suggests that the perisylvian language circuit, from the Heschl gyri to Wernicke's area to Broca's area, is functioning. Lesions can be in the angular gyrus area, where they are also associated with alexia, agraphia, right-left confusion, acalculia, and finger agnosia ("Gerstmann syndrome"). Tumors of the deep left temporal white matter may produce isolated anomia. Anomic aphasia may also be the last stage in recovery in a variety of aphasic syndromes, including conduction aphasia, Wernicke's aphasia, and even Broca's aphasia. Anomia can be a sign of less localized disorders such as subdural hematoma, acute confusional states, and dementing illnesses such as Alzheimer disease (AD) and Pick disease.

Transcortical Aphasias

Lichtheim used the term "transcortical aphasias" to indicate that the lesion is not in the primary language cortex, but rather in adjacent areas of cortex, which he called the "area of concepts." The sparing of the perisylvian language circuit is responsible for the intact repetition, the hallmark of these aphasia syndromes. The features of the three transcortical aphasia syndromes are presented in Table 17-7.

Transcortical Motor Aphasia. Transcortical motor aphasia (TCMA) resembles Broca's aphasia, except that repetition is preserved. The patient speaks little, after a delay, or in a whisper. In contrast to the paucity of spontaneous speech, the patient can repeat long sentences fluently. Naming performance may vary, but auditory comprehension and reading are usually preserved. Writing may share some of the same hesitancy as speaking. Most patients have at least a partial right hemiparesis. The Russian neuropsychiatrist Luria called the same aphasia syndrome "dynamic aphasia," referring to the lack of initiation of speech.

TCMA represents a frontal lobe syndrome affecting language. Frontal lobe disorders generally involve a lack of movement or a difficulty with the initiation of movement; in this case, a localized left frontal lesion causes the patient to have reduced initiation of speech. Lesions causing transcortical motor aphasia virtually always involve the left frontal lobe, often within the territory of the anterior cerebral artery. The site of damage may be anterior to Broca's area, deep in the subcortical frontal white matter, or on the medial surface of the frontal lobe, in the vicinity of the supplementary motor area. The hemiparesis in an anterior cerebral artery stroke is different from that of the more typical left middle cerebral artery stroke, in that the leg is affected more than the arm, and the shoulder is affected more than the hand. Some patients demonstrate an involuntary grasp response in the affected hand. Because TCMA involves a separate vascular territory and a separate lobar anatomy from the aphasia syndromes of the middle cerebral artery, it tends to be relatively pure, with little overlap with other aphasia syndromes.

Albert and colleagues (1989) compared the hesitant speech of TCMA to the motor akinesia of Parkinson disease and treated three patients with the dopaminergic drug, bromocriptine, to increase speech fluency. Although this approach to the pharmacotherapy of aphasia has remained of doubtful benefit, it has opened a new field of language rehabilitation.

Transcortical Sensory Aphasia. The syndrome of transcortical sensory aphasia (TCSA) resembles Wernicke's aphasia, except that repetition is spared. Speech is fluent and paraphasic, naming is also paraphasic, and auditory and reading comprehension is severely impaired. Associated signs may be absent. TCSA is uncommon as a stroke syndrome, though a few cases have been reported with lesions near the temporo-occipital junction, classically sparing Wernicke's area itself. Boatman and colleagues (2000), in studies of electrical stimulation of the superior temporal region, found nearby areas in which stimulation could produce either Wernicke's or transcortical sensory aphasia. TCSA has also been described in AD.

TABLE 17-7. Features of Transcortical Aphasias

Characteristic	Transcortical motor aphasia	Transcortical sensory aphasia	Mixed transcortical aphasia
Speech	Nonfluent	Fluent	Nonfluent
Naming	Impaired	Impaired	Impaired
Repetition	Preserved	Echolalic	Echolalic
Comprehension	Preserved	Impaired	Impaired
Reading	Preserved	Impaired	Impaired
Writing	Reduced	Paragraphic	Poor
Associated signs	Right leg > arm weakness, abulia	Variable, often none	Right or bilateral hemiparesis

Mixed Transcortical Aphasia (Isolation of the Speech Area, Mixed TCA). Mixed transcortical aphasia is similar to global aphasia, except for the sparing of repetition, which can even be echolalic. Patients are nearly mute, cannot name, cannot follow commands or comprehend yes/no questions, and cannot read or write. Another name for the syndrome is "the syndrome of isolation of the speech area."

One of the best-described cases of this syndrome was a 13-year-old girl described by Geschwind and colleagues (1968), who suffered carbon monoxide poisoning, with large infarctions in the watershed distribution of both hemispheres. The patient repeated echolalically and sang songs. She completed familiar phrases begun by the examiner, and she could learn the lyrics of new songs, despite the fact that she could not produce any prepositional speech or follow any commands. The only language system this patient had was the circuit from Wernicke's to Broca's area, and even connections to the limbic system to recall lyrics of new songs, but no connection to the other association cortices ("areas of concepts") of the brain. This syndrome, like TCSA, has been described as a late stage in the language deterioration of AD.

Subcortical Aphasias

Aphasia has traditionally been assumed to involve damage to the left hemisphere language cortex. In recent years, many cases of aphasia from subcortical lesions have been reported, and a new category of "subcortical aphasia" has been added to the aphasia classification. It should not be surprising that subcortical sites that project up or down from portions of the language cortex might themselves produce aphasic symptomatology when damaged. As the name implies, subcortical aphasias are defined more by the anatomy of the brain lesion than by specific language characteristics. Several patterns of language disorder have been defined in patients with subcortical lesions. The common theme is that these syndromes are atypical for the classical cortical aphasia syndromes.

Thalamic Aphasia. The first type of subcortical aphasia is thalamic aphasia, first described in patients with thalamic hemorrhage. The aphasia pattern usually associated with thalamic damage is fluent, often with paraphasic errors, but with better comprehension and repetition than Wernicke's aphasia. A "dichotomous" state has been described, in which patients alternate between an alert state, with coherent speech, and a somnolent state, in which speech is mumbled, unintelligible, and paraphasic. Luria called thalamic aphasia a "quasi-aphasic disturbance of vigilance," theorizing that this disorder arises from a reduced alerting mechanism for the language cortex. The posterior thalamus has exten-sive projections to Wernicke's area, and the anterior and paramedian thalamic nuclei connect to structures involved in memory and attention.

More precise anatomic localization in thalamic aphasia has come from cases of ischemic infarction of the thalamus, because ischemic strokes have less swelling and mass effect than hemorrhages. Bogousslavsky and colleagues (1988) correlated thalamic aphasia with ischemic infarctions within the territories of the tuberothalamic artery, which supplies the anterior thalamus, including the ventral anterior and part of the ventral lateral nuclei, and the thalamoperforating artery. Common features were hypophonia, verbal paraphasias, impaired comprehension, and intact repetition.

Anterior Subcortical Aphasia Syndrome. Lesions of the caudate nucleus, putamen, and adjacent white matter have also been associated with aphasia. As in thalamic aphasia, the first cases of anterior basal ganglia lesions with aphasia were patients with hemorrhages of the left capsuloputamenal area. These patients were often mute initially, but later fluent, with some paraphasias and relatively preserved comprehension and repetition. Better definition of the subcortical aphasia syndromes has come with study of patients with basal ganglia infarctions. The most common is the "anterior subcortical aphasia syndrome" secondary to infarction of the head of the caudate nucleus, anterior limb of internal capsule, and anterior putamen, in the territory of lenticulostriate branches of the middle cerebral artery. The aphasia syndrome is nonfluent, usually with dysarthria; language abnormalities are usually mild (Alexander et al., 1987). Many patients have an associated right hemiparesis. Recovery is typically good. The neuroanatomy of this syndrome likely involves disruption in the caudate nucleus or anterior limb of fibers projecting to the caudate from the temporal cortex, and from the caudate to the globus pallidus, ventrolateral thalamus, and premotor cortex. Figure 17-4 shows a CT scan from a patient with the anterior subcortical aphasia syndrome.

Subcortical aphasia syndromes are complex and incompletely classified. Alexander and colleagues (1987) systematically examined language deficits in patients with subcortical lesions. Lesions restricted to the putamen or head of the caudate nucleus did not produce language disturbance, or at worst mild word-finding difficulty. Lesions involving the more posterior putamen were associated with hypophonia. There was still no language disturbance with involvement of the anterior limb of the internal capsule, except when this involved extensive injury to the caudate, putamen, and anterior limb of internal capsule, in which case the patients had the full anterior subcortical aphasia syndrome. Dysarthria was also associated if the damage

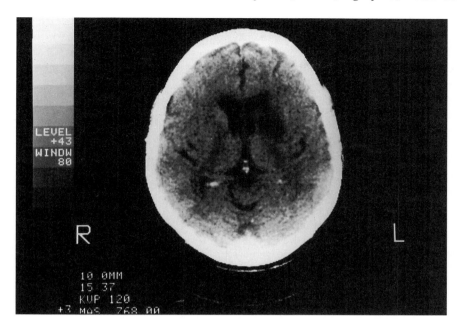

FIGURE 17-4. CT scan from a patient with anterior subcortical aphasia syndrome. The lesion is an infarction involving the anterior caudate, putamen, and anterior limb of the left internal capsule.

extended to the white matter of the periventricular region or the genu of the internal capsule. Lesions located more posteriorly, converging on the temporal isthmus, produced fluent aphasia, neologisms, and impaired comprehension. Lesions involving both areas, including the anterior caudate and putamen, internal capsule, periventricular white matter, and temporal isthmus, produced global aphasia. Finally, lesions more laterally placed, involving the insular cortex, extreme capsule, claustrum, and internal capsule, were associated with fluent aphasia, mild word-finding difficulty, and phonemic paraphasias, which increased on repetition and reading aloud. This last syndrome is a subcortical version of conduction aphasia. Hence, nearly the full spectrum of cortical aphasia types can be seen with subcortical lesions. These syndromes, however, are uncommon, and for the most part it remains true that aphasia usually signifies cortical pathology.

Other features of subcortical aphasias include disproportionate impairment of writing (Tanridag & Kirshner, 1985) with capsular lesions, and "frontal lobe" syndromes in patients with lesions of the left caudate nucleus, involving impaired attention, sequencing, and planning (Mendez et al., 1989).

Aphasia in Left-Handed Persons

In general, left-handed persons are more likely to develop aphasia regardless of the side of the stroke, suggesting that left-handed patients have some language representation in both cerebral hemispheres. Although aphasia is more common in left-handers, recovery may be better, suggesting greater plasticity of either hemisphere to permit language recovery. Naeser and Borod

(1986) reported a series of 31 left-handed aphasic patients, 27 with left and 4 with right hemisphere lesions. Most patients showed similar aphasia syndromes to those of a matched group of right-handed aphasic patients with left hemisphere lesions. Two patients, however, had destruction of the right frontal, temporal, and parietal cortices with nonfluent speech output but preserved comprehension, suggesting a left hemisphere Wernicke's area but a right hemisphere Broca's area. Basso and colleagues (1990) also found only minor differences between matched right-handed and non–right-handed patients with aphasia; the one exception was a left-handed patient with conduction aphasia, whose matched right-handed patient with a similar lesion had global aphasia. In summary, most left-handed patients have relative left hemisphere dominance for language, though they may have a higher percentage of mixed hemispheric dominance for language or pure right hemisphere dominance than right-handed patients.

Crossed Aphasia in Dextrals

More than 99% of right-handed patients with aphasia have left hemisphere lesions, but occasional right-handed patients develop aphasia after right hemisphere lesions, a phenomenon called "crossed aphasia." As in left-handed people, the majority of crossed aphasia cases resemble those of left hemisphere strokes in the analogous areas. Alexander and colleagues (1989) distinguished "mirror image" syndromes, those analogous to left hemisphere lesions, from "anomalous" cases. In their literature review, 22 of 34 cases had "mirror image" syndromes, whereas 12 cases had anomalous deficits. A common "anomalous" aphasia syndrome was the preservation of fluent speech despite large lesions that would be expected to produce nonfluent aphasia in the left hemisphere. Overall, the "anomalous" cases suggest that dominance for specific language functions may lie in separate hemispheres. For example, the left hemisphere may be necessary for fluent speech production, the right hemisphere for language comprehension.

New techniques such as Wada testing, SPECT, and PET functional brain imaging are beginning to be applied to crossed aphasia. With Wada testing, the injection of sodium amytal into the left carotid artery has not worsened the language performance of "crossed aphasia" patients (Alexander et al., 1989), confirming the complete lateralization of language to the right hemisphere. Studies with SPECT or PET imaging have confirmed the atypical finding of reduced cerebral blood flow in the right hemisphere (Bakar et al., 1996), but some studies have found reduced blood flow or metabolism in the left hemisphere as well, corresponding to "diaschisis" or reduced blood flow and metabolism in synaptically connected but undamaged areas. In one recent case, left hemisphere metabolism recovered while the aphasia remained severe (Bakar et al., 1996). Crossed aphasia likely results not from diaschisis, but from atypical cerebral dominance for language.

Aphasia in Polyglots

The effect of acquired aphasia on different languages has interested aphasiologists for generations. Early theories stated that patients would perform better in their native languages than in newly acquired languages after a stroke (Ribot law, 1895), but a rival theory stated that the language used most before the stroke would recover better (Pitres law, 1906). Obler and Albert (1977) found that the Ribots law applied no more than half the time, whereas the Pitres rule appeared to apply more regularly in younger aphasic patients. Studies from Canada, where many people speak both English and French, have shown that subjects who learn both languages simultaneously in childhood (compound bilinguals) have similar patterns of aphasia in both languages, whereas subjects who learn one language and then the other (coordinate bilinguals) show greater differences between languages. Occasionally, the aphasia types in bilingual patients can be different in one language versus another; for example, a Russian immigrant to Israel developed global aphasia in the newly learned Hebrew language, but only a mild, anomic aphasia in Russian (Obler & Albert, 1977). Recently, PET imaging has been applied to the study of bilingual patients. Perani and coworkers (1998) found that subjects with very high proficiency for two languages showed similar patterns of brain activation in response to language tasks, but those with different levels of proficiency showed differences in activation patterns. These authors concluded that the level of proficiency, and not the time of acquisition, determines the cerebral organization of a second language.

ALEXIAS AND AGRAPHIAS

Alexias and agraphias are acquired disorders of reading and writing secondary to brain damage (Alexander & Benson, 1999). Because reading and writing are language modalities, alexias and agraphias are aphasic disorders, but ones in which the comprehension and production of written language are affected more than spoken language modalities. The term "alexia" signifies an acquired reading disorder, just as "aphasia" means an acquired language disorder. Developmental or congenital reading disorders are referred to as dyslexias. In Europe and in some neuropsychological and neurolinguistic writings, "dyslexia" is used to denote partial as opposed to complete loss of reading.

Like the aphasias, the alexias and agraphias are defined by the bedside language examination. Without deliberate testing of reading and writing, these disorders cannot be detected. A history of intact premorbid reading and writing skills is also required.

Alexias

Traditionally, the alexias are divided into three categories: pure alexia with agraphia, pure alexia without agraphia, and alexia associated with aphasia ("aphasic alexia"). We shall first discuss these syndromes. The ability to read may be compromised by attentional impairments or problems with sequencing, as well as by speech or language disorders. Reading involves several distinct steps in cognitive processing: the visuospatial perception of individual letters and word shapes, the learned correspondence between letters and sounds, the recognition of groups of letters to the spoken form of words, and the association of meaning to these letter strings. We shall discuss how these stages in reading have led to new, neurolinguistic classifications of alexias.

Pure Alexia with Agraphia

The syndrome of alexia with agraphia, described by the French physician Dejerine in 1891, is in effect an acquired illiteracy. Reading and writing are both disrupted without significant dysfunction of other language modalities. Features of the bedside examination are presented in Table 17-8. Most patients with alexia with agraphia have some paraphasic speech, and naming errors are also common. Repetition and auditory comprehension are preserved. Occasional cases of

TABLE 17-8. Features of Pure Alexia with Agraphia

Spontaneous speech	Fluent, often paraphasic
Naming	Often impaired
Auditory comprehension	Intact
Repetition	Intact
Reading	Impaired
Writing	Impaired
Associated signs	Gerstmann syndrome, right visual field defect
Localization	Left inferior parietal

TABLE 17-9. Features of the Angular Gyrus Syndrome

Anomia
Alexia
Agraphia
Acalculia
Right-left disorientation
Finger agnosia
Constructional apraxia
± Mild, fluent aphasia
Right visual field defect

alexia with agraphia evolve from an initial deficit of Wernicke's aphasia, with some impairment of auditory comprehension as well as reading. Both reading words aloud and reading comprehension are abnormal. The patient usually cannot understand words spelled orally. This difficulty with letters is generally reflected in number tasks (acalculia) and may also be seen in other symbolic forms of notation such as musical notation. Occasionally patients may have some preserved ability to spell words or to comprehend words spelled orally. Writing is usually affected totally, such that the patient cannot write or spell even single words. Some patients can copy but cannot write sentences spontaneously or to dictation. Synonyms for this syndrome include parietal-temporal alexia, angular alexia, central alexia, and semantic alexia.

Other, associated neurologic deficits are variable and may be completely absent. A right visual field defect, or right inferior quadrant defect, is often present. Right-sided sensory and motor signs are usually mild if present at all. Other features of the Gerstmann syndrome (acalculia, finger agnosia, and right-left confusion) may also be present.

The lesion in alexia with agraphia involves the left inferior parietal lobule, and in particular the left angular gyrus. The syndrome may be seen in strokes involving the inferior division of the left middle cerebral artery or a "watershed" infarct between the left middle and posterior cerebral arteries. Isolated left parietal lesions such as tumors, traumatic injuries, hemorrhages, and arteriovenous malformations can also result in this syndrome.

Gerstmann and Angular Gyrus Syndromes

In 1930, Gerstmann described four deficits associated with left parietal lesions: agraphia, right-left confusion, disorientation, acalculia, and finger agnosia. Finger agnosia refers to a topographic and lateral difficulty with body parts, of which identification of fingers on the patient's own or the examiner's hand is perhaps the most sensitive index.

The four elements of the Gerstmann syndrome do not necessarily all occur together; any combination of three items would indicate a left inferior parietal lesion, and other, related deficits including alexia and mild aphasia may be combined. Morris and colleagues (1984) documented that the four deficits could be produced by electrical stimulation in the left angular and supramarginal gyrus of an adolescent with epilepsy. Benson and colleagues (1982) described the "angular gyrus syndrome" as a variant of Gerstmann syndrome and a mimicker of dementia. This vital confluence of the temporal and parietal lobe involves multiple cortical functions within a small anatomic territory. A patient with a single lesion in the left angular gyrus, documented by PET scan but not by CT, had combined deficits of anomia, fluent aphasia, alexia, agraphia, acalculia, right-left disorientation, finger agnosia, and constructional apraxia. The sheer multiplicity of these deficits resembled a dementia syndrome such as AD. The features of the angular gyrus syndrome are shown in Table 17-9.

The role of the angular gyrus in alexia with agraphia, Gerstmann syndrome, and the "angular gyrus" syndrome relates to larger, theoretical issues concerning the functions of this important brain region. Whereas Dejerine conceived of the angular gyrus as a visual word center, analogous to Wernicke's area as an auditory word center, the contemporary concept of the parietal "heteromodal" association cortex holds that this region is crucial for the transfer and integration of information from different sensory modalities. A clear example is the translation of visual into auditory language symbols that is so important to reading.

Pure Alexia without Agraphia

Dejerine described the second acquired alexia syndrome, pure alexia without agraphia, in 1892. The syndrome has been referred to as occipital alexia, pure alexia, posterior alexia, pure word blindness, and letter-by-letter alexia. These patients have no gross aphasia, and they can write, either spontaneously or to dictation.

The hallmark of this syndrome is the paradoxical inability of the patients to read words they have just written. Pure alexia is a true "word blindness," in which printed words have lost their meaning, though the patient is not blind. In other words, the patient has acquired not a total illiteracy as in alexia with agraphia, but rather a linguistic blindfold.

The features of alexia without agraphia are shown in Table 17-10. Spontaneous speech is usually normal, without paraphasias. Naming may be mildly impaired, especially for colors (see below). Auditory comprehension and repetition are typically intact, and most patients can spell words orally and comprehend words dictated in spelled form. Oral spelling and comprehension of orally spelled words is impaired in almost all other alexic syndromes and is therefore useful in the diagnosis of pure alexia without agraphia. Reading may be completely impossible at first, but over time the patient becomes able to recognize and name letters and to spell words out, letter-by-letter, first aloud and then silently. Reading remains slow and effortful, and reading for pleasure is impossible. Sometimes, the patient will make errors in reading aloud; the beginnings of words are typically correct but the endings may be guessed. For example, the patient may read "medical" as "medicine." Writing remains intact, except that patients cannot read their own written productions.

Associated symptoms and signs are quite different from those of alexia with agraphia. Primary motor and sensory deficits are usually absent. Occasionally patients have partial right hemiparesis or hemisensory loss. Most patients have a visual field deficit, either a hemianopia or a right upper quadrant defect. Rare patients have intact visual fields; some of these lose color vision in the right visual field (hemiachromatopsia; Damasio & Damasio, 1983). These visual deficits are important to test for, because they may be the only elementary neurologic deficits to aid in the detection of this syndrome.

Associated behavioral deficits in pure alexia include color anomia, visual agnosia, and memory loss. The inability of these patients to name colors is not a perceptual problem; as described by Geschwind and Fusillo (1966), they can match and sort colors normally, indicating that the deficit is not a problem of visual perception. They can also name colors in the abstract, such as the color of the inside of a watermelon, so the problem is not an anomia. The deficit is an inability to associate a perceived color with its name; this might be better termed "color agnosia." Occasionally, the deficit in naming colors may extend even to pictures and objects, in which case the patient has visual agnosia. Deficits in memory may manifest initially as an acute confusional state; as the sensorium clears, a pure short-term memory impairment remains. Immediate memory and memory for remote events are preserved. Patients with pure alexia typically have no parietal lobe signs such as calculation difficulty or the other elements of the Gerstmann and angular gyrus syndromes.

Alexia without agraphia is specific for a consistent lesion site, the left posterior cerebral artery distribution in the medial occipital and medial temporal lobes, often including the splenium of the corpus callosum. The left occipital lobe lesion produces a right homonymous hemianopia, whereas the lesion in the corpus callosum prevents visual information from the right occipital lobe from reaching left hemisphere language centers (Fig. 17-5, which is adapted from a similar figure in Dejerine's 1892 article). Alexia without agraphia, like conduction aphasia, is an example of a "disconnection syndrome." The features of pure alexia without agraphia correlate with specific branches of the posterior cerebral artery; alexia correlates with the medial occipital and splenial lesion; motor and sensory involvement, when present, correlates with involvement of proximal branches to the thalamus and cerebral peduncle. The short-term memory loss seen in some pure alexic patients correlates with medial temporal involvement, especially the hippocampus. This deficit may contribute to the inability of patients with pure alexia to be able to read a sentence they have just written. Patients with more lateral occipital infarctions, sparing the splenium and medial occipital and temporal regions, have a more partial or transient alexia, sparing letters and often sparing memory, color-naming, and visual field deficits (Damasio & Damasio, 1983).

Aphasic Alexia

Many patients with aphasia have associated alexia. Wernicke's aphasia, for example, frequently affects reading. In common usage, however, the term *aphasic*

TABLE 17-10. Characteristics of Pure Alexia without Agraphia

Spontaneous speech	Normal
Naming	Color-naming difficulty
Auditory comprehension	Intact
Repetition	Intact
Reading	Impaired
Writing	Intact
Associated signs	Right hemianopia; short-term memory loss; occasionally, motor, sensory signs
Localization	Left occipital lobe, splenium, medial temporal lobe

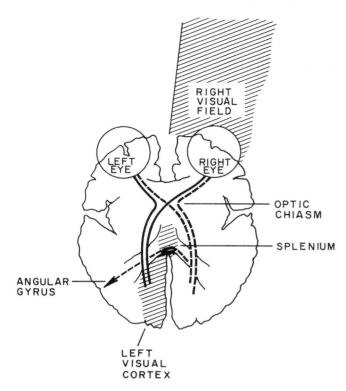

FIGURE 17-5. Disconnection model of alexia without agraphia, based on Dejerine's 1892 schema. Damage to the left visual cortex produces right hemianopia. Visual information from the left visual field, perceived in the intact right occipital cortex, cannot reach the left angular gyrus because of damage to the splenium of the corpus callosum.

alexia refers to the alexia associated with left frontal lesions and global or Broca's aphasia. Benson (1977) termed this the "third alexia," following the two classical syndromes of alexia with and without agraphia. Aphasic alexia is also referred to as anterior or frontal alexia. Most patients with Broca's aphasia have difficulty in reading out of proportion to auditory comprehension. Of Benson's series of 61 Broca's aphasia patients, all but 10 had significant reading deficits. As in both the expressive speech and auditory comprehension modalities, patients with Broca's aphasia often have difficulty with syntactic relationships in written sentences.

In some patients the reading disorder affects even more elementary aspects of the ability to derive meaning from printed symbols. In such severely impaired patients, naming individual letters may be difficult, a phenomenon first described in 1900 by Hinshelwood as "letter blindness." Whereas patients with occipital lesions and pure alexia can read individual letters but not words, patients with frontal lesions can often recognize familiar words but not name letters or read words by grapheme-phoneme conversion. Patients with frontal

alexia have been reported who can read "be" but not "b" and "ambulance" but not "am." In addition, these patients cannot read phonetically pronounceable nonwords such as "fod" or "mip" (Kirshner & Webb, 1982).

The syndrome of aphasic alexia suggests that there are at least two ways in which an individual can read: by translation from graphemes to phonemes and by direct word recognition. We shall return to this analysis in discussion of the psycholinguistic classifications of reading.

Psycholinguistic Alexia Syndromes

Psycholinguists approach reading by defining the sequential cognitive steps required for reading; they test individual patients with tasks that probe these specific steps and find where the deficit lies (Newcombe & Marshall, 1981; Lorch, 1995). Part of this analysis involves the classification of reading errors and the use of specific types of words, varying in length, frequency of occurrence, concreteness or "imageability," part of speech (nouns, verbs, etc.), and regularity of spelling ("boat" is a regular word, "yacht" an irregular word). These analyses permit classification of the alexias into a number of syndromes.

Letter-by-Letter Reading

"Letter-by letter alexia" is the same syndrome as the traditional alexia without agraphia (Patterson & Kay, 1982). By this analysis, pure alexia or "letter-by-letter reading" is a failure of a specific reading function, the ability to take in a word at a glance. Warrington and Shallice (1980) referred to this type of alexia as "visual word-form dyslexia." The ability to take in a word at a glance appears to reside in the left occipital lobe; some investigators have related this deficit to an inability to perceive more than one stimulus at a time, called "simultanagnosia." Such explanations of pure alexia involve a concept of limited visual immediate memory span; note the similarity to the discussion of conduction aphasia as a deficit of immediate auditory-verbal memory. It is clear that normal, rapid reading requires the perception of whole words at a glance; laborious, letter-by-letter or grapheme-phoneme reading is too slow and effortful.

Deep Alexia (Dyslexia)

Deep alexia is similar to aphasic alexia, as defined above, with regard to frontal lobe lesions and Broca's or global aphasia. Patients read familiar words by direct recognition and knowledge of their meaning. They cannot read phonetically, as in nonsense syllables, and they cannot name letters. Both letter naming and grapheme-phoneme reading appear to require the left frontal language cortex. Errors in deep alexia tend to be semantic ("boat" for "ship") or visual ("perform for perfume"). The patient's ability to read a word is directly related to its frequency, its concreteness or imageability, and its part of speech (nouns and verbs are read more readily than adjectives or adverbs). Word length is not an important variable. Most patients with deep dyslexia have large left hemisphere lesions and nonfluent aphasia (Coltheart et al., 1980).

The ability to read familiar words by direct recognition of their meaning implies a separate mechanism of reading from the usual technique taught in elementary school, namely, the ability to transform a printed letter string ("grapheme") into a sound (or "phoneme"), and then to interpret its meaning. This is a rapid reading technique, but in deep dyslexia, the words the subject can read are so limited that reading as a practical mode of communication is not possible.

Theories of the residual recognition or reading of familiar words have involved either spared areas of the left hemisphere or perhaps the right hemisphere (Coltheart et al., 1980). A recent study using PET scanning has shown activation predominantly in adjacent left hemisphere cortical areas during reading of familiar words in two patients with deep alexia (Price et al., 1998).

Phonological Alexia (Dyslexia)

Phonological alexia is similar to deep alexia, with a loss of ability to read phonetically or to read nonwords (Friedman, 1995). In phonological dyslexia, however, single words are read relatively normally, and semantic errors are rare. The syndrome is less severe than deep dyslexia, because phonological alexics can read most words, and they can read aloud. They appear to read real words by a direct conversion of printed word to phonemes, without necessary access to meaning. This is called the lexical-phonological path to reading. Phonological dyslexia thus provides evidence of a third route to reading (Fig. 17-6).

Surface Alexia (Dyslexia)

Surface alexia is opposite to deep alexia, in that subjects can read only phonetically. They read nonsense syllables normally but cannot read irregularly spelled words such as "colonel," "yacht," or "wrench." They may read "pint" and "lint" as if they rhyme, or they may read "bough" and "rough" with the same vowel sound. If they mispronounce a word, they interpret the meaning of the word pronounced in error. Patients with surface alexia can read laboriously, but they cannot recognize words at a glance; they are like elementary school children learning to read.

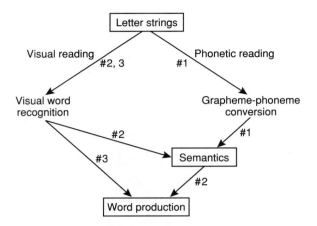

FIGURE 17-6. Three-part model of the reading system. There are three routes to reading: (1) direct grapheme-phoneme translation, (2) direct visual recognition-semantics (meaning), and (3) visual recognition-phonology, without necessary access to semantics.

Psycholinguistic Model of Reading

The syndromes of deep, phonological, and surface dyslexia suggest that there are three separate pathways used in reading: (1) a grapheme-phoneme route, (2) a grapheme-semantics-phonology route, and (3) a grapheme-word-phonology route. These three routes to reading are shown in Figure 17-6. The grapheme-phoneme route is the laborious method by which we all learn to read, by sounding out each printed syllable, but more rapid reading requires the other two pathways. If grapheme-phoneme reading is the only method available, the patient has surface dyslexia. If it is lost, but both of the other two pathways are available, the patient has phonological dyslexia. If only the semantic route is available, the patient has deep dyslexia and can read only a few, common, imageable words.

Agraphia: The Neurology of Writing

Agraphia is defined as the disruption of previously intact writing skills by brain damage. Writing is generally very sensitive to impairment with acquired brain lesions, and it is sensitive to disorders of spelling. In dementing illness and in acute confusional states, writing may be the most abnormal language function (Chedru & Geschwind, 1972).

Writing involves several elements: language processing, spelling, visual perception, visual-spatial orientation for graphic symbols, motor planning, and motor control of writing. A disturbance of any of these processes can impair writing. Agraphia may occur by itself or in association with aphasia, alexia, agnosia, and apraxia. Agraphia can also result from "peripheral" involvement of the motor act of writing.

Classification of Agraphia

There are several classifications of agraphia (Lorch, 1995). First, writing disorders can be classified by the underlying cognitive deficits: aphasic agraphia, apraxic agraphia, and spatial agraphia. In addition, "pure agraphia" indicates the absence of any other language or cognitive disorder. Another way of classifying agraphias is to divide writing into its component psycholinguistic steps and to analyze writing disorders according to the specific step that is disrupted, as in the classification of the alexias. In the psycholinguistic classification of agraphias, we first distinguish between "central" agraphia, resulting from disorders of central language processing, versus "peripheral" agraphia, resulting from disorders of the motor aspect of writing. Central agraphias thus affect lexical (word choice), semantic (word meaning), and phonological processes, after which a "graphemic" (written) version of the word is generated. The peripheral portion of writing involves selection of the proper letter string and the motor output to write it. The distinction between peripheral and central should not be taken as literal, neuroanatomic truth.

The agraphias are very complex, and it is not necessary for the average neurologist to commit all of the types of agraphia to memory. The principal classifications are included here for reference.

Central Agraphias

Aphasic Agraphia

For aphasic patients, writing is often the most severely impaired language modality. In aphasic patients, written language typically mirrors spoken language expression; thus, in nonfluent aphasias such as Broca's, global, and TCMA, writing resembles speech: brief, effortful, and lacking in syntax. The fluent aphasias, especially Wernicke's aphasia, also produce fluent errors in writing, and spelling errors are a sensitive measure of mild deficits. Occasional aphasic patients have dissociations between spoken and written language patterns, such as a patient with fluent, paraphasic speech but agrammatical written output with preserved nouns and verbs.

As in the alexias, agraphias have been classified according to the specific language-processing step that is deranged. The types of agraphia by this classification include phonological, deep, and surface agraphia.

Lexical (Surface, Orthographic) Agraphia. Surface or lexical agraphia is characterized by regularized spellings of words and phonologically plausible errors. Lexical agraphic patients typically make errors in which words are misspelled but are phonologically plausible, such as "spaid" for "spade" or "flud" for "flood." Lexical agraphia is associated with temporoparieto-occipital lesions and posterior aphasia (Wernicke's, TCSA, or anomic aphasia). The cognitive deficit of lexical or surface agraphia is an impairment in the ability to spell by access to word meanings; instead, words are accessed by knowledge of sound to spelling correspondence, and spelling is phonetic.

Phonological Agraphia. The patient with phonological agraphia can write irregular words or words with ambiguous spellings but cannot spell nonwords. In addition, patients cannot spell words they did not know before their stroke or brain injury. Patients with phonological agraphia can spell and write words they know semantically, but they cannot use sound to spelling correspondences. Phonological agraphia is seen in patients with lesions of the left supramarginal gyrus or underlying insula. The type of aphasia varies with the exact size and location of lesion; phonological agraphia may be associated with Broca's, conduction, Wernicke's, or anomic aphasia (Alexander et al., 1992).

Deep Agraphia. Deep agraphia parallels deep dyslexia. As in phonological agraphia, patients have difficulty spelling nonwords, but deep agraphics also show deficits in spelling certain classes of words. The patient can write words with concrete, imageable meanings better than those with abstract meanings and semantic words (nouns and verbs) better than syntactic words (prepositions and conjunctions). Errors may involve semantically related words, such as "chair" for "desk." Lesions in deep agraphia generally involve the left parietal region, often including the supramarginal gyrus or insula but sparing the angular gyrus.

Semantic Agraphia. Patients with semantic agraphia have a selective inability to spell and write meaningful words, though they can spell irregular words and nonwords. Often associated are aphasic deficits in comprehension. Semantic agraphics confuse homonyms in writing to dictation, even when given semantic information that should lead to the correct homonym (e.g., "doe" instead of "dough").

Other Types of Agraphia

There are several other types of agraphia, which we shall not discuss because of space limitations. These include unilateral or callosal agraphia, seen in patients with corpus callosum lesions; peripheral agraphias such as graphemic buffer agraphia, in which the number of letters in the memory store seems to be the crucial problem; allographic agraphia, in which the shapes of letters seem to be forgotten; apraxic agraphia, in which failure to produce written words is part of a more general disorder of learned motor acts; and spatial agraphia, a disorder of the spatial ordering of writing, usually seen in patients with right hemisphere lesions. In these rare types of agraphia, the patient can retrieve a word and know how to spell it, but subsequent stages in the writing process such as the number of letters kept in memory store, the selection of letter shapes, and the production of legible handwriting cause difficulty. The chapter by Lorch (1995) provides further information on these agraphia syndromes.

The final type of agraphia is *pure agraphia*, a loss of ability to write without other language deficits. Pure agraphia is sometimes used to refer to writing disturbances arising from focal lesions, in contrast to isolated agraphia, which refers to writing disturbances arising from multifocal or diffuse disorders. Isolated agraphia has been reported in diffuse encephalopathies and in confusional states associated with acute right middle cerebral artery infarctions (Chedru & Geschwind, 1972).

Pure agraphia is often found as the only residual language disturbance after the recovery of a more general aphasia. At one time, a writing area was thought to exist in the middle frontal gyrus, termed Exner's area. Lesions in the left middle frontal gyrus have occasionally been associated with pure agraphia, as have parasagittal parietal and even subcortical lesions. Pure agraphia following superior parietal damage may be associated with a defect of visually guided hand movements.

The patient's native language also influences pure agraphia. Italian, for example, is entirely regular in spelling, whereas English has many irregularly spelled words. Surface agraphia would thus be much easier to detect in English than in Italian. Japanese writing has two separate systems of pictograms, kanji (pictorial ideograms) and kana (phonograms more similar to English writing). A patient with pure kanji agraphia had a lesion in the foot of the middle frontal gyrus and adjacent portion of the precentral gyrus, whereas the patient with pure agraphia for kana had a lesion in the posterior two thirds of the middle frontal gyrus only (Sakurai et al., 1997). The selectivity of these deficits parallels the separate processes of morphologic (word recognition) and phonological (grapheme-phoneme) reading, as we saw in the syndromes of deep and surface alexia. These separate processes are more evident in Japanese than in English, because of the two systems of writing. Although the basic cognitive processes involved in producing meaningful graphic language are universal, different languages reveal the underlying mechanisms of agraphia.

ACALCULIA

Acalculia is the loss of ability to calculate, either mentally or with paper and pencil. Acalculia can be divided into three types: (1) inability to read and write numbers; (2) spatial acalculia, or difficulty lining up the numbers correctly or keeping them in columns; and (3) anarithmetia, or true loss of ability to perform mental arithmetic, not explained by writing or spatial difficulties. The first and third types correlate with left parietal lesions (Jackson & Warrington, 1986), whereas spatial acalculia correlates more with right hemisphere lesions. Patients with aphasia may be unable to verbalize calculations, yet some can perform silent calculations and indicate the correct answer by pointing to one of a series of choices. Occasional patients with severe aphasic deficits can play bridge or comprehend complex business ledgers and spreadsheets. Isolated left parietal lesions can impair calculations in the absence of aphasia. This syndrome is a true "anarithmetia" or loss of the concept of numbers (Grafman et al., 1982). Other studies have confirmed that calculation disorders are most common in posterior left hemisphere lesions, though they occur with lesions in other, varied sites.

CONCLUSION

Language disorders are highly complex in their clinical phenomenology and in the psycholinguistic classifications and models reviewed above. Detailed analysis of such disorders may seem to go beyond the limits of practical usefulness. This is an area of neurology, however, in which careful testing of individual patients at the bedside can truly generate new research information. The most important aspect of language disorders is the necessity of testing these functions to detect deficits. Language deficits, including those of reading and writing, are important in the practical localization of brain lesions. In addition, they impair patients' ability to function in the world. If we are to understand our patients' difficulties, and to use them both to diagnose illnesses and to help them cope in the world, we must pay attention to language disorders.

■ KEY POINTS

□ Aphasias are acquired disorders of language secondary to brain disease.

□ Alexias and agraphias are acquired disorders of reading and writing secondary to brain disease.

□ There are three separate pathways used in reading: (1) a grapheme-phoneme route, (2) a grapheme-semantics-phonology route, and (3) a grapheme-word-phonology route.

□ Acalculia is the loss of the ability to calculate, either mentally or with paper and pencil.

□ The most important aspect of language disorders is the necessity of testing these functions to detect deficits.

□ If we are to understand our patients' difficulties, and to use them both to diagnose illnesses and to help them cope in the world, we must pay attention to language disorders.

KEY READINGS

Alexander MP, Benson DF: The aphasias and related disturbances, in Joynt RJ (ed): Clinical Neurology. Philadelphia, PA: Lippincott Williams & Wilkins, 1999, pp. 1–58.

Benson DF, Ardila A: Aphasia. A Clinical Perspective. New York, NY: Oxford University Press, 1996.

Kirshner HS: Behavioral Neurology. Practical Science of Mind and Brain. Boston, MA: Butterworth Heinemann, 2002.

REFERENCES

Albert ML, Bachman DL, Morgan A, et al: Pharmacotherapy for aphasia. Neurology 38:877–879, 1988.

Alexander MP, Benson DF: The aphasias and related disturbances, in Joynt RJ (ed): Clinical Neurology. Philadelphia, PA: Lippincott Williams & Wilkins, 1999, pp. 1–58.

Alexander MP, Fischette MR, Fischer RS: Crossed aphasias can be mirror image or anomalous. Brain 112:953–973, 1989.

Alexander MP, Friedman RB, Loverso F, et al: Lesion localization in phonological agraphia. Brain Lang 43:83–95, 1992.

Alexander MP, Naeser MA, Palumbo CL: Correlations of subcortical CT lesion sites and aphasia profiles. Brain 110:961–991, 1987.

Alexander MP, Naeser MA, Palumbo CL: Broca's area aphasias: Aphasia after lesions including the frontal operculum. Neurology 40:353–362, 1990.

Bakar M, Kirshner HS, Wertz RT: Crossed aphasia: Functional brain imaging with PET or SPECT. Arch Neurol 53:1026–1032, 1996.

Basso A, Farabola M, Pia Grassi M, et al: Aphasia in left handers: Comparison of aphasia profiles and language recovery in non-right-handed and matched right-handed patients. Brain Lang 38:233–252, 1990.

Benson DF: The third alexia. Arch Neurol 34:327–331, 1977.

Benson DF, Ardila A: Aphasia: A Clinical Perspective. New York: Oxford University Press, 1996.

Benson DF, Cummings JC, Tsai SI: Angular gyrus syndrome simulating Alzheimer's disease. Arch Neurol 39:616–620, 1982.

Boatman D, Gordon B, Hart J, et al: Transcortical sensory aphasia: Revisited and revised. Brain 123:1634–1642, 2000.

Bogousslavsky J, Regli F, Uske A: Thalamic infarcts: Clinical syndromes, etiology, and prognosis. Neurology 38:837–848, 1988.

Caplan D, Alpert N, Waters G: Effects of syntactic structure and number of propositions on patterns of regional cerebral blood flow. Brain Lang 60:66–69, 1997.

Chedru F, Geschwind N: Writing disturbances in acute confusional states. Neuropsychologia 10:343–354, 1972.

Coltheart M, Patterson K, Marshall JC: Deep Dyslexia. London, UK: Routledge & Kegan Paul, 1980.

Damasio H, Damasio AR: The anatomical basis of conduction aphasia. Brain 103:337–350, 1980.

Damasio AR, Damasio H: The anatomic basis of pure alexia. Neurology 33:1573–1583, 1983.

Demonet J-F, Chollet F, Ramsay S, et al: The anatomy of phonological and semantic processing in normal subjects. Brain 115:1753–1768, 1992.

Docherty NM, DeRosa M, Andreasen NC: Communication disturbances in schizophrenia and mania. Arch Gen Psychiatry 53:358–364, 1996.

Friedman RB: Two types of phonological alexia. Cortex 31:397–403, 1995.

Geschwind N, Fusillo M: Color-naming defects in association with alexia. Arch Neurol 15:137–146, 1966.

Geschwind N, Quadfasel F, Segarra J: Isolation of the speech area. Neuropsychologia 6:327–340, 1968.

Grafman J, Passafiume D, Faglioni P, et al: Calculation disturbances in adults with focal hemispheric damage. Cortex 18:37–50, 1982.

Jackson M, Warrington EK: Arithmetic skills in patients with unilateral cerebral lesions. Cortex 22:611–620, 1986.

Kertesz A, Lau WK, Polk M: The structural determinants of recovery in Wernicke's aphasia. Brain Lang 44:153–164, 1993.

Kirshner HS, Alexander M, Lorch MP, et al: Disorders of speech and language. Continuum 5:61–79, 1999.

Kirshner HS, Casey PF, Henson J, et al: Behavioural features and lesion localization in Wernicke's aphasia. Aphasiology 3:169–176, 1989.

Kirshner HS, Webb WG: Word and letter reading and the mechanism of the third alexia. Arch Neurol 39:84–87, 1982.

Lazar RM, Marshall RS, Prell GD, et al: The experience of Wernicke's aphasia. Neurology 55:1222–1224, 2000.

Lesser RP, Luders H, Morris HH, et al: Electrical stimulation of Wernicke's area interferes with comprehension. Neurology 36:658–663, 1986.

Lorch MP: Disorders of writing and spelling, in Kirshner HS (ed): Handbook of Neurological Speech and Language Disorders. New York: Marcel Dekker, 1995, pp. 295–324.

Mendez MF, Adams NL, Lewandowski KS: Neurobehavioral changes associated with caudate lesions. Neurology 39:349–354, 1989.

Mohr JP, Pessin MS, Finklestein S, et al: Broca aphasia: Pathologic and clinical. Neurology 28:311–324, 1978.

Morris HH, Luders H, Lesser RP, et al: Transient neuropsychological abnormalities (including Gerstmann syndrome) during cortical stimulation. Neurology 34:877–883, 1984.

Naeser MA, Borod JC: Aphasia in left-handers: Lesion site, lesion side, and hemispheric asymmetries on CT. Neurology 36:471–488, 1986.

Naeser MA, Gaddie A, Palumbo CL, et al: Late recovery of auditory comprehension in global aphasia: Improved recovery observed with subcortical temporal isthmus lesion vs Wernicke's cortical area lesion. Arch Neurol 47:425–432, 1990.

Naeser MA, Helm-Estabrooks N, Haas G, et al. Relationship between lesion extent in "Wernicke's area" on CT scan and predicting recovery of comprehension in Wernicke's aphasia. Arch Neurol 44:73–82, 1987.

Naeser MA, Palumbo CL, Helm-Estabrooks N, et al: Role of the medial subcallosal fasciculus and other white matter pathways in recovery of spontaneous speech. Brain 112:1–38, 1989.

Newcombe F, Marshall JC: On psycholinguistic classifications of the acquired dyslexias. Bull Orton Soc 31:29–46, 1981.

Obler LK, Albert ML: Influence of aging on recovery from aphasia in polyglots. Brain Lang 4:460–463, 1977.

Patterson K, Kay J: Letter-by-letter reading: Psychological descriptions of a neurological syndrome. Q J Exp Psychol 34A:411–441, 1982.

Perani D, Paulesu E, Galles NS, et al: The bilingual brain: Proficiency and age of acquisition of the second language. Brain 121:1841–1852, 1998.

Price CJ, Howard D, Patterson K, et al: A functional neuroimaging description of two deep dyslexic patients. J Cogn Neurosci 10:303–315, 1998.

Robinson RG: An 82-year-old woman with mood changes following a stroke. Clinical crossroads. JAMA 283:1607–1614, 2000.

Robinson RG, Kubos KL, Starr LB, et al: Mood disorders in stroke patients: Importance of location of lesion. Brain 107:81–93, 1984.

Sakurai Y, Matsumura K, Iwatsubo T, et al: Frontal pure agraphia for kanji or kana: Dissociation between morphology and phonology. Neurology 49:946–952, 1997.

Takahasi N, Kawamura M, Shinotou H, et al: Pure word deafness due to left hemisphere damage. Cortex 28:295–303, 1992.

Tanridag O, Kirshner HS: Aphasia and agraphia in lesions of the posterior internal capsule and putamen. Neurology 35:1797–1801, 1985.

Warrington EK, Shallice T: Word-form dyslexia. Brain 103:99–112, 1980.

Whurr M, Lorch M: The use of a prosthesis to facilitate writing in aphasia and right hemiplegia. Aphasiology 5:411–418, 1991.

Apraxia

Anna M. Barrett
Anne L. Foundas

Apraxia
Disability
Functional activities
Motor programming
Motor rehabilitation
Neurodegenerative disease
Stroke
Tool use

INTRODUCTION: DEFINITIONS
AND GENERAL CONSIDERATIONS

Clinicians seeking to understand apraxia may quickly find themselves with more questions than answers. Their first difficulty may be in understanding exactly what the term *apraxia* means, when it is used to describe a number of abnormal behaviors in patients with brain injuries. In general, disorders labeled apraxic are motor disorders attributed to dysfunction of cortical association areas rather than lower motor systems. However, different apraxic patients may evince quite different motor performance errors. These include disordered drawing ability (constructional apraxia; Guerin et al., 1999; see also Chapter 12), inability to orient clothing appropriately with respect to the body (dressing apraxia; Brain, 1941), phonemic dysarticulation or disintegration (apraxia of speech; Buckingham, 1998; see also Chapter 49), abnormal directed eye movements or eyelid opening (oculomotor apraxia; Bálint,1909; see also Chapter 12), apraxia of eyelid opening (Defazio et al., 1998), gait disorders (gait apraxia; Fisher, 1977; see also Chapter 29), and disorders of learned skilled purposive movements (limb apraxia and apractic agraphia; see Chapter 17). Practitioners also use apraxia or dyspraxia to describe abnormal visuomotor function after right hemisphere stroke, though this disorder may not be primarily motor in character but spatial-perceptual (Patten, 2000). Difficulty with carrying out motor actions independently (e.g., self-care) when these actions can be carried out under explicit instruction is also sometimes called apraxic. This deficit may be due to a problem affecting other, nonmotor behaviors such as initiation failure or even psychological factors resulting in poor effort (Ballard & Stoudemire, 1992).

In this chapter, we will use the term *apraxia* specifically to refer to limb apraxia, a disorder of learned skilled purposive movement not caused by elemental neurologic dysfunction such as weakness; sensory impairment; abnormal posture, tone, or movement; or lack of understanding/cooperation (Heilman & Rothi, 1993). We refer only to acquired disorders of movement in individuals with previously normal ability to use the limbs, not to disorders that occur developmentally. Although most patients with apraxia have cortical brain dysfunction, apraxia occurs in neurological conditions affecting other brain structures. Therefore, our definition should be regarded as primarily operational rather than neuroanatomic.

THE FUNCTIONAL IMPACT OF LIMB APRAXIA

A second question facing the clinician wishing to learn about limb apraxia regards its functional importance. How much weight should it be assigned in the overall clinical picture, relative to other cognitive and noncognitive deficits?

It is commonly believed that apraxia demonstrated by a behavioral clinician on examination probably does not affect the patient's life. Poeck (1985) wrote that limb apraxia appears "only under testing conditions.... This makes therapy in most instances unnecessary." Although it is true that many patients with limb apraxia perform better while holding a tool in a natural context, holding a tool constrains a patient's behavior and can thus reduce errors (see Assessment of Apraxia, below). Though their performance may improve when holding a tool, patients with limb apraxia perform abnormally even with a tool in hand (Ochipa et al., 1989; McDonald et al., 1994; Poizner et al., 1989, cited in Maher & Ochipa, 1997).

Even if it affects performance with tools, it is still tempting to regard limb apraxia as an artifact of testing that does not affect daily activities. However, if we consider the purpose of the praxis system, it is hard to imagine that limb apraxia would not affect environmental competence. The praxis system allows access to previously constructed complex action programs, so as to confer a processing advantage on the behaving organism in its environment. Without a functioning praxis system, one would need new action programs for each behavioral situation, no matter how familiar (Rothi et al., 1991). Limb apraxia should thus increase attentional demands for actions and should have an especially devastating effect on actions involved in performing everyday tasks.

Consistent with this reasoning, a number of investigators report that limb apraxia has pragmatic conse-quences. These studies are summarized in Table 18-1. Limb apraxia can impair activities of daily living such as toileting and bathing, leading to a loss of independence (Bjorneby & Reinvang, 1985; Sundet et al., 1988; Hanna-Pladdy et al., 2002). Apraxic individuals are commonly unaware of their deficit (anosognosia), and this may prevent them from using compensatory strategies. Limb apraxia may predict poorer recovery following stroke (Giaquinto et al., 1999), and stroke patients with limb apraxia are more likely to have other cognitive deficits (van Heugten et al., 2000).

Limb apraxia may have an adverse effect on higher-level functions as well as self-care. It may impair the use of communicative gestures in patients with post-stroke aphasia (Feyereisen et al., 1988; Borod et al., 1989). Apraxia after stroke can cause agraphia, making writing ineffective for communication even when oral language is not impaired (apractic agraphia; Ogle, 1867). Apractic agraphia is associated with limb apraxia but may also occur independently (Coslett et al., 1986; see also Chapter 17). Subjects with neurodegenerative disease (e.g., Alzheimer disease [AD]) also often suffer from limb apraxia. These people are also reported to be functionally disabled by abnormal skilled movements. In the neurodegenerative disorder corticobasal ganglionic degeneration, limb apraxia may be a presenting complaint and may be quite disabling (Riley et al., 1990; Rinne et al., 1994).

In summary, we feel that the published literature suggests limb apraxia is a major risk factor for disability. This problem thus has considerable functional importance and is not simply of intellectual interest. Detecting apraxia may improve our ability to provide appropriate safety guidelines, counseling, and prognostic information for our patients with stroke or neurodegenerative disease.

PREVALENCE OF APRAXIA

A third question facing the clinician is how commonly apraxia occurs. Uncommon disorders are less likely to affect the typical patient and may be assigned lesser priority. A recent study of patients admitted to rehabilitation in The Netherlands for a first, left hemisphere stroke found that approximately one third met criteria for limb apraxia (Donkervoort et al., 2000). DeRenzi (1989) reported similar findings. A recent review of studies reporting prevalence of limb apraxia after stroke (van Heughten, 2002) reported that in 13 studies of left- and right-sided stroke, 28% to 57% of the group with left hemisphere damage had apraxia, as did 0% to 34% of the patients with right hemisphere damage. Although its prevalence in this disorder is not yet fully defined, ideomotor limb apraxia is also common in neurodegenerative dementia of the Alzheimer type (Foster et al., 1986; Rapscack et al., 1989; Ochipa et al., 1992;

TABLE 18-1. Impact of Limb Apraxia in Stroke and Neurodegenerative Disease

Increases caregiver burden (stroke)	Sundet et al., 1988
Adversely affects tasks relevant to activities of daily living (stroke)	Sundet et al., 1988; Foundas et al., 1995b; Goldenberg & Hagmann, 1998; van Heugten et al., 2000; Goldenberg et al., 2001; Hanna-Pladdy et al., 2002
Adversely affects tasks relevant to activities of daily living (AD)	Della Sala et al., 1987; Edwards et al., 1991; LeClerc et al., 1998; Derouesne et al., 2000
Adversely affects tasks relevant to activities of daily living (traumatic brain injury)	Mayer et al., 1992
Predicts posthospitalization dependency (stroke)	Bjorneby & Reinvang, 1985
Impairs return to work (stroke)	Saeki et al., 1993
Predicts increased fall risk (stroke)	Teasell et al., 2002
Associated with abnormal unskilled, simple movements (stroke)	Sunderland et al., 1999
Associated with abnormal unskilled, simple movements (AD, CBGD)	Caselli et al., 1999
Associated with abnormal motor learning (stroke)	Heilman et al., 1975

AD, Alzheimer disease; CBGD, corticobasal ganglionic degeneration.

Travniczek-Marterer et al., 1993; Foundas et al., 1999, Blondel et al., 2001; Ruiz et al., 2001). Kompoliti and coworkers (1998) reported that 82% of 147 patients diagnosed with corticobasal ganglionic degeneration, an atypical parkinsonian neurodegenerative disorder, had limb apraxia. Limb apraxia has been observed to occur in subjects with traumatic brain injury, like other cognitive syndromes associated with focal brain damage. Pachalska and colleagues (2002) reported that 60% of 40 patients recovering from post-traumatic coma had pathologic limb praxis assessment scores, but comprehensive information about the prevalence of limb apraxia in the traumatic brain injury population is not currently available.

Both stroke and neurodegenerative diseases are disorders more common in the aged, and as the median age of the US population increases, we may expect the population prevalence of limb apraxia to increase as well.

NATURAL HISTORY OF APRAXIA

A fourth question the clinician may have when learning about limb apraxia is how long the disorder may last. For example, if apraxia after stroke is transient, then those who primarily see patients in an outpatient setting may not need to learn about it in detail. It is also more important to master treatments for a disorder not expected to resolve spontaneously. Maher and Ochipa (1997) reviewed the natural history of apraxia and noted that though some writers maintain that apraxia spontaneously improves (Basso et al., 1987), many investigators report persistent apraxic deficits (Foundas et al., 1993; Maher et al., 1995). The disorder may

be irreversible even in treated patients (van Heugten et al., 1998).

THEORETICAL BACKGROUND

The final questions facing a clinician are whether limb apraxia definitely indicates that a patient is suffering from focal brain dysfunction, and, if so, how detailed an assessment is needed to inform diagnosis. A large body of neuropsychological research in brain-injured patients, published over nearly a century ago, suggests that apraxia is robust evidence of abnormality in the left cortical hemisphere. Some recent research suggests that apraxia caused by different brain disorders may differ in its characteristics.

Liepmann (1905) is credited with the first description of the neuropsychological mechanisms that mediate learned, skilled movements. In a group of 89 patients with brain injuries, he reported that left hemispheric stroke patients with aphasia had the highest incidence of apraxia. There was a lower frequency of apraxia among right hemispheric stroke patients without aphasia, and no evidence of apraxia among right hemispheric stroke patients. He posited that the performance of skilled limb movements required the acquisition of "movement formulae" (Liepmann, 1920). Geschwind (1975) elaborated on Liepmann's model by defining a neural network that mediates skilled movements. He proposed that pantomime to command requires that auditory input via primary auditory cortex (Heschl's gyrus) project to auditory association cortex (Wernicke's area), which in turn flows to motor association cortex (area 6). Motor association cortex, in turn, activates the primary motor areas (area 4). When gestures are performed by the left hand, motor programs from the left motor association area cortex cross the corpus callosum to the contralateral premotor cortex and then activate the primary motor cortex for gesture production. Heilman and colleagues (1982) suggested that this neural network contained movement representations or "visuokinesthetic engrams." These representations or engrams are thought to be represented in the left inferior parietal lobule of right-handed people. Heilman and colleagues (1982) and Rothi and associates (1985) proposed that there are at least two types of mechanisms that could account for performance deficits associated with ideomotor apraxia: a praxis production system and a praxis reception system. Heilman and colleagues (1982) tested 20 patients with unilateral left hemisphere stroke using a gesture to command and a gesture discrimination task and found a relationship between task and lesion location. Whereas the patients with lesions to left parietal cortex were impaired in their production and discrimination of gestures, patients with frontal lesions were impaired in their gesture production but were not impaired in gesture discrimination. Rothi and colleagues (1991) proposed a model of praxis processing that accounts for the reception and production of skilled movements of the right and left limbs in response to auditory, tactile, or visual input. Learned skilled movement is also dependent on the conceptual knowledge of tools, objects, and actions. Thus, the representational nature of gesture means that there is some interaction between semantics and the action lexicon. Based on this model, the syndrome of ideomotor apraxia would result from a praxis production defect, whereas loss of knowledge of tool use would result in ideational or conceptual apraxia.

Based on these models and support from lesion studies, it has been well established that the frontal and parietal cortices are involved in the representation of goal-directed movements, but the crucial neuroanatomic sites have not been completely established in humans. Lesion location studies have supported the notion that multiple parallel frontoparietal circuits are required to support the computations needed to translate an action goal into a movement (Basso et al., 1980; Kertesz & Ferro, 1984; Heilman & Rothi, 1993; Barrett et al., 1998; Poizner et al., 1998). Sensory input must be integrated with the central representations of movement based on prior experience. To identify these sites more precisely, Haaland and colleagues (2000) studied unilateral stroke patients with and without limb apraxia. Magnetic resonance imaging (MRI) or computed tomography (CT) scans were used for lesion localization, and areas of overlap were compared in those patients with and without limb apraxia. Patients with ideomotor limb apraxia had damage lateralized to a left hemispheric network involving the middle frontal gyrus and intraparietal sulcus region. Thus, the results of this study revealed that discrete areas in the left hemisphere of humans are critical for the control of complex goal-directed movements. Apraxia can also result from brain damage restricted to subcortical white matter, including the corpus callosum (Kertesz & Ferro, 1984; Hanna-Pladdy et al., 2001b; see also Chapter 19). Studies supporting a left hemisphere locus for praxis investigated praxis laterality by comparing patients with unilateral left and right hemisphere damage (Liepmann, 1905; Haaland & Flaherty, 1984; Rapscak et al., 1993; Maher, et al., 1997; Roy et al., 2000; Hanna-Pladdy et al., 2001a) and by studying praxis performance during selective hemispheric anesthesia or Wada testing (Foundas et al., 1995a; Meador et al., 1999). Moll and colleagues (2000) also studied brain activation with functional MRI while subjects pantomimed tool use with either hand and imagined tool-use gestures. During both real and imagined tool-use pantomimes, as compared with a nonsymbolic limb movement task, the left intraparietal cortex and posterior dorsolateral frontal cortex were activated. This is consistent with dysfunctional left cortical regions in brain-damaged patients with apraxia.

Based on the information above, we recommend classifying limb apraxia by the nature of the errors a patient makes and the pathways through which these errors are elicited. We base our classification on a two-system model for the organization of action: a production system and a conceptual system (Heilman & Rothi, 1993; Rothi et al., 1997). Apraxia can thus be classified in a manner analogous to the classification of speech-language disorders, because production and comprehension can be separately impaired. Dysfunction of the production system with intact function of the conceptual system would cause *ideomotor* apraxia. Dysfunction of the conceptual system, with or without dysfunction of the production system, induces *conceptual* (also called ideational) apraxia. Patients with ideomotor apraxia are thought to have deficits in the control or programming of the spatial organization, sequencing, or timing of goal-directed movements. Patients with conceptual apraxia have deficits affecting action semantics (meaning systems underlying actions), internal representations of movements (movement imagery), or both.

An additional category of limb apraxia involves functional disconnection between conceptual and production systems involved in limb praxis (see Chapter 19). Callosal apraxia classically affects only the hand ipsilateral to the hemisphere specialized for language. Other types of disconnection apraxia may functionally disconnect meaning representations for action from one sensory modality; for example, the patient may have difficulty visually recognizing gestures but may be able to recognize them tactually.

Classifying a patient's apraxia as ideomotor, conceptual, or of both types may not only aid in localizing brain dysfunction (conceptual difficulties implicate posterior left hemisphere dysfunction; see below), but may help in identifying the underlying disorder. Patients with apraxia caused by neurodegenerative disease appear to have more conceptual impairment. These patients appear to make frequent content errors (wrong tool) compared with apraxic stroke patients and produce gestures with reduced conceptual complexity (Foundas et al., 1999; Glosser et al., 1998). Additionally, Foundas and colleagues (1999) reported that patients with AD were significantly more impaired than stroke patients when performing intransitive limb movements (gestures not using a tool, such as waving goodbye; see below under Assessment). The authors suggested that intransitive limb movements might be highly dependent on input from action semantics (meaning systems used to plan gestures), because semantic impairment is known to occur in patients with AD. AD patients may typically have gestural recognition impairments, which is evidence of conceptual dysfunction (Dumont & Ska, 2000). A substantial subgroup of AD subjects may have difficulty with tool-action concepts (features of conceptual apraxia) and still gesture accurately to command (Ochipa et al., 1992). This presentation of conceptual without ideomotor apraxia is uncommon in patients with stroke that causes left hemispheric dysfunction. It is possible that abnormal gesture/action concepts (action semantics) may be an early sign of AD.

ASSESSMENT OF APRAXIA

Why Assess?

As discussed above, apraxia can be considered common, can persist rather than improving spontaneously, and can be functionally relevant. Detecting apraxia, then, like identifying any other neurologic symptom, may aid in localizing a disease process, determining its severity, and planning treatments. The presence of apraxia may also be helpful in diagnosing the etiology of brain dysfunction. For example, patients with both memory loss and limb apraxia may be more likely to have early Alzheimer disease and less likely to have cognitive impairment due to depression (Crowe et al., 2000).

As summarized above, in right-handed individuals with limb apraxia, dysfunction of the left cortical hemisphere should be strongly suspected. Sudden onset of impairment suggests stroke, and the clinician should pay special attention to investigating for a possible source of cerebral embolus. If the onset of the disorder is gradual and accompanied by other cognitive deficits such as amnesia, this suggests left hemispheric dysfunction due to neurodegenerative disease (Foster et al., 1986).

Detailed Assessment Versus Screening

Apraxia is typically assessed by having patients pantomime a series of gestures to verbal command, with the nonparalyzed (ipsilesional) hand (see below, Which Hand Should We Test?). This pantomime to command task is considered the most sensitive test of apraxia, because many apraxic patients improve when gesturing to imitation and improve further when performing gestures with the actual tool (Liepmann, 1905, 1920; Geschwind, 1975; DeRenzi, 1985; Heilman & Rothi, 1993). However, a brief screen (asking a patient to pantomime three to four gestures) may be normal in patients with mild apraxia. Of more concern, patients with isolated conceptual apraxia (no ideomotor apraxia) will perform well when gesturing to command but poorly in natural situations when they themselves must decide what tools to use and how.

Unfortunately, there is no widely used standardized test for limb apraxia. An ideal evaluation of limb apraxia would include all of these tasks: gesture to command, gesture imitation, and gesture recognition/discrimination. Using testing items that require patients to draw on action concepts to generate gestures is probably best. Requiring that patients activate action concepts means patients are asked to infer the appropriate tool and movement rather than simply generating a gesture after being told what tool and movement to generate. An example of this type of conceptual-gesture test is the Florida Action Recall Test (FLART; Schwartz et al., 2000), which has several standardized short versions (Schwartz & Santschi, 2000). In this test, subjects look at a picture of an object (e.g., a nail in a piece of wood) and have to generate the gesture for the tool to be used in this situation (e.g., hammering).

The typical clinical practitioner, however, does not have access to this test and also works within very limited time constraints. A compromise in such a situation may be to ask the patient to generate 12 to 15 gestures to command as a screen for ideomotor apraxia. If no abnormality of learned skilled movements to command is identified, this does not eliminate the possibility of an isolated conceptual impairment. Concepts can be tested separately by asking patients to name gestures or give other information based on action semantics. Figure 18-1 presents a flow chart outlining our recommendations for apraxia testing when no standardized instrument is available. Table 18-2 contains a more comprehensive list of methods of apraxia testing for situations in which more testing can be performed.

Pantomiming tool use to verbal command is not an easy task. Stroke patients tested on an instrument we and our collaborators use to assess praxis, the Florida Apraxia Screening Test, revised (FAST-R; Rothi et al., 1997), can make up to 50% errors and still score in an unimpaired range. Interestingly, few normal or

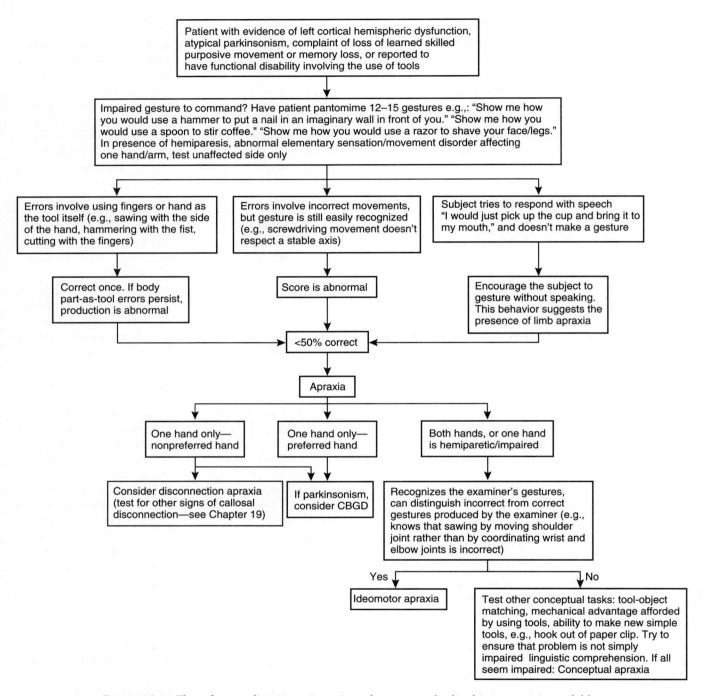

FIGURE 18-1. Flow chart outlines apraxia testing when no standardized instrument is available.

neurologically impaired subjects judge gesture to command to be a difficult task. Normal aged subjects tested on this task, in fact, reliably overestimated their performance (Barrett et al., 2002b).

When testing gestures made to command, it is important to include both transitive and intransitive gestures. Transitive gestures are those that involve the manipulation of an object, often a tool. Some examples

of transitive gestures include showing the examiner how to use a hammer, how to use a key to unlock a door, and how to hold a cup to drink water. Intransitive gestures do not require the use of an object but are more abstract representational movements. Examples of intransitive gestures include demonstrating how to salute, how to wave goodbye, and how to make a gesture that someone should "be quiet."

TABLE 18-2. Methods of Limb Apraxia Assessment

Apraxia testing	Patient's response	Error type
Gesture to command: Transitive gestures (tool use on object) *"Show me how you would use a fork to beat eggs in a bowl in your lap."* *"Show me how you would use a pair of scissors to cut a piece of paper out in front of you."* Intransitive gestures (no tool use) *"Show me how you would gesture to tell someone 'come here.'"*	1. Patient generates a recognizable gesture, but the movement is incorrect (too large, incorrectly timed, wrong joint moved). 2. Patient generates a recognizable gesture, but the hand is not positioned properly for the tool (e.g., in showing how to use a salt shaker, the hand is closed and there would be no room to hold it).	1. Spatial (movement) error (most common type). Suggestive of ideomotor limb apraxia. 2. Spatial (hand or internal configuration) error. Suggestive of ideomotor limb apraxia.
Gesture imitation *"Can you do this?"* (Examiner mimes using hammer, scissors, screwdriver, etc. Examiner uses the same hand, e.g., left, that the patient is expected to use for response.)	3. Patient generates a recognizable gesture, but its component movements are sequenced incorrectly (e.g., pantomimes peeling a banana after starting to eat it).	3. Temporal (sequencing) error. Suggestive of ideomotor limb apraxia.
Gesture while viewing real object *"Show me how you would use this piece of chalk to write on an imaginary chalk board in front of you."* (Object is positioned neutrally so as not to give hand posture cues.)	4. Patient generates a gesture with the wrong number of movement cycles (e.g., rotating the wrist over and over when showing how to use a key to unlock a door).	4. Temporal (occurrence) error. Suggestive of ideomotor limb apraxia.
Gesture with real object *"Show me how you would use this (examiner indicates neutrally positioned toothbrush) to clean your teeth."*	5. Patient generates perseverative movements (e.g., from previous testing).	5. Content (perseveration) error. May occur in either conceptual or ideomotor limb apraxia or in patients with combined deficits.
Gesture recognition/ discrimination *"I'm going to make three gestures. Tell me which one of these is correct for hammering."* (Examiner makes three gestures. Two gestures are incorrect—either content, temporal, or spatial errors.)	6. Patient generates an incorrect but related gesture (e.g., combing hair for using a razor).	6. Content (related item) error. May occur in either conceptual or ideomotor limb apraxia or in patients with combined deficits.
Tool-object matching *"Which of these tools would act on this object?"* (Examiner indicates picture of roast turkey, patient picks from a tool array.)	7. Patient cannot pick correct gesture from three choices. 8. Patient cannot match tools and objects reliably above chance.	7. Gesture recognition error. Consistent with conceptual apraxia. 8. Tool-object semantic error. Consistent with conceptual apraxia.
Knowledge of tool affordances *"Which of these tools could you use, in an emergency, to pound a nail?"* (Examiner indicates an array of tools and objects from which hammer is absent, containing an object of the requisite weight and flatness, e.g., brick.)	9. Patient indicates no knowledge of how to use common objects as tools or indicates secondary use of a tool incorrectly (e.g., states scissors could be used to pound nail).	9. Tool semantic error. Consistent with conceptual apraxia.

Which Hand Should We Test?

In unilateral stroke patients, it is critical that the unaffected ipsilesional limb is used when assessing praxis performance. This procedure controls for sensorimotor deficits or movement disorders, some of which may be so mild as to escape notice on brief motor or sensory screening but may still affect performance. Given that dystonia and rigidity in corticobasal degeneration is often asymmetrical, it is best if the least affected limb is assessed in these patients. In patients without identified neurologic disease, or in patients with early AD, either limb can be tested, because sensorimotor systems are presumed to be spared.

If a patient with a suspected stroke has apraxia affecting the ipsilesional, nonpreferred hand, performance with the preferred hand should also be briefly tested if possible. Some patients with anterior cerebral artery stroke will have markedly asymmetrical apraxia with the ipsilesional, nonpreferred hand affected and the contralesional, preferred hand spared. This pattern can help to localize the responsible brain lesion (to the anterior corpus callosum; see also Chapter 19; Heilman & Rothi, 1993).

Error Types

Rothi and colleagues (1988) developed a qualitative approach to analyze errors in limb apraxia and broadly classified errors into three types: *spatial errors, temporal errors*, and *content errors*. Common *spatial errors* include movement and body part as tool (object) errors. When acting on an object with a tool, there are movements characteristic of the action and movements necessary to perform the action. Any disturbance of these characteristic movements reflects a movement error. For example, when asked to pantomime using a screwdriver, a subject may orient the imagined screwdriver correctly to the imagined screw, but instead of stabilizing the shoulder and wrist and twisting at the elbow, the subject stabilizes at the elbow and twists at the wrist or shoulder. This gesture would be considered a movement error. When pantomiming a transitive movement, the fingers-hand-arm and the imagined tool must be oriented in a specific relationship to the "object" receiving the action. Errors that involve the incorrect positioning of the limb in relation to the "object" or in placing the "object" in space are called external and internal configuration errors, respectively. For example, the subject might pantomime brushing teeth by holding his hand next to his mouth without reflecting the distance necessary to accommodate an imagined toothbrush. Another example would be when asked to hammer a nail the subject might hammer in differing locations in space reflecting difficulty placing the imagined nail in a stable orientation. *Temporal*

errors include sequencing and timing errors. Some pantomimes require that the limb be placed in multiple positions with these movements performed in a characteristic sequence. Sequencing errors involve any perturbation of this sequence including addition, deletion, or transposition of movement elements. Timing errors reflect alterations from the typical timing or speed of a pantomime and may include abnormally increased, decreased, or an irregular rate of production. Content errors include related and unrelated content errors. That is, an individual may substitute another action (e.g., key) for the target action (e.g., screwdriver).

Goodglass and Kaplan (1963) were the first to describe body part as tool errors (described by them as "body part as object" errors). They found that when pantomiming to command, patients with left hemisphere brain damage (LBD) often produced errors in which they used a body part as if it were the tool (BPT), and suggested that this error type may be pathognomonic of limb apraxia. Some clinicians have questioned the significance of this error type because some individuals without brain damage may make BPT responses. To investigate the significance of BPT errors, Raymer and colleagues (1997) analyzed this type of error in a group of LBD patients and normal subjects who were reinstructed to modify the inappropriate BPT responses when they occurred. Errors in normal subjects who were not reinstructed if a BPT error occurred were also analyzed. Whereas LBD subjects who were reinstructed produced significantly more BPT errors than normals who were also reinstructed, LBD subjects were not different from normals who were not reinstructed. When reinstructed, the normal control subjects correctly modified virtually all BPT errors, whereas LBD subjects did not modify BPT errors. These findings underscore the need for reinstruction when a BPT error occurs to determine whether it represents a true BPT error in a patient with ideomotor apraxia or whether it represents a nonsignificant error. These data offer support for the hypothesis that a true BPT error may be pathognomonic of limb apraxia. Ideomotor apraxia should be suspected in a patient who makes BPT errors that are not corrected with reinstruction. When evaluating error types it is also important to note that content errors have been found to distinguish ideomotor apraxia from conceptual apraxia (Ochipa et al., 1989, 1992).

The Patient Who Will Not Stop Talking

Based on the casual observation that patients with apraxia respond verbally instead of gesturally when tested for gestures to command, Barrett and coworkers (2002a) examined the relationship between gesture to command performance and spontaneous speech in a group of aged adults without neurologic disease. Although none met criteria for apraxia, subjects who spoke more words had lower FAST-R scores (Rothi et al., 1997). Because all of these subjects were specifically instructed not to speak, their speech may have been involuntary. It is possible that spontaneous speech during praxis testing may be a pathologic sign. Instruct subjects not to speak while gesturing, reminding them as necessary, because dual-tasking would be expected to distract them and adversely affect their performance.

Ideomotor Versus Conceptual Apraxia

Detailed assessment of praxis may include, as above, gesture imitation, gesture discrimination (e.g., distinguishing erasing a chalkboard from ironing a shirt), comprehension of gestures (verbal naming of gestures, tool-gesture matching), and even conceptual tasks not involving gesture, such as tool-object matching (for a review, see Rothi et al., 1997). By testing these different functions, isolated abnormality of the production system (as would occur in ideomotor apraxia) can be separated from deficits affecting both comprehension and production of gestures (ideomotor and conceptual apraxia) or conceptual apraxia in isolation. The chief reason to distinguish ideomotor from conceptual apraxia is that the latter would be expected to be more disabling, although empirical evidence of this is currently limited to single-patient investigations (e.g., Ochipa et al., 1989). As above, isolated conceptual apraxia may also suggest the etiology of apraxia is neurodegenerative disease.

TREATMENT OF APRAXIA

Although completely restoring normal function in the natural environment for patients with limb apraxia due to stroke or neurodegenerative disease is unlikely, management and treatment of apraxia is still very important. As the population ages, more and more people with stroke and neurodegenerative syndromes may be identified. We can thus expect apraxia to increase in prevalence. The negative impact of apraxia on daily activities may increase patients' need for home services or even a supervised setting. Thus, clinical practitioners with aged patients should be familiar with basic management and treatment options.

Maher and Ochipa (1997) and van Heugten (2002) comprehensively reviewed management and treatment of limb apraxia. Underdiagnosis of apraxia is probably the major stumbling block in offering care for this symptom. Limb apraxia may go undetected in a hospital setting where daily needs are provided by staff and opportunities for independent tool use are limited. Patients are unlikely to draw the clinical team's attention to the disorder because they are typically unaware of it (anosognosia) or may attribute it to weakness or clumsiness. Thus it may only be by formal apraxia assessment, described above, that the team becomes aware of a patient's apraxia and its attendant disability and safety risk.

Once a patient is diagnosed with limb apraxia, ability to perform self-care and independent activities of daily living must be assessed. The most efficient way to perform this assessment may be with the help of experienced speech and occupational therapists, who can also share responsibility for management and treatment. Therapy professionals are rarely consulted to participate in the care of people with neurodegenerative disease. However, limb apraxia may be one of several situations in which a limited course of therapy with defined goals is of benefit to people with neurodegenerative disease. This remains to be examined in controlled studies.

Therapeutic approaches to limb apraxia discussed in this section are also summarized in Table 18-3.

The cornerstone of apraxia management is modifying the patient's interaction with the home environment, a restructuring that may include (Maher & Ochipa, 1997):

- Removing tools that could be dangerously misused, e.g., guns, power tools
- Replacing tasks performed with tools with tasks performed without tools whenever possible, e.g., finger foods instead of meals requiring silverware
- Educating and instructing family members or caregivers, e.g., teaching them to provide cues, limiting tool access, having patients perform only familiar tasks

Treatment, rather than simply adapting others or the environment, attempts to improve the deficit itself. Maher and Ochipa (1997) and van Heugten (2002) reviewed the literature on treatment of apraxia and concluded that direct treatment of abnormal gestures might improve performance. Available studies on treatment of apraxia are of three types: case studies using systematic multiple assessments with control variables (Code & Gaunt, 1986; Wilson, 1988; Cubelli et al., 1991; Maher et al., 1991; Bergego et al., 1994; Pilgrim & Humphreys, 1994; Ochipa et al., 1995; Butler, 1997; Maher & Ochipa, 1997), group studies in which all subjects received treatment (Goldenberg & Hagman, 1998; van Heugten et al., 1998), and group studies in which both conventional-treatment controls and special-intervention subjects were included (Smania et al., 2000; Donkevoort et al., 2001; Pachalska et al., 2002). Unfortunately, all of the studies except for that of Pachalska and coworkers (who studied patients recovering from post-traumatic coma) address the effects of training on apraxia after stroke. No studies are available examining the efficacy of therapies in apraxia due to neurodegenerative disease or the impact of such therapies on everyday activities.

TABLE 18-3. Therapeutic Approach to Limb Apraxia

Management	Environmental modification Family/caregiver education
Conventional speech and occupational therapy referral	Techniques are not standardized or theoretically based. Methods such as external and self-cuing may be introduced based on observations of the patient's performance on simulated activities of daily living. Patients may be taught alternative strategies if unable to use tools safely.
Theoretically based treatment	Direct treatment to improve abnormal gestures or action performance based on deficits observed during systematic assessment (conceptual, representational, production).
Evidence-based treatment	No treatment methods are available that are shown to benefit patients with apraxia of single or mixed etiologies at the population level. Theoretically based treatment strategies reported to confer greater benefit than conventional therapy, although only one study reported improvement on activities of daily living (Donkervoort et al., 2001).

In single-case studies of apraxia treatment, direct training of abnormal gestures had a modest beneficial effect (Code & Gaunt, 1986; Wilson, 1988; Cubelli et al., 1991; Maher et al., 1991; Bergego et al., 1994, cited in van Heugten, 2002; Pilgrim & Humphreys, 1994; Ochipa et al., 1995; Butler, 1997; Maher & Ochipa, 1997 [11 patients total]). In one patient, gestural improvement after treatment was not maintained over 2 weeks of follow-up (Maher et al., 1991). More critically, in a number of these studies (Ochipa et al., 1995; Maher et al., 1997 [eight patients]), there was no improvement of untreated gestures after treatment. Thus, therapy did not have a generalized effect but only improved targeted gestures.

The results of three group studies of apraxia treatment in which all apraxic subjects were treated (Goldenberg & Hagman, 1998; van Heugten et al., 1998; Goldenberg et al., 2001) appear to support the results of single-patient studies. Gestural training resulted in gestural improvement in the study of Goldenberg and colleagues of 6 patients, Goldenberg and Hagman's study of 15 patients, and van Heugten and colleagues' study of 33 patients. Goldenberg and colleagues did not observe generalization to untreated gestures in either study. Goldenberg and Hagman (1998), however, reported that treatment benefits persisted over 6 months in subjects who were compliant with home training after treatment.

Many patients with apraxia after brain injury receive multidisciplinary rehabilitation. Clinicians may feel that this conventional therapy is sufficient to address their deficits. However, often occupational or speech therapies geared toward improving fundamental motor problems (weakness, incoordination) may not be effective for disorders of learned skilled movements. Smania and colleagues (2000) and Donkervoort and colleagues (2001) examined whether administering therapy to apraxic patients that incorporated training methods specifically directed at improving gesture resulted in more gains than conventional poststroke treatment. In both of these studies (Smania et al. included 13 patients, Donkervoort et al., 113 patients), apraxia improved more after patients received specific therapy programs. In the study by the Donkervoort group, treated patients also improved more on activities of daily living, and level of function was maintained over a 20-week follow-up period. Pachalska and colleagues (2002) studied whether a therapy program focused on improving motor programming would be more beneficial to patients with traumatic brain injury and apraxia if this program incorporated semantic and verbal cues. Their subjects receiving semantic and verbal cuing made greater gains on post-treatment neuropsychological assessment, although the functional impact of these gains was not assessed. These studies suggest that simply referring patients with apraxia for poststroke therapy may not be sufficient treatment. We would recommend that clinicians discuss targeted therapy of apraxia with treating therapists, referring them to Smania and colleagues (2000), Donkervoort and colleagues (2001), and Pachalska and associates (2002) for a review of specific methods.

Because preliminary data suggest that direct treatment of apraxia may not generalize (Ochipa et al., 1995; Maher et al., 1997; Goldenberg et al., 1998, 2001), we recommend that it should always be combined with management strategies in a therapeutic plan. Direct gestural treatment should be limited to gestures considered of great functional value to the patient (e.g., oral hygiene, toileting). For patients with neurodegenerative disease, periodic reassessment should include an assessment of home safety and retraining as indicated. It is possible that this may help to maintain function and keep patients in a home environment longer.

SUMMARY AND CONCLUSIONS

In this chapter, we attempted to address the important issues facing a clinician who wants to learn about limb apraxia. A distinct disorder affecting learned skilled movements, limb apraxia can have a devastating impact on activities of daily living, patient safety, and other pragmatic outcomes in home, community, and vocational settings. Limb apraxia has considerable and probably growing prevalence and is persistent in many patients. We presented an overview of the robust neuropsychological evidence supporting limb apraxia as a symptom of left hemisphere dysfunction and discussed subclassification of limb apraxia into ideomotor and conceptual types. Although acknowledging that clinical tools for apraxia assessment are sometimes unwieldy and incomplete, we made recommendations on assessment of apraxia and briefly summarized principles of management and treatment. Although it is probably unrealistic to think that people with limb apraxia can perform normally after therapy, environmental modification, caregiver education, and treatment focused on improving gestures of highest priority may improve the patient's abilities and functional status. A wise clinician involves other professionals such as speech and occupational therapists in apraxia assessment and treatment, so that its disturbing and costly associated disability can be quickly addressed and preventive action taken as appropriate.

■ KEY POINTS

☐ Limb apraxia is a specific cognitive disorder of skilled, learned, purposive movement, associated with functional disability.

☐ Limb apraxia may affect as many as one third to one half of stroke survivors.

☐ Limb apraxia is common in neurodegenerative Alzheimer disease and other neurodegenerative syndromes.

☐ Limb apraxia appears to result from dysfunction of discrete left hemisphere regions critical for the control of complex goal-directed movements.

☐ A therapeutic approach for limb apraxia based on systematic assessment, and integrating management as well as treatment, may confer maximal benefit.

KEY READINGS

Geschwind N: The apraxias: Neural mechanism of disorders of learned movement. Am Scientist 63:188–195, 1975.

Heilman KM, Rothi LJG: Apraxia, in Heilman KM, Valenstein E (eds): Clinical Neuropsychology, ed 3. New York: Oxford University Press, 1993, pp. 141–164.

Rothi LJG, Heilman KM (eds): Apraxia: The Neuropsychology of Action. East Sussex, United Kingdom: Psychology Press, 1997.

REFERENCES

Balint R: Seelenlähmung des "Schauens," optische Ataxie, räumliche Storung der Aufmerksamkeit. Monatshrift der Psychiatrie und Neurologie 25:51–58, 1909.

Ballard RS, Stoudemire A: Factitious apraxia. Int J Psychiatry Med 22:275–280, 1992.

Barrett AM, Dore LS, Hansell KA, et al: Speaking while gesturing: The relationship between spontaneous speech and limb praxis. Neurology 58:499–500, 2002a.

Barrett AM, Muniz KJ, Eslinger PJ, et al: Unawareness of cognitive deficit (cognitive anosognosia) in subjects with probable Alzheimer disease and matched controls [abstract]. Neurology 58:A354, 2002b.

Barrett AM, Schwartz RL, Raymer AM, et al: Dyssynchronous apraxia: Failure to combine simultaneous preprogrammed movements. Cogn Neuropsychol 15:685–704, 1998.

Basso A, Capitani E, Sala SD, et al: Recovery from ideomotor apraxia. Brain 110:747–760, 1987.

Basso A, Luzzatti C, Spinnler H: Is ideomotor apraxia the outcome of damage to well-defined regions of the left hemisphere? J Neurol Neurosurg Psychiatry 43:118–126, 1980.

Bergego C, Pradat-Diehl P, Taillefer C, et al: Evaluation et reeducation de l'apraxie d'utilisation des objets, in El Gall D, Aubin G (eds): L'apraxie. Marseille, France: Solal, 1994.

Bjorneby ER, Reinvang IR: Acquiring and maintaining self-care skills after stroke. The predictive value of apraxia. Scan J Rehabil Med 17:75–80, 1985.

Blondel A, Desgranges B, de la Sayette V, et al: Disorders in intentional gestural organization in Alzheimer's disease: Combined or selective impairment of the conceptual and production systems? Eur J Neurol 8:629–641, 2001.

Borod JC, Fitzpatrick PM, Helm-Estebrooks N, et al: The relationship between limb apraxia and the spontaneous use of communicative gesture in aphasia. Brain Cogn 10:121–131, 1989.

Brain WR: Visual orientation with special reference to lesions of the right cerebral hemisphere. Brain 64:244–272, 1941.

Buckingham HW: Explanations for the concept of apraxia of speech, in Sarno MT (ed): Acquired Aphasia. New York: Academic Press, 1998, pp. 269–300.

Butler J: Intervention effectiveness: Evidence from a case study of ideomotor apraxia. Br J Occup Ther 60:491–497, 1997.

Caselli RJ, Stelmach GE, Caviness JN, et al: A kinematic study of progressive apraxia with and without dementia. Move Disord 14:276–287, 1999.

Code C, Gaunt C: Treating severe speech and limb apraxia in a case of aphasia. Br J Dis Commun 21:11–20, 1986.

Coslett HB, Rothi LJG, Valenstein E, et al: Dissociations of writing and praxis: Two cases in point. Brain Lang 28:357–369, 1986.

Crowe SF, Hoogenraad K: Differentiation of dementia of the Alzheimer's type from depression with cognitive impairment on the basis of a cortical versus subcortical pattern of cognitive deficit. Arch Clin Neuropsychol 15:9–19, 2000.

Cubelli R, Trentini P, Mantagna CG: Re-education of gestural communication in a case of chronic global aphasia and limb apraxia. Cogn Neuropsychol 8:369–380, 1991.

Defazio G, Livrea P, Lamberti P, et al: Isolated so-called apraxia of eyelid opening: Report of 10 cases and a review of the literature. Eur Neurol 39:204–210, 1998.

Della Sala S, Lucchelli F, Spinnler H: Ideomotor apraxia in patients with dementia of the Alzheimer type. J Neurol 234:91–93, 1987.

DeRenzi E: Apraxia, in Boller F, Grafman J (eds): Handbook of Neuropsychology. Amsterdam: Elsevier Science, 1989, Vol. 2, pp. 245–263.

Derouesne C, Lagha-Pierucci S, Thibault S, et al: Apraxic disturbances in patients with mild to moderate Alzheimer's disease. Neuropsychologia 38:1760–1769, 2000.

Donkervoort M, Dekker J, van den Ende E, et al: Prevalence of apraxia among patients with a first left hemisphere stroke in rehabilitation centres and nursing homes. Clin Rehabil 14:130–136, 2000.

Donkervoort M, Dekker J, Stehmann-Saris FC, et al: Efficacy of strategy training in left hemisphere stroke patients with apraxia: A randomised clinical trial. Neuropsychol Rehabil 11:549–566, 2001.

Dumont C, Ska B: Pantomime recognition impairment in Alzheimer's disease. Brain Cogn 43:177–181, 2000.

Edwards DF, Deuel RK, Baum CM, et al: A quantitative analysis of apraxia in senile dementia of the Alzheimer type: Stage-related differences in prevalence and type. Dementia 2:142–149, 1991.

Feyereisen P, Barter D, Goossens M, et al: Gestures and speech in referential communication by aphasic subjects: Channel use and efficiency. Aphasiology 2:21–32, 1988.

Fisher CM: The clinical picture in occult hydrocephalus. Clin Neurosurg 24:270–284, 1977.

Foster NL, Chase TN, Patronas NJ, et al: Cerebral mapping of apraxia in Alzheimer's disease by positron emission tomography. Ann Neurol 19:139–143, 1986.

Foundas AL, Henchey R, Gilmore RL, et al: Apraxia during Wada testing. Neurology 45:1379–1383, 1995a.

Foundas AL, Macauley BL, Raymer AM, et al: Ecological implications of limb apraxia: Evidence from mealtime behavior. J Int Neuropsychol Soc 1:62–66, 1995b.

Foundas AL, Macauley BL, Raymer AM, et al: Ideomotor apraxia in Alzheimer disease and left hemisphere stroke: Limb transitive and intransitive movements. Neuropsychiatry Neuropsychol Behav Neurol 12:161–166, 1999.

Foundas AL, Raymer AM, Maher LM, et al: Recovery in ideomotor apraxia [abstract]. J Clin Exp Neuropsychol 15:44, 1993.

Geschwind N: The apraxias: Neural mechanism of disorders of learned movement. Am Scientist 63:188–195, 1975.

Giaquinto S, Buzzelli S, Di Francesco L, et al: On the prognosis of outcome after stroke. Acta Neurol Scand 100:202–208, 1999.

Glosser G, Wiley MJ, Barnoski EJ: Gestural communication in Alzheimer's disease. J Clin Exp Neuropsychol 20:1–13, 1998.

Goldenberg G, Daumuller M, Hagmann S: Assessment and therapy of complex activities of daily living in apraxia. Neuropsychol Rehabil 11:147–169, 2001.

Goldenberg G, Hagmann S: Therapy of activities of daily living in patients with apraxia. Neuropsychol Rehabil 8:123–141, 1998.

Goodglass H, Kaplan E: Disturbances of gesture and pantomime in aphasia. Brain 86:703–720, 1963.

Guerin F, Ska B, Belleville S: Cognitive processing of drawing abilities Brain Cogn 40:464–478, 1999.

Haaland KY, Flaherty D: The different types of limb apraxia errors made by patients with left vs. right hemisphere damage. Brain Cogn 3:370–384, 1984.

Haaland KY, Harrington DL, Knight RT: Neural representations of skilled movement. Brain 123:2306–2313, 2000.

Hanna-Pladdy B, Daniels SK, Fieselman MA, et al: Praxis lateralization: Errors in right and left hemisphere stroke. Cortex 37:219–230, 2001a.

Hanna-Pladdy B, Heilman KM, Foundas AL: Cortical and subcortical contributions to ideomotor apraxia: Analysis of task demands and error types. Brain 124:2513–2527, 2001b.

Hanna-Pladdy B, Heilman KM, Foundas AL: Ecological implications of ideomotor apraxia: Evidence from activities of daily living [abstract]. J Int Neuropsychol Soc 7:248, 2002.

Heilman KM, Rothi LJG: Apraxia, in Heilman KM, Valenstein E (eds): Clinical Neuropsychology, ed 3. New York: Oxford University Press, 1993, pp. 141–164.

Heilman KM, Rothi LJG, Valenstein E: Two forms of ideomotor apraxia. Neurology 32:342–346, 1982.

Heilman KM, Schwartz HD, Geschwind N: Defective motor learning in ideomotor apraxia. Neurology 25:1018–1020, 1975.

Kertesz A, Ferro JM: Lesion size and location in ideomotor apraxia. Brain 107:921–933, 1984.

Kompoliti K, Goetz CG, Boeve BF, et al: Clinical presentation and pharmacological therapy in corticobasal degeneration. Arch Neurol 55:957–961, 1998.

LeClerc CM, Wells DL: Use of a content methodology process to enhance feeding abilities threatened by ideational apraxia in people with Alzheimer's-type dementia. Geriatr Nurs 19:261–268, 1998.

Liepmann, H: Die linke Hemisphare und das Handeln. Muenchner Medizinische Wochenschrift 49:2322–2326, 2375–2378, 1905.

Liepmann H: Apraxie. Ergebnisse der gesamten medizin 1:516–543, 1920.

Maher LM, Ochipa C: Management and treatment of limb apraxia, in Rothi LJG, Heilman KM (eds): Apraxia: The Neuropsychology of Action. Hove, East Sussex, United Kingdom: Psychology Press, 1997, pp. 75–92.

Maher LM, Raymer AM, Foundas A, et al: Patterns of recovery in ideomotor apraxia [abstract]. J Int Neuropsychol Soc 1:351, 1995.

Maher LM, Rothi LJG, Greenwald ML: Treatment of gesture impairment: A single case [abstract]. Am Speech Hear Assoc 33:195, 1991.

Maher LM, Rothi LJG, Heilman KM: Praxis performance with left versus right hemisphere lesions. Neuro Rehabilitation 9:45–47, 1997.

Mayer NH, Reed E, Schwartz MF, et al: Buttering a hot cup of coffee: An approach to the study of errors of action in patients with brain damage, in Tupper DE, Cicerone CE (eds): The Neuropsychology of Everyday Life. Assessment and Basic Competencies, Vol. 2. Boston: Kluwer Academic Publishing, 1992, pp. 259–284.

McDonald S, Tate RC, Rigby J: Error types in ideomotor apraxia: A qualitative analysis. Brain Cogn 25:250–270, 1994.

Meador KJ, Loring DW, Lee K, et al: Cerebral lateralization: Relationship of language and ideomotor praxis. Neurology 53:2028–2031, 1999.

Moll J, de Oliveira-Souza R, Passman LJ, et al: Functional MRI correlates of real and imagined tool-use pantomimes. Neurology 54:1331–1336, 2000.

Ochipa C, Maher LM, Rothi LJG: Treatment of ideomotor apraxia [abstract]. J Int Neuropsychol Soc 2:149, 1995.

Ochipa C, Rothi LJG, Heilman KM: Ideational apraxia: A deficit in tool selection and use. Ann Neurol 25:190–193, 1989.

Ochipa C, Rothi LJG, Heilman KM: Conceptual apraxia in Alzheimer's disease. Brain 115:1061–1071, 1992.

Ogle JW: Aphasia and agraphia. Report of the Medical Research Council of Saint-George's Hospital (London) 2:83–122, 1867.

Pachalska M, Talar J, MacQueen B: Role of semantic control of action in the comprehensive rehabilitation of patients recovering from prolonged post-traumatic coma. Med Sci Monit 8:CR576–586, 2002.

Patten J: The cerebral hemispheres: The lobes of the brain, in Patten J (ed): Neurological Differential Diagnosis, ed 2. New York: Springer-Verlag, 2000, p. 107.

Pilgrim E, Humphreys GW: Rehabilitation of a case of ideomotor apraxia, in MJ Riddoch MJ, Humphreys GW (eds): Cognitive Neuropsychology and Cognitive Rehabilitation. Hove, United Kingdom: Lawrence Erlbaum, 1994, pp. 99–107.

Poeck K: Clues to the nature of disruptions to limb praxis, in Roy EA (ed): Neuropsychological Studies of Apraxia and Related Disorders. New York: North-Holland, 1985, pp. 99–107.

Poizner H, Soechting JF, Bracewell M, et al: Disruption of hand and joint kinematics in limb apraxia. Soc Neurosci Abstr 15:481, 1989.

Poizner H, Merians AS, Clark MA, et al: Left hemispheric specialization for learned, skilled, and purposeful action. Neuropsychology 12:163–182, 1998.

Rapcsak SZ, Croswell SC, Rubens AB: Apraxia in Alzheimer's disease. Neurology 39:664–669, 1989.

Rapcsak SZ, Ochipa C, Beeson PM, et al: Praxis and the right hemisphere. Brain Cogn 23:181–202, 1993.

Raymer AM, Maher LM, Foundas AL, et al: The significance of body part as tool errors in limb apraxia. Brain Cogn 34:287–292, 1997.

Riley DE, Lang AE, Lewis A, et al: Cortical-basal ganglionic degeneration. Neurology 40:1203–1212, 1990.

Rinne JO, Lee MS, Thompson PD, et al: Corticobasal degeneration. A clinical study of 36 cases. Brain 117:1183–1196, 1994.

Rothi LJG, Heilman KM, Watson RT: Pantomime comprehension and ideomotor apraxia. J Neurol Neurosurg Psychiatry 48:207–210, 1985.

Rothi LJG, Mack L, Verfaellie M, et al: Ideomotor apraxia: Error pattern analysis. Aphasiology 2:381–388, 1988.

Rothi LJG, Ochipa C, Heilman KM: A cognitive neuropsychological model of limb praxis. Cogn Neuropsychol 8:443–458, 1991.

Rothi LJG, Raymer AM, Heilman KM: Limb praxis assessment, in Rothi LJG, Heliman KM (eds): Apraxia: The Neuropsychology of Action. East Sussex, United Kingdom: Psychology Press, 1997, pp. 61–73.

Roy EA, Heath M, Westwood D, et al: Task demands and limb apraxia in stroke. Brain Cogn 20:44, 253–279, 2000.

Ruiz SL, Adair JC, Schwartz RL: Assessment of ideomotor apraxia in patients with Alzheimer's disease [abstract]. Neurology 56 (8, Suppl. 3):A175, 2001.

Saeki S, Ogata H, Okubo T, et al: Factors influencing return to work after stroke in Japan. Stroke 24:1182–1185, 1993.

Schwartz RL, Adair JC, Raymer AM, et al: Conceptual apraxia in probable Alzheimer's disease as demonstrated by the Florida Action Recall Test. J Int Neuropsychol Soc 6:265–270, 2000.

Schwartz RL, Santschi C: Early cognitive deficits and conceptual apraxia in Alzheimer's disease [abstract]. J Int Neuropsychol Soc 6:180, 2000.

Smania N, Girardi F, Domenicali C, et al: The rehabilitation of limb apraxia: A study in left-brain damaged patients. Arch Phys Med Rehabil 81:379–388, 2000.

Sunderland A, Bowers MP, Sluman SM, et al: Impaired dexterity of the ipsilateral hand after stroke and the relationship to cognitive deficit. Stroke 30:949–955, 1999.

Sundet K, Finset A, Reinvang I: Neuropsychological predictors in stroke rehabilitation. J Clin Exp Neuropsychol 10:363–379, 1988.

Teasell R, McRae M, Foley N, Bhardwaj A: The incidence and consequence of falls in stroke patients during inpatient rehabilitation: Factors associated with high risk. Arch Phys Med Rehabil 83:329–333, 2002.

Travniczek-Marterer A, Danielczyk W, Simanyi M, et al: Ideomotor apraxia in Alzheimer's disease. Acta Neurol Scand 88:1–4, 1993.

van Heugten CM: Apraxia, in Eslinger PJ (ed): Neuropsychological Interventions: Clinical Research and Practice. New York: Guilford, 2002, pp. 222–245.

van Heugten CM, Dekker J, Deelman BG, et al: Rehabilitation of stroke patients with apraxia: The role of additional cognitive and motor impairments. Disabil Rehab 22:547–554, 2000.

van Heugten CM, Dekker J, Deelman BG, et al: Outcome of strategy training in stroke patients with apraxia: A phase II study. Clin Rehabil 12(4):294–303, 1998.

Wilson B: Sarah: Remediation of apraxia following an anaesthetic accident, in West J, Spinks P (eds): Case Studies in Clinical Psychology. Bristol, United Kingdom: John Wright, 1988.

The Corpus Callosum and Callosal Disconnection Syndromes: A Model for Understanding Brain Connectivity, Asymmetry, and Function

Zoe Arvanitakis

Neill R. Graff-Radford

Alexia

Apraxia

Callosal disconnection

Callosotomy

Corpus callosum

Integration of information

Lateralization of function

INTRODUCTION

The brain is composed of a complex network of neuronal pathways with almost infinite connections, both intrahemispheric and interhemispheric, which are not yet fully described. The corpus callosum (CC) is the largest commissural tract (white matter tract crossing the midline) and connects the cerebral hemispheres to one another. Callosotomized animal studies of cats, monkeys (Butler, 1966; Pandya et al., 1971), and chimpanzees, as well as studies of patients with intractable epilepsy who underwent therapeutic sectioning of the corpus callosum (Akelaitis, 1941; Geschwind, 1965; Gazzaniga et al., 1962; Milner, 1972) and of patients who have acquired a callosal lesion (e.g., stroke), allow for a better understanding of the functions of the CC and of the brain as a whole. In recognition of his lifelong work, R.W. Sperry was one of the recipients of the Nobel Prize for Medicine and Physiology in 1981, for studies of the functions of the cerebral commissures in split-brain experiments. The importance of these discoveries relates not only to the elucidation of the functions played by the CC, but also to the understanding of brain asymmetry and lateralized brain function. Indeed, the two cerebral hemispheres do not appear to be anatomically or functionally equivalent, as first discussed at the end of the 19th century regarding Broca's aphasic patient with a left posterior frontal lesion. The CC appears to play a role in the ontogenesis of this asymmetry; asymmetrical cortical areas are associated with a loss of callosal connections (Witelson & Nowakowski, 1991).

This chapter will first review the normal anatomy, functions, and lesions of the CC, followed by a presentation of a case with a callosal disconnection syndrome. Congenital callosal lesions, such as agenesis of the CC, will be only briefly discussed. We will address specific cerebral functions affected by callosal lesions, with an emphasis on language, but we will also discuss motor, memory, and sensory functions. Finally, we will present possible roles of the CC in attention and in human consciousness. The chapter will conclude with comments on hemispheric asymmetry and cerebral function. We hope to demonstrate the key role played by the CC in the integration of specialized cerebral function and of human behavior.

ANATOMY, FUNCTIONS, AND LESIONS OF THE CORPUS CALLOSUM

Corpus Callosum Anatomy

The CC is the largest neocortical commissural pathway, with the anterior commissure being the second largest. The CC is a broad, C-shaped arched band containing approximately 300 million fibers, which connect the right to the left hemisphere. It is largest in the mammalian brain, in proportion to the volume of neocortex. The CC is approximately 10 cm long and is divided into four main portions: most posteriorly is the splenium, followed by the trunk, then the genu, and finally the rostrum. The latter is the smallest part of the CC, connecting the temporal lobes, and is continuous with the lamina terminalis, which forms the anterior wall of the third ventricle. The splenium followed by the genu are the largest portions of the CC. The blood supply to the CC is via both anterior cerebral arteries, arising from the anterior cerebral circulation. In rare instances, both anterior cerebral arteries may arise from a single trunk.

The CC lies in the floor of the central region of the great longitudinal fissure, within the midsagittal plane, and forms the roof of the lateral ventricles. Inferiorly, the fornix runs on its undersurface. The CC is in contact anteriorly with the anterior cerebral vessels and posteri-

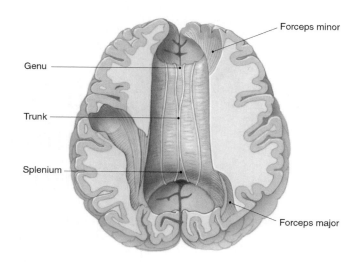

FIGURE 19-1. The corpus callosum (CC), axial view from above, with partial removal of the superior aspect of the cerebral hemispheres. Three midline portions of the CC are seen (the genu, trunk, and splenium). The forceps minor and forceps major are shown more laterally.

orly with the falx cerebri. Laterally, the CC merges with fibers from the internal capsule, corona radiata, and other intrahemispheric tracts. The fibers emanating from the genu form the forceps minor, and those from the splenium, the forceps major (Fig. 19-1).

Functions of the Corpus Callosum

The role of the CC is to connect functionally related cortical areas from one hemisphere to the other. Two types of callosal connections are described and are highly specific: homotopic and heterotopic connections. The first type links corresponding cortices. It is noteworthy that these homotopic connections concern cerebral regions with predominantly midline representation, such as the central vision and somatosensory information from the trunk. The second type of connection (heterotopic connections) links anatomically different areas that may serve a similar function (e.g., the connection of the right occipital cortex to the left language cortex for reading). Pandya and colleagues (1971) described the interhemispheric connectivity of the CC in seven rhesus monkeys with either total (n = 1) or partial callosotomies, affecting the genu (n = 2), splenium (n = 2), or body (n = 2) of the CC. The anterior commissure was spared in all cases. The animals underwent detailed histologic analysis looking for evidence of cortical fiber and terminal bouton degeneration. The topography of the CC respects an anterior to posterior and superior to inferior representation of fibers (Fig. 19-2). The rostral half of the CC subserves the frontal cortical structures, and the caudal half subserves the parietal, temporal, and occipital lobes (most posteriorly), as well as the insulo-opercular regions. Further-

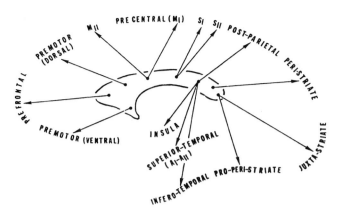

FIGURE 19-2. Connectivity of the CC. (Reprinted from Pandya DN, Karol EA, Heilbronn D: The topographical distribution of interhemispheric projections in the corpus callosum of the rhesus monkey. Brain Res 32:31–43, 1971, Figure 5, with permission from Elsevier Science.)

more, within these callosal regions, the more superior and inferior fibers have connections to superior and inferior structures, respectively. In the human, a similar topographic representation may be observed. For instance, the rostrum carries semantic and sensory-motor information, whereas the splenium carries visual information (Gazzaniga, 2000).

As we will discuss below in the section on callosal disconnection syndromes, lesional studies of callosotomized animals and humans have allowed for a better understanding of brain function. In essence, the CC participates in the transmission of several types of information including those concerning language, memory and motor learning, and sensory information. It is worth mentioning that, although lesional studies have proved very useful in elucidating CC function, inferring function based on such studies is not without several important weaknesses. The CC may indeed play a different role under normal conditions. For instance, a normal brain may have a different localization for language processing than a commissurotomized brain, which may have undergone changes secondary to neuroplasticity. The neuroplasticity could be from the disease (epilepsy) for which the person is undergoing surgery or from the surgery itself. Furthermore, the normal variability of CC function may not be taken into account in commissurotomy studies; for example, left-handed persons or patients with brain damage or epilepsy may have a different pattern of callosal connectivity as compared to a typical right-handed person.

Lesions of the Corpus Callosum

Natural, pathologic, and therapeutic (e.g., callosotomy for intractable epilepsy) events may lead to a disconnection syndrome. Lesions of the CC and its outflow tracts can be either congenital or acquired (Table 19-1). Surprisingly, congenital conditions such as absence or agenesis of the CC may be entirely asymptomatic or associated with few clinical signs.

An important example of an acquired iatrogenic/therapeutic event leading to callosal disconnection is the performance of callosotomy for intractable primary or secondary generalized epilepsies in debilitated patients who do not respond to medical therapy. This neurosurgical procedure was pioneered in the first half of the 20th century by Penfield at the Montreal Neurological Institute, Quebec, and Bogen from the White Memorial Medical Center, Los Angeles. This procedure is now rarely performed but has allowed for a better understanding of lateralization hemispheric function. Currently, partial callosotomies are favored because this seems to be associated with fewer neurologic sequelae. However, this partial sectioning may not provide as good seizure control.

CASE STUDY

A 39-year-old right-handed woman presented with a sudden neurologic deficit and was found to have suffered from a left pericallosal aneurysmal rupture, as demonstrated by cerebral angiogram (Graff-Radford et al., 1987). She underwent emergency clipping of the aneurysm, and by postoperative week 4, she dramatically improved; she was ambulating independently, had no focal deficits, and had a fluent speech. However, she displayed an alien hand syndrome. A brain magnetic resonance imaging (MRI) scan was obtained at week 4 and week 16 after the aneurysmal rupture (Fig. 19-3). The genu and most of the body but not the splenium of the CC were affected. The supplementary motor areas were spared. Detailed neurologic and neuropsychological studies were performed. Although the patient was mildly impaired on tests of intelligence and visual memory at week 4, her scores normalized at week 16. Using the left hand, she could not write to dictation. Standardized praxis testing was carried out at 4, 6, and 16 weeks. The patient performed normally with the right hand. Using the left hand, she could not mime a gesture to auditory command but improved when asked to imitate the same gesture. She could not demonstrate the use of an object by looking at it or by touching it blindfolded. The apraxia was attributed to the lesion of the CC and not to an abnormality of the supplementary motor areas as suggested in other studies. This case demonstrates that (1) the left hemisphere is dominant for praxis in both hands, and (2) the variability in performance depends on the type of praxis test used.

Callosal apraxia will be discussed further in the section on motor function (see below).

TABLE 19-1. Examples of Lesions of the CC and Its Outflow Tracts

Congenital lesions

Agenesis of the CC	Isolated agenesis: complete or partial (usually affecting posterior portion of CC)
	In association with other abnormalities: malformations (e.g., holoprosencephaly), migrational disorders, lesions (lipoma)
	Specific syndromes: Aicardi syndrome, Meckel syndrome, MASA syndrome
Stroke	Germinal matrix hemorrhage with extension into surrounding structures

Acquired lesions

Stroke	Infarction: anterior cerebral artery territory, superior sagittal sinus thrombosis
	Hemorrhage: aneurysmal rupture of anterior communicating artery or pericallosal artery
Trauma	Diffuse axonal injury (in acceleration/deceleration injuries)
	Hemorrhagic lesions of CC
Tumor	Glioma, lymphoma
Toxic/nutritional	Marchiafava-Bignami disease
Demyelination	Multiple sclerosis
Degenerative	Amyotrophic lateral sclerosis, Alzheimer disease
Psychiatric	Schizophrenia

COGNITIVE FUNCTIONS IN CALLOSAL DISCONNECTION

Language Functions

By the late 19th century, the work of Broca and Wernicke showed that each cerebral hemisphere is not equivalent and that lesions of a particular part of the brain, such as the left posterior frontal or left superior parietal areas, may be associated with a particular type of aphasia. A more detailed discussion on left hemisphere (LH) language function and aphasia is presented elsewhere (see Chapter 17). Since then, scientists have come to view the LH as the language-dominant hemisphere (Geschwind, 1965). Sodium amytol testing suggests little or no right hemisphere (RH) language in most patients (Rasmussen & Milner, 1977). This has led some to regard the RH as playing at most a minimal role in language processing; the RH has been referred to as the "minor" and "subordinate" hemisphere (Gazzaniga & Sperry, 1967; Levy et al., 1971),

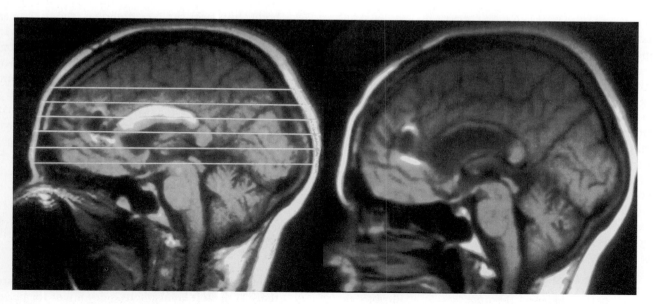

FIGURE 19-3. MRI showing callosal damage at week 4 (left panel) and week 16 (right panel) after pericallosal aneurysmal rupture. Arrows indicate areas of callosal sparing. (Reprinted from Graff-Radford NR, Welsh K, Godersky J: Callosal apraxia. Neurology 37:100–105, 1987, with permission from Lippincott Williams & Wilkins.)

and, more recently, as the "nondominant" hemisphere. Some have erroneously come to view the RH as playing only a minor role not only in language but also in other cognitive functions.

It was not until detailed work on comissurotomized patients in the mid-20th century that the concept of independent RH language skills emerged. The LH of callosotomized patients appears to retain the ability for speech, reading, and comprehension. As of 1977, only five commissurotomized patients had systematic language testing, allowing the demonstration of RH language abilities. These abilities are variable from subject to subject. Gazzaniga and coworkers have clearly shown that the RH is capable of processing nouns, verbs, rhymes, and superordinate concepts, and even of producing verbal responses, such as writing (Gazzaniga et al., 1977). The RH appears to have semantic and conceptual processing skills and a variable ability for processing phonetic and syntactic information and for producing verbal responses (Sidtis et al., 1981; Gazzaniga et al., 1984). In a paper presenting a 20-year perspective on RH language, only 3 of 28 callosotomized patients had a right hemispheric lexicon (Gazzaniga, 1983), suggesting that RH linguistic representation is uncommon.

The degree of complexity for which the RH can process language may be limited compared to that of the LH. Researchers have proposed that a continuum of generative capacity exists between the two hemispheres and that the difference in language abilities is quantitative rather than qualitative (Sidtis et al., 1981). The RH is no longer viewed as a minor hemisphere nor as simply a relay hemisphere for language (transmitting left visual field information to the left language centers via the CC), but as a structure possibly involved in language processing. Nevertheless, these observations have been based on callosotomized patients and the extent to which they may be extrapolated to explain normal brain function is controversial.

Cerebral dominance for language and handedness appear intricately associated. Handedness may be determined by genetic or acquired factors. During gestational development, normally occurring CC axonal loss may influence handedness, hemispheric anatomy, and functional asymmetry (Witelson & Nowakowski, 1991). In the first RH-dominant commissurotomy case carefully studied for language skills, researchers found that only the RH performed active voice syntax and that this hemisphere showed better performance for oral naming and reading as compared to the left (Lutsep et al., 1995). The study concluded that, in this case, the right brain performs grammar tasks and the left is able to access speech and comprehend single words. Complex grammatical manipulation appears to be a function of the dominant hemisphere.

Alexia can occur as a manifestation of a more global language disorder or may occur in relative isolation (see Chapter 8).

We will briefly discuss disturbances of reading and writing in the context of callosal dysfunction. Pure alexia (or alexia without agraphia) was first described by Déjerine at the end of the 19th century (1892); a lesion of the splenium of the CC, of the left medial occipital cortex, and the occipital horn periventricular white matter region caused disconnection of the right visual cortex from the left angular gyrus (containing word forms). More recently, Coslett and Saffran (1989) studied language function in four pure alexia cases with a lesion involving either the splenium of the CC or the left forceps major. They found that three of the four patients regained the ability to explicitly identify briefly presented words, being more accurate with nouns and words of high imageability. Furthermore, all four patients had the ability for tacit reading (reading without awareness), as demonstrated by better-than-chance performance on lexical decisions (word versus nonword identification) and forced-choice semantic categorization tasks. The authors argued that reading was mediated by the RH in these patients. This observation had been made previously when a patient recovered from alexia due to a left hemispheric stroke but then suffered from a right stroke leaving the patient permanently alexic (Heilman et al., 1979). Also, word superiority effect (better performance at identifying a letter when it is in the context of a real word) was found in both the LH and the RH testing of a callosotomized patient (Reuter-Lorenz & Baynes, 1992). Furthermore, the RH of this case may have an independent visual lexicon and provide an alternative but less efficient route for reading.

Although the RH is literate, normal and diseased brain may vary in their capacity for RH language function, as suggested by the wide variability in performance in subjects. This variability may be attributed to the use of different strategies. Traditional therapy with letter-by-letter reading may be counterproductive, and some support the concept that allowing the alexic subject to rely on "gestalt" reading strategies may be more beneficial (see Chapter 49).

A case with isolated agraphia of only the left hand was reported in a Japanese patient, following a lesion of the posterior half of the CC trunk (Sugishita et al., 1980). Apraxia, alexia, and anomia were absent. Interestingly, the patient performed worse while writing in kana characters (phonograms: each character has no meaning in itself and corresponds to a syllable in Japanese) than while writing in kanji characters (ideograms: each character has one or more meanings and pronunciations). This may be similar to the word superiority effect for reading observed in alexics. The anatomic explanation for the unilateral agraphia may be attributed to a disconnection of the right motor cortex from the left language cortex.

In summary, the callosal studies have provided a framework for understanding the language capacity of each half brain; the RH may play a role in comprehension (particularly auditory comprehension) more so than in expression (speech), whereas the LH is equally capable of both comprehension and expression. Also, in some patients with 2 years or more since their commissurotomy in whom neuroplasticity changes have taken place, the RH may develop the ability to produce speech, and the LH to interpret meaning (Gazzaniga et al., 1996).

Motor Functions

This section will present data on motor function, both of the limbs and the face (as an example of axial movement), after partial or total callosotomy (see Chapter 18). Liepmann and Maas first described apraxia in 1907 in patient Ochs who had callosal and pontine lesions; he was unable to pantomime with the left upper limb (Liepman & Maas, 1907). The right limb was untestable because of hemiparesis. The patient also had difficulty with imitation of gestures, thus implicating pathways outside the left language–right motor cortex regions. This was the first time that the notion of an LH dominance for praxis arose; the LH was postulated to contain information on movements (motor engrams) for both hemibodies.

Results of subsequent studies have supported the notion of LH dominance for learned motor movements (Geschwind 1975; Watson & Heilman 1983; Graff-Radford et al., 1987). Also, in a recent study on patients undergoing presurgical sodium amytol testing, anesthesia of the LH was associated with equal loss of deftness (dexterity) of both the right and left upper limb (Heilman et al., 2000). When the RH was anesthetized, only left-hand but not right-hand apraxia was noted. Interestingly, for the group of patients who were not right-handed or without left hemisphere language dominance, each hemisphere controlled deftness of the contralateral hand. However, in a left-handed patient who suffered from a near-total callosal infarction, the clinical disconnection syndrome was similar to that found in right-handed cases; motor dominance was felt to be in the LH (Lausberg et al., 1999).

In a study of eight patients who had undergone a commissurotomy 5 to 10 years before and had detailed praxis testing performed, Zaidel and Sperry (1977) found that movements were remarkably free of noticeable clumsiness. The patients performed poorly on tasks requiring speed, which may, at least in part, be attributed to anticonvulsive medication usage. The patients had severe agraphia, but minimal left-sided ideomotor apraxia. These authors proposed that motor control of the ipsilateral limb might involve both ipsilateral and contralateral pathways via the CC, in contradiction to the position that the LH is dominant for motor control. Another study found that either hemisphere might have the capacity to perform a range of sequential distal movements in the contralateral limb, without contribution of the opposite hemisphere (Volpe et al., 1982). Motor coordination was felt to be controlled exclusively by the contralateral hemisphere.

Patients with callosal lesions may manifest an alien limb phenomenon, whereby the limb carries out an involuntary action which is contrary to the individual's intent. Two types of alien hand syndrome (AHS) have been defined: a frontal AHS (attributable to a lesion in the right supplementary motor cortex) and a callosal AHS (Feinberg et al., 1992). The latter differs from the frontal AHS by the presence of frequent intermanual conflicting movements, which affect the left limb. The syndrome is caused by a lesion in the anterior CC.

In patients with callosal damage, apraxia may be associated with deficits, such as agraphia. In a patient who had undergone resection for a frontal glioblastoma multiform, a peculiar cerebral disconnection syndrome was described (Geschwind & Kaplan, 1962). With regards to left hand praxis, the patient was unable to write both spontaneously and to dictation (although drawing was intact) and was unable to name objects placed in the left hand (although he could select the object by touch). Demonstration of object use in the left hand was intact. The authors suggested that this case provides evidence that the two hemispheres were disconnected and attributed the syndrome to a callosal lesion, following intraoperative clipping of a large branch of the anterior cerebral artery. The dissociation between faulty naming yet preserved object use may be reversed in other callosal patients, such as the one presented here, who demonstrate intact naming but inability to demonstrate object use (Graff-Radford et al., 1987). In another observation, a dissociation between agraphia and preserved praxis in the left hand suggested to authors that praxis and writing fibers travel at a different level of the CC (Gersh & Damasio, 1981).

Finally, abnormal facial movement may be the most common syndrome following callosal damage (Geschwind, 1975). The LH appears to be dominant for voluntary facial movements. In three split-brain patients with normal spontaneous facial expression (Gazzaniga & Smylie, 1990), the LH was able to generate voluntary lower facial movements for both sides of the face, yet the RH was unable to do so. Left hemisphere dominance for praxis thus appears to exist for both limb and facial movements.

Memory Functions

Memory is a complex cognitive function involving activation of several important cerebral structures (see

Chapter 11). Sperry first explored the role of the CC in memory by conducting experiments on transfer of learning in the 1950s (Sperry, 1961). In a nonverbal memory study comparing 7 commissurotomy patients with 10 patients with a cortical lesion, Milner and Taylor (1972) tested delayed matching of tactile patterns consisting of wire figures. In six of seven commissurotomy patients, left-hand performance was superior to that of the right hand, demonstrating that the RH specializes in perception and recall of spatial patterns. The finding that the individuals with a cortical lesion were more proficient at the task suggested that both hemispheres normally participate, but that the RH plays a more important role in tactile pattern recognition.

Although persons with a long-standing cerebral disconnection secondary to a commissurotomy may appear overall cognitively normal in everyday life, severe and persistent short-term memory difficulty is noted by family and friends. To assess the long-term effects of commissurotomy on memory, Zaidel and Sperry (1974) administered six standardized tests to eight patients with complete and two with partial commissurotomies. As compared to norms and IQ-matched controls, patients performed markedly worse on testing for visual reproduction, temporal sequential relations, verbal and logical retention, and free picture recall; regardless of the sensory modality involved, both verbal and nonverbal memory was impaired. Because long-term memory was relatively preserved, the authors proposed that the CC plays a role not only in making memory engrams accessible to the contralateral hemisphere, but also in the initial encoding of memory. It is the anterior CC that appears to be implicated in memory function. Other neuroscientists have argued that concurrent extracallosal lesions, particularly to the fornix and its connections, may be important in the pathogenesis of recent memory loss observed over time in callosotomy patients (Clark & Geffen, 1989).

In an effort to clarify the effect the specific type of callosotomy (anterior, posterior, or complete section) has on the pattern of memory deficit, Phelps and colleagues (1991) carried out presurgical and postsurgical testing of neuropsychological tasks. A posterior section often included damage to the hippocampal commissure, whereas the anterior section did not. In the patients who had undergone a posterior section but not an anterior section, visual and verbal recall was impaired. Verbal recognition was spared in patients with various types of callosotomies.

In a small series of callosotomy patients, both hemispheres respond differently to a task consisting of facial recognition; whereas the LH is unable to match faces, the RH could clearly perform facial recognition (Gazzaniga & Smylie, 1983). The right temporal lobe appears to be particularly important for the retrieval of information related to faces. In another paper, memory tasks of pictures with consistent or inconsistent distracters were administered to two split-brain patients (Phelps & Gazzaniga, 1992). The LH performed below chance on consistent distracter pictures (not being able to distinguish between previously seen and new pictures consistent with the original scene shown), whereas the RH performed above chance. LH recognition is more strongly influenced by expectation than is the RH; the LH has a better ability to make inferences and interpret events and may act as the interpreter in memory tasks. More recently, a series of six experiments administered to a callosotomy patient showed that it was the RH that has a more veridical memory system as compared to the LH. The RH maintains an accurate record of information, whereas the LH may interfere with this record because of its capacity for interpretation and inferences (Metcalfe et al., 1995).

Sensory Functions

The CC plays a role in various perceptual experiences. We will be focusing on visual perception as an example of one of these experiences. Although initial CC studies found no cerebral dominance for visual perception and no disturbance in orientation, discrimination of size, or recognition of color and objects in callosotomy patients (Akelaitis, 1941), it soon became clear that the RH may in fact play the dominant role for certain visuospatial tasks (Bogen & Gazzaniga, 1965). With the understanding of the uniqueness of visual perception and the visual pathways (the right hemifields of both eyes projects to the LH and vice versa), Sperry outlined novel experiments for vision testing in callosotomy patients, using chimeric stimuli (Sperry, 1970). Researchers demonstrated the independent and simultaneous processing of conflicting visual information by the disconnected hemispheres (Levy et al., 1972; Holtzman & Gazzaniga, 1985). Furthermore, the RH superiority for tasks involving recognition and comparison of visual form was confirmed. Finally, in a dual task where two different spatial patterns are presented to both hemispheres independently, the performance of a commissurotomy patient was surprisingly superior to that of two neurologically normal controls (Holtzman & Gassaniga, 1985). The authors proposed that competition for common internal processing mechanisms interferes with overall processing efficiency.

The LH also plays an important role for processing of visually based information. A split-brain patient was able to perform mental imagery tasks (classifying letters from memory according to their height in lowercase form) with the LH but not the RH (Farah et al., 1985). This patient performed normally with both hemispheres tested independently on two control tasks involving the same skills except the imagery component.

Other Observations

As shown above, the CC plays a role in the transfer and integration of information related to higher cognitive functions, such as language, motor skills, memory, and sensory experiences. The brain, partly through the action of the CC, has the capacity to perform complex functions via the integration of multimodal information, both at the cortical and subcortical levels. Several authors have synthesized the problem of the "unity of consciousness" or of "conscious awareness" and the integration of the self, particularly as this relates to the callosotomy patient, but also as this would relate to the experience of an individual with normal brain function (Geschwind, 1965; Sperry, 1968). The topic of consciousness and altered states of consciousness are covered in detail elsewhere (see Chapter 30).

Several functions are integral to the experience of consciousness and a particular disorder may affect any part of the necessary components. For instance, a disturbance in the ability to maintain and shift attention (see Chapter 10) can present as neglect or extinction. This is frequently attributed to a lesion of the right parietal cortex, but, in three commissurotomy patients in whom the LH was aware of the left hemibody and space, this was attributed to a loss of the compensatory LH function (Plourde & Sperry, 1984). In another split-brain study, the hemispheres appear to have independent but asymmetrical abilities for attentional skills, with the RH responding to stimuli throughout the visual space (left and right sided), but the LH selectively biased toward events in the contralateral visual field (Mangun et al., 1994).

Other functions that participate in consciousness are recognition (failure of this function may lead to various forms of agnosia), memory, emotions, and thought (see Chapter 10). Language is, some may argue, a defining human characteristic that also greatly influences our sense of self and consciousness. In a unique split-brain patient who had extensive bilateral linguistic skills, LeDoux and coworkers (1977) described a "divided mind" whereby the patient seemed to possess two separate consciousnesses, one for each hemisphere. Furthermore, in another split-brain patient, the RH was capable of speech, possibly by the unconscious transfer of information between both hemispheres (Gazzaniga et al., 1987).

In a recent review on human cognition, the CC, and cerebral specialization, Gazzaniga (2000, p. 1293) summarized over 40 years of work in this field. With regard to the sense of self, he stated: "even though each cerebral hemisphere has its own set of capacities, with the left hemisphere specialized for language and speech and major problem-solving capacities and the right hemisphere specialized for tasks such as facial recognition and attentional monitoring, we all have the subjective experience of feeling totally integrated." In general, even split-brain patients maintain a unified sense of the self, despite both hemispheres functioning independently and not communicating via the CC. This state of single consciousness may be attributable to the action of the LH, which acts as the interpreter of events that are processed not only in the LH but also in the RH. The LH interpreter allows for the creation of theories about the relationships between perceived events, actions, and feelings. This may arguably lay the foundation for a state of consciousness.

Several mechanisms have been postulated to explain integration of behavior into purposeful actions in commissurotomized patients. Information may be duplicated in the two disconnected hemispheres (Sperry, 1984). The cerebral hemispheres may elaborate crosscueing strategies between one another (Baynes et al., 1995). One hemisphere may acquire homolateral control over the ipsilateral hemibody (Zaidel & Sperry, 1977; LeDoux et al., 1978) (e.g., the RH controls the right hand for a block design performance) or acquire a cerebral function that was previously carried out by the opposite hemisphere (Baynes et al., 1995) (e.g., the RH controlling motor speech after callosotomy). Subcortical pathways may provide a common stem for both hemispheres (Sergent, 1986, 1990). However, the answer to this problem remains elusive, and researchers have proposed arguments for and against each of these mechanisms. For instance, some argue against the presence of subcortical pathways. Others postulate that transfer of information via the anterior commissures, which may be spared, allows for preservation of communication between both hemispheres.

CONCLUSION

In summary, the study of the CC and of its associated lesions has led to a better understanding of brain connectivity, asymmetry, and function. Hemispheric asymmetry occurs because it presents an evolutionary advantage: It maximizes function within the limits of anatomy (e.g., skull volume and number of neurons) allowing for further specialization of cerebral function. This results in ontological progress but does not come without a cost. After a unilateral hemispheric lesion, the preserved hemisphere might not be able to perform the necessary behavior because it no longer possesses the ability to perform all cognitive skills. For instance, after a left hemispheric stroke, language becomes impaired and the patient is aphasic. Thus, the LH and the RH may be dominant for different cerebral functions (Table 19-2).

However helpful the callosal studies are in providing insight into brain function, these studies are not without several limitations. Callosal studies assume that certain brain capacities are functioning normally and

TABLE 19-2. Hemispheric Asymmetry and Specialization: Examples of Lateralized Cognitive Functions

Function	Left hemisphere (LH)	Right hemisphere (RH)
Language	Most aspects of language	May have a RH lexicon
	Speech, generative phonology, and syntax	Extremely rare ability for speech
Sensory function	Volitional attention	Attentional monitoring: orienting, focusing, and automatic shifting of attention
	Attention to stimuli in right visual field only	Attention to stimuli in both visual fields
	Crude visuospatial processing	Complex visuospatial processing and spatial discrimination
	Some facial recognition: familiar faces	Facial recognition: upright faces, unfamiliar faces
Motor function	Bilateral motor planning and control	Sensory motor tasks (e.g., block design)
	Voluntary facial expression	
Memory	Semantic memory: word and object knowledge, semantic elaboration and judgment (which may lead to some errors)	Episodic memory: much more veridical knowledge
	Less material-specific memory	Material-specific: encoding of visual material (e.g., faces)
Problem solving	LH dominance for problem solving	Crude problem-solving skills
Complex functions	Interpreter of information from both LH and RH	Emotions: comprehension and expression

Information presented in this table is based in part on a review article by Gazzaniga MS: Cerebral specialization and interhemispheric communication: Does the corpus callosum enable the human condition? Brain 123:1293–1326, 2000.

that they maintain normal connectivity to select surrounding brain structures. Caution must be taken when extrapolating function from callosal studies to the developmentally normal and unlesioned brain (Baynes et al., 1992). Also, normal variation in brain function in a given individual over time (e.g., early development and aging) and between individuals (anatomic and physiologic variability) may be overlooked.

Understanding of normal and abnormal human cognitive function is expanding with improved technology leading to the advances in brain imaging (see Chapters 6 and 7), biochemistry, molecular biology, and genetic studies. Finally, research may allow for the elucidation of the mechanisms leading to neuroplasticity (Baynes et al., 1995), a potential target for treatment of individuals with brain lesions.

■ KEY POINTS

☐ The corpus callosum is the largest white matter tract in the brain and connects the cerebral hemispheres to one another.

☐ The corpus callosum relays information between the hemispheres via two major types of connections: homotopic connections and heterotopic connections.

☐ Lesional studies of the corpus callosum allow for a better understanding of brain connectivity, brain function, and brain asymmetry.

☐ Such studies suggest that the left hemisphere plays an important role in most aspects of language, in bilateral motor planning and control, and in semantic memory. The right hemisphere plays an important role in attention to stimuli in both visual fields, facial recognition, and episodic memory.

☐ The integrational capacity of the corpus callosum may lay the foundation for a consciousness and a sense of the self.

KEY READINGS

Gazzaniga MS: Cerebral specialization and interhemispheric communication: Does the corpus callosum enable the human condition? Brain 23:1293–1326, 2000.

Graff-Radford NR, Welsh K, Godersky J: Callosal apraxia. Neurology 37:100–105, 1987.

Sperry R: Consciousness, personal identity and the divided brain. Neuropsychologia 22:661–673, 1984.

REFERENCES

Akelaitis AJ: Studies on the corpus callosum II. The higher visual functions in each homonymous field following complete section of the corpus callosum. Arch Neurol Psychiatry 45:788–796, 1941.

Baynes K, Tramo MJ, Gazzaniga MS: Reading with a limited lexicon in the right hemisphere of a callosotomy patient. Neuropsychologia 30:187–200, 1992.

Baynes K, Wessinger CM, Fendrich R, et al: The emergence of the capacity to name left visual field stimuli in a callosotomy patient: Implications for functional plasticity. Neuropsychologia 33:1225–1242, 1995.

Bogen JE, Gazzaniga MS: Cerebral commissurotomy in man. J Neurosurg 23:394–399, 1965.

Butler CR: Cortical lesions and interhemispheric communication in monkeys (*Macaca mulatta*). Nature 209:59–61, 1966.

Clark CR, Geffen GM: Corpus callosum surgery and recent memory. A review. Brain 112:165–175, 1989.

Coslett HB, Saffran EM: Evidence for preserved reading in 'pure alexia'. Brain 112:327–359, 1989.

Dejerine J: [Contribution à l'étude anatomo-pathologique et clinique de différentes variétés de cécites verbale] Mémoires de la Société de biologie 4:61–90, 1892.

Farah MJ, Gazzaniga MS, Holtzman JD, et al: A left hemisphere basis for visual mental imagery? Neuropsychologia 23:115–118, 1985.

Feinberg TE, Schindler RJ, Flanagan NG, et al: Two alien hand syndromes. Neurology 42:19–24, 1992.

Gazzaniga MS: Right hemisphere language following brain bisection. A 20-year perspective. Am Psychol 38:525–537, 1983.

Gazzaniga MS: Cerebral specialization and interhemispheric communication: Does the corpus callosum enable the human condition? Brain 123:1293–1326, 2000.

Gazzaniga MS, Bogen GM, Sperry RW: Some functional effects of sectioning the cerebral commissures in man. Proc Natl Acad Sci U S A 48:1765–1769, 1962.

Gazzaniga MS, Eliassen JC, Nisenson L, et al: Collaboration between the hemispheres of a callosotomy patient. Emerging right hemisphere speech and the left hemisphere interpreter. Brain 19:1255–1262, 1996.

Gazzaniga MS, Holtzman JD, Smylie CS: Speech without conscious awareness. Neurology 37:682–685, 1987.

Gazzaniga MS, LeDoux JE, Wilson DH: Language, praxis, and the right hemisphere: Clues to some mechanisms of consciousness. Neurology 27:1144–1147, 1977.

Gazzaniga MS, Smylie CS: Facial recognition and brain asymmetries: Clues to underlying mechanisms. Ann Neurol 13:536–540, 1983.

Gazzaniga MS, Smylie CS: Hemispheric mechanisms controlling voluntary and spontaneous facial expressions. J Cogn Neurosci 2:239–245, 1990.

Gazzaniga MS, Smylie CS, Baynes K, et al: Profiles of right hemisphere language and speech following brain bisection. Brain Lang 22:206–220, 1984.

Gazzaniga MS, Sperry RW: Language after section of the cerebral commissures. Brain 90:131–148, 1967.

Gersh F, Damasio AR: Praxis and writing of the left hand may be served by different callosal pathways. Arch Neurol 38:634–636, 1981.

Geschwind N: Disconnexion syndromes in animals and man. I. Brain 88:237–294, 1965.

Geschwind N: Disconnexion syndromes in animals and man. II. Brain 88:585–644, 1965.

Geschwind N: The apraxias: Neural mechanisms of disorders of learned movement. Am Sci 63:188–195, 1975.

Geschwind N, Kaplan E: A human cerebral deconnection syndrome: A preliminary report. Neurology 12:675–685, 1962.

Graff-Radford NR, Welsh K, Godersky J: Callosal apraxia. Neurology 37:100–105, 1987.

Heilman KM, Meador KJ, Loring DW: Hemispheric asymmetries of limb-kinetic apraxia: A loss of deftness. Neurology 55:523–526, 2000.

Heilman KM, Rothi L, Campanella D, et al: Wernicke's and global aphasia without alexia. Arch Neurol 36:129–133, 1979.

Holtzman JD, Gazzaniga MS: Enhanced dual task performance following corpus commissurotomy in humans. Neuropsychologia 23:315–321, 1985.

Lausberg H, Gottert R, Munssinger U, et al: Callosal disconnection syndrome in a left-handed patient due to infarction of the total length of the corpus callosum. Neuropsychologia 37:253–265, 1999.

LeDoux JE, Wilson DH, Gazzaniga MS: A divided mind: Observations on the conscious properties of the separated hemispheres. Ann Neurol 2:417–421, 1977.

LeDoux JE, Wilson DH, Gazzaniga MS: Block design performance following callosal sectioning. Observations on functional recovery. Arch Neurol 35:506–508, 1978.

Levy J, Nebes RD, Sperry RW: Expressive language in the surgically separated minor hemisphere. Cortex 7:49–58, 1971.

Levy J, Trevarthen C, Sperry RW: Reception of bilateral chimeric figures following hemispheric deconnexion. Brain 95:61–78, 1972.

Liepman H, Maas O: Fall von linksseitiger Agraphie und Apraxie bei rechtsseitiger Lähmung. Z Psycho Neurol 10:214–227, 1907.

Lutsep HL, Wessinger CM, Gazzaniga MS: Cerebral and callosal organisation in a right hemisphere dominant "split brain" patient. J Neurol Neurosurg Psychiatry 59:50–54, 1995.

Mangun GR, Luck SJ, Plager R, et al. Monitoring the visual world: Hemispheric asymmetries and subcortical processes in attention. J Cogn Neurosci 6:267–275, 1994.

Metcalfe J, Funnell M, Gazzaniga MS: Right-hemisphere memory superiority: Studies of a split-brain patient. Psychol Sci 6:157–164, 1995.

Milner B, Taylor L: Right-hemisphere superiority in tactile pattern-recognition after cerebral commissurotomy: Evidence for nonverbal memory. Neuropsychologia 10:1–15, 1972.

Pandya DN, Karol EA, Heilbronn D: The topographical distribution of interhemispheric projections in the corpus callosum of the rhesus monkey. Brain Res 32:31–43, 1971.

Phelps EA, Gazzaniga MS: Hemispheric differences in mnemonic processing: The effects of left hemisphere interpretation. Neuropsychologia 30:293–297, 1992.

Phelps EA, Hirst W, Gazzaniga MS: Deficits in recall following partial and complete commissurotomy. Cereb Cortex 1:492–498, 1991.

Plourde G, Sperry RW: Left hemisphere involvement in left spatial neglect from right-sided lesions. Brain 107:95–106, 1984.

Rasmussen T, Milner B: The role of early left-brain injury in determining lateralization of cerebral speech functions. Ann N Y Acad Sci 299:355–369, 1977.

Reuter-Lorenz PA, Baynes K: Modes of lexical access in the callosotomized brain. J Cogn Neurosci 4:155–164, 1992.

Sergent J: Furtive incursions into bicameral minds. Integrative and coordinating role of subcortical structures. Brain 113:537–568, 1990.

Sergent J: Subcortical coordination of hemisphere activity in commissurotomized patients. Brain 109:357–369, 1986.

Sidtis JJ, Volpe BT, Wilson DH, et al: Variability in right hemisphere language function after callosal section: Evidence for a continuum of generative capacity. J Neurosci 1:323–331, 1981.

Sperry R: Consciousness, personal identity and the divided brain. Neuropsychologia 22:661–673, 1984.

Sperry RW: Cerebral organization and behavior. Science 133:1749–1757, 1961.

Sperry RW: Hemisphere deconnection and unity in conscious awareness. Am Psychol 3:723–733, 1968.

Sperry RW: Perception in the absence of the neocortical commissures. Res Publ Assoc Res Nerv Ment Dis 48:123–138, 1970.

Sugishita M, Toyokura Y, Yoshioka M, et al: Unilateral agraphia after section of the posterior half of the truncus of the corpus callosum. Brain Lang 9:215–225, 1980.

Volpe BT, Sidtis JJ, Holtzman JD, et al: Cortical mechanisms involved in praxis: Observations following partial and complete section of the corpus callosum in man. Neurology 32:645–650, 1982.

Watson RT, Heilman KM: Callosal apraxia. Brain 106:391–403, 1983.

Witelson SF, Nowakowski RS: Left out axons make men right: A hypothesis for the origin of handedness and functional asymmetry. Neuropsychologia 29:327–333, 1991.

Zaidel D, Sperry RW: Memory impairment after commissurotomy in man. Brain 97:263–272, 1974.

Zaidel D, Sperry RW: Some long-term motor effects of cerebral commissurotomy in man. Neuropsychologia 15:193–204, 1977.

Frontal Lobe and Executive Functions

Paul J. Eslinger

Freeman Chakara

Acquired sociopathy

Akinesia and mutism

Dorsolateral frontal cortex

Dysexecutive syndrome

Executive functions

Orbitofrontal cortex

Prefrontal cortex

Premotor cortex

INTRODUCTION

The frontal lobes have been portrayed in poetic terms as the organ of civilization, a riddle, an enigma, and the brain region that makes humans unique from all other species. Modern scientific and clinical interest in the frontal lobe dates back to the famous "crowbar" case of Phineas Gage described by Harlowe (1848, 1868), which has continued to be discussed in clinical and theoretical terms (Stuss et al., 1992; Damasio et al., 1994). Though Gage's survival and enigmatic change in personality after frontal lobe damage was more of a curiosity at the time, investigators have continued to probe frontal lobe functions through the eras of functional localization, mass action–equipotentiality, psychosurgery, the cognitive revolution, the rise of modern neuroscience, and the current systems approach to brain organization (see Benton, 1991a, and Eslinger, 1999, for summaries). The frontal lobes are considered so vital to the coordination, monitoring, and management of behavioral-brain systems that they have been touted as the "executive" of the brain and "conductor" of the

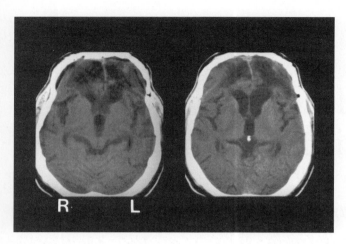

FIGURE 20-1. Brain magnetic resonance imaging (MRI) scan showing extensive bilateral frontal lobe damage from a penetrating injury that required surgical debridement. This patient continues to experience disabling executive function, behavioral, and emotional impairments 7 years after the incident.

brain's symphony. With extensive damage to the prefrontal region (Fig. 20-1, for example), patients develop *frontal lobe syndromes* that are disabling and unusually problematic for caregivers. The frontal lobes also play a critical role in child development and adult psychological maturation that has added further to its importance for human lifespan adaptation (Ackerly & Benton, 1948; Ackerly, 1964; Benton, 1991b; Eslinger et al., 1997; Tranel & Eslinger, 2000). These descriptors, while intriguing, do not precisely characterize what the frontal lobes do, how they develop, their interaction with other brain areas, assessment of frontal-mediated functions, how their damage changes behavior, and treatment of the ensuing clinical syndromes (e.g., Nauta, 1971; Tranel et al., 1994).

While there are no comprehensive survey data on the incidence of frontal lobe syndromes, we do know that this cortical region can be damaged by several commonly occurring diseases and conditions. These include traumatic brain injury (TBI), stroke, ruptured aneurysm, tumor, neurodegenerative diseases, schizophrenia, major depression, bipolar disorder, autism, attention deficit hyperactivity disorder (ADHD), hydrocephalus, and many others. Thus, presentation of frontal lobe syndromes is common enough to be encountered by most practitioners.

This chapter reviews the anatomic and functional organization of the frontal lobe along with the diseases, clinical deficits, assessment approaches, and interventions to treat and manage associated neurobehavioral impairments. More comprehensive reviews of these topics can be found in several recent books and special journal issues devoted solely to the frontal lobe (e.g., Stuss & Benson, 1986; Uylings et al., 1990; Eslinger & Grattan, 1991; Fuster, 1991; Levin et al., 1991;

Grafman, 1995a, 1995b; Krasnegor et al., 1997; Miller & Cummings, 1999; Eslinger, 1999; Tranel & Eslinger, 2000; Stuss & Knight, 2002).

A FRAMEWORK FOR FRONTAL LOBE ORGANIZATION

Anatomic and Physiologic Aspects

The modern understanding of anatomy and physiology has been derived from animal and human studies of neural cytoarchitecture, pathways, electrophysiology, diverse diseases, pharmacologic interventions, and functional brain imaging (e.g., Porrino et al., 1981; Barbas & Pandya, 1989; Neafsey, 1990; Barbas & Pandya, 1991; Bogousslavsky, 1994; Mega & Cummings, 1994; Barbas 1995; Price et al., 1996; Wharton et al., 2000). This section first describes organizational and operational features of the frontal lobes, followed by major neurobehavioral syndromes associated with frontal lobe disease, particularly affecting the prefrontal cortex.

Gross Anatomy and Frontal-Cortical Projections

The frontal lobe is grossly divided into *primary motor*, *premotor*, and *prefrontal* regions. These cortical areas are anatomically and functionally distinct (Fig. 20-2A, B).

The primary motor area is composed of agranular cortex that is closely linked with premotor cortex, primary somatosensory cortex and basal ganglia in the generation and control of movement. It is the center of the pyramidal motor system and gives rise to the substantial pyramidal tracts that descend subcortically through the internal capsule, through brainstem and spinal cord to body musculature.

The premotor area is dysgranular cortex that is located just rostral to primary motor cortex. It receives extensive projections from other cortical regions and is a critical convergence zone for primary motor cortex activation, including motor planning, anticipation, programming, and memory. Broca's area is located in the lower portion of premotor cortex in the left hemisphere, in the region of the pars triangularis. Both primary motor and premotor cortices are functionally organized in a *homuncular* pattern, with representation of perioral areas in the most inferior lateral region, ascending through the face, upper extremities, upper body, and then trunk, lower extremity, and genital areas along the superior mesial surface.

The prefrontal area is composed of granular cortex and is quite different from motor and premotor regions in its anatomy, physiology, and functional organization. Although it is a cortical association area, it does not receive any primary sensory input (except for olfaction in a small portion of the orbital surface), but

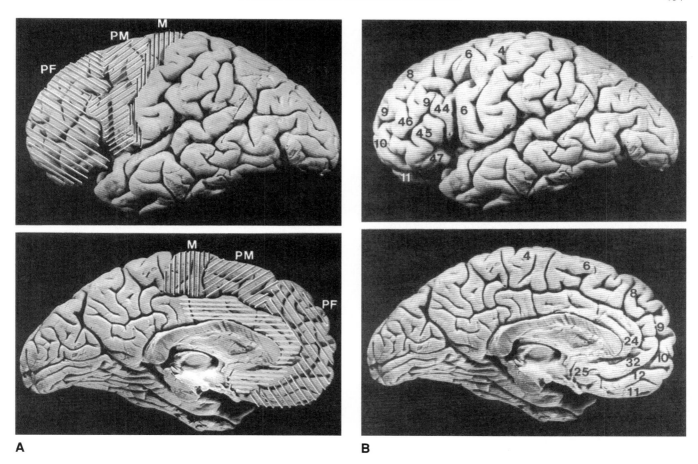

FIGURE 20-2. (*A*) Lateral and medial views of the human frontal lobe with demarcation of the primary motor, premotor and prefrontal cortical regions (yellow on the medial surface denotes limbic cortex). (*B*) Lateral and medial views of the human brain with Brodmann's areas notated within the frontal lobe. Anatomic and functional correlates to these areas are summarized in Tables 20-1 & 20-2. (Reproduced with permission from Damasio H: Neuroanatomy of frontal lobe in vivo: A comment on methodology, in Levin HS, Eisenberg HM, Benton AL (eds): Frontal Lobe Function and Dysfunction. New York: Oxford University, 1991.)

rather extensive projections from virtually all other association cortices. These encompass sensory-perceptual systems and unimodal and multimodal cortical association areas for vision, audition, somatosensory, olfaction, and gustation. In addition, the prefrontal cortex receives extensive projections from limbic system structures mediating memory and emotion, and from diencephalic-brainstem regions related to visceral-autonomic, hormonal, vegetative, and cognitive functions. These projection systems are dynamic and multidimensional. That is, rather than comprising a single pathway, say from the auditory association cortex to prefrontal cortex, these cortical-cortical connections consist of several pathways. For example, earlier auditory association areas target certain prefrontal neurons, whereas later auditory association areas project to prefrontal areas with a different laminar pattern. Reciprocating projections from prefrontal cortex to auditory association areas follow a similar scheme. This feature may allow for greater efficiency and complexity in elaboration of auditory-related information and its associative processing with prefrontal mechanisms. Furthermore, it may permit the prefrontal cortex to access and in turn influence auditory perceptual, memory and long-term knowledge systems (see Barbas & Pandya, 1991, for a summary). These connectional patterns may provide an anatomic bases for so-called 'bottom-up" and "top-down" processing emanating, respectively, from the increasingly detailed perception and analysis of incoming information versus the directed search for specific auditory information in order to accomplish a specific goal (Eslinger & Geder, 2000). There are similar reciprocating projections for the somatosensory and visual systems. Most importantly, because of these projection patterns, the prefrontal cortex can readily activate several effector systems including motor, hormonal, visceral-autonomic, and diverse aspects of cognition (e.g., sensory-perceptual alterations, memory, directed attention) that can lead to specific actions and behavioral responses.

Cytoarchitecture

Cytoarchitecture refers to the combined anatomic features of cell types, cell layers, and cell densities that characterize a particular cortical area. The primary motor (area 4) and premotor (areas 6, 44, 45) cortices each have relatively homogeneous cytoarchitectural patterns (see Fig. 20-2A, B). In contrast, the prefrontal cortex shows a heterogeneous cytoarchitecture (including areas 8, 9, 10, 11, 12, 13, 14, 24, 25, 32, 46, and 47) that varies from the 6-layered neocortical pattern to the 3–4-layered paralimbic pattern (see Damasio, 1991, for a summary). These cellular aspects of organization may reflect different architectonic stages and evolutionary trends in both the development and complexity of this cortical region (Barbas & Pandya, 1989, 1991; Barbas, 1995). The neocortical areas of prefrontal cortex provide a neural framework for associative processing, such as temporary mental representations (working memory), long-term memory storage, and operations such as decision making. The paralimbic areas permit significant influences from primary reinforcers (e.g., taste, smell, touch, pain) as well as emotion, vegetative, and autonomic-visceral processing regions (Rolls, 1990, 1999; Eslinger, 1999). The neocortical and paralimbic streams of the prefrontal cortex, therefore, are very important for the integrative processing of cognition and emotion (Barbas, 1995).

Prefrontal-Limbic System Connections

The prefrontal cortex is also interconnected with several other limbic and paralimbic structures. These include the amygdala, hippocampus, anterior and dorsomedial nuclei of the thalamus, temporal polar cortex, parahippocampal gyrus, insula, and cingulate gyrus (Porrino et al, 1981; Goldman-Rakic & Friedman, 1991; Price, 1999). The paralimbic areas of prefrontal cortex, located in the orbital and inferior medial regions, receive the strongest projections, although other areas also receive and reciprocate projections. Prefrontal-limbic interactions have been implicated in learning and memory, decision making, cognitive-emotional appraisal, and diverse social processing such as empathy, moral emotions, theory of mind, and interpersonal judgment (e.g., Eslinger & Damasio, 1985; Bechara et al., 1994; Moll et al., 2003).

Prefrontal-Subcortical Networks

In addition to limbic systems interconnections, there are two other major cortical-subcortical networks that prominently involve the frontal lobe: the thalamo-frontal and the frontal-striatal (e.g., Alexander et al., 1990; Chow & Cummings, 1999). The thalamus and basal ganglia operate in concert with the frontal lobe, including motor, premotor, and prefrontal regions. The pathways form loops that either emanate from or terminate on prefrontal neurons in specific clusters (see Chapter 25 on Subcortical Disorders and Chapter 24 on Movement Disorders for further details). These cortical-subcortical networks provide vital input-output, convergence, filtering, and coactivation processing that are necessary for cortical regions to operate effectively. When there is damage to the basal ganglia and thalamus, frontal-type impairments can result, including disinhibition, perseveration, loss of initiative and motivation, environmental dependency, hemispatial neglect and attentional disorders, disorganization, emotional blunting, and decreased memory.

Prefrontal Cortex and Behavior

The prefrontal cortex is one of the most important cortical regions involved in cognition, behavior, and emotion. As a multimodal convergence and cortical association area, it has been associated with diverse aspects of behavior that are difficult to place within a single construct or process. Study of patients with pathophysiology of the prefrontal cortex, investigations in animal models, and the more recent findings from functional brain imaging studies point to three areas of behavioral mediation: *long-term knowledge storage, learning and short-term representational knowledge, and executive functions and self-regulation.*

Long-Term Knowledge Storage

One of the enigmas about prefrontal cortex function has centered on characterizing the types of long-term memory, knowledge, and other representations that are stored there. The prefrontal cortex has anatomic and physiologic properties similar to those of other cortical association regions that store long-term memory. For example, neurons in the premotor and primary somatosensory cortex appear to contribute to motor programming, motor memory, and sensory-motor transformations (see Chapter 14 on the Somatosensory System). Premotor cortex damage leads to impairments such as ideomotor apraxia, melokinetic apraxia, nonfluent (Broca's type) aphasia, and motor learning deficits. Hence, it appears reasonable that long-term motor-related knowledge underlying skilled movements, bimanual coordination, and speech is represented in the premotor cortex.

The prefrontal cortex is also thought to store substantial amounts of acquired knowledge that are important for decision making and adaptation. One of the most intriguing observations has been that patients with prefrontal cortex damage often do not demonstrate deficits in measured intelligence (e.g., Ardila, 1999). Except in cases of massive frontal lobe damage, most patients perform within the average range on standard tests of intelligence such as the Wechsler scales. Normal range of intelligence quotient (IQ) scores occurs despite the fact that they may show other significant executive function deficits such as impaired planning, organization, working memory, and sequencing. For example, patient E.V.R. had superior IQ scores after orbitofrontal meningioma resection, yet he could not organize himself to get out to work in the morning or maintain a job he had held for many years (Eslinger & Damasio, 1985). This is one of the reasons that patients with prefrontal cortex damage may be difficult to assess in brief office visits. That is, while family members report concerns about the patient's everyday functioning, judgment, and behavior, he or she may be quite articulate, attentive, and detailed in verbal responses to a variety of orientation, reasoning, language, memory, and judgment questions. This chasm between "real-life" report and clinical assessment can be puzzling.

The lack of statistical correlation between IQ and executive functions has also been demonstrated in cognitive development studies in typical children (Welsh et al., 1991; Archibald & Kerns, 1999). Thus, the "knowledge domain" of the prefrontal cortex may not be that measured by general intelligence tests, but rather that associated with being a well-organized and goal-directed executive of one's own behavior and life.

Grafman (1995b) has suggested that the prefrontal cortex is specialized for acquisition and storage of more complex types of knowledge and operations than the more general and routine knowledge and processes associated with temporal, parietal, and occipital cortices. These entail sequences of action, relational reasoning, and open-ended schemas, scripts, and plans that are typically goal-directed and contextually dependent. He proposed that prefrontal mechanisms can be conceptualized as managerial knowledge units that encapsulate goals, sequences of action, and response options that extend over periods of time, sometimes a few minutes (getting a drink of water) and others over several years (e.g., becoming a doctor, raising a family). Managerial knowledge units are proposed to be large units of memory that comprise the mental models that guide our actions over time, space, and changing circumstances, so as to achieve necessary personal, professional, family, financial, social, and other tasks in organized, timely and appropriate ways. Sirigu and colleagues (1995) demonstrated that patients with frontal lobe damage show specific impairments in managerial knowledge. Within an office setting, it is obviously difficult to observe and assess these executive functions, but reports of real-life behaviors can be fraught with examples. Furthermore, this managerial knowledge is acquired over long periods of time, extending well into adulthood and underlying continuing adult development, psychological adjustment, and many aspects of achievement and creativity throughout life (Grattan & Eslinger, 1991; Eslinger et al., 1997). Children who suffer early damage to the prefrontal cortex do not develop adequate executive function skills and often fare poorly in school, work, and adult adaptation (see Eslinger et al., in press, for a summary of these cases).

Learning and Short-Term Representational Knowledge

The prefrontal cortex has an important influence on learning, related to its roles in attention, analytical processing, and working memory. These processes are necessary for the acquisition of new information and separate active from passive learning. One telling example of this influence is provided by study of *depth of processing* in relationship to verbal learning and memory (Craik & Lockhart, 1972). In this paradigm, subjects are asked to make judgments about words and then, unbeknownst to them, to recall those words later. Words with equated physical and semantic properties are used, but the orienting question for each set is different. These orienting questions ask for decisions regarding either: (1) a physical feature of the printed word, (2) its phonemic structure, or (3) a semantic categorical judgment. More specifically, questions include, respectively, (1) Is the word printed in uppercase letters? (2) Does the word rhyme with _____? (3) Is the word a type of _____? For each orienting question, one half of the target words will generate a *yes* response and one half a *no* response. Results have consistently shown that subjects typically remember words processed at the semantic-categorical level best, then the phonemic level, and finally the physical feature level. The interpretation of this finding is that semantically judged words are thought to be processed more *deeply* (i.e., requiring more semantic associations or elaborative processing in order to be judged accurately). Hence, semantic level of processing requires more analytical brain-related activity and generates a stronger trace for later memory recall. In contrast, judgment about a physical feature of the word is thought to generate the least semantic processing and a lesser trace for later memory recall. Kapur (1994) demonstrated further that the more deeply processed words selectively activated left prefrontal cortex in functional imaging of normal volunteers.

Tulving and colleagues (1994) have also demonstrated in functional imaging studies that normal persons selectively activate left prefrontal cortex in verbal learning (or encoding) operations but the right prefrontal cortex in verbal retrieval processes. These studies support the important influence of the prefrontal cortex in mediating diverse cognitive and attentional aspects of learning and memory. This complements the purported role of the hippocampus and medial temporal lobe in memory consolidation processes (see Chapter 11 on Memory and Learning). These functional correlates would also be consistent with the observation that patients with frontal lobe damage typically do not demonstrate the clinical amnesias associated with medial temporal lobe damage, but develop inefficiencies and disorganization in learning and memory retrieval processes (such as "forgetting to remember"). Rather than primary memory dysfunction, these kinds of memory impairment are manifested in the impaired natural or spontaneous use of memory in daily activities and tasks. Frontal lobe damage has also been linked to impaired source memory (i.e., remembering the original spatial-temporal context of specific memories) as well as memory for temporal order and frequency. Hence, the learning capacities associated with frontal lobe damage have been found to be altered in ways that tend to be more disorganized, more shallow in level of processing, and atypical in learning curve characteristics.

The other important aspect of frontal lobe and memory concerns *working memory*. Working memory refers to the temporary and changing representations of knowledge that permit us to keep new information active or *in mind* for purposes of comprehension, problem solving, sequencing, and multitasking (see Chapter 10). Baddeley (1992) has suggested that working memory encompasses two components: (1) limited capacity, temporary storage sites for rapidly changing verbal and visuospatial information that include left and right hemisphere temporal, parietal, and occipital lobe structures; and (2) central executive mechanisms in the prefrontal cortex that mediate operations on the information such as manipulation, computation, and associative imagery. Goldman-Rakic and colleagues (1987, 1991) and Wilson and colleagues (1993) have provided consistent data from the nonhuman primate model that the dorsolateral prefrontal cortex has a large role in working memory operations, in coordination with posterior sensory association areas. In a sense, working memory has been conceptualized as the mental workspace for decision making and executive functions because the latter necessarily entail keeping information in mind to guide actions toward achievement of goals over time. Without working memory capacities, patients quickly become dependent on immediate environmental circumstances and external cues to guide their behavior, leading to problematic clinical syndromes of utilization behavior and environmental dependency (Eslinger, 2002). However, many important goals in daily life are not immediately in front of us at home and at work, and require that we maintain internal representations (working memory) of these in preparing and executing actions over time. Functional imaging studies have shown consistent evidence that the prefrontal cortex along with posterior sensory association areas become active during diverse working memory tasks (e.g., Jonides et al., 1993; Petrides et al., 1993; Ungerleider et al., 1998).

Executive Functions and Self-Regulation

The operations of the frontal lobe, particularly the prefrontal cortex, have been conceptualized in different ways (see Grafman, 1995b for a recent summary). Many aspects of prefrontal functioning have been assembled under the rubric of *executive functions and self-regulation*. Executive functions can be defined as the diverse psychological processes that:

- Control the activation and inhibition of response sequences that are guided by internal neural representations (e.g., verbal rules, biologic needs, somatic states, emotions, goals, mental models),
- For the purpose of meeting a balance of immediate situational, short-term, and long-term goals and demands,
- That span physical-environmental, cognitive, behavioral, emotional, and social domains of functioning (Eslinger, 1996).

In addition to what is described above, three other ideas are important to highlight. First, Shallice (1988) has introduced the construct of a supervisory attentional system (SAS) mediated via prefrontal mechanisms. The role of the SAS is to intentionally select and guide behavior responses that are not the usual or prepotent responses that constitute habits and well-practiced routines. This necessarily involves components of self-awareness, working memory, goal-directed behavior, inhibition, and self-monitoring. This is an important and useful construct in evaluating patients' clinical impairments. Second, Damasio and colleagues (1991) proposed that behavior can also be guided by somatic markers that emanate from the visceral-autonomic states that become associated with reward, punishment, and other emotion- and somatic-based experiences. Patients with ventromedial frontal lobe damage show both impaired autonomic responses and decision-making skills, particularly around risk-taking and social judgment. Finally, Fuster (1991) has suggested that complex behavior is organized over time by cross-temporal contingencies. Actions are sequenced within perception-action cycles and coded within prefrontal neurons. These become elaborated into temporally based sequences that interrelate events and actions in stable knowledge structures.

Levine and colleagues (1999) have used the term self-regulatory disorder to describe *pathologica* of previously inhibited behavior, impulsivity and perseveration that can occur after frontal damage.

DISEASES CAUSING FRONTAL LOBE DAMAGE

There are many kinds of pathophysiology that compromise the frontal lobe, either in an isolated and focal manner or more diffuse and multilobar. Common causes include:

- Tumors of benign and malignant nature (e.g., orbitofrontal meningioma)
- Traumatic brain injury from blunt and acceleration-deceleration forces as well as projectile wounds. These are associated with diffuse axonal shearing of white matter pathways, cerebral contusions, lacerations, and hemorrhagic (e.g., petechial, subdural, and intraparenchymal) lesions, most commonly involving frontal and anterior temporal lobes.
- Ischemic and hemorrhagic infarctions of the anterior cerebral artery and rostral branches of the middle cerebral artery.
- Ruptured aneurysms of the anterior communicating and anterior cerebral artery.
- Arteriovenous malformations at cortical and subcortical levels that can become hemorrhagic and require surgical resection.
- Multiple sclerosis with demyelinating plaques located in deep frontal white matter.
- Mass effects from hydrocephalus, including normal pressure hydrocephalus.
- Necrotic lesions from herpes simplex encephalitis.
- Anoxic brain injury that compromises frontal *watershed* regions located between the anterior and middle cerebral arteries.
- Degenerative disorders including frontotemporal dementias (progressive nonfluent aphasia and behavioral disorder–dysexecutive subtypes), frontal lobe dementia, Pick's disease, and Alzheimer disease.

Many of the above-mentioned etiologies occur not only in adults but also in children, the latter including perinatal cerebrovascular disease.

Other developmental forms of frontal lobe dysfunction include:

- Attention deficit hyperactivity disorder
- Autism spectrum disorders, including Asperger syndrome and autism

Psychiatric disorders in which frontal lobe dysfunction is suspected include:

- Schizophrenia
- Major depression
- Bipolar disorder
- Obsessive-compulsive disorder
- Reactive attachment disorder
- Oppositional defiant disorder

Not all cases with the same etiology necessarily present with the same symptoms and course. This is related, in part, to different effects of pathophysiology on anatomy, physiology, and chemistry of brain tissue. Disease processes can differ in *momentum* of lesion (sudden onset, rapidly progressive, slow growing), *location* throughout frontal regions (unilateral vs. bilateral, single vs. multiple, white matter vs. cortex), *physiology* (e.g., epileptic, edematous), *mass effects*, and *compensatory processes* (e.g., collateral flow).

CLINICAL PRESENTATION AND SPECIALIZED REGIONS OF THE FRONTAL LOBE

Tables 20-1 and 20-2 provide a comprehensive summary of frontal lobe regions that have distinctive anatomy and lead to specific neurobehavioral syndromes when damaged. These have been derived from extensive animal model studies and clinical studies of patients with frontal lobe disease.

Primary Motor and Premotor

These specialized motor-related cortices mediate the learning, memory and execution of skilled motor movements, bimanual coordination, and specific interactions with sensory-perceptual cortices that contribute to sensory-motor transformations. Damage to primary motor cortex causes contralateral limb and facial weakness, varying from mild hemiparesis to hemiplegia, expressed according to the homuncular representation of the body. Dysarthria (or impaired articulation of speech) is a specific type of perioral weakness and alteration from lower motor strip damage. Lesions to premotor cortex are associated with limb and buccofacial forms of apraxia. These refer to impairments of skilled motor movements that are not explainable by weakness and that affect transitive and intransitive upper extremity actions (e.g., using a toothbrush, hammer, or spoon; making hand signals for hitchhiking, thumbs up, OK, and waving) and perioral actions (e.g., lip, tongue, and facial movements such as whistling, sucking in through a straw, etc.). Damage to the left anterior-inferior premotor region causes Broca's aphasia in the left hemisphere and aprosodia in the right hemisphere.

Superior Medial

This region is the superior and medial extent of the premotor cortex, located in the interhemispheric fissure, and comprises the supplementary motor area (SMA) primarily but also aspects of the anterior cingulate

TABLE 20-1. Anatomical Features of Specialized Frontal Lobe Regions

Cortical regions	Prominent anatomic landmarks	Brodmann's cytoarchitectonic areas	Neural systems
Lateral frontal region			
Primary motor and premotor	Central sulcus/precentral gyrus Broca's area (left)	4, 6 (lateral), 44, 45	Motor Premotor
Lateral prefrontal (dorsal and ventral)	Frontal pole & frontal gyri (inferior, middle, superior)	8, 9, 10, 11, 46, 47	Prefrontal
Mesial frontal region			
Superior mesial	Central sulcus/precentral gyrus Supplementary motor area Anterior cingulate gyrus	4, 6 (mesial) 24	Motor Premotor Limbic
Inferior mesial	Subcallosal gyrus Mesial gyrus rectus	25, 32, 14, 11, 12	Paralimbic Prefrontal
Ventral frontal region			
Basal forebrain	Septal nuclei Precommissural fornix Nucleus accumbens Substantia innominata Diagonal band of Broca		Limbic
Orbital	Gyrus rectus Olfactory tracts Orbital gyri Medial Middle Lateral	10, 11, 13, 14, 47	Paralimbic Prefrontal
Deep white matter	Periventricular (rostral, lateral, inferior, superior to frontal horns)		Frontal-striatal Frontal-thalamic Frontal-limbic Frontal-cortical pathways

gyrus. Unilateral and bilateral forms of damage occur with anterior cerebral artery stroke, head trauma and parasagittal tumors. Clinically, patients can exhibit loss of behavioral initiation and spontaneity affecting speech and goal-directed behaviors. The most severe presentation, usually associated with bilateral lesions, is akinesia and mutism, in which patients fail to respond to their environment, including other persons, despite being awake, alert, and capable of both movement and speech. Such individuals are unable to initiate and maintain responsiveness, and have profound loss of motivation, emotional expression, and emotional experience (Lhermitte, 1983; Bogousslavsky, 1994; Eslinger & Geder, 2000). Although akinetic and mute, patients can briefly generate appropriate responses such as answering the telephone, but do not continue the conversation. This would indicate that motor, perceptual, and language systems are still functional but insufficiently activated to maintain behavioral responding. Inability to generate and sustain behavioral responses has been

likened to a "whole-body apraxia." Unilateral lesions, even those restricted to underlying white matter, tend to cause less severe impairments that can nevertheless include transcortical motor aphasia, emotional blunting, and a spectrum of motor release disorders such as alien hand (also described as "anarchic" hand), grasping and groping, and utilization behavior (Della Sala et al., 1994; Ishihara et al., 2002). Utilization behavior refers to the acquired disorder of needless and excessive use of objects encountered in the patient's immediate environment, regardless of whether they intend to use the objects or whether it is socially appropriate (Eslinger, 2002). A recent case study suggested that utilization behavior can be conceptualized as bilateral anarchic hands and is related to bilateral medial premotor cortex lesions and can emerge either as akinesia and mutism resolve or as a direct effect of a limited SMA lesion (Boccardi et al., 2002). An example of a superior medial frontal lesion is shown in Figure 20-3. Trial treatments with dopamine agonists such as bromocrip-

TABLE 20-2. Prominent Impairments Associated with Damage to Specific Frontal Lobe Regions

Region	Clinical impairments	Clinical impairments
Lateral frontal region		
Primary motor and premotor	Hemiparesis	Apraxia (oral and limb kinetic)
	Dysarthria	Motor impersistence
	Aprosodia	Nonfluent aphasia (left)
Lateral prefrontal (dorsal and ventral)	Disorganized thinking and behavior	Impaired working memory
	Perseveration	Cognitive rigidity
	Poor planning	Intentional disorders
	Impulsive responding	Inattention/distractibility
	Stimulus-boundedness	Lack of empathy
	Poor self-regulation	Conjugate eye deviation
	(Right lateral prefrontal	(Left lateral prefrontal
	Left hemispatial neglect	Transcortical motor aphasia
	Poor spatial cognition)	Word finding difficulties
		Discourse)
Mesial frontal region		
Superior mesial	Akinesia/bradykinesia	Mutism
	Apathy	Loss of motivation
	Apraxia	Aspontaneity
	Utilization behavior	Alien hand
	Grasping/groping	Altered self-regulation
	Intentional disorders	Callosal disconnection signs
Inferior mesial	Disinhibition	Lack of motivation
	Altered self-regulation	Altered emotional processing
Ventral frontal region		
Basal forebrain	Amnesia	Confabulations
	Reduced motivation	Delusions (Capgras syndrome, reduplicative paramnesia)
Orbital cortices	Personality change	Impulsive actions
	Poor social judgment	Reduced empathy
	Lack of goal-directed behavior	Altered self-regulation
	Environmental dependency	
Deep white matter	Personality change	Poor empathy
	Emotional lability	Irritability

tine have been reported to be helpful in lessening symptoms (Eslinger & Geder, 2000).

Inferior Medial

This region is located rostral and inferior to the genu of the corpus callosum (Brodmannn's areas 10 medial, 12, parts of areas 14, 24, 25, and 32—including the most rostral cingulate gyrus, subcallosal gyrus, and medial gyrus rectus) and has strong connections with limbic and paralimbic structures. Tract tracing experiments in the nonhuman primate model have revealed a medial prefrontal network that is distinctive from orbital prefrontal cortex (Price, 1999). The inferior medial prefrontal cortex is strongly interconnected within its cytoarchitectonic areas and also interconnects with the most ventromedial sector of the frontal lobe and the superior temporal sulcus that has been implicated in social signal detection. Its output projections target visceral control structures in the hypothalamus and brainstem. It has been implicated in emotional processing, motivation, memory, and emotional self-regulation, including depression and bipolar disorder (Eslinger & Damasio, 1984; Drevets et al., 1997; Eslinger & Geder, 2000). Damage to inferior medial prefrontal regions can often occur together with medial orbital damage, for example, from ruptured anterior communicating artery aneurysm and orbital tumors. However, damage can also occur without orbital involvement, as in case B.Y. summarized below.

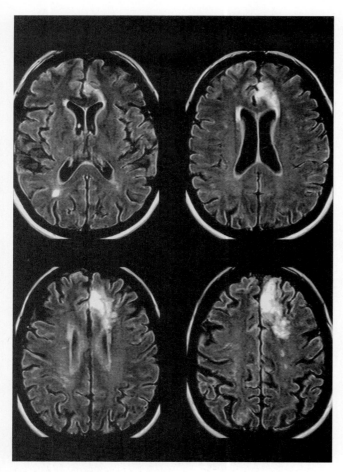

FIGURE 20-3. T2 brain magnetic resonance imaging (MRI) scan illustrating right superior medial frontal lobe ischemic stroke causing damage to the anterior cingulate gyrus and supplementary motor area (right on right). This lesion was associated with bradykinesia, blunting of emotional expression, and decreased motivation. Note the disconnection of crossing callosal fibers in the upper left image, leading to ideomotor apraxia in left upper extremity.

Case Illustration

A 56-year-old woman was surgically treated for ruptured left pericallosal artery aneurysm in 1995, with very good medical recovery but persistent personality change. The latter included reduced and labile emotional expression, loss of motivation in usual goal-directed and recreational activities, and disinhibition in social discourse. Two years later she underwent surgical treatment for a ruptured anterior communicating artery aneurysm that resulted in additional symptoms of forgetfulness and slower reading. Brain magnetic resonance imaging (MRI) scan at that time revealed bilateral inferior medial prefrontal damage with sparing of superior medial and orbital regions (Fig 20-4).

Neuropsychological examination revealed deficits in working memory, cognitive flexibility, and memory retrieval in an otherwise alert, articulate, and well-oriented woman. Her greatest personal concerns centered around her memory difficulties, lack of motivation, and reduced emotional intensity in her relationships with family members. Her memory difficulties were addressed through compensatory, self-cuing strategies tailored for her work and daily activities. A trial of the dopamine agonist bromocriptine 2.5 mg twice daily resulted in gradual improvement of motivation and emotional responsiveness (Eslinger & Geder, 2000).

Anatomic and functional data have suggested that significant differences in the inferior medial prefrontal region exist in patients with depression and bipolar disorder. Cerebral blood flow and cerebral glucose metabolism alterations have also been reported in inferior medial prefrontal regions in major depressive disorder and bipolar-depressed patients. Morphometric analysis has indicated that left subgenual cortical volumes were reduced by 39% in bipolar subjects and 48% in unipolar depression subjects compared with controls. These reductions may be related to a marked decrease in the number and density of glia that typically affect neuronal transmission and sustain receptors for serotonin and corticosteroids (Drevets et al., 1998).

Basal Forebrain

The basal forebrain encompasses several nuclei clustered along the inferior and medial aspects of the posterior frontal lobe, including the septum, nucleus basalis of Meynert, precommissural fornix, nucleus accumbens, and nucleus of the diagonal band of Broca. This region has strong limbic system input, being interconnected with the amygdala, hippocampus, and ventral striatum. Basal forebrain damage is most often from ruptured anterior communicating artery aneurysms, and causes a clinical amnesia with prominent confabulations. These memory deficits are differentiated from the impaired consolidation and rapid forgetting associated with medial temporal lobe amnesia (see Chapter 11 on Memory and Learning). Basal forebrain amnesia is characterized by temporal and spatial context confusion that not only limits accuracy of memory but also may give rise to spontaneous confabulations (Ptak & Schnider, 1999).

Orbitofrontal

Damage to the orbitofrontal region has been linked to prominent personality changes in the form of disinhi-

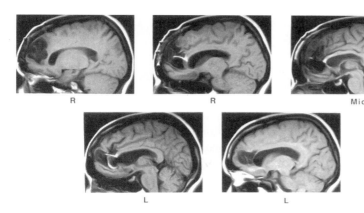

FIGURE 20-4. Brain magnetic resonance imaging (MRI) scan illustrating bilateral inferior medial frontal lobe damage from ruptured aneurysms, but preserved superior and orbital regions. Changes in motivation, emotional expression, empathy, and memory were evident.

bition and impaired social judgment, emotion-based learning, and self-awareness (Eslinger & Damasio, 1985; Grafman et al., 1986). This region is strongly interconnected with both cognitive and emotion processing areas and contains paralimbic as well as neocortical tissue. The most posterior and medial area is considered to be one of the main cortical regions for autonomic mediation and forms a network with other limbic cortices such as the insula as well as the amygdala, temporal polar cortex, hypothalamus, and brainstem. Bechara and colleagues (1994) have linked this area to risk-taking behavior and alterations in judgment that depend upon learning from contingency-based outcomes. Damasio and colleagues (1991) have conceptualized such a defect as involving loss of somatic markers of experiences and contingencies that impair patients' anticipation of future consequences. Along a similar vein, Rolls and colleagues (Rolls, 1990; Rolls et al., 1994; Hornak et al., 1996; Rolls, 1999) have investigated contingency-based learning involving primary and emotional reinforcers. They reported that patients with orbitofrontal damage were impaired in such emotion-based learning and the guidance of their responses based on these contingencies. These accumulated data indicate that medial orbitofrontal damage can cause impulsive actions and poor social judgment despite the lack of change in intellect, memory, attention, perception and language. Interpersonal behaviors are further affected by reduced empathy, Theory of Mind capacities, and self-awareness (Eslinger, 1998). An example of orbitofrontal damage after traumatic brain injury is shown in Figure 20-5.

Deep White Matter

As mentioned previously, the deep white matter of the frontal lobe includes many prominent pathways that link frontal regions with other regions of the cortex, basal ganglia, thalamus, and limbic and brainstem structures. These have been conceptualized as frontal-cortical and frontal-subcortical circuits that are critical to adaptive behavior across motor, cognitive, and emo-

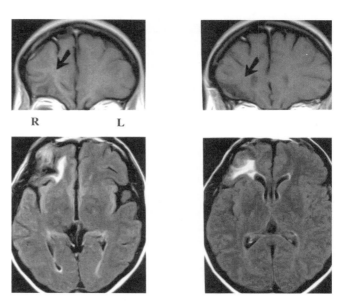

FIGURE 20-5. Brain magnetic resonance imaging (MRI) scan demonstrating residual right orbitofrontal lesion from traumatic brain injury. The upper images are T1 coronal sections and the lower images are T2 axial cuts. The patient showed impairments in working memory, multitasking, regulation of attention, and emotional processing.

tional domains (Alexander et al., 1990; Cummings, 1993; Mega & Cummings, 1994). Disconnection of these pathways can occur from various diseases that affect the white matter such as multiple sclerosis, stroke, traumatic brain injury, and ruptured aneurysms (an example is presented in Fig. 20-6). Patients develop changes in emotion, personality, cognition, and interpersonal processes, leading to irritability and reduced empathy, motivation, and self-awareness.

Dorsolateral

This multimodal convergence area is closely interconnected with other cortical association areas and correlated with higher cognitive processes of attentional control, planning, organization, working memory, and

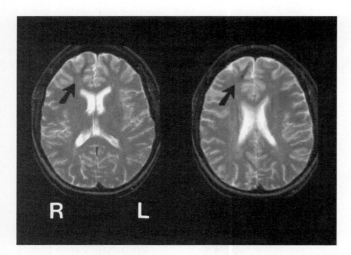

FIGURE 20-6. Brain magnetic resonance imaging (MRI) scan illustrating residual white matter shear injury after traumatic brain injury. These bilateral white matter scars were associated with hypomania and disinhibited behavior in the chronic recovery phase.

decision making. In functional brain imaging studies, the dorsolateral prefrontal cortex appears to frequently activate in paradigms that require making a decision, analyzing the interrelationship of task elements (relational reasoning), and keeping information temporarily in mind (working memory) until used in behavioral responses. Patients with dorsolateral prefrontal damage show a wide variety of executive function and behavioral deficits (see Table 20-2 for summary) that vary according to side of lesion. An example of right dorsolateral prefrontal cortex lesion is shown in Figure 20-7.

Frontal Pole

Functions of the frontal polar cortex remain minimally understood. Hebb (1945) linked this region to planning and future-oriented thinking. Moll and colleagues (2003) reported frontal polar activation in healthy participants during a cognitive task of social-moral judgment.

ASSESSMENT OF FRONTAL LOBE DISORDERS

Approaches to the assessment of frontal-related functions are diverse and depend in part on how the cognitive, social-emotional, and behavioral processes subserved by frontal systems are conceptualized. There are several models of frontal-related executive functions, yet consensus on what comprises these functions is lacking and there is no universal definition of executive functions (Grafman, 1995b; Eslinger, 1996). Despite limited agreement many clinicians and researchers consider fundamental executive processes to include working memory, inhibition and self-regulation, sequencing of behavior, cognitive flexibility, planning, and organization of behavior. Recent research and clinical approaches to the assessment of executive functions have tried to match neuroanatomic substrates to functional behavioral constructs. For example, Malloy & Aloia (1998) examined the links between apathy and the medial frontal lobes, disinhibition and the orbital prefrontal cortex, and cognitive executive functions and the dorsolateral prefrontal cortices. Similarly, Sarazin and colleagues (1998) distinguished between the dorsolateral prefrontal cortices and the orbitomedial prefrontal cortex on the basis of cognitive and social/behavioral measures, respectively. These proposed structure/function relationships rely on observations of patient behavior in the laboratory and in real-life settings. Kimberg & Farah (1993) caution, however, that our current understanding of prefrontal cortical functions does not allow a comprehensive explanation of the neuroanatomic basis of executive functions because performance on standard measures of executive functions does not necessarily translate or generalize to "real-life" quantifiable deficits (Anderson, 1991; Levine et al., 2000). Satish and

FIGURE 20-7. Chronic brain magnetic resonance imaging (MRI) scan of a 7-year-old male illustrating a right dorsolateral prefrontal cortex lesion after surgical treatment of a deep hemorrhagic arteriovenous malformation. Acute effects on spatial-related executive functions were evident, but showed remarkable recovery over a 4-year period. Residual symptoms of attention deficit remained after 8 years with otherwise excellent recovery.

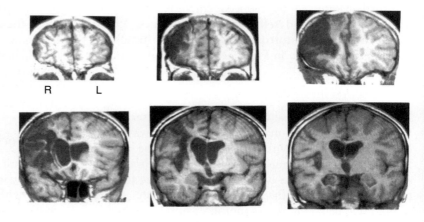

TABLE 20-3. Instruments for Assessment of Frontal-Related Functions

Test	Publisher/s	Function	Strengths	Weaknesses
TMT	Reitan Lab PAR	Sequencing Flexibility Motor speed Visual scan	Sensitivity to brain injury (higher in Trails B)	Questionable specificity to FL
TOH	WPS	Inhibition Strategy formation	Sensitivity Specificity to FL	Limited norm data Planning validity Questionable
TOL	CNT	Planning & problem solving	Sensitivity & specificity to FL left dorsolateral	Normative data not robust
WCST	PAR	Flexibility Abstraction Inhibition	Sensitivity to brain injury (with 19+ perseverative errors)	Specificity is low; high false negative
CT	WPS	Concept formation & flexibility	Very sensitive to brain injury (more anterior)	Can be cumbersome & time-consuming
COWA	PsyCorp	Flexibility, inhibition	Sensitivity; left hemisphere & good normative data	Gender effects: Males perform less well than females
RFFT	PAR	Flexibility	Sensitivity & ® FL Specificity	Weak norms
CVLT	PsyCorp	Planning organization & flexibility	Sensitivity & rich data; good norms	Gender effects as COWA
RCFT	PAR	Organization Inhibition Flexibility	Sensitivity with some specificity for ® FL functions	Nonunified scoring (qualitative vs. quantitative data)
KAS-R	WPS	Disinhibition awareness & regulation	Extensive normative data. Sensitivity to brain injury	Lack of specificity Evaluator bias may be a concern
FRSBE	PAR	Apathy & disinhibition	Sensitive & specific Extensive data	Accuracy of baseline behaviors questionable
Brock	Dywan	Disinhibition & apathy	Face validity; some research support	Cumbersome scoring Norms limited as yet
MEPS	Shure	Flexibility & self-regulation	"Ecological" real-world validity	Limited specificity & sensitivity data

(From Psychological Assessment Resources [PAR], Lutz, FL; www.parinc.com; Western Psychological Service [WPS], Los Angeles, CA, www.wpspublish.com; The Psychological Corporation [PsyCorp], San Antonio, TX, www.PsychCorp.com.)

colleagues (1999) and Burgess (1997) both emphasized the need for evaluative procedures that most closely approximate the real-life challenges of patients.

There are various procedures designed to measure executive functions, consistent with the dorsolateral, medial, orbital and other regional substrates noted above (Table 20-3). In keeping with the wide body of literature supporting the primary role of working memory in executive functions, all of the measures discussed below depend, to some degree, on the relative integrity of working memory capacity. There are numer-

ous tests and procedures available on the market, thus only brief descriptions will be provided. The relative strengths and weaknesses of these procedures will be reviewed with some consideration of the executive functions assessed by these measures. Detailed descriptions of administration, scoring, interpretation, reliability, and validity data are usually available from test publishers as well as compendia and texts on measures of neuropsychological assessment.

The Trailmaking Test (TMT A & B) and the Color Trails Test require connecting 25 encircled numbers

(Trails A) or 25 encircled numbers and letters in an alternating pattern. The trail making test requires attention, working memory, sequencing, alternating responses, and self-monitoring. It is fairly simple to administer and may be completed within 10 minutes.

The Tower of Hanoi (TOH) task is a puzzle consisting of three equal-length pegs and several disks of varying size. Given a start state, in which the disks are stacked on one or more pegs, the task is to reach a goal state in which the disks are stacked in descending order on a specified peg. Only one disk may be moved at a time; any disk not currently being moved must remain on a peg; and a larger disk may not be placed on a smaller disk (Goel & Grafman, 1995). A relatively similar task, the Tower of London, requires participants to move colored beads from their initial position on upright but different-length pegs to attain new predetermined patterns, using the fewest moves possible. As with the TOH, the computer version of the TOL is available with 3, 4, or 5 disks/beads in different colors and shapes. The TOL, a simpler task than the TOH, is designed to assess planning and it has been highly correlated to the left dorsolateral prefrontal area (Morris et al., 1993; Denckla, 1994; Owen, 1997).

The Wisconsin Card Sorting Test (WCST) requires participants to sort cards into stacks matching four reference cards. The examiner does not inform the examinee of the sorting principle; thus, the participants infer the sorting principle primarily from examiner feedback. The sorting principle is changed following the completion of one set (10 cards matching a predetermined sorting principle), and the task is considered complete when the participant either completes six categories or sorts through all 128 cards (Milner, 1963; Anderson et al., 1998). There is also a 64-card version available.

Another very sensitive, but not specific, measure of cerebral dysfunction, the Category Test (CT) (full and shortened versions) requires participants to examine various figures and identify something about the shape that reminds them of one number between one and four; that is, in this task, examinees respond by identifying (pointing or verbally) one of four numbers (I, II, III, or IV) printed on a response card. The examiner provides feedback as to whether the response was correct or incorrect.

The Controlled Oral Word Association Test (COWA) is part of the Multilingual Aphasia Examination. In this task, participants are asked to produce (either orally or in written form) as many words as they can that begin with a given letter of the alphabet. Examinees are given one minute for each letter, usually with a maximum of three letters, e.g., F, A, and S. This measure assesses rapid phonetic associative fluency rather than verbal naming per se.

Perhaps a nonverbal analogue to verbal generative fluency measures, Ruff Figural Fluency Test (RFFT) measures generative figural fluency by having examinees create as many unique designs as they can by connecting dots in a five-dot matrix. Participants are exposed to five separate pages, and they are asked to create unique designs on each new page, thus unique designs used on page one may be used again on pages two and three, etc. (Lee et al., 1997). Patients are allowed only 60 seconds per page, allowing a total of 5 minutes for test administration.

The California Verbal Learning Test–2nd Edition (CVLT-II) requires participants to listen to the examiner reading a list of words, and they are then asked to recite the list. This process is repeated four additional times, and then examinees are given an alternative (distracter) list for recall. Following these trials, participants are then asked to recite the original list, first without cueing and then with categorical cues. Following a 20-minute delay, participants are then asked to repeat the original list without cues and following cues. Finally they are requested to discriminate words from the original list from a group of related and unrelated distracter items (Spreen & Strauss, 1998).

In the Rey Complex Figure and Recognition Test (RCFT) participants must copy (in some cases visually observe) a complex geometric shape with 18 pieces of discrete detail (Fastenau, 2001). Once completed, the original template and the examinee's copy are immediately removed from view. The examinee is then required to reproduce the shape from memory at 3- and 30-minute intervals. The latter recall task is immediately followed by a recognition task in which the participant is asked to circle items belonging to the original shape from a group of 24 shapes, 12 of which are distracters.

Other batteries designed to assess "practical" presentations of dysexecutive functions are also available from various sources. Perhaps the best known among such batteries is the Behavioral Assessment of the Dysexecutive Syndrome (BADS). This battery involves six subtests that assess most of the popular notions associated with the concept of executive functioning (Spreen & Strauss, 1998). The BADS and related batteries have been associated with moderate to high levels of practical/ecological validity. That is, they closely approximate the patient's "real-world" difficulties, thereby providing clinicians with concrete descriptions of the difficulties patients and care providers or employers are likely to experience. As beneficial as these self-contained batteries may be, clinicians should consider assembling assessment protocols based on the patient's needs and resources available for devising intervention strategies.

As noted, patients with orbitofrontal damage can perform within the normal range of expectancy on common measures of executive functioning (Eslinger & Damasio, 1985). Nonetheless, they can exhibit real-life impairments in decision making and interpreting social situations, some of which are detectable with simulation-based assessment (Satish et al., 1999) as well as various gambling and risk-factor paradigms (Bechara et al., 1994). Other aspects are reported by caregivers and significant associates of these patients, with accounts that are quite different from the "unremarkable" profiles that can be observed on cognitive testing and self-report behavioral inventories.

Certain frontal lobe inventories are available that may help in assessing lack of inhibition, declines in empathy, and changes in personality and behavioral self-regulation in everyday life (Grafman et al., 1986; Barrash et al., 2000; Levine et al., 2000; Grace & Malloy, 2001). An instrument that has enjoyed prominent use in assessing socioemotional and personality change after traumatic brain injury (TBI) is the Katz Adjustment Scale–Relatives (KAS-R) form. Relatives of TBI patients are asked to rate patients on various behaviors, based on premorbid presentation as well as behaviors following the injury. Five advantages of the KAS-R have been observed (Jackson et al., 1992):

- Clearly worded; reduced psychological denial in rater (relative)
- Simple wording of items adequate for use by nonprofessionals
- Face validity for cognitive, socioemotional, psychiatric, and behavioral issues
- Items assess behavior in community rather than structured (laboratory) setting
- Extensive normative data

Barrash et al. (2000) recently described the development and validation of the Iowa Rating Scales of Personality Change. The Frontal Systems Behavior Scale (FRSBE) was developed to assess orbital dysfunction (Grace & Malloy, 2001). As such, TBI patients with injuries to the orbital prefrontal cortices are likely to display disinhibition, socially inappropriate behavior along with several other difficulties. The FRSBE additionally assesses behavioral apathy that is more closely associated with the mesial prefrontal lobes. The task requires relatives and caregivers of TBI patients to rate examinees on several behaviors and compare these socioemotional characteristics to observed functioning prior to injury.

The Brock Adaptive Functioning Questionnaire (Dywan et al., 1995) provides a wealth of data regarding patient functioning. This instrument, which has been used in a few research protocols, is currently available for the cost of shipping from Jayne Dywan, PhD, at Brock University, St. Catharines, Ontario, Canada. The Brock exists in two forms, a self-report version and another one completed by a care provider or companion. The patient's scores are then compared with profiles endorsed by caregivers.

An adaptation of the Means–Ends Problem Solving (MEPS) task has been demonstrated to differentiate social executive dysfunctions in TBI patients. The MEPS has been used widely with adolescents and adults, with recent applications to patients with frontal lobe injuries. This measure, initially developed by George Spivak and Myrna Shure, provides a stem (starting point) and conclusion (ending) to five different social scenarios that require problem solving. The patient is then asked to tell a story that best "fills in the blank" to the one provided by the examiner . . . Despite insignificant differences in the length of the stories told, patients with frontal lobe injuries consistently produced stories with implausible and generally poor solutions to the interpersonal challenges posed (Chakara, 2000). MEPS is available for the cost of shipping from Myrna Shure at Hahnemann University, Philadelphia, PA.

The social, emotional, and behavioral deficits associated with frontal lobe dysfunction may not receive sufficient attention in daily clinical practice, particularly among nonspecialists. Unfortunately, these impairments often cause significant distress to patients and their care providers. Consequently, it is important for examiners to integrate multiple measures that speak to issues of validity as well as comprehensiveness with regards to the various spheres in which the patient's life has been disrupted or altered.

RECOVERY PATTERNS AND INTERVENTION

Recovery of Function

Recovery of function after frontal lobe damage is highly variable, and there is a substantial role for health care providers in advancing patient outcomes. Clearly defined, evidenced-based approaches remain to be identified. Rehabilitation services usually involve multidisciplinary treatment services. derived from comprehensive assessments of neurologic, neuropsychological, and everyday functional capacities of patients (Cicerone & Giacino, 1992; Mateer, 1997). To date, few studies have specifically followed frontal damaged patients through their various stages of recovery. Studies of head trauma, hemispatial neglect, aphasia, and stroke-related motor deficits provide some relevant data, but are generally not geared specifically toward frontal damage. The available rehabilitative services appear to be most beneficial for well-defined functional goals, and are quite helpful to patients and families in many daily living challenges. Cognitive rehabilitation has also shown some beneficial effects when targeted at specific skills and situations (see further description in section following). However, these common therapy approaches are least able to identify and intervene on the notable motivational, emotional, executive, self-awareness, and interpersonal deficits that are significant barriers to rehabilitation, recovery, and reintegration after frontal lobe injury.

Predictors of Outcome

A case control study of unilateral frontal lesion patients identified four variables that differentiated positive from negative outcomes after a 2- to 4-year follow-up period (see Eslinger & Geder, 2000, for summary). The variables spanned anatomy, cognition, emotion, and personality as follows:

- Favorable outcome was associated with frontal lesions that *spared* deep white matter pathways, the ventrolateral frontal cortex, and extension of lesions to the anterior insula and basal ganglia. The decisive deep white matter lesions that contributed to negative outcomes were thought to involve frontal-limbic, -striatal and -thalamic pathways traversing subjacent and adjacent to the frontal horns, and involved with self-regulatory, emotional, and cognitive processes. The insula has been linked to emotional and prosocial affiliative tendencies (Mesulam & Mufson, 1982), whereas ventrolateral frontal cortex participates in emotional and linguistic communication proficiency. Hence, frontal lesions that affect these areas exacerbated the more evident cognitive deficits.
- Favorable outcome depended upon a normal range of certain executive functions, particularly in measures of cognitive flexibility.
- The preserved ability to relate to others in empathic ways distinguished favorable from unfavorable outcome. Normal range of empathy scores was associated with social adjustment, continued supportive relationships and positive attitudes from others. Low empathy was correlated with hostile treatment of others, marital strain, social withdrawal, and resentment from others.
- Premorbid personality characteristics of being agreeable, flexible, and sensitive to others was also associated with favorable outcomes. Patients with unfavorable outcomes were described with different premorbid personality characteristics, such as controlling, antagonistic, and rigid.

Although much more extensive research is needed to elucidate recovery patterns and treatment effects, the aforementioned data do raise questions about the potential role of neurologic, cognitive, and psychological "protective factors" in recovery. The findings also indicate areas of potential intervention. An equally important issue is whether pharmacologic treatment can contribute further to such remediation.

Pharmacologic Considerations

Although there are no Food and Drug Administration (FDA)-approved medications for treatment of frontal lobe impairments, at least three classes of drugs can potentially have therapeutic benefits. These include (1) dopamine agonists, (2) antidepressant-anxiolytics, and (3) low-dose stimulants. Dopamine agonists have been evaluated in very limited open-label trials. Some benefits have been noted for nonfluent aphasia, hemispatial neglect, akinesia-mutism, and other deficits in initiation, motivation, and affect (Fleet et al., 1987; Gupta & McCoch, 1992; Eslinger & Geder, 2000). These effects may be mediated via increased postsynaptic activation from the ascending dopaminergic nigrostriatal and mesocorticolimbic pathways to the basal ganglia and mesial frontal regions. Selective serotonergic reuptake inhibitors and newer generation compounds are also helpful in relief of the blunted affect, low mood, irritability, and other emotional alterations. Buspirone is a nonsedating anxiolytic that can be used in isolation or together with antidepressants. Divalproex sodium and carbamazepine have been used in treatment of hypomania after frontal lobe damage. Finally, low-dose stimulants can potentially improve the attentional deficits and distractibility that are common after dorsolateral frontal lesions. Medication treatment in frontotemporal dementias remains uncertain. There are no definitive studies to date on whether these conditions might benefit from cholinesterase inhibitors, as used in Alzheimer disease (see Chapter 22), but our clinical observations suggest caution and a treatment trial approach.

Cognitive-Behavioral Interventions

Neuropsychological evaluation often leads to recommendations for the management of deficits evident from assessment. Patients with executive dysfunction are commonly prescribed cognitive or neuropsychological rehabilitation as part of their treatment package. The cognitive and functional benefits of neuropsychological rehabilitation have been supported by a respectable body of studies (Cicerone et al., 2000). A brief review of rehabilitation will follow; a thorough discussion is provided in section VI of this volume.

Cognitive rehabilitation generally entails assisting patients in their attempts to return to premorbid levels of functioning or the closest approximation thereof. Thus, patients can be provided with methods to improve functional capacity in sustained attention or expressive language, whereas more creative solutions may be needed to enhance impaired memory (Wilson,

2000). *Neuropsychological rehabilitation* is a term that is more comprehensive in that it integrates patient recovery with adjunctive support services aimed at enhancing global "improvements" in overall functioning. Prigatano (1997) proposes five key components to comprehensive neuropsychological rehabilitation: (1) cognitive rehabilitation, (2) psychotherapy, (3) the establishment of a therapeutic milieu, (4) education and working alliance with the patient and family, and (5) a protected work trial. The multisystemic nature of such a model requires clinical judgment as well as facility with interdisciplinary relationships. Ben-Yishay and Prigatano (1990) observed that this holistic approach to neuropsychological rehabilitation has benefits that often transcend cognitive, emotional, and motivational issues; in addition, it is cost-efficient. Prigatano (1997) reports that while the overall cost of neuropsychological rehabilitation is between US$50,000 and US$60,000, the financial and emotional returns to society are manifold if the patient can return to work and maintain productivity.

At a functional level, neuropsychological rehabilitation roughly takes one of three forms: (1) prosthetic/orthotic devices, (2) compensatory strategies, and (3) restitution or remediation of function (Ben-Yishay & Prigatano, 1990). Prosthetics encompass environmental supports and individualized mechanisms designed to carry out some functions for the patient. These devices include lists, appointment books, key rings with beepers; watches with alarms to remind patients to take medications, computer-aided visual magnifiers, etc. As noted, orthotic aids are modifications designed to help patients adapt to their environmental challenges. The clinician will need to assist patients in setting up use of these devices and providing family members, school staff, and employers with tools for monitoring effective use of such strategies. The following vignette illustrates a clinical application of orthotic devices.

Case Illustration

The patient is a 53-year-old right-hand-dominant male who presented for neuropsychological evaluation after a right cerebrovascular accident involving the distribution of the middle cerebral artery. Assessment revealed mild hemispheric neglect, moderately impaired visual scanning and attention, severe difficulties with both auditory and visual consolidation/encoding of new information, impulsivity, and heightened anxiety. He reported that his anxiety was elevated due, most likely, to the impending possibility of losing his job of 23 years. The patient was employed by a TV station as a production manager, where his primary role was to play prerecorded commercials at predetermined times during the course of a program. On several occasions after his stroke the patient failed to "run" the commercials at these preset times, which led to customer complaints and loss of revenue for his employer. The patient indicated that such gross lapses in memory were evident elsewhere in his life. For example, he completely forgot to attend a function that he and his fiancée had been planning for several weeks. Despite the anxiety related to the possible loss of employment, the patient generally considered himself to be functioning as efficiently as he always had. Thus, his lack of appreciation for his deficits further complicated initial rehabilitation efforts.

The management of the patient's neuropsychological deficits required an individualized plan to be carried out mainly within the setting of his place of employment. Assistance from his employer and his fiancée were key assets to the success of the intervention prescribed. We focused on educating his employer as well as his fiancée about the nature of his deficits, with particular emphasis on the impairments in cognitive and social executive functions. The patient's supervisor temporarily assigned him to tasks with fewer demands for precision, and threats of loss of employment were removed from his file. His employer understood that lack of insight into cognitive and socioemotional deficits is a common feature in the disruption of executive functions following right hemisphere injuries. We devised an individualized rehabilitation plan for the patient because his financial obligations and manifest anxiety would have made a comprehensive rehabilitation program a frustrating experience. While the ideal context for rehabilitative efforts might be the clinical setting where the clinician provides close supervision, there are times when the employment setting or the classroom would be more reasonable in order to reduce disruptions in the patient's routines and to observe the functional merits of neuropsychological interventions.

Compensatory strategies are techniques used by patients to work around their limitations (Sohlberg & Mateer, 1989). Kazdin (1975) points out that in order to develop a successful set of compensatory strategies one needs to identify the function that is compromised by brain injury. Thus attention, memory, language, visual tracking, language, reading, and other skills can be broken down into their individual components for the purposes of identifying "where" in the global task/process the limitation is most pronounced. For example, a patient with predominately encoding/consolidation memory deficits will need different strategies than someone whose impairments are characterized by recall difficulties. Most neuropsychological functions are admittedly complex, involving various systems. Therefore, it is necessary to analyze the functional components of important tasks in order to identify where and how rehabilitation should be focused. Restitution is the process of enhancing functional skills that have been partially impaired. This step may involve repetition of various exercises aimed at improving impaired skills, be it attention, visual neglect, reading, etc. (Wilson, 2000).

From a neurobiological perspective, rehabilitation presumes internal processes such as neuroanatomic reparative mechanisms and other compensatory modifications (Prigatano, 1997). For example, Kolb & Whishaw (1995) list the following neuroanatomic reparative processes: (1) regeneration, (2) sprouting, (3) denervation supersensitivity, and (4) disinhibition of potential compensatory zones. Regeneration occurs when damaged cells (often in the peripheral nervous system), previously deprived of oxygen, regrow new connections to areas they previously innervated. Sprouting involves the growth of nerve fibers to innervate new targets, particularly those vacated by other terminals. Supersensitivity often entails a heightened sensitivity of postsynaptic neurons to neurotransmitters in order to compensate for inefficiencies in the presynaptic neurons. Disinhibition of compensatory zones suggests that other areas of the brain can potentially mediate functions that were compromised by damage.

Prigatano (1997) observed that the mechanisms of recovery and deterioration are necessarily superimposed upon the processes of normal aging and development. As such, patient recovery is likely to present a dynamic pattern that often eludes simplistic expectations of linear, predictable changes in patients' cognition and behavior. Thus at a functional level, rehabilitation processes and outcomes can be conceptualized in terms of impairment, disability, and handicap (WHO, 2000). Wilson (1997) further defines impairment as damage to physical or mental structures; disability refers to particular problems resulting from impairment (e.g., forgetting to take medication following compromise to one's memory system); handicap implies problems in societal participation because of someone's disability (see Chapter 50). These distinctions help guide the timing and intensity of rehabilitative efforts.

The successes of rehabilitative efforts ultimately depend upon the efficient deployment of clinical skills by those assessing and treating such patients. That is, the remarkable data on the efficacy of neuropsychological rehabilitation are less likely to have a significant impact on the functioning of patients if treating/assisting professionals are unable to "operationalize" theoretical constructs into "real-life" solutions for patients and care providers.

CONCLUSIONS

The frontal lobe is a heterogeneous region of the cerebral cortex that subserves a wide variety of behavioral processes. The primary and premotor areas are closely linked and necessary for the initiation, coordination and maintenance of movements. These areas are also critically involved in motor learning and sensory-motor transformations that underlie efficient and accurate motor responses. The prefrontal cortex is comprised of lateral, medial, and orbital regions that have both limbic and neocortical properties for processing and storage of information and experiences. Many of the cognitive and integrated cognitive-emotional operations of the prefrontal cortex are described under the construct of executive functions. Whereas posterior cortical regions might be considered more hard-wired and linear in their detection, processing and organization of the environment and acquired knowledge systems, the prefrontal cortex appears to be comparatively more dynamic, interactive, and interwoven with parallel systems processing. The latter, in particular, can include cognitive, emotional, and autonomic-visceral systems that are used in learning, decision making, planning, judgment, and the formulation and pursuit of goals. Frontal lobe impairments are among the most difficult to assess and manage, due to the their complex, *real-life* character, and the interplay of neurologic, cognitive, emotional, social, and personality factors. Rehabilitation entails multidisciplinary approaches by functionally based therapies together with select pharmacologic trials, family education, and adjustments made to patient's home setting, vocational activities, and social interactions.

■ KEY POINTS

☐   The frontal lobes comprise approximately 30% of the entire cortical surface and can be grossly divided into dorsolateral, medial, orbital, and polar regions. These regions are anatomically and functionally organized into networks that include subcortical, cortical, and limbic structures.

☐   The frontal lobes, in particular the prefrontal regions, undergo the longest postnatal maturational change, which extends well into the second decade of a person's life, and likely are necessary for ongoing adaptation, achievement, and growth in cognitive, social, and emotional domains.

☐   The frontal lobes are involved in a broad array of behavior-related processes, including response selection, working memory, self-regulation (e.g., initiation and inhibition) planning, self-monitoring, self-awareness, Theory of Mind, emotion, and organization of goal-directed behavior.

☐ A wide variety of diseases affect the frontal lobes, some of which are treatable. Neurobehavioral effects can range from subtle changes in personality, cognition, and emotion to devastating impairments of response initiation, cognitive organization, judgment, social behavior, and self-regulation.

☐ Remediation of frontal-related impairments in executive function, social behavior, and emotion is very challenging and typically draws upon a combination of behavioral, cognitive, medical, and environmental interventions.

KEY READINGS

Chow TW, Cummings JL: Frontal-subcortical circuits, in Miller BL, Cummings JL (eds): The Human Frontal Lobes. New York: Guilford, 1999, pp. 3–26.

Grafman J (ed): Similarities and distinctions among current models of prefrontal cortical functions. Ann N Y Acad Sci 769:337-368, 1995b.

Stuss DT, Knight RT: Principles of Frontal Lobe Function. Oxford, UK: Oxford University Press, 2002.

REFERENCES

Ackerly SS: A case of paranatal bilateral frontal lobe defect observed for thirty years, in Warren JM, Albert K (eds): The Frontal Granular Cortex and Behavior. New York: McGraw-Hill, 1964, pp. 192–194.

Ackerly SS, Benton AL: Report of a case of bilateral frontal lobe defect. Proc Assoc Res Nerv Ment Dis 27:479–504, 1948.

Alexander GE, Crutcher MD, DeLong MR: Basal ganglia-thalamo-cortical circuits: Parallel substrates for motor, oculomotor, "prefrontal" and "limbic" functions. Prog Brain Res 85:119–146, 1990.

Anderson SW, Damasio H, Jones RD, et al: Wisconsin Card Sorting Test as a Measure of Frontal Lobe Damage. J Clin Exp Neuropsychol 13:909–922, 1991.

Archibald SJ, Kerns KA: Identification and description of new tests of executive functioning in children. Child Neuropsychol 5:115–129, 1999.

Ardila A, Pineda D, Rosselli M: Correlation between intelligence test scores and executive function measures. Arch Clin Neuropsychol 15:31–36, 2000.

Baddeley A: Working memory. Science 255:556–559, 1992.

Barbas H: Anatomic basis of cognitive-emotional interactions in the primate prefrontal cortex. Neurosci Biobehav Rev 19:499–510, 1995.

Barbas H, Pandya DN: Architecture and intrinsic connections of the prefrontal cortex in the rhesus monkey. J Comp Neurol 286:353–375, 1989.

Barbas H, Pandya DN: Patterns of connections of the prefrontal cortex in the rhesus monkey associated with cortical architecture, in Levin HS, Eisenberg HM, Benton AL (eds): Frontal Lobe Function and Dysfunction. New York: Oxford University Press, 1991, pp. 35–58.

Barrash J, Tranel D, Anderson SW: Acquired personality disturbances associated with bilateral damage to the ventromedial prefrontal region. Dev Neuropsychol 18:355–382, 2000.

Bechara A, Damasio AR, Damasio H, et al: Insensitivity to future consequences following damage to human prefrontal cortex. Cognition 50:7–15, 1994.

Ben-Yishay Y, Prigatano GP: Cognitive remediation, in Griffith E, Rosenthal M, Bond MR, et al. (eds): Rehabilitation of the Adult and Child with Traumatic Brain Injury. Philadelphia, PA: Davis, 1990, pp. 393–409.

Benton AL The prefrontal region: Its early history, in Levin HS, Eisenberg, Benton AL (eds): Frontal Lobe Function and Dysfunction. New York: Oxford University Press, 1991a, pp. 3–32.

Benton AL: Prefrontal injury and behavior in children. Dev Neuropsychol 7:276–281, 1991b.

Boccardi E, Della-Sala S, Motto C, et al: Utilisation behaviour consequent to bilateral SMA softening. Cortex 38:289–308, 2002.

Bogousslavsky J: Frontal stroke syndromes. Eur Neurol 34:306–315, 1994.

Burgess PW: Theory and methodology in executive function research, in Rabbitt P (ed): Methodology of Frontal and Executive Function. Hove, UK: Psychology Press, pp. 81–111.

Chakara FM: The Impairment of Interpersonal Problem Solving Skills in TBI Patients [dissertation]. Chester, PA: Widener University, 2000.

Chow TW, Cummings JL: Frontal-subcortical circuits, in Miller BL; Cummings JL (eds): The Human Frontal Lobes. New York: Guilford, 1999, pp. 3–26.

Cicerone KD, Giacino JT: Remediation of executive function deficits after traumatic brain injury. NeuroRehabilitation 2:12–22, 1992.

Cicerone, KD, Dahlberg C, Kalmar K, et al: Evidence-based Cognitive Rehabilitation: Recommendations for Clinical Practice. Arch Phys Med Rehabil 81:1596–1615, 2000.

Craik FIM, Lockhart RS: Levels of processing: A framework for memory research. J Verb Learn Verb Behav 11:671–684, 1972.

Cummings JL: Frontal-subcortical circuits and human behavior. Arch Neurol 50:873–880, 1993.

Damasio H: Neuroanatomy of frontal lobe in vivo: A comment on methodology, in Levin HS, Eisenberg HM, Benton AL (eds): Frontal Lobe Function and Dysfunction. New York: Oxford University, 1991, pp. 92–121.

Damasio AR, Tranel D, Damasio HC: Somatic markers and the guidance of behavior: Theory and preliminary testing, in HS Levin, HM Eisenberg, Benton AL (eds): Frontal Lobe Function and Dysfunction. New York: Oxford University Press, 1991, pp. 217–229.

Damasio H, Grabowsky T, Frank R, et al: The return of Phineas Gage: Clues into the brain from the skull of a famous patient. Science 264:1102–1105.

Della Sala S, Marchetti C, Spinnler H: The anarchic hand: A fronto-mesial sign, in Boller F, Grafman J (eds): Handbook of Neuropsychology, Vol. 9. Amsterdam, The Netherlands: Elsevier, 1994, pp. 233–255.

Denckla MB: Measurement of executive function, in Lyon GR (ed): Frames of Reference for the Assessment of Learning Disabilities: New Views on Measurement Issues. Baltimore, MD: Paul H. Brookes, pp. 117–142.

Drevets WC, Price JL, Simpson JR Jr, et al: Subgenual prefrontal cortex abnormalities in mood disorders. Nature 386:824–827, 1997.

Drevets WC, Ongur D, Price DL: Neuroimaging abnormalities in the subgenual prefrontal cortex: Implications for the pathophysiology of familial mood disorders. Mol Psychiatry 3:220–226, 1998.

Eslinger PJ: Conceptualizing, describing and measuring components of executive functions, in Lyon GR, Krasenger DA (eds): Attention, Memory, and Executive Function. Baltimore, MD: Paul H. Brookes, 1996, pp. 367–395.

Eslinger PJ: Neurological and neuropsychological bases of empathy. Eur Neurol 39:193–1998.

Eslinger PJ: Orbital frontal cortex: Historical and contemporary views about its behavioral and physiological significance. Neurocase 5:225–230, 1999.

Eslinger PJ: The anatomic basis of utilization behaviour: A shift from frontal-parietal to intra-frontal mechanisms. Cortex 38:273–276, 2002.

Eslinger PJ, Biddle KR, Grattan LM: Cognitive and social development in children with prefrontal cortex lesions, in Krasnegor NA, Lyon GR, Goldman-Rakic PS (eds): Development of the Prefrontal Cortex: Evolution, Neurobiology, and Behavior. Baltimore: Paul H. Brookes, 1997, pp. 225–335.

Eslinger PJ, Damasio AR: Behavioral disturbances associated with rupture of anterior communicating artery aneurysms. Semin Neurol 4:385–389, 1984.

Eslinger PJ, Damasio AR: Severe disturbance of higher cognition after bilateral frontal lobe ablation: Patient EVR. Neurology 49:764–769, 1985.

Eslinger PJ, Flaherty-Craig CV, Benton AL: Cognitive, social, and moral development after early prefrontal cortex damage: Review of Clinical cases. Brain Cogn, in press.

Eslinger PJ, Geder L: Behavioral and emotional changes after focal frontal lobe damage, in Bogousslavsky J, Cummings JL (eds): Focal Brain Lesions and Emotion. Cambridge UK: Cambridge University Press, 2000, pp. 217–260.

Eslinger PJ, Grattan LM (eds): Special Issue: Developmental consequences of early frontal lobe damage. Dev Neuropsychol 7:257–419, 1991.

Fastenau PS: The Extended Complex Figure Test. National Academy of Neuropsychology 21st Annual Conference, Course 19, San Francisco, CA, 2000.

Fleet WSH, Valenstien E, Watson RT, et al: Dopamine agonist therapy for neglect in humans. Neurology 37:1765–1770, 2001.

Fuster JM: Role of prefrontal cortex in delay tasks: Evidence from reversible lesion and unit recording in monkey, in Levin HS, Eisenberg HM, Benton AL (eds): Frontal Lobe Function and Dysfunction. New York: Oxford University Press, 1991, pp. 66–71.

Goel V, Grafman J: Are frontal lobes implicated in "planning" functions? Interpreting data from the Tower of Hanoi. Neuropsychologia 33:623–642, 1995

Goldman-Rakic PS: Circuitry of primate prefrontal cortex and regulation of behavior by representational memory, in: Mountcastle VB (ed): Handbook of Physiology, the Nervous System V. New York: Raven Press, 1987, pp. 373–417.

Goldman-Rakic PS, Friedman HR: The circuitry of working memory revealed by anatomy and metabolic imaging, in Levin HS, Eisenberg HM, Benton AL (eds): Frontal Lobe Function and Dysfunction. New York: Oxford University Press, 1991, pp. 72–91.

Grace J, Malloy PF: Assessment of Frontal Behavioral Syndrome with the Frontal Systems Behavior Scale (FRSBE). National Academy of Neuropsychology 21st Annual Conference, Course 30, San Francisco, CA, 2000.

Grafman J (ed): Structure and function of the human prefrontal cortex. Ann N Y Acad Sci 769, 1995.

Grafman J (ed): Similarities and distinctions among current models of prefrontal cortical functions. Ann N Y Acad Sci 769:337–368, 1995.

Grafman J, Vance SC, Weingartner H, et al: The effects of lateralized frontal lesions on mood regulation. Brain 109:1127–1148, 1986.

Grattan Lm, Eslinger PJ: Frontal lobe damage in children and adults: A comparative review. Dev Neuropsychol 7:283–326, 1991.

Gupta SR, McCoch AG: Bromocriptine treatment of non-fluent aphasia. Arch Phys Med Rehabil 73:373–376, 1992.

Harlowe JM: Passage of an iron bar through the head. Boston Med Surg J 39:389–393, 1848.

Harlowe JM: Recovery from passage of an iron bar through the head. Pub Mass Med Soc 2:327–347, 1868.

Hebb DO: Man's frontal lobes: A critical review. Arch Neurol Psychiatry 54:10–24, 1945.

Hornak J, Rolls ET, Wade D: Face and voice expression identification in patients with emotional and behavioral changes following ventral frontal lobe damage. Neuropsychologia 34:247–261, 1996.

Ishihara K, Nishino H, Maki T, et al: Utilization behavior as white matter disconnection syndrome. Cortex 38:379–387, 2002.

Jackson HF, Hopewell C A, Glass C A, et al: The Katz Adjustment Scale: Modification for use with victims of traumatic brain and spinal injury. Brain Injury 6:109–127, 1992

Jonides J, Smith EE, Koeppe RA et al: Spatial working memory in humans as revealed by PET. Nature 363:623–625, 1993.

Kazdin AE: Behavior Modification in Applied Settings. Homewood, IL: Dorsey Press, 1975.

Kimberg DY, Farah MJ: A unified account of cognitive impairments following frontal lobe damage: The role of working memory in complex, organized behavior. J Exper Psychol Gen 122:411–428, 1993.

Kolb B, Whishaw IQ: Fundamentals of Human Neuropsychology. New York: F. H. Freeman & Co., 1995, pp. 539–564.

Krasnegor NA, Lyon GR, Goldman-Rakic PS (eds): Development of the Prefrontal Cortex, Evolution, Neurobiology, and Behavior. Baltimore: Paul H. Brookes, 1997.

Lee GP, Strauss E, Loring D W et al: Sensitivity of figural fluency on the Five-point Test to focal neurological disease. Clin Neuropsychol 11:59–68, 1997.

Levin HS, Eisenberg HM, Benton AL (eds): Frontal Lobe Function and Dysfunction. New York: Oxford University Press, 1991.

Levine B, Freedman M, Dawson D, et al: Ventral frontal contribution to self-regulation: Convergence of episodic memory and inhibition. Neurocase 5:263–275, 1999.

Levine B, Dawson D, Boutet I, et al: Strategic self-regulation in traumatic brain injury: Its relationship to injury severity and psychological outcome. Neuropsychology 14: 491–500, 2000.

Lhermitte F: Utilization behavior and its relation to lesions of the frontal lobes. Brain 106:237–255, 1983.

Malloy PF, Aloia M: Frontal lobe dysfunction in traumatic brain injury. Semin Clin Neuropsychiatry 3:186–194, 1998.

Milner B: Effects of different brain lesions on card sorting. Arch Neurol 9:90–100, 1963.

Morris RG, Ahmed GM, Syed GM, et al: Neural correlates of planning ability: Frontal lobe activation during the Tower of London Test. Neuropsychologia 31:1367–1378, 1993.

Mateer CA: Rehabilitation of individuals with frontal lobe impairments, in Leon-Carrion J (ed): Neuropsychological Rehabilitation: Fundamentals, Innovations and Directions. Delray Beach, FL: GR/St Lucia Press, 1997, pp. 285–300.

Mega MS, Cummings JL: Frontal-subcortical circuits and neuropsychiatric disorders. Neuropsychiatry Clin Neurosci 6:358–370, 1994.

Mesulam MM, Mufson EJ: Insula of the old world monkey. I. Architectonics in the insulo-orbito-temporal component of the paralimbic brain. J Comp Neurol 212:1–22, 1982.

Miller BL, Cummings JL: The Human Frontal Lobes: Functions and Disorders. New York: Guilford Press, 1999.

Moll J, Oliveira-Souza R, Eslinger PJ: Morals and the human brain: A working model. NeuroReport 14:299–305, 2003.

Nauta WJH: The problem of the frontal lobe: A reinterpretation. J Psychiatr Res 8:167–187, 1971.

Neafsey EJ: Prefrontal cortical control of the autonomic nervous system: Anatomical and physiological observations. Prog Brain Res 85:147–165, 1990.

Owen A M: Cognitive planning in humans: Neuropsychological, neuroanatomical and neuropharmacological perspectives. Prog Neurobiol 53:431–450, 1997.

Petrides M, Alivisates B, Meyer E, et al: Functional activation of the human frontal cortex during the performance of verbal working memory tasks. Proc Natl Acad Sci U S A 90:878–882, 1993.

Prigatano GP: Learning from our successes and failures: Reflections and comments on Cognitive rehabilitation: How it is and how it might be. J Int Neuropsychol Soc 3:497–499, 1997.

Porrino LJ, Crane AM, Golman-Rakic PS: Direct and indirect pathways from the amygdala to the frontal lobe in the rhesus monkey. J Comp Neurol 198:121–136, 1981.

Price JL: Networks within the orbital and medial prefrontal cortex. Neurocase 5:231–241, 1999.

Price JL, Carmichael ST, Drevets WC: Networks related to the orbital and medial prefrontal cortex: A substrate for emotional behavior? Prog Brain Res 107:523–536, 1996.

Ptak R, Schnider A: Spontaneous confabulations after orbitofrontal damage: The role of temporal context confusion and self-monitoring. Neurocase 5:243–250, 1999.

Rolls ET: A theory of emotion, and its application to understanding the neural basis of emotion. Cogn Emotion 4:161–190, 1990.

Rolls ET: The functions of the orbitofrontal cortex. Neurocase 5:301–312, 1999.

Rolls ET, Hornak J, Wade D, et al: Emotion-related learning in patients with social and emotional changes associated with frontal lobe damage. J Neurol Neurosurg Psychiatry 57:1518–1524, 1994.

Sarazin M, Pillon B, Giannakopoulos P, et al: Clinicometabolic dissociation of cognitive functions and social behavior in frontal lobe lesions. Neurology 51:142–147, 1998.

Satish U, Streufert S, Eslinger PJ: Complex decision making after orbitofrontal damage: Neuropsychological and strategic management simulation assessment. Neurocase 5:355–364, 1999.

Sohlberg MM, Mateer C: Training use of compensatory memory books: A three-stage behavioral approach. J Clin Exp Neuropsychol 11:871–891, 1989.

Shallice T: From Neuropsychology to Mental Structure. New York: Cambridge University Press, 1988.

Sirigu A, Zalla T, Pillon J, et al: Selective impairments in managerial knowledge following prefrontal cortex damage. Cortex 31:301–316, 1995.

Spreen O, Strauss E: A Compendium of Neuropsychological Tests. New York: Oxford University Press, 1998.

Stuss D, Benson DF: The Frontal Lobes. New York: Raven Press, 1986.

Stuss DT, Gow CA, Hetherington CR: "No longer Gage": Frontal lobe dysfunction and emotional changes. J Consult Clin Psychol 60:349–359, 1992.

Stuss DT, Knight RT: Principles of Frontal Lobe Function. Oxford: Oxford University Press, 2002.

Tranel D, Anderson SW, Benton A: Development of the concept of "executive function" and its relationship to the frontal lobes, in Boller F, Grafman J (eds): Handbook of Neuropsychology, Vol. 9. Amsterdam: Elsevier Science BV, 1994, pp. 125–148.

Tranel D, Eslinger PJ (eds): Effects of early onset damage on the development of cognition and behavior. Dev Neuropsychol 18:273–454, 2000.

Tulving E, Kapur S, Craik FIM, et al: Hemisphere encoding/retrieval symmetry in episodic memory: Positron emission tomography findings. Proc Natl Acad Sci U S A 91:2016–2020, 1994.

Ungerleider LG, Courtneyi SM, Haxbry JV: A neural system for human visual working memory. Proceedings Nat Acad Sci U S A 95:883–890, 1998.

Uylings HBM, Van Eden CG, DeBruin JPC, et al (eds): The prefrontal cortex: Its structure, function and pathology. Prog Brain Res 85, 1990.

Welsh MC, Pennington BF, Grossier DB: A normative-developmental study of executive function: A window on prefrontal function in children. Dev Neuropsychol 7:131–149, 1991.

Wharton CM, Grafman J, Flitman SS, et al: Toward neuroanatomical models of analogy: A positron emission tomography study of analogical mapping. Cog Psychol 40:173–197, 2000.

Wilson BA: Cognitive rehabilitation: How it is and how it might be. J Int Neuropsychol Soc 3:487–496, 1997.

Wilson BA: Compensating for cognitive deficits following brain injury. Neuropsychol Rev 10:223–243, 2000.

Wilson FAW, Oscalaidhe SP, Goldman-Rakic PS: Dissociation of object and spatial processing domains in primate prefrontal cortex. Science 260:1955–1958, 1993.

World Health Organization. The World Health Report. Geneva: Author, 2000.

Emotion

Ralph Adolphs
Daniel Tranel

Amygdala
Emotion
Facial expression
Fear
Mood
Orbitofrontal cortex

INTRODUCTION

Emotion is a topic of paramount importance both from the viewpoint of basic research on the nervous system as well as from clinical neurosciences. Nearly all cognitive functions are modulated in important ways by emotion; emotion influences how we think, what we pay attention to, what we remember, and what we decide to do. Emotion also figures prominently in neurologic diseases, including Alzheimer disease, head injury, stroke, and seizure disorders; in neuropsychiatric disorders such as schizophrenia and autism; and of course in bona fide mood disorders such as depression, anxiety disorders, or phobias. No less importantly, emotion influences our functioning outside the realm of pathology in how individuals adapt to situations in everyday life. An increasing research effort is being aimed at understanding how individual differences in emotional style contribute to coping styles, career success, and interpersonal relationships, and how they reflect components of personality.

The important role played by emotion in both health and disease is mirrored by a number of tracks of scientific investigations that are currently underway; basic research in animals and humans is complemented by a large literature on studies in clinical populations. This chapter gives an overview of these diverse approaches and attempts to tie some of the findings from basic research to their relevance to diagnosis, management, and treatment strategies in clinical disease.

WHAT IS AN EMOTION?

When the psychologist and philosopher William James wrote a paper with the eponymous title in the 19th century, he proposed an account of emotion that has resurfaced in modern times (James, 1884; Damasio, 1994). Somewhat counter to how we might intuitively think about emotion, current research supports a theoretical framework with the following components. Suppose you see an emotional stimulus—say, as James did, you see a bear chasing after you. First, of course, your brain needs to construct a perceptual representation of the bear; that is, you have to perceive it visually. This relies on neural activity in visual and visual association cortices. Subsequent to perceiving the bear, your brain needs to link the perception to the elicitation of behaviors and cognitive processes that will provide an adaptive response to the bear. For instance, in terms of behaviors, your heart rate would accelerate, your blood pressure would rise, and blood would be diverted from your digestive system toward large leg muscles so that you can sprint away. No less importantly, in terms of cognitive changes, your general wakefulness and arousal would increase, your attention to the bear would increase, and you would probably stop thinking about anything other than the bear! All of this, the changes in your body, and the changes in cognitive processes, constitutes the emotional response to the bear. Note that it consists of many different components, but that all the components are concerted and executed together so as to generate a coherent, adaptive overall response that will maximize your survival chances. So, we have the perception of the bear, the emotional response to the bear, and subsequent to this emotional response (or at least to some components of it), you also feel the emotion—typically, you feel afraid. This was the key insight provided by William James—he proposed that we run away from the bear first and feel the fear only afterward. Of course, this is not entirely accurate because common experience tells us that we often feel an emotion prior to exhibiting emotional behaviors. But the key point is that at least some early, rapid components of an emotional response (or, perhaps, even just a central representation of such a response) needs to occur prior to feeling the emotion. This is because feeling the emotion is precisely that: we feel the emotional response. There has to be something there first, some emotional response, for us to feel it. This scheme is depicted in Figure 21-1.

In some ways this view just pushes the question of what an emotion is one step further back. Now the question becomes: what counts as an emotional response, or in other words, what is it that makes a response *emotional*? The answer to this question is somewhat more complicated because it boils down to

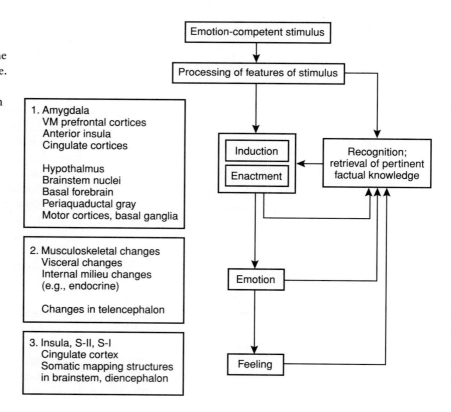

FIGURE 21-1. Schematic framework for the processing of emotion. On the left are candidate neural structures; to the right are the component processes in which they participate. A key question concerns the separation of the different processes shown. To what degree can those different processes be functionally or anatomically separated? For instance, could one apportion some structures in box 1 to "induction" but not "enactment"? Can damage to particular structures impair the processes from one aspect of emotion while leaving other processes relatively unaffected? Answers to these questions depend on the grain of the investigation. Our working assumption is that there will be some separation of processes and of structures, at the systems level, but that a considerable functional overlap should also be expected. That is why some of the structures in box 1 reappear in box 3.

"semantic" issues over what we mean by the word "emotion." Roughly, as indicated in the example above, an emotional response is a response that (1) involves multiple physiologic systems in a concerted manner; (2) depends on the detection, appraisal, or evaluation in some way of the significance or value of the stimulus to the organism; and (3) maximizes the long-term survival of the organism, that is, it is adaptive. The complexity arises in that there is a very large class of responses that satisfy all three criteria (the majority of behaviors perhaps do so, but we might not want to call all of them emotional). In attempting to further restrict our notion of emotion, it is useful to begin with a phylogenetic view of emotions. The most primitive class of responses that satisfy the above criteria are those linked to processing basic homeostatic information, such as brainstem and hypothalamic circuits for regulating blood pressure, oxygen saturation, or fluid balance. This constitutes the core of an emotional response—those responses that regulate immediate survival and homeostasis. All organisms possess such mechanisms in some form or other, although in the simplest cases they may not rely on neural mechanisms. Somewhat more phylogenetically advanced is what we might call "motivation," classes of responses that regulate an organism's survival to external stimuli that are rewarding or punishing. Layered still on top of this are finer differentiations: stimuli are not all aversive in the same way, for instance. At some stage in this hierarchical scheme, we finally encounter differentiations in value-related sets of reactions to stimuli that correspond to what we would call emotions: happiness, fear, anger, disgust, sadness, and so on. It remains an open question precisely at what point we want to call a motivated behavior an "emotional" behavior and what emotion categories we want to specify. Typically, researchers working in animal research have taken a simpler scheme in which reward and punishment are the only two "emotions," whereas basic research in humans has often used so-called basic emotions like fear, disgust, or anger, and research in psychiatry or in social psychology has used even more complex states such as jealousy, embarrassment, or other "social" emotions. A list of some of the ways of categorizing emotional states is given in Table 21-1.

In whatever way we divide up emotions, we can draw some other boundaries depending on the stage of processing. One useful division is three-part: (1) input processing—the perception and recognition of emotional stimuli; (2) output processing—emotional reaction/ expression on the part of the subject; and (3) subjective experience of emotion—the feeling of the emotion. All three of these sets of processes, while to some extent distinct, are closely related and depend in part on one another. It is thus often the case that impairments in one of them are correlated with impairments in another— many patients who experience or express emotions abnormally are also impaired in recognizing emotions in other people, for example. This has implications for clinical approaches to emotion; it may be useful to consider not just emotion perception, or emotional expression, or feeling, in isolation, but rather to consider all three of them together, both for purposes of diagnosis as well as treatment. In some sense, one might say that the clinical approach to emotions should be more "holistic," which is not to say that one cannot focus on certain core processes or structures that are dysfunctional, or that some of the more reductionist findings from basic research, especially in animals, are not useful, but one typically needs to consider the patient's functioning in a complex social setting, their interaction with other people, their perceptions of and behaviors toward others, and their internal emotional lives as one

TABLE 21-1. Classes of Emotional States

Behavioral states	Motivational state	Moods, Background emotions	Basic emotions	Social emotions
Approach	Reward	Depression	Happiness	Pride
Withdrawal	Punishment	Anxiety	Fear	Embarrassment
		Mania	Anger	Guilt
	Thirst		Disgust	Shame
	Hunger	Cheerfulness	Sadness	Maternal Love
	Pain	Contentment	(Surprise)	Jealousy
	Craving	Worry	(Contempt)	Infatuation
		.		Admiration
		.		Sexual Love
		.		(Awe)
				(Submission)
				(Dominance)

complex package, no part of which can be entirely ignored.

HISTORICAL STUDIES IN ANIMALS

We begin with a brief overview of basic research in animals. Early studies of the neural substrates of emotion-related behavior in nonhuman animals used both lesion and stimulation methods. In the 1920s, Philip Bard and Walter Cannon observed behaviors in decorticate cats that appeared similar to extreme anger or rage. Brain transections produced behaviors including tail lashing, limb jerking, biting, clawing, and increased autonomic activity. They termed this *sham rage* because they thought it occurred without conscious emotional experience (i.e., without feeling the emotion) and because it was elicited by very mild stimuli, such as light touches. Further research showed that when the lateral hypothalamus was included in the transected region, sham rage was not observed. More focal lesions of the lateral hypothalamus were found to result in placidity, and lesions of medial hypothalamus to result in irritability. This observation correlated with the results of stimulation experiments performed around the same time by Walter Hess. Hess implanted electrodes into different areas of the hypothalamus and observed different constellations of behaviors depending on electrode placement. Stimulation of the lateral hypothalamus in cats resulted in increased blood pressure, arching of the back, and other autonomic and somatic responses associated with anger. These results led to a concept of the hypothalamus as an organizer and integrator of the autonomic and behavioral components of emotional responses.

A second key neuroanatomic finding in animals was the observation by Klüver and Bucy in 1937, who showed that large bilateral lesions of the temporal lobe, including the amygdala, produced a syndrome in monkeys such that the animals appeared unable to recognize the emotional significance of stimuli (Klüver & Bucy, 1939). For instance, the monkeys would be unusually tame and approach and handle stimuli, such as snakes, of which normal monkeys are afraid.

On the basis of these animal findings, as well as on the basis of findings in humans, early theorists proposed several neural structures as important components of a system that processes emotion. One of the most influential of these, put forth by Paul MacLean in the 1940s and 1950s, was the notion of a so-called "limbic system," encompassing the amygdala, septal nuclei, and orbitofrontal and cingulate cortices, which was interposed between, and mediated between, neocortical systems concerned with perceiving, recognizing, and thinking, on the one hand, and brainstem and hypothalamic structures concerned with emotional reaction and homeostasis, on the other hand (MacLean, 1955).

While the concept of a specific limbic system is debated, the idea is useful to distinguish some of the functional components of emotion, as we have done in the above sections. A key insight is the need for specific structures that can link sensory processing (e.g., the perception of a stimulus) to autonomic, endocrine, and somatomotor effector structures in hypothalamus, periaqueductal gray, and other midbrain and brainstem nuclei. In the next section, we discuss various structures that play a role either in linking sensory processing to emotional behavior, or in effecting the body-state changes of emotion.

NEURAL STRUCTURES THAT PROCESS EMOTION IN HUMANS

Right Cerebral Hemisphere

Both clinical and experimental studies have suggested that the right hemisphere is preferentially involved in processing emotion in humans and other primates. Lesions in right temporal and parietal cortices have been shown to impair emotional experience, arousal, and imagery for emotion. It has been proposed that the right hemisphere contains specific structures important for nonverbal affect computation, which may have evolved to subserve aspects of social cognition (Bowers et al., 1993).

Recent functional imaging studies have corroborated the role of the right hemisphere in emotion recognition from facial expressions and from prosody. There is currently some argument over the extent to which the right hemisphere participates in emotion. Is it specialized to process all emotions (the *right hemisphere hypothesis*), or is it specialized only for processing emotions of negative valence while the left hemisphere is specialized for processing emotions of positive valence (the *valence hypothesis*)? It may well be that an answer to this issue will depend on more precise specification of which components of emotion are under consideration (Borod, 1992; Davidson & Hugdahl, 1995; Canli, 1999; Davidson & Irwin, 1999).

Recognition of emotional facial expressions can be selectively impaired following damage to cortical sectors in right hemisphere, and both positron emission tomography (PET) and neuronal recordings corroborate the importance of right parietal cortex for processing facial expressions of emotion. For example, lesions restricted to the right somatosensory cortex result in impaired recognition of emotion from visual presentation of face stimuli, and this impairment seems to hold across all basic emotions, consistent with the right hemisphere hypothesis mentioned above.

In contrast to recognition of emotional stimuli, emotional experience appears to be lateralized in a pattern supporting the valence hypothesis, in which the left hemisphere is more involved in positive emotions and the right hemisphere more involved in negative emotions. Richard Davidson (1992) has posited an approach/withdrawal dimension, correlating increased right hemisphere activity with increases in withdrawal behaviors (including emotions such as fear or sadness, as well as depressive tendencies), and increased left hemisphere activity with increases in approach behaviors (including emotions such as happiness).

Regions in the right hemisphere most critical for the recognition of emotions in other people (e.g., from facial expressions) include the cortex that represents somatosensory information. A study of over 100 patients with focal brain damage demonstrated that subjects with lesions that included somatosensory cortices were, on average, more impaired in their ability to recognize emotion in facial expressions than could be expected by chance (Adolphs et al., 2000). This finding is evidence that the recognition of emotion in others requires the reconstruction in the perceiver of somatosensory representations that simulate what the signaled emotion would feel like. That is, the reconstruction of knowledge about emotions expressed by other people might rely on a simulation of how the emotion would feel in the perceiver (the subject may be unaware of the process of simulation, which could operate covertly). The notion that somatosensory simulation is important to retrieve knowledge about emotions signaled by other individuals is related to the idea that mental simulation guides our knowledge of what goes on in the minds of others, a proposal that has been put forth by philosophers and cognitive scientists. The proposal has received recent attention from the finding of so-called *mirror neurons* in monkey prefrontal cortex that respond when the monkey observes another individual performing an action (Gallese & Goldman, 1999). The idea that we may draw on simulation to obtain information about other people's feelings is part of a broader debate: do we have a theory about other people's mental states (the so-called Theory of Mind view), or do we know about other people's mental states by analogy to our own states, that is, by empathy and simulation (the so-called Simulation view)? The issue has been explored in detail in patients with certain neuropsychiatric disorders, notably autism, in which the patients have difficulty in their social and emotional interaction with other people (see Baron-Cohen, 1995, for a review).

Amygdala

The amygdala is a collection of nuclei deep in the anterior temporal lobe that receive highly processed sensory information from all sensory modalities (with the exception of direct input from the olfactory bulb) and that has extensive, reciprocal connections with a large number of other brain structures whose function can be modulated by emotion (for a review, see Amaral et al., 1992). Specifically, the amygdala has massive connections, both directly and via the thalamus, with the orbitofrontal cortices, which are known to play a key role in planning and making decisions (see below). The amygdala connects with hippocampus, basal ganglia, and basal forebrain, structures that all participate in various aspects of memory and attention. In addition, the amygdala projects to structures, such as the hypothalamus, that are involved in controlling homeostasis and visceral and neuroendocrine output. Consequently, the amygdala is situated so as to link information about external stimuli conveyed by sensory cortices, on the one hand, with modulation of decision-making, memory, and attention, as well as somatic, visceral, and endocrine processes, on the other hand.

Although it has become clear that the amygdala participates in a diverse array of emotional and social behaviors, the mechanisms that underlie this function remain poorly understood. In general terms, the amygdala can participate in emotion in three different ways: (1) it can link perception of stimuli to an emotional response, by virtue of its inputs from sensory cortices and its outputs to control structures such as the hypothalamus, brainstem nuclei, and periaqueductal gray matter; (2) it can link perception of stimuli to modulation of cognition, by virtue of its connections with structures involved in decision making, memory, and attention; and (3) it can link early perceptual processing of stimuli with modulation of such perception via direct feedback. The participation of the amygdala in all three of these mechanisms puts it in the position to globally contribute to affective processing in a concerted manner, by modulating multiple processes simultaneously.

Although the work of Klüver and Bucy mentioned above had already implicated the amygdala in mediating behaviors triggered by the emotional and social relevance of stimuli, by far the most numerous studies of the amygdala in animals have investigated emotion not at the level of social behavior, but at the level of responses to reward and punishment. These studies have demonstrated the role of the amygdala in one type of associative memory: the association between a stimulus and the survival-related value that the stimulus has for the organism. The amygdala is essential to link initially innocuous stimuli with emotional responses on the basis of the apparent causal contingencies between the stimulus and a reinforcer. Although such a mechanism is in principle consistent with the broad role of the amygdala in real-life social and emotional behaviors, it has been best studied in the laboratory as *fear conditioning*. Fear conditioning uses the innate response to danger, which is similar in many mammals and includes freezing in place, increase in blood pressure and heart rate, and release of stress hormones. This response is elicited in fear conditioning by a noxious stimulus such as an electric shock to the foot. If this shock is preceded by an innocuous stimulus, such as a bell, the bell comes to be associated with the shock, and eventually the subject will exhibit the fear response to the bell (for a review, see LeDoux, 1996). The role of the amygdala in associating sensory stimuli with emotional behaviors is supported also by findings at the single-cell level. Neurons within the amygdala modulate their responses on the basis of the rewarding or punishing contingencies of a stimulus (for a review, see Rolls, 1999). Likewise, the responses of neurons in primate amygdala are modulated by socially relevant visual stimuli, such as faces and videos of complex social interactions. It is important to realize that the amygdala is but one component of a distributed neural system that links stimuli with emotional response. Several other structures, all intimately connected with the amygdala, subserve similar roles and together function to regulate emotional and social aspects of behavior (Brothers, 1990; Adolphs, 1999) (Figs. 21-1 and 21-2).

Studies of the amygdala in humans have come primarily from lesion studies and from functional imaging studies (e.g., PET or functional magnetic resonance imaging [fMRI]). These studies have provided evidence that the amygdala responds to emotionally salient stimuli in the visual, auditory, olfactory, and gustatory modalities. Lesion studies involve patients who have had amygdala damage because of encephalitis (such as herpes simplex encephalitis) or other rare diseases, or who have had neurosurgical resection of the amygdala on one side of the brain to ameliorate epilepsy.

As in animals, the human amygdala appears to be important for fear conditioning; amygdala lesions impair the ability to acquire conditioned autonomic responses to stimuli that have been paired with unconditioned aversive stimuli (Bechara et al., 1995), and acquisition of such conditioned responses in normal subjects activates the amygdala in functional imaging studies (Buechel et al., 1998). A variety of neuropsychological tasks have been used in humans to investigate in more detail both the recognition of emotion from stimuli (such as from viewing facial expressions of other people) as well as the experience of emotion triggered by emotional stimuli or emotional memories. Studies of the role of the amygdala in emotion recognition have primarily used photographs of emotional facial expression. One subject with selective bilateral amygdala damage has been studied extensively with regard to her recognition of emotion in these photographs of facial expressions (Fig. 21-3). This subject, 046, has been shown in several different tasks to be specifically and severely impaired in regard to faces of fear (Adolphs & Tranel, 2000). When rating the intensity of emotions in facial expressions, 046 consistently failed to rate the emotions of surprise, fear, and anger as very intense. She was particularly impaired in rating the intensity of fear, on several occasions failing to recog-

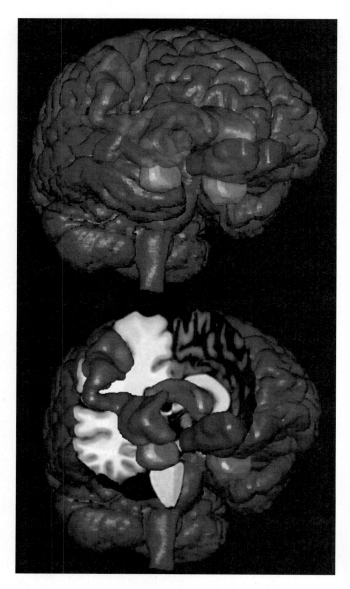

FIGURE 21-2. Neuroanatomy of a few of the structures implicated in processing emotion. Three-dimensional renderings of the amygdala (yellow), ventromedial prefrontal cortex (red), right somatosensory cortices (S-I, S-II, and insula; green) and for orientation the lateral ventricles (light blue) were obtained from segmentation of these structures from serial magnetic resonance images of a normal human brain. The structures were corendered with a three-dimensional reconstruction of the normal brain (top) and a reconstruction of the brain with the anterior right quarter removed to clearly show location of the internal structures (bottom). Images prepared by Ralph Adolphs, Hanna Damasio, and John Haller, Human Neuroimaging and Neuroanatomy Laboratory. (See Color Plate 8)

nize any fear whatsoever in prototypical facial expressions of fear (Adolphs et al., 1995).

046's spontaneous naming of the emotions shown in faces, in a labeling experiment using identical stimuli, was impaired, relative to normal controls; she virtually

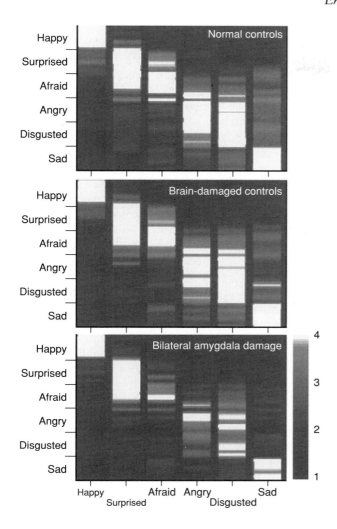

FIGURE 21-3. Bilateral amygdala damage impairs recognition of multiple negative emotions. Raw rating scores of facial expressions of emotion are shown from 7 normal controls, from 16 brain-damaged controls with no amygdala damage, and from 8 subjects with bilateral amygdala damage (Adolphs et al., 1999). The emotional stimuli (36 faces; 6 each of the 6 basic emotions indicated) are ordered on the y-axis according to their perceived similarity (stimuli perceived to be similar, for example, happy and surprised faces, are adjacent; stimuli perceived to be dissimilar, e.g., happy and sad faces, are distant). The six emotion labels on which subjects rated the faces are displayed on the x-axis. Grayscale brightness encodes the mean rating given to each face by a group of subjects, as indicated in the scale. Thus, a darker line would indicate a lower mean rating than a brighter line for a given face; a thin bright line for a given emotion category would indicate that few stimuli of that emotion received a high rating, whereas a thick bright line would indicate that many or all stimuli within that emotion category received high ratings. Because very few mean ratings were less than 1 or more than 4, we truncated the graphs outside these values. Data from subjects with bilateral amygdala damage indicate abnormally low ratings of negative emotions (thinner bright bands across any horizontal position corresponding to an expression of a negative emotion). (From Adolphs R, Tranel D, Hamann S, et al: Recognition of facial emotion in nine subjects with bilateral amygdala damage. Neuropsychologia 37:1111–1117, 1999; copyright Elsevier Science Publishers, 1999.)

never used the label "fear," typically mislabeling such faces as surprised, angry, or disgusted. Thus, subject 046's impairment in recognizing emotional facial expressions is disproportionately severe with respect to fear. However, she also has lesser impairments in recognition of highly arousing emotions that are similar to fear, such as anger. This is consistent with a more general impairment in recognition of negative emotions observed in other subjects with bilateral amygdala damage (Adolphs et al., 1999) (Fig. 21-3), and leads to the question of how specific the amygdala's role is in recognition of certain emotions. Interestingly, subject 046 is also impaired in her ratings of the degree of arousal present in facial expressions of emotion. Asked to place photographs of emotional facial expressions on a grid with valence (positive/negative) and arousal (low/high) as orthogonal axes, subject 046 was normal in her valence ratings, but abnormal in the level of arousal that she assigned to negative facial expressions. The amygdala may thus play a role in recognizing highly arousing, unpleasant emotions—in other words, emotions that signal potential harm to the organism— and in triggering rapid physiologic states related to these stimuli. In animals, the amygdala may trigger pre-

dominantly behavioral reactions; in humans it may trigger both behavior and conscious knowledge that the stimulus predicts something "bad."

Functional imaging studies in normal individuals have corroborated the lesion studies implicating the amygdala in recognition of signals of unpleasant and arousing emotions (Morris et al., 1996). Visual, auditory, olfactory, and gustatory stimuli have all been reported to engage the amygdala when signaling unpleasant and arousing emotions, although the evidence is strongest for aversive olfactory stimuli (Royet et al., 2000). The functional imaging studies have examined the encoding and recognition of emotional stimuli, as well as emotional experience and emotional response (for a review, see Davidson & Irwin, 1999), but it has been exceedingly difficult to disentangle all these different components. Although there is now clear evidence of amygdala activation during encoding of emotional material (Cahill et al., 1996; Hamann et al., 1999), it is less clear whether the amygdala is also activated during retrieval.

A further insight has come from studies that used stimuli that could not be consciously perceived. Amygdala activation has been observed when subjects viewed facial expressions of fear that were presented so briefly they could not be consciously recognized, showing that the amygdala plays a role in nonconscious processing of emotional stimuli (Whalen et al., 1998). Such nonconscious processing may rely on visual inputs to the amygdala via the superior colliculus and pulvinar thalamus, rather than the usual route via visual cortices (Morris et al., 1999). In summary, an important function of the amygdala may be to trigger responses and to allocate processing resources to stimuli that may be of special importance or threat to the organism, and ecological considerations as well as the data adduced above all appear to argue for such a role, especially in regard to rapid responses that need not involve conscious awareness.

The automaticity of emotional reactions triggered by the amygdala also has important clinical implications. It is likely that phobias and post-traumatic stress disorder include as part of their neurobiologic pathology dysfunction within the amygdala. A functional imaging study found that the amygdala was activated when subjects with social phobia viewed other people's faces, even though the faces showed neutral expressions (Birbaumer et al., 1998).

The amygdala also plays a more pervasive role in social behavior, extending to making complex social judgments of other people. For instance, subjects with bilateral amygdala damage are impaired in judging when other people look untrustworthy (Adolphs et al., 1998), and when normal subjects view faces of another race, they show amygdala activations that correlate with implicit measures of race stereotyping (Phelps et al., 2000). Several studies point toward an involvement of amygdala pathology in autism, and it is possible that some of the impaired social functioning seen in subjects with autism can be attributed to amygdala dysfunction. Taken together, the findings to date clearly show that the amygdala is important for social cognition and point to a relatively disproportionate role in regard to rapid processing of ambiguous, potentially threatening or dangerous stimuli.

Orbitofrontal Cortex

In animals, lesions of the orbitofrontal cortex can produce impairments quite similar to those seen following amygdala damage. As in the amygdala, single-neuron responses in the orbitofrontal cortex are modulated by the emotional significance of stimuli, such as their rewarding and punishing contingencies, although the role of the orbitofrontal cortex may be more general and less stimulus-bound than that of the amygdala. Amygdala and orbitofrontal cortex are bidirectionally connected, and lesion studies have shown that disconnecting the two structures results in impairments similar to those following lesions of either structure, providing further support that they function as components of a densely connected network.

Prefrontal and anterior cingulate cortices have been implicated in emotional behaviors in humans for some time; the prefrontal region was first highlighted by the famous case of Phineas Gage (Damasio, 1994), and the anterior cingulate cortex has been the topic of a large number of recent functional imaging studies that have assigned to it emotional, attentional, and "executive" functions (Bush et al., 2000). Both regions appear to participate in response selection, decision making, and volitional control of behavior, a collection of processes that figures prominently in emotional and social behaviors.

Damage to the frontal lobes, particularly to orbitofrontal cortex, results in impaired social behavior in primates (see Chapter 20). In humans, the impairment is notable for an inability to organize and plan future activity, a diminished capacity to respond to punishment, stereotyped and sometimes inappropriate social manners, and an apparent lack of concern for other individuals, all in the face of otherwise normal intellectual functioning. Recent functional imaging studies, as well as studies in nonhuman primates, have confirmed a role for the ventral prefrontal cortices in linking interoceptive and exteroceptive information (Cavada & Schultz, 2000), a function in which it participates together with a network of other structures, notably the amygdala and ventral striatum. A study in a rare neurosurgical patient found single-unit responses in the orbitofrontal cortex that were selective for socially and emotionally aversive visual stimuli (pictures of mutilations and war scenes) (Kawasaki et al., 2001), findings complementing those obtained from recordings in the orbitofrontal cortex of animals (Rolls, 1999).

Studies using a gambling task have shown that subjects with damage to the ventromedial frontal cortex are unable to represent choice bias in the form of an emotional hunch (Bechara et al., 1994), findings consistent with prior reports that subjects with such damage are unable to trigger normal emotional responses to socially relevant stimuli. These data have corroborated the somatic marker hypothesis (Damasio, 1994, 1996), which proposes that the prefrontal cortex participates in implementing a particular mechanism by which we acquire, represent, and retrieve the values of our actions. This mechanism relies on generating somatic states, or representations of somatic states, that correspond to the anticipated future outcome of decisions. Such "somatic markers" steer the decision-making process toward those outcomes that are advantageous for the individual, based on the individual's past experience with similar situations. Such a mechanism may be of special importance in the social domain, where the enormous complexity of the decision space typically precludes an exhaustive analysis.

The cingulate cortex, including both anterior and posterior sectors (as well as the posteriorly adjacent retrosplenial cortex), plays a key role in emotion and in social behavior. Damage to the anterior cingulate cortex can result in a gross loss of motivation (akinetic mutism), and this region is activated in normal subjects by emotional versions of the Stroop task (Bush et al., 2000), supporting the idea that it helps monitor errors and response conflicts.

Basal Ganglia

A long history of studies shows that the basal ganglia, especially on the right, participate in emotion. Lesions to the basal ganglia in either hemisphere can result in impaired recognition of emotion from a variety of stimuli (Cancelliere & Kertesz, 1990). Functional imaging studies have reported differential activation in the right basal ganglia when comparing the perception of happy faces to fearful faces (Morris et al., 1996), or when comparing sad to neutral faces (Phillips et al., 1997). Both lesion and functional imaging studies suffer from their relatively poor spatial resolution in investigations of the basal ganglia, which consist of many different nuclei and white matter tracts in close spatial proximity. Additional insights are offered by diseases that preferentially damage certain sectors of the basal ganglia.

Three diseases that involve the basal ganglia have been investigated in some detail regarding emotion processing: obsessive-compulsive disorder, Parkinson disease (PD), and Huntington disease (HD). Subjects with obsessive-compulsive disorder (OCD) experience abnormal feelings of disgust and are impaired also in the recognition of facial expressions of disgust (Sprengelmeyer et al., 1997), and one of the neural correlates of this impairment may be the dysfunction of sectors of the basal ganglia affected in this disease. PD first damages the motor components of the basal ganglia and results in impaired emotional expression; but impaired feeling of the emotion and impaired recognition of emotion in other people may also result from this disease. There is a curious finding in patients with HD: a disproportionate impairment in recognizing disgust from facial expressions (Jacobs et al., 1995; Sprengelmeyer et al., 1996). Especially intriguing is the finding that subjects who carry the gene for HD show impairments in recognition of disgust prior to the onset of any other symptoms (Gray et al., 1997), possibly making the recognition impairment one of the earliest phenotypic markers of the disease. As with other evidence accrued in the discussions above, the basal ganglia point to the close involvement of emotional experience, of the motor expression of facial expressions of emotion, and of their recognition from visual stimuli. It is of interest to note here that electrical stimulation of the basal ganglia (probably primarily in the substantia nigra) in a neurosurgical patient resulted in the acute and intense experience of emotion (a feeling of sadness, in this case) as well as of its expression in the face (Dejjani et al., 1999).

Other Structures

Several other structures link stimulus perception to emotional response. Work in rats has highlighted nuclei situated very close to the amygdala, such as the bed nucleus of the stria terminalis, and emphasized their role in anxiety (Davis et al., 1997); the neuropeptide corticotropin-releasing factor plays a key role in this system. Other nuclei in the vicinity, such as the substantia innominata and nuclei in the septum, are also important and may mediate their effects through the neurotransmitter acetylcholine.

There are collections of nuclei in the brainstem that can modulate brain function in a rather global fashion by virtue of very diverse projections. The locus ceruleus, a very small set of nuclei, provides the brain with its sole source of noradrenergic innervation. Similarly, the Raphe nuclei provide a broad innervation of serotonergic terminals. These neuromodulatory nuclei, together with the dopaminergic and cholinergic nuclei mentioned above, are thus in a position to alter information processing globally in the brain. It is important to emphasize again that these changes in the brain's information processing mode are just as important as the somatic components of an emotional reaction—and just as noticeable when we feel the emotion.

Another important region is the ventral striatum. Structures such as the nucleus accumbens receive input from the amygdala and appear to be especially important for processing rewarding stimuli and for engaging the behaviors that cause an organism to seek stimuli that predict reward. The amygdala, ventral striatum, and orbitofrontal cortex all participate jointly in guiding an organism's expectation of reward on the basis of prior experience. Recent single-unit studies in animals dissect some of the specific component processes subserved by these different structures and have pointed to an important neurochemical system subserving the functional connectivity between ventral striatum and frontal cortex: the neurotransmitter dopamine. This system and the specific neurotransmitters involved are currently intensively investigated as models of drug addiction (Everitt et al., 1999), and they likely play a role also in psychiatric disorders ranging from depression to schizophrenia.

The structures involved in emotional reaction and behavior include essentially all structures that control motor, autonomic, and endocrine output. Some of these structures have further internal organization that permits them to trigger a coordinated set of responses. For instance, motor structures in the basal ganglia control some of the somatic components of emotional response, and distinct regions in the hypothalamus trigger concerted emotional reactions of fear or aggression, as we mentioned at the beginning of this chapter. Another important structure is the periaqueductal gray (PAG), which consists of multiple columns of cells surrounding the aqueduct in the midbrain. Stimulation of these areas has long been known to produce panic-like behavioral and autonomic changes, as well as reports of panic-like feelings in humans. Moreover, different columns within the PAG appear to be important for different components of emotional response (see Panksepp, 1998, for a review).

NEUROPSYCHIATRIC ASPECTS OF EMOTION

Emotion is a topic of paramount importance to the diagnosis, treatment, and theoretical understanding of many neuropsychiatric disorders. The amygdala has received considerable attention in this regard, and this structure has been shown to be especially involved in disorders that center around fear and anxiety. Moreover, specific neurotransmitters, acting within the amygdala and surrounding structures, have been shown to contribute importantly to fear and anxiety. Anxiolytic drugs such as Valium, for instance, bind to γ-aminobutyric acid A (GABA-A) receptor subtypes in the amygdala and alter the neuronal excitability there. Corticotropin-releasing factor is an anxiogenic peptide that appears to act in the amygdala and adjacent nuclei. Several functional imaging studies have demonstrated that phobic and depressive symptoms rely on abnormal activity within the amygdala, together with abnormalities in other brain structures. Another region that has been implicated in many psychiatric conditions is the frontal lobes. Below, we review some of the most prevalent neuropsychiatric manifestations of abnormal emotion processing, and some of their putative neuroanatomic correlates, with particular emphasis on the amygdala and frontal lobes.

Depression and Mania

The development of major depression has been associated with damage to the frontal lobes. Starkstein and Robinson (1991) identified several factors that seem to play a consistent role in the relationship between depression and frontal lobe injury: (1) side of lesion: major depression is more strongly associated with *left* frontal lesions. In contrast, right frontal lesions tend to produce a sort of apathetic indifference or even cheerfulness; (2) proximity of the lesion to the frontal pole: lesions closer to the pole are associated with more severe depression; (3) depression has been associated with lesions to the frontal opercular region and to the dorsolateral prefrontal sector. By contrast, depression following ventromedial prefrontal lesions is extremely uncommon (see Barrash et al., 2000). In fact, it has been suggested that ventromedial lesions may sometimes

produce conditions that are more akin to mania, although this issue has not been studied sufficiently.

Functional imaging studies have begun to provide some corroborative evidence regarding the relationships between prefrontal lobe structures and depression and mania. Drevets and colleagues (1997), using PET, found that a region under the genu of the corpus callosum—termed the "subgenual" region—was consistently *under*activated in patients with either unipolar (who suffer depression only) or bipolar (who alternate between depression and mania) depression. By contrast, the subgenual region was activated during periods of mania. Drevets and colleagues also found that the *size* of this region (gray matter volume) was consistently reduced in the left hemisphere of depressive patients compared with normal controls. This result is broadly consistent with the ideas proposed by Starkstein and Robinson (1991), reviewed above. The importance of the finding by Drevets and colleagues is underscored when placed in the context of the fact that this region has been implicated in the modulation of neurotransmitters such as serotonin, noradrenaline, and dopamine. Interestingly, the activity of these neurotransmitter systems is often blunted in patients with major depression and is augmented by antidepressant drugs (Goodwin & Jamison, 1990).

Schizophrenia

Schizophrenia has also been linked to dysfunction of frontal lobe structures (Weinberger et al., 1991), among a number of other brain regions (Andreasen et al., 1992, 1994). For a number of years, investigators have noted that many of the neuropsychological abnormalities seen in patients with schizophrenia bear a striking resemblance to those evidenced by patients with frontal lobe lesions. For example, both types of patients fail complex neuropsychological decision-making tasks such as the Wisconsin Card Sorting Test and the Tower of Hanoi (Andreasen et al., 1992). More direct support comes from studies using functional imaging approaches, which have shown, for example, that schizophrenic patients have decreased regional cerebral blood flow (rCBF) in prefrontal regions (Ingvar & Franzen, 1974). This pattern of "hypofrontality" has been found in a number of studies, particularly activation paradigms in which patients were engaged in a cognitive task that normally activates frontal lobe structures (Andreasen et al., 1992). Structural brain abnormalities in the frontal lobes may be most strongly related to what is known as the "negative" symptomatology of schizophrenia, such as apathy, blunted affect, social withdrawal, and impaired attention (Malloy & Duffy, 1994).

Neural Correlates of Violent Behavior

The neural correlates of violent and aggressive behavior include various "limbic" structures, such as the amygdala, hypothalamus, cingulate gyrus, septal nucleus, anterior thalamus, and anterior temporal lobe (Moyer, 1976; Volavka, 1995). Another region that has received considerable attention in connection with violent and aggressive behavior is the frontal lobes, especially the orbital and lower mesial portions.

Hypothalamus

Older reviews of the nonhuman animal literature documented the relationship between damage to the ventromedial hypothalamic region and the development of aggressive, ragelike behavior (Moyer, 1976; Valzelli, 1981), as we mentioned earlier. A similar relationship has been hinted at in humans (Weiger & Bear, 1988). According to Malamud (1967), most destructive lesions in the hypothalamic region associated with aggressive behavior and rage reactions are neoplastic in nature, and most are bilateral.

Amygdala and Anterior Temporal Lobe

The importance of the amygdala and nearby anterior temporal lobe structures in the modulation of aggressive behavior has been emphasized in a number of studies, in humans and other animals, and these findings are very consistent with other data showing the importance of these regions for a wide range of emotional behaviors, as reviewed earlier. Dysfunction of these structures has been associated with violent and aggressive behavior in psychiatric patients and patients with a history of epilepsy (Volkow & Tancredi, 1987; Garyfallos et al., 1988; Tonkonogy, 1991). Convergent evidence comes from studies that have shown that electrical stimulation of the amygdala sometimes produces rage outbursts and other aggressive behavioral manifestations (Mark & Ervin, 1970; Egger & Flynn, 1981; see Kling, 1986, for a review). In fact, the anterior temporal lobes in general have been associated with violent behavior. Volkow and Tancredi (1987), using PET, found that in four patients with repetitive acts of violence, there were blood flow and metabolic abnormalities in the left temporal lobe. Two of the patients also had abnormalities in the frontal cortex. Unilateral or bilateral amygdalotomy has been used to control aggressive behavior, often with favorable outcomes (for reviews, see Goldstein, 1974; Lee et al., 1988). Lee and colleagues have published data on two patients with bilateral amygdalotomy, both of whom showed significant improvement of uncontrollable aggressive behavior following their surgeries (Lee et al., 1988, 1995).

However, the well-studied neurologic cases with bilateral amygdala lesions that we mentioned earlier (see "Amygdala") have actually been shown to have *less* aggression than normal (Adolphs et al., 1994, 1995, 1998). We have studied three patients with extensive bilateral mesial temporal lobe lesions (which include the amygdala), all of whom have a remarkable preference for positive affect and an equally impressive inclination to avoid negative affect. The patient known as Boswell, who has complete bilateral damage to the entire mesial temporal region, provides a striking illustration. For example, when asked to explain what is happening in a picture showing people leaping off a burning ship into the ocean, Boswell said that the people are "swimming, going for a dip." Shown a film clip in which military persons are gunning down a fleeing crowd of civilians, Boswell said that the people are "jogging, exercising." Boswell's behavior in other situations is similar; for example, he is very uncomfortable when placed in situations of social conflict (e.g., when asked to decide which of two experimenters is "nicer").

The findings reviewed here emphasize the fact that it is not possible to draw simple conclusions about cause-and-effect relationships between amygdala dysfunction and violent behavior (Garza-Trevino, 1994; Treiman, 1991). Nonetheless, the weight of the evidence points to a close relationship between amygdala function and modulation of emotion, including regulation of at least some aspects of aggressive behavior. It is interesting to note in this context, as we mentioned earlier, that the role of the amygdala in emotional processing appears to be heavily weighted to negatively valenced emotions, especially fear and anger (Adolphs et al., 1998). These findings are quite consistent with the idea that the amygdala is a critical part of neural systems on which the modulation of aggressive behavior, especially in response to aversive or threatening stimuli, depends.

The Frontal Lobes

A number of lines of evidence have supported the idea that the frontal lobes are related to violent and aggressive behavior, although, as with the case for the amygdala, the relationship is far from simple.

A critical review of the literature was published by Kandel and Freed (1989, p. 410), who concluded that "the evidence for the association between specifically violent criminal behavior and frontal-lobe dysfunction is weak at best." Nevertheless, the authors note that in *all* studies that have explored brain-behavior relationships in regard to violent and psychopathic behavior, it has been concluded that the anterior regions of the brain, including the frontal lobes and anterior temporal lobes, are the most likely neuroanatomic correlates. The fact that there are no exceptions to this pattern supports the conclusion that there is probably at least some credibility to the idea that dysfunction of anterior brain regions (frontal/temporal) could be related to the development of violent and aggressive behavior, provided the needed catalysts are in place.

Another clue comes from studies of patients who sustained frontal lobe injuries early in life, and then went on to have severe impairments in comportment (Grattan & Eslinger, 1991; Anderson et al., 1999, 2000; Eslinger et al., 2000). For example, two cases of this type published by Price and colleagues (1990) both exhibited significant aggressive and violent behavior. However, as we mentioned in regard to adult-onset damage to frontal lobe, it is important to keep in mind that the principal focus of abnormality in these cases, and in virtually all like cases published to date, is in the realm of *social conduct*: the patients make very poor decisions regarding friends, sexual encounters, and occupational pursuits (see review in Tranel, 1994). As Price and colleagues note, the behavioral features of these developmental cases seem to be qualitatively similar to, but quantitatively more severe than, those exhibited by patients who acquire bilateral prefrontal lesions in adulthood. This same point was also emphasized by Anderson and colleagues (1999, 2000) in their report of two developmental cases. Specifically, social misconduct is a central feature, but blatant violence and aggression are not necessarily the predominant manifestations.

Another source of evidence comes from studies of patients with head injuries. Head injuries often produce damage to orbital prefrontal cortices, and such injuries have been associated with a very high incidence of aggressive behavior (see Silver & Yudofsky, 1994, for a review). Silver and Yudofsky (1994) argued that this condition should be classified as a special form of psychiatric disorder, namely, *organic aggressive syndrome*, rather than as a "personality change" as currently designated in the DSM-IV (American Psychiatric Association, 1994) nosology. In general, deficits in emotional processing are extremely common in patients with head injuries. Moreover, such deficits have been postulated to play a fundamental role in the broader impairments that head-injured patients manifest in regard to social conduct and social communication (e.g., Newton & Johnson, 1985). For example, reduced sensitivity to the emotional reactions of others in head-injured individuals has been hypothesized to contribute to poor social functioning (e.g., Cicone et al., 1980; Prigatano & Pribram, 1982; Pettersen, 1991). Newton and Johnson (1985) reported that patients with head injuries had very poor social adjustment following their injury; in fact, this social maladjustment was reminiscent of that typically manifested by psychiatric patients. Also, it has long been noted that the relatives of head-injured patients consider the emotional changes to be greater burdens than either physical or cognitive impairments (Oddy et al., 1978; Brooks & Aughton, 1979). It goes without saying that such impairments are a profound obstacle for rehabilitation efforts, and often, they represent the most debilitating residua of head injury.

Patients with head injuries have been shown to be impaired in their ability to recognize emotional facial expressions and emotionally toned postures (Jackson & Moffat, 1987), and to be impaired in perception of and memory for facial affect (Prigatano & Pribram, 1982). Injury to the right frontal lobe in particular may interfere with affective functioning (Lishman, 1968) and has been implicated specifically in difficulty using facial expression cues (Prigatano & Pribram, 1982). Deficits in emotional processing, including the recognition and interpretation of facial affect, have also been demonstrated in children with head injuries (Pettersen, 1991).

The ventromedial prefrontal region is important for regulation of behavior—social conduct in particular—and it plays a critical role in making decisions. There is little question that dysfunction of this region often leads to maladaptive behavior. However, the vast majority of patients with ventromedial prefrontal damage do *not* engage in violent or aggressive behavior. In fact, many of these patients become rather placid and affectively flat. The reason so many patients with head injury develop aggressive and violent behavior may have to do with a *combination* of orbital prefrontal injury and anterior temporal lobe injury (Relkin et al., 1996; Tranel, 2001). Another possibility is that, while prefrontal cortex, especially in its medial and orbital sectors, broadly participates in regulating emotional and social behaviors, the precise nature of impairments following dysfunction in this region depends on the details of the dysfunction (e.g., hypofunctionality due to the lesion, hyperfunctionality due to other pathology, functional diaschisis in other related neural systems), on the details of the premorbid personality of the affected individual, and on the details of the particular social situation in which the behavior is assessed. Given the complex control of social behavior, and the sensitivity to background personality and environmental circumstances, it should not be too surprising that the way in which dysfunction of the prefrontal cortex actually plays out in terms of real-life behavior is difficult to predict precisely.

Alexithymia

The term *alexithymia* was introduced several decades ago as a descriptor for the condition in which an individual is unable to experience, regulate, and label accurately his or her emotions and feelings (Sifneos, 1972). It is generally considered a personality construct, nosologically akin to traits such as "extraverted" or "narcissistic." From the beginning, the construct has been a rather ambiguous conflation of various aspects of personality traits, emotions and feelings, and verbal labeling abilities, and not surprisingly, the construct has proved highly elusive to empirical investigation. In one of the clearest definitions currently available for alexithymia (Bagby & Taylor, 1997), it is considered to be comprised of the following features: (1) difficulty identifying feelings and distinguishing between feelings and the bodily sensations of emotional arousal; (2) difficulty describing feelings to other people; (3) constricted imaginal processes, as evidenced by a paucity of fantasies; and (4) a stimulus-bound, externally oriented cognitive style. Bagby and Taylor (1997) also emphasize that alexithymia is conceptualized as a dimensional construct, one that is distributed normally in the general population. Accordingly, it is at the extreme ends of the distribution that the construct takes on special importance—in particular, persons who are high on the trait of alexithymia are considered to be at elevated risk for certain medical and psychiatric diseases (Lumley & Norman, 1996).

The initial conceptualizations of alexithymia placed primary emphasis on the individual's inability to put emotions into words. This stress, however, has been questioned by Lane and colleagues (1997a), who have suggested a broader conceptualization, namely, that alexithymia is characterized by a deficit in emotional processing, which may include but is not limited to a difficulty in putting emotions into words. A number of recent studies have provided empirical support for this broader approach to the construct of alexithymia. For example, Lane and colleagues (1996) showed that on a task requiring matching of emotion stimuli to emotion responses, alexithymic individuals were deficient, relative to nonalexithymic individuals, at purely nonverbal matching, purely verbal matching, and mixed verbal-nonverbal matching, suggesting that alexithymia is associated with impaired verbal *and* nonverbal recognition of emotion stimuli.

Lane and colleagues (1997a) have proposed that the fundamental deficit in alexithymia is a limited ability to experience emotion consciously; in extreme cases, the ability may be completely nonexistent. In fact, the authors have gone so far as to propose that alexithymia (at least in extreme form) is an emotional equivalent of blindsight—that is, "blindfeel." Specifically, when alexithymic persons are emotionally aroused, they will manifest behavioral and autonomic responses (which may even be exaggerated), but because of their impaired interoceptive awareness, they will say that they are not feeling anything, or that they do not know how they are feeling. Lane and colleagues (1997b) have proposed that the neurologic basis for this

deficit may involve defective activation of the anterior cingulate cortex.

A recent functional imaging study by Lane and colleagues (1998) provided some support for this idea. Using PET, the investigators found that blood flow changes in the anterior cingulate cortex (ACC), in response to recalling emotional experiences or viewing emotion-inducing films, were correlated with subjects' scores on a level of emotional awareness scale, which measures the capacity to experience emotion in a differentiated and complex fashion. Lane and colleagues suggest that the ability to detect emotional signals, either interoceptively or exteroceptively, may be a function of the degree to which the ACC participates in the experiential processing and response to emotion cues. In other words, ACC activity may provide a neural basis for the conscious experience of emotion. There are other recent functional imaging findings that are consistent with this idea (Lane et al., 1997b; Damasio et al., 1999).

A number of other interesting findings have been reported in studies of alexithymic individuals. Jessimer and Markham (1997) showed that alexithymic subjects were relatively poor at recognizing emotional facial expressions and manifested a weaker leftward perceptual bias in processing chimeric faces (made up of conjoined emotive and nonemotive face halves); the authors argued that their results support a "right hemisphere dysfunction" model of alexithymia. A similar idea has been proposed by Parker and associates (1993), and additional empirical support was provided by Berenbaum and Prince (1994), although both of these studies also reported complicating effects of gender differences. Emotional face recognition deficiencies have been reported in other studies of alexithymic subjects (Parker et al., 1993). Another study showed that alexithymic individuals were inferior to nonalexithymic individuals in an interhemispheric transfer task (tactile finger localization), suggesting that poor integration of information processing of the two cerebral hemispheres plays a role in the alexithymic cognitive style (Parker et al., 1999). This finding was partially replicated by Lumley and Sielky (2000), who found that inefficient interhemispheric transfer was characteristic of male alexithymic subjects, but not female ones.

ASSESSMENT OF MOOD AND EMOTION

It is important in assessing patients with cognitive disturbances caused by neurologic or psychiatric disease to include a careful investigation of the emotional status of the patients. Emotional factors can influence profoundly many aspects of cognition, as has been emphasized repeatedly throughout this chapter, and thus it is absolutely crucial to assess such factors to interpret validly the cognitive performances of a patient. A number of instruments provide reliable and valid means with which to assess mood and emotion in patients, and the most widely used and well researched of these are reviewed briefly here. It should be noted before we begin this review that many of these instruments provide considerable information about personality, as well as mood and emotion, reflecting the large extent to which many personality characteristics overlap with mood and emotion. Our focus here, though, is on mood and emotion, rather than the broader domain of personality.

The Minnesota Multiphasic Personality Inventory

The Minnesota Multiphasic Personality Inventory (MMPI) is a self-report personality inventory developed in the late 1930s by a psychologist (Hathaway) and psychiatrist (McKinley) as a means of measuring various personality traits and states (Hathaway & McKinley, 1940, 1943). A key concept behind the development of the MMPI was that the items were selected on the basis of their ability to discriminate clinical groups from normal populations, in what is termed *criterion keying test construction*. In 1989, the MMPI was revised and updated, and new normative data were published (Butcher et al., 1989); the revised version was termed the MMPI-2. The MMPI-2 is the most widely used personality test in existence, and it has been subjected to literally thousands of research studies (Butcher, 1999; Graham, 2000). Its popularity owes in considerable measure to its enormous success in achieving the original objectives of its creators, namely, distinguishing reliably between individuals with a clinical psychiatric or psychological disorder and normal persons.

Insofar as emotion is concerned, the MMPI-2 is a highly useful test, although it should be kept in mind that the MMPI-2 is aimed at a much broader survey of personality and psychological functioning than simply emotion. Also, the usefulness of the MMPI-2 is rather dependent on the savvy of the clinician who is interpreting the results; hence, it is recommended that the MMPI-2 be kept in the hands of clinical psychologists and other similarly qualified persons who can extract the most valid and meaningful data from the instrument. In this context, the MMPI-2 can profile a wealth of information about the personality makeup of individuals, their psychological strengths and weaknesses, their coping mechanisms and whether such coping mechanisms are effective, behavioral proclivities, and the degree and nature of their socialization. For many personality dimensions, including emotion and mood, information will be available for both *traits* and *states*, traits referring to relatively enduring personality char-

acteristics, and states referring to conditions under which the individual is currently operating, and which may tend to vary considerably from day to day or depending on other vicissitudes.

It is our position that the MMPI-2 should be considered more or less mandatory in the evaluation of any person in the context of assessment of mood and emotion, whether for clinical reasons or for research purposes. The valuable information generated by the MMPI-2 is indispensable to a complete analysis of the mood and emotion of a person and is critical to the interpretation of performances on all manner of other tests, or experiments aimed at assessing aspects of emotional processing. MMPI-2 results are often crucial for determining whether potential subjects meet or do not meet exclusion and inclusion criteria for experiments. In short, the MMPI-2 should be considered carefully as part of the armamentarium of the emotion researcher, not to mention the clinician.

The Beck Scales

Two self-report inventories written by Aaron Beck have gained widespread popularity as convenient and informative measures of important aspects of mood and emotion. The Beck Depression Inventory (BDI; Beck, 1987) provides an easy and quick method for measuring various signs and symptoms of depression, including a wide range of cognitive, behavioral, and somatic problems. The BDI is very useful in determining the presence and severity of depressive symptoms, although it does not yield information about duration. The Beck Anxiety Inventory (BAI) is parallel in construction to the BDI, and focuses in particular on symptomatology related to anxiety. Like the BDI, the BAI is easy and quick to administer. It can yield useful information about patients and research participants in regard to their current state of anxiety and general susceptibility to anxiety.

The Iowa Rating Scales of Personality Change

The Iowa Rating Scales of Personality Change (IPSPC, aka Iowa Scales) were developed as a sensitive and reliable means to measure changes in emotional functioning and personality that occur following brain injury (Barrash et al., 2000). The Iowa Scales use an informant (i.e., someone who knows the patient well, both before and after lesion onset) to rate the patient on various aspects of emotional functioning, behavioral control, social and interpersonal behavior, real-world decision making, and insight. Research on patients with bilateral ventromedial prefrontal lesions has demonstrated that the Iowa Scales identify a core set of disturbances in such patients (Barrash et al., 2000; Tranel, 2002):

(1) general dampening of emotional experience (impoverished emotional experience, low emotional expressiveness, apathy, and inappropriate affect); (2) poorly modulated emotional reactions (poor frustration tolerance, irritability, lability); (3) disturbances in decision making, especially in the social realm (indecisiveness, poor judgment, inflexibility, social inappropriateness, and insensitivity or lack of empathy); (4) disturbances in goal-directed behavior (problems in planning, initiation, persistence, and behavioral rigidity or nonspontaneity); and (5) a striking lack of insight into these personality changes. We have termed this set of characteristics "acquired sociopathy" and have noted parallels between this condition and developmental sociopathy (Barrash et al., 2000). The Iowa Scales have not been researched as extensively as some of the more traditional instruments such as the MMPI, but they show considerable promise as a means of assessing *changes* in emotional functioning as a consequence of brain injury. Perhaps of greatest importance, because they rely on a collateral rather than on the patient, the Iowa Scales are an effective means of circumventing problems associated with self-report instruments, when the individual completing the instrument has major limitations of insight, defects in self-awareness, and the like.

Millon Clinical Multiaxial Inventory

The Millon Clinical Multiaxial Inventory (MCMI; Millon, 1977) is a self-report test that measures a variety of personality traits and states, including aspects of emotional functioning. The MCMI is especially well suited for psychiatric populations and, in general, for individuals with fairly pronounced disturbances of emotion. The test has been updated to reflect the current nosology and nomenclature of DSM-IV (Millon & Davis, 1997). Also, the factor structure of the MCMI has been investigated in some detail, making the test well suited for application to experimental populations (Craig & Bivens, 1998). Like the MMPI-2, the MCMI has been the focus of a considerable amount of research, and its general utility in measuring emotion and personality has been well established (Craig, 1999).

CONCLUDING COMMENTS

It is clear that emotion has now become a major topic of research in cognitive neuroscience and that the methods available to study it, as well as the theoretical frameworks in which the findings can be interpreted, are rapidly gaining sophistication. Future directions in research on the psychological and neurologic bases of facial emotion recognition will build on the findings to date, extend them to broader issues, and attempt to resolve some of the current discrepancies and difficulties. Of special value will be attempts to extend the current findings, almost all of which come from adult humans, to developmental and comparative approaches; studies in infants and in nonhuman primates will provide valuable insights into the ontogenetic and phylogenetic background of emotion recognition. These issues will also relate closely to the investigation of emotions other than the basic ones, on which we have focused in this chapter. Very little is known regarding how we process social/moral emotions, such as shame, pride, or embarrassment.

Another important avenue for further studies is the development of stimuli and tasks with more ecological validity. For instance, nearly all studies of visual emotion recognition to date have used static images of facial expressions, whereas one would want to use dynamic facial expressions, and perhaps also extend their presentation to viewing in specific social contexts that include other social information. After all, we do not make judgments about basic emotions shown in pictures of single faces in real life; we make complex social judgments about fleeting, dynamic facial signals encountered together with body posture and voice stimuli in a certain situation with a social background. Needless to say, approaches to the full complexity of emotional signals available in real life need to tackle this issue in small stages.

Although there is much to be said for having diverse stimuli and tasks, there is also a lot to be said for having a uniform set of stimuli and tasks that could be used across different studies. This seems especially valuable given the burgeoning functional imaging literature on emotion, where quite different tasks often make comparisons between different studies problematic. An ideal situation would be a set of stimuli and tasks that could be used in functional imaging and lesion studies with adult humans, and that might have straightforward analogues that could also be administered to infants and nonhuman primates. Even better would be a set of tasks that could be used not only for research studies, but that would also have diagnostic value in the clinic.

As we reviewed above, several neuropsychiatric disorders, especially autism, phobias, and depression, involve alterations in the ability to perceive, recognize, express, or experience emotions. It is important to emphasize that, especially in the domain of emotion, many such alterations of course fall within the normal variability, and an additional intriguing issue is the investigation of individual differences in the ability to process emotions, and the possible correlations of such differences with personality and with social functioning. That is, the study of emotion is of great importance not only to our understanding of pathologies that might be studied by a psychiatrist or neurologist, but also to the well being of healthy people, a topic that has been studied considerably within social psychology, but for which there is as yet little research linking it to the neural underpinnings. As with other domains of cognitive neuroscience, the exploration of emotion is bringing together psychologists, psychiatrists, neurobiologists, computer scientists, and philosophers. One of the main challenges is much more practical than any of those mentioned above: the difficulty of integrating knowledge from such disparate fields into a unified framework. It is our hope that the present review has at least sketched some directions in which such integration might proceed.

■ KEY POINTS

☐   Emotions are adaptive, phasic, multisystem patterns of coordinated response within the body.

☐   Feeling an emotion depends on a neural representation of the emotional response pattern.

☐   Key structures that process emotions are the amygdala, orbitofrontal cortex, regions of right hemisphere, and nuclei in the hypothalamus and brainstem.

☐   Most psychiatric disorders involve impairments in emotion processing.

KEY READINGS

Adolphs R: Recognizing emotion from facial expressions: Psychological and neurological mechanisms. Behav Cogn Neurosci Rev 1:21–61, 2002.

Damasio AR: Descartes' Error: Emotion, Reason, and the Human Brain. New York: Grosset/Putnam, 1994.

LeDoux J: The Emotional Brain. New York: Simon and Schuster, 1996.

Panksepp J Affective Neuroscience. New York: Oxford University Press, 1998.

REFERENCES

Adolphs R: Social cognition and the human brain. Trends Cogn Sci 3:469–479, 1999.

Adolphs R, Damasio H, Tranel D, et al: A role for somatosensory cortices in the visual recognition of emotions as revealed by three-dimensional lesion mapping. J Neurosci 20:2683–2690, 2000.

Adolphs R, Tranel D: Emotion recognition and the human amygdala, in Aggleton JP (ed): The Amygdala: A Functional Analysis. New York: Oxford University Press, 2000, pp. 587–630.

Adolphs R, Tranel D, Damasio AR: The human amygdala in social judgment. Nature 393:470–474, 1998.

Adolphs R, Tranel D, Damasio H, et al: Fear and the human amygdala. J Neurosci 15:5879–5892, 1995.

Adolphs R, Tranel D, Damasio H, et al: Impaired recognition of emotion in facial expressions following bilateral damage to the human amygdala. Nature 372:669–672, 1994.

Adolphs R, Tranel D, Hamann S, et al: Recognition of facial emotion in nine subjects with bilateral amygdala damage. Neuropsychologia 37:1111–1117, 1999.

Amaral DG, Price JL, Pitkanen A, et al: Anatomical organization of the primate amygdaloid complex, in Aggleton JP (ed): The Amygdala: Neurobiological Aspects of Emotion, Memory, and Mental Dysfunction. New York: Wiley-Liss, 1992, pp. 1–66.

American Psychiatric Association: Diagnostic and Statistical Manual of Mental Disorders, ed 4 (DSM-IV). Washington, DC: Author, 1994.

Anderson SW, Bechara A, Damasio H, et al: Impairment of social and moral behavior related to early damage in human prefrontal cortex. Nat Neurosci 2:1032–1037, 1999.

Anderson SW, Damasio H, Tranel D, Damasio AR: Long-tem sequelae of prefrontal damage acquired in early childhood. Dev Neuropsychol 18:281–296, 2000.

Andreasen NC, Arndt S, Swayze V, et al: Thalamic abnormalities in schizophrenia visualized through magnetic resonance image averaging. Science 266:294–298, 1994.

Andreasen NC, Rezai K, Alliger R, et al:. Hypofrontality in neuroleptic-naïve patients and in patients with chronic schizophrenia: Assessment with xenon 133 single-photon emission computed tomography and the Tower of London. Arch Gen Psychiatry 49:943–958, 1992.

Bagby M, Taylor G: Affect dysregulation and alexithymia, in Taylor GJ, Bagby RM, Parker JDA (eds): Disorders of Affect Regulation: Alexithymia in Medical and Psychiatric Illness. Cambridge, MA: Cambridge University Press, 1997, pp. 26–45.

Barrash J, Tranel D, Anderson SW: Acquired personality disturbances associated with bilateral damage to the ventromedial prefrontal region. Dev Neuropsychol 18:355–381, 2000.

Baron-Cohen S: Mindblindness: An Essay on Autism and Theory of Mind. Cambridge, MA: MIT Press, 1995.

Bechara A, Damasio AR, Damasio H, et al: Insensitivity to future consequences following damage to human prefrontal cortex. Cognition 50:7–15, 1994.

Bechara A, Tranel D, Damasio H, et al: Double dissociation of conditioning and declarative knowledge relative to the amygdala and hippocampus in humans. Science 269:1115–1118, 1995.

Beck AT: Beck Depression Inventory. San Antonio, TX: The Psychological Corporation, 1987.

Berenbaum H, Prince JD: Alexithymia and the interpretation of emotion-relevant information. Cogn Emotion 8:231–244, 1994.

Birbaumer N, Grodd W, Diedrich O, et al: fMRI reveals amygdala activation to human faces in social phobics. Neuroreport 9:1223–1226, 1998.

Borod J: Interhemispheric and intrahemispheric control of emotion: A focus on unilateral brain damage. J Consult Clin Psychol 60:339–348, 1992.

Bowers D, Bauer RM, Heilman KM: The nonverbal affect lexicon: Theoretical perspectives from neuropsychological studies of affect perception. Neuropsychology 7:433–444, 1993.

Brooks DN, Aughton ME: Psychological consequences of blunt head injury. Intern Rehabilitation Med 1:160–165, 1979.

Brothers L: The social brain: A project for integrating primate behavior and neurophysiology in a new domain. Concepts Neurosci 1:27–51, 1990.

Buechel C, Morris J, Dolan RJ, et al: Brain systems mediating aversive conditioning: An event-related fMRI study. Neuron 20:947–957, 1998.

Bush G, Luu P, Posner MI: Cognitive and emotional influences in anterior cingulate cortex. Trends Cogn Sci 4:215–222, 2000.

Butcher JN: A Beginner's Guide to the MMPI-2. Washington, DC: American Psychological Association, 1999.

Butcher JN, Dahlstrom WG, Graham JR, et al: Minnesota Multiphasic Personality Inventory-2 (MMPI-2): Manual for Administration and Scoring. Minneapolis: University of Minnesota Press, 1989.

Cahill L, Haier RJ, Fallon J, et al: Amygdala activity at encoding correlated with long-term, free recall of emotional information. Proc Natl Acad Sci U S A 93:8016–8021, 1996.

Cancelliere AEB, Kertesz A: Lesion localization in acquired deficits of emotional expression and comprehension. Brain Cogn 13:133–147, 1990.

Canli T: Hemispheric asymmetry in the experience of emotion. Neuroscientist 5:201–207, 1999.

Cavada C, Schultz W (eds): The mysterious orbitofrontal cortex. Cereb Cortex 10, 2000.

Cicone M, Wapner W, Gardner H: Sensitivity to emotional expressions and situations in organic patients. Cortex 16:145–158, 1980.

Craig RJ: Testimony based on the Millon Clinical Multiaxial Inventory: Review, commentary, and guidelines. J Pers Assess 73:290–304, 1999.

Craig RJ, Bivens A: Factor structure of the MCMI-III. J Pers Assess 70:190–196, 1998.

Damasio AR: Descartes' Error: Emotion, Reason, and the Human Brain. New York: Grosset/Putnam, 1994.

Damasio AR: The somatic marker hypothesis and the possible functions of the prefrontal cortex. Philos Trans R Soc Lond B Biol Sci, 351:1413–1420, 1996.

Davidson RJ: Anterior cerebral asymmetry and the nature of emotion. Brain Cogn 6:245–268, 1992.

Davidson RJ, Hugdahl K: Brain Asymmetry. Cambridge, MA: MIT Press, 1995.

Davidson RJ, Irwin W: The functional neuroanatomy of emotion and affective style. Trends Cogn Sci 3:11–22, 1999.

Davis M, Walker DL, Lee Y: Amygdala and bed nucleus of the stria terminalis: Differential roles in fear and anxiety measured with the acoustic startle reflex. Philos Trans R Soc Lond B Biol Sci 352:1675–1687, 1997.

Dejjani B-P, Damier P, et al: Transient acute depression induced by high-frequency deep-brain stimulation. N Engl J Med 340:1476–1480, 1999.

Drevets WC, Price JL, Simpson JR, et al: Subgenual prefrontal cortex abnormalities in mood disorders. Nature 386:824–827, 1997.

Egger MD, Flynn JP: Effects of electrical stimulation of the amygdala on hypothalamically elicited attack behavior in cats. J Neurophysiol 26:705–720, 1981.

Eslinger PJ, Biddle KR: Adolescent neuropsychological development after early right prefrontal damage. Dev Neuropsychol 18:281–296, 2000.

Everitt BJ, Parkinson JA, Olmstead MC, et al: Associative processes in addiction and reward: The role of amygdala-ventral striatal subsystems. Ann N Y Acad Sci 877:412–438, 1999.

Gallese V, Goldman A: Mirror neurons and the simulation theory of mind-reading. Trends Cogn Sci 2:493–500, 1999.

Garyfallos G, Manos N, Adamopoulou A: Psychopathology and personality characteristics of epileptic patients: Epilepsy, psychopathology and personality. Acta Psychiatr Scand 78:87–95, 1988.

Garza-Trevino ES: Neurobiological factors in aggressive behavior. Hosp Community Psychiatry 45:690–699, 1994.

Goldstein M: Brain research and violent behavior. Arch Neurol 30:1–35, 1974.

Goodwin FK, Jamison KR: Manic-Depressive Illness. New York: Oxford University Press, 1990.

Grattan LM, Eslinger PJ: Frontal lobe damage in children and adults: A comparative review. Dev Neuropsychol 7:283–326, 1991.

Graham JR: MMPI-2: Assessing Personality and Psychopathology, ed 3. New York: Oxford University Press, 2000.

Gray JM, Young AW, Barker WA, et al: Impaired recognition of disgust in Huntington's disease gene carriers. Brain 120:2029–2038, 1997.

Hamann SB, Ely TD, Grafton ST, et al: Amygdala activity related to enhanced memory for pleasant and aversive stimuli. Nat Neurosci 2:289–293, 1999.

Hathaway SR, McKinley JC: A multiphasic personality schedule (Minnesota): I. Construction of the schedule. J Psychol 10:249–254, 1940.

Hathaway SR, McKinley JC: The Minnesota Multiphasic Personality Schedule. Minneapolis: University of Minnesota Press, 1943.

Ingvar DH, Franzen G:. Distribution of cerebral activity in chronic schizophrenia. Lancet 2:1484–1486, 1974.

Jackson HF, Moffat NJ: Impaired emotional recognition following severe head injury. Cortex 23:293–300, 1987.

Jacobs DH, Shuren J, Heilman KM: Impaired perception of facial identity and facial affect in Huntington's disease. Neurology 45:1217–1218, 1995.

James W: What is an emotion? Mind 9:188–205, 1884.

Jessimer M, Markham R: Alexithymia: A right hemisphere dysfunction specific to recognition of certain facial expressions? Brain Cogn 34:246–258, 1997.

Kandel E, Freed D: Frontal-lobe dysfunction and antisocial behavior: A review. Clin Psychol 45:404–413, 1989.

Kawasaki H, Adolphs R, Kaufman O, et al: Single-unit responses to emotional visual stimuli recorded in human ventral prefrontal cortex. Nat Neurosci 4:15–16, 2001.

Kling AS: The anatomy of aggression and affiliation, in Plutchik R, Kellerman H (eds): Emotion: Theory, Research, and Experience. New York: Academic Press, 1986, Vol. 3, pp. 237–264.

Klüver H, Bucy PC: Preliminary analysis of functions of the temporal lobes in monkeys. Arch Neurol Psychiatry 42:979–997, 1939.

Lane RD, Ahern GL, Schwartz GE, et al: Is alexithymia the emotional equivalent of blindsight? Biol Psychiatry 42:834–844, 1997a.

Lane RD, Reiman EM, Ahern GL, et al: Neuroanatomical correlates of happiness, sadness, and disgust. Am J Psychiatry 154:926–933, 1997b.

Lane RD, Reiman EM, Axelrod B, et al: Neural correlates of levels of emotional awareness: Evidence of an interaction between emotion and attention in the anterior cingulate cortex. J Cogn Neurosci 10:525–535, 1998.

Lane RD, Sechrest L, Reidel R, et al: Impaired verbal and nonverbal emotion recognition in alexithymia. Psychosom Med 58:203–210, 1996.

LeDoux J. The Emotional Brain. New York: Simon and Schuster, 1996.

Lee GP, Arena JG, Meador KJ, et al: Changes in autonomic responsiveness following bilateral amygdalotomy in humans. Neuropsychiatry Neuropsychol Behav Neurol 1:119–129, 1988.

Lee GP, Reed MF, Meador KJ, et al: Is the amygdala crucial for cross-modal association in humans? Neuropsychology 9:236–245, 1995.

Lishman WA Brain damage in relation to psychiatric disability after head injury. Br J Psychiatry 114:373–410, 1968.

Lumley MA, Norman S: Alexithymia and health care utilization. Psychosom Med 58:197–202, 1996.

Lumley MA, Sielky K: Alexithymia, gender, and hemispheric functioning. Compr Psychiatry 41:352–359, 2000.

MacLean PD: The limbic system ("visceral brain") and emotional behavior. Arch Neurol Psychiatry 73:130–134, 1955.

Malamud N: Psychiatric disorder with intracranial tumors of limbic system. Arch Neurol 17:113–123, 1967.

Malloy P, Duffy J: The frontal lobes in neuropsychiatric disorders, in Boller F, Grafman J (eds). Handbook of Neuropsychology. Amsterdam: Elsevier, 1994, Vol. 9, pp. 203–232, 1994.

Mark VH, Ervin FR: Violence and the Brain. New York: Harper & Row, 1970.

Millon T: Manual for the Millon Clinical Multiaxial Inventory (MCMI). Minneapolis, MN: National Computer Systems, 1977.

Millon T, Davis RD: The MCMI-III: Present and future directions. J Pers Assess 68:69–85, 1997.

Morris JS, Frith CD, Perrett DI, et al: A differential neural response in the human amygdala to fearful and happy facial expressions. Nature 383:812–815, 1996.

Morris JS, Ohman A, Dolan RJ: A subcortical pathway to the right amygdala mediating "unseen" fear. Proc Natl Acad Sci U S A 96:1680–1685, 1999.

Moyer KE: The Psychobiology of Aggression. New York: Harper & Row, 1976.

Newton A, Johnson DA: Social adjustment and interaction after severe head injury. Br J Clin Psychol 24:225–234, 1985.

Oddy M, Humphrey M, Uttley D: Stresses upon the relatives of head injury patients. Br J Psychiatry 133:507–513, 1978.

Panksepp J: Affective Neuroscience. New York: Oxford University Press, 1998.

Parker JDA, Keightley ML, Smith CT, et al: Interhemispheric transfer deficit in alexithymia: An experimental study. Psychosom Med 61:464–468, 1999.

Parker JDA, Taylor GJ, Bagby RM: Alexithymia and the recognition of facial expressions of emotion. Psychother Psychosom 59:197–202, 1993.

Pettersen L: Sensitivity to emotional cues and social behavior in children and adolescents after head injury. Percept Mot Skills 73:1139–1150, 1991.

Phelps EA, O'Connor KJ, Cunningham WA, et al: Performance on indirect measures of race evaluation predicts amygdala activation. J Cogn Neurosci 12:729–738, 2000.

Phillips ML, Bullmore E, Howard R, et al: Investigation of facial processing using functional MRI [abstract]. Neuroimage 5:S611, 1997.

Price BH, Daffner KR, Stowe RM, et al: The comportmental learning disabilities of early frontal lobe damage. Brain 113:1383–1393, 1990.

Prigatano GP, Pribram KH: Perception and memory of facial affect following brain injury. Percept Mot Skills 54:859–869, 1982.

Relkin N, Plum F, Mattis S, et al: Impulsive homicide associated with an arachnoid cyst and unilateral frontotemporal cerebral dysfunction. Semin Clin Neuropsychiatry 1:172–183, 1996.

Rolls ET: The Brain and Emotion. New York: Oxford University Press.

Royet J-P, Zald D, Versace R, et al: Emotional responses to pleasant and unpleasant olfactory, visual, and auditory stimuli: A positron emission tomography study. J Neurosci 20:7752–7759, 2000.

Sifneos PE: Short-term Psychotherapy and Emotional Crisis. Cambridge, MA: Harvard University Press, 1972.

Silver JM, Yudofsky SC: Aggressive disorders, in Silver JM, Yudofsky SC, Hales RE (eds): Neuropsychiatry of Traumatic Brain Injury. Washington, DC: American Psychiatric Press, 1994, pp. 313–353.

Sprengelmeyer R, Young AW, Calder AJ, et al: Loss of disgust: Perception of faces and emotions in Huntington's disease. Brain 119:1647–1666, 1996.

Sprengelmeyer R, Young AW, Pundt I, et al: Disgust implicated in obsessive-compulsive disorder. Proc R Soc Lond B Biol Sci 264:1767–1773, 1997.

Starkstein SE, Robinson RG: The role of the frontal lobes in affective disorder following stroke, in Levin HS, Eisenberg HM, Benton A (eds): Frontal Lobe Function and Dysfunction. New York: Oxford University Press, 1991, pp. 288–303.

Tonkonogy JM: Violence and temporal lobe lesion: Head CT and MRI data. J Neuropsychiatry 3:189–196, 1991.

Tranel D: "Acquired sociopathy": The development of sociopathic behavior following focal brain damage, in Fowles DC, Sutker P, Goodman SH (eds): Progress in Experimental Personality and Psychopathology Research. New York: Springer, 1994, Vol. 17, pp. 285–311.

Tranel D: Neural correlates of violent behavior, in Bogousslavsky J, Cummings J (eds): Behavior and Mood Disorders in Focal Brain Lesions. Cambridge, England: Cambridge University Press, 2000, pp. 399–418.

Tranel D: Emotion, decision-making, and the ventromedial prefrontal cortex, in Stuss DT, Knight RT (eds): Frontal Lobes. New York: Oxford University Press, 2002.

Treiman DM: Psychobiology of ictal aggression. Adv Neurol 55:341–356, 1991.

Valzelli L: Psychobiology of Aggression and Violence. New York: Raven Press, 1981.

Volavka J: Neurobiology of Violence. Washington, DC: American Psychiatric Press, 1995.

Volkow ND, Tancredi L: Neural substrates of violent behavior: A preliminary study with positron emission tomography. Br J Psychiatry 151:668–673, 1987.

Weiger WA, Bear DM: An approach to the neurology of aggression. J Psychiatr Res 22:85–98, 1988.

Weinberger DR, Berman KF, Daniel DG: Prefrontal cortex dysfunction in schizophrenia, in Levin HS, Eisenberg HM, Benton A (eds): Frontal Lobe Function and Dysfunction. New York: Oxford University Press, 1991, pp. 275–287.

Whalen PJ, Rauch SL, Etcoff NL et al: Masked presentations of emotional facial expressions modulate amygdala activity without explicit knowledge. J Neurosci 18:411–418, 1998.

Cognition/ Behavior and Disease

Degenerative Diseases

Norman R. Relkin

Gregg L. Caporaso

Acetylcholinesterase

Alzheimer disease (AD)

Amnestic dementia

Anti-inflammatory

Antioxidant

β-Amyloid

Degenerative disorders

Dementia

Dementia with Lewy bodies (DLB)

Donepezil

Estrogen replacement therapy

Frontotemporal dementia (FTD)

Galantamine

Huntington disease (HD)

Mild cognitive impairment (MCI)

Neurofibrillary tangles

Parkinson disease (PD)

Primary progressive aphasia (PPA)

Progressive supranuclear palsy (PSP)

Rivastigmine

Senile plaques

Spongiform encephalopathy

Tau

Tacrine

Vitamin E

OVERVIEW

Degenerative disorders of the central nervous system (CNS) progressively destroy the primary fabric of the brain and/or spinal cord, resulting in the disruption of neuronal function and intercellular communication. Cognitive disturbances are among the most dreaded manifestations of several degenerative disorders. These disorders cause a progressive decline in cognition, comportment, and functional abilities, thereby diminishing the quality of life and frequently shortening the life span of those affected. In the second half of the 20th century, degenerative disorders became the most common cause of dementia in the elderly, and their prevalence is increasing as the world's population ages.

Degenerative disorders of the brain present enormous challenges to the scientists who study their underlying biology, to the clinicians who attempt to diagnose and treat these maladies, and, most importantly, to the patients and families who must cope with chronic, progressive afflictions that ravage mind, behavior, and emotional well-being. Just three decades ago, most cases of dementia were believed to be a variable consequence of aging or of cerebrovascular disease (i.e., arteriosclerosis or "hardening of the arteries"). Recent years, however, have witnessed an explosion in our recognition of the role that primary degenerative diseases play in dementia. Accompanying this neurologic epiphany have been the classification and subclassification of these diseases based on clinical, pathologic, and molecular features, the results of interdisciplinary efforts by behavioral neurologists, neuropsychologists, pathologists, radiologists, epidemiologists, geneticists, and cell biologists.

The diseases discussed in this chapter increase in incidence and prevalence with age. Taking Alzheimer disease (AD) as the prototype for this group of disorders, prevalence has increased precipitously over the past century as human life expectancy has lengthened. Between two and four million individuals now suffer from AD in the United States alone, resulting in annual health care expenditures in excess of $100 billion (Meek

et al., 1998). The enormity of this and other dementia-associated degenerative diseases will presumably worsen in coming years until effective disease-modifying treatments and preventions are found.

Rather than presenting an exhaustive discussion of the degenerative disorders that produce cognitive and behavioral symptoms, this chapter provides a practical framework for clinicians, neuropsychologists, neuroscientists, and students to understand and approach these disorders. First, we present a classification scheme that guides diagnosis based on initial disease features, affected neuroanatomic systems, and biological underpinnings. Next, we describe a biological model that attempts to unify common genetic and molecular themes of degenerative diseases, focusing on AD. This is followed by more detailed discussions of the major dementing degenerative diseases, focusing on clinical presentation, demographics, cognitive and neurologic profile, genetic associations, pathology, and specific diagnostic aids. We then present a general scheme for the evaluation of these disorders. Lastly, we discuss both pharmacologic and nonpharmacologic treatments for degenerative diseases.

CLASSIFICATION

Neurologic disorders produce a range of cognitive deficits during their course. In the earliest stages of disease, cognitive deficits may be so subtle as to go undetected or to be mistaken for normal, day-to-day fluctuations in mental abilities. A prodromal state or transition period between normal cognition and full-blown dementia is referred to as "mild cognitive impairment" (MCI) (Petersen et al., 2001). The symptoms present at the onset of a degenerative disorder provide specific clues to diagnosis. For example, MCI in which memory impairment is the sole cognitive disturbance is associated with an increased risk of subsequently developing AD. As these diseases advance, though, patterns of cognitive impairment tend to become more global and less distinctive.

When one suspects a degenerative dementia, it is helpful to classify the general features of the dementia and work deductively towards a more specific etiology. Dementias have been classified according to several nosologic schemes. One framework classifies dementias based on the predominant domain of cognitive or behavioral impairment present at the onset of symptoms (Fig. 22-1). This system recognizes subtypes such as *amnestic dementia* (i.e., affecting memory, as in AD), *comportmental dementia* (i.e., affecting behavior, as in dementia of the frontal lobe type), *linguistic dementia* (i.e., affecting language, as in primary progressive aphasia [PPA]), and *dementia associated with movement disorders* (i.e., affecting pyramidal or extrapyramidal systems, as in Parkinson disease [PD] or Huntington's disease [HD]).

FIGURE 22-1. Classification of degenerative diseases of the brain based on presenting symptoms and underlying pathophysiology (see text for explanation). AD, Alzheimer disease; CBD, corticobasal degeneration; DLB, dementia with Lewy bodies; HD, Huntington's disease; PD, Parkinson disease; PPA, primary progressive aphasia; PSP, progressive supranuclear palsy.

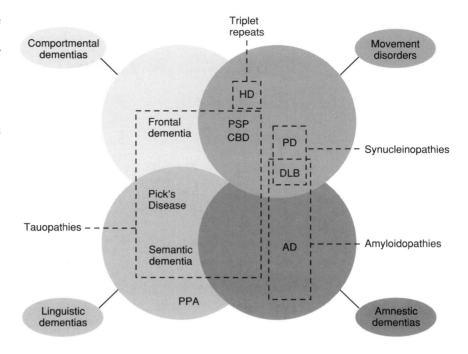

Another strategy focuses on the rate of disease progression, differentiating between dementias that progress *rapidly* (e.g., spongiform encephalopathy), *step-wise* (e.g., vascular dementia), or *insidiously* (e.g., AD). Anatomic classification systems distinguish *cortical dementias* (e.g., AD) from *subcortical dementias* (e.g., PD) (Cummings, 1990) or relate focal symptoms to *lobar* degenerations of the brain (e.g., dementia of the frontal type or posterior cortical atrophy [PCA] (Neary, 1990). Other distinctions include age of onset and mode of inheritance. *Presenile* dementia and *senile* dementia typically refer to whether the age of onset is before or after age 65, respectively. AD is the prototypical senile dementia, but it is also the most common degenerative cause of presenile dementia, followed in prevalence by HD, frontotemporal dementia (FTD), and the parkinsonian dementias such as corticobasal degeneration (CBD) and progressive supranuclear palsy (PSP) (Ratnavalli et al., 2002). *Familial* dementias occur among two or more members of a given family and often span multiple generations, whereas *sporadic* dementias show no discernible pattern of inheritance among family members. These various classification systems are not mutually exclusive and are useful in narrowing down the many potential causes of degenerative dementias.

It is important to understand the distinction between clinically defined dementia syndromes and pathologically defined degenerative diseases. A single clinically defined dementia syndrome can arise from several different underlying diseases. For example, a patient with behavioral disinhibition, perseveration, and aphasia may be diagnosed on clinical grounds with FTD.

Postmortem examination of the patient's brain might show specific neuropathologic changes within the frontal and/or temporal lobes indicative of Pick disease, CBD, PSP, or another degenerative disorder associated with frontal and temporal lobe symptoms. In all of these cases, the clinical diagnosis of FTD would be considered accurate as long as the autopsy indicates that there is relevant degenerative neuropathology within the frontal and/or temporal lobes of the brain, and/or their functional connections.

Distinctive clinical features and specific biological markers can often permit the accurate diagnosis of dementia without resorting to invasive procedures such as a brain biopsy. For example, in a patient with a rapidly progressive dementia and startle myoclonus, the combined findings of periodic discharges on electroencephalography (EEG), "ribbon-like" cortical hyperintense lesions on diffusion-weighted magnetic resonance imaging (MRI), and the detection of 14-3-3 protein in cerebrospinal fluid (CSF) would strongly suggest a diagnosis of spongiform encephalopathy secondary to Creutzfeldt-Jakob disease (CJD). Many cases of AD can now be diagnosed before death with an accuracy approaching that of autopsy, especially when the clinical presentation is characteristic of AD and the course is uncomplicated by other disorders. Diagnosis of AD depends on recognizing its common presenting symptoms and excluding other forms of dementia. By correlating clinical features with the likelihood of neuropathologic findings, the National Institute of Neurological and Communicative Disorders and Stroke and the Alzheimer's Disease and Related Disorders Association (NINCDS-ADRDA) Work Group delineated criteria for "definite," "probable," "possible," and "unlikely" AD (McKhann et al., 1984). These criteria were developed for research purposes but may be used clinically to help clarify and convey the clinician's level of diagnostic certainty.

Emerging theories on the etiology of degenerative disorders of the brain have converged on common genetic and biochemical underpinnings, prompting a reclassification of these diseases, which had originally been classified according to clinical and neuropathological characteristics. The altered expression, misfolding, and abnormal deposition of certain brain proteins (β-amyloid, tau, α-synuclein, ubiquitin, huntingtin, prion protein, etc.) appear to underlie several major degenerative disorders (see next section). Tests for genetic mutations in some of these proteins permit antemortem diagnosis reflective of the molecular underpinnings of a particular disorder, such as "tauopathy," "α-synucleinopathy," or "β-amyloidopathy" (see Fig. 22-1). Although discrete genetic mutations are found in a relatively small number of patients with degenerative dementias, the discovery of disease-causing and risk-enhancing genetic factors has been an important step toward understanding the pathophysiology of these conditions and in designing effective treatments (Table 22-1).

BIOLOGICAL UNDERPINNINGS OF DEGENERATIVE DISEASES

Although progress has been made in understanding the biology underlying several neurodegenerative disorders, actual causal pathways have yet to be fully elucidated. Traditional methods of studying these diseases relied on microscopic and chemical analyses of pathologic specimens. Indeed, much of the disease nomenclature reflects the efforts of investigators like Drs. Alzheimer, Pick, and Lewy, who identified the characteristic pathologic lesions of distinct clinical syndromes. Though informative, such techniques could provide only limited insights into disease etiology. The introduction of molecular bio-

logical techniques has extended the pathologic classification of these diseases and implicated several proteins in their pathogenesis.

Our understanding of AD and related degenerative dementia syndromes has benefited from genetic linkage studies. The identification of families with inherited degenerative diseases of the brain, combined with genetic linkage analysis, cloning, molecular biology, and biochemistry, has enabled the isolation of many molecules that appear to play causative or supportive roles in these disorders. Experiments in transgenic mice have helped define the contributions of these proteins to disease and have provided systems to test potential therapies. In most degenerative dementias, it appears that disease-related genetic and epigenetic factors lead to the abnormal folding or clearance, of specific proteins that, by forming multimers or aggregates, disrupt cell function and lead to the death of selected neuronal populations.

Amyloid Cascade Hypothesis

Nearly a hundred years ago, the German physician Alois Alzheimer characterized two types of neuropathological structures in the brain of an institutionalized woman (identified as Auguste D.) who had died from a progressive dementing illness. The lesions—intracellular neurofibrillary tangles (NFTs) and extracellular senile (or neuritic) plaques—are now recognized as important features of the disease that bears Alzheimer's name. NFTs are composed of paired helical filaments (PHFs), the principal constituent of which is the microtubule-associated protein tau (for an overview, see Buee et al., 2000). In the NFTs associated with AD, several abnormally phosphorylated forms of tau have been identified. In vitro studies have demonstrated that these posttranslational modifications disrupt the normal ability of tau to bundle microtubules. The formation of PHFs or NFTs within neurons presumably interferes with cellular function and probably contributes to cell death.

TABLE 22-1. Proteins Associated with the Formation of Pathological Lesions in Degenerative Diseases of the Brain

Diseases	Pathological lesions	Principal protein constituents
Alzheimer disease	Senile plaques	Aβ
	Neurofibrillary tangles	Tau
Frontotemporal dementia	Pick bodies	Tau
Corticobasal degeneration	Intraneuronal inclusions	Tau
Progressive supranuclear palsy	Neurofibrillary tangles	Tau
Dementia with Lewy bodies	Lewy bodies	α-Synuclein
Parkinson disease	Lewy bodies	α-Synuclein
Huntington's disease	Intranuclear inclusions	Huntingtin
Creutzfeldt-Jakob disease	Plaques	Prion (PrP^{sc})

Much of our knowledge of the pathogenesis of AD, though, has come from the study of senile plaques. The cores of senile plaques are composed of "amyloid" material, a term coined by Rudolph Virchow to describe the "starch-like" staining properties of this class of protein deposits. The numerous amyloid proteins that have been implicated in both systemic and neurologic diseases are unrelated by sequence. However, they all share β-pleated sheet structures and exhibit birefringence when stained with the dyes Congo red or thioflavin-S. The latter property refers to the yellow-green appearance of amyloid deposits when viewed with polarized light under a microscope.

The isolation and amino acid sequencing of the β-amyloid peptide, called Aβ, from vascular amyloid deposits in the brains of Alzheimer's patients represented a major breakthrough in understanding the etiology of AD (Glenner & Wong, 1984). This discovery led to the cloning of the gene for a large transmembrane protein, called the amyloid precursor protein (APP), from which Aβ is proteolytically cleaved (for recent reviews on the biology of APP and Aβ, see Selkoe, 2000; Hardy & Selkoe, 2002). Subsequent studies demonstrated that several isoforms of APP result from alternative splicing of APP transcripts, which are encoded by a single gene on chromosome 21. Experiments revealed that most APP molecules are secreted after being cleaved within the Aβ domain by a protease called α-secretase, thus precluding formation of the Aβ peptide itself. A relatively minor pathway is responsible for cleavage of APP at the amino- and carboxyl-termini of the Aβ domain by proteases called β-secretase (or BACE, for "β-site APP-cleaving enzyme") and γ-secretase, respectively, to release intact Aβ. However, the precise physiological functions of full-length APP, the splice variants, secreted APP, or Aβ are not yet known.

Localization of APP to chromosome 21 accorded with the earlier observation that virtually all patients with Down syndrome (trisomy 21) are at risk for developing clinical and pathologic features of AD with advancing age. This implied that an extra copy of APP is sufficient to cause AD. Stronger evidence suggesting that abnormal Aβ processing could cause AD came from the identification of several mutations in the APP gene in families with rare, autosomal dominant forms of the disease (Price & Sisodia, 1998). When these mutant forms of APP are expressed in cultured cells, one finds an increase in secretion of the 42-amino acid form of Aβ (Aβ42) relative to the 40-amino acid peptide (Aβ40) normally secreted by cells. In addition, transgenic mice bearing APP mutations develop β-amyloid deposits similar to those seen in the brains of AD patients; however, no NFTs are formed. All of the discovered AD-producing APP mutations lie at or near the cleavage sites for Aβ release and seem to enhance the ability of β- or γ-secretase to cleave APP. [The one exception to date is the recently described "Arctic mutation" present in a Swedish family with autosomal dominant AD (Nilsberth et al., 2001). This mutation in APP seems to affect the rate of formation of Aβ fibrils rather than APP proteolysis by secretases.]

Subsequent genetic studies of familial AD identified mutations in the genes encoding presenilin 1 (PS1) and presenilin 2 (PS2), proteins that bear homology to molecules identified in the Notch-1 signal transduction pathway. This signaling pathway is important for the normal regulation of neural cell proliferation and differentiation in early development. As is seen with APP mutations, expression of the presenilin gene mutations in cultured cells results in increased production of Aβ42. Mice expressing PS1 mutations also develop Aβ-amyloid deposits, a phenotype that is augmented by co-expression of mutant APP (Price et al., 1998). It remains to be determined whether either presenilin is actually the catalytic component or merely a necessary component of γ-secretase, which appears to be a large complex of several distinct proteins.

The seminal observation that all genetic mutations associated with inherited AD seem to alter the processing of Aβ led to the "amyloid cascade hypothesis" (Hardy & Higgins, 1992; Hardy, 1997) (Fig. 22-2). In brief, this theory posits that genetic factors (e.g., trisomy 21 in Down syndrome or mutations in APP, PS1, or PS2 in AD) and epigenetic factors (e.g., age, head trauma, menopause) lead to an alteration in APP proteolysis and Aβ processing that favors the formation of Aβ42 over Aβ40. As will be discussed below, the Aβ42 isoform gives rise to enhanced β-amyloid fibril production and β-amyloid deposition in the brain. Although its precise mechanism of action is not yet known, β-amyloid triggers impaired neuronal function, synapse loss, and cell death. These pathologic changes in the brain correlate with and are likely responsible for the symptoms observed during the course of AD.

Conformational Diseases

Biochemical findings in AD, other degenerative diseases of the brain, and several nonneurologic disorders support the idea that a multitude of diseases are caused by abnormal folding and aggregation of proteins (Carrell & Lomas, 1997). Such "conformational diseases" would include sickle-cell anemia, α1-antitrypsin deficiency (resulting in emphysema and cirrhosis), systemic amyloidoses, and degenerative dementias like AD. In these diseases, changes in the size or shape of a protein appear to result in its self-association, formation of aggregates, and tissue deposition (Taubes, 1996).

In 1972, Christian Anfinsen won the Nobel Prize in chemistry for demonstrating that a protein's three-dimensional structure is determined by its primary amino acid sequence (Anfinsen, 1973). More recent work has

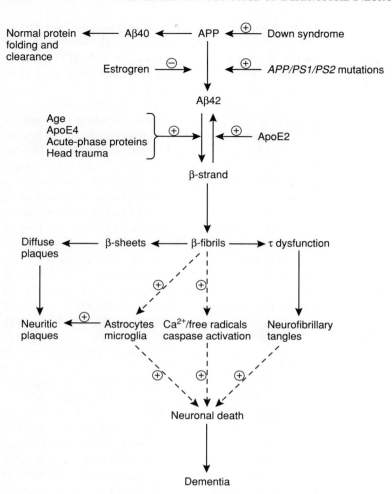

FIGURE 22-2. The amyloid cascade hypothesis (see text for explanation). More speculative pathways in the cascade are indicated by dashed arrows.

shown that in some cases protein folding depends on proteins called chaperonins to direct the conformational folding process of nascent peptides (Wickner et al., 1999). Chaperonins prevent newly formed proteins from folding into intermediate structures that self-assemble, a process that is concentration-dependent and facilitated by the presence of hydrophobic amino acid residues. Amino acid mutations or peptide-peptide interactions overcome subtle difference in free energies of stabilization (e.g., between α-helices and β-strands). These changes prevent or overwhelm normal intrinsic or chaperonin-mediated protein folding, thereby resulting in misfolded peptides. Under appropriate conditions, even the native folded state of highly globular proteins like myoglobulin can be destabilized enough to form β-strands similar to those comprising amyloid deposits (Fandrich et al., 2001).

For proteins like immunoglobulin light chains, which are associated with systemic amyloidoses, single amino acid mutations can alter peptide folding and cause aggregation. In others, such as *APP*, mutations affect the production or availability of peptides that are more susceptible to aggregation (i.e., Aβ42 in contrast to Aβ40). A whole group of disorders, of which HD is the best known, is characterized by abnormally long glutamine

repeats at the amino-termini of proteins (e.g., huntingtin), which result in intraneuronal inclusions. In the "prionoses," disease-causing prion proteins (PrP^{sc}) seem to induce normal cellular prions (PrP^c) to assume the same abnormal, pro-aggregative conformation, a reiterative process that may grow exponentially (Prusiner, 1998). Prions have been implicated in the class of disorders known as spongiform encephalopathies (e.g., CJD and kuru in humans, and "mad cow" disease, scrapie, and chronic wasting disease of elk and deer in other mammals).

Additional genetic and epigenetic factors modify the risk for developing a degenerative disorder of the brain. A genetic linkage between AD and chromosome 19 led to the discovery that a particular allele of the apolipoprotein E gene (*APOE*) increases the risk for developing the more common sporadic form of AD (Roses, 1998). There are three different alleles for this gene (called ε2, ε3, and ε4), which encodes a protein (ApoE) important for the transport and cellular uptake of lipids and cholesterol. Having one or two copies of the ε4 allele increases an individual's risk for developing AD and results in an earlier age of onset, though the ε4 allele does not affect the rate of disease progression. In familial AD associated with *APP* mutations, the *APOE* genotype of affected individuals modifies the age of symptoms onset, with one copy of an ε4 allele producing earlier onset, one copy of an ε2 allele producing later onset, and homozygosity for ε3 producing an intermediate age of onset (Sorbi et al., 1995). In vitro data suggest that the ApoE protein encoded by the ε4 allele (ApoE4) causes Aβ-amyloid to aggregate more readily than the ApoE protein associated with either of the other two alleles (i.e., ApoE2 or ApoE3). In this sense, ApoE may act as a chaperonin for Aβ-amyloid, although it does not possess enzymatic activity, as do many other prokaryotic and eukaryotic chaperonins.

For most degenerative diseases that cause dementia, age is perhaps the greatest risk factor (see Chapter 36). Over its life span, an organism accumulates proteins damaged by oxidization, and its cells lose particular enzymatic activities (Friguet et al., 2000). The association of disease-related protein aggregation and age may thus be the result of increased oxidative damage and decreased peptide folding or protease activity. Immunoreactivity for ubiquitin can be demonstrated in most of the lesions that characterize degenerative diseases, including senile plaques, NFTs, and Lewy bodies. This small peptide is normally added to cellular proteins that are "tagged" for destruction by proteasomes, which are large, multimeric, barrel-like intracytoplasmic structures that degrade misfolded and other abnormal proteins (Wickner et al., 1999). The presence of ubiquitin in most brain lesions comprised of protein aggregates may represent a neuron's unsuccessful attempts to rid itself of or sequester damaging proteins such as Aβ.

Finally, several retrospective studies have shown a negative correlation between estrogen use in postmenopausal women and the development of AD. Studies in cell cultures have demonstrated that estrogen can regulate the secretion of *APP* by a pathway that diverts the protein from amyloidogenic processing (Jaffe et al., 1994; Xu et al., 1998), suggesting a mechanism by which estrogen might prevent the development or slow the progression of AD. Estrogen may also support neuronal survival, as it appears to regulate dendrite formation and synaptic growth in hippocampal neurons (Woolley & McEwen, 1993). The possibility that estrogen may thus protect against the development of AD is being examined in clinical trials.

Protein Aggregates

A salient feature of degenerative diseases of the brain is the presence of intracellular or extracellular protein aggregates. Certain lesions such as senile plaques or Pick bodies seem to be relatively disease-specific (for AD and Pick disease, respectively). Others, such as NFTs or Lewy bodies, occur in several diseases, including AD, PSP, CBD, and some cases of FTD (see Table 22-1), and

appear to reflect a general neuronal response to degenerative disease rather than a mechanism of causation in AD or any other degenerative disease. In support of a primary role for β-amyloid deposits in the pathogenesis of AD and a secondary role for NFTs, autopsy studies of individuals with Down syndrome show β-amyloid deposition and senile plaque formation early in life, whereas NFTs are found primarily in the brains of older subjects. Several mutations have been found in *APP* in familial cases of AD, but no mutations have been found in the gene encoding the microtubule-associated protein tau, which is the primary component of NFTs. This too argues against a primary role for NFTs in AD. A mutation in the tau gene, however, was recently found in familial cases of FTD with parkinsonism (Lee & Trojanowski, 1999). Furthermore, transgenic mice expressing mutated tau develop motor and behavioral signs accompanied by NFTs in the brainstem and multiple subcortical nuclei (Lewis et al., 2000).

Transgenic mice have also been instructive in studying HD (see Chapter 24). HD is characterized by the presence of intranuclear inclusions composed of huntingtin within neurons of the striatum. In transgenic mice expressing huntingtin with expanded amino-terminal glutamine repeats, identical inclusions form, and the animals develop tremor and abnormal movements (Price et al., 1998). This suggests that the expanded glutamine repeats might affect protein conformation and aggregation. However, little neuronal loss is seen, raising the possibility that the intranuclear inclusions inhibit normal neuronal function and might have a lethal toxic effect that is seen only over prolonged time. Consistent with this hypothesis, mice expressing a gene for a mutated fragment of huntingtin develop both neuronal inclusions and motor signs that are reversed when the gene is turned off (Yamamoto et al., 2000). It is therefore possible that at least some of the pathologic and clinical effects seen in HD could be therapeutically halted or reversed.

Most of the pathologic lesions in degenerative diseases are not composed of a single protein. The presence of ubiquitin in many lesions has already been described above. Other proteins associated with pathologic lesions might play a causative or supportive role. For example, the acute-phase inflammatory protein α1-antichymotrypsin (ACT) is found in senile plaques. This protein has been shown in vitro to promote Aβ-amyloid polymerization, and double transgenic mice bearing *APP* mutations along with a gene that expresses ACT in astrocytes have more β-amyloid deposits than mice bearing the *APP* mutations alone (Nilsson et al., 2001).

Oxidative Damage

Disruption of normal cellular metabolic pathways and associated oxidative damage have been found in many of the degenerative diseases (Beal, 2000). In some diseases, such findings seem to represent a common downstream consequence of specific processes that initially trigger the pathogenic cascade. In others, evidence suggests that abnormal cellular energetics play a more upstream, causal role. Although our understanding of these pathogenic mechanisms is limited at present, the identification of oxidative and free-radical processes in degenerative disorders of the brain has been a fruitful source for developing therapies aimed at preventing or slowing the progression of disease.

Normal cellular metabolism and energy homeostasis begin with the conversion of large, complex molecules—carbohydrates, lipids, and proteins—into smaller molecules, with concomitant generation of compounds containing high-energy molecular bonds, like those of adenosine 5'-triphosphate (ATP) and nicotinic adenine dinucleotide phosphate. Protein complexes within the inner membrane of mitochondria perform the electron transfer reactions that lead to ATP production. Several mechanisms can disrupt or overwhelm a cell's ability to maintain a proper energy balance, including: impaired mitochondrial function; depletion of ATP; elevated intracellular calcium levels; generation of free radicals (e.g., superoxide and hydroxyl radicals, and peroxynitrite); oxidation of cellular lipids, proteins, and nucleic acids, and activation of both necrotic and apoptotic cell death pathways (i.e., caspase activation). For example, excessive activation of N-methyl-D-aspartate (NMDA) receptors by glutamate results in harmful calcium influx, a mechanism commonly invoked in neuronal death due to stroke that could also play a role in degenerative diseases. NMDA receptors may indeed mediate some aspect of the neuronal toxicity of Aβ in AD (Mattson et al., 1992).

Several types of mitochondrial dysfunction have been implicated in degenerative diseases. Mitochondrial proteins are encoded by nuclear or mitochondrial deoxyribonucleic acid (mDNA), and mutations in either genomic subset can produce neurologic disease. In Wilson disease, a neurologic disorder characterized by abnormal copper metabolism and progressive dementia, psychosis, and extrapyramidal signs, mutations in the nuclear gene for a P-type ATPase might be responsible for elevated concentrations of mitochondrial copper and oxidative damage (Beal, 2000). Though not associated with dementia per se, several degenerative diseases, including MELAS (*m*itochondrial *e*ncephalopathy, *l*actic *a*cidosis, and *s*trokes) and Leigh disease, are caused by mutations in mDNA. It remains to be seen whether mDNA mutations will be found in dementing illnesses.

As mentioned above, transgenic mice expressing huntingtin protein with expanded amino-terminal glutamine repeats develop a phenotype similar to that seen in HD. These animals have decreased levels of N-acetylaspartate, a neuronal marker produced within mitochondria, suggesting that huntingtin might disrupt normal mitochondrial function. A dramatic illustration of the effects of altered mitochondrial function in producing neurologic disease came accidentally when several young people developed a condition similar to PD after injecting a synthetic opiate contaminated with 1-methyl-4-phenyl-1,2,3,6-tetrahydropyridine (MPTP) (Langston et al., 1984). A metabolite of MPTP selectively inhibits complex I of the electron transport chain in dopaminergic cells of the substantia nigra, thus reducing mitochondrial ATP production and causing neuronal death. No convincing candidate has yet been found for an environmental toxin that can be traced to the majority of cases of idiopathic PD, but decreased complex I activity in the substantia nigra has been found in several studies of this disease.

Selective Cell Death

One of the most puzzling questions in the study of degeneration in the brain is why certain populations of neurons are specifically susceptible in each disease. In AD, neurons of the basal forebrain and hippocampal formation are affected early. PD is characterized by loss of dopaminergic neurons in the substantia nigra pars compacta. Gamma-aminobutyric acid (GABA)-producing neurons in the head of the caudate nucleus are the first to die in HD. Although this selective vulnerability correlates well with clinical symptoms and signs (e.g., tremor and rigidity in PD due to basal ganglia pathology), the mechanisms underlying cell-specific vulnerability remain unknown. Any understanding of the basis for selective cell death must consider lesion type, affected neurons and brain regions, changes seen over time, variation in disease phenotype, and overlap—both clinical and pathologic—between diseases.

Different groups of neurons can be affected during different stages of a degenerative disease. Pathologic changes in AD begin in the basal forebrain and entorhinal cortex, but eventually extend to involve temporal and parietal cortices (Braak & Braak, 1996). The types of lesions manifested during the course of an illness can also vary. Pathologic studies of brains from Down syndrome patients show that the earliest lesions, present even in adolescence, are diffuse β-amyloid deposits, followed over time by senile plaques with surrounding dystrophic neurites (degenerating axons and dendrites), and then by NFTs. NFTs are most abundant in the basal forebrain of AD patients, whereas senile plaques are more commonly found in cortical structures (Braak & Braak, 1998).

In addition, some AD patients can develop symptoms of PD, reflecting basal ganglia involvement. Conversely, patients with PD often develop dementia as a result of cortical disease. Overlapping pathologies further blur the distinction between diseases, such as the identification of Lewy bodies (intracytoplasmic aggregates of the protein α-synuclein in affected neurons) in PD, dementia with Lewy bodies (DLB), and in some forms of AD and prion disease. Selective vulnerability may reflect the interplay between a global pathologic process that affects neurons to different degrees over time and the ability of different brain systems to compensate until threshold neuronal loss occurs and symptoms develop (Hardy & Gwinn-Hardy, 1998).

Particular molecular features of a given cell type might confer selective vulnerability, but synaptic connections between neurons and contacts with surrounding glial cells could also modify susceptibility. The identification of relatively few types of lesions (i.e., NFTs and Lewy bodies) in several different disorders suggests that a neuron has a limited range of pathologic responses to a wide range of disease processes (Hardy & Gwinn-Hardy, 1998). That is, NFTs can form as a result of tau gene mutations in certain forms of FTD, but are often secondary manifestations of AD, DLB, PSP, or prion diseases.

There seems to be an inverse correlation between the cortical density of NFTs in AD and the sequence of cortical myelination during development (Braak & Braak, 1998). Greater myelination of certain populations of projection neurons may protect them against oxidative stress, NFT formation, and neuronal death (Braak et al., 2000). Another theory emphasizes the predilection in AD for early lesions in the hippocampal formation and other areas that may be important for neuronal "plasticity" (i.e., the capacity of synaptic connections and neuronal signaling to be modified in response to varying degrees of activity). The ability of brain networks to remain plastic decreases with age, and damaging processes (e.g., triggered by Aβ) eventually overwhelm the brain's capacity to adapt (Mesulam, 1999). One group of neurons after another degenerates, with AD pathology spreading over time from the basal forebrain and hippocampal structures to their projections in neocortical regions.

Clinical Correlation

Any biological theory for degenerative diseases of the brain must correlate underlying cellular defects and pathologic lesions with particular cognitive and behavioral manifestations over time. A detailed discussion of brain anatomy, neuronal networks, and the cognitive properties that arise from them (e.g., attention, memory, language) are beyond the scope of this chapter (an introduction to this topic may be found in Mesulam, 1990). However, we can illustrate the effects of synaptic impairment, neuronal function, and brain pathology on cognition by focusing on the clinical course of AD. There is a good correlation between the progressive symptoms encountered in AD and the gross structural changes of the brain seen by computed tomography (CT), MRI, or autopsy. Changes in the activity of different brain regions can also be detected during life by cerebral blood flow or

metabolic studies using positron emission tomography (PET) and other techniques. Short-term memory loss manifesting as rapid forgetting is the usual presenting symptom of AD, and this corresponds in time to the atrophy of the entorhinal cortex and hippocampus—structures important for the induction and consolidation of episodic memories, and affected early in the course of AD. In contrast, impairments in visuospatial function and praxis are seen in a somewhat later stage of the illness, at a time when atrophy of higher-level cortical association areas important for these functions, such as the posterior temporal and inferior parietal lobes, becomes apparent.

As mentioned earlier, the stereotyped spatial progression of atrophy and pathologic changes observed in AD may represent selective neuronal vulnerability based on levels of synaptic plasticity or axonal myelination (Mesulam, 1999; Braak et al., 2000). One apparent paradox, however, has plagued those who believe that abnormal Aβ processing is central to the pathogenesis of AD and who support the amyloid cascade hypothesis—namely, that despite the overwhelming genetic evidence pointing to Aβ's role in initiating the disease, extracellular β-amyloid deposition correlates only to a limited extent with the symptoms and gross structural changes that are routinely observed. In contrast, the distribution of NFTs correlates more strongly with the clinical and gross pathologic features. The degree of dementia severity is related to the number of NFTs, but not senile plaques, in neocortical areas, and NFTs are found in the entorhinal cortex and hippocampus early in the disease, whereas plaques are not (Arriagada et al., 1992). At present, no solid explanation can account for this apparent discrepancy. However, recent evidence suggests that levels of soluble Aβ, present well before the peptide forms β-amyloid deposits in senile plaques, do indeed correlate with disease severity, suggesting that dysequilibrium between soluble and insoluble pools of Aβ may underlie the pathogenesis of AD (McLean et al., 1999).

MAJOR DEGENERATIVE DISEASES

A review of all of the degenerative disorders that affect cognition would be encyclopedic and is beyond the scope of this chapter. Instead, we will focus on the four major subtypes of degenerative dementias defined in Section II (amnestic, comportmental, linguistic, and movement disorder–related) and provide illustrative examples of disorders in each category.

Alzheimer Disease—An Amnestic Dementia

Epidemiology

AD is the most common cause of dementia in the industrialized world. The typical course is one of insidious memory loss and progressive cognitive, behavioral, and emotional decline lasting on average from 5 to 9 years (Molsa et al., 1986; Walsh et al., 1990). Women are more often affected than men, and the risk for developing AD increases with age, with one clinical study suggesting that approximately 10% of individuals over age 65 and 47% of those over age 85 have probable AD (Evans et al., 1989). However, several other clinical studies have reported slightly lower rates of prevalence, and one investigation reported a prevalence of clinically diagnosed AD at 16% and pathologically diagnosed AD at 33% for a population aged 85 years or older (Polvikoski et al., 2001). Such discrepancies are presumably due to differences in study populations and the criteria used in diagnosis. Most studies employ the diagnostic criteria set by the NINCDS-ADRDA, which require deficits in at least two areas of cognition and progressive worsening of memory (McKhann et al., 1984). Nonetheless, these criteria do not always allow for the distinction between AD and other degenerative dementias, so many studies include more stringent diagnostic features based on structural imaging (CT or MRI) or even pathology.

Most cases of AD occur after the age of 65 years, but approximately 2% of cases are inherited in an autosomal dominant fashion and present at a much younger age. As described in the previous section (summarized in Table 22-2), mutations in the genes for *APP* and the presenilin proteins account for most of familial AD, with *PS1* mutations comprising the largest fraction of inherited early-onset cases, usually occurring before 50 years of age. Possession of one or two *APOE* ε4 alleles increases one's susceptibility to the more common late-onset, sporadic form of the disease.

In addition to advancing age, several other possible risk factors and risk modifiers have been identified, though none have been conclusively confirmed. For example, head trauma appears to increase the likelihood of developing AD, and the blows to the head sustained by boxers are associated with cognitive impairment ("dementia pugilistica") and pathologic changes similar to those seen in AD (Tokuda et al., 1991). Boxers who possess the *APOE* ε4 allele and have lengthier professional careers appear to be more susceptible to the neurologic impairments associated with dementia pugilistica (Jordan, 1997).

Considerable effort is being expended in attempts to identify preventative measures that offer some degree of protection against AD. Given the long prodromal period in which AD neuropathology develops in the brain before dementia becomes evident, there is a large window of opportunity for pre-emptive interventions. A retrospective study of dementia in nuns demonstrated that intellectual ability in early adulthood was inversely correlated with risk of development of AD in later life (Snowdon et al., 1996). Similarly, a higher level of education or occupational attainment is associated with a lower incidence of AD (Stern et al., 1994), which has led to the "use it or lose it" theory. Based on the working model of the amyloid cascade hypothesis (Fig. 22-2), several putative pharmaceutical approaches to AD prevention are under study, including antioxidants, anti-inflammatories, hormonal replacement, statins, and antiamyloid therapies.

Pathology

At the gross level, brains from patients with AD predominantly exhibit atrophy of the medial temporal and posterior parietal lobes. The hippocampal formation is especially affected, eventually becoming a mere tissue remnant in the most severe cases (Fig. 22-3A). A variable amount of lateral temporal and prefrontal lobe atrophy can be seen, whereas the occipital lobes and primary motor and sensory cortices are relatively spared. Large pyramidal neurons that participate in cortico-cortical association networks show particular vulnerability to AD pathology, with other cell types being affected to varying degrees.

As described in the previous section, the two principal pathologic lesions in AD are NFTs and senile plaques. NFTs are flame-shaped intraneuronal inclusions that can be visualized by silver or hematoxylin-eosin staining (Fig. 22-3C). They are most often found in neurons of the cerebral cortex, hippocampus, amygdala, basal forebrain, and brainstem. NFTs are not restricted to AD, but are also found in PSP, dementia pugilistica, and several other disorders. It is widely believed that the density of NFTs in affected areas of the brain correlates with the severity of dementia in AD and is thus used in the pathologic staging of the disease (Blessed et al., 1968; Braak & Braak, 1996).

TABLE 22-2. Genetic Associations in Alzheimer Disease

Protein	Gene	Chromosome	Genotype	Effect
Amyloid precursor protein	*APP*	21	Point mutations	Increased Aβ production
			Extra copy (trisomy 21)	Increased Aβ production
Presenilin 1	*PS1*	14	Point mutations	Increased Aβ production
Presenilin 2	*PS2*	1	Point mutations	Increased Aβ production
Apolipoprotein E	*APOE*	19	ε4 allele	Enhanced Aβ fibril formation

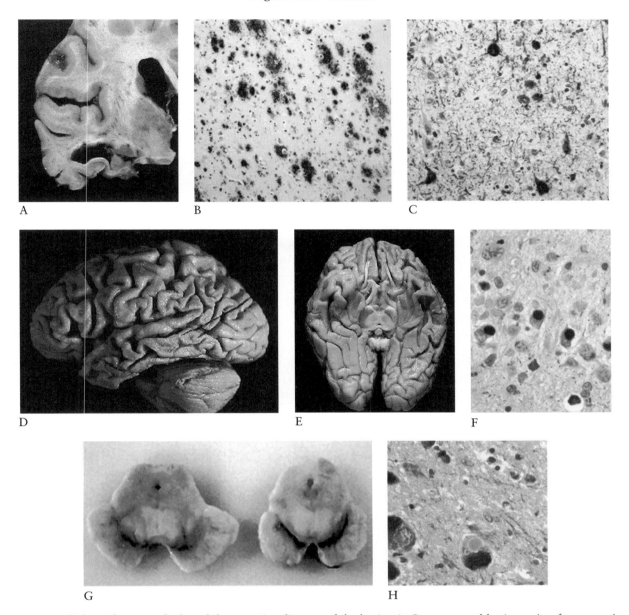

FIGURE 22-3. Pathologic features of selected degenerative diseases of the brain. *A,* Gross coronal brain section from a patient with Alzheimer disease (AD) showing marked hippocampal atrophy and ventricular dilation secondary to cerebral atrophy. *B,* Immunohistochemistry for Aβ revealing extracellular senile plaques and β-amyloid deposits in AD. *C,* Silver staining of intracellular neurofibrillary tangles in AD. *D* and *E,* Gross lateral and ventral whole brain images from a patient with Pick disease demonstrating marked frontal and temporal lobe atrophy. *F,* Silver staining of intracellular Pick bodies in Pick disease. *G,* Gross midbrain sections from a normal subject (*right*) and a patient with Parkinson disease (PD) (*left*). *H,* Hematoxylin and eosin staining of a Lewy body within a pigmented neuron of the substania nigra in PD.   *Continued*

When examined by electron microscopy, NFTs are found to be composed of PHFs, ~10 nm fibrils twisted in a double helix. The principal component of the PHFs is the neuron-specific microtubule-associated protein tau (Kosik et al., 1986). Six protein isoforms arise by alternative splicing of transcripts from the single tau gene. Tau is abnormally phosphorylated in AD, which inhibits its normal ability to bundle microtubules and causes it to aggregate into filaments.

Senile plaques (Fig. 22-3B) are extracellular deposits of β-amyloid surrounded by dystrophic neurites—the degenerating processes of nearby neurons—and reactive glial cells. Plaques can be visualized by any of several staining methods, including silver impregnation, Congo red, or thioflavin-S, or by immunohistochemistry for Aβ. Other proteins have been found to be associated with plaques, including ubiquitin, tau, ACT, and α2-macroglobulin. Congophilic angiopathy, in which

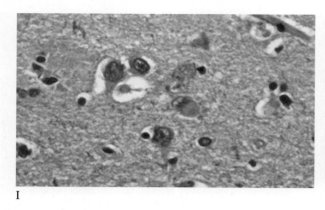
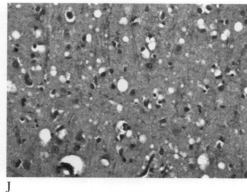

I   J

FIGURE 22-3, *cont'd. I,* Hematoxylin and eosin staining of a cortical Lewy body in dementia with Lewy bodies. *J,* Hematoxylin and eosin staining showing cortical spongiform changes in Creutzfeldt-Jakob disease. (Images of gross brain and microscopic specimens courtesy of Dr. Mark Edgar, Department of Neuropathology, New York-Presbyterian Hospital.)

β-amyloid fragments are deposited in the walls of brain blood vessels, is a common associated feature of AD, but can occur independently of AD symptoms. Amyloid deposition in cerebral blood vessels weakens the integrity of their walls and can lead to their catastrophic rupture, producing so-called lobar hemorrhages in temporal and parietal regions.

Cognitive Symptoms

AD is considered an "amnestic dementia" because its most common presenting symptom is the rapid forgetting of recently learned material. AD patients are generally capable of learning new material at the onset of the disease, but characteristically fail to recall this information spontaneously within minutes of its initial presentation. Memory for recent events is preferentially affected early in the course of the illness, whereas memories for more remote events (e.g., those of childhood) are relatively preserved until more advanced stages of the disease. The initial involvement of episodic memory is thought to reflect the particular vulnerability of medial temporal lobe structures, particularly the hippocampal formation, in the nascent disease process.

In addition to memory loss, disturbances in verbal fluency, attention, insight, and other executive functions are often among the earliest symptoms of AD (Hodges, 1998; Collette et al., 1999; Perry & Hodges, 1999). A characteristic loss of awareness of one's impairment (anosognosia) renders AD patients unable to fully appreciate the scope and magnitude of their deficits. As the disease progresses to involve cortical association areas in the temporal and parietal lobes, language comprehension, visuospatial function, and arithmetic skills are affected. Symptoms at this time may be relatively mild, but nonetheless impair social function and the ability to live independently.

In the stages of moderate AD, patients may require assistance with routine daily functions but usually retain the capacity to participate in their own care. They develop worsening visuospatial difficulties and impairments of skilled movements (apraxias) that limit their ability to perform tasks such as operating household appliances, dressing, and writing. Spatial and temporal disorientation worsen as the disease progresses, often leading to wandering and sleep disturbances. These symptoms, as well as impaired toileting and other indications of reduced personal hygiene, place increasing burdens on caregivers.

With further progression of the disease, disturbances in cognition, emotion, and behavior become global and more profound. At this stage, the patient usually develops urinary or frank incontinence, as well as complete dependency on a caregiver for survival. Eventually, neurologic functions that had originally been spared, including primary motor and sensory abilities, become affected, and the patient becomes bed-bound. AD invariably reduces the quality of life and often shortens life span. Progressive loss of cognitive function in AD eventually deprives the individual of livelihood, independence, thought, and identity, and causes great distress for the patient's family, friends, and caregivers. Although many AD patients are cared for at home for the full duration of their illness, care difficulties sometimes mandate institutionalization. Nursing home placement is an emotionally and financially difficult step for most caregivers. Symptoms increase over the course of a decade, leading to a state in which only vegetative neurologic functions are retained. Death is typically the result of secondary causes, most commonly systemic infections, rather than brain degeneration itself (Katzman, 1986).

Behavioral Symptoms

AD is associated with neuropsychiatric symptoms and functional impairment that are at least partially independent of memory, language, visuospatial, and other cognitive disturbances (Chen et al., 1998). Behavioral disturbances can be broadly divided into "positive" symptoms (paranoia, agitation, aggression, anxiety, delusions, and hallucinations) and "negative" symptoms (disinterest, social withdrawal, reduced speech output, and apathy) (Doody et al., 1995). In one study of 63 AD patients, the most frequent behavioral disturbances were anxiety (65%), apathy (58%), and dysphoria (58%) (Benoit et al., 1999). Another study of 50 patients with AD reported apathy (72%), agitation (60%), anxiety (48%), and dysphoria or aberrant motor activity (38%); all of these symptoms except for anxiety correlated with cognitive impairment (Mega et al., 1996).

The "positive" behavioral symptoms are troubling for family members and caregivers of AD patients, especially when they affect comportment and personality. There is also evidence that psychotic features are associated with more rapid cognitive decline (Stern et al., 1987; Burns et al., 1990; Rosen & Zubenko, 1991). Agitation and behavioral unrest are frequent precipitants of institutionalization, particularly when they are associated with verbal or physical aggression that is poorly controlled by medication.

Emotional Symptoms

Changes in emotion are a significant component of AD and can be expressed in many different ways, such as social withdrawal, loss of motivation, lessening of long-standing family relationships, and the loss of sense of humor or other pleasurable aspects of sensory and perceptual experiences. Major depression affects many patients with AD and may be underdiagnosed (Greenwald, 1995). The prevalence of depression in AD varies depending on study methods, with a median of 41% experiencing depressed mood and 19% having a major depressive disorder (Wragg & Jeste, 1989). In some patients, depression is a reaction to a loss of function (i.e., reactive depression), but in many others the cause may be progressive damage to subcortical, limbic and cortical structures mediating diverse aspects of emotion (organic depression) (Borson & Raskind, 1997). The high prevalence of depression and other behavioral disturbances in AD has been attributed to the loss of forebrain serotonergic innervation from the dorsal raphe nucleus (Meltzer et al., 1998). PET analysis has suggested a reduction in serotonin receptors in cerebral cortices of individuals with AD compared with age-matched controls (Blin et al., 1993). Also, reduced levels of serotonin and its major metabolite were found in the superior frontal gyrus, anterior and inferior temporal lobes, and fusiform gyrus in the brains from patients with AD compared with controls (Palmer et al., 1988).

Apathy, which may be defined as a lack of motivation or drive not caused by an alteration of consciousness or emotional distress, is common in AD and can be difficult to distinguish from depression. AD is also often accompanied by anosodiaphoria, an emotional indifference or lack of affective response to one's illness. Investigations into the pathophysiological substrates for apathy in patients with AD have yielded conflicting results but overall suggest the involvement of frontal and temporal brain systems. Apathetic AD patients score lower on tests of verbal memory, verbal fluency, naming, and set shifting (Kuzis et al., 1999), suggesting some involvement of frontal brain networks. In a single-photon emission computed tomography (SPECT) study of 40 patients with AD, apathy was correlated with decreased cerebral blood perfusion in the right temporal-parietal region (Ott et al., 1996). Another SPECT study of 31 AD patients with apathy showed severe prefrontal and anterior temporal lobe hypoperfusion (Craig, 1996). Decreased perfusion in the right cingulate gyrus was shown in 20 patients with AD and apathy (Benoit et al., 1999). Pathologic results have shown greater NFT pathology in the parahippocampal gyrus and frontal, and parietal cortices; and greater neuronal loss was seen in the hippocampus and basal nucleus in AD patients with higher composite scores for apathy, physical disability, and communication failure (Forstl et al., 1993).

Central Autonomic Involvement

Patients with AD may show central autonomic dysfunction, such as postural hypotension or impaired autonomic responses to strong emotional stimuli (Algotsson et al., 1995; Chu et al., 1994). Recently, widespread pathologic involvement of the central autonomic system has been described in AD. The ventral medial frontal cortex appears to play an important role in modulating central autonomic function (Neafsey, 1990). Closely apposed posterior orbital and anterior insular cortices are affected early in AD, almost to the same degree as the medial temporal cortices (Chu et al., 1997). The parabrachial nucleus in AD also shows marked pathologic changes compared with control brains (Parvizi et al., 1998). This brainstem nucleus is thought to be involved in relay and integration of visceral information (including vagal signals by way of the nucleus of the solitary tract) and in homeostatic control.

Frontotemporal Dementia— A Comportmental Dementia

Epidemiology

The average age of onset of FTD is between 50 and 60 years, making FTD a presenile disorder (i.e., usually occurring before age 65). FTD is thought to represent approximately 15% of all presenile dementias, in contrast to AD, which accounts for about 25% (Ratnavalli et al., 2002). The disease is much more common in men than women. Survival with FTD is variable, ranging from as few as 2 years to greater than 10 years in some cases. As in AD, death is usually a secondary complication of aspiration pneumonia, sepsis, or other complications of diminished ability for self-care.

Although most FTD appears to occur sporadically, the disease is familial in perhaps 40% of cases, with an autosomal dominant pattern of inheritance demonstrated in around 89% of these (Stevens et al., 1998; Chow et al., 1999). The first of several missense mutations in the tau gene was recently identified in an autosomal dominant familial form of FTD associated with parkinsonism and genetic linkage to chromosome 17 (FTDP-17) (Hutton et al., 1998). As noted above, tau protein is a central component of the NFTs found in AD and other degenerative diseases. However, disease-causing mutations in the tau gene have so far only been identified in FTD, though specific tau polymorphisms are a risk factor for the development of PSP (Conrad et al., 1997; Baker et al., 1999). Their precise pathogenetic role in the disease is not known, but the majority of missense mutations in FTDP-17 affect the ability of tau to bind and polymerize microtubules in vitro (for a review, see Hutton, 2000). The various mutations in the familial "tauopathies," as these genetically linked diseases are sometimes called, are associated with different patterns of brain microscopic pathology. It should be noted that most cases of familial FTD and the vast majority of sporadic cases are not associated with tau mutations (Houlden et al., 1999; Rizzu et al., 1999).

Pathology

The distribution of pathology in FTD is more heterogeneous than AD, resulting in more varied clinical presentations. The gross changes in brain volume affect frontal and temporal lobes bilaterally in many cases, but may be relatively unilateral (Fig. 22-3D, E). The dorsolateral prefrontal, orbitofrontal, temporal polar, and medial temporal cortices are predominantly affected, as are some subcortical structures, including the striatum and substantia nigra. Variant forms may show relative sparing of the dorsolateral prefrontal cortex. CBD, PSP, semantic dementia, dementia of the frontal lobe type, and Pick disease may represent different expressions of a single disease in that they can all give rise to forms of

dementia that would be characterized clinically as FTD, and they share similar pathologic features (Kertesz et al., 2000). An important feature that distinguishes FTD from AD is the relative lack of the progression along neuroanatomical projections within affected areas (e.g., from the hippocampus to neocortical association areas in AD). FTD typically involves worsening of initial symptoms and the development of new symptoms attributable to increasing cell death and pathologic changes within the frontal, temporal, and, sometimes, parietal areas. The progression of symptoms in FTD is also somewhat less predictable than in AD.

Microscopic pathology varies in sporadic FTD. Ballooned neurons containing silver-staining inclusions known as Pick bodies are occasionally seen. Their presence, however, is necessary for the pathologic diagnosis of Pick disease. Pick bodies, which are primarily composed of tau and ubiquitin, are found within the cytoplasm of affected neurons (Fig. 22-3F). Punctate "holes" sometimes appear in certain cortical layers, a condition called "status spongiosus." Nonspecific neuronal loss and astrocytic gliosis are commonly seen in cortical layers I through III in regions of brain atrophy. In contrast to AD, there is an absence of senile plaques and tangles. The pattern of frontal and temporal atrophy is an important defining feature, and can sometimes be diagnosed antemortem on structural and functional brain imaging studies.

Clinical Features

Consensus criteria for the diagnosis of FTD were originally established by groups of specialists in Lund, Sweden, and Manchester, United Kingdom (Lund and Manchester Groups, 1994). More recently, three principal syndromes of FTD have been described based on the presenting symptoms: frontal variant FTD, semantic dementia, and progressive nonfluent aphasia (Hodges, 2001). The last two syndromes, which represent primary language disturbances, will be discussed in the next section on PPA. Frontal variant FTD typically presents with altered personality and behavior that results from orbitobasal and ventromedial frontal disease. As in AD, relatives, friends, or co-workers usually bring the patient to medical attention, as the affected individual has little or no insight into his or her affliction. Occasionally, criminal behaviors bring patients with FTD to the attention of the justice system (see Chapter 54). Myriad signs of a frontal system disturbance can be seen, including a loss of normal social comportment, withdrawal from the company of others, impulsivity, disinhibited behavior (e.g., inappropriate joking or unrestrained sexuality), garrulousness, depression, anxiety, emotional lability, and appetitive disturbances (e.g., cravings for sweet foods). Language disturbances include logorrhea (excessive speech output), palilalia (repetition of the patient's own sounds), and echolalia (repetition of sounds made by others). Diametrically opposed behavioral abnormalities—apathy and agitation, depression and mania, gregariousness and social withdrawal—may affect the same patient at different times or stages of the disease. Later in the disease, he or she may demonstrate stereotyped, perseverative, or utilization behaviors, the last referring to an environmental "stickiness" in which the patient becomes bound to any attended stimulus—visual, auditory, or tactile.

Neurologic examination may show "frontal release" signs, such as grasp, palmomental, snout, root, and glabellar reflexes that indicate the loss of normal frontal lobe motor inhibition. Some of these reflexes reflect, in essence, the return of automatic protective or feeding responses that are present during early infancy. Movement disorders are not usually presenting symptoms of FTD, but, as the disease advances, patients may develop gait disturbances, bradykinesia, rigidity, and other extrapyramidal signs suggestive of PD. Cognitive testing in FTD tends to show impairments of executive function, language, attention, and working memory (e.g., serial recitation of numbers or the months of the year, forward and in reverse), response inhibition (Go/No-Go Test), and perseverance (e.g., Trail Making Tests). Encoding of new information may be impaired in the early stages of FTD, but delayed recall, calculation, and visuospatial abilities are generally intact (refer to Chapters 1–3 on cognitive testing).

Primary Progressive Aphasia— A Linguistic Dementia

Mesulam (1982) reported a progressive aphasic syndrome in the absence of superimposed dementia in a series of six right-handed patients. All had a presenile onset of language disturbances. One patient presented with pure word deafness, while the others showed anomic aphasia. Only two of the six patients developed more generalized dementias within a 5- to 11-year period of follow-up (Weintraub et al., 1990). The others developed worsening language abilities but did not become demented. Neuroimaging and postmortem findings implicated the left perisylvian areas (i.e., the frontal, temporal, and parietal neocortices surrounding the left Sylvian fissure) but did not reveal any specific pathologic findings indicative of a particular degenerative disease.

In subsequent decades, many examples of PPA have been documented in the medical literature, with the average age of onset of PPA usually around 60 years. As in FTD, the clinical manifestations can be quite variable within the affected domain of language. Anomia is a common presenting symptom, and progression to mutism is also frequently described. Some reported cases exhibit predominantly receptive disturbances at onset, whereas others demonstrate nonfluent aphasia with relative retention of semantic knowledge. No specific neuropathology has emerged, though some reports have linked PPA to focal presentations of AD or FTD.

The semantic dementia and progressive nonfluent aphasia variants of FTD are characterized by primary language disturbances (Hodges, 2001) and therefore overlap with some cases of PPA reported in the literature. Semantic dementia is a progressive loss of knowledge for words and objects and reflects predominant involvement of the left anterior-lateral temporal lobe. Patients have problems with more complex words early in their illness, often substituting simpler words or phrases. Language is fluent with normal grammar. In contrast, predominant involvement of the left perisylvian areas characterizes progressive nonfluent aphasia, typified by effortful speech and grammatical errors, along with word-finding difficulty. In later stages, patients may develop hypophonic speech or muteness. These variants of FTD probably account for some cases of PPA. More than half of patients with progressive nonfluent aphasia have FTD-like pathology with neuronal loss, gliosis, and status spongiosus in superficial cortical layers, a smaller fraction having Pick bodies, whereas the remainder have pathologic features typical of AD (Kertesz et al., 2002).

Instruments for evaluating aphasia, such as the Boston Diagnostic Aphasia Examination, can be applied in suspected cases of PPA, in combination with nonlinguistic testing instruments, to help distinguish PPA from other neurodegenerative disorders. Structural brain imaging often shows lobar atrophy in the perisylvian area, whereas functional neuroimaging may show hypometabolism or hypoperfusion confined to the language-related areas of the left frontal and temporal lobes. There is no proven medical treatment for PPA. In early stages of PPA, speech and language therapy are sometimes helpful. Assisted communication strategies, in which visual or verbal cues are provided, may be more effective later in the disease.

Parkinson Disease—A Dementia with Movement Disorders

Epidemiology

PD is estimated to afflict about one percent of the population (see Chapter 24). Most cases develop in adults over the age of 65 years, but juvenile cases can occur in early adulthood. The majority of cases are sporadic. Rare autosomal dominant forms of PD have been linked to mutations in the α-synuclein gene, whereas autosomal recessive cases of PD have been linked to mutations in the gene for parkin (Gwinn-Hardy, 2002). The precise normal function of neither protein is known at present.

Pathology

Few if any gross changes are found in the brains of patients with PD, but a striking loss of pigmented neurons in the substantia nigra, and in some cases the locus ceruleus, can be seen with the naked eye on freshly sectioned autopsy material (Fig. 22-3G). Cell loss in the substantia nigra is mirrored by the depletion of dopamine axon terminals in the striatum. Intracytoplasmic inclusions of α-synuclein and ubiquitin, called Lewy bodies, can be found in the pigmented, melanin-rich neurons of the substantia nigra pars compacta. With hematoxylin-eosin staining, Lewy bodies appear as pink spherical inclusions with a pale halo (Fig. 22-3H). Less distinct Lewy bodies can also be found in the neocortex (Fig. 22-3I), but these are more easily demonstrated by immunohistochemistry for α-synuclein or ubiquitin. Such cortical Lewy bodies may be responsible for many of the symptoms seen in the related disease DLB, including cognitive impairment and hallucinations (Gomez-Tortosa et al., 1999). In addition, NFTs and senile plaques can be found in cases of PD with dementia. Given the overlap between conditions, PD, AD, and DLB may represent a spectrum of illness, in which PD exhibits predominantly motor symptoms, AD cognitive symptoms, and DLB a combination of the two (see Fig. 22-1) (Kotzbauer et al., 2001).

Clinical Features

The clinical triad necessary for the diagnosis of PD is tremor, rigidity, and bradykinesia. Other common signs include an expressionless, mask-like face with drooling and bradyphrenia (slowness of thought). Patients with PD have a characteristic gait with stooped posture; short, shuffling steps; and absent arm swing. They have difficulty initiating steps, and a visual cue, such as a series of stripes taped on the floor, can enhance their walking. In addition, the gait usually quickens with subsequent steps, a process termed *festination*, from the Latin *festinare*, to hurry up.

Dementia is frequently seen later in the course of the illness, though it can sometimes occur earlier, afflicting perhaps 20% to 30% of patients with PD. Patients with PD have a sixfold increased risk of developing dementia relative to persons of a comparable age without PD (Aarsland et al., 2001). The distinction between PD with dementia, AD with parkinsonism, and dementia with Lewy bodies can be difficult (see Chapter 24). Dementia in PD may have features that distinguish it from disorders such as AD and FTD, such as accentuated disturbances of visuospatial function and attention, as might be expected with nondominant hemisphere involvement (Bodis-Wollner & Paulus, 1999). Advanced age may also be a risk factor for dementia in PD, as cognitive impairment is more common in PD patients with onset after 70 years of age (Levy et al., 2002). Lastly, there is an increased predilection for affective disorders in PD, particularly depression, which occurs in up to 31% of patients (Slaughter et al., 2001).

The cognitive symptoms of PD, with the possible exception of bradyphrenia, do not tend to respond very dramatically to treatment with dopaminergic agents (Kulisevsky, 2000). Indeed, demented PD patients may be more prone to develop symptoms of psychosis, including paranoia and frank hallucinations, when treated with this class of medications (Okada et al., 1999). Recently reported clinical case series have suggested a possible future role for cholinesterase inhibitors in the treatment of dementia in PD (Werber & Rabey, 2001; Bullock & Cameron, 2002).

CLINICAL EVALUATION OF SUSPECTED DEGENERATIVE DEMENTIAS

Currently, the diagnosis of a degenerative dementia implies an incurable condition with limited opportunity to slow its progression. The physician should make every effort to establish a correct diagnosis and exclude possible medically treatable conditions that can mimic a degenerative process or contribute to debilitation. A carefully obtained history will often narrow the differential diagnosis down to a few probable conditions. Laboratory tests can then be selected to support or refute the diagnostician's clinical hypothesis. This section provides a guide to evaluation of patients with cognitive, behavioral, or motor problems suggestive of a degenerative disease. Additional relevant material can be found elsewhere in this textbook and in review articles (e.g., Fleming et al., 1995; Geldmacher & Whitehouse, 1996).

History and Caregiver's Report

The patient with cognitive impairment is often unable to provide a reliable history of his or her illness. The examiner should attempt to gather as much information as possible from the patient, but often the evaluating physician or neuropsychologist must rely on a patient's spouse, family, friends, home attendants, or nursing staff to obtain an accurate medical history. Medical records from the primary care physician, prior neurologic evaluations, or nursing care facility can provide valuable data on the course of the disease and help minimize the unproductive repetition of laboratory tests.

By definition, dementia is a decline in mental function from an individual's premorbid level of performance that involves two or more cognitive domains. The degree of cognitive or behavioral impairment in dementia is sufficient to interfere with normal daily functioning. Relevant history should address whether cognitive deterioration is due to dementia, delirium, psychiatric illness, or systemic medical conditions. As a rule, illnesses characterized by depressed arousal at their earliest stages will likely be due to delirium from a toxic or metabolic process, stroke, intracranial hemorrhage, or epilepsy, and not the result of degenerative disease.

The onset of AD and most other degenerative disorders is insidious, with symptoms initially going almost unnoticed—misplacing one's keys or eyeglasses, a tendency to repeat questions, or forgetting the details of recent events. As these disorders inevitably progress, the patient or those around him or her will suspect a problem. The onset of vascular dementia is more abrupt than in AD and seems to fluctuate more. In addition, an acute illness or stressor can make a degenerative disorder appear abrupt in onset. Acute cognitive deterioration can also be seen with infections (both neurologic and systemic), metabolic disturbances, stroke, neoplastic and paraneoplastic disorders, subdural hematomas, hydrocephalus, and changes in medications.

Most informants will supply specific examples in response to an inquiry about the patient's memory capacity; but focused questions can bring to light deficits overlooked by the patient's spouse, family member, or friend. Does the patient misplace things or forget recent events, birthdays, anniversaries, or the names of familiar persons? In conversation, does the patient have trouble finding words, as if they were on the tip of the tongue? Cognitive and behavioral changes will hinder a range of activities of daily living (ADLs), which is relevant to staging of AD (see below). For example, if the patient is still employed, has job performance declined?

Changes in personality, indifference towards others, apathy, regression, impulsivity, social withdrawal, disinhibited behavior, suspicion of caregivers, outbursts, and violence are characteristic of dementia of the frontal lobes, but can surface in other dementias, often as a latent manifestation of premorbid personality traits. Delusions and hallucinations are prominent features early in the course of DLB, but might be seen in middle and later stages of AD or PD and with side effects of medications.

The patient's mood should be assessed because depression can produce cognitive symptoms as in "pseudodementia" and also frequently accompanies AD and PD. Depression is associated with feelings of hopelessness, tearfulness, somatic delusions, poor appetite, and disturbed sleep. It is important to ask whether the depressed patient has passive wishes of death, or ideas, or tangible plans of committing suicide. In depression, daily functions such as dressing ability and orientation tend to be preserved. To assist in the diagnosis, the clinician should inquire about past psychiatric illness, alcohol use, and drug abuse.

The clinician should obtain a routine history of other medical conditions, such as hypertension or heart disease, and also inquire about head trauma, seizures, and stroke. Gait problems or urinary incontinence might suggest normal pressure hydrocephalus (NPH) or vascular disease. Many medications, both prescription and nonprescription, can impair brain function. These include analgesics, anticholinergics (e.g., antispasmodics for urinary incontinence), antihypertensives (betablockers in particular), diuretics, psychotropic agents, and sedative-hypnotics. A family history might reveal an inherited condition or a genetic predisposition to AD, PD, or stroke. The social history should address the patient's living conditions, network of family and friends, need for home services, marital status, employment, source of income, management of finances, and assessment of home safety.

Neurologic Examination

Each patient who presents with complaints of cognitive, behavioral, or motor impairment should undergo a thorough neurologic evaluation. Specific neurologic findings can be highly useful in distinguishing one disorder from another. The patient's general appearance will serve as a rough measure of his or her ability to perform ADLs, such as bathing, grooming, and dressing. It might also indicate a spouse's or other caregiver's ability or inability to assist adequately the more dependent patient.

The general medical examination should address factors that can predispose to cerebrovascular disease, including cardiac arrhythmia, hypertension, hypotension (e.g., due to antihypertensive medications), carotid bruits, and heart murmurs. Heart rate and blood pressure measurements should be recorded, both with the patient lying down and standing, in any patient who has episodic or positional changes in mental state, or a degenerative disease associated with autonomic dysfunction (e.g., AD, DLB, PD or multiple system atrophy [MSA]). Skin changes and joint deformities might represent an autoimmune or rheumatological illness that can produce or contribute to cognitive impairment.

The neurologic examination can show signs that are common to several or specific to only certain degenerative diseases. One should test smell whenever a disturbance in the frontal lobes is suspected, although sense of smell may diminish with normal aging or following head trauma (see Chapter 15). Visual fields can be assessed by a confrontational technique such as finger counting in the four visual quadrants (see Chapter 12). Hemispatial neglect can be detected by looking for extinction of stimuli presented simultaneously in the two visual hemifields. Extinction usually indicates contralateral parietal lobe dysfunction (see Chapter 10).

The clinician should also be vigilant for the presence of simultanagnosia, the inability to perceive an entire visual composition and in which only individual components can be seen at a given moment. This is a result of bilateral disturbances in the occipitoparietal region and can be seen in AD (especially the PCA variant), boundary zone vascular insults (so-called "watershed" infarcts) between the anterior and posterior cerebral arterial systems, CJD, or CBD (Rizzo & Vecera, 2002). It is not uncommon for a caregiver to state that the patient has trouble finding eating utensils on the table in front of him. The patient usually is subjected to extensive optometric evaluations and might be prescribed new eyeglasses to no avail. Simultanagnosia can be assessed by asking the patient to circle each letter "A" on a sheet of paper randomly covered by these and other letters of varying sizes. The patient with simultanagnosia will be unable to find the largest "A"s as a result of an inability to perceive anything but fragments of an entire visual scene.

Simultanagnosia may occur as part of Balint syndrome, a clinical triad that also includes optic ataxia and ocular apraxia. The latter is an ability to voluntarily direct one's gaze to the periphery despite a full range of ocular rotations. It can be evaluated by comparing a patient's saccadic eye movements (e.g., eliciting the patient to look left or right) with his or her smooth pursuit eye movements (e.g., following a target such as a finger or picture), which should be preserved. Optic ataxia is a disturbance in directing limb movements to a target under visual guidance. This could be assessed by asking the patient to reach for and touch a small object with his or her finger; the examiner should be suspicious of even subtle errors in finding the target.

Intrusions of tiny saccadic movements during smooth eye pursuit and a slight limitation of upgaze are common findings in the elderly, but more significant impairment in eye movements, especially in downgaze, can suggest brainstem microinfarcts, PSP, Wernicke's disease, or cerebellar disease. Pupillary abnormalities may suggest a general autonomic disturbance or a more localized process such as neurosyphilis. Subtle facial asymmetries, such as not burying the eyelashes on one side upon eye closure, can indicate contralateral cerebrovascular disease. The tongue should be examined for atrophy or fasciculations characteristic of motor neuron disease. The quality of the patient's voice and speech patterns can point to either bulbar disease (e.g., amyotrophic lateral sclerosis [ALS] or MSA) or pseudobulbar disease (e.g., PSP or frontal lobe infarcts).

In the absence of gross muscle weakness, a pronator drift can be a useful indicator of stroke, as can changes in deep tendon reflexes. One should remember that a patient with ALS often has evidence of disease of upper motor neurons (increased muscle tone and hyperreflexia) and lower motor neurons (atrophy and fasciculations). Extrapyramidal signs, seen in the parkinsonian disorders (PD, DLB, MSA, PSP, and CBD), may include resting tremors of the hands and sometimes lower extremities, rigidity—either of the "lead pipe" or "cogwheeling"

type—bradykinesia, impoverished facial expression, reduced eye blinking, and slowness or difficulty in arising from a chair. A Babinski sign or variant of extensor plantar reflex indicates corticospinal tract disease.

The sensory examination will be most useful if attention is paid to modalities requiring large nerve fiber integrity and cortical sensory areas. Vitamin B_{12} deficiency usually affects vibration and position sense. The patient might complain of numbness and paresthesias. Tests of cortical sensory areas include double simultaneous sensory stimulation (looking for extinction), graphesthesia, and stereognosis.

Signs of corticospinal weakness or cerebellar dysfunction can be elicited by asking the patient to rapidly pat his hands on his lap, alternating the palm and dorsal sides. Cerebellar integrity can be further assessed by finger-to-nose and heel-to-shin testing.

No neurologic examination is complete without an assessment of gait, both as a diagnostic tool and as an indicator of a patient's risk for falls. Slow, shuffling types of gait are often associated with idiopathic PD, but can also be seen in other disorders like PSP and CBD, NPH, and cerebrovascular disease. Romberg's sign should be looked for as an indicator of disease in the posterior columns of the spinal cord, such as might be seen with neurosyphilis or vitamin B_{12} deficiency.

Lastly, several signs demonstrate disease usually involving the frontal lobes. They can be seen early in the course of FTD but can often be seen in most dementias by the later stages. Grasp and palmomental reflexes, snouting and rooting, and Meyerson's sign (glabellar reflex) are thus useful but nonspecific findings.

Cognitive Testing

The cognitive assessment of the patients with a suspected degenerative disorder is important for documenting the presence of mental impairment, inferring the underlying cause, gauging the severity of symptoms, monitoring disease progression, and assessing response to treatment. Delineating the presenting symptoms and pattern of progression is a key part of the degenerative dementia evaluation. Each degenerative disease has different affinities for structures and pathways within the brain, resulting in idiosyncratic symptoms and pattern of progression that are sufficiently stereotyped to provide potent indications of the most likely underlying disorder. Recognizing these characteristic patterns of presentation and progression is currently the most important means of diagnosing degenerative diseases. Any deviation from the expected course of progression may indicate the presence of another co-morbid condition or an error in the primary diagnosis. While the first evaluation provides a "snapshot" of the patient's condition, annual or biannual reevaluations add longitudinal details that allow estimates of the rate of decline. In well-studied diseases such as AD, initial amnestic symptoms are attributable to involvement of the hippocampal formation. The disease then progresses along the afferent and efferent connections of the hippocampus to other limbic structures and to neocortical association areas. By understanding the functions of the affected structures and their combined actions as part of neural systems, clinicians can effectively follow the course of the illness as it affects the various brain regions in sequence.

Cognitive testing should begin with general clinical screening using standardized testing instruments (see Chapter 1). These are useful to determine whether dementia is present, to grade the severity of any cognitive disability, to identify the cognitive domains that are most affected, and to provide a baseline by which to gauge, quantitatively, changes over time or in response to treatment. If dementia cannot clearly be demonstrated at this first evaluation, yet the main complaints and history suggest the possibility of a cognitive disorder, the clinician may proceed in one of two ways. The patient could be referred to a clinical neuropsychologist or behavioral neurologist for a more detailed evaluation. Alternatively, the patient could be asked to return for repeat testing in 6 to 12 months to see if a decline in function suggestive of a degenerative illness is present. This decision will depend upon the clinician's level of expertise or familiarity with these disorders, the strength of suspicion of a cognitive disorder, and compelling circumstances in the patient's life, such as employment, financial, or legal issues.

Several screening instruments are in common use including the Mini-Mental State Exam (MMSE) (Folstein et al., 1975), the Blessed Dementia Scale (Blessed et al., 1968), the Mattis Dementia Rating Scale (Mattis, 1988), and the Consortium to Establish a Registry for Alzheimer's Disease battery (Welsh et al., 1992) (see Chapter 1). The MMSE is a 30-point assessment and is probably the most widely used and easiest to administer. It tests attention, recall, orientation, naming, written and oral comprehension, writing, and drawing. A modified form of the MMSE (referred to informally as the 3MS) uses a 100-point rating scale and allows for graded scaling, as well as assessments of verbal fluency and abstract thinking (Teng & Chui, 1987). These two tests can be administered concurrently and usually take only five to ten minutes to complete. Normative tables for different ages and levels of education are available for the MMSE (Crum et al., 1993). However, a single cutoff value of 23 or less has been demonstrated in an internal medicine practice to have a sensitivity of 69% and a specificity of 99% for detecting dementia (Tangalos et al., 1996).

The clinical history and screening test results should provide some indication of which cognitive systems might be affected or spared. More comprehensive testing can then be directed at these areas. The interpretation of a patient's test performance must take into context his or her age, education, career, lifestyle, and primary or secondary language. A general clinician can perform an initial screening test (as outlined below) during an office evaluation, but in many cases referral to a behavioral neurologist or neuropsychologist is warranted for more definitive testing. These would include patients with subtle deficits that could escape the detection of screening instruments. For example, referral to a neuropsychologist would be indicated for patients with an advanced level of education or high-performance job who recognize that they are not functioning up to their normal standards but who would score normally on all but the most challenging cognitive tasks. The testing instruments used by neuropsychologists have normative tables for different ages, level of education, and estimated premorbid intelligence. Neuropsychological testing also allows for longitudinal evaluation when following a patient with possible incipient dementia (e.g., in MCI or age-related cognitive decline). It is also very useful when the differential diagnosis is difficult (e.g., atypical disease presentations) or when the clinical picture is clouded by the presence of depression or premorbid cognitive disability (e.g., dyslexia). Neuropsychological testing is described in detail in Chapter 2. Here we will limit our discussion of the cognitive assessment to tests that can be performed at the bedside or that are part of the MMSE or modified MMSE.

Reliable cognitive testing cannot be performed unless the patient is alert, so *arousal* should be initially assessed. Arousal can be decreased by metabolic disturbances, medication toxicity, raised intracranial pressure, infection (either systemic or primary nervous system), epileptic and postictal states (e.g., complex partial seizures), or advanced degenerative state.

A disturbance in *attention* is rarely the sole manifestation of mental impairment, as it will also impact other areas of cognitive performance (see Chapter 10). Attention can be tested by asking the patient to perform a task that requires ongoing focused concentration such as reciting a numerical sequence or the months of the year in reverse. The ability to repeat increasingly longer series of digits forward and then in reverse tests attention and working memory; it provides a quantitative measure that can be used for future reference. A more difficult test for working memory is to ask the patient to alternate numbers and letters in sequence out loud: one, A, two, B, etc. In the Go/No-Go test, the patient sits with the dominant hand flat on a table or desk opposite the examiner. The clinician first asks the subject to tap his hand once in response to the examiner's single taps on the underside of the desk or table. If the patient can perform this task, the test is made more difficult by asking the patient to tap once if the examiner taps once and not to tap at all if the examiner taps twice. Errors of omission (i.e., not tapping when required) and commission (i.e., tapping when not indicated) should be noted.

Orientation to time is affected earlier in AD than is orientation to place, and largely represents the prominent disability in short-term memory in this illness. Three-item memory tests are a component of the MMSE and other general screening batteries (e.g., "shirt, brown, honesty" or "John Brown, 42 Market St., Chicago"), but patients with mild amnestic impairments might perform normally on this limited task, so a longer list of items might be more instructive. On the modified MMSE, spontaneous recall and, if necessary, recognition of missed words from a list are assessed immediately and then at one and ten minutes with intervening distracting tasks (e.g., giving a figure to copy or a clock to draw). This type of memory test allows for the distinction of disturbances in the three components of memory, namely registration or encoding, recall, and recognition. For example, the pseudodementia of depression is characterized by impaired encoding but normal recall, whereas encoding will be normal but spontaneous recall impaired in early AD. A test of long-term memory retrieval might assess the ability of the patient to recall his or her own date of birth or birthplace.

An initial impression of the patient's *language* ability will be formed during the history interview. Is speech fluent, with normal cadence and prosody? Does the patient seem to have trouble finding words and substitute circumlocutions (e.g., "the thing you talk with" instead of "telephone") or make paraphasic errors (e.g., "this is my *wafe*" instead of "wife")? *Naming* of objects is often impaired early in the course of AD. The MMSE asks the patient to name simple objects such as a pencil and a watch. The 3MS is a more demanding test that asks the names of several body parts. The examiner must always distinguish between an impairment in naming, which implies preserved recognition of the object (i.e., true anomia), versus impairment in object recognition or agnosia. The patient with anomia, but not agnosia, should still be able to verbally describe an item or demonstrate its use.

Verbal comprehension can begin with simple "yes-no" types of question and progress to more difficult questions, such as, "Point to the receptacle in the room used for discarding waste," or, "Which relation is the mother of your first cousin?" The examiner should take care not to mistake hearing deficits or apraxia for comprehension problems. *Reading comprehension* is part of the MMSE ("Close your eyes"), but performance impairment might be due to a refractive error, visual field defect, spatial neglect, or simultanagnosia. Writing to dictation and spontaneous production of a written sentence are both part of the 3MS.

Word *fluency* assesses attention, working memory, and language. Deficits in semantic or categorical fluency (e.g., the number of animals the patient can list in one minute) are often a sign of impairment in temporal and inferior parietal lobe disease and may be affected early in the course of AD. *Executive function* can be assessed by the patient's ability to think abstractly. A normal, abstract answer to the question, "What do an apple and an orange have in common?" would be that they are both fruits or round objects, whereas a very concrete patient might say that they have nothing in common. The subject can also be asked about differences between items such as a river and a canal.

Copying a figure of two interlocking pentagons is a test of *visuospatial function* from the MMSE. In patients with mild to moderate dementia, pentagon copying is more impaired in DLB than in AD (Ala et al., 2001). More subtle impairments can be detected by asking the patient to copy a picture of a solid cube (not the transparent Necker cube used in tests of Gestalt psychology, which is easier to draw). Providing a circle and requesting that the patient draw in all the numbers of a clock and insert the hands to indicate a specific time (e.g., 2:45) tests both executive planning ability as well as visuospatial skills. Simply asking the patient to copy a completed clock face relies more on visuospatial function and is usually associated with a disturbance in the nondominant posterior parietal area. Improved performance on the copy part of the test relative to the drawing part is seen in AD and PD, whereas patients with DLB perform equally poorly on both tasks (Gnanalingham et al., 1997).

When testing for *apraxia*, the clinician must determine whether the patient has impairment in the ability to conceive of a complex task (ideational apraxia), the ability to translate an understood task into a motor action (ideomotor apraxia), or selective impairment in fine-skilled hand movements (kinetomotor or limb-kinetic apraxia) (see Chapter 18). Remember that apraxia can be accurately assessed only in the setting of normal primary motor function and comprehension. Ideomotor apraxia is most commonly tested by ordering the patient to pantomime how he combs his hair, brushes his teeth, or lights a match. Substitution of a body part for the pantomimed object (e.g., using her or his index finger to simulate a toothbrush) is a subtle sign of apraxia. With ideomotor apraxia, the patient can usually correctly imitate the task if demonstrated by the examiner or if provided with the actual tool or implement (e.g., a comb). Differences in praxic ability can sometimes be seen for midline tasks (e.g., "stick out your tongue") compared with appendicular tasks (e.g., "wave good-bye"). Kinetomotor apraxia can be demonstrated by asking the patient to pick up a small coin from a tabletop or to roll a coin between her or his index finger and thumb. These types of apraxia are associated with disturbances in the dominant hemisphere, but dressing apraxia is most often seen with nondominant parietal lobe lesions. Turning the sleeve of a patient's coat or jacket inside out without his knowledge and then asking him to put it on is a sensitive test of this type of praxis.

A disturbance in the ability to *calculate* or perform arithmetic is by itself suggestive of a lesion in the angular gyrus of the dominant hemisphere (see Chapter 17). However, impaired attention or working memory can distort the interpretation of abnormal calculating ability. Thus, the examiner may need to assess this task both verbally and in writing to discriminate between these possibilities. Testing should begin with simple tasks (i.e., addition and subtraction) and increase to more difficult problems (e.g., multiplication and division).

Staging

By their nature, neurodegenerative diseases are progressive illnesses, and accurate staging is important in discussing a patient's prognosis, needs, and treatment. Assessment of functional ability should address a patient's ability to perform ADLs. These include basic care—washing, bathing, dressing, continence, eating, grooming, and using the toilet—as well as more complex tasks such as choosing clothes and dressing, which tend to be affected earlier than simple ones. There is little cultural bias in ADLs in contrast to instrumental activities of daily living (IADLs), which are more complex integrative tasks and social skills: preparing meals, shopping, using money, telephoning, performing household chores, and using public transportation or driving a car (see Chapter 36). These are invariably affected earlier in a degenerative disease than are ADLs.

An accurate assessment of the patient's functional status can usually be obtained by interviewing a spouse or other caregiver. This will allow the physician to gauge how much the patient's illness has affected normal life, and whether the disease is in the early, middle, or late stage. One can also use established grading scales that correlate functional status with the stage of dementia. The Functional Assessment Staging (FAST) system distinguishes seven different phases of dementia (Auer & Reisberg, 1997). Stages 1 through 3 characterize function associated with neurologically normal elderly individuals and those with age-associated memory impairment. Stage 4 represents early dementia in which the patient still functions relatively independently despite some difficulty with IADLs. In stage 5, the patient has trouble choosing her or his clothes; for example, she or he may wear the same clothes every day or dress inappropriately for the season. By stage 6, the patient exhibits dressing apraxia, needs help dressing, and requires constant supervision of other activities. Finally, in stage 7, the patient is mute and bedridden, and requires full-time care (see Chapter 1 for further details of deterioration and dementia rating scales).

Blood Tests

Several routine blood tests should be included in the initial evaluation of every patient suspected of having a degenerative disorder, though such screening might only detect a reversible etiology for dementia in 5% to 10% of cases (Larson et al, 1986; Weytingh et al., 1995). The reason to perform blood screens is twofold: some medical conditions can mimic degenerative disease and others can contribute to the impairment posed by degenerative disease (Fleming et al., 1995).

A complete blood cell count and erythrocyte sedimentation rate (ESR) will rule out anemia, myeloproliferative disease, infection, and inflammatory conditions. Routine blood chemistry tests should assess electrolytes, liver enzymes, renal function, and serum glucose. Testing of parathyroid hormone levels should be performed if a calcium abnormality is detected. A history of acute or fluctuating cognitive decline accompanied by gastrointestinal pain, "surgical abdomen," urinary retention or incontinence, autonomic dysfunction, and neuropathy should raise the possibility of acute intermittent porphyria and lead to a search for urinary porphyrins.

Hypothyroidism is a common disease of the elderly characterized by depression, irritability, and mental slowness, which can be the primary cause of dementia or worsen the cognitive impairment of another illness. Testing should include a thyrotropin (thyroid-stimulating hormone) and free thyroxine (T_4) level. Hashimoto's thyroiditis, in addition to being the most common etiology of hypothyroidism, especially in women, can also be associated with an encephalopathy characterized by acute cognitive decline and decreased arousal, myoclonus, and seizures. If it is suspected, blood tests for antithyroid antibodies should be performed.

Along with large-fiber neuropathy and posterior column myelopathy, vitamin B_{12} or folate deficiency can produce cognitive and psychiatric manifestations. Recent evidence suggests that vitamin B_{12} and folate deficiency may contribute to the development of AD (Wang et al., 2001). If blood levels for both vitamins are normal despite clinical suspicion, methylmalonic acid and homocysteine levels should be checked since patients with these vitamin deficiencies may have normal blood counts (i.e., anemia or macrocytosis) and vitamin levels early in the illness (Lindenbaum et al., 1988). Although elevated plasma homocysteine levels may possibly be a risk factor for the development of AD (Seshadri et al., 2002), routine screening of homocysteine levels is not recommended as part of the dementia evaluation.

Neurosyphilis was once a prevalent illness but is a rare cause of dementia nowadays. In addition, the serum Venereal Disease Research Laboratories test (VDRL), rapid plasmin reagin test (RPR), and free treponemal antibody test (FTA) all have problems with sensitivity and specificity. Therefore, routine screening for neurosyphilis is now recommended only in areas where the disease is still prevalent (Knopman et al., 2001). Lyme disease can be associated with cognitive symptoms (usually attentional disturbances) and should be tested for if the patient lives in an endemic area, is aware of tick exposure, or has systemic symptoms or signs suggestive of this illness, such as a ring-forming rash, arthralgias, and fatigue.

Rheumatologic illnesses, including systemic lupus erythematosus, rheumatoid arthritis, Sjögren syndrome, and sarcoidosis, can produce cognitive and psychiatric illness. They can be examined by blood testing for antinuclear antibodies, rheumatoid factor, anti-Ro and anti-La antibodies, and angiotensin-converting enzyme (ACE) levels. Appropriate tests should likewise be performed if the patient has risk factors for human immunodeficiency virus (HIV) or exposure to toxic substances, including heavy metals (e.g., arsenic, lead, and mercury), carbon monoxide, or illicit drugs.

Structural Imaging

The initial evaluation should include a structural assessment of the brain by CT or MRI. These tests will help exclude stroke, tumor, hydrocephalus, congenital anomalies, and demyelinating disease. So-called "silent strokes" might contribute to the cognitive or motor effects of degenerative diseases.

The pattern of atrophy seen on structural imaging can be useful in supporting a clinical diagnosis of brain degeneration (see Chapter 4). Early in the illness, AD is associated with medial temporal lobe atrophy, which progresses over time. FTD is characterized by frontal lobe atrophy along with variable shrinkage of the polar and medial temporal lobe. Midbrain atrophy is seen with PSP, and the head of the caudate nucleus is markedly reduced in volume in HD.

CT is an x-ray-based technique with a resolution of 1.5 to 2.0 mm. Intravenous contrast can be administered to visualize neoplasms, vasculitic lesions, and infections such as abscesses. However, even without contrast, atrophy, ventriculomegaly, hematomas, and infarcts can be seen. CT has the advantages of being inexpensive, rapid, and excellent for the detection of hemorrhage, but suffers from poor resolution of tissues in proximity to bone (especially the structures of the posterior fossa) and limited differentiation between gray and white matter regions.

MRI uses a magnetic field and pulsed radio waves to produce brain images based upon changes in proton dipole moments. It has a resolution of 1.0 to 1.5 mm with standard 1.5 Tesla magnets. Several types of images are routinely generated. T1 images are useful for studying brain anatomy and CSF spaces. T2 is excellent for detecting pathology such as effacement of the gray

and white matter borders, edema, infarcts, and vasculitis. Fluid attenuation inversion recovery (FLAIR) imaging is a very sensitive technique for white matter changes such as microinfarcts. Infarcts that are from 30 minutes to one week old can be seen by diffusion-weighted imaging (DWI). Gradient spin echo is a technique sensitive to deposits of hemosiderin, which are indicative of old hemorrhages such as those due to amyloid angiopathy. The disadvantages of MRI include cost, long testing periods in an enclosed space (which might be intolerable to claustrophobic subjects or impractical in agitated patients), and prohibitive in patients with implanted cardiac pacemakers or defibrillators. However, it remains the structural imaging tool of choice due to its detailed information and resolution, sensitivity to changes in hippocampal size, its ability to produce images in axial, coronal, and sagittal planes, and visualization of the brainstem and cerebellum.

Functional Imaging

The majority of diagnoses for patients with degenerative disorders of the brain will be relatively straightforward. For cases in which the diagnosis is uncertain, functional brain imaging may be helpful in detecting an early stage of a disease or distinguishing one disorder from another. However, functional brain imaging remains an experimental study and is not a diagnostic test. Two techniques are commonly used: SPECT and PET (see Chapter 6). In the future, functional MRI (fMRI) techniques that correlate cellular oxygen states with regional brain activity may be used in the clinical assessment of dementia (see Chapter 7).

SPECT employs radionuclide-labeled agents to demonstrate cerebral blood flow and is therefore an indirect measure of metabolism and brain activity. Distinct patterns of reduced blood flow help to discriminate between different disorders. AD is characterized by temporal and parietal lobe hypoperfusion. Frontal and temporal lobe reductions are seen with FTD. Like AD, DLB is associated with reduced temporal and parietal blood flow, but the medial temporal lobes tend to be spared and involvement of occipital areas is notable (Lobotesis et al., 2001). Vascular disease, such as multiple infarcts, is distinguished by scattered gray and white matter areas of hypoperfusion. However, a similar pattern may be seen with CJD. Superior frontal hypoperfusion with relative sparing of inferior areas can be demonstrated in PSP (Johnson et al., 1992). One should not be misled by the phenomenon of diaschisis—decreased perfusion or metabolism in an unaffected brain area that receives nerve projections from an affected area.

PET transforms the coincident detection of positrons emitted by radionuclides such as ^{19}F-glucose to produce high-resolution maps that directly measure metabolic activity. It is more expensive than SPECT and less widely available because of the necessity of an on-site cyclotron to produce the labeled tracers. Similar patterns of hypometabolism are seen as with SPECT, but it is generally more sensitive to such changes.

Genetic Testing

At this time, routine genetic testing is not recommended for most degenerative disorders of the brain. There is relative acceptance of presymptomatic genetic testing for illnesses such as HD that are associated with deterministic autosomal dominant mutations. That is, an individual with a parent who has HD has a 50% chance of developing the disease. HD is a "triplet repeat" disease in which repetitive CAG-nucleotide sequences at the 5′-end DNA coding region of the protein huntingtin are expanded. The highly expanded repetitive sequences associated with the disease can be detected by a blood test. Autosomal dominant FTD with mutations in the gene for tau have been recently discovered (for a review, see Hutton, 2000), as have familial forms of PD with mutations in the genes for α-synuclein and parkin (for a review, see Gwinn-Hardy, 2002). Genetic testing for *APP*, *PS1*, or *PS2* mutations associated with AD is warranted when the disease presents in individuals below the age of 50 and when there is an autosomal dominant pattern of inheritance.

There are certain instances in which testing for genetic mutations or polymorphisms can be useful in diagnosis. The vast majority of cases of AD are sporadic in nature or have an inheritance pattern that does not obey a classical Mendelian pattern of inheritance. Possession of either one or two copies of the *APOE* ε4 allele increases the risk that an individual will develop AD and lowers the likely age of onset. Genetic testing for *APOE* alleles can be useful in *supporting* a diagnosis of AD, particularly when an individual is in the range of 55 to 70 years of age. However, possession of an ε4 allele does not necessarily mean an otherwise asymptomatic individual will develop AD. Presymptomatic testing for AD based on *APOE* status is thus not currently recommended (Relkin et al., 1996), although this recommendation may change when disease-modifying or preventative treatments for AD become available.

Electroencephalography

EEG can provide useful information for several conditions (see Chapter 8). In dementias such as AD, background slowing, manifested as reduced alpha (8 to 13 Hz) and beta (14 to 25 Hz), and increased delta (< 4 Hz) and theta (4 to 7 Hz) brain electrical activity can be seen, but may be absent or unapparent early in the illness. These findings can also be seen in encephalopathy due to metabolic or toxic insults. Focal abnormalities (slowing, reduced amplitude, sharp waves, spikes, or slow waves) should raise the suspicion of processes such as infarction, hemorrhage, neoplasm, or epilepsy. Epilepsy has an increasing incidence in the elderly and can occur late in the course of AD, but is unusual in FTD. Affected patients may have complex partial epilepsy characterized by behavioral changes, automatisms, or fugue states.

Whenever the diagnosis of CJD is suspected or when confronted with a rapidly progressive dementia, an EEG is warranted. The characteristic EEG findings in CJD are triphasic waves and one-per-second synchronous periodic sharp waves. However, these are sometimes seen only late in the disease and are not diagnostic findings. Triphasic waves can be seen in toxic-metabolic encephalopathy, and synchronous bilateral sharp wave activity can be seen in herpes simplex encephalitis, subacute sclerosing panencephalitis, and during or following status epilepticus.

Lumbar Puncture

The analysis of CSF by lumbar puncture is most useful for evaluating atypical dementias, those that present in young patients (less than 55 years of age), in patients with known connective tissue disease, and when there is the possibility of CNS infections, neoplasms, or primary vasculitis. Contraindications for lumbar puncture include raised intracranial pressure with mass effect, in which brain herniation is a risk, and infections in the vicinity of the puncture site, which can seed the infectious agent into the CNS.

Infections are generally characterized by elevated white blood cell counts and high protein levels. Similar profiles will be seen with vasculitis. It should be noted that primary CNS vasculitis is often accompanied by a normal ESR, in contrast to most systemic vasculitides. Studies for specific antibody markers (e.g., neurosyphilis, Lyme disease, and viral encephalitis), antigens (e.g., cryptococcus), and cultures (e.g., for bacteria, tuberculosis, and fungal infections) are widely used. The patient with HIV might have a primary dementing illness or one secondary to an opportunistic infection and, in the absence of a mass-occupying brain lesion, should undergo CSF analysis.

Monoclonal or oligoclonal antibodies can be seen with neoplastic, paraneoplastic, and demyelinating disorders. Antibody markers are especially useful for illnesses characterized by cerebellar degeneration (anti-Yo), opsoclonus-myoclonus (anti-Ri), or encephalopathy (anti-Hu) (Dalmau & Posner, 1999). The presence of any of these markers demands an investigation for an underlying neoplasm. Cytology should also be examined whenever neoplastic disease is suspected, and specific chemical markers should be considered (e.g., β2-microglobulin for carcinomas and lymphoma, lactic acid dehydrogenase isoenzyme 5, and β-glucoronidase for various neoplasms) (Jaeckle, 1985).

An elevated level of 14-3-3 protein in the CSF has good sensitivity and specificity for CJD, but brain hypoxia, infections, and neoplasms can produce false-positive results, as can other causes of dementia (Zerr et al., 1998; Burkhard et al., 2001). In questionable cases of AD, a combination of elevated tau levels and decreased Aβ levels in the CSF can help support the diagnosis (Galasko et al., 1998). Lastly, no specific test has yet proven reliable by itself in diagnosing NPH, but an improvement in cognitive or motor symptoms following the removal of 40 to 50 cc of CSF ("tap test") has been demonstrated to predict responsiveness to ventriculoperitoneal shunting in this condition (see Chapter 29).

Miscellaneous Testing

Several other tests might be ordered to help exclude or establish various medical conditions associated with cognitive changes. Patients with suspected stroke or infarcts demonstrated on CT or MRI might undergo an electrocardiogram, Holter monitoring, or event recording to rule out an arrhythmia. Carotid Doppler ultrasound can assess the presence of carotid atheromatous plaques and help in determining whether endarterectomy is warranted. Magnetic resonance angiography has been demonstrated to be an accurate tool to image the cervical and cerebral vasculature that has supplanted conventional angiography in many medical centers due to its greater safety. Lastly, electromyography (EMG), nerve conduction studies, and evoked potentials (EPs) are useful for the diagnosis of ALS, metachromatic leukodystrophy, and vitamin B_{12} deficiency–related disease.

Legal Issues Regarding Competency

The clinician caring for the patient with a degenerative disease of the brain is often asked to provide an evaluation regarding the patient's competency to make legal or financial decisions. A quantitative assessment of the degree of the patient's dementia should be provided with specific comments about what cognitive domains are most and least affected. The patient's insight into his or her illness and degree of impairment must be evaluated. Psychiatrists and neuropsychologists may be enlisted to help support the determination of competency, and other professionals may be needed to assess capacity to operate a motor vehicle, carry firearms, or take part in other potentially dangerous activities. These issues are outlined in detail in Chapters 52 and 55.

GENERAL TREATMENT RECOMMENDATIONS

Medical therapies directed at the degenerative dementias can be directed at symptoms of the disease or at the underlying disease mechanisms in an attempt to prevent or modify the course of the disease (Table 22-3). Once again, our discussion of treatments will focus on AD, since most dementia treatments have been developed and tested in this disorder. Nonetheless, many of the principles of AD treatment, in particular those directed at behavioral and emotional symptoms, may be extrapolated to caring for patients with other degenerative diseases.

Symptomatic Medications

Relatively specific neurochemical alterations occur early in the course of AD owing to the disproportionate involvement of certain deep gray matter nuclei in the

TABLE 22-3. Established and Potential Medical Treatments for Alzheimer Disease

Symptomatic medications	Disease-modifying agents
Cholinesterase inhibitors[1] (see Table 22-4)	Vitamin E[1]
Psychotropic drugs[1] (see Table 22-5)	Memantine[1]
	Ginkgo biloba[2]
	Nonsteroidal anti-inflammatory drugs[3,4]
	Estrogen[3,4]
	Histamine H_2 receptor antagonists[3,4]
	Statins (HMG-CoA-red inhibitors)[3,4]
	Aβ vaccines[4]
	β- and γ-secretase inhibitors[4]
	Clioquinol[4]

[1] Efficacy established by controlled clinical trial(s).
[2] Unclear efficacy.
[3] Possible efficacy based on epidemiologic evidence.
[4] Under development or in clinical trial(s).
HMG-CoA-red, 3-hydroxy-3-methylglutaryl coenzyme A reductase.

disease process. One such structure is the basal nucleus of Meynert, which is the primary source of cholinergic innervation for the cerebral cortex. The neurotransmitter acetylcholine plays a fundamental role in the modulation of attention and memory formation (Mesulam, 1996). Although there is a small decrease in cortical cholinergic innervation with life span that might produce age-related memory decline (Geula et al., 1989), there is a marked degree of NFT pathology in the basal nucleus and a profound depletion of cholinergic innervation in AD (Geula et al., 1994). This decrease in cholinergic activity occurs early in the course of the disease and correlates somewhat with memory and attentional impairments in AD (Francis et al., 1999; Winkler et al., 1998). The "cholinergic hypothesis" that grew out of these observations stimulated development of the first class of pharmacologic therapies for AD. Although acetylcholine deficiency is no longer considered the primary cause of the disease, acetylcholinesterase inhibitors (AChEIs) have become the mainstay of treatment for AD in the United States and throughout a large part of the developed world. Symptomatic (or palliative) therapies, such as AChEIs, target the clinical manifestations of the disease without altering the underlying pathogenetic mechanisms. They may act by remedying neurochemical, physiologic, or other functional disturbances that are related to the disease but that are not necessarily causal.

Four AChEIs have received approval from the Food and Drug Administration (FDA) in the United States for the treatment of AD (Table 22-4). These agents inhibit the enzyme responsible for the breakdown of acetylcholine in the synaptic cleft, thereby increasing the quantity of this neurotransmitter available to bind and activate postsynaptic receptors. Early attempts at increasing acetylcholine levels by providing cholinergic precursors, such as lecithin or choline, were unsuccessful in producing improvements in the symptoms of AD (Etienne et al., 1981; Thal et al., 1981). Direct cholinergic receptor agonists have had intolerable side effects and are therefore not used (Mayeux & Sano, 1999).

Tacrine was the first medication shown to produce a modest improvement in cognitive function in patients with AD (Summers et al., 1981; Kaye et al., 1982). In a multicenter, double-blind, randomized, placebo-controlled crossover study of 632 subjects with probable AD, tacrine produced a small but statistically significant improvement of 2.4 units on the Alzheimer's Disease Assessment Scale (ADAS, scale range 0 to 70 units) over a six-week period (Davis et al., 1992). Longer-term effects of higher dosages of tacrine were investigated in a multicenter trial of 663 patients (Knapp et al., 1994). Only 42% of subjects completed the study, with most of those withdrawing (74%) citing adverse effects, predominantly abnormalities of serum liver function tests. Of the subjects who completed the trial, there was a significant dose-dependent improvement in the scores of several cognitive measures, including a 4.1-unit mean increase on the ADAS in the group receiving 160 mg tacrine/day compared with a placebo group. However, in another 36-week trial of tacrine, there was little evidence of significant improvement on a battery of cognitive and functional instruments (Maltby et al., 1994). Nevertheless, tacrine became the first medication approved by the FDA for the specific indication of symptomatic treatment of AD.

Within two years of tacrine's approval, donepezil emerged as an alternative AChEI that lacked most of it predecessor's problematic toxicity. In a multicenter, double-blind, randomized, placebo-controlled study of 141 subjects with AD, donepezil

TABLE 22-4. Comparison of Cholinesterase Inhibitors Approved by the Food and Drug Administration for the Treatment of Alzheimer Disease

Drug	Principal study	Daily dosage	Change in ADAS-Cog		Adverse event–related dropouts (%)		Principal adverse events
			Drug	Placebo	Drug	Placebo	
Tacrine (Cognex)	Knapp, 1994	160 mg (4 divided doses)	−2.1	2.0	55	11	Elevated LFTs, nausea, vomiting
Donepezil (Aricept)	Rogers, 1998a	5–10 mg	−1.06	1.82	16	7	Diarrhea, nausea, vomiting
Rivastigmine (Exelon)	Rösler, 1999	6–12 mg (2 divided doses)	−0.26	1.34	23	7	Nausea, vomiting, dizziness
Galantamine (Reminyl)	Raskind, 2000	24 mg (2 divided doses)	−1.9	2.0	23	8	Nausea, vomiting, anorexia

ADAS-Cog, Alzheimer disease assessment scale, cognitive subscale (intent-to-treat analyses); LFTs, liver function tests. Trade names of drugs are given in parentheses.

Data from Cummings JL: Cholinesterase inhibitors: A new class of psychotropic compounds. Am J Psychiatry 157:4–15, 2000.

produced dose-dependent improvements on the cognitive subscale of the ADAS and the MMSE (Rogers et al., 1996). Side effects, primarily diarrhea, nausea, and vomiting, were mild and transitory, although more common with higher dosages. The same study also demonstrated improvements on the Clinician's Interview Based Impression of Change (CIBIC)-Plus and Clinical Dementia Rating Scale (CDRS) (Rogers et al., 1998a). In an expanded trial of 468 patients treated at 23 centers in the United States, donepezil produced statistically significant higher outcome scores using the same testing instruments (Rogers et al., 1998b). Even at the higher 10-mg dose, the reported improvements were modest, amounting to a mean of 3.1 units on the ADAS, 0.4 units on the CIBIC-Plus (scale range 1 to 7 units), and 1.3 units on the MMSE (scale range 0 to 30 units).

More recently, pivotal studies have established the safety and efficacy of two other AChEIs, rivastigmine and galantamine, for the symptomatic treatment of mild to moderate AD. Although rivastigmine may have additional antagonistic actions against butyrylcholinesterase and galantamine against nicotinic acetylcholine receptors, these drugs have been approved by the FDA only as AChEIs. A randomized, double-blind trial of 725 patients with mild to moderately severe probable AD demonstrated significant improvements for high-dose rivastigmine (6 to 12 mg/day) compared with placebo on the cognitive subscale of the ADAS (1.6 units, intention to treat analysis), CIBIC-Plus (0.47 units), and progressive deterioration scale (PDS, 2.23 units, scale range 0 to 100 units), which assesses ADLs (Rösler et al., 1999). More impressive benefits for high-dose rivastigmine over placebo were seen in a similar study of 699 AD patients: 3.78 units on the ADAS cognitive subscale, 0.29 units on the CIBIC-Plus, and 3.38 units on the PDS (Corey-Bloom et al., 1998). The predominant adverse events in both studies included anorexia, nausea, vomiting, diarrhea, dizziness, headache, abdominal pain, and fatigue, predominantly seen at higher doses.

Comparable efficacy on the ADAS cognitive subscale (3.4 units, intention to treat analysis) was found for galantamine in a study of 636 patients with mild to moderately severe AD who received 32 mg/day drug compared with placebo (Raskind et al., 2000). The type of adverse effects seen with galantamine was similar to those occurring in the donepezil and rivastigmine trials. A separate study of 978 patients demonstrated similar benefits on the ADAS cognitive subscale (3.1 units, intention-to-treat analysis) but greater drug tolerability by using a more gradual dose-escalation regimen and slightly lower maximal daily dosage (24 mg/day) (Tariot et al., 2000). Both studies demonstrated comparable benefits of galantamine on global function and ADLs.

The AChEIs have also shown early promise in the treatment of MCI, a possible dementia prodrome, and in the symptomatic treatment of other neurodegenerative disorders such as DLB. At present, clinical trials have failed to demonstrate any advantage on cognitive performance measures of any one AChEI over another. With the exception of tacrine, these drugs are relatively safe with few contraindications (e.g., certain cardiac conduction abnormalities or arrhythmias). Whether to choose donepezil, rivastigmine, or galantamine as the first-line AChEI for a patient with AD will depend on the treating physician's familiarity in using these agents, adverse effects that might be encountered (e.g., severe nausea), and evidence of efficacy in the individual patient. These three AChEI medications, though, should be used at the dosages recommended by their manufacturers and should not be combined. However, they can usually be combined with other classes of noncholinergic medications used for treating other medical conditions or behavioral and emotional symptoms associated with AD (see next section). Nonetheless, it is important that the treating physician make a careful record of all the medications taken by a patient, including nonprescription drugs and herbal remedies, since some of these (in particular, the herbal AChEI huperzine) can produce potentially dangerous interactions.

Medications Targeting Emotional and Behavioral Symptoms

Other extremely important targets for symptomatic therapy of AD are the emotional and behavioral disturbances of the disease, including depression, agitation, insomnia, and psychosis (Table 22-5). Most agents employed for the treatment of these conditions have been approved for use in patients without dementia and have not been specifically approved or thoroughly evaluated for use in AD patients. The model most commonly used in the treatment of behavioral disturbances in dementia patients is the "analogous symptom" approach. This entails treating dementia patients as though they were suffering from a primary psychiatric disturbance, such as depression or psychosis, despite the likelihood that their symptoms arise from different underlying disease mechanisms.

Several classes of medications are in common use for the treatment of depression in AD, although data on efficacy in this population are limited. Tricyclic antidepressant agents (TCAs), such as amitriptyline, nortriptyline, imipramine, and desipramine, inhibit the presynaptic uptake of norepinephrine and serotonin, thereby increasing the half-lives of these neurotransmitters in the synaptic cleft. Anticholinergic symptoms are the most common adverse effects encountered with TCAs and usually consist of dry mouth, blurring of vision, light-headedness, constipation, urinary retention, and orthostatic hypotension. In disorders with depressed cholinergic reserves such as AD, the anticholinergic effects of these agents can worsen cognitive

TABLE 22-5. Medical Treatment of Behavioral and Emotional Symptoms in Dementia

Depression	Agitation
SSRIs	Antipsychotic drugs
Sertraline (Zoloft)	SSRIs
Paroxetine (Paxil)	Benzodiazepines
Citalopram (Celexa)	Lorazepam (Ativan)
SNRIs	Clonazepam (Klonopin)
Venlafaxine (Effexor)	Anticonvulsant "mood stabilizers"
	Carbamazepine (Tegretol)
Psychosis	Divalproex (Depakote)
Risperidone (Risperdal)	
Olanzapine (Zyprexa)	**Apathy**
Quetiapine (Seroquel)	Amantadine (Symmetrel)
	Dextroamphetamine (Dexedrine)
Sleep disturbances	Bromocriptine (Parlodel)
Melatonin	Methylphenidate (Ritalin)
Zolpidem (Ambien)	Pemoline (Cylert)
Trazodone (Desyrel)	

SSRIs, selective serotonin reuptake inhibitors; SNRIs, serotonin-norepinephrine reuptake inhibitors. Trade names of drugs are in parentheses.

Data from Borson S, Raskind MA: Clinical features and pharmacologic treatment of behavioral symptoms of Alzheimer's disease. Neurology 48(Suppl. 6):S17–S24, 1997.

functioning (Sunderland et al., 1987), and they should thus be avoided whenever possible. Selective serotonin reuptake inhibitors (SSRIs), such as fluoxetine, paroxetine, sertraline, and citalopram, are effective in treating depression in the elderly and may be better tolerated. They can, however, produce fatigue, insomnia, gastrointestinal upset, and anorexia, and they might increase the risk of falls.

A clinical trial in 61 AD patients with ($N = 28$) or without ($N = 33$) depression demonstrated no difference between imipramine and placebo in alleviating depression (Reifler et al., 1989). In a randomized trial comparing fluoxetine and amitriptyline in 37 patients with AD and depression, both drugs were equally effective in relieving depression, but 58% of patients receiving amitriptyline dropped out of the study as a result of adverse effects, in contrast to 22% of those receiving fluoxetine (Taragano et al., 1997). Paroxetine was shown to be as effective as and better tolerated than imipramine in a group of 198 subjects with both dementia and depression (Katona et al., 1998). In a multicenter, placebo-controlled study, citalopram was demonstrated to be effective in reducing the symptoms of depression and improving cognitive function in patients with AD (Nyth & Gottfries, 1990; Nyth et al., 1992). Although there are no reports in the medical literature on the efficacy of the serotonin-norepinephrine reuptake inhibitor venlafaxine in treating depression in patients with dementia, we have found this drug to be safe and effective in patients with AD or related dementias.

Neuroleptic agents (or antipsychotics) have been the mainstay of treatment for paranoia, delusions, hallucinations, and agitation in the demented population (Borson & Raskind, 1997). These drugs act as antagonists at dopamine D2 receptors. Their sites of action are believed to be the limbic striatum—composed of the ventral tegmental area, olfactory bulb, and nucleus accumbens—and the frontal lobe. Although medications such as chlorpromazine and haloperidol have long been used effectively in controlling psychotic symptoms in the elderly (Seager, 1955; Sugarman et al., 1964), they have the potential to cause serious neurologic side effects, including parkinsonism, dystonia, tardive dyskinesia, neuroleptic malignant syndrome, akathisia, and anticholinergic symptoms.

Parkinsonism is most commonly seen and is manifested as axial and limb rigidity, tremor, and bradykinesia. Tardive dyskinesia is associated with disfiguring involuntary movements that often persist despite the discontinuation of therapy. Neuroleptic malignant syndrome is a combination of altered consciousness, muscular rigidity, and autonomic instability that can be fatal if untreated. These side effects put the patient at greater risk for falls and can be a significant source of morbidity in elderly individuals. Extrapyramidal symptoms are thought to be due to the nonselective binding of antipsychotic agents to dopamine D1 receptors in the caudate and putamen. Newer-generation neuroleptics with greater selectivity for the D2 class of dopamine receptors (e.g., risperidone and olanzapine) have fewer extrapyramidal side effects than do traditional agents. However, like their earlier counterparts, they can produce parkinsonism, as well as excessive sedation and psychomotor slowing.

Based on their effectiveness in treating hyperactive and aggressive behaviors in individuals with bipolar disorder, anticonvulsant agents have been used to manage agitation and hostility in demented patients. Several studies have demonstrated the efficacy of carbamazepine in treating agitated or aggressive demented elderly patients (Gleason & Schneider, 1990; Tariot et al., 1994, 1998). Carbamazepine must be used with caution in the elderly population, however, since it can produce ataxia and increase the risk for falls. Valproic acid or divalproex may be safer to use and has been shown to reduce behavioral disturbances in demented patients, including some who had received no prior benefit from neuroleptics (Mellow et al., 1993; Herrmann, 1998).

A variety of psychostimulant medications have been used for the treatment of apathy and other "negative" behavioral symptoms occurring in neurologic disorders. Amantadine, dextroamphetamine, bromocriptine, methylphenidate, and pemoline are all agents that activate dopaminergic and/or noradrenergic receptors in forebrain systems. Half of all the brain's noradrenergic innervation arises from the locus ceruleus, a midbrain nucleus which projects to the hypothalamus, thalamus, and most regions of the cerebral cortex, including the hippocampus. Neurons of the locus ceruleus are often severely depleted in the brains of AD patients studied at autopsy. In addition to modulating arousal and attention through its effects on diencephalic and frontal lobe neurons, the locus ceruleus also influences memory formation, presumably by activation of noradrenergic receptors in the hippocampus. Indeed, memory performance has been shown to be impaired in hypertensive patients who received beta-blockers (Lichter et al., 1986; Richardson & Wyke, 1988). However, *peripheral* epinephrine also enhances memory consolidation; it does not easily cross the blood-brain barrier and appears to mediate its effects on memory by stimulating vagal afferent fibers projecting to the nucleus of the solitary tract (McGaugh, 2000).

Both mesolimbocortical and ventral mesostriatal dopaminergic pathways have been implicated to explain dopamine's effects on attention, drive, and executive functions. An age-associated decline in dopamine receptors in the striatum has been correlated with performance on neuropsychological tasks involving frontal systems, such as attention, response inhibition, abstraction, and mental flexibility (Volkow et al., 1998). However, no pathologic studies have described a specific loss of dopaminergic neurons in AD.

Most of the evidence for the usefulness of dopaminergic agents in demented patients is based on small clinical trials, case studies, anecdotal reports, and extrapolation from other neuropsychiatric disorders. In a study of eight patients with vascular or degenerative dementia, bromocriptine reduced perseverative responses on attentional tasks but had no effects on general attention or overall cognitive function (Imamura et al., 1998). Methylphenidate was shown to improve the reaction time of a patient with prominent apathy due to multiple subcortical frontal infarcts (Watanabe et al., 1995). This agent was also demonstrated to improve negative behavioral symptoms in a clinical study of 12 patients with AD and 15 patients with vascular dementia (Galynker et al., 1997). Amantadine was reported to improve muteness and immobility in three patients with pathologically confirmed advanced AD (Erkulwater & Pillai, 1989). These medications have not been accepted for routine use in the dementia population owing to limited efficacy and unacceptable side effects, including the precipitation of psychosis in susceptible patients. In particular, these agents should be avoided in patients with a history of hallucinations or delusions or in patients with DLB.

Cholinergic agents have also demonstrated some efficacy in treating behavioral symptoms in AD, suggesting that behavioral disturbances relate at least in part to decreased cholinergic innervation from the basal nucleus (Cummings & Back, 1998). In a study of 86 patients with AD who were receiving donepezil, 41% experienced an improvement in behavior, 28% worsened, and 31% exhibited no change in behavior (Mega et al., 1999). For those responding, there were statistically significant improvements in symptoms of delusions, agitation, anxiety, disinhibition, and irritability. It has been postulated that cholinergic systems are involved in "low-level" aspects of attention, such as orienting, whereas dopaminergic systems are involved in more "executive" aspects, such as working memory (Coull, 1998). While behavioral improvements occur in some patients receiving cholinergic therapy, the magnitude of the response is usually insufficient to replace neuroleptics in all but the mildest cases.

Potential Disease-Modifying Therapies

The features delineated in the model for the pathogenesis of degenerative diseases (Section III, Biological Underpinnings of Degenerative Diseases) have allowed for the development of treatments directed at prevention, slowing of progression, or reversal of disease effects. Such neuroprotective therapies contrast with treatments that are designed to ameliorate specific symptoms or improve overall function for the patient with degenerative disease. With the exception of copper-chelating therapy in Wilson's disease, the evidence that any treatment modifies the course of any of the degenerative disorders is limited and sometimes controversial (Shoulson, 1998a). Nevertheless, data from epidemiologic studies and clinical trials have demonstrated some potential benefits of treatments already in use. Several classes of investigational treatments, including anti-inflammatory, antioxidant, hormonal, and anti-amyloid therapies, are currently under study.

Several pharmacologic and nonpharmacologic medical treatments have been proven effective in slowing the course of AD, are being tested in clinical trials, or are under development (see Table 22-3). For example, an inverse association between the use of histamine H_2 receptor antagonists (cimetidine, ranitidine, famotidine, and nizatidine) and AD has been observed retrospectively (Anthony et al., 2000), raising the possibility that treatment with these agents may be beneficial in preventing or slowing the progression of the disease. Similarly, epidemiologic evidence suggests that the lipid-lowering 3-hydroxy-3-methylglutaryl coenzyme A (HMG-CoA) reductase inhibitors, or statins (e.g., lovastatin and pravastatin), may reduce the risk of AD (Wolozin et al., 2000; Jick et al., 2000). Whether the putative ability of these agents to prevent AD lies in their antiamyloidogenic abilities (Fassbender et al., 2001) or in cholesterol-lowering properties (Burns & Duff, 2002), clinical trials are under way to determine prospectively if they can affect the course of AD.

Free radicals are generated by activated microglia, and various forms of oxidative stress are believed to play a role in the pathogenesis of the AD (Smith et al., 1991; Smith et al., 1996). The antioxidant agents selegiline (deprenyl), a monoamine oxidase inhibitor, and α-tocopherol (vitamin E), a scavenger of free-radical compounds, were each shown to delay progression in patients with AD (Sano et al., 1997). Prospective studies have suggested that high-dose vitamin E or vitamin C supplementation may reduce the risk in the elderly of developing AD (Morris et al, 1998) and vascular dementia (Masaki et al., 2000). Therefore, unless there is a risk of gastrointestinal bleeding, all patients with AD should probably receive 2000 IU of vitamin E a day. Other vitamin supplements are of unproven value in degenerative dementias, though the minimal risk posed by supplementation makes it reasonable to consider a daily multivitamin or vitamin C.

Antioxidant therapies have been used in other neurodegenerative diseases, with their use in PD being most intensely studied. A large, randomized placebo-controlled study of selegiline in PD demonstrated a significant delay in disability, defined as the time when symptomatic treatment with levodopa was needed (Parkinson Study Group, 1989, 1993). However, selegiline treatment did not prolong survival or reduce the adverse effects of levodopa treatment. Some have therefore raised the possibility that selegiline has dopaminergic effects that provide symptomatic benefits as opposed to disease-modifying effects (Shoulson, 1998b). Strategies targeting antioxidant (vitamin E) and anti-excitotoxic (riluzole and gabapentin) pathways have been attempted in transgenic animal models of ALS, but with mixed results (Gurney et al., 1996). Vitamin E was demonstrated to delay disease onset and slow progression, but had no effect on survival. In contrast, riluzole or gabapentin, both of which are believed to antagonize the glutamate system, prolonged survival without affecting the time of onset of symptoms.

Gonadal hormone therapy has been proposed as a potential treatment for AD, based on experimental data showing neurotrophic and antiamyloid effects of agents such as estrogen and on epidemiologic evidence demonstrating a lower risk of AD in postmenopausal women who have received estrogen replacement therapy (Tang et al., 1996; Gandy & Duffy, 2000). Prospective trials using estrogen have failed to slow the progression of disease in women with AD. High-dose estradiol administered by skin patch produced small, but significant, improvements in attention and memory in postmenopausal women with AD (Asthana et al., 2001). However, a sizable clinical trial in hysterectomized women with AD failed to discern any positive effects from 1 year of estrogen therapy compared with placebo (Mulnard et al., 2000). It might be that the effects of estrogen are primarily preventative, and that the hormone is ineffective once the disease has reached a critical point. The type of estrogen used, dosage, and route of administration are other variables that might be important.

As noted above, a mutation in the P-type ATPase has been found in some cases of Wilson disease (Beal, 2000). All patients share a defect in copper transport that can be identified by reduced copper incorporation in ceruloplasmin, the principal copper transport protein. The consequence of altered copper transport is the excessive deposition of copper in affected organs, including the brain and liver. Chelation of circulating copper by D-penicillamine has been the mainstay of treatment for this disease. It can reverse some of the symptoms and pathology of patients who have already manifested symptoms as well as prevent development of the disease in homozygotic gene carriers.

Recently, another chelating agent, the antibiotic clioquinol, has been examined as a potential treatment for AD. Chelation of copper and zinc ions solubilizes Aβ deposits in postmortem AD brain tissue (Cherny et al., 1999). Clioquinol was subsequently demonstrated to reduce the brain deposition of Aβ in a transgenic mouse model of AD (Cherny et al., 2001). This was accompanied by an improvement in general behavior. Clioquinol had been previously withdrawn from the market due to a serious adverse effect, subacute myelo-optic neuropathy, which resembles subacute combined degeneration due to vitamin B_{12} deficiency. It is believed that clioquinol precipitated this condition in patients who had been vitamin B_{12} deficient and would otherwise be safe. Clioquinol is now being tested in patients with AD who are also being supplemented with vitamin B_{12}.

A potentially promising treatment involving an immunologic "chelation" of sorts was recently developed for AD. Intraperitoneal Aβ vaccination of transgenic mice expressing a mutant form of human *APP* resulted in prevention of amyloid deposition, neuritic dystrophy, and gliosis in the brain (Schenk et al., 1999). More surprisingly, administration of the vaccine at an age after pathologic changes were known to occur resulted in reduced amyloid deposits, suggesting that immunization actually reversed lesion development. A Phase 2 clinical trial examining the efficacy of Aβ42 immunization in AD patients (called AN-1792) was undertaken in 2001, but was halted in 2002 when a number of participants developed meningoencephalitis. Several other concerns have been raised about this treatment approach. These include the potential risk of vaccinating individuals against a protein that is normally made by the human body. In the mice expressing human *APP*, human Aβ was used as the immunogen. Also, it may not be possible to achieve high enough antibody titers within the CNS or an immune response that can adequately cross the blood-brain barrier. Lastly, in patients who already have AD, there is little reason to expect any degree of cognitive or behavioral improvement in patients who have already experienced substantial neuronal death in regions such as the basal forebrain and hippocampus. Nonetheless, immunization therapy may help prevent the disease in susceptible individuals or slow the progression of AD. Following suspension of the initial human trials of the active vaccination approach, other strategies have been proposed such as passive immunization and immunization with coincident administration of agents to suppress brain edema (Schenk, 2002; Sigurdsson et al., 2002).

The actual role of the immune system in AD and the potential utility of medications to modulate the immune response in AD are poorly understood and controversial. Studies in the transgenic mice demonstrated that vaccination produced microglial activation, which appears to be a potential mechanism by which β-amyloid is cleared. The presence of activated microglia and inflammation-related proteins such as α2-macroglobulin surrounding or within senile plaques was previously taken as evidence that a harmful immune response contributed to the pathogenesis of AD (Eikelenboom et al., 2000). Microglia migrate to insoluble Aβ deposits and become intensely activated by them. The action of microglia appears to be essential for the conversion of diffuse amyloid deposits into senile plaques. Cytokines, as well as other oxidative inflammatory intermediates produced by microglia, may cause neuronal injury and thereby propagate their damaging effects along axonal projection pathways throughout the brain. In light of the Aβ vaccine data, though, it is possible that such pathologic findings reflect an attempt by the immune system to clear the brain of pathogenic β-amyloid.

Nevertheless, earlier epidemiologic and clinical data suggested that inhibition of immune system pathways could be beneficial in AD. There is an inverse relationship between the use of anti-inflammatory medications and the development of AD (McGeer et al., 1996; Aisen & Davis, 1997; in t' Veld, 2001), and a lower incidence of AD is found in patients with inflammatory disorders such as rheumatoid arthritis who chronically use these drugs (Jenkinson et al., 1989). Nonsteroidal anti-inflammatory drugs have shown mild benefits in preserving cognitive function in AD (Rogers et al., 1993). Several trials now in progress are examining whether selective cyclooxygenase-2 inhibitors are effective in slowing the progression of AD. Initial findings suggest that anti-inflammatory approaches may have an impact in reducing the risk of AD but have questionable value in the treatment of individuals already affected by dementia.

Many AD patients (as well as some normal adults) currently take ginkgo extract on an over-the-counter basis. This compound is derived from the leaves of the *Ginkgo biloba* tree and is reported to exert both antioxidant and anti-inflammatory effects (Kanowski et al., 1996). Two caveats in recommending *Gingko biloba* to patients are the lack of uniform standards in the production of extract and a potential increased risk of gastrointestinal bleeding. A meta-analysis examined the objective benefits of gingko extract on cognition in patients with AD and found a small but significant improvement, which would translate to a 3% gain on the cognitive subscale of the ADAS (Oken et al., 1998). However, a recent randomized, double-blind, placebo-controlled clinical trial failed to find any improvement by ginkgo extract on cognitive and clinical measures in 214 nursing home residents with mild to moderate dementia (both AD and vascular dementia) or with age-associated memory impairment (van Dongen et al., 2000).

As mentioned above, excitotoxicity triggered by glutamate has been postulated as a mechanism for neuronal death in degenerative diseases, including AD (Greenamyre, 1991). The glutamate NMDA receptor antagonist memantine has been shown in several European clinical trials to have beneficial effects on various clinical measures in patients with moderate to severe dementia. Most studies, though, have preferentially examined memantine in patients with vascular dementia. A randomized, double-blind trial involving 166 subjects with either AD or vascular dementia demonstrated functional improvement of memantine compared with placebo (Winblad, 1999). The sole clinical trial conducted to date in the United States also showed a significant benefit of memantine over placebo on overall function, as well as cognition, in a population of 252 patients with moderate to severe AD (Reisberg et al., 2000). Another phase 3 clinical trial is currently under way in the United States and the drug awaits FDA approval.

Finally, perhaps no potential medical therapy has been as greatly anticipated as agents that will inhibit production of Aβ from *APP* and thereby prevent or slow the progression of AD. As described previously in Section III, Aβ is released from *APP* by the sequential proteolytic cleavage of β- and γ-secretase (for a review, see Sinha & Lieberburg, 1999). Because inhibition of either protease would prevent Aβ production, the development of pharmacologic β- or γ-secretase inhibitors has been a major goal of academic researchers and the pharmaceutical industry (Tsai et al., 2002; Citron, 2002; Xu et al., 2002). Although inhibition of β-secretase could theoretically also affect the Notch signaling pathway in the brain, γ-secretase is believed to be unique to the amyloidogenic pathway and might be a more specific therapeutic target. However, the development of soluble, nonpeptide β-secretase inhibitors that can cross the blood-brain barrier has not yet been reported. Soluble chemical γ-secretase inhibitors, though, have entered into phase 1 clinical trials.

SCOPE OF THE PROBLEM

Across several randomized, double-blind, placebo-controlled studies, AChEIs have been shown to stabilize symptom progression in mild to moderate AD patients for a period of at least 30 weeks (see above). Actual symptomatic improvement occurred in less than half of those treated and was commensurate on average with reversing 6 to 8 months of disease progression. Although there is emerging evidence that the symptomatic benefits of AChEIs relative to placebo persist beyond 1 year, in most cases patients decline below their pretreatment baseline within 6 to 12 months of initiating therapy. There is little convincing evidence to show that AChEIs alter the underlying pathology of AD. Patients discontinuing AChEI therapy rapidly decline to a level of cognitive function comparable to untreated controls, indicating that these agents exert little or no effect on modifying the mechanisms of the underlying disease.

AChEIs were approved by the FDA as the first symptomatic therapy for AD despite their relatively limited and transient effects on cognition and behavior in AD patients. This may in part be attributable to the lack of alternative treatments at this time. However, the value of AChEIs in the symptomatic treatment of AD has been well substantiated by the assessments of treating physicians and caregivers, as well as by other measures. In the pivotal clinical trials cited above, donepezil-treated patients were judged by their doctors and caregivers to fare significantly better than placebo-treated controls over double-blinded periods of 12 to 30 weeks (Fillit et al., 2000).

From an economic standpoint, symptomatic treatment with AChEIs can be potentially cost-effective by reducing the burden of care. For example, tacrine treatment has been shown to delay significantly the time until nursing home admission in AD patients (Knopman et al., 1996), a potential saving of thousands of dollars per year required for institutionalization. Since the expense of caring for a patient with AD tends to increase as the severity of cognitive impairment worsens, the cost of care can theoretically be reduced by treatments that improve the patient's mental status. For an AD patient in a severe stage of dementia (MMSE score of around 5), improving cognition by the equivalent of five points on the MMSE is estimated to provide a potential cost savings of approximately $8600 per year (Ernst et al., 1997). In comparison, the annual cost of treatment with donepezil is between $1400 and $2000. In a disease as prevalent as AD, future symptomatic therapies must be cost-effective. They can do this by improving mentation sufficiently to reduce caregiver dependency and by prolonging the time that the AD patient can be cared for at home.

A variety of symptomatic therapies are available to treat the behavioral symptoms of AD. Unfortunately, not every patient responds favorably to these agents, and adverse effects from such medications are particularly problematic in this population. The use of psy-choactive medications in elderly patients with dementia is fraught with special dangers. Increased susceptibility to falls, cardiac arrhythmias, and parkinsonism are among the more troublesome adverse effects of currently available medications. Many elderly patients require the use of multiple medications, and "polypharmacy" creates a greater tendency for drug interactions, as well as added compliance and cost problems. Nevertheless, the morbidity associated with the behavioral symptoms of AD can be so profound that it is justifiable in many circumstances to prescribe psychoactive medications despite their potential risks. One measure of the success of any potential nonpharmacologic treatment for behavioral symptoms of AD will be the extent to which it reduces the dependence on psychoactive medications and their attendant adverse effects.

Although antiamyloid agents and other promising lines of therapy have recently entered into human trials, it is likely to take several years or more before disease-arresting treatments for AD are discovered, comprehensively tested, approved, and made available to the population at risk for the disease. It is likely to take even longer to develop a means of restoring function to AD-degenerated brains through strategies such as neuronal regeneration and transplantation. In the meantime, millions of individuals worldwide will develop AD and progress to stages of impairment for which there is currently little available means of palliation. It is therefore of the utmost importance that we develop more effective symptomatic treatments for AD in parallel with testing promising new disease-modifying and preventative therapies.

■ KEY POINTS

☐ Degenerative diseases impair cognition and behavior by disrupting the microscopic, cellular and integrative organization of the brain. Among many conditions that cause dementia in adults, degenerative disorders such as AD are currently the most prevalent.

☐ Understanding the biological mechanisms underlying degenerative dementias provides a rational basis for their diagnosis and treatment. Neurodegenerative disorders arise from the combined effects of multiple genetic and environmental factors. A common feature of these conditions is the abnormal accumulation of specific proteins within the brain as part of a cascade of events that ultimately results in neuronal dysfunction and death.

☐ Degenerative processes tend to be slowly deleterious to the brain, often over a considerable portion of the life span. Cognitive symptoms become evident when the burden of disease reaches a critical threshold within the brain. The neuropathologic changes associated with individual degenerative disorders tend to affect particular brain regions in sequence, giving rise to characteristic constellations of symptoms and patterns of progression.

☐ Clinical diagnosis of dementia is facilitated by direct identification of the general class of symptoms (e.g., amnestic, comportmental, linguistic, movement-related) that predominates during the initial years of disease presentation and subsequent progression. Exclusion of other causes of impairment increases diagnostic certainty and assists in identifying comorbid conditions. Intelligent use of diagnostic tests, including neuropsychological assessments, blood tests, spinal fluid analysis, brain imaging, and other tests, can increase the accuracy of the clinical diagnosis and staging.

☐ Treatment of neurodegenerative dementias has advanced sufficiently to make medical therapy part of the standard of care. Medications that ameliorate the cognitive and behavioral symptoms of dementia are now available, and should be administered as early as possible in the course of the illness. Nonpharmacologic interventions can also help to preserve the health and well-being of the affected individuals and their caregivers. Several promising therapies and preventative interventions are under development that target underlying degenerative mechanisms. New techniques for presymptomatic identification of those at risk for degenerative dementias should assist in the implementation of future dementia prevention programs.

KEY READINGS

Braak H, Braak E: Evolution of the neuropathology of Alzheimer's disease. Acta Neurol Scand 165(Suppl.):3–12, 1996.

Doody RS, Stevens JC, Beck C, et al: Practice parameter: Management of dementia (an evidence-based review). Report of the Quality Standards Subcommittee of the American Academy of Neurology. Neurology 56:1154–1166, 2001.

Knopman DS, De Kosky ST, Cummings JL, et al: Practice parameter: Diagnosis of dementia (an evidence-based review). Report of the Quality Standards Subcommittee of the American Academy of Neurology. Neurology 56:1143–1153, 2001.

Petersen RC, Doody R, Kurz A, et al: Current concepts in mild cognitive impairment. Arch Neurol 58:198–1992, 2001.

Weintraub S, Mesulam M: Four neuropsychological profiles in dementia. Handbook of Neuropsychology 8:253–282, 1993.

REFERENCES

Aarsland D, Andersen K, Larsen JP, et al: Risk of dementia in Parkinson's disease: A community-based prospective study. Neurology 56:730–736, 2001.

Aisen PS, Davis, KL: The search for disease-modifying treatment for Alzheimer's disease. Neurology 48(Suppl. 6):S35–S41, 1997.

Ala TA, Hughes LF, Kyrouac GA, et al: Pentagon copying is more impaired in dementia with Lewy bodies than in Alzheimer's disease. J Neurol Neurosurg Psychiatry 70:483–488, 2001.

Algotsson A, Viitanen M, Winbald B, Soldiers G: Autonomic dysfunction in Alzheimer's disease. Acta Neurol Scand 91:14–18, 1995.

Anfinsen CB: Principles that govern the folding of protein chains. Science 181:223–230, 1973.

Anthony JC, Breitner JC, Zandi PP, et al: Reduced prevalence of AD in users of NSAIDs and H2 receptor antagonists: The Cache County Study. Neurology 54:2066–2071, 2000.

Arriagada PV, Growdon JH, Hedley-Whyte ET, Hyman BT: Neurofibrillary tangles but not senile plaques parallel duration and severity of Alzheimer's disease. Neurology 42:631–639, 1992.

Asthana S, Baker LD, Craft S, et al: High-dose estradiol improves cognition for women with AD: Results of a randomized study. Neurology 57:605–612, 2001.

Auer S, Reisberg B: The GDS/FAST staging system. Int Psychogeriatr 9(Suppl. 1):167–171, 1997.

Baker M, Litvan I, Houlden H, et al: Association of an extended haplotype in the tau gene with progressive supranuclear palsy. Hum Mol Genet 8:711–715, 1999.

Beal MF: Energetics in the pathogenesis of neurodegenerative diseases. Trends Neurosci 23:298–304, 2000.

Benoit M, Dygai I, Migneco O, et al: Behavioral and psychological symptoms in Alzheimer's disease: Relation between apathy and regional cerebral perfusion. Dement Geriatr Cogn Disord 10:511–517, 1999.

Blessed G, Tomlinson BE, Roth M: The association between quantitative measures of dementia and of senile change in the cerebral grey matter of elderly subjects. Br J Psychiatry 114:797–811, 1968.

Blin J, Baron JC, Dubois B, et al: Loss of brain 5-HT2 receptors in Alzheimer's disease: In vivo assessment with positron emission tomography and (^{18}F)setoperone. Brain 116(Pt 3):497–510, 1993.

Bodis-Wollner IG, Paulus W: Visual and visual-cognitive dysfunction in Parkinson's disease: Spatial and chromatic vision. Adv Neurol 80:383–388, 1999.

Borson S, Raskind MA: Clinical features and pharmacologic treatment of behavioral symptoms of Alzheimer's disease. Neurology 48(Suppl. 6):S17–S24, 1997.

Braak H, Braak E: Evolution of the neuropathology of Alzheimer's disease. Acta Neurol Scand Suppl 165:3–12, 1996.

Braak H, Braak E: Evolution of neuronal changes in the course of Alzheimer's disease. J Neural Transm Suppl 53:127–140, 1998.

Braak H, Del Tredici K, Schultz C, Braak E: Vulnerability of select neuronal types to Alzheimer's disease. Ann N Y Acad Sci 924:53–61, 2000.

Buee L, Bussiere T, Buee-Scherrer V, et al. Tau protein isoforms, phosphorylation and role in neurodegenerative disorders. Brain Res Rev 33:95–130, 2000.

Bullock R, Cameron A: Rivastigmine for the treatment of dementia and visual hallucinations associated with Parkinson's disease: A case series. Curr Med Res Opin 18:258–264, 2002.

Burkhard PR, Sanchez JC, Landis T, Hochstrasser DF: CSF detection of the 14-3-3 protein in unselected patients with dementia. Neurology 56:1528–1533, 2001.

Burns A, Jacoby R, Levy R: Psychiatric phenomena in Alzheimer's disease. II: Disorders of perception. Br J Psychiatry 157:76–81, 1990.

Burns M, Duff K: Cholesterol in Alzheimer's disease and tauopathy. Ann N Y Acad Sci 977:367–375, 2002.

Carrell RW, Lomas DA: Conformational disease. Lancet 350: 134–138, 1997.

Chen ST, Sultzer DL, Hinkin CH, et al: Executive dysfunction in Alzheimer's disease: Association with neuropsychiatric symptoms and functional impairment. J Neuropsychiatry Clin Neurosci 10:426–432, 1998.

Cherny RA, Legg JT, McLean A, et al: Aqueous dissolution of Alzheimer's disease Abeta amyloid deposits by biometal depletion. J Biol Chem 274:23223–23228, 1999.

Cherny RA, Atwood CS, Xilinas ME, et al: Treatment with a copper-zinc chelator markedly and rapidly inhibits beta-amyloid accumulation in Alzheimer's disease transgenic mice. Neuron 30:665–676, 2001.

Chow TW, Miller BL, Hayashi VN, Geschwind DW: Inheritance of frontotemporal dementia. Arch Neurol 56:817–822, 1999.

Chu CC, Tranel D, Damasio ARl: Impaired autonomic responses to emotionally significant stimuli in Alzheimer's disease. Soc Neurosci Abs 20:1006, 1994.

Chu CC, Tranel D, Damasio AR, Van Hoesen GW: The autonomic-related cortex: Pathology in Alzheimer's disease. Cereb Cortex 7:86–95, 1997.

Citron M: Beta-secretase as a target for the treatment of Alzheimer's disease. J Neurosci Res 70:373–379, 2002.

Collette F, Van der Linden M, Salmon E, et al: Executive dysfunction in Alzheimer's disease. Cortex 35:57–72, 1999.

Conrad C, Andreadis A, Trojanowski JO, et al: Genetic evidence for the involvement of tau in progressive supranuclear palsy. Ann Neurol 41:277–281, 1997.

Corey-Bloom, J, Anand R, Veach J, et al: A randomized trial evaluating the efficacy and safety of ENA 713 (rivastigmine tartrate), a new acetylcholinesterase inhibitor, in patients with mild to moderately severe Alzheimer's disease. Intl J Geriatr Psychopharmacol 1:55–65, 1998.

Coull JT: Neural correlates of attention and arousal: Insights from electrophysiology, functional neuroimaging and psychopharmacology. Prog Neurobiol 55:343–361, 1998.

Craig AH, Cummings JL, Fairbankd L, et al: Cerebral blood flow correlates of apathy in Alzheimer disease. Arch Neurol 53:1116–1120, 1996.

Crum RM, Anthony JC, Bassett SS, Folstein MF: Population-based norms for the Mini-Mental State Examination by age and educational level. JAMA 269:2386–2391, 1993.

Cummings JL: Cholinesterase inhibitors: A new class of psychotropic compounds. Am J Psychiatry 157:4–15, 2000.

Cummings JL (ed): Subcortical Dementia. New York: Oxford University Press, 1990.

Cummings JL, Back C: The cholinergic hypothesis of neuropsychiatric symptoms in Alzheimer's disease. Am J Geriatr Psychiatry 6 (Suppl. 1):S64–S78, 1998.

Dalmau JO, Posner, JB: Paraneoplastic syndromes. Arch Neurol 56:405–408, 1999.

Davis KL, Thal LJ, Gamzu ER, et al: A double-blind, placebo-controlled multicenter study of tacrine for Alzheimer's disease. The Tacrine Collaborative Study Group. N Engl J Med 327:1253–1259, 1992.

Doody RS, Massman P, Mahurin L, Law S: Positive and negative neuropsychiatric features in Alzheimer's disease. J Neuropsychiatry Clin Neurosci 7:54–60, 1995.

Doody RS, Stevens JC, Beck C, et al: Praactice parameter: Management of dementia (an evidence-based review). Report of the Quality Standards Subcommittee of the American Academy of Neurology. Neurology 56:1154–1166, 2001.

Eikelenboom P, Rozemuller AJ, Hoozemans JJ: Neuroinflammation and Alzheimer's disease: Clinical and therapeutic implications. Alzheimer Dis Assoc Disord 14(Suppl. 1):S54–S61, 2000.

Erkulwater S, Pillai R: Amantadine and the end-stage dementia of Alzheimer's type. South Med J 82:550–554, 1989.

Ernst RL, Hay JW, Fenn C, et al: Cognitive function and the costs of Alzheimer disease: An exploratory study. Arch Neurol 54:687–693, 1997.

Etienne P, Dastoor D, Gauthier S, et al: Alzheimer disease: Lack of effect of lecithin treatment for 3 months. Neurology 31:1552–1554, 1981.

Evans DA, Funkenstein HH, Albert MS, et al: Prevalence of Alzheimer's disease in a community population of older persons: Higher than previously reported. JAMA 262:2551–2556, 1989.

Fandrich M, Fletcher MA, Dobson CM: Amyloid fibrils from muscle myoglobin. Nature 410:165–166, 2001.

Fassbender K, Simons M, Bergmann C, et al: Simvastatin strongly reduces levels of Alzheimer's disease β-amyloid peptides Aβ42 and Aβ40 in vitro and in vivo. Proc Natl Acad Sci U S A 98:5856–5861, 2001.

Fillit HM, Gutterman EM, Brooks RL: Impact of donepezil on caregiving burden for patients with Alzheimer's disease. Int Psychogeriatr 12:389–401, 2000.

Fleming KC, Adams AC, Petersen RC: Dementia: Diagnosis and evaluation. Mayo Clin Proc 70:1093–1097, 1995.

Folstein MF, Folstein SE, McHugh PR: Mini-mental state: A practical method for grading the cognitive state of patients for the clinician. J Psychiatr Res 12:189–198, 1975.

Forstl H, Burns A, Levy R, et al: Neuropathological correlates of behavioural disturbance in confirmed Alzheimer's disease. Br J Psychiatry 163:364–368, 1993.

Francis PT, Palmer AM, Snape M, Wilcock GK: The cholinergic hypothesis of Alzheimer's disease: A review of progress. J Neurol Neurosurg Psychiatry 66:137–147, 1999.

Friguet B, Bulteau AL, Chondrogianni N, et al: Protein degradation by the proteasome and its implications in aging. Ann N Y Acad Sci 908:143–154, 2000.

Galasko D, Chang L, Motter R, et al: High cerebrospinal fluid tau and low amyloid beta42 levels in the clinical diagnosis of Alzheimer disease and relation to apolipoprotein E genotype. Arch Neurol 55:937–945, 1998.

Galynker I, Ieronimo C, Miner C, et al: Methylphenidate treatment of negative symptoms in patients with dementia. J Neuropsychiatry Clin Neurosci 9:231–239, 1997.

Gandy S, Duffy K: Post-menopausal estrogen deprivation and Alzheimer's disease. Exp Gerontol 35:503–511, 2000.

Geldmacher DS, Whitehouse PJ: Evaluation of dementia. N Engl J Med 335:330–336, 1996.

Geula C, Mesulam MM: Cortical cholinergic fibers in aging and Alzheimer's disease: A morphometric study. Neuroscience 33:469–481, 1989.

Geula C, Mesulam MM: Cholinergic systems and related neuropathological predilection patterns in Alzheimer disease, in Terry RD, Katzman R, Bick KL (eds). Alzheimer Disease. New York: Raven Press, 1994, pp. 263–294.

Gleason RP, Schneider LS: Carbamazepine treatment of agitation in Alzheimer's outpatients refractory to neuroleptics. J Clin Psychiatry 51:115–118, 1990.

Glenner GG, Wong CW: Alzheimer's disease: Initial report of the purification and characterization of a novel cerebrovascular amyloid protein. Biochem Biophys Res Commun 120: 885–890, 1984.

Gnanalingham KK, Byrne EJ, Thornton A, et al: Motor and cognitive function in Lewy body dementia: Comparison with Alzheimer's and Parkinson's diseases. J Neurol Neurosurg Psychiatry 62:243–252, 1997.

Gomez-Tortosa E, Newell K, Irizarry MC, et al: Clinical and quantitative pathologic correlates of dementia with Lewy bodies. Neurology 53:1284–1291, 1999.

Greenamyre JT: Neuronal bioenergetic defects, excitotoxicity and Alzheimer's disease: "Use it and lose it." Neurobiol Aging 12:334–336, 1991.

Greenwald BS: Depression in Alzheimer's disease and related dementias, in Lawlor BA (ed): Behavioral Complications of Alzheimer's Disease. Washington, D.C.: American Psychiatric Press, 1995, pp. 19–53.

Gurney ME, Cutting FB, Zhai P, et al: Benefit of vitamin E, riluzole, and gabapentin in a transgenic model of familial amyotrophic lateral sclerosis. Ann Neurol 39:147–157, 1996.

Gwinn-Hardy K: Genetics of parkinsonism. Mov Disord 17:645–656, 2002.

Hardy J: Amyloid, the presenilins and Alzheimer's disease. Trends Neurosci 20:154–159, 1997.

Hardy J, Gwinn-Hardy K: Genetic classification of primary neurodegenerative disease. Science 282:1075–1079, 1998.

Hardy J, Selkoe DJ: The amyloid hypothesis of Alzheimer's disease: Progress and problems on the road to therapeutics. Science 297:353–356, 2002.

Hardy JA, Higgins GA: Alzheimer's disease: The amyloid cascade hypothesis. Science 256:184–185, 1992.

Herrmann N: Valproic acid treatment of agitation in dementia. Can J Psychiatry 43:69–72, 1998.

Hodges J: The amnestic prodrome of Alzheimer's disease. Brain 121:1601–1602, 1998.

Hodges JR: Frontotemporal dementia (Pick's disease): Clinical features and assessment. Neurology 56(Suppl. 4):S6–S10, 2001.

Houlden H, Baker M, Adamson J, et al: Frequency of tau mutations in three series of non-Alzheimer's degenerative dementia. Ann Neurol 46:243–248, 1999.

Hutton M, Lendon CL, Rizzu P, et al: Association of missense and 5'-splice-site mutations in tau with the inherited dementia FTDP-17. Nature 393:702–705, 1998.

Hutton M: Molecular genetics of chromosome 17 tauopathies. Ann N Y Acad Sci 920:63–73, 2000.

Imamura T, Takanashi M, Hatton N, et al: Bromocriptine treatment for perseveration in demented patients. Alzheimer Dis Assoc Disord 12:109–113, 1998.

in 't Veld BA, Ruitenberg A, Hofman A, et al: Nonsteroidal antiinflammatory drugs and the risk of Alzheimer's disease. N Engl J Med 345:1515–1521, 2001.

Jaeckle KA: Assessment of tumor markers in cerebrospinal fluid. Clin Lab Med 5:303–315, 1985.

Jaffe AB, Toran-Allerand CD, Greengard P, Gandy SE: Estrogen regulates metabolism of Alzheimer amyloid beta precursor protein. J Biol Chem 269:13065–13068, 1994.

Jenkinson ML, Bliss MR, Brain AT, Scott DL: Rheumatoid arthritis and senile dementia of the Alzheimer's type. Br J Rheumatol 28:86–88, 1989.

Jick H, Zornberg GL, Jick SS, et al: Statins and the risk of dementia. Lancet 356:1627–1631, 2000.

Johnson KA, Sperling RA, Holman BL, et al: Cerebral perfusion in progressive supranuclear palsy. J Nucl Med 33:704–709, 1992.

Jordan DB, Relkin NR, Ravdin LD, et al: Apolipoprotein E epsilon4 associated with chronic traumatic brain injury in boxing. JAMA 278:136–140, 1997.

Kanowski S, Herrmann WM, Stephan K, et al: Proof of efficacy of the ginkgo biloba special extract EGb 761 in outpatients suffering from mild to moderate primary degenerative dementia of the Alzheimer type or multi-infarct dementia. Pharmacopsychiatry 29:47–56, 1996.

Katona CL, Hunter BN, Bray J: A double-blind comparison of the efficacy and safety of paroxetine and imipramine in the treatment of depression with dementia. Int J Geriatr Psychiatry 13:100–108, 1998.

Katzman R: Alzheimer's disease. N Engl J Med 314:964–973, 1986.

Kaye WH, Sitaram N, Weingartner H, et al: Modest facilitation of memory in dementia with combined lecithin and anticholinerestase treatment. Biol Psychiatry 17:275–280, 1982.

Kertesz A, Martinez-Lage P, Davidson W, Munoz DG: The corticobasal degeneration syndrome overlaps progressive aphasia and frontotemporal dementia. Neurology 55:1368–1375, 2000.

Kertesz A, Munoz DG:. Primary progressive aphasia: A review of the neurobiology of a common presentation of Pick complex. Am J Alzheimer's Dis Other Demen 17:30–36, 2002.

Knapp MJ, Knopman DS, Solomon PR, et al: A 30-week randomized controlled trial of high-dose tacrine in patients with Alzheimer's disease: The Tacrine Study Group. JAMA 271:985–991, 1994.

Knopman D, Schneider L, Davis K, et al: Long-term tacrine (Cognex) treatment: Effects on nursing home placement and mortality. Tacrine Study Group. Neurology 47:166–177, 1996.

Knopman DS, De Kosky ST, Cummings JL, et al: Practice parameter: Diagnosis of dementia (an evidence-based review). Report of the Quality Standards Subcommittee of the American Academy of Neurology. Neurology 56:1143–1153, 2001.

Kosik KS, Joachim CL, Selkoe DJ: Microtubule-associated protein tau (tau) is a major antigenic component of paired helical filaments in Alzheimer disease. Proc Natl Acad Sci U S A 83:4044–4048, 1986.

Kotzbauer PT, Trojanowski JQ, Lee VM: Lewy body pathology in Alzheimer's disease. J Mol Neurosci 17:225–232, 2001.

Kulisevsky J: Role of dopamine in learning and memory: Implications for the treatment of cognitive dysfunction in patients with Parkinson's disease. Drugs Aging 16:365–379, 2000.

Kuzis G, Sabe L, Tiberti C, et al: Neuropsychological correlates of apathy and depression in patients with dementia. Neurology 52:1403–1407, 1999.

Langston JW, Langston EB, Irwin I: MPTP-induced parkinsonism in human and non-human primates—clinical and experimental aspects. Acta Neurol Scand 100(Suppl.):49–54, 1984.

Larson EB, Reifler BV, Sumi SM, et al: Diagnostic tests in the evaluation of dementia: A prospective study of 200 elderly outpatients. Arch Intern Med 146:1917–1922, 1986.

Lee VM, Trojanowski JQ: Neurodegenerative tauopathies: Human disease and transgenic mouse models. Neuron 24:507–510, 1999.

Levy G, Schupf N, Tang MX, et al: Combined effect of age and severity on the risk of dementia in Parkinson's disease. Ann Neurol 51:722–729, 2002.

Lewis J, McGowan E, Rockwood J, et al: Neurofibrillary tangles, amyotrophy and progressive motor disturbance in mice expressing mutant (P301L) tau protein. Nat Genet 25:402–405, 2000.

Lichter I, Richardson PJ, Wyke MA: Differential effects of atenolol and enalapril on memory during treatment for essential hypertension. Br J Clin Pharmacol 21:641–645, 1986.

Lindenbaum J, Healton EB, Savage DG, et al: Neuropsychiatric disorders caused by cobalamin deficiency in the absence of anemia or macrocytosis. N Engl J Med 318:1720–1728, 1988.

Lobotesis K, Fenwick JD, Phipps A, et al: Occipital hypoperfusion on SPECT in dementia with Lewy bodies but not AD. Neurology 56:643–649, 2001.

Lund and Manchester Groups. Clinical and neuropathological criteria for frontotemporal dementia. J Neurol Neurosurg Psychiatry 57:416–418, 1994.

Maltby N, Broe GA, Creasey H, et al: Efficacy of tacrine and lecithin in mild to moderate Alzheimer's disease: Double blind trial. BMJ 308:879–883, 1994.

Masaki KH, Losonczy KG, Izmirlian G, et al: Association of vitamin E and C supplement use with cognitive function and dementia in elderly men. Neurology 54:1265–1272, 2000.

Mattis S: Dementia Rating Scale: Professional Manual. Odessa, Florida: Psychological Assessment Resources, 1988.

Mattson MP, Cheng B, Davis D, et al: Beta-amyloid peptides destabilize calcium homeostasis and render human cortical neurons vulnerable to excitotoxicity. J Neurosci 12:376–389, 1992.

Mayeux R, Sano M: Treatment of Alzheimer's disease. N Engl J Med 341:1670–1679, 1999.

McGaugh JL: Memory: A century of consolidation. Science 287:248–251, 2000.

McGeer PL, Schulzer M, McGeer EG: Arthritis and anti-inflammatory agents as possible protective factors for Alzheimer's disease: A review of 17 epidemiologic studies. Neurology 47:425–432, 1996.

McKhann G, Drachman D, Folstein M, et al: Clinical diagnosis of Alzheimer's disease: Report of the NINCDS-ARDA Work Group under the auspices of Department of Health and Human Services Task Force on Alzheimer's disease. Neurology 34:939–944, 1984.

McLean CA, Cherny RA, Fraser FW, et al: Soluble pool of Aβ amyloid as a determinant of severity of neurodegeneration in Alzheimer's disease. Ann Neurol 46:860–866, 1999.

Meek PD, McKeithan K, Schumock GT: Economic considerations in Alzheimer's disease. Pharmacotherapy 18:68–73, 1998.

Mega MS, Cummings JL, Fiorello T, Gornbein J: The spectrum of behavioral changes in Alzheimer's disease. Neurology 46:130–135, 1996.

Mega MS, Masterman DM, O'Connor SM, et al: The spectrum of behavioral responses to cholinesterase inhibitor therapy in Alzheimer disease. Arch Neurol 56:1388–1393, 1999.

Mellow AM, Solano-Lopez C, Davis S: Sodium valproate in the treatment of behavioral disturbance in dementia. J Geriatr Psychiatry Neurol 6:205–209, 1993.

Meltzer CC, Smith G, DeKoskey ST, et al: Serotonin in aging, late-life depression, and Alzheimer's disease: The emerging role of functional imaging. Neuropsychopharmacology 18:407–430, 1998.

Mesulam MM: Large-scale neurocognitive networks and distributed processing for attention, language, and memory. Ann Neurol 28:597–613, 1990.

Mesulam MM: Neuroplasticity failure in Alzheimer's disease: Bridging the gap between plaques and tangles. Neuron 24:521–529, 1999.

Mesulam MM: Slowly progressive aphasia without generalized dementia. Ann Neurol 11:592–598, 1982.

Mesulam MM: The systems-level organization of cholinergic innervation in the human cerebral cortex and its alterations in Alzheimer's disease. Prog Brain Res 109:285–297, 1996.

Molsa PK, Marttila RJ, Rinne UK: Survival and cause of death in Alzheimer's disease and multi-infarct dementia. Acta Neurol Scand 74:103–107, 1986.

Morris MC, Beckett LA, Scherr PA, et al: Vitamin E and vitamin C supplement use and risk of incident Alzheimer disease. Alzheimer Dis Assoc Disord 12:121–126, 1998.

Mulnard RA, Cotman CW, Kawas C, et al: Estrogen replacement therapy for treatment of mild to moderate Alzheimer disease: A randomized controlled trial. Alzheimer's Disease Cooperative Study. JAMA 283:1007–1015, 2000.

Neafsey EJ: Prefrontal cortical control of the autonomic nervous system: Anatomical and physiological observations. Prog Brain Res 85:147–165, 1990.

Neary D: Non Alzheimer's disease forms of cerebral atrophy. J Neurol Neurosurg Psychiatry 53:929–931, 1990.

Nilsberth C, Westlind-Danielsson A, Eckman CB, et al: The "Arctic" APP mutation (E693G) causes Alzheimer's disease by enhanced Abeta protofibril formation. Nat Neurosci 4:859–860, 2001.

Nilsson LN, Bales KR, DiCarlo G. et al: α-1-Antichymotrypsin promotes β-sheet amyloid plaque deposition in a transgenic mouse model of Alzheimer's disease. J Neurosci 21:1444–1451, 2001.

Nyth AL, Gottfries CG: The clinical efficacy of citalopram in treatment of emotional disturbances in dementia disorders: A Nordic multicentre study. Br J Psychiatry 157:894–901, 1990.

Nyth AL, Gottfries CG, Lyby K, et al: A controlled multicenter clinical study of citalopram and placebo in elderly depressed patients with and without concomitant dementia. Acta Psychiatr Scand 86:138–145, 1992.

Okada K, Suyama N, Oguro H, et al: Medication-induced hallucination and cerebral blood flow in Parkinson's disease. J Neurol 246:365–368, 1999.

Oken BS, Storzbach DM, Kaye JA: The efficacy of Ginkgo biloba on cognitive function in Alzheimer disease. Arch Neurol 55:1409–1415, 1998.

Ott BR, Noto RB, Fogel BS: Apathy and loss of insight in Alzheimer's disease: A SPECT imaging study. J Neuropsychiatry Clin Neurosci 8:41–46, 1996.

Palmer AM, Stratmann GC, Procter AW, Bowen DM: Possible neurotransmitter basis of behavioral changes in Alzheimer's disease. Ann Neurol 23:616–620, 1988.

Parkinson Study Group: Effect of deprenyl on the progression of disability in early Parkinson's disease. N Engl J Med 321:1364–1371, 1989.

Parkinson Study Group: Effects of tocopherol and deprenyl on the progression of disability in early Parkinson's disease. N Engl J Med 328:176–183, 1993.

Parvizi J, Van Hoesen GW, Damasio A: Severe pathological changes of parabrachial nucleus in Alzheimer's disease. Neuroreport 9:4151–4154, 1998.

Perry RJ, Hodges JR: Attention and executive deficits in Alzheimer's disease: A critical review. Brain 122(Pt 3):383–404, 1999.

Petersen RC, Doody R, Kurz A, et al: Current concepts in mild cognitive impairment. Arch Neurol 58:1985–1992, 2001.

Polvikoski T, Sulkava R, Myllykangas L, et al: Prevalence of Alzheimer's disease in very elderly people. Neurology 56:1690–1696, 2001.

Price DL, Sisodia SS: Mutant genes in familial Alzheimer's disease and transgenic models. Annu Rev Neurosci 21:479–505, 1998.

Price DL, Sisodia SS, Borchelt DR: Genetic neurodegenerative diseases: The human illness and transgenic models. Science 282:1079–1083, 1998.

Prusiner SB: Prions. Proc Natl Acad Sci U S A 95:13363–13383, 1998.

Raskind MA, Peskind ER, Wessel T, Yuan W: Galantamine in AD: A 6-month randomized, placebo-controlled trial with a 6-month extension. Neurology 54:2261–2268, 2000.

Ratnavalli E, Brayne C, Dawson K, Hodges JR: The prevalence of frontotemporal dementia. Neurology 58:1615–1621, 2002.

Reifler BV, Teri L, Raskind M, et al: Double-blind trial of imipramine in Alzheimer's disease patients with and without depression. Am J Psychiatry 146:45–49, 1989.

Reisberg B, Ferris S, Sahin K, et al: Results of a placebo-controlled 6-month trial with memantine in moderate to severe Alzheimer's disease (AD). Eur Neuropsychopharm 10(Suppl. 3):S363–S364, 2000.

Relkin NR, Kwon YJ, Tsai J, Gandy S: The National Institute on Aging/Alzheimer's Association recommendations on the application of apolipoprotein E genotyping to Alzheimer's disease. Ann N Y Acad Sci 802:149–176, 1996.

Richardson PJ, Wyke MA: Memory function: Effects of different antihypertensive drugs. Drugs 35(Suppl. 5): 80–85, 1988.

Rizzo M, Vecera SP: Psychoanatomical substrates of Bálint's syndrome. J Neurol Neurosurg Psychiatr 72:162–178, 2002.

Rizzu P, Van Swieten JC, Joosse M, et al: High prevalence of mutations in the microtubule-associated protein tau in a population study of frontotemporal dementia in The Netherlands. Am J Hum Genet 64:414–421, 1999.

Rogers J, Kirby LC, Hempelman SR, et al: Clinical trial of indomethacin in Alzheimer's disease. Neurology 43: 1609–1611, 1993.

Rogers SL, Farlow MR, Doody RS, et al: A 24-week, double-blind, placebo-controlled trial of donepezil in patients with Alzheimer's disease. Donepezil Study Group. Neurology 50:136–145, 1998a.

Rogers SL, Farlow MR, Mohs RC, Friedhoff LT: Donepezil improves cognition and global function in Alzheimer disease: A 15-week, double-blind, placebo-controlled study. Donepezil Study Group. Arch Intern Med 158:1021–1031, 1998b.

Rogers SL, Friedhoff LT, Doody RS, et al: The efficacy and safety of donepezil in patients with Alzheimer's disease: Results of a US multicentre, randomized, double-blind, placebo-controlled trial: The Donepezil Study Group. Dementia 7:293–303, 1996.

Rosen J, Zubenko GS: Emergence of psychosis and depression in the longitudinal evaluation of Alzheimer's disease. Biol Psychiatry 29:224–232, 1991.

Roses AD: Apolipoprotein E and Alzheimer's disease: The tip of the susceptibility iceberg. Ann N Y Acad Sci 855:738–743, 1998.

Rösler M, Anand R, Cicin-Sain A, et al: Efficacy and safety of rivastigmine in patients with Alzheimer's disease: International randomised controlled trial. BMJ 318:633–638, 1999.

Sano M, Ernesto C, Thomas RGet al: A controlled trial of selegiline, alpha-tocopherol, or both as treatment for Alzheimer's disease. The Alzheimer's Disease Cooperative Study. N Engl J Med 336:1216–1222, 1997.

Schenk D, Barbour R, Dunn W, et al: Immunization with amyloid-beta attenuates Alzheimer-disease-like pathology in the PDAPP mouse. Nature 400:173–177, 1999.

Schenk D: Amyloid-beta immunotherapy for Alzheimer's disease: The end of the beginning. Nat Rev Neurosci 3:824–828, 2002.

Seager CP: Chlorpromazine in treatment of elderly psychotic women. Br Med J 1: 882–885, 1955.

Selkoe DJ: The genetics and molecular pathology of Alzheimer's disease: Roles of amyloid and the presenilins. Neurol Clin 18:903–922, 2000.

Seshadri S, Beiser A, Selhub J, et al: Plasma homocysteine as a risk factor for dementia and Alzheimer's disease. New Engl J Med 346:476–483, 2002.

Shoulson I: Experimental therapeutics of neurodegenerative disorders: Unmet needs. Science 282:1072–1074, 1998a.

Shoulson I: DATATOP: A decade of neuroprotective inquiry. Parkinson Study Group. Deprenyl and Tocopherol Antioxidative Therapy of Parkinsonism. Ann Neurol 44(Suppl. 1):S160–S166, 1998b.

Sigurdsson EM, Wisniewski T, Frangione B: A safer vaccine for Alzheimer's disease? Neurobiol Aging 23:1001–1008, 2002.

Sinha S, Lieberburg I: Cellular mechanisms of beta-amyloid production and secretion. Proc Natl Acad Sci U S A 96:11049–11053, 1999.

Slaughter JR, Slaughter KA, Nichols D, et al: Prevalence, clinical manifestations, etiology, and treatment of depression in Parkinson's disease. J Neuropsychiatry Clin Neurosci 13:187–196, 2001.

Smith CD, Carney JM, Starke-Reed P, et al: Excess brain protein oxidation and enzyme dysfunction in normal aging and in Alzheimer disease. Proc Natl Acad Sci U S A 88:10540–10543, 1991.

Smith MA, Perry G, Richey PL, et al: Oxidative damage in Alzheimer's. Nature 382:120–121, 1996.

Snowdon DA, Kemper SJ, Mortimer JA, et al: Linguistic ability in early life and cognitive function and Alzheimer's disease in late life: Findings from the Nun Study. JAMA 275:528–532, 1996.

Sorbi S, Nacmias B, Forleo P, et al: Epistatic effect of APP717 mutation and apolipoprotein E genotype in familial Alzheimer's disease. Ann Neurol 38:124–127, 1995.

Stern Y, Mayeux R, Sano M, et al: Predictors of disease course in patients with probable Alzheimer's disease. Neurology 37(10): 1649–1653, 1987.

Stern Y, Gurland B, Tatemichi TK, et al: Influence of education and occupation on the incidence of Alzheimer's disease. JAMA 271:1004–1010, 1994.

Stevens M, van Duijn CM, Kamphorst W, et al: Familial aggregation in frontotemporal dementia. Neurology 50:1541–1545, 1998.

Sugarman AA, Williams BH, Adlerstein AM et al: Haloperidol in the psychiatric disorders of old age. Am J Psychiatry 121: 1190–1192, 1964.

Summers WK, Viesselman JO, Marsh GM, Candelora K: Use of THA in treatment of Alzheimer-like dementia: Pilot study in twelve patients. Biol Psychiatry 16:145–153, 1981.

Sunderland T, Tariot PN, Cohen RM, et al: Anticholinergic sensitivity in patients with dementia of the Alzheimer type and age-matched controls: A dose-response study. Arch Gen Psychiatry 44:418–426, 1987.

Tang MX, Jacobs D, Stern Y, et al: Effect of oestrogen during menopause on risk and age of onset of Alzheimer's disease. Lancet 348:429–432, 1996.

Tangalos EG, Smith GE, Ivnik RJ, et al: The Mini-Mental State Examination in general medical practice: Clinical utility and acceptance. Mayo Clin Proc 71:829–837, 1996.

Taragano FE, Lyketsos CG, Mangone CA, et al: A double-blind, randomized, fixed-dose trial of fluoxetine vs. amitriptyline in the treatment of major depression complicating Alzheimer's disease. Psychosomatics 38:246–252, 1997.

Tariot PN, Erb R, Leibovici A, et al: Carbamazepine treatment of agitation in nursing home patients with dementia: A preliminary study. J Am Geriatr Soc 42:1160–1166, 1994.

Tariot PN, Erb R, Podgorski CA, et al: Efficacy and tolerability of carbamazepine for agitation and aggression in dementia. Am J Psychiatry 155:54–61, 1998.

Tariot PN, Solomon PR, Morris JC, et al: A 5-month, randomized, placebo-controlled trial of galantamine in AD. The Galantamine USA-10 Study Group. Neurology 54:2269–2276, 2000.

Taubes G: Misfolding the way to disease. Science 271:1493–1495, 1996.

Teng EL, Chui HC: The Modified Mini-Mental State (3MS) Examination. J Clin Psychiatry 48:314–318, 1987.

Thal LJ, Rosen W, Sharpless NS, Crystal H: Choline chloride fails to improve cognition of Alzheimer's disease. Neurobiol Aging 2:205–208, 1981.

Tokuda T, Ikeda S, Yanagisawa N, et al: Re-examination of ex-boxers' brains using immunohistochemistry with antibodies to amyloid beta-protein and tau protein. Acta Neuropathol 82:280–285, 1991.

Tsai JY, Wolfe MS, Xia W: The search for gamma-secretase and development of inhibitors. Curr Med Chem 9:1087–1106, 2002.

van Dongen MC, van Rossum E, Kessels AG, et al: The efficacy of ginkgo for elderly people with dementia and age-associated memory impairment: New results of a randomized clinical trial. J Am Geriatr Soc 48:1183–1194, 2000.

Volkow ND, Gur RC, Wang GJ, et al: Association between decline in brain dopamine activity with age and cognitive and motor impairment in healthy individuals. Am J Psychiatry 155:344–349, 1998.

Walsh JS, Welch HG, Larson EB: Survival of outpatients with Alzheimer-type dementia. Ann Intern Med 113:429–434, 1990.

Wang HX, Wahlin A, Basun H, et al: Vitamin B(12) and folate in relation to the development of Alzheimer's disease. Neurology 56:1188–1194, 2001.

Watanabe MD, Martin EM, DeLeon OA, et al: Successful methylphenidate treatment of apathy after subcortical infarcts. J Neuropsychiatry Clin Neurosci 7:502–504, 1995.

Weintraub S, Rubin NP, Mesulam MM: Primary progressive aphasia: Longitudinal course, profile, and language features. Arch Neurol 47:1329–1335, 1990.

Weintraub S, Mesulam M: Four neuropsychological profiles in dementia. Handbook of Neuropsychology 8:253–282, 1993.

Welsh KA, Butters N, Hughes JP, et al: Detection and staging of dementia in Alzheimer's disease: Use of the neuropsychological measures developed for the Consortium to Establish a Registry for Alzheimer's Disease. Arch Neurol 49:448–452, 1992.

Werber EA, Rabey JM: The beneficial effect of cholinesterase inhibitors on patients suffering from Parkinson's disease and dementia. J Neural Transm 108:1319–1325, 2001.

Weytingh MD, Bossuyt PM, van Crevel H: Reversible dementia: More than 10% or less than 1%? A quantitative review. J Neurol 242:466–471, 1995.

Wickner S, Maurizi MR, Gotesman S: Posttranslational quality control: Folding, refolding, and degrading proteins. Science 286:1888–1893, 1999.

Winblad B, Poritis N: Memantine in severe dementia: Results of the 9M-Best Study (Benefit and efficacy in severely demented patients during treatment with memantine). Int J Geriatr Psychiatry 14:135–146, 1999.

Winkler J, Thal LJ, Gage FH, Fisher LJ: Cholinergic strategies for Alzheimer's disease. J Mol Med 76:555–567, 1998.

Wolozin B, Kellman W, Ruosseau P, et al: Decreased prevalence of Alzheimer disease associated with 3-hydroxy-3-methyglutaryl coenzyme A reductase inhibitors. Arch Neurol 57:1439–1443, 2000.

Woolley CS, McEwen BS: Roles of estradiol and progesterone in regulation of hippocampal dendritic spine density during the estrous cycle in the rat. J Comp Neurol 336:293–306, 1993.

Wragg RE, Jeste DV. Overview of depression and psychosis in Alzheimer's disease. Am J Psychiatry 146:577–587, 1989.

Xu H, Gouras GK, Greenfield GP, et al: Estrogen reduces neuronal generation of Alzheimer beta-amyloid peptides. Nat Med 4:447–451, 1998.

Xu M, Lai MT, Huang O, et al: Gamma-secretase: Characterization and implication for Alzheimer disease therapy. Neurobiol Aging 23:1023–1030, 2002.

Yamamoto A, Lucas JJ, Hen R: Reversal of neuropathology and motor dysfunction in a conditional model of Huntington's disease. Cell 101:57–66, 2000.

Zerr I, Bodemer M, Gefeller O, et al: Detection of 14-3-3 protein in the cerebrospinal fluid supports the diagnosis of Creutzfeldt-Jakob disease. Ann Neurol 43:32–40, 1998.

Brain Infections

Karen L. Roos

Bacterial meningitis

Brain abscess

Fungal meningitis

HIV-associated dementia complex

Lyme disease

Neurosyphilis

Prion diseases

Viral encephalitis

INTRODUCTION

Cognitive impairment and behavioral abnormalities may be a presenting sign of or a consequence of central nervous system (CNS) infection. Herpes simplex virus encephalitis is the classic CNS infection that presents with behavioral abnormalities. Historically, syphilis was the most common CNS infection with dementia as a prominent feature. At the present time, human immunodeficiency virus (HIV) and prion diseases are more often implicated as infectious causes of cognitive difficulty. This chapter reviews the clinical presentation, diagnosis, and neuropsychological sequelae of bacterial meningitis, viral encephalitis, HIV-associated dementia complex, neurosyphilis, Creutzfeldt-Jakob disease (CJD), Lyme disease, brain abscess, and fungal meningitis.

BACTERIAL MENINGITIS

The clinical presentation of bacterial meningitis consists of fever, stiff neck, headache, nausea, vomiting, and photophobia. An altered level of consciousness, ranging from lethargy to stupor or coma, and seizure activity can be associated with or follow the initial symptoms. The most common etiologic organisms of community-acquired bacterial meningitis in children and adults are *Streptococcus pneumoniae* and *Neisseria meningitidis*. Prior to the routine use of the *Haemophilus influenzae* type b (Hib) conjugate vaccine, Hib was the most common causative organism of bacterial meningitis in children. The incidence of Hib invasive disease among children 4 years of age and younger has declined 98% since the introduction of the Hib conjugate vaccine. Hib remains a causative organism of bacterial meningitis in older adults, immunocompromised patients, and patients with chronic lung disease, splenectomy, leukemia, and sickle cell disease. Gram-negative bacilli cause meningitis in older adults, neurosurgical patients, alcoholics, and adults with underlying diseases, such as cancer, diabetes, congestive heart failure, chronic pulmonary disease, and hepatic or renal disease. *Listeria monocytogenes* is a causative organism of meningitis in individuals with impaired cell-mediated immunity from acquired immunodeficiency syndrome (AIDS), organ transplantation, pregnancy, malignancy, chronic illness, or immunosuppressive therapy. *Staphylococcus aureus* and coagulase-negative staphylococci are predominant organisms causing meningitis as a complication of a neurosurgical procedure, particularly shunting procedures for hydrocephalus, and as a complication of lumbar puncture for the administration of intrathecal chemotherapy. *Streptococcus agalactiae* or group B streptococcus is a leading cause of bacterial meningitis and sepsis in neonates and is increasingly seen in two groups of adults, puerperal women and older adults with chronic diseases.

The diagnosis of bacterial meningitis is made by examination of the cerebrospinal fluid (CSF). The classic CSF abnormalities in bacterial meningitis are as follows: (1) increased opening pressure; (2) a pleocytosis of polymorphonuclear leukocytes (10–10,000 cells/mm^3); (3) decreased glucose concentration (<45 mg/dL and/or CSF/serum glucose ratio of <0.31); and (4) an increased protein concentration. The specific meningeal pathogen can be identified by Gram stain or grown in culture. The polymerase chain reaction (PCR) technique is available to detect bacterial DNA in CSF, but the sensitivity and specificity of this test have not been defined. The latex particle agglutination (LA) test can detect bacterial antigens of *S. pneumoniae*, *N. meningitidis*, Hib, group B streptococcus, and *Escherichia coli* K1 strains in CSF.

Mortality and neurologic morbidity, specifically cognitive outcome, are related to a number of factors, but most importantly, the time from onset of symptoms to initiation of therapy and the patient's underlying medical condition. In a series that examined cognitive function in adult patients months after acute bacterial meningitis, the principal abnormalities on psychometric tests were decreased speed of cognitive and psychomotor performance, decreased visual memory, reduced concentration, reduced visuoconstructive capacity, diminished nonverbal and logical memory, and impaired associative learning. No clear, cortical-type cognitive deficits were seen. The abnormalities were suggestive of a subcortical type of cognitive impairment (Merkelbach et al., 2000).

Cerebral ischemia and infarction are major neurologic complications of bacterial meningitis. The large arteries at the base of the brain are narrowed due to encroachment on the vessel wall by the inflammatory subarachnoid purulent exudate and infiltration of the arterial wall by inflammatory cells, and there is narrowing of medium-sized arteries and thrombotic or stenotic occlusion of branches of the middle cerebral artery (Opfister et al., 1991). When cerebrovascular disease complicates bacterial meningitis, the patient may be left with an aphasia or a hemiparesis.

Twenty-five percent of children with bacterial meningitis have functionally important disabilities years later, including mild to moderate hearing loss, learning disabilities, and behavioral problems (Grimwood et al., 1995). Approximately 10% of children who survive bacterial meningitis have major neurologic sequelae including seizures, hydrocephalus, spasticity, blindness, or severe to profound hearing loss (Grimwood et al., 1994). The causative organism of the meningitis appears to be significantly associated with outcome in children. Pneumococcal meningitis is reported to have the highest frequency of later sequelae, followed by *H. influenzae* and meningococcal meningitis (Baraff et al., 1993; Kaaresen & Flaegstad, 1995). Neurologic sequelae including hearing loss, hydrocephalus, seizure activity, and mental retardation have been reported in 29% to 56% of children with pneumococcal meningitis (Kornelisse et al., 1995). The most precisely quantitated sequela of bacterial meningitis in children is hearing loss (Kabani & Jadavji, 1002). This loss may have a role in developmental delay and cognitive deficits.

ENCEPHALITIS

Encephalitis is an acute infection of brain parenchyma that presents with fever, headache, and an altered level of consciousness. There may also be focal or multifocal neurologic deficits and focal or generalized seizure activity. The major causes of encephalitis are herpes simplex virus type 1 (HSV-1), herpes simplex virus type 2 (HSV-2) in neonates, and the arthropod-borne viruses, including La Crosse virus, St. Louis encephalitis (SLE) virus, Japanese encephalitis virus, West Nile virus, eastern equine encephalitis virus, western equine encephalitis virus, Venezuelan equine encephalitis virus, tick-borne encephalitis virus, Powassan virus, and Colorado tick fever.

Primary infection with HSV-1 usually occurs in the oropharyngeal mucosa, typically during childhood, and is asymptomatic or characterized by fever, pain, and an inability to swallow due to lesions on the buccal and gingival mucosa (Whitley et al., 1998). After primary infection, HSV-1 is transported to the CNS by retrograde transneuronal spread of the virus along a division of the trigeminal nerve. The trigeminal ganglion becomes colonized and the virus then establishes latent infection in the trigeminal ganglion. Reactivation of latent ganglionic infection with replication of the virus leads to viral encephalitis with infection in the temporal cortex and limbic system structures (Barnett et al., 1994). The clinical presentation of HSV-1 encephalitis is typically a subacute presentation of fever, hemicranial or generalized headache, behavioral abnormalities, focal seizure activity, and focal neurologic deficits, most often dysphasia or hemiparesis. The diagnosis of HSV-1 encephalitis is made by neuroimaging, electroencephalography (EEG), and examination of the CSF. Magnetic resonance imaging (MRI) scan is the neuroimaging procedure of choice. The characteristic abnormality on MRI scan of HSV-1 encephalitis is a high signal intensity lesion on T2-weighted and fluid-attenuated inversion recovery (FLAIR) images in the medial and inferior temporal lobe extending up into the insula. A normal T2-weighted and FLAIR MRI scan is evidence against the diagnosis of HSV-1 encephalitis. The classic EEG abnormality in HSV encephalitis consists of periodic, stereotyped, sharp-and-slow wave complexes that occur at regular intervals of 2 to 3 seconds and are expressed maximally over the involved temporal lobe. Examination of the CSF reveals an increased opening pressure, a lymphocytic pleocytosis of 5 to 500 cells/mm³, a mild to moderate elevation of the protein concentration, and a normal or mildly decreased glucose concentration. CSF viral cultures for HSV-1 are almost always negative. PCR has become the gold standard for making a diagnosis of HSV encephalitis. CSF PCR for HSV DNA is most likely to be positive within the first 24 to 48 hours of infection, but then may begin to decline and can be falsely negative 10 to 14 days after the onset of infection. In addition, PCR should not be performed on bloody CSF. Porphyrin compounds derived from the degradation of heme in erythrocytes may inhibit the PCR, giving a false-negative result (Aurelius et al., 1991). HSV DNA in CSF precedes the appearance of HSV antibodies by several days. CSF and serum samples should be obtained to determine if there is intrathecal synthesis of antibodies against HSV. Antibodies against HSV do not appear in the CSF until approximately 8 to 12 days after the onset of disease and increase significantly during the first 2 to 4 weeks of infection. A serum/CSF antibody ratio of less than 20:1 is considered diagnostic of HSV infection.

The primary neurocognitive deficits in patients who survive HSV encephalitis are related to language. Speech is fluent, but the patient has verbal paraphasias, difficulty finding words, and dysnomia. Comprehension typically remains intact. Patients also demonstrate cognitive slowing, decreased memory, and emotional lability or personality changes. Both the cognitive and psychiatric problems improve with the passage of time, and predictions should not be made on the permanency of these deficits until the patient is at least 2 years from the acute illness.

The symptoms of encephalitis due to an arthropod-borne virus are often preceded by an influenza-like prodrome of malaise, myalgias, and fever. This is followed by symptoms of headache, nausea, vomiting, confusion, disorientation, stupor, tremors, and convulsions. The laboratory diagnosis of arthropod-borne viral encephalitis has been established by the Centers for Disease Control and Prevention. A confirmed case of arthropod-borne viral encephalitis is defined as a febrile illness with encephalitis during a period when mosquito or tick transmission is likely to occur, plus at least one of the following: (1) fourfold or greater rise in viral antibody titer between acute and convalescent sera; (2) viral isolation from tissue, blood, or CSF; or (3) specific immunoglobulin M (IgM) antibody in CSF. A presumptive case is defined as a compatible illness plus either a stable elevated antibody titer to an arthropod-borne virus (≥320 by hemagglutination inhibition, ≥128 by complement fixation, ≥256 by immunofluorescent assay, or ≥160 by plaque-reduction neutralization test) or specific IgM antibody in serum by enzyme immunoassay (Centers for Disease Control and Prevention, 1995). Neuroimaging in arthropod-borne viral encephalitis may be normal or show hyperintense lesions on T2-weighted images in the basal ganglia and thalami or small hyperintense lesions in the cortical gray matter on T2-weighted and FLAIR images. Examination of the CSF demonstrates a lymphocytic pleocytosis, a normal glucose concentration, and a moderately elevated protein concentration.

Neurologic sequelae from arthropod-borne viral encephalitis depend on the specific virus. Encephalitis due to eastern equine encephalitis virus has the highest mortality rate of the arthropod-borne viral encephalitides and the highest morbidity, especially in children under 10 years of age. Neurologic sequelae include mental retardation, convulsions, and emotional problems (Feemster, 1957). The fatality rate from SLE is highest in patients over 55 years of age and is approximately 5% to 10%. Most survivors recover completely, but emotional instability and behavioral difficulties have been reported in elderly survivors (Lawton et al., 1966). La Crosse virus encephalitis is predominantly a childhood disease. Seventy-five percent of cases occur in children under 10 years of age (McJunkin et al., 1998). The most common neurologic sequelae following La Crosse virus encephalitis are decreased short-term memory and behavioral problems, especially attention-deficit/hyperactivity disorder (McJunkin et al., 2001).

Subacute sclerosing panencephalitis (SSPE) is an inflammatory and degenerative disease caused by the measles virus. It is characterized by progressive mental deterioration beginning several years after measles infection in early childhood. In children, the earliest symptoms consist of behavioral changes affecting school performance, lethargy, malaise, and occasionally seizures. This is associated with or followed by myoclonic jerks. Dementia progresses as the myoclonic jerks diminish, culminating in a state of akinetic mutism and death. Visual symptomatology occurs in 50% or more of patients and includes papilledema, papillitis, retinitis, chorioretinitis, optic nerve pallor, homonymous visual field defects, and cortical blindness. The EEG demonstrates classic periodic complexes associated with myoclonus. Elevated measles antibody titers can be found in serum and CSF (Singer et al., 1997).

Rasmussen encephalitis is characterized by intractable focal seizures; radiologic evidence of slowly progressive, usually unilateral, brain atrophy with histopathologic evidence of perivascular inflammation; and gliotic changes suggestive of chronic encephalitis (Rasmussen & Andermann, 1991; Hennessy et al., 2001). Evidence for a viral etiology has been thoroughly investigated in patients with Rasmussen encephalitis, but to date a virus has not been identified.

HUMAN IMMUNODEFICIENCY VIRUS

HIV is one of the leading causes of dementia in young people. Dementia is rarely the first AIDS-defining illness. More often, dementia develops after immune deficiency and systemic opportunistic infections have been recognized. The term HIV-associated dementia complex is preferred over HIV dementia and HIV encephalopathy because of the high prevalence of upper motor neuron signs and behavioral abnormalities in addition to the features of dementia. Typical symptoms of HIV-associated dementia include forgetfulness, difficulty with concentration, loss of libido, apathy, inertia, loss of interest in work and hobbies, impaired short-term memory, and blunting of emotional responses. Motor complaints include trouble with coordination, a tendency to drop things, and difficulty with gait. HIV-associated dementia is a subcortical dementia, and the abnormalities on neuropsychological testing are characterized by memory loss selective for impaired retrieval, impaired manipulation of acquired knowledge, and a general slowing of psychomotor speed and thought processes. Attention, calculations, and language are usually not initially affected in HIV-associated dementia. The most useful tests for screening for HIV-associated dementia are those that examine psychomotor speed—Trailmaking, Grooved Pegboard, and Symbol-Digit (McArthur et al., 1999).

Neurologic examination in the early stages of HIV-associated dementia may only be remarkable for hyperreflexia. In patients with an associated HIV-related myelopathy there may be spastic paraparesis with a variable sensory ataxia and bladder involvement. Focal neurologic signs suggest a CNS opportunistic process rather than HIV-associated dementia (McArthur et al., 1999). Cranial MRI scan demonstrates central and cortical atrophy and deep white matter diffuse hyperintensities. The white matter abnormalities are sometimes confused with progressive multifocal leukoencephalopathy. Examination of the CSF may reveal a mild lymphocytic pleocytosis with an increased protein concentration, but similar CSF abnormalities are found in neurologically normal HIV seropositive patients. Lumbar puncture is important in these patients to rule out cryptococcal or histoplasma meningitis, cytomegalovirus (CMV) encephalitis, and neurosyphilis. HIV RNA levels in the CSF correlate with the severity of dementia (McAruthur et al., 1999).

TABLE 23-1. Clinical Features Useful for Diagnosis of HIV-1–Related Dementia

HIV-1 seropositivity

History of *progressive* cognitive/behavioral decline with apathy, memory loss, slowed mental processing

Neurologic exam: diffuse CNS signs including slowed rapid eye/limb movements, hyperreflexia, hypertonia, and release signs

Neuropsychological assessment: impairment in at least two areas including frontal lobe, motor speed, and nonverbal memory

CSF analysis: exclusion of neurosyphilis and cryptococcal meningitis

Imaging studies: diffuse cerebral atrophy with ill-defined white matter hyperintensities on MRI, exclusion of opportunistic processes

Absence of major psychiatric disorder or intoxication

Absence of metabolic derangement, e.g., hypoxia, sepsis

Absence of active CNS opportunistic processes

Reproduced with permission from McArthur JC, Sacktor N, Selnes O: Human immunodeficiency virus-associated dementia. Semin Neurol 19:129–150, 1999.

Progressive symptoms of HIV-associated dementia with high CSF HIV RNA levels and low plasma HIV RNA levels in a patient on highly active antiretroviral therapy (HAART) are frequently recognized. The clinical features useful for the diagnosis of dementia related to HIV-1 are listed in Table 23-1.

NEUROSYPHILIS

Prior to the availability of penicillin, syphilis was a common cause of dementia. Today the most common forms of neurosyphilis are asymptomatic neurosyphilis and acute syphilitic meningitis. Dementia paralytica or general paresis is a slow and subtle deterioration in cognitive functioning, with impaired memory and loss of insight and judgment. As the disease progresses, typically over a period of 3 to 4 years, there is loss of appendicular strength; pupillary abnormalities, including Argyll-Robertson pupils (loss of the pupillary reaction to light, with preservation of pupillary constriction to accommodation); tremor of the tongue and hands; and loss of bowel and bladder control.

Traditionally, as part of the work-up for treatable causes of dementia, a serum nontreponemal test, typically the Venereal Disease Research Laboratory test (VDRL) or the rapid plasma reagin test (RPR) is obtained. When either of these tests is positive, consideration is given to the possibility that syphilis is the cause of the dementia. Serologic tests for syphilis are divided into two categories, treponemal and nontreponemal. The VDRL and RPR are nontreponemal tests. They detect antibodies to lipids found on the membrane of *Treponema pallidum* using antigens such as cardiolipin, lecithin, or cholesterol. Nontreponemal tests become positive 5 to 6 weeks after inoculation, and their titers are highest during the secondary and latent stages of syphilis. In the absence of treatment, titers tend to decline spontaneously; in one quarter of untreated patients, the VDRL becomes negative. A transient (<6 months) false-positive nontreponemal test may be due to *Mycoplasma pneumoniae*, enterovirus infection, infectious mononucleosis, tuberculosis, or viral pneumonia. A chronic false-positive nontreponemal test (lasting >6 months) can be due to systemic lupus erythematosus and other connective tissue disorders, intravenous drug use, rheumatoid arthritis, age, reticuloendothelial malignancy, or Hashimoto thyroiditis. Ten percent of individuals over the age of 80 have a low-titer false-positive VDRL test. Most false-positive VDRL tests have a titer of 1:8 or less (Roos, 1996).

Treponemal tests are more specific than nontreponemal tests and become positive earlier in the course of infection. They remain positive for life. Treponemal tests detect specific antibody to *T. pallidum* antigen and include the following: (1) fluorescent treponemal antibody absorption test (FTA-ABS) and (2) *T. pallidum* microhemagglutination assay (MHA-TP). Treponemal tests can be falsely positive in Lyme disease, nonvenereal treponematoses, genital herpes simplex virus infection, pregnancy, systemic lupus erythematosus, alcoholic cirrhosis, scleroderma, and mixed connective tissue disease (Johnson & White, 1992). Screening for syphilis in individuals infected with HIV-1 should be performed by the serum FTA-ABS test.

The diagnosis of neurosyphilis is made by examination of the CSF. A reactive serum treponemal test and a CSF lymphocytic or mononuclear pleocytosis and an elevated protein concentration are diagnostic of neurosyphilis. A reactive CSF VDRL is diagnostic of neurosyphilis. False-positive results are rare but may be obtained when the CSF is visibly blood tinged (Johnson & White, 1992). A negative CSF VDRL does not rule out neurosyphilis. A negative CSF FTA-ABS or MHA-TP rules out neurosyphilis. A reactive CSF FTA-ABS is not definitive evidence of neurosyphilis. The CSF FTA-ABS can be falsely positive from blood contamination without the CSF being visibly tinged with blood (Davis & Sperry, 1979).

Neurosyphilis is treated with 18 to 24 million units of aqueous penicillin G intravenously for 10 to 14 days.

PRION DISEASES

Creutzfeldt-Jakob disease (CJD) is one of the human prion diseases also referred to as transmissible subacute spongiform encephalopathy. The prion diseases are caused by an infectious agent, termed a "prion" by Prusiner to emphasize its infectious and protein-like properties (Prusiner & Hsiao, 1994). The prion protein exists in two major isoforms: the nonpathogenic or normal cellular isoform, designated PrP^c, and the pathogenic or scrapie-like form, designated PrP^{Sc} (Mastrianni & Roos, 2000). A fundamental event in prion diseases is a conversion of the normal cellular prion protein into the scrapie isoform. The normal cellular isoform (PrP^c) of the protein is rich in α helices and is virtually devoid of β-sheet content. The scrapie isoform (PrP^{Sc}) differs physically from PrP^c by its high β-sheet content, insolubility in detergents, propensity to aggregate, and relative resistance to proteolysis (Prusiner & Hsiao, 1994). Infectious prions are composed almost entirely of PrP^{Sc}. PrP^{Sc} interacts with PrP^c to cause its conversion to PrP^{Sc}. The conversion of PrP^c into PrP^{Sc} involves the unfolding of α helices and their refolding into β sheets. Accumulation of pathogenic protein is a critical step in cellular dysfunction (Mastrianni & Roos, 2000).

Sporadic CJD generally presents in the seventh decade or later and has a relatively short course of 4 to 6 months. The disease starts with confusion, forgetfulness, and memory loss that progress to a severe cortical dementia in association with ataxia, myoclonus, and an abnormal EEG. The clinical characteristics of new-variant CJD, associated with exposure to bovine spongiform encephalopathy prions, are psychiatric and sensory symptoms, most often dysesthesias, progressing to dementia and ataxia.

Iatrogenic CJD occurs when a prion disease is transmitted through a surgical procedure, a diagnostic procedure, or human growth hormone or pooled plasma derivatives. The first case of iatrogenic CJD was reported in 1974 in a corneal transplant recipient whose symptoms began 18 months after surgery (Duffy et al., 1974). Shortly thereafter CJD was reported in two patients after they had a stereotactic EEG depth recording. The same electrodes had previously been used in a patient with CJD in an attempt to localize the origin of her myoclonus (Brown et al., 1992). There have been a number of cases of CJD transmitted by cadaveric dura mater grafts and by growth hormone derived from pools of human cadaver pituitary glands (Brown 1988). Recently there has been concern about the risk of CJD from pooled plasma derivatives, specifically from intravenous immunoglobulin.

In addition to CJD and new-variant CJD, there are three other major subtypes of prion diseases: Kuru, Gerstmann-Straussler-Scheinker disease, and fatal insomnia. Kuru was the first recognized prion disease and was confined to the Fore people in the highlands of New Guinea who practiced ritualistic cannibalism (Mastrianni & Roos, 2000). Gerstmann-Straussler-Scheinker disease is characterized by ataxia and dysarthria with dementia developing later (Mastrianni & Roos, 2000). Fatal insomnia begins with weeks of insomnia followed by symptoms of autonomic nervous system dysfunction, ataxia, and dementia.

In sporadic CJD disease, the EEG is very helpful in making the diagnosis. The classic EEG demonstrates periodic or pseudoperiodic paroxysms of triphasic or sharp waves of 0.5 to 2.0 Hz with a slow background. The combination of dementia, myoclonus, and periodic complexes on the EEG has been considered diagnostic for sporadic CJD. New-variant CJD begins with psychiatric symptoms, and the typical EEG periodic complexes of CJD are not seen in patients with new-variant CJD. Neuroimaging is usually normal; however, in less than 10% of cases of sporadic CJD, hyperintensities are seen on T2-weighted images in the basal ganglia (Mastrianni & Roos, 2000). A positive CSF 14-3-3 protein is sensitive but not specific for CJD (Zerr et al., 2000). False-positive CSF 14-3-3 protein results have been reported in patients with cerebral anoxia, stroke, metabolic encephalopathy, multiple myeloma, Alzheimer disease, and herpes simplex encephalitis (Zerr et al., 2000).

LYME DISEASE

Lyme disease is caused by the spirochete *Borrelia burgdorferi*. Infection is acquired by the bite of a tick of the *Ixodes ricinus* complex. The first sign of infection is the characteristic skin lesion, erythema migrans, a centrifugally expanding annular lesion present in 80% of cases. Neurologic abnormalities can occur within the first 3 months of infection and include headache, unilateral or bilateral facial nerve palsy, motor or sensory radiculoneuropathies, and lymphocytic meningitis, or more than a year after infection and present as a subacute encephalopathy affecting memory and concentration associated with fatigue. In these patients, neuropsychological tests will demonstrate evidence of memory impairment, attention, concentration, and problem solving. The diagnosis of Lyme disease is made by serologic tests, consisting of an enzyme-linked immunosorbent assay followed by a Western blot. The limitation of the serologic tests is that they do not distinguish between active and inactive infection. Patients may remain seropositive for years, even after adequate antibiotic treatment (Steere, 2001). Examination of the CSF reveals a lymphocytic pleocytosis, an elevated protein concentration, and anti-*B. burgdorferi* antibodies. The neurocognitive problems improve with antibiotic therapy.

BRAIN ABSCESS

A brain abscess is a focal, suppurative process within the brain parenchyma. A brain abscess may develop by direct spread from a contiguous site of infection, such as paranasal sinusitis, otitis media, or dental infection; as a result of hematogenous dissemination from a remote site of infection, such as the lungs; or following head trauma or a neurosurgical procedure. A brain abscess can be caused by bacteria, fungi, or parasites. The most common symptoms of a brain abscess are headache and a focal neurologic deficit. Fever is present in 50% of patients, and new-onset focal or generalized seizure activity is a presenting sign in 25% to 30% of patients with a bacterial brain abscess. A focal seizure is the most common presenting symptom of neurocysticercosis.

The presenting clinical signs of a brain abscess are determined by the location of the abscess in the brain and the complication of cerebral edema and increased intracranial pressure. Hemiparesis is the most common localizing sign of a frontal lobe abscess, dysphasia of a temporal lobe abscess, and nystagmus and ataxia of a cerebellar abscess. Signs of increased intracranial pressure are papilledema, nausea and vomiting, and an altered level of consciousness.

The diagnosis of a brain abscess is made by cranial MRI or computed tomography (CT) scanning, and the organism is identified by CT-guided stereotactic aspiration. An exception to this rule is brain abscess in an immunosuppressed individual from either HIV infection or solid organ, bone marrow, or stem cell transplantation. In these individuals, *Toxoplasma gondii* may be the etiologic organism of the brain abscess. The characteristic appearance on CT or MRI of a brain abscess or abscesses due to *T. gondii* is a lesion or lesions in the basal ganglia or at the hemispheric gray-white junction that enhance after the administration of contrast. In these patients, if there is detectable anti-*Toxoplasma* IgG in serum, a treatment trial of pyrimethamine and sulfadiazine is initiated. Treatment is also initiated for neurocysticercosis without biopsy when MRI scan demonstrates the classic cystic lesion, the *Taenia solium* scolex, and parenchymal brain calcifications.

Specific antimicrobial therapy and the duration of treatment are determined by the etiologic organisms. Due to the risk of focal or generalized seizures, prophylactic anticonvulsant therapy is recommended. Response to therapy is followed by serial CT or MRI scans on a monthly or bimonthly basis. Most patients have a good prognosis and typically do not have cognitive or behavioral problems. Seizures occur in as many as 70% but can resolve over time so that long-term anticonvulsant therapy is usually not indicated.

FUNGAL MENINGITIS

The most common fungi that cause meningitis are *Cryptococcus neoformans* and *Histoplasma capsulatum*. Fungal meningitis occurs in both immunosuppressed and immunocompetent individuals and is usually the result of hematogenous dissemination from a pulmonary focus. Headache, fever, nausea, and vomiting may be present for weeks before cranial nerve palsies, cognitive dysfunction, and signs of increased intracranial pressure develop. The formation of a purulent exudate in the basilar cisterns obstructs the flow and resorption of CSF. The result is communicating and obstructive hydrocephalus and increased intracranial pressure. A clinical course of subacute meningitis with headache, fever, and cranial nerve palsies that progresses to an altered level of consciousness with pathologically brisk reflexes is typical of fungal meningitis.

The typical neuroimaging abnormality in fungal meningitis is enhancement of the basilar meninges following the administration of contrast and progressive hydrocephalus. Examination of the CSF reveals an increased opening pressure, a lymphocytic pleocytosis, an elevated protein concentration, and a decreased glucose concentration. The cryptococcal polysaccharide antigen test is the most sensitive and specific test for cryptococcal meningitis. The organism may be demonstrated on India ink examination of the CSF and grown in culture. Similarly, *H. capsulatum* may be demonstrated by microscopy and culture of CSF or the *Histoplasma* polysaccharide antigen may be detected in CSF. The studies on CSF to determine infectious causes of cognitive dysfunction are listed in Table 23-2.

Fungal meningitis is treated with a course of amphotericin B or amphotericin B lipid complex (AmBisome) with or without flucytosine. Most patients develop increased intracranial pressure due to altered CSF hemodynamics and require a CSF diversion device, such as a ventriculostomy or ventriculoperitoneal shunt, or serial lumbar punctures. This is followed by oral fluconazole therapy for months to years depending on the immune status of the patient. With aggressive therapy of the infection and the increased intracranial pressure, patients make a good recovery, but many are left with cranial nerve palsies and a spastic gait.

TABLE 23-2. Diagnostic Studies for Infectious Causes of Cognitive Dysfunction

---

Cell count with differential

Glucose and protein concentration

Gram stain and bacterial culture

India ink and fungal culture

Cryptococcal polysaccharide antigen

Histoplasma polysaccharide antigen

PCR for HIV RNA and CMV DNA

VDRL

FTA-ABS

Anti-*B. burgdorferi* antibodies

ENCEPHALOPATHY: THAT WHICH IS REAL AND THAT WHICH IS IMAGINED

Elderly patients with seemingly clinically mild urinary tract infections can have cognitive difficulty that takes weeks to resolve after treatment of the infection. This is real. Chronic fatigue associated with difficulty with concentration and memory has been attributed to chronic Epstein-Barr virus (EBV) infection of the CNS. This is not real. EBV can reactivate in the CNS and, when it does, causes one of four well-defined clinical syndromes: (1) aseptic meningitis, (2) encephalomyelitis, (3) primary CNS lymphoma, and (4) lymphoproliferative disease. Headache is the predominant symptom of aseptic meningitis due to EBV. This will resolve over weeks to months. EBV encephalomyelitis presents with an altered level of consciousness, multifocal neurologic deficits, or new-onset seizure activity. EBV DNA can be detected in CSF by PCR. EBV DNA found in peripheral blood mononuclear cells can contaminate spinal fluid during a bloody tap giving a false-positive result. Primary CNS lymphoma is one of the most common CNS malignancies in HIV-infected individuals. Neuroimaging demonstrates multiple enhancing lesions surrounded by edema. EBV lymphoproliferative disease occurs in immunosuppressed patients due to reactivation of latent virus with a subsequent monoclonal B-cell proliferation.

Patients who have the perception that they are having memory trouble due to a chronic CNS viral infection are sometimes only reassured by a thorough work-up including serologies and CSF analysis. Clinicians are advised not to send PCR on CSF for human herpesvirus 6 (HHV-6) DNA or HSV DNA (when the laboratory does not use primers to distinguish HSV-1 from HSV-2) in the evaluation of difficulty with memory and concentration in immunocompetent patients. Individuals with latent HSV-2 infections from genital herpes can have a positive CSF PCR for HSV DNA. HHV-6 is the causative agent of the common childhood infection, sixth disease. The majority of the population is exposed to HHV-6 in infancy, and most adults are seropositive. The virus invades the brain during primary infection, establishes latency, and can reactivate in the setting of immunosuppression to cause encephalitis. It does not cause chronic fatigue and trouble with memory. CSF PCR for HHV-6 can be positive in otherwise healthy latently infected individuals.

A 69-year-old right-handed gentleman presents with a 1-week history of hemicranial headache and word-finding difficulty. His family complains he has been intermittently confused. On examination, he is febrile, has word-finding difficulty, and has poor short-term memory. Facial strength and sensation is symmetrical. There is no meningismus. Appendicular strength is symmetrical. Deep tendon reflexes are symmetrical. There is an equivocal right Babinski sign. Gait and stance are normal.

The presence of fever, headache, and focal neurologic deficits (dysphasia and impaired short-term memory) warrants immediate empirical therapy for HSV-1 encephalitis and bacterial meningoencephalitis before a diagnostic evaluation is begun. Blood cultures are obtained as treatment is begun with a third- or fourth-generation cephalosporin plus vancomycin and acyclovir. During tick season, doxycycline is added to the empirical regimen to treat for tick-borne bacterial diseases.

Given the presence of fever and focal neurologic deficits on examination, neuroimaging should be done prior to lumbar puncture. MRI scan is preferred over CT scan because MRI is much more sensitive for HSV encephalitis than is CT. The characteristic abnormality on MRI scan of HSV-1 encephalitis is a high signal intensity lesion on T2-weighted images in the medial and inferior temporal lobe extending up into the insula (Fig. 23-1).

Examination of the CSF reveals an increased opening pressure, a lymphocytic pleocytosis of 5 to 500 cells/mm^3, a mild to moderate elevation of the protein concentration, and a normal or mildly decreased glucose concentration. CSF is also sent for PCR assay to detect HSV-1 DNA. CSF PCR for HSV DNA is most likely to be positive within the first 24 to 48 hours of infection but may become falsely negative 10 to 14 days or more after the onset of infection. CSF and serum samples should be obtained to determine if there is intrathecal synthesis of antibodies against HSV. Antibodies against HSV appear in the CSF 8 to 12 days after the onset of disease and may remain for as long as 3 months. There is a classic EEG abnormality in HSV encephalitis consisting of periodic, stereotyped, sharp-and-slow wave complexes that occur at regular intervals of 2 to 3 seconds and are expressed maximally over the involved temporal lobe. As the infection progresses, patients develop focal seizures that may become secondarily generalized.

HSV encephalitis is treated with 3 weeks of intravenous acyclovir 10 mg/kg every 8 hours. There are ongoing clinical trials to determine if a several-week course of oral valacyclovir following a 3-week course of intravenous acyclovir is beneficial in preventing recurrence and improving outcome. The severity of the neurologic sequelae is related to the level of consciousness at the time when treatment is initiated. Neurologic sequelae include word-finding difficulty, impaired short-term memory, behavioral problems, and seizure disorder.

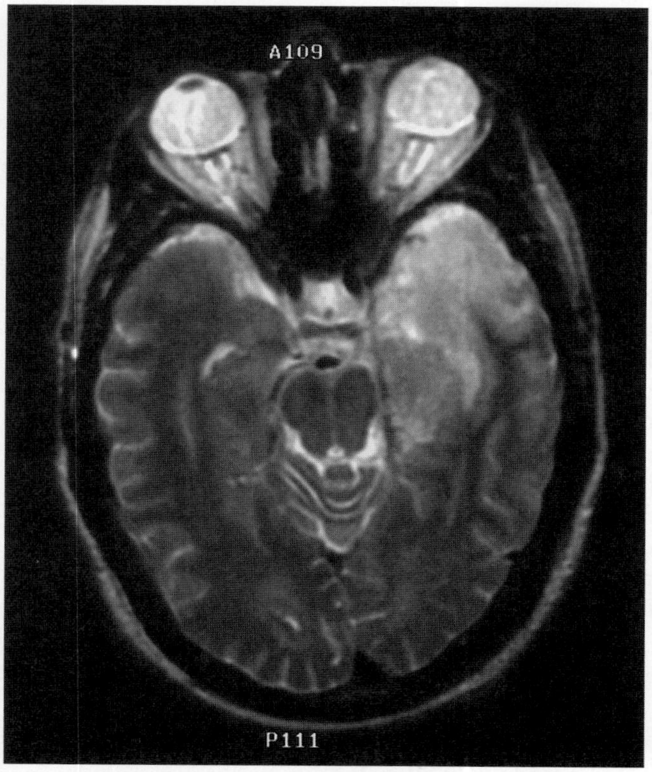

FIGURE 23-1. MRI scan demonstrates the classic lesion of HSV-1 encephalitis.

■ KEY POINTS

☐   The principal abnormalities of cognitive function in adult patients months after acute bacterial meningitis are decreased speed of cognitive and psychomotor performance, decreased visual memory, reduced concentration, diminished nonverbal and logical memory, and impaired associative learning.

☐   The primary neurocognitive deficits in patients who survive HSV encephalitis are verbal paraphasias, word-finding difficulty, and dysnomia.

☐   HIV-associated dementia is a subcortical dementia characterized by memory loss selective for impaired retrieval, impaired manipulation of acquired language, and a general slowing of psychomotor speed and thought processes. Attention, calculations, and language are usually not initially affected in HIV-associated dementia.

☐   The classic clinical triad of CJD is dementia, myoclonus, and ataxia.

KEY READINGS

Mastrianni JA, Roos RP: The prion diseases. Semin Neurol 20:337–352, 2000.

Mathisen GE, Johnson JP: Brain abscess. Clin Infect Dis 25:763–781, 1997.

Roos KL: Encephalitis. Neurol Clin 17:813–834, 1999.

REFERENCES

Aurelius E, Johansson B, Skoldenberg B, et al: Rapid diagnosis of herpes simplex encephalitis by nested polymerase chain reaction assay of cerebrospinal fluid. Lancet 337:189–192, 1991.

Baraff LJ, Lee SI, Schriger DL: Outcomes of bacterial meningitis in children: A meta-analysis. Pediatr Infect Dis J 12:389–394, 1993.

Barnett EM, Jacobsen G, Evans G, et al: Herpes simplex encephalitis in the temporal cortex and limbic system after trigeminal nerve inoculation. J Infect Dis 169:782–786, 1994.

Brown P: The clinical neurology and epidemiology of Creutzfeldt-Jakob disease, with special reference to iatrogenic cases: Novel infectious agents and the central nervous system. Ciba Found Symp 135:3–23, 1988.

Brown P, Pierce MA, Will RG: "Friendly fire" in medicine: Hormones, homografts, and Creutzfeldt-Jakob disease. Lancet 340:24–27, 1992.

Centers for Disease Control and Prevention: Arboviral disease—United States, 1994. Morb Mortal Wkly Rep 44:641–644, 1995.

Davis LE, Sperry S: The CSF-FTA test and the significance of blood contamination. Ann Neurol 6:68–69, 1979.

Duffy P, Wolf J, Collins G, et al: Possible person-to-person transmission of Creutzfeldt-Jakob disease. N Engl J Med 290:692–693, 1974.

Feemster RF: Equine encephalitis in Massachusetts. N Engl J Med 257:701–704, 1957.

Grimwood K, Anderson VA, Bond L, et al: Adverse outcomes of bacterial meningitis in school-age survivors. Pediatrics 95:646–656, 1995.

Hennessy MJ, Koutroumanidis M, Dean AF, et al: Chronic encephalitis and temporal lobe epilepsy—a variant of Rasmussen's syndrome? Neurology 56:678–681, 2001.

Johnson RA, White M: Syphilis in the 1990s: Cutaneous and neurologic manifestations. Semin Neurol 12:287–298, 1992.

Kaaresen PI, Flaegstad T: Prognostic factors in childhood bacterial meningitis. Acta Paediatr 84:873–878, 1995.

Kabani A, Jadavji T: Sequelae of acute bacterial meningitis in children, in Schonfeld H, Helwig H (eds): Bacterial Meningitis: Antibiotic Chemotherapy. Basel, Switzerland: Karger, 1992, Vol. 45, pp. 209–217.

Kornelisse RF, Westerbeek CML, Spoor AB, et al: Pneumococcal meningitis in children: Prognostic indicators and outcome. Clin Infect Dis 21:1390–1397, 1995.

Lawton AH, Seaburg C, Branch LC, et al: Follow-up studies of St. Louis encephalitis in Florida: Comparison of 1964 and 1965 health question findings. South Med J 59:1409–1414, 1966.

Mastrianni JA, Roos RP: The prion diseases. Semin Neurol 20:337–352, 2000.

McArthur JC, Sacktor N, Selnes O: Human immunodeficiency virus-associated dementia. Semin Neurol 19:129–150, 1999.

McJunkin JE, de los Reyes EC, Irazuzta JE, et al: La Crosse encephalitis in children. N Engl J Med 344:801–807, 2001.

McJunkin JE, Khan RR, Tsai TF: California-La Crosse encephalitis. Infect Dis Clin North Am 12:83–93, 1998.

Merkelbach S, Sittinger H, Schweizer I, et al: Cognitive outcome after bacterial meningitis. Acta Neurol Scand 102:118–123, 2000.

Pfister HW, Borasio GD, Dirnagl U, et al: Cerebrovascular complications of bacterial meningitis in adults. Neurology 42:1497–1504, 1992.

Prusiner SB, Hsiao KK: Human prion diseases. Ann Neurol 35:385–395, 1994.

Rasmussen T, Andermann F: Rasmussen's syndrome: Symptomatology of the syndrome of chronic encephalitis and seizures: 35-year experience with 51 cases, in Luders H (ed): Epilepsy Surgery. New York: Raven Press, 1991, pp. 173–182.

Roos KL: Syphilitic meningitis, in Roos KL (ed): Meningitis: 100 Maxims in Neurology. London: Oxford, 1996, pp. 171–181.

Singer C, Lang AE, Suchowersky O: Adult-onset subacute sclerosing panencephalitis: Case reports and review of the literature. Move Disord 12:342–353, 1997.

Steere AC: Lyme borreliosis, in Braunwald E, Fauci AS, Kasper DL, et al (eds): Harrison's Principles of Internal Medicine, ed 15. New York: McGraw-Hill, 2001, pp. 1061–1065.

Whitley RJ, Kimberlin DW, Roizman B: Herpes simplex viruses. Clin Infect Dis 26:541–555, 1998.

Zerr I, Pocchiari M, Collins S, et al: Analysis of EEG and CSF 14-3-3 proteins as aids to the diagnosis of Creutzfeldt-Jakob disease. Neurology 55:811–815, 2000.

Basal Ganglia and Movement Disorders

Jane S. Paulsen

Carissa Nehl

Mark Guttman

Basal ganglia circuitry
Cognition
Huntington disease
Neuropsychiatry
Neuropsychology
Parkinson disease
Progressive supranuclear palsy
Tourette syndrome

INTRODUCTION

It has been known for some time that basal ganglia pathology is associated with cognitive and behavioral deficits, yet tradition has emphasized motor abnormali-ties. A reappraisal of nonmotor aspects of movement disorders has been prompted by observations of cognitive and mood disorders associated with the basal ganglia as well as significant advances in neuroanatomy resulting in the refined description of cortico-striatal-pallidal-thalamic brain circuits (Middleton & Strick, 2001). The disorders described in this chapter are considered subcortical, by definition, although the cognitive and psychiatric characteristics of each movement disorder vary. For example, Huntington disease is virtually always associated with cognitive impairment, which occurs early in the course of the disease and eventually develops into dementia. Parkinson disease is also associated with cognitive dysfunction, yet progression of the disease coincides with the development of dementia in only a subset of persons. In contrast, Tourette syndrome is rarely associated with dementia and in most cases, cognitive decline is difficult to substantiate. This chapter provides an overview of basal ganglia circuitry and its relevance to cognition and behavior in movement disorders.

RATIONALE FOR COGNITIVE AND BEHAVIORAL CHANGES IN MOVEMENT DISORDERS OF THE BASAL GANGLIA

A series of discrete, parallel circuits have been described that link regions of the frontal lobes to subcortical structures in functional systems (Alexander et al., 1986). The earliest models of basal ganglia function emphasized motor abnormalities and addressed the differential circuit alterations leading to hypokinetic movement disorders (e.g., Parkinson disease [PD]) and hyperkinetic movement disorders (e.g., Huntington disease [HD]). These "classic" motor models predicted two circuits through the basal ganglia: (1) a "direct" reinforcing cortico-striatal-medial pallidal-thalamo-cortical circuit and (2) an "indirect" suppressing cortico-striatal-lateral pallidal-subthalamo-medial pallidal-thalamo-cortico circuit. Dopamine was excitatory on the former (via dopamine D1 receptors) and inhibitory (via dopamine D2 receptors) on the latter. Overall, the direct pathway facilitates the flow of information, whereas the indirect pathway inhibits it. Hypokinetic movement disorders are believed to result from a relative preponderance of activity of the indirect pathway, leading to an increase of the normal inhibitory basal ganglia output to the thalamus. Conversely, hyperkinetic disorders are thought to reflect a shift of the balance toward the direct pathway, leading to reduced inhibitory basal ganglia output and increased thalamocortical activation (Young & Penney, 1998).

Several efforts to link functional domains with distinct basal ganglia architecture have been developed. Stahl (1988) proposed that the basal ganglia be divided into a neurologist's, a psychologist's, and a psychiatrist's portion responsible for motor, cognitive, and emotional disorders, respectively. In this schema, the neurologist's circuit is the putamen-based motor circuits (i.e., yellow in bottom of Fig. 24-1), the psychologist's emphasis is on the caudate-dorsolateral prefrontal circuit (i.e., blue in bottom of Fig. 24-1), and the psychiatrist's pathway is the ventral striatopallidal system (i.e., red in bottom of Fig. 24-1), especially the nucleus accumbens. In a somewhat similar vein, McHugh (1989) suggested a triadic syndrome in basal ganglia disorders with distinct impairments in the motor-sensory (dyskinesia), cognitive (dementia), and affective (depression) domains. Cummings (1993) reviewed neurobehavioral literature and described three syndromes corresponding to three prefrontal-subcortical circuits. The dorsolateral (i.e., blue in bottom of Fig. 24-1) prefrontal syndrome was characterized primarily by executive function deficits and motor programming abnormalities. The orbitofrontal (i.e., green in bottom of Fig. 24-1) syndrome featured personality changes with irritability, lability, euphoria, and disinhibition. The anterior cingulate (i.e., red in bottom of Fig. 24-1) syndrome was comprised of patients with apathy and akinesia. Another perspective of this circuitry is shown in Figure 24-2. Although such models may be heuristic in developing function-structure hypotheses, it is unlikely that any current model is sufficient to explain the complex interface of behavior and the basal ganglia.

Recent work involving physiologic recording in awake trained primates (Fuster, 1997) and functional imaging studies in humans (Jueptner et al., 1997) suggest that individual output channels are involved in different functions, which resemble those of the cortical area they innervate. At least 11 so-called nonmotor circuits have been recently described (Middleton & Strick, 2001), although distinct cognitive and behavioral correlates of these circuits have not yet been established. Research involving both animal and human subjects has revealed specific cognitive performances that are distinctly associated with specific frontal striatal brain circuitry (Fig. 24-3).

HYPOKINETIC DISORDERS

Parkinson Disease

Demographic and Clinical Characteristics

Parkinson disease (PD) is a movement disorder that is characterized by the presence of a pill-rolling resting tremor, rigidity, and bradykinesia (slowed voluntary motor movements). Having a good response to levodopa often confirms the PD diagnosis, although approximately 20% of cases diagnosed as PD are incorrectly diagnosed (Adler, 1999). In addition to motor symptoms, PD is associated with increased levels of depression and other emotional disturbances as well as cognitive impairments. The mean age of PD onset is 60 years of age. Incidence of PD rises with increasing age from 4.1/100,000 between ages 30 and 54 to 209/100,000 between ages 75 and 84. It is estimated that approximately one million individuals are currently suffering from PD in the United States. Although family history remains the strongest risk factor for the disease (Maher et al., 2002), epidemiologic studies have reported increased risk for PD associated with farming, rural living, drinking well water, pesticide exposure, head trauma, and pollutants. To date, specific mutations have been identified in three separate genes (a-synuclein, Parkin, UCH-L1) and four additional loci have been linked to inherited PD (for a review, see Mouradian, 2002). Clinical ratings based on the level of clinical disability have become the standard method of measuring PD-related functioning. The Unified Parkinson's Disease Rating Scale (Fahn et al., 1987) is the most widely used scale today and incorporates the Hoehn-Yahr clinical disability stages as well as the Schwab and England activities of daily living into scores

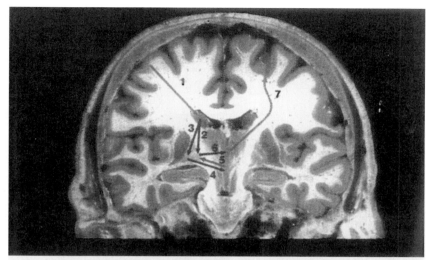

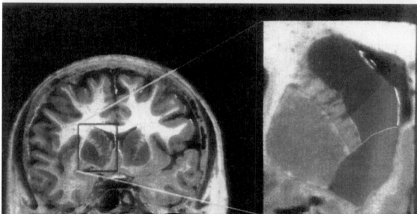

FIGURE 24-1. Frontal-striatal projections. Brain sections illustrating the frontal-subcortical circuits. Top, The direct and indirect circuits (red arrows indicate excitatory connections and blue arrows indicate inhibitory connections). (1) Excitatory glutamatergic corticostriatal fibers. (2) Direct inhibitory g-aminobutyric acid (GABA)/substance P fibers (associated with D1 dopamine receptors) from the striatum to the globus pallidus interna/substantia nigra pars reticulata. (3) Indirect inhibitory GABA/enkephalin fibers (associated with D2 dopamine receptors) from the striatum to the globus pallidus externa. (4) Indirect inhibitory GABA fibers from the globus pallidus externa to the subthalamic nucleus. (5) Indirect excitatory glutamatergic fibers from the subthalamic nucleus to the globus pallidus interna/substantia nigra pars reticulata. (6) Basal ganglia inhibitory outflow via GABA fibers from the globus pallidus interna/substantia nigra pars reticulata to specific thalamic sites. (7) Thalamic excitatory fibers returning to the cortex (shown in the contralateral hemisphere for convenience). Bottom, The general segregated anatomy of the oculomotor (purple), dorsolateral prefrontal (blue), orbitofrontal (green), anterior cingulated (red), and motor (yellow) circuits in the striatum. (From Litvan I, Paulsen JS, Mega MS, et al: Neuropsychiatric assessment of patients with hyperkinetic and hypokinetic movement disorders. Arch Neurol 55:1313–1319, 1998. Copyright 1998 by the American Medical Association. Reprinted by permission.) (See Color Plate 9)

that are used to assess treatments and measure disease stages.

Pathology

PD is associated with significant loss of pigmented cells in the substantia nigra with additional loss of pigmented cells in the locus ceruleus, raphe, and the dorsal motor nucleus of the vagus. The loss of these cells results in a significant deficit of the neurotransmitter dopamine. The gold standard for neuropathologic diagnosis of PD is the presence of Lewy bodies in the substantia nigra with loss of dopaminergic neurons.

Although the Parkinson Study Group recently used in vivo single photon emission computed tomography (SPECT) imaging with the dopamine transporter to successfully identify parkinsonian patients (Parkinson Study Group, 2000), no biomarker for PD currently exists. The absence of a specific biologic marker for PD limits our ability to answer the critical question of whether PD is a single, clinical pathologic disease or a syndrome with diverse etiologies.

Cognition

Claims about the status of cognition in PD have ranged from intact functions to pervasive impairments. Disparate views emerged before the cognitive heterogeneity of PD was appreciated. At present, cognitive performances are known to vary in concert with other disease factors such as onset age, symptom severity, motor pattern, depression comorbidity, and medication treatment. Although cognitive impairment is the rule

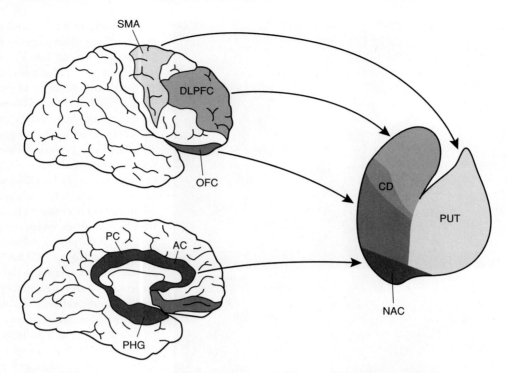

FIGURE 24-2. Frontal-striatal projections. AC, anterior cingulate gyrus; CD, caudate nucleus; DLPFC, dorsal lateral prefrontal cortex; PUT, putamen; NAC, nucleus accumbens; OFC, orbital frontal cortex; PC, posterior cingulate gyrus; PHG, parahippocampal gyrus; SMA, supplementary motor area. (From Brody AL, Saxena S: Brain imaging in obsessive-compulsive disorder: Evidence for the involvement of frontal-subcortical circuitry in the mediation of symptomatology. CNS Spectrums 1:27–41, 1996. Copyright 1996 by MBL Communications. Reprinted by permission.)

rather than the exception in PD, there is heterogeneity in presentation and progression of cognitive deficits. The neuropsychological profile of PD includes cognitive slowing, memory impairment, visuospatial deficits (e.g., problems with pattern completion and facial recognition), and a range of executive deficits including impairments in decision making, planning, shifting, and monitoring of goal-directed behaviors (Robbins et al.,

1994). Nearly all individuals with PD suffer from a general cognitive slowing, or bradyphrenia, although measures of psychomotor speed are correlated with rigidity and hypokinesia measures making it difficult to interpret whether the cause of the slower performance is due to cognitive or motor speed. Most studies now attempt to control for reduced speed and continue to report cognitive impairments (Robbins et al., 1994).

FIGURE 24-3. Basal ganglia circuitry. GPi, globus pallidus interna; SNpr, substantia nigra pars reticulata; VApc, nucleus ventralis anterior, parvocellular portion; VAmc, nucleus ventralis anterior, magnocellular division. (From Middleton FA, Strick PL: Basal ganglia output and cognition: Evidence from anatomical, behavioral, and clinical studies. Brain Cogn 42:188, 2000. Copyright 2000 by Academic Press. Reprinted by permission.)

	Cognitive			Sensory
Function	Planning, working memory	Spatial working memory	Object working memory	Visual recognition, discrimination
Cortical area	9	46	12	TE
Thalamic nuclei	VApc VAmc	VApc MDmf	VAmc MDmf	VAmc
Output nucleus	GPi SNpr	GPi SNpr	SNpr	SNpr

In addition to slowed processing, however, evidence indicates that patients with PD experience problems in pattern completion, facial recognition, and map reading. Although individuals with PD traditionally show decreased performance on the nonverbal subtests of the Wechsler Adult Intelligence Scales, nonstandard administration of tests and hypothesis-testing neuropsychological techniques can be used to better determine whether deficits are due to speed or other cognitive impairments. For instance, increased time can be allowed to better determine whether items can be completed when the time limitation is removed. Analyses of error types can also be helpful to evaluate problem-solving strategies and to illuminate perceptual and planning deficits.

Several studies suggest that changes in executive functioning may be one of the earliest signs of cognitive decline in PD. Individuals with PD often report problems with decision making, planning, and monitoring of goal-directed behaviors. Using traditional and computerized neuropsychological tests, even nondemented individuals with PD show impaired ability to shift between sets (Robbins et al., 1994).

Up to 80% of individuals with PD experience speech problems beyond production problems related to motor symptoms. Individuals experience problems comprehending and producing syntactically complex sentences. Unlike cognitive changes associated with Alzheimer disease (AD), individuals with PD do not generally experience problems with name finding.

Memory problems are also commonly reported among individuals with PD. In particular, individuals report difficulty in the recall of effortful information, but exhibit intact recognition (Appollonio et al., 1994). Several studies have demonstrated that learning and retrieval deficits exist in PD patients without frank dementia (e.g., Robbins et al., 1994).

Dementia

Dementia occurs in up to 25% of individuals with PD (Mayeux et al., 1990). A number of factors have been implicated as risk factors for dementia in PD, including older age, lower education, and the presence of depression and confusion or psychosis following levodopa treatment (Caparros-Lefebvre et al., 1995). The E4 allele of apolipoprotein E, a known risk factor for AD, is not a risk factor for dementia in PD. The impact of depression on cognitive decline has been studied the most, with increasing evidence that depression is associated with greater cognitive decline and exaggeration of decline in activities of daily living (Starkstein et al., 1992). Data in Figure 24-4 show that PD patients with depression show a faster progression along the stages of the illness defined on the Hoehn and Yahr scale (Hoehn & Yahr, 1967). These data suggest that PD patients who develop demen-

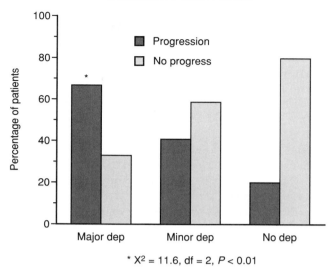

PROGRESSION TO THE NEXT HOEHN AND YAHR STAGE IN A 1-YEAR PERIOD

* $X^2 = 11.6$, df = 2, $P < 0.01$

FIGURE 24-4. Faster progression of PD in patients with major depression (dep). (From Starkstein SE, Mayberg HS: Depression in Parkinson disease, in Starkstein SE, Robinson RG (eds): Depression in Neurologic Disease. Baltimore, MD: Johns Hopkins University Press, 1993, pp. 97–116. Copyright 1993 by The Johns Hopkins University Press. Reprinted by permission.)

tia may have additional pathology and more diffuse impairment of their neurotransmitter systems, whereas all PD patients have dysfunction of frontal-striatal circuitry resulting in mild cognitive impairments.

Medication Effects on Cognitive Function

There is a lack of consensus regarding the effect of pharmacologic treatment on cognition in PD. Levodopa treatment has been shown to improve performance in delayed verbal memory, choice reaction time, and attention, as well as interfere with tasks associated with frontal lobe function. Gotham and colleagues (1988) assessed cognitive function in PD patients either "on" or "off" levodopa therapy and found a variable pattern of results. Patients were impaired in verbal fluency while off levodopa and impaired in associative learning while on levodopa. Cooper and colleagues (1992) reported that anticholinergic medication impaired short-term memory, whereas dopaminergic therapy improved working memory performance. When levodopa treatment was temporarily withdrawn from PD patients, performances in planning and problem solving worsened above and beyond that expected by motor disability. In summary, it is clear that for some PD patients, the typical "gold standard" treatment (i.e., levodopa therapy) may exert a highly selective and deleterious effect on cognitive function. This is particularly salient given that the cognitive decline observed in PD remains a major source of disability and mortality in PD.

Neuropsychiatric Aspects

Neuropsychiatric deficits are commonly associated with PD. Aarsland and colleagues (1999) report that 38% of individuals with PD suffer from depression, 27% experience hallucinations, 20% experience anxiety, 16.5% become agitated, and 16.5% become apathetic. Depression is the most frequent psychiatric disturbance in persons with PD (Starkstein et al., 1990). Cross-sectional studies have demonstrated that approximately 20% of patients have major and another 20% minor depression. Longitudinal studies show that more than 50% of PD patients will develop depression at some point in the disease, and several studies suggest that the frequency of depression is greater than expected when compared with other diseases producing physical limi-

tations. As a result, it is well accepted that the high prevalence of depression in PD is likely a component of the disease process due to biochemical changes in the brain. Mayberg and Solomon (1995) proposed a model for the pathophysiology of depression in PD whereby degeneration of dopaminergic neurons causes dysfunction of orbitofrontal cortex, which secondarily affects serotonergic connections of the dorsal raphae nucleus. This model of depression is illustrated in Figure 24-5. Paralimbic hypometabolism appears to be common to patients with primary and secondary depression. Positron emission tomography (PET) studies using ^{18}F-fluoro-2-deoxyglucose (FDG) in patients with secondary depression demonstrate bilateral ventral frontal, anterior temporal, and anterior cingulate hypometabolism that characterizes the depressive syndrome independent of the underlying disease etiology.

One of the most important issues in the study of PD is the reliability with which depression can be

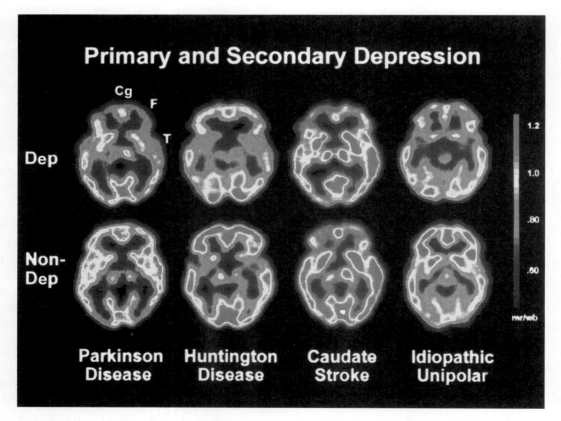

FIGURE 24-5. Depression in movement disorders. Paralimbic hypometabolism common to patients with primary and secondary depression. ^{18}F-fluoro-2-deoxyglucose (FDG) positron emission tomography (PET) studies of patients with secondary depression identify the bilateral ventral frontal (F), anterior temporal (T), and anterior cingulated (Cg) hypometabolism that characterizes the depressive syndrome, independently of underlying disease etiology. Images are individual patients. (From Mayberg HS: Depression and frontal-subcortical circuits: Focus on prefrontal-limbic interactions, in Lechter DG, Cummings JL (eds): Frontal-Subcortical Circuits in Psychiatric and Neurological Disorders. New York: Guilford Press, 2001, pp. 177–206. Copyright 2001 by The Guilford Press. Reprinted by permission.) (See Color Plate 10)

diagnosed. Difficulties in concentration, slowness in movement, and low energy may be frequent features of both PD and depression. To improve the specificity of depressive symptoms in PD, Starkstein and colleagues (1990) assessed the frequency of symptoms in PD patients both with and without depressed mood. The Diagnostic and Statistical Manual (DSM) of Psychiatric Disorders (American Psychiatric Association, 1994) criteria for depression (including early morning awakening, anergia, and motor retardation) were not related to the severity of the illness in PD. The presence of at least three affective and three autonomic symptoms of depression had a sensitivity of 96% and a specificity of 100% in PD. Findings indicated that modified DSM criteria were most appropriate for the determination of major and minor depression in PD (Table 24-1). Affective symptoms are similarly frequent throughout the disease, whereas autonomic symptoms are observed more typically in later stages of PD.

The duration of depression is longer than 1 year in the majority of PD patients with major depression, but the course is shorter for patients identified with only minor depression. Starkstein and colleagues (1990) suggested that PD patients with minor depression could not be separated from normal comparison subjects, whereas PD patients with major depression had impaired cognitive functioning and more rapid disease progression. Given the association between depression severity and course it is critical to identify and aggressively treat minor depression in PD. Nearly 20% of PD patients

without depression will develop depression within a year, and depression onset can predate the onset of motor symptoms in a subset of PD patients. Risk factors for depression in PD have included greater cognitive impairment, presence of a thought disorder, and earlier disease onset (Tandberg et al., 1997). Findings indicate that rapid identification and early treatment of depression in PD is critical and might lessen the duration and severity of the illness. Depression in PD is currently undertreated; a large survey of more than 20,000 patients with PD revealed that only 26% were receiving pharmacotherapy for depression (Richard & Kurlan, 1997). A recent review by Cummings and Masterman (1999) reported only four controlled clinical trials of antidepressant therapy in PD. Selective serotonin reuptake inhibitors (SSRIs) are considered first-line therapy for depression in PD patients despite case reports that SSRIs can worsen motor symptoms. Double-blind prospective studies are needed to evaluate the safety and efficacy of antidepressants in PD.

Treatment

The current mainstay of PD therapy is levodopa, a precursor to dopamine that readily crosses the blood-brain barrier and is converted into dopamine. Levodopa is typically administered in conjunction with the dopa-decarboxylase inhibitor carbidopa to minimize peripheral side effects. Direct-acting dopamine agonists stimulate dopamine receptors without requiring conversion to

TABLE 24-1. Criteria for Major Depression and Dysthymia

Major depression	*Dysthymia ("minor depression")*
• Depressed mood for most of the day, nearly every day and/or	• Depressed mood for most of the day, nearly every day
• Diminished interest or pleasure in all or almost all activities most of the day, nearly every day	
Presence of at least four of the following symptoms:	Presence of at least two of the following symptoms:
• Significant weight loss without dieting, or weight gain, or decrease or increase of appetite	• Poor appetite or overeating
• Insomnia or hypersomnia	• Insomnia or hypersomnia
• Psychomotor agitation or retardation, nearly every day	
• Fatigue or loss of energy, nearly every day	• Low energy or fatigue
• Feelings of worthlessness or excessive or inappropriate guilt, nearly every day	• Low self-esteem
• Diminished ability to think or concentrate, or indecisiveness, nearly every day	• Poor concentration or difficulty making decisions
• Recurrent thoughts of death, recurrent suicidal ideation without a specific plan, or a specific plan for committing suicide, or a suicide attempt	• Feelings of hopelessness

Copyright 1997 by the American Psychiatric Association. Reprinted by permission.

active drugs. Many agents are available including bromocriptine, pergolide, pramipexole, and ropinirole. A number of agents may affect the metabolism of levodopa to improve its therapeutic efficacy. Selegiline is a monoamine oxidase (MAO) inhibitor that reduces the metabolism of dopamine. Entacapone and tolcapone are catechol-O-methyltransferase (COMT) inhibitors that reduce levodopa metabolism in the periphery to increase the bioavailability to the brain. Amantadine acts by releasing dopamine into the synaptic cleft and inhibiting acetylcholine receptors. There are many anticholinergic agents including trihexyphenidyl and benztropine mesylate (Cogentin) that are used to treat PD. For an extensive review, see the article by Lang and Lozano (1998). The American Academy of Neurology recently published practice guidelines on the medical treatment of PD. Conclusions are as follows: "1) Selegiline has very mild symptomatic benefit (level A, class II evidence) with no evidence for neuroprotective benefit (level U, class II evidence). 2) For PD patients requiring initiation of symptomatic therapy, either levodopa or a DA [Dopamine agonist] can be used (level A, class I and class II evidence). Levodopa provides superior motor benefit but is associated with a higher risk of dyskinesia. 3) No evidence was found that initiating treatment with sustained-release levodopa provides an advantage over immediate-release levodopa (level B, class II evidence)" (Miyasaki et al., 2002).

Most individuals with PD show significant improvement in neurologic symptoms following the use of levodopa. With time, however, some patients may develop dyskinesias when taking levodopa, whereas rigidity, bradykinesia, and tremors occur when patients stop taking levodopa. The addition of other drugs including dopamine agonists, COMT inhibitors, MAO inhibitors, or amantadine is often successful in reducing these response fluctuations (see review article by Guttman et al., 2003). Many patients experience abrupt changes in mobility described as "on-off" phenomena. It has been estimated that up to 50% of individuals experience fluctuations after use of levodopa for 5 years. Individuals in the "off" stage exhibit severe parkinsonian symptoms, whereas in the "on" stage individuals experience increased mobility and involuntary movements. As these differences initially occur, patients experience a "wearing off" effect of L-dopa, which progresses to rapid and unpredictable changes between "on" and "off." Treatment of this phenomenon remains difficult with the use of dopamine agonists the most frequently used treatment.

If medical treatment fails, patients may benefit from a number of surgical techniques. Pallidotomy (surgical lesioning of the globus pallidus) was initially performed in the 1960s and was the first procedure to gain acceptance for the treatment of PD in the 1990s. This procedure may provide relief of motor symptoms (Rettig et al., 2000) and improves ability to perform activities of daily living. Although a few studies have reported no cognitive decline following pallidotomy, others report transient impairments resolving within 3 months, and some have found consistent cognitive impairments 1 year following surgery (verbal fluency and vocabulary; Junque et al., 1999). Variables associated with poorer cognitive outcome following pallidotomy include later Hoehn and Yahr stages (greater disability), later disease onset, bilateral (versus unilateral) procedures, and the presence of other neurologic complications, such as infarction (Rettig et al., 2000). In general, factors found to improve following pallidotomy include mood, obsessive-compulsive symptoms, and quality of life (Junque et al., 1999; Lombardi et al., 2000).

Most surgical centers have shifted from pallidotomy to deep brain stimulation (DBS) of the subthalamic nucleus or globus pallidum (Eskandar et al., 2001) with improved efficacy and lower risk of complications. To date, it does not appear that DBS of the subthalamic nucleus is associated with significant cognitive decline. Mild impairments in verbal fluency, verbal memory, visuospatial ability, and executive functioning have been noted (Alegret et al., 2001), although cognitive decline following DBS is more likely to occur in elderly patients (Saint-Cyr et al., 2000).

Dementia with Lewy Bodies

Demographic and Clinical Characteristics

Disorders associated with the presence of Lewy bodies in areas of the brain outside of the substantia nigra have been identified for over 30 years, although the designation "Dementia with Lewy Bodies" (DLB) was only recently accepted as a descriptive and all-encompassing label (McKeith et al., 1996). With the growing realization that the various forms of DLB are most likely the second leading cause of dementia after AD, considerable research on the disorder has been carried out over the past 10 years. Although debate regarding distinction between disorders remains, the clinical presentation of DLB includes spontaneous motor features of parkinsonism, recurrent and well-formed visual hallucinations, and fluctuating cognition with pronounced variations in attention or alertness. Probable DLB is diagnosed if two of these features are present and possible DLB if only one is present.

Differential diagnosis of DLB from other disorders is becoming clearer. Patients with DLB have disproportionately severe deficits relative to patients with AD in visuospatial, executive, and attentional functions. Rate of progression is most rapid in DLB, followed by AD, and finally, PD. Order of symptom presentation may be helpful in diagnosis. Parkinsonism typically precedes the onset of dementia in PD, whereas the cognitive decline in DLB typically precedes or co-occurs with the onset of parkinsonism (Litvan et al., 1998b). Patients with DLB are more likely to experience hallucinations, lack a balance disorder at onset (Litvan et al., 1998b), be older at onset of disease, and have a shorter disease duration than persons with PD.

Progressive Supranuclear Palsy

Demographic and Clinical Characteristics

Progressive supranuclear palsy (PSP), also called Steele-Richardson-Olszewski syndrome, is the most common misdiagnosis for PD (Adler, 1999). Individuals with PSP experience bradykinesia, postural instability, rigidity (most notably in the neck and trunk), and visual disturbances due to vertical gaze paresis. PSP patients experience less resting tremor and more gait difficulties than individuals with PD. Clinical research criteria for the diagnosis of PSP were recently established in a workshop sponsored by the National Institute of Neurological Disorders and Stroke (NINDS) and the Society for PSP (Litvanet al., 1996a). Diagnosis of PSP is made when individuals who are over the age of 40 experience both a vertical supranuclear gaze palsy and prominent postural instability with falls within the first year of disease onset. Additionally, the diagnosis of PSP is strengthened if the patient does not respond well to levodopa treatment or shows early cognitive impairments. Onset of this disorder generally occurs late in life with onset most common in the sixth decade of life, with an average length of survival being 6 years. It is estimated that the prevalence of PSP in the United States is 1.39/100,000 individuals (Golbe et al., 1988). Progression of PSP occurs quite rapidly, with at least 70% of individuals experiencing frequent falls, slow performance of activities of daily living, inability of reading, and slurring of speech within the first year of diagnosis (Santacruz et al., 1998). One study reported risk factors for more rapid progression including older age, male gender, and greater severity in motor symptoms (Santacruz et al., 1998).

Pathology

Neuropathologic examination remains the "gold standard" for diagnosis of PSP. Abundant neurofibrillary tangles and neurophil threads in the pallidum, subthalamus, substantia nigra, and pons, with accompanying neuronal loss and gliosis, characterize typical PSP. Less dense neurofibrillary tangles are found in the striatum, oculomotor complex, medulla, or dentate nucleus.

Cognition

Cognitive impairment is common in PSP, with over 50% of individuals reporting impairments in concentration and word finding within 2 years of diagnosis and 50% reporting memory impairments within 3 years of diagnosis (Santacruz et al., 1998). Dementia is diagnosed in about 50% of individuals with PSP (Pahwa, 1999). Research investigating the association of cognitive impairment and disease severity has been mixed. Some research suggests that cognitive impairment is not associated with severity of disease (oculomotor dysfunction), whereas others report that memory impairment is correlated with disease duration. Consistent with all basal ganglia disorders, general cognitive slowing is prominent in PSP. Dubois and colleagues (1988) reported that individuals with PSP showed increased cognitive processing time for cognitively complex tasks beyond that of controls or individuals with PD.

Impairment in frontal functioning is quite often noted in individuals with PSP. Deficits have been shown on most traditional tasks including letter and category fluency, the Stroop task, the Cambridge Automated Neuropsychological Test Assessment Battery (CANTAB) set-shifting task, and the Similarities subtest of the Wechsler Adult Intelligence Test (WAIS) (Robbins et al., 1994). Performance on the Wisconsin Card Sorting Task (WCST) is associated with fewer categories achieved and increased numbers of perseverative errors (Dubois et al., 1988).

Individuals with PSP exhibit memory deficits on various tests including visual memory, verbal memory, and working memory (Dubois et al., 1988). When compared to other basal ganglia patient groups, PSP patients perform most similarly to PD patients, whereas individuals with HD show poorer use of semantic clustering. Although individuals with PSP exhibit accelerated forgetting, PSP patients demonstrate much better retention than patients with AD. In combination, findings indicate that the memory deficit of PSP can be best characterized by a primary encoding deficit with a prominent retrieval deficit and a mild impairment in forgetting.

Neuropsychiatric Symptoms

Psychiatric and behavioral symptoms are common in PSP. Nearly all (>90%) PSP patients show high levels of apathy (Litvan et al., 1996b), whereas about half of PSP patients exhibit a change in personality and less than half suffer from depression (Santacruz et al., 1998). Disinhibition, or loss of control for emotions, is noted in 30% to 36% of PSP patients (Litvan et al., 1996b).

Corticobasal Degeneration

Demographic and Clinical Characteristics

Corticobasal degeneration (CBD), a neurodegenerative disorder affecting the basal ganglia as well as the cortex, shows some overlap in symptomatology with other disorders such as PD, PSP, Pick disease, and AD. CBD generally presents in late adulthood with mean age of onset occurring at 63 years of age. Current observations suggest no distinct genetic basis for CBD, although a particular genetic background may be a risk factor for both CBD and PSP (Di Maria et al., 2000). Although accurate estimates of the prevalence of CBD are difficult to ascertain, the prevalence is considered rare (<1/200,000).

Individuals with CBD typically present with symptoms of limb clumsiness, although dementia may be the presenting symptom in cases with minimal motor involvement (Grimes et al., 1999). Common motor signs of CBD include asymmetrical presentation of dystonia, myoclonus, rigidity, postural tremor, and akinesia with postural disturbances and increased horizontal saccadic latencies. Cortical involvement is evident 1 to 3 years following disease onset and includes apraxia, aphasia, cortical sensory loss, alien limb phenomenon, and dementia. Changes in speech can also occur in CBD with individuals exhibiting slow speech, dysphonia, echolalia, and palilalia.

Pathology

CBD is associated with asymmetrical atrophy of the frontal lobes as well as in subcortical regions of the brain, typically the thalamus, caudate, and midbrain tegmentum with a loss of pigmentation in the substantia nigra. In comparison with other neurodegenerative diseases, PSP is associated with atrophy of the midbrain, whereas CBD is not (Soliveri et al., 1999). AD is associated with atrophy of the hippocampus and temporal lobe, whereas CBD is not.

Cognition

The majority of individuals with CBD will experience dementia as the disease progresses (Kertesz et al., 2000). Impairments in memory are commonly noted in CBD although not as severe as those occurring in AD. Executive functioning impairments are typical of those found in other basal ganglia disorders with impairments on the WCST (Pillon et al., 1995). In contrast to other subcortical disorders, more than 50% of individuals with CBD experience aphasia with both naming and word fluency impairments, and severity of aphasic impairment is correlated with severity of dementia (Kertesz et al., 2000).

Neuropsychiatric Symptoms

Neuropsychiatric symptoms in CBD have received less study than motor and cognitive symptoms although evidence suggests that neuropsychiatric symptoms are common in CBD. The current literature notes three distinct types of symptoms occurring in CBD: depression, frontal lobe–type behaviors, and obsessive-compulsive behaviors. One study documented symptoms of depression in 74% of persons with CBD (Litvan et al., 1998a).

Multiple System Atrophy

Demographic and Clinical Characteristics

Multiple system atrophy (MSA) is the term for previously separated disorders: olivopontocerebellar atrophy (OPCA), Shy-Drager syndrome (SDS), and striatonigral degeneration (SND). Individuals with MSA exhibit classic parkinsonian symptoms (rigidity, bradykinesia, postural instability) commonly in an asymmetrical manner. Approximately 50% of individuals with MSA exhibit these symptoms at onset with the majority of individuals exhibiting these symptoms during the disease progression (Wenning et al., 1997). Resting tremor, however, is less common in MSA than PD. Autonomic dysfunction is a common presenting symptom in MSA (41%) with approximately 97% experiencing autonomic dysfunction during the course of disease progression. Impotence in men and incontinence in women are the most common autonomic dysfunction symptoms. The striatonigral degeneration subtype of MSA is the most common and presents with more tremor, pyramidal signs, and myoclonus than the other subtypes of MSA. Although cognitive impairment, particularly frontal dysfunction, may occur in individuals with MSA, dementia is uncommon. MSA is slightly more common in men than women (1.3:1) with a median age of onset of 55 years. Disease progression is faster than in PD with mean survival in MSA of 6 to 7 years.

Wilson Disease

Demographic and Clinical Characteristics

Wilson disease (WD) is an autosomally recessive disorder associated with abnormal accumulation of copper in the liver or brain (or both), particularly the basal ganglia. Additionally, the copper accumulates in the corneal limbus, forming Kayser-Fleischer rings (KF rings), which have been shown to correlate with disease severity (Rodman et al., 1997). WD is rare with an estimated incidence of 12 to 30 per million (Hoogenraad & Houwen, 1996). Individuals with WD generally present with symptoms in childhood or early adulthood with a mean age of onset of 17 years of age. The gene associated with WD is located on chromosome 13. Approximately one third of individuals with WD will present with liver disease due to the accumulation of copper within the liver. A second third of individuals present with neurologic signs, dysarthric speech, impaired fine motor skills, tremor, dystonia, or abnormal gait. The final group of patients presents with psychiatric or behavioral symptoms such as affective disorders and personality change.

Pathology

WD most commonly affects the putamen and pons. Computed tomography (CT) findings in WD show ventricular dilation, basal ganglia hyperintensities, and atrophy of cerebral cortex, brainstem, or cerebellum. Functional imaging studies suggest that WD is associated with hypometabolism in the cerebellum, striatum, cerebral cortex, and thalamus.

Treatment

Treatment of WD involves copper chelation therapy with penicillamine or trientine or therapy to reduce copper absorption. In extreme cases when the liver has been severely damaged, a liver transplant may be necessary.

Cognition

Cognitive impairment has been reported in many cases of WD, although the impairment is generally mild (Rathbun, 1996). Cognitive impairments noted include impairments in memory, verbal fluency, and psychomotor speed.

Neuropsychiatric Symptoms

The presence of psychiatric symptoms is common in individuals with WD, with estimated lifetime prevalence ranging from 30% to 100% (Dening & Berrios, 1989). Common psychiatric symptoms in WD include personality changes, depression, anxiety, and psychosis. Personality changes (e.g., irritability, emotionality) have been reported to occur in over 71% of individuals with WD, whereas depression is found in over 60% (Oder et al., 1991). The relationship between psychiatric symptoms and degree of copper deposits is not currently understood although psychiatric symptoms may be more common in individuals presenting with neurologic symptoms or KF rings.

Fahr Disease

Demographic and Clinical Characteristics

Bilateral striopallidodentate calcinosis, commonly known as Fahr disease (FD), is another movement disorder affecting the basal ganglia. A diagnosis of FD is given to any disorder in which calcium deposits occur bilaterally within the brain, particularly in the dentate nucleus and the basal ganglia. FD is quite rare in the general population. Although the etiology of FD is disputed, a study pooling data from several case studies suggests that the disease is often, but not always, inherited in an autosomally dominant manner (Manyam et al., 2001) with some evidence that the responsible gene is found on chromosome 14q.

Cognition

The most common symptom of FD is movement disorder, particularly parkinsonism (55%) and chorea (19%), with some individuals exhibiting tremor, dystonia, athetosis, and dyskinesia. Although more comprehensive studies have not been conducted, it is estimated that at least one third of patients display cognitive impairments, including psychomotor slowing, visual spatial misperception, poor learning, and executive dysfunction (Lopez-Villegas et al., 1996).

Neuropsychiatric Symptoms

Psychiatric symptoms in FD are correlated with increased calcification and subarachnoid space dilation. Mood disorders are the most common psychiatric symptom with one fifth experiencing a mood disorder at presentation and about two thirds experiencing a mood disorder during the course of disease progression. Specifically, depression occurs in approximately 40% of individuals with FD, and mania occurs in up to 20% of individuals with FD. Obsessive-compulsive disorder (OCD) is common, occurring in up to one third of individuals (Lopez-Villegas et al., 1996).

HYPERKINETIC DISORDERS

Huntington Disease

Demographic and Clinical Characteristics

Huntington disease (HD) is a genetically transmitted neurodegenerative disease of the basal ganglia that is characterized by a triad of clinical symptoms including choreoathetosis, cognitive decline, and psychiatric features. The prevalence of HD is 7 to 10/100,000. Despite the availability of a genetic test (i.e., 37 or more cytosine-adenine-guanine [CAG] repeats on the IT-15 gene on chromosome 4), the diagnosis of symptomatic HD is based on a neurologic evaluation and requires the presence of an unequivocal movement disorder. The motor disorder of HD changes over time. Early signs often include involuntary movements, a change in saccadic eye movements, an inability to suppress reflexive glances to novel visual stimuli, tongue motor impersistence, impaired rapid alternating movements, balance problems, and akathisia (Siemers et al., 1996). Epilepsy is rare in adult-onset HD, though more common in juvenile-onset HD. Choking is an increasing hazard in middle and later stages of HD, as it becomes harder to coordinate chewing, swallowing, and breathing. Early chorea may be suppressed or masked by purposeful movements, but as the disease progresses, the choreic movements become larger and less easy to conceal. The severity of the chorea tends to plateau and then decline, while rigidity, spasticity, dystonia, and bradykinesia become more prominent (Penney et al., 1990). In later stages, dystonia and bradykinesia are prominent and patients become immobile and bedridden.

The clinical characteristics of HD are assessed using the Unified Huntington's Disease Rating Scale (UHDRS; Huntington's Study Group, 1996). The UHDRS assesses four components of HD: motor function, cognition, behavior, and functional abilities. The instrument has been used since 1994, and data have been collected prospectively on more than 4000 patients with symptomatic HD and 500 individuals at risk for HD.

Cognition

Zakzanis (1998) recently conducted an effect-size analysis incorporating meta-analytic principles to summarize neuropsychological performances from 760 patients with HD and 943 healthy controls. Results indicated that patients with HD are most deficient in the acquisition of new information, delayed recall, cognitive flexibility, manual dexterity, attention, speed of processing, and verbal skill. Cognitive functions have been shown to be useful predictors of total functional capacity (Marder et al., 2000). For instance, Rothlind and Brandt (1993) examined motor and cognitive measures as predictors of independence in activities of daily living and reported that cognitive measures were more highly correlated with functioning than were other clinical measures of disease. Similarly, Hamilton and her colleagues (2003) found that cognitive and behavioral aspects of HD were highly predictive of instrumental and physical activities of daily living, even after controlling for limitations secondary to motor dysfunction and abnormal movements (Fig. 24-6).

It is well established that among the most prominent cognitive impairments in HD are the so-called "executive functions." These fundamental abilities can affect performance in many cognitive areas including reasoning, planning, judgment, decision making, attention, learning, memory, flexibility, and timing. Several studies have demonstrated that HD patients are impaired on tests that require executive functions, such as the WCST (Paulsen, 1995b) and the Stroop Color Word Test (Paulsen, 1996a), as well as clinical rating scales of executive dyscontrol (Paulsen et al., 1996b; Paulsen et al., 1997). In fact, brief tests of executive functions have been suggested as sensitive tools for identification of subcortical dysfunction. That is, the Serial Sevens item on the Mini-Mental Status Exam (Folstein et al., 1975), the Initiation and Perseveration subtest of the Dementia Rating Scale (Mattis, 1976), and an abbreviated battery of frontal lobe tests have been demonstrated to be distinctly sensitive to patients with HD (Paulsen et al., 1995).

Some recent research has evaluated HD patients' performance on clinically relevant, face-valid tests of

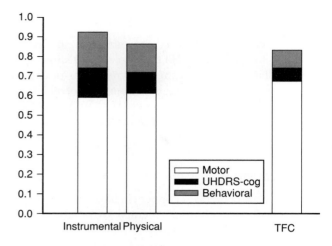

FIGURE 24-6. Relationship between functional capacity and HD symptoms. (Reproduced with permission from Hamilton JM, Salmon DP, Corey-Bloom J, et al: Behavioral abnormalities contribute to functional decline in Huntington's disease. J Neurol Neurosurg Psychiatry 74:120–122, 2003.)

judgment and decision making. Stout and colleagues (2001) used a simulated gambling task to quantify decision-making deficits in HD patients. Findings showed that HD patients made fewer advantageous selections than age- and education-matched healthy controls and dementia severity-matched patients with PD. Impairments on tasks requiring decision making may be due to various cognitive decrements, including learning, attention, inhibition, or appreciation for future consequences. Findings can also be interpreted as further evidence that HD patients are less able to benefit from feedback and have difficulty varying output based on performance (Paulsen et al., 1993). Despite evidence of explicit knowledge for the tasks, HD patients were unable to update existing "programs" based on new experience and to alter their responses. Numerous wide-ranging consequences of these types of executive deficits are self-evident.

Early neuropsychological studies reported that HD patients perform poorly on subtests requiring attention and working memory (Boll et al., 1974). More recent studies have emphasized dysfunction in unique aspects of attention, including resource allocation, response flexibility, and vigilance. For instance, Lawrence and colleagues (1996) reported that HD patients are able to maintain attention for a previously learned response set but have difficulty shifting attention to a new set. Sprengelmeyer and colleagues (1995) reported that HD patients are able to maintain alertness when the task involves an external cue but fail when internal self-generated vigilance is required. The clinical implications of the attentional impairment in HD are significant. Many people with HD perform better when they avoid tasks involving divided attention. Patients and families agree that trying to divide the already-compromised attentional resources can contribute to discomfort and increased safety risks. For instance, driving a car while listening to the radio, talking to the children in the back seat, or talking on the cell phone is not recommended. To reduce choking risk, the environment should be quiet and calm at mealtimes to emphasize concentration on chewing and swallowing, rather than the TV, doorbell, and conversation.

Deficits in learning and memory are the most frequently reported cognitive complaints from people with HD and their family members. HD patients exhibit verbal learning deficits even in the earliest stages of the illness (Delis et al., 1991). The majority of studies have described the memory impairment as a primary encoding and retrieval deficit because recognition memory is often preserved (Delis et al., 1991). That is, most studies show that people with HD consistently have problems learning new information and also experience difficulty when asked to use free recall to remember what they have learned; in contrast, they perform near normal when a less-effortful memory strategy is used, such as offering choices of, or recognizing, possible learned items. HD patients manifest relatively intact retention over a delay period (Jacobs et al., 1990), indicating no abnormal forgetting or rapid loss of information. When tested on memory for information acquired long ago, they demonstrate no temporal gradient in performance, indicating that memory performance is equivalent for all periods of their lives.

Research in HD has made significant contributions to our understanding of memory over the past few decades. Briefly, observations that skill learning is intact in patients with medial-temporal and diencephalic damage and deficient in patients with HD led to an explosion of research investigating the existence of multiple, independent memory systems in the brain.

Although it has become accepted that skill learning is dependent on the integrity of the basal ganglia, Gabrieli and colleagues (1997) documented dissociable skill learning performances in HD, suggesting separable neural circuits for skill learning. Consistent with this interpretation is the finding by Paulsen and colleagues (1993) that skill learning was impaired in HD patients only when external feedback was no longer available. Similarly, Willingham and colleagues (1996) showed intact skill learning when visual feedback was available to HD patients, but showed defective performance when not allowed feedback. In summary, the memory impairment of HD is characterized by a mild encoding deficit (likely due to impaired organization of the to-be-learned information and ineffective working memory), moderately impaired retrieval in the context of relatively intact memory storage when measured with a less effortful strategy (recognition). Skill learning can be acquired when external feedback is allowed, but motor programs are not stored for later usage possibly due to the dependence of the striatum in "chunking" components of the motor program.

Several studies have shown olfaction impairments in HD using the University of Pennsylvania Smell Identification Test (UPSIT; Doty, 1991). In the most comprehensive research to date, Nordin and colleagues (1995) assessed absolute detection, intensity discrimination, quality discrimination, short-term recognition memory, and lexical- and picture-based identification for odor, using taste and vision as comparison modalities. Results suggested that although odor-recognition memory is not affected in HD patients, absolute detection, intensity discrimination, quality discrimination, and identification were significantly impaired. Poor detection sensitivity explained performance on several other olfactory tasks where odor identification was the function most impaired.

Deficits in the ability to copy simple geometric designs, to copy block designs, and to put together puzzles are evident in HD. Although some of these impairments likely reflect motor abnormalities, performance is also impaired on motor-free untimed perceptual tasks. Mohr and colleagues (1997) recently examined whether visuospatial deficits in basal ganglia disease are a nonspecific function of dementia severity or whether they reflect disease-specific impairments. Findings suggested that general visuospatial processing capacity is impaired as a nonspecific dementia effect in both HD and PD, whereas only patients with HD showed specific impairment in person-centered spatial judgment. For instance, people with HD (but not PD) experience difficulty with map reading, directional sense, and varying their motor responses following alterations in space. Individuals with HD typically misjudge distances and the relationship of their body to walls, curbs, and other potential obstacles. Although the underlying basis for these impairments is not fully understood, disruptions in corticostriatal circuitry make it difficult to update spatial relations based on feedback. Cortico-cortico connections to the parietal cortex may also be compromised secondary to disruption of the prefrontal cortex.

One of the most prominent features of HD is the motor speech impairment, or dysarthria, that is characteristic of the illness. Early speech changes may include insufficient breath support, varying prosody, increased response latencies, and mild misarticulations. As HD progresses, phrase length becomes reduced and pauses in speech output lengthen. Performances on tasks of letter and category fluency are impaired early in the disease, although the integrity of word associations remains relatively intact with little evidence of intrusion or perseveration errors. Despite significant impairments in verbal fluency, speed of output, and complexity, syntactic structure remains intact and speech content is usually appropriate (Illes, 1989). Although there are some reports in late-stage HD of mild deterioration in semantic knowledge structure, several other studies have shown that errors in confrontation naming are more likely due to visual-perceptual deficits (Hodges et al., 1991) and retrieval slowing (Rohrer et al., 1999). Speech output becomes severely impaired as the disease progresses, typically resulting in a profound communication deficit. Assistive devices for language expression are recommended early in the disease to ensure that preferences are understood and needs are met in later stages when traditional communication is no longer possible. Computer devices are useful for a brief period, after which lack of motor control limits use of a keyboard or joystick. Infrared detectors are often prone to error due to involuntary movements. Alphabet boards and pictures that summarize frequently requested needs are adaptive and can be used throughout the illness. Simple computer response keys and large YES-NO cards are critical in late stages of HD. Although motor output of speech is the primary impairment, several more subtle language impairments are associated with HD. Comprehension of conversational speech is limited by its length and complexity. Poor executive control impairs the ability to sequence and organize the information communicated. In addition, some evidence indicates that people with HD cannot benefit from affective and propositional prosody (Speedie et al., 1990).

Recent findings have suggested that people with basal ganglia dysfunction, and specifically people with HD, have difficulty with the estimation and production of time. These findings are corroborated clinically; people often complain that their once-punctual spouse becomes frequently late and makes errors in estimating how long activities will take. The clinical relevance of these findings to daily activities, such as driving, is unknown, but research is underway to better characterize these observations.

Psychiatric and Behavioral Symptoms

Psychiatric and behavioral symptoms are common in HD and have been reported as the presenting disease manifestations in up to 79% of patients (Morris, 1991). Research on the incidence of psychiatric symptoms in HD is variable, however, encumbered by limitations within and across studies. Some limitations of the available research are: (1) affected people are often medicated to minimize abnormal involuntary movements; such treatment may mask psychiatric and behavioral symptoms; (2) most available neuropsychiatric assessment tools use conventional psychiatric terminology based on idiopathic psychiatric illness, which fails to distinctly reflect the symptoms associated with striatal deterioration; and (3) most research has emphasized the motor and cognitive impairments associated with HD, despite

family reports that psychiatric disturbances are most strongly associated with stress, disability, and placement decisions. Data from 1857 Huntington Study Group (HSG) subjects with a diagnosis of symptomatic HD are presented in Table 24-2. Subjects are grouped into disease stages according to ratings obtained on the Total Functional Capacity Scale (Shoulson & Fahn, 1979).

Depression is one of the most common concerns for individuals and families with HD, occurring in up to 63% of patients. It has been suggested that depression can precede the onset of neurologic symptoms in HD by 2 to 20 years, although formal research has been minimal. Recent data from the HSG indicate that depression is most common immediately prior to diagnosis, when neurologic soft signs and other subtle abnormalities become evident. Following a definite diagnosis of HD, however, depression is most prevalent in the middle stages of the disease (i.e., Shoulson-Fahn stages 2 and 3) and may diminish in the later stages. PET studies of HD patients with depression show hypermetabolism in the inferior frontal cortex and thalamus relative to nondepressed HD patients or normal, age-comparable controls (Mayberg et al., 1992). Although less well studied, mania episodes occur in 2% to 12% of HD patients (see Morris, 1991, for an overview).

Suicide is more common in HD than in other neurologic disorders with high rates of depression, such as stroke and PD. Most studies have found a fourfold to sixfold increase of suicide in HD, and some studies have reported it to be 8 to 20 times higher than in the general population (Almqvist et al., 1999). Suicidal ideation, as measured by the behavioral rating scale on the UHDRS, is highly prevalent throughout the disease, with 8% of all individuals diagnosed with HD having active ideation. Suicidal ideation was recently examined in 4342 individuals in the HSG database. All subjects were grouped according to the standardized neurologic exam from 0 (i.e., normal exam) to 3 (unquestionable HD). Patients with an unequivocal diagnosis of HD were further divided into stage of disease (stage 1 to stage 5). The proportion of persons with suicidal ideation varied significantly by risk status and HD stage. Two primary "critical periods" were evident, during which suicidal ideation in HD increased dramatically. The frequency of suicidal ideation doubled from 10.4% in at-risk persons with a normal neurologic exam to 20.5% in at-risk persons with soft neurologic signs. In persons with a diagnosis of HD, 16% had suicidal ideation in stage 1, whereas nearly 21% had suicidal ideation in stage 2. Although the underlying mechanisms for suicidal risk in HD is poorly understood, it may be beneficial for health care providers to be aware of periods during which patients may be at an increased risk for suicide (Ferneyhough et al., 2002).

Psychosis occurs with increased frequency in HD, with estimates ranging from 3% to 12%. Although the

TABLE 24-2. Percentage of HD Patients Endorsing Psychiatric Symptoms by TFC Stage

Symptom	Stage 1 (n = 432)	Stage 2 (n = 660)	Stage 3 (n = 520)	Stage 4 (n = 221)	Stage 5 (n = 84)
Depression	57.5%	62.9%	59.3%	52.1%	42.2%
Suicide	6.0%	9.7%	10.3%	9.9%	5.5%
Aggression	39.5%	47.7%	51.8%	54.1%	54.4%
Obsessions	13.3%	16.9%	25.5%	28.9%	13.3%
Delusions	2.4%	3.5%	6.1%	9.9%	2.2%
Hallucinations	2.3%	4.2%	6.3%	11.2%	3.3%

TFC = total functional capacity.

Reproduced with permission from Huntington Study Group: Unified Huntington's Disease Rating Scale: Reliability and consistency. Mov Disord 11:136–142, 1996.

majority of the research has been conducted using the Johns Hopkins sample, data are consistent with others' clinical experience, suggesting that psychosis in HD is broad and similar to that seen in other psychiatric disorders. Psychosis is more common among early adult-onset cases than among those whose disease begins in middle or late adulthood. Psychosis associated with HD is more resistant to treatment than psychosis in schizophrenia. HSG data suggest that psychosis may increase somewhat as the disease progresses (see Table 24-2), although psychosis can become difficult to measure in the later stages of disease.

Although true OCD is not often reported in HD (Cummings & Cummingham, 1992), obsessive and compulsive behaviors are prevalent (i.e., 13%–30%). Obsessional thinking often increases with proximity to disease onset and then remains somewhat stable throughout the illness. Obsessional thinking associated with HD is reminiscent of perseveration, such that individuals get "stuck" on a previous occurrence or need and are unable to shift. For instance, patients often emphasize a time in the past when they felt wronged (e.g., divorce, job loss) and maintain discussion on this topic for several years. Another example of obsessional thinking in HD is when patients get fixated on a specific need, such as needing a cigarette, soda, sweater, or specific kind of juice.

A spectrum of behaviors ranging from irritability to intermittent explosive disorders occurs in 19% to 59% of HD patients. Although aggressive outbursts are often the principal reason for admission to a psychiatric facility (Shiwach & Patel, 1993), research on the prevalence and incidence of irritability and aggressive outbursts in HD is sparse. The primary limitation in summarizing these symptoms in HD is the varied terminology used to describe this continuum of behaviors. A recent survey of several clinicians as well as HD family members suggested that difficulty with placement, due to aggression, was among the principal obstacles to providing an effective continuum of care for people with HD. Table 24-3 shows what percentage of skilled nursing

TABLE 24-3. Ratings by Nursing Home Staff of Problematic Behaviors in Patients with HD

Behavior problem	Percentage	Rank
Agitation	76%	2.0
Irritability	72%	2.9
Disinhibition	59%	3.3
Depression	51%	4.2
Anxiety	50%	4.4
Appetite	54%	5.1
Delusions	43%	5.5
Sleep disorders	50%	5.5
Apathy	32%	6.8
Euphoria	40%	6.9

From unpublished data from Dr. Jane Paulsen, University of Iowa, and Dr. Joanne Hamilton, University of California at San Diego.

facilities surveyed rated behaviors as problematic in caring for an individual with HD. The final column represents the overall rank of each behavior from most problematic (1) to least problematic (10) in providing care for HD. Findings reveal that agitation is the most prominent behavior problem cited. Irritability, disinhibition, and depression were the next most common behavior problems cited by the facilities surveyed.

Early signs of HD may include withdrawal from activities and friends, decline in personal appearance, lack of behavioral initiation, decreased spontaneous speech, and constriction of emotional expression. Often, however, these symptoms are considered merely reflective of depression, and more conclusive evaluations are precluded. Although difficult to distinguish, apathy is defined as diminished motivation not attributable to cognitive impairment, emotional distress, or decreased level of consciousness. Depression involves considerable emotional distress, evidenced by tearfulness, sadness, anxiety, agitation, insomnia, anorexia, feelings of worthlessness and hopelessness, and recurrent thoughts of death (American Psychiatric Association, 1994). Levy and colleagues (1998) recently examined the relationship of apathy and depression in 34 people with HD and concluded that apathy is common (59%) in HD and is separable from depression (70%). Fifty-three percent of HD patients had mutually exclusive apathy or depression, and the two symptoms were not correlated ($r = -0.15$, $P = .40$). Apathy was correlated with lower cognitive function, however, replicating previous research indicating relationships between apathy and dementia. Although the frequency of complaints from patients and family members about apathy may be low, the prevalence of this behavior is not. The consequences of apathy are rarely problematic (in contrast to temper outbursts, which are less frequent but highly distressing), but effective treatment of apathy is typically appreciated by patients and family members.

One of the most frequent behavioral complaints about HD from family members is that the affected individual "refuses to accept" or "denies" the disease and its consequences. Ample evidence suggests that the apparent "denial" represents a neurologically based unawareness or anosognosia (Snowden et al., 1998). Past research has emphasized the presence of unawareness and the difficulty in assessment with available unawareness tools. One recent study (Deckel & Morrison, 1996) administered an 8-item self-rating scale to 19 individuals with HD and 15 consecutive patients referred for neuropsychological assessment with non-HD diagnoses. Two staff members also independently rated each subject's deficits in cognitive and motor abilities. Inconsistencies between the two ratings indicated anosognosia. HD patients showed higher anosognosia than the comparison patients. In addition, performances on the WCST and the visuospatial subtests of the WAIS-R were significantly associated with levels of anosognosia for the HD patients. These findings suggest that unawareness in HD is likely to reflect circuitry dysfunction affecting the frontoparietal lobes and their connections, not merely unwillingness to face the diagnosis.

Longitudinal Research

Several studies have relied on the Total Functional Capacity (TFC) Scale to quantify disease stages and functional dependence associated with HD. Research has been largely consistent, with most studies demonstrating an average decline of 0.63 ± 0.75 U/yr on the TFC Scale. Although controversial, some evidence indicates that rate of progression is more rapid in juvenile onset and more gradual in late onset. Marder and colleagues (2000) recently examined the annual rate of functional decline in 960 prospective HD patients followed an average of 18 months at 43 sites in the HSG. Findings were consistent with previous research, suggesting TFC decline of 0.72 U/yr and independent-scale decline of 4.52 U/yr. Better cognitive status at baseline, lower baseline TFC, and longer disease duration were associated with a less rapid rate of decline, whereas depressive symptoms were associated with more rapid functional decline. Bamford and colleagues (1996) conducted neuropsychological evaluations, functional capacity ratings, and CT scans on 29 HD patients at 18, 30, and 42 months. Results indicate that tests of psychomotor skills showed the greatest amount of consistent decline among the cognitive functions assessed; memory did not deteriorate until advanced stages. Rich and colleagues (1999) assessed flexibility and language functions over 5 years and reported stable semantic clustering (language) performances in HD patients despite a progressive reduction in shifting. Findings are consistent with a cross-sectional study of 75 HD patients divided into three stages of illness: early, middle, and advanced (Fig. 24-7). These findings suggested that memory, receptive language, and simple attention remain relatively intact throughout the stages of HD (Paulsen et al., 1995b). It is important for professionals and family members to educate staff at care facilities regarding the pattern of impaired and preserved cognitive functions in later stages of HD, when verbal output is severely limited.

Tourette Syndrome

Demographic and Clinical Characteristics

Tourette syndrome (TS) is an inherited neuropsychiatric disorder characterized by motor and phonic tics. Diagnostic criteria for TS include the presence of multiple motor tics and one or more vocal tics, both of which must exceed a year's duration. Onset of this disorder occurs in childhood with an average onset age of 6 to 7 years, although ages of onset have been reported from 1 to 19 years. The prevalence of TS is between 1 and 10/10,000 individuals (Singer, 2000) and is more common in boys than in girls, with a 3:1 ratio. Although evidence suggests a genetic transmission of TS, identification of a gene has not yet occurred. Although the etiology of TS remains unknown, some recent reports confirm the utility of D8/17 cell overexpression as a peripheral blood marker in TS patients; these data are compatible with a streptococcus-related pathogenesis for at least a subgroup of patients with tic disorders (Cardona & Orefici, 2001). Course of illness is variable, with some individuals experiencing spontaneous remission or significant decrease of symptom severity, whereas others experience lifelong presence of symptoms.

Comorbidity

Comorbidity is common among individuals with TS. Attention-deficit/hyperactivity disorder (ADHD) co-occurs in 50% to 60% of those with TS, with ADHD

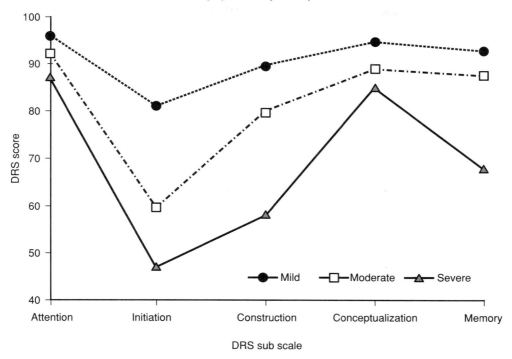

FIGURE 24-7. Dementia Rating Scale (DRS) in HD by impairment. (Reproduced with permission from Paulsen JS, Butters N, Sadek JR, et al: Distinct cognitive profiles of cortical and subcortical dementia in advanced illness. Neurology 45:951–956, 1995.)

symptoms commonly preceding the onset of TS by 2 to 3 years. Between 30% and 60% of individuals with TS experience obsessive-compulsive symptoms generally occurring several years following the onset of tics. It is often difficult to distinguish between a complex motor tic and a compulsive ritual, but accurate diagnosis is vital, because treatment for these disorders is vastly different.

Pathology

Although the neuropathology of TS remains somewhat unclear, current evidence indicates that the basal ganglia and related cortical and thalamic structures are the most likely sites of underlying abnormality in TS. Imaging studies have shown that individuals with TS tend to have decreased basal ganglia volume as well as asymmetrical basal ganglia (a reversal of the expected left larger than right lenticular region of the basal ganglia) and a larger than expected corpus callosum (Schuerholz et al., 1998).

Treatment

Drug therapy is reserved for patients with tics that are functionally disabling because none of the available pharmacotherapies are curative and all are associated with side effects. A number of nonpharmacologic treatments (relaxation training, biofeedback hypnosis, acupuncture conditioning) have been proposed, but few have been adequately evaluated. Several groups are currently conducting efficacy trials of cognitive-behavioral therapy. Tics can be suppressed by the use of α-adrenergic agonists, neuroleptics, and dopamine-depleting agents including tetrabenazine. These medications can cause sedation, apathy, depression, and rigidity. Sedative side effects can affect academic performance and have been associated with cognitive decline. Of promise, however, is a report by Bornstein and Yang (1991) showing that performances on a wide range of neuropsychological tests were not significantly different between a group of medicated (with neuroleptics) and unmedicated TS patients. One recent study noted a dose-related effect of the opioid antagonist, naloxone, on tic behavior in patients with TS; a low dose (30 mg) caused a significant decrease in tics, whereas a high dose (300 mg) caused a significant increase in tics (van Wattum et al., 2000). Despite the best psychopharmacologic and behavioral therapeutic efforts, a few patients have residual debilitating symptoms, including self-injurious behavior. The management of this malignant manifestation of TS remains controversial and some patients are referred for surgery. Babel and colleagues (2001) recently reported effective control of tics after infrathalamic and thalamic lesioning. Dystonia and dysarthria were the most common complications, although only 6 of 11 cases were seen for follow-up. Thalamic deep brain stimulation has been used successfully in case studies. Although stereotactic techniques have several advantages over other neurosurgical approaches, treatment protocols have not yet been developed.

Cognition

Up to 68% of children with TS function below expectations in school. The neuropsychology of TS is incomplete, however, in part because there have been insufficient experimental studies of primary psychological systems, and in part because most studies that have been carried out have included a mix of subjects. Because comorbidity in TS is high, subject samples are often heterogeneous with regard to obsessive-compulsive symptoms, ADHD, mood disorders, coprolalia, age, medication usage, illness duration, and age of onset. In addition, TS children are sometimes distracted by their various motor and vocal tics, or use a great deal of resources to suppress these tics, taking attention from their studies. Motor tics may interfere with writing of homework, taking notes, or performance on written exams. Children with TS are clearly seen as different from other children in the classroom, and often experience psychological and emotional burdens associated with being perceived as different. Despite these limitations, some preliminary conclusions may be drawn.

Although some findings suggest that children with TS have executive dysfunction, other reports show that children with pure TS (no comorbid diagnoses) have normal performances on neuropsychological measures (de Groot et al., 1997) or nearly normal performances with only subtle slowing or disinhibition. It has been suggested that TS demonstrates a "weaker version" of the HD response pattern in dysexecutive functions (Georgiou et al., 1995). Cirino and colleagues (2000) used a novel approach to teasing apart the heterogeneity of TS. Rather than try to segregate TS with and without OCD and ADHD, this study compared groups with high and low ADHD symptoms and found no differences in card-sorting performances. This finding suggests that poor executive functions, including weak self-monitoring and reduced inhibition, and impulse control may be common in all subtypes of TS. When considered together, findings suggest that cognitive impairments in pure TS are mild and not easily captured with gross measures. More comprehensive executive evaluations and novel study designs (Cirino et al., 2000) are probably required to better differentiate the core cognitive component of TS from the cognitive deficits associated with its comorbid disorders.

Children with TS and a comorbid diagnosis of ADHD demonstrate dysexecutive performances and increased perseverative errors (de Groot et al., 1997) as well as increased incidence of learning disability. Primary cognitive dysfunction associated with frontal systems may impair the planning, organization, and execution of behavioral output for children with TS and ADHD. Compensatory strategies that might be useful involve increased structure for problem solving. Although psychostimulant medications are generally regarded as the treatment of choice for ADHD, their use in children with TS has been controversial. Early reports suggested that stimulant medications could provoke or intensify tics, although recent evidence suggests that low doses of stimulants are beneficial for ADHD symptoms in TS. Children with TS and comorbid obsessive-compulsive symptoms show dysexecutive performances as well; however, performance is most severely impaired in children with TS, ADHD, and obsessive-compulsive symptoms (de Groot et al., 1997). Even after controlling for tic severity, TS children with comorbid ADHD and OCD demonstrated the most severe cognitive impairments and poorer academic achievement (de Groot et al., 1997).

CLINICAL ASSESSMENT OF MOVEMENT DISORDERS OF THE BASAL GANGLIA

Unidimensional assessment of movement disorders is a tradition of the past that has long outlived its usefulness. Clinical assessment of movement disorders requires a multifaceted approach involving assessments of neurologic abnormalities, functional capacity, cognitive impairments, and psychiatric symptoms. Omission of any one of these features results in an incomplete evaluation and can lead to increasing disability and morbidity.

Common referrals for cognitive and behavioral assessment of patients with movement disorders typically emphasize the following questions:

1. What cognitive strengths and weaknesses are present and how can findings be used to maximize function?
2. How has cognitive function changed over time?
3. At what stage of disease is this patient currently functioning and what can assessment findings tell us about prognosis and course?
4. Has cognitive performance been affected by treatment?

Referrals for cognitive and behavioral assessments are not typically made for assistance in differential diagnoses, because these are primarily determined by the motor examination and history. Most recently, neuropsychological evaluations are being requested to detect early disease in persons who are at known risk for developing specific neurologic illness. Table 24-4 provides a list of specific cognitive instruments commonly used and offers recommendations for adaptation in the assessment of persons with movement disorders.

Motor Examination

Many movement disorders have distinct assessment tools to assist the neurologist in the characterization of the motor abnormalities associated with specific disease. For instance, the Parkinson and Huntington study groups (under the leadership of Ira Shoulson) have developed the UPDRS and the UHDRS to standardize the neurologic examination best suited to each disorder. Formal motor examination remains critical to thorough characterization of the movement disorder and is paramount for its diagnosis and treatment. Details of the motor examination are provided in numerous other texts and are beyond the scope of this chapter.

Cognitive Evaluation

Not surprisingly, standard assessment protocols are less readily available for the cognitive and psychiatric evaluations of movement disorders of the basal ganglia. Although the specific tools used to evaluate cognitive deficits in movement disorders may be a matter of personal preference, the content areas specified in Table 24-4 may be helpful in the design of clinical batteries. Guidelines critical to test selection include the presence of alternate forms, the availability of normative performance data in age-, race-, and gender-matched normal individuals, and established reliability in persons with movement disorders. Thorough assessment of basal ganglia movement disorders will involve a combination of traditional neuropsychological measures, measures adapted for clinical use from cognitive neuroscience, and informal assessments. Formal assessment practices often require adaptation for use in patients with movement disorders of the basal ganglia. Some common accommodations that may be required in standardized assessment protocols include increased time allowance for completion of tasks, limited use of manual responses to tests (drawing, writing, speaking) with increased usage of multiple choice formats, amplification of speech for hearing or understanding output, and abbreviated testing protocols or extended assessment times spread over days to accommodate fatigue.

There are ample standardized measures to assess basic cognitive abilities such as attention, working memory, learning, memory, visual perception, constructional praxis, speech and language, establishing and shifting cognitive sets, abstract thinking, speed of processing, motor dexterity, and estimated premorbid intellect. Specific tasks for executive functions are often created by cognitive scientists and require intensive reliability and validity research prior to usage in clinical neuropsychology. To allow assessment of tasks that may be available only in experimental paradigms, several options are available for less standardized assessment of important functions sensitive to basal ganglia involvement. The Cambridge Automated Neuropsychological Test Assessment Battery (CANTAB) is a computerized assessment of set-shifting, planning, speed of processing, timing, and reaction time that is commercially available for clinical use. Unfortunately, the battery is quite expensive. Similar tasks have been programmed by other academicians, however, and psychometric tests of new executive measures are in development. The Frontal Assessment Battery involves informal bedside assessment of executive functions, whereas the Delis Kaplan Executive Function battery was recently normed and published for clinical use. Some tasks such as smell can be informally assessed using peanut butter held under the nostrils with eyes closed or formally assessed with purchase of the UPSIT. Timing impairments can be readily elicited by interview when asking about the punctuality of the individual and any changes in time estimation. Sequencing can be assessed using the Luria three-step, which appears sensitive to subtle movement abnormalities and possibly cognitive organization as well. Previous reports have not, in general, found associations between cognitive performance and the severity of the movement disorder in HD, although it is possible that certain motor symptoms may affect cognitive performances. Tests used should allow a separation of motor skill from the processing time component by recording movement time and down time separately.

Psychiatric Examination

Evaluation of patients with movement disorders typically involves assessment of the features listed in Table 24-5. Research on the psychiatric manifestations of movement disorders is in its infancy, but some excellent measures have emerged as helpful in the measurement of psychiatric symptoms and their treatment. The Neuropsychiatric Inventory (NPI; Cummings et al., 1994) assesses the frequency (4-point rating scale) and severity (3-point scale) of 10 neuropsychiatric disturbances (delusions, hallucinations, agitation, dysphoria, anxiety, euphoria, apathy, disinhibition, irritability, aberrant motor behavior). The NPI is standardized, has adequate reliability and validity, and is not influenced by normal aging. Research with the NPI has previously demonstrated distinctive neuropsychiatric profiles for various neurologic disorders (Litvan et al., 1996b, 1998c). The NPI has also been used in transcultural studies, as a measure of treatment response for neurodegenerative disorders, and in investigations of the biologic correlates of neuropsychiatric symptoms. The

TABLE 24-4. Neuropsychological Tests and Adaptations for Movement Disorders

Test and description	Motor demands	Possible adaptations
PREMORBID IQ ESTIMATE		
ANART: Assesses reading ability as an estimate of IQ; difficult for individuals with dysarthria	Speech output—clear pronunciation is important	Clarify pronunciations if necessary
WASI/WAIS Vocabulary subtest: Assesses vocabulary knowledge as estimate of IQ	Speech output	Clarify pronunciations if necessary
Barona: Uses demographic and education/occupation information to calculate premorbid IQ	None	Good alternative if speech output is severely impaired
STAGING/DEMENTIA SEVERITY		
Mattis Dementia Rating Scale (DRS)	Copying drawings, writing, repeating bimanual movements, speech output	Important to have an awareness of what each item is meant to measure, for example, liberal scoring on visuo-construction items is allowed (i.e., do not take off points for sloppiness due to chorea)
Mini-Mental Status Exam (MMSE): Less demanding than DRS, but less sensitive	Copying drawings, writing, speech output	Important to have an awareness of what each item is meant to measure, score accordingly
COGNITIVE SCREENING		
CERAD (includes MMSE): Assesses basic attention, category fluency, visual and verbal memory	Copying drawings, writing, speech output	Important to have an awareness of what each item is meant to measure, score accordingly; liberal scoring on visual construction items is allowed
VERBAL MEMORY AND LEARNING		
CVLT-II, CVLT: CVLT-II alternate: Two versions and a short form, computerized scoring program	Speech output	Ask for repetitions of responses if necessary, extra time for responses if needed; do not assume the patient is finished (always ask)
Logical Memory (WMS-R, WMS-III): Assesses ability to recall short stories, immediate and delayed recall scores	Speech output	Ask for repetitions of responses if necessary, extra time for responses if needed; do not assume the patient is finished (always ask)
Hopkins Verbal Learning Test-Revised: 6 versions—good choice for repeat evaluations, somewhat easier than CVLT (shorter list)	Speech output	Ask for repetitions of responses if necessary, extra time for responses if needed; do not assume the patient is finished (always ask)
VISUAL MEMORY AND LEARNING		
Rey Complex Figure Test (RCFT): Assesses immediate and delayed visual memory, visuo-construction, planning/organizational abilities	Copying and free recall of a detailed drawing, difficult (not a good choice) for people with moderate to severe tremor or chorea	Disregard the timing aspect and allow breaks if needed, this is often used as a "process approach" task—examiner can gain information about strategy, visuo-construction, and visual memory even if normative data are not applicable

TABLE 24-4. Neuropsychological Tests and Adaptations for Movement Disorders—cont'd

Test and description	Motor demands	Possible adaptations
WMS-III Visual Reproduction: Assesses immediate and delayed visual memory, and visuo-construction	Drawing of five figures, while not as detailed or demanding as RCFT but still difficult for those with tremor or chorea	Liberal scoring; this is a measure of memory—it is not intended to assess drawing ability
Brief Visuospatial Memory Test: Assesses memory of both location and form. Three trials—adds a learning component; recognition trial—visual only (no motor component); simple drawings—not as reliant on visuo-construction	Drawing of simple shapes required	Liberal scoring of responses
Memory for Faces (from Warrington Recognition Memory Test or WMS-III): No motor demands, visual recognition format only	None, other than pointing to or stating correct response	None needed
Continuous Recognition Memory Test (CRMT): Assesses visual memory in a recognition format	None, other than indicating that an item is old or new	None needed

MEASURES OF EXECUTIVE FUNCTIONS

Wisconsin Card Sorting Test (WCST): Assesses set shifting, problem solving, perseveration nonverbal only—good for those with speech output problems	Moving cards from stack to one of four response locations	Assist patient with handling of cards: Examiner can stack cards in front of patient and then ask patient to point to the stack where the top one should be moved; examiner can move cards for the patient
Stroop Color Word Interference Test: Assesses ability to inhibit a dominant response; also used as a measure of processing speed (first two trials)	Speech output, visual tracking	Place the card on a table so patient does not have to hold it; allow him to point to items to mark their place
Trailmaking B: Assesses ability to shift between two sets of stimuli, maintain response set; also relies on visual scanning and speeded motor movement	Speeded motor movements, visual scanning	Normative data may not be worthwhile if movement is particularly slow If the goal is to assess ability to maintain and shift set, then evaluate this in a process-oriented manner (i.e., not using the timed norms)
Self-Ordered Pointing Test: Assess working memory and strategy abilities; lack of normative data	None, other than pointing	Ask patient to touch the selected item each time, as pointing may be difficult to interpret due to tremor/chorea
WAIS-III similarities: Assesses verbal abstraction abilities	Speech output	Ask patient to repeat if necessary

LANGUAGE TESTS

Boston Naming Test: Assesses naming ability	Speech output	Clarify responses if necessary
Verbal Fluency/Controlled Oral Word Association: Assesses production of specific word list	Rapid speech output	Clarify responses if necessary

Continued

TABLE 24-4. Neuropsychological Tests and Adaptations for Movement Disorders—cont'd

Test and description	Motor demands	Possible adaptations
Peabody Picture Vocabulary Test-III: Assesses vocabulary and comprehension; good choice when speech is severely impaired	Pointing	Ask patient to touch the selected response—pointing may be difficult to interpret due to tremor/chorea
Token Test: Assesses comprehension; good choice when speech is severely impaired	Pointing or touching token	Ask patient to touch the selected token—pointing may not be accurate due to tremor/chorea. May not be possible to administer the items that require moving and picking up tokens—in this case use this test in a process approach to assess integrity or impairment of comprehension
AUDITORY ATTENTION		
Digit Span: Assesses verbal working memory	Speech output	Clarify responses if necessary
Brief Test of Attention: Assesses divided auditory attention	None	None required
VISUAL ATTENTION		
WMS-III Spatial Span: Assesses visual working memory	Pointing to a set of blocks in a specified pattern	Ask patient to touch the blocks—pointing may be difficult to interpret due to tremor/chorea
PERCEPTUAL ABILITY		
Hooper Visual Organization Test (HVOT): Assesses perception and ability to integrate nonverbal material; requires naming—not a good choice if BNT or other tests of word retrieval indicate impairment	Speech output—single-word naming	For patients with word retrieval/naming problems, examiner can attempt to determine if the perceptual aspect of the task is intact by detecting related words or gestures that indicate the patient accurately recognizes the item
Test of Visual-Perceptual Skills: Designed for children/adolescents, but norms for adults are available; seven subtests assess a variety of visual spatial abilities in the absence of motor demands	Pointing to responses	Examiner can select individual tests that are relevant to the evaluation question(s). Ask patient to touch the selected item, as pointing may not be accurate due to tremor/chorea

Frontal Systems Behavioral Evaluation (FrSBe; (Grace et al., 1999), previously known as the Frontal Lobe Personality Scale (FloPS), is a 46-item scale which assesses dysfunction in frontal behavioral systems. The FrSBe is composed of three subscales: apathy (14 items), disinhibition (15 items), and executive dysfunction (17 items). Each item is rated on a 5-point Likert scale. Additionally, the FrSBe quantitatively measures change over time from a retrospective baseline to the present. Community-based norms are provided in the manual.

Data from patients with frontal-temporal dementia, frontal lesion, nonfrontal stroke, head injury, AD, HD, and PD are also provided. Given the high frequency of unawareness in persons with basal ganglia dysfunction, it is possible to have the FrSBe completed by the person with the movement disorder as well as a companion or family member. Differences between endorsed items can be used as a measure of anosognosia. Psychiatric measures should be formally evaluated in all persons with basal ganglia dysfunction. Findings from the NPI or a

TABLE 24–5. Evaluation of Patients with Movement Disorders

Assessment	Components
Demographics	Age, education, onset age, patient and family history
Appearance	Grooming, posture, poise
Language	Coherence, goal-directedness, perseveration
Speech	Quantity, spontaneity, rate, rhythm, volume, prosody, articulation
Effort	Attitude, effort
Voluntary movement	Speed, dexterity, timing
Involuntary movement	Tremor, chorea
	With divided attention
	With dual tasks
	Under stress
Psychiatric symptoms	Depression, psychosis, anxiety, obsessions, delusions, hallucinations
Insight	Awareness of movements
	Awareness of psychiatric symptoms
	Awareness of cognitive skill
	Awareness of impaired functions
Functional capacity	Employment, fiscal responsibility, relationships, domestic chores, self-care

structured psychiatric rating scale must be used to interpret cognitive and functional performances as well as to guide when referrals to mental health professionals are necessary. The little research conducted in this area has suggested that psychiatric disorders are undertreated in persons with movement disorders, and proper treatment can increase functional capacity, maintain independence in living, delay institutionalization, and minimize caregiver stress.

■ KEY POINTS

☐ The observation of cognitive and emotional dysfunction in persons with movement disorders is theoretically supported by research describing circuitry connecting discrete areas of frontal cortex with the striatum.

☐ Cognitive impairments associated with movement disorders are often considered "subcortical" syndromes and include slowed cognitive processing, poor learning, decreased working memory, inefficiency in cognitive shifting, and poor executive control.

☐ The presence of dementia in movement disorders varies widely from being absent in TS to nearly 100% in persons with HD.

☐ Referral for cognitive and psychiatric assessment of patients with movement disorders is common and typically involves nonstandard administration of tests and interpretation of performance in the context of the motor abnormality.

☐ Virtually all patients with PD have cognitive impairments, although fewer than 25% exhibit progressive decline and dementia.

☐ Depression is common in PD and occurs in nearly half of PD patients. Rapid identification and treatment is critical because depression increases the severity and progression of the illness.

☐ Dementia is diagnosed in 50% of persons with PSP, whereas high levels of apathy are found in over 90%.

☐ Patients with corticobasal degeneration show higher rates of aphasia (50%) than other basal ganglia disorders.

☐ Approximately one third of patients with Wilson disease present with psychiatric disorders and one third present with cognitive disorders, although cognitive impairments are typically mild.

☐ Cognitive and psychiatric dysfunction may be the presenting symptoms in many movement disorders and has been reported as the first symptoms in up to 70% of persons with Huntington disease.

☐ Cognitive and psychiatric deficits in persons with TS vary with comorbidity. ADHD co-occurs in 50% to 60% and OCD co-occurs in 30% to 60% of patients.

☐ Assessment of movement disorders requires formal evaluation of motor abnormalities, cognitive deficits, psychiatric symptoms, and functional capacity; omission of any area can affect prognosis and course.

KEY READINGS

Guttman M, Kish SJ, Furukawa Y: Parkinson's disease. Can Med Assoc J 263:293–301, 2003.

Lechter DG, Cummings JL: Frontal-Subcortical Circuits in Psychiatric and Neurological Disorders. New York: Guilford Press, 2001.

Paulsen JS, Robinson RG: Huntington's disease, in Hodges J (ed): Early-Onset Dementia. New York: Oxford University Press, 2001, pp. 338–366.

REFERENCES

Aarsland D, Larsen JP, Lim NG, et al: Range of neuropsychiatric disturbances in patients with Parkinson's disease. J Neurol Neurosurg Psychiatry 67: 492–496, 1999.

Adler C: Differential diagnosis of Parkinson's disease. Med Clin North Am 83:349–367, 1999.

Alegret M, Junque C, Valldeoriola F, et al: Effects of bilateral subthalamic stimulation on cognitive function in Parkinson's disease. Arch Neurol 58:1223–1227, 2001.

Alexander GE, DeLong MR, Strick PI: Parallel organization of functionally segregated circuits linking basal ganglia and cortex. Annu Rev Neurosci 9:357–381, 1986.

Almqvist EW, Bloch M, Brinkman R, et al: A worldwide assessment of the frequency of suicide, suicide attempts and psychiatric hospitalizations following predictive testing for Huntington disease. Am J Hum Genet 64:1293–1304, 1999.

American Psychiatric Association: Diagnostic and Statistical Manual of Mental Disorders, ed 4. Washington, DC: Author, 1994.

Appollonio I, Grafman J, Clark K, et al: Implicit and explicit memory in patients with Parkinson's disease with and without dementia. Arch Neurol 51:359–367, 1994.

Babel TB, Warnke PC, Osterag CB: Immediate and longterm outcome after infrathalamic and thalamic lesioning for intractable Tourette's syndrome. J Neurol Neurosurg Psychiatry 70:666–671, 2001.

Bamford KA, Caine ED, Kido DK, et al: A prospective evaluation of cognitive decline in early Huntington's disease: Functional and radiographic correlates. Neurology 45:1867–1873, 1996.

Boll TJ, Heaton R, Reitan R: Neuropsychological and emotional correlates of Huntington's disease. J Ment Nerv Disord 158:61–69, 1974.

Bornstein RA, Yang V: Neuropsychological performance in medicated and unmedicated patients with Tourette's disorder. Am J Psychiatry 148:468–471, 1991.

Brody AL, Saxena S: Brain imaging in obsessive-compulsive disorder: Evidence for the involvement of frontal-subcortical circuitry in the mediation of symptomatology. CNS Spectrums 1:27–41, 1996.

Caparros-Lefebvre D, Pecheux N, Petit V, et al: Which factors predict cognitive decline in Parkinson's disease? J Neurol Neurosurg Psychiatry 58:51–55, 1995.

Cardona F, Orefici G: Group A streptococccal infections and tic disorders in an Italian pediatric population. J Pediatr 138:71–75, 2001.

Cirino P, Chapieski M, Massman P: Card sorting performance and ADHD symptomatology in children and adolescents with Tourette syndrome. J Clin Exp Neuropsychol 22:245–256, 2000.

Cooper J, Sagar H, Doherty S, et al: Different effects of dopaminergic and anticholinergic therapies on cognitive and motor function in Parkinson's disease. A follow-up study of untreated patients. Brain 115:1701–1725, 1992.

Cummings J, Masterman D: Depression in patients with Parkinson's disease. Int J Geriatr Psychiatry 14:711–718, 1999.

Cummings JL: Frontal-subcortical circuits and human behavior. Neurol Rev 50:873–880, 1993.

Cummings JL, Cummingham K: Obsessive-compulsive disorder in Huntington's disease. Biol Psychiatry 31:263–270, 1992.

Cummings JL, Mega M, Gray K, et al: The neuropsychiatric inventory: Comprehensive assessment of psychopathology in dementia. Neurology 44:2308–2314, 1994.

de Groot CM, Yeates KO, Baker GB, et al: Impaired neuropsychological functioning in Tourette's syndrome subjects with co-occurring obsessive-compulsive and attention deficit symptoms. J Neuropsychiatry Clin Neurosci 9:267–272, 1997.

Deckel AW, Morrison D: Evidence of a neurologically based "denial of illness" in patients with Huntington's disease. Arch Clin Neurol 11:295–302, 1996.

Delis DC, Massman PJ, Butters N, et al: Profiles of demented and amnesic patients on the California Verbal Learning Test: Implications for the assessment of memory disorders. Psychol Assess 3:19–26, 1991.

Dening TR, Berrios GE: Wilson's disease: Psychiatric symptoms in 195 cases. Arch Gen Psychiatry 46:1126–1134, 1989.

Di Maria E, Tabaton M, Vigo T, et al: Corticobasal degeneration shares a common genetic background with progressive supranuclear palsy. Ann Neurol 47:374–377, 2000.

Doty RL: Olfactory dysfunction in neurodegenerative disorders, in Getchell TV, Doty RL, Bartoshuk LM, et al (eds): Smell and Taste in Health and Disease. New York: Raven Press, 1991, pp. 735–751.

Dubois B, Pillon B, Legault F, et al: Slowing of cognitive processing in progressive supranuclear palsy. Arch Neurol 45:1194–1199, 1988.

Eskandar EN, Cosgrove GR, Shinobu LA: Surgical treatment of Parkinson disease. JAMA 286:3056–3059, 2001.

Fahn S, Elton RL, members of the UPDRS Development Committee: The Unified Parkinson's Disease Rating Scale, in Fahn S, Marsden CD, Calne DB, et al (eds): Recent Developments in Parkinson's Disease. Florham Park, NJ: Macmillan Healthcare Information, 1987, pp. 153–163, 293–304.

Ferneyhough K, Steirman L, Turner B, et al: Critical periods of suicide risk in Huntington's disease [abstract]. J Neuropsychiatry Clin Neurosci 14:104, Winter 2002.

Folstein MF, Folstein SE, McHugh PR: Mini-Mental State: A practical method for grading the cognitive state of patients for the clinician. J Psychiatr Res 12:189–198, 1975.

Fuster JM: The Prefrontal Cortex. New York, Raven Press, 1997.

Gabrieli JD, Stebbins GT, Singh J, et al: Intact mirror-tracing and impaired rotary-pursuit skill learning in patients with Huntington's disease: Evidence for dissociable memory systems in skill learning. Neuropsychology 11:272–281, 1997.

Georgiou N, Bradshaw JL, Phillips JG, et al: The Simon effect and attention deficits in Gilles de la Tourette's syndrome and Huntington's disease. Brain 118:1305–1318, 1995.

Golbe LI, Davis PH, Schoenberg BS, et al: Prevalence and natural history of progressive supranuclear palsy. Neurology 38:1031–1034, 1988.

Gotham AM, Brown RG, Marsden CD: "Frontal" cognitive function in patients with Parkinson's disease on and off levodopa. Brain 111:299–321, 1988.

Grimes DA, Lang AE, Bergeron CB: Dementia as the most common presentation of cortical-basal ganglionic degeneration. Neurology 53:1969–1974, 1999.

Grace J, Stout JC, Malloy PF: Assessing frontal lobe behavioral syndromes with the frontal lobe personality scale. Assessment 6:269–284, 1999.

Guttman M, Kish SJ, Furukawa Y: Parkinson's disease. Can Med Assoc J 168:293–301, 2003.

Hamilton JM: Cognitive, motor, and behavioral correlates of functional decline in Huntington's disease, in Clinical Psychology. San Diego: University of California, 1998, p. 58.

Hamilton JM, Salmon, DP, Corey-Bloom, J, et al: Behavioral abnormalities contribute to functional decline in Huntington's disease. J Neurol Neurosurg Psychiatry 74:120–122, 2003.

Hodges JR, Salmon DP, Butters N: The nature of the naming deficit in Alzheimer's and Huntington's disease. Brain 114:1547–1558, 1991.

Hoehn M, Yahr MD: Parkinsonism: Onset, progression, and mortality. Neurology 17:427–442, 1967.

Hoogenraad TU, Houwen R: Prevalence and genetics, in Hoogenraad TU (ed): Wilson's Disease. London: WB Saunders, 1996, pp. 14–24.

Huntington Study Group: Unified Huntington's Disease Rating Scale: Reliability and consistency. Mov Disord 11:136–142, 1996.

Illes J: Neurolinguistic features of spontaneous language production dissociate three forms of neurodegenerative disease: Alzheimer's, Huntington's, and Parkinson's. Brain Lang 37:628–642, 1989.

Jacobs D, Salmon DP, Troester AI, et al: Intrusion errors in the figural memory of patients with Alzheimer's and Huntington's disease. Arch Clin Neuropsych 5:49–57, 1990.

Jueptner M, Frith CD, Brooks DJ, et al: Anatomy of motor learning. II. Subcortical structures and learning by trial and error. J Neurophysiol 77:1325–1337, 1997.

Junque C, Alegret M, Nobbe F, et al: Cognitive and behavioral changes after unilateral posteroventral pallidotomy: Relationship with lesional data from MRI. Mov Disord 14:780–789, 1999.

Kertesz A, Martinez-Lage P, Davidson W, et al: The corticobasal degeneration syndrome overlaps progressive aphasia and frontotemporal dementia. Neurology 55:1368–1375, 2000.

Lang A, Lozano A: Medical progress: Parkinson's disease—second of two parts. N Engl J Med 339:1130–1143, 1998.

Lawrence AD, Sahakian BJ, Hodges JR, et al: Executive and mnemonic functions in early Huntington's disease. Brain 119:1633–1645, 1996.

Levy ML, Cummings JL, Fairbanks LA, et al: Apathy is not depression. J Neuropsychiatry Clin Neurosci 10:314–319, 1998.

Litvan I, Agid Y, Galne D, et al: Clinical research criteria for the diagnosis of progressive supranuclear palsy (Steele-Richardson-Olszewski syndrome): Report of the NINDS-SPSP International Workshop. Neurology 47:1–9, 1996.

Litvan I, Cummings JL, Mega M: Neuropsychiatric features of corticobasal degeneration. J Neurol Neurosurg Psychiatry 65:717–721, 1998a.

Litvan I, MacIntyre A, Goetz CG, et al: Accuracy of the clinical diagnoses of Lewy body disease, Parkinson disease and dementia with Lewy bodies. Arch of Neurol 55:969–978, 1998b.

Litvan I, Mega MS, Cummings JL, et al: Neuropsychiatric aspects of progressive supranuclear palsy. Neurology 47:1184–1189, 1996.

Litvan I, Paulsen JS, Mega MS, et al: Neuropsychiatric assessment of patients with hyperkinetic and hypokinetic movement disorders. Arch Neurol 55:1313–1319, 1998c.

Lombardi W, Growss R, Trepanier L, et al: Relationship of lesion location to cognitive outcome following microelectrode-guided pallidotomy for Parkinson's disease. Brain 123:746–758, 2000.

Lopez-Villegas D, Kulisevsky J, Deus J, et al: Neuropsychological alterations in patients with computer tomography-detected basal ganglia calcification. Arch Neurol 53:251–256, 1996.

Maher NE, Golbe LI, Lazzarini AM, et al: Epidemiologic study of 203 sibling pairs with Parkinson's diease: The *Gene*PD study. Neurology 58:79–84, 2002.

Manyam BV, Walters AS, Narla KR: Bilateral striopallidodentate calcinosis: Clinical characteristics of patients seen in a registry. Mov Disord 16:258–264, 2001.

Marder K, Zhao H, Myers RH, et al and The Huntington Study Group: Rate of functional decline in Huntington's disease. Neurology 54:452–458, 2000.

Mattis S: Mental status examination for organic mental syndrome in the elderly patient, in Bellak L, Karasu TB (eds): Geriatric Psychiatry. New York: Grune & Stratton, 1976, pp. 77–122.

Mayberg HS, Solomon DH: Depression in Parkinson's disease: A biochemical and organic viewpoint. Adv Neurol 65:49–60, 1995.

Mayberg HS, Starkstein SE, Peyser CE, et al: Paralimbic frontal lobe hypometabolism in depression associated with Huntington's disease. Neurology 42:1791–1797, 1992.

Mayeux R, Chen J, Mirabello E, et al: An estimate of the incidence of dementia in idiopathic Parkinson's disease. Neurology 40:1513–1517, 1990.

McHugh PR: The neuropsychiatry of basal ganglia disorders. Neuropsychiat Neuropsychol Behav Neurol 2:239–247, 1989.

McKeith IG, Galasko D, Kosaka K, et al: Consensus guidelines for the clinical and pathologic diagnosis of dementia with Lewy bodies (DLB): Report of the consortium on DLB international workshop. Neurology 47:1113–1124, 1996.

Middleton FA, Strick PL: A revised neuroanatomy of frontal-subcortical circuits, in Lichter DG, Cummings, JL (eds): Frontal-Subcortical Circuits in Psychiatric and Neurological Disorders. New York: The Guilford Press, 2001, pp. 44–58.

Middleton FA, Strick PL: Basal ganglia output and cognition: Evidence from anatomical, behavioral, and clinical studies. Brain Cogn 42:188, 2000.

Miyasaki JM, Martin W, Suchowersky O, et al: Practice parameter: Initiation of treatment for Parkinson's disease: An evidence-based review: Report of the quality standards subcommittee of the American Academy of Neurology. Neurology 58:11–17, 2002.

Mohr E, Claus JJ, Brouwers P: Basal ganglia disease and visuospatial cognition: Are these disease-specific impairments? Behav Neurol 10:67–75, 1997.

Morris M: Psychiatric aspects of Huntington's disease, in Harper PS (ed): Huntington's Disease. London: WB Saunders, 1991, pp. 81–126.

Mouradian M: Recent advances in the genetics and pathogenesis of Parkinson's disease. Neurology 58:308–310, 2002.

Nordin S, Paulsen JS, Murphy C: Sensory- and memory-mediated olfactory dysfunction in Huntington's disease. J Int Neuropsychol Soc 1:271–280, 1995.

Oder W, Grimm G, Kollegger H, et al: Neurological and neuropsychiatric spectrum of Wilson's disease: A prospective study of 45 cases. J Neurol 238:281–287, 1991.

Pahwa R: Progressive supranuclear palsy. Med Clin North Am 83:369–379, 1999.

Parkinson Study Group: A multicenter assessment of dopamine transporter imaging with DOPASCAN/SPECT in parkinsonism. Neurology 55:1540–1547, 2000.

Paulsen JS, Butters N, Sadek JR, et al: Distinct cognitive profiles of cortical and subcortical dementia in advanced illness. Neurology 45:951–956, 1995a.

Paulsen JS, Butters N, Salmon DP, et al: Prism adaptation in Alzheimer's and Huntington's disease. Neuropsychology 7:73–81, 1993.

Paulsen JS, Como P, Rey G, et al. and The Huntington Study Group: The clinical utility of the Stroop test in a multicenter study of Huntington's disease [abstract]. J Int Neuropsychol Soc 2:35, 1996a.

Paulsen JS, Mega MS, Cummings JL: The spectrum of behavioral changes in Huntington's disease. J Neurospychiatry 9:655–656, 1997.

Paulsen JS, Salmon DP, Monsch AU, et al: Discrimination of cortical from subcortical dementias on the basis of memory and problem-solving tests. J Clin Psychol 51:48–58, 1995b.

Paulsen JS, Stout JC, Delapena J, et al: Frontal behavioral syndromes in cortical and subcortical dementia. Assessment 3:327–337, 1996b.

Penney JB Jr, Young AB, Shoulson I, et al: Huntington's disease in Venezuela: 7 years of follow-up on symptomatic and asymptomatic individuals. Mov Disord 5:93–99, 1990.

Pillon B, Blin J, Vidailhet M, et al: The neuropsychological pattern of corticobasal degeneration: Comparison with progressive supranuclear palsy and Alzheimer's disease. Neurology 45:1477–1483, 1995.

Rathbun JK: Neuropsychological aspects of Wilson's disease. Int J Neurosci 85:221–229, 1996.

Rettig G, York M, Lai E, et al: Neuropsychological outcome after unilateral pallidotomy for the treatment of Parkinson's disease. J Neurol Neurosurg Psychiatry 69:326–336, 2000.

Rich JB, Troyer AK, Bylsma FW, et al: Longitudinal analysis of phonemic clustering and switching during word-list generation in Huntington's disease. Neuropsychology 13:525–531, 1999.

Richard IH, Kurlan R: A survey of antidepressant drug use in Parkinson's disease: Parkinson Study Group. Neurology 49:1168–1170, 1997.

Robbins TW, James M, Owen AM, et al: Cognitive deficits in progressive supranuclear palsy, Parkinson's disease, and multiple system atrophy in tests sensitive to frontal lobe dysfunction. J Neurol Neurosurg Psychiatry 54:79–88, 1994.

Rodman R, Burnstine M, Esmaeli B, et al: Wilson's disease: Presymptomatic patients and Kayser-Fleischer rings. Ophthalmic Genet 18:79–85, 1997.

Rohrer D, Salmon DP, Wixted JT, et al: The disparate effects of Alzheimer's disease and Huntington's disease on semantic memory. Neuropsychology 13:381–388, 1999.

Rothlind JC, Brandt J: A brief assessment of frontal and subcortical functions in dementia. J Neuropsychiatry Clin Neurosci 5:73–77, 1993.

Saint-Cyr JA, Trepanier LL, Kumar R, et al: Neuropsychological consequences of chronic bilateral stimulation of the subthalamic nucleus in Parkinson's disease. Brain 123:2091–2108, 2000.

Santacruz P, Uttl B, Litvan I, et al: Progressive supranuclear palsy. Neurology 50:1637–1647, 1998.

Schuerholz LJ, Singer HS, Denckla MB: Gender study of neuropsychological and neuromotor function in children with Tourette syndrome with and without attention-deficit hyperactivity disorder. J Child Neurol 13:277–282, 1998.

Shiwach RS, Patel V: Aggressive behaviour in Huntington's disease: A cross-sectional study in a nursing home population. Behav Neurol 6:43–47, 1993.

Shoulson I, Fahn S: Huntington's disease: Clinical care and evaluation. Neurology 29:1–3, 1979.

Siemers E, Foroud T, Bill DJ, et al: Motor changes in presymptomatic Huntington disease gene carriers. Arch Neurol 53:487–492, 1996.

Singer HS: Current issues in Tourette syndrome. Mov Disord 15:1051–1063, 2000.

Snowden JS, Craufurd D, Griffiths HL, et al: Awareness of involuntary movements in Huntington's disease. Arch Neurol 55:801–805, 1998.

Soliveri P, Monza D, Paridi D, et al: Cognitive and magnetic resonance imaging aspects of corticobasal degeneration and progressive supranuclear palsy. Neurology 53:502–507, 1999.

Speedie LJ, Brake N, Folstein SE, et al: Comprehension of prosody in Huntington's disease. J Neurol Neurosurg Psychiatry 53:607–610, 1990.

Sprengelmeyer R, Lange H, Homberg V: The pattern of attentional deficits in Huntington's disease. Brain 118:145–152, 1995.

Stahl SM: Basal ganglia neuropharmacology and obsessive-compulsive disorder: The obsessive compulsive disorder hypothesis of basal ganglia dysfunction. Psychopharmacol Bull 24:370–374, 1988.

Starkstein SE, Bolduc PL, Mayberg HS, et al: Cognitive impairments and depression in Parkinson's disease: A follow up study. J Neurol Neurosurg Psychiatry 53:597–602, 1990.

Starkstein SE, Mayberg HS: Depression in Parkinson disease, in Starkstein SE, Robinson RG (eds): Depression in Neurologic Disease. Baltimore, MD: Johns Hopkins University Press, 1993, pp. 97–116.

Starkstein SE, Mayberg HS, Leiguarda R, et al: A prospective longitudinal study of depression, cognitive decline, and physical impairments in patients with Parkinson's disease. J Neurol Neurosurg Psychiatry 55:377–382, 1992.

Stout JC, Rodawalt WC, Siemers ER: Risky decision making in Huntington's disease. J Int Neuropsychol Soc 7:92–101, 2001.

Tandberg E, Larsen JP, Aarsland D, et al: Risk factors for depression in Parkinson disease. Arch Neurol 54:625–630, 1997.

van Wattum PJ, Chappell PB, Zelterman D, et al: Patterns of response to acute naloxone infusion in Tourette's syndrome. Mov Disord 15:1252–1254, 2000.

Wenning G, Tison F, Ben Shlomo Y, et al: Multiple system atrophy: A review of 203 pathologically proven cases. Mov Disord 12:133–147, 1997.

Willingham DB, Koroshetz WJ, Peterson EW: Motor skills have diverse neural bases: Spared and impaired skill acquisition in Huntington's disease. Neuropsychology 10:315–321, 1996.

Young AB, Penney JB Jr: Biochemical and functional organization of the basal ganglia, in Tolosa JJE (ed): Parkinson's Disease and Movement Disorders. Baltimore, MD: Williams & Wilkins, 1998, pp. 1–12.

Zakzanis KK: The subcortical dementia of Huntington's disease. J Clin Exp Neuropsychol 20:565–578, 1998.

Subcortical Deficits

Jeremy D. Schmahmann

Affect
Behavior
Cerebellum
Cerebrocerebellar
Cognition
Diaschisis
Disconnection syndrome
Distributed neural circuit
Dysmetria of thought
Fiber pathways
Thalamocortical
Thalamus
Universal cerebellar transform

INTRODUCTION*

Higher-order functions, such as intellect, memory, and reasoning, have long been held to be exclusively within the domain of the cerebral cortex. Clinical-anatomic correlations in behavioral neurology have been instrumental in developing this notion, and anatomic studies and experimental observation in animals have further solidified this relationship. Along with the deepening understanding of the functions of the cerebral cortex, there has been a line of investigation pointing to the importance of subcortical structures in cognition,

---

*A list of abbreviations used in this chapter appears on pages 585–587.

personality, and mood. This is most readily appreciated in the investigations of the limbic system, including such "subcortical" structures as the amygdala, septal nuclei, and fornix, which are integrally involved in emotion. Studies of the thalamus, basal ganglia (discussed elsewhere in this volume), cerebellum, and cerebral white matter have also indicated that cognitive processing and the regulation of mood are not confined to the cerebral cortex. Clinical and anatomic observations have supported the hypothesis that nervous system function is subserved by distributed neural circuits comprised of distinct nodes geographically separated in the brain (see Mesulam, 1981). This concept is predicated on the intrinsic architecture of different brain regions, as well as the highly organized connections that link them. In this view, subcortical structures are involved in both sensorimotor and complex behaviors, in a manner determined by both their intrinsic anatomic organization as well as their links with the cerebral cortex. In this chapter we discuss the role of thalamus, cerebellum, and white matter pathways in supporting cognition and emotion. We attempt to understand the relationship between cognitive disorders and these neural structures beneath the cerebral cortex, in light of the anatomic principles that subserve the concept of distributed neural circuits.

THALAMUS

Prion diseases such as the thalamic form of Creutzfeldt-Jakob disease and fatal familial insomnia, and thalamic involvement in system degenerations, are known to be associated with impaired cognitive performance (Martin, 1997). Fisher (1959) reported confusion and language impairment following pathologically documented thalamic hemorrhage, and the early thalamotomy and thalamic stimulation studies, discussed below, indicated a role for the thalamus in linguistic expression. The consistent involvement of the medial dorsal nucleus of the thalamus, along with the medial mamillary bodies, in the thiamine-deficient amnestic-confabulatory syndrome of Korsakoff (Victor et al., 1971) further established that disorders of higher-order behavior are associated with focal thalamic lesions. More widespread attention to the behavioral consequences of thalamic lesions was prompted by the early computed tomography (CT) scan demonstration of ischemic or hemorrhagic lesions in thalamus as the anatomic correlate of cognitive impairment, by the elucidation of the

anatomy of thalamic interrelations with cerebral cortex, and by the development of the concept that cognition is subserved by interconnected neural circuits, or networks, geographically distributed throughout the nervous system. It is now apparent that thalamic lesions are associated with a complex range of deficits that mimic many of those witnessed following lesions of the cerebral cortex. These include deficits in sensorimotor functions and in cognitive domains such as language, memory, attention, and executive function, as well as in autonomic and emotional systems. Some questions that arise from this recognition include how these deficits manifest, which nuclei are accountable for the different impairments, and how the disorders are grouped into syndromes as a consequence of common vascular supply. Additionally, why do thalamic lesions produce behavioral changes at all, and what are the fundamental functions of thalamic nuclei?

Thalamic Nuclear Topography and Connections

Much of the knowledge of thalamic anatomy, connections, and function has been derived from work in nonhuman primates. Previously accepted nomenclature of the human thalamus (Hassler 1959; Van Buren & Borke, 1972) is quite different from that used in the monkey (Olszewski, 1952; Jones 1981, 1985; Ilinsky & Kultas-Ilinsky, 1987), presenting a challenge to the further understanding of the human thalamus. More recent histologic analyses have resolved these dissimilarities (Jones, 1997; Macchi & Jones, 1997) and made it possible to describe the human thalamus using nomenclature readily interchangeable with that of other species in which experimental work has been performed (Fig. 25-1).

The thalamic nuclei have well-defined cytoarchitectonic features, and the connections with the cerebral cortex as well as with basal ganglia and peripheral sensorimotor afferents are organized with great respect for topography. With the exception of the reticular nucleus, the connections with the cerebral cortex are reciprocal. The laminar termination and origination of thalamocortical and corticothalamic connections are determined by the pattern of the connections, and these in turn reflect the putative functions of the nuclei. Diffuse, or nonspecific, projections to cortex from intralaminar nuclei terminate in layer I, with regional zones of dominance. Some limbic and associative nuclei

---

FIGURE 25-1. Diagram illustrating the nuclei of the human thalamus, according to Jones (1997). Horizontal sections are seen above, from ventral to dorsal. Coronal sections below proceed from rostral to caudal. The revised nomenclature correlates with terminology used in the monkey. The earlier nomenclature of Hassler (1959) is presented in parentheses and is not further described. See List of Abbreviations. (From Jones EG: A description of the human thalamus, in Steriade M, Jones EG, McCormick DA [eds]: Thalamus: Experimental and Clinical Aspects. New York: Elsevier, 1997, Vol. II, pp. 425–499.)

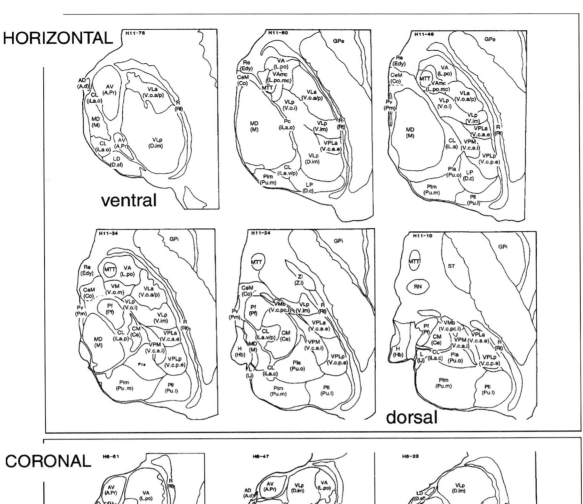

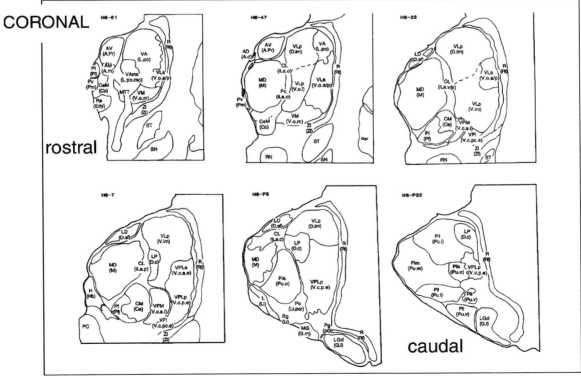

also project to layer I, but in areas in which they have more focal or specific projections in the deeper layers as well. Specific projections arise from most of the remaining thalamic nuclei and terminate in layer III, although projections to the somatosensory and auditory cortices terminate more heavily in layer IV than in layer III, and those to the primary visual cortex terminate only in layer IV. Additionally, thalamocortical fibers to most cortical areas have some terminations at the junction of layers V and VI. The laminar origin of cortical projections to the thalamus also varies. Cortical layer V neurons project to thalamic nuclei that have diffuse cortical projections, whereas cortical layer VI neurons project to the somatosensory nuclei (Jones, 1985). Each cortical area has a unique connectional pattern within the thalamus, and the topographic organization within nuclei is precisely arranged. The corticothalamic projections to the associative nuclei, in particular, are not necessarily limited by nuclear boundaries, however. Further, there is a rod-to-column pattern of the thalamocortical interrelationship: a single vertically oriented cortical column is linked with one or more "rods" of thalamic neurons or neuronal dentritic arborizations oriented in the rostrocaudal or mediolateral dimension (Jones, 1985).

Behavioral Role of Thalamic Nuclei

The functions of some thalamic nuclei are now quite well established, although conclusions regarding a number of others are still tentative. The thalamus is extensively interconnected with all regions of the cerebral cortex, and nuclear and intranuclear topography of reciprocal thalamocortical connections is exquisitely maintained throughout. Focal lesions would be expected to disrupt discrete thalamocortical and thalamosubcortical circuits that are part of a more widespread neural system, and the resulting neurologic deficit should theoretically be specific to each thalamic nuclear subregion. Conclusions about the function of thalamic nuclei are presently based on two main sources of information: (1) direct evidence from studies of the thalamus, including physiology and focal pathology, and the consequences of these lesion or physiologic studies on neurologic function; and (2) indirect, derivative evidence from knowledge of the functional attributes of the cortical or subcortical areas with which the different thalamic nuclei have been shown to be anatomically linked in anatomic and physiologic studies in experimental animals. Before discussing the clinical syndromes resulting from thalamic lesions, it may be helpful to review a clinically directed synopsis of the chief functional properties of the major thalamic nuclei as currently conceptualized (Table 25-1).

Reticular/Intralaminar

The reticular nucleus surrounds the thalamus and conveys afferents from the cerebral cortex exclusively into the thalamus. It is critical for arousal and attention, maintains normal rhythmicity of thalamic neuronal firing, and is central in the consideration of the pathophysiology of epilepsy and related disorders (Huguenard & Prince, 1997) and in the discussion of the neural substrates of conscious awareness (Llinas & Ribary, 2001).

The intralaminar nuclei include the paracentral (Pcn), central lateral (CL), centromedian (CM), parafascicular (Pf), and a number of "midline" nuclei, such as the paraventricular, rhomboid, and reunions. These nuclei play a role in autonomic drive, and they may provide the striatum with attention-specific sensory information important for conditional responses. They receive afferents from the brainstem, spinal cord, and cerebellum and have reciprocal connections with cerebral hemispheres. They project diffusely to the first layer of cortex throughout the cerebral hemispheres. Additionally, CM and CL have focused projections to the third layer. The CM/Pf nuclei have strong reciprocal connections with the basal ganglia, arranged as tightly connected functional circuits. According to Sidibe and colleagues (2002), a "sensorimotor" circuit links the putamen with the CM through the ventrolateral part of the internal segment of the globus pallidus (GPi); a "limbic" circuit links the ventral striatum with the Pf through the rostromedial GPi; and cognitive circuits link the caudate with the Pf through the dorsal GPi and through the pars reticulata of the substantia nigra. The midline nuclei that receive input from the periaqueductal gray as well as the spinothalamic tract constitute the medial thalamic system involved in processing the motivational-affective components of nociceptive information (Bentivoglio et al., 1993; Lenz & Dougherty, 1997; Willis, 1997).

Limbic

The limbic thalamic nuclei are defined by their reciprocal anatomic connections with limbic structures in the cingulate gyrus, hippocampus, parahippocampal formation, entorhinal cortex, retrosplenial cortex, orbitofrontal and medial prefrontal cortices, and with subcortical structures including the mamillary bodies and amygdala (Yakovlev et al., 1960; Locke et al., 1961; Yeterian & Pandya, 1988). They include the anterior nuclear group—anteroventral (AV), anteromedial (AM), and anterodorsal (AD) nuclei, and the dorsally and more posteriorly situated lateral dorsal (LD) nucleus. The mamillothalamic tract and ventral amygdalothalamic tract, which link the anterior nuclei with other limbic regions, pass through the anterior thalamus. Other nuclei, not traditionally thought of as

TABLE 25-1. Behavioral Role of Thalamic Nuclei

Major functional grouping	Thalamic nuclei	Putative functional attributes
Reticular	Reticular	Arousal, rhythmicity, role in epileptogenesis
Intralaminar	CM, Pf, CL, Pcn, midline (reunions, paraventricular, rhomboid)	Arousal, attention, motivation, affective components of pain
Limbic	Anterior nuclear group (AD, AM, AV) Lateral dorsal nucleus Other—MDmc, medial pulvinar, ventral anterior	Learning, memory, emotional experience and expression, drive, motivation
Sensory	Medial geniculate	Auditory
	Lateral geniculate	Visual
	Ventroposterior – Lateral (VPL)	Somatosensory body and limbs
	– Medial (VPM)	Somatosensory head and neck
	– Medial, parvicellular (VPMpc)	Gustatory
	– Inferior (VPI)	Vestibular
Effector	Ventral anterior – Reticulata recipient	Complex behaviors
	– Pallidal recipient	Motor programming
	Ventral medial	Motor
	Ventral lateral – Ventral part	Motor
	– Dorsal part	Language (dominant hemisphere)
Associative	Lateral posterior	High-order somatosensory and visuospatial integration—spatial cognition
	Medial dorsal – Medial, magnocellular (MDmc)	Drive, motivation, inhibition, emotion
	– Intermediate, parvicellular (MDpc)	Executive functions, working memory
	– Lateral, multiform (MDmf)	Attention, horizontal gaze
	Pulvinar – Medial	Supramodal, high-level association region across multiple domains
	– Lateral	Somatosensory, visual association
	– Inferior	Visual association
	– Anterior (pulvinar oralis)	Intramodality somatosensory association, pain appreciation

From Schmahmann JD: Vascular syndromes of the thalamus. Stroke 34: 2264–2278, 2003.

limbic, have subcomponents that are reciprocally interconnected with the cingulate gyrus and other structures in the limbic system, and thus should be considered limbic as well. These are the magnocellular (large-celled) division of the medial dorsal nucleus (MDmc), and parts of the medial pulvinar and ventral anterior (VA) nuclei. Like their cortical and other subcortical counterparts (Mesulam, 1988; Devinsky & Luciano, 1997), the limbic thalamic nuclei are critical for learning and memory, emotional experience and expression, and drive and motivation.

Sensory Nuclei

The sensory nuclei include the medial geniculate nucleus (MGN), lateral geniculate nucleus (LGN), and ventroposterior nuclear group (lateral, medial, and inferior—VPL, VPM, VPI).

The functions of the medial geniculate nucleus are confined to the auditory realm. By virtue of its connections with both primary and association auditory cortices, it is likely to play a role in higher-level auditory processing as well as in simple audition (Mesulam & Pandya, 1973; Pandya et al., 1994; Hackett et al., 1998).

The lateral geniculate nucleus, a critical component of the visual system, projects in a highly ordered manner to the primary and secondary visual cortices (Kennedy & Bullier, 1985). It also receives projections back from the visual areas (Shatz & Rakic, 1981), indicating that higher-order processing can influence visual perception at an early stage.

The VPL and VPM nuclei are reciprocally interconnected with the primary somatosensory cortices. VPL serves body and limbs, and VPM serves head and neck (Jones & Powell, 1970). Gustatory function is subserved by VPMpc, the parvicellular (small cell) division of VPM (Pritchard et al., 1986). The somatotopy of these nuclei is highly precise, and lesions of VPL and VPM produce focal sensory deficits in the affected regions. The VPI nucleus has anatomic connections with the rostral inferior parietal lobule and SII, that is, the second somatosensory area in the parietal operculum (Yeterian & Pandya, 1985; Schmahmann & Pandya, 1990). By virtue of its anatomic connections with the frontal operculum and physiologic studies, VPI is also implicated in vestibular functions (Deecke et al., 1977).

Spinothalamic and trigeminothalamic inputs, and the presence of topographically organized wide dynamic neurons and nociceptive-specific, or high-threshold, neurons in the ventroposterior nuclei (VPL, VPM, and VPI) facilitate the role of the sensory nuclei in the lateral, or specific, component of the pain system (Willis, 1997).

Effector

The effector, or more commonly, "motor" nuclei, include the VA, ventromedial (VM), and ventral lateral (VL) nuclei. The VA nucleus, according to Ilinsky and Kultas-Ilinsky (1987), incorporates the VLa of Jones (1997). Afferents to precise and segregated subregions within VA are derived from the pars reticulata of the substantia nigra (Jones, 1985; Francois et al., 2002) and from the internal globus pallidus (Ilinsky & Kultas-Ilinsky, 1987). The reticulata recipient VA nucleus is linked with premotor, supplementary motor (Schell & Strick, 1984), and prefrontal cortices (Goldman-Rakic & Porrino, 1985), as well as with the caudal parts of the posterior parietal cortices (Schmahmann & Pandya, 1990) and the rostral cingulate gyrus (Vogt et al., 1987). The pallidal recipient VA is linked with premotor cortices (Jones, 1997). The functions of the VA nucleus are not well established. It is possible that the dystonic component of motor syndromes from some rostral thalamic lesions may be accounted for by involvement of nuclear groups in VA that are linked with motor and premotor cortices, whereas complex behavioral syndromes seen in lesions of the anterior thalamus may be accounted for by the VA regions linked with the cingulate, prefrontal and posterior parietal association, and paralimbic cortices.

The VL nucleus, like the cerebellum from which it receives its input, has traditionally been thought of as a relay nucleus from cerebellum to motor cortex. This is not the case in its entirety. The posterior part of VL (VLp according to Jones, 1997; VL according to Ilinsky & Kultas-Ilinsky, 1987) has complex connec-

tions. Its ventral part is linked with the motor cortex, whereas the dorsal part has projections through its caudal and pars postrema subdivisions to the posterior parietal cortices (Schmahmann & Pandya, 1990), prefrontal cortices (Kievit & Kuypers, 1977; Künzle & Akert, 1977; Middleton & Strick, 1994), and upper bank of the superior temporal sulcus (Yeterian & Pandya, 1989). Lesions in the VL nucleus are responsible for the ataxic component of the motor syndrome following thalamic lesions and probably for the mild motor weakness seen in lesions that avoid the adjacent posterior limb of the internal capsule. It is likely, although not proven, that the ventral part of VL is responsible. Given the consistent involvement of the VL nucleus in language processing (Johnson & Ojemann, 2000), and the recent elucidation of the role of the cerebellum in linguistic disorders (Leiner et al., 1986; Molinari et al., 1997; Schmahmann & Sherman, 1998a; Riva & Giorgi, 2000), it is likely that the cerebellar-recipient dorsal sectors of VL that project to prefrontal, superior temporal, and posterior parietal areas play a role in language.

Associative

The associative thalamic nuclei include the lateral posterior, medial dorsal, and pulvinar nuclei.

The lateral posterior (LP) nucleus has strong anatomic connections with the posterior parietal cortices (Weber & Yin, 1984; Yeterian & Pandya, 1985; Schmahmann & Pandya, 1990), medial and dorsolateral extrastriate cortices (Yeterian & Pandya, 1997), and paralimbic regions in the posterior cingulate and medial parahippocampal regions (Yeterian & Pandya, 1988). Anatomic studies suggest that its role is an integrative one in the intramodal and multimodal associative somatosensory and visual systems. It may be expected to participate in higher-order somatosensory and visual-spatial function, such as in goal-directed reaching (Acuña et al., 1990), and possibly in conceptual and analytical thinking.

The medial dorsal (MD) nucleus has strong reciprocal connections with the prefrontal cortex (Tobias, 1975; Goldman-Rakic & Porrino, 1985; Giguere & Goldman-Rakic, 1988; Barbas et al., 1991; Siwek & Pandya, 1991). The frontal behavioral syndromes following thalamic lesions routinely involve MD, but the unique architectonic features of the different MD sectors that are linked with different regions of the prefrontal cortex are likely to determine the precise nature of the behavioral deficit.

The medial part (magnocellular MDmc) is linked with paralimbic regions—medial and orbital prefrontal cortices, as well as with the amygdala, basal forebrain, and olfactory and entorhinal cortices (Russchen et al., 1987; Graff-Radford et al., 1990). Apathy, abulia, disinhibition, and failure to inhibit inappropriate behaviors are likely to result from MDmc lesions, but the extent to which the amnestic (Victor et al., 1971) and aphasic disorders (Bogousslavsky et al., 1988) following medial thalamic lesions are a result of MDmc involvement is unresolved, because lesions are seldom confined to this subnucleus.

The intermediate part of MD (the parvicellular MDpc) is linked with the dorsolateral and dorsomedial prefrontal cortices, areas 9 and 46. The properties of these cortical areas suggest that the dysexecutive problems stemming from MD lesions, including poor working memory and perseveration, are a result of involvement of MDpc.

The laterally placed multiformis part (MDmf) is linked with area 8 in the arcuate concavity, and therefore the impairments of volitional horizontal gaze, as well as deficits in attention, are possibly related to involvement of this sector of MD.

The pulvinar, like the MD nucleus, has subcomponents with unique architecture and connectional properties. Pulvinar, however, is even more diverse than MD with respect to its connections, and possibly with respect to its functional attributes as well.

Different subregions within the medial pulvinar (PM) are linked with the prefrontal cortex (Asanuma et al., 1985; Yeterian & Pandya, 1988; Romanski et al., 1997), posterior parietal lobe (Asanuma et al., 1985; Yeterian & Pandya, 1985; Schmahmann & Pandya, 1990), auditory-related (Pandya et al., 1994) and multimodal cortices of the superior temporal region (Yeterian & Pandya, 1991), paralimbic cingulate and parahippocampal cortices (Yeterian & Pandya, 1988), and the limbic insula (Mufson & Mesulam, 1984). Some reports have suggested that pulvinar contributes to language processing (Ojemann et al., 1968) and that pulvinar lesions result in spatial neglect (Karnath et al., 2002) and affective and psychotic manifestations (Guard et al., 1986). These anatomic connections and clinical features suggest that the medial pulvinar is truly an "associative" thalamus.

The lateral pulvinar (PL) is linked with posterior parietal (Asanuma et al., 1985; Schmahmann & Pandya, 1990), superior temporal (Yeterian & Pandya, 1991), and medial and dorsolateral extrastriate cortices (Yeterian & Pandya, 1997), as well as with the superior colliculus (Robinson & Cowie, 1997). It may contribute to the integration of somatosensory and visual information.

The inferior pulvinar (PI) is a strongly visual region, linked both with temporal lobe areas concerned with visual feature discrimination, and with ventrolateral and ventromedial extrastriate areas concerned with the analysis of visual motion (Cusick et al., 1993; Yeterian & Pandya, 1997). It also receives direct visual input from retinal ganglion cells (Cowey et al., 1994) and from the visual neurons of the superior colliculus (Robinson & Cowie, 1997).

The anterior pulvinar, or pulvinar oralis (PO), is interconnected with the intramodality somatosensory association cortices in the rostral part of the posterior parietal region, and with SII, the second somatosensory region (Asanuma et al., 1985; Yeterian & Pandya, 1985; Acuña et al., 1990; Schmahmann & Pandya, 1990). The PO nucleus may also be important in the appreciation of pain, among other possible functions.

Other nuclei such as the suprageniculate, limitans, and posterior nuclei are small in size, but may be important constituents of the "posterior nuclei of thalamus" (Jones, 1985) thought to be responsible for the perception of pain in the animal model.

Specificity of Thalamocortical Connections

The sensorimotor, effector, limbic, and associative regions of cerebral cortex are linked with distinctly different sets of thalamic nuclei. The thalamic projections to the posterior parietal lobe will serve here to exemplify this concept (Schmahmann & Pandya, 1990), although a similar general schema can be discerned from a number of anatomic studies. All architectonic areas within both the superior and inferior parietal lobules are linked with neuronal populations within the LP and PL nuclei, and to a lesser degree with CL and the pars postrema of the ventral lateral nucleus (VLps). This suggests that there are subpopulations of thalamic neurons in LP and PL, in particular, which in essence "define" the posterior parietal cortex. Superimposed on this overall thalamic-posterior parietal system, the connections of the superior parietal lobule versus the inferior parietal lobule differ from each other with respect to their input from pulvinar. Thus, PO projects preferentially to the superior parietal lobule, PM to the inferior parietal lobule. Furthermore, the thalamic connections become progressively elaborated as one moves from rostral to caudal within both the superior and the inferior parietal lobules. More rostral areas are related to modality-specific thalamic nuclei, whereas more caudal regions, concerned with complex functions, derive their input from multimodal and limbic nuclei (Fig. 25-2). Within the thalamus, a rostrocaudal difference is reflected within the LP and PO nuclei that project to both superior and inferior parietal lobules. Rostral parietal subdivisions receive projections from ventral regions within these thalamic nuclei, caudal parietal afferents arise from the dorsal parts of these nuclei, and the intervening cortical levels receive projections from intermediate positions within the nuclei. A similar topographic arrangement is present in the medial pulvinar projections to the inferior parietal lobule (Fig. 25-3).

This precise arrangement of thalamocortical connections, exemplified here by the thalamic projections to the posterior parietal cortices, suggests that thalamic

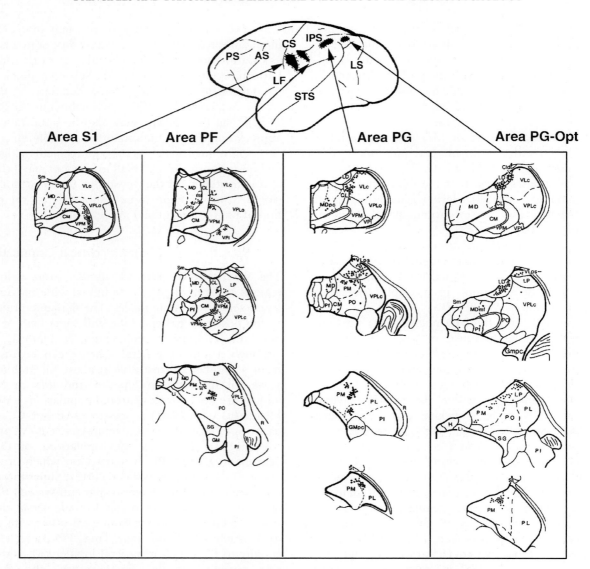

FIGURE 25-2. Diagrammatic representation (*above*) of thalamic projections to the posterior parietal cortices in the rhesus monkey. Wheat germ agglutinated horseradish peroxidase or fluorescent retrograde tracer injections (shown as blackened areas), injected into the inferior parietal lobule, resulted in labeled neurons in thalamus (shown as black dots). Projections to primary somatosensory cortex S1, area PF, area PG, and area PG-Opt are shown in thalamic nuclei in selected representative rostral to caudal levels of thalamus. (Thalamic nomenclature according to Olszewski, 1952. Parietal lobe nomenclature according to Pandya & Seltzer, 1982.)

subpopulations of neurons may together represent the functional equivalent of the cortical architectonic regions with which they are reciprocally interconnected. Further, the heterogeneity of thalamic nuclear cyto-architecture suggests that each nucleus uses its own fundamental mechanism to contribute a particular neural transform to the neural circuit in which it participates. The higher-order deficits resulting from lesions of thalamus may then be viewed within the context of each thalamic nuclear region participating in a unique manner in the elaboration of different behaviors. The focused link between primary somatosensory cortex,

S1, and the VPM and CL nuclei, stands in contrast to the connections of caudal inferior parietal lobule, area PG-Opt, that is interconnected with multiple thalamic nuclei, each imbued with different functional attributes, that is, the LD nucleus as well as LP, PL, CL, VLps, PM, and MDpc. Complex, cognitive modalities such as those reflected in the caudal inferior parietal lobule, may thus require the contribution of the neural transforms unique to each of these thalamic nuclei. Focal thalamic lesions involving different thalamic nuclei, then, should result in distinct behavioral syndromes. Further, thalamic lesions should mimic the "parent cortical syndrome" in

Parietal cortical region	S1	Area PF	Area PG	Area PG-Opt
Principal thalamic nuclear afferents	**Sensory** VPM	**Sensory** VPM VPI **Associative** Pulvinar oralis Lateral posterior Pulvinar medialis	**Associative** Pulvinar medialis Lateral posterior **Effector** Ventral lateral (caudal and pars postrema)	**Associative** Pulvinar medialis Lateral posterior **Effector** Ventral lateral (pars postrema) **Intralaminar** Paracentralis **Limbic** Lateral dorsal Anterior nuclei
Putative functional properties	Primary unimodal somatosensory	Intramodality association within somatosensory domain; for graphesthesia and stereognosis	Multimodal somatosensory and visual: for integration of visual and cutaneokinesthetic spatial information	Multimodal associative and paralimbic: visual spatial and somesthetic stimuli invested with emotional and motivational valence

FIGURE 25-2. *(Continued)* The table *(above)* summarizes the areas injected with tracer, the principal thalamic nuclei demonstrating retrogradely labeled neurons, and the putative functional attributes of the cortical areas studied. See List of Abbreviations. (Derived from Schmahmann JD, Pandya DN: Anatomical investigation of thalamic projections to the posterior parietal cortices in rhesus monkey. J Comp Neurol 295:299–326, 1990.)

terms of hemispheric specialization—impairments in linguistic function arise from lesions of the left thalamus, spatial impairments and neglect syndromes from lesions of the right thalamus.

A Note on Thalamic Fiber Systems

In attempting to understand the effects of thalamic lesions on behavior, it is necessary to consider the roles of the fiber systems that link thalamic nuclei with other brain regions, and of fiber systems that pass through the thalamus.

The mamillothalamic tract (of Vicq d' Azyr) connects the anterior thalamic nuclear group with the mamillary body, which in turn is linked with the hippocampus and entorhinal cortex. This tract, along with the fornix, tightly binds the anterior thalamic nuclei into the neural system that subserves learning and memory.

The ventral amygdalofugal pathway links the amygdala with the medial part of MD, and damage may, therefore, contribute to emotional dysregulation and amnesia.

Lesions of the medial thalamus disrupt the corticofugal fibers that lead from motor and premotor cortices to the nucleus of Darkschewitz and the interstitial nucleus of Cajal in the midbrain that are concerned with vertical gaze (up and down). They also disrupt the fibers to the rostral nucleus of the medial longitudinal fasciculus in the tectal region that is concerned chiefly with downgaze (Leigh & Zee, 1983). It has been sug-

gested that disruption of these pathways produces the aberrations of oculomotor control in thalamic lesions, rather than damage to the nuclei themselves.

The thalamic "peduncles" at the superior, medial and inferior, and lateral aspects of the thalamus convey information in and out of the thalamus. Lesions restricted to these small white matter tracts occur rarely, if at all, but their trajectory to the cerebral cortex and basal ganglia are relevant in considering the anatomic basis of thalamic effects on behavior.

The anterior limb of the internal capsule conveys the bulk of the prefrontal and anterior cingulate interaction with the thalamus (mostly the medial dorsal and the anterior thalamic nuclei), and focal lesions of the anterior limb, or genu, of the capsule essentially disconnect these nuclei from their cortical targets, producing a complex behavioral syndrome (Schmahmann, 1984; Tatemichi et al., 1992; Chukwudelunzu et al., 2001). The anterior limb also conveys prefrontal input to the cerebrocerebellar system, so the effects of this lesion are not exclusively on the thalamocortical interaction.

Physiologic Evidence

Early evidence for the role of thalamus in cognition was provided by the demonstration of anomia following stimulation of the pulvinar (Ojemann et al., 1968). In a series of physiologic studies spanning over three decades (Ojemann et al., 1968; Ojemann & Ward 1971; summarized in Johnson & Ojemann, 2000), electrical

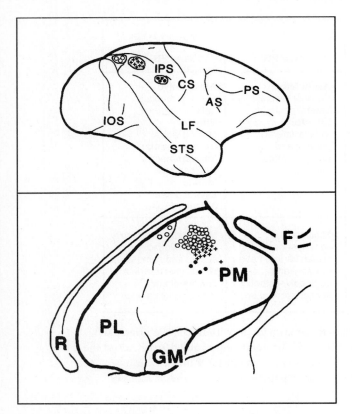

FIGURE 25-3. Diagrammatic representation of the topographic organization of projections from the medial pulvinar thalamic nucleus (PM) to the posterior parietal region of the rhesus monkey. Fluorescent retrograde tracers were placed in area PF (*filled circles*), area PG (*crosses*), and area PG-Opt (*open circles*) in a rhesus monkey, and the resulting retrogradely labeled neurons were identified in the PM nucleus. See List of Abbreviations. (Adapted from Schmahmann JD, Pandya DN: Anatomical investigation of thalamic projections to the posterior parietal cortices in rhesus monkey. J Comp Neurol 295:299–326, 1990.)

stimulation of the VL nucleus in the hemisphere dominant for language produced impairment of speech articulation, as well as deficits in language processing that varied depending on the precise location within the VL itself. Stimulation of anterior VL resulted in production of a repeated erroneous word; medial VL produced perseveration; posterior VL and anterior pulvinar resulted in misnaming and omissions. These investigators also studied the effects of VL stimulation on verbal and nonverbal short-term memory. In the left thalamus, VL stimulation during retrieval of previously learned verbal material degraded the performance, a finding noted also by Hugdahl and Wester (2000). In contrast, VL stimulation during the process of verbal memory encoding actually enhanced the subsequent recall. Further, in agreement with the notion that the thalamus is "true to

hemisphere" in its behavioral manifestations, stimulation of VL thalamus in the hemisphere nondominant for language (right thalamus in right-handed individuals) produced a similar result with encoding and retrieving nonverbal information. That is, stimulation of VL during recall of previously learned material worsened the performance; stimulation during encoding of nonverbal material enhanced subsequent recall. Furthermore, stimulation of the left pulvinar disrupted verbal memory processing, as opposed to right pulvinar stimulation that disrupted nonverbal memory processing.

Thalamotomy Reports

Early systematic reports of the effects of thalamic lesions on nonmotor functions were derived from thalamotomy in patients with Parkinson disease or tremor. Therapeutic lesions were directed toward the VL thalamus, but the precision of the early lesion placement is open to question, because in Bell's (1968) series, the postoperative course was complicated by impaired consciousness, "chronic organic brain syndrome," or dementia, monoparesis, hemiparesis, lateropulsion, impaired gait, and hemiballismus. Speech and language disorders fell into three categories: (1) hypophonia was noted particularly after bilateral lesions; (2) dysarthria was more prominent after left-sided lesions and included impaired articulation, nasal intonation, stuttering, and abnormalities of rhythm and modulation; and (3) "dysphasia" was noted following left-sided lesions only. The aphasic syndromes ranged from mild anomia to incomprehensible speech and reduced verbal output. Semantic and phonemic paraphasic errors, agrammatism, perseveration, and impaired reading were evident, but comprehension was relatively preserved and repetition was normal. These findings were in general agreement with the earlier reports. (For a review, see Bell, 1968; Ojemann & Ward, 1971; Lhermitte, 1984; Hugdahl & Wester, 2000). Thalamic lesions have become more precise since the resurgence of this modality as a therapeutic option. They are guided by magnetic resonance imaging (MRI), and aim for the posterior part of VL and the anterior part of the VP nucleus (Atkinson et al., 2002). In patients with Parkinson disease, these focused lesions are reported to be quite benign, with no apparent worsening of pre-existent cognitive deficits (Lund-Johansen et al., 1996) or only mild decline in verbal fluency and in executive functions measured by the Stroop interference test (Schuurman et al., 2002).

Functional Imaging

A comprehensive review of the thalamic activations seen in cognitive, affective, psychiatric, sensory, and nociceptive studies is beyond the scope of this discussion (see e.g., Cabeza & Nyberg, 2000). Suffice it to say that thalamic activation in all these areas of human brain function have been reported. The thalamus is activated by vestibular activity during caloric stimulation, along with insular cortex, intraparietal sulcus, superior temporal gyrus, hippocampus, and cingulate gyrus (Suzuki et al., 2001). Nociceptive stimulation is accompanied by activation of a widely distributed network of cerebral structures, including the thalamus and the somatosensory, insular, and anterior cingulate cortices (Rainville et al., 2001). Verbal stimulation activated the thalamus in an early positron emission tomography (PET) study (Mazziotta et al., 1984), providing evidence implicating subcortical structures in the processing of language and auditory information. The role of the thalamus as an integral component of the distributed neural circuitry subserving both elementary and high-level cognitive and emotional processing is amenable to further study using the new imaging modalities. Greater understanding of the anatomy of the thalamic nuclei, together with the increased detail of subcortical structures visible with the new techniques, holds great promise for future investigations.

Functional Mechanisms of Thalamic Nuclei

Conclusions regarding the mechanisms of the contribution of the thalamus to the wide range of behaviors enumerated above remain necessarily speculative. Penfield and Roberts (1959) suggested that thalamus is involved in integrative processing of neural information. Based on the results of their stimulation experiments, Johnson and Ojemann (2000) conclude that the thalamus provides a "specific alerting response" (Ojemann, 1983), increasing the input to memory of category-specific material, while simultaneously inhibiting retrieval from memory. In the area of language, Schaltenbrand (1975) proposed that the thalamus controls the release and inhibition of preformed speech patterns. Crosson's analysis (1999) of patients with focal thalamic lesions led to the conclusion that thalamus contributes a "selective engagement mechanism" to language processing and working memory (Crosson, 1985; Nadeau & Crosson, 1997) involving the frontal lobes, inferior thalamic peduncle, and reticular and possibly centromedian nucleus. This mechanism selectively engages those cortical areas required to perform a cognitive task, while maintaining other areas in a state of relative disengagement. These authors cite cases of pulvinar lesions that produce category-specific anomias, and visual processing problems in the early stages of reading, to conclude that there may be multiple thalamic processes that support cortical (language) functions. This would be in agreement with the notion that each thalamic nucleus may subserve a unique neural transform based on its architecture, similar to the concept of a universal cerebellar transform (UCT; Schmahmann, 2000b), discussed below. In the limbic system, Bentivoglio and colleagues (1993) describe the limbic thalamus as conveying to the cingulate gyrus (and other limbic structures) the integrated inputs necessary for the control of emotional, motivational, and autonomic aspects of behavior, limbic inputs subserving memory and learning processes, and motor inputs for appropriate control of behavior. The physiologic view of Steriade and colleagues (1997) is that the thalamus and neocortex function as a unified oscillatory machine. Rhythmic fast (mainly 30–40 Hz) and slow (<15 Hz) brain oscillations, which play a role in highly integrative processes, including consciousness, are determined by the intrinsic properties of thalamic and neocortical neurons. Further, certain aspects of brain rhythms, such as the coherent expression of oscillations in large populations of neurons, and the altered patterns and frequencies noted during shifts in the state of vigilance, depend on synchronizing devices provided by "complex synaptic articulations among neurons forming the building blocks of thalamocortical networks, and by generalized regulatory systems implicated in behavioral state control (p. 213)." In this view, the cellular properties of the thalamus, and the network organization of the thalamocortical connections, are not dissociable.

These hypotheses concerning the possible mechanisms of thalamic function (the "thalamic transform") have been offered for the thalamus as a whole. It is our contention that the fundamental transform may vary from one thalamic nucleus to another, as dictated by the architecture of each nucleus. Thus, each anatomic thalamic region (i.e., each nucleus) performs a particular transform to make its contribution to the overall behavior. What those transforms are, how they resemble each other within an overall thalamic framework, and how they differ from each other in terms of their heterogeneous architecture, still remains to be determined.

Focal Thalamic Lesion Analysis

In the first detailed account of the behavioral consequences of thalamic hemorrhage, Fisher (1959) described data on 13 patients of a total of 102 cases of intracerebral hemorrhage pathologically studied. He noted that sensory deficit may be associated with neglect ("modified anosognosia and hemiasomatognosia") and that "dysphasia is global and only moderate in severity." Confusion, delirium, visual hallucinations, and peduncular hallucinosis taking the form of colorful objects, animals, and flowers were described. Fisher's description of the abnormal eye movements following lesions of the thalamic-subthalamic region remains valid.

When the hemorrhage extends medially to the region of the posterior commissure and subthalamus, a series of abnormal ocular signs may appear. Vertical gaze upwards and downwards may be in abeyance; or gaze upwards is absent, while gaze downwards is only impaired. The eyes may be tonically deviated downwards, seeming to peer at the tip of the nose. The pupils may be small and fixed to light, although the patients respond rather clearly. The pupil on the side of the lesion is slightly smaller and may be combined with mild ptosis. Skew deviation of the eyes is common. Conjugate horizontal gaze may be impaired on voluntary effort mimicking palsy of the lateral rectus or even a conjugate gaze disturbance and irregular nystagmoid jerks are seen as well; however lateral excursions will be full on head rotation or caloric testing or a combination thereof. Convergence is absent and Bell's phenomenon cannot be elicited. (p. 57)

Some of these features (e.g., Horner syndrome) are surely accounted for by hypothalamic involvement, as suggested by subsequent ischemic stroke studies. Later reports of thalamic hemorrhage confirmed and extended the relationship between thalamic lesions and cognitive deficits beyond the aphasia and neglect described by Fisher (Watson & Heilman, 1979; Kumral et al., 1995; Chung et al., 1996; Manabe et al., 1999). Hemorrhage is seldom confined to the thalamus itself, however, and the remote effects of intracranial blood include pressure effects of the hemorrhagic mass, the effects of edema surrounding the hemorrhage on adjacent structures, and local toxic effects of the blood products. Similarly, accounts of the deficits in adults (Ziegler et al., 1977) and children (Nass et al., 2000) with tumors of the thalamus are useful, and have helped shape the understanding of the behavioral manifestations of thalamic lesions. As with hemorrhage, however, the issues that arise in structure-function analysis with tumors are too complex to establish with certainty that the behavior witnessed is a consequence of the involvement of the thalamus alone.

Lesion-deficit correlations in patients with focal infarction are generally described in terms of the affected vascular territories as determined by morphologic analysis of neuroimaging studies, and the thalamic nuclei involved are ascertained with reference to established maps of the human thalamus. The relationship of the observed behavior to individual thalamic nuclei is necessarily imprecise using this method, as the different ischemic syndromes usually destroy more than one thalamic nucleus. Nevertheless, there is enough consistency in the reports of the clinical presentations to permit statements about the manifestations of the particular vascular infarction and to allow cautious conclusions to be drawn about the functions in humans of the thalamic nuclei affected (Table 25-2).

Thalamic Blood Supply

The detailed understanding of the vascular supply of the thalamus has been limited by complex nomenclatures and seemingly incompatible conclusions from different studies. First evaluated by Duret (1874) and Foix and Hillemand (1925), and subsequently by Lazorthes (1961) and Plets and colleagues (1970), Percheron (1973, 1976a,b, 1977a,b) made a concerted attempt to delineate the vasculature of the thalamus and confirmed some of the essential principles of its arrangement. Subsequent clinical and anatomic evaluations (Castaigne et al., 1981; Graff-Radford et al., 1984, 1985; Von Crammon et al., 1985; Bogousslavsky et al., 1986, 1988; Caplan et al., 1988; Clarke et al., 1994; Tatu et al., 1998; Ghika-Schmid & Bogousslavsky, 2000) helped clarify and simplify the clinical-anatomic considerations. The details of the vascular supply are important in interpreting the conclusions in the literature about the functions of the thalamic nuclei based on their destruction in stroke. There are four major vascular territories in the thalamus, each with a predilection for supplying particular groups of thalamic nuclei. In the nomenclature used here, these are the (a) tuberothalamic, (b) inferolateral, (c) paramedian, and (d) posterior choroidal vessels (Figs. 25-4 and 25-5). The thalamic blood vessels may vary between individuals with respect to the parent vessel from which each thalamic branch arises, the number of tributaries that constitute each named vessel, the position of the medium and small-sized arteries that penetrate the thalamus, the

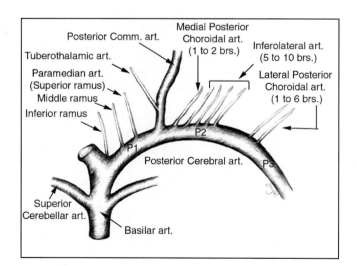

FIGURE 25-4. Artist's rendition of the origin of the arteries to the thalamus arising from the vertebrobasilar system. Note that the medial posterior choroidal artery may arise before (P1) or after (P2) the origin of the posterior communicating artery. The inferolateral arteries may arise individually or from a common pedicle. (From Schmahmann JD: Vascular syndromes of the thalamus. Stroke 34: 2264–2278, 2003.)

TABLE 25-2. Thalamic Arterial Supply and Principal Clinical Features of Local Infarction

Thalamic blood vessel	Prior designations	Nuclei irrigated	Clinical features reported
Tuberothalamic artery (arises from middle third of P. Comm)	Premamillary branch of thalamotuberian pedicle Polar artery Premamillary branch of posterior communicating artery Anterior internal optic artery Inferior thalamic peduncle Anterior thalamoperforating artery Anterior thalamosubthalamic paramedian artery	Reticular, VA, rostral VL, ventral pole of MD, anterior nuclei (AD, AM, AV), ventral internal medullary lamina, ventral amygdalofugal pathway, mamillothalamic tract	Fluctuating arousal and orientation Impaired learning, memory, autobiographical memory Superimposition of temporally unrelated information Personality changes, apathy, abulia Executive failure, perseveration True to hemisphere—language if VL involved on left; hemispatial neglect if right sided Emotional facial, acalculia, apraxia
Paramedian artery (arises from P1)	Thalamoperforating pedicle Retromamillary pedicle Posterior thalamo-subthalamic artery Interpeduncular profundus artery Superior ramus of interpeduncular artery	MD, intralaminar (CM, Pf, CL), posteromedial VL, ventromedial pulvinar, paraventricular, LD, dorsal internal medullary lamina	Decreased arousal (coma vigil if bilateral) Impaired learning and memory, confabulation, temporal disorientation, poor autobiographical memory Aphasia if left-sided, spatial deficits if right-sided Altered social skills and personality, including apathy, aggression, agitation
Inferolateral artery (arises from P2)	Thalamogeniculate pedicle Posterior and external arteries of thalamus		
Principal inferolateral branches		Ventroposterior complex—VPM, VPL, VPI Ventral lateral nucleus, ventral (motor) part	Sensory loss (variable extent, all modalities) Hemiataxia Hemiparesis Postlesion pain syndrome (Dejerine-Roussy)—right hemisphere predominant
Medial branches		Medial geniculate	Auditory consequences
Inferolateral pulvinar branches		Rostral and lateral pulvinar, LD nucleus	Behavioral
Posterior choroidal artery (arises from P2)			
Lateral branches		LGN, LD, LP, inferolateral parts of pulvinar	Visual field loss (hemianopsia, quadrantanopsia)
Medial branches		MGN, posterior parts of CM and CL, pulvinar	Variable sensory loss, weakness, aphasia, memory impairment, dystonia, hand tremor

From Schmahmann JD: Vascular syndromes of the thalamus. Stroke 34: 2264–2278, 2003.

FIGURE 25-5. Thalamic vascular supply. Schematic diagram of the lateral (A) and dorsal (B) views of the four major thalamic arteries, and the nuclei they irrigate, according to Bogousslavsky and colleagues (1988). 1, carotid artery; 2, basilar artery; 3, P1 region of the posterior cerebral artery (mesencephalic artery); 4, posterior cerebral artery; 5, posterior communicating artery; 6, tuberothalamic artery; 7, paramedian artery; 8, inferolateral artery; 9, posterior choroidal artery; DM, dorsomedial nucleus; IL, intralaminar nuclear complex; P, pulvinar; VP, ventral posterior complex. The diagram in (C) is Percheron's (1976b) representation of the varying patterns of origin of the paramedian artery off the mesencephalic/P1 artery. The illustrations in (D) and (E) from De Freitas and Bogousslavsky (2002) are an adapted version of the conclusions of von Cramon and colleagues (1985) regarding the patterns of irrigation by the thalamic arterial supply to the thalamic nuclei. Thalamic terminology in this diagram is from Hassler (1959); see Figure 25-1. (A and B from Bogousslavsky J, Regli F, Uske A: Thalamic infarcts: Clinical syndromes, etiology, and prognosis. Neurology 38:837–848, 1998; C from Percheron G: Les artères du thalamus humain. II. Artères et territoire thalamiques paramédians de l'artère basilaire communicante. Rev Neurol [Paris] 132:309–324, 1976; D and E from De Freitas GR, Bogousslavsky J: Thalamic infarcts, in Donnan G, Norving B, Bamford J, et al [eds]: Subcortical Stroke: Oxford: Oxford University Press, 2002, pp. 255–285.)

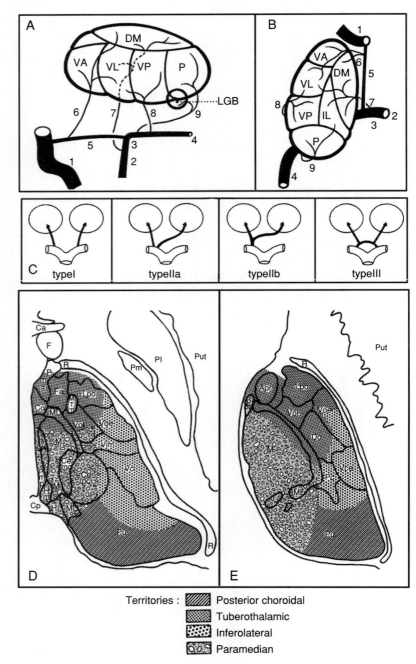

number and position of the arterioles off these small arteries that irrigate the thalamus, and the nuclei that are supplied by each blood vessel and its tributaries (Fig. 25-6). This situation is analogous to the lenticulostriate branches of the middle cerebral artery that irrigate the basal ganglia and internal capsule (Castaigne et al., 1981; Caplan et al., 1988). Neuroimaging has become increasingly sophisticated, exemplified by diffusion-weighted imaging that can detect infarcts, millimeters in size, within minutes of occurrence (Weber et al., 2000), and apparent diffusion coefficient maps and perfusion scans can determine whether neural tissue is at risk but not infarcted (e.g., Desmond et al., 2001).

Further, knowledge of stroke pathophysiology has improved, revealing that emboli in large or medium-sized vessels can fragment or move downstream, and that lacunar infarcts may be confined to minute territories (Brandt et al., 2000). With these technical and conceptual advances, the functional properties of thalamic nuclei, as determined by lesion-deficit analysis, will likely be established more clearly in the future.

Tuberothalamic Artery Infarction

The tuberothalamic artery originates from the middle third of the posterior communicating artery. (Previous

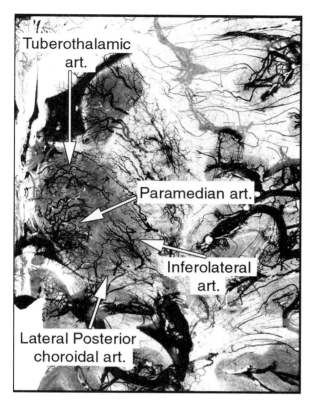

FIGURE 25-6. Illustration of the thalamic vascular complexity within the four major vascular territories, as shown by the injection of dye into the posterior circulation post-mortem. (Adapted from Salamon G: Atlas of Arteries of the Human Brain. Paris: Sandoz, 1971.)

names include the anterior internal optic artery [Duret, 1874], polar artery [Percheron, 1973], premamillary branch of the thalamo-tuberian peduncle [Foix & Hillemand, 1925], inferior thalamic peduncle [Lazorthes & Salomon, 1971], premamillary branch of the posterior communicating artery [Pedroza et al., 1987], anterior thalamoperforating artery, and anterior thalamo-subthalamic paramedian artery [see Castaigne et al., 1981; Graff-Radford et al., 1984; Bogousslavsky et al., 1986]). Within the thalamus it follows the course of the mamillothalamic tract. It is absent in approximately one third of the normal population, in which case its territory is supplied by the paramedian artery (Bogousslavsky et al., 1986).

The tuberothalamic artery irrigates the reticular nucleus, VA, rostral part of VL, ventral pole of MD, the mamillothalamic tract, the ventral amygdalofugal pathway, the ventral part of the internal medullary lamina, and the anterior thalamic nuclei—AM, AV, AD. Percheron (1973) concludes that the anterior nuclear group is not supplied by this tuberothalamic artery, but rather by the posterior choroidal artery, an assertion reflected in the discussion of Von Crammon and colleagues (1985). This relationship is questionable,

however, given the anatomic proximity of the tuberothalamic artery and the mamillothalamic tract to the AM/AV/AD nuclei, and by the demonstration (Clarke et al., 1994; Ghika-Schmid & Bogousslavsky, 2000) of involvement of the anterior nuclei along with the VA, VL, mamillothalamic tract, and internal medullary lamina that are known to be supplied by the tuberothalamic artery.

The clinical syndrome resulting from infarction in the territory of the tuberothalamic artery (Fig. 25-7) is characteristic, with severe and wide-ranging neuropsychological deficits. Graff-Radford and colleagues (1984, 1985) reported that in the early stages of infarction patients exhibit fluctuating levels of consciousness and appear withdrawn. They are disoriented in time and place and may develop persistent personality changes, including euphoria, lack of insight, and apathy. Memory for recent events is impaired, new learning markedly deficient, and temporal disorientation present. Language disturbances occur in left hemisphere lesions, characterized by anomia, impairment of comprehension, and fluent paraphasic speech, which may be diminished in quantity, lacking meaningful content, and replete with perseveration. Reading may be relatively preserved, although the comprehension of what is being read may be poor. In striking contrast, repetition is well preserved. These general characteristics of language impairment are consistent in different reports of thalamic aphasia, although the component features may vary between individuals, and the contribution of each thalamic nucleus to the impaired linguistic elements remains unresolved. Left-sided lesions are accompanied by impairment of both verbal and visual memory, constructional apraxia, and a decline in both verbal and visual IQ. Right-sided lesions have less pervasive cognitive impairment, with deficits in visual memory, nonverbal intellect, and constructional apraxia, but preservation of language functions. The clinical feature of emotional central facial paralysis is observed, characterized by good facial movement with volition, but pronounced facial asymmetry during laughing or crying. The elementary findings of sensory disturbances are rare, minimal, and transient.

Neuropsychological disturbance was also the principal manifestation in patients with tuberothalamic infarction described by Bogousslavsky and colleagues (1986, 1988). Patients with left-sided lesions had hyopophonia and language impairments characterized by reduced verbal output, anomia, semantic and phonemic paraphasias, occasional neologisms, moderate impairment of comprehension, and preserved repetition. Amnestic syndromes were prominent: verbal and visual memory impairments were seen in left-sided lesions, visual memory impairments and disturbed visual-spatial processing in right-sided lesions. Acalculia followed left thalamic lesions. Right thalamic lesions

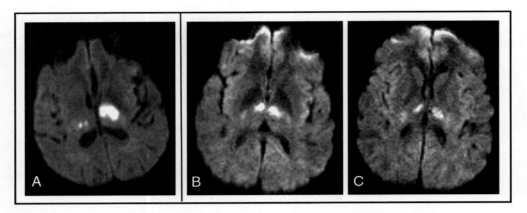

FIGURE 25-7. Diffusion-weighted MRI of acute thalamic infarction in two patients. (A) Extensive tuberothalamic artery territory infarction on the left (right of diagram), as well as small lesions in the territory of the inferolateral arteries on the right. The images in B and C reveal bilateral infarction in a teenager with patent foramen ovale. The infarcted region is in the tuberothalamic artery territory, although this pattern of bilateral stroke is more usually seen following paramedian artery infarcts. This case is likely to be an example of the paramedian artery irrigating both the paramedian as well as the tuberothalamic "territories." The patient made a complete recovery, and follow-up MRI scans revealed only minute lesions. (From Schmahmann JD: Vascular syndromes of the thalamus. Stroke 34: 2264–2278, 2003.)

were associated with hemispatial neglect, impaired visual spatial processing, and constructional apraxia. Apathy and lack of spontaneity were prominent. Lower facial weakness was also present only for "emotional movements," and sensory deficits were present but not prominent. Mild to moderate contralateral weakness or clumsiness was seen in most of their cases. Lisovoski and colleagues (1993) describe data on a patient with left thalamic infarction in whom the major feature of the presentation was lack of spontaneity and emotional unconcern, along with severe verbal memory impairment. The patient of Warren and colleagues (2000) with a lesion involving the tuberothalamic distribution developed buccofacial and limb apraxia in addition to severe anterograde amnesia. Von Crammon and associates (1985) considered the amnestic syndrome in their patients with tuberothalamic infarction to represent a disconnection between anterior thalamic nuclei and hippocampal formation, by virtue of the disruption of the mamillothalamic tract, and between amygdala and anterior nuclei by damage to the amygdalothalamic projections passing through the internal medullary lamina. This conclusion was supported by Graff-Radford and colleagues (1990) who described a patient with a severe amnestic syndrome following infarction involving the internal medullary lamina. These authors used a monkey tract tracing study to confirm that the ventral amygdalofugal pathway that links the amygdala with the medial dorsal thalamic nucleus runs through the internal medullary lamina.

By virtue of the variation in vascular architecture in normal states and in the distribution of the lipohya-linosis that characterizes lacunar infarction (Fisher, 1982), the VL and MD nuclei appear to be entirely spared in some patients with tuberothalamic infarction. Rather, the lesion involves the anterior nuclei, VA, paramedian nuclei, mamillothalamic tract, and the internal medullary lamina. The presentation in these patients is different from those with the larger tuberothalamic infarctions, in that memory is impaired, but language is spared, except for decreased verbal fluency. The patient of Clarke and colleagues (1994) developed global amnesia, more for verbal than nonverbal memory. Autobiographical memory and newly acquired information were disorganized with respect to temporal order. There was inattention, disorientation, anomia, perseveration, and acalculia. Apart from decreased verbal fluency, there was no aphasia. Some months later, verbal memory functions remained poor, and the patient's emotional engagement remained impaired. Hypometabolism in the posterior cingulate cortex was demonstrated on PET.

Ghika-Schmid and Bogousslavsky (2000) studied 12 patients with lesions (8 left, 4 right) restricted to the anterior thalamic regions supplied by the tuberothalamic artery. In the domain of speech and language, patients were dysarthric (8 of 12) and hypophonic (5 of 12). All, including those with right thalamic lesions, had word-finding difficulties and poor initiation of speech. In contrast, comprehension, writing, and reading were normal, as was repetition. The domain most affected was that of new learning and memory. All patients had abnormal anterograde memory with poor delayed recall. Perseveration, impaired planning, and motor sequencing were evident, and many were apathetic, with decreased verbal and nonverbal fluency. The impaired anterograde memory, word-finding difficulty, and apathy were persistent. A hallmark in these patients was the presence of severe perseverative behaviors in thinking, spontaneous speech, and all memory and executive tasks. Patients displayed superimposition of temporally unrelated information, producing a state of parallel expression of mental activities that the authors term *palipsychism*.

Paramedian Artery Infarction

The retromamillary or thalamoperforating pedicle of Foix and Hillemand (1925), or the interpeduncular profundus artery of Schlesinger (1976), was considered by Percheron (1973) to be composed of several paramedian arteries "that represent a special differentiation of the highest of the group of paramedian arteries which can be found all along the neuraxis." They arise from the P1 section of the posterior cerebral artery, to which the term *mesencephalic artery* may correctly be applied, because it is "the proximal stretch of the posterior cerebral artery from the bifurcation of the basilar to its junction with the posterior communicating" artery (Segarra, 1970). Tatu and colleagues (1998) adopt a useful approach of grouping the interpeduncular branches that arise from the mesencephalic, or P1 artery, into inferior, middle, and superior rami. The inferior ramus of the interpeduncular arteries that arises from the basilar bifurcation, and the middle ramus, that Percheron (1973) together called the paramedian mesencephalic pedicle, irrigate the pons and midbrain (Castaigne et al., 1981; Tatu et al., 1998) and can produce the "locked in" component of the "top of the basilar" infarction (Caplan, 1980). The superior ramus that irrigates the thalamus, corresponds to the posterior thalamosubthalamic paramedian artery of Percheron (1973), or in the nomenclature adopted here, the paramedian artery. The paramedian arteries can arise as a pair from each P1, but they may equally arise from a common trunk off one P1, thus supplying the thalamus bilaterally (Fig. 25-5C).

The paramedian artery ascends within the thalamus from its medial and ventral aspect to its lateral and dorsal part. It supplies a variable extent of the thalamus, but principally the dorsomedial nucleus, internal medullary lamina, and intralaminar nuclei (CL, CM, Pf). The paraventricular nuclei, posteromedial part of VL, and ventromedial part of the pulvinar may also be supplied. The LD, LP, and VA have been involved in some instances. When the tuberothalamic artery is absent, the paramedian artery may assume that territory as well, and thus infarction in this vascular territory can be devastating.

Unilateral thalamic infarction in the territory of the paramedian artery (Fig. 25-8) produces neuro-

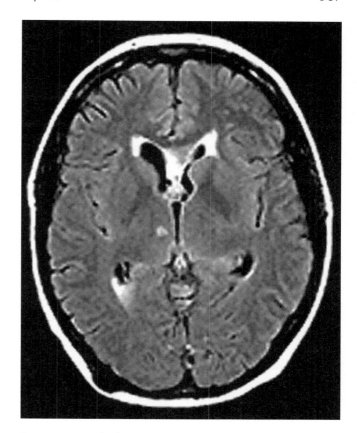

FIGURE 25-8. Fluid-attenuated inversion recovery (FLAIR) MRI revealing right paramedian thalamic infarction in a patient with abrupt-onset confusion, confabulation, and autobiographical memory impairment in the setting of underlying ventriculitis following placement of a ventriculoperitoneal shunt for hydrocephalus. (From Schmahmann JD: Vascular syndromes of the thalamus. Stroke 34:2264–2278, 2003.)

psychologic disturbances predominantly in the areas of arousal and memory. A left-right asymmetry is evident in language versus visual-spatial deficits. Impairment of arousal with decreased and fluctuating level of consciousness is a conspicuous feature in the early stages, lasting for hours to days. Confusion, agitation, aggression, and apathy may be persistent features (Castaigne et al., 1981; Graff-Radford et al., 1984, 1985; Bogousslavsky et al., 1988). Speech and language impairments are characterized by hypophonia and dyprosodia, with frequent perseveration, markedly reduced verbal fluency, but generally preserved syntactic structure with occasional paraphasic errors and normal repetition—the *adynamic aphasia* of Guberman and Stuss (1983).

Bilateral infarction in the paramedian artery territory may result in an acutely ill and severely impaired patient. Disorientation, confusion, hypersomnolence, deep coma, "coma vigil" or akinetic mutism (awake unresponsiveness), and severe memory impairment with perseveration and confabulation are prominent behavioral features, often accompanied by eye movement abnormalities (Castaigne et al., 1981; Graff-Radford et al., 1984; 1985; Reilly et al., 1992). The anterograde and retrograde memory deficit and the apathy can be severe and persistent. The syndrome may be accompanied in the late stages by inappropriate social behaviors, impulsive aggressive outbursts, emotional blunting, loss of initiative, and a reported absence of spontaneous thoughts or mental activities (see Guberman & Stuss, 1983, for case reports and early literature), conceptualized as loss of psychic self-activation (Bogousslavsky et al., 1991; Engelborghs et al., 2000). In one case, Hodges and colleagues (1993) noted a severe and systematic distortion of personally relevant autobiographical memory, but relative sparing of knowledge of famous people and public events, suggesting a "thematic retrieval" memory disorder resulting from disconnection of frontal and medial temporal memory systems. Prominent disorientation in time is observed (Castaigne et al., 1981; Graff-Radford et al., 1990), similar to the report of Spiegel and colleagues (1956) that introduced the term *chronotaraxis* to describe the phenomenon. Apraxia and dysgraphia are noted in some cases (Castaigne et al., 1981). Complete recovery from bilateral paramedian thalamic infarction has occasionally been reported (Krolak-Salmon et al., 2000).

The amnestic syndrome resulting from paramedian territory infarction is similar to the thiamine-deficient Korsakoff syndrome that destroys the medial dorsal thalamic nuclei along with the mamillary bodies (Victor et al., 1971), but the addition of the other behavioral features produces a constellation that led to the term "thalamic dementia" (Segarra, 1970) used also to describe the behavioral and cognitive consequences of thalamic involvement in Creutzfeldt-Jakob disease and fatal familial insomnia (Martin, 1997). The phenomenon of transient global amnesia is thought to be related to transient ischemia in the paramedian thalamus, but with the exception of rare case reports supporting this assertion anatomically (Goldenberg et al., 1991; Chen et al., 1996; Pradalier et al., 2000), there is no pathologic verification of this association.

A number of elementary neurologic signs are evident also in lesions of the paramedian artery, including asterixis, complete or partial vertical gaze paresis, loss of convergence, pseudo-sixth nerve palsies, bilateral internuclear ophthalmoplegia, miosis, and even intolerance to bright light (Guberman & Stuss, 1983; Bogousslavsky et al., 1988). These are among the findings reported initially by Fisher (1959) in his cases of medially situated thalamic hemorrhage and are likely to result from lesions involving midbrain nuclei supplied by the inferior and middle rami of the interpeduncular arteries that arise from P1 medial to the paramedian artery to thalamus.

A cautionary note is warranted in deriving precise anatomic-functional correlations with regard to the behavioral and motor consequences of paramedian artery infarctions. First, these strokes are not limited to the dorsomedial nucleus in the majority of cases reported to date, and second, as documented in the autopsy study of Castaigne and colleagues (1981), thalamic infarcts may be accompanied by lesions outside the thalamus, such as in the midbrain. Involvement of nonthalamic structures occurs in the setting of basilar artery emboli, because the embolus can fragment and lodge in small distal vessels, or produce ischemia prior to moving further distally within the artery. Further, the distribution of lacunar infarction within the paramedian artery territory is not constant, because of the anatomic variability of the end vessels within thalamus, so some cases will be more restricted than others (Caplan et al., 1988; Brandt et al., 2000).

Inferolateral Artery Infarction

The inferolateral arteries (Percheron, 1973; Bogousslavsky et al., 1988) are equivalent to the thalamogeniculate pedicle of Foix and Hillemand (1925), and the posterior and external arteries of the optic thalamus of Duret (1874). They are comprised of 5 to 10 arteries that arise from the P2 branch of the posterior cerebral artery, that is, after the origin of the posterior communicating artery. According to Percheron (1973), the inferolateral arteries are comprised of three main groups: the medial geniculate, the principal inferolateral, and the inferolateral pulvinar arteries.

1. The medial branch supplies the external half of the medial geniculate nucleus.
2. The principal inferolateral arteries, the "most voluminous, longest, most vertical of the short branches of the posterior cerebral artery," penetrate between the geniculate bodies, ascend in the lateral medullary lamina, and supply the major part of the ventral posterior nuclei (VPL, VPM, VPI), as well as the ventral and lateral parts of the VL nucleus more rostrally. In Percheron's material, the CM nucleus is not supplied by these vessels, as suggested by Foix and Hillemand (1925) and Plets and colleagues (1970).
3. The inferolateral pulvinar branches are posteriorly situated among the inferolateral arterial group, and supply dorsal and posterolateral regions, including the rostral and lateral parts of the pulvinar, and the LD nucleus (Percheron, 1973; Caplan et al., 1988; Bogousslavsky et al., 1988; Tatu et al., 1998).

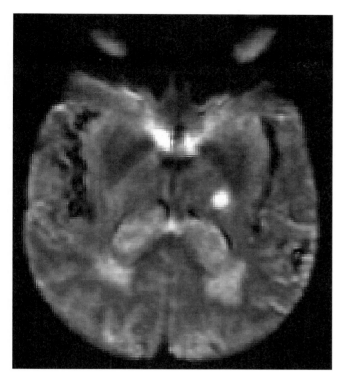

FIGURE 25-9. Diffusion-weighted MRI of acute infarction in the left inferolateral artery territory causing the clinical triad of ataxia, mild hemiparesis, and hemisensory loss on the contralateral side. (From Schmahmann JD: Vascular syndromes of the thalamus. Stroke 34:2264–2278, 2003.)

Patients with inferolateral artery infarction present with the thalamic syndrome described by Dejerine and Roussy (1906), namely, sensory loss to a variable extent, with impaired extremity movement, sometimes with postlesion pain. The details of this presentation have been explored in numerous reports (Garcin & Lapresle, 1954, 1969; Fisher, 1978; Lapresle & Haguenau, 1973; Caplan et al., 1988). In the report of Bogousslavsky and colleagues (1988), for example, sensory loss included all modalities, but not necessarily in the same patient. Touch, temperature, and pin sense were decreased in 5 of 17 patients, whereas the remainder also had impairment of position and vibration sense. Ataxia with hemiparesis is also noted in this group (Dejerine & Roussy, 1906; Foix & Hillemand, 1925; Garcin, 1955; Caplan et al., 1988; Gutrecht et al., 1992), and, indeed, the combination of sensory loss with ataxic hemiparesis is strongly indicative of a thalamic lesion, although not pathognomonic (Fig. 25-9). The thalamic pain syndrome of Dejerine and Roussy occurs following lesions of this region of the thalamus, but more complex behavioral syndromes have not been reported. The "thalamic hand" of Foix and Hillemand (1925), produced by lesions of the inferolateral artery, is flexed and pronated, with the thumb buried beneath the other fingers.

The complexity of the penetrating arteries that constitute the inferolateral arteries explains why small vessel disease in this territory can have distinctly different presentations. Pure sensory stroke affecting face, arm, and leg in whole or in part results from variable involvement of the VPM (head and neck) or VPL nuclei (trunk and extremities). Infarction in those VL regions that convey cerebellar fibers to the motor related cortices adds an ataxic component to the presentation. Cognitive and psychiatric presentations are notably missing from the descriptions of infarction restricted to the ventral posterior nuclei. The pulvinar is strongly associative, and LD is related to limbic cortices, although reports of the clinical manifestations of infarction in the inferolateral pulvinar vessels restricted to, or predominantly involving, these nuclei have yet to appear. Similarly, whereas the VL nucleus receives some supply from the inferolateral arteries, it is mostly supplied by the tuberothalamic artery territory, as described above. Incoordination is noted in patients with inferolateral territory infarction when it involves the VL, but the language disturbances that accompany VL lesions in tuberothalamic artery infarction are not commonly seen following stroke in the inferolateral artery territory. Karussis and colleagues (2000) reported that two patients with inferolateral territory infarcts (no neuroimaging published) had aphasia with impaired fluency, comprehension, and naming, and Graff-Radford and colleagues (1985) described impaired fluency in patients with thalamocapsular infarction. This only occasional involvement of language in inferolateral territory lesions may reflect the fact that different nuclei may be involved within the territory of the infarcted inferolateral arteries. This is to be expected based on the number of vessels that constitute the inferolateral constellation, normal variability in the arteriolar and capillary supply within thalamus, and the effect of slowly evolving lipohyalinosis on the zone of supply of the remaining intact blood vessels. The involvement of the different subcomponents of the VL, in particular, that link deep cerebellar nuclei (DCN) with motor, premotor, prefrontal, and posterior parietal regions of the cerebral hemispheres, may also have markedly different clinical consequences.

Posterior Choroidal Artery Infarction

The posterior choroidal arteries, like the inferolateral, arise from the P2 segment of the posterior cerebral artery, and are made up of a number of branches. One to two medially placed branches arise adjacent to the take-off of the posterior communicating artery (i.e., at the distal P1 or proximal P2 segment of the posterior cerebral artery). These supply the subthalamic nucleus and midbrain, the medial half of the medial geniculate nucleus, the posterior parts of the intralaminar nuclei CM and CL (MDdc [medial dorsal thalamic nucleus, densocellular part] in the terminology of Olszewski, CL in the terminology of Jones), and the pulvinar nuclei (Percheron, 1973, 1977b; Castaigne et al., 1981; Bogousslavsky et al., 1988; Tatu et al., 1998). Percheron's (1973) conclusion that it also supplies the AD, AV, and AM components of the anterior nuclear group is not universally shared (Tatu et al., 1998). In the lateral group of posterior choroidal arteries, one to six branches arise from the distal P2 segment of the posterior cerebral artery. Some of these supply medial temporal structures, but the thalamic arteries are destined for the lateral geniculate nucleus, the inferolateral region of the pulvinar, the lateral dorsal nucleus, and the lateral posterior nucleus. The LGN may also receive supply from the anterior choroidal artery (Tatu et al., 1988), although Percheron (1973, 1977b) could not confirm this in his material, and the thalamus was not involved in the series of anterior choroidal artery infarcts reported by Decroix and colleagues (1986).

There is only limited information on the clinical manifestations of infarction confined to the thalamus in the distribution of the posterior choroidal arteries. The Lausanne group (Bogousslavsky et al., 1988) reported data on three patients with lateral geniculate nucleus infarcts in whom quadrantanopsia was detected, along with impaired fast phase of the optokinetic response to the side opposite the lesion. One patient had contralateral hemibody numbness and mild aphasia. These authors (Neau & Bogousslavsky, 1996) subsequently described data on 20 patients (10 personal, 10 previously published) in which lateral posterior choroidal artery territory infarcts were associated with homonymous quadrantanopsia or horizontal "sectoranopsia," hemisensory loss, transcortical aphasia, and memory deficits, whereas medial infarcts produced eye movement disorders not suggestive of thalamic involvement. Three of their patients (Ghika et al., 1994) with infarcts reportedly restricted to the pulvinar developed a delayed complex hyperkinetic motor syndrome, including ataxia, rubral tremor, dystonia, myoclonus, and chorea, a constellation they termed "the jerky dystonic unsteady hand." Sensory dysfunction in all three patients and a thalamic pain syndrome in two raise the question as to whether the lesion involved other nuclei in addition to the pulvinar, however. The observation of incongruous homonymous hemianopic scotoma after lateral posterior choroidal artery stroke was also reported by Wada and colleagues (1999). Spatial neglect was associated with lesions located mostly in the right pulvinar, in the study of Karnath and colleagues (2002), although the LD and VL were involved as well.

Recovery of Function Following Thalamic Lesions

Prognosis following stroke confined to the thalamus is generally regarded as being rather good compared to lesions of the cerebral cortex or other subcortical structures, both in adults (Buttner et al., 1991; Steinke et al., 1992) and children (Garg & DeMyer, 1995; Brower et al., 1996). This generally applies to the low incidence of mortality and the good recovery from motor deficit, however. Persistence of cognitive and psychiatric manifestations following infarction of limbic, reticular, and associative thalamic nuclei (i.e., in the territory of the tuberothalamic or paramedian arteries) is commented on routinely in reports of thalamic stroke, but systematic longitudinal analyses have not been performed. Similarly, whereas the characteristics of poststroke pain have been studied, including higher incidence after lesions of the right thalamus (Nasreddine & Saver, 1997), the overall incidence and long-term outcome of poststroke thalamic pain is not well established. The prognosis following thalamic hemorrhage is more complicated and is correlated with the volume of the hematoma, level of consciousness at onset, extent of motor weakness at presentation, and the presence of intraventricular extension and hydrocephalus (Chung et al., 1996; Kase, 2002).

CEREBELLUM

The cerebellum is "subcortical" only in that it is distinct from the cerebral cortex. The traditional view of cerebellar function is that it is confined to the coordination of voluntary motor activity. This view has evolved in recent years. As with the discussion of the thalamus and basal ganglia, the anatomic organization of the cerebellar linkage with the association areas of the cerebral hemispheres has been at the core of this reevaluation. The cerebellar linkage with the cerebral cortex has traditionally been regarded as consisting in large part of motor-related cortices projecting through basilar pontine nuclei to the cerebellum, and the cerebellar dentate nucleus sending efferents back through the VL thalamus to the motor cortex. More recent anatomic examination of the cerebrocerebellar system, however, reveals that this system is far more intricately organized, and is indeed well constructed to subserve a multitude of sensorimotor as well as higher-order behavior patterns.

Anatomic Considerations

Cerebellar connections with the reticular system support arousal (e.g., Andrezik et al., 1984; Qvist, 1989); the hypothalamus, important for autonomic function (Haines & Dietrichs, 1984); and the limbic system that subserves the experience and expression of emotion (e.g., Whiteside & Snider, 1953; Heath & Harper, 1974).

The associative and paralimbic regions of the cerebral cortex have topographically organized feedforward projections through the nuclei in the basilar pons into the cerebellum, as well as feedback projections from the cerebellum (Fig. 25-10). These projections arise from

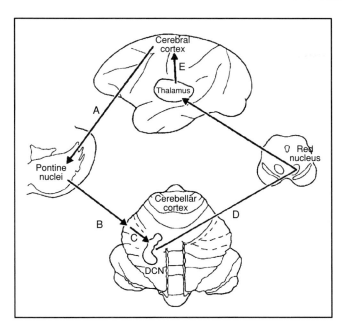

FIGURE 25-10. Diagrammatic representation of the cerebrocerebellar circuit. The two-stage feedforward limb consists of (*A*) the corticopontine projection, and (*B*) the pontocerebellar pathway. The feedback limb originates in the cerebellar corticonuclear projection (*C*). The two-stage feedback from cerebellum to cerebral cortex continues through the cerebellothalamic projection (*D*) via the red nucleus. The thalamocortical projection (*E*) completes the circuit. (From Schmahmann JD: The cerebellum in autism: clinical and anatomic perspectives, in Bauman ML, Kemper TL [eds]: The Neurobiology of Autism. Baltimore, MD: Johns Hopkins University Press, 1994, pp. 195–226).

the prefrontal (Schmahmann & Pandya, 1997), posterior parietal (Brodal, 1978; Glickstein et al., 1985; May & Andersen, 1986; Schmahmann & Pandya, 1989), superior temporal visual and polymodal regions (Ungerleider et al., 1984; Schmahmann & Pandya, 1991), and dorsal parastriate cortices (Fries, 1990; Schmahmann & Pandya, 1993). Paralimbic projections arise from the posterior parahippocampal cortex (Schmahmann & Pandya, 1993), limbic regions (Devinsky et al., 1995; Paus, 2001) of the cingulate gyrus (Vilensky & Van Hoesen, 1981), and the anterior insular cortex (Glickstein et al., 1985) involved in autonomic and pain modulation systems (Mesulam & Mufson, 1985). These associative and paralimbic corticopontine pathways (Fig. 25-11) appear to be funneled through the cerebrocerebellar circuit within multiple parallel but partially overlapping loops (Schmahmann & Pandya, 1992), converging with topographic ordering throughout the pons, whereas the motor corticopontine projections are mostly in the caudal half of the pons (Schmahmann, 1996).

A precise pattern of organization is probably present also in the pontine projections to the cerebellar cortex, although this still remains to be demonstrated. The cerebellar anterior lobe receives input from medial parts of the caudal pons; the vermal visual area from the dorsomedial and dorsolateral pons; vermal lobule VIIIB from the intrapeduncular nucleus; crus I of the ansiform lobule from medial parts of the rostral pons; and crus II from the medial, ventral, and lateral pons (Brodal, 1979). These anatomic studies, together with physiologic investigations (Allen & Tsukahara, 1974; Sasaki et al., 1975), suggest that the anterior lobe receives afferents from motor, premotor, and rostral parietal cortices; the prefrontal cortices are linked with crus I of the ansiform lobule, and with crus II to a lesser extent; and the parietal association cortices are linked with crus I, crus II, and lobule VIIB. A more complete exploration of the pontocerebellar pathways is still needed to better understand the relationship between the cerebral cortex and cerebellum.

Once conveyed to the cerebellar cortex, these streams of information are acted on by the cerebellar corticonuclear microcomplexes (Ito, 1982), and then transmitted via the DCN to the thalamus, on their way back to the cerebral cortex.

Cerebellar projections to the thalamus arise from fastigial and interpositus nuclei as well as from the dentate nucleus and are directed not only to the cerebellar recipient VL, but also to centralis lateralis (CL), paracentralis (Pcn), centromedian-parafascicular (CM-Pf) complex, and pars multiformis (MDmf) of the medial dorsal nucleus (Strick, 1976; Batton et al., 1977; Thach & Jones, 1979; Stanton, 1980; Kalil, 1981; Wiesendanger & Wiesendanger, 1985; Ilinsky & Kultas-Ilinsky, 1987; Orioli & Strick, 1989). The associative connections of these thalamic nuclei are discussed above. Furthermore, the dorsal parts of the VL nucleus itself are reciprocally interconnected with the prefrontal periarcuate areas (Kievit & Kuypers, 1977; Stanton et al., 1988; Künzle & Akert, 1977), the multimodal cortex in the upper bank of the superior temporal sulcus (Yeterian & Pandya, 1989), and the posterior parietal cortices (Schmahmann & Pandya, 1990) (Fig. 25-12).

Trans-synaptic retrograde tracer studies using attenuated herpesvirus (Middleton & Strick, 1994, 1997) demonstrate more directly that the cerebellar dentate nucleus sends projections through the thalamus to different areas of the frontal lobe in the monkey. The dorsomedial part of the dentate nucleus sends its projections to the motor cortex, whereas the ventrolateral and ventromedial parts of the dentate nucleus are connected with the prefrontal cortex, including area 9/46 (Fig. 25-13). It is likely that this degree of organization in the feedback from the cerebellum to the cerebral hemispheres is reproduced throughout the cerebrocerebellar system, but this remains to be demonstrated.

The cerebrocerebellar system in this view then consists of discretely organized parallel anatomic subsystems that serve as the substrates for differentially

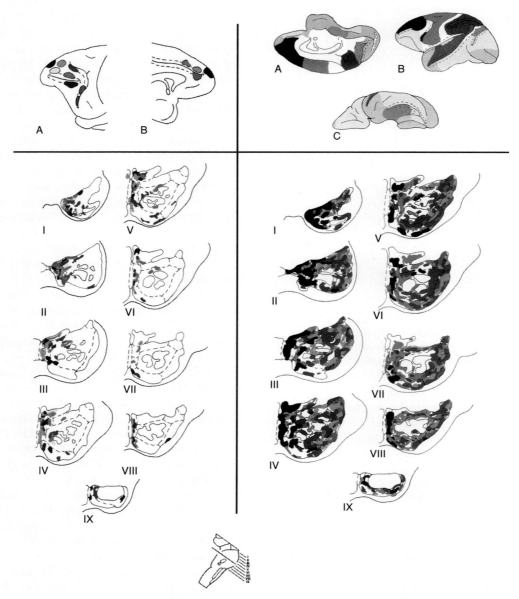

FIGURE 25-11. Color-coded summary diagrams of the corticopontine projections from associative, paralimbic, and motor cortices in the rhesus monkey. (*Left*) Tract tracers (tritiated amino acids) were injected into selected architectonic regions of the prefrontal cortices of rhesus monkeys, and the termination patterns of the anterogradely transported label in the nuclei of the basilar pons were identified. Each color represents a single case. Terminations are mostly in the medial part of the pons, and each cortical area has its own unique set of terminations in the basilar pontine nuclei. Lateral prefrontal cortex in *A*, medial surface in *B*. Levels I (rostral) through IX (caudal) of the basilar pons are shown, as seen in the schematic of the brainstem below. (*Right*) In this composite diagram, corticopontine projections are seen from the prefrontal cortices (purple), posterior parietal area (blue), superior temporal region (red), posterior parahippocampal and parastriate cortices (orange), and motor and supplementary motor cortices (green). Each cortical area has its own region of termination in the pons. The associative and paralimbic projections are not overshadowed by the motor projections. Areas in the cerebral hemispheres in yellow and gray do not project to the pons (yellow, as shown by anterograde and retrograde techniques; gray as shown by retrograde techniques). Medial surface of the rhesus monkey brain is shown in *A*, lateral surface in *B*, orbital surface in *C*. (*Left* From Schmahmann JD, Pandya DN: Anatomic organization of the basilar pontine projections from prefrontal cortices in rhesus monkey. J Neurosci 17:438–458, 1997. *Right* From Schmahmann JD: From movement to thought: Anatomic substrates of the cerebellar contribution to cognitive processing. Hum Brain Mapping 4:174–198, 1996.) (See Color Plate 11)

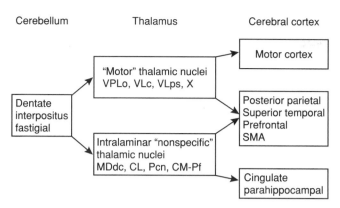

FIGURE 25-12. Diagram depicting the feedback system from cerebellar nuclei through the thalamus to the cerebral cortex, derived from a review of multiple single-tract tracer studies in rhesus monkey. All cerebellar nuclei participate in this circuit and terminate on traditionally motor as well as intralaminar nuclei. Both sets of thalamic nuclei then provide projections to motor as well as to associative cerebral areas. (From Schmahmann JD: The cerebellum in autism: Clinical and anatomic perspectives, in Bauman ML, Kemper TL [eds]: The Neurobiology of Autism. Baltimore, MD: Johns Hopkins University Press, 1994, pp. 195–226.)

organized functional subsystems (or loops) within the framework of distributed neural circuits. The hypothesis derived from this anatomic model is that disruption of the neural circuitry linking the cerebellum with the associative and paralimbic cerebral regions prevents the cerebellar modulation of functions subserved by the affected subsystems, thus producing the behavioral deficits observed in both early and recent accounts and discussed below more comprehensively (Snider, 1950; Dow, 1974; Heath, 1977, Leiner et al., 1986; Schmahmann & Pandya, 1987, 1989; Botez et al., 1989; Schmahmann, 1991, 1996).

The interaction between the mossy fiber system input to the cerebellum from the pons and the climbing fibers derived exclusively from the inferior olivary nucleus has served as the substrate for hypotheses concerning the cerebellar role in both motor and nonmotor behaviors (Marr, 1969; Albus, 1971; Ito, 1993). The inferior olive receives little, if any, direct input from the cerebral cortex. Its major source of descending afferents arises from the red nucleus that carries mostly sensorimotor information (Kuypers & Lawrence, 1967; Humphrey et al., 1984; Kennedy et al., 1986). It does, however, also receive some associative cortical input indirectly from brainstem reticular nuclei and from the zona incerta (ZI; Saint-Cyr & Courville, 1980). The ZI receives input from the rostral cingulate cortex (area 24); the prefrontal cortex (areas 9/46d at the dorsolateral convexity and area 9 at the medial convexity); the posterior parietal cortex (areas PF and PG in the inferior parietal lobule and area PGm at the medial con-

vexity of the superior parietal lobule); and from the medial prestriate cortex (Shah et al., 1997). The detection of associative projections to the ZI, which in turn projects to the inferior olivary nucleus, maintains the possibility that interaction between the mossy fiber and climbing fiber systems may be relevant for higher function, in addition to tasks related to motor performance and motor learning.

Clinical Studies

Early anecdotal reports of neuropsychiatric presentations in patients with cerebellar anomalies (see Schmahmann, 1991, 1997) were followed by studies of patients with hereditary ataxia who demonstrated emotional lability, irritability, loss of comprehension, poverty of association, and general intellectual impairment (Knoepfel & Macken, 1947), and of patients with olivopontocerebellar degeneration who displayed deficits in verbal and nonverbal intelligence, memory, and frontal system function including concept formation (Kish et al., 1988; Bracke-Tolkmitt et al., 1989). Impaired executive function was demonstrated in patients with cerebellar cortical atrophy as shown by increased planning times when performing the Tower of Hanoi test (Grafman et al., 1992),

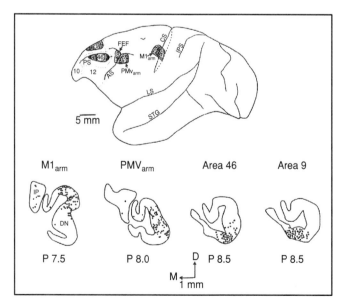

FIGURE 25-13. Lateral view of a cebus monkey brain (*top*) to show the location of injections of McIntyre-B strain of herpes simplex virus type 1 in the primary motor cortex, ventral premotor cortex, and areas 9 and 46. The resulting retrogradely labeled neurons in the cerebellar dentate nucleus (*bottom*) are indicated by solid dots. (From Middleton FA, Strick PL: Cerebellar output channels, in Schmahmann JD [ed]: The Cerebellum and Cognition. International Review of Neurobiology, Vol. 41. San Diego, CA: Academic Press, 1997, pp. 61–82.)

and by poor performance on tests of fluency and the initiation/perseveration subtest of the Mattis Dementia Rating Scale (Appollonio et al., 1993). Most of the genetically identified spinocerebellar ataxias have now been reported to have cognitive decline as part of the clinical spectrum at some point in the course (Geschwind, 1999). Neuropsychological studies in patients with focal cerebellar injuries have revealed visual spatial deficits following focal left hemisphere lesions such as tumor excision (Wallesch & Horn, 1990) and left superior cerebellar artery territory infarction (Botez-Marquard et al., 1994), and agrammatism (Silveri et al., 1994) and impaired error detection and practice-related learning of a verb-for-noun generation task (Fiez et al., 1992) following right cerebellar infarction. These accounts did not resolve the question whether focal lesions of the cerebellum produce cognitive or other behavioral deficits that are clinically relevant. The report of a cerebellar cognitive affective syndrome (Schmahmann & Sherman, 1998a) resulting from lesions confined to the cerebellum appears to have added this previously missing important clinical description to the discussion.

The Cerebellar Cognitive Affective Syndrome

In our series (Schmahmann & Sherman, 1998a), 20 patients had pathology confined to the cerebellum on clinical and neuroimaging grounds. Thirteen patients suffered stroke, three had postinfectious cerebellitis, three had cerebellar cortical atrophy, and one had a midline cerebellar tumor resected.

On bedside mental state testing, all patients were awake, cooperative, and able to give an account of their history, although the level of attention was variable. Eighteen patients demonstrated problems with executive functions. Working memory was poor in 11 (of 16 tested), motor or ideational set shifting in 16 (of 19), and perseveration of actions or drawings was noted in 16 (of 20). Verbal fluency was impaired in 18 patients, and in some this was clinically evident as telegraphic speech. In two patients, speech output was so limited as to resemble mutism. Decreased verbal fluency was unrelated to dysarthria. Some patients with minimal dysarthria in the setting of acute lesions performed more poorly on fluency tests than others with severe dysarthria and disease of greater duration.

Visuospatial disintegration, most marked in attempting to draw or copy a diagram, was found in 19 patients, regardless of lesion acuity or severity of the dysmetria (Fig. 25-14). The sequential approach to the drawing of the diagrams and the conceptualization of the figures was disorganized. Four patients demonstrated simultanagnosia.

Naming was impaired in 13 patients, generally being spared in those with smaller lesions. Six patients

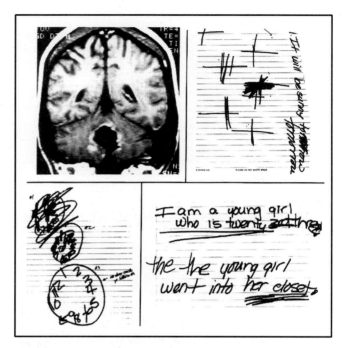

FIGURE 25-14. T1-weighted coronal MRI of the brain of a young woman showing the site of excision of a cerebellar ganglioglioma and her responses when asked to draw a clock, bisect a line, and write a sentence. This performance captures some essential elements of the cerebellar cognitive affective syndrome, including perseveration, impulsivity and disinhibition, visual-spatial disorganization, and agrammatism. (From Schmahmann JD, Sherman JC: The cerebellar cognitive affective syndrome. Brain 121:561–579, 1998.)

had agrammatic speech, most notably in those with bilateral acute disease. Elements of abnormal syntactic structure were noted in others, but less prominently. Prosody was abnormal in 8 patients, with tone of voice characterized by a high-pitched, whining, childish, and hypophonic quality.

Mental arithmetic was deficient in 14 patients. Verbal learning and recall were mildly abnormal in 11, and visual learning and recall were impaired in 4 of 13 patients tested. Ideational apraxia was evident in 2 individuals.

A prominent feature of the bedside mental state examination in 15 patients was the presence of difficulty in modulation of behavior and personality style. The notable exception was those patients whose strokes were either very limited in size or confined to the anterior lobe. Flattening of affect and disinhibition were manifested as overfamiliarity, flamboyant and impulsive actions, and humorous but inappropriate and flippant comments. Behavior was regressive and childlike, particularly following large or bilateral posterior inferior cerebellar artery (PICA) territory infarcts, and in the patient with surgical excision of the vermis and paravermian structures. Obsessive-compulsive traits were occasionally observed.

TABLE 25-3. Clinical Features of the Cerebellar Cognitive Affective Syndrome in Adults

- Executive function deficits
  Planning, set-shifting, verbal fluency, abstract
    reasoning, working memory
- Spatial cognition impairments
  Visual-spatial organization and memory
- Personality changes
  Blunting of affect or disinhibited and inappropriate
    behavior
- Language disorders
  Agrammatism and aprosodia

Data from Schmahmann JD, Sherman JC: The cerebellar cognitive affective syndrome. Brain 121: 561–579, 1998.

Autonomic changes were the central feature in one patient, whose stroke in a medial branch of the right PICA involved the fastigial nucleus and paravermian cortex region. This manifested as spells of hiccuping and coughing that precipitated bradycardia and syncope.

The findings on neuropsychological testing were in agreement with the observations from the bedside mental state evaluation with respect to the nature of the deficits detected. The distribution of patients' scores differed significantly from normal, with the most marked deviation evident in the categories of executive and visual-spatial function. Attention and orientation and language functions more closely approximated a normal distribution of scores. In addition, performance on the Porteus Mazes Task (a test of visual-spatial planning) was very poor, with all subjects scoring at or below a test age of 12 years. Patients with bilateral lesions and posterior lobe lesions were most impaired, and those with small lesions, or in whom disease was confined to the anterior lobe of the cerebellum, were least affected.

The essential features of the cerebellar cognitive affective syndrome (CCAS; executive, spatial, linguistic, psychiatric) are outlined in Table 25-3. The net effect of these disturbances in cognitive functioning is a general lowering of overall intellectual function.

These deficits were clinically relevant, noted by family members and nursing and medical staff, and were associated with detectable abnormalities in the bedside mental state examination. The neurobehavioral presentation in our patients was more pronounced and generalized in patients with large, bilateral, or pancerebellar disorders, and particularly in those with acute-onset cerebellar disease. It was less evident in patients with more insidious disease, in the recovery phase (3–4 months) after acute stroke, and in those with restricted cerebellar pathology. Lesions of the posterior lobe were particularly important in the generation of the disturbed cognitive behaviors, and the vermis was

consistently involved in patients with pronounced affective presentations. The anterior lobe seemed to be less prominently involved in the generation of these cognitive and behavioral deficits. The one patient with an autonomic syndrome had a lesion involving the medial posterior lobe, including the fastigial nucleus.

The clinical relevance of the CCAS has been emphasized in subsequent clinical reports. Young adults (ages 18–44) with cerebellar strokes have delayed return to the workforce because of cognitive limitations, not motor incapacity (Malm et al., 1998). The cognitive deficits described in this group of patients was similar to those with the CCAS, proportional to the size of the infarct, and included deficits in attention, working memory, the temporary storage of complex information, visuospatial skills, and cognitive flexibility. Performance on the block design task in the early post-stroke period predicted maximal working capacity at 12 months. Similarly, Neau and colleagues (2000) studied 15 patients with cerebellar infarcts (10 PICA, 4 superior cerebellar artery [SCA], and 1 anterior inferior cerebellar artery [AICA]), and reported findings consistent with the CCAS as defined above. These included deficits in executive function as revealed by poor performance on phonemic and alternate categorical fluency, naming with and without interference, and a paced auditory serial addition task; and visual spatial deficits with low scores on the Wechsler Adult Intelligence Scale-Revised (WAIS-R) block design.

Parvizi and colleagues (2001) explored the dysequilibrium inherent in the emotional display of some patients with cerebellar lesions, by considering the phenomenon of pathologic laughter and crying in a patient in whom the cerebellum was partially deafferented by multiple infarcts in the left lateral cerebral peduncle, midline rostral basilar pons, right middle cerebellar peduncle, and white matter of right cerebellar crus II (inferior semilunar lobule). Cognitive testing also revealed deficits in executive function and visual memory and relative weakness in abstract reasoning. The authors concluded that pathologic laughter and crying arise from lesions of the cerebro-ponto-cerebellar pathways. In their view, the normal cerebellum automatically adjusts the execution of laughter or crying to the cognitive and situational context of a potential stimulus. Loss of the cerebellar input requires that the cerebellum operate on the basis of incomplete information about that context, the result of which is inadequate or chaotic behavior. One study of patients with cerebellar lesions failed to detect neuropsychological deficits (Gomez Beldarrain et al., 1997). The control population had limited education and poor mini-mental state score, however, that may have limited the ability of the investigators to detect significant behavioral impairments in the study group (Schmahmann & Sherman, 1998b). Further, the study included patients with lesions that were more than 6 months old, and the CCAS from unilateral lesions has been shown to recover with time (Botez-Marquard et al., 1994; Schmahmann & Sherman, 1998a; Neau et al., 2000).

Cerebellar Cognitive Affective Syndrome in Children

Impairments in intelligence, memory, language, attention, academic skills, and psychosocial function have been reported in children following resection of cerebellar tumors (Dennis et al., 1996), but these have been observed in groups that have undergone cerebellar resection as well as cranial radiation or chemotherapy or both. This is problematic because radiation necrosis is associated with deficits in general intelligence, academic achievement, verbal knowledge and reasoning, and perceptual motor abilities, and methotrexate causes substantial neurologic and neurobehavioral impairment (Dennis et al., 1996; Duffner et al., 1983; Glauser & Packer, 1991; Radcliffe et al., 1992).

To determine whether the CCAS is observed in children, Levisohn and colleagues (2000) performed a retrospective record review of the results of standardized neuropsychological tests in 19 children with cerebellar tumors who received neither methotrexate nor radiation therapy prior to testing (Table 25-4). Eleven had medulloblastoma, 7 astrocytoma, 1 an ependymoma. The children ranged in age from 3 to 14 years at the time of tumor resection. The time between surgery and neuropsychological testing ranged from 1 to 22 months (mean 5.1, SD 6.4). Eight children received chemotherapy prior to neuropsychological testing. Two patients had hydrocephalus that required shunting.

Seven of the 19 patients (37%) met criteria for expressive language deficits. Another 4 demonstrated word-finding difficulties detected in testing (difficulty

TABLE 25-4. Clinical Features of Cerebellar Cognitive Affective Syndrome in Children Following Tumor Resection

- Problem-solving
  Fail to organize verbal or visual-spatial material

- Visual-spatial
  Impaired planning and organization

- Regulation of affect (vermis lesions)
  Irritable, impulsive, disinhibited, labile affect

- Expressive language
  Poor initiation and lack of elaboration, impaired word finding and naming

- Memory
  Impaired for stories. Retrieval better with multiple-choice

Data from Levisohn L, Cronin-Golomb A, Schmahmann JD: Neuropsychological consequences of cerebellar tumor resection in children: Cerebellar cognitive affective syndrome in a pediatric population. Brain 123: 1041–1050, 2000.

naming objects in the Picture Completion test) or in spontaneous conversation in the context of otherwise intact language abilities. Seven (37%) had deficits in visual-spatial functions. Three (16%) had deficits in both expressive language and visual-spatial functions. In addition to these deficits in expressive language and visual-spatial functions, of 14 children administered the Digit Span test, 8 (57%) performed poorly. Additionally, some with average scores on Digit Span showed perseveration and difficulties establishing set. Five of 15 tested (33%) had verbal memory deficits along with other deficits in visual-spatial or language function. Standard measures used to evaluate executive/prefrontal function in this group were limited.

Six patients (32%) had deficits in affect regulation, and they all had extensive vermis damage. In contrast, none of the patients without affect problems had extensive vermis damage. Children with prominent vermis damage were more likely to exhibit changes in affect regulation than those with intact vermis or only minimal vermis damage. Five of nine children who sustained extensive vermis damage (56%) exhibited the posterior fossa syndrome postoperatively. Patients who were older at the time of testing were more likely to show neuropsychological deficits. Eight of the 10 patients older than 7 years had deficits (80%), whereas 3 of the 9 children (33%) younger than 7 years were impaired. These age effects may have been confounded by tumor type because medulloblastomas were more common in the older children, and astrocytomas or ependymomas were more common (75%) in the younger children.

Other investigators have replicated the observation that children with cerebellar tumor excision manifest high-level cognitive and emotional deficits. Riva and Giorgi (2000) evaluated 26 such children and reported that those with right cerebellar hemisphere tumors presented with disturbances of auditory sequential memory and language processing, whereas those with left hemisphere tumors showed deficits on tests of spatial and visual sequential memory. These investigators also found that vermal lesions led to postsurgical mutism, which evolved into speech disorders or language disturbances similar to agrammatism, and behavioral disturbances including irritability, decreased ability to tolerate the company of others, and a general tendency to avoid physical and eye contact. Complex repetitive and rhythmic rocking movements, stereotyped linguistic utterances, and general lack of empathy in one patient met DSM-IV criteria for a diagnosis of autism.

The Posterior Fossa Syndrome

An intriguing neurobehavioral syndrome has been observed in children who undergo resection of midline tumors of the cerebellum (Wisoff & Epstein, 1984;

Pollack, 1997; Catsman-Berrevoets et al., 1999). The phenomenon is marked by the development of mutism within 48 hours following surgical approach involving the cerebellar vermis, and in the recovery phase over a period of months it is accompanied by dysarthria and buccal and lingual apraxia. There is no involvement of equilibrium, gait, or appendicular movements, although motor tone is decreased. In addition to the mutism, these children display a behavioral syndrome that includes regressive personality changes, apathy, and poverty of spontaneous movement. Emotional lability is marked, and there is rapid fluctuation of expression of emotion that gravitates between irritability with inconsolable crying and agitation, to giggling and easy distractibility. Not all children with the CCAS pass through the stage of the posterior fossa syndrome, because the CCAS develops following unilateral or bilateral damage to the posterior lobes with or without vermal involvement, whereas the posterior fossa syndrome occurs only following midline lesions. Children with the CCAS whose damage includes the vermis, however, have prominent mood dysregulation, and some of these pass initially through the phase of postoperative mutism. Postoperative mutism has been observed in some adults (Dunwoody et al., 1997). Restriction of verbal fluency, almost to the point of mutism, was present in some patients in the original CCAS series, but was less marked than in the children with posterior fossa syndrome.

Developmental Cognitive Abilities

Recent observations suggest a relationship between developmental anomalies of the cerebellum and neurobehavioral syndromes. Quantitative morphometry of the cerebellum in attention-deficit/hyperactivity disorder (ADHD) reveals smaller posterior lobes of the vermis (lobules VIII through X) in both boys (Berquin et al., 1998; Mostofsky et al., 1998) and girls (Castellanos et al., 2001), and early evidence suggests that the size of the vermis is related to the severity of the ADHD.

Allin and colleagues (2001) set out to establish whether cognitive and motor impairments in adolescents born very preterm (before 33 weeks of gestation) are associated with abnormalities of the cerebellum as revealed by volumetric analysis of brain MRI scans. In their longitudinal study cognitive and neurologic evaluations are performed from ages 1 through 15. The MRI scans of 67 children born very preterm and 50 age-matched, full-term-born controls were studied. The preterm-born subjects had significantly reduced cerebellar volume compared with term-born controls ($P < .001$). This difference was present after controlling for potential confounders. There was no association between cerebellar volume and motor neurologic signs. However, there were significant associations between cerebellar volume and several cognitive test scores. These included impaired executive and visual-spatial functions as revealed by the Similarities, Block Design, and Object Assembly subtests of the Wechsler Intelligence Scale for Children-Revised; impaired language skills as revealed by Schonnel reading age; and difficulty decoding and understanding the Kaufman Assessment Battery for Children. The similarity between the major findings of this study and the CCAS in adults and children provides a concordance of information from different spheres of clinical investigation.

Acquired dyslexia was also noted in patients with lesions of the vermis and paravermian region (Moretti et al., 2002). These observations are of interest in the light of the report that individuals with dyslexia demonstrate lower cerebellar activation on PET scans compared to controls when performing motor tasks (Nicolson et al., 1999). Activation was significantly lower for the dyslexic adults than for the controls in the right cerebellar cortex and the left cingulate gyrus when executing a prelearned sequence of finger movements, and in the right cerebellar cortex when learning a novel sequence. These findings on traditional tests of cerebellar motor coordination in dyslexics suggest a possible cerebellar role in this high-level cognitive skill.

Cerebellar tumors were found to have an adverse effect on the developmental cognitive profile of seven right-handed children studied by Scott and colleagues (2001), in whom the mean age at diagnosis was 3 years and the mean age at first assessment was 7 years. Greater damage to right cerebellum resulted in a plateauing in verbal and literacy skills, whereas predominantly left cerebellar damage was associated with delayed or impaired nonverbal/spatial skills. This kind of analysis indicates the importance of future long-term follow-up studies of children with acquired cerebellar pathology to evaluate the cognitive and, possibly, psychiatric implications of the cerebellar pathology.

Cerebellar agenesis is rare, and until recently was considered to be asymptomatic. Glickstein (1994) challenged the accepted notion that cerebellar agenesis is asymptomatic from the perspective of motor control, and uncovered historical accounts of children with agenesis showing impairments of coordination, speech, and oromotor faculties along with delay of motor milestones. Additionally, clinical reports of cerebellar agenesis from the 19th century describe a variety of higher-order deficits, including "subnormal intelligence," "mental retardation," and "idiocy" (Schmahmann, 1991). Gardner and colleagues (2001) evaluated three patients with near-total absence of the cerebellum, and reported delayed milestones, mild motor impairments, and intellectual handicap. Chheda and colleagues (2002) found that near-complete or partial cerebellar agenesis was accompanied by behavioral and motor deficits in six children and two adults,

TABLE 25-5. Clinical Presentation of Cerebellar Agenesis

Motor impairments
- Impaired saccades and vestibulo-ocular reflex cancellation (VORC)
- Oral motor apraxia
- Gross and fine motor delay
- Mild clumsiness and ataxia

Cognitive and affective deficits
- Executive impairments
    Perseveration, disinhibition, impaired abstract reasoning, working memory and verbal fluency
- Spatial cognition
    Poor perceptual organization, copying, and recall
- Language
    Expressive language delay—some requiring sign language. Impaired prosody. Over-regularization of past-tense verbs
- Psychiatric/affective
    Autistic-like stereotypical performance, obsessive rituals, difficulty understanding social cues

Data from Chheda M, Sherman J, Schmahmann JD: Neurologic, psychiatric, and cognitive manifestations in cerebellar agenesis [abstract]. Neurology 58 (Suppl.3):356, 2002.

and the location and extent of the agenesis was correlated with the severity and range of the motor, cognitive, and psychiatric impairments (Table 25-5). The children presented with gross and fine motor delay, oral motor apraxia, impaired saccades and vestibulo-ocular reflex cancellation, clumsiness, and mild ataxia. Behavioral features included autistic-like stereotypical performance, obsessive rituals, and difficulty understanding social cues. Tactile defensiveness (avoidance of, and adverse reaction to touch) was a prominent feature in four children. Executive impairments included perseveration, disinhibition, and poor abstract reasoning, working memory, and verbal fluency. Spatial cognition was impaired for perceptual organization, visual-spatial copying, and recall. Some children presented with expressive language delay as the principal manifestation, in two instances so severe as to require instruction in sign language. Impaired prosody was evident in all cases, and over-regularization of past-tense verbs was noted. In longitudinal follow-up, extensive rehabilitation enhanced motor, linguistic, and cognitive performance. Of the two adults with partial agenesis in this study, one with vermal predominant agenesis suffered from lifelong psychotic depression, and the other with subtotal right hemisphere agenesis experienced a psychotic episode in adolescence.

It is our own clinical experience that patients with nonprogressive cerebellar ataxia ("cerebellar cerebral palsy" of earlier times) are associated with cognitive

impairments, including language delay. This was documented by Steinlin and colleagues (1998). There were 34 patients in their cohort. Fifteen of 27 had normal MRI scans. Some had spasticity, focal dystonia, and epilepsy, so the degree to which the disorder was purely confined to the cerebellum in all cases is uncertain. Nevertheless, all patients had delayed motor and speech development, and cognitive impairment was present in 22. Indeed, in the majority of their cases, cognitive impairment proved to be the major problem, rather than the "neurologic" symptoms.

The Cerebellum and Psychosis

The CCAS includes as part of its spectrum of manifestations the alterations in behavior that extend beyond cognition. Adults and children experience altered regulation of mood and personality, display obsessive-compulsive tendencies, and demonstrate psychotic thinking. The mother of one patient (unpublished) who underwent resection of a midline astrocytoma reported her surprise at witnessing a prominent and persistent behavior change in her son. His personality style had been characterized by impulsiveness and assertiveness to the point of aggression from age 5. The tumor declared itself with nausea, vomiting, vertigo, and ataxia, and at age 12 it was resected. The patient's personality changed from the moment that he recovered from anesthesia. He became passive, immature, and childlike and showed no hint of the previous aggressive behavior. He has remained unchanged for 6 years. Another patient (Schmahmann, Sherman, Weilburg, unpublished) who underwent resection of a midline tumor at age 6, has slipped in early adulthood into a state of paranoid ideation, bizarre illogical thinking (at times of psychotic proportions), depressed mood, obsessional preoccupation, and personal stereotypical rituals. He became inaccessible to family and friends and unable to organize his thoughts and plan his life. He improved on neuroleptic medication. Systematic investigations of this putative relationship between acquired cerebellar pathology and the subsequent development of psychosis are much needed.

Anecdotal examples from selected patients may be purely coincidental, and a prospective study to evaluate the presence and nature of immediate or delayed postcerebellectomy psychosis has yet to be performed. The disturbances of behavior and emotion that have declared themselves in the series of patients with the CCAS, however, emphasize the relevance of the cerebellum for the psychiatric population, and for clinicians and investigators interested in understanding psychiatric diseases. The descriptions of cognitive and emotional influences in patients with cerebellar diseases are complemented by the investigations of conditions that are defined by their behavioral features, and in which cerebellar anomalies have subsequently been defined.

Publications in the 1800s noted deviant and aberrant behaviors in individuals with cerebellar anomalies. These reports were strengthened by later clinical observations of a relationship between the cerebellum and personality, aggression, and emotion, and that linked psychosis, and schizophrenia in particular, with cerebellar structural abnormalities. Heath and colleagues (1979) described pathology such as cysts and tumors in the midline cerebellum in patients diagnosed with psychosis. Pollak and associates (1996) also described data on seven patients with posterior fossa structural abnormalities who presented with neuropsychiatric symptomatology. Two patients had tumors, two mega-cisterna magna, two Dandy-Walker variants, and in one patient a fourth ventricle tumor was removed in childhood. Psychiatric diagnoses that met DSM-IV criteria were psychosis (two patients), major depression (one), personality disorders (one), and somatoform disorders (one).

Pathologic anatomic findings have been reported in schizophrenia including enlargement of the fourth ventricle, smaller cerebellar vermis, and cerebellar atrophy (Lippmann et al., 1981; Moriguchi, 1981). More recently, Loeber and colleagues (2001) used MRI to measure the volume of individual cerebellar lobules in 19 patients with schizophrenia and 19 healthy comparison subjects. They found that compared to the controls, patients with schizophrenia had a significantly smaller inferior vermis, and significantly less cerebellar hemispheric asymmetry. In an MRI study of schizophrenic patients who had no history of using neuroleptic medication, Ichimiya and colleagues (2001) found significantly reduced vermis volume in the schizophrenic group, and no significant differences in the volumes of other cerebellar structures or cerebral hemispheres. Furthermore, reduction in the vermal volume correlated with the Depression and Paranoia subscores of the Brief Psychiatric Rating Scale. Volz and colleagues (2000) undertook a morphometric study in order to explore the dysmetria of thought hypothesis (Schmahmann, 1991, 1994, 1996, 2000b) as it has been applied to schizophrenia (Andreasen et al., 1996). They found reduced volumes in patients with schizophrenia in the left cerebellar hemisphere and the right cerebellar vermis as well as in the frontal lobe, the temporal lobe, and thalamus. Not all studies, however, have demonstrated the smaller cerebellar volumes (Staal et al., 2001), but this may reflect differences in methodologic approach.

Quantitative MRI morphometry (Courchesne et al., 1988; Murakami et al., 1989) and postmortem analysis of early infantile autism (Kemper & Bauman, 1998), that was once classified as juvenile schizophrenia have revealed abnormalities in the midline DCN, the cortex in the posterior lobes, and the vermis. These contemporary observations lend credence to the notion that midline structures of the cerebellum in patients and monkeys play a role in emotion, aggression, and psychosis (Snider, 1950; Reis et al., 1973; Heath, 1977; Berman et al., 1978; Cooper et al., 1978). The activation of midline cerebellar structures on functional imaging studies of panic (Reiman et al., 1989) and sadness (Lane et al., 1997; Beauregard et al., 1998) add to the clinical evidence implicating the vermis in the regulation of emotion.

Functional Imaging and the Human Cerebellum

Since Petersen and colleagues (1989) demonstrated midline and right cerebellar activation by a linguistic task (verb-for-noun generation paradigm) in the absence of an overt motor act, a large and growing literature has demonstrated cerebellar activation on PET and functional (fMRI) of a wide variety of sensory, cognitive, autonomic, and cognitive paradigms (Table 25-6). A review of functional neuroimaging experiments dating back to 1985 (Schmahmann et al., 1998; Schmahmann, 2000a; see also Desmond & Fiez, 1998) demonstrates that there appears to be a general topographic organization of function in the human cerebellum. The "sensorimotor cerebellum" is located in lobules III through V in the anterior lobe (rostral to the primary fissure), with a secondary representation in lobules VIII/IX. The "cognitive cerebellum" is predominantly in the posterior lobe, that is, in lobules VI and VII and their hemispheric extensions into lobule VI, crus I and II of lobule VIIA (ansiform lobe), and lobule

TABLE 25-6. Partial List of Paradigms Across Multiple Domains that Activate Cerebellum in Functional Imaging Studies

- Sensorimotor activation
- Sensory processing and discrimination
- Mental imagery
- Motor learning
- Classical conditioning
- Nonmotor learning and memory
- Linguistic processing
- Attentional modulation
- Timing estimation
- Emotion perception and experience
- Visual-spatial memory
- Executive function
  Verbal working memory
  Strategy, reasoning, verbal fluency
- Autonomic function
  Pain, thirst, hunger, smell, hypoxemia

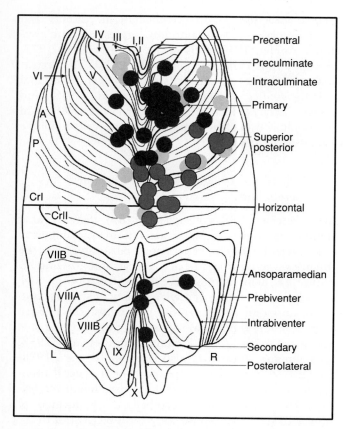

FIGURE 25-15. Diagram illustrating cerebellar activation sites from functional imaging studies represented on a semi-flattened map of the human cerebellum. Motor activation sites are depicted by black circles, motor imagery tasks by light gray circles, and linguistic processing tasks by the outlined gray circles. (From Schmahmann JD, Loeber RT, Marjani J, et al: Topographic organization of cognitive function in the human cerebellum. A meta-analysis of functional imaging studies. Neuroimage 7:S721, 1998; and Schmahmann JD: Cerebellum and brainstem, in Toga A, Mazziotta J [eds]: Brain Mapping: The Systems. San Diego, CA: Academic Press, 2000, pp. 207–259.)

VIIB (nomenclature according to Schmahmann et al., 1999, 2000). Language tasks activate lobule VI and crus I at the vermis and right hemisphere (Fig. 25-15). Verbal working memory tasks activate lobule VI and crus I on the right, in a location slightly rostral to language processing. Attentional modulation is more heavily concentrated in lobule VI on the left; and nonmotor learning is focused particularly in crus I and crus II bilaterally. Activation predominantly in the vermis or paravermian regions by emotional experience (Lane et al., 1997), pain (Coghill et al., 1999), thirst (Parsons et al., 2000), hunger (Tataranni et al., 1999), and smell (Sobel et al., 1998) provide some support for the hypothesis that the phylogenetically older cerebellar vermis and fastigial nucleus may be the equivalent of the "limbic cerebellum."

These studies are in agreement with early physiologic and connectivity studies in nonhuman primates and cats (Snider, 1952; Hampson et al., 1952; Henneman et al., 1952; Chambers & Sprague, 1955a,b) showing a primary sensorimotor region in the anterior lobe and a "secondary" (Woolsey, 1952) representation in the posterior lobe, and with the observation that lesions of the cerebellar anterior lobe are associated with the motor impairments of ataxia, dysmetria, and disordered eye movements (Holmes, 1917). The imaging studies are in accord also with the anatomy of the cerebellar cognitive affective syndrome, which is associated mostly with lesions of the posterior lobe. Further, the disordered affective regulation is linked particularly with involvement of the vermis (Schmahmann & Sherman, 1998a), as suggested by studies in other patients and animals (Heath et al., 1979; Snider, 1982; Pollack et al., 1995; Schmahmann, 1991, 1997; Levisohn et al., 2000; Riva & Giorgi, 2000).

Thus, cerebellar activation by cognitive and other nonmotor tasks helps bring the cerebellum squarely into the realm of behavioral neuroscience. The apparent topographic organization of cognition in the cerebellum is consistent with the hypothesis that the cerebellum is an essential node in the distributed neural circuitry subserving cognitive operations, and the multiple discrete channels of information in the cerebrocerebellar system provide the anatomic substrate to support the findings in these imaging studies.

Functional Topography in the Human Cerebellum

Topographic organization of motor function in the cerebellum was proposed by Bolk (1906) and further supported by clinical (Holmes, 1917), physiologic (Snider, 1950), and anatomic investigations (Chambers & Sprague, 1955a,b). It now appears that there are also neurobehavioral syndromes associated with cerebellar lesions and that the cerebellum is topographically organized with respect to these higher order functions as well (Table 25-7). The sensorimotor cerebellum is located in the anterior lobe, with a secondary representation (after Woolsey, 1952, and Snider, 1950, 1952) in lobules VIII/IX. The vermis and midline fastigial nucleus constitute the "limbic cerebellum," and may be considered an extension of Papez (1937) circuit concerned with emotional modulation and autonomic function. These regions are thought to be concerned with primitive defense mechanisms including the autonomic manifestations of the fight-or-flight response, as well as with emotion and affect, and possibly also with affectively important memory. In contrast, the lateral cerebellar hemispheres and associated dentate and emboliform nuclei constitute the "cognitive cerebellum," linked with association areas and paralimbic cortices. These regions are concerned with high-level,

TABLE 25-7. Postulated Topography of Function in the Human Cerebellum

Anterior-Posterior Organization
Sensorimotor
Predominantly anterior lobe (lobules I–V)
"Secondary" representation in lobules VIII/IX

Cognitive, affective
Predominantly neocerebellum (vermal and hemispheric components of lobules VI, VII)

Medial–Lateral Organization
Vermis and fastigial nucleus
Autonomic regulation, affect, emotionally important memory

Cerebellar hemispheres and dentate nucleus
Executive, visual-spatial, linguistic, learning and memory

Data from Schmahmann JD: From movement to thought: Anatomic substrates of the cerebellar contribution to cognitive processing. Hum Brain Mapping 4: 174–198, 1996.

cognitive operations, including the modulation of thought, planning, strategy formation, spatial and temporal parameters, learning, memory, and language (Schmahmann, 1991, 1996).

Theoretical Considerations

The Dysmetria of Thought Hypothesis

The clinical descriptions and this putative functional topography are consistent with a broad vision of cerebellar function, encapsulated by the *dysmetria of thought* hypothesis (Schmahmann, 1991, 1994, 1996, 2000b). Immunohistochemistry has identified that the cerebellar cortex contains anatomically identifiable parasagittal bands (Gravel & Hawkes, 1990) that appear to have connectional and physiologic specificity (Hallem et al., 1999), but there are no "Brodmann areas" in the cerebellum. The cerebellar cortex has an essentially uniform, monotonously repetitive architecture, suggesting that the transformations performed by the cerebellum are invariant throughout the structure. There is, however, anatomic specificity linking each segment of the cerebrocerebellar pathway, that is, cerebral cortex, pontine nuclei, cerebellar cortex, cerebellar nuclei, and thalamus. There is thus a unitary principle of architecture but a localizationist principle of connectivity. The dysmetria of thought hypothesis draws on these anatomic features and proposes that the cerebellar contribution to the nervous system is embodied in a universal cerebellar transform (UCT) applied to multiple domains of neurologic function. The nature of the transform is constant because of the uniform architecture, but the information modulated by different regions within the cerebellum varies because of the connectional topography.

TABLE 25-8. Dysmetria of Thought Hypothesis

The **universal cerebellar transform (UCT)** is a fundamental function distributed throughout the cerebellum that **modulates behavior automatically around a homeostatic baseline.** Anatomic specificity within the cerebrocerebellar system permits the cerebellum to contribute to multiple domains of neurologic function.

By corollary, there is **a universal cerebellar impairment (UCI)**, namely, **dysmetria**. This includes dysmetria of movement—*ataxia*, and dysmetria of thought and emotion—the *cerebellar cognitive affective syndrome.*

Data from Schmahmann JD: The role of the cerebellum in affect and psychosis. J Neurolinguistics 13:189–214, 2000.

The cerebellum thus performs its UCT on the information to which it has access, whether that information subserves arousal, autonomic functions, affective behaviors, cognitive operations, or sensorimotor processes (Table 25-8).

In this hypothesis, the cerebellar contribution to the multiple different functions is to modulate behaviors and serve as an oscillation dampener, automatically maintaining function around a homeostatic baseline, smoothing out performance in all domains. The cerebellum compares the consequences of actions with the intended outcome, and matches reality with perceived reality. It facilitates actions harmonious with the goal, appropriate to context, and judged accurately and reliably according to the strategies mapped prior to, and during, the behavior. In this view, the cerebellum detects, prevents, and corrects mismatches between intended outcome and perceived outcome of the organism's interaction with the environment. In the same way that the cerebellum regulates the rate, force, rhythm, and accuracy of movements, so does it influence the speed, capacity, consistency, and appropriateness of mental or cognitive processes. In this model, the cerebellar contribution to cognition is one of modulation rather than generation. The dysmetria of thought hypothesis is in accord with the suggestions of Snider (1950) that the cerebellum is the great modulator of neurologic function, of Heath (1977) that the cerebellum is an emotional pacemaker for the brain, and of Ito (1993) that the cerebellum serves to prevent, detect, and correct errors of thought in the same way as it does so for errors of movement.

If there is a UCT, then cerebellar damage must, by corollary, lead to a universal cerebellar impairment (UCI). Following a cerebellar lesion, the cerebellar component of the distributed neural circuit is lost or disrupted, and the loss of the UCT implies that the oscillation dampener is removed. The hypothesis holds that the UCI is characterized by dysmetria. The UCI from lesions in the sensorimotor cerebellum is incoordination, that is, gait ataxia and dysmetria, or incoordination, of the extremities; articulation; and eye movements. The UCI in the behavioral realm is dysmetria of thought, manifesting as the various components of the CCAS (Schmahmann & Sherman, 1998a; Levisohn et al., 2000; Schmahmann, 2000b). Mental processes are imperfectly conceived, erratically monitored, and poorly performed. There is unpredictability to social and societal interaction, a mismatch between reality and perceived reality, and erratic attempts to correct the errors of thought or behavior. The overshoot and inability in the motor system to check parameters of movement may be equated, in the behavioral realm, with a mismatch between reality and perceived reality, and erratic attempts to correct the errors of thought or behavior. Cognitive deficits result from lesions of the cognitive cerebellum in the cerebellar hemispheres, and emotional and psychiatric disturbances follow lesions of the limbic cerebellum in the vermis and fastigial nucleus.

This dysmetria of thought hypothesis helps explain the observed clinical phenomena in the CCAS and its different cognitive and psychiatric variants, including psychosis. It has provided a testable model for the evaluation of the anatomic substrates of major psychiatric illnesses such as schizophrenia (e.g., Andreasen et al., 1996), and it helps predict observations and guide experiments directed toward elucidating the anatomic substrates and clinical manifestations of neurobehavioral and psychiatric phenomena. Further neuropsychological and psychiatric observations in patients with known cerebellar lesions and morphometric and functional imaging studies of the cerebellum in psychiatric patients will be important as investigators further evaluate the manifestations of the CCAS, test the dysmetria of thought hypothesis, and extend the understanding of the cerebellar role in the nervous system.

Other Theories

Other hypotheses about the role of the cerebellum in cognitive and emotional behaviors have been proposed, some of which are briefly summarized here.

The Marr (1969)-Albus (1971) hypothesis (subsequently modified by others including Ito, 1982) proposed that the cerebellum is involved in motor learning. The hypothesis draws on the synaptic organization within the cerebellar cortex and holds that the parallel fiber-Purkinje cell synapse is modifiable, that the mossy fiber system conveys to the cerebellum the context in which an action is taking place, and the climbing fibers convey an error signal that through the mechanism of long-term depression results in the learning of adaptive and predictive responses. The introduction of this concept proposing plasticity and learning in the cerebellum was a major innovation at the time, although it does not now account for the multiple other functions attributed to the cerebellum.

Ivry and colleagues (1997) have maintained that the problems of coordination and mental functions that patients with cerebellar lesions experience can be understood as a problem in controlling and regulating the temporal patterns of movement and behavior. Thus, the timing capabilities of the cerebellum are not limited to the motor domain but are used in perceptual tasks that require the precise representation of temporal information.

In the view of Courchesne and colleagues (Courchesne & Allen, 1997), the cerebellum is a master computational system able to anticipate and adjust responsiveness in a variety of brain systems to achieve goals determined by cerebral and other subcortical systems. These investigators have supported their view that the cerebellum is important for direction of selective attention by demonstrating impairments in this function in cerebellar patients and in autism.

The notions of Bower (1997) that the cerebellum is involved in monitoring and adjusting the acquisition of most of the sensory data on which the rest of the nervous system depends has prompted functional imaging studies that have provided support for this view. This concept holds that rather than being responsible for any particular behaviorally related function, the cerebellum instead facilitates the efficiency with which other brain structures perform their own function.

In an analogous but slightly different view, Paulin (1993) has stated that cerebellar function can be explained by assuming that it is involved in constructing neural representations of moving systems. Thus, the cerebellum could be a neural analog of a dynamic state estimator, and this would explain the participation of the cerebellum in controlling, perceiving, and imagining systems that move.

Thach (1997) proposed that the cerebellum performs context response linkage in motor and nonmotor areas of behavior and is involved in shaping of responses to trial-and-error learning. Through practice, an experiential context automatically evokes a certain mental action plan that may be in the realm of thought, but would not necessarily lead to execution.

In Ito's view (1993, 1997) the cerebellum uses its unique, error-driven adaptive control mechanism, and the model-building capability that is based on it, to function as a regulatory organ subserving different executive functions. The cerebellar corticonuclear microcomplex may represent a dynamic, or inverse dynamic, model of mental representations.

Leiner and colleagues (1986, 1997) regard the cerebrocerebellar system like the circuitry in a versatile computer, in which the cerebellum performs a wide repertoire of computations on a wide range of information to which it has access. The bundling of cerebrocerebellar fibers enables a high level of discourse to take place between the cerebellum and cerebral cortex, using internal languages capable of conveying complex information about what to do and when to do it.

Houk (1997) has proposed that in the sensorimotor domain, a diversity of sensorimotor memories are stored in the cerebellum, and during practice these programs are exported to premotor networks for more efficient execution. According to this hypothesis, cognitive functions could also be exported to the cerebral cortex to improve the efficiency of thinking.

Molinari and colleagues (2002) suggest that the cerebellum influences the neurobiologic substrate for implicit learning. It does this by modulation of cerebral cortical excitability in a discrete topographic manner, thus inducing coupling between significant sensory inputs and definite motor outputs, and hence controlling plastic changes in the cerebral cortex. Doyon and colleagues (2002) suggest that for motor sequence learning to occur, intrinsic modulation must occur within the cerebellum in conjunction with activity in motor-related cerebral cortical regions. This sets up a procedurally acquired sequence of movements that is then maintained elsewhere in the brain. Passingham and colleagues view the function of the cerebellum as being involved in the process by which motor tasks become automatic (Jenkins et al., 1994), and that its role in motor sequence learning reflects a more general operation in preparing responses to predictable sensory events (Nixon & Passingham, 2001).

The notion that the cerebellum performs its unique computations in a topographically precise manner on diverse streams of information relating to almost all aspects of behavior has brought to life the ideas and contributions of earlier investigators and opened the way to a new era of cognitive neuroscience.

CEREBRAL WHITE MATTER

The ability of different brain regions to communicate with each other over long distances is a fundamental premise inherent in the concept of distributed neural circuits subserving nervous system function. This communication occurs by virtue of the white matter pathways that link cortico-cortical and cortico-subcortical structures. The clinical significance of white matter systems is evident in the motor consequences of lesions of the posterior limb of the internal capsule and the spinal cord and is a well-established entity within clinical neurology. The importance of white matter fiber systems for behavioral neurology and psychiatry has been recognized in selected circumstances. Prefrontal leucotomy, for example, was designed to interrupt fiber systems within the frontal lobe in an attempt to ameliorate psychosis (Meyer et al., 1947); callosal section, designed to disconnect the cerebral hemispheres from each other, has provided a fruitful avenue for exploration of issues of consciousness and hemispheric specialization

(Gazzaniga, 2000); and cingulotomy has re-emerged as a valid technique in the management of obsessive-compulsive disorder (Dougherty et al., 2002).

Norman Geschwind (1926–1984), in his 1965 papers, underscored the relevance of the disconnection syndromes to the understanding of human behavior and the neural substrates of higher function. He re-emphasized the syndrome described by Dejerine of alexia without agraphia in cases of infarction of both the splenium of the corpus callosum and the left occipital lobe. In this circumstance, visually perceived information in the intact right occipital lobe is unable to pass through the lesioned splenium to reach the preserved posterior temporal language area in the left hemisphere. Geschwind also credited Wernicke (1874) with proposing conduction aphasia as a type of language disorder (Benson et al., 1973), characterized by impairment of repetition out of proportion to deficits in comprehension and output. Wernicke's notion, developed further by Goldstein (1911), and supported by the anatomic studies of von Monakow (according to Benson et al., 1973), was that conduction aphasia results from disruption of the suprasylvian region containing the arcuate fasciculus that links the language areas in the posterior temporal cortex (now Wernicke's area), with Broca's area in the inferior prefrontal cortices.

The concept of disconnection syndromes has been further applied to lesions of the mamillothalamic tract and of the fornix that lead to amnestic disturbances, as discussed earlier in the chapter. But the true extent of the importance of the concept of disconnection syndromes is only starting to be appreciated, and it appears likely that the "behavioral neurology of white matter" (Filley, 2001) is destined to be a field of major importance within the disciplines of behavioral neurology and psychiatry.

At present, reports concerning diseases of the white matter are essentially descriptive and somewhat amorphous in their attempt to understand the relationship between white matter systems and the clinical manifestations. Patients develop "white matter dementia" from ischemic cerebrovascular disease, as occurs in progressive subcortical ischemic leukoencephalopathy (Binswanger disease), multiple subcortical lacunes, and CADASIL (cerebral autosomal dominant arteriopathy with strokes and ischemic leukoencephalopathy; Fig. 25-16); from demyelinating lesions as occurs in multiple sclerosis (Fig. 25-17), the Creutzfeldt-Jakob (CJ) virus induced progressive multifocal leukoencephalopathy, and from human immunodeficiency virus (HIV) infection of the white matter itself; from leukodystrophies (adrenoleukodystrophy); small vessel disease as occurs in cerebral vasculitis and postradiation obliterative endarteritis; toxic disorders including methotrexate chemotherapy and organic solvent exposure; and mitochondrial disorders such as MELAS

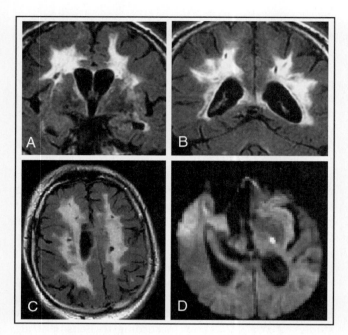

FIGURE 25-16. Rostral (*A*) and caudal (*B*) coronal FLAIR MRI in a 52-year-old man with progressive cognitive and motor decline from cerebral autosomal dominant arteriopathy with strokes and ischemic leukoencephalopathy (CADASIL). A horizontal view is presented in *C*. Acute infarction in the posterior limb of the left internal capsule, superimposed on the underlying disease, is evident on the difusion-weighted image seen in *D*.

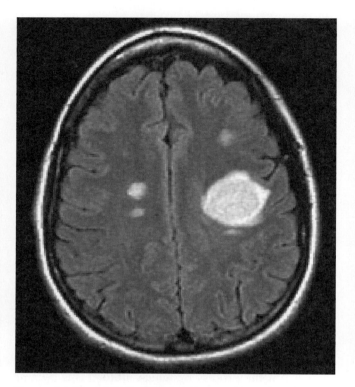

FIGURE 25-17. Multiple areas of abnormal signal in the white matter, with a large focal lesion in the left hemisphere, in a patient with the tumefactive variant of multiple sclerosis.

(mitochondrial encephalopathy with lactic acidosis and stroke-like episodes) and Leigh disease, among others. All these disorders are encountered, some frequently, some less often, in busy clinical practices, and their association with cognitive dysfunction is generally well recognized and reported in case series or anecdotal observations. What is less well appreciated is the frequency of white matter change both in the cerebral cortex itself and in the hemispheric parenchyma in degenerative conditions such as Alzheimer disease (Englund et al., 1988) and in normal aging (Peters et al., 1994). In these conditions, the white matter changes, which are associated with slowing of electrophysiologic conduction time, may be related to some of the intellectual decline (Mochizuki et al., 1998).

The cognitive decline in "white matter dementia" includes poorly sustained attention, impaired memory and visual-spatial skills, and alterations in personality and emotion (Filley, 2001), attesting to the strong "frontal" component of the disorder. Our own clinical experience with this patient population is in general agreement with this overall assessment and with the conclusions of other investigators in a now vast literature on this topic (see Pantoni et al., 1999; Filley, 2001), although restricted neurologic deficits resulting from focal lesions do occur, and some patients may commence their decline with different forms of language dis-

turbance, apraxia, and neglect. The time course and characteristic features of the decline are determined by the underlying pathology. Thus, progressive accumulation of stroke burden produces, typically, a stepwise deterioration, whereas the decline in patients with chronic progressive multiple sclerosis, or toxicity from methotrexate or organic solvent exposure, may have a more linear progression, with variable rapidity.

The description of the clinical effects of white matter lesions remains somewhat general and overarching, with no lucid and detailed explanation of anatomic-functional correlations yet possible. This situation has come about because there is an essential missing component in the consideration of the disorders of white matter. That is, there is, at present, no detailed account in humans or monkeys of the normal organization of the white matter association fiber systems or the information conveyed by these fiber systems. The anatomic detail that presently exists for the cerebral cortex and other subcortical structures, with respect to both architecture and connections, does not exist for the white matter fiber systems. The most comprehensive and authoritative account of this complex and vital neural system is that of Joseph Jules Dejerine (1849–1917) published in 1895. As extraordinary as that work is, it is based on postmortem normal human material, supported by analysis of degeneration following large lesions in some cases. Dejerine demonstrated many of the major fiber bundles that he and earlier investigators had described (most notably Karl Friedrich Burdach [1776–1847]), but given the methodology available at that time, it is not possible to appreciate with certainty what neural systems are linked by which white matter structure. Useful investigations of white matter association systems have been undertaken over the past century (e.g., Yakovlev & Locke, 1961), but a comprehensive analysis of the information conveyed by these fiber bundles has not yet been performed.

It is hoped that the development of a more comprehensive and detailed understanding of the fiber pathways of the brain will enable more sophisticated structure-function correlations using diffusion tensor magnetic resonance imaging in patient lesion studies, in functional imaging experiments, and in behavioral investigations in animal models. That would facilitate the ongoing elucidation of the disconnection syndromes in animal and man, as conceptualized and foreseen in Geschwind's seminal work.

A FINAL COMMENT CONCERNING THE ISSUE OF DIASCHISIS

The concept of nervous system function being subserved by discrete, architectonically and functionally distinct structures, or nodes, geographically distributed through the brain but linked by white matter fiber pathways, is predicated on the functional interaction of each of these nodes in the circuit. Loss of one part produces functional disability in the circuit as a whole, detectable both by virtue of loss of the behavior subserved by that circuit and also by physiologic parameters that evaluate the integrity of the circuit. Depending on the nature of the effect of one nodal region on another, that is, whether the synaptic activity leads to positive or negative feedback, the physiologic manifestation will be reflected in either an increase or a decrease in metabolic activity of the interconnected region. The understanding of basal ganglia and thalamic circuitry, for example, and the clinical utility of pallidotomy, thalamotomy, and deep brain stimulation, is predicated on this fundamental notion. The change in metabolic activity leads, *pari passu*, to a change in the blood flow to that brain region. This dynamic change in metabolic activity and blood flow in the interconnected regions of a circuit are the detectable underpinnings of Constantin von Monakow's (1853–1930) hypothesis of "diaschisis" (von Monakow, 1911). Fundamentally, changes in blood flow are the consequence, not the cause, of the altered function of a node in a system that has been lesioned elsewhere. This diaschisis may occur in cortical areas following subcortical lesions, or in subcortical (including cerebellar) regions following damage to the cerebral cortex.

The demonstration of metabolic and blood flow changes is convincing evidence in favor of the phenomenon of diaschisis and the distributed neural circuitry hypothesis. The challenge to the concept (Hillis et al., 2002) draws on evidence of true ischemia, that is, primary blood flow abnormalities, in regions supposedly suffering diaschisis. The conclusion thus reached is that cognitive deficits result from subcortical lesions when cerebral cortical areas are hypoperfused as well, but not when the hypoperfusion spares the cerebral cortex. This assertion is counterbalanced by evidence from different spheres of investigation. In the case of the thalamus, and even more so for the cerebellum, the vascular supply (vertebrobasilar system) is quite separate from that of most of the cerebral cortex. Cerebellar infarcts lead to reversed diaschisis in the cerebral cortex (Baron et al., 1980; Pantano et al., 1986; Botez et al., 1991; Schmahmann, 1991; Schmahmann & Sherman, 1998a), and cerebral hemispheric lesions lead to diaschisis in the cerebellum (Kushner et al., 1984; Metter et al., 1987). Further, in the case of diaschisis following thalamic infarction (Szelies et al., 1991; Baron et al., 1992) or thalamotomy (Baron et al., 1992), the large vessels are unaffected, and the lesion is quite localized (see also Fisher, 1982). There is no pathophysiologic support for the view that a lacune in a deep structure is associated with a primary ischemic event in considerable areas of overlying cerebral cortex. In addition, the presence of increased activity seen in areas to which affected regions send inhibitory signals, such as the thalamus in some cases of cerebellar infarction, indicate that the physiologic changes are not always hypoactive, and the direction of change is in accordance with the known or postulated inhibitory-excitatory interaction. Moreover, focal lesions of cortical areas 4 and 6 in monkeys produce a significant decrease of glucose metabolic activity in the ipsilateral caudate nucleus, putamen, globus pallidus, substantia nigra, and subthalamic nucleus, along with a decrease in the blood flow in the same structures (Dauth et al., 1985), reflecting the diaschisis in the interconnected structures (decreased metabolic activity because of disruption of connections, leading to decreased blood flow). In these clinical and experimental situations, the primary ischemia, or hypoperfusion, hypothesis is untenable.

The phenomenon of diaschisis does not, therefore, present a problem for the interpretation of effects-at-a-distance in the cerebral hemispheres, brainstem, and cerebellum. Rather, diaschisis provides compelling, physiologic evidence corroborating the hypothesis of distributed neural circuits, and it is a useful tool that may help further understand the organization of the nervous system in the performance of its multiple and varied responsibilities.

LIST OF ABBREVIATIONS *

AD	anterior dorsal thalamic nucleus
ADHD	attention-deficit/hyperactivity disorder
AICA	anterior inferior cerebellar artery

AM	anteromedial thalamic nucleus
Art.	artery
AS	arcuate sulcus
AV	anteroventral thalamic nucleus
CADASIL	cerebral autosomal dominant arteriopathy with strokes and ischemic leukoencephalopathy
CCAS	cerebellar cognitive affective syndrome
CeM	central medial thalamic nucleus
CL	central lateral thalamic nucleus
CM	centromedian thalamic nucleus
CS	central sulcus
Csl	centralis superior lateralis thalamic nucleus
CT	computed tomography
DCN	deep cerebellar nuclei
DSM-IV	Diagnostic and Statistical Manual of Mental Disorders-IV
DWI	diffusion-weighted imaging
F	fornix
FLAIR	fluid-attenuated inversion recovery
fMRI	functional magnetic resonance imaging
GM	medial geniculate nucleus
GMpc	medial geniculate nucleus, parvicellular part
GPe	globus pallidus, external segment
GPi	globus pallidus, internal segment
H	habenula
HIV	human immunodeficiency virus
IML	internal medullary lamina of thalamus
IOS	inferior occipital sulcus
IPS	inferior parietal sulcus
IQ	intelligence quotient
L/Li	limitans thalamic nucleus
LD	lateral dorsal thalamic nucleus
LF	lateral fissure
LGN/LGd/LGB	lateral geniculate thalamic nucleus
LP	lateral posterior thalamic nucleus
MD	medial dorsal thalamic nucleus
MDdc	medial dorsal thalamic nucleus, densocellular part
MDmc	medial dorsal thalamic nucleus, magnocellular part
MDmf	medial dorsal thalamic nucleus, multiform part
MDpc	medial dorsal thalamic nucleus, parvicellular part
MELAS	mitochondrial encephalopathy with lactic acidosis and stroke-like episodes
MGN/MG	medial geniculate thalamic nucleus
MRI	magnetic resonance imaging
MTT	mamillothalamic tract
P.Comm	posterior communicating artery
P1,P2,P3	first, second, and third divisions of the posterior cerebral artery
Pcn	paracentral thalamic nucleus
PET	positron emission tomography
Pf	parafascicular thalamic nucleus
PI	inferior pulvinar thalamic nucleus
PICA	posterior inferior cerebellar artery
PL/Pll	lateral pulvinar thalamic nucleus
PM/Plm	medial pulvinar thalamic nucleus
PO/Pla	anterior pulvinar (pulvinar oralis) thalamic nucleus
Po	posterior thalamic nucleus (Jones)
PS	principal sulcus
Pt	paratenial thalamic nucleus
Pv	paraventricular thalamic nucleus
R	reticular thalamic nucleus
Re	reunions thalamic nucleus
RN	red nucleus
SCA	superior cerebellar artery
SG, Sg	suprageniculate thalamic nucleus
SII	second somatosensory area
Sm	stria medullaris
SN	substantia nigra
ST	subthalamic nucleus
STS	superior temporal sulcus
UCI	universal cerebellar impairment
UCT	universal cerebellar transform
VA	ventral anterior thalamic nucleus
VAF	ventral amygdalofugal pathway
VL	ventral lateral thalamic nucleus

VLa	ventral lateral anterior nucleus (Jones) = VLo (Olszewski)
VLc	ventral lateral thalamic nucleus, pars caudalis (Olszewski) = VLp (dorsal part) [Jones]
VLo	ventral lateral thalamic nucleus, pars oralis (Olszewski) = VLa (Jones)
VLp	ventral lateral posterior nucleus (Jones)
VLps	ventral lateral thalamic nucleus, pars postrema (Olszewski) = VLp (posterodorsal part) [Jones]]
VM	ventromedial thalamic nucleus
VMb	ventromedial thalamic nucleus, basal part
VP	ventral posterior thalamic nucleus
VPI	ventral posterior inferior thalamic nucleus
VPL	ventral posterolateral thalamic nucleus
VPLa	ventral posterolateral nucleus, anterior division (Jones) = VPLc (Olszewski)
VPLc	ventral posterolateral thalamic nucleus, pars caudalis (Olszewski) = VPLa (Jones)
VPLo	ventral posterolateral thalamic nucleus, pars oralis (Olszewski) = VLp (ventral part), [Jones]
VPM	ventral posteromedial thalamic nucleus
VPMpc	ventral posteromedial thalamic nucleus, parvicellular part
WAIS-R	Wechsler adult intelligence scale revised
ZI	zona incerta

* Comparisons of nomenclature for ventral tier thalamic nuclei according to Olszewski (1952) and Jones (1997).

Acknowledgments

The invaluable assistance of Charlene DeMong, B.A. is gratefully acknowledged. This work was supported in part by the McDonnell Pew Program in Cognitive Neuroscience and the Birmingham Foundation.

■ KEY POINTS

☐ Cognition, emotion, and sensorimotor functions are subserved by distributed neural systems comprising anatomically unique regions (nodes) that are geographically distributed throughout the brain, and linked together in a precise and highly ordered manner by white matter fiber pathways.

☐ Lesions of the subcortical nodes, or the fiber systems that link them with the cerebral cortex, produce behavioral syndromes that resemble those arising from lesions of the cerebral cortices with which the subcortical regions are linked.

☐ The nature of the resulting behavioral syndrome is determined by two central factors—the histology of the lesioned structure and the corticosubcortical circuit that has been interrupted.

☐ Thalamic nuclei are comprised of five major functional classes—reticular and intralaminar nuclei that subserve arousal and pain sensation, sensory nuclei in all major domains, effector nuclei concerned with motor function as well as aspects of language, associative nuclei that participate in high-level cognitive functions, and limbic nuclei concerned with mood states and motivation. Vascular lesions destroy these nuclei in different combinations and produce sensory and behavioral syndromes depending on which nuclei are involved.

☐ The incorporation of the associative and paralimbic cerebral cortices into the cerebrocerebellar system is the anatomic underpinning of the cerebellar contribution to cognition and emotion.

☐ Topography of function has been postulated for the cerebellum. Sensorimotor function is subserved by the anterior lobe and lobules VIII and IX of the posterior lobe, whereas cognitive and emotional function is subserved by the cerebellar posterior lobe (lobules VI and VII). The midline posterior vermis is important for affect, the lateral posterior hemisphere is important for cognitive operations.

☐ The cerebellar cognitive affective syndrome (CCAS) is characterized by deficits in executive, visual spatial, and linguistic performance, with affective dysregulation produced by midline lesions.

☐ The dysmetria of thought hypothesis holds that there is a universal cerebellar transform applied by the cerebellum to information to which it has access. Lesions of the sensorimotor cerebellum produce ataxia of movement; lesions of the cognitive and affective parts of the cerebellum produce the CCAS.

☐ White matter fiber pathways are the essential connecting link in the distributed neural circuit. Lesions of white matter fiber bundles produce deficits in sensorimotor as well as high-level function, depending on the fiber system that is lesioned.

☐ Diaschisis is the physiologic correlate of lesions of subcortical structures and cerebellum causing high-level behavioral deficits. Hypometabolism and secondary hypoperfusion are observed in anatomically normal regions of the cerebral cortex that are interconnected with the lesioned subcortical regions.

KEY READINGS

Bogousslavsky J, Regli F, Uske A: Thalamic infarcts: Clinical syndromes, etiology, and prognosis. Neurology 38:837–848, 1988.

Filley CM: The Behavioral Neurology of White Matter. New York: Oxford University Press, 2001.

Graff-Radford NR, Tranel D, Van Hoesen GW, et al: Diencephalic amnesia. Brain 113(Pt 1):1–25, 1990.

Schmahmann JD (ed): The Cerebellum and Cognition. International Review of Neurobiology, Vol. 41, 1997, San Diego, CA: Academic Press.

Schmahmann JD, Sherman JC: The cerebellar cognitive affective syndrome. Brain 121:561–579, 1998.

Steriade M, Jones EG, McCormick DA (eds): Thalamus: Experimental and Clinical Aspects. New York: Elsevier, 1997, Vol. II, pp. 617–651, 1997.

REFERENCES

Acuña C, Cudeiro J, Gonzalez F, et al: Lateral-posterior and pulvinar reaching cells—comparison with parietal area 5a: A study in behaving *Macaca nemestrina* monkeys. Exp Brain Res 82:158–166, 1990.

Albus JS: A theory of cerebellar function. Math Biosc 10:25–61, 1971.

Allen GI, Tsukahara N: Cerebrocerebellar communication systems. Physiol Rev 54:957–1008, 1974.

Allin M, Matsumoto H, Santhouse AM, et al: Cognitive and motor function and the size of the cerebellum in adolescents born very pre-term. Brain 124(Pt 1):60–66, 2001.

American Psychiatric Association: Diagnostic and Statistical Manual of Mental Disorders, ed 4. Washington, DC: Author, 1994.

Andreasen NC, O'Leary DS, Cizadlo T, et al: Schizophrenia and cognitive dysmetria: A positron-emission tomography study of dysfunctional prefrontal-thalamic-cerebellar circuitry. Proc Natl Acad Sci U S A 93:9985–9990, 1996.

Andrezik JA, Dormer KJ, Foreman RD, et al: Fastigial nucleus projections to the brain stem in beagles: Pathways for autonomic regulation. Neuroscience 11:497–507, 1984.

Appollonio IM, Grafman J, Schwartz V, et al: Memory in patients with cerebellar degeneration. Neurology 43:1536–1544, 1993.

Asanuma C, Andersen RA, Cowan WM: The thalamic relations of the caudal inferior parietal lobule and the lateral prefrontal cortex in monkeys: Divergent cortical projections from cell clusters in the medial pulvinar nucleus. J Comp Neurol 241:357–381, 1985.

Atkinson JD, Collins DL, Bertrand G, et al: Optimal location of thalamotomy lesions for tremor associated with Parkinson disease: A probabilistic analysis based on postoperative magnetic resonance imaging and an integrated digital atlas. J Neurosurg 96:854–866, 2002.

Barbas H, Henion TH, Dermon CR: Diverse thalamic projections to the prefrontal cortex in the rhesus monkey. J Comp Neurol 313:65–94, 1991.

Baron JC, Bousser MG, Comar D, et al: "Crossed cerebellar diaschisis" in human supratentorial brain infarction. Trans Am Neurol Assn 105:459–461, 1980.

Baron JC, Levasseur M, Mazoyer B, et al: Thalamocortical diaschisis: Positron emission tomography in humans. J Neurol Neurosurg Psychiatry 55:935–942, 1992.

Batton RR III, Jayaraman A, Ruggiero D, et al: Fastigial efferent projections in the monkey: An autoradiographic study. J Comp Neurol 174:281–306, 1977.

Beauregard M, Leroux JM, Bergman S, et al: The functional neuroanatomy of major depression: An fMRI study using an emotional activation paradigm. Neuroreport 9:3253–3258, 1998.

Bell DS: Speech functions of the thalamus inferred from the effects of thalamotomy. Brain 91:619–638, 1968.

Benson DF, Sheremata WA, Bouchard R, et al: Conduction aphasia: A clinicopathological study. Arch Neurol 28:339–346, 1973.

Bentivoglio M, Kultas-Ilinsky K, Ilinsky I: Limbic thalamus: Structure, intrinsic organization, and connections, in Vogt BA, Gabriel M (eds): Neurobiology of Cingulate Cortex and Limbic Thalamus. Boston: Birkhäuser, 1993, pp. 71–122.

Berquin PC, Giedd JN, Jacobsen LK, et al: Cerebellum in attention-deficit hyperactivity disorder: A morphometric MRI study. Neurology 50:1087–1093, 1998.

Berman AF, Berman D, Prescott JW: The effect of cerebellar lesions on emotional behavior in the rhesus monkey, in Cooper IS, Riklan M, Snider RS (eds): The Cerebellum, Epilepsy and Behavior. New York: Plenum Press, 1978, pp. 277–284.

Bogousslavsky J, Regli F, Assal G: The syndrome of unilateral tuberothalamic artery territory infarction. Stroke 17:434–441, 1986.

Bogousslavsky J, Regli F, Delaloye B, et al: (1991) Loss of psychic self-activation with bithalamic infarction. Neurobehavioural, CT, MRI and SPECT correlates. Acta Neurol Scand 83:309–316, 1991.

Bogousslavsky J, Regli F, Uske A: Thalamic infarcts: Clinical syndromes, etiology, and prognosis. Neurology 38:837–848, 1988.

Bolk L: Das Cerebellum der Säugetiere. Haarlem: De Erven F. Bohn, 1906.

Botez MI, Botez T, Elie R, et al: Role of the cerebellum in complex human behavior. Ital J Neurol Sci 10:291–300, 1989.

Botez MI, Léveillé J, Lambert R, et al: Single photon emission computed tomography (SPECT) in cerebellar disease: Cerebello-cerebral diaschisis. Eur Neurol 31:405–421, 1991.

Botez-Maquard T, Leveille J, Botez MI: Neuropsychological functioning in unilateral cerebellar damage. Can J Neurol Sci 21:353–357, 1994.

Bower JM: Control of sensory data acquisition, in Schmahmann JD (ed): The Cerebellum and Cognition. International Review of Neurobiology, Vol. 41. San Diego, CA: Academic Press, 1997, pp. 489–513.

Bracke-Tolkmitt R, Linden A, Canavan AGM, et al: The cerebellum contributes to mental skills. Behav Neurosci 103:442–446, 1989.

Brandt T, Steinke W, Thie A, et al: Posterior cerebral artery territory infarcts: Clinical features, infarct topography, causes and outcome: Multicenter results and a review of the literature. Cerebrovasc Dis 10:170–182, 2000.

Brodal P: The corticopontine projection in the rhesus monkey: Origin and principles of organization. Brain 101:251–283, 1978.

Brodal P: The pontocerebellar projection in the rhesus monkey: An experimental study with retrograde axonal transport of horseradish peroxidase. Neuroscience 4:193–208, 1979.

Brower MC, Rollins N, Roach ES: Basal ganglia and thalamic infarction in children. Cause and clinical features. Arch Neurol 53:1252–1256, 1996.

Buttner T, Schilling G, Hornig CR, et al: Thalamic infarcts—clinical aspects, neuropsychological findings, prognosis. Fortschr Neurol Psychiatr 59:479–487, 1991.

Cabeza R, Nyberg L: Imaging cognition II: An empirical review of 275 PET and fMRI studies. J Cogn Neurosci 12:1–47, 2000.

Caplan LR: "Top of the basilar" syndrome. Neurology 30:72–79, 1980.

Caplan LR, DeWitt LD, Pessin MS, et al: Lateral thalamic infarcts. Arch Neurol 45:959–964, 1988.

Castaigne P, Lhermitte F, Buge A, et al: Paramedian thalamic and midbrain infarct: Clinical and neuropathological study. Ann Neurol 10:127–148, 1981.

Castellanos FX, Giedd JN, Berquin PC, et al: Quantitative brain magnetic resonance imaging in girls with attention-deficit/hyperactivity disorder. Arch Gen Psychiatry 58:289–295, 2001.

Catsman-Berrevoets CE, Van Dongen HR, Mulder PG, et al: Tumour type and size are high risk factors for the syndrome of "cerebellar" mutism and subsequent dysarthria. J Neurol Neurosurg Psychiatry 67:755–757, 1999.

Chambers WW, Sprague JM: Functional localization in the cerebellum. I. Organization in longitudinal corticonuclear zones and their contribution to the control of posture, both extrapyramidal and pyramidal. J Comp Neurol 103:105–130, 1955a.

Chambers WW, Sprague JM: Functional localization in the cerebellum. II. Somatotopic organization in cortex and nuclei. Arch Neurol Psychiatry 653–780, 1955b.

Chen WH, Liu JS, Wu SC, et al: Transient global amnesia and thalamic hemorrhage. Clin Neurol Neurosurg 98:309–311, 1996.

Chheda M, Sherman J, Schmahmann JD: Neurologic, psychiatric and cognitive manifestations in cerebellar agenesis [abstract]. Neurology 58(Suppl 3):356, 2002.

Chukwudelunzu FE, Meschia, JF, Graff-Radford NR, et al: Extensive metabolic and neuropsychological abnormalities associated with discrete infarction of the genu of the internal capsule. J Neurol Neurosurg Psychiatry 71:658–662, 2001.

Chung CS, Caplan LR, Han W, et al: Thalamic haemorrhage. Brain 119:1873–1886, 1996.

Clarke S, Assal G, Bogousslavsky J, et al: Pure amnesia after unilateral left polar thalamic infarct: Topographic and sequential neuropsychological and metabolic (PET) correlations. J Neurol Neurosurg Psychiatry 57:27–34, 1994.

Coghill RC, Sang CN, Maisog JM., et al: Pain intensity processing within the human brain: A bilateral, distributed mechanism. J Neurophysiol 82, 1934–1943, 1999.

Cooper IS, Riklan M, Amin I, et al: A long term follow-up study of cerebellar stimulation for the control of epilepsy, in Cooper IS (ed): Cerebellar Stimulation in Man. New York: Raven Press, 1978, pp. 19–38.

Courchesne E, Allen G: Prediction and preparation, fundamental functions of the cerebellum. Learn Mem 4:1–35, 1997.

Courchesne E, Yeung-Courchesne R, Press GA, et al: Hypoplasia of cerebellar vermal lobules VI and VII in autism. N Engl J Med 318:1349–1354, 1988.

Cowey A, Stoerig P, Bannister M: Retinal ganglion cells labelled from the pulvinar nucleus in macaque monkeys. Neuroscience 61:691–705, 1994.

Crosson B: Subcortical aphasia: A working model. Brain Lang 25:257–292, 1985.

Crosson B: Subcortical mechanisms in language: Lexical-semantic mechanisms and the thalamus. Brain Cogn 40:414–438, 1999.

Cusick CG, Scripter JL, Darensbourg JG, et al: Chemoarchitectonic subdivisions of the visual pulvinar in monkeys and their connectional relations with the middle temporal and rostral dorsolateral visual areas, MT and DLr. J Comp Neurol 336:1–30, 1993.

Dauth GW, Gilman S, Frey KA, et al: Basal ganglia glucose utilization after recent precentral ablation in the monkey. Ann Neurol 17:431–438, 1985.

Decroix JP, Graveleau P, Masson M, et al: Infarction in the territory of the anterior choroidal artery: A clinical and computerized tomographic study of 16 cases. Brain 109:1071–1085, 1986.

Deecke L, Schwarz DW, Fredrickson JM: Vestibular responses in the rhesus monkey ventroposterior thalamus. II. Vestibuloproprioceptive convergence at thalamic neurons. Exp Brain Res 30:219–232, 1977.

De Freitas GR, Bogousslavsky J: Thalamic infarcts, in Donnan G, Norving B, Bamford J, et al (eds): Subcortical Stroke. Oxford: Oxford University Press, 2002, pp. 255–285.

Dejerine J: Des différentes variétiés de cécité verbale. Mem Soc Biol 4: 61, 1892. (Referenced in Geschwind, 1965).

Dejerine J: Anatomie des Centres Nerveux. Paris: Rueff et Cie, 1895.

Dejerine J, Roussy G: Le syndrome thalamique. Rev Neurol 14:521–532, 1906.

Dennis M, Spiegler BJ, Hetherington CR, et al: Neuropsychological sequelae of the treatment of children with medulloblastoma. J Neurooncol 29:91–101, 1996.

Desmond JE, Fiez JA: Neuroimaging studies of the cerebellum: Language, learning and memory. Trends Cog Sci 2:355–362, 1998.

Desmond PM, Lovell AC, Rawlinson AA, et al: The value of apparent diffusion coefficient maps in early cerebral ischemia. Am J Neuroradiol 22:1260–1267, 2001.

Devinsky O, Luciano D: The contributions of cingulate cortex to human behavior, in Vogt BA, Gabriel M (eds): Neurobiology of Cingulate Cortex and Limbic Thalamus. Boston: Birkhäuser, 1997, pp. 527–556.

Devinsky O, Morrell MJ, Vogt BA: Contributions of anterior cingulate cortex to behaviour. Brain 118:279–306, 1995.

Dougherty DD, Baer L, Cosgrove GR, et al: Prospective long-term follow-up of 44 patients who received cingulotomy for treatment-refractory obsessive-compulsive disorder. Am J Psychiatry 159:269–275, 2002.

Dow RS: Some novel concepts of cerebellar physiology. Mt Sinai J Med 41:103–119, 1974.

Doyon J, Song AW, Karni A, et al: Experience-dependent changes in cerebellar contributions to motor sequence learning. Proc Natl Acad Sci U S A 99:1017–1022, 2002.

Duffner PK, Cohen ME, Thomas P: Late effects of treatment on the intelligence of children with posterior fossa tumors. Cancer 51:233–237, 1983.

Dunwoody GW, Alsagoff ZS, Yuan SY: Cerebellar mutism with subsequent dysarthria in an adult: Case report. Br J Neurosurg 11:161–163, 1997.

Duret H: Recherches anatomiques sur la circulation de l'encephale. Arch Physiol Norm Pathol 1:60–91;316–354;915–957, 1874.

Engelborghs S, Marien P, Pickut BA, et al: Loss of psychic self-activation after paramedian bithalamic infarction. Stroke 31:1762–175, 2000.

Englund E, Brun A, Alling C: White matter changes in dementia of Alzheimer's type—biochemical and neuropathological correlates. Brain 111:1425–1439, 1988.

Fiez JA, Petersen SE, Cheney MK, et al: Impaired non-motor learning and error detection associated with cerebellar damage. Brain 115:155–178, 1992.

Filley CM: The Behavioral Neurology of White Matter. New York: Oxford University Press, 2001.

Fisher CM: The pathologic and clinical aspects of thalamic hemorrhage. Trans Am Neurol Assoc 33:56–59, 1959.

Fisher CM: Thalamic pure sensory stroke: A pathologic study. Neurology 28:1141–1144, 1978.

Fisher CM: Lacunar strokes and infarcts: A review. Neurology 32:871–876, 1982.

Foix C, Hillemand P: Les artères de laxe encéphalique jusqu'au diencéphale inclusivement. Rev Neurol 2:705–739, 1925.

Francois C, Tande D, Yelnik J, et al: Distribution and morphology of nigral axons projecting to the thalamus in primates. J Comp Neurol 447:249–260, 2002.

Fries W: Pontine projection from striate and prestriate visual cortex in the macaque monkey: An anterograde study. Vis Neurosci 4:205–216, 1990.

Garcin R: Syndrome cérébello-thalamique par lésion localisée du thalamus avec une digression sur le "signe de la main creuse" et son intérêt séméiologique. (Jubilé du Doctor André-Thomas.) Rev Neurol 93:143–149, 1955.

Garcin R, Lapresle J: Syndrome sensitif de type thalamique et a topographie chéiro-orale par lésion localisée du thalamus. Rev Neurol 90:124–129, 1954.

Garcin R, Lapresle J: Incoordination cérébelleuse du membre inférieur par lésion localisée dans la région interne du thalamus controlatéral. Rev Neurol 120:5–13, 1969.

Gardner RJ, Coleman LT, Mitchell LA, et al: Near-total absence of the cerebellum. Neuropediatrics 32:62–68, 2001.

Garg BP, DeMyer WE: Ischemic thalamic infarction in children: Clinical presentation, etiology, and outcome. Pediatr Neurol 13:46–49, 1995.

Gazzaniga MS: Cerebral specialization and interhemispheric communication: Does the corpus callosum enable the human condition? Brain 123:1293–326, 2000.

Geschwind N: Disconnexion syndromes in animals and man. Brain 88:237–294, and 88:585–644, 1965.

Geschwind DH: Focusing attention on cognitive impairment in spinocerebellar ataxia. Arch Neurol 56:20–22, 1999.

Ghika J, Bogousslavsky J, Henderson J, et al: The "jerky dystonic unsteady hand": A delayed motor syndrome in posterior thalamic infarctions. J Neurol 241:537–542, 1994.

Ghika-Schmid F, Bogousslavsky J: The acute behavioral syndrome of anterior thalamic infarction: A prospective study of 12 cases. Ann Neurol 48:220–227, 2000.

Giguere M, Goldman-Rakic PS: Mediodorsal nucleus: Areal, laminar, and tangential distribution of afferents and efferents in the frontal lobe of rhesus monkeys. J Comp Neurol 277:195–213, 1988.

Glauser TA, Packer RJ: Cognitive deficits in long-term survivors of childhood brain tumors. Childs Nerv Syst 7:2–12, 1991.

Glickstein M: Cerebellar agenesis. Brain 117:1209–1212, 1994.

Glickstein M, May JG, Mercier BE: Corticopontine projection in the macaque: The distribution of labelled cortical cells after large injections of horseradish peroxidase in the pontine nuclei. J Comp Neurol 235:343–359, 1985.

Goldenberg G, Podreka I, Pfaffelmeyer N, et al: Thalamic ischemia in transient global amnesia: A SPECT study. Neurology 41:1748–1752, 1991.

Goldman-Rakic PS, Porrino LJ: The primate mediodorsal (MD) nucleus and its projection to the frontal lobe. J Comp Neurol 242:535–560, 1985.

Goldstein K: Über die amnestiche und centrale aphasie. Arch Psychiat Neurol 48:408, 1911.

Gomez Beldarrain M, Garcia-Monco JC, Quntana JM, et al: Diaschisis and neuropsychological performance after cerebellar stroke. Eur Neurol 37(2):82–89, 1997.

Graff-Radford NR, Damasio H, Yamada T, et al: Nonhaemorrhagic thalamic infarction. Clinical, neuropsychological and electrophysiological findings in four anatomical groups defined by computerized tomography. Brain 108(Pt 2):485–516, 1985.

Graff-Radford NR, Eslinger PJ, Damasio AR, et al: Nonhemorrhagic infarction of the thalamus: Behavioral, anatomic, and physiologic correlates. Neurology 34:14–23, 1984.

Graff-Radford NR, Tranel D, Van Hoesen GW, et al: Diencephalic amnesia. Brain 113(Pt 1):1–25, 1990.

Grafman J, Litvan I, Massaquoi S, et al: Cognitive planning deficit in patients with cerebellar atrophy. Neurology 42:1493–1496, 1992.

Gravel C, Hawkes R: Parasagittal organization of the rat cerebellar cortex: Direct comparison of Purkinje cell compartments and the organization of the spinocerebellar projection. J Comp Neurol 291:79–102, 1990.

Guard O, Bellis F, Mabille JP, et al: Demence thalamique apres lesion hemorragique unilaterale du pulvinar droit. Rev Neurol (Paris) 142:759–765, 1986.

Guberman A, Stuss D: The syndrome of bilateral paramedian thalamic infarction. Neurology 33:540–546, 1983.

Gutrecht JA, Zamani AA, Pandya DN: Lacunar thalamic stroke with pure cerebellar and proprioceptive deficits. J Neurol Neurosurg Psychiatry 55:854–856, 1992.

Hackett TA, Stepniewska I, Kaas JH: Thalamocortical connections of the parabelt auditory cortex in macaque monkeys. J Comp Neurol 400:271–286, 1998.

Haines DE and Dietrichs E: An HRP study of hypothalamo-cerebellar and cerebello-hypothalamic connections in squirrel monkey (Saimiri sciureus). J Comp Neurol 229:559–575, 1984.

Hallem JS, Thompson JH, Gundappa-Sulur G, et al: Spatial correspondence between tactile projection patterns and the distribution of the antigenic Purkinje cell markers anti-zebrin I and anti-zebrin II in the cerebellar folium crus IIA of the rat. Neuroscience 93:1083–1094, 1999.

Hampson JL, Harrison CR, Woolsey CN: Cerebrocerebellar projections and somatotopic localization of motor function in the cerebellum, in Bard P (ed): Patterns of Organization in the Central Nervous System. Res Publ Assoc Nerv Ment Dis 30:299–316, 1952.

Hassler R: Anatomy of the thalamus, in Schaltenbrand G, Bailey P (eds): Introduction to Stereotaxis with an Atlas of the Human Brain. Stuttgart: Thieme, 1959, pp. 230–290.

Heath RG: Modulation of emotion with a brain pacemaker. J Nerv Ment Dis 165:300–317, 1977.

Heath RG, Franklin DE, Shraberg D: Gross pathology of the cerebellum in patients diagnosed and treated as functional psychiatric disorders. J Nerv Ment Dis 167:585–592, 1979.

Heath RG, Harper JW: Ascending projections of the cerebellar fastigial nucleus to the hippocampus amygdala and other temporal lobe sites: Evoked potential and histological studies in monkeys and cats. Exp Neurol 45:2682–2687, 1974.

Henneman E, Cooke PM, Snider RS: Cerebellar projections to the cerebral cortex, in Bard P (ed): Patterns of Organization in the Central Nervous System. Res Publ Assoc Nerv Ment Dis 30:317–333, 1952.

Hillis AE, Wityk RJ, Barker PB, et al: Subcortical aphasia and neglect in acute stroke: The role of cortical hypoperfusion. Brain 125:1094–1104, 2002.

Hodges JR, McCarthy RA: Autobiographical amnesia resulting from bilateral paramedian thalamic infarction. A case study in cognitive neurobiology. Brain 116(Pt 4):921–940, 1993.

Holmes G: The symptoms of acute cerebellar injuries due to gunshot wounds. Brain 40:461–535, 1917.

Houk JC: On the role of the cerebellum and basal ganglia in cognitive signal processing. Prog Brain Res 114: 545–554, 1997.

Hugdahl K, Wester K: Neurocognitive correlates of stereotactic thalamotomy and thalamic stimulation in parkinsonian patients. Brain Cogn 42:231–252, 2000.

Huguenard JR, Prince DA: Basic mechanisms of epileptic discharges in the thalamus, in Steriade M, Jones EG, McCormick DA (eds): Thalamus: Experimental and Clinical Aspects. New York: Elsevier, 1997, Vol. II, pp. 295–330.

Humphrey DR, Gold R, Reed DJ: Sizes, laminar and topographic origins of cortical projections to the major divisions of the red nucleus in the monkey. J Comp Neurol 225:75–94, 1984.

Ichimiya T, Okubo Y, Suhara T, et al: Reduced volume of the cerebellar vermis in neuroleptic-naive schizophrenia. Biol Psychiatry 49:20–27, 2001.

Ilinsky IA, Kultas-Ilinsky K: Sagittal cytoarchitectonic maps of the *Macaca mulatta* thalamus with a revised nomenclature of the motor-related nuclei validated by observations on their connectivity. J Comp Neurol 262:331–364, 1987.

Ito M: Questions in modeling the cerebellum. J Theor Biol 99:81–86, 1982.

Ito M: Movement and thought: Identical control mechanisms by the cerebellum. Trends Neurosci 16:448–450, 1993.

Ito M: Cerebellar microcomplexes, in Schmahmann JD (ed): The Cerebellum and Cognition. International Review of Neurobiology, Vol. 41. San Diego, CA: Academic Press, 1997, pp. 475–489.

Ivry R: Cerebellar timing systems, in Schmahmann JD (ed): The Cerebellum and Cognition. International Review of Neurobiology, Vol. 41. San Diego, CA: Academic Press, 1997, pp. 556–571.

Jenkins IH, Brooks DJ, Nixon PD, et al: Motor sequence learning: A study with positron emission tomography. J Neurosci 14:3775–3790, 1994.

Johnson MD, Ojemann GA: The role of the human thalamus in language and memory: Evidence from electrophysiological studies. Brain Cogn 42:218–230, 2000.

Jones EG: Functional subdivision and synaptic organization of the mammalian thalamus. Int Rev Physiol 25:173–245, 1981.

Jones EG: The Thalamus. New York: Plenum Press, 1985, pp. 378–396.

Jones EG: A description of the human thalamus, in Steriade M, Jones EG, McCormick DA (eds): Thalamus: Experimental and Clinical Aspects. New York: Elsevier, 1997, Vol. II, pp. 425–499.

Jones EG, Powell TP: Connexions of the somatic sensory cortex of the rhesus monkey. 3. Thalamic connexions. Brain 93:37–56, 1970.

Kalil K: Projections of the cerebellar and dorsal column nuclei upon the thalamus of the rhesus monkey. J Comp Neurol 195:25–50, 1981.

Karnath HO, Himmelbach M, Rorden C: The subcortical anatomy of human spatial neglect: Putamen, caudate nucleus and pulvinar. Brain 125:350–360, 2002.

Karussis D, Leker RR, Abarmsky O: Cognitive dysfunction following thalamic stroke: A study of 16 cases and review of the literature. J Neurol Sci 172:25–29, 2000.

Kase CS: Subcortical hemorrhages, in Donnan G, Norving B, Bamford J, et al (eds): Subcortical Stroke. Oxford: Oxford University Press, 2002, pp. 347–377.

Kemper TL, Bauman M: Neuropathology of infantile autism. J Neuropathol Exp Neurol 57:645–652, 1998.

Kennedy H, Bullier J: A double-labeling investigation of the afferent connectivity to cortical areas V1 and V2 of the macaque monkey. J Neurosci 5:2815–2830, 1985.

Kennedy PR, Gibson AR, Houk JC: Functional and anatomic differentiation between parvicellular and magnocellular regions of red nucleus in the monkey. Brain Res 364:124–136, 1986.

Kievit J, Kuypers HGJM: Organization of the thalamocortical connections to the frontal lobe in the rhesus monkey. Exp Brain Res 29:299–322, 1977.

Kish SJ, El-Awar M, Schut L, et al: Cognitive deficits in olivopontocerebellar atrophy: Implications for the cholinergic hypothesis of Alzheimer's dementia. Ann Neurol 24:200–206, 1988.

Knoepfel HK, Macken J: Le syndrome psycho-organique dans les hérédo-ataxies. J Belge Neurol Psychiat 47:314–323, 1947.

Krolak-Salmon P, Croisile B, Houzard C, et al: Total recovery after bilateral paramedian thalamic infarct. Eur Neurol 44:216–218, 2000.

Kumral E, Kocaer T, Ertubey NO, et al: Thalamic hemorrhage: A prospective study of 100 patients. Stroke 26:964–970, 1995.

Künzle H, Akert K: Efferent connections of cortical area 8 (frontal eye field) in *Macaca fascicularis*: A reinvestigation using the autoradiographic technique. J Comp Neurol 173:147–164, 1977.

Kushner M, Alavi A, Reivich M, et al: Contralateral cerebellar hypometabolism following cerebral insult: A positron emission tomographic study. Ann Neurol 15:425–434, 1984.

Kuypers HGJM, Lawrence DG: Cortical projections to the red nucleus and the brainstem in the rhesus monkey. Brain Res 4:151–188, 1967.

Lane RD, Reiman EM, Ahern GL, et al: Neuroanatomical correlates of happiness, sadness, and disgust. Am J Psychiatry 154:926–933, 1997.

Lapresele J, Haguenau M: Anatomico-chemical clinical in focal thalamic lesions. Z Neurol 205:29–46, 1973.

Lazorthes G: Vascularisation et circulation cérébral. Paris: Masson, 1961.

Lazorthes G, Salamon G: The arteries of the thalamus: An anatomical and radiological study. J Neurosurg 34:23–26, 1971.

Leigh RJ, Zee DS: The neurology of eye movements. Philadelphia: F.A. Davis, 1983.

Leiner HC, Leiner AL, Dow RS: Does the cerebellum contribute to mental skills? Behav Neurosci 100:443–454, 1986.

Leiner HC, Leiner AL: How fibers subserve computing capabilities: Similarities between brains and machines, in Schmahmann JD (ed): The Cerebellum and Cognition. International Review of Neurobiology, Vol. 41. San Diego, CA: Academic Press, 1997, pp. 535–553.

Lenz FA, Dougherty PM: Pain processing in the human thalamus, in Steriade M, Jones EG, McCormick DA (eds): Thalamus: Experimental and Clinical Aspects. New York: Elsevier, 1997, Vol. II, pp. 617–651.

Levisohn L, Cronin-Golomb A, Schmahmann JD: Neuropsychological consequences of cerebellar tumor resection in children: Cerebellar cognitive affective syndrome in a pediatric population. Brain 123:1041–1050, 2000.

Lhermitte F: Language disorders and their relationship to thalamic lesions. Adv Neurol 42:99–113, 1984.

Lippmann S, Manshadi M, Baldwin H: Cerebellar vermis dimensions on computerized tomographic scans of schizophrenic and bipolar patients. Am J Psychiatry 139:667–668, 1981.

Lisovoski F, Koskas P, Dubard T, et al: Left tuberothalamic artery territory infarction: Neuropsychological and MRI features. Eur Neurol 33:181–184, 1993.

Llinas R, Ribary U: Consciousness and the brain. The thalamocortical dialogue in health and disease. Ann N Y Acad Sci 929:166–175, 2001.

Locke S, Angevine JB Jr, Yakovlev PI: Limbic nuclei of thalamus and connections of limbic cortex. II. Thalamo-cortical projection of the lateral dorsal nucleus in man. Arch Neurol 4:355–366, 1961.

Loeber RT, Cintron CM, Yurgelun-Todd DA: Morphometry of individual cerebellar lobules in schizophrenia. Am J Psychiatry 158:952–954, 2001.

Lund-Johansen M, Hugdahl K, Wester K: Cognitive function in patients with Parkinson's disease undergoing stereotaxic thalamotomy. J Neurol Neurosurg Psychiatry 60:564–571, 1996.

Macchi G, Jones EG: Toward an agreement on terminology of nuclear and subnuclear divisions of the motor thalamus. J Neurosurg 86:670–685, 1997.

Malm J, Kristensen B, Karlsson T, et al: Cognitive impairment in young adults with infratentorial infarcts. Neurology 51:433–440, 1998.

Manabe Y, Kashihara K, Ota T, et al: Motor neglect following left thalamic hemorrhage: A case report. J Neurol Sci 171:69–71, 1999.

Marr D: A Theory of cerebellar cortex. J Physiol 202:437–470, 1969.

Martin JJ: Degenerative diseases of the human thalamus, in Steriade M, Jones EG, McCormick DA (eds): Thalamus: Experimental and Clinical Aspects. New York: Elsevier, 1997, Vol. II, pp. 653–687.

May JG, Andersen RA: Different patterns of corticopontine projections from separate cortical fields within the inferior parietal lobule and dorsal prelunate gyrus of the macaque. Exp Brain Res 63:265–278, 1986.

Mazziotta JC, Phelps ME, Carson RE: Tomographic mapping of human cerebral metabolism: Subcortical responses to auditory and visual stimulation. Neurology 34:825–828, 1984.

Mesulam MM: A cortical network for directed attention and unilateral neglect. Ann Neurol 10:309–325, 1981.

Mesulam M-M: Patterns in behavioral neuroanatomy: Association areas, the limbic system, and hemispheric specialization, in Mesulam M-M (ed): Principles of Behavioral Neurology. Contemporary Neurology Series. Philadelphia: F.A. Davis, 1988, pp. 1–70.

Mesulam M-M, Mufson EJ: The insula of Reil in man and monkey. Architectonics, connectivity, and function, in Peters A, Jones EG (eds): Cerebral Cortex. New York: Plenum Press, 1985, Vol. 4, pp. 179–226.

Mesulam MM, Pandya DN: The projections of the medial geniculate complex within the sylvian fissure of the rhesus monkey. Brain Res 60:315–333, 1973.

Metter EJ, Kempler D, Jackson CA, et al: Cerebellar glucose metabolism in chronic aphasia. Neurology 37:1599–1606, 1987.

Meyer A, Beck E, McLardy T: Prefrontal leucotomy: A neuroanatomical report. Brain 70:19–49, 1947.

Middleton FA, Strick PL: Anatomical evidence for cerebellar and basal ganglia involvement in higher cognitive function. Science 266:458–451, 1994.

Middleton FA, Strick PL: Cerebellar output channels, in Schmahmann JD (ed.): The Cerebellum and Cognition. International Review of Neurobiology, Vol. 41. San Diego, CA: Academic Press, 1997, pp. 61–82.

Mochizuki Y, Oishi M, Takasu T: Central motor conduction time and regional cerebral blood flow in patients with leuko-araiosis. J Neurol Sci 160:60–63, 1998.

Molinari M, Filippini V, Leggio MG: Neuronal plasticity of interrelated cerebellar and cortical networks. Neuroscience 111:863–870, 2002.

Molinari M, Leggio MG, Silveri MC: Verbal fluency and agrammatism, in Schmahmann JD (ed): The Cerebellum and Cognition. International Review of Neurobiology, Vol. 41. San Diego, CA: Academic Press, 1997, pp. 325–339.

Monakow C von: Lokalisation der Hirnfunktionen. J Psychol Neurol 17:185–200, 1911.

Moretti R, Bava A, Torre P, et al: Reading errors in patients with cerebellar vermis lesions. J Neurol 249:461–468, 2002.

Moriguchi I: A study of schizophrenic brains by computerized tomography scans. Folia Psychiat Neurol Jpn 35:55–72, 1981.

Mostofsky SH, Reiss AL, Lockhart P, et al: Decreased cerebellar posterior vermis size in fragile X syndrome: Correlation with neurocognitive performance. Neurology 50:121–130, 1998.

Mufson EJ, Mesulam MM: Thalamic connections of the insula in the rhesus monkey and comments on the paralimbic connectivity of the medial pulvinar nucleus. J Comp Neurol 227:109–120, 1984.

Murakami JW, Courchesne E, Press GA, et al: Reduced cerebellar hemisphere size and its relationship to vermal hypoplasia in autism. Arch Neurol 46:689–694, 1989.

Nadeau SE, Crosson B: Subcortical aphasia. Brain Lang 58:355–402; discussion 418–423, 1997.

Nasreddine ZS, Saver JL: Pain after thalamic stroke: Right diencephalic predominance and clinical features in 180 patients. Neurology 48:1196–1199, 1997.

Nass R, Boyce L, Leventhal F, et al: Acquired aphasia in children after surgical resection of left-thalamic tumors. Dev Med Child Neurol 42:580–590, 2000.

Neau JP, Arroyo-Anllo E, Bonnaud V, et al: Neuropsychological disturbances in cerebellar infarcts. Acta Neurol Scand 102:363–370, 2000.

Neau JP, Bogousslavsky J: The syndrome of posterior choroidal artery territory infarction. Ann Neurol 39:779–788, 1996.

Nicolson RI, Fawcett AJ, Berry EL, et al: Association of abnormal cerebellar activation with motor learning difficulties in dyslexic adults. Lancet 353:1662–1667, 1999.

Nixon PD, Passingham RE: Predicting sensory events: The role of the cerebellum in motor learning. Exp Brain Res 138:251–257, 2001.

Ojemann GA: Brain organization for language from the perspective of electrical stimulation mapping. Behav Brain Sciences 6:189–230, 1983.

Ojemann GA, Fedio P, Van Buren JM: Anomia from pulvinar and subcortical parietal stimulation. Brain 91:99–116, 1968.

Ojemann GA, Ward AA Jr: Speech representation in ventrolateral thalamus. Brain 94:669–680, 1971.

Olszewski J: The Thalamus of the Macaca mulatta. Basel: Karger, 1952.

Orioli PJ, Strick PL: Cerebellar connections with the motor cortex and the arcuate premotor area: An analysis employing retrograde transneuronal transport of WGA-HRP. J Comp Neurol 288:621–626, 1989.

Pandya DN, Rosene DL, Doolittle AM: Corticothalamic connections of auditory-related areas of the temporal lobe in the rhesus monkey. J Comp Neurol 345:447–471, 1994.

Pandya DN, Selzter B: Intrinsic connections and architectonics of posterior parietal cortex in the rhesus monkey. J Comp Neurol 204:196–210, 1982.

Pantano P, Baron JC, Samson Y, et al: Crossed cerebellar diaschisis. Further studies. Brain 109:677–694, 1986.

Pantoni L, Leys D, Fazekas F, et al: Role of white matter lesions in cognitive impairment of vascular origin. Alzheimer Dis Assoc Disord 13(Suppl 3):S49–S54, 1999.

Papez JW: A proposed mechanism of emotion. Arch Neurol Psychiatry 38:725–744, 1937.

Parsons LM, Denton D, Egan G, et al: Neuroimaging evidence implicating cerebellum in support of sensory/cognitive processes associated with thirst. Proc Natl Acad Sci U S A 97:2332–2336, 2000.

Parvizi J, Anderson SW, Martin CO, et al: Pathological laughter and crying: A link to the cerebellum. Brain 124(Pt 9):1708–1719 2001.

Paulin M: The role of the cerebellum in motor control and perception. Brain Behav Evolut 41:39–50, 1993.

Paus T: Primate anterior cingulate cortex: Where motor control, drive and cognition interface. Nat Rev Neurosci 2:417–424, 2001.

Pedroza A, Dujovny M, Artero JC, et al: Microanatomy of the posterior communicating artery. Neurosurgery 20:228–235, 1987.

Penfield W, Roberts L: Speech and Brain Mechanisms. Princeton, NJ: Princeton University Press, 1959.

Percheron G: The anatomy of the arterial supply of the human thalamus and its use for the interpretation of the thalamic vascular pathology. Z Neurol 205:1–13, 1973.

Percheron G: Les artères du thalamus humain. I. Artère et territoire thalamiques polaires de l'artère communicante postérieure. Rev Neurol 132:297–307, 1976a.

Percheron G: Les artères du thalamus humain. II. Artères et territoire thalamiques paramédians de l'artère basilaire communicante. Rev Neurol 132:309–324, 1976b.

Percheron G: Les artères du thalamus humain. Les artères choroïdiennes. I. Étude macroscopique des variations individuelles. II. Systématisation. Rev Neurol 133:533–545, 1977a.

Percheron G: Les artères du thalamus humain. Les artères choroïdiennes. III. Absence de territoire thalamique constitué de l'artère choroïdien antérieure. IV. Artères et territoires thalamique du système artériel choroïdien et thalamique postéromédian. V. Artères et territoires thalamique du système artériel choroïdien et thalamique postérolatéral. Rev Neurol 133:547–558,1977b.

Peters A, Leahu D, Moss MB, et al: The effects of aging on area 46 of the frontal cortex of the rhesus monkey. Cereb Cortex 4: 621–635, 1994.

Petersen SE, Fox PT, Posner MI, et al: Positron emission tomographic studies of the processing of single words. J Cognit Neurosci 1:153–170, 1989.

Plets C, De Reuck J, Vander Eecken H, et al: The vascularization of the human thalamus. Acta Neurol Belg 70:687–770, 1970.

Pollack IF: Posterior fossa syndrome, in Schmahmann JD (ed): The Cerebellum and Cognition. International Review of Neurobiology, Vol. 41. San Diego, CA: Academic Press, 1997, pp. 411–432.

Pollack IF, Polinko P, Albright AL, et al: Mutism and pseudobulbar symptoms after resection of posterior fossa tumors in children: Incidence and pathophysiology. Neurosurgery 37:885–893, 1995.

Pollak L, Klein C, Rabey JM, et al: Posterior fossa lesions associated with neuropsychiatric symptomatology. Int J Neurosci 87:119–126, 1996.

Pradalier A, Lutz G, Vincent D: Transient global amnesia, migraine, thalamic infarct, dihydroergotamine, and sumatriptan. Headache 40:324–327, 2000.

Pritchard TC, Hamilton RB, Morse JR, et al: Projections of thalamic gustatory and lingual areas in the monkey, *Macaca fascicularis*. J Comp Neurol 244:213–228, 1986.

Qvist H: Demonstration of axonal branching of fibres from certain precerebellar nuclei to the cerebellar cortex and nuclei: A retrograde fluorescent double-labelling study in the cat. Exp Brain Res 75:15–27, 1989.

Radcliffe J, Packer RJ, Atkins TE, et al: Three- and four- year cognitive outcome in children with noncortical brain tumors treated with whole-brain radiotherapy. Ann Neurol 32:551–554, 1992.

Rainville P, Bushnell MC, Duncan GH: Representation of acute and persistent pain in the human CNS: Potential implications for chemical intolerance. Ann N Y Acad Sci 933:130–141, 2001.

Reilly M, Connolly S, Stack J, et al: Bilateral paramedian thalamic infarction: A distinct but poorly recognized stroke syndrome. Q J Med 82:63–70, 1992.

Reiman EM, Raichle ME, Robins E, et al: Neuroanatomical correlates of a lactate-induced anxiety attack. Arch Gen Psychiatry 46, 493–500, 1989.

Reis DJ, Doba N, Nathan MA: Predatory attack, grooming and consummatory behaviors evoked by electrical stimulation of cat cerebellar nuclei. Science 182, 845–847, 1973.

Riva D, Giorgi C: The cerebellum contributes to higher function during development: Evidence from a series of children surgically treated for posterior fossa tumors. Brain 123:1051–1061, 2000.

Robinson DL, Cowie RJ: The primate pulvinar: Structural, functional and behavioral components of visual salience, in Steriade M, Jones EG, McCormick DA (eds): Thalamus. Experimental and Clinical Aspects. New York: Elsevier, 1997, Vol. II, pp. 53–92.

Romanski LM, Giguere M, Bates JF, et al: Topographic organization of medial pulvinar connections with the prefrontal cortex in the rhesus monkey. J Comp Neurol 379:313–332, 1997.

Russchen FT, Amaral DG, Price JL: The afferent input to the magnocellular division of the mediodorsal thalamic nucleus in the monkey, *Macaca fascicularis*. J Comp Neurol 256:175–210, 1987.

Saint-Cyr JA, Courville J: Projections from the motor cortex, midbrain, and vestibular nuclei to the inferior olive in the cat: Anatomical and functional correlates, in Courville J, de Montigny C, Lamarre Y (eds): The Inferior Olivary Nucleus: Anatomy and Physiology. New York: Raven Press, 1980, pp. 97–124.

Salamon G: Atlas of Arteries of the Human Brain. Paris: Sandoz, 1971.

Sasaki K, Oka H, Matsuda Y, et al: Electrophysiological studies of the projections from the parietal association area to the cerebellar cortex. Exp Brain Res 23:91–102, 1975.

Schaltenbrand G: The effects on speech and language of stereotactical stimulation in thalamus and corpus callosum. Brain Lang 2:70–77, 1975.

Schell GR, Strick PL: The origin of thalamic inputs to the arcuate premotor and supplementary motor areas. J Neurosci 4:539–560, 1984.

Schlesinger B: The Upper Brainstem in the Human: Its Nuclear Configuration and Vascular Supply. New York: Springer, 1976.

Schmahmann JD: Hemi-inattention from right hemisphere subcortical infarction. Boston Society of Neurology and Psychiatry, 1984.

Schmahmann JD: An emerging concept: The cerebellar contribution to higher function. Archiv Neurol 48:1178–1187, 1991.

Schmahmann JD: The cerebellum in autism: Clinical and anatomic perspectives, in Bauman ML, Kemper TL (eds): The Neurobiology of Autism. Baltimore, MD: Johns Hopkins University Press, 1994, pp. 195–226.

Schmahmann JD: From movement to thought: Anatomic substrates of the cerebellar contribution to cognitive processing. Hum Brain Mapping 4:174–198, 1996.

Schmahmann JD (ed): The Cerebellum and Cognition. International Review of Neurobiology, Vol. 41. San Diego, CA: Academic Press, 1997.

Schmahmann JD: Cerebellum and brainstem, in Toga A, Mazziotta, J (eds): Brain Mapping. The Systems. San Diego, CA: Academic Press, 2000a, pp. 207–259.

Schmahmann JD: The role of the cerebellum in affect and psychosis. J Neurolinguistics 13:189–214, 2000b.

Schmahmann JD: Vascular syndromes of the thalamus. Stroke 34:2264–2278, 2003.

Schmahmann JD, Doyon J, McDonald D, et al: Three-dimensional MRI atlas of the human cerebellum in proportional stereotaxic space. Neuroimage 10:233–260, 1999.

Schmahmann JD, Doyon J, Toga A, et al: MRI Atlas of the Human Cerebellum. San Diego, CA: Academic Press, 2000.

Schmahmann JD, Loeber RT, Marjani J, et al: Topographic organization of cognitive function in the human cerebellum: A meta-analysis of functional imaging studies [abstract]. Neuroimage 7:S721, 1998.

Schmahmann JD, Pandya DN: Posterior parietal projections to the basis pontis in rhesus monkey: Possible anatomical substrate for the cerebellar modulation of complex behavior? [abstract]. Neurology 37(Suppl. 1):291, 1987.

Schmahmann JD, Pandya DN: Anatomical investigation of projections to the basis pontis from posterior parietal association cortices in rhesus monkey. J Comp Neurol 289:53–73, 1989.

Schmahmann JD, Pandya DN: Anatomical investigation of thalamic projections to the posterior parietal cortices in rhesus monkey. J Comp Neurol 295:299–326, 1990.

Schmahmann JD, Pandya DN: Projections to the basis pontis from the superior temporal sulcus and superior temporal region in the rhesus monkey. J Comp Neurol 308:224–248, 1991.

Schmahmann JD, Pandya DN: Fiber pathways to the pons from parasensory association cortices in rhesus monkey. J Comp Neurol 326:159–179, 1992.

Schmahmann JD, Pandya DN: Prelunate, occipitotemporal, and parahipppocampal projections to the basis pontis in rhesus monkey. J Comp Neurol 337:94–112, 1993.

Schmahmann JD, Pandya DN: Anatomic organization of the basilar pontine projections from prefrontal cortices in rhesus monkey. J Neurosci 17:438–458, 1997.

Schmahmann JD, Sherman JC: The cerebellar cognitive affective syndrome. Brain 121:561–579, 1998a.

Schmahmann JD, Sherman JC: The cerebellar cognitive affective syndrome [letter]. Brain 121:2203–2205, 1998b.

Schuurman PR, Bruins J, Merkus MP, et al: A comparison of neuropsychological effects of thalamotomy and thalamic stimulation. Neurology 59:1232–1239, 2002.

Scott RB, Stoodley CJ, Anslow P, et al: Lateralized cognitive deficits in children following cerebellar lesions. Dev Med Child Neurol 43:685–691, 2001.

Segarra JM: Cerebral vascular disease and behavior. I. The syndrome of the mesencephalic artery (basilar artery bifurcation). Arch Neurol 22:408–418, 1970.

Shah VS, Schmahmann JD, Pandya DN, et al: Associative projections to the zona incerta: Possible anatomic substrates for extension of the Marr-Albus hypothesis to non-motor learning. Soc Neurosci 23:1829, 1997. (Abstract)

Shatz CJ, Rakic P: The genesis of efferent connections from the visual cortex of the fetal rhesus monkey. J Comp Neurol 196:287–307, 1981.

Sidibe M, Pare JF, Smith Y: Nigral and pallidal inputs to functionally segregated thalamostriatal neurons in the centromedian/parafascicular intralaminar nuclear complex in monkey. J Comp Neurol 447: 286–992, 2002.

Silveri MC, Leggio MG, Molinari M: The cerebellum contributes to linguistic production: A case of agrammatic speech following a right cerebellar lesion. Neurology 44:2047–2050, 1994.

Siwek DF, Pandya DN: Prefrontal projections to the mediodorsal nucleus of the thalamus in the rhesus monkey. J Comp Neurol 312:509–524, 1991.

Snider RS: Recent contributions to the anatomy and physiology of the cerebellum. Arch Neurol Psychiatry 64:196–219, 1950.

Snider RS: Interrelations of cerebellum and brainstem, in Bard P (ed): Patterns of organization of the central nervous system. Res Publ Ass Nerv Ment Dis 30:267–281, 1952.

Snider SR: Cerebellar pathology in schizophrenia—cause or consequence? Neurosci Behav Rev 6:47–53, 1982.

Sobel N, Prabhakaran V, Hartley CA, et al: Odorant-induced and sniff-induced activation in the cerebellum of the human. J Neurosci 18:8990–9001, 1998.

Spiegel EA, Wycis HT, Orchinik C, et al: Thalamic chronotaraxis. Am J Psychiatry 113:97–105, 1956.

Staal WG, Hulshoff Pol HE, Schnack HG, et al: Structural brain abnormalities in chronic schizophrenia at the extremes of the outcome spectrum. Am J Psychiatry 158:1140–1142, 2001.

Stanton GB: Topographical organization of ascending cerebellar projections from the dentate and interposed nuclei in *Macaca mulatta*: An anterograde degeneration study. J Comp Neurol 190:699–731, 1980.

Stanton GB, Goldberg ME, Bruce CJ: Frontal eye field efferents in the macaque monkey: II. Topography of terminal fields in midbrain and pons. J Comp Neurol 271:493–506, 1988.

Steinke W, Sacco RL, Mohr JP, et al: Thalamic stroke. Presentation and prognosis of infarcts and hemorrhages. Arch Neurol 49:703–710, 1002.

Steinlin M, Zangger B, Boltshauser E: Non-progressive congenital ataxia with or without cerebellar hypoplasia: A review of 34 subjects. Dev Med Child Neurol 40:148–154, 1998.

Steriade M, Contreras D, Amzica F: The thalamocortical dialogue during wake, sleep and paroxysmal oscillations, in Steriade M, Jones EG, McCormick DA (eds): Thalamus: Experimental and Clinical Aspects. New York: Elsevier, 1997, Vol. II, pp. 213–294.

Strick PL: Anatomical analysis of ventrolateral thalamic input to primate motor cortex. J Neurophysiol 39:1020–1031, 1976.

Suzuki M, Kitano H, Ito R, et al: Cortical and subcortical vestibular response to caloric stimulation detected by functional magnetic resonance imaging. Brain Res Cogn 12:441–419, 2001.

Szelies B, Herholz K, Pawlik G, et al: Widespread functional effects of discrete thalamic infarction. Arch Neurol 48:178–182, 1991.

Tataranni PA, Gautier JF, Chen K, et al: Neuroanatomical correlates of hunger and satiation in humans using positron emission tomography. Proc Natl Acad Sci U S A 96:4569–4574, 1999.

Tatemichi TK, Desmond DW, Prohovnik I, et al: Confusion and memory loss from capsular genu infarction: A thalamocortical disconnection syndrome? Neurology 42:1966–1979, 1992.

Tatu L, Moulin T, Bogousslavsky J, Duvernoy H. (1998) Arterial territories of the human brain: Cerebral hemispheres. Neurology 50(6):1699–708.

Thach WT: Context-response linkage, in Schmahmann JD (ed): The Cerebellum and Cognition. International Review of Neurobiology, Vol. 41. San Diego, CA: Academic Press, 1997, pp. 599–611.

Thach WT, Jones EG: The cerebellar dentatothalamic connection: Terminal field, lamellae, rods and somatotopy. Brain Res 169:168–172, 1979.

Tobias TJ: Afferents to prefrontal cortex from the thalamic mediodorsal nucleus in the rhesus monkey. Brain Res 83:191–212, 1975.

Ungerleider LG, Desimone R, Galkin TW, et al: Subcortical projections of area MT in the macaque. J Comp Neurol 223:368–386, 1984.

Van Buren JM, Borke RC: Variations and Connections of the Human Thalamus. Berlin: Springer, 1972.

Victor M, Adams RD, Collins GH: The Wernicke-Korsakoff syndrome. A clinical and pathological study of 245 patients, 82 with postmortem examinations. Contemp Neurol Ser 7:1–206, 1971.

Vilensky JA, Van Hoesen GW: Corticopontine projections from the cingulate cortex in the rhesus monkey. Brain Res 205:391–395, 1981.

Vogt BA, Pandya DN, Rosene DL: Cingulate cortex of the rhesus monkey: I. Cytoarchitecture and thalamic afferents. J Comp Neurol 262:256–270, 1987.

Volz H, Gaser C, Sauer H: Supporting evidence for the model of cognitive dysmetria in schizophrenia: A structural magnetic resonance imaging study using deformation-based morphometry. Schizophr Res 46:45–56, 2000.

von Cramon DY, Hebel N, Schuri U: A contribution to the anatomical basis of thalamic amnesia. Brain 108(Pt 4):993–1008, 1985.

Wada K, Kimura K, Minematsu K, et al: Incongruous homonymous hemianopic scotoma. J Neurol Sci 163:179–182, 1999.

Wallesch C-W, Horn A: Long-term effects of cerebellar pathology on cognitive functions. Brain Cogn 14:19–25, 1990.

Warren JD, Thompson PD, Thompson PD: Diencephalic amnesia and apraxia after left thalamic infarction. J Neurol Neurosurg Psychiatry 68:248, 2000.

Watson RT Heilman KM: Thalamic neglect. Neurology 29:690–694, 1979.

Weber J, Mattle HP, Heid O, et al: Diffusion-weighted imaging in ischaemic stroke: A follow-up study. Neuroradiology 42:184–191, 2000.

Weber JT, Yin TCT: Subcortical projections of the inferior parietal cortex (area 7) in the stump-tailed monkey. J Comp Neurol 224:206–230, 1984.

Wernicke C: Der aphasische Symptomencomplex. Bresalu: Cohn and Weigert, 1874. (Referenced in Benson et al., 1973)

Whiteside DG, Snider RS: Relation of cerebellum to upper brain stem. J Neurophysiol 16:397–413, 1953.

Wiesendanger R, Wiesendanger M: The thalamic connections with medial area 6 (supplementary motor cortex) in the monkey (*Macaca fascicularis*). Exp Brain Res 59:91–104, 1985.

Willis WD Jr: Nociceptive functions of thalamic neurons, in Steriade M, Jones EG, McCormick DA (eds): Thalamus: Experimental and Clinical Aspects. New York: Elsevier, 1997, Vol. II, pp. 373–424.

Wisoff JH, Epstein FJ: Pseudobulbar palsy after posterior fossa operation in children. Neurosurgery 15:707–709, 1984.

Woolsey CN: Summary of papers on the cerebellum, in Bard P (ed): Patterns of Organization in the Central Nervous System. Res Publ Ass Nerv Ment Dis 30:334–336, 1952.

Yakovlev PI, Locke S: Limbic nuclei of thalamus and connections of limbic cortex. III. Corticocortical connections of the anterior cingulate gyrus, the cingulum, and the subcallosal bundle in monkey. Arch Neurol 5:34–70, 1961.

Yakovlev PI, Locke S, Koskoff DY, et al: Limbic nuclei of thalamus and connections of limbic cortex. I. Organization of projections of the anterior group of nuclei and of the midline thalamic nuclei of the thalamus to the anterior cingulate gyrus and hippocampal rudiment in the monkey. Arch Neurol 3:620–641, 1960.

Yeterian EH, Pandya DN: Corticothalamic connections of the posterior parietal cortex in the rhesus monkey. J Comp Neurol 237:408–426, 1985.

Yeterian EH, Pandya DN: Corticothalamic connections of paralimbic regions in the rhesus monkey. J Comp Neurol 269:130–146, 1988.

Yeterian EH, Pandya DN: Thalamic connections of the cortex of the superior temporal sulcus in the rhesus monkey. J Comp Neurol 282:80–97, 1989.

Yeterian EH, Pandya DN: Corticothalamic connections of the superior temporal sulcus in rhesus monkeys. Exp Brain Res 83:268–84, 1991.

Yeterian EH, Pandya DN: Corticothalamic connections of extrastriate visual areas in rhesus monkeys. J Comp Neurol 378:562–585, 1997.

Ziegler DK, Kaufman A, Marshall HE: Abrupt memory loss associated with thalamic tumor. Arch Neurol 34:545–548, 1977.

Cerebrovascular Disease

Ashok Devasenapathy
Vladimir Hachinski

Brain attack
Brain at risk
Cerebral leukoaraiosis
Cerebrovascular disease
Multi-infarct dementia
Vascular cognitive impairment

INTRODUCTION

Stroke can be broadly defined as a sudden attack of a specific neurologic deficit, caused by thrombosis or hemorrhage in the cerebral circulation. The arcane term *cerebrovascular accident* suggests that all strokes share a nonspecific, deterministic mechanism, and has fallen out of favor. Figure 26-1 depicts the most common causes of stroke and Table 26-1 provides a classification scheme for stroke subtypes. Specific diagnoses for coding purposes are listed in the International Classification of Diseases (ICD) and the Centers for Medicare and Medicaid Service (CMS) (WHO, 1991).

A stroke may produce circumscribed deficits in specific cognitive domains. Multiple strokes may procedure more pervasive cognitive deficits, and may lead to vascular dementia (Hachinski et al., 1992), which may be the second most common cause of dementia in the elderly, behind Alzheimer disease (AD) (see Chapter 22 on Degenerative Disease for more details). Vascular dementia is a terminal stage of a potentially preventable cognitive syndrome, for it is estimated that up to 75% of all strokes can be prevented. Yet, despite recent advances in stroke prevention, only about 5% to 10% of acute stroke victims in the United States receive thrombolytic therapy. Cognitive impairments associated with both cardiovascular risk factors and treatable cerebrovascular disease have recently been labeled vascular cognitive impairment (VCI).

This chapter reviews basic concepts in cerebrovascular disease. After initial description of cerebrovascular anatomy, we emphasize recent advances in VCI

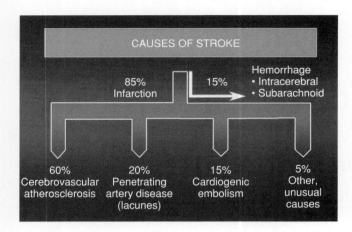

FIGURE 26-1. Predominant causes of stroke.

epidemiology, pathophysiology, pathology, diagnosis, and treatment. Modern clinical trials aim to develop preventive approaches to cardiovascular and cerebrovascular disease that can be applied to VCI.

CEREBROVASCULAR ANATOMY

Lesion location is a prime determinant of clinical presentations and functional and behavioral consequences of stroke. The following section reviews essential features of cerebrovascular anatomy and their relationship to cerebrovascular pathology.

Extracranial Cerebral Vessels

The brain receives its blood supply from the heart by way of the aortic arch. The latter gives rise to the innominate artery (brachycephalic) on the right side, which branches into the common carotid and subclavian vessels. On the left side the arch branches directly into the left common carotid and subclavian arteries. The vertebral vessels are usually derived from the first branches of the subclavian arteries. In the neck, the two common carotid arteries (CCAs) usually divide into internal and external branches at the level of the angle of the mandible (Fig. 26-2).

The internal carotid arteries (ICAs) run directly into the skull. The external branches terminate as the superficial temporal artery and the occipital artery. The external carotid provides an important collateral source of blood supply to the brain when the internal carotid artery becomes stenotic or occluded. Important collateral branches also include ethmoidal and lacrimal branches of the ophthalmic artery. Dural-based collaterals arise from ascending pharyngeal, maxillary, and occipital arteries. However, the most important meningeal-based collateral arises from the maxillary artery.

TABLE 26-1. TOAST Classification of Stroke Subtypes

Large-artery arteriosclerosis

Significant stenosis (0.50%) or occlusion of a large cerebral vessel—either the major cerebral vessels or branch cortical vessel—presumably on the basis of atherosclerosis.

Cardioembolism

Cardiac embolism is divided into high-, medium-, and low-risk groups based on their relative propensity for embolism. Evidence of TIA or strokes involving more than one vascular territory is suggestive. A stroke from a medium-risk cardioembolic source with no other apparent source for stroke is classified as probable cardioembolic stroke.

Small-artery occlusion (lacuna)

This category includes patients with the classic lacunar syndromes without any clinical evidence of cerebral cortical dysfunction. The patient should have either a normal CT or MRI examination or a subcortical hemispheric lesion with a diameter of less than 1.5 cm demonstrated. Potential cardiac sources of embolism should be excluded, and the large extracranial cerebral vessel on the ipsilateral side should not demonstrate stenosis in excess of 50%.

Acute stroke of other determined etiology

Category includes rare causes of stroke such as nonatherosclerotic vasculopathies, hypercoagulable states, or hematological disorders. CT or MRI studies should show an acute ischemic stroke, and diagnostic studies should reveal one of the unusual causes of stokes. Cardiac sources of embolism and large-artery atherosclerosis should be excluded by other studies.

Strokes of undetermined etiology

In several instances the cause for the stroke cannot be determined with any degree of confidence, even after an extensive work-up. This category also includes two or more potential causes of stroke so that the physician is unable to make a final diagnosis.

CT, computed tomography; MRI, magnetic resonance imaging; TIA, transient ischemic attack; TOAST, Trial of Org 10172 in Acute Stroke Treatment.

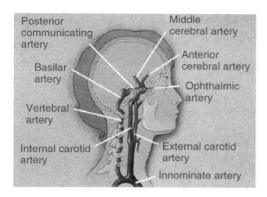

FIGURE 26-2. Major arterial vessels providing blood supply to the brain.

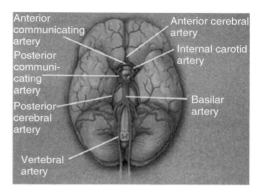

FIGURE 26-3. Vascular artery of the circle of Willis.

In the back of the neck, the two vertebral arteries (VAs) ascend to join each other and form the basilar artery. One vertebral artery is almost always larger than the other and this vessel is therefore referred to as dominant. The vertebral artery is anatomically defined into three different segments. The first part (V1 segment) is the segment from its origin to the C6 vertebra. The vessel then penetrates into the transverse foramina of C6 to C1 (V2 segment). After exiting the foramina of the C1 vertebra (V3 segment), the artery passes through the foramen magnum and subsequently unites ventral to the medulla to form the basilar artery.

Important collateral from the vertebral arteries includes a rather large constant branch at C5 level that anastomoses with the anterior spinal artery. In the suboccipital triangle, the vessel is covered only by soft tissue; free anastomosis occurs with the occipital branches of the external carotid artery.

Intracranial Cerebral Vessels

The ICA penetrates the base of the skull through the carotid canal and the petrous portion of the temporal bone. Thereafter, it travels between the layers of the dura, supplying the adjacent important structures as it ascends to lie in the sella turcica and enters the cavernous sinus. The ophthalmic artery arises from the dorsal aspect of the carotid siphon just above the diaphragm sellae and beneath the optic nerve. This artery supplies the orbital contents and anastomoses with the above-mentioned branches of the external carotid artery.

Common anatomic variants of the circle of Willis occur in about one half of normal individuals (Fig. 26-3). An incomplete circle becomes most significant when there is hemodynamic compromise of cerebral blood flow. The rate of hemodynamic alterations in cerebral blood flow is also important for the establishment of cerebral collateral pathways.

The internal carotid artery bifurcates into the anterior and middle cerebral arteries. The anterior cerebral

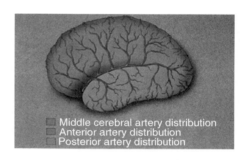

FIGURE 26-4. Distribution of the major cerebral vascular territories.

artery (ACA) runs anteromedially. The most clinically significant branches of the ACA include the medial striate artery (i.e., recurrent artery of Heubner) (Fig. 26-4). This vessel arises from the ACA, just after the anterior communicating artery (ACOA), and supplies the anterior portion of the caudate nucleus, adjacent portions of the basal ganglia, and the anterior limb of internal capsule. The two ACAs run a parallel course around the genu of the corpus callosum. Small anastomoses from either side occur at irregular intervals. Other clinically significant branches of the ACA include the frontopolar and callosomarginal arteries that supply the intrahemispheric or medial aspects of the frontal and parietal lobes.

The two ACAs are united in the midline, just above the optic chiasm, by the ACOA. This vessel may be absent, but otherwise serves as an important collateral pathway between the two carotid circulations. It is also a common site of aneurysm. The middle cerebral artery (MCA), which is the largest of all cerebral vessels, supplies important cortical regions including motor, somatosensory, auditory, language, visuospatial, and multimodal cortices as well as subcortical nuclei such as the basal ganglia and white matter corticospinal tracts. The deep penetrating lenticulostriate vessels of the MCA, along with other vessels of similar caliber, form the basilar circulation for the so-called *vascular centroencephalon*. The walls of these vessels are prone to damage from hypertension due to their inability to autoregulate blood flow and are therefore predisposed to lacunar strokes and hypertensive hemorrhages.

Relationships between lesions in specific arterial territories, the resulting focal damage in cytoarchitectonic areas, and specific neurobehavioral deficits are illustrated by Damasio and Damasio (1989) and by Damasio (1992). Multiple lesions in multiple territories can produce increasing cognitive deficits, leading to dementia.

VASCULAR COGNITIVE IMPAIRMENT

Definition

Vascular dementia is a generic term that neither identifies a specific etiology nor recognizes the broad clinical spectrum of acquired cognitive impairments (Hachinski, 1992; 1994). An alternate approach is desirable, one that identifies individuals across the entire spectrum of VCI, from high risk, with no clinical symptoms ("brain at risk" stage), to full-blown dementia (Hachinski, 1991, 1992).

The concept of VCI leading to dementia might seem to suggest a degenerative etiology for the increasing deficits of memory and cognition, as in AD. However, in contrast to AD, strokes have more clearly identified etiology that respond better than AD to preventive and acute therapeutic measures (Bowler & Hachinski, 1995) such as thrombolytic therapy (reviewed later in this chapter).

Population-based studies show that cognitive deficits are detectable in at least 10% of individuals over age 65 years and in 25% of those over age 85 (Heyman et al., 1984; see Chapter 36 on Aging and the Brain). Although AD accounts for up to two thirds of all dementias, vascular causes form the second largest group, with a prevalence of 15% to 20% (Ebly et al., 1994). Epidemiology studies suggest that up to one quarter of stroke patients may go on to develop VCI (Tatemichi et al., 1992). The lack of standardized criteria for identifying VCI hinders diagnosis and recruitment of participants for research protocols. In addition, the widespread use of short-term memory-oriented screening tests for cognitive deficits in patients with cerebrovascular disease may underestimate the true clinical magnitude of VCI, in which cognitive impairments tend to be more diverse than in AD (Devasenapathy, 1997).

VCI is a clinical syndrome, not a single disease (Bowler & Hachinski, 1995). Multiple large infarcts from ischemic strokes form the severe end of a clinical continuum associated with this syndrome. However, the majority of patients with VCI will have subtle cognitive deficits within the context of vascular risk factors (such as hypertension, obesity, tobacco abuse, and atrial fibrillation) and/or clinically "silent" strokes from under-

treated risk factors. This constitutes the so-called "brain at risk" stage, in which preventive measures and treatments are most effective (Bowler & Hachinski, 1995).

Age-related cognitive impairment may be unavoidable (see Chapter 36) and may produce a clinical syndrome of mild cognitive impairment or MCI that may announce the onset of a neurodegenerative or cerebrovascular disorder (Myers et al., 2002; see Chapter 22 on Degenerative Disease). Elderly patients who have a non-neurodegenerative cause for their cognitive deficits may have early manifestations of cardiovascular and cerebrovascular disease, which may eventually produce ischemic and hemorrhagic strokes (Ferruci et al., 1996). Despite advances in the early identification and treatment of vascular risk factors for heart disease and strokes, the relative risk for developing VCI associated with known vascular risk factors remains poorly characterized, perhaps due to the heterogeneous nature of VCI (Devasenapathy, 1997).

Epidemiology

VCI accounts for 15% to 20% of all dementias (Heyman et al., 1984). Its prevalence increases with age, ranging from 1.2% to 4.2% in people over age 65 years (Brayne, 1995). In Western countries, up to 30% of patients with cognitive impairment (as shown in clinical studies of dementia that have autopsy series) have a "mixed dementia," usually due to a combination of vascular and degenerative processes (Ebly et al., 1994; Devasenapathy, 1997). The prevalence of mixed dementias is unclear, as no standard clinical or pathologic criteria yet exist for diagnosis of this condition.

Up to one quarter of stroke patients develop some form of cognitive impairment, and this risk becomes especially high in patients over 70 years of age (Tatemichi et al., 1992). The relative risk of VCI is higher in certain racial groups and in demographic regions such as China and Japan (Kasahara & Sasahara, 1993). Stroke subtypes and risk factors may carry differing relative risk factor for VCI. Patients with lacunar strokes have a four- to fivefold increased risk of developing cognitive deficits, compared with nonstroke control groups (Loeb, 1995). Further research is needed to define the risk of VCI in other stroke subtypes. A better understanding of risk factors and pathogenic mechanisms, especially in lacunar strokes and subcortical white matter infarcts, would presumably improve the ability to treat and prevent VCI.

Pathophysiology

AD and VCI are different disorders, yet several pathologic neurochemical processes induced by cerebral ischemia are also seen in AD (Devasenapathy, 1997). Patients with strokes are prone to develop Alzheimer-type histopathology (Bowen, 1991). One possibility is that vascular damage to the brain activates or accelerates degenerative mechanisms (Sulzer et al., 1995). Ischemia-induced inflammation, microglial activation, glutamate toxicity, and neuronal death are common to AD and VCI (Mcgeer & Rojers, 1992). Inflammatory processes in AD and VCI are associated with proliferation of microglial cells and production of cytokines (mainly interleukin-1-β, tumor necrosis factor-β, and neurotoxic free radicals) (Djuricic et al., 1989). The neurotoxic free radicals promote aggregation of β-amyloid peptides (an important component of amyloid plaques), which is a key pathologic feature of AD (Jarett, 1993). Ischemia/degenerative processes cause mature astrocytes that normally produce nerve growth factor (NGF) to produce abnormal NGF subtypes that have a reduced capacity to maintain extracellular homeostasis (Beal & Flint, 1991). Furthermore, neuronal death from ischemia or degeneration provokes excessive glutamate release, with an increase in extracellular calcium concentration (Beal & Flint, 1991). Astrocytes have a physiologic role as scavengers of excess extracellular calcium. Intracellular "calcium overload" results in astrocyte death, which leads to the production of neuritic (astrocytic) plaques, another hallmark of AD (Beal & Flint, 1991).

Deposition of amyloid in cerebral vessel walls causes congophilic angiopathy (based on staining of the vessels with Congo Red), leading to vessel necrosis, microaneurysm formation, and lobar hemorrhage. Patients with congophilic angiopathy (also termed *amyloid angiopathy*) are prone to develop dementia (Ghiso & Frangione, 2001).

A fraction of patients with VCI seem to show delayed onset and insidious evolution of cognitive deficits during the months after a stroke, without the usual acute onset of cognitive deficits (Tatemichi et al., 1992). Impaired activity of cholinergic neurons in the forebrain (i.e., basal nucleus of Meynert) has been implicated in slowly progressive cognitive deficits and behavioral disturbance associated with AD (Palmer & Gershon, 1990). Similar biochemical mechanisms may help explain insidious evolution of cognitive impairments in VCI.

Pathologic Subtypes of VCI

The following section describes the clinical spectrum of VCI, from the asymptomatic "brain at risk" stage to severe dementia, with emphasis on neuropsychological and neuroradiologic evidence.

Brain at Risk Stage

Longitudinal follow-up of asymptomatic patients with isolated vascular risk factors indicate these patients are at risk for strokes and cognitive impairment. Some develop clinically evident strokes; in others, "silent" strokes are hypothesized to contribute to the cognitive deficits (Ferruci et al., 1996).

Patients without demonstrable strokes may have chronic ongoing brain ischemia and even ischemia-induced degeneration due to one or more risk factors. Long-term effects of vascular risk factors or cerebral arteriosclerosis may impair cerebral autoregulation, leading to chronic cerebral hypoperfusion (Sulzer, 1995). This phenomenon has been termed *misery perfusion* in positron emission tomography (PET) studies that show a sharp drop in oxygen extraction values in individuals with VCI (Sulzer, 1995). Cerebral ischemia may directly or indirectly influence neurochemical pathways involved in cognition, activate degenerative mechanisms (as described above), and diminish activity of important neurotransmitters (Bowen & Davison, 1986; Palmer & Gershon, 1990).

Early and aggressive treatment of all identified vascular risk factors may help prevent VCI (Henderson, 1997). This approach has been supported by studies that support the cognitive benefits of primary and secondary prevention of strokes. The use of postmenopausal estrogen replacement therapy was suggested as possible prevention for vascular morbidity and AD in women (Henderson, 1997). Longitudinal, population-based studies of dementia are needed to more clearly assess the benefits of treating vascular risk factors and shed light on the pathogenesis of VCI (Skoog et al., 1993; Bryne, 1995; Devasenapathy, 1997).

However, the presumed benefits of estrogen in the secondary prevention of AD are clear. In the Alzheimer's Disease Cooperative Study, women older than 60 years who had undergone a hysterectomy were randomized to receive estrogen if they had a diagnosis of probable AD. The authors concluded that estrogen did not improve outcomes (cognitive or functional) in women with mild to moderate AD who receive this treatment for 1 year. A slight benefit seen at 2 months with 0.625 mg per day of estrogen does not persist if treatment continues (Mulnard et al., 2000; Shaywitz & Shaywitz, 2000).

Strategic Infarct Dementia

Ischemic or hemorrhagic strokes that damage diverse cortical association areas and subcortical nuclei (e.g., thalamus, basal ganglia) have long been associated with the abrupt onset of clinically evident and very characteristic patterns of cognitive deficits (Damasio & Damasio, 1989). The "strategic" location of this infarct or infarcts determines the pattern of VCI. For the anterior cerebral artery, these neurobehavioral syndromes are described in the chapter on frontal lobe syndromes (see Chapter 20) and include aphasia, akinesia-mutism, social-emotional impairments and executive dysfunction. Syndromes associated with middle cerebral artery stroke include aphasias (see Chapter 17), hemispatial neglect (see Chapter 10), apraxia (see Chapter 18), auditory processing (see Chapter 13), and somatosensory functions (see Chapter 14). Neurobehavioral syndromes associated with posterior cerebral artery stroke include visual disorders (see Chapter 12) and thalamic syndromes (see Chapter 25). Small strategic infarcts in key cortical areas (e.g., Broca's area), the thalamus, or basal ganglia may also produce diverse neurologic and neuropsychological symptoms (Tatemichi et al., 1995). The severity of cognitive deficits associated with such strokes are often dependent on the patient's age, presence of premorbid cognitive deficits, location of the stroke, underlying etiology for the stroke, and the extent of associated cerebrovascular disease. Of note, patients with acute unilateral strokes may show more pervasive findings than expected given apparent lesion size and location, possibly due to acute effects of damage to long-range connections with the injured area, in line with the century-old diaschesis hypothesis of von Monakow (Pearce, 1994). The resulting cognitive deficits can show variable outcomes, ranging from slow improvement to quick recovery.

Cognitive Impairment after a Single Stroke

Single, large strokes involving either cerebral hemisphere or the frontal lobes may produce acute and profound cognitive impairment, behavioral changes and complex neuropsychological deficits. In such instances, the site and volume of cerebral infarction may predict the severity of the cognitive impairment (Tatemichi et al., 1995). Some individuals develop subtle cognitive impairments after an isolated nondebilitating stroke (clinically evident or silent). As mentioned above, cerebral ischemia may activate or accelerate mechanisms that lead to the development of cerebral histopathology typically seen in AD, including neurofibrillary tangles and senile plaques.

In addition, patients with stroke may become depressed because of damage in frontal and limbic system structures, catastrophic reaction to illness, side effects of medications, and other illnesses. Hence, the combination of stroke effects and depression may produce a picture resembling dementia (see Chapters 3 and 22 for further details).

Multi-infarct Dementia

The term multi-infarct dementia generally refers to cognitive impairment associated with multiple large strokes or recurrent lacunar strokes (so-called *lacunar state*) (Hachinski, 1994). The resulting pattern of cognitive deficit has been described as stepwise in its progression (Loeb, 1995). The Hachinski Ischemic Scale (Table 26-2) has been validated for use in the diagnosis of multi-infarct dementia and provides a reliable

TABLE 26-2. The Ischemic Scale[*]

Feature	Value
Abrupt onset	2
Stepwise deterioration	1
Fluctuating course	2
Nocturnal confusion	1
Relative preservation of personality	1
Depression	1
Somatic complaints	1
Emotional incontinence	1
History or presence of hypertension	1
History of strokes	2
Evidence of associated atherosclerosis	1
Focal neurologic symptoms	2

[*]Scores of 7 or more suggest a vascular etiology for dementia; scores of 4 or less do not support a vascular etiology.
(Data from Hachinski VC, Lliff LD, Zilkha E, et al: Cerebral blood flow in dementia. Arch Neurol 32:632–637, 1975.)

measure for differentiating multi-infarct dementia from AD (Loeb, 1995). This tool does not differentiate VCI from mixed dementias, although the vascular component is a key treatable element of both conditions (Chui, 1989).

Cerebral Leukoariosis and White Matter Dementia

The cerebral white matter is perfused by superficial cortical penetrating blood vessels and by deep terminal perforating vessels. By virtue of this endarterial pattern of blood supply, the white matter is a vulnerable "watershed" zone that is susceptible to ischemia from many different causes.

Current brain imaging techniques cannot definitely differentiate cerebral white matter ischemia from nonischemic pathology. Brain magnetic resonance imaging (MRI) is highly sensitive to white matter abnormalities (see Chapter 7 on fMRI and Related Techniques). Leukoariosis refers to nonspecific MRI signal alterations (hyperintensity) in the cerebral white matter (Hachinski et al., 1986). It is commonly found in individuals with normal cognition (associated with or without vascular risk factors), clinically probable AD, and ischemic cerebrovascular disease. This term makes no reference to the underlying pathology or neurologic/cognitive deficits (Hachinski et al., 1986).

In patients with normal neurologic examination results and cognition, the most likely causes for leukoariosis include: (1) dilated perivascular space (état crible) that surrounds the penetrating cerebral blood vessels (commonly observed in individuals with poorly controlled hypertension) (Devasenapathy, 2000), and/or (2) "ventricular caps" and "rims" that surround the cerebrospinal fluid cavity of the brain (Willin & Blenow, 1991) (also termed *Virchow-Robin spaces*). The latter observation is often observed in young individuals and can be misinterpreted as being pathologic (Rizzo & Tranel, 1996).

Patients who meet clinical criteria for probable AD often demonstrate leukoariosis on MRI scans. The underlying basis for this observation includes the presence of hypertensive arteriopathy, amyloid angiopathy and cerebral small artery disease (Willin & Blenow, 1991). Ischemic white matter disease may reflect the effects of longstanding vascular risk factors such as hypertension, diabetes, and impaired cerebral autoregulation (Raiha et al., 1993). An impaired cerebral autoregulatory mechanism may accompany normal aging but is more pronounced in individuals with arteriosclerosis of the cerebral vessels (Skoog, 1994). Patients with dementia and other neurodegenerative disorders that are associated with cell loss in the midbrain/brainstem autonomic nuclei, often have more pronounced postural hypotension with a predisposition for recurrent acute drops in cerebral perfusion (Skoog, 1994). Postural drops in blood pressure from low cardiac output states (e.g., angina, atrial fibrillation, etc.) and ischemic heart disease can accompany normal aging and may worsen preexisting white matter ischemia (Raiha et al., 1993).

Patients with clinical evidence of diffuse (bilateral) or focal neurologic deficits may also have leukoariosis. Some have cognitive deficits that reflect different stages of ischemic injury to the white matter tracts, with resultant disconnection of the association pathways to the overlying cerebral cortex, between the hemispheres and the subcortical grey nuclei (Djurici et al., 1989). Additionally, such patients often have radiological evidence of strokes in the thalamus/basal ganglia (vascular centroencephalon) that may compound the observed cognitive deficits (Sulzer, 1995). Gait problems and bowel/bladder incontinence may accompany later stages of this process (Hennerici et al., 1994). Emotional incontinence (e.g., pseudobulbar phenomena) usually suggests bilateral damage to pathways between the brainstem, frontal association cortex, and thalamus (Hennerici et al., 1994). Hypertension-induced microvascular infarcts (lacunar strokes) with recurrent subcortical ischemic strokes (known as "lacunar state") may be a rare cause for such symptoms. Other conditions recently identified with these symptoms include central autosomal dominant arteriopathy with subcortical strokes and ischemic leukoencephalopathy (CADASIL) (Tournier-Lesserve et al., 1993), lupus anticoagulant/antiphospholipid antibody syndrome, and systemic autoimmune disease (Brayne, 1995).

Subcortical vascular dementias have a general pattern of cognitive deficits that includes slowing of information processing and impaired memory with poor sustained attention. Expressive language deficits are often evident and include poor word list generation, impaired verbal fluency, and impaired motor programming with impersistence and preservation. Additionally, reduced concentration and immediate memory result in difficulties with set shifting that may be characterized by the poor retrieval of information but intact recognition (Hennerici et al., 1994).

There is little evidence to suggest that "Binswanger disease" is a distinct pathologic entity. The clinical features of Binswanger disease (i.e., cognitive problems, gait disorder, emotional incontinence, bowel/bladder incontinence) are common to all subcortical vascular dementias (Pantoni & Garcia, 1995).

The pathologic lesions in the subcortical vascular dementias are thought to affect the circuitry interconnecting the caudate nucleus, globus pallidus, thalamus, and frontal lobes (see Chapter 25 for a discussion of these circuits). Gait problems often accompany the cognitive impairment and are the result of the involvement of frontal subcortical and periventricular white matter with the disruption of the thalamocorticomediocapsular pathways (Hennerici et al., 1994).

Vasculitis

Vasculitis of the brain is a relatively uncommon cause of stroke, and encompasses a variety of autoimmune conditions (Table 26-3). The anatomical and physiologic barrier between the cardiovascular and cerebrovascular systems includes a heterogenous group of immune mechanisms, so that antigen-antibody responses against nervous system tissue are clinically heterogeneous. The patterns of impairment in vasculitis are influenced by variables such as age, gender, premorbid personality, psychological status and concurrent medial diseases.

Cognitive impairments are well known to occur in patients with central nervous system (CNS) vasculitis. For example, a study of 43 neurologically asymptomatic patients with antineutrophil cytoplasmic antibody (ANCA)-related systemic vasculitis showed that 30% of patients had neuropsychological impairment, characterized by mild abstract reasoning loss, mental speed reduction, and nonverbal memory impairment. MRI findings in impaired patients were consistent with the subcortical microvascular damage (Mattioli et al., 2002).

Temporal arteritis should be considered in the differential diagnosis of psychosis and affective disorders in the elderly. The erythrocyte sedimentation rate is a valuable parameter in the assessment of old-age psychiatric patients presenting both with functional and neurologic disorders (Johnson et al., 1997).

TABLE 26-3. Classification of Cerebral Vasculitis

Infectious vasculitis	Sarcoidosis
Spirochetal (syphilis)	Relapsing polychondritis
Mycobacterial	Kohlmeier-Degos disease
Fungal	Giant cell arteritides
Bacterial (purulent) meningitis	Takayasu arteritis
Viral (e.g., HIV)	Temporal (cranial) arteritis
Other organisms	Hypersensitivity vasculitides
Necrotizing vasculitis	Henoch-Schönlein purpura
Classic polyarteritis nodosa	Drug-induced vasculitis (e.g., cocaine, amphetamines)
Wegener granulomatosis	Chemical vasculitides
Allergic angitis and granulomatosis (Churg-Strauss)	Essential mixed cryoglobulinimeia
Necrotizing systemic vasculitis—overlap syndrome	Miscellaneous
Lymphomatoid granulomatosis	Vasculitis associated with neoplasm
Vasculitis associated with collagen vascular diseases	Vasculitis associated with radiation
Systemic lupus erythematosus	Cogan syndrome
Rheumatoid arthritis	Dermatomyositis-polymyositis
Scleroderma	X-linked lymphoproliferative syndrome
Sjogren syndrome	Thromboangiitis obliterans
Vasculitis associated with other systemic disorders	Kawasaki syndrome
Behçet disease	Primary central nervous system angitis
Ulcerative colitis	

Systemic lupus erythematosus (SLE) is an autoimmune disease characterized by frequent neuropsychiatric manifestations. At least two different pathogenetic mechanisms have been proposed for neuropsychiatric and cognitive symptoms, including vasculitis and antibodies against neurons, from serum lymphocytotoxic antibodies (LCAs). The pattern of cognitive impairment in LCA-positive patients included defective visuospatial functions (Denburg et al., 1988).

The use of methamphetamines and cocaine is regrettably common, particularly among younger adults, and can produce a picture of vasculitis with associated cognitive impairment (Margolis & Newton, 1971). Nonvasculitic autoimmune inflammatory meningoencephalitis is reviewed in Chapter 37.

Risk Factors

Stroke(s) and age are the most important independent predictors of VCI. A racial predilection for VCI remains unproven (Bowler & Hachinski, 1995; Devasenapathy et al., 1997). Although Asians may have a higher prevalence of VCI compared with whites, the lack of uniformly accepted criteria for the diagnosis of VCI may result in an underestimation of its prevalence (Devasenapathy et al., 1997). Risk factors for VCI should mirror those for cerebrovascular disease, yet the relative risk associated with any individual risk factor remains unclear (Skoog, 1994). Systolic hypertension

may be an important risk factor, although a meta-analysis of the different population-based prevalence studies in VCI shows inconclusive results (Munson et al., 1998).

Clinical Criteria

The last three decades have witnessed an increased interest in prevention and early treatment of cerebrovascular disease. Researchers have tried to develop clinical criteria for the diagnosis of VCI that can be applied to both research and clinical practice that goes beyond a fatalistic approach to dementia as an unavoidable and untreatable "hardening of the arteries."

In the 1970s, widespread understanding that cerebrovascular disease was preventable prompted the development of the Ischemic Scale (see Table 26-2). This helped to differentiate multi-infarct dementia as a distinct disorder from the degenerative dementias and has since been applied to operationalize clinical criteria for vascular dementia. This scoring system has been validated for use in the differentiation of pure AD from definitive vascular dementia, but lacks sensitivity in the diagnosis of mixed dementia (Chui, 1989). Five clinical criteria are commonly used in clinical research for the diagnosis of vascular dementia. These may be categorized into two groups. The first set of criteria are the DSM-IV (American Psychiatric Association, 1994) criteria for multi-infarct dementia and AD (Table 26-4a,b).

TABLE 26-4a. Diagnostic Criteria for Vascular Dementia According to the DSM-IV

A. The development of multiple cognitive deficits manifested by both:

1. Memory impairment (impaired ability to learn new information or recall previously learned information)

2. One (or more) of the following cognitive disturbances:
   a. Aphasia
   b. Apraxia
   c. Agnosia
   d. Disturbance in executive functioning

B. The memory and other cognitive deficits each cause significant impairment in social or occupational functioning and represent a significant decline from a previous level of functioning.

C. Focal neurologic signs and symptoms (e.g., exaggeration of deep tendon reflexes, extensor plantar response, pseudobulbar palsy, gait abnormalities, weakness of an extremity) or laboratory evidence indicative of cerebrovascular disease (e.g., multiple infarctions involving cortex and underlying white matter) that are judged to be etiologically related to the disturbance.

D. The deficits do not occur exclusively during the course of a delirium.

Modified from Diagnostic and Statistical Manual of Mental Disorders, 4th ed. Washington, DC: American Psychiatric Association, 1994.

TABLE 26-4b. Diagnostic Criteria for Alzheimer Disease According to the DSM-IV

A. The development of multiple cognitive deficits manifested by both:

1. Memory impairment

2. One (or more) of the following cognitive disturbances:
   a. Aphasia
   b. Apraxia
   c. Agnosia
   d. Disturbance in executive functioning

B. The cognitive deficits in Criteria A1 and A2 each cause significant impairment in social or occupational functioning and represent a significant decline from a previous level of functioning.

C. The course is characterized by gradual onset and continuing cognitive decline.

D. The memory and other cognitive deficits are not due to any of the following:

1. Other central nervous conditions that cause progressive deficits in memory and cognition.

2. Systemic conditions that are known to cause dementia.

3. Substance-induced conditions.

E. The deficits do not occur exclusively during the course of a delirium.

F. The disturbance is not better accounted for by another disorder.

Modified from Diagnostic and Statistical Manual of Mental Disorders, 4th ed. Washington, DC: American Psychiatric Association, 1994.

Both are similar and emphasize "long tract signs" and focal neurologic deficits as key diagnostic elements. The second set includes those developed by the California Alzheimer's Disease Diagnostic and Treatment Centers (CADDTC), the National Institute of Neurological Disease and Stroke (NINDS), and the Association International pour la Research et l'Enseignement en Neuroscience (AIREN) (Table 26-5) (Chui et al., 1992; Roman et al., 1993) (see Table 26-4). The NINDS and AIREN criteria have arisen from the DSM-IV and recent ICD criteria to better facilitate operationality of the clinical criteria. NINDS and AIREN are each based on clinical and neuroimaging features of cerebral infarct but fail to acknowledge cerebral hemorrhage and anoxic injuries. These clinical criteria do not identify patients at the "brain-at-risk" stage in which intervention would be most desirable (Chui et al., 1992; Roman et al., 1993; Bowler & Hachinski, 1995). The NINDS-AIREN and the CADDTC clinical criteria categorize the certainty of diagnosis of vascular dementia as "probable," "possible," and "definite." A definite diagnosis requires tissue diagnosis either from autopsy or brain biopsy. All of the clinical criteria require a causal role for stroke(s) in cognitive impairment (Chui et al., 1992;

Roman et al., 1993). None of the criteria recognize the mixed dementias (which become increasingly common with advancing age and are seen in up to one third of patients with cognitive impairment) (Devasenapathy et al., 1997).

Neurology and Neuropsychology

Clinicians should use caution in relating the presence or absence of neurologic signs found on examination to a diagnosis of VCI. Patients with a diagnosis of VCI need not have multifocal neurologic deficits or bilateral corticospinal tract signs. Bilateral corticospinal signs may be caused by brainstem strokes or cervical disk disease in patients with normal cognition (Bowler & Hachinski, 1995; Devasenapathy et al., 1997).

Although patients with strategic cerebral infarct(s) and multi-infarct dementia may have diverse neurologic signs and neuropsychological deficits, many patients with VCI have neurologic examination results and cognitive deficits that suggest a subcortical dementia

Table 26-5. Criteria for Vascular Dementia from the State of California Alzheimer's Disease Diagnostic and Treatment Centers

1. Dementia. Dementia is a deterioration from a known or estimated prior level of function sufficient to interfere broadly with the conduct of the patient's customary activities of daily living, which is not isolated to a single narrow category of intellectual performance, and which is independent of level of consciousness.

   This deterioration should be supported by historical evidence and documented by either bedside mental status testing or ideally by more detailed neuropsychological examination, using tests that are available.

2. Probable IVD

   A. The criteria for the clinical diagnosis of PROBABLE IVD include ALL of the following:

      1. Dementia;

      2. Evidence of two or more ischemic strokes by history, neurologic signs, and/or neuroimaging studies (CT or T1-weighted MRI) or occurrence of a single stroke with a clearly documented temporal relationship to the onset of dementia;

      3. Evidence of at least one infarct outside the cerebellum by CT or T1-MRI.

   B. The diagnosis of probable IVD is supported by

      1. Evidence of multiple infarcts in brain regions known to affect cognition.

      2. A history of multiple transient ischemic attacks.

      3. History of vascular risk factors (e.g., hypertension, heart disease, diabetus mellitus).

      4. Elevated Hachinski Ischemic Scale (original or modified versions).

   C. Clinical features that are thought to be associated with IVD, but await further research include

      1. Relatively early appearance of gait disturbance and urinary incontinence;

      2. Periventricular and deep white matter changes on T2-weighted MRI that are excessive for age;

      3. Focal changes in electrophysiological studies (e.g. EEG, evoked potentials) or physiologic neuroimaging studies (e.g., SPECT, PET, NMR, spectroscopy).

   D. Other clinical features that do not constitute strong evidence either for or against a diagnosis of PROBABLE IVD include

      1. Periods of slowly progressive symptoms;

      2. Illusion, psychosis, hallucinations, delusions;

      3. Seizures.

   E. Clinical features that cast doubt on a daignosis of PROBABLE IVD include

      1. Transcortical sensory aphasia in the absence of corresponding focal lesions on neuroimaging studies;

      2. Absence of central neurological symptoms/signs, other than cognitive disturbances;

      3. Possible IVD

3. A clinical diagnosis of POSSIBLE IVD may be made where there is

   1. Dementia;
      and one or more of the following:

   2.a. A history or evidence of a single stroke (but not multiple strokes) without a clearly documented temporal relationship to the onset of dementia;

      or

   2.b. Binswanger syndrome (without multiple strokes) that includes all of the following:

      1. Early-onset urinary incontinence not explained by urologic disease; gait disturbance (e.g., parkinsonian, magnetic, apraxia, or "senile" gait) not explained by peripheral cause;

      2. Vascular risk factors;

      3. Extensive white matter change on neuroimaging.

TABLE 26-5. Criteria for Vascular Dementia from the State of California Alzheimer's Disease Diagnostic and Treatment Centers—cont'd

4. Definite IVD

A diagnosis of DEFINITE IVD requires histopathologic examination of the brain, as well as

A. Clinical evidence of dementia;

B. Pathologic confirmation of multiple infarcts, some outside the cerebellum.

Note: If there is evidence of Alzheimer disease or some other pathologic disorder that is thought to have contributed to the dementia, a diagnosis of mixed dementia should be made.

5. Mixed dementia

A diagnosis of MIXED dementia should be made in the presence of one or more other systemic or brain disorders that are thought to be causally related to dementia.

The degree of confidence in the diagnosis of IVD should be specified as possible, probable, or definite, and other disorders(s) contributing to the dementia should be listed. For example: mixed dementia due to probable IVD and possible Alzheimer disease, or mixed dementia due to definite IVD and hypothyroidism.

Location: Cortical white matter, periventricular, basal ganglia, thalamus

Size: Volume

Distribution: Large, small, or microvessel.

Severity: Chronic ischemia versus infarction

Etiology: Embolism, atherosclerosis, arteriosclerosis, cerebral amyloid angiopathy, hypoperfusion.

CT, computed tomography; IVD ischemic vascular dementia; NMR, nuclear magnetic resonance; PET, positron emission tomography; SPECT, single proton emission computed tomography.

(Data from Chui HC, Victoroff JI, Margolin D, et al: Criteria for the diagnosis of ischemic vascular dementia proposed by the State of California Alzheimer's Disease Diagnostic and Treatment Centers. Neurology 42:473–480, 1992.)

(Roman et al., 1993). Some of these patients may develop short-term memory problems or worsening of ongoing memory problems (Kertesz & Clydesdale, 1994).

Neuropsychological tests, such as the Mini-Mental Status Examination (MMSE) are insensitive screening tests for VCI. The MMSE places greater emphasis on memory and language than on visuoperception (see Chapter 1 on Mental Status Screening). This task penalizes patients with aphasia who may not be demented, and may fail to detect visuoperceptual processing deficits in patients with VCI. Studies show that patients with vascular dementia typically do poorly on test items that are influenced by frontal and subcortical mechanisms that are involved in executive functions, verbal fluency, attention, and motor performance (Kertesz & Clydesdale, 1994).

Psychometric tests sensitive in identifying the spectrum of cognitive deficits associated with VCI include the Mattis Dementia Rating Scale (MDRS), motor performance subsets; the Wechsler Adult Intelligence Scale-Revised (WAIS-R); and the Western Aphasia Battery (WAB).

The cognitive deficits that are associated with the mixed dementias remain poorly characterized, primarily due to limited studies and underestimation of the clinical magnitude of this disorder (Roman et al., 1993).

STROKE EPIDEMIOLOGY AND PREVENTION

Vascular Cognitive Impairment in the Spectrum of Cardiovascular Disease

Patients with ischemic cerebrovascular disease or hypertensive intracranial hemorrhage have varying cardiovascular disorders and risk factors that are amenable to primary and secondary prevention measures (Fig. 26-5 and Table 26-6). Rare causes of stroke (hypercoagulable states, vasculitides, CADASIL, etc.), generally occur in younger adults (generally ≤55 years old), as a result of noncardiovascular risk factors.

Addressing cardiovascular and cerebrovascular risk factors is important because patients with clinically symptomatic or silent stroke may develop additional deficits that result in vascular dementia. Such patients are at greater risk for strokes and cardiovascular death (Skoog et al., 1994).

Longitudinal follow-up of asymptomatic patients with isolated vascular risk factors also indicates that these patients develop symptomatic or silent strokes that may contribute to cognitive decline. Older patients with multiple vascular risk factors are more likely to suffer silent strokes revealed on neuroimaging studies, and meet criteria for probable AD, compared with those without such risk factors (Fig. 26-6).

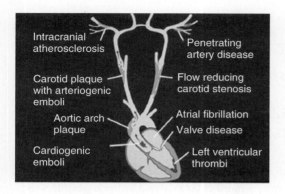

FIGURE 26-5. Summary of the main causes of stroke.

Our current understanding of coronary heart disease exceeds that of stroke, due to the heterogeneity of cerebrovascular disease and complexity of the brain compared with the heart. Guidelines are available for treating coronary risk factors that can be applied to help mitigate the risk of stroke. These include the National Cholesterol Education Program–Adult Treatment Panel (NCEP-ATP III) guidelines (see Fig. 26-6 for a summary of these risk data). A similar scale exists for stroke, derived from the Framingham study cohort risk factor scale. However, the stroke risk stratification scale fails to take into account the influences of lipids and smoking. Additionally, the Framingham risk factor scales show a sampling bias toward white populations and do not consider individual risk factors related to diabetes and family history of premature cardiovascular mortality.

Newly identified demographic factors may help identify individuals at the earliest possible stage of cardiovascular disease, when preventive measures would be most effective. These factors include assays for homocystine, apolipoprotein B-100, lipoprotein A, high-sensitivity C-reactive protein levels, non–high-density lipoprotein (HDL) cholesterol level (in patients with hypertriglyceridemia), small dense low-density lipoprotein (LDL), and clinical criteria for the metabolic syndrome (syndrome X).

The incidence and prevalence of all forms of cardiovascular disease including stroke become more

TABLE 26-6. Stroke Risk Factors

Treatment specifically effective	Treatment of associated factors effective
Established factors	Established factors
Hypertension	Age
Cardiac disease	Sex
Transient ischemic attacks	Familial heredity
Cigarette smoking	Race
Alcohol abuse	Prior strokes
Illicit drug abuse	Diabetes mellitus
Elevated lipids	Factors not well established
Probable risk factors	Migraine and migraine equivalents
Homocystine	Treatment of factors in combination
Factors not well established	Elevated hematocrit
Oral contraceptives	Elevated fibrinogen
Sedentary lifestyle	Sickle cell disease
Obesity	Lupus anticoagulant
Hyperuricemia	Asymptomatic structural lesions (bruits)
Infection	Treatment not possible
	Factors not well established
	Geographic location
	Season and climate
	Socioeconomic factors
	Personality type

(Data from Dyken ML: Stroke risk factors, in Norris JW, Hachinski VC [eds]: Prevention of Stroke. New York: Springer-Verlag, 1991, pp. 83–101, with permission.)

ESTIMATE OF 10-YEAR RISK FOR MEN	ESTIMATE OF 10-YEAR RISK FOR WOMEN

(Framingham point scores)

Men

Age	Points
20–34	−9
35–39	−4
40–44	0
45–49	3
50–54	6
55–59	8
60–64	10
65–69	11
70–74	12
75–79	13

Total cholesterol	Points				
	Age 20–39	Age 40–49	Age 50–59	Age 60–69	Age 70–79
<160	0	0	0	0	0
160–199	4	3	2	1	0
200–239	7	5	3	1	0
240–279	9	6	4	2	1
≥280	11	8	5	3	1

	Points				
	Age 20–39	Age 40–49	Age 50–59	Age 60–69	Age 70–79
Non-smoker	0	0	0	0	0
Smoker	8	5	3	1	1

HDL (mg/dL)	Points
≥60	−1
50–59	0
40–49	1
<40	2

Systolic BP	If untreated	If treated
<120	0	0
120–129	0	1
130–139	1	2
140–159	1	2
≥160	2	3

Point total	10-year risk %
<0	<1
0	1
1	1
2	1
3	1
4	1
5	2
6	2
7	3
8	4
9	5
10	6
11	8
12	10
13	12
14	16
15	20
16	25
≥17	≥30

10-year risk ___%

Women

(Framingham point scores)

Age	Points
20–34	−7
35–39	−3
40–44	0
45–49	3
50–54	6
55–59	8
60–64	10
65–69	12
70–74	14
75–79	16

Total cholesterol	Points				
	Age 20–39	Age 40–49	Age 50–59	Age 60–69	Age 70–79
<160	0	0	0	0	0
160–199	4	3	2	1	1
200–239	8	6	4	2	1
240–279	11	8	5	3	2
≥280	13	10	7	4	2

	Points				
	Age 20–39	Age 40–49	Age 50–59	Age 60–69	Age 70–79
Non-smoker	0	0	0	0	0
Smoker	9	7	4	2	1

HDL (mg/dL)	Points
≥60	−1
50–59	0
40–49	1
<40	2

Systolic BP	If untreated	If treated
<120	0	0
120–129	1	3
130–139	2	4
140–159	3	5
≥160	4	6

Point total	10-year risk %
<9	<1
9	1
10	1
11	1
12	1
13	2
14	2
15	3
16	4
17	5
18	6
19	8
20	11
21	14
22	17
23	22
24	27
≥25	≥30

10-year risk ___%

U.S. DEPARTMENT OF HEALTH AND HUMAN SERVICES
Public Health Service
National Institutes of Health
National Heart, Lung, and Blood Institute

NIH Publication No. 01-3305
May 2001

FIGURE 26-6. Framingham coronary risk assessment scale.

common with aging. This burden of VCI is increasing with the incidence and prevalence of stroke. People in the Western world are living longer, but not necessarily healthier. Stroke is the second leading cause of mortality worldwide and a leading global cause of disability, including dementia. In the Framingham Study, the 10-year probability for stroke in the 65-to-79-year-old group was 11% to 19% for men and 7.2% to 15.5% for women. In the 80-to-84-year-old group, it was 22.3% for men and 23.9% for women. Currently, in North America, 10% to 15% of the population are over 65 years of age. This number is expected to escalate to 20% to 25% by 2025, with the incidence of stroke and attendant vascular dementia escalating at the fastest rate in women, African Americans, and Hispanics.

In the nonwhite and Asian population groups in the United States, the incidence and prevalence of AD and vascular dementia are less clear than in whites, mainly due to inadequate epidemiologic screening and assessment tools. Available psychometric measures have been validated primarily with English language versions, in white samples, and may lack sensitivity and specificity in identifying dementia in other populations. Several other factors, such as culture and education, also influence the sensitivity of such tests. However, the incidence of dementia in all groups should be reduced by the prevention of strokes and the treatment of vascular risk factors. Such findings argue for the development of appropriate instruments for early recognition of VCI in populations that are at greatest risk for cardiovascular disease.

Despite a trend toward lower mortality from cardiovascular disease, there has been a trend towards a higher prevalence of stroke and stroke survivors (Fig. 26-7). In the United States the annual incidence of stroke is about 600,000 cases, with 500,000 new and 100,000 recurrent cases. Stroke killed 167,366 people in 1999, accounting for about 1 out of 14.3 deaths. This makes stroke the third leading cause of death, behind cardiovascular disease and cancer (Arias et al., 2003). Approximately, 7.6% of ischemic and 36% of cerebral hemorrhagic strokes result in death within the first 30 days. The most common stroke subtype is atherothrombosis, accounting for 61% of all strokes. Cerebral embolism is the next major subtype, accounting for 21%. In 1999 there were 4,600,000 stroke survivors (almost equally divided between the sexes), many with disabilities and cognitive impairments. According to the National Heart, Lung, and Blood Institute (NHLBI) Framingham Heart Study, 28% of people who suffer stroke in a given year are under 65 years of age. For people over age 55, the incidence of stroke more than doubles in each successive decade. In most age groups, stroke is more common in men than women (Figs. 26-8 and 26-9). Curiously, this trend reverses in the older age range, the incidence of stroke becoming higher in women. Over the past decade and a half, the incidence of mortality after stroke has been slightly increasing in women but declining in men. Mortality rates from stroke for all ages are also higher for African Americans, who have two to three times the risk of ischemic stroke and are more likely to die from stroke. Racial and ethnic minority population in some age groups have a higher relative risk of stroke death when compared with the white population. In Hispanics, the risk of stroke is about 1.3 times higher at ages 35 to 64 years, but slightly lower at ages 65 to 74 years. The risk is about one half that of non-Hispanic whites at age 75 years and older.

DIAGNOSIS AND TREATMENT

Patients with either silent or symptomatic cerebrovascular disease and vascular risk factors warrant treatment of all modifiable risk factors regardless of whether these risk factors are symptomatic. These patients appear to

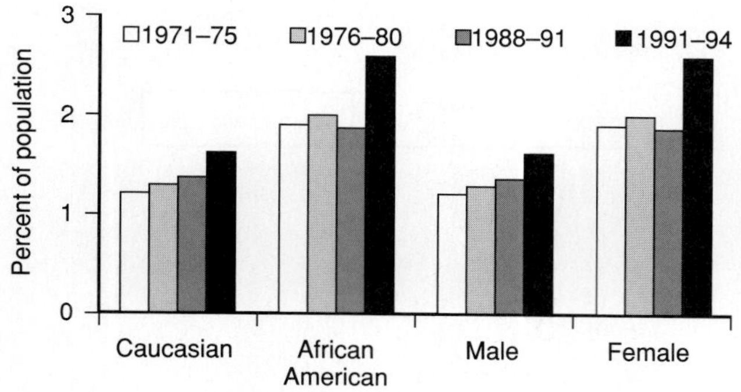

FIGURE 26-7. Stroke prevalence from 1971 through 1994 in Caucasians, African Americans, males, and females.

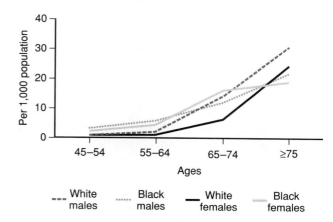

FIGURE 26-8. Annual rate of first and recurrent strokes by age, gender, and race.

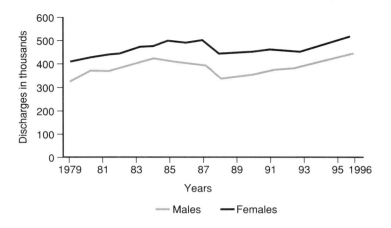

FIGURE 26-9. Hospital discharge of stroke patients by sex.

be at considerable risk for not only stroke but also for VCI (Hachinski, 1994; Bowler & Hachinski, 1995; Devasenapathy et al., 1997; Devasenapathy & Hachinski, 2000).

Regardless of whether vascular risk factors are causal or "casual" in the development of vascular dementia, their treatment remains the only means of preventing "premature senility" from cerebrovascular disease. Although epidemiologic studies show conflicting results for the relative importance of individual vascular risk factors that may contribute to the development of VCI, all studies show that the prevention of stroke(s) (either clinical or "silent") may be the only means of preventing VCI. Other than hemorrhagic strokes from vascular malformations and amyloid angiopathy that have no primary prevention, most ischemic stroke(s) are the result of longstanding, poorly controlled, and/or treated risk factors (Tatemichi et al., 1995). Therefore, it is recommended that aggressive and early treatment of all major risk factors (especially in all individuals older than 50 years) be undertaken in order to prevent or reduce the incidence and severity of VCI.

A rational approach toward the optimal treatment of all patients with nondebilitating strokes should include periodic neuropsychological assessments to determine the individual stroke patient's rehabilitation requirements. Functional MRI (fMRI) may be an important research tool in this regard and may serve as a "physiological" instrument that can assess neuronal plasticity and functional recovery in the brain regions of interest (Reukert et al., 1994; Goldman-Rakic, 1995; see Chapter 7). fMRI techniques may also aid in assessing the beneficial effects of novel pharmacologic agents and rehabilitation techniques that may potentially enhance functional recovery from strokes (Reukert et al., 1994).

Pharmacologic agents may serve as a future adjuvant to standard rehabilitation protocols. Amphetamines have been shown to accentuate learning and improve functional recovery in stroke patients. Synthetic compounds with pharmacologic effects on dopamine receptors similar to the parent drug, with less potential for abuse and tolerance, and currently in development for use in stroke rehabilitation (Hornstein et al., 1996).

Stroke as a "Brain Attack": Use of Tissue Plasminogen Activator (tPA)

The thrombolytic agent tissue plasminogen activator (tPA) was approved by the Federal Drug Administration in June 1996. In December, 1995, results of the NINDS (NIH) tPA trial showed that the administration of tPA within 3 hours of onset of ischemic stroke substantially improved long-term functional outcome compared WITH placebo (Horowitz, 1998). Improvement was evident even when tPA-associated intracerebral hemorrhage was included. The NINDS trial has been the only positive trial of intravenous thrombolytic therapy for acute stroke. A summary of key outcomes for tPA treatment is presented in Figure 26-10. Patients were considered to have a full recovery if they scored 95 or 100 on the Barthel index of activities of daily living such as eating, bathing, walking, and using the toilet. Improvement was defined as a score of 0 to 1 on the Rankin scale (0 = absence of symptoms; 5 = severe disability), meaning the patient recovered to prestroke functions (occupational, social, and personal). An improved patient also had to score 0 or 1 on the NIH stroke scale. These scores allow either a mild facial droop, mild dysarthria, or slight arm drift as the only deficit. TPA is associated with an increased rate of brain hemorrhage (6.4% with tPA vs. 0.6% with placebo within 36 hours). Nevertheless, the highly selected patients given tPA had better neurologic outcomes. Fatal intracranial hemorrhage occurred in 2.9% of tPA-treated patients versus 0.3% of placebo-treated patients. There was no significant difference in death overall between the groups (17% with tPA vs. 21% with placebo).

The benefit of tPA compared with other trials of thrombolytic therapy for acute stroke may be due to

NINDS tPA STUDY KEY OUTCOMES

	tPA	Placebo	Absolute difference
Good outcome			
• Barthel 95–100	50%	38%	12%*
• Rankin 0–1	39%	26%	13%
Death	17%	21%	−4%
Brain hemorrhage	6%	1%	+5%

*12 extra patients/100 given tPA regained normal function.

FIGURE 26-10. National Institute of Neurological Disease and Stroke (NINDS) tissue plasminogen activator (tPA) study outcomes.

several factors: the specific agent (i.e., tPA instead of streptokinase), the dose, and the 3-hour time-to-treatment limit. tPA must be used according to the strict guidelines of the NINDS study in order to limit the incidence of hemorrhage. Although 1 person in 15 receiving tPA suffered serious brain hemorrhage, the overall incidence of neurologic deterioration from all causes during the first 24 hours was similar in both treatment and placebo groups (17.4% in the tPA group vs. 18.3% in the placebo group). This suggests that neurologic deterioration from hemorrhage associated with tPA is counterbalanced in the placebo group by neurologic deterioration from other causes, such as brain edema and progressing ischemia.

Use of tPA is not justified for very mild symptoms of stroke or for rapidly improving symptoms. If nitroprusside or more than two doses of an intravenous antihypertensive agent are required to lower the blood pressure below a systolic blood pressure of 185 or a diastolic blood pressure of 110 mm Hg, the patient is generally not a thrombolytic candidate. Antiplatelet therapy is not an exclusionary criterion. However, any cause of International Normalized Ratio (INR) >1.3 or 1.4, such as liver disease, warfarin, etc. is an exclusionary criterion.

Guidelines for management of acute stroke are outlined in the April 2003 issue of *Continuum* and can be found at the AAN website at URL: http://www.aan.com/publications/continuum/index.cfm.

CONCLUSIONS

Stroke produces a range of cognitive impairments, from focal deficits in specific cognitive domains to dementia. VCI comprises a range of impairments and is potentially preventable. VCI may be prevented and treated by instituting appropriate interventions (against cardiovascular disorders and risk factors) at the asymptomatic "brain-at-risk" stage.

In a minority of cases, acute "brain attacks" can be treated with thrombolytic therapy. There is overlap

between the pathophysiology and clinical symptoms associated with VCI and AD. Vascular risk factors and disorders should be addressed and treated in all patients with dementia.

Research in the basic medical sciences has led to the development of pharmacologic agents that act on ischemia-induced excitotoxic mechanisms that may underlie some forms of VCI. Transitional research aimed at bringing these developments to the clinic is needed and warrants the development of clinical criteria that will aid in the early identification of VCI.

■ KEY POINTS

☐ Cerebrovascular disease is a common cause of cognitive impairment, the second most common cause of dementia after AD, and the third leading cause of death behind cardiovascular disease and cancer.

☐ Vascular cognitive impairment refers to cognitive, behavioral, and emotional deficits that are caused by treatable and preventable cardiovascular and cerebrovascular disease. The deficits can be subtle and progressive with need for early detection, treatment of risk factors, and continued management.

☐ The term *vascular dementia* is considered vague and obsolete and its use is discouraged.

☐ Primary and secondary prevention of coronary artery disease and strokes will likely prevent a substantial number of acquired dementias in the elderly.

KEY READINGS

Hachinski V: Vascular dementia: A radical redefinition. Dementia 5:130–132, 1994.

Devasenapathy A, Hachinski VC: Vascular cognitive impairment. Curr Treat Options Neurol 2:61–72, 2000.

Appelros P, Nydevik I, Seiger A, et al: Predictors of severe stroke: Influence of preexisting dementia and cardiac disorders. Stroke 33:2357–2362, 2002.

REFERENCES

American Psychiatric Association: Diagnostic and Statistical Manual of Mental Disorders, ed. 4. Washington, DC: Author, 1994.

Appelros P, Nydevik I, Seiger A, et al: Predictors of severe stroke: Influence of preexisting dementia and cardiac disorders. Stroke 33:2357–2362, 2002.

Beal M, Flint M: Mechanisms of excitotoxicity in neurological disease. FASEB J 6:3338–3334, 1991.

Bowen DM, Davison AN: Can the pathophysiology of dementia lead to rational therapy?, in Crook T, Bartus R, Ferris S, et al (eds): Treatment Development Strategies for Alzheimer's Disease. Madison, CT: Mark Powley Associates, 1986, pp. 36–66.

Bowler JV, Hachinski V: Vascular cognitive impairment: A new approach to vascular dementia. Baillieres Clin Neurol 4:357–376, 1995.

Brayne, HR: Epidemiology of vascular dementia. Neuroepidemiology 14:240–257, 1995.

Chui HC: Dementia: A review emphasizing clinico-pathological correlations and brain-behavior relationships. Arch Neurol 46:806–814, 1989.

Chui HC, Victoroff JI, Margolin D, et al: Criteria for the diagnosis of ischemic vascular dementia proposed by the State of California Alzheimer's Disease Diagnostic and Treatment Centers. Neurology 42:473–480, 1992.

Damasio H, Damasio A: Lesion Analysis in Neuropsychology. New York: Oxford University Press, 1989.

Damasio AR: Neuropsychology, dementia and aging. Curr Opin Neurol Neurosurg 5:63–64, 1992.

Denburg SD, Carbotte RM, Long AA, et al: Neuropsychological correlates of serum lymphocytotoxic antibodies in systemic lupus erythematosus. Brain Behav Immun 2:222–234, 1988.

Devasenapathy A, Hachinski VC: Vascular cognitive impairment: A new approach in Advances in Old Age Psychiatry. Lechtworth, UK: Wrightson Biomedical Publishing, 1997, pp. 790–795.

Devasenapathy A, Hachinski VC: Vascular cognitive impairment. Curr Treat Options Neurol 2:61–72, 2000.

Djuricic BM, Kostic VS, et al: Prostanoids and ischemic brain edema: Human and animal study. Ann N Y Acad Sci 559:435–437, 1989.

Dyken ML: Stroke risk factors, in Norris JW, Hachinski VC (eds): Prevention of Stroke. New York: Springer-Verlag, 1991, pp. 83–101.

Ebly EM, Parhad IM, Hogan DB, et al: Prevalence and types of dementia in the very old: Results from the Canadian Study of Health and Aging. Neurology 44:1563, 1999.

Ferruci L, Guralnik JM, Salive ME, et al: Cognitive impairment and the risk of stroke in the older population. J Am Geriatr Soc 44, 237–241, 1996.

Ghiso J, Frangione B: Cerebral amyloidosis, amyloid angiopathy, and their relationship to stroke and dementia. J Alzheimer Dis 3:65–73, 2001.

Goldman-Rakic PS: Cellular basis of working memory. Neuron 14:477–485, 1995.

Hachinski VC, Potter P, Merskey H: Leukoariosis: An ancient term for a new problem. Can J Neurol Sci 13 (Suppl. 4):533–534, 1986.

Hachinski V: Preventable senility: A call for action against the vascular dementias. Lancet :340:645–648, 1992.

Hachinski V: Vascular dementia: A radical redefinition. Dementia 5:130–132, 1994.

Henderson VW: Estrogen, cognition and a woman's risk of Alzheimer's disease. Am J Med 103:11S–18S, 1997.

Hennerici MG, Oster M, Cohen S, et al: Are gait disturbances and white matter degeneration early indicators of vascular dementia? Dementia 5:197–202, 1994.

Heyman A, Wilkinson WE, Stafford JA, et al: Alzheimer's disease: A study of epidemiological aspects. Ann Neurol 15:335–341, 1984.

Hornstein A, Lennihan L, Seliger G, et al: Amphetamines in recovery from brain injury. Brain Inj 10:145–148, 1996.

Horowitz SH: Thrombolytic therapy in acute stroke: Neurologists, get off your hands! Arch Neurol 55:155–157, 1998.

Johnson H, Bouman W, Pinner G: Psychiatric aspects of temporal arteritis: A case report and review of the literature. J Geriatr Psychiatry Neurol 10:142–145, 1997.

Kasahara H, Sasahara R: Diagnostic criteria of cerebral vascular dementia: DSM-III-R, ICD-10-JCM, ischemic score and vascular score for differential diagnosis from SDAT. Nippon Rinsho 51(Suppl.):443–451, 1993.

Kertesz A, Clydesdale S: Neuropsychological deficits in vascular dementia vs Alzheimer's disease. Frontal lobe deficits prominent in vascular dementia. Arch Neurol 51:1226–1231, 1994.

Loeb C. Dementia due to lacunar infarctions: A misnomer or a clinical entity? Eur Neurol 35:187–192, 1995.

Margolis MT, Newton TH: Methamphetamine {"speed") arteritis. Neuroradiology 2:179–182, 1971.

Mattioli F, Capra R, Rovaris M, et al: Frequency and patterns of subclinical cognitive impairment in patients with ANCA-associated small vessel vasculitides. Neurol Sci 195:161–166, 2002.

Mcgeer PL, Rojers J: Anti-inflammatory agents as a therapeutic approach for Alzheimer's disease. Neurology 42:447–449, 1992.

Mulnard RA, Cotman CW, Kawas C, et al: Estrogen replacement therapy for treatment of mild to moderate Alzheimer disease. A randomized controlled trial. JAMA 283:1007–1015, 2000.

Munson RJ, Bowler J, et al: The importance of quantification of risk factors for stroke and dementia. Stroke 1:321, 1998.

Myers JS, Xu G, Chowdhury MH, et al: "Is mild cognitive impairment prodromal for vascular dementia like Alzheimer's disease?" Stroke 33:1981–1985, 2002.

Palmer AM, Gershon S: Is the neuronal basis of Alzheimer's disease cholinergic or glutamatergic? FASEB J 4:2745–2752, 1990.

Pantoni L, Garcia JH: The significance of cerebral white matter abnormalities 100 years after Binswanger's report. A review. Stroke 26:1293–1301, 1995.

Pearce JM: Von Monakow and diaschisis. J Neurol Neurosurg Psychiatry 57:197, 1994.

Raiha I, Tarvonen S, Kurki T, et al: Relationship between vascular factors and white matter low attenuation of the brain. Acta Neurol Scand 87:286–289, 1993.

Reukert L, Appollonio I, Grafman J, et al: Magnetic resonance imaging functional activation of prefrontal cortex during covert word production. J Neuroimaging 4:67–70, 1994.

Rizzo M, Tranel D: Overview of head injury and postconcussive syndrome, in Rizzo M, Tranel D (eds): Head Injury and Postconcussive Syndrome. New York: Churchill Livingstone, 1996, pp. 1–18.

Roman GC, Tatemichi TK, Erkinjuntii T, et al: Vascular dementia diagnostic criteria for research studies. Report of the NINDS-AIREN international workshop. Neurology 43:250–260, 1993.

Shaywitz BA, Shaywitz SE: Estrogen and Alzheimer disease. Plausible theory, negative clinical trial [editorial]. JAMA 283:1055–1056, 2000.

Skoog I, Nilsson L, Palmertz B, et al: A population-based study of dementia in 85-year-olds. N Engl J Med 328:153–158, 1993

Skoog I: Risk factors for vascular dementia: A review. Dementia 5:137–144, 1994.

Sulzer DL, Mahler ME, Cunnings JL, et al: Cortical abnormalities associated with subcortical lesions in vascular dementia. Clinical and positron emission tomography findings. Arch Neurol 52:773–780, 1995.

Tatemichi TK, Desmond DW, Mayeux R, et al: Dementia after stroke: Baseline frequency, risks and clinical features in a hospitalized cohort. Neurology 42:1185–1193, 1992.

Tatemichi TK, Desmond DW, Prohovnik I: Strategic infarcts in vascular dementia. A clinical and brain imaging experience. Arzneimittelforschung 45:371–385, 1995.

Tournier-Lasserve E, Joutel A, Melki J, et al: Cerebral autosomal dominant arteriopathy with subcortical infarcts and leukoencephalopathy maps to chromosome 19q12. Nature Genet 3:256–259, 1993.

Willin A, Blenow K: Pathogenetic basis of vascular dementia. Alzheimer Dis Assoc Disord 15:91–102, 1991.

World Health Organization (WHO): The Neurological Adaptation of the International Classification of Disease (ICD-10NA). Geneva: Author, 1991.

Head Trauma and Traumatic Brain Injury

R. D. Jones
Matthew Rizzo

Acceleration-deceleration injury

Anosmia

Anosognosia

Axonal injury

Concussion

Executive dysfunction

Glasgow Coma Scale

Head injury

Postconcussive syndrome

Post-traumatic amnesia (PTA)

Traumatic brain injury (TBI)

OVERVIEW

Traumatic brain injury (TBI) is a major public health problem in terms of financial cost and human suffering (Thurman & Guerrero, 1999; Adekoya et al., 2002; Langlois et al., 2002). Estimates of its incidence and prevalence depend on how TBI is defined (Frankowski et al., 1985; Marshall et al., 1991; see Torner & Schootman, 1996 for an overview). In general, TBI risk is greatest in the late teens and early twenties, most injuries are in the "mild" category, and males outnumber females about two to one (Frankowski et al., 1985). Approximately one half of all TBI occurs in motor vehicle crashes, 20% are the result of falls to the ground (particularly in the young and elderly), and the remainder are attributable to assaults, sports-related injuries, and other causes. Work-related causes may account for approximately 4% to 5% of cases. Approximately 45,000 deaths in the United States are attributed to TBI each year, most occurring before arrival at the hospital. Direct and indirect costs of TBI are measured in the tens of billions of dollars (Torner & Schootman, 1996). This chapter reviews the range of deficits in TBI, associated cognitive sequelae, means of assessment, and management.

SPECTRUM OF THE DISORDER

Head trauma and TBI are not equivalent; unfortunately the terms are sometimes used interchangeably. Although head trauma is the usual antecedent of TBI, it must be distinguished from TBI because head trauma, particularly trauma with limited force, often results in no brain injury. Also, the acute fear that is often associated with a traumatic event (e.g., a car crash or an assault) that leads to head trauma or TBI must be distinguished from post-traumatic stress disorder, an emotional/psychiatric syndrome that may follow extreme threat or psychological stress (American Psychiatric Association, 1994; Bryant, 2001).

TBI is typically classified into two types: open and closed. In open head injury (also known as penetrating head injury) a foreign object penetrates the skull and may damage underlying brain. In closed head injury, which is far more common, there is no penetration of the skull. Deformation of the skull by a blow to the head can transmit destructive energy to the underlying brain and cause a focal contusion (a bruise) without penetrating or fracturing the skull. Another common type of closed head injury is associated with rapid deceleration of the head and continued movement of the brain resulting from inertia. This type of injury is associated with motor vehicle collisions. Direct impact of the brain against the inner surfaces of the skull may result in a brain injury beneath the site of impact, known as a coup injury. Contrecoup injury to the brain may occur opposite the site of impact (e.g., frontal lobe damage after an occipital coup injury), possibly caused by rebound of the brain within the skull or to vacuum effects. In acceleration-deceleration circumstances, inertial forces acting on the brain can produce torque that can shear white matter fibers, often described as axonal injury.

Potential behavioral outcomes of TBI range from complete recovery to permanent coma (see Chapters 30 and 40). Postconcussive syndrome (PCS) lies at the mild end of the spectrum and refers to a range of cognitive and physical complaints following trauma with brief loss of consciousness (LOC) or post-traumatic amnesia (PTA). These complaints may include symptoms of headache, dizziness, memory impairment, concentration and attention deficits, or other cognitive difficulties, insomnia, fatigue, apathy, loss of motivation, visual complaints, anhedonia, depression, pain, dizziness, and personality change. These types of complaints are not specific to PCS, should be interpreted against the complaint base rate in the general population, and are increased in stressful situations such as litigation (Lees-Haley & Brown, 1993). Further, nonneurologic factors may be playing a role in patients whose complaints fail to resolve, because complete recovery following other-wise uncomplicated concussion is usually expected (Ruff et al., 1989; Dikmen et al., 2001; Griffenstein & Baker, 2001; Suhr & Gunstad, 2002). Improvement in acute symptoms and signs is the rule in survivors of moderate and severe TBI, although chronic residua are more likely (as in the case example discussed later).

The severity of the initial injury is often graded using the Glasgow Coma Scale (GCS) score (Teasdale & Jennett, 1974). The GCS is widely used by paramedics and emergency personnel and provides a more reliable index of initial impairment than simple judgments of "conscious" versus "unconscious" (Teasdale et al., 1978). GCS scores range from 3 to 15, and depend on ratings of motor functions, verbal output, and eye opening (Table 27-1). Mild injury is typically characterized by acute GCS scores of 13–15, moderate injury by scores of 8–12, and severe injury by scores of 3–7 (e.g., van der Naalt, 2001). Lower scores are associated with worse coma and higher fatality rates (Teasdale & Jennett, 1974). However, there is heterogeneity among these groups. Rarely, a GCS score of 13–15 may be associated with radiologic evidence of brain injury and abnormal neuropsychological tests scores (Levin et al., 1990; Dikmen et al., 2001). Examples include cases of a focal penetrating brain injury (e.g., caused by a small-caliber bullet or ice pick), or a temporal bone fracture that tears the middle meningeal artery, producing an epidural hematoma with mass effect. Mild head trauma may cause a subdural hematoma with secondary brain damage in an elderly person. In these patients the bridging veins are more susceptible to being torn by torque because they have a longer course to reach an atrophic brain. Note also that the GCS is used only to characterize the initial sequelae of the trauma, and following recovery there may be little or no permanent effects of an injury that was initially characterized as severe. Other factors to consider in evaluating TBI severity include nature of the injury (acceleration-deceleration, blow to the head, whether or not the head was struck), presence of altered consciousness, retrograde amnesia, PTA, duration of time elapsed after injury to resume following commands, initial neurologic findings, initial laboratory findings (neuroimaging, toxicology screens), and seizure (presence/number/proximity to injury).

Other scales besides the GCS may be used to characterize recovery and outcome from TBI. The Rancho Los Amigos Scale (developed by Hagan et al., 1972) is sometimes used to broadly characterize the stages of recovery from TBI. The scale has eight levels, from "no response" to "purposeful and appropriate." Also, the Glasgow Outcome Scale (GOS) (Jennett & Bond, 1975) is a simple rating scale that has been used in research on chronic outcome of TBI and relies on subjective ratings of social and occupational functioning (Table 27-2).

TABLE 27-1. Glasgow Coma Scale

Eye opening	
Spontaneously	4
To verbal command	3
To pain	2
No eye opening	1
Best motor response	
Obeys commands	6
Localizes pain	5
Flexion-withdrawal	4
Decorticate posturing	3
Decerebrate posturing	2
No response	1
Best verbal response	
Oriented, converses	5
Disoriented, converses	4
Verbalizes	3
Vocalizes	2
No response	1
Total (3–15):	

Modified from Teasdale G, Jennett B: Assessment of coma and impaired consciousness. Lancet ii:81–84, 1974.

More detailed tools are needed to investigate the chronic real-world consequences of TBI (van der Naalt, 2001).

CASE REPORT 1

Patient 1 is a 27-year-old right-handed factory employee with 12 years of education who was injured in a motor vehicle crash. He had no significant prior medical, neurologic, or psychiatric problems, and no substance abuse or school difficulties. He sustained multiple skull fractures including frontal, left orbital, and right parietal bones. He was asleep at the time of the injury, which occurred in the late afternoon, and had no recall of that day. Post-traumatic amnesia, based on extensive interview with the patient, was approximately 4 weeks. He was initially ambulatory at the scene, then became obtunded. Pupils were unequal, and he had an oval, nonreactive left pupil, according to acute records. Computed tomography showed right frontal hemorrhage and bilateral occipital hemorrhages. He was intubated and ventilated. A ventricular drain was placed on the day of the injury. In the subsequent several days he showed improvement, and was extubated 10 days after the

TABLE 27-2. Glasgow Outcome Scale

1. Dead
2. Vegetative state
    Unable to interact with environment
    Unresponsive
3. Severe disability
    Able to follow commands/unable to live independently
4. Moderate disability
    Able to live independently/unable to return to work or school
5. Good recovery
    Able to return to work or school

injury. The next day he was characterized as alert and responsive, but with continued memory problems. He was admitted to rehabilitation and noted to be alert but confused and easily agitated. He was fully oriented 3 weeks after his injury and 1 week later was discharged home, in the care of his family. According to family reports he made steady progress in the ensuing months.

Neuropsychological assessment was completed 22 months after the injury. In general, his performances reflected a very strong recovery, particularly given the nature and severity of the initial injury. Specifically, he performed in the average to high average range on tests of verbal and nonverbal intellect. Performances were within broad expectations of normal on tests of memory, orientation, constructional praxis, language, spatial judgment, executive functions, fine motor skills, and cognitive speed. A mild impairment was observed on a test of visual discrimination (Facial Recognition Test), and there was anosmia. There was a mild, relative weakness on selected tests of attention. At the time of the neuropsychological assessment he had returned to work, and by report was doing well in his job.

This case demonstrates excellent recovery from severe initial injury that might have been fatal, and underscores that prediction of recovery can be hazardous when based on early clinical parameters (see Table 27-6).

SEQUELAE OF TRAUMATIC BRAIN INJURY

Cognitive impairments are a core feature of TBI and can impair all manner of daily activities, depending on the patterns of impairment. This section describes effects of TBI on memory, attention and information processing, intellect, language, visuoperceptual and visuoconstructional functions, executive control and personality, and social functioning.

Memory

Memory impairment is one of the most common complaints in TBI (Van Zomeren & Van Denberg, 1985; Levin, 1989; Tate et al., 1991; Arcia & Gualtieri, 1993). Estimates of its prevalence vary depending on factors such as injury severity, preinjury factors (such as prior concussive or other neurologic injury or psychiatric disease), postinjury complications (e.g., seizures), and demographic characteristics (Schacter & Crovits, 1977; Oddy et al., 1985; Ruff et al., 1989). Memory impairments are associated with blunt trauma and acceleration-deceleration injury affecting temporal and frontal lobe regions that are vital to attention, learning, and memory systems (Levin et al., 1988; Eisenberg & Levin, 1989; Levin, 1989; Levin et al., 1990; Hamm et al., 1992; see Chapter 11).

Retrograde amnesia refers to inability to remember events prior to trauma and typically shows a temporal gradient. That is, events nearer to the time of injury are more likely to be forgotten, whereas remote events (e.g., of childhood) are more likely to be retained (Levin et al., 1985; Capruso & Levin, 1992). Retrograde amnesia is typically briefer than post-traumatic amnesia and tends to recede or "shrink" over time. As patients emerge from their initial confusion and disorientation, retrograde events (that are closer in time to the occurrence of the injury) will be recalled (Levin et al., 1985). Of note, inability to recall circumstances before or during a traumatic event may be related to other factors. For example, the person may have been asleep, impaired by drugs or alcohol, distracted by different thoughts or tasks, or simply too excited to realize what was happening.

Following resumption of consciousness there is often post-traumatic amnesia (PTA). Patients with PTA do not make a coherent permanent record of ongoing events, and may seem disoriented and confused (Russell, 1971). The staging of PTA has been debated (see Gronwall, 1989a; Levin et al., 1982), but a prospective study of 84 patients with TBI sufficient to cause disorientation showed that orientation to personal information usually recovered before orientation to place and time (High et al., 1990). Evidence of PTA may be found in medical records (e.g., from paramedics, police, ambulance personnel, and hospital emergency room personnel) that describe a patient who is awake and responsive, but repeating questions or disoriented. By definition, PTA subsides when "continuous" memory returns.

Some research suggests that memory problems can be detected after mild TBI despite no loss of consciousness (Leininger et al., 1990). However, other studies suggest that most patients with mild TBI recover cognitive capacities completely, including memory (Levin et al., 1987b; Ruff et al., 1989). In part, discrepant findings may be due to how "mild" is defined. For example, Dikmen et al. (2001) found that injury patients with GCS scores of 13–15, normal brain computed tomography (CT) scan, inability to follow commands <1 hour, and PTA <24 hours showed no memory impairments relative to controls. This and other studies suggest that most patients with injuries that are characterized as mild in the acute phase can be expected to recover fully from initial problems with memory (see Levin et al., 1989).

In sum, the best available scientific evidence indicates: (1) the likelihood of memory impairment is greater the more severe the TBI; (2) most patients with mild TBI and no other risk factors and complications recover to normal or near-normal levels of memory functioning; and (3) retrograde amnesia following TBI can shrink over time and is usually brief relative to post-traumatic anterograde amnesia.

Executive Functions and Personality

Executive functions (EF) refer to higher-level abilities such as judgment, decision making, social conduct, organizational skills, and planning. Decision-making impairments may reflect failure to respond to changing contingencies, inhibit responses, and appreciate future consequences of actions (Bechara et al., 1994; Rolls et al., 1994; Best et al., 2002). These functions depend in large part on prefrontal cortical areas that are the most susceptible to effects of brain trauma (Benton, 1991; Eslinger et al., 1996). Damage to the orbital surface of the frontal lobes can cause severe impairments of social conduct, rational judgment, and planning (e.g., Eslinger

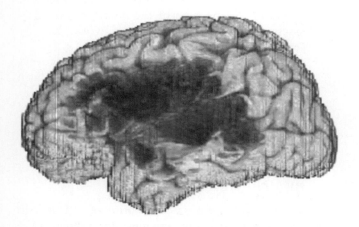

FIGURE 27-1. Three-dimensional MRI reconstruction of the lateral left hemisphere of patient 2. (Courtesy of Dr. Hanna Damasio, University of Iowa, Department of Neurology.)

et al., 1985; Damasio & Anderson, 1993; Damasio, 1994). These patients should be carefully assessed with standardized neuropsychological tests of EFs (Tranel et al., 1994). Clinical assessment is also important because some patients with frontal lobe lesions may perform well on tests of EFs and some patients with lesions outside of the frontal lobes may not (Anderson et al., 1991; Damasio & Anderson, 1993). Patients should be interviewed directly for symptoms of executive impairment. Collateral informants (e.g., a spouse, family members or friends) can provide ancillary information on a patient's social behavior, judgment, and decision making.

Another aspect of executive dysfunction is anosognosia, or deficient self-awareness of impairment (Anderson & Tranel, 1989). Anosognosia poses a challenge to health and safety management because TBI patients who are unaware of their deficits are less likely to take compensatory steps to mitigate their difficulties, are seldom willing to participate in rehabilitation or other key interventions, may fail to take needed medications, and create additional burden for family members and other caregivers. Anosognosia can vary in severity and is associated with anosodiaphoria, the lack of mood-appropriate emotional reaction to acquired deficits, often expressed as indifference to deficits. Severe anosognosics may deny all medical impairments (e.g., orthopedic as well as cognitive). Anosognosia follows a course of recovery similar to other cognitive functions; i.e., most patients recover some awareness of their medical condition and cognitive impairments, although the likelihood of unawareness of defects increases with increased severity of TBI.

Patients with executive dysfunction often develop associated personality changes. Families and patients may report changes in the patient's judgment, organization, initiation, and regulation of behavior, in association with apathy, depression, and irritability. Many of these changes are direct effects of TBI-associated brain damage (e.g., to limbic system and frontal lobe structures that are associated with mood and emotional regulation). These changes can be accompanied by stress associated with a serious medical injury and disability, financial strain, and other factors. Assessment of personality changes is difficult, and each patient's premorbid personality characteristics, social and vocational history, and current stressors must be considered. Also, the effects of TBI must be taken into account in interpreting psychological profiles (Gass, 1991; Gass & Wald, 1997). Some patients (including those with TBI) show modest elevations on clinical scales of the Minnesota Multiphasic Personality Inventory (MMPI) associated with somatizing tendencies. Interpretation of the MMPI and similar clinical instruments should consider this possibility in patients with multitrauma, physical symptoms as in PCS, post-traumatic stress, depression, and adjustment reaction.

Laboratory tests of executive functions (Table 27-3) have shown mixed success in detecting, characterizing, and indicating prognosis and course in recovery from TBI. This is perhaps due to conceptual and methodological limitations in how EF are assessed, as well as the wide range of functions subsumed by this category. For example, measures of "fluency" (e.g., semantic fluency, letter fluency, design fluency) aim to characterize a patient's ability to generate, quickly and strategically, novel and appropriate responses from existing knowledge. Other measures that address perseverative responses (e.g., Wisconsin Card Sorting Test, Benton Visual Retention Test), are designed to inform clinical decisions relevant to the patient's ability to conceptualize and modify response sets. However, a limitation is that these measures may show a relatively high rate of false negative and false positive results if interpreted in isolation. For example, some widely used tests of EFs (e.g., Wisconsin Card Sorting Test, Trailmaking Test) may produce results that fail to validate the expected relation between frontal lobe injury and EF (Anderson et al., 1991). These tests have value in a neuropsychological battery and may aid decisions relevant to management and rehabilitation, but further evidence is needed for how well these tests predict success or failure in activities of daily living and their relationship to behavioral inventories of everyday executive functioning. Newer tests have been developed that may be more sensitive to specific aspects of executive dysfunction (see, e.g., Bechara et al., 1996, 1997).

Attention and Information Processing

Information processing, the ability to synthesize and utilize sequential information on an ongoing basis, depends on perceptual memory and attentional systems (Van Zomeren, 1981; Stuss et al., 1985). Selective defects can be demonstrated with neuropsychological methods (Gentilini et al., 1989; Gronwall, 1989). Attention is a complex topic and can be broken into several subcomponents (see Chapter 10). These include "automatic" processes (Schiffrin & Schneider, 1977) that are "fast" or "effortless," and "controlled" processes that are "slow" and "effortful" (Parasuraman & Davies, 1984). Controlled processes are more vulnerable to TBI and include sustained, divided, and selective attention. Sustained attention (related to vigilance) refers to ability to maintain concentration on a task over a period of time. Divided attention refers to ability to attend to two or more tasks simultaneously. Selective attention refers to ability to focus on a specific target or task amid distracters. Impairments of attention in TBI are more marked for cognitive tasks that require processing of multiple stimuli or tasks. Along these lines, Hugenholtz and colleagues (1988) emphasized the greater degree of "central" processing in divided

Table 27-3. Tests Commonly Used in the Benton Neuropsychological Laboratory

Orientation
  Time
  Personal information
  Place
  Recent presidents
  Recent news events
Intellect/academic achievement
  WAIS-III
    Information
    Digit Span
    Vocabulary
    Arithmetic
    Comprehension
    Similarities
    Letter-Number Sequencing
    Picture Completion
    Picture Arrangement
    Matrix Reasoning
    Object Assembly
    Digit Symbol
  Wide Range Achievement Test
    Reading
    Spelling
    Arithmetic
  National Adult Reading Test—Revised
  Stanford Binet
Memory
  Auditory Verbal Learning Test
    Trials 1–5
    Delayed Recall
    Delayed Recognition
  Complex Figure Test
    Copy
    Recall
  Benton Visual Retention Test
    Copy of Design #E10
    Number Correct
    Number Errors
  Wechsler Memory Scale–III
    Verbal
    Visual
    General
    Attention/Concentration
    Delayed Recall

Warrington Recognition Memory Test
  Words
  Faces
Forced Choice Memory Assessment
Iowa Autobiographical Memory Questionnaire
Iowa Famous Faces
Boston Remote Memory Battery
Attention and concentration
  PASAT
  WAIS-III Digit Span
    Digit Symbol
    Digit Span
    Letter Number Sequencing
  WMS-III
    Mental Control
  Brief Test of Attention
  Visual Search and Attention Test
  Continuous Performance Test
Speech and language
  Fluency
  Paraphasias
  Articulation
  Prosody
  Comprehension
  Writing
    Copy
    Dictation
    Spontaneous
  Gestural praxis
  Multilingual Aphasia Exam (MAE)
    Controlled Oral Word Association (COWA)
    Visual Naming
    Sentence Repetition
    Token Test
    Reading Comprehension of Word and Phrases
    Aural Comprehension of Words and Phrases
    Spelling
      Oral
      Written
  Boston Naming Test
  Boston Diagnostic Aphasia Exam (BDAE)
    Automatized Sequences
    Complex Ideational Material
    Reading Sentences and Paragraphs

TABLE 27-3. Tests Commonly Used in the Benton Neuropsychological Laboratory—cont'd

Boston Diagnostic Aphasia Exam (BDAE) (*Continued*)	Executive functions
Repeating Phrases	Trailmaking Test
High Probability	Wisconsin Card Sorting Test
Low Probability	Design Fluency
Responsive Naming	Booklet Category Test
Verbal Agility	Tower of Hanoi/London
Chapman Speed of Reading	Stroop Test
Action Naming Test	Gambling Test (experimental)
Visual perception/construction/motor	Mood/personality
Facial Recognition Test	Beck Depression Inventory
Judgment of Line Orientation	Beck Anxiety Inventory
Line Cancellation	MMPI
Left	Iowa Rating Scales of Personality Change
Center	Rorschach
Right	Miscellaneous
Hooper VOT	Dementia ratings
Useful Field of View	Right-left discrimination
Starry Night	Self
Drawing	Confrontation
Clock ("20 to 4")	Finger localization
House	Dichotic listening
Bicycle	
3-D Block Construction	
Mirror Tracing Grooved Pegboard Test	

attention tasks, and subtle defects in attention may occur even in mild TBI (see Stuss et al., 1989). Parasuraman et al. (1991) found normal attentional performances in mild TBI on visual "vigilance" testing, but performance worsened when stimuli were degraded (see Chapter 10).

Information processing in TBI has been assessed extensively by the Paced Auditory Serial Addition Test (PASAT) (Gronwall et al., 1977; Gronwall, 1989). In this task the subject is presented auditorily with a series of single digits at different speeds, and is asked to add the first to the second, the second to the third, and so forth. The test can discriminate between mildly brain-injured subjects and normal controls and is a gauge of recovery in mild TBI (Gronwall, 1989). Ponsford and Kinsella (1992) reported that TBI affects speed of processing more than it affects "focused" attention or "sustained" attention, and that the PASAT, Symbol Digit Modality Test, and Stroop Color-Word test discriminate between TBI patients and controls. A variety of additional clinical tests are available for assessing attention in patients with TBI, e.g., WAIS-III subtests such as Digit Span and Letter-Number Sequencing, WMS-III Mental Control,

and the Brief Test of Attention (see Spreen & Strauss, 1998).

Intellect

Intellectual abilities in TBI patients are generally assessed with the Wechsler Adult Intelligence Scale (WAIS) or its later editions (WAIS-R, WAIS-III). This test consists of eleven subscales, including six "Verbal," and five "Performance" subtests, and supplementary subtests are available for the current version (WAIS-III). Resultant summary scores are designated as Verbal IQ (VIQ), Performance IQ (PIQ), and Full Scale IQ (FSIQ). VIQ relates more strongly to well-learned or "crystallized" information (such as fund of information). PIQ is based on nonverbal and generally novel tasks and does not rely as heavily on well-learned skills. Summary IQ scores, while more statistically reliable, reflect a collection of performances on disparate tasks (Lezak, 1988; 1995; Kaplan et al., 1991).

Useful information on specific intellectual abilities from individual subtest scores may be lost by relying on summary scores alone. For example, evidence of a large discrepancy between a Vocabulary subtest performance (generally thought to be resistant to brain damage) and a Digit Symbol subtest score (shown to be sensitive to TBI) may be lost in a FSIQ score that reflects "average" overall performance. However, in general, lower summary IQ scores on the WAIS and later versions of the test appear to correlate with more severe TBI. (Mandelberg & Brooks, 1975; Barth et al., 1983; Tabaddor et al., 1984; Dikmen et al., 1986a; Mayes et al., 1989). Compared to controls, subjects with mild TBI show little if any impairments on formal tests of intellect (e.g., Drudge et al., 1984), whereas more severely injured patients show clear defects, both acutely and chronically (Mandelberg & Brooks, 1975; Tabaddor et al., 1984; Mayes et al., 1989).

Intellectual functions improve over time after TBI, from the acute stages following trauma to the chronic epoch (Jones et al., 1996). For example, Mandleberg and Brooks (1975) studied 40 men with TBI of varying severity, defined by the duration of PTA. Initial scores on most subscale tests of the WAIS were below those of a control group; however, there was no significant difference in VIQ between the groups after 10 months. Performance subscale scores of the TBI group showed slower improvement, and did not approach those of the control group until a 3-year follow-up assessment. In short, initial scores on the Verbal tests were not as low as scores on the Performance tests, and improved to normal levels more quickly. This pattern may reflect the relative novelty of Performance subscale tasks, which are generally more sensitive to brain dysfunction than Verbal subscale tasks (Mayes et al., 1989; Lezak, 1995; Jones et al., 1992).

In sum, patients with TBI show intellectual deficits that generally correlate with the severity of the trauma. Assessment of overall intellectual functioning is of interest, but understanding of specific cognitive abilities relies on analyses of performances on specific subscales.

Language

Language complaints are relatively common in patients with TBI sufficient to cause at least 10 to 15 minutes loss of consciousness (Sarno, 1980). However, it is relatively rare to acquire a "pure" language disorder or aphasia following TBI because the neural substrates of language are seldom injured selectively (but see Case Report 2 following).

The most prevalent language-related complaints following TBI are impairments in word finding or retrieval (Heilman et al., 1971; Levin et al., 1976, 1981). Such impairments may not be immediately evident in conversational speech but may be detected on standardized tests such as in the Boston Diagnostic Aphasia Battery or the Multilingual Aphasia Examination. These language deficits may reflect the

susceptibility to injury to the temporal poles. The left temporal pole is outside perisylvian language-related areas of the brain, but may be crucial for naming of unique entities (Grabowski et al., 2001). Because TBI patients may have impairments in language comprehension, these abilities should be assessed in detail with standardized neuropsychological tests. This assessment is especially critical when there is a question of a patient's ability to understand information relevant to informed consent, decision making, and planning germane to his or her medical treatment, legal affairs, and living arrangements (see Chapter 52).

In patients with aphasia after TBI, fluent aphasias are more common than nonfluent aphasias (Heilman et al., 1971; Basso & Scarpa, 1990). Global aphasia is rare and usually transient, and is associated with severe generalized cognitive defects and with older age at the time of trauma (Luria, 1970; Sarno, 1980; Levin et al., 1981). Even when most aspects of language are well preserved, TBI patients may have significant impairments in discourse and pragmatic use of language, such as understanding indirect requests or hints (McDonald & van Sommers, 1993).

Recovery of language abilities tends to be strong following TBI, and often exceeds recovery of other cognitive abilities (Levin et al., 1990). This may reflect the fact that language is a highly practiced skill mediated by structures not typically damaged in TBI. More detailed aspects of aphasia and associated language impairments can be found in Chapter 17.

CASE REPORT 2

Patient 2 is a 39-year-old former sales manager with a high school education who suffered loss of consciousness in a multivehicle collision. Acute CT scan of the brain showed a depressed left temporal skull fracture and epidural and subdural hematomas that were evacuated via left frontotemporal craniotomy. He was supported on a ventilator with drug-induced coma, hyperventilation, and antiedema agents for 11 days.

As he awakened it became clear that he had severe expressive and receptive language difficulties associated with right-sided weakness. Following discharge from acute care, he spent 2 months at a rehabilitation hospital where he was noted to make a "remarkable recovery." Nevertheless, he was unable to continue his job, because of language difficulties and behavior changes. He divorced his wife and moved into a supervised living situation. Because of continued chronic difficulties, he moved back in with his parents. By 1 year after the injury, he could cook simple meals for himself, but reportedly had defects in attention as well as language. He took no medicine, but subsequently had a grand mal seizure that was treated with phenytoin. Speech therapy screening from 1 and 2 years after the injury showed a nonfluent, Broca-type aphasia ("speech apraxia") with relative preservation of comprehension and nonverbal abilities. Results on the Western Aphasia Battery 3 years after the injury suggested stable performances compared with prior assessments 1 and 2 years after the injury, consistent with continued aphasia. He could read at the ninth-grade level, given adequate time.

Five years after the TBI, the patient moved near our facility and sought consultation in our clinic for language and social deficits. His seizures were well controlled on phenytoin. He reported depression that was being managed with a serotonin reuptake inhibitor.

On neurologic exam Patient 2 was alert and oriented, and in no acute distress. He had a marked aphasia and reading difficulties, and buccofacial apraxia was noted. He had minimal right hemiparesis and showed relatively normal gait, balance, and rapid alternating movements. He denied anosmia. The neurologist felt that the principal finding on the examination was the patient's aphasia, and that post-traumatic seizures were adequately controlled. Neuropsychological testing was recommended to assess the patient's level of cognitive functioning in anticipation of cognitive therapy to address activities of daily living.

The results of neuropsychological testing are shown in Table 27-7. Patient 2 showed a profound residual aphasia, most closely resembling a severe Broca type. His reading and aural comprehension were spared relative to range of expression, although comprehension was not entirely spared. Formal testing disclosed defects of language, including associative fluency, repetition, comprehension of grammatically complex materials, and reading. Visuoperceptual abilities, motor coordination, speed of information-processing, and rapid cognitive shifting, and most nonverbal intellectual skills were normal. Neuroimaging showed a large left hemisphere perisylvian lesion that included frontal, temporal, and parietal cortices. There was no evidence of white matter shearing. Figure 27-1 is a three-dimensional reconstruction of the magnetic resonance imaging (MRI) scan that shows the extent of the lesion on the lateral surface of the left hemisphere.

The patient had previously undergone extensive speech therapy, but had never participated in neuropsychological rehabilitation. With this in mind, the patient was referred for consultation with a cognitive rehabilitation specialist, with the aim of addressing means by which he could deal with the practical implications of his profound aphasia.

This case is a demonstration of a focal language deficit with TBI. Striking is the lack of nonlinguistic defects and preservation of awareness despite severe TBI. While the patient had marked difficulties with emotional, social, and occupational adjustment, his awareness of impairment permitted him to participate in rehabilitation programs and to recover a measure of self-esteem and independence. Despite his severe injury he was not anosmic, and he was not incapacitated by headaches, diplopia, or vertigo. At the time of our last contact with him, he had assumed independent living arrangements in the same town as his parents. He was continuing to participate in outpatient neuropsychological rehabilitation, received supplemental security income (SSI), and performed supervised work for wages on a farm. He was able to resume shopping, handling money, and paying bills. Although he had a seizure as a result of his TBI, this was successfully managed with phenytoin. He resumed automobile driving and has had no moving violations or subsequent crashes (Fig. 27-1).

Visual Functions

TBI can damage virtually all components of the visual system (Mishra & Digre, 1996). Impaired vision is among the most commonly reported long-term symptoms of TBI (Carlsson et al., 1987), and visual dysfunction may affect 50% or more of patients with severe TBI (Gianutsos et al., 1988; Schlageter et al., 1993). These impairments are usually at early anatomic or peripheral levels of the visual system (e.g., optic neuropathy, ocular motor palsy), but there can also be damage to cerebral areas that process vision (see Chapter 12).

The occipital lobes and adjacent temporal and parietal areas, which contain primary and secondary visual cortices, can be damaged by direct trauma to the occiput, or indirectly from a contrecoup injury. Damage to primary visual cortex and optic radiations in the occipital lobes produces a variety of visual field defects. Alexia, visual agnosia, prosopagnosia, and achromatopsia may result with occipitotemporal lesions, and components of Balint syndrome with occipitoparietal lesions. The attention problems in TBI (noted earlier) include impairments of visual attention (Parasuraman et al., 1991; Heinze et al., 1992).

A neuro-ophthalmological evaluation may need to be performed on TBI patients with visual difficulties (see Chapter 12). Furthermore, visual acuity should be tested in the neuropsychology clinic, given the detrimental effect of visual impairment on neuropsychological test performance (Kempen et al., 1994; Mishra & Digre, 1996).

There has been limited investigation of recovery and rehabilitation of higher-order visuoperceptual defects following TBI, although some studies have indicated generally good recovery (Levin et al., 1977, 1990). Models for rehabilitation of visuoperceptual impairments in brain-injured individuals are being actively explored (Anderson, 2002).

Social and Emotional Outcome

Social and emotional deficits have been described as a "subtle and yet most handicapping" feature of TBI (Lezak, 1989), and are, perhaps, the most underappreciated aspect of TBI. TBI can impair family life, marriage, social activity and competency, and vocational outcome (Dikmen et al., 1986a, 1986b; see Chapter 50). Spouses of TBI patients are at greater risk of emotional and marital problems (Peters et al., 1990; 1992; O'Carroll et al., 1991; Kreutzer et al., 1992), which may underlie the reported increased likelihood of divorce (Panting & Merry, 1972; Thomsen, 1984; Kreutzer et al., 1992) and sexual dissatisfaction or dysfunction after brain injury (O'Carrol et al., 1991; see Chapter 32). Marital discord is often accompanied by decline in numbers of friends, visits with friends, involvement in social groups, and stability of ongoing relationships (Oddy et al., 1985; for review see Dikmen, 1986b). Social interaction style and social relationships are more likely to be impaired in severe TBI. Additional research is needed on social and emotional outcome in mild TBI that controls for effects of injuries to other systems (e.g., orthopedic) (Dikmen et al., 1986a). Intervention approaches for rehabilitation of social deficits associated with TBI are described in Grattan and Ghahramanlou (2002).

Depression and other disorders of emotion are common in TBI, particularly in moderate and severe cases in which frontal and limbic cortices are damaged. Emotional disruption that increases over time may occur as the consequences of an injury sink in and a patient begins to recognize and react to personal limitations and lifestyle changes that have resulted from the injury. Also, a number of stressors associated with TBI may contribute to depression, such as litigation, unemployment, marital discord, and medication side effects.

Return to Work and Sports

Return to work is a critical measure of outcome, given the costs of disability and lost income following TBI. Current research is aimed at addressing specific predictors of return to work, which includes demographic factors, neurologic status, and domain of cognitive impairments (see Chapter 50).

Younger patients (Crepeau & Scherzer, 1993; Dikmen et al., 1994) and skilled workers with longer work histories (Brooks et al., 1987; Dikmen et al., 1994) are more likely to resume employment after TBI. Gender has not been a reliable predictor of return to work following TBI (Crepeau & Scherzer, 1993). Patients are less likely to return to work if there is severe TBI (measured by GCS score, duration of PTA, or length of hospitalization) (Fraser et al., 1988; Rao et al., 1990) or radiologic evidence of brain abnormality (e.g., contusion, hematoma) (Eide & Tysnes, 1992).

Notwithstanding methodologic limitations of current research, neuropsychological assessment may be helpful in predicting return to work (Sherer et al., 2002). In a meta-analysis of variables predictive of return to work, Crepeau and Scherzer (1993) indicated that performances on tests of EFs, as well as emotional health, are important factors in post-trauma employment status. Memory, attention, visuospatial impairments, and language defects also influence return to work (Brooks et al., 1987; Fraser, et al., 1988; Schwab et al., 1993). Schwab and colleagues (1993) and Dikmen and colleagues (1994) performed two large-scale studies (n = 520 and 366 patients, respectively) that used multivariate models predicting return to work. The study by Schwab and colleagues (1993) provided a means to calculate a "disability score" based on seven neurologic, neuropsychological, and social/emotional variables. The model of Dikmen and colleagues (1994) used a number of weighted variables (e.g., GCS score, preinjury job stability, injury to other systems such as orthopedic injuries, and neuropsychological performance on the Halstead-Reitan Neuropsychological Battery). The advantage of such models is the potential to accurately advise patients, families, employers, and insurance companies about expected work status following recovery. Accurate predictions can help all concerned parties to prepare emotionally and financially for altered living arrangements (Dikmen et al., 1994).

Effective planning for return to work must consider work-related stress, employee safety, productivity demands, and decision-making burden. These considerations are aided, when possible, by employer allowance such as a part-time schedule or modified duty, and by vocational rehabilitation and training. Effective planning will not only optimize the transition back to the workplace, but will also improve the general well-being and self-esteem of the TBI patient.

Return to sports activity following TBI is being actively investigated, and some consistent findings have emerged from this literature. First, there appears to be a relationship between performance on neuropsychological measures and the number of traumas to the head, even in the absence of loss of consciousness (Matser et al., 2001). Also, there are findings to suggest that a second mild TBI occurring shortly after an initial mild TBI may have significant deleterious effects. Thus, if a concussion is experienced, return to sports should be delayed for some period after recovery of normal mental status, rather than immediately after resumption of normal mental status. The basis of reports of so-called "second impact syndrome" is a topic of active research (McCrory & Berkovic, 1998). Practitioners should follow established guidelines (e.g., those established by the Quality Standards Subcommittee of the American Academy of Neurology, 1997).

METHODS OF ASSESSMENT OF TRAUMATIC BRAIN INJURY

Neurologic Assessment

There are multiple means to assess consequences of TBI. Here, we consider neurologic assessment, neuropsychological assessment, and neuroimaging, although other means of assessment are also appropriate in given cases (e.g., electrophysiological studies).

Management of severe head injury is covered in neurosurgery and acute care neurology texts (e.g., Ropper, 1993). There is a need to assess and maintain airway, breathing, and circulation, and treatment of potential metabolic disturbances must be addressed (Table 27-4). Features of the acute examination include testing for cerebrospinal fluid leaks and for Battle's sign and raccoon eyes (discoloration behind the ears and around the eyes, respectively, caused by blood seepage from a basilar skull fracture). Patients with signs of increased intracranial pressure or focal neurologic signs receive an emergent CT scan (without contrast). Patients with GCS score of 13 or less at the scene of the injury should also receive a CT scan, even if they have recovered by the time they arrive in an emergency treatment setting. Guidelines for performing CT in milder cases (GCS >13) are unclear, particularly in children because of concerns of exposure of growing brains to unnecessary radiation. We recommend obtaining a CT whenever there is suspicion of brain injury. It is better to err on the side of safety. If the CT is negative and axonal injury is suspected, a nonemergent brain MRI can be helpful (Levin et al., 1987a).

Physical Examination

The neurologic examination is a cornerstone in the evaluation of patients with continuing complaints and takes a head-to-toe approach as described in several excellent reviews (e.g., Gilman, 2000; Van Allen & Rodnitzky, 1988; Haerer, 1992). The first cranial (olfactory) nerve may be sheared as it passes through the cribriform plate

TABLE 27-4. Medical Management of Acute Traumatic Brain Injury

Assess and maintain airway, breathing, and circulation
Administer
Oxygen
Thiamine 100 mg IV for potential Wernicke-Korsakoff syndrome
D50 1 ampule IV for potential hypoglycemia
Naloxone 0.4–2 mg IV or flumazenil 0.2 mg IV to reverse opiate intoxication
Draw blood
To assess sodium, potassium, calcium, phosphate, glucose, SGPT, SGOT, ammonia
For toxicology screen (blood and urine)
Assess for and treat increased intracranial pressure
Hyperventilate to pCO$_2$ of 25–30 mm Hg
Administer mannitol 0.5–1 gram per kg IV
Consider furosemide 20 mg IV
Perform CT scan

CT, computed tomography; IV, intravenously; SGPT, serum glutamate pyruvate transaminase; SGOT, serum glutamic oxalo-acetic transaminase.

of the ethmoid bone. Olfaction may also be disturbed by damage to the olfactory cortex at the base of the frontal lobe (see Chapter 15). Patients who have trouble identifying aromatic compounds (such as clove oil) can be tested in detail on a standardized smell identification task. However, olfactory defects may also be related to smoking, congestion, age, medications, sinus disease, or even a deviated septum. Complete anosmia is uncommon and is not expected in mild head injury.

Motor examination should include testing of muscle strength, tone, station and gait, and functional maneuvers such as toe, heel, and tandem walking, and hopping on each foot. Coordination can be assessed by finger-on-thumb tapping, rapid alternating pronation and supination of the hand, pointing movements between the examiner's finger and the patient's nose, and heel-to-knee-to-shin testing. Tendon reflexes and the presence of pathologic reflexes (Babinski, Glabellar, snout, root, suck) should be assessed as usual. The sensory examination requires the patient to detect, discriminate, identify, and report on different sensory stimuli (e.g., sharp, dull, vibration, joint position; see Chapter 14). The examination is susceptible to error in patients without optimal cooperation.

A general medical examination will help identify any treatable systemic factors (see Chapter 28) that could be causing chronic malaise and help guide referrals to other specialists. Auscultation of carotid bruits may suggest ischemic headache (see Chapter 26) and help explain complaints of "spells" (see Chapters 8 and 45). A high blood pressure reading may suggest hypertensive headache. The assessment of chronic headache should also check for dental caries, tenderness over the frontal and maxillary sinus areas, restricted range of motion or point tenderness of the neck, and reduced visual acuity. Pupillary, ocular motility, and visual field defects can be screened using a flashlight, a Snellen card or magazine, and an ophthalmoscope (see Chapter 12). The Dix-Hallpike maneuver can be used to screen for a neuro-otological disturbance (see Chapter 16).

The mental status screening assessment is essential in the neurologic assessment of the brain-injured patient and should address disturbances of perception, attention, language, memory, decision making and implementation, mood, and self-awareness. The examiner can make useful observations throughout the interview and examination, and even in waiting areas. Mental status screening can include a variety of tests such as the Mini Mental Status Examination (MMSE) (see Chapter 1). The findings may help direct a referral for a detailed neuropsychological assessment (see below).

A patient's complaints may sometimes defy expected physiology and suggest a patient's symptoms are not due to TBI or are exacerbating the effects of TBI (Table 27-5). In such cases, alternative diagnostic possibilities include psychological or psychiatric conditions such as somatoform, conversion, post-traumatic stress,

personality, and adjustment disorders, and malingering. Also, a patient with suspected TBI may instead have an unrelated neurologic condition (e.g., primary progressive dementia, multiple sclerosis, or cerebrovascular disease).

Neuropsychological Assessment

Neuropsychological assessment aims to characterize the cognitive, emotional, and behavioral sequelae of TBI. Neuropsychological consequences of TBI are often the most distressing and salient features of the syndrome, and in the case of mild injury may be the only evidence of brain dysfunction (i.e., when other procedures such as the neurologic examination, electroencephalography [EEG], or neuroimaging are negative). In severe TBI, neuropsychological assessment may not be needed to establish the diagnosis, but can guide rehabilitation and management decisions (e.g., determine placement needs, establish guardianship). Neuropsychological results are sensitive to depression, fatigue, drugs, chronic pain, and other factors, and require expert interpretation.

A core feature of clinical neuropsychological assessment is the administration of standardized, objective neuropsychological tests. Such tests directly assess memory, attention, decision making, language, higher-order visual functions, and other abilities that may be compromised by TBI. Most neuropsychologists use tests

TABLE 27-5. Unexpected Complaints after Traumatic Brain Injury

"Anosmia" with insensitivity to trigeminal irritants such as ammonia

Astasia-abasia, in which a person presents an unsteady gait yet demonstrates good balance by not falling

Failure to provide direct answers to questions

Forgetting one's own name

Ganser's syndrome, in which the patient is always slightly off, e.g., one off on counting fingers

Hemianesthesia, splitting the body midline

Hoover's (heel) sign in which the patient shows good strength in a "paralyzed" leg by planting its heel firmly against the examiner's underlying palm in lifting the good leg off the examining table

La belle indifférence, or an apparent uncaring attitude toward one's own disabilities

Report of diffuse pain, e.g., moaning to slight touch of the skin without specific localization

Lack of effort on strength testing, e.g., breakaway weakness

MMSE scores in the range of severe dementia in a person with a history of mild trauma

Monocular polyopia, unexplained by abnormalities of the eye

Nonepileptic seizure activity

Selective memory, e.g., dense amnesia with convenient islands of recall

Retrograde amnesia without anterograde amnesia

Tunnel vision that defies the laws of optics, i.e., objects not seen close-up remain unseen no matter how far away they are removed

Variable findings, e.g., the patient walks easily into the waiting room, but seems unable to walk on direct examination

MMSE, Mini-Mental State Examination.

TABLE 27-6. Case 1: 27-Year-Old Right-Handed (+100) Male Factory Worker with 12 Years of Education; TBI Suffered during Motor Vehicle Crash, Neuropsychological Evaluation Completed 22 Months after Injury

Orientation		
Date and time	Normal	
Place	Normal	
Personal information	Normal	

Intellect	*Scaled scores (SS)*	*Interpretation*
WAIS-III		
Vocabulary	11	63rd percentile = Average
Similarities	12	75th percentile = High average
Arithmetic	15	95th percentile = Superior
Digit Span	08	25th percentile = Average
Information	10	50th percentile = Average
Comprehension	14	91st percentile = Superior
Letter-Number Sequencing	09	37th percentile = Average
Picture Completion	11	63rd percentile = Average
Digit Symbol-Coding	11	63rd percentile = Average
Block Design	15	95th percentile = Superior
Matrix Reasoning	13	84th percentile = High average
Picture Arrangement	10	50th percentile = Average
VIQ	110	75th percentile = High average
PIQ	113	81st percentile = High average
FSIQ	112	79th percentile = High average
VCI	105	63rd percentile = Average
POI	118	88th percentile = High average
WMI	104	61st percentile = Average

Memory		
Rey AVLT		
Learning Trials	5-10-12-14-15	
30-Minute Delay Recall	14	
30-Minute Recognition Hits	15/15	
30-Minute Recognition False Positives	0/15	
Rey-Osterrieth Complex Figure Test		
Copy Score	31/36	
30-Minute Delay Recall	24.5/36	
Benton VRT		
No. of Correct	10	
No. of Errors	0	

Speech and language		
Clinician's description	"Fluent, prosodic, well-articulated speech, with no evidence of word-finding problems, paraphasic errors, or comprehension defect."	
COWA corrected raw score	35+3 (56th percentile = Average)	
Boston Naming Test raw score	53 (within normal limits)	

Continued

TABLE 27-6. Case 1: 27-Year-Old Right-Handed (+100) Male Factory Worker with 12 Years of Education; TBI Suffered During MVA, Neuropsychological Evaluation Completed 22 Months After-Injury—cont'd

Test	Score/interpretation
Visual perception/construction	
Benton Facial Discrimination Test corrected raw score	39 + 0 (8th percentile = Mild impairment)
Benton Judgment of Line Test corrected raw score	28 + 0 (74th percentile = High normal)
Motor and olfaction	
Grooved Pegboard Test	
Dominant Hand	65″ (SS = 10; t = 47)
Nondominant Hand	67″ (SS = 10; t = 46)
Smell ID Test (10-item screen)	
5/10 ("defective")	
Executive function	
Trailmaking Test	
Trails-A	21″ (Ssa = 12; t = 55)
Trails-B	46″ (Ssa = 13; t = 61)
Wisconsin Card Sorting Test	
No. of errors	08 (95th percentile)
No. of correct	62
No. of perseverative errors	04 (>99th percentile)
No. of categories completed	06 (>16th percentile)
Mood/personality	
BDI-II	17 (10–18 = mild–moderate)
BAI	0 (0–9 = none–minimal)
MMPI-2	

that are reliable and valid and relevant to the clinical question. However, there are differing approaches to the neuropsychological examination. (See Jones & Butters, 1983; Golden et al., 1985; Milberg et al., 1996; Reitan & Wolfson, 1996; Tranel, 1996, for more detailed information regarding major schools of neuropsychological assessment.)

Neuropsychologists may use "fixed" or "flexible" test batteries. In the fixed battery approach, test selection does not vary, as in the Halstead-Reitan Neuropsychological Battery (Reitan & Wolfson, 1996). Flexible test batteries are specifically tailored for each patient and depend on the patient's condition, the referral question, and the examination findings, and may vary from case to case.

There are advantages and disadvantages to each approach. For example, because the fixed battery approach typically employs a comprehensive set of measures, impairments that might not have been expected are less likely to be overlooked. However, fixed batteries are often quite long, and may be inefficient if unnecessary tests are administered. A flexible battery usually offers brevity, but may sacrifice comprehensiveness, so that impairments may be missed that would have been detected with a fixed set of tests (see Chapter 2).

The Iowa-Benton approach takes advantages of both fixed and flexible batteries (Tranel, 1996; Jones, 1996). A small, core battery is administered, and the remaining examination is guided by referral questions, patient complaints and condition, the underlying disease or condition, and results of the core battery and other tests (e.g., neuroimaging). In a severely brain-injured patient the assessment can proceed rapidly, taking as little as 30–45 minutes. A large set of tests is available (see Table 27-3) to assess complex cases (e.g., in which legal questions arise). Such comprehensive assessment may take six hours or more (see Chapter 2).

Most neuropsychological measures rely on empirical normative data from individuals with no known neurologic condition or cognitive impairments (Spreen & Strauss, 1998), and are interpreted in the context of known statistical and psychometric properties such as reliability (test-retest, inter-rater, internal consistency) and validity (face, construct, predictive, concurrent). Performances on specific tests are adjusted for age,

TABLE 27-7. Case 2: 39-Year-Old Former Sales Manager who Suffered Loss of Consciousness in a Multivehicle Crash

Intellect and academic achievement test	Score	Interpretation
Wechsler Adult Intelligence Scale—III (scaled scores)		
Performance IQ	91	Average
Picture Completion	9	Average
Digit Symbol-Coding	6	Low average
Block Design	9	High average
Matrix Reasoning	11	Average
Picture Arrangement	9	Average
Wide Range Achievement Test—III (standard scores)		
Reading	45	Defective
Arithmetic	81	Low average

Nonverbal anterograde memory test (raw scores)		
Complex Figure 30' recall (#/36)	18	Normal
BVRT (correct/errors)	8/3	Normal

Speech and language test		
Multilingual Aphasia Examination (percentiles)		
Controlled Oral Word Association	<1st percentile	Defective
Visual Naming	<1st percentile	Defective
Sentence Repetition	<1st percentile	Defective
Token Test	<1st percentile	Defective
Aural Comprehension	20th percentile	Low normal
Reading Comprehension	59th percentile	Normal
Boston Diagnostic Aphasia Examination (raw scores)		
Automatized Sequences (#/8)	1	Defective
Responsive Naming (#/30)	7	Defective
Reading Sentences and Paragraphs (#/10)	10	Normal
Boston Naming (#/60)	3	Defective
Iowa-Chapman Speed of Reading (#/25)	3	Defective

Visual perception/construction test		
Facial Discrimination	15th percentile	Low normal
Judgment of Line Orientation	74th percentile	High normal
Hooper Visual Organization Test	$t = 46$	Normal
Complex Figure Copy (#/36)	34	Normal

Executive function/motor test		
Wisconsin Card Sorting Test		
Categories completed	1	Defective
Perseverative errors	37	Defective
Trailmaking Test A	37″ ($t = 35$)	Low average
Trailmaking Test B	113″ ($t = 31$)	Borderline
Grooved Pegboard—right hand	75″ ($t = 35$)	Low average
Grooved Pegboard—left hand	84″ ($t = 35$)	Low average

education, and other relevant demographic factors that bear on performance, and a given patient's scores are compared with the normative data. In patients with TBI, assessments typically include measures of orientation, intellect, attention, memory, higher visual functions, nonverbal skills and praxis, executive functions, personality and mood, and motor skills.

Neuropsychological test scores must be interpreted in the context of the patient's history, and in the case of TBI, the facts of the incident or trauma. For example, poor memory test scores in a patient who was in coma for 1 month are likely caused by trauma. But the same poor memory performances in an elderly patient with no loss of consciousness, no amnesia, acute GCS of 15, normal neuroimaging, and a history of slowly progressive premorbid memory decline, is more likely to indicate a primary progressive dementia than TBI.

In short, the diagnosis of TBI-related cognitive defects must consider the relationship between the facts of the trauma, neuropsychological and other test results, and the patient's history. If suboptimal effort or malingering is suspected, tests aimed at assessing these possibilities may be administered (e.g., Portland Digit Recognition Test or other two-alternative forced choice test, the Symptom Validity Test).

Neuroimaging

Neuroimaging is a valuable tool that is routinely used in diagnosis and management of TBI and can show contusions, intraparenchymal hemorrhage, subdural and epidural hematomas, ischemic infarcts, cerebral edema, white matter lesions associated with axonal injury, and herniation from increased intracranial pressure.

The main structural imaging techniques used currently are CT and MRI. CT is often used acutely, given its widespread availability and sensitivity to detect hematomas. Images can be acquired in as little as 15–20 minutes, and cost is relatively low. It is reasonable to use CT acutely, even in mild head injury cases (GCS 13–15), to help address any questions of brain lesion or the development of hematoma (Miller et al., 1990; Borczuk, 1995; Haydel et al., 2000; Dikmen et al., 2001; McAllister et al., 2001). MRI should be considered particularly in cases of patients who have normal CT scans, but continued clinical complaints that are suggestive of brain damage, or whose initial clinical picture suggested significant trauma. MRI is more sensitive than CT in detecting axonal injury. However, it is important not to confuse nonspecific white matter changes, microvascular disease, or normal perivascular anatomy (Virchow-Robin spaces) with axonal injury.

There are few consistent data on validity and reliability of functional imaging techniques in clinical cases of TBI. The main techniques in use, positron emission tomography (PET) and functional MRI (fMRI), have as yet been applied in single cases or small group studies (Herscovitch, 1996; McAllister et al., 2001). PET is relatively cumbersome, expensive, time-consuming, and invasive and requires generation and administration of radioisotopes (see Chapter 6). fMRI and related techniques hold promise as a clinical tool, but further experimental investigation is needed, and clinical results should be interpreted cautiously (see Chapter 7).

INTERVENTIONS AND MANAGEMENT

Intervention and rehabilitation approaches to patients with cognitive impairments resulting from brain lesions can be referenced in section VI and are applicable to patients with TBI. In general, patients with TBI benefit from multidisciplinary approaches to treatment including neuropsychological rehabilitation, psychological counseling, and medical/pharmacologic intervention (Eslinger, 2002). In more complicated case, such as those with multisystem trauma, consultation with services such as pain management, physical therapy, occupational therapy, and other services may be valuable. Patients with TBI are often treated with medications, as indicated, for conditions such as pain or depression. Treatment of cognitive complaints and motivational or emotional symptoms is less clear-cut. Single cases and small series of TBI cases have provided preliminary and inconclusive evidence on the use of psychostimulants (such as methylphenidate), dopamine agonists, selective serotonin reuptake inhibitors (SSRIs), anticonvulsants (such as valproate), and even cognitive activators such as the cholinesterase inhibitor, donepezil. However, "off-label" use of drugs (i.e., for other than FDA-approved indications) may be ineffective and even dangerous. Polypharmacy, from adding one ineffective drug to others, may result in harm, and should be avoided.

Current surveillance data on TBI as well as current information on research, diagnosis, and treatment can be found through the Centers for Disease Control and Prevention, and from head injury association sources (e.g., Langlois et al., 2003; see also URL: http://www.cdc.gov/mmwr/ and go to "MMWR Search") A key public health strategy addresses prevention of injury by emphasizing safety interventions such as helmets, lap belts, shoulder belts, playground safety, delayed return to sports after head injury, and bans on very high-risk activities (e.g., boxing). Current progress includes development of trauma centers, emergency services, neuroprotective agents, physical and occupational therapy, cognitive rehabilitation, and treatment of ancillary disorders such as epilepsy, depression, and balance disturbances. Families should be educated about risks, safety interventions, and management of a family member with TBI. Methods of education include support groups, public awareness campaigns, and direct counseling of the family by rehabilitation team members.

SUMMARY AND CONCLUSIONS

TBI is an important public health problem, and knowledge of the pathophysiology, diagnosis, and treatment of TBI continues to evolve. Active areas of contemporary research include the spectrum of deficits and recovery in postconcussive syndrome, course of recovery, potential clinical utility of fMRI and PET, and evidence-based interventions for alleviation of TBI symptoms. Structural neuroimaging has improved dramatically since introduction of the CT, and recent advances in high-resolution MRI have only added to the value of structural imaging as a diagnostic tool. Neuropsychological examination sometimes provides the only evidence of abnormality in mild head injury, but can be influenced by factors other than TBI and must be carefully interpreted. An important question is how deficits measured in a neuropsychology clinic map onto instrumental activities of daily living, such as holding a job and participating in family life. Clearer understanding of the term *recovery* is needed vis-à-vis return to real-world activities such as work, school, automobile driving, and social activities, which may differ from the rate and course of medical recovery.

Acknowledgment

The authors thank Carol Devore for her effort in the production of this chapter, and also thank Ken Manzel and Stephen Cross for their assistance in the development of the case examples.

This work was supported by Program Project Grant NINDS NS19632 and NIA AG15071.

■ KEY POINTS

☐ Retrograde amnesia, for events immediately preceding head trauma, is typically briefer than post-traumatic amnesia.

☐ The incidence of head injury is greatest in the mid-teens to mid-twenties, but increased risk is also found in the very young and very old.

☐ Most head injuries are due to motor vehicle crashes, and falls are the second most common cause. Protective measures such as seat belts and lap belts, helmets for certain sports, and avoidance of high-risk activities have demonstrable effects in decreasing the incidence of TBI.

☐ The initial sequelae of head trauma (e.g., duration of loss of consciousness, duration of amnesia) are helpful, albeit imperfect predictors of eventual outcome.

☐ Deficits in memory, attention, and word finding are among the most prevalent cognitive impairments associated with traumatic brain injury.

KEY READINGS

Dikmen S, Machamer J, Temkin N: Mild head injury: Facts and artifacts. J Clin Exp Neuropsychol 23:729–738, 2001.

Eslinger PJ (ed): Neuropsychological Interventions. New York: Guilford Press, 2002.

Levin HS, Eisenberg HM, Benton AL (eds): Mild Head Injury. New York: Oxford, 1989.

Rizzo M, Tranel D (eds): Head Injury and Postconcussive Syndrome. New York: Churchill Livingstone, 1996.

Teasdale G, Jennett B: Assessment of coma and impaired consciousness. Lancet ii:81–84, 1974.

REFERENCES

Adekoya N, Thurman DJ, White DD, Webb KW: Surveillance for traumatic brain injury deaths-United States, 1989–1998. MMWR Surveill Summ 51(SS-10):1–14, 2002.

American Psychiatric Association: Diagnostic and Statistical Manual of Mental Disorders, ed 4. Washington, DC: Author, 1994.

Anderson SW: Visuoperceptual impairments, in Eslinger PJ (ed): Neuropsychological Interventions. New York: Guilford Press, 2002.

Anderson SW, Damasio H, Jones RD, Tranel D: Wisconsin Card Sorting Test performance as a measure of frontal lobe damage. J Clin Exp Neuropsychol 13:909–922, 1991.

Anderson SW, Tranel D: Awareness of disease states following cerebral infarction, dementia, and head trauma: Standardized assessment. Clin Neuropsychol 3:327–339, 1989.

Arcia E, Gualtieri CT: Association between patient report of symptoms after mild head injury and neurobehavioural performance. Brain Injury 7:481–489, 1993.

Barth JT, Macciocchi SN, Giordani B, et al: Neuropsychological sequelae of minor head injury. Neurosurgery 13:529–533, 1983.

Basso A, Scarpa MT: Traumatic aphasia in children and adults: A comparison of clinical features and evolution. Cortex 26:501–514, 1990.

Bechara A, Tranel D, Damasio H, Damasio AR: Failure to respond autonomically to anticipated future outcomes following damage to prefrontal cortex. Cerebral Cortex 6:215–225, 1996.

Bechara A, Damasio H, Tranel D, Damasio AR: Deciding advantageously before knowing the advantageous strategy. Science 275:1293–1295, 1997.

Bechara A, Damasio AR, Damasio H, Anderson SW: Insensitivity to future consequences following damage to human prefrontal cortex. Cognition 50:7–15, 1994.

Benton AL: The prefrontal region: Its early history, in Levin HS, Eisenberg HM, Benton AL (eds): Frontal Lobe Function and Dysfunction. New York: Oxford University Press, 1991.

Best M, Williams JM, Coccaro EF: Evidence for a dysfunctional prefrontal circuit in patients with an impulsive aggressive disorder. Proc Nat Acad Sci U S A 99:8448–8853, 2002.

Brooks N, McKinlay W, Symington C, et al: Return to work within the first seven years of severe head injury. Brain Injury 1:5–19, 1987.

Bryant RA: Posttraumatic stress disorder and mild brain injury: Controversies, causes, and consequences. J Clin Exp Neuropsychol 23:718–728, 2001.

Capruso DX, Levin HS: Cognitive impairment following head injury. Neurol Clin 10:879–893, 1992.

Carlsson GS, Svardsudd K, Welin L: Long-term effects of head injuries sustained during life in three male populations. J Neurosurg 67:197–205, 1987.

Crepeau F, Scherzer P: Predictors and indicators of work status after traumatic brain injury: A meta-analysis. Neuropsychol Rehab 3:5–35, 1993.

Damasio AR: Descartes' Error: Emotion, Reason, and the Human Brain. New York: Grosset/Putnam, 1994.

Damasio AR, Anderson SW: The frontal lobes, in Heilman K, Valenstein E (eds): Clinical Neuropsychology, ed 3. New York: Oxford University Press, 1993.

Dikmen S, Machamer J, Temkin N: Mild head injury: Facts and artifacts. J Clin Exp Neuropsychol 23:729–738, 2001.

Dikmen S, McLean A, Temkin N: Neuropsychological and psychosocial consequences of minor head injury. J Neurol Neurosurg Psychiatry 49:1227–1232, 1986b.

Dikmen S, McLean A, Temkin NR, Wyler AR: Neuropsychological outcome at one month postinjury. Arch Phys Med Rehab 67:507–513, 1986a.

Dikmen SS, Temkin NR, Machamer JE, et al: Employment following traumatic head injuries. Arch Neurol 51:177–186, 1994.

Drudge OW, Williams JM, Kessler M, Gomes FB: Recovery from severe head injuries: Repeat testing with the Halstead-Reitan Neuropsychological Battery. J Clin Psychol 40:259–265, 1984.

Eide PK, Tysnes OB: Early and late outcome in head injury patients with radiological evidence of brain damage. Acta Neurol Scand 86:194–198, 1992.

Eisenberg HM, Levin HS: Computed tomography and magnetic resonance imaging in mild to moderate head injury, in Levin HS, Eisenberg HM, Benton AL (eds): Mild Head Injury. New York: Oxford, 1989.

Eslinger PJ (ed): Neuropsychological Interventions. New York: Guilford Press, 2002.

Eslinger PJ, Damasio AR, Benton AL, Van Allen M: Neuropsychological detection of abnormal mental decline in older persons. JAMA 253:670–674, 1985.

Eslinger PJ, Grattan LM, Geder L: Neurological and neuropsychological aspects of frontal lobe impairments in post concussive syndrome, in Rizzo M, Tranel D (eds): Head Injury and Post Concussive Syndrome. New York: Churchill Livingstone, 1996, pp. 415–440.

Frankowski RF, Annegers JF, Whitman S: Epidemiological and descriptive studies. Part I: The descriptive epidemiology of head trauma in the United States, in Becker DP, Povlishock JT (eds): Central Nervous System Trauma Status Report 1985. Bethesda, MD: NINDS, 1985, pp. 33–43.

Fraser R, Dikmen S, McLean A, et al: Employability of head injury survivors: First year post-injury. Rehab Counsel Bull 31:276–288, 1988.

Gass CS: MMPI-2 Interpretation and closed head injury: A correction factor. Psychol Assess 3:27–31, 1991.

Gass CS, Wald HS: MMPI-2 Interpretation and closed-head trauma: Cross-validation of a correction factor. Arch Clin Neuropsychol 12:199–205, 1997.

Gentilini M, Nichelli P, Schoenhuber R: Assessment of attention in mild head injury, in Levin HS, Eisenberg HM, Benton AL (eds): Mild Head Injury. New York: Oxford, 1989.

Gianutsos R, Ramsey G, Perlin RR: Rehabilitative optometric services for survivors of acquired brain injury. Arch Phys Med Rehab 69:573–578, 1988.

Gilman S (ed): Clinical Examination of the Nervous System. New York: McGraw-Hill, 2000.

Golden CJ, Purisch AD, Hammeke TA: Luria Nebraska Neuropsychological Battery: Forms I and II Manual. Los Angeles, CA: Western Psychological Services, 1985.

Grabowski TJ, Damasio H, Tranel D, et al: A role for left temporal pole in the retrieval of words for unique entities. Hum Brain Map 13:199–212, 2001.

Grattan LM, Ghahramanlou M: The rehabilitation of neurologically based social disturbances, in Eslinger PJ (ed): Neuropsychological Interventions. New York: Guilford Press, 2002.

Griffenstein MF, Baker WJ: Comparison of premorbid and postinjury MMPI-2 profiles in late postconcussion claimants. Clin Neuropsychol 15:162–170, 2001.

Gronwall D: Behavioral assessment during the acute stages of traumatic brain injury, in Lezak MD (ed): Assessment of the Behavioral Consequences of Head Trauma. Vol. 1. Frontiers of Neuroscience. New York: Liss, 1989a, pp. 19–36.

Gronwall D (ed): Cumulative and Persisting Effects of Concussion on Attention and Cognition, in Levin HS, Eisenberg HM, Benton AL (eds): Mild Head Injury. New York: Oxford University Press, 1989b, pp. 153–162.

Gronwall D: Paced auditory serial addition task: A measure of recovery from concussion. Percept Motor Skills 44:367–373, 1977.

Haerer AF: Dejong's The Neurologic Examination, ed 5. Philadelphia, PA: Lippincott, 1992.

Hagan C, Malkmus D, Durham P: Rancho Los Amigos Scale of Cognitive Functioning. Communication Disorders Service, Rancho Los Amigos Hospital, CA, 1972.

Hamm RJ, Dixon CE, Gbadebo DM, et al: Cognitive deficits following traumatic brain injury produced by controlled cortical impact. J Neurotrauma 9:11–20, 1992.

Heilman KM, Safran A, Geschwind N: Closed head trauma and aphasia. J Neurol Neurosurg Psychiatry 34:265–269, 1971.

Heinze H-J, Munte TF, Gobiet W, et al: Parallel and serial visual search after closed head injury: Electrophysiological evidence for perceptual dysfunctions. Neuropsychologia 30:495–514, 1992.

Herscovitch P: Functional brain imaging: Basic principles and application to head trauma, in Rizzo M, Tranel D (eds): Head Injury and Postconcussive Syndrome. New York: Churchill Livingstone, 1996, pp. 89–118.

High WM Jr, Levin HS, Howard EG Jr: Recovery of orientation following closed head injury. J Clin Exp Neuropsychol 12:703–714, 1990.

Hugenholtz H, Stuss DT, Stethem LL, Richard MT: How long does it take to recover from a mild concussion? Neurosurgery 22:853–858, 1988.

Jennett B, Bond M: Assessment of outcome after severe brain damage: A practical scale. Lancet 1:480–484, 1975.

Jones BP, Butters N: Neuropsychological assessment, in Hersen M, Kazdin AE, Bellack AS (eds): The Clinical Psychology Handbook. New York: Pergamon Press, 1983.

Jones RD: Neuropsychological assessment of patients with traumatic brain injury: The Iowa-Benton approach, in Rizzo M, Tranel D (eds): Head Injury and Postconcussive Syndrome. New York: Churchill Livingstone, 1996, pp. 375–393.

Jones RD, Anderson SW, Cole T, Hathaway-Nepple J: Neuropsychological sequelae of traumatic brain injury, in Rizzo M, Tranel D (eds): Head Injury and Postconcussive Syndrome. New York: Churchill Livingstone, 1996, pp. 395–414.

Jones RD, Tranel D, Benton AL, Paulsen J: Differentiating dementia from "pseudodementia" early in the clinical course: Utility of neuropsychological tests. Neuropsychology 6:13–21, 1992.

Kaplan E, Fein D, Morris R, Delis DC: The Wechsler Adult Intelligence Scale-Revised as a Neuropsychological Instrument. San Antonio, TX: The Psychological Corporation, 1991.

Kempen JH, Kritchevsky M, Feldman S: Effect of visual impairment on neuropsychological test performance. J Clin Exp Neuropsychol 16:223–231, 1994.

Kreutzer J S, Marwitz JH, Kepler K: Traumatic brain injury: Family response and outcome. Arch Phys Med Rehab 73:771–778, 1992.

Langlois J, Kegler SR, Buttler JA, et al: Traumatic brain-injury-related hospital discharges: Results from a fourteen-state surveillance system, 1997. MMWR 52:1–18, 2003.

Lees-Haley PR, Brown RS: Neuropsychological complaint base rates of 170 personal injury claimants. Arch Clin Neuropsychol 8:185–202, 1993.

Leininger BE, Gramling SE, Farrel AD, et al: Neuropsychological deficits in symptomatic minor head injury following concussion and mild concussion. J Neurol Neurosurg Psychiatry 53:293–296, 1990.

Levin HS: Memory deficit after closed head injury. J Clin Exp Neuropsychol 12:129–153, 1989.

Levin HS, Amparo E, Eisenberg HM, et al: Magnetic resonance imaging and computerized tomography in relation to the neurobehavioral sequelae of mild and moderate head injuries. J Neurosurg 66:706–13, 1987a.

Levin HS, Benton AL, Grossman RG: Neurobehavioral Consequences of Closed Head Injury. New York: Oxford, 1982.

Levin HS, Eisenberg HM, Benton AL (eds): Mild Head Injury. New York: Oxford, 1989.

Levin HS, Gary HE, Eisenberg HM, et al: Neurobehavioral outcome 1 year after severe head injury: Experience of the Traumatic Coma Data Bank. J Neurosurg 73:699–709, 1990.

Levin HS, Goldstein FC, High WM, Eisenberg HM: Disproportionately severe memory deficit in relation to normal intellectual functioning after closed head injury. J Neurol Neurosurg Psychiatry 51:1294–1301, 1988.

Levin HS, Grossman RG, Kelly PJ: Aphasic disorder in patients with closed head injury. J Neurol Neurosurg Psychiatry 39:1062–1070, 1976.

Levin HS, Grossman RG, Kelly PJ: Impairment of facial recognition after closed head injuries of varying severity. Cortex 13:119–130, 1977.

Levin HS, Grossman RG, Sarwar M, Meyers CA: Linguistic recovery after closed head injury. Brain Lang 12:360–374, 1981.

Levin HS, High WM, Meyers CA, et al: Impairment of remote memory after closed head injury. J Neurol Neurosurg Psychiatry 48:556–563, 1985.

Levin HS, Mattis S, Ruff R, et al: Neurobehavioral outcome following minor head injury: A three center study. J Neurosurg 66:234–243, 1987b.

Lezak MD: Assessment of psychosocial dysfunctions resulting from head trauma, in Lezak MD (ed): Assessment of the Behavioral Consequences of Head Trauma. New York: Alan R. Liss, 1989, pp. 113–143.

Lezak MD: IQ: R.I.P. J Clin Exp Neuropsychol 10:351–361, 1988.

Lezak MD: Neuropsychological Assessment, ed 3. New York: Oxford University Press, 1995.

Mandelberg IA, Brooks DN: Cognitive recovery after severe head injury. 1. Serial testing on the Wechsler Adult Intelligence Scale. J Neurol Neurosurg Psychiatry 38:1121–1126, 1975.

Marshall LF, Marshall SB, Klauber MR, et al: A new classification of head injury based on computerized axial tomography. J Neurotraum 9(Suppl. 1):S287–S292, 1991.

Matser JT, Kessels AGH, Lezak MD, Troost A: A dose-response relation of headers and concussions with cognitive impairment in professional soccer players. J Clin Exp Neuropsychol 23:770–774, 2001.

Mayes SD, Pelco LE, Campbell CJ: Relationships among pre- and post-injury intelligence, length of coma and age in individuals with severe closed-head injuries. Brain Injury 3:301–313, 1989.

McCrory R, Berkovic SF: Second impact syndrome. Neurology 50:677–683, 1998.

McDonald S, van Sommers P: Pragmatic language skills after closed head injury: Ability to negotiate requests. Cognit Neuropsychol 10:297–315, 1993.

Milberg WP, Hebben N, Kaplan E: The Boston process approach to neuropsychological assessment, in Grant I, Adams K (eds): Neuropsychological Assessment of Neuropsychiatric Disorders. New York: Oxford, 1996.

Miller JD, Murray LS, Teasdale GM: Development of a traumatic intracranial hematoma after a "minor" head injury. Neurosurgery 27:669–673, 1990.

Mishra AV, Digre KB: Neuro-ophthalmologic disturbances in head injury, in Rizzo M, Tranel D (eds): Head Injury and Postconcussive Syndrome. New York: Churchill Livingstone, 1996.

O'Carroll RE, Wooodrow J, Maroun F: Psychosexual and psychosocial sequelae of closed head injury. Brain Injury 5:303–313, 1991.

Oddy M, Coughlan T, Tyerman A, Jenkins D: Social adjustment after closed head injury: A further follow-up seven years after injury. J Neurol Neurosurg Psychiatry 48:564–568, 1985.

Panting A, Merry PH: The long-term rehabilitation of severe head injuries with particular reference to the need for social and medical support for the patient's family. Rehabilitation 38:33–37, 1972.

Parasuraman R, Davies DR: Varieties of Attention. Orlando, FL: Academic Press, 1984.

Parasuraman R, Mutter SA, Molloy R: Sustained attention following mild closed-head injury. J Clin Exp Neuropsychol 13:789–811, 1991.

Peters LC, Stambrook M, Moore AD, et al: Differential effects of spinal cord injury and head injury on marital adjustment. Brain Injury 6:461–467, 1992.

Peters LC, Stambrook M, Moore AD, Esses L: Psychosocial sequelae of closed head injury: Effects on the marital relationship. Brain Injury 4:39–47, 1990.

Ponsford J, Kinsella G: Attentional deficits following closed head injury. J Clin Exp Neuropsychol 14:822–838, 1992.

Quality Standards Subcommittee Practice Parameter: The Management of Concussion in Sports (Summary Statement). Neurology 48:581–585, 1997.

Rao N, Rosenthal M, Cronin-Stubbs D, et al: Return to work after rehabilitation following traumatic brain injury. Brain Injury 4:49–56, 1990.

Reitan RM, Wolfson D: The Halstead-Reitan Neuropsychological Test Battery: Theory and Clinical Interpretation. Tucson, AZ: Neuropsychology Press, 1996.

Rizzo M, Tranel D (eds): Head Injury and Postconcussive Syndrome. New York: Churchill Livingstone, 1996.

Rolls ET, Hornak J, Wade D, McGrath J: Emotion-related learning in patients with social and emotional changes associated with frontal lobe damage. J Neurol Neurosurg Psychiatry 57:1518–1524, 1994.

Ropper AH: Neurological and Neurosurgical Intensive Care, ed 3. New York: Raven Press, 1993.

Ruff RM, Levin HS, Mattis S, et al: Recovery of memory after mild head injury, in Levin HS, Eisenberg HM, Benton AL (eds): Mild Head Injury. New York: Oxford, 1989.

Russell WR: The Traumatic Amnesias. New York: Oxford University Press, 1971.

Sarno MT: The nature of verbal impairment after closed head injury. J Nerv Ment Dis 168:685–692, 1980.

Schacter DL, Crovits HF: Memory function after closed head injury: A review of the quantitative research. Cortex 13:150–176, 1977.

Schiffrin RM, Schneider W: Controlled and automatic information processing II. Perceptual learning and automatic attending, and a general theory. Psycholog Rev 84:127–190, 1977.

Schlageter K, Gray B, Hall K, et al: Incidence and treatment of visual dysfunction in traumatic brain injury. Brain Injury 7:439–448, 1993.

Schwab K, Grafman J, Salazar AM, Kraft J: Residual impairments and work status 15 years after penetrating head injury: Report from the Vietnam Head Injury Study. Neurology 43:95–103, 1993.

Sherer M, Novack TA, Sander AM, et al: Neuropsychological assessment and employment outcome after traumatic brain injury: A review. Clin Neuropsychol 10:157–178, 2002.

Spreen O, Strauss E: A compendium of neuropsychological tests: Administration, norms, and commentary, ed 2. New York: Oxford University Press, 1998.

Stuss DT, Ely P, Hugenholtz H, et al: Subtle neuropsychological deficits in patients with good recovery after closed head injury. Neurosurgery 17:41–47, 1985.

Stuss DT, Stethem LL, Hugenholtz H, et al: Reaction time after head injury: Fatigue, divided and focused attention, and consistency of performance. J Neurol Neurosurg Psychiatry 52:742–748, 1989.

Suhr JA, Gurstad J: Postconcussive symptom report: The relative influence of head injury and depression. J Clin Exp Neuropsychol 24 981–993, 2002.

Tabaddor M, Mattis S, Zazula T: Cognitive sequelae and recovery course after moderate and severe head injury. Neurosurgery 14:701–708, 1984.

Tate RL, Fenelson B, Manning ML, Hunter M: Patterns of neuropsychological impairment after severe blunt head injury. J Nerv Ment Dis 179:117–126, 1991.

Teasdale G, Jennett B: Assessment of coma and impaired consciousness. Lancet ii:81–84, 1974.

Teasdale G, Knill-Jones R, Van Der Sand J: Observer variability in assessing impaired consciousness and coma. J Neurol Neurosurg Psychiatry 41:603–610, 1978.

Thomsen IV: Late outcome of very severe blunt head trauma: A 10–15 year second follow-up. J Neurol Neurosurg Psychiatry 47:260–268, 1984.

Thurman DJ, Guerrero J: Trends in hospitalization associated with traumatic brain injury. JAMA 282:954–957, 1999.

Torner JC, Schootman Mario: Epidemiology of closed head injury, in Rizzo M, Tranel D (eds): Head Injury and Postconcussive Syndrome. New York: Churchill Livingstone, 1996, pp. 19–46.

Tranel D: The Iowa-Benton school of neuropsychological assessment, in Grant I, Adams KM (eds): Neuropsychological Assessment of Neuropsychiatric Disorders, ed 2. New York: Oxford University Press, 1996, pp. 81–101.

Tranel D, Anderson SW, Benton A: Development of the concept of "executive function" and its relationship to the frontal lobes, in Boller F, Grafman J (eds): Handbook of Neuropsychology, Vol. 9. New York: Elsevier, 1994, pp. 125–148.

Van Allen MW, Rodnitzky RL: Pictorial Manual of Neurologic Tests: A Guide to the Performance and Interpretation of the Neurologic Examination. Chicago, IL: Yearbook Medical Publishers, 1988.

Van der Naalt J: Prediction of outcome in mild to moderate head injury. J Clin Exp Neuropsychol 23:837–851, 2001.

Van Zomeren AH: Reaction time and attention after closed head injury. Lisse, The Netherlands: Swets & Zeitlinger, 1981.

Van Zomeren AH, Van Denburg W: Residual complaints of patients two years after severe head injury. J Neurol Neurosurg Psychiatry 48:21–28, 1985.

Wechsler D: WAIS-R Manual. New York: Psychological Corporation, 1981.

Encephalopathies

Christopher M. Filley

Acute confusional state

Attention

Encephalopathy

Metabolic disorders

Toxic disorders

Toxic leukoencephalopathy

CONCEPTUAL FRAMEWORK

Encephalopathy is a broad concept referring to a clinical syndrome caused by any disorder of the brain. This syndrome can be acute or chronic, inherited or acquired, and reversible or irreversible. A wide range of disturbances may produce encephalopathy, including those that arise within the central nervous system (CNS) and those related to systemic diseases, and either altered function or structural lesions of the brain may prove to be responsible. In this chapter, the focus is on acquired encephalopathy resulting from systemic toxic and meta-bolic disorders. Discussions of other forms of encephalopathy can be found elsewhere in this volume.

Toxic and metabolic disorders affecting the brain are common in clinical practice. The brain is highly dependent on the maintenance of the internal milieu, and is thus vulnerable to many toxic and metabolic insults that disrupt homeostatic equilibrium. Fortunately, most of these disorders can be treated effectively if they are recognized early and the underlying problem is promptly addressed. For this reason, many patients with this syndrome are cared for by emergency room physicians, internists, or primary care physicians. Nevertheless, the many diverse clinical manifestations of encephalopathy often call for the services of behavioral neurologists and neuropsychologists. In addition, this syndrome is instructive in theoretical terms because of the important neurobehavioral effects that toxic and metabolic disturbances may produce.

The most common neurobehavioral syndrome in patients with encephalopathy arising in the setting of toxic and metabolic disorders is the acute confusional state (Filley, 2001). Up to 25% of adults over 65 can be expected to develop an acute confusional state during admission to a general hospital, most often secondary to a toxic or metabolic insult (Mesulam, 2000). Confusion, defined as the inability to maintain a coherent line of thought, is the salient feature of the acute confusional state and results from a profound deficit in attentional function (Mesulam, 2000; Filley, 2001). An alternate term for the acute confusional state is *toxic-metabolic encephalopathy*, which emphasizes the most common etiologies of the syndrome. Another frequently used word for this syndrome is *delirium*, which denotes a florid state of agitation and autonomic dysfunction combined with confusion. However, it should be emphasized that acute confusional states often manifest as hypoarousal (lethargy, drowsiness, or somnolence) in contrast to hyperarousal, so that the term *delirium* fails to capture the entire range of arousal disturbances that can occur. The term *acute confusional state* is preferred by many because it refers to the temporal dimension of the illness as well as identifies its most prominent clinical feature. The archaic term *acute organic brain syndrome* has been discarded because it is not specific enough to be useful.

Encephalopathy from toxic and metabolic disturbances can also take the form of subacute or chronic cognitive impairment that qualifies as dementia. This syndrome resembles the hypoaroused variety of the acute confusional state, but evolves over a longer time period, and may therefore be considered a "chronic confusional state" (Mesulam, 2000; Filley, 2001). The same toxic and metabolic insults that lead to acute encephalopathy may also produce dementia, and recognition of this syndrome is important in the evaluation of dementia patients because toxic and metabolic disorders may be partially or completely reversible even at this stage.

A primary disorder of attention, typically commingled with variable alterations in arousal, can be seen as the unifying characteristic of all the toxic and metabolic encephalopathies (Filley, 2001). As a general rule, the clinical features of encephalopathic patients reflect transient or permanent dysfunction in the attentional structures of the thalamus and cerebral hemispheres, and the arousal system that originates in the reticular formation of the brainstem (Mesulam, 2000). Acute and chronic confusional states thus represent an interference with the operations of neural networks devoted to critical neurobehavioral domains that participate in all aspects of higher mental activity (Mesulam, 2000). Thus, although the encephalopathies discussed in this chapter cannot be localized in the usual neurologic sense, they nevertheless offer important insights into fundamental brain-behavior relationships.

DIAGNOSIS

Encephalopathy is a clinical diagnosis, as there is no single test that either rules in or excludes this syndrome (Table 28-1). The essential process in the diagnosis of acute or chronic encephalopathy is the history and physical examination, with special attention to the mental state. Additional useful information can be obtained from laboratory tests, neuroimaging, lumbar puncture, electroencephalography (EEG), and a variety of special procedures.

A thorough history, as in neurology generally, is the cornerstone of the evaluation. The patient is usually unable to provide many details, and so the history must usually be obtained from or confirmed by relatives, friends, or caregivers. Evidence that the patient has had an acute or chronic decline in mental function is central, and typical features include inattention, confusion, and disorientation, often with personality change, delusions, hallucinations, lethargy, and drowsiness. An altered sleep pattern is also characteristic, and interference with the normal circadian rhythm exacerbates the confusion because of continuing patient fatigue (see Chapter 31). Chronic neurodegenerative disorders such as Alzheimer disease (AD) share some of these features, but alterations in consciousness are decidedly uncharacteristic. The history should also probe whether focal disorders of the brain have developed to account for confusion, as suggested by such features as limb weakness, focal sensory loss, visual dysfunction, and convulsive movements. In the case of toxic and metabolic disorders, identification of potential toxic and metabolic disturbances is crucial. Data on the patient's medications (prescription and over-the-counter), medical and surgical diseases, habits such as the use of alcohol and other drugs, occupation, and home situation may all be relevant. Care should be taken to ensure that a psychiatric problem is not the explanation of the presenting syndrome. Depression, for example, typically produces inattention, forgetfulness, and cognitive slowing, and careful clinical assessment may be required to separate this syndrome from chronic toxic or metabolic encephalopathies.

TABLE 28-1. Diagnosis of Encephalopathy

History
Examination (physical, neurologic, mental status)
Laboratory tests (electrolytes, glucose, blood urea nitrogen, creatinine, liver function tests, calcium, complete blood count)
Chest roentgenogram
Electrocardiogram (EKG)
Urinalysis
Brain imaging (computed tomography, magnetic resonance imaging)
Lumbar puncture
Electroencephalogram (EEG)
Special tests (toxicology screens, arterial blood gases, carboxyhemoglobin, plasma cholinesterase, metal screens)
Neuropsychological testing

The physical examination may disclose evidence of intoxication, such as the odor of alcohol or solvents, or of metabolic imbalance, such as the asterixis that often accompanies hepatic, renal, and pulmonary disease. Abnormal vital signs may indicate possible infection, hypertensive crisis, or major cardiopulmonary disease. Physical signs of acute or chronic systemic illness such as cyanosis, tachypnea, or jaundice may be evident. On the elemental neurologic examination, focal signs are generally absent in toxic and metabolic encephalopathy, although some disorders such as uremia can produce transient focal motor findings as a concomitant feature.

The mental status examination is a key component of the diagnostic process. As inattention is the core deficit of acute and chronic encephalopathy, assessment of orientation, the forward and reverse digit span, and serial sevens can provide a convenient survey of the nature and depth of this disturbance. Altered consciousness is often present, either as a hypoaroused or hyperaroused state, and fluctuations in the level of consciousness are common. Delusions, illusions, and hallucinations may often be present. In many cases, the disturbances of attention and arousal found early in the examination are severe enough to interfere with the evaluation of any memory, language, or other cognitive domains, and further testing may be an exercise in futility. In some mildly affected patients, however, deficient memory retrieval, dysgraphia, and visuospatial disturbances may be evident. In those with preexisting dementing disease, the examination may disclose a "beclouded dementia" that represents an acute confusional state superimposed on underlying cognitive loss (Mesulam, 2000). In these individuals, determining the relative contribution of the confusional state compared with the prior dementia can only be approximated, but treatment of the acute process can allow the baseline syndrome to reemerge.

Laboratory testing is useful to screen for a wide range of medical diseases. Electrolytes, glucose, renal and hepatic function tests, calcium, and a complete blood count are routine blood tests that are always helpful. A chest roentgenogram, electrocardiogram (EKG), and urinalysis can offer additional information about potential systemic diseases. A brain image may disclose an acute structural lesion, and either computed tomography (CT) or magnetic resonance imaging (MRI) may be used for this purpose. In the absence of focal neurologic findings, a localized structural lesion is unlikely to be revealed by neuroimaging. Neuroimaging is unremarkable or shows only nonspecific cerebral atrophy in most toxic and metabolic encephalopathies. An exception to this rule is the toxic leukoencephalopathies (Filley & Kleinschmidt-DeMasters, 2001), in which diffuse or focal white matter hyperintensity can detected; MRI is superior to CT for evaluat-

ing the effects of many toxins on the cerebral white matter. Lumbar puncture is essential if any infection in the central nervous system is suspected, but the optic fundi should first be examined in order to avoid tapping a patient with papilledema and increased intracranial pressure who may be at risk for herniation. An EEG can be helpful in the evaluation of many cases of encephalopathy, because diffuse intermixed slow activity is typical of toxic and metabolic dysfunction (Mesulam, 2000). Special tests include blood and urine toxicology screens, arterial blood gases, carboxyhemoglobin, plasma cholinesterase, and metal screening.

Finally, neuropsychological testing may be of value in some patients with encephalopathy. Many individuals who are delirious or somnolent will not be able to comply with the procedures of the evaluation, and the utility of neuropsychological referral is limited in the acute setting. However, those patients with less dramatic syndromes can often be usefully tested. Neuropsychological evaluation will be most helpful in those with chronic encephalopathy, and deficits in sustained attention and memory retrieval will typically emerge, consistent with the attentional and memory deficits apparent on the mental status examination (Filley, 2001). Documentation of lasting deficits in those individuals with chronic encephalopathy can serve as a baseline for future evaluations, and often assist with a number of treatment and disability issues.

TOXIC DISORDERS

Toxic encephalopathy is becoming increasingly common as new therapeutic agents are introduced, illicit drugs gain more popularity, and environmental toxins are recognized. The understanding of these intoxications is typically limited, however, as details of exposure dose and duration, pathophysiology, and natural history are often obscure. Nevertheless, these syndromes underscore the vulnerability of the brain to a wide range of toxic insults, and emphasize the need to consider intoxications in the differential diagnosis of acute and chronic encephalopathies.

Therapeutic Agents

Therapeutic advances in medicine, while clearly beneficial, frequently involve significant toxicities. Table 28-2 lists the therapeutic agents most implicated in encephalopathy. Drugs given for the treatment of medical, psychiatric, and neurologic disorders are common sources of cognitive impairment (Meador, 1998), and almost any drug can cause encephalopathy (Moore & O'Keefe, 1999). Up to 30% of cases of the acute confusional state are the result of drug toxicity (Moore & O'Keefe, 1999), and drug-induced dementia is the most common cause of reversible dementia (Katzman et al., 1988). Older persons taking prescription drugs are particularly vulnerable to encephalopathy because of age-related changes in drug metabolism, increased medication use, and preexisting cognitive impairment (Meador, 1998). Polypharmacy, the use of more than one drug to treat symptoms or disease, is another factor that probably contributes to encephalopathy in this age group, as the number of medications, both prescribed and over-the-counter, increases with advancing age (Stewart & Hale, 1992). Moreover, drugs often exacerbate preexisting cognitive impairment, and the presence of dementia increases the risk of acute confusional state by two- to threefold (Meador, 1998). A thorough assessment of exposure to all kinds of drugs is thus crucial in the evaluation of acute confusional states and dementia.

Licit Drugs

A wide variety of prescription and over-the-counter drugs have been implicated in the etiology of acute and chronic encephalopathy. The most commonly reported drugs are the anticholinergics, benzodiazepines, barbiturates, narcotics, neuroleptics, and antiepileptic drugs, which all produce clinical changes by their prominent

TABLE 28-2. Therapeutic Agents Associated with Encephalopathy

Drugs

Anticholinergics (tricyclic antidepressants, antihistamines, meclizine, atropine, scopolamine, benztropine, trihexyphenidyl)

Benzodiazepines (diazepam, chlordiazepoxide)

Barbiturates (butalbital, secobarbital)

Narcotics (morphine, hydrocodone, oxycodone, codeine, meperidine)

Neuroleptics (phenothiazines, butyrophenones)

Antiepileptic drugs (phenobarbital, clonazepam, phenytoin, carbamazepine)

Antihypertensive drugs (methyldopa, clonidine, reserpine)

Cardiac drugs (digoxin, quinidine, disopyramide, lidocaine)

H_2 receptor antagonists (cimetidine, ranitidine)

Corticosteroids (prednisone, methylprednisolone)

Nonsteroidal antiinflammatory drugs (ibuprofen, naproxen, diclofenac)

Antibiotics (penicillin, cephalosporins, quinolones, amphotericin B)

Cancer chemotherapy drugs (methotrexate, BCNU)

Immunosuppressive drugs (cyclosporine, tacrolimus)

Cranial irradiation

BCNU, 1,3-bis(2-chloroethyl)-1-nitrosourea.

effects on central neurotransmitter function (Meador, 1998; Moore & O'Keefe, 1999). Particular attention should be paid to anticholinergic drugs and benzodiazepines because they are so commonly prescribed. The central anticholinergic effects of tricyclic antidepressants such as amitriptyline are commonly implicated in cognitive loss among depressed patients, and confusion from anticholinergic drugs used for the treatment of parkinsonism is common (Meador, 1998). Similarly, the benzodiazepines may induce attention and memory deficits, especially in older patients who are more sensitive to their effects (Meador, 1998).

Less common but often unrecognized causes of encephalopathy are other drugs widely employed in medical practice. These include certain antihypertensives, cardiac drugs, H_2 receptor antagonists, corticosteroids, nonsteroidal anti-inflammatory drugs, and antibiotics (Meador, 1998). Each of these drugs, while often well tolerated when given individually, may contribute to encephalopathy in a patient with multiple medical problems who is taking several medications. The possibility of adverse drug-drug interactions increases substantially with the addition of each new medication, and the benefits of adding new drugs to a patient's regimen must be carefully balanced against the risks involved.

Whereas most drugs that cause encephalopathy do so by interfering with functional aspects of the brain and are not associated with a recognized neuropathology, some medications have the capacity to produce structural change as determined neuroradiologically or neuropathologically. The cerebral white matter is particularly vulnerable to many toxins. An increasingly common neurotoxic syndrome is leukoencephalopathy, which can follow treatment with many antineoplastic and immunosuppressive drugs (Filley & Kleinschmidt-DeMasters, 2001). Methotrexate and 1,3-bis(2-chloroethyl)-1-nitrosourea (BCNU) are the most commonly implicated antineoplastic agents, and among the immunosuppressive drugs, cyclosporine and tacrolimus (FK506) have been linked most securely with leukoencephalopathy (Filley & Kleinschmidt-DeMasters, 2001). Clinical features may range from mild inattention to coma, and the degree of clinical involvement is commensurate with the severity of leukoencephalopathy as assessed neuroradiologically (Filley & Kleinschmidt-DeMasters, 2001). Recovery also depends largely on the extent of white matter toxicity; patients with mild white matter hyperintensity usually recover uneventfully with drug discontinuation, whereas those with white matter necrosis usually have a poor or even fatal outcome (Filley & Kleinschmidt-DeMasters, 2001).

Cranial Irradiation

Radiation to the brain is often used in the treatment of primary and metastatic malignancies, and leukoencephalopathy can appear that is clinically, neuroradiologically, and neuropathologically similar to that produced by cancer chemotherapy drugs (Filley & Kleinschmidt-DeMasters, 2001). Radiation leukoencephalopathy has come to be one of the major limiting side effects of this often very effective form of treatment. Three types of cerebral white matter injury can occur after cranial irradiation (Sheline et al., 1980). First, an acute reaction with confusion or worsening of preexisting neurologic signs can develop during and immediately after treatment; this syndrome is attributed to transient edema, and is typically self-limited (Sheline et al., 1980). Next, an early delayed reaction, the so-called "somnolence syndrome," may appear within weeks to months after treatment, and probably relates to cerebral demyelination; this problem is also self-limited, although recovery is less prompt (Sheline et al., 1980). Most serious is the late delayed reaction, which presents 6 months to 2 years after treatment with progressive dementia; widespread demyelination and necrosis are often present, and an irreversible course and fatal outcome may ensue (Sheline et al., 1980). The pathophysiology of radiation leukoencephalopathy is thought to involve a primary effect on blood vessels, which undergo thrombosis or fibrinoid necrosis that can impair blood flow; this effect is especially evident in long penetrating arterioles supplying the hemispheric white matter. The combined effects of chemotherapy and irradiation are particularly injurious to the cerebral white matter, as there is an additive toxic effect (Filley & Kleinschmidt-DeMasters, 2001).

Drugs of Abuse

Although the use of intoxicating substances has been known since antiquity, the abuse of such agents is currently an enormous and growing problem in our society. Many of these drugs have been associated with encephalopathy (Table 28-3), whether as an acute effect of intoxication, a withdrawal syndrome, or a chronic dementia. Although precise characterization of the clinical syndromes produced by specific drugs is hampered by the fact that drug abusers often use more than one substance simultaneously, information on the cognitive effects of these agents is gradually accumulating.

Ethanol

The abuse of ethanol has been abundantly documented in literature and the arts as well as in medical writings. Alcoholism continues to be a major worldwide problem with staggering morbidity and mortality. The intended site of action of alcohol is the brain, and among the many organ systems at risk for damage from the effects of excessive ethanol, the nervous system ranks high. Any level of the peripheral or CNS can be affected, and the syndromes of myopathy, peripheral neuropathy,

TABLE 28-3. Drugs of Abuse Associated with Encephalopathy

Ethanol
Sedative-hypnotics (benzodiazepines, barbiturates)
Opiates (heroin, prescription opiates)
Stimulants (dextroamphetamine, methamphetamine)
Cocaine
MDMA ("Ecstasy")
Hallucinogens (LSD, psilocybin, mescaline)
Phencyclidine
Marijuana
Inhalants (toluene, other volatile agents)

myelopathy, and cerebellar dysfunction can result, but most disabling are the myriad neurobehavioral syndromes associated with alcoholism.

The commonplace occurrence of alcohol intoxication should not obscure the fact that inebriation is in fact an acute confusional state, one that the general public witnesses at least as much as medical professionals do. This syndrome produces a range of familiar behavioral changes, including euphoria, impaired concentration, and disinhibition (Brust, 1998). Encephalopathy typically appears at blood ethanol levels of 50–300 mg/dL; stupor occurs at 300 mg/dL; coma at 400 mg/dL; and death at 500 mg/dL (Brust, 1998), although considerable individual variability exists because of tolerance that can develop in chronic abusers. Alcoholic "blackouts"—periods of the drinking bout for which patients have no memory—also occur in the context of heavy alcohol use (Brust, 1998). An acute confusional state may also represent Wernicke's encephalopathy, and the possibility of coexisting Wernicke-Korsakoff syndrome from thiamine deficiency should always be remembered in any patient who exhibits excessive alcohol use (see discussion following).

Several additional neurologic syndromes are well known in the context of alcohol withdrawal. Individuals who have recently desisted from the acute intake of alcohol may experience a coarse tremor that may impel them to drink more so that the involuntary movement is suppressed. Alcohol withdrawal seizures—generalized tonic-clonic convulsions occurring within 2 days of the last drink—are common events in heavy drinkers, and a postictal lethargic confusional state of variable length is typical. The syndrome of alcoholic hallucinosis is less common, but the persistent auditory hallucinations in affected patients can be troubling. However, the most dangerous withdrawal syndrome is delirium tremens, a dramatic, agitated, acute confusional state with visual hallucinations, fever, tachycardia, diaphoresis, and hypotension (Brust, 1998). Benzodiazepines are used for sedation, but even with optimal management, mortality from delirium tremens may be as high as 15% because of the associated medical problems experienced by many alcoholic patients (Brust, 1998).

Another concern in the context of alcohol and the brain is the dementia seen in many patients between drinking bouts or in long-term follow-up. The chronic effects of alcohol abuse on the brain are disputed, because although there is no doubt that many alcoholics do indeed develop dementia, a direct toxic effect of ethanol on the brain is difficult to establish. Some authorities maintain that dementia in alcoholics can be explained by the many concomitant problems to which alcoholics are predisposed, including traumatic brain injury, hepatic disease (see discussion following), and thiamine deficiency causing the prominent amnesia of Korsakoff's psychosis (Victor, 1993). Alternatively, many alcoholics have a pervasive dementia syndrome that appears to be unrelated to any of these complications, and a toxic effect of ethanol on the brain has been postulated (Lishman, 1981). Whereas neuropathologists have not previously been convinced of unequivocal toxic effects on the cerebrum, more recent neuropathologic and neuroradiologic examination of the cerebral white matter has suggested that the white matter may be the target of ethanol (Filley & Kleinschmidt-DeMasters, 2001). This possibility is supported by the fact that some alcoholics can show clinical improvement and a reduction in ventriculomegaly on neuroimaging scans with abstinence, implying that a restoration of white matter volume may have taken place (Filley & Kleinschmidt-DeMasters, 2001). Further support for the idea that ethanol may be leukotoxic can be derived from considering Marchiafava-Bignami disease, an unusual dementing disease characterized by degeneration of the corpus callosum and other white matter regions, which is strongly associated with chronic alcoholism (Brust, 1998). To summarize, the origin of dementia in alcoholics is a complex issue; although its etiology is likely multifactorial, primary damage to cerebral white matter is an increasingly likely contributor (Filley & Kleinschmidt-DeMasters, 2001).

Sedative-Hypnotics

Many commonly prescribed sedative-hypnotics— among them the benzodiazepines, barbiturates, chloral hydrate, zolpidem, and buspirone—can also be taken as drugs of abuse (Brust, 1998). All the sedative-hypnotics are CNS depressants, although their potency differs widely. Barbiturates, for example, have pronounced acute effects and are commonly used to attempt suicide, whereas buspirone is in general far less hazardous. Long-term cognitive effects of sedative-hypnotics have not been emphasized, but the many problems associated with drug dependence with these drugs are of major concern.

The benzodiazepines are used as tranquilizers and anxiolytics (e.g., diazepam, chlordiazepoxide, chlorazepate, alprazolam, and lorazepam), hypnotics (e.g., flurazepam, temazepam, triazolam), anticonvulsants (clonazepam), and for anesthesia induction (midazolam); a benzodiazepine antagonist (flumazenil) is also available (Brust, 1998). Recreational use of the benzodiazepines is common, and confusion, amnesia, anxiety, panic, agitation, and panic can result; drug dependence is frequent in long-term users (Brust, 1998). The acute effects of the barbiturates, sedative drugs used as anticonvulsants (e.g., phenobarbital), analgesics (e.g., butalbital), soporifics (e.g., secobarbital), and anesthetics (e.g., thiopental) resemble ethanol intoxication, and respiratory depression and hypothermia can develop in those with barbiturate overdose; dependence is even more likely with these drugs than with the benzodiazepines (Brust, 1998). Chloral hydrate and zolpidem are soporific drugs, and buspirone is used for the treatment of anxiety; the abuse potential for these drugs is relatively low (Brust, 1998).

Sedative-hypnotics as a group, particularly the benzodiazepines, have some cross-tolerance with ethanol, and the clinical features of withdrawal from these drugs may closely resemble alcohol withdrawal. Benzodiazepines are in fact routinely used in the treatment of alcohol withdrawal syndromes (see discussion following). Withdrawal from alcohol or sedative-hypnotics should always be considered as a potential cause of the acute confusional state (Chan & Brennan, 1999).

Opiates

The drug in this group most commonly used for recreational purposes is heroin (diacetylmorphine), which is traditionally injected either intravenously or subcutaneously. More recently, since the acquired immunodeficiency syndrome (AIDS) epidemic has raised fears of parenteral use, heroin is increasingly snorted (inhaled intranasally) or smoked (Brust, 1998). Although its intoxicating and withdrawal effects do not usually induce confusion, heroin (and other narcotics) can sometimes cause memory loss and precipitate an acute confusional state (Brust, 1998). Heroin has also been recognized as a cause of leukoencephalopathy. The intravenous use of the drug can cause hypoxic-ischemic white matter damage, and inhalation of heroin pyrolysate after heating the drug on aluminum foil ("chasing the dragon") can result in severe and irreversible toxic leukoencephalopathy (Filley & Kleinschmidt-DeMasters, 2001).

Stimulants

This group includes some drugs used for therapeutic purposes (e.g., dextroamphetamine, methylphenidate, pemoline, ephedrine, pseudoephedrine, and phenylpropanolamine), and some for recreational purposes (e.g., dextroamphetamine, methamphetamine). In general, these drugs produce increased alertness and euphoria, but overdose can produce an acute confusional state with headache, hypertension, fever, cardiac dysfunction, and psychosis (Brust, 1998). Metabolic acidosis, rhabdomyolysis, disseminated intravascular coagulation, myocardial infarction, seizures, coma, and death may ensue (Brust, 1998). Paranoia and hallucinations can develop in chronic users of these drugs. In addition, cerebral vasculitis and stroke have been reported, most notably with the amphetamines (Brust, 1998).

Cocaine

Effects similar to those of the amphetamines are produced by cocaine, a local anesthetic that has stimulant properties. This drug can be taken intranasally or parenterally, and its alkaloidal form, known as crack, is smoked. Metabolic complications of acute cocaine overdose can be severe, and hypoxic-ischemic injury can impede recovery (Brust, 1998). Seizures can occur in chronic users of cocaine, putatively related to a kindling effect of repeated subconvulsant doses (Brust, 1998). The long-term cognitive effects of cocaine are unknown, although the drug has been associated with both ischemic and hemorrhagic stroke (Brust, 1998).

Ecstasy

The drug, methylenedioxymethamphetamine or MDMA, aka "Ecstasy," has recently been used extensively by young people at dance parties known as "raves." MDMA is taken orally and has a combination of stimulant and hallucinogenic properties. Despite the widespread perception that it is a relatively safe drug of abuse, evidence for selective serotonin neurotoxicity has been derived from animal studies, and memory deficits in humans have also been linked with serotonin toxicity in users of MDMA (Bolla et al., 1998).

Hallucinogens

Drugs of this group produce visual and auditory illusions and hallucinations, although frequent, adverse symptoms such as paranoia and panic usually resolve within 24 hours (Brust, 1998). The major hallucinogenic drugs are the ergot lysergic acid diethylamide (LSD), the indolealkylamine psilocybin (derived from the mushroom *Psilocybe mexicana*), and the phenylalkylamine mescaline (derived from peyote cactus) (Brust, 1998). With high doses, confusion and seizures can occur, but fatalities typically result from accident or suicide rather than neurologic toxicity (Brust, 1998). Chronic encephalopathy is not described, although the spontaneous recurrence of hallucinations weeks or months later (flashbacks) is reported by some users of hallucinogens.

Phencyclidine

Also known as angel dust, phencyclidine (PCP) can be smoked, sprinkled on tobacco or marijuana, eaten, snorted, or injected. PCP is an anesthetic drug with N-methyl-D-aspartate receptor antagonist action, and its variable acute effects include euphoria, dysphoria, emotional lability, illusions, hallucinations, agitation, amnesia, catatonia, seizures, coma, and death (Brust, 1998). Psychotic features may last for weeks after a single dose, and some authorities believe that lasting psychosis can follow the use of this drug (Brust, 1998).

Marijuana

Marijuana (cannabis) is the most widely used illicit drug in the United States (Brust, 1998). Typical acute effects of this drug, the active ingredient of which is tetrahydrocannabinol (THC), are euphoria and anxiety, but high doses can produce illusions, hallucinations, agitation, memory impairment, and depression (Brust, 1998). The disinhibition typical of alcohol intoxication is not seen. Evidence is as yet insufficient to support a lasting effect of cannabis on cognition (Pope et al., 1995). Although a "drug residue" effect on neuropsychological performance may last 12 to 24 hours after acute intoxication, there are no data clearly implicating a toxic effect on the brain beyond this period (Pope et al., 1995).

Inhalants

The recreational inhalation of volatile fumes is common among children and adolescents who can easily gain access to many commercial products that are legal and relatively inexpensive. Some examples of these abusable substances are aerosols, dry-cleaning fluids, degreasers, glues, petroleum products, and paints (Brust, 1998). In general, the effect of these vapors is to produce dose-related euphoria and relaxation that are transient, but high doses can produce toxic psychosis, and death from cardiac arrhythmia (Brust, 1998). One of the most thoroughly studied inhalants is toluene (methyl benzene), an organic hydrocarbon that comprises the major solvent in spray paint. Intense daily exposure to toluene over a period of months to years can result in severe leukoencephalopathy characterized by dementia, ataxia, and other neurologic deficits (Hormes et al., 1986). Autopsy study of demented toluene abusers discloses selective loss of myelin in the cerebrum and cerebellum, with sparing of cell bodies and axons (Rosenberg et al., 1988). The dementia is the most disabling aspect of the syndrome (Hormes et al., 1986), and the severity of the cognitive impairment is correlated with the degree of white matter involvement on MRI scans (Filley et al., 1990).

Environmental Toxins

The nervous system is vulnerable to a wide spectrum of environmental toxins. Many of these intoxications are evident only in the peripheral nervous system, as the culpable substances lack the capacity to enter the CNS. However, a number of toxic agents have been associated with brain damage and cognitive sequelae (Table 28-4); support for a toxic effect of these agents on the brain is strong in some cases and equivocal in others.

Solvents

Exposure to many solvents (e.g., toluene, methanol, benzene, xylene, styrene, trichloroethylene, methylene chloride, carbon disulfide) occurs among workers in a variety of occupations, and may also be significant in the home setting. Toluene leukoencephalopathy (see above) may thus serve as a model for neurobehavioral toxicity in solvent-exposed individuals, but the relevance of this syndrome to occupational or home solvent exposure is uncertain. Since the 1970s, some investigators have claimed that toxic encephalopathy ("the painters' syndrome") can be detected in many workers chronically exposed to solvents (Arlien-Soborg et al., 1979). However, firm evidence that this low-level exposure leads to encephalopathy has been difficult to secure, because the details of the degree and duration of exposure are unclear, individuals may be exposed to multiple solvents, and symptoms could be explained by other problems such as alcohol abuse and psychiatric dysfunction (Albers & Berent, 2000). Despite this uncertainty, it may be that a threshold of exposure can be determined above which leukoencephalopathy develops (Filley & Klineschmidt-DeMasters, 2001), but this level can be established only by prospective studies of workers at risk using sensitive neuropsychological and neuroimaging techniques.

Carbon Monoxide

Carbon monoxide (CO) is a gas produced by vehicular fuel combustion, and by home and industrial energy consumption. Poisoning from CO is common, either from accidental exposure or suicide attempt. CO binds avidly to the hemoglobin in erythrocytes, and the result-

ing carboxyhemoglobin cannot normally transport oxygen to tissues. In the brain, which is extremely sensitive to oxygen deprivation, the acute result is encephalopathy related to anemic hypoxia (Ginsburg, 1985). This syndrome may range from an acute confusional state with inattention, memory loss, and incoordination to irreversible coma and the vegetative state. Similar to other forms of hypoxia, the damage is mainly in the cerebral cortex, hippocampus, basal ganglia, and cerebellum (see discussion following). A unique syndrome that has also been recognized in survivors of CO poisoning is delayed posthypoxic demyelination, which appears within a few weeks of the exposure incident, when recovery appears to be progressing well (Filley & Kleinschmidt-DeMasters, 2001). For unknown reasons, individuals with this complication develop extensive cerebral demyelination that may foreshadow a fatal outcome.

Metals

A number of metals have been implicated in encephalopathy. In clinical practice, a careful history to elicit any accidental or occupational exposure to metals can often be helpful. Lead poisoning has long been recognized as a problem in children with pica, or the compulsive ingestion of leaded paint. In adults, lead poisoning is less common, but can be seen in industrial workers exposed to the metal. Encephalopathy is the prominent neurologic syndrome in poisoned children, whereas adults with lead intoxication are more likely to manifest peripheral neuropathy. In children, acute encephalopathy may be fatal, and cognitive dysfunction is common in those who survive. Even low-level exposure to lead has been shown to be inversely related to neuropsychological development in childhood (Baghurst et al., 1992). Arsenic poisoning is uncommon in the present era, but occasional cases are seen, and both acute and chronic neurobehavioral dysfunction have been associated with leukoencephalopathy (Filley & Kleinschmidt-DeMasters, 2001). Mercury intoxication can be devastating to the cerebrum and cerebellum, causing persistent dementia, visual loss, and ataxia; lasting neuropsychological deficits can also be seen in those with less severe intoxication (Yeates & Mortensen, 1994). Poisoning with manganese occurs mainly in miners of the ore, and an initial confusional state may be followed by chronic parkinsonism and dementia (Yamada et al., 1986). Finally, aluminum has been identified as the cerebral toxin in the encephalopathy associated with dialysis dementia, a progressive disease of renal dialysis patients who were shown to have markedly high levels of aluminum in the brain (see discussion following). This syndrome resembles the dementia of AD in some respects, and it was hypothesized that aluminum could also be responsible for this very

TABLE 28-4. Environmental Toxins Associated with Encephalopathy

Solvents (toluene, other organic solvents)
Carbon monoxide
Metals (lead, arsenic, mercury, manganese, aluminum)
Pesticides (organophosphates, carbamates)

common disorder; however, current opinion generally concurs that genetic factors are probably more important in pathogenesis (Filley, 2001).

Pesticides

Pesticides are widely used throughout the world for insect control in agriculture, and in many homes and businesses. The most commonly used pesticides are the organophosphate compounds and the carbamates, which all act by inhibiting acetylcholinesterase and thereby increasing the available acetylcholine at cholinergic synapses. The organophosphates have become the principal means of agricultural pest control worldwide (Stephens et al., 1995), and are particularly concerning because they irreversibly inhibit acetylcholinesterase; in contrast, drugs commonly used for the treatment of myasthenia gravis, such as pyridostigmine, are reversible inhibitors of the enzyme. Organophosphates are in fact used as chemical warfare agents because of their severe neurotoxicity. Acute cholinergic effects of organophosphate intoxication include headache, vomiting, abdominal cramping, weakness, muscle twitching, diaphoresis, miosis, and bronchial spasm, and a low plasma cholinesterase level can be diagnostic (Jamal, 1997). It is also acknowledged that organophosphates can have both intermediate and delayed effects on the peripheral nervous system (Jamal, 1997). Encephalopathy in exposed persons has been more difficult to establish, although an entity termed chronic organophosphate induced neuropsychiatric disorder (COPIND) has been introduced (Jamal, 1997). Controversy exists concerning the validity of the syndrome, which has reportedly produced a wide range of neurobehavioral and psychiatric syndromes, but for which the mechanism is unknown (Jamal, 1997). Concern appears justified on the basis of controlled studies showing deficits in sustained attention and speed of information processing in farmers exposed to organophosphates in sheep dip (Stephens et al., 1995). However, it is worthwhile recalling that centrally active irreversible acetylcholinesterase inhibitors such as metrifonate have actually been of some benefit for the cognitive loss associated with AD (Cummings et al., 1998). More study of this question is in order in view of the large numbers of individuals throughout the world who are exposed to these compounds.

The issue of organophosphate neurotoxicity is also relevant to the controversial "Gulf War syndrome" reported in many United States military personnel who participated in the Persian Gulf War of 1990 and 1991. Among the many postulated causes of this controversial syndrome is organophosphate exposure, but to date no neurobehavioral syndrome can be plausibly linked with any toxic exposure in the Persian Gulf War (Albers & Berent, 2000).

METABOLIC DISORDERS

The brain is often secondarily affected by primary disease in other organs, including the heart, lungs, liver, kidneys, and endocrine glands. Multisystem involvement is particularly likely to be associated with secondary brain dysfunction. The syndrome of metabolic encephalopathy may thus arise as a general phenomenon in patients with a wide range of medical and surgical diseases (Table 28-5). Although the pathogenesis of brain dysfunction related to metabolic disturbances is poorly understood, and each visceral disease has unique effects on the brain, sufficient similarity exists between these disorders to justify their inclusion under the heading of metabolic encephalopathy.

Circulatory Disturbances

The constant delivery of well-oxygenated blood to the brain is essential for its normal function. Even momentary interruption of this process may prove devastating. A number of cardiopulmonary disorders may compromise cerebral blood flow and oxygenation, leading to various forms of encephalopathy.

Hypoxia-Ischemia

Clinicians routinely use this concept in describing patients with encephalopathy after cardiac arrest, respiratory arrest, or other causes of diminished cerebral oxygenation or blood flow. Although it is often difficult

TABLE 28-5. Metabolic Causes of Encephalopathy

Circulatory disturbances (hypoxia-ischemia, hypertensive encephalopathy)

Pulmonary disease

Disorders of glucose metabolism (hypoglycemia, hyperglycemia)

Endocrinopathies (hypothyroidism, hyperthyroidism, hypoparathyroidism, hyperparathyroidism, Addison disease, Cushing syndrome)

Fluid and electrolyte disturbances (hyponatremia, hypernatremia, central pontine myelinolysis, hypercalcemia)

Hepatic encephalopathy

Renal failure (uremic encephalopathy, dialysis dysequilibrium syndrome, dialysis dementia, transplantation complications)

Vitamin deficiency (thiamine, cobalamin, niacin)

Septic encephalopathy

Organ failure

Postsurgical encephalopathy

to determine whether hypoxia or ischemia predominates, affected patients may have cognitive disturbances ranging from transient acute confusional states to coma, and the severity of the syndrome reflects the degree of cerebral injury. Hypoxia is known to affect certain brain areas preferentially, notably the hippocampus, cerebral cortex, basal ganglia, and cerebellum. Ischemia may affect these and other areas in a variable fashion depending on the adequacy of arterial blood supply. Because of the improved resuscitation of patients with acute cardiovascular disease that has been possible in recent years, hypoxic-ischemic encephalopathy is one of the common causes of vegetative and minimally conscious states (Giacino et al., 1997). Another less common syndrome, considered above as a sequela of carbon monoxide poisoning, is delayed posthypoxic demyelination, which develops days to weeks after the hypoxic event in patients who are apparently recovering from acute encephalopathy (Filley & Kleinschmidt-DeMasters, 2001; Ginsburg, 1985). The pathogenesis of this syndrome is unknown, and recovery is variable.

Hypertensive Encephalopathy

Hypertension is increasingly regarded as damaging to the brain. Acute hypertension is clearly deleterious, and clinicians have long recognized the syndrome of hypertensive encephalopathy as a medical emergency. This disorder is an acute confusional state that results from rapidly developing and severe arterial hypertension. Headache, lethargy, papilledema, visual dysfunction, and seizures are common features of this disease. The pathophysiology involves a breakdown in normal cerebral autoregulation with secondary hyperemia, and edema develops primarily in the cerebral white matter. Neuroimaging with CT and especially MRI can reveal these white matter changes, which are particularly prominent in the parietal and occipital regions (Vaughn & Delanty, 2000). With prompt treatment of elevated blood pressure, the clinical and neuroradiologic features can both resolve. The prognosis for full recovery is thus generally good, but death can occur in untreated cases.

The effects of chronic hypertension have also received considerable attention as a result of recent advances in neuroimaging. Hypertension is now understood to be a strong risk factor for the development of leukoaraiosis, a term referring to the appearance of low-density CT or high-signal MRI changes in the cerebral white matter of older persons (van Gijn, 1998). Although some controversy still prevails, much evidence indicates that leukoaraiosis is associated with cognitive decline, probably when a certain threshold of area is involved (Filley, 1998). Moreover, many believe that leukoaraiosis is likely to be a precursor of the frank dementia seen in Binswanger's disease, a subcortical white matter encephalopathy strongly associated with hypertension (Filley, 1998; van Gijn, 1998). These considerations contribute to an emerging understanding that cerebral white matter disorders of any type can cause cognitive loss or dementia if the degree of involvement is sufficiently extensive (Filley, 1998).

Pulmonary Disease

Respiratory insufficiency from any cause can lead to acute or chronic encephalopathy through a combination of hypoxia, hypercapnia, and respiratory acidosis (Jozefowicz, 1989). Headache and asterixis are common features, and mental status changes usually include drowsiness, inattention, confusion, and forgetfulness. As pulmonary failure advances, stupor and coma may develop. Anoxia that lasts more than four minutes produces irreversible hippocampal damage (Jozefowicz, 1989). Hypercapnia may be revealed by the presence of papilledema, a sign of cerebral edema and increased intracranial pressure; reduction of the PCO_2 by hyperventilation can often prevent irreversible brain damage. In patients with chronic lung disease, renal and other compensatory mechanisms mitigate metabolic derangements, and respiratory insufficiency can exist for protracted periods with minimal neurologic morbidity. Many individuals with chronic obstructive pulmonary disease, for example, do not show significant neuropsychological decline as a feature of their illness, particularly if they are being treated with oxygen (Kozora et al., 1999). Oxygen therapy should be closely monitored, however, because high flow rates may suppress the hypoxic respiratory drive and produce significant carbon dioxide retention (Jozefowicz, 1989).

Disorders of Glucose Metabolism

Glucose is an important metabolic substrate for brain function, and maintenance of a steady supply of glucose is essential. Both hypoglycemia and hyperglycemia have been associated with encephalopathy.

Hypoglycemia

When blood glucose levels fall below normal, a wide range of neurologic symptoms and signs may develop, although a close correlation between hypoglycemia and severity of the clinical syndrome is not always apparent (Malouf & Brust, 1985). Hypoglycemia typically results from overtreatment with insulin or certain oral hypoglycemic agents, and rarely from insulin-secreting tumors of the pancreas. The most common presentation of hypoglycemia is an alteration in mental status, which may be confusion, behavioral change, stupor, or coma (Malouf & Brust, 1985). Coma and even death may occur with extreme hypoglycemia (10 mg/dL or less), and brain damage may be irreversible if the blood sugar level is not promptly corrected. Areas of the brain affected by hypoglycemia are similar to those damaged by hypoxia, although the cerebellum is somewhat less affected (Malouf & Brust, 1985).

Hyperglycemia

Elevated blood glucose may cause several forms of encephalopathy. Diabetic ketoacidosis and nonketotic hyperosmolar coma are well-known complications of diabetes mellitus. A lethargic acute confusional state is typical of diabetic ketoacidosis, which is commonly precipitated by cessation of insulin use (Kaminski & Ruff, 1989). In contrast, focal signs and seizures tend to dominate in the nonketotic hyperosmolar coma, a syndrome that often follows an infection (Kaminski & Ruff, 1989). The neurologic problems caused by these syndromes typically resolve with appropriate treatment. Neuropsychological dysfunction has also been detected in stable diabetic individuals, and impaired performance tends to be associated with severity of disease (Skenazy & Bigler, 1984). Most of the damage to the brain appears to relate to cerebral infarction; diabetes mellitus accelerates atherosclerosis, and the risk of stroke is increased two- to fourfold in diabetic individuals (Kaminski & Ruff, 1989). Increasing evidence also indicates that hyperglycemia may adversely affect the outcome from stroke; conversely, insulin may reduce ischemic damage by lowering peripheral blood glucose, and also by a direct neuroprotective effect on the brain (Auer, 1998).

Endocrinopathies

Diabetes mellitus is the most common endocrine disease capable of producing encephalopathy, but this syndrome is also well known to accompany disorders of the thyroid, parathyroid, and adrenal glands. Many of these syndromes are fully reversible if recognized early and treated appropriately.

Hypothyroidism

Diminished thyroid function has a plethora of adverse neurologic effects, including myopathy, peripheral neuropathy, cranial nerve dysfunction, cerebellar ataxia, psychosis, dementia, coma, and seizures. Changes in mental state are common; apathy, inattention, and cognitive slowing may occur with mild hypothyroidism, prompting the routine evaluation of thyroid function in the evaluation of dementia (Kaminski & Ruff, 1989). With more severe hypothyroidism, dementia can appear as well as frank psychosis and even coma (Kaminski & Ruff, 1989). Myxedema coma has a poor prognosis, with death in at least 50% of those individuals affected

(Kaminski & Ruff, 1989). Recovery of mental function in individuals with dementia from hypothyroidism is variable, but more likely and more complete if the thyroid dysfunction has been of short duration.

Hyperthyroidism

Similar to its counterpart of low secretion, excessive production or ingestion of thyroid hormone may lead to many neurologic disturbances, including myopathy, peripheral neuropathy, movement disorders, optic neuropathy, and exophthalmic ophthalmoplegia. Neurobehavioral manifestations are common. Patients with this disorder may be restless, irritable, and hypervigilant, and with more prolonged disease, psychosis, dementia, and coma can appear. Especially in the elderly, so-called "apathetic hyperthyroidism" can develop, misleading the clinician and potentially obscuring the diagnosis (Kaminski & Ruff, 1989). Thyroid storm is a severe hyperaroused acute confusional state that is usually fatal if left untreated (Kaminski & Ruff, 1989).

Hypoparathyroidism

This disorder results from deficient secretion of parathyroid hormone. The parathyroid glands are centrally involved in calcium metabolism, and parathyroid dysfunction results in prominent hypocalcemia (see below), hypophosphatemia, and often hypomagnesemia (Kaminski & Ruff, 1989). Calcification of the basal ganglia with parkinsonism and choreoathetosis can be seen. Intellectual impairment, dementia, mania, and schizophrenia have all been described in primary hypoparathyroidism (Kaminski & Ruff, 1989). Similar clinical sequelae can follow the onset of pseudohypoparathyroidism, in which hypocalcemia results from defective tissue responsiveness to parathyroid hormone.

Hyperparathyroidism

Excessive secretion of parathyroid hormone occurs because of primary parathormone excess or ectopic parathormone production from neoplasms of the lung, kidney, ovary, uterus, and pancreas. Some hyperparathyroid patients present with an acute confusional state, and others may have cognitive slowing and psychiatric dysfunction (Kaminski & Ruff, 1989). Hypercalcemia (see discussion following) is present, and alertness decreases with a rising calcium level; however, the severity of encephalopathy is not fully explained by the degree of calcium elevation (Kaminski & Ruff, 1989). If the syndrome is severe and prolonged, the confusional state may advance into stupor and coma.

Addison Disease

Primary adrenal insufficiency, or Addison disease, is a presumed autoimmune disorder of the adrenal glands that causes lowered serum cortisol, pigmentation of the skin, hypotension, hyponatremia, muscle weakness, and mental status alterations. Tuberculosis was a common cause of Addison disease in the past, and occasionally metastatic tumors can be responsible. Adrenal insufficiency also occurs in adrenoleukodystrophy, an X-linked disease mostly seen in children that also involves dysmyelination of the brain, spinal cord, and peripheral nerves. Addison disease may produce an acute confusional state that progresses to stupor and coma or, less dramatically, symptoms of irritability, depression, and psychosis (Kaminski & Ruff, 1989). Seizures may occur because of associated hyponatremia (see below).

Cushing Syndrome

Cushing syndrome is a term referring to cases of hypercortisolism secondary to prescribed corticosteroids, adenomas of the adrenal cortex, and pulmonary carcinomas that produce adrenocorticotrophin (ACTH). In contrast, Cushing disease results from a pituitary adenoma secreting excessive ACTH. Cushing syndrome can lead to numerous psychiatric complications—mania, depression, psychosis—in up to 70% of patients, and many patients may also have cognitive disturbances (Kaminski & Ruff, 1989). In practice, these features are most commonly seen in patients receiving high doses of corticosteroids for other medical problems who develop so-called "steroid psychosis." Cognitive dysfunction can also occur in Cushing syndrome. Recent evidence has implicated glucocorticoid excess as a cause of hippocampal atrophy, and this finding has been correlated with deficits in explicit memory; treatment is crucial, as it appears that this atrophy is reversible with normalization of the serum cortisol (Sapolsky, 2000).

Fluid and Electrolyte Disturbances

In general, fluid and electrolyte disturbances may affect both central and peripheral nervous systems, but disturbances of sodium and calcium metabolism are specifically associated with encephalopathy (Riggs, 1989). In most cases, these abnormalities represent functional alterations in nervous system function, and recovery is complete with prompt therapy. Severe derangements, however, can be associated with a poor outcome and, in some cases, structural brain disease.

Hyponatremia

Hyponatremia is the most frequent electrolyte disturbance in clinical medicine (Gross et al., 1996), and an alteration of mental status is its most common manifestation (Riggs, 1989). Most patients with hyponatremia are also hypo-osmolar, and the causes of hypo-osmolar hyponatremia include the syndrome of inappropriate secretion of antidiuretic hormone (SIADH), various drugs including carbamazepine, and acute or chronic renal failure (Riggs, 1989). The encephalopathy may range from a mild acute confusional state to coma. Symptoms and signs are more frequent and severe if the lowering of sodium is acute; thus, a patient with an abrupt onset of a sodium level of 130 meq/L may experience more neurologic symptoms than one who has had a gradual decline to a level of 115 meq/L. However, seizures are always more likely at very low sodium levels (less than 115 meq/L), and may portend a mortality of 50% (Riggs, 1989); in such cases, immediate treatment with hypertonic saline to produce a level of 120–125 meq/L is appropriate (Riggs, 1989). In cases of less severe hyponatremia, fluid restriction is generally the preferred strategy.

Central Pontine Myelinolysis

Aggressive treatment of hyponatremia can also, however, have an adverse effect. Central pontine myelinolysis (CPM) is a syndrome of osmotic demyelination that affects the central pons, and often extrapontine areas as well, as a result of overly rapid correction of hyponatremia (Laureno & Karp, 1997). The disorder affects those individuals with alcoholism and malnutrition primarily, although not all cases have these predisposing factors. Clinical manifestations may include mild confusion, spastic quadriparesis, pseudobulbar palsy, and coma (Laureno & Karp, 1997). Recovery is now possible in a substantial proportion of patients, reflecting improved treatment that has evolved with a better understanding of pathogenesis. A consensus has gradually developed that CPM can be avoided by limiting correction of chronic hyponatremia to less than 10 meq/L in any 24-hour period (Laureno & Karp, 1997).

Hypernatremia

Symptoms and signs of hypernatremia are most often referable to the CNS, and typically appear with serum levels above 160 meq/L (Riggs, 1989). Changes in mental status ranging from lethargy to coma are the most common manifestations of this disorder (Riggs, 1989). Hypernatremia results from dehydration, and patients are typically hyperosmolar as well. This disorder is most common in the very young (often from gastroenteritis) and the very old (who may be unable to obtain adequate water because of disability). Rehydration is indicated, although seizures may occur during this process (Riggs, 1989). Diabetes insipidus, which results from low levels of antidiuretic hormone, can also cause hypernatremia, although ordinarily this is averted by sufficient water intake.

Hypocalcemia

Hypocalcemia occurs in patients with hypoparathyroidism, recent parathyroid or thyroid surgery, renal failure, and acute pancreatitis (Riggs, 1989). Changes in mental status and seizures are the most common neurologic manifestations. Mental alterations are numerous, and may include irritability, confusion, delusions, hallucinations, depression, and dementia (Riggs, 1989). Chorea and parkinsonism can be seen in the setting of chronic hypocalcemia, possibly explained by the deposition of calcium in the basal ganglia (Riggs, 1989).

Hypercalcemia

This syndrome usually occurs in patients with malignant neoplasms and in those with hyperparathyroidism (Riggs, 1989). The tumors most implicated in hypercalcemia are breast cancer, lung cancer, and multiple myeloma; elevated calcium is a result of either osteolytic skeletal metastases or elevated levels of circulating parathormone. In primary hyperparathyroidism, excessive release of parathyroid hormone produces the syndrome. Elevations of serum calcium above 14 mg/dL commonly give rise to an acute lethargic confusional state that progresses to stupor and coma if left untreated. If the serum albumin is low and the ionized calcium increased, the same features can appear at calcium levels of 10–12 mg/dL (Riggs, 1989).

Hepatic Encephalopathy

This syndrome, also known as portal-systemic encephalopathy, is a major neurobehavioral complication of cirrhosis of the liver (Butterworth, 2000). Hepatic encephalopathy characteristically appears in individuals with severe liver disease who receive an oral load of protein, sustain gastrointestinal bleeding, or take sedative medications (Butterworth, 2000). Affected patients develop insidious or abrupt onset of personality change, inattention, altered sleep, and confusion, and progression to stupor and coma may occur; asterixis and rigidity are common. Even in cirrhotic patients who have a normal neurologic examination, neuropsychological deficits have been shown in up to 84% (Butterworth, 2000), highlighting the potential for major neurobehavioral effects of hepatic disease. The pathophysiology of hepatic encephalopathy involves the accumulation of excessive ammonia in the brain (Butterworth, 2000), but the details of pathogenesis are still unclear. Manganese toxicity may play a role; the most common finding on brain MRI scans of cirrhotic patients is T1 hyperintensity in the globus pallidus bilaterally that may represent manganese deposition. Neuropathologically, no consistent neuronal change has been documented in hepatic encephalopathy, and the most significant finding is hyperplasia of abnormal glial cells known as Alzheimer type II astrocytes (Butterworth, 2000). Astrocytes are the only cells in the brain that can metabolize ammonia, and they appear to be its major cerebral target (Butterworth, 2000). Changes in neurotransmitter function may relate to the astrocytic "gliopathy" and explain the neurologic features of this disorder (Butterworth, 2000). Treatment involves ammonia-lowering strategies that include restricting dietary protein, and the use of lactulose, neomycin, sodium benzoate, and L-ornithine-aspartate (Butterworth, 2000). Liver transplantation is also an option for some individuals, and can result in significant clinical improvement.

Repeated episodes of hepatic encephalopathy, especially with coma, can eventuate in a lasting dementia syndrome with prominent extrapyramidal features, the so-called acquired (non-Wilsonian) hepatocerebral degeneration (Brust, 1998). The neuropathology of this dementia features necrosis and neuronal death in the cortex and basal ganglia—regions also affected by astrocytic hyperplasia in hepatic encephalopathy—suggesting that repeated episodes of encephalopathy can lead to structural damage that supersedes functional derangements.

Renal Failure

The systemic complications of renal failure are protean, and the nervous system is no exception. Uremia may affect both the peripheral and central nervous systems, and in the brain, the effects can manifest as a wide variety of acute and chronic syndromes (Burn & Bates, 1998).

Uremic Encephalopathy

As is true of many metabolic disorders, uremic encephalopathy usually begins insidiously and may be subtle in its early stages. Fatigue, apathy, impaired attention and concentration, and clumsiness may not be clinically evident at first, but they may progress, or other symptoms soon develop, to clarify the picture (Burn & Bates, 1998). A frontal lobe syndrome with personality change, impaired abstract reasoning, emotionally lability, and frontal release signs can be seen, and with further progression, agitated confusional states, stupor, and coma can appear (Burn & Bates, 1998). A wide range of motor signs can occur in uremia, including multifocal myclonus, asterixis, rigidity, focal weakness, hyperreflexia, ankle clonus, and extensor plantar responses, and seizures, either focal or generalized, are frequent (Burn & Bates, 1998). On neuropsychological testing, deficits in sustained attention and cognitive speed are most typically detected (Burn & Bates, 1998). The pathophysiology of uremic encephalopathy is uncertain; initially, a defect in neurotransmission at the synaptic level is likely, and in later stages, it is possible that aluminum accumulation contributes to the deposition of amyloid in the cerebral cortex (Burn & Bates, 1998). Uremic encephalopathy is unrelated to AD, however, as neurofibrillary tangles are not commonly found in the brains of patients with uremia (Burn & Bates, 1998).

Dialysis Dysequilibrium Syndrome

This is a syndrome of headache, restlessness, muscle cramps, and nausea that develops in the setting of either peritoneal dialysis or hemodialysis; usually arising at the end of the dialysis session, it resolves over several hours (Burn & Bates, 1998). In more severe cases, myoclonus and an agitated confusional state can persist for days (Burn & Bates, 1998). The syndrome develops because of an osmotic gradient between plasma and the brain during rapid dialysis, and prevention can usually be achieved by a "slow" dialysis (Burn & Bates, 1998).

Dialysis Dementia

Also known as dialysis encephalopathy, this is a progressive dementing disease of hemodialysis patients now known to be a result of cerebral aluminum toxicity (Alfrey et al., 1976; Burn & Bates, 1998). Early features include dysarthria, apathy, depression, aphasia, and apraxia, and as the disease progresses, ataxia, myoclonus, seizures, and psychosis become evident (Burn & Bates, 1998). Aluminum in the dialysate water supply was determined to be responsible; reduction of this concentration prevents the onset of dialysis dementia, and may improve established cases that still occasionally appear (Burn & Bates, 1998). The disease is now thought to relate to the use of phosphate-binding gels such as aluminum hydroxide and other factors (Burn & Bates, 1998). This syndrome has also proved relevant to the study of AD, as it appeared to support other evidence that aluminum toxicity might be pathogenetic; however, whereas neurofibrillary tangles do appear in the brains of patients with dialysis dementia, these tangles are morphologically and regionally distinct from those of AD (Burn & Bates, 1998), and excess neuritic plaques are not found.

Transplantation Complications

Renal transplantation has become an increasingly common procedure as surgical techniques and immunosuppressive therapies continue to improve. With this advance, however, comes the increased risk of two diseases to which the chronically immunosuppressed are vulnerable: progressive multifocal leukoencephalopathy and primary central nervous system lymphoma (Burn & Bates, 1998). Another neurobehavioral complication of uremia is the leukoencephalopathy that occurs in some renal transplant patients who receive the immunosuppressive drugs cyclosporine or tacrolimus (Burn & Bates, 1998; Filley & Kleinschmidt-DeMasters, 2001). This is typically a posterior leukoencephalopathy that is well seen on MRI scans, and patients manifest confusion, visual disturbances, and sometimes seizures; recovery is the rule after the responsible drug is discontinued (Filley & Kleinschmidt-DeMasters, 2001).

Vitamin Deficiency

A number of nutritional disorders can produce acute or chronic encephalopathy, or in some cases both. These examples point out the potential impact that primary care may have, as adequate nutrition and medical care can in most cases easily prevent these complications.

Thiamine

Deficiency of thiamine, vitamin B_1, is common in chronic alcoholics who unknowingly rely on alcohol for their caloric intake and thus do not receive adequate nutrition (Victor, 1993). The Wernicke-Korsakoff syndrome, which results from dietary thiamine deficiency, is well recognized in neurology and emergency medicine as a cause of an acute encephalopathy with confusion, ophthalmoplegia, and ataxia (Wernicke's encephalopathy) followed by a chronic amnestic state (known as Korsakoff's psychosis). The features of Wernicke's encephalopathy improve within hours if thiamine is given early, but if this therapy is not provided, permanent dysfunction may develop. The amnesia of Korsakoff's psychosis may be disabling, although some patients can experience considerable improvement.

Cobalamin

This vitamin, commonly known as vitamin B_{12}, is classically associated with pernicious anemia and megaloblastosis. However, more recent information indicates that clinically significant cobalamin deficiency can occur with no evidence of hematologic abnormality (Lindenbaum et al., 1988). Neurologic manifestations of cobalamin deficiency include dementia and neuropsychiatric dysfunction (Lindenbaum et al., 1988), as well as familiar subacute combined degeneration of the spinal cord. Cobalamin levels are thus commonly measured in the evaluation of dementia, and levels below 300 pg/mL should be considered suspicious. Deficiency of folate is less likely to produce nervous system complications, but on rare occasions it can produce a dementia similar to that of cobalamin deficiency.

Niacin

A deficiency of niacin (nicotinic acid) is rare but occasionally occurs in diseases characterized by chronic dietary neglect, such as alcoholism, or from other causes of poor nutrition. Pellagra is the disease state produced by niacin deficiency, and in addition to dermatitis, diarrhea, and glossitis, both acute and chronic encephalopathy have been described (Brust, 1998).

Septic Encephalopathy

Clinicians have long recognized that acute infectious diseases such as pneumonia and urinary tract infections can have detrimental effects on mentation, particularly in older persons. This observation is still more apparent in those with sepsis. Patients who are acutely ill with septicemia develop encephalopathy, but relatively little attention has been devoted to this problem. Most individuals with proven sepsis have an acute confusional state, which may include inattention, disorientation, dysgraphia, inappropriate behavior, paratonia, and obtundation (Young et al., 1990). Focal neurologic signs are uncommon (Young et al., 1990). Encephalopathy has been suspected of being one of the earliest and most common manifestations of sepsis (Young, 1995). A diffuse effect on the brain that parallels systemic disease is suspected, but the pathogenesis of septic encephalopathy is unknown (Young et al., 1990; Young, 1995). This issue is complicated by the fact that septic patients always have one or more of several other possible causes of encephalopathy, including dysfunction of multiple organs and a variety of centrally acting medications.

Organ Failure

As discussed above, dysfunction of many different organs in critically ill patients may also produce encephalopathy (Young, 1995). When many organs are involved, the secondary effects on the brain are amplified. Encephalopathy as a complication of organ failure is extremely common, as would be expected from the fact that the homeostatic equilibrium of the patient is compromised by many factors. Acute confusional states frequently herald the onset of multiorgan failure, and in some cases may represent a preterminal event. This complication can also significantly retard recovery. For example, septic encephalopathy in combination with critical illness polyneuropathy can interfere with the vital task of weaning patients off the ventilator (Young, 1995).

Postsurgical Encephalopathy

A frequent setting in which acute confusional states are seen is in the postoperative period (Dyer et al., 1995).

This complication usually arises within the first few days of surgery, but may appear any time in the first 2 weeks. Although the incidence of this problem is uncertain, postoperative delirium may occur in as many as 37% of surgical patients (Dyer et al., 1995). Many factors contribute to this syndrome, including hypoxia during surgery, infection, electrolyte imbalance, atelectasis with hypoxemia, loss of sleep, and analgesic and sedative medications. Age, preoperative cognitive impairment, and the use of anticholinergic drugs all appear to be particularly important (Dyer et al., 1995).

Long-term neurobehavioral effects of surgery are also beginning to be examined. One of the emerging areas of interest in recent years is the cognitive syndrome that develops after coronary artery bypass graft surgery (Llinas et al., 2000; Newman et al., 2001). In addition to toxic-metabolic encephalopathy, cardiac surgery in general can result in hemispheric strokes and hypoxic injury that cause lasting encephalopathy (Llinas et al., 2000). Formal study of the long-term effects of coronary artery bypass graft surgery has been initiated, and one group has reported that 53% of patients had cognitive decline at discharge, many of whom had continuing cognitive dysfunction 5 years later (Newman et al., 2001). The mechanism of the perioperative injury is uncertain, but the data imply that neurobehavioral disturbances can persist for years in many patients after major surgery.

PATHOPHYSIOLOGY

Encephalopathy is a syndrome of diffuse brain involvement. Although some encephalopathies can present with focal neurologic features, the neurobehavioral aspects of encephalopathy result from widespread functional or structural disruption of cerebral areas. The domains of arousal and attention are typically the most vulnerable to toxic and metabolic disturbances. Patients with encephalopathy manifest fluctuations in level of consciousness that stem from dysfunction in brainstem and thalamic regions responsible for arousal. Simultaneously, they show signs of confusion that likely reflect dysfunction in thalamo-cortical systems and their white matter connections (Filley, 2001). Because some patients with subtle encephalopathy have no disturbance in arousal but still show impaired attention, the attentional deficit is considered the most consistent—even the defining—feature of encephalopathy (Mesulam, 2000; Filley, 2001).

It is possible to speculate at this point that the pathophysiology of acute encephalopathy can be distinguished from the chronic alterations of mental status that have been described as a chronic confusional state. The early phase may be related to functional changes in neurotransmission or synaptic function, whereas chronic encephalopathy may imply a greater degree of structural damage. Considerable evidence suggests that acute encephalopathy may result from alterations in neurotransmitter function (Chan & Brennan, 1999). Among the neurotransmitters implicated are acetylcholine, dopamine, serotonin, gamma-aminobutyric acid, and beta-endorphin (Chan & Brennan, 1999). Acetylcholine appears to be the most culpable because of the well-known propensity of anticholinergic drugs to produce confusion; patients with AD, the most common irreversible dementia, are especially susceptible to anticholinergic effects because of the profound central cholinergic deficit that characterizes this disease (Chan & Brennan, 1999). Dopamine may also be important in view of the improvement in confusion that can be seen with dopamine-blocking agents such as the neuroleptics (Chan & Brennan, 1999). These considerations suggest that pharmacologic manipulation of various neurotransmitter systems may have therapeutic value.

Conversely, lasting structural damage may help explain the chronic encephalopathy that develops when toxic or metabolic insults are severe or prolonged (Filley & Kleinschmidt-DeMasters, 2001). Many patients so affected develop a dementia syndrome that resembles subcortical dementia (Filley, 2001), implying that toxic and metabolic disorders can exert lasting structural effects on deep cerebral regions mediating arousal and attention. Numerous examples of this phenomenon can be found in the toxic leukoencephalopathies; toluene, radiation, and cancer chemotherapeutic agents can all produce permanent structural injury in the subcortical white matter (Filley & Kleinschmidt-DeMasters, 2001), justifying the term white matter dementia in these cases (Filley, 1998). In addition, neuropathologic changes in the cortex may also appear. In hepatic encephalopathy, for example, the initial episodes of ammonia intoxication that interfere with neurotransmitter function are then succeeded by astrocytic and neuronal injury that conspire to produce the lasting dementia of hepatocerebral degeneration.

TREATMENT

The treatment of encephalopathy begins with accurate diagnosis. In the acute setting, the first imperative is to identify neurologic and neurosurgical emergencies for which immediate treatment is critical. These include meningitis, encephalitis, elevated intracranial pressure from a variety of mass lesions, acute stroke, and status epilepticus (Feske, 1998). When these etiologies can be excluded, a toxic or metabolic cause becomes more likely. If the encephalopathy arises subacutely or over a protracted period, structural lesions must still be excluded, but toxic and metabolic disorders are generally more likely to be responsible.

Encephalopathy from toxic and metabolic causes requires both medical and neurologic attention (Table 28-6).

The principles of treatment, which formally apply to the management of the acute confusional state (Feske, 1998; Chan & Brennan, 1999), are equally useful in the care of individuals with chronic encephalopathy. In all encephalopathic patients, the goal is to address the relevant medical issues while simultaneously attending to the special problems raised by the neurobehavioral dysfunction associated with confusion.

Prevention of the problem is crucial when possible, and involves effective primary care and management of chronic medical problems to prevent the development of encephalopathy. This approach is clearly the most cost-effective way to deal with this increasingly prevalent problem because it can often avert the substantial costs of hospitalization that may otherwise be necessary. In younger persons, primary prevention of alcohol and drug abuse is an enormous challenge, but efforts in this regard can have lasting benefits. Particularly in older individuals, minimization of the number of prescription drugs is critical, and a periodic review of the medication list is recommended. Alcohol and over-the-counter drug use should also be monitored in older patients, as amounts of these substances that seem innocuous in younger healthy persons may have significant adverse effects in older or chronically ill individuals. Equally important is the maintenance of normal metabolic homeostasis by regular follow-up

TABLE 28-6. Treatment of Encephalopathy

Medical
  Prevention
    Management of chronic medical problems
    Minimization of drug regimen and medication doses
    Avoidance of other toxins
  Attention to the primary disorder
    Complete history and physical examination
    Laboratory tests, brain imaging (CT or MRI), LP, and EEG
    Specific treatment (e.g., naloxone, flumazenil, thiamine, glucose, oxygen)
Neurologic
  Environmental changes
    Clock, calendar, television, radio
    Visits from family members or friends
    Night light
  Medications
    Haloperidol 0.5 to 2.0 mg PO or IM every 4 hours PRN
    Risperidone 0.5 to 1.0 mg PO twice daily PRN
    Lorazepam 0.5 to 2.0 mg PO, IM, or IV every 1–4 hours PRN
    Chloral hydrate 500–1000 mg PO QHS PRN

of chronic metabolic disorders such as diabetes mellitus, cardiac disease, pulmonary insufficiency, renal dysfunction, hepatic disease, and various endocrinopathies.

When toxic-metabolic encephalopathy does occur, accurate evaluation is the key, followed by immediate attention to the causative insult. Little need be added to the recommendation that rapid diagnosis and treatment of the primary problem is essential. Many disorders causing encephalopathy can be readily corrected or improved with prompt recognition, and details of these interventions can be found in standard medical textbooks. Examples of immediate treatments that may be effective are naloxone and flumazenil for opiate and benzodiazepine overdose, respectively, glucose for hypoglycemia, thiamine for Wernicke-Korsakoff syndrome, and oxygen for hypoxia (Feske, 1998). A key point to remember is that the recovery from encephalopathy may be less rapid than expected even when the cause is discovered and treated. Older persons and those who have multiple causes of their syndrome may require substantially longer to recover than other patients. Thus considerable patience may be necessary in the treatment of encephalopathy. It may also be the case that more impaired individuals may have a less-than-complete recovery.

More relevant to the behavioral neurologist and neuropsychologist are the challenges presented by patients who have encephalopathy that has not responded satisfactorily to initial interventions. Examples include the delirious patient on a detoxification unit and the mildly confused individual referred for neuropsychological evaluation. These cases may have as yet undetermined etiologies of their encephalopathy, diseases for which there is no curative treatment, or encephalopathies that have not yet responded to the appropriate treatment. Many issues of management at this stage are important. It is crucial to optimize treatment so that the evaluation can proceed efficiently and the causes of the syndrome accurately identified. Some patients will remain encephalopathic for days to weeks before a clear understanding of their syndrome emerges.

A broad range of nonpharmacologic and pharmacologic interventions are available for the treatment of encephalopathic individuals (see Table 28-6). Often overlooked are the environmental changes that can substantially improve the agitation of acutely confused patients. These measures may also find use in the longer-term management of those with chronic encephalopathy. Because patients are typically disoriented, constant reminders such as clocks, calendars, television, and radio are useful, and frequent visits from family and friends are desirable. These simple procedures are especially important in older persons who may have baseline sensory deprivation because of visual loss, poor hearing, and sensory neuropathy. To deal with the frequent problem of "sundowning," or the deterioration in mental status during the evening hours,

a night light can help prevent excessive confusion and ensure a better sleep.

The need for effective pharmacologic intervention must always be balanced by the risk of exacerbating the problem by the therapy. As a general rule, the use of drugs for encephalopathy, particularly in the acute setting, should be limited to the lowest effective dose and the shortest possible duration of therapy. A standing order of a potent drug may inadvertently result in cumulative neurotoxicity, and frequent review of the need for ongoing treatment is imperative. The most effective and least hazardous group of medications in this setting is the neuroleptics. Haloperidol is a high-potency antipsychotic agent that has been used extensively for acute encephalopathy (Chan & Brennan, 1999). A newer drug of this group is risperidone, a welcome advance in the field because its relatively low risk of extrapyramidal side effects permit its use in individuals with Parkinson disease (PD) or parkinsonism from some other cause (Feske, 1998). Benzodiazepines such as lorazepam are most useful in the short-term treatment of alcohol or benzodiazepine withdrawal, but long-term use of these drugs is not recommended because of the risks of oversedation and drug dependence. Chloral hydrate can be an effective soporific drug.

PROGNOSIS

The prognosis for patients with encephalopathy is unknown with certainty. Some individuals with acute confusional state may have easily reversible disorders and recover within days, whereas others may exhibit deficits lasting for months or years (Chan & Brennan, 1999). The issue is complex because of the heterogeneity of this syndrome; a widely variable prognosis may be expected, depending on the magnitude of the acute insult, the promptness with which treatment is provided, patient age, associated medical problems, and the degree of premorbid cognitive impairment. Studies on prognosis reflect this variablity; in some patient groups, full recovery has been reported to occur within a single day in two thirds of patients, but, in other groups, less than one fifth of the patients will have complete resolution at 6 months after hospital discharge (Chan & Brennan, 1999).

The prognosis for prolonged encephalopathy is still less certain. Whereas this syndrome may result from structural brain damage (Filley & Kleinschmidt-DeMasters, 2001), the pathogenesis of this kind of impairment is often unclear. It can also be difficult to distinguish lasting encephalopathy from subcortical (PD) or cortical (AD) degenerative dementias that frequently coexist in older persons. Despite every reasonable effort to find and treat reversible causes of encephalopathy, some individuals will not exhibit substantial recovery. It can generally be stated that chronic encephalopathy from toxic and metabolic insults becomes increasingly less reversible with a greater number of insults, a longer duration of the offending problem(s), and an older patient age.

CONCLUSION

Encephalopathy is a common neurologic syndrome seen in a variety of medical, surgical, and psychiatric settings. In this chapter, encephalopathy resulting from toxic and metabolic disorders has been emphasized, and the number of such disorders is large and expanding. Affected individuals may present with florid delirium, or, more commonly, signs of lethargy, drowsiness, and somnolence. In either instance, the unifying feature of encephalopathy is confusion, which fundamentally results from disturbed attention. Most causes of encephalopathy can be addressed effectively if they are detected, and this syndrome is one of the most reversible in neurology. Even patients with dementia (the chronic confusional state) from toxic and metabolic derangements can often be significantly improved, although, as a general rule, the longer the encephalopathy has been present, the less likely full recovery will be. In any case, early diagnosis and treatment are essential.

The pathogenesis of encephalopathy is poorly understood, and the mechanism of brain dysfunction in the many varieties of this syndrome remain to be elucidated. In neurobehavioral terms, however, the recognition that prominent disruption in arousal and particularly attention is central to the syndrome offers the opportunity to develop a deeper understanding of these basic brain functions. Evidence increasingly points to functional derangements as pathogenetic in acute encephalopathy—at the level of the synapse and neurotransmitter function—and to structural change as important in chronic encephalopathy. In this regard, encephalopathy illuminates many aspects of the normal and abnormal operations of neural networks that are indispensable for normal neurobehavioral function.

◼ KEY POINTS

☐ Encephalopathy may result from a wide range of toxic and metabolic disorders that disturb brain function by disrupting the homeostatic equilibrium of the internal milieu.

☐ The most common neurobehavioral syndrome in patients with encephalopathy from toxic and metabolic disorders is the acute confusional state.

☐ The diagnosis of encephalopathy rests on an accurate history, physical and neurologic examination with emphasis on the mental state, and selected laboratory and neuroimaging tests.

☐ Treatment of encephalopathy involves prevention when possible, prompt attention to the primary disorder, and management of the acute syndrome with appropriate environmental and pharmacologic interventions.

☐ The progress of encephalopathy is usually favorable, but the outcome may be influenced by the severity of the insult(s), promptness of treatment, patient age, associated medical problems, and the degree of premorbid cognitive impairment.

KEY READINGS

Brust JCM: Acute neurologic complications of drug and alcohol abuse. Neurol Clin N Am 16:503–19, 1998.

Feske SJ: Coma and confusional states: Emergency diagnosis and management. Neurol Clin N Am 16:237–56, 1998.

Meador KJ: Cognitive side effects of medications. Neurol Clin N Am 16:141–55, 1998.

REFERENCES

Albers JW, Berent S: Controversies in neurotoxicology: Current status. Neurol Clin 18:741–763, 2000.

Alfrey AC, Legendre GR, Kaehny WD: The dialysis encephalopathy syndrome: Possible aluminum intoxication. N Engl J Med 294:184–188, 1976.

Arlien-Soborg P, Bruhn P, Glydensted C, Melgarrd B: Chronic painters' syndrome: Chronic toxic encephalopathy in house painters. Acta Neurol Scand 60:149–156, 1979.

Auer RN: Insulin, blood glucose levels, and ischemic brain damage. Neurology 51(Suppl. 3):S39–S43, 1998.

Baghurst PA, McMichael AJ, Wigg NR, et al: Environmental exposure to lead and children's intelligence at the age of seven years: The Port Pirie Cohort Study. N Engl J Med 327:1279–1284, 1992.

Bolla KI, McCann UD, Ricaurte GA: Memory impairment in abstinent MDMA ("Ecstasy") users. Neurology 51:1532–1537, 1998.

Brust JCM: Acute neurologic complications of drug and alcohol abuse. Neurol Clin N Am 16:503–519, 1998.

Burn DJ, Bates D: Neurology and the kidney. J Neurol Neurosurg Psychiatry 65:810–821, 1998.

Butterworth RF: Complications of cirrhosis III: Hepatic encephalopathy. J Hepatol 32(Suppl. 1):171–180, 2000.

Chan D, Brennan NJ: Delirium: Making the diagnosis, improving the prognosis. Geriatrics 54:28–42, 1999.

Cummings JL, Cyrus PA, Bieber F, et al: Metrifonate treatment of the cognitive deficits of Alzheimer's disease. Metrifonate Study Group. Neurology 50:1214–1221, 1998.

Dyer CB, Ashton CM, Teasdale TA: Postoperative delirium: A review of 80 primary data collection studies. Arch Intern Med 13:461–465, 1995.

Feske SK: Coma and confusional states: Emergency diagnosis and management. Neurol Clin N Am 16:237–256, 1998.

Filley CM: The behavioral neurology of cerebral white matter. Neurology 50:1535–1540, 1998.

Filley CM, Rosenberg NL, Heaton RK: White matter dementia in chronic toluene abuse. Neurology 40:532–534, 1990.

Filley CM: Neurobehavioral Anatomy, ed 2. Boulder, CO: University Press of Colorado, 2001.

Filley CM, Kleinschmidt-DeMasters BK: Toxic leukoencephalopathy. N Engl J Med 345:425–432, 2001.

Giacino JT, Zasler ND, Katz DI, et al: Development of practice guidelines for assessment and management of the vegetative and minimally conscious states. J Head Trauma Rehab 12:79–89, 1997.

Ginsburg MD: Carbon monoxide intoxication: Clinical features, neuropathology and mechanisms of injury. J Toxicol Clin Toxicol 23:281–288, 1985.

Gross P, Wehrle R, Bussemaker E: Hyponatremia: Pathophysiology, differential diagnosis, and new aspects of treatment. Clin Nephrol 46:273–276, 1996.

Hormes JT, Filley CM, Rosenberg NL: Neurologic sequelae of chronic solvent vapor abuse. Neurology 36:698–702, 1986.

Jamal GA: Neurological syndromes of organophosphorus compounds. Adverse Drug React Toxicol Rev 16:133–170, 1997.

Jozefowicz RF: Neurologic manifestations of pulmonary disease. Neurol Clin 7:605–616, 1989.

Kaminski HJ, Ruff RL: Neurologic complications of endocrine diseases. Neurol Clin 7:489–508, 1989.

Katzman R, Lasker B, Bernstein N: Advances in the diagnosis of dementia: Accuracy of diagnosis and consequences of misdiagnosis of disorders causing dementia. Aging Brain 32:17–62, 1988.

Kozora E, Filley CM, Julian LJ, Cullum CM: Cognitive functioning in patients with mild chronic obstructive pulmonary disease and mild hypoxemia compared with patients with mild Alzheimer's disease and normal controls. Neuropsychiatry Neuropsychol Behav Neurol 12:178–183, 1999.

Laureno R, Karp BI: Myelinolysis after correction of hyponatremia. Ann Intern Med 126:57–62, 1997.

Lindenbaum J, Healton EB, Savage DG, et al: Neuropsychiatric disorders caused by cobalamin deficiency in the absence of anemia or macrocytosis. N Engl J Med 318:1720–1728, 1988.

Lishman WA: Cerebral disorder in alcoholism: Syndromes of impairment. Brain 104:1–20, 1981.

Llinas R, Barbut D, Caplan LR: Neurologic complications of cardiac surgery. Prog Cardiovasc Dis 43:101–112, 2000.

Malouf R, Brust JCM: Hypoglycemia: Causes, neurological manifestations, and outcome. Ann Neurol 17:421–430, 1985.

Meador KJ: Cognitive side effects of medications. Neurol Clin N Am 16:141–155, 1998.

Mesulam MM: Attentional networks, confusional states, and neglect syndromes, in Mesulam MM (ed): Principles of Behavioral and Cognitive Neurology, ed 2. Oxford, UK: Oxford University Press, 2000, pp. 174–256.

Moore AR, O'Keefe ST: Drug-induced cognitive impairment in the elderly. Drugs Aging 15:15–28, 1999.

Newman MF, Kirchner JL, Phillips-Bute B, et al: Longitudinal assessment of neurocognitive function after coronary-artery bypass surgery. N Engl J Med 344:395–402, 2001.

Pope HG, Gruber AJ, Yurgelan-Todd D: The residual neuropsychological effects of cannabis: The current status of research. Drug Alcohol Depend 38:25–34, 1995.

Riggs JE: Neurologic manifestations of fluid and electrolyte disturbances. Neurol Clin 7:509–523, 1989.

Rosenberg NL, Kleinschmidt-DeMasters BK, Davis KA, et al: Toluene abuse causes diffuse central nervous system white matter changes. Ann Neurol 23:611–614, 1988.

Sapolsky RM: Glucocorticoids and hippocampal atrophy in neuropsychiatric disorders. Arch Gen Psychiatry 57:925–935, 2000.

Sheline GE, Wara WM, Smith V: Therapeutic irradiation and brain injury. Int J Radiation Oncology Biol Phys 6:1215–1228, 1980.

Skenazy JA, Bigler ED: Neuropsychological findings in diabetes mellitus. J Clin Psychol 40:246–258, 1984.

Stephens R, Spurgeon A, Calvert IA, et al: Neuropsychological effects of long-term exposure to organophosphates in sheep dip. Lancet 345:1135–1139, 1995.

Stewart RB, Hale WE: Acute confusional states in older adults and the role of polypharmacy. Annu Rev Publ Health 13:415–430, 1992.

Van Gijn J: Leukoaraiosis and vascular dementia. Neurology 51 (Suppl. 1):S3–S8, 1998.

Vaughn CJ, Delanty N: Hypertensive emergencies. Lancet 356:411–417, 2000.

Victor M: Persistent altered mentation due to ethanol. Neurol Clin 11:639–661, 1993.

Yamada M, Ohno S, Okayasu I, et al: Chronic manganese poisoning: A neuropathological study with determination of manganese distribution in the brain. Act Neuropathol 70:273–278, 1986.

Yeates KO, Mortensen ME: Acute and chronic neuropsychological consequences of mercury vapor poisoning in two early adolescents. J Clin Exp Neuropsychol 16:209–222, 1994.

Young GB: Neurologic complications of systemic critical illness. Neurol Clin 13:645–658, 1995.

Young GB, Bolton CF, Austin TW, et al: The encephalopathy associated with septic illness. Clin Invest Med 13:297–304, 1990.

Neurosurgical Perspectives

Jeremy D. W. Greenlee
Meryl A. Severson III
Matthew A. Howard III

Functional neurosurgery
Epilepsy surgery
Traumatic brain injury
Brain tumor
Stroke
Hydrocephalus
Cerebrovascular disease
Brain death
Deep brain stimulation

INTRODUCTION

This chapter reviews a variety of neurosurgical conditions that involve disturbances of cognitive and behavior functions (Table 29-1). The typical neurosurgery patient often first encounters an emergency room physician, primary care physician or medical specialist, with cognitive impairment alone as the presenting complaint. Physicians who are well versed in evaluating this patient population are best positioned to make accurate and timely referrals that could save the patient's life. In addition, many neurosurgery patients have well-circumscribed lesions.

TABLE 29-1. Neurosurgical Conditions That May Involve Cognitive/Behavioral Impairment

Condition	Incidence per 100,000 population
Traumatic brain injury	95
Brain tumors	65
Epilepsy	500–800
Hydrocephalus, congenital	100
Stroke	210

Studies of this patient population have greatly increased understanding of the biologic basis of human cognition and behavior.

Many conditions covered in the other chapters in this textbook may require neurosurgical evaluation and treatment. This chapter focuses on representative neurosurgical conditions that are particularly salient to behavioral neurology, neuropsychology, and cognitive neuroscience.

TRAUMATIC BRAIN INJURY

Direct Injuries

Traumatic brain injuries (TBIs) are ubiquitous, require skilled neurosurgical management, and are a major topic of neurosurgery research. (Chapter 27 by Jones and Rizzo reviews nonsurgical details.) There can be direct mechanical injuries to the brain at the time of impact as well as secondary injuries.

Traumatic forces impacting on the skull cause a wide range of tissue injuries. The severity of injury is influenced by the cumulative energy being delivered, the duration of time in which energy is transferred, and angular incidence of impact (Gennaralli & Thibault, 1985; Graham et al., 1988). In general, the higher the energy and the shorter the duration of energy transfer to the brain, the more severe the injury. In the case of a penetrating gunshot wound, there is a correlation between bullet velocity and magnitude of brain injury. A 22-caliber shell is only slightly larger in cross-sectional diameter than a therapeutic ventricular catheter. A catheter introduced slowly by hand through frontal lobe tissue results in no significant functional damage to the brain. A bullet delivered at the muzzle velocity of a handgun transfers large amounts of kinetic energy into the tissue, often resulting in a fatal brain injury (Fig. 29-1).

The pattern of energy distribution within the brain after gunshot wounds is complex. The same is true of high-energy blunt injuries to the brain. Gross tissue disruption with associated hemorrhage can be visualized easily on brain imaging studies and postmortem inspection, although axonal injuries may be more difficult to detect and are better seen on ultra-

structural inspection of the post-mortem brain using special axonal staining methods (Adams et al., 1982; Povlishock, 1992). In patients who survive high-energy injuries with diffuse damage throughout the brain, it is difficult to correlate the extent of systems disruption with the patient's postinjury cognitive deficit.

This is not the case for low-energy penetrating injuries whose deleterious effects are confined to discrete brain regions. Consider Phineas Gage, who suffered an injury to both frontal lobes when a tamping rod penetrated his skull. This was a case of a low-velocity injury with parenchymal injuries confined to a well-defined track. The behavioral disturbances displayed by Phineas Gage were clearly referable to the bifrontal injury sites. This rare case study has fueled extensive investigative work, even more than a century after the original injury (Damasio, 1994).

At the beginning of the 21st century, there are no clinical means available for directly repairing injured brain tissue. Numerous attempts have been made to use steroids (Bullock et al., 1995), calcium channel blockers, and other agents to mitigate the effects of direct brain injury. To date, none have proven to be convincingly effective. For this reason a key neurosurgical treatment strategy is to prevent secondary injuries to the brain.

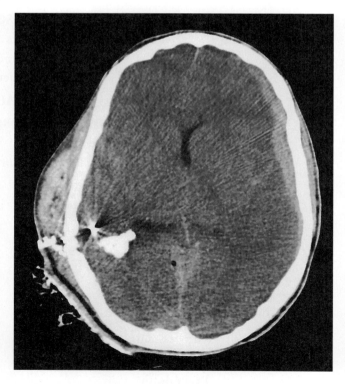

FIGURE 29-1. Gunshot wound, computed tomography (CT) scan. Demonstrates intraparenchymal shrapnel and bone fragments with bilateral injury.

Secondary Brain Injuries

To function properly, brain tissue must be perfused by blood carrying a continuous supply of oxygen, glucose, and electrolytes (Powers et al., 1985). In the clinical setting of injury, a host of factors threaten this critical flow of nutrients. The patient with multiple organ system injuries may become anemic and/or hypotensive as consequence of systemic injuries. The injured brain is particularly intolerant of this type of perturbation, and initial resuscitative efforts are directed at ensuring that airway, breathing, and cardiac function needs are met. Other organ systems can recover from periods of sustained ischemia or hypoxia, but the injured brain cannot (Jones et al., 1994).

The skull can be thought of as a rigid box with minimal compliance. If pressures within this box rise to levels approaching systemic arterial pressure, there is insufficient pressure gradient to drive blood into the cerebral circulation (Miller et al., 1972). Increased intracranial pressure (ICP) can result from a variety of pathologic conditions, and is a constant source of concern in the critically ill neurosurgery patient. Injured brain is prone to swell and thereby trigger a cascade of adverse events. Frequently ICP monitors are placed in head-injured patients to enable the surgeon to objectively quantify dangerous trends and to guide interventions. Medical measures to reduce ICP include hyperventilation (Grubb et al., 1974) and administration of diuretics (Barry et al., 1961).

A common etiology for increased ICP after head injury is the development of intracranial hemorrhage. Different injuries tend to cause different types of hemorrhages, with distinctly different outcomes. A sharp transient blow to the skull can cause a temporal bone skull fracture, but no immediate direct brain injury. A tear in the middle meningeal artery results in the formation of a steadily growing blood clot in the extradural space. Over time, the patient can develop headaches, nausea, and vomiting followed by loss of consciousness. If the epidural hematoma is rapidly surgically evacuated, the recovery can be excellent. Because there is no direct injury to the brain, and the dura separates the hematoma from the brain parenchyma, the critical pathologic process is the steady elevation in ICP. The key is to recognize and surgically address this process immediately (McKissock et al., 1960; Rivas et al., 1988) (Fig. 29-2).

Hematomas that form acutely in the subdural space are a different entity. In most instances, acute subdural hematomas occur after high-energy injuries that damage the brain directly as well as blood vessels on the surface of the brain. Patients with this type of injury typically display significant neurologic deficits immediately after the injury, which worsen as blood accumulates in the subdural space. Urgent surgical evacuation

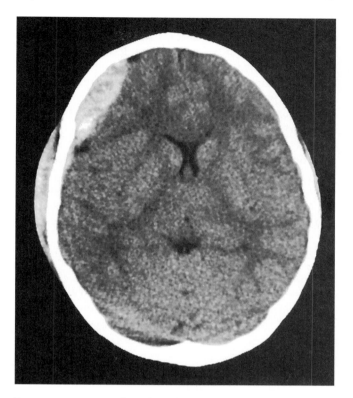

FIGURE 29-2. Frontal epidural hematoma, computed tomography scan. Note mass effect and midline shift.

is indicated, but unfortunately the results of treatment are less encouraging than with epidural hematomas (Wilberger et al., 1991).

A different type of subdural hematoma develops gradually in older patients (Howard et al., 1989). Anatomic changes of aging predispose this group of patients to bleed after minimal or no apparent injury. Cortical atrophy results in an enlargement of the subdural space and a stretching of the bridging veins that span from the brain surface and insert into the rigid venous sinuses attached to the skull. In addition, these bridging veins are not as structurally sound as those of younger patients. Even slight jarring of the head can cause the brain to shift relative to the venous sinus and cause a bridging vein to rupture. Chronic subdural hematomas have even been reported to result from sitting down too quickly. Many patients diagnosed with this condition have no recollection of a traumatic event preceding the onset of symptoms.

These vessels are typically small and under low pressure, so that the rate of blood accumulation in the subdural space is slow. Often blood products accumulate over a period of weeks to months before a diagnosis is made. During this time period, the hematoma liquefies, presenting a characteristic low-density appearance on the head computed tomography (CT) scan. In the absence of clear history of trauma, these patients can be difficult to diagnose. Although the chronic subdural hematoma is a focal mass lesion overlying a specific brain region, the presenting symptoms can be those of diffuse brain dysfunction, including dementia and lethargy. A detailed neurologic exam often reveals subtle localizing signs (e.g., unilateral arm drift). With a sufficient index of suspicion, the diagnosis can be arrived at rapidly with a head CT scan. The surgical treatment involves creating burr holes in the skull overlying the hematoma, and washing the liquefied clot out of the subdural space. This approach is usually successful, and dramatic symptomatic relief is frequently noted (Fig. 29-3).

Traumatic Brain Injury Sequelae

Two million people suffer TBIs every year, 4% of whom develop chronic disability (Frankowski, 1986). The likelihood of cognition sequela depends on severity of injury and this is often indexed acutely by the Glasgow Coma Scale Score (see Chapter 27). In addition to cognitive disorders, patients may exhibit depression, mania, anxiety, apathy, and psychosis (Rao & Lyketsos, 2002). Despite the high incidence of neuropsychiatric sequelae, cognitive rehabilitation has been shown to improve memory, attention, communication, and decision making in TBI patients (Cicerone et al., 2000).

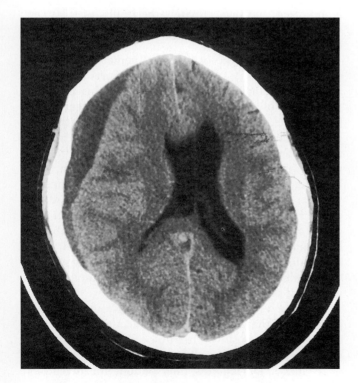

FIGURE 29-3. Frontoparietal chronic subdural hematoma, computed tomography scan.

Endocrinologic sequelae are also common to TBI patients. The syndrome of inappropriate antidiuretic hormone secretion (SIADH) occurs in approximately 5% of head trauma patients. These patients secrete excess ADH, causing their kidneys to conserve water. As a result, serum sodium levels are diluted to below normal limits. This extra water then diffuses into cells throughout the body, including the brain, resulting in more swelling in an already injured brain. Restricting these patients to less than one liter of water per day is usually sufficient to treat SIADH. In some patients, however, hypertonic saline may need to be administered in addition to a diuretic to restore the body's normal serum sodium level. If the level is corrected too quickly, central pontine myelinolysis (CPM) (demyelination of pontine white matter tracts) results, leaving the patient neurologically devastated.

Diabetes insipidus (DI) results from lower-than-normal levels of ADH and is much less common than SIADH. TBI patients suffer from neurogenic DI caused by hypothalamic-pituitary injury, which differs from nephrogenic DI. The kidneys of patients with nephrogenic DI are resistant to ADH and, therefore, waste water, resulting in severe dehydration and hypotension. These patients crave ice water and benefit from administration of desmopressin or arginine vasopressin.

Injury to the hypothalamic-pituitary axis can produce hypopituitarism (PHTH), endocrinologic derangements ranging from pan-hypopituitarism to selective pituitary hormone deficiencies (Benvenga et al., 2000). In PHTH syndrome, approximately 48% of patients have a prolactin (PRL) increase, 24% a growth hormone (GH) decrease, 53% a decrease in adrenocorticotropic hormone (ACTH), 44% an increase in thyroid-stimulating hormone (TSH), and almost 100% suffer a decrease in gonadotropin levels (Benvenga et al., 2000).

Hypopituitarism, specifically decreases in GH, has been reported to result in cognitive impairment in both men and women (Deijen et al., 1996; Bulow et al., 2002). Patients suffering from endocrinologic dysfunction should be evaluated by an endocrinologist to address the need for hormone supplementation.

Medications in Traumatic Brain Injury

One of the risks of TBI is a seizure. Acute head injury patients are often given phenytoin, an antiepileptic drug, for 1 week after injury to prevent the occurrence of acute seizures. The early use of antiepileptic drugs in head injury patients is not to prevent the development of post-traumatic epilepsy; rather, such drugs are administered to prevent the occurrence of acute seizures secondary to the acute brain injury. If the patient develops seizures while taking phenytoin it will be continued for an additional 6 to 12 months. Seizures are not expected, and anticonvulsants are not administered to those patients with normal head CT scans.

Cellular influx of calcium is one of the hypothesized mechanisms of neuronal injury in head trauma, and therapy with calcium channel blockers may be useful (Langham et al., 2000). Pentobarbital is used to induce coma in cases where ICP cannot be controlled with other medical and surgical measures. The goal of pentobarbital coma is to dramatically reduce cerebral metabolism and achieve an ICP value of less than 24 mm Hg.

Corticosteroids have long been used in TBI. Randomized-controlled trials have been inconclusive regarding their effectiveness in TBI, and there is now a large randomized controlled study under way, the CRASH (Corticosteroid Randomization After Significant Head Injury) trial, to examine their use in the early period after injury (Yates & Roberts, 2000). Adverse effects include immunosuppression and neuropsychiatric disorders, including mania, impaired logic, memory difficulty, and mood disturbances (Brown et al., 1999; Belanoff et al., 2001).

Informed Consent/Brain Death/Organ Donation

To provide informed consent for treatment, a patient must be of legal age and clinically competent, receive adequate information, and voluntarily consent to the procedure (Nora & Benvenuti, 1998). Exceptions to obtaining consent include emergencies, therapeutic privileges, and patient waiver (Nora & Benvenuti, 1998). Therapeutic privilege refers to situations in which a physician does not fully inform the patient for fear that such information will be to the detriment of the patient, given the physical, mental, or emotional condition of the patient.

Neurosurgery patients with severe intracranial pathology are often unable to give informed consent for potentially lifesaving neurosurgical procedures because of impaired cognition, obtundation, or coma. In these instances the courts and state legislatures have outlined steps for designating an appropriate surrogate decision maker. First it must be determined if the patient has an executed advanced directive (Miller & Marin, 2000). Advanced directives (also known as living wills) may indicate the patient's wishes with regard to heroic life-sustaining treatment (Miller & Marin, 2000)(see Chapter 52). In the absence of an advanced directive a surrogate decision maker who has durable power of attorney for health care will make decisions about treatment for the patient. In cases of emergency the physician becomes the surrogate decision maker; otherwise, depending on the state, the following groups are arranged in a hierarchy to make decisions for the patient: legal guardian, spouse, adult children, parents, and adult siblings (Miller & Marin, 2000) (see Chapter 52).

The phrase "brain death" refers to a normothermic, nonsedated patient without metabolic abnormalities who has irreversibly lost higher cortical function, including brainstem reflexes, motor function, and respiratory drive. These criteria are outlined in the U.S. Uniform Determination of Death Act (Wijdicks, 2002). Most hospitals in the United States now have specially trained personnel in specific organ procurement departments to discuss with families the option of organ donation in instances of brain death. Unfortunately, the supply of organs in the United States has leveled off, while the number of patients needing transplants has increased; one third of patients eligible for transplantation will die awaiting a new organ (Arnold et al., 1996).

VASCULAR DISORDERS

Cerebrovascular diseases encompass a vast array of pathologic conditions and clinical presentations, many of which manifest with behavioral and neuropsychological dysfunction (see Chapters 26 and 37). Many of these conditions are managed by neurosurgeons. The most common entities in this category are reviewed below.

Ischemic Infarcts

Ischemic strokes account for the majority of cerebrovascular accidents and are the result of an interruption in blood flow to the brain. In most instances, the interruption occurs within a specific cerebral blood vessel as a result of intraluminal thrombus or occlusion of the vessel by embolic material (Cerebral Embolism Task Force, 1986; Del Zoppo et al., 1992). If the brain tissue served by the occluded vessel does not receive blood supply from collateral vessels, the tissue infarcts and dies. The clinical consequence of the infarct relates to many factors, including the specific brain region involved, the age of the patient, and the size of the infarct.

The primary treatment modality for ischemic stroke is medical management. Systemic thrombolytics such as tissue plasminogen activator (tPA) have been shown to improve outcome (Kwiatkowski et al., 1999; NINDS rtPA Stroke Study Group, 1995). Intra-arterial administration of thrombolytics is an emerging therapy that holds promise for select patients (Furlan et al., 1999). Medical optimization to reduce the likelihood of recurrent stroke is important (Hankey et al., 2002).

Despite aggressive medical therapy, large infarcts can require surgical treatment as a result of life-threatening increased ICP caused by edematous, infarcted brain tissue. These large infarctions result from either internal carotid or middle cerebral artery occlusions, and result in death in 80% of patients (Hacke et al., 1996). Surgical treatment in these difficult situations may be viewed as lifesaving. However, a patient who survives the acute stroke but is left vegetative or in a severely cognitively disabled state is clearly not well served. Consideration of many variables is required when decisions on surgical intervention are made, such as the clinical condition of the patient and medical comorbidities, advanced directives and any previously expressed views on quality of life by the patient, and, most importantly, estimates of functional recovery for the patient beyond the acute stroke. Typically, better indications for surgical decompression include younger patients with non-language-dominant hemisphere infarcts.

Decompressive craniectomy with resection of non-viable brain tissue is the primary surgical treatment for massive cerebral infarction. The procedure consists of removing a large portion of the skull overlying the infarct, removal of necrotic brain, and dural enlargement using a patch graft. This combination allows for expanding brain edema with less transmitted increase in intracranial pressure (Fig. 29-4).

Small, uncontrolled case series show the procedure reduces mortality, from approximately 80% to 20% to 30% (Carter et al., 1997; Schwab et al., 1998). Fewer data exist for functional outcome improvement, but reports suggest that even for language-dominant hemi-

sphere middle cerebral artery stroke, up to 50% of patients can achieve a functional outcome with only mild or moderate aphasia (Carter et al., 1997; Kondziolka & Fazl, 1988). An important issue that is not yet adequately addressed is the timing of surgical intervention. Some authors have shown that patients treated within the first 24 hours of stroke fare better than those operated on later, after neurological decline (Schwab et al., 1998). It is hoped that, as the knowledge base increases with controlled studies, identification of the best candidates for surgery will be more straightforward.

Intracranial Hemorrhage

Intracranial hemorrhage can be caused by trauma, hemorrhagic strokes, rupture of vascular lesions such as aneurysms or vascular malformations, vasculopathies, tumors, and hypertensive hemorrhage. A detailed review of these specific conditions is beyond the scope of this chapter, but a discussion focusing on cognitive and behavioral consequences of intracranial hemorrhage is worthwhile.

Subarachnoid Hemorrhage

Subarachnoid hemorrhages (SAH) are a distinct form of cerebrovascular disease with unique clinical, pathologic, and management features. Each year in the United States, approximately 6 per 100,000 people suffer from SAH from a ruptured cerebral aneurysm (Broderick et al., 1993). More than half of these patients die or become severely disabled. Aneurysms are acquired over time as pulsatile arterial flow impacts on an abnormal portion of the blood vessel lumen. This process typically occurs at the branch point of a major intracerebral vessel in close proximity to the skull base. As the aneurysm expands away from the parent vessel, the tissue forming the dome of the aneurysm becomes thin and lacks the histologic structure of a normal arterial vessel. At a critical point, the dome bursts and blood extravasates into the subarachnoid space, and in certain situations can result in hematoma formation in the brain tissue immediately adjacent to the aneurysm. Presenting symptoms include a stiff neck, nausea and vomiting, and sudden severe headaches; often there is sudden loss of consciousness. In severe cases the patient can rapidly progress to respiratory or cardiac arrest and death (Fig. 29-5).

The management of patients with SAH is complex, and one of the critical treatment objectives is to secure the aneurysm to eliminate the chance of rebleeding. Unlike the situation with ruptured arteriovenous malformations, the risk of early rebleeding from an aneurysm is very high (Inagawa et al., 1987). The traditional strategy to secure a ruptured aneurysm is to perform a craniotomy and place a metal clip around the neck of the aneurysm, flush

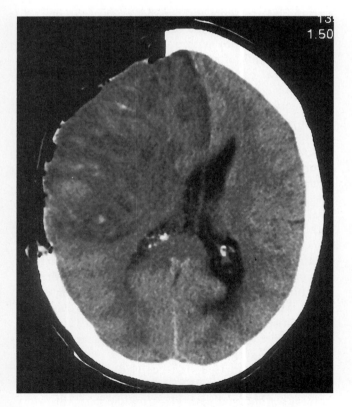

FIGURE 29-4. Decompressive craniectomy for large infarct with edema and mass effect, computed tomography (CT) scan.

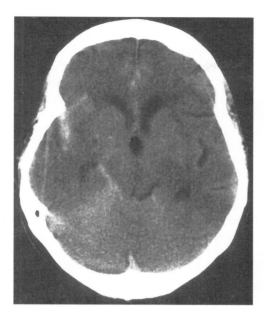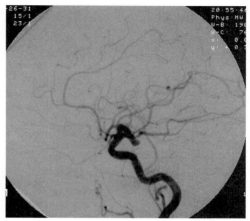

FIGURE 29-5. Subarachnoid hemorrhage, computed tomography scan (*left*). Diffuse blood in interhemispheric and sylvian fissures, and along tentorium cerebelli. Angiogram in same patient showing aneurysm at origin of posterior communicating artery, oblique view of internal carotid injection (*right*).

with the parent vessel, thus eliminating the aneurysm from the circulation. These are dangerous procedures, with significant risks of complications, but if the aneurysm is successfully secured the risk of rebleeding is essentially eliminated. A newer treatment involves using endovascular techniques to achieve the same objectives. With this approach, interventional neuroradiologists advance a catheter up to the mouth of the aneurysm and carefully deploy fine metal coils inside the aneurysm (McDougall & Spetzler, 1998; Brilstra et al., 1999). As more coils are deployed, the aneurysm becomes "packed" with these foreign bodies, and the blood within the aneurysm forms a wire-filled thrombus. This approach is rapidly becoming more refined, and in skilled hands is a safe and effective procedure. The one disadvantage of this approach relates to the significant incidence of recanalization of the coiled aneurysm over time. This potential for recanalization necessitates regular follow-up angiograms and repeat coiling if indicated. As the methods continue to improve, it is likely coils will be perfected that permanently and consistently obliterate the aneurysm.

There are often significant neuropsychological sequelae in survivors of SAH, and these have been examined extensively in clinical studies (Hop et al., 1997). Up to 36% of patients report depression, and 23% report physical disability (Carter et al., 2000). Neurobehavioral impairment is likely to be observed and reported as more severe by patients and their relatives than by operating surgeons (Buchanan et al., 2000). Neuropsychological testing following convales-

cence after SAH reveals deficiencies in verbal fluency, pattern recognition, and spatial working memory (Mavaddat et al., 1999). Generally these data have been used in the context of an important clinical endpoint that must be evaluated to examine the efficacy of new therapeutic agents. Particularly in poor-grade SAH patients, meaning those patients who are most ill at the time of presentation (comatose), it is difficult to correlate neuropsychological deficits with specific regional brain dysfunction due to the nature of the illness. It is presumed that the severe neurologic injuries in poor-grade patients are a consequence of severe intracranial hypertension and the resulting diffuse brain injury during the time immediately surrounding the bleed. More localizable deficits can be detected in patients who do not sustain diffuse injuries initially, but develop clearly defined focal brain injuries as a consequence of strokes caused by post-SAH vasospasm, or tissue injury sustained during surgery.

An example of the latter category is patients with anterior communicating artery aneurysms. Most surgeons approach these lesions from a pterional or anterior lateral exposure, and remove a portion of the ipsilateral gyrus rectus to gain access to the aneurysm. In these instances, the region of brain that has been removed can be accurately delineated anatomically and correlated with findings from neuropsychological testing.

Nimodipine, a calcium-channel blocking medication, is considered a standard-of-care treatment for aneurysmal SAH patients, because it improves outcome (Barker & Ogilvy, 1996). The drug is given for 3 weeks, beginning when SAH is diagnosed. The benefits of the medication are possibly caused by cerebral protection, as the incidence of radiographic vasospasm is not altered (Allen et al., 1983). Vasospasm is a devastating but finite entity, which can occur with other types of hemorrhage, but is most commonly encountered after aneurysmal rupture. Cerebral arteries and arterioles constrict in a delayed manner, beginning days after the rupture, and persisting up to a few weeks. Neurologically symptomatic vasospasm occurs in 20% to 30% of patients (Kassell et al., 1985). Although vasospasm always resolves, patients can die or be left severely disabled if infarction results from reduced cerebral blood flow caused by the narrowed vessels. Up to 7% of patients who survive obliteration of the aneurysm will suffer strokes as a result of vasospasm (Kassell et al., 1985). Treatment therefore is aggressive and includes elevating systemic blood pressure and blood volume, bed rest, and intra-arterial therapy with angioplasty and vasodilators.

HYDROCEPHALUS

Hydrocephalus denotes a range of conditions, all having the common feature of excessive intracranial accumulation of cerebrospinal fluid (CSF). CSF is constantly generated by the choroid plexus, ependymal cells, and brain parenchyma at a rate of approximately 30 mL per hour in adults. Under normal conditions, CSF flows unimpeded through the ventricular system and out of the apertures of the fourth ventricle into the subarachnoid space in the posterior fossa. The CSF then disperses over the convexities of the hemispheres and is absorbed into the venous sinuses through specialized fluid transport structures known as arachnoid granulations (Barlow, 1984). Disorders of CSF dynamics are among the most common conditions faced by neurosurgeons, and yet continue to be poorly understood and difficult to treat definitively (Fig. 29-6).

As might be expected for any hydraulic-like system, disturbances can occur at any level of the production-reabsorption pathway (Hamid & Newfield, 2001). Tumors of the choroid plexus that secrete CSF can develop (choroid plexus papillomas), resulting in excessive production of fluid. Nonsecretory tumors or congenital strictures can mechanically block a critical CSF conduit in the brain (e.g., cerebral aqueduct). This is a particularly dangerous form of obstructive hydrocephalus because CSF production continues, there is no route for egress of the fluid, and pressure can build up rapidly within the closed, noncompliant cavity of the skull. Symptoms of increased pressure include headaches, nausea, vomiting, visual disturbances, and decreased level of consciousness. Acute obstructive hydrocephalus can be fatal.

Disruption of the arachnoid granulations can cause hydrocephalus as a result of impaired absorption of CSF

into the venous system. This is often referred to as communicating hydrocephalus because there is no mechanical impediment blocking flow of fluid from the ventricular system into the subarachnoid space. This form of hydrocephalus can complicate any brain disorders that incite reactive changes in the subarachnoid space, such as subarachnoid hemorrhage and meningitis.

Hydrocephalus is encountered in all age groups, and symptoms vary depending on the age of the patient. Infants can experience progressive head enlargement because the cranial sutures have not fused, resulting in sometimes massive degrees of macrocephaly. As a result of the skull expandability, however, the infant may be otherwise asymptomatic. More commonly, the primary symptoms of infantile hydrocephalus include irritability, vomiting, failure to thrive, eye deviation (especially paresis of upgaze or lateral gaze), bulging fontanelle, and enlarged scalp veins.

Physical problems such as epilepsy and motor, visual, or auditory deficits affect approximately one fourth of treated children with congenital hydrocephalus, and 40% have IQs below 70 (Hoppe-Hirsch et al., 1998). The majority (60%) of treated hydrocephalic children attend normal schools, but half have some difficulties or lag behind their age group, and behavioral disorders are frequent (Hoppe-Hirsch et al., 1998). Speech impairment and deficits in memory, concentration, and shifting and sustaining of attention are often seen (Lumenta & Skotarczak, 1995; Brewer et al., 2001).

The cranial sutures fuse at approximately 2 years of age, and cranial growth is effectively complete at age 7. In older children and adults excess accumulation of CSF is not tolerated, and symptoms of increased intracranial pressure can develop rapidly.

The least understood form of hydrocephalus, normal pressure hydrocephalus (NPH) (Hebb et al., 2001), is seen in elderly patients. Initial observations showed that elderly patients with a triad of clinical symptoms (gait disturbance, bladder incontinence, dementia), and enlarged ventricles demonstrated clinical improvement after spinal fluid drainage, even though the spinal fluid pressures were not elevated. Patients whose gait and bladder symptoms precede the onset of cognitive symptoms are much more likely to experience clinical improvement after CSF drainage. Patients whose cognitive symptoms are more severe, and predate the onset of bladder and gait symptoms, respond poorly (Fig. 29-7).

The pathophysiology of NPH and mechanisms of improvement with CSF diversion procedures are still unclear. Magnetic resonance imaging (MRI) demonstrates enlarged ventricles, yet baseline intracranial pressures are not elevated. Patients with Alzheimer disease have diffuse cortical atrophy, with ex vacuo enlargement of the ventricles—i.e., the ventricles appear enlarged because the cortex around them has atrophied.

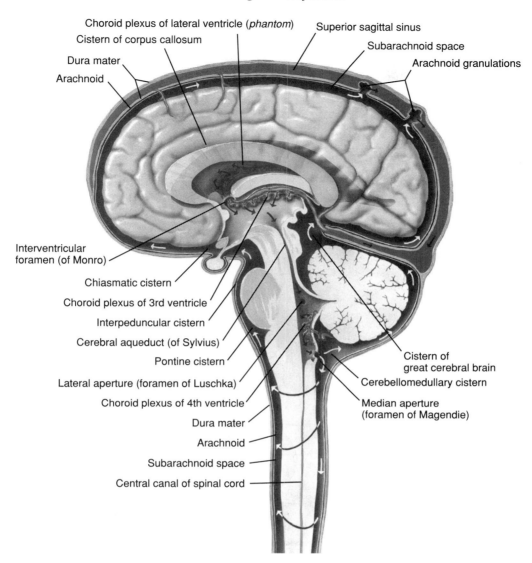

FIGURE 29-6. Schematic of normal cerebrospinal fluid flow pattern. (Reprinted with permission from Netter F: Atlas of Human Anatomy. Summit, NJ: CIBA-Geigy Corp, ed 1, 1989.)

These patients will not benefit from shunting. It is necessary to differentiate a lesser degree of cortical atrophy relative to ventricular enlargement to identify patients with NPH. NPH patients who are most likely to respond favorably to shunting have minimal cortical atrophy relative to ventricular enlargement.

Intracranial pressure monitoring in NPH (Hebb et al., 2001) is a safe and simple diagnostic procedure, but the interpretation is subjective and the ability of this test to predict which patients will benefit from shunt placement is debated. Some authors believe that the key diagnostic findings during ICP monitoring are periodic, moderate elevations in pressure during sleep. Transient abnormal surges of pressure on the distended walls of the ventricles may disrupt function of the leg and bladder axonal fibers that course immediately adjacent to the ventricle as they pass from the cerebral cortex to the spinal cord. Ventricular distention might also affect a variety of cognitive systems.

The treatment of hydrocephalus at any age is surgical and depends on the mechanism (e.g., communicating vs. noncommunicating). CSF can be diverted around obstructions by different techniques: ventriculoperitoneal shunting, lumboperitoneal shunting, and third ventriculostomy.

For example in cases of transient communicating hydrocephalus after subarachnoid hemorrhage it is often appropriate to place a lumbar subarachnoid drain while the intracranial arachnoid granulations recover from temporary dysfunction induced by the hemorrhage. In contrast, a lumbar puncture in a patient with symptomatic hydrocephalus secondary to a cystic mass

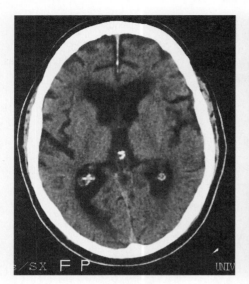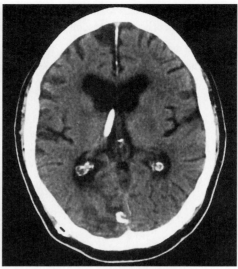

FIGURE 29-7. Preoperative computed tomography scan of patient with normal pressure hydrocephalus (*left*). Computed tomography scan after placement of ventriculoperitoneal shunt. Although the clinical condition of the patient improved, the size of the ventricles did not change (*right*).

blocking the foramen of Monro will not provide egress for the trapped CSF. In fact, a lumbar puncture in this setting will further exacerbate the pressure gradient between the intracranial and spinal compartments, and may cause brainstem herniation and death.

The surgical treatment strategies for hydrocephalus are conceptually simple and technically straightforward, and yet are associated with the highest reported incidence of complications of any procedure performed by neurosurgeons (Hebb et al., 2001). The tantalizing simplicity of the hydrodynamic problem has made the failure to develop definitive treatments all the more frustrating. The objective of all current surgical treatments is to continuously remove an appropriate amount of CSF from the cerebrospinal space in a safe and reliable manner, for an indefinite period of time. The failure rate of shunts is significant. Half of all ventriculoperitoneal shunts implanted in children will fail within 3 years of placement (Kestle et al., 2000). This number is higher than that of shunt systems implanted in adults, which require revision in 10% to 40% of cases (Black, 1980; Lund-Johansen et al., 1994). Infections occur in 7% to 11% of shunt implantations (Drake et al., 1998).

In some cases of communicating hydrocephalus, CSF can be diverted from the lumbar cistern, but lumbar catheters have significant occlusion rates and they are not used as commonly as ventricular shunts (Aoki, 1990). Ventricular catheters are placed using a variety of techniques, from both the frontal and occipital approaches, with the common desired endpoint being to position the tip of the catheter in the anterior horn of the lateral ventricle. There is no choroid plexus in this region of the ventricular system, thus reducing the chance of mechanical obstruction of the catheter (Howard et al., 1995). Perhaps the most challenging aspect of shunt function is to regulate the amount of CSF drained out of the ventricular catheter. Excessive CSF drainage can cause disabling headaches and predispose older patients to develop life-threatening subdural hematomas. That is why a simple drainage tube cannot be used. Conversely, inadequate CSF drainage will not relieve the patient's symptoms.

The major technological breakthrough in shunt technology was the development of flow-controlling valves. The CSF from the ventricular catheter enters the valve, where flow is regulated, and the outflow from the valve is carried away in the distal catheter. The fact that dozens of valves have been designed and marketed speaks to the fact that an ideal valve has yet to be developed. To date, engineers have been unable to develop a valve that always allows the appropriate amount of CSF to pass, year after year. The most common shortcoming of valves is for them to become mechanically obstructed. Although CSF is a clear fluid with minimal viscosity, under certain conditions deposits form on the valve mechanism. This can result in partial malfunction or complete obstruction (Fig. 29-8).

The distal, or outflow, catheter of shunt systems has been placed in a wide range of body cavities, again reflecting the imperfections of our current approach. The most common site for distal catheter placement is the peritoneal cavity. The catheter is introduced into the cavity through an opening in the peritoneal lining, and

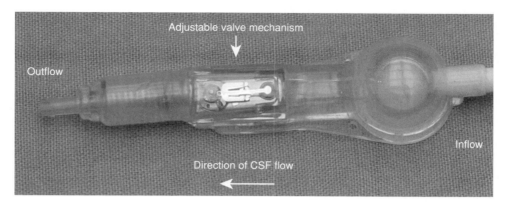

FIGURE 29-8. Schematic of an adjustable ventriculoperitoneal shunt valve (Codman Hakim programmable valve). (Reprinted with permission from Codman & Shurtleff, Inc., Raynham, MA.)

the distal end lies within the intra-abdominal cavity, constantly secreting spinal fluid. Under most conditions, the peritoneal cavity is well suited to absorb the entire CSF output from the cerebrospinal system. This is not a suitable solution when the peritoneal cavity is infected. In that case, alternative distal drainage sites include the right atrium, the pleural cavity, and even the gallbladder. These are less desirable sites than the peritoneal cavity and are used only when the more preferred option is not available.

Third ventriculostomy entails using an endoscope to create a connection between the floor of the third ventricle and the interpeduncular cistern, thus providing a bypass for CSF from lateral and third ventricles to the subarachnoid space without passing through the aqueduct of Sylvius and the fourth ventricle. Accordingly, the most common diagnosis treated by this technique is aqueductal stenosis. The surgery is effective, with 33% to 85% of patients requiring no further treatment, and can avert the need for mechanical shunt systems, which are more prone to complications (Hopf et al., 1999; Javadpour et al., 2001). Revision necessitated by occlusion of the artificially created stoma is necessary in 10% to 18% of cases (Cinalli et al., 1999). The risk of significant morbidity from third ventriculostomy resulting from damage to adjacent critical structures is approximately 5% (Abtin et al., 1998).

BRAIN TUMORS

Brain tumor patients are a mainstay of neurosurgical practice. Clinical presentations vary widely, and patients often present to a primary care physician (see Chapter 38). Because of the widespread availability of diagnostic brain scanning in community centers, most brain tumors are diagnosed before a neurosurgeon is called. The variable, and frequently subtle, clinical presentations often delay a definitive diagnostic study.

Benign Tumors

Two key variables influencing a patient's presentation and course outcome are tumor location and histologic characteristics. Slow-growing, benign tumors in nondominant areas of the brain may be incidentally diagnosed and cured with surgical resection. The same histologically benign tumor in a more critical brain location may be incurable and cause death. Malignant brain tumors are generally associated with a poor prognosis regardless of their location within the brain.

The most frequently encountered histologically benign brain tumor is the meningioma. This tumor evolves from neoplastic cells of the arachnoid, and can be found in any location in the brain and spinal cord, where these progenitor cells arise (Mahmood et al., 1993). Meningiomas often have a spherical shape and are located over the cerebral hemispheres or adjacent to the falx cerebri. These tumors are usually well encapsulated and displace surrounding brain tissue as they grow. Because of their slow growth characteristics, and due to the remarkable capacity of the brain to compensate for slowly growing masses, patients can present with intracranial meningiomas several centimeters in diameter, with no detectable pathologic signs or symptoms. Generally speaking, these convexity meningiomas can be effectively and safely treated by surgically removing the entire lesion (Fig. 29-9).

Meningiomas located in the skull base, and involving cranial nerves or the cavernous sinus, are much more difficult lesions to manage. Even though the histologic characteristics of these skull base lesions may be consistent with a slowly growing, benign neoplasm, the clinical consequences can be devastating. Tumor tissue can encase vital vascular structures and cranial nerves, making it impossible to completely remove the tumor without damaging critical structures. Surgery in this setting can be complicated by strokes and disabling

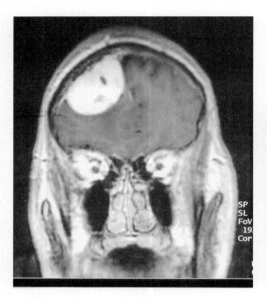
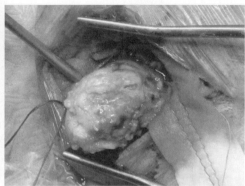

FIGURE 29-9. Frontal convexity meningioma, coronal T1-weighted magnetic resonance image after contrast administration (*left*). Intraoperative photo of meningioma removal (*right*).

cranial nerve palsies. Focused radiation therapy (Wara et al., 1975) with modern techniques is becoming a more safe and attractive option.

Another histologically benign lesion that can cause disabling symptoms and even sudden death is a colloid cyst of the third ventricle (Little & MacCarty, 1974). These lesions are less common than meningiomas, but are being diagnosed more often with the widespread availability of MRI and CT scans. These spherically shaped cystic structures are attached to the roof of the third ventricle and extend partially into the lateral ventricles via the foramen of Monro. Colloid cysts may be detected incidentally when patients undergo brain imaging for closed head injury, or to evaluate complaints unrelated to the cyst. They can be asymptomatic for many years, and then without warning cause sudden death from acute obstructive hydrocephalus (Ryder et al., 1986). It appears that there is a point of obstruction beyond which there is sudden catastrophic decompensation. The only intervention that can save the patient at this point is emergent placement of catheters into both lateral ventricles. The fact that many patients with these cysts have no evidence of hydrocephalus and live a full life without developing any symptoms related to the lesion whereas others experience obstructed ventricles and sudden death presents a difficult management challenge for patients with asymptomatic lesions. A variety of surgical approaches have been developed to remove the lesions safely. They involve entering the ventricular system and detaching the cyst from its point of attachment in the roof of the third ventricle. One of the potentially devastating complications that can occur during this procedure involves

damaging the columns of the fornix as they course adjacent to the foramen of Monro. At this point in their course both fornices are abutting each other, and a destructive lesion at this location can functionally disconnect the critical pathways between the ventral forebrain and hippocampal formations. Profound memory disturbances result.

Malignant Tumors

The most common form of brain tumor is malignant. The progenitor cells for primary malignant brain tumors are glial in origin. Glial cells outnumber neurons and are capable of reacting and dividing even in mature adults. After malignant transformation the glial cells lose many of their identifying cellular characteristics and take on the appearance of poorly differentiated, pleomorphic cells with high rates of mitotic activity. The most common primary brain tumor is called a glioblastoma multiforme (Blumenthal & De Angelis, 1998).

Malignant cells within the brain are capable of streaming along the billions of fiber tracks that connect all regions of the brain. A dense concentration of malignant cells accumulates at the site of tumor origin, destroying the normal brain cells and transforming the histologic characteristics of blood vessels in that brain region. Normal brain blood vessels form part of a functional barrier, referred to as the blood-brain barrier, which prevents charged molecules from passing from the bloodstream into the brain parenchyma. Vessels within the core region of a malignant tumor lose this filtering property and become leaky, allowing large charged molecules to pass into the surrounding tissue.

This abnormal property is exploited for diagnostic purposes during brain imaging studies such as CT and MRI. When carrying out a brain imaging study to rule out a malignant brain tumor, baseline images are obtained, and then the same study is repeated after an intravenous contrast agent is administered. The high-density charged contrast molecules do not pass through the normal, intact blood-brain barrier, but will pass through abnormal leaking blood vessels and into malignant brain tumor tissue. Regions of brain that are heavily infiltrated by malignant tumor cells and contain transformed blood vessels will enhance brightly on the contrast study. Surrounding brain regions with histologically normal blood vessels will not enhance.

Unfortunately, the focal area of brain enhancement noted on imaging studies does not provide an accurate reflection of the true extent of malignant disease. By the time imaging studies demonstrate a focal area of enhancement, small numbers of malignant glial cells have already migrated to distant sites in the brain. These isolated distant cells do not destroy the brain parenchyma or transform the blood vessels in the region, but they survive and divide behind the blood-brain barrier, impervious to every therapeutic intervention attempted to date. Chemotherapeutic agents that are highly effective in controlling or curing hematologic malignancies are largely ineffective in treating malignant brain tumors. Over many decades, hundreds of scientific papers have been published describing how dozens of different chemical agents destroy malignant glioma cells in culture, or in experimental animals injected with tumor cells. None have been consistently effective in human subjects (Darling & Thomas, 2001).

Whereas chemotherapy has evolved into a highly effective and, in some cases, definitive treatment for many cancers, the dismal long-term survival prognosis for patients with malignant gliomas is essentially the same now as it was when the disease was first characterized more than a century ago. The average length of survival for a patient newly diagnosed with a glioblastoma is approximately 1 year (Lacroix et al., 2001). Resection of the tumor bulk defined on imaging studies prolongs survival but does not address the malignant cells that have migrated elsewhere in the brain. Even attempts to surgically remove an entire hemisphere in patients with presumed unilateral malignant gliomas have been ineffective: tumors cells expand into fatal masses in the contralateral hemisphere. Radiation treatment prolongs survival, but the doses required to eradicate all tumor cells are not tolerated by the central nervous system and cause unacceptable radiation-induced morbidity and mortality (see Chapter 38).

Future hopes are pinned on therapies that selectively attack malignant cells throughout the brain. The blood-brain barrier is a major obstacle to treatment. Promising macromolecular agents, such as antibody conjugates and gene therapy viruses, as well as smaller molecules that are charged, do not cross from the bloodstream into the brain. One alternative strategy being pursued by investigators at the National Institutes of Health involves pumping antineoplastic agents directly into brain tissue via parenchymal catheters (de Guzman et al., 2000). By driving agents into the extracellular space with hydraulic pressure, malignant cells throughout the brain might be reached.

Immunotherapy is another potential treatment for malignant brain tumors. Although no tumor-specific antigens (TSAs) have yet been found, there are numerous tumor-associated antigens (TAAs) that may allow researchers to attack malignant gliomas (Virasch & Kruse, 2001). Serologic analysis of recombinant cDNA expression libraries (SEREX) and microarray analysis are helping to identify new TAAs (Rosenberg, 1999).

EPILEPSY SURGERY

Overview

One in ten Americans has experienced a seizure (Son et al., 1994). Most of these events occur with high fevers in infants (Verity & Golding, 1991). Epilepsy, a series of seizures unrelated to fevers, affects more than 1 million adults in the United States. The majority of these patients are effectively treated using anticonvulsant medications. A minority of patients with epilepsy, those who fail medical management, are potential candidates for surgical treatment (see Chapter 34).

Surgical treatments of medically refractory epilepsy can be grouped into three general categories: resection surgery, disconnection surgery, and chronic electrical stimulation. A thorough preoperative evaluation process that is directed at clearly identifying the nature of the individual's seizure disorder is essential to identify the appropriate surgical treatment.

Preoperative Evaluation

In many epilepsy surgery centers, neuropsychologists and cognitive neuroscientists play an integral role in the preoperative evaluation of surgical candidates. One of the primary preoperative objectives is to identify the brain region from which seizures begin. Studies carried out when the patient is not actively seizing are referred to as interictal examinations. Neuropsychological testing can generate results that suggest specific lobar abnormalities. A patient's pattern of impaired performance might, for example, be consistent with left mesial temporal lobe dysfunction. This information, in conjunction with other concordant diagnostic information, can enable physicians to conclude that seizures emanate from that brain region, and that the patient would benefit from having that region of the brain resected.

Brain imaging studies are also routinely obtained, making use of a similar diagnostic strategy. Anatomic MRI images might demonstrate that one hippocampus is atrophied, and thus aid in the seizure localization process (see Chapter 4). Interictal positron emission tomography (PET) scans may demonstrate areas of decreased metabolic activity, which can be of equally useful diagnostic value (see Chapter 6). It is generally accepted that brain regions showing decreased levels of function between seizures (interictal studies) often include the region from which seizures originate (Henry et al., 1993). Studies obtained during an actual seizure event (ictal studies) provide even more useful localizing information. It is sometimes possible to obtain brain metabolic imaging data during a seizure. The ictal single photon emission computed tomography (SPECT) study necessitates infusing radioactive tracers during or soon after a seizure. Activity from these short duration isotopes is measured in the brain and can provide additional useful evidence of where seizures originate. SPECT scanning does not provide the level of anatomic detail observed with MRI or CT imaging (Berkovic et al., 1993).

The most important of all preoperative diagnostic studies are electrophysiological recordings. Seizures occur when large numbers of neurons fire in an abnormal, synchronous pattern. The gold standard for identifying this activity is an electroencephalogram (EEG) taken during the seizure. Brain electrical activity is most often recorded using scalp electrodes. Signals generated within brain tissue propagate outwards through the lining of the brain, skull, and scalp. The EEG can provide a large amount of useful information despite the distance separating the recording contacts from the neurons that generate the electrical signals.

All patients who are candidates for epilepsy surgery will have had one or more interictal EEGs. The most important finding on an interictal EEG study is periodic epileptic spikes. These episodic synchronous discharges often identify the site of seizure onsets (Gloor, 1975). The episodic discharges recorded on the interictal exam can be thought of as a smoldering electrophysiological process that can abruptly convert to full-blown seizure activity under certain conditions (Fig. 29-10).

Interictal EEG studies are extremely useful, but in most surgical cases initial recordings are also needed. For this purpose patients are admitted to an Epilepsy Monitoring Unit for chronic monitoring. Scalp recording electrodes are placed, and the patient is housed in a hospital room that is equipped to relay and record the EEG signals continuously, and to capture video images of the patient. When the patient experiences a seizure, the epileptologist can examine the EEG activity that

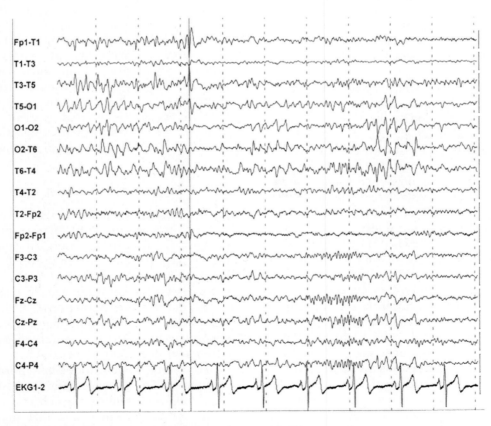

FIGURE 29-10. Scalp electroencephalogram activity; note spike as marked by vertical cursor.

coincides with the onset of the seizure event together with the clinical manifestations of the seizure captured on the video recording. Data from the ictal video-EEG, diagnostic imaging, and neuropsychological data allow the epileptologist to recommend surgical resection.

Intracranial, or phase II, epilepsy monitoring is reserved for patients in whom the noninvasive data are inconclusive. In these cases the evidence suggests that seizures are originating from a discrete seizure focus that cannot be pinpointed with scalp recordings. As stated earlier, scalp recording contacts can be remote from the locus of seizure activity especially deep structures of the temporal lobe, which are frequently implicated in refractory seizure cases. Specifically, the amygdala and hippocampus are more than 5 centimeters from the nearest scalp recording contact, and a large volume of electrically active and inactive biologic tissue is positioned in between. It is very difficult to capture the spread of electrical activity from one amygdala to the other using noninvasive techniques. Because it is imperative that the correct side of origin be identified, more direct studies must be undertaken.

Chronic intracranial recording procedures often provide this critical clinical information, as well as a unique scientific opportunity for neuroscience researchers (Howard et al., 1997, 2000). The diagnostic strategy is to place an array of electrodes on the surface of the brain, and into targeted deep structures, to capture the earliest electrical events that herald the onset of seizure. Typically, the epilepsy team formulates a general hypothesis of where the seizure onsets are likely to occur based on the available clinical data, and then strives to place recording contacts throughout the targeted region. Some electrodes consist of small, flat recording discs embedded in a flexible silicon sheet. Large numbers of such recording contacts can be positioned within a single sheet that is placed over the brain surface of interest. Deep brain sites are accessed using small-diameter, cylindrical, multicontact, depth electrodes. These electrodes are usually less than 3 mm in cross-sectional diameter, and have recording sites positioned at intervals along the shaft.

The depth electrodes are placed using a stereotactic neurosurgical technique. Before surgery a rigid head frame is placed on the patient. The patient is then brought to the MRI scanner, where images of the brain are obtained that provide precise geometric information regarding the location of target sites in the brain relative to the rigid head frame. During surgery, a special electrode-positioning device is mounted on the rigid frame, and a target trajectory is calculated based on the MRI imaging data. Typical target sites include the amygdala and hippocampus. The cylindrical electrode is gently advanced through brain tissue to the target site. Cumulatively, the surface grid arrays and multiple depth electrodes may provide more than 100 intracranial recording contacts. After recovery from general anesthesia, the patient is transported to the video-EEG monitoring facility, the intracranial electrode leads are connected (as would be the case with scalp recording devices), and continuous video-EEG monitoring ensues. Typically this monitoring period lasts 2 weeks, after which the electrodes are removed. If a clear seizure focus has been identified, that brain region is resected at that time (Fig. 29-11).

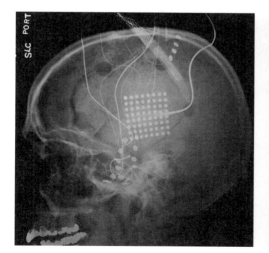
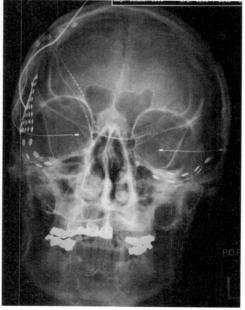

FIGURE 29-11. Lateral (*left*) and anteroposterior (*right*) skull x-rays showing location of implanted surface and depth electrodes.

The intercranial electrodes that have been placed on and into the brain for clinical purposes are also capable of recording data that are highly useful to scientists who study information processing in the human brain. The epilepsy patients undergoing chronic intracranial recordings are awake, alert, and fully capable of participating in complex neuroscience experiments. By directly examining the brain activity during these experiments, it is possible to gain unique and important insights into the basic mechanisms of human brain function. For example, this approach has been used extensively to identify how auditory information is represented in the human brain (Howard et al., 1996, 1997, 2000; Steinschneider et al., 1999; Fishman et al., 2001) (Fig. 29-12).

One additional diagnostic study that is frequently used in the evaluation of epilepsy surgery patients, and has implications for neuropsychological research, is the intra-arterial amobarbital sodium test. This procedure, often referred to as the Wada exam (Wada & Rasmussen, 1960) is an outpatient study that involves cannulation of a femoral artery under local anesthesia to introduce a catheter into the internal carotid artery of a subject. Amobarbital sodium is then infused and diffuses throughout the ipsilateral hemisphere's cerebral circulation. The amobarbital causes the cerebral tissue supplied by the carotid circulation to become temporarily dysfunctional. As a result, the subject experiences a transient hemiparesis, as well as possible speech, language, and memory deficits. In most instances, the Wada test is used for two purposes: to determine which hemisphere subserves speech functions and to determine how important each hemisphere is for memory function. During the speech testing procedure, the patient is asked to verbally identify objects while the amobarbital is being infused. When amobarbital is infused into the "speech-dominant" hemisphere, which is usually the left side, disruption of speech function is noted. Infusion into the non–speech-dominant hemisphere causes no disruption. The patient's memory is evaluated by testing the ability to recall objects presented during the procedure.

Resection Surgery

The best results obtained in the surgical treatment of epilepsy are seen in patients with a mesial temporal lobe seizure focus. Resection of the lateral temporal neocortex and anterior portion of hippocampus provides excellent seizure control in approximately 75% to 85% of patients. A large percentage of these patients are seizure-free after surgery (NIH, 1990; Son et al., 1994).

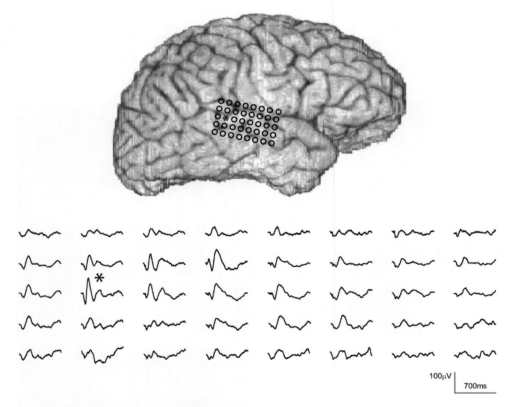

FIGURE 29-12. Sample recording of auditory evoked potentials recorded from a multicontact cortical grid, located as shown in the magnetic resonance imaging surface reconstruction. Note maximal response at site indicated by asterisk.

Some patients are found to have onset of epileptic activity from locations outside the temporal lobe. This may occur in cases of anatomic lesions, such as brain tumors, traumatic brain injury or stroke, or congenital anomalies. Although seizure control after resection of an extratemporal seizure focus is often effective, the results fall short of those obtained from temporal resection (Dogali, 1998).

Disconnection Surgery

Patients who have refractory epilepsy, but without a resectable focus, may benefit from disconnecting the site of seizure onset from the surrounding brain that is recruited secondarily. Examples of such treatment include corpus callosotomy, hemispherectomy, and multiple subpial transection (MSPT). Callosotomy may be either partial or complete. Both techniques have been shown beneficial for atonic and generalized tonic-clonic seizures (Gates et al., 1987). MSPT is used in cases in which seizure onset is from eloquent cortical regions. It takes advantage of the columnar anatomic organization of the neocortex. Horizontal cortical connections are disrupted around the focus, using a cutting instrument, in order to prevent spread of epileptic activity, while the vertical or columnar fibers are spared, thus preserving function of the region. The procedure appears to be effective, with 71% of patients with generalized seizures and 63% of those with partial epilepsy achieving excellent outcomes (Gross & Dogali, 1998; Spencer et al., 2002). New neurologic deficits after MSPT have been seen in approximately 20% of patients (Spencer et al., 2002).

Chronic Electrical Stimulation

A recent surgical development in epilepsy treatment has been the use of electrical stimulation. Implantation of a subcutaneous pulse generator below the clavicle with stimulating electrodes wrapped around the cervical portion of the vagus nerve, or vagal nerve stimulator (VNS), is now increasingly used. This treatment is technically easy to perform, and can be done with low risk of serious morbidity and without disruption of viable brain tissues. For these reasons, the device is a reasonable treatment possibility for almost any patient with medically refractory epilepsy that does not harbor a resectable focus. The literature concerning long-term seizure reduction efficacy is evolving. but the data thus far show significantly reduced frequency of seizures in 20% to 45% of patients. Interestingly, the efficacy of these devices appears to improve with time (DeGiorgio et al., 2000).

FUNCTIONAL NEUROSURGERY

Functional neurosurgery is currently one of the fastest-growing areas within the neurosurgical realm. Conti-nually expanding technologic advances offer the neurosurgeon a large armamentarium with which to treat a diverse range of pathologies including movement disorders, pain syndromes, dystonia, and spasticity, plus offering functional mapping techniques that allow for improved treatments such as brain tumor excision with reduced morbidity.

Movement Disorders

Surgical treatment of movement disorders is not a new phenomenon. Cortical resection was undertaken as early as 1909 to treat athetosis (Horsley, 1909). A variety of different techniques and targets involving the cerebrum, basal ganglia, brainstem, and spinal cord have been attempted since then, with varying degrees of success. While the early results were generally encouraging, the development of detailed neuroimaging techniques, improved stereotactic targeting, and reduction of overall surgical risk now make invasive treatments even more attractive options.

The most common movement disorders now treated by neurosurgeons are Parkinson disease (PD) and tremor (see Chapter 24). Deep brain stimulation (DBS) is becoming the primary surgical modality for medically refractory PD, and is gradually replacing ablative procedures. Implantation of DBS systems is a two-stage procedure. The first stage involves placing a small stimulating electrode through a small hole in the skull to a target near the center of the brain. Usual targets for PD include the subthalamic nucleus, globus pallidus interna, and thalamus. The tip of the electrode has four contacts that allow for fine-tuning the stimulus location and thereby optimizing the clinical response. Patients are typically under local anesthesia for electrode placement, so as to confirm proper location by the clinical effects experienced by the patient. The final stage of the operation is performed under general anesthesia. This entails tunneling the electrode subcutaneously from the scalp to the upper chest, and connecting it to a small pulse generator, which is implanted in a subcutaneous pocket created just below the patient's clavicle.

Once the patient has recovered from surgery, the pulse generator can be programmed transcutaneously using a magnetic programmer held over the generator. The movement disorder specialist can then use different stimulation parameters including contacts stimulated, polarity, frequency, amplitude, and pulse width to obtain maximal symptom reduction. The adjustments are made on an ongoing basis, in the outpatient clinic setting.

The advantages of DBS over ablative or lesioning surgeries are the above-mentioned response optimization capabilities and the reversibility of effects by turning the pulse generator off, although an extremely small lesion is created by the positioning of the electrode in brain tissue. Additionally, bilateral DBS treatments are well tolerated, whereas lesion procedures have increased risks of complications if performed on both sides (Favre et al., 2000; Intemann et al., 2001). Drawbacks of DBS therapy are that the expense is much higher than lesioning and pulse generators have a finite battery life span, usually 2 to 4 years, depending on the stimulation parameters used. Replacement of depleted pulse generators requires another operation.

Target selection is guided by the clinical effects desired, regardless of whether the planned operation is DBS or ablative. The patient population of PD is diverse, with tremor predominating in some patients, whereas rigidity or drug-induced dyskinesias are the chief complaints of others. Subthalamic stimulation is primarily used to treat L-dopa–induced dyskinesias, but, in comparison with the other targets, is most effective in improving all of the cardinal symptoms of PD (tremor, rigidity, bradykinesia, postural instability). Thermal lesions placed in the subthalamic nucleus, or subthalamotomy, are reported to have a higher incidence of contralateral hemiballism than found with lesioning or stimulation of other targets (Guridi & Obeso, 2001).

The treatment directed at the ventroposterior portion of the globus pallidus interna (GPi) is successful in treating PD as well. Unilateral and bilateral lesions improve drug-induced dyskinesias and motor performance off medication (Alkhani et al., 2001; Counihan et al., 2001). Tremor, rigidity, and bradykinesia improve off medication (Fine et al., 2000). Deep brain stimulation of the GPi is similarly effective, but both DBS and pallidotomy are slightly less effective overall than subthalamic nucleus DBS (Deep-Brain Stimulation for PD Study Group, 2001).

The ventrointermediate thalamic nucleus (V_{im}) is an excellent target choice for patients with debilitating tremor. Both lesioning and DBS of V_{im} provides effective control of contralateral tremor in 75% to 90% of patients and is a procedure with low morbidity (Benabid et al., 1996; Pahwa et al., 2001). The risk of complications increases with bilateral V_{im} procedures, whether lesioning or DBS, but DBS offers the advantage of adjusting the response or intermittently stimulating (Ondo et al., 2001).

Cognitive decline can occur after surgery for movement disorders, in up to 25% of patients (Trepanier et al., 2000). Specifically, patients with preoperative cognitive impairment and older patients appear to be at highest risk (Trepanier et al., 2000). Although DBS can produce cognitive impairment, the severity and incidence of these have been shown to be less than those produced by bilateral ablative procedures (Ardouin et al., 1999; Fields et al., 1999; Ghika et al., 1999; Dujardin et al., 2001). Executive function, fluency, mood, and behavior can all be affected. For further description of the cognitive effects of subcortical lesions, see Chapters 21 and 25.

Pain

Chronic pain is a significant public health problem, and arises from many diseases and conditions, including peripheral nerve injury, degenerative conditions, spasticity, and amputations (see Chapter 33). Pain syndromes such as complex regional pain syndrome and trigeminal neuralgia can often be successfully treated with surgical techniques. Modern techniques include dorsal column spinal cord stimulation, implanted intrathecal medication systems, lesioning of peripheral nerves or dorsal root entry zones, and nerve decompression.

The primary advantages of surgical treatment in chronic pain are in reducing the use of medications that have adverse cognitive effects. For example, narcotic use can produce sedation or behavioral impairment, as can anticonvulsants used commonly for trigeminal neuralgia. Microvascular decompression and radiofrequency rhizotomy are both effective in achieving lasting pain-free outcomes for trigeminal neuralgia (Barker et al., 1996; Kanpolat et al., 2001). Implanted electrodes that chronically stimulate primary motor cortex are an emerging technology that holds promise for facial or extremity pain (Carroll et al., 2000; Saitoh et al., 2000).

Medications may be delivered intrathecally in order to minimize systemic side effects. Similar to DBS, where changes and titration of the drug delivery can be made transcutaneously, these systems offer flexibility. The intrathecal system requires implantation of a small catheter in usually the thoracolumbar spinal subarachnoid space. The catheter is then tunneled subcutaneously and connected to a combined pump and reservoir implanted in the abdominal wall. The pump is programmable to allow for variable dosing regimens. The reservoir may be accessed using a transdermic needle to refill or change medications.

These systems are beneficial in treating pain. Specifically, both cancer pain and noncancer pain (neuropathic, nociceptive) respond to intrathecal morphine in approximately 50% to 100% of patients after 2 years of treatment (Penn & Paice, 1987; Anderson & Burchiel, 1999; Gilmer-Hill et al., 1999). Patients report reduced use of other analgesics, and improved level of activity (Leavens et al., 1982).

Spasticity

Spasticity describes motion-induced resistance of motion. It can result from several central nervous system insults, including multiple sclerosis, spinal cord injury, traumatic brain injury, cerebral palsy, or stroke. The patient is afflicted with muscle spasms, which can be painful, and difficulties with nursing care, mobility, and transfers. Oral medications, including baclofen and benzodiazepines, are first-line therapy. However, some patients experience unacceptable toxicities from the medications, such as sedation or confusion. In these patients, surgical treatment becomes a possibility.

Surgical options for treating spasticity include intrathecal medicine delivery devices, nerve block or removal, rhizotomy (cutting of spinal nerve roots), myelotomy (cutting of spinal cord) or cordectomy (removal of a portion of spinal cord). A fundamental difference in choosing specific surgical techniques is whether or not any muscle tone is preserved, which can allow for ambulation. When anterior spinal roots or peripheral nerves are sectioned, muscles become flaccid. This obviously impacts those patients who depend on some level of muscle tone to ambulate or transfer.

Intrathecal delivery of baclofen has been shown to improve quality of life. In particular, mobility improves, spasm-related pain improves, and functional improvements such as sitting up out of bed are likely in carefully selected patients (Sampson et al., 2002). Complications do occur in 20% of patients however, and pump batteries need replacement every 3 to 5 years, depending on usage.

SURGERY FOR PSYCHOLOGICAL DISEASE

Psychiatric diseases have been treated with contemporary surgical treatments since the first half of the 20th century. Their history, however, has been filled with stigma. Sometimes referred to as *psychosurgery*, a term that has fallen out of favor recently because of such negative connotations, operations intending to treat schizophrenia, mania, depression, obsessive-compulsive disorder (OCD), and others fall into this category (see Chapter 3).

Anterior cingulotomy is the most common neurosurgical operation for psychiatric disease. It is primarily used to treat refractory affective disorders and OCD. Although the procedure is uncommon, the results can be satisfying. Significant symptom relief is seen in approximately 30% to 50% of patients. Patients with affective disorders tend to do slightly better after surgery than do those with OCD. Originally the lesions were made in the anterior, supracallosal cingulate gyrus and its fibers using open, transcortical techniques. Stereotactic thermal lesioning has largely replaced that technique, however. Adverse events following surgery are low (Feldman et al., 2001).

Subcaudate tractotomy evolved from techniques including orbital undercutting. Disruption of white matter between the orbitofrontal cortex and the head of the caudate interrupts connections between the striatum, thalamus, and basal frontal cortex. The indications for the operation are similar to those of cingulotomy: OCD,

affective disorders, chronic pain, and anxiety. Results are similar to cingulotomy as well, with 36% to 60% of patients achieving good results. Cognitive impairment after surgery is not common. Stereotactic radiofrequency lesioning is used to create bilateral lesions. The combination of tractotomy and cingulotomy is called limbic leucotomy. It is even less commonly reported in the literature, but the results are effective in up to 89% of patients (Feldman et al., 2001).

Anterior capsulotomy involves lesioning the anterior limb of the internal capsule. This destroys connections between the medial thalamus and frontal lobe. Lesions may be created with focused radiation, or with radiofrequency thermal ablation. Symptomatic improvement for patients with OCD or affective disorders can result in 45% to 70% of cases. Schizophrenia is not as responsive (Feldman et al., 2001).

There is still a role for modern neurosurgery to treat medically refractory psychiatric disease. As understanding of pathophysiology of both the diseases and the treatments is refined, the ability to interrupt the disease process with focused interventions will hopefully be enhanced. Nevertheless, randomized, controlled studies are difficult to perform with the small application of these techniques across different centers.

BRAIN BIOPSY

This neurosurgical procedure is performed to provide a definitive diagnosis in cases of unexplained neurodegenerative disease. These patients present with organic cognitive and neurologic disturbances, the cause of which evades noninvasive diagnostic strategies. In these instances a brain biopsy is performed to obtain abnormal neural tissue for pathologic examination and diagnosis. The procedure frequently aids in the diagnosis of Creutzfeld-Jakob disease, herpes simplex encephalitis, and various vasculitides, as well as neurosarcoidosis. Unfortunately, brain biopsies performed for unknown neurodegenerative disease produce a diagnosis in only 20% of cases and are nonspecifically abnormal 66% of the time (Javedan & Tamargo, 1997). In patients with acquired immunodeficiency syndrome (AIDS), brain biopsy is used to diagnose low-density lesions of unknown cause seen on head CT scan. These lesions may be due to progressive multifocal leukoencephalopathy, toxoplasmosis, tuberculosis, cryptococcal infection, or lymphoma of the CNS.

It is extremely important to sample noneloquent, or not functionally critical, areas of the brain when performing a brain biopsy procedure. Some important structures to be avoided if at all possible include the internal capsule, speech-dominant areas, thalamus and basal ganglia, and auditory and visual cortex, as well as the motor and sensory gyri. Thus, neurosurgeons prefer to biopsy the frontal lobe or the inferior temporal gyrus.

To improve the likelihood of sampling abnormal tissue the neurosurgeon must (1) take a large enough piece of tissue, (2) take from the abnormal area as seen on CT or MRI, (3) sample both gray and white matter, and (4) handle the specimen carefully to avoid creating tissue artifacts (Groves & Moller, 1966). Brain biopsy is not without significant risk of complication, which can include bleeding, infection, permanent neurologic deficit, and, although rare, death. It is therefore used only in patients in whom a treatable diagnosis is suspected that cannot be diagnosed by less invasive means (Sandson & Price, 1997).

SUMMARY

Neurosurgeons are a vital part of the neuroscience team in the treatment of a wide variety of clinicopathologic conditions. In conjunction with neurologists, neuropsychologists, psychiatrists, psychologists, and others, neurosurgeons can contribute to improvement of quality of life for many patients. Additionally, a multidisciplinary approach to basic research in the various disciplines of neuroscience holds a wealth of promise to enhance the understanding of the nervous system, in both normal and pathologic conditions.

◼ KEY POINTS

☐   Cognitive impairment is common in the neurosurgical patient population and can result from a wide variety of underlying conditions.

☐   A prompt, multidisciplinary approach to the treatment and rehabilitation of brain-injured patients is critical to the achievement of optimal outcomes.

☐   Surgical treatment of medically refractory epilepsy is a safe and effective option that can profoundly improve patients' lives.

☐   Hydrocephalus can be seen in all ages and its presentation can differ between the age groups.

☐   Stroke is, unfortunately, common, and a subset of stroke patients may benefit from early neurosurgical evaluation.

KEY READINGS

National Institutes of Health (NIH). Surgery for epilepsy. NIH Consensus Statement 1990 [online]. Mar 19–21; 8:1–20. Retrieved from http:consensus.nih.gov/cons/077/077_statement.htm.

The Deep-Brain Stimulation for Parkinson's Disease Study Group: Deep-brain stimulation of the subthalamic nucleus or the pars interna of the globus pallidus in Parkinson's disease. N Engl J Med 345:956–963, 2001.

Feldman RP, Alterman RL, Goodrich JT: Contemporary psychosurgery and a look to the future. J Neurosurg 95:944–56, 2001.

REFERENCES

Abtin K, Thompson BG, Walker ML: Basilar artery perforation as a complication of endoscopic third ventriculostomy. Pediatr Neurosurg 28:35–41, 1998.

Adams JH, Graham DI, Murray LS, Scott G: Diffuse axonal injury due to non-missile head injury in humans: An analysis of 45 cases. Ann Neurol 12:557–563, 1982.

Alkhani A, Lozano AM. Pallidotomy for Parkinson disease: A review of contemporary literature. J Neurosurg 94:43–49, 2001.

Allen GS, Ahn HS, Preziosi TJ, et al: Cerebral arterial spasm: A controlled trial of nimodipine in patients with subarachnoid hemorrhage. N Engl J Med 308:619–624, 1983.

Anderson VC, Burchiel KJ: A prospective study of long-term intrathecal morphine in the management of chronic non-malignant pain. Neurosurgery 44:289–300, 1999.

Aoki N: Lumboperitoneal shunt: Clinical applications, complications, and comparison with ventriculoperitoneal shunt. Neurosurgery 26: 998–1003, 1990.

Ardouin C, Pillon B, Peiffer E, et al: Bilateral subthalamic or pallidal stimulation for Parkinson's disease affects neither memory nor executive functions: A consecutive series of 62 patients. Ann Neurol 46:217–223, 1999.

Arnold RM, Siminoff LA, Frader JE: Ethical issues in organ procurement: A review for intensivists. Crit Care Clin 12:29–48, 1996.

Barker FG 2nd, Jannetta PJ, Bissonette DJ, et al: The long-term outcome of microvascular decompression for trigeminal neuralgia. N Engl J Med 334:1077–1083, 1996.

Barker FG, Ogilvy CS: Efficacy of prophylactic nimodipine for delayed ischemic deficit after subarachnoid hemorrhage: A meta-analysis. J Neurosurg 84:405–414, 1996.

Barlow CF: CSF dynamics in hydrocephalus—with special attention to external hydrocephalus. Brain Dev 6:119–127, 1984.

Barry KG, Berman AR: Mannitol infusion. Part III. The acute effect of the intravenous infusion of mannitol on blood and plasma volume. N Engl J Med 254:1085–1088, 1961.

Belanoff JK, Gross K, Yager A, Schatzberg AF: Corticosteroids and cognition. J Psychiatr Res 35:127–145, 2001.

Benabid AL, Pollak P, Gao D, et al: Chronic electrical stimulation of the ventralis intermedius nucleus of the thalamus as a treatment of movement disorders. J Neurosurg 84:203–214, 1996.

Benvenga S, Campenni A, Ruggeri R, Trimarchi F: Clinical review 113: Hypopituitarism secondary to head trauma. J Clin Endocrinol Metab 85:1353–1361, 2000.

Berkovic SF, Newton MR, Chiran C, et al: Single photon emission computed tomography, in Engel J (ed): Surgical Treatment of the Epilepsies, ed 2. New York: Raven Press, pp. 233–243, 1993.

Black PM: Idiopathic normal-pressure hydrocephalus. J Neurosurg 52:371–377, 1980.

Blumenthal DT, DeAngelis LM: Aging and primary central nervous system neoplasms. Neurol Clin 16:671–686, 1998.

Brewer VR, Fletcher JM, Hiscock M, et al: Attention processes in children with shunted hydrocephalus versus attention deficit-hyperactivity disorder. Neuropsychology 15:185–198, 2001.

Brilstra EH, Rinkel GJE, van der Graaf Y, et al: Treatment of intracranial aneurysms by embolization with coils: A systematic review. Stroke 30:470–476, 1999.

Broderick JP, Brott TG, Tomsick T, et al: Intracerebral hemorrhage more than twice as common as subarachnoid hemorrhage. J Neurosurg 78:188–191, 1993.

Brown ES, Khan DA, Nejtek VA: The psychiatric side effects of corticosteroids. Ann Allergy Asthma Immunol 83:495–503; 1999.

Buchanan KM, Elias LJ, Goplen GB: Differing perspectives on outcome after subarachnoid hemorrhage: The patient, the relative, the neurosurgeon. Neurosurgery 46:831–838, 2000.

Bullock R, Chestnut R M, Clifton G, et al: Guidelines for the Management of Severe Head Injury. New York: Brain Trauma Foundation, 1995.

Bulow B, Hagmar L, Orboek P, et al: High incidence of mental disorders, reduced mental well-being and cognitive function in hypopituitary women with GH deficiency treated for pituitary disease. Clin Endocrin 56:183–193, 2002.

Carroll D, Joint C, Maartens N, et al: Motor cortex stimulation for chronic neuropathic pain: A preliminary study of 10 cases. Pain 84:431–437, 2000.

Carter BS, Buckley D, Ferraro R, et al: Factors associated with reintegration to normal living after subarachnoid hemorrhage. Neurosurgery 46:1326–1333, 2000.

Carter BS, Ogilvy CS, Candia GJ, et al: One-year outcome after decompressive surgery for massive non-dominant hemispheric infaction. Neurosurgery 40:1168–1175, 1997.

Cerebral Embolism Task Force: Cardiogenic brain embolism. Arch Neurol 43:71–84, 1986.

Cicerone KD, Dahlberg C, Kalmar K, et al: Evidence-based cognitive rehabilitation: Recommendations for clinical practice. Arch Phys Med Rehabil 81:1596–1615, 2000.

Cinalli G, Sainte-Rose C, Chumas P, et al: Failure of third ventriculostomy in the treatment of aqueductal stenosis in children. J Neurosurg 90:448–54, 1999.

Counihan TJ, Shinobu LA, Eskandar EN, et al: Outcomes following staged bilateral pallidotomy in advanced Parkinson's disease. Neurology 56:799–802, 2001.

Damasio AR: Descartes' Error. Emotion, Reason, and the Human Brain. New York: Avon Books, 1994.

Darling JL, Thomas DG: Response of short-term cultures derived from human malignant glioma to aziridinylbenzoquinone, etoposide and doxorubicin: An in vitro phase II trial. Anticancer Drugs 12:753–60, 2001.

DeGiorgio CM, Schachter S, Handforth A, et al: Prospective long-term study of vagus nerve stimulation for the treatment of refractory seizures. Epilepsia 41:1195–1200, 2000.

de Guzman AF, Tatter SB, Shaw EG, et al: Brachytherapy of re-resected malignant glioma cavity margins utilizing a novel delivery system—The GliaSite Radiotherapy System. Presented at: 2000 AAPM. Med Phys 27:1443, 2000.

Deijen JB, de Boer H, Blok GJ, van der Veen EA: Cognitive impairments and mood disturbances in growth hormone deficient men. Psychoneuroendocrinology 21:313–322, 1996.

Del Zoppo GJ, Poeck K, Pessin MS, et al: Recombinant tissue plasminogen activator in acute thrombotic and embolic stroke. Ann Neurol 32:78–86, 1992.

Dogali M: Cortical and lesion resection in the control of epilepsy, in Gildenberg PL, Tasker RR (eds): Textbook of Stereotactic and Functional Neurosurgery. New York: McGraw-Hill, 1998, pp. 1889–1891.

Drake JM, Kestle JRW, Milner R, et al: Randomized trial of cerebrospinal fluid shunt valve design in pediatric hydrocephalus. Neurosurgery 43:294–305, 1998.

Dujardin K, Defebvre L, Krystkowiak P, et al: Influence of chronic bilateral stimulation of the subthalamic nucleus on cognitive function in Parkinson's disease. J Neurol 248:603–611, 2001.

Favre J, Burchiel KJ, Taha JM, Hammerstad J: Outcome of unilateral and bilateral pallidotomy for Parkinson's disease: Patient assessment. Neurosurgery 46:344–353, 2000.

Feldman, RP, Alterman RL, Goodrich JT: Contemporary psychosurgery and a look to the future. J Neurosurg 95:944–956, 2001.

Fields JA, Troster AI, Wilkinson SB, et al: Cognitive outcome following staged bilateral pallidal stimulation for the treatment of Parkinson's disease. Clin Neurol Neurosurg 101:182–188, 1999.

Fine J, Duff J, Chen R, et al: Long-term follow-up of unilateral pallidotomy in advanced Parkinson's disease. N Engl J Med 342:1708–1714, 2000.

Fishman YI, Volkov IO, Noh MD, et al: Consonance and dissonance of musical chords: Neural correlates in auditory cortex of monkeys and humans. J Neurophysiol 86:2761–2788, 2001.

Frankowski RF: Descriptive epidemiologic studies of head injury in the United States. Adv Psychosom Med 16:153–172, 1986.

Furlan A, Higashida R, Wechsler L, et al: Intra-arterial prourokinase for acute ischemic stroke. The PROACT II study: A randomized controlled trial. Prolyse in Acute Cerebral Thromboembolism. JAMA 282:2003–2011, 1999.

Gates JR, Rosenfeld WE, Maxwell RE: Response of multiple seizure types to corpus callosum sectioning. Epilepsia 28:28–34, 1987.

Gennaralli TA, Thibault LE: Biological models of head injury, in Becker JP, Povlishock JT (eds): Central Nervous System Trauma Status Report. Bethesda, MD: NINCDS, 1985, pp. 391–404.

Ghika J, Ghika-Schmid F, Fankhauser H, et al: Bilateral contemporaneous posteroventral pallidotomy for the treatment of Parkinson's disease: Neuropsychological and neurological side effects. Report of four cases and review of the literature. J Neurosurg 91:313–321, 1999.

Gilmer-Hill HS, Boggan JE, Smith KA, et al: Intrathecal morphine delivered via subcutaneous pump for intractable cancer pain: A review of the literature. Surg Neurol 51:12–15, 1999.

Gloor P. Contributions of electroencephalography and electrocorticography to the neurosurgical treatment of the epilepsies, in Purpura DP, Penry JK, Walter RD (eds): Neurosurgical Management of the Epilepsies: Advances in Neurology, Vol. 8. New York: Raven Press, 1975, pp. 59–105.

Graham DI, Adams JH, Gennarelli TA: Mechanisms of nonpenetrating head injury, in Bond RF (ed): Perspectives in Shock Research: Progress in Clinical and Biological Research, Vol. 264. New York: Liss, 1988, pp. 159–168.

Gross JD, Dogali M: Subpial transactions for the surgical management of epilepsy, in Gildenberg PL, Tasker RR (eds): Textbook of stereotactic and functional neurosurgery. New York: McGraw-Hill, 1998, pp. 1893–1901.

Groves R, Moller J: The value of cerebral cortical biopsy. Acta Neurol Scand 42:477–82, 1966.

Grubb RL, Raichle ME, Eichling JO, et al: The effects of changes in $PaCO_2$ on cerebral blood volume, blood flow, and vascular mean transit time. Stroke 5:630–639, 1974.

Guridi J, Obeso JA: The subthalamic nucleus, hemiballismus, and Parkinson's disease: Reappraisal of a neurosurgical dogma. Brain 124:5–19, 2001.

Hacke W, Schwab S, Horn M, et al: Malignant middle cerebral artery territory infarction: Clinical course and prognostic signs. Arch Neurol 53:309–315, 1996.

Hamid RKA, Newfield P: Pediatric neuroanesthesia: Hydrocephalus. Anesthesiol Clin N Am 19:207–218, 2001.

Hankey GJ, Jamrozik K, Broadhurst RJ, et al: Long-term disability after first-ever stroke and related prognostic factors in the Perth Community Stroke Study, 1989–1990. Stroke 33:1034–1040, 2002.

Hebb AO, Cusimano MD: Idiopathic normal pressure hydrocephalus: A systematic review of diagnosis and outcome. Neurosurgery 49:1166–1184; 2001.

Henry TR, Chugani HT, Abou-Khalil BW, et al: Positron emission tomography, in Engel J (ed): Surgical Treatment of the Epilepsies, ed 2, New York: Raven Press, 1993, pp. 211–232.

Hop JW, Rinkel GJ, Algra A, et al: Case-fatality rates and functional outcome after subarachnoid hemorrhage: A systematic review. Stroke 28:660–664,1997.

Hopf NJ, Grunert P, Fries G, et al: Endoscopic third ventriculostomy: Outcome analysis of 100 consecutive procedures. Neurosurgery 44:795–804, 1999.

Hoppe-Hirsch E, Laroussinie F, Brunet L, et al: Late outcome of the surgical treatment of hydrocephalus. Childs Nerv Syst 14:97–99, 1998.

Horsley V: The function of the so-called motor area of the brain. Br Med J 2:125–132, 1909.

Howard MA 3rd, Volkov IO, Abbas PJ, et al: A chronic microelectrode investigation of the tonotopic organization of human auditory cortex. Brain Res 724:260–264, 1996.

Howard MA, Srinivasan J, Bevering CG, et al: A guide to placement of parietooccipital ventricular catheters: Technical note. J Neurosurg 82:300–304, 1995.

Howard MA, Gross AS, Dacey RG, et al: Acute subdural hematomas: An age-dependent clinical entity. J Neurosurg 71:858–863, 1989.

Howard MA, Volkov IO, Mirsky R, et al: Auditory cortex on the human posterior superior temporal gyrus. J Comp Neurol 416:79–92, 2000.

Howard MA, Volkov IO, Noh MD, et al: Chronic microelectrode investigations of normal human brain physiology using a hybrid depth electrode. Stereotact Funct Neurosurg 68:236–242, 1997.

Inagawa T, Kamiya K, Ogasawara H, et al: Rebleeding of ruptured intracranial aneurysms in the acute stage. Surg Neurol 28:93–99, 1987.

Intemann PM, Masterman D, Subramanian I, et al: Staged bilateral pallidotomy for treatment of Parkinson disease. J Neurosurg 94:437–444, 2001.

Javadpour M, Mallucci C, Brodbelt A, et al: The impact of endoscopic third ventriculostomy on the management of newly diagnosed hydrocephalus in infants. Pediatr Neurosurg 35:131–135, 2001.

Javedan SP, Tamargo RJ: Diagnostic yield of brain biopsy in neurodegenerative disorders. Neurosurgery 41:823–830, 1997.

Jones PA, Andrews PJD, Midgley S, et al: Measuring the burden of secondary insults in head injured patients during intensive care. J Neurosurg Anesth 6:4–14, 1994.

Kanpolat Y, Savas A, Bekar A, et al: Percutaneous controlled radiofrequency trigeminal rhizotomy for the treatment of idiopathic trigeminal neuralgia: A 25-year experience with 1,600 patients. Neurosurgery 48:524–532, 2001.

Kassell NF, Sasaki T, Colohan ART, et al: Cerebral vasospasm following aneurysmal subarachnoid hemorrhage. Stroke 16:562–572, 1985.

Kestle J, Drake J, Milner R, et al: Long-term follow-up data from the shunt design trial. Pediatr Neurosurg 33:230–236, 2000.

Kondziolka D, Fazl M: Functional recovery after decompressive craniectomy for cerebral infarction. Neurosurgery 23:143–147, 1988.

Kwiatkowski TG, Libman RB, Frankel M, et al: Effects of tissue plasminogen activator for acute ischemic stroke at one year. National Institute of Neurological Disorders and Stroke Recombinant Tissue Plasminogen Activator Stroke Study Group. N Engl J Med 340:1781–1787, 1999.

Lacroix M, Abi-Said D, Fourney DR, et al: A multivariate analysis of 416 patients with glioblastoma multiforme: Prognosis, extent of resection, and survival. J Neurosurg 95:190–198, 2001.

Langham J, Goldfrad C, Teasdale G, et al: Calcium channel blockers for acute traumatic brain injury. Cochrane Database Syst Rev (2):CD000565, 2000.

Leavens ME, Hill CS, Cech DA, et al: Intrathecal and intraventricular morphine for pain in cancer patients: Initial study. J Neurosurg 56:241–245, 1982.

Little JR, MacCarty CS: Colloid cysts of the third ventricle. J Neurosurg 39:230–25, 1974.

Lumenta CB, Skotarczak U: Long-term follow-up in 233 patients with congenital hydrocephalus. Childs Nerv Syst 11:173–175, 1995.

Lund-Johansen M, Svendsen F, Wester K: Shunt failures and complications in adults as related to shunt type, diagnosis, and the experience of the surgeon. Neurosurgery 35:839–844, 1994.

Mahmood A, Caccamo DV, Tomecek FJ, et al: Atypical and malignant meningiomas: A clinicopathological review. Neurosurgery 33:955–963, 1993.

Mavaddat N, Sahakian BJ, Hutchinson PJ, Kirkpatrick PJ: Cognition following subarachnoid hemorrhage from anterior communicating artery aneurysm: Relation to timing of surgery. J Neurosurg 91:402–407, 1999.

McDougall CG, Spetzler RF: Cerebral aneurysms: Clip or coil? Surg Neurol 50:395–397, 1998.

McKissock W, Taylor JC, Bloom WH, et al: Extradural hematoma: Observations on 125 cases. Lancet 2:167–172, 1960.

Miller JD, Stanek AE, Langfitt TW: Concepts of cerebral perfusion pressure and vascular compression during intracranial hypertension, in Meyer JS, Schade J (eds): Progress in Brain Research, Vol. 35: Cerebral Blood Flow. Amsterdam: Elsevier, 1972, pp. 411–432.

Miller SS, Marin DB: Assessing capacity. Emerg Med Clin North Am 18:233–242, 2000.

National Institutes of Health (NIH). Surgery for epilepsy. NIH Consensus Statement 1990 [online]. Mar 19–21; 8:1–20. Retrieved from http:consensus.nih.gov/cons/077/077_statement.htm.

The National Institute of Neurological Disorders and Stroke rt-PA Stroke Study Group: Tissue plasminogen activator for acute ischemic stroke. N Engl J Med 333:1581–1587, 1995.

Nora LM, Benvenuti RJ: Medicolegal aspects of informed consent. Neurol Clin 16:207–216, 1998.

Ondo W, Almaguer M, Jankovic J, et al: Thalamic deep brain stimulation: Comparison between unilateral and bilateral placement. Arch Neurol 58:218–222, 2001.

Pahwa R, Lyons KE, Wilkinson SB, et al: Comparison of thalamotomy to deep brain stimulation of the thalamus in essential tremor. Mov Disord 16:140–143, 2001.

Penn RD, Paice JA: Chronic intrathecal morphine for intractable pain. J Neurosurg 67:182–186, 1987.

Povlishock JT: Traumatically induced axonal injury: Pathogenesis and pathobiological implications. Brain Pathol 2:1–12, 1992.

Powers WJ, Grubb RL, Darriet D, et al: Cerebral blood flow and cerebral metabolic rate of oxygen requirements for cerebral function and viability in humans. J Cereb Blood Flow Metab 5:600–608, 1985.

Rao V, Lyketsos CG Psychiatric aspects of traumatic brain injury. Psychiatr Clin North Am 25:43–69, 2002.

Rivas JJ, Lobato RD, Sarabia R, et al: Extradural hematoma: Analysis of factors influencing the courses of 161 patients. Neurosurgery 23:44–51, 1988.

Rosenberg SA: A new era for cancer immunotherapy based on the genes that encode cancer antigens. Immunity 10:281–287, 1999.

Ryder JW, Kleinschmidt BK, Keller TS: Sudden deterioration and death in patients with benign tumors of the third ventricle area. J Neurosurg 64:216–223, 1986.

Saitoh Y, Shibata M, Hirano S, et al: Motor cortex stimulation for central and peripheral deafferentation pain. Report of eight cases. J Neurosurg 92:150–155, 2000.

Sampson FC, Hayward A, Evans G, et al: Functional benefits and cost/benefit analysis of continuous intrathecal baclofen infusion for the management of severe spasticity. J Neurosurg 96:1052–1057, 2002.

Sandson TA, Price BH: Diagnostic testing and dementia. Neurol Clin 14:823–830, 1997.

Schwab S, Steiner T, Aschoff A, et al: Early hemicraniectomy in patients with complete middle cerebral artery infarction. Stroke 29:1888–1893, 1998.

Son EI, Howard MA, Ojemann GA, et al: Comparing the extent of hippocampal removal to the outcome in terms of seizure control. Stereotact Funct Neurosurg 62:232–237, 1994.

Spencer SS, Schramm J, Wyler A, et al: Multiple subpial transection for intractable partial epilepsy: An international meta-analysis. Epilepsia 43:141–145, 2002.

Steinschneider M, Volkov IO, Noh MD, et al: Temporal encoding of the voice onset time phonetic parameter by field potentials recorded directly from human auditory cortex. J Neurophysiol 82:2346–2357, 1999.

The Deep-Brain Stimulation for Parkinson's Disease Study Group. Deep-brain stimulation of the subthalamic nucleus or the pars interna of the globus pallidus in Parkinson's disease. N Engl J Med 345:956–963, 2001.

Trepanier LL, Kumar R, Lozano AM, et al: Neuropsychological outcome of Gpi pallidotomy and Gpi or STN deep brain stimulation in Parkinson's disease. Brain Cogn 42:324–347, 2000.

Verity CM, Golding J: Risk of epilepsy after febrile convulsion: A national cohort study. BMJ 303:1373–1376, 1991.

Virasch N, Kruse CA: Strategies using the immune system for therapy of brain tumors. Hematol Oncol Clin North Am 15:1053–1071, 2001.

Wada J, Rasmussen T: Intracarotid injection of sodium amytal for the lateralization of cerebral speech dominance experimental and clinical observations. J Neurosurg 17:266–282, 1960.

Wara WM, Sheline GE, Newman H, et al: Radiation therapy of meningiomas. Am J Roentgenol Radium Ther Nucl Med 123:453–458, 1975.

Wijdicks EF: Brain death worldwide: Accepted fact but no global consensus in diagnostic criteria. Neurology 58:20–25, 2002.

Wilberger JE, Harris M, Diamond DL: Acute subdural hematoma: Morbidity, mortality, and operative timing. J Neurosurg 74:212–28, 1991.

Yates D, Roberts I: Corticosteroids in head injury: It's time for a large simple randomized trial. CRASH trial management group. Corticosteroid randomisation after significant head injury. BMJ 321:128–129, 2000.

Disorders of Consciousness

Douglas I. Katz

Joseph T. Giacino

Ascending reticular activating system (ARAS)

Brain death

Coma

Consciousness

Confusional state

Locked-in state

Minimally conscious state (MCS)

Vegetative state (VS)

DISORDERS OF CONSCIOUSNESS

One of the most challenging tasks in clinical practice is the assessment of patients with impaired consciousness. Faced with a person with severely limited or degraded responsiveness, the clinician must decipher whether there is any evidence of cognitive awareness. The assessment includes recognizing the clinical condition, applying the appropriate diagnostic label, and determining the cause, location and severity of brain dysfunction. The purpose of this chapter is to present information necessary for clinicians to understand and diagnose disorders of consciousness based on presently understood diagnostic nomenclature and pathophysiology. The accuracy of this assessment may be crucial to prognosis, treatment decisions, and ethical issues surrounding whether or not to continue a treatment. The following sections will elaborate some of conceptual issues and problems in defining consciousness, the anatomic substrate of consciousness, and the pathologic causes of altered consciousness. Some information from functional neuroimaging is presented that may shed new light on our concepts of unconsciousness with partially preserved cerebral functioning. Subsequent sections discuss the definitions and diagnostic criteria for various conditions of impaired consciousness and related disorders, issues in assessment of patients with profound impairments of consciousness, prognosis, and treatment options.

The Problem of Defining Consciousness

Defining consciousness has been a longstanding, elusive challenge, engaging disciplines ranging from neuroscientists to psychologists to philosophers. Dualist philosophers separated mind and body, presenting consciousness as a mysterious interaction of spiritual and physical realms. Most modern neuroscientists approach the problem from a tacit foundation that consciousness exists as a biologic brain function. The challenge of explaining consciousness at a neural level remains formidable, but is increasingly available to scientific study. There has been a surge of interest in neuroscience for the study of consciousness and impairments of consciousness, spurred further by the field of artificial intelligence and the prospect of powerful computers that may some day possess characteristics of consciousness.

Widely accepted definitions of consciousness usually include some reference to *awareness* of self and the environment (James, 1890; Plum & Posner, 1980). Hobson (1997) defines consciousness as the brain's ability to form a unified representation of the world, our bodies, and ourselves. William James (1890) (and more recently others such as John Searle [1992], Thomas Nagel [1986], and Antonio Damasio [1999]) emphasized several properties of consciousness including its *personal* aspects, unique to the point of view of the conscious individual; its *constantly changing* characteristics, stable for only short periods of time; its *continuity*, linking consciousness of the past with consciousness of the present; its *selectivity* and *finite* capacity to attend to the array of stimuli presenting to the nervous system at any moment.

These definitions of consciousness provoke further questions, including what constitutes "awareness" and what level of awareness is sufficient for attribution of "conscious awareness." The complexity of processing from basic sensation to cognition of self and environment over time varies considerably from lower animals to humans, from infants to adults, and even, at different times, in fully conscious adult humans. Are infants or nonhuman animals fully conscious? What qualities or complexity of processing constitute "full consciousness"? These are among the provocative, frequently debated questions encountered in discussions of the definition of the nature of consciousness.

Various authors have proposed hierarchical levels of consciousness and awareness that highlight distinctions from gross wakefulness, to elemental perception, to highly processed multimodal perceptions, integrated with a sense of self. At the highest levels, consciousness encompasses an individual's awareness of his or her internal state and external world, integrated with a comprehensive sense of self, and includes perspective of the past and anticipated future. One such hierarchy (Block, 1996; Young, 1998) includes the terms *crude consciousness, phenomenal consciousness,* and *access consciousness.* Crude consciousness refers to alertness and wakefulness but does not imply awareness of self or the environment. Phenomenal consciousness is the basic registration of external and internal phenomena—perception at the simplest levels, not necessarily at a level of awareness apparent to the person. Access consciousness is awareness at a level available for directing attention, decision making, and action, and includes both external and self-awareness. Damasio (1999) argues that awareness of self and awareness of objects in the environment are neurobiologically intertwined. He proposes two levels of awareness of self with respect to objects, referred to as *core* and *extended consciousness.* Core consciousness provides the individual with a sense of self in the here and now. It is the simplest sense of self within the environment, without a sense of past or future, and without any requirement for memory or linguistic capacity. (Core consciousness is present in lower animals.) Extended consciousness, which itself has many gradations, refers to an elaborated sense of self in the world, within the context of an individual's history and future.

These gradations of consciousness are further illustrated by the evidence of mental operations and neural encoding that occur outside of explicit conscious awareness in persons capable of full consciousness. Brain activity during sleep and dreaming is the most obvious example. Other examples include "blindsight" in persons with hemianopia (Weiskrantz et al., 1974), preserved implicit memory in patients with severe amnesia (Schacter,1990), procedural learning (Cohen & Squire, 1980), and "covert" recognition in patients with prosopagnosia (Tranel & Damasio, 1985). The process of "unconsciously" tying one's shoe while simultaneously engaged in another activity qualifies as one of the many normal lapses in awareness that occur routinely in quotidian reality.

The problem of defining consciousness is compounded further by the property of subjectivity. This has been referred to as the "hard problem" of consciousness (Chalmers, 1996). It is an issue not only in how the brain forms a sense of self but also that one's consciousness is an entirely personal representation, one that cannot be fully objectified. It is accessible only through report of that person, analogy to one's own experience, or inference based on behavior. This lack of an objective probe of consciousness creates one of the main challenges for clinicians who assess patients with severely impaired consciousness.

The Problem of Defining Impaired Consciousness

Compromise in the capacity for full conscious awareness is a common consequence of neurologic disorders. There are numerous acute and chronic causes of impaired consciousness (Table 30-1). Impairments range from complete unconsciousness to alterations of consciousness at various quantitative and qualitative levels. There may be only minimal evidence of sensory cognitive integration or there may be a deficit in a particular capacity (such as attention, memory, or executive functioning) that affects the quality of conscious awareness. Further, there may be a deficit in conscious awareness of particular classes or properties of stimuli, such as semantic awareness in patients with Wernicke's aphasia or hemispatial awareness is some patients with large right hemisphere lesions. Conversely, recent evidence demonstrates there may be loss of consciousness for all but an isolated class of responses (see discussion of modular phenomena in section following).

Assessment of impaired consciousness and accurate diagnosis are confounded by three inherent problems. The first concerns applying labels to different levels of impairment and recognizing that boundaries between conditions may be somewhat arbitrary. Evaluation and the proper application of diagnostic labels is often a difficult clinical challenge, fraught with inaccuracy and inconsistency (Childs et al., 1993; Andrews, 1996). Diagnostic labels have been developed for conditions of impaired consciousness (e.g., coma, vegetative state (VS), minimally conscious state (MCS), confusional state, or delirium) depending on the quantity and quality of the disturbance. Conditions that resemble unconsciousness, such as those that limit capacity to respond, combined with relatively preserved cognition (locked-in syndrome) add to the diagnostic challenge. Block's (1996) conceptual levels of consciousness, described above, provide a heuristic model for differentiating among states of impaired consciousness (Table 30-2). The absence of *crude consciousness* corresponds to *coma;* the absence of *phenomenal consciousness* corresponds to the *vegetative state;* without *access consciousness*, the individual is left in a *minimally conscious state* (see definitions in section following).

The second inherent problem of assessment and diagnosis is that judgments concerning the presence or absence of consciousness are based on indirect evidence. Plum and Posner (1980) acknowledged this dilemma nearly two decades ago, noting that "the limits of consciousness are hard to define satisfactorily and quantitatively and we can only infer the self-awareness of others by their appearance and their acts." There is currently no specific biologic probe for consciousness and the assessment of conscious awareness is necessarily indirect. Functional neuroimaging provides another window on the nature of consciousness and disorders of consciousness, albeit still indirect. Assessment of level of consciousness relies primarily on behavioral observation, but behavior is often nonspecific. The same behavior may reflect reflexive, involuntary, or intentional activity. For example, episodes of "smiling" in a noncommunicative patient with impaired consciousness could be due to facial dystonia (i.e., reflexive), pseudobulbar release syndrome (i.e., involuntary), or

TABLE 30-1. Causes of Impaired Consciousness—Coma/ Vegetative/Minimally Conscious States

Acute causes	Subacute/chronic causes
Traumatic injury	Degenerative diseases
Nontraumatic injury	Tumors
Hypoxic-ischemic disturbances	Developmental malformations
Stroke	Metabolic dysfunction
Central nervous system infection	
Metabolic/toxic disturbances	

TABLE 30-2. Conceptual Levels of Consciousness, Anatomy and Clinical-Pathologic Consequences

Level of consciousness	Anatomy	Pathologic consequence
Crude	Brainstem/ diencephalon	Coma
Phenomenal	Partial cortical	Vegetative state
Access	Integrated cortical	Minimally conscious state

(From Block N, Flanagan O, Guzeldere [eds]: The Nature of Consciousness: Philosophical Debates. Cambridge, MA: MIT Press, 1997; and Young GB: Consciousness, in Young GB, Ropper AH, Bolton CF; Coma and Impaired Consciousness: A Clinical Perspective. New York: McGraw–Hill, 1998.)

amusement (i.e., intentional). Valid interpretation of behavioral responses in patients with disturbances in consciousness frequently requires repeated evaluation and, in some cases, may not be possible. Cognitive awareness or conscious intent may be difficult to interpret when responses are extremely inconsistent or simple. There is an inverse relationship between the dimensions of *complexity* and *consistency* when judging whether behavior is evidence of consciousness. When a behavior is more complex, such as a verbalization, fewer instances of the response are sufficient to diagnose consciousness. When a behavior is less complex, such as a finger movement, a greater number of occurrences are necessary to establish a link to stimulus awareness or conscious intention.

A third problem that militates against the establishment of consensual definitions of impaired consciousness involves the issue of temporal flux. Consciousness is a dynamic process. Diurnal fluctuations in normal consciousness are well recognized but little is known about the process of recovery from states of unconsciousness. Figure 30-1 depicts theoretic temporal variations in the progression from unconsciousness to consciousness. The *linear* model conceptualizes consciousness as a dichotomous phenomenon in which unconsciousness resolves across progressively decreasing gradations until a specific, albeit undefined, threshold is crossed and consciousness is recovered. The Glasgow Coma Scale (GCS) (Teasdale & Jennett, 1974), which was designed to measure the depth and duration of unconsciousness, is built upon this framework. The linear model reflects traditional notions of consciousness and is the model adhered to by the medicolegal system.

The *stochastic* model maintains that there are random fluctuations in consciousness, particularly during the early stages of recovery from coma or the VS. These fluctuations may occur on a day-to-day or moment-to-moment basis, and may account for the

inconsistency in responsiveness that typifies patients with disorders of consciousness.

Consciousness may also be construed as a *modular* phenomenon with no clear boundary demarcating consciousness and unconsciousness. This model suggests that one can retain fragments of conscious behavior while remaining unconscious. This seemingly radical view is supported by recent functional neuroimaging studies. Schiff and colleagues (1999) studied a series of patients diagnosed with persistent VS who demonstrated stereotypical fragments of organized behavior. Cerebral metabolic function was investigated in these patients by co-registering positron emission tomography with [18]fluorodeoxyglucose (FDG-PET) images with magnetic resonance imaging (MRI) data. Functional neuroimaging findings were subsequently analyzed relative to the behaviors of interest. Among the patients studied, the authors reported results obtained from a woman who was in a VS of 20 years' duration following multiple ruptures of an arteriovenous malformation. Despite the absence of any evidence of command following, communication, or other purposeful behavior, videotaped observation revealed intelligible verbalization of single words every 24 to 72 hours. MRI findings were indicative of severe bilateral posterior subcortical hemorrhagic changes and destruction of the right thalamus, posterior left thalamus, and right basal ganglia. The results of the PET studies showed that average global cerebral metabolism was reduced to 43% of normal. Of particular interest, the left frontal operculum, left superior temporal gyrus and left basal ganglia remained active at 50% to 60% of normal. The authors concluded that the patient's capacity to generate words represented a "fixed motor action pattern" mediated by remnant circuits of the speech module and was unrelated to intentional language function. Figure 30-2 shows the PET regions of interest coregistered on MRI. Similar results showing preserved auditory (Laureys et al., 2000) and visual processing (Menon et al., 1998) in the VS have also been reported. These findings suggest that isolated modular operations may be retained in the absence of consciousness after catastrophic brain injury.

Although these problems in establishing consensual definitions of impaired consciousness represent significant obstacles to the study of normal and altered states of consciousness, they also offer potentially fruitful directions for research. To date, very little clinical research has addressed the issues raised in the preceding discussion. It is likely that the ever-expanding range of functional neuroimaging techniques will contribute significantly to the study of consciousness. At the same time, it is essential that terminology and experimental methods be standardized to facilitate comparison of results across studies.

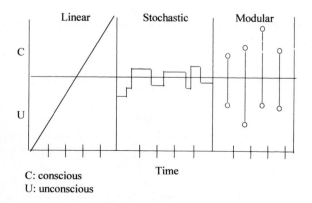

FIGURE 30-1. Temporal models illustrating theoretical temporal variations in the progression from unconsciousness to consciousness.

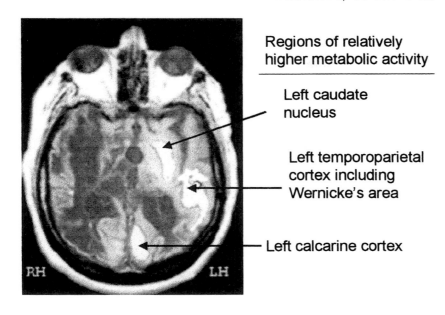

Regions of relatively higher metabolic activity

Left caudate nucleus

Left temporoparietal cortex including Wernicke's area

Left calcarine cortex

FIGURE 30-2. Coregistered image of positron emission tomography with [18]fluorodeoxyglucose (FDG-PET) with magnetic resonance imaging (MRI) of a woman in a vegetative state for more than 20 years after arteriovenous malformation hemorrhages. The patient had no evidence of command following, communication, or other purposeful behavior, but she displayed intelligible verbalization of single words every 24 to 72 hours. The FDG-PET study indicated that average global cerebral metabolism was reduced to 43% of normal; however the left frontal operculum, left superior temporal gyrus, and left basal ganglia remained active at 50% to 60% of normal. Regions of relatively higher metabolism are bright areas (*arrows*). The patient's capacity to generate words may represent a "fixed motor action pattern" mediated by remnant circuits of the speech module but unrelated to intentional language function. (Reproduced with permission from Schiff ND, Ribary U, Plum F, et al: Words without mind. J Cogn Neurosci 11:650–656, 1999.)(See Color Plate 12)

Impaired Consciousness: Clinical Conditions and Definitions

Coma (Unarousable Unconsciousness)

Coma is a state of unconsciousness without capacity for arousal (Plum & Posner, 1980). Patients in coma lack any sign of spontaneous or stimulus-induced arousal, and there are no signs of sleep-wake cycles. They exhibit neither signs of consciousness nor purposeful movement. When occurring as a result of acquired damage, such as after traumatic brain injury (TBI) or anoxic brain injury, coma is an acute or subacute condition that usually evolves to the VS or to a higher level of consciousness within 2 to 4 weeks in patients who survive (Plum & Posner, 1980; Multi-Society Task Force on PVS, 1994). Other terms are used to describe disorders of arousability and wakefulness, including *somnolence, obtundation,* and *stupor.* These terms do not define either level of consciousness or the capacity for conscious awareness. They simply describe the present state of arousal and are not interchangeable with the terms that define disorders of consciousness.

Vegetative State (Arousable Unconsciousness)

The *vegetative state* (VS) is a term that was introduced by Jennett and Plum (1972) to describe a condition of absence of signs of conscious awareness but with capacity for spontaneous or stimulus-induced arousal and sleep-wake cycles. There is complete or partial preservation of brainstem and hypothalamic functions. The condition may be part of the evolving course of a disorder from coma to VS to higher levels of consciousness, such as the *minimally conscious state* and *confusional state*; or the end stage of a deteriorating condition such as dementia (Volicer et al., 1997); it may also be a prolonged or permanent condition. The Multi-Society Task Force on PVS (1994) proposed the term *permanent vegetative state* (PVS) in cases where the probability of recovery from unconsciousness is extremely low (12 months for patients with TBI and 3 months for patients with non-TBI). The use of the term permanent remains controversial because there are occasional reports of patients who recover consciousness after these cutoffs (Childs & Mercer, 1996). The Task Force also proposed use of the term *persistent* vegetative state when the condition lasts longer than 1 month. This term is even more controversial and confusing because it has been used in a variety of ways, at different intervals post onset, sometimes implying permanence. The term *persistent vegetative state* probably should not be used because of these ambiguities. Instead, the diagnosis, *vegetative state* might be described by the time from onset to indicate the level of chronicity, as recommended by the Aspen

Workgroup on Vegetative and Minimally Conscious States (Giacino et al., 1997).

The diagnostic criteria for VS include all the following (Multi-Society Task Force on PVS, 1994):

- No evidence of awareness of self or environment
- No evidence of sustained, reproducible, purposeful, or voluntary behavioral responses to visual, auditory, tactile, or noxious stimuli
- No evidence of language comprehension or expression
- Intermittent wakefulness manifested by the presence of sleep–wake cycles
- Sufficiently preserved hypothalamic and brainstem autonomic functions to permit survival with medical and nursing care
- Bowel and bladder incontinence
- Variably preserved cranial nerve reflexes and spinal reflexes

Patients in vegetative states may move in a non-purposeful manner. Smiling, grimacing, tearing, grunting, and moaning may occur, but without any apparent relation to external or internal stimuli. Patients in the VS generally do not track or fixate on objects, a capacity requiring some preservation of the cortical-subcortical visual network. Often, fixation and sustained visual pursuit are early signs of the transition to low levels of conscious awareness, such as the MCS. Giacino and Kalmar (1997) found that visual tracking did occur in as many as 20% of patients who otherwise fit the criteria for the VS.

Minimally Conscious State

The MCS is a recently defined diagnostic condition to describe patients who have clinical signs of awareness beyond the criteria for the VS but still have profoundly impaired consciousness (Giacino et al., 2002). It has been widely recognized that many patients display such a clinical condition (Andrews, 1996; ACRM, 1995). This clinical state may occur during the transition between unconsciousness and higher levels of consciousness, or as a fixed, persistent condition in those with very severe brain damage. A number of clinical scales address the transition to these levels (e.g., the Rancho Los Amigos Scale [Hagen et al., 1972], Glasgow Coma Scale [Teasdale & Jennett, 1974], Coma–Near Coma Scale [Rappaport et al., 1992], Coma Recovery Scale [Giacino et al., 1991], neurologic recovery stages of diffuse brain injury [Alexander, 1982; Katz, 1992; Katz & Mills, 1999]. Several workgroups have recently grappled with defining this clinical state: American Congress of Rehabilitation Medicine (ACRM) Interdisciplinary Special Interest Group for Head Injury (1995), International Working Party on the Manage-

ment of the Vegetative State (Andrews, 1996), and the Aspen Neurobehavioral Conference Workgroup (Giacino et al., 1997). All these groups recognized the need for more precision in the diagnosis of different levels of impaired consciousness. The ACRM group (ACRM, 1995) proposed the term *minimally responsive state* and the International Working Party used *inconsistent low awareness state* in addition to various gradations of the VS (Andrews, 1996). More recently, the Aspen Workgroup recommended the term *minimally conscious state* (Giacino et al., 1997, 2002).

The *minimally conscious state* is defined as "a condition of severely altered consciousness in which minimal but definite behavioral evidence of self or environmental awareness is demonstrated" (Giacino et al., 2002).

The diagnostic criteria for *minimally conscious state* include limited but clearly discernible evidence of self or environmental awareness demonstrated on a reproducible or sustained basis by one or more of the following behaviors (Giacino et al., 2002):

- Simple command following
- Gestural or verbal "yes/no" responses (regardless of accuracy)
- Intelligible verbalization
- Purposeful behavior, including movements or affective behaviors that occur in contingent relation to relevant environmental stimuli and are not the result of reflexive activity.

Any of the following behavioral examples provide sufficient evidence for "purposeful behavior." This list is not meant to be exhaustive:

a. Smiling or crying in response to the linguistic or visual content of emotional but not neutral topics or stimuli
b. Vocalizations or gestures that occur in direct response to the linguistic content of questions
c. Reaching for objects in a manner that demonstrates a clear relationship between object location and direction of reach
d. Touching or holding objects in a manner that accommodates the size and shape of the object
e. Pursuit eye movement or sustained fixation that occurs in direct response to moving or salient stimuli

Criteria for the upper boundary, distinguishing MCS from higher levels of consciousness, are required to complete the definition of MCS. This clinical boundary is somewhat more arbitrary because there is no single clinical dimension that easily delineates higher levels of consciousness. This problem points out the difficulty in defining all of these clinical states, trying to apply distinct clinical borders to a process that occurs along a continuum of arousal and cognition. Nevertheless, the Aspen Workgroup proposed the following clinical criteria for emergence from the MCS (Giacino et al., 2002). One or both of the following should be present:

- Functional interactive communication (at least, ability to answer six out of six basic yes/no questions on two separate occasions regarding personal or environmental orientation (e.g., Are you sitting down?) using verbalization, writing, signaling or augmentative communication devices), or
- Functional use of objects (demonstrating the ability to appropriately use two different objects on two consecutive evaluations (e.g., bringing comb to head or pencil to paper).

It should be apparent that the ability to communicate or use objects may be affected by loss of certain capacities such as language and praxis in a person who is otherwise fully conscious. The ability to communicate or manipulate objects may also be constrained by impairments in speech or motor abilities. In such cases, evaluation of communication and object use should be tailored to the person's preserved motor abilities, or enhanced by compensatory strategies or augmentative devices.

The distinction between *vegetative* and *minimally conscious states* is important because prognosis and treatment choices may be different for these two conditions. Decisions regarding withdrawing fluid and nutrition, continuing medical or rehabilitative treatment, or managing pain and suffering might hinge on the differentiation of unconsciousness and minimal consciousness. Further, scientific study of severe alterations of consciousness requires uniform and precise definitions of these clinical states to allow replication and comparisons across studies. Diagnostic accuracy for the *vegetative state*, distinguishing it from the *minimally conscious state* and other related conditions, has been less than ideal (Childs et al., 1993; Andrews et al., 1996). Figure 30-3 provides an algorithm for distinguishing coma, VS, MCS, and related disorders.

Acute Confusional State

Acute confusional state is a condition of global cognitive impairment primarily related to a deficit in attention (Lipowski, 1990; Mesulam, 2000). *Delirium* is another commonly used term for this condition. Abilities to focus, sustain, select, and shift attention are compromised, and the coherence of perception and thought may be lost because of distractibility and mental intrusions. Patients

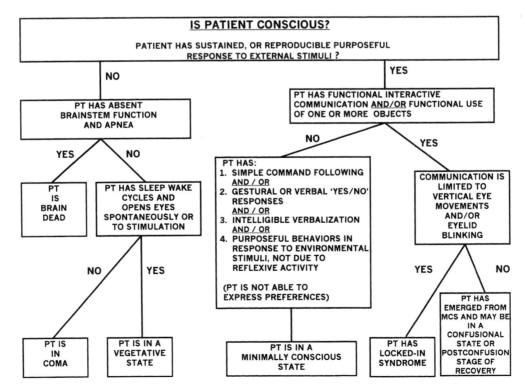

FIGURE 30-3. Algorithm for determining appropriate diagnostic category for patients with impaired consciousness and limited responsiveness. MCS, minimally conscious state; PT, patient. (Adapted with permission from Ashwal S, Cranford R: The minimally conscious state in children. Semin Pediatr Neurol 9:19–34, 2002.)

in confusional states are usually disoriented, have difficulty sustaining mental activity, have disrupted sleep-wake cycles, and have heightened or reduced levels of psychomotor activity. Confusion compromises all cognitive domains to variable extents, in large part because of the disruption of attention. Patients in confusional states are frequently confabulatory or delusional, and they may experience auditory, visual, or tactile hallucinations. Perseveration and impersistence of thought and movement are other common signs. Emotion, behavior, drive, and motor activity may range from a hypokinetic, apathetic, amotivational syndrome (abulia) to a hyperkinetic, agitated, impulsive, irritable, combative syndrome. Patients may display one or the other of these extremes, or may shift between syndromes as their conditions evolve, or even in the course of a day.

There are numerous causes of confusion, including systemic, toxic, and metabolic disturbances as well as diffuse, multifocal, and focal neurologic disturbances (Table 30-3). Older persons or those with underlying neurologic conditions, such as dementia, are particularly prone to confusional states. By definition, onset is acute or subacute and fluctuations in impairments and behaviors are typical. Some individuals, especially the elderly, may display diurnal variations ("sundowning"). Acute confusional states may be a self-limited problem related to a particular neurologic insult, such as a seizure or a toxic/metabolic disturbance, or may be part of the evolving natural history of a disorder such as TBI. When part of the natural history of a disorder, acute confusional states may be a transitional stage between unconsciousness, minimal consciousness and higher levels of consciousness and cognitive functioning. Several scales, such as the Rancho Los Amigos Levels of Cognitive Functioning and Braintree Neurological Stages of Recovery, have been developed to track these transitions (Table 30-4). There is a proportional relationship between the time to evolve through the stages of unconsciousness and the acute confusional state in persons with diffuse TBI; both are largely a function of the severity of diffuse traumatic pathology (Katz & Alexander, 1994). Confusional states generally resolve in hours to weeks, but some patients may develop more persistent attentional and global cognitive disturbances. When chronic, other diagnostic labels, such as dementia, may be used.

Other Related Terms and Conditions

A number of related neurologic conditions and terms may be included in, or must be distinguished from, the conditions defined above.

Akinetic Mutism: Originally described by Cairns and colleagues (1941), this refers to a condition of wakefulness with an absence or paucity of speech and spontaneous movement. There is usually some evidence of conscious behavior in these patients but these behaviors are inconsistent, incomplete, and usually ineffective. It is usually the drive or intent to speak or move that is severely compromised in these patients. The syndrome may be incomplete or fluctuating; some patients display varying levels of speech, movement, and interaction.

A number of clinical and pathological variations of this condition have been described. In general, akinetic mutism involves bilateral damage to reticular-cortical or limbic-cortical connections in the central neuraxis, from paramedian reticular areas of the midbrain and diencephalon to basal or medial frontal areas (Plum & Posner, 1980). Damage to dopaminergic projections may be key and the condition has been partially reversed using dopaminergic agents (Anderson, 1992).

Most patients with this condition will fit the diagnostic criteria of MCS. There are some who may not, highlighting the possible discrepancy between cognitive awareness (consciousness) and the drive to move and speak (responsiveness). There may be a spectrum of this condition ranging from patients with primarily motor initiation deficits to those with both motor to cognitive deficits.

Dementia: This term refers to a persistent or progressive impairment of intellectual function involving a number of cognitive spheres. It is a general term that may or may not imply a compromise in consciousness. Sometimes consciousness is compromised in later stages

TABLE 30-3. Causes of Confusional States

Systemic causes	Diffuse/multifocal CNS causes	Focal CNS causes
Metabolic conditions	Traumatic brain injury	Right hemisphere
Systemic infection	Anoxic brain injury	Occipitotemporal lobe
Endocrine dysfunction	Meningoencephalitis	Caudate
Nutritional deficiency	Epileptic seizures	Thalamus
Intoxications	Vasculitis	Midbrain
	Hypertensive encephalopathy	

CNS, central nervous system.

of progressive dementias. Therefore, patients with chronic impairments of consciousness may be considered demented but not all patients with dementia have impaired consciousness.

Brain death: This is an irreversible condition of complete absence of brain function, including brainstem function. Cranial nerve function and brainstem reflexes are absent. There may be some preservation of spinal cord reflex activity. Respirations cease without external ventilator support, though the heart may continue to beat. There are prescribed criteria for diagnosing brain death, including flatline electroencephalogram (EEG) or absence of metabolic activity on PET scanning, or excluding confounds such as hypothermia and central nervous system (CNS) depressants (Beecher, 1968).

Locked-in syndrome: This is a condition of loss of voluntary motor control in the setting of preserved consciousness. The classic syndrome involves damage to corticospinal and corticobulbar pathways in the *basis pontis*. Other conditions that cause bilateral profound damage to these pathways or diffuse compromise to peripheral nerves (e.g., Guillain-Barré syndrome) or neuromuscular junction (e.g. neuromuscular blocking agents) can cause the syndrome.

It is important to distinguish impairments of consciousness from locked-in syndrome because classical locked-in syndrome implies fully preserved consciousness. It should be recognized, however, that many patients in vegetative or minimally conscious states have profound loss of motor abilities because of concomitant damage to motor control areas. It may be difficult to demonstrate conscious behavior as it emerges in these patients because of limited motor output capabilities. Clinicians must be vigilant for signs of cognitive awareness in patients with very limited motor response capabilities, because consciousness may emerge, masked by the loss of motor ability.

Anatomy of Consciousness

Two basic anatomic principles underlie the anatomy of consciousness: the upper brainstem is critical for arousal, and thalamic-cortical activity is necessary for the content of consciousness.

The prerequisite of consciousness is arousal and the anatomic substrate for arousal is the widespread

TABLE 30-4. Scales to Track Progression through Stages of Impaired Consciousness

Rancho Los Amigos Levels of Cognitive Functioning*

I.	No response
II.	Generalized responses
III.	Localized responses
IV.	Confused—agitated
V.	Confused—inappropriate
VI.	Confused—appropriate
VII.	Automatic—appropriate
VIII.	Purposeful and appropriate

Braintree Stages of Neurologic Recovery (Diffuse Brain Injury)†

1. Coma/unarousable unconsciousness: unresponsive, eyes closed

2. Vegetative state/arousable unconsciousness: no cognitive responsiveness, gross wakefulness, sleep-wake cycles

3. Minimally conscious state: inconsistent response to commands, inconsistent but definite signs of purposeful behavior

4. Confusional state: recovered communication, amnesic (PTA), severe attentional deficits, agitated, hypoaroused or labile behavior

5. Postconfusional/evolving independence: resolution of PTA, cognitive improvement, achieving independence in daily self-care, improving social interaction; developing independence at home

6. Social competence/community reentry: safety and independence in the home, recovering cognitive abilities, goal-directed behaviors, social skills, personality; developing independence in community; returning to academic or vocational pursuits

PTA, post-traumatic amnesia.

* From Hagen C, Malkmus D, Durham P: Levels of Cognitive Functioning. Downey, CA: Rancho Los Amigos Hospital, 1972.

† From Katz DI, Neuropathology and neurobehavioral recovery from closed head injury. J Head Trauma Rehab 7:1–15, 1992; and Katz DI, Mills VM: Traumatic brain injury: Natural history and efficacy of cognitive rehabilitation, in Stuss DT, Winocur G, Robertson IH (eds): Cognitive Neurorehabilitation. New York: Cambridge University Press, 1999, pp. 175–187.

FIGURE 30-4. Ascending reticular activating system. (Reproduced with permission from Young GB, Ropper AH, Bolton CF: Coma and Impaired Consciousness: A Clinical Perspective. New York: McGraw-Hill, 1998, pp. 3–38.)

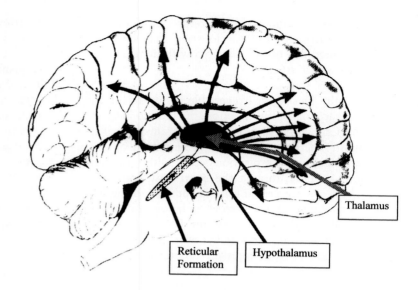

innervation of cortex by small groups of neurons in the brainstem, diencephalon (principally the hypothalamus and thalamus) and basal forebrain. These projections are collectively known as the ascending reticular activating system (ARAS). The projections reach the cortex either directly or by way of a thalamic relay (Fig. 30-4). A number of neurotransmitters are involved including acetylcholine, monoamines and gamma-aminobutyric acid (GABA).

The importance of the ARAS to arousal was made clear by Moruzzi and Magoun (1949), who demonstrated that electrical stimulation of the brainstem reticular formation could produce long-lasting cortical activation. This was further supported with the observation that destruction of the rostral ARAS led to coma in laboratory animals.

There are three sources of interconnected ascending projections to the cortex that make up the ARAS (Fig. 30-5). The first, the reticulothalamic pathway, originates in the brainstem and projects a dorsal pathway to the thalamus, particularly the reticular and intralaminar nuclei. A ventral pathway bypasses the thalamus and projects to the basal forebrain by way of the lateral hypothalamus. The second source is the thalamus itself, the specific nuclei, under the influence of the intralaminar and reticular nuclei, projecting somatotopically to specific cortical regions. The third source of cortical projections is extrathalamic and originates in the basal forebrain (cholinergic), and the posterior hypothalamus (histaminergic).

Specific neurochemicals play key roles in arousal. The cholinergic pathway arising in the brainstem reticular formation (mesopontine in *pedunculopontine, laterodorsal tegmental* nuclei) that project to the reticular and intralaminar nuclei of the thalamus makes up the reticulothalamic pathway. The direct source of the cortical cholinergic pathway is from the *nucleus basalis* in

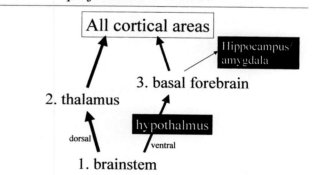

FIGURE 30-5. The ascending reticular activating system projects to the cortex by way of three interconnected sources: (1) brainstem; (2) thalamus; (3) basal forebrain.

the basal forebrain projecting to all cortical areas but more intensely within limbic areas (Mesulum, 2000, Chapter 1). A noradrenergic pathway originates in the *locus ceruleus* and has a diffuse cortical projection, but particularly dense in primary sensory areas (Mesulum, 2000). Other neurotransmitter pathways include a histaminergic pathway from the posterior hypothalamus (*tuberomammillary nucleus)* to the cortex; dopaminergic pathways from the *substantia nigra* and *ventral tegmental areas* of the midbrain projecting to the striatum, limbic, basal frontal, and medial frontal cortical areas; and a serotonergic pathway arising from the *raphe nuclei* in the midline of the brainstem, from the midbrain to medulla, largely synapsing on inhibitory interneurons.

The thalamus, at the apex of the brainstem reticular activating system (RAS), plays a key role as a distributor and relay of activating functions (Fig. 30-6).

Thalamic Reticular Nucleus:
gating reticular activation to cortex

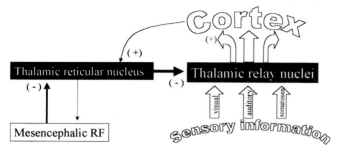

FIGURE 30-6. The reticular nucleus of the thalamus has a tonic inhibitory influence on the thalamus. The mesencephalic reticular formation inhibits the inhibitory influence of the reticular nucleus, allowing enhanced activation of the thalamic nuclei and consequently, the cortex. Inhibitory influence (*minus signs*); excitatory influence (*plus signs*).

The specific thalamic relay nuclei can selectively activate particular areas of cortex, promoted by specific sensory inputs. The reticular nucleus of the thalamus serves as an inhibitory gate to thalamic activation. The mesencephalic reticular formation inhibits the inhibitory influence of the reticular nucleus, allowing enhanced activation of the thalamic nuclei and as a consequence, the cortex. Thalamocortical neurons become tonically activated by these cholinergic, noradrenergic and histaminergic inputs from the brainstem and hypothalamic RAS projections. During sleep and in some pathological states there is a simultaneous disinhibition of the reticular nucleus of the thalamus and reduction of cholinergic input from the brain stem, allowing GABAergic inhibitory influences on thalamocortical neurons. The hyperpolarization of these cells sets them into a mode of rhythmic, periodic bursts of action potentials reaching cortical neurons to produce a characteristic synchronized slow-wave pattern on EEG. This slow wave activity indicates that the thalamus is not enabled to relay sensory information to the cortex and is characteristic of deep sleep, some seizure types, and pathologic states that block thalamocortical transmission. During normal wakefulness, when the thalamus is in the transmission mode under the influence of cholinergic inputs, the cortex is activated, reflected by a fast, low-voltage, desynchronized EEG pattern. (Mesulum, 2000, Chapter 3). Global arousal and attention depend on the ascending inframodal influence of the ARAS and the descending supramodal influence of prefrontal, parietal, and cingulate cortices. These supramodal and inframodal components of the attentional matrix influence each other by way of cortical projections to the reticular nucleus of the thalamus and to nuclei of the transmitter-specific pathways in the extrathalamic ARAS, and reciprocal projections from the ARAS by way of intralaminar thalamic nuclei and neurotransmitter-specific brainstem nuclei (Mesulum, 2000, Chapter 3).

While the ARAS is clearly involved in wakefulness, attentiveness and sleep, the ARAS alone does not account for the full spectrum of consciousness and the various hierarchical levels of conscious awareness. The biological correlates of consciousness remain one of the most challenging problems in neuroscience. The basic components of consciousness are derived from the conjoining of self-awareness with perception of the external world. These components require activity in cortical and subcortical areas beyond the ARAS. Expanding this connection of self-awareness and perception to realms of memory and autobiographical awareness makes up even higher levels of conscious awareness which require yet other distributed neural systems. How consciousness, especially the aspect of subjectivity, derives from the activity in various cortical-subcortical networks remains unclear. Damasio (1999) proposes that the more basic level of conscious awareness that he terms *core consciousness* (a basic sense of self in the here and now) requires activity beginning in brainstem nuclei, hypothalamus and basal forebrain, and coordinating with the cingulate, thalamus and superior colliculi that create second-order representations of objects with respect to the organism. Damage to structures outside of these areas leaves core consciousness preserved. Damasio further proposes that higher levels of conscious awareness, which he terms *extended consciousness*, require coordinated activity in other brain areas such as temporal and prefrontal cortices, including areas involved in working memory, and subcortical areas, including the amygdala and thalamus.

Pathophysiology of Impaired Consciousness

Coma is caused by structural or metabolic disruption of the arousal system. Coma may occur with damage to the ARAS in the brainstem from the midpontine level upward. More prolonged coma requires somewhat larger lesions that involve bilateral reticular structures in midbrain and diencephalon (hypothalamus and thalamus) or midbrain and upper pontine tegmentum (Plum & Posner, 1980; Plum, 1991). Coma may also occur with diffuse cortical dysfunction, perhaps by secondarily depressing ARAS functioning (Feeney & Baron, 1986, Young, 1998). More restricted lesions in the brainstem, diencephalons or cortex may cause transient coma. For instance, bilateral paramedian thalamic lesions (Castaigne et al., 1981, Katz et al., 1987) and unilateral, dominant hemisphere lesions (Albert et al., 1976) may cause transient coma.

Vegetative state is related to diffuse cortical damage, often with laminar necrosis as seen in patients with anoxia, white matter damage, such as patients with diffuse axonal injury after trauma, or thalamic damage. Often these structures are damaged in combination. Relatively isolated damage to the brainstem as a cause of prolonged VS is uncommon; most of those patients do not survive (Adams et al., 2000). There have been reports of relatively isolated damage to the thalamus, bilaterally as a cause of prolonged VS (Kinney et al., 1994), and when the cortex and brainstem are spared there is usually profound damage to the subcortical white matter or thalamus, bilaterally (Adams et al., 2000). Damage to thalamic relay nuclei or damage to thalamic-cortical connections is central in many cases of prolonged VS.

There is limited information regarding pathologic damage for patients in the *minimally conscious state*. It is likely that prolonged MCS is associated with the same pathologic types and distributions as that associated with prolonged VS. Theoretically, the difference in clinical conditions may be related to some additional preservation of thalamocortical or cortical activity in the minimally conscious state compared with the VS. Adams and colleagues (2000) point out that patients who remain at a level of recovery just beyond VS, which they term *severe disability* (presumably including those who may fit the criteria of MCS), have similar pathology to patients who remained vegetative. They speculate that the damage may, in general, be less severe in patients with MCS but note that there are not yet good quantitative methods to measure damage such as diffuse axonal injury. In a subsequent study (Jennett et al., 2001) researchers compared pathology in patients who were vegetative versus those who were severely disabled at death. All patients who were vegetative had either severe grades of diffuse axonal injury or thalamic damage or both; half of patients who recovered to the severe disability level had neither severe grades of diffuse axonal injury nor thalamic damage. It is not known, however, how many of those patients defined as severely disabled would have fit the criteria for MCS.

One special case is the subset of patients with *akinetic mutism*. This syndrome is usually associated with bilateral mesial prefrontal, thalamic or midbrain damage (Cairns et al., 1941). Interruption of mesencephalic cortical dopaminergic projections may be an important cause of the syndrome.

The acute confusional state is related to damage or dysfunction in structures related to arousal and attention. Confusional states may occur with focal lesions involving the attentional matrix, including supramodal (limbic, prefrontal, and parietal areas) and inframodal (ARAS), or with multifocal lesions that affect domain specific attentional modulations (Mesulum, 2000, Chapter 3).

CLINICAL ASSESSMENT

Assessment procedures designed specifically for use in patients with chronic disorders of consciousness have proliferated and improved during the last decade. Many of the newer generation of assessment strategies were developed by clinicians working in rehabilitation settings in order to address the limitations of the GCS in detecting subtle changes in neurobehavioral function and predicting postacute outcome. Two different behavioral approaches to assessment have been devised. Standardized methods rely on fixed administration and scoring criteria to generate a global profile of cerebral function. The primary indications for use of standardized measures include monitoring rate of recovery, predicting outcome and disposition needs, facilitating interdisciplinary treatment planning, and evaluating the efficacy of rehabilitative interventions. Alternatively, individualized quantitative assessment protocols based on single-subject design principles have been developed to address case-specific questions.

Standardized Behavioral Assessment Methods

Standardized assessment measures designed for patients with disorders of consciousness include the Coma Recovery Scale (CRS) (Giacino et al., 1991), the Coma–Near Coma Scale (CNC) (Rappaport et al., 1992) and the Western NeuroSensory Stimulation Profile (WNSSP) (Ansell & Keenan, 1989). Although item content varies across measures, all elicit auditory, visual, motor, and communication responses following administration of specific types of sensory stimuli. Adequate reliability and validity have been demonstrated for each measure (O'Dell et al., 1996). Only the CRS has been shown to meet requirements for equal interval measurement of neurobehavioral function (Kalmar & Giacino, 2000). These instruments appear to represent improvements over the GCS in evaluating level of consciousness over time; however, their diagnostic and prognostic sensitivity and specificity remain unknown.

Individualized Behavioral Assessment Methods

The major limitation of standardized approaches is that they cannot be modified to address case-specific questions without jeopardizing validity and reliability. As discussed previously, it is often difficult to interpret behavioral responses in patients with disorders of consciousness because their response repertoire is typically diminished, inconsistent, or qualitatively ambiguous. For this reason, individualized quantitative behavioral assessment strategies have been developed. In this technique, clinical questions are individually tailored, stimuli and target responses are operationalized a priori, and efforts are made to control for examiner and examinee response biases. Target behaviors are recorded during repeated trials administered under varying conditions (e.g., at rest, to command, to an unrelated command). This technique has been used to differentiate command following (Whyte et al., 1999a), visual attention (Whyte & DiPasquale, 1995), and gestural communication responses (Whyte et al., 1999b) from random motor activity. McMillan (1996) employed a single-subject design to determine whether a minimally responsive traumatically brain-injured patient could reliably communicate a preference concerning withdrawal of life-sustaining treatment. Responses to questions were executed using a button press. Results indicated that the number of affirmative responses to "wish to live" questions was significantly greater than chance suggesting that the patient could participate in end-of-life decision making.

Strategies to Enhance Behavioral Assessment

When behavioral responses are equivocal on bedside examination, additional steps may be taken to facilitate detection of consciousness. The following recommendations should be considered when response ambiguity is encountered:

- Provide sensory stimulation (e.g., tactile, deep pressure, vestibular) prior to assessment to ensure that arousal level is maximized
- Screen for subclinical seizure activity
- Administer a broad range of stimuli and test more than one response modality
- Use motor commands that are within the patient's neuromuscular capacity
- Perform serial reassessments to increase the likelihood of detecting volitional responses and to establish response consistency
- Incorporate observations of family members and paraprofessionals into assessment procedures
- Discontinue potentially sedating medications
- Eliminate unnecessary sources of distraction
- Avoid multiunit and syntactically complex commands
- Avoid commands that rely on behaviors that may be difficult to differentiate from generalized or reflexive motor activity (e.g., hand squeeze, eye blinks)

Special care must be taken when evaluating young children with disturbances in consciousness. Immature language and motor development may confound interpretation of command-following and communicative responses. It is also important to consider the potential influence of aphasia, apraxia, and other higher cortical disorders when evaluating adults and children.

PROGNOSIS

Outcome of Vegetative State

The Multi-Society Task Force on PVS (1994) reviewed the available outcome data for patients in the VS. They considered two dimensions of recovery: regaining consciousness and functional outcome based on Glasgow Outcome Scale (Jennett & Bond, 1975). They analyzed data on 434 adults and 106 children with TBI, and 169 adults and 45 children with non-TBI—primarily anoxic brain injury and stroke. Of adults with TBI who were unconscious at least 1 month, 33% recovered consciousness by 3 months postinjury and 52% by 1 year. If patients were still unconsciousness at 3 months, 35% regained consciousness by 1 year. The probability of regaining consciousness was considerably lower for adults with nontraumatic brain injuries. Of those unconscious for 1 month, only 11% recovered consciousness at 3 months and 15% at 6 months. There were no additional recoveries after 6 months for those with nontraumatic injuries. Children fared only a little better, with up to 62% regaining consciousness at 1 year after TBI; after nontraumatic injury, recovery of consciousness was observed mostly within the first 3 months (11%), but a very small percentage (2%) regained consciousness between 6 and 12 months. (Table 30-5 summarizes these outcome data.) The Task Force concluded that prognosis for recovery of consciousness was very poor 12 months after traumatic injuries and 3 months after non-TBI for both adults and children. They deemed that VS is *permanent* if there is no sign of consciousness by these intervals after injury.

Some caution is warranted in the use of the term *permanent* VS at 3 and 12 months, because the number of patients with TBI observed for follow-up after 12 months is limited, and there are several reports of patients who regain consciousness after these times (Multi-Society Task Force on PVS, 1994; Childs & Mercer, 1996). Although probability of recovery of consciousness is very low after 12 months, the chance of recovery is not absolutely lost.

TABLE 30-5. Prognosis and Functional Outcome for Adults after Prolonged Unconsciousness in Patients with Traumatic Brain Injury (TBI) or Nontraumatic Brain Injury (Non-TBI)

Unconscious at least 1 month

   TBI: 33% death, 15% VS, 28% SD, 17% MD, 7% GR

   non-TBI: 53% death, 32% VS, 11% SD, 3% MD, 1% GR

Unconscious at least 3 months

   TBI: 35% death, 30% VS, 19% SD, 16% MD or GR

   non-TBI: 46% death, 47% VS, 6% SD, 1% MD or GR

Unconscious at least 6 months

   TBI: 32% death, 52% VS, 12% SD, 4% MD or GR

   non-TBI: 28% death, 72% VS, 0% SD, 0% MD or GR

VS, vegetative state; SD, severe disability; MD, moderate disability; GR, good recovery.

(From Multi-Society Task Force on PVS: Medical aspects of the vegetative state. N Engl J Med 330: 1499–1508, 1572–1579, 1994.)

Functional outcome in those patients who regain consciousness is summarized in Table 30-5. Of adults who recover consciousness by 12 months after TBI, more than half were *severely disabled,* nearly one third were *moderately disabled,* and a little more than one in eight patients were at a *good recovery* level. After nontraumatic brain injury, nearly three quarters of those who regained consciousness remained severely disabled at 12 months. Children fared a little better for nontraumatic injuries in that over half were severely disabled and nearly half achieved a good recovery level. Adults over age 40 had a considerably worse prognosis, rarely better than the severe disability level of recovery.

Mortality rates were relatively high for patients in vegetative states at least 1 month, with 82% at 3 years, and 95% at 5 years (Multi-Society Task Force on PVS, 1994). These figures do not consider somewhat better life expectancy in those that survive the first year and do not account for recent improvements in survival with better medical care.

The rate of early improvement is a significant factor in predicting recovery from a prolonged impairment of consciousness. A recent multicenter study of patients with severely impaired consciousness demonstrated that improvement in level of consciousness in the first 2 weeks after rehabilitation admission accounted for half the variance of outcome at 4 months after TBI (Whyte et al., 1999a).

Neuroimaging and electrophysiologic studies may aid in determining prognosis. Kampfl and colleagues (1998) found that location of brain lesions after trauma was a better predictor of recovery from prolonged unconsciousness than Glasgow Coma Scale scores, age and papillary abnormalities. Patients who did not recover consciousness by 12 months had a significantly higher frequency of corpus callosum, corona radiata, and dorsolateral brainstem lesions than those who did regain consciousness. Somatosensory evoked potential studies may be useful in predicting outcome of VS after anoxic brain injury. Absence of the N20 potential in the presence of the earlier N14 potential is a very poor prognostic sign for recovery of consciousness (Zegers et al., 1986).

Outcome of Minimally Conscious State

There is very little specific information about the prognosis of the MCS. Rappaport and colleagues (1992) reported improvement in 25% of a small group of patients with impaired consciousness followed over a 4-month period. Only those in MCS (referred to as "near-coma") improved; none in VS improved in the follow-up period.

Giacino and Kalmar (1997) compared outcomes of patients in VS versus MCS. In this study 55 patients in VS were compared with 49 patients in MCS when they were first evaluated an average of 9.6 weeks postinjury. Causes of injury were traumatic (n = 70) and nontraumatic (n = 34) (mostly anoxic brain injury and stroke). Using the Disability Rating Scale (DRS) s the outcome measure at 1, 3, 6, and 12 months postinjury, they reported the following findings:

1. Patients initially in MCS fared better than those initially in VS, the differences becoming progressively more apparent at 3, 6, and 12 months postinjury.
2. The probability of a more favorable outcome (moderate or no disability) by 1 year was much greater for the MCS group (38%) than for the VS group (2%), and occurred only in those patients with TBI.
3. Forty-three percent of the MCS group remained severely disabled or worse (1/10 of the nontraumatic MCS group was vegetative and 2/10 died) at 12 months.
4. So-called "borderzone" clinical signs (visual tracking, motor agitation) were much more prevalent among patients in MCS than those in VS. Seventy-three percent of patients in VS who displayed tracking recovered consciousness, whereas 45% without tracking recovered consciousness.

Impaired Consciousness in the Natural History of Recovery after Brain Injury

Coma, VS, minimally conscious state, and acute confusional state should be viewed as a part of the natural history of diffuse and multifocal brain injury. The majority of patients with diffuse brain injury (traumatic and nontraumatic) pass through a series of stages that are qualitatively similar across a wide range of severity (see Table 30-4). The duration of these stages and severity of impairments vary in proportion to injury severity (Katz & Alexander, 1994; Katz, 1997). Most patients with brain injury severe enough to cause unconsciousness, probably progress through stages of unconsciousness, with eyes closed (*coma*), to unconsciousness with eyes open (*vegetative state*), to a stage of inconsistent, erratic responsiveness (*minimally conscious state*). Once consciousness is clearly established, patients enter a stage of impaired attention and anterograde amnesia (e.g., post-traumatic amnesia [PTA]) (*confusional state*) followed by a post-confusion phase of recovery. In patients with diffuse TBI (diffuse axonal injury) there is a predictable, proportional relationship between the duration of unconsciousness (coma and VS) and the duration of the confusional state (PTA) (Katz & Alexander, 1994; Katz et al., 1999).

In patients with very severe damage, recovery may stall at one or another stage (e.g., *"permanent" vegeta-*

tive state or minimally conscious state). Patients with less severe injuries may transition through the early stages quickly and discrete stages may not be clinically apparent. It remains to be established what proportion of patients recovering from unconsciousness at different severities of injury evolve through discernible coma, vegetative, and minimally conscious stages.

Viewed in this way, the transition from unconsciousness to consciousness is a continuum without distinct boundaries. As the transition progresses, and cortical function resumes, the consistency and complexity of behavior increases. The first signs of the transition may be an increase in alertness and spontaneous movement with lower levels of stimulation, such as the arrival of the examiner (Wilson et al., 1996). At the "borderzone," behaviors such as tracking, emotional expressions, and nonstereotyped motor sequences resume, heralding higher-level cognitive behaviors (Multi-Society Task Force on PVS, 1994; Ansell, 1995; Giacino & Kalmar, 1997). A small number of patients will recover these borderzone behaviors without resuming any other cognitive behavior, such as following commands (Giacino & Kalmar, 1997).

TREATMENT INTERVENTIONS AND THEIR EFFECTIVENESS

Despite the daily demands on clinicians in acute, subacute and postacute settings to provide treatment for patients with disorders of consciousness, there are no standards of care. This stems from the dearth of well-designed empirical investigations of treatment effectiveness in this population. The majority of studies completed to date represent class III evidence (Woolf, 1992), which includes case reports, uncontrolled case series, and retrospective data analyses. Few prospective randomized controlled trials have been conducted. Consequently, clinical decision making is often idiosyncratic across patients and between centers. In the remainder of this section, treatment methods commonly employed in patients with severe disturbances in consciousness will be reviewed with attention to the effectiveness of these interventions.

Physical Management Strategies

Basic medical and physical management strategies are routinely used in patients with disorders of consciousness to maintain comfort, reduce complications, and maximize the opportunity for functional recovery (Giacino, et al., 1997). These interventions typically include pharmacologic stabilization of autonomic dysreflexia, range of motion exercises to prevent spasticity and contractures, positioning protocols to minimize positional hypotension and skin breakdown, nutritional supplementation to maintain optimal body weight and management of abnormal muscle tone to facilitate voluntary movement.

There is some evidence that formal physical management programs may decrease inpatient rehabilitation length of stay (Mackay et al., 1992) and reduce residual functional disability through the postacute period of recovery (Tanheco & Kaplan, 1982; Timmons et al., 1987; Gray & Burnham, 2000). Based on a retrospective review of 349 "slow-to-recover" Canadian patients (mean initial GCS score = 5.9) admitted to a long-term rehabilitation unit (mean time to rehab admission >12 months), Gray and Burnham (2000) found significant improvements in functional outcome from admission to discharge (mean length of stay = 359 days) on the DRS (Rappaport et al., 1982) and in combined Functional Independence Measure/ Functional Assessment Measure scores (Hall, 1997). Specifically, motor and cognitive subscores significantly improved across treatment with 85% of patients admitted from inpatient facilities discharged to community-based settings. Interestingly, there was no significant difference in degree of improvement between patients with TBI and non-TBI, although late TBI admissions showed significantly less improvement than those admitted earlier.

Sensory Stimulation

Sensory stimulation (SS) typically involves the controlled application of specific types and intensities of sensory stimuli determined by measurement of response thresholds. SS is almost universally employed in rehabilitation centers that offer services for patients with disorders of consciousness. Some trauma centers also provide SS, although modifications may be instituted to prevent iatrogenic effects (e.g., elevated intracranial pressure, abnormal posturing, dysautonomia). Despite the widespread use of SS, its efficacy remains controversial. In addition to the fact that most of the existing literature on the effectiveness of SS is based on class III evidence, interpretation of the results of these studies is compromised by nonuniform use of diagnostic terms, failure to control for spontaneous recovery, reliance on outcome measures with limited external validity, and lack of attention to enduring changes in behavior.

The effectiveness of SS has been investigated by multiple reviewers during the last 10 years. In their 1991 review, Zasler and colleagues (1991) selected eight studies frequently cited by proponents of coma stimulation programs. These investigators opined that "the present knowledge and literature when taken as a whole do not support the utility of structured sensory stimulation as a means of altering the course of neurological recovery after severe brain injury." Based on this conclusion, they suggested that sensory stimulation should not be relied upon as the primary component of rehabilitative intervention. The same conclusion was reached by the Multi-Society Task Force on the PVS (1994) as part of their review of the world literature on PVS. The Task Force acknowledged published reports of improvement induced by stimulation programs but noted the absence of any verified controlled studies. They stated, "Overall, there is no published evidence that coma sensory stimulation improves the clinical outcome in patients in a persistent vegetative state." Wilson and McMillan (1993) reviewed 14 studies published between 1978 and 1992 that included patients in coma and the VS. These authors concluded, "In relatively few studies where attention has been given to extraneous factors, the balance of evidence suggests that SS can alter behavior in the unconscious patient and can reduce the duration of acute coma." In 1996, Giacino completed an evidence-based review of seven "representative" studies concerning the effectiveness of SS. Citing the weakness of published research in this area, the author argued that "it is difficult to draw any definitive conclusions regarding the utility of SS as a rehabilitative intervention capable of influencing patient outcome." In light of the lack of sufficient negative evidence disproving the effectiveness of SS, Giacino concluded that SS could be considered a treatment option with the admonition that clinicians have a duty to clearly discuss with family and caretakers the degree of uncertainty associated with this type of treatment.

In one of the few studies published in the United States subsequent to completion of the reviews described above, Gruner and Terhaag (2000) reported "significant changes" during administration of multimodal stimulation in 16 patients admitted to a neurosurgical intensive care unit (mean GCS = 6.56, range = 3–9). Using a single-subject ABA design, these investigators found significant increases in heart and respiratory rates during application of tactile and auditory stimuli relative to baseline measures. The authors reported that 14 of the 16 patients were reevaluated 2 years later. Of these, one patient remained vegetative, two were completely dependent on care, six had severe functional disability but were able to perform self-care, and three regained independence. The degree to which stimulation-induced changes in physiologic parameters predicted later recovery of function cannot be determined from the data reported, which obviously limits the significance of the study.

Pharmacologic Interventions

The rationale underlying the use of pharmacologic interventions for patients with disorders of consciousness involves the exogenous regulation of targeted neurotransmitter systems thought to underlie dysfunctional neurophysiologic processes. Stimulants, dopamine ago-

nists, and tricyclic antidepressants are frequently prescribed to enhance arousal (i.e., wakefulness), expedite recovery of consciousness, facilitate behavioral initiation, and promote communication in patients diagnosed with VS and MCS. Published evidence supporting the effectiveness of these agents is relatively sparse and varies according to diagnosis and target behavior.

Although there are a number of case reports suggesting that stimulants (e.g., methylphenidate, dextroamphetamine, pemoline) and dopamine agonists (e.g., amantadine, bromocriptine, levodopa-carbidopa) can facilitate recovery of consciousness in comatose and vegetative patients (Haig & Ruess, 1990; Worzniak et al., 1997; Chatham-Showalter & Netsky-Kimmel, 2000; Passler & Riggs, 2001), none provide compelling evidence. Chatham-Showalter and Netsky-Kimmel (2000) reported that they were able to stimulate improvement in consciousness and cognition in a cohort (n = 13) of Rancho level I to III patients after initiation of the anticonvulsant lamotrigine. This finding was based on retrospective comparison of lamotrigine-treated and untreated patients who completed a course of rehabilitation within the authors' facility. Based on progress notes, the authors concluded that 75% of the treated patients showed shorter lengths of stay (72 vs. 117 days), more cognitive improvement, and better discharge dispositions (community vs. facility) than the untreated group. The report does not specify how many, if any, of the subjects were in coma or VS at the time lamotrigine was introduced and states only that the mean Rancho level was 2.6. The authors' "index case" for the study was, in fact, a 53-year-old man who had sustained a ruptured anterior communicating artery aneurysm and was "following one- to two-step repetitive directions" prior to receiving lamotrigine. In addition, there was no attempt to control for spontaneous recovery even though some subjects were included as early as 2 weeks postinjury.

Passler and Riggs (2001) reported greater functional recovery on the DRS in five consecutive traumatic VS patients treated with bromocriptine (2.5 mg twice daily) relative to a comparison group of 33 TBI VS patients previously described by Giacino and Kalmar (1997). Giacino and Kalmar reported that all five of their patients treated with bromocriptine emerged from VS and that mean DRS scores at 12 months postinjury (mean = 4.4, standard deviation [SD] = 4.4) were lower than the scores of the comparison group (mean = 19.0, SD = 4.5). From these data, Passler and Riggs concluded that recovery of the five treated patients "exceeded predicted levels of recovery based on the results of Giacino and Kalmar." This conclusion is tempered by methodological confounds in the design of Passler and Riggs' study. First, it is not clear that severity of injury was equivalent in the two groups of patients. Passler and Riggs' subjects were approximately 5 weeks postinjury at the time they were diagnosed with VS. In comparison, Giacino and Kalmar's subjects were almost 10 weeks postinjury at the time of diagnosis. Given the small number of subjects and shorter time postinjury, it is possible that Passler and Riggs' patients were less severely injured which may have accounted for a more rapid rate of recovery and less functional disability at 1 year.

In contrast to published findings concerning recovery of consciousness, there is reasonably good evidence that stimulants and dopaminergic agents can improve arousal in patients with VS and MCS. Using well-controlled single-subject designs, Whyte and colleagues have shown increases in duration of eye-opening with (DiPasquale & Whyte, 1996) and without (Whyte et al., 1999b) concomitant improvements in cognition following administration of methylphenidate and amantadine, respectively.

There is some evidence that pharmacologic interventions may be more effective for patients who have recovered at least basic signs of consciousness. Zafonte and colleagues (1998) used a single-subject design to explore the effectiveness of amantadine in a patient who remained in MCS for 5 months following a traumatic subdural hematoma. There was a strong dose–response relationship between amantadine and performance on the CNC scale. CNC performance gradually improved to the "no-coma" level as the amantadine was increased to a maximum dose of 400 mg/day. When the amantadine was reduced to 100 mg/day, CNC scores subsequently declined over a 2-week period; however, they recovered to the no-coma level after retitration up to the maximum dose.

Powell and colleagues (1996) recorded significant improvements in behavioral spontaneity and treatment participation in 10 consecutive patients with severe motivational deficits treated with bromocriptine (maximum dose = 10 mg/day) following admission to a rehabilitation unit. Improvements in behavioral initiative were maintained in eight of the subjects after the medication was discontinued. Reinhard and colleagues (1996) also reported significant improvements in behavioral and verbal initiation in three severely brain-injured patients with MCS who received tricyclic antidepressants (e.g., amitriptyline, desipramine) using an ABAB protocol. Other investigators have reported re-emergence of spontaneous speech and increased verbal fluency in MCS patients treated with dopaminergic agents (Barrett, 1991; Powell, Al-Adawi, Morgan et al., 1996). Adverse side effects including agitation (Giacino et al., 1992), perseveration (Giacino et al., 1992), and exacerbation of neglect (Barrett et al., 1999) have also been noted in association with the use of dopaminergic agents, suggesting the need for careful behavioral monitoring.

In sum, pharmacologic interventions appear to be most effective for enhancing verbal and behavioral expression in patients who have recovered consciousness but continue to demonstrate markedly diminished response repertoires. Although these agents appear to effectively improve behavioral initiation in some cases, concurrent increases in behavioral dysregulation have also been noted. It remains uncertain whether pharmacologic intervention can alter the natural history of recovery for patients with impaired consciousness.

Hyperbaric Oxygen Therapy

Hyperbaric oxygen therapy (HBOT) involves the inhalation of highly concentrated oxygen. This is accomplished by administering oxygen in a pressurized chamber filled with compressed air. This enhances the amount of arterial oxygen to more than 200% of normal, which produces vasoconstriction and reduces cerebral blood flow (CBF). A concomitant decrease in intracranial pressure ensues and there is improved glucose metabolism. In patients with severe brain injury, it has been hypothesized that HBOT may promote revascularization of the ischemic penumbra that surrounds the necrotic core, thereby restoring cellular function in damaged but still viable neurons. This process has been termed the "idling neuron" theory (Neubauer et al., 1990). HBOT-related changes in CBF detected on SPECT imaging have been reported to support this theory (Neubauer et al., 1992; Barrett et al., 1998). Rockswold and colleagues (2001) recently demonstrated significant increases in cerebrospinal fluid (CSF) and cerebral oxygen metabolism lasting up to 6 hours after HBOT in comatose patients with reduced or normal pre-treatment CBF. CSF lactate, a marker for ischemic brain injury, was also found to be significantly lower following HBOT. The effects of HBOT were no longer apparent 24 hours after treatment. These findings were thought to be indicative of sustained improvement in aerobic metabolism brought about by HBOT.

There are a few published reports of significant improvement in mortality and morbidity in acutely brain injured patients who received HBOT. Rockswold and colleagues (1992) conducted a large (n = 168) randomized, controlled trial of HBOT in a group of patients with severe closed head injury (CHI). There was a 50% reduction in mortality in those patients treated with HBOT (17%), compared with matched controls (32%). There was no significant difference in morbidity between groups based on GOS (Jennett & Bond, 1975) scores. An earlier study by Holbach and colleagues (1977) also compared GOS scores in HBOT-treated and untreated patients. Thirty-three percent of the HBOT-treated group met criteria for good recovery, compared with 6% of the untreated group.

A few tentative conclusions can be drawn about the effectiveness of HBOT based on the studies reviewed above. There is reasonably good evidence that HBOT can improve survival in severely brain-injured patients. At best, the evidence for functional improvement following HBOT is equivocal. Finally, there are no controlled studies indicating that HBOT significantly improves mortality or morbidity when utilized after the acute period of injury.

Deep Brain Stimulation

The classic animal studies of Moruzzi and Magoun (1949) and of Magoun (1965) mainly conducted in the 1950s first demonstrated that arousal is not dependent upon sensory input. These researchers were able to produce behavioral and electrophysiologic evidence of wakefulness in deeply anesthetized cats by electrically stimulating the brainstem reticular formation. They also showed preserved arousal reactions following auditory stimulation (i.e., whistle blast) in cats with bilateral ablation of the auditory and somatic afferent pathways of the rostral midbrain. Despite the animals' inability to hear or experience tactile sensation, they awakened to the whistle blast. EEG studies indicated that wakefulness was induced indirectly via excitation of the intact tegmental pathway located in the ARAS. These findings provided convincing evidence that arousal reactions were not triggered through direct activation of the cortex by sensory discharge, but rather by indirect excitation of the brainstem reticular formation.

Based on the findings of Moruzzi and Magoun, a number of investigators have attempted to facilitate recovery of consciousness in patients diagnosed with persistent VS by administering chronic deep brain stimulation (DBS). In these studies, DBS was applied through the dorsal column of the spine (Kanno et al., 1987), midbrain reticular formation (Tsubokawa et al., 1990; Katayama et al., 1991), or nonspecific thalamic nuclei (Tsubokawa et al., 1990; Katayama et al., 1991; Cohadon & Richer, 1993). Electrical pulses, delivered daily at various intensities on a recurring fixed schedule, were maintained for as long as 8 months. The results of these studies have been inconsistent. DBS has reportedly elicited a broad spectrum of responses ranging from reflexive (e.g., eye-opening, meaningless vocalizations, random limb movement) to purposeful (e.g., command following, verbal communication, self-feeding) behavior. In some cases, clinical recovery has reportedly been accompanied by improvements in EEG (Kanno et al., 1987; Tsubokawa et al., 1990), CBF (Tsubokawa, et al., 1990), cerebral metabolism (Tsubokawa et al., 1990) and evoked responses (Tsubokawa et al., 1990; Katayama et al., 1991). DBS trials have not been conducted in the United States because of the invasive nature of this treatment and the lack of convincing efficacy data. There are important methodological flaws and omissions in all the aforementioned studies, including insufficient documentation to confirm the diagnosis of VS, reliance on crude assessment and outcome measures, and failure to control for spontaneous recovery.

More recently, Schiff and colleagues (2000) have described a redesigned strategy for use of DBS that exploits modern advances in neuroimaging and neurosurgical intervention. In reviewing the earlier generation of DBS studies, these investigators identified some important limitations that may have decreased the effectiveness of the DBS. They note that previous studies targeted the nonspecific thalamic activating system in an effort to increase arousal in catastrophically brain-injured patients with no apparent sign of consciousness. They go on to point out that the likelihood of a favorable response to DBS is presumably lower when it is applied diffusely to the brains of patients who may not have adequate residual cortex (or cognitive function) to harness the DBS. Therefore, significant revisions to the original DBS protocol have been proposed.

In view of these concerns, Schiff and colleagues (2000) have suggested that eligibility criteria be modified to include only patients who demonstrate clear, albeit diminished, signs of consciousness. Second, they recommend that structural and functional neuroimaging studies be completed to identify patients who have sufficiently spared cortical fields to serve as a substrate for DBS. Finally, stereotactically guided surgical procedures would be performed to ensure that electrodes are placed within specific subdivisions of the thalamic nuclei that project to regions of preserved cortex. This procedure is intended to amplify residual cortical circuits and facilitate reemergence of coordinated cognitive and behavioral activity. The overarching goal of this approach is to restore functional capacity, not simply to promote arousal. This work is now in the preliminary stages.

Although formal programs for treatment of patients with disorders of consciousness have been in existence for approximately 25 years, there are still no standards of care for this population. As noted previously, empirical investigations of treatment efficacy in this area are surprisingly sparse, and most published studies have significant metholodologic weaknesses that compromise the strength of existing evidence. Thus, clinical decision making remains arbitrary and tends to be guided by subjective factors.

CONCLUSIONS

Disorders of consciousness present some of the most perplexing and difficult challenges for neurologic assessment. Our understanding of the nature of consciousness and the pathophysiology and clinical presentation of disorders of consciousness is still developing. New technologies, including functional imaging, may provide an added window on the anatomy and pathophysiology of consciousness and impaired consciousness. Treatment is another area where research is needed to develop guidelines for interventions, such as sensory stimulation, pharmacologic interventions, and unconventional procedures, such as DBS and HBOT. All these efforts, as well as good clinical diagnosis and prognosis, require a clearly defined, well-understood nomenclature, describing the clinical conditions and natural history observed in individuals with impaired consciousness. The recent surge in interest in consciousness and disorders of consciousness among a wide range of disciplines creates promise for progress in these areas in the near future.

■ KEY POINTS

☐ Defining consciousness has been an elusive challenge but most definitions include some reference to awareness of the environment and awareness of self. There are hierarchical levels of consciousness and awareness from gross wakefulness, to elemental perception, to highly processed multimodal perceptions integrated with a sense of self. At the highest levels, conscious awareness encompasses a comprehensive sense of self within the world and in the context of the individual past and future.

☐ Defining impaired consciousness is a challenge with regard to accurately applying diagnostic labels to a continuum of conditions with arbitrary boundaries, using indirect evidence based on varying, inconsistent, and often ambiguous behaviors.

☐ Several clinical conditions define different levels of impaired consciousness. *Coma* is a state of unconsciousness without signs of wakefulness. *Vegetative state* (VS) is unconsciousness with periods of gross wakefulness. The *minimally conscious state* (MCS) is a recently introduced term for patients with very limited or inconsistent signs of conscious awareness, but lacking capacity for functional communication or functional use of objects. *Acute confusional state* or *delirium* is a temporary condition of global impairment of cognitive functioning, primarily related to deficits in attention.

☐ Two anatomic principles underlie the anatomy of consciousness: the upper brainstem (ascending reticular activating system [ARAS]) is critical for arousal, and thalamic-cortical activity is necessary for the content of consciousness. Cortical arousal is facilitated by reticular brainstem-thalamic, brainstem-basal forebrain and specific thalamic-cortical projections. The anatomy of cognitive awareness is less understood and requires activity in various cortical-subcortical networks.

☐ The pathophysiology of coma involves damage to the ARAS or diffuse cortical dysfunction. The VS is caused by severe diffuse cortical or subcortical damage or profound damage to the thalamic nuclei or thalamic-cortical connections. The MCS is associated with less severe diffuse damage and significantly less chance of thalamic-cortical damage.

☐ Clinical assessment of patients with impaired consciousness can employ standardized scales to measure and track different levels of consciousness or individualized evaluations, including quantitative assessment of responses to statistically distinguish conscious volitional responses from reflexive or random automatic responses.

☐ Limited evidence for treatment effectiveness indicates that patients with severely impaired consciousness benefit from physical and medical management such as treating spasticity and contracture, and reducing autonomic dysfunction. There is little evidence to support sensory stimulation programs. Pharmacologic management using stimulants, dopamine agonists or other catecholamine agonists promote arousal and may improve responsiveness in patients who have regained some level of consciousness. It remains to be proven whether these agents can promote recovery of consciousness in unconscious patient. Deep brain stimulation to promote consciousness is an area of ongoing investigation.

☐ Prognosis for regaining consciousness and ultimate level of recovery is much worse for nontraumatic than traumatic brain injury (TBI). Children fare only a little better than adults. Prospects for recovery of consciousness are very poor if still unconscious at 12 months after TBI and only 3 months after non-TBI. Patients in the MCS have a significantly better prognosis than patients in the VS evaluated at a similar period after injury.

☐ Recovery of consciousness from coma to the VS to the MCS and higher levels of consciousness is a continuum without distinct boundaries. Severity of brain damage largely determines the rate of progression through this continuum and the potential to stall at one or another stage of recovery.

KEY READINGS

Damasio A: The Feeling of What Happens: Body and Emotion in the Making of Consciousness. San Diego, CA: Harcourt, 1999.

Giacino JT, Ashwal S, Childs N, et al: The minimally conscious state: definition and diagnostic criteria. Neurology 58:349–353, 2002.

Multi-Society Task Force on PVS: Medical aspects of the persistent vegetative state. N Engl J Med 330:1499–1508, 1994.

Plum F, Posner J: The Diagnosis of Stupor and Coma, ed 3. Philadelphia, PA: Davis, 1980.

Whyte J, Laborde A, DiPasquale MC: Assessment and treatment of the vegetative and minimally conscious patient, in Rosenthal M, Griffith ER, Kreutzer J, Pentland B (eds): Rehabilitation of the Adult and Child with Traumatic Brain Injury, ed 3. Philadelphia, PA: Davis, 1999, pp. 435–452.

Young GB, Ropper AH, Bolton CF: Coma and impaired consciousness: A clinical perspective. New York: McGraw-Hill, 1998.

REFERENCES

Adams JH, Graham DI, Jennett B: The neuropathology of the vegetative state after an acute brain insult. Brain 123:1327–1338, 2000.

Albert ML, Silverberg R, Reches A, et al: Cerebral dominance for consciousness. Arch Neurol 33:453–454, 1976.

Alexander MP: Traumatic brain injury, in Benson DF, Blumer D (eds): Psychiatric Aspects of Neurological Disease. New York: Grune and Stratton, 1982.

American Congress of Rehabilitation Medicine: Recommendations for the use of uniform nomenclature pertinent to patients with severe alterations in consciousness. Arch Phys Med Rehabil 76:205–209, 1995.

Anderson B: Relief of akinetic mutism from obstructive hydrocephalus using bromocriptine and ephedrine. J Neurosurg 76:152–155, 1992.

Andrews K: International Working Party on the management of the vegetative state: Summary report. Brain Injury 10:797–806, 1996.

Ansell B: Visual tracking behavior in low functioning head-injured adults. Arch Phys Med Rehabil 76:726–731, 1995.

Ansell BJ, Keenan JE: The Western Neuro Sensory Stimulation Profile: A tool for assessing slow-to-recover head-injured patients. Arch Phys Med Rehabil 70:104–108, 1989.

Ashwall S, Cranford R: The minimally conscious state in children. Semin Pediatr Neurol 9:19–34, 2002.

Barrett AM, Crucian GP, Schwartz RL, et al: Adverse effect of dopamine agonist therapy in a patient with motor-intentional neglect. Arch Phys Med Rehabil 80:600–603,1999.

Barrett K: Treating organic abulia with bromocriptine and lisuride: Four case studies. J Neurol Neurosurg Psychiatry 54:718–721, 1991.

Barrett KG, Masel BE, Harch PG, et al: Cerebral blood flow changes and cognitive improvement in chronic stable traumatic brain injuries treated with hyperbaric oxygen therapy. Paper presented at the American Academy of Neurology Annual Meeting, Minneapolis, MN, 1998.

Beecher HK: A definition of irreversible coma: Report of the Ad Hoc Committee of the Harvard Medical School to examine the definition of brain death. JAMA 205:85, 1968.

Block N: How can we find the neural correlate of consciousness. Trends Neurosci 19:456–459, 1996.

Cairns H, Oldfield RC, Pennybacker JB, et al: Akinetic mutism with an epidermoid cyst of the 3rd ventricle. Brain 64:273–290, 1941.

Castaigne P, Lhermitte F, Buge A, et al: Paramedian thalamic and midbrain infarcts: Clinical and neuropathological study. Ann Neurol 10:127, 1981.

Chalmers DJ: The Conscious Mind. New York: Oxford University Press, 1996.

Chatham-Showalter PE, Netsky-Kimmel D: Stimulating consciousness and cognition following severe brain injury: A new potential clinical use for lamotrigine. Brain Injury 14:997–1001, 2000.

Childs NL, Mercer WN, Childs HW: Accuracy of diagnosis of persistent vegetative state. Neurology 43:1465–1467, 1993.

Childs NL, Mercer WN: Brief report: Late improvement in consciousness after post-traumatic vegetative state. N Engl J Med 334:24–25, 1996.

Cohadon F, Richer E: Deep cerebral stimulation in patients with post-traumatic vegetative state: 25 cases. Neurochirurgie 39:281–292, 1993.

Cohen NJ, Squire LR: Preserved learning and retention of pattern analyzing skill in amnesia: Dissociation of knowing how and knowing that. Science 210:207–209, 1980.

Damasio A: The Feeling of What Happens: Body and Emotion in the Making of Consciousness. San Diego, CA: Harcourt, 1999.

DiPasquale MC, Whyte J: The use of quantitative data in treatment planning for minimally conscious patients. J Head Trauma Rehabil 11:9–17, 1996.

Feeney DM, Baron J-C: Diaschisis. Stroke 17:817–830, 1986.

Giacino JT, Ashwal S, Childs N, et al: The minimally conscious state: Definition and diagnostic criteria. Neurology 58:349–353, 2002.

Giacino JT, Kalmar K: The vegetative and minimally conscious states: A comparison of clinical features and functional outcome. J Head Trauma Rehabil 12:36–51,1997.

Giacino JT, Kezmarsky MA, DeLuca J, et al: Monitoring rate of recovery to predict outcome in minimally responsive patients. Arch Phys Med Rehabil 72:897–901, 1991.

Giacino JT, Zasler ND, Katz DI, et al: Development of practice guidelines for assessment and management of the vegetative and minimally conscious states. J Head Trauma Rehabil 12:79–89, 1997.

Giacino J: Sensory stimulation: Theoretical perspectives and the evidence for effectiveness. Neurorehabilitation 6:69–78, 1996.

Giacino JT, Rodriguez M, Cicerone KD: Exacerbation of frontal release behaviors with use of amantadine following traumatic brain injury [abstract]. Arch Phys Med Rehabil 73:975, 1992.

Gray DS, Burnham RS: Preliminary outcome analysis of a long-term rehabilitation program for severe acquired brain injury. Arch Phys Med Rehabil 81:1447–1456, 2000.

Gruner ML, Terhaag D: Multimodal early onset stimulation (MEOS) in rehabilitation after brain injury. Brain Injury 14:585–594, 2000.

Hagen C, Malkmus D, Durham P: Levels of Cognitive Functioning. Downey, CA: Ranchos Los Amigos Hospital, 1972.

Haig AJ, Ruess JM: Recovery from vegetative state of six months duration associated with Sinemet (levodopa/carbidopa). Arch Phys Med Rehabil 71:1081–1083, 1990.

Hall K: The functional assessment measure (FAM). J Rehabil Outcomes Measurement 1:63–65, 1997.

Holbach KH, Caroli A, Wassman H: Cerebral energy metabolism in patients with brain lesions at normo- and hyperbaric oxygen pressures. J Neurol 217:17–30, 1977.

James W: The Principles of Psychology. New York: Holt, 1890.

Jennett B, Bond M: Assessment of outcome after severe brain damage: A practical scale. Lancet 1:480–484, 1975.

Jennett B, Plum F: Persistent vegetative state after brain damage: A syndrome in search of a name. Lancet 1:734, 1972.

Jennett B, Adams JH, Murray LS, et al: Neuropathology in vegetative and severely disabled patients after head injury. Neurology 56:486–489, 2001.

Kalmar K, Giacino JT: Rating scale analysis of the JFK Coma Recovery Scale: Measurement properties [abstract]. Arch Phys Med Rehabil 81:619, 2000.

Kampfl A, Schmutzhard E, Franz G, Pfausler B, et al: Prediction of recovery from post-traumatic vegetative state with cerebral magnetic-resonance imaging. Lancet 351:1763–1767, 1998.

Kanno T, Kamei Y, Yokoyama T, et al: Neurostimulation for patients in vegetative status. Pacing Clin Electrophysiol 10:207–208, 1987.

Katayama Y, Tsubokawa T, Yamamoto T, et al: Characterization and modification of brain activity with deep brain stimulation in patients in a persistent vegetative state: Pain-related late positive component of cerebral evoked potential. Pacing Clin Electrophysiol 14:116–121, 1991.

Katz DI, Alexander MP: Predicting outcome and course of recovery in patients admitted to rehabilitation. Arch Neurol 51:661–670, 1994.

Katz DI, Alexander MP, Mandell AM: Dementia following strokes in the diencephalon and mesencephalon. Arch Neurol 44:1127–1133, 1987.

Katz DI, Mills VM: Traumatic brain injury: natural history and efficacy of cognitive rehabilitation, in Stuss DT, Winocur G, Robertson IH (eds): Cognitive Neurorehabilitation. New York: Cambridge University Press, 1999, pp. 175–187.

Katz DI, Otto RM, Agosti RM, et al: Factors affecting duration of posttraumatic amnesia after traumatic brain injury [abstract]. J Intl Neuropsychol Soc 5:139, 1999.

Katz DI: Neuropathology and neurobehavioral recovery from closed head injury. J Head Trauma Rehabil 7:1–15, 1992.

Katz DI: Traumatic brain injury, in Mills VM, Cassidy JW, Katz DI (eds): Neurologic Rehabilitation: A Guide to Diagnosis, Prognosis and Treatment Planning. Cambridge MA: Blackwell Science, 1997.

Kinney HC, Korein J, PanigrahyA, et al: Neuropathological findings in the brain of Karen Ann Quinlan: The role of the thalamus in the persistent vegetative state. N Engl J Med 330:1469–1475, 1994.

Laureys S, Faymonville ME, Degueldre C, et al: Auditory processing in the vegetative state. Brain 123:1589–1681, 2000.

Lipowski ZJ: Delirium. Acute Confusional States. New York: Oxford University Press, 1990.

Mackay LE, Bernstein BB, Chapman PE, et al: Early intervention in severe head injury: Long-term benefits of a formalized program. Arch Phys Med Rehabil 73:635–641,1992.

Magoun HW: The Waking Brain, ed 2. Springfield, IL: Charles C Thomas, 1965.

McMillan TM: Neuropsychological assessment after extremely severe head injury in a case of life or death. Brain Injury 11:483–490, 1996.

Menon DK, Owen AM, Williams EJ, et al: Cortical processing in persistent vegetative state. Lancet 352:200, 1998.

Mesulam MM: Attentional networks, confusional states and neglect syndromes, in Mesulam MM (ed): Principles of Behavioral and Cognitive Neurology. New York: Oxford, 2000, pp. 174–256.

Moruzzi G, Magoun HW: Brain stem reticular formation and activation of the EEG. EEG Clin Neurophysiol 1:455–473, 1949.

Multi-Society Task Force on PVS: Medical aspects of the persistent vegetative state. N Engl J Med 330:1499–1508; 1572–1579, 1994.

Nagel T: What is the mind-brain problem? in: Experimental and Theoretical Studies of Consciousness. New York: Wiley Interscience/CIBA Foundation, 1986, pp. 61–80.

Neubauer RA, Gottlieb SF, Kaga RL: Enhancing "idling neurons." Lancet 1:335–342, 1990.

Neubauer RA, Gottlieb SF, Miale A: Identification of hypometabolic areas in the brain using brain imaging and hyperbaric oxygen. Clin Nucl Med 17:477–481, 1992.

O'Dell MW, Jasin P, Stivers M, et al: Interrater reliability of the Coma Recovery Scale. J Head Trauma Rehabil 11:61–66, 1996.

Passler MA, Riggs RV: Positive outcomes in traumatic brain injury-Vegetative state: Patients treated with bromocriptine. Arch Phys Med Rehabil 82:311–315, 2001.

Plum F: Coma and related global disturbances of the human conscious state, in Peters A, Jones EG (eds): Cerebral Cortex: Normal and Altered States of Function. New York: Plenum Press, 1991.

Plum F, Posner J: The Diagnosis of Stupor and Coma, ed 3. Philadelphia: Davis, 1980.

Powell JH, Al-Adawi S, Morgan J, et al: Motivational deficits after brain injury: Effects of bromocriptine in 11 patients. J Neurol Neurosurg Psychiatry 60:416–421, 1996.

Rappaport M, Dougherty AM, Kelting DI: Evaluation of coma and vegetative states. Arch Phys Med Rehabil 73:628–634, 1992.

Rappaport M, Hall KM, Hopkins K, et al: Disability rating scale for severe head trauma: Coma to community. Arch Phys Med Rehabil 73:628–634, 1982.

Reinhard DL, Whyte J, Sandel ME: Improved arousal and initiation following tricyclic antidepressant use in severe brain injury. Arch Phys Med Rehabil 77:80–83, 1996.

Rockswold GL, Ford SE, Anderson DC, et al: Results of a prospective randomized trial for treatment of severely brain-injured patients with hyperbaric oxygen. J Neurosurg 76:929–934, 1992.

Rockswold SB, Rockswold GL, Vargo JM, et al: Effects of hyperbaric oxygenation therapy on cerebral metabolism and intracranial pressure in severely brain injured patients. J Neurosurg 94:403–411, 2001.

Schacter DL: Toward a cognitive neuropsychology of awareness: Implicit knowledge and anosognosia. J Clin Exp Neuropsychol 12:155–178, 1990.

Schiff ND, Rezai AR, Plum FP: A neuromodulation strategy for rational therapy of complex brain injury states. Neurolog Res 22:267–272, 2000.

Schiff ND, Ribary U, Plum F, et al: Words without mind. J Cogn Neurosci 11:650–656, 1999.

Searle JR: The problem of consciousness, in Experimental and Theoretical Studies of Consciousness. New York: Wiley Interscience/CIBA Foundation, 1992, pp. 61–80.

Tanheco J, Kaplan PE: Physical and surgical rehabilitation of patient after 6-year coma. Arch Phys Med Rehabil 63:36–38, 1982.

Teasdale G, Jennett B: Assessment of coma and impaired consciousness. Lancet 2:81–84, 1974.

Timmons M, Gasquoine L, Scibak JW: Functional changes with rehabilitation of very severe traumatic brain injury survivors. J Head Trauma Rehabil 2:64–67, 1987.

Tranel D, Damasio A: Knowledge without awareness: An autonomic index of facial recognition by prosopagnosics. Science 228:1453–1454, 1985.

Tsubokawa T, Yamamoto T, Katayama Y, et al: Deep brain stimulation in a persistent vegetative state: Follow up results and selection of candidates. Brain Injury 4:315–327, 1990.

Weiskrantz L, Warrington EK, Sanders MD, et al: Visual capacity in the hemianopic field following a restricted occipital ablation. Brain 97:709–728, 1974.

Whyte J, DiPasquale MC: Assessment of vision and visual attention in minimally responsive brain-injured patients. Arch Phys Med Rehabil 76:804–810, 1995.

Whyte J, DiPasquale MC, Katz DI, et al: Predicting recovery in patients with severely impaired consciousness after traumatic brain injury (TBI): A multicenter study [abstract]. Neurorehabil Neural Repair 13:44–45, 1999a.

Whyte J, DiPasquale MC, Vaccaro M: Assessment of command-following in minimally conscious brain injured patients. Arch Phys Med Rehabil 80:653–660, 1999b.

Whyte J, Laborde A, DiPasquale MC: Assessment and treatment of the vegetative and minimally conscious patient, in Rosenthal M, Griffith ER, Kreutzer J, et al (eds): Rehabilitation of the Adult and Child with Traumatic Brain Injury, ed 3. Philadelphia, PA: Davis, 1999, pp. 435–452.

Wilson SL, Powell GE, Brock D, et al: Behavioural differences between patients who emerged from vegetative state and those who did not. Brain Injury 10:509–516, 1996.

Wilson SL, McMillan TM: A review of the evidence for the effectiveness of sensory stimulation treatment for coma and vegetative states. Neuropsycholog Rehabil 3:149–160, 1993.

Woolf SH: Practice guidelines, a new reality in medicine. II. Methods of developing guidelines. Arch Intern Med 152:946–952, 1992.

Worzniak M, Fetters MD, Comfort M: Methylphenidate in the treatment of coma. J Family Practice 44:495–498, 1997.

Young GB: Consiousness, in Young GB, Ropper AH, Bolton CF: Coma and Impaired Consciousness: A Clinical Perspective. New York: McGraw-Hill, 1998, pp. 3–38.

Zafonte RD, Watanabe T, Mann NR: Amantadine: A potential treatment for the minimally conscious state. Brain Injury 12:617–21, 1998.

Zasler ND, Kreutzer JS, Taylor D: Coma recovery and coma stimulation: A critical review. Neurorehabilitation 1:33–40, 1991.

Zegers De Beryl D, Brunko E: Prediction of chronic vegetative state with somatosensory evoked potentials. Neurology 36:134, 1986.

Disorders of Sleep and Arousal

Mark W. Mahowald

Circadian rhythm abnormalities

Narcolepsy

Shift work

Sleep apnea

Sleep deprivation

Sleepiness

Sleep inertia

"Sleepiness is important in that it is both a transition state between sleep and performance and a modifier of the two." (Monk, 1991)

INTRODUCTION

Sleepiness has prominent, and often severe, neuropsychiatric behavioral consequences, primarily in the arenas of impaired mood, attention, and performance, with serious ramifications in the family, classroom, workplace, and behind the wheel. The repercussions of sleepiness are identical, whether the result of one of a number of primary sleep disorders or of voluntary sleep deprivation, which is rampant in our society, and tending to worsen as individuals increasingly pursue more activities at the expense of sleep, and as more employees become engaged in shift work.

OVERVIEW OF NORMAL SLEEP

Until relatively recently, it was thought that sleep was a unitary phenomenon—the passive absence of wakefulness. In the first half of this century, it was discovered that sleep is an active state. In 1953, it was discovered that sleep is actually consists of two completely different states: non–rapid-eye movement (NREM) and rapid-eye movement (REM) sleep. Human beings, like most mammals, spend our lives in three completely different states of being: wakefulness (W), REM sleep, and NREM sleep. Each of these states has its unique neuroanatomic, neurophysiologic, neurochemical, and neuropharmacologic correlates (Jones, 2000).

It is now apparent that there are no single specific areas in the nervous system that control all the manifestations of the states of wakefulness, REM sleep, and NREM sleep. Most of the state-determining mechanisms that result in the declaration of a given state depend upon the brainstem (especially the pons) and basal forebrain regions. In general, the generators of W are diffusely located in the brainstem, particularly in the reticular activating system, those of NREM in the medulla and basal forebrain, and those of REM in the pons. The components of the waking, REM, and non-REM states are undoubtedly recruited and orchestrated by very complex phenomena, involving many levels of the neuraxis, different neurotransmitters, and circulating "sleep factors." It is also apparent that areas involved in some elements of a given state are uninvolved in the generation of other elements of that state, confirming the multiplicity of neuronal networks involved in state declaration. The fact that no one part of the central nervous system (CNS) is responsible for the appearance of any state of sleep is underscored by lesion studies in animals: any stage of NREM sleep which is eliminated by a nonlethal lesion will eventually reappear—indicating that multiple parts of the CNS are capable of generating sleep.

The number of neuroanatomic regions, neurotransmitters, and neuropeptides involved in wake/sleep regulation are being identified at an astonishing rate, making any listing obsolete within months. Common neurotransmitters such as Ach serotonin, GABA, NE, 5-HT are clearly involved in the generation/modulation of state. Important new neurotransmitters and neuropeptides involved in wakefulness and sleep continue to be identified (i.e., the role of adenosine in NREM sleep induction, and that of hypocretin (orexin) in the control of REM sleep). Others include progesterone, nerve growth factor, nitric oxide, and histamine. The roles of glial cells and extrasynaptic transmission are also of growing importance. It may be that different sleep-promoting substances acting on different neuronal networks are responsible for generating sleep under different conditions, such as sleep deprivation, systemic infection, and others. The fact that two-headed conjoined twins with a common circulatory system sleep independently speaks against a primary role of circulating sleep-inducing substances (Lahmeyer, 1988).

Just as interesting as the concept of sleep/wake promoting regions/factors is that of how sleep debt is remembered. During make-up sleep following sleep deprivation, all lost deep NREM and 50% of lost REM sleep are recovered. The brain structures responsible for keeping track of the accumulating sleep debt and for discharging that debt during make-up sleep are not known. There is growing evidence that adenosine accumulation in the basal forebrain during wakefulness may play a role in promoting sleep in the setting of sleep deprivation (Basheer et al., 2000).

CIRCADIAN RHYTHMS

Major advances have been made in the field of circadian rhythms. Most living creatures follow a relentless and pervasive daily rhythm of activity and rest that is ultimately linked to the environmental light/dark cycle. Plants, animals, and even unicellular organisms show daily variations in metabolic activity, locomotion, feeding, and many other functions. When isolated from time cues such as sunlight, many creatures show intrinsic rhythms of nearly, but rarely exactly, 24 hours. This intrinsic rhythm is unmasked by isolation studies, in which subjects are sequestered from all time cues while being monitored for activity, core temperature, electroencephalogram (EEG) results, and other physiologic variables. All circadian rhythms share two features: 1) they free-run (persist at a not-quite 24-hour period) in the absence of light/dark or time cues, and 2) they are normally entrained to the external light/dark cycle. The biologic clock regulates numerous functions in addition to the wake/sleep cycle, including fatigue, alertness, and cognitive performance (Van Dongen & Dinges, 2000).

In humans and other mammals the suprachiasmatic nucleus (SCN) of the hypothalamus controls most circadian rhythms. The biologic clock has an inherent rhythm that is entrained by the environmental light/dark cycle. Proof that the SCN is the "biologic clock" is compelling: 1) lesions of the SCN in humans and animals result in a random, irregular wake/sleep pattern, and 2) lesioning of the SCN in one strain of hamster with a given wake/sleep cycle and transplanting it with the SCN of another strain with a different cycle results in the recipient's developing the cycle of the donor (Ralph et al., 1990). There is good evidence that the SCN promotes wakefulness, and not sleep, because animals whose SCN have been destroyed display an increase in total sleep time (Edgar et al., 1993).

The discovery of a retinohypothalamic tract in animals indicated that the biologic clock may be directly influenced by environmental light. It is clear that timed light exposure can both synchronize and reset the phase of the circadian pacemaker in a predictable manner. This has led to the application of bright light to reset rhythms of activity in animal studies and the wake/sleep cycle in humans. The timing of exposure to bright light with respect to the intrinsic rhythm controls the nature of the resetting. Light at the beginning of the conventional sleep period will delay, and light at the end of the conventional sleep period will advance, the sleep period. Light administered in the middle of the day will have no effect. This variability of the effect of light on the wake/sleep cycle led to the concept of the phase response curve (PRC), which indicates the various responses of advance, "dead zone," and delay of the cycle. The PRC may differ substantially among individuals, and will differ systematically with the intensity of the light or pharmacologic stimulus (Terman & Terman, 2000). Although light exposure is the primary determinant of the phase of the biologic clock, other factors, such as exercise, may also affect the biologic clock (Kas & Edgar, 2001).

Circadian rhythm disorders, discussed below, are of more than academic interest; they affect alertness, concentration, and performance, which may be crucial for safety in certain occupations such as transportation and manufacturing. The recently released Report of the National Commission on Sleep Disorders Research has underscored the startling socioeconomic consequences of sleepiness in our society—at a personal, national, and international level (National Commission on Sleep Disorders Research, 1992). The wake/sleep scheduling conditions may play a major role in these disastrous events. Job-related and social demands on the wake/sleep schedules of individuals may result in circadian rhythm disorders that can be life-threatening. Studies have shown a circadian pattern of motor vehicle and industrial accidents, with severalfold higher incidence in early morning hours, and with a lesser peak in the afternoon (Mitler et al., 1988). Other circadian rhythm disorders may not have any obvious cause, but can nevertheless result in significant impairment if affected individuals are required to perform when sleepy or fatigued as they attempt to adjust to the geophysical world.

FUNCTION OF SLEEP

Although the function(s) of sleep remain unknown, there is clear evidence that sleep deprivation has severe physiologic consequences. In rats, total (both NREM and REM) sleep deprivation is fatal within about 3 weeks (similar to the survival time associated with total food deprivation), and isolated REM sleep deprivation is fatal in about 6 weeks. Preterminally, there is a marked increase in energy expenditure (Rechtschaffen, 1998). The mechanism of death remains completely unknown. Interestingly, if rescued "at the brink," many sleep-deprived animals survive and apparently return to normal (Everson et al., 1989). Numerous theories of the function of sleep exist. The intuitively attractive theories such as "restoration" or "energy conservation" are not supported by scientific data. One of the most attractive theories is that of maintenance of neuronal integrity. Inasmuch as neural structure and function are influenced by the frequency and nature of neural activity, there is good reason to believe that the periodic and systematic stimulation of neural networks is necessary to preserve CNS function. REM and NREM sleep may serve to maintain neural integrity to assure long-term optimal waking function, particularly at the neuronal group level (Krueger & Obal, 1993). Neural plasticity results from the fact that neural networks are use-dependent. Long-lasting maintenance of synaptic efficacy is probably achieved by repetitive activations (dynamic stabilization), which may have been the evolutionary impetus to the development of neurons and neuronal circuits with oscillatory capacities to serve as a source of repetitive spontaneous activations to maintain synaptic efficacy in infrequently used circuits (Kavanau, 1997).

DETERMINANTS OF SLEEP/WAKEFULNESS

Multiple factors interact to determine the degree of sleepiness or alertness at any given point in time. The two most important are homeostatic and chronobiologic (i.e., circadian).

Homeostatic and Circadian Determinants

The homeostatic factor is related to the duration of prior wakefulness: the longer the duration of wakefulness, the greater the pressure to sleep. The "opponent process" model of the biologic clock suggests that the initiation and maintenance of wakefulness that opposes the homeostatic sleep tendency is generated by the biologic clock (Edgar et al., 1993). Studies of inbred mice clearly indicate a genetic influence on sleep regulation (Franken et al., 1999).

The human biologic clock has two "sleepy" times: the primary is between midnight and 6 AM, with a secondary period of sleepiness in the early to mid-afternoon (Monk et al., 1966). The circadian peaks of motor vehicle crashes (MVCs) and virtually all other industrial/workplace errors follows this bimodal period of sleepiness (Mitler et al., 1988).

Age

Some studies indicate that older adults are sleepier than their younger counterparts, as determined by objective measures of daytime sleepiness. This suggests that older individuals sleep less because there is a deterioration in quality and/or quantity of sleep, rather than that the total sleep requirement diminishes with age. If the sleep need declined, there should be no compromise in daytime alertness. There is also evidence that tolerance to shift work diminishes with increasing age (Monk, 2000a; Reid & Dawson, 2001).

Drugs

Many medications induce drowsiness, sleepiness, or insomnia. The effects of drugs show a wide variation among different individuals. To date there are very few objective studies evaluating these medication effects, either in isolation or, as is more commonly encountered in clinical practice, in combination.

Central Nervous System Pathology

Inasmuch as sleep is generated by the brain, it would be expected that CNS pathology could result in a wide variety of sleep/wake complaints. Formal study of large numbers of patients with given types of acquired neurologic disorders will provide important information about wakefulness/sleep and CNS function (Mahowald, 2000). For instance, the deterioration of the wake/sleep pattern in Alzheimer disease results in a major burden on caregivers (Moe et al., 1995; McCurry et al., 1999). The high prevalence of sleep complaints following traumatic brain injury warrants further study, the results of which will undoubtedly have important rehabilitation implications (Masel et al., 2001). Two primary neurologic conditions resulting in excessive daytime sleepiness (EDS), narcolepsy and idiopathic central nervous system hypersomnia, are discussed below.

Sleep Disorders

Numerous primary sleep disorders result in EDS. The most common of these are discussed in the sections following.

Somnotypes

In addition to the above-mentioned factors, it is apparent that the basic level of sleepiness/alertness in a given individual is also genetically influenced and stable over time. Some people are inherently sleepier or more alert than others, resulting in two "somnotypes": "alert" and "sleepy." This inherent "sleepiness propensity" affects both the ability to sleep at night and to remain alert during the daytime. Daytime levels of sleepiness are systematically related to nocturnal sleep parameters: those who are the "best" sleepers at night are the sleepiest during the day, and those who are the most "fragile"

sleepers during the night are less apt to fall asleep during the day (Lavie & Zvuluni, 1992).

BEHAVIORAL CONSEQUENCES OF SLEEPINESS/SLEEP DEPRIVATION

Humans cannot ethically be deprived of sleep for sufficient periods of time to result in any known medical consequence, because sleep eventually supervenes regardless of the technique of sleep deprivation. Therefore, to the extent that sleep deprivation is possible in humans, the only known consequences are severe sleepiness, irritability, negative affect on mood, and impaired performance, particularly in tasks resulting in sustained attention (Pilcher & Huffcutt, 1996).

The consequences of sleep deprivation may be subtle, but interfere with some of the most important cognitive processes, including those pertaining to creativity, abstract thinking, control of attention and emotion, and suggestibility (Dahl, 1996; Harrison & Horne, 1998; Randazzo et al., 1998; Blagrove & Akehurst, 2000; Harrison & Horne, 2000). The impaired performance during sleepiness may be thought of as "state instability" (Doran et al., 2001). Functional neuroimaging studies demonstrate global and regional changes in cerebral metabolic activity caused by sleep deprivation (Thomas et al., 2000). Workplace consequences include communication problems, lack of innovation, distraction, unwillingness to try new strategies, unreliable memory, and mood changes, including loss of empathy and the inability to deal with surprise and the unexpected (Horne, 1999). Subtle but important decrements include interference with novel responses and the ability to suppress routine answers (Harrison & Horne, 1998).

Many are raised to believe that sleep deprivation should be worn as a "badge of honor," reflecting the pervasive societal attitude that sleepiness is a minor annoyance that can be overcome by motivation, commitment, dedication, or sheer will. This is simply not true. The consequences of sleep deprivation are relentlessly cumulative; the performance and mood ramifications escalate (Dinges et al., 1997). One does not "get used to" sleepiness: accumulated sleep debt is dissipated *only* by catch-up sleep. To make matters worse, the relentless move toward a 24-hour society increasingly encourages and promotes chronic sleep deprivation. Although fatigue-related impairment may be appreciated by the individual, there can be a potentially dangerous discrepancy between the objective performance decrements and the subjective perception of sleepiness (VanDongen et al., 1999; Dorrian et al., 2000). (As an aside, the previously held concept that REM sleep deprivation in humans results in psychiatric or psychological problems is not true [Vogel, 1975]). In keeping with the concept that the brain is the only organ of the body benefitting from or requiring sleep is the fact that sleep deprivation results in CNS impairments, but not physical ailments (Reed et al., 2000).

Two meta-analysis studies of sleep deprivation have been performed, one of which concluded that longer periods of sleep deprivation had increasingly greater impact upon performance, and that speed of performance was affected more than accuracy; the other concluded that mood measures were more affected than cognitive, and that cognitive effects were greater than performance effects (Koslowski & Babkoff, 1992; Pilcher & Huffcutt, 1996). Tasks most adversely affected by sleep deprivation are long, monotonous, without feedback, externally paced, newly learned, and those with a memory component (Bonnet, 2000). The general public, employers, and policy makers are generally unaware of the relationship between sleepiness and accidents (Mitler et al., 2000). There is growing evidence that sleep deprivation is as impairing to performance as having a legally intoxicated blood alcohol level of 0.1% (Dawson & Reid, 1997; Powell et al., 1999; Weiler et al., 2000; Williamson & Feyer, 2000).

"Adult attention deficit disorder (ADD)" is becoming an increasingly popular diagnosis, often based upon computer-generated sustained attention tasks. It is likely that some patients who perform poorly on such tests do so on the basis of sleepiness impairment of sustained attention. Indeed, a number of patients evaluated who had been previously diagnosed as "ADD" seen at our center were found to have severe underlying primary sleep disorders which, in retrospect, explained the "attention deficit."

Many people think that sleepiness-related decrements in performance are the result of frank "microsleep" episodes. It is clear that impairment of vigilance and reaction time precedes the appearance of true physiologic sleep; someone who is sleepy may appear to be "awake," but is actually significantly impaired (Dinges, 1995). In the setting of sleep deprivation, errors occur during the absence of electrophysiologically defined sleepiness, and in the setting of one night's sleep deprivation, the brain is functioning at a lower level at *all* times (Gillberg & Akerstedt, 1998). Amplitude reduction in visual event-related potentials resulting from sleep deprivation exemplifies fundamental changes in neurophysiologic mechanisms, indicating variability and reduction of alertness mechanisms and changes in thalamocortical gating affecting attention, discrimination, and decision-making (Corsi-Cabrera et al., 1999). The lack of awareness of the extent to which sleep deprivation impairs cognitive tasks has been well documented (Pilcher & Walters, 1997).

SLEEP INERTIA

Sleep inertia refers to a period of impaired performance and reduced vigilance following awakening from the regular sleep episode or from a nap (Ferrara & De Gennaro, 2000; Tassi & Muzet, 2000). This impairment may be extreme, last from minutes to hours, and be accompanied by polygraphically recorded microsleep episodes (Roth et al., 1981; Dinges, 1989; Dinges, 1990). Recent studies have clearly proven that sleep inertia is a potent phenomenon, resulting in impaired performance and vigilance, averaging one hour, and requiring up to 2–4 hours to dissipate, in normal, non–sleep-deprived individuals, and is worse following sleep deprivation (Achermann et al., 1995; Jewett et al., 1999; Wright & Czeisler, 1999). Basic science support of a gradual disengagement from sleep to wakefulness comes from neurophysiologic studies in animals (Horner et al., 1997) and cerebral blood flow studies in humans (Koboyama et al., 1997; Balkin et al., 1998; Winter et al., 1999). The persistent reduction, lasting minutes, of the photomyoclonic response upon awakening from NREM sleep is further confirmation of a less than immediate transition from sleep to wakefulness (Meier-Ewert & Broughton, 1967). Impaired performance during the transition from sleep to wake has important implications for rapid decision-making upon forced awakenings (such as a middle-of-the-night telephone call) and for performance following scheduled naps in the workplace (Sallinen et al., 1998; Ferrara et al., 2000). There appears to be great interindividual variability in the extent and duration of sleep inertia, both following spontaneous awakening after the major sleep period, and following naps.

TREATMENT OF SLEEPINESS-IMPAIRED PERFORMANCE

There is evidence that administration of stimulants such as caffeine, methylphenidate, and other stimulants, as well as modafinil, may counteract some of the consequences of sleepiness-impaired function; however, more systematic study is needed (Pigeau et al., 1995; Baranski & Pigeau, 1997; Brun et al., 1998; Nicholson & Turner, 1998; Bonnet, 2000).

EVALUATION OF EXCESSIVE DAYTIME SLEEPINESS

Evaluation of Sleep Physiology

Polysomnography (PSG) is the technology used for the physiologic diagnosis of sleep and sleep disorders employs standard electrophysiologic recording systems and techniques (Carskadon, 2000; Mitler et al., 2000).

Subjective Evaluation: Sleepiness Scales

Subjective introspective alertness/sleepiness scales such as the Stanford Sleepiness Scale and the Epworth Sleepiness Scale (ESS) have been developed (Johns,

1991; Carskadon & Dement, 1994). The ESS is frequently used as a screening tool for identifying EDS, and generally correlates with other measures of sleep propensity (Johns, 1993; Johns, 1994). It must be remembered that such instruments are limited by their lack of sensitivity: there may be a striking discrepancy between the self-perceived sleepiness and the underlying true physiologic sleepiness in a given individual (Benbadis et al., 1997; Chervin et al., 1997). Subjective sleepiness scales may be an inaccurate surrogate for true daytime sleepiness.

Objective Evaluation

Numerous methods have been developed to measure physiologic sleepiness during the waking period. The most commonly employed are the Multiple Sleep Latency Test (MSLT) and the maintenance of wakefulness test (Mitler & Miller, 1996).

Multiple Sleep Latency Test

The MSLT is a standardized and well-validated measure of physiologic sleepiness. Parameters monitored are the same parameters as for basic PSG: (usually two eye movement and two EEG [central and occipital] channels, in addition to electrocardiogram [EKG], airflow, and submental electromyogram [EMG]). The MSLT consists of 4–5 20-minute nap opportunities offered at 2-hour intervals (Carskadon et al., 1986). The MSLT is designed 1) to quantitate sleepiness by measuring how quickly an individual falls asleep on sequential naps during the day (Roehrs et al., 1989), and 2) to identify the abnormal occurrence of REM sleep during a nap. For each nap, the latency between "lights out" and sleep onset is recorded. Pathologic ranges of sleep latency have been carefully defined. A mean latency of 5 minutes or less indicates severe excessive sleepiness. The number of naps during which REM sleep appears is also noted. Many factors can affect sleep latency during the daytime: prior sleep deprivation, sleep continuity, age, time of day, and medication (Carskadon et al., 1986; American Sleep Disorders Association, 1992; Roehrs et al., 1992). Proper interpretation requires a PSG the preceding night to measure the quality and quantity of sleep obtained immediately prior to the MSLT. The MSLT is a most useful tool in quantifying daytime sleepiness and in differentiating the subjective complaints of "sleepiness," "tiredness," and "fatigue."

It must be remembered that falsely negative MSLTs can and do occur, and that there may be a discrepancy between the subjective complaint of sleepiness and the results of the MSLT (Rosenthal et al., 1994; Chervin et al., 1995). Stating that a patient does not have EDS on the basis of a "normal" MSLT is analogous to stating that a patient with chest pain does not have cardiac disease on the basis of a normal EKG. Importantly, REM sleep may also occur during daytime naps in subjects with no complaints of EDS (Bishop et al., 1996).

Maintenance of Wakefulness Test

The Maintenance of Wakefulness Test (MWT) is a variation of the MSLT. The subject during the MWT is asked to resist sleep while sitting in a chair, rather than asked to fall asleep lying in bed, as in the MSLT (Mitler et al., 1982). The MWT appears to offer no specific advantage over the MSLT (Roth et al., 1994).

It is clear that all currently available subjective and objective measures of sleepiness have limitations, and, as with many other tests in medicine, the results of either must be interpreted in light of the specific clinical situation (Johns, 1994; Aldrich et al., 1997).

CAUSES OF EXCESSIVE DAYTIME SLEEPINESS

Sleep Deprivation

Most population survey studies indicate that the prevalence of EDS is 5% to 15% (Partinen & Hublin, 2000). By far, the most common cause of EDS in our society is chronic sleep deprivation. We sleep 25% less that our forefathers one century ago. There is no evidence that they required more sleep than we do, nor is there any reason to believe that we require less sleep than they. This sleep deprivation is volitional, often driven by social or economic factors. For instance, approximately 20% of workers in industrialized countries are employed in shift work, and it has been shown that night shift workers obtain, on the average, 8 hours less sleep per week than day workers (Moore-Ede, 1993; Akerstedt, 1995). That amounts to the loss of an entire night's sleep, every week. The growing availability of 24-hour businesses and stock markets, all-night TV, e-mail, and the Internet encourage sleep deprivation.

Sufficient sleep is not measured in terms of absolute hours of sleep obtained, but, rather, by the ability to achieve enough sleep to awaken rested and restored. The total genetically-determined sleep requirement for some individuals is 10 hours nightly. Therefore, those 10-hour sleepers who receive 8 hours of sleep nightly may become severely sleep deprived, and therefore severely hypersomnolent. This sleep deprivation is cumulative. One does not "get used to it," nor does sleep deprivation–induced sleepiness diminish without make-up sleep (Dinges et al., 1997).

Sleep-Disordered Breathing

Sleep-disordered breathing takes many different forms, including obstructive sleep apnea (OSA), central sleep apnea, and Cheyne-Stokes respiration.

OSA is extraordinarily prevalent in the general population, affecting at least 2% of adult women and 4% of adult men (Young et al., 1993). The stereotype of having to be male, middle-aged, and overweight is erroneous. OSA affects women, children, and thin individuals. OSA is readily diagnosable and treatable (Kryger, 2000). The daytime sleepiness in patients with OSA may be severe, resulting in marked neuropsychological impairment of vigilance, concentration, memory, and executive function, with dire consequences in the workplace or on the highway (Kim et al., 1997; Day et al., 1999; Bassiri & Guilleminault, 2000). Even mild sleep-disordered breathing compromises psychomotor efficiency (Kim et al., 1997). For instance, the incidence of motor vehicle crashes is more than 6 times higher in patients with OSA (Teran-Santos et al., 1999).

Narcolepsy

Narcolepsy is a relatively frequent disorder, with a prevalence of 0.09%, affecting between 125,000 to 250,000 Americans. The prevalence approximates that of Parkinson disease or multiple sclerosis. EDS is the primary symptom of narcolepsy. Ancillary symptoms include: cataplexy (sudden loss of muscle tone often triggered by emotionally laden events), hypnagogic hallucinations (dreaming beginning during relaxed wakefulness during the transition between wake and sleep), and sleep paralysis (awakening to find the entire body paralyzed with the exception of the diaphragm). Notably, fewer than half of people with narcolepsy will report all four symptoms of sleep attacks, cataplexy, hypnagogic hallucinations, and sleep paralysis (Aldrich, 1992).

EDS is the primary symptom of narcolepsy. Unwanted or unanticipated sleep episodes that last seconds to minutes occur at inappropriate times, particularly during periods of reduced environmental stimulation, such as reading, watching television, during classes or meetings, or while riding in or operating a motor vehicle. Such feelings of sleepiness are often dramatically, but briefly, reversed by a brief nap. Patients with narcolepsy often complain of memory impairment. This is not due to memory impairment per se, but to the adverse effects of impaired alertness on complex cognitive tasks (Hood & Bruck, 1996). Aggressive treatment is in order, as the psychosocial and socioeconomic consequences of narcolepsy are significant (Broughton et al., 1983; Broughton & Broughton, 1994). Quality of life surveys have indicated that disability in narcolepsy is similar to that caused by epilepsy or Parkinson disease (Beusterien et al., 1999).

Narcolepsy is the only sleep disorder known to specifically affect the generation and organization of sleep. The underlying pathophysiology of narcolepsy results in impaired control of the boundaries that normally separate the states of wakefulness from REM and NREM sleep (Broughton et al., 1986). The total sleep time per 24 hours in people with narcolepsy is similar to that in those without narcolepsy (Nobili et al., 1996). However, the control of the onset/offset of both REM and non-REM sleep is impaired. Moreover, there is a clear dissociation of various components of the individual wake and sleep states. Cataplexy and sleep paralysis simply represent the isolated and inappropriate intrusion or persistence of REM sleep-related atonia (paralysis) into wakefulness. The hypnagogic hallucinations are (REM sleep-related) dreams occurring during wakefulness (Aldrich, 1992).

A genetic factor has long been suspected. A multigenetic and environmentally induced model has been proposed: familial cases have been identified, but most are sporadic in nature. There is a clear genetic component, with over 85% of individuals with narcolepsy carrying the chromosome 6 allele *HLA DQB1*0602* (found in less than 30% of the general population). This association is present in the different ethnic populations to varying degrees, and represents the highest disease-HLA linkage known in medicine. Recently, the neuropeptide hypocretin (orexin) has been implicated in the pathophysiology of narcolepsy (Mignot, 2000; Krahn et al., 2001). The finding of selective destruction of the hypocretin-containing neurons of the lateral hypothalamic region in humans with narcolepsy suggests an immune-mediated phenomenon (Siegel, 1999).

The diagnosis of narcolepsy may be indicated by history. In view of the nature and duration of treatment with stimulant medications, objective sleep laboratory diagnosis is imperative. Formal sleep studies in narcolepsy include both PSG and MSLT. An all-night PSG must be performed the night before the MSLT to determine the quality and quantity of the preceding night's sleep. During the MSLT, patients with narcolepsy typically fall asleep in 5 minutes or less and usually display REM sleep on two or more of the daytime naps, an occurrence rarely seen in normals. The MSLT results must be interpreted in light of the patient's clinical symptoms and in view of the results of the preceding night's PSG. In one large study, the combination of a mean latency of less than 5 minutes and REM sleep on two or more naps had a specificity of 97% for narcolepsy, but the sensitivity was only 70%, meaning that 30% of individuals with those MSLT values did not have narcolepsy (Aldrich et al., 1997). Conversely, a "negative" MSLT (or maintenance of wakefulness test) does not absolutely rule out the possibility of narcolepsy. False-negative MSLTs do occur (Jahnke & Aldrich, 1990; Mitler et al., 1998).

To date, there is no reliable objective measure of the compliance with or response to stimulant medication in patients with narcolepsy (American Sleep

Disorders Association, 1994). The response must be evaluated by the patient's subjective report.

Stimulant medications such as mazindol, methylphenidate, methamphetamine, dextroamphetamine sulfate (SmithKline Beecham Pharmaceuticals, Philadelphia, PA), or modafinil are used to control the hypersomnia. (The recent announcement by the manufacturer of pemoline regarding hepatic necrosis limits its utility). These stimulants all appear to increase presynaptic activation of dopamine (Nishino et al., 1998). No pharmacokinetic studies have been performed, rendering stated "maximum doses" arbitrary and without scientific basis. Many practitioners will titrate the medications to maximally control the symptoms (Nishino & Mignot, 1997). The abuse potential for these agents in the bona fide patient populations for which they are therapeutic has been greatly overrated, as have the cardiovascular and psychiatric consequences (American Sleep Disorders Association, 1994; Pawluk et al., 1995; Nishino & Mignot, 1997; Goldman et al., 1998; Wallin & Mahowald, 1998). Treatment of the ancillary symptoms includes tricyclic antidepressants, serotonin-specific reuptake inhibitors, and gamma-hydroxy butyrate (Guilleminault, 1994b).

Nonpharmacologic management includes the use of strategically timed naps. Studies have demonstrated improvement in performance on days with naps compared with days without naps. Close cooperation with employers is desirable, because manipulation of the work environment/schedule will be beneficial to both employer and employee. Shift work, which is very poorly tolerated by those with narcolepsy, should be discouraged. The Narcolepsy Network and local narcolepsy support groups are a valuable resource for patients and their families.

Idiopathic Central Nervous System Hypersomnia

Idiopathic CNS hypersomnia may represent a number of different conditions that present as unexplained EDS. This condition is characterized by EDS in the absence of sleep deprivation or other identifiable abnormality during sleep such as obstructive sleep apnea (Bassetti & Aldrich, 1997; Billiard, 1996; Guilleminault, 1994a). In some cases, the total sleep requirement may be extraordinary, underscoring the heterogeneity of this condition (Voderholzer et al., 1998). The pathophysiology is unknown.

The diagnosis may be suspected by the history of unexplained EDS in the absence of symptoms suggestive of OSA, narcolepsy, or sleep deprivation. Formal studies are mandatory to confirm the absence of unsuspected sleep-related pathologies and to confirm the subjective complaint of EDS. Chronic sleep deprivation must be aggressively ruled out as an explanation for EDS . As with narcolepsy, the treatment implications (stimulant

medications indefinitely) require formal, objective diagnosis. In idiopathic CNS hypersomnia, the all-night PSG is unremarkable, and the MSLT reveals objective hypersomnia, usually without the occurrence of REM sleep during the naps (Guilleminault, 1994a). It is becoming clear that there is great overlap of symptoms and confusion in establishing a diagnosis between narcolepsy and idiopathic CNS hypersomnia (Moscovitch et al., 1993; Bruck & Parkes, 1996).

Treatment of idiopathic CNS hypersomnia involves the use of the same stimulants used in narcolepsy.

Circadian Rhythm Abnormalities

Circadian rhythm disorders can be classified into two categories: primary (disorders of the biologic clock per se) and secondary (disorders resulting from adopting sleep-wake patterns at variance with the underlying clock).

Primary Circadian Dysrhythmias

Delayed Sleep Phase Syndrome (DSPS). In DSPS, the patient falls asleep late and rises late. There is a striking inability to fall asleep at an earlier, more desirable time. For example, a college student is habitually unable to fall asleep until 2 AM, and has great difficulty getting up in time for her 8 AM classes Monday through Friday. She finds herself dozing off during morning classes. On Saturday and Sunday she sleeps in until about 10 AM, and feels rested upon arising, with no episodes of dozing during the day. This disorder may represent 5% to10% of cases with presenting complaints of insomnia at some sleep disorders centers (Diagnostic Classification Steering Committee, 1990). Onset is often during adolescence, but some patients report onset in childhood. A history of DSPS in family members has been noted clinically. DSPS may follow head trauma (Patten & Lauderdale, 1992).

Some individuals may suffer serious disruption of school and work. The complications depend partly on the tolerance of the patient's environment. A lenient employer and flexible schedule may allow a person to perform unimpaired if permitted to begin and end work a few hours later than others. More demanding or rigid work or school regimens may not allow this, and will require the patient to drop out if treatment is not possible. Disrupted family life may also result, if other family members do not have a similar schedule. The pervasive misperception that "sleeping in" is an undesirable personality characteristic such as laziness, slothfulness, or avoidance behavior often leads to interpersonal stress and hostility. Driving or operating machinery when sleepy can result in accidents. Persons with DSPS may use alcohol and sedative–hypnotics in an attempt to induce sleep earlier, sometimes developing alcohol or drug dependence (Institute of Medicine, 1971).

Bright light exposure upon awakening (toward the end of the PRC) has been shown to be effective in advancing sleep onset as well as in advancing temperature rhythm in a placebo-controlled study. The patient is asked to sit near a bright light, furnishing 5000–10000 lux, for about an hour upon awakening every day. The response may not be evident for 2 weeks, and the treatment may have to be continuous (Rosenthal et al., 1990).

Other treatment for DSPS includes chronotherapy and schedule change. For example, the patient goes to sleep at 2 AM the first night, then at 5 AM, then at 8 AM, and so on, until reaching 10 AM. Once adjusted, the wake/sleep cycle must be rigidly kept.

DSPS may be difficult to treat, and tends to relapse if the treatment is suspended. It may be that a combination of approaches such as chronotherapy, phototherapy, and pharmacotherapy will provide better treatment results (Alvarez et al., 1992; Ito et al., 1993; Regestein & Monk, 1995; Regestein & Pavlova, 1995). From a practical standpoint, the most effective means of dealing with DSPS is for the patient to accommodate his/her academic or employment activities to fit the underlying clock pattern.

Advanced Sleep Phase Syndrome (ASPS). Individuals suffering from ASPS fall asleep early and awaken early. They are unable to remain awake until the desired time, falling asleep in the early evening and awakening in the very early hours of the morning.

There are no studies of the prevalence and incidence of this disorder, but clinical experience suggests that it may be far less common than DSPS. However, it may also be the case that ASPS is more common than generally appreciated, but less likely to come to medical attention, because the consequences in the classroom or workplace are much less than with DSPS.

Patients complain of interruption of evening activities by their sleepiness. They may avoid evening social activities, fearing the intrusive sleepiness. They are also distressed by the very early awakenings. Driving and operation of machinery while sleepy (particularly in the evening) can result in accidents.

Bright light administered in the late afternoon or early evening (at the early portion of the PRC) has been reported effective in delaying both sleep onset and temperature rhythm (Murphy & Campbell, 1996). The technique is the same as that for DSPS, except for the timing of exposure. Chronotherapy, with a 3-hour advance every other day until the desired sleep-onset time has been reached, may also be effective (Moldofsky et al., 1986).

Other circadian dysrhythmias include the "non–24-hour sleep/wake disorder" (hypernychthemeral syndrome) and the "irregular sleep/wake pattern." These conditions appear to be rare and poorly understood, and are beyond the scope of this chapter. Individuals suffering from these conditions are unable to be entrained, or synchronized, by the usual time cues such as sunlight and social activity. Patients may complain of insomnia or excessive sleepiness, cognitive disturbance, and fatigue. Complications include severe disruption of work or studies, and accidents when attempting to drive or operate machinery while sleepy (Mahowald & Ettinger, 1999).

Secondary Circadian Dysrhythmias

In contrast to the primary circadian dysrhythmias, which represent malfunctioning of the biologic clock within the conventional geophysical environment, the secondary circadian dysrhythmias occur *because* the biologic clock is working properly—but functioning out of phase due to an imposed shift in the geophysical environment. Technological advances such as electric lights and the jet planes have allowed us to override or intentionally ignore our physiologic biologic rhythms. The numbers of people involved in transmeridian flight and shift work are startling (nearly one fifth of all workers in industrialized countries work unconventional shifts). This situation, coupled with the well-documented impairment of performance and judgment attendant with trying to buck the biologic clock, has staggering implications at the personal, national, and international level (National Commission on Sleep Disorders Research, 1992). The changes associated with time-zone crossing are transient and self-limited; those with shift work persist as long as the shift work. The symptoms of these disorders have been experienced by most of us, and are well-reviewed elsewhere (Loat et al., 1989; U. S. Congress Office of Technology Assessment, 1991). Schedule-induced decrements in alertness and performance have enormous implications for shuttle diplomats, traveling athletic teams, and shift workers.

Jet Lag. The consequences of jet lag are variable on an individual basis. Most travelers who cross many time zones will experience transient impaired performance resulting from circadian factors of alertness and performance. Countermeasures such as bright light exposure, sedative-hypnotic medications, and the use of melatonin require further study (Arendt et al., 2000).

Shift Work. The primary consequence of shift work is impaired performance (Akerstedt, 1991). In addition, there is some evidence to link shift work with increased cardiovascular morbidity and mortality, and with gastrointestinal disease (Harrington, 1994; Kawachi et al., 1995). Disruption of circadian organization in animals and insects has a deleterious effect on longevity (Hurd & Ralph, 1998; Klarsfeld & Rouyer, 1998). There is a high degree of variability in the short- and long-term adjustment to shift work (Quera-Salva et al., 1996;

Costa, 1997; Monk, 2000a). This is in part due to the exposure to bright light on the drive home in the morning. This exposure can impair or prevent circadian adaptation (Mitchell et al., 1997).

Night shift workers rarely develop circadian adaptation to the night shift. In the past, one approach to improving adjustment to shift work has been to use sedative-hypnotic agents to promote sleep. Inasmuch as the human circadian pacemaker promotes alertness, it has been suggested that emulation of the biologic function of the circadian pacemaker by administering wake-promoting agents may be more effective in combating the sleepiness experienced during working hours in shift workers (Edgar, 1996). Shift work schedules should be individualized to accommodate the goals of the employer, the desires of the employee, and ergonomic recommendations for the design of shift systems (Knauth, 1997; Monk, 2000b). The effect of napping during work for shift workers remains to be documented, and is complicated by sleep inertia experienced by some individuals (Akerstedt, 1989; Naitoh & Angus, 1989).

Effective treatment to reduce or minimize the devastating consequences of the secondary circadian dysrhythmias is in the developmental stage and includes chronotherapy (Czeisler et al., 1982), benzodiazepines (Bonnet et al., 1988; Walsh et al., 1988; Cohen et al., 1991), phototherapy (Czeisler et al., 1990), and melatonin administration (Samel et al., 1991; Petrie et al., 1993; Redfern et al., 1994; Arendt, 1997). Such chronobiologic, phototherapeutic, and pharmacologic manipulations are promising, but require further study.

SUMMARY

Sleepiness from whatever cause, with its predictable impairment of mood, attention, and performance, extracts a formidable toll at both personal and societal levels. Individuals, employers, and policy makers are learning that sleep is not "negotiable" or "a waste of time," but rather, is a biologic imperative. Sleep deprivation and sleep disorders resulting in excessive sleepiness are readily identifiable, and more importantly, are treatable. As this fact is more widely appreciated, sleepiness-related catastrophes may become less frequent. Close collaboration among basic researchers, clinicians, and public policy makers dealing with the causes, consequences, and management of sleepiness will provide great benefit to both individuals and to society as a whole.

■ KEY POINTS

☐   Sleepiness has prominent, and often severe, neuropsychiatric behavioral consequences, primarily in the arenas of impaired mood, attention, and performance, with serious ramifications in the family, classroom, workplace, and behind the wheel.

☐   Most population survey studies indicate that the prevalence of EDS is 5% to 15%. By far, the most common cause of EDS in our society is chronic volitional sleep deprivation.

☐   Wake/sleep scheduling conditions may play a major role in many motor vehicle crashes and workplace "accidents." Job-related and social demands on the wake/sleep schedules of individuals may result in circadian rhythm disorders that can be life-threatening. Studies have shown a circadian pattern of motor vehicle and industrial accidents, with severalfold higher incidence in early morning hours, and with a lesser peak in the afternoon.

☐   There is evidence that administration of stimulants such as caffeine, methylphenidate, and other stimulants, as well as modafinil, may counteract some of the consequences of sleepiness-impaired function; however, more systematic study is needed.

☐   The primary consequence of shift work is impaired performance.

KEY READINGS

Costa G: The problem: Shiftwork. Chronobiol Int 14:89–98, 1997.

Doran SM, Van Dongen HPA, Dinges DF: Sustained attention performance during sleep deprivation: Evidence of state instability. Arch Ital Biol 139:253–276, 2001.

Williamson AM, Feyer A-M: Moderate sleep deprivation produces impairments in cognitive and motor performance equivalent to legally prescribed levels of alcohol intoxication. Occup Environ Med 57:649–655, 2000.

REFERENCES

Achermann P, Werth E, Dijk D-J, Borbely AA: Time course of sleep inertia after nighttime and daytime sleep episodes. Arc Ital Biol 134:109–119, 1995.

Akerstedt T: Shift work and napping, in Dinges DF, Broughton RJ (eds): Sleep and Alertness: Chronobiological, Behavioral, and Medical Aspects of Napping. New York: Raven Press, 1989, pp. 205–220.

Akerstedt T: Sleepiness at work: Effects of irregular work hours, in Monk TH (ed): Sleep, Sleepiness and Performance. Chichester: John Wiley & Sons; 1991, pp. 129–152.

Akerstedt T: Work hours and sleepiness. Neurophsiol Clin 25:367–375, 1995.

Aldrich MS: The neurobiology of narcolepsy. Prog Neurobiol 41:538–541, 1992.

Aldrich MS, Chervin RD, Malow BA: Value of the multiple sleep latency test (MSLT) for the diagnosis of narcolepsy. Sleep 20:620–629, 1997.

Alvarez B, Dahlitz MJ, Vignau J, Parkes JD: The delayed sleep phase syndrome: Clinical and investigative findings in fourteen subjects. J Neurol Neurosurg Psychiatry 55:665–670, 1992.

American Sleep Disorders Association: The clinical use of the multiple sleep latency test. Sleep 15:268–276, 1992.

American Sleep Disorders Association: Practice parameters for the use of stimulants in the treatment of narcolepsy. Sleep 17:348–351, 1994.

Arendt J, Deacon S: Treatment of circadian rhythm disorders—melatonin. Chronobiol Int 14:185–204, 1997.

Arendt J, Stone B, Skene D: Jet lag and sleep disruption, in Kryger MH, Roth T, Dement WC (eds); Principles and Practice of Sleep Medicine, ed 3. Philadelphia: Saunders, 2000, pp. 591–599.

Balkin TJ, Wesensten NJ, Braun AR, et al: Shaking out the cobwebs: changes in regional cerebral blood flow (rCBF) across the first 20 minutes of wakefulness. J Sleep Res 21:411.A, 1998.

Baranski JV, Pigeau RA: Self-monitoring cognitive performance during sleep deprivation: effects of modafinil, d-amphetamine, and placebo. J Sleep Res 6:84–91, 1997.

Basheer R, Porkka-Heiskanen T, Strecker RE, et al: Adenosine as a biological signal mediating sleepiness following prolonged wakefulness. Biol Signals Recept 9:319–327, 2000.

Bassetti C, Aldrich MS: Idiopathic hypersomnia: A series of 42 patients. Brain 120:1423–1435, 1997.

Bassiri AG, Guilleminault C: Clinical features and evaluation of obstructive sleep apnea-hypopnea syndrome, in Kryger MH, Roth T, Dement WC (eds): Principles and Practice of Sleep Medicine, ed 3. Philadelphia: Saunders, 2000, pp. 869–878.

Benbadis SR, Perry MC, Mascha E, et al: Subjective vs. objective measures of sleepiness: correlation between Epworth sleepiness scale and MSLT. Sleep Res 26:641, 1997.

Beusterien KM, Rogers AE, Walsleben JA, et al: Health-related quality of life effects of modafinil for treatment of narcolepsy. Sleep 22:757–765, 1999.

Billiard M: Idiopathic hypersomnia. Neurol Clin 14:573–582, 1996.

Bishop C, Rosenthal L, Helmus T, et al: The frequency of multiple sleep onset REM periods among subjects with no excessive daytime sleepiness. Sleep 19:727–730, 1996.

Blagrove M, Akehurst L: Effects of sleep loss on confidence-accuracy relationships for reasoning and eyewitness memory. J Exp Psychol Appl 6:59–73, 2000.

Bonnet MH. Sleep deprivation, in Kryger MH, Roth T, Dement WC (eds): Principles and Practice of Sleep Medicine, ed 3. Philadelphia: Saunders, 2000, pp. 53–71.

Bonnet MH, Dexter JR, Gillin JC, et al: The use of triazolam in phase-advanced sleep. Neuropsychopharmacology 1:225–234, 1988.

Broughton R, Ghanem Q, Hishikawa Y, et al: Life effects of narcolepsy: relationships to geographic origin (North American, Asian, or European) and to other patient and illness variables. Can J Neurol Sci 10:100–104, 1983.

Broughton R, Valley A, Agguirre M, et al: Excessive daytime sleepiness and the pathophysiology of narcolepsy–cataplexy: a laboratory perspective. Sleep 9:205–215, 1986.

Broughton WA, Broughton RJ: Psychosocial impact of narcolepsy. Sleep 17:S45–S49, 1994.

Bruck D, Parkes JD: A comparison of idiopathic hypersomnia and narcolepsy–cataplexy using self report measures and sleep diary data. J Neurol Neurosurg Psychiatry 60:576–578, 1996.

Brun J, Chamba G, Khalfallah Y, et al: Effect of modafinil on plasma melatonin, cortisol and growth hormone rhythms, rectal temperature and performance in healthy subjects during a 36 h sleep deprivation. J Sleep Res 7:105–114, 1998.

29. Carskadon MA, Dement WC: Normal human sleep: An overview, in Kryger MH, Roth T, Dement WC (eds): Principles and Practice of Sleep Medicine, ed 3. Philadelphia: Saunders, 1994, pp. 16–25.

Carskadon MA, Dement WC, Mitler MM, Westbrook PR, Keenan S: Guidelines for the multiple sleep latency test (MSLT): a standard measure of sleepiness. Sleep 9:519–524, 1986.

Carskadon MA, Rechtschaffen A: Monitoring and staging human sleep, in Kryger MH, Roth T, Dement WC (eds): Principles and Practice of Sleep Medicine, ed 3. Philadelphia: Saunders, 2000, pp. 1197–1215.

Chervin RD, Aldrich MS, Pickett R, Guilleminault C: Comparison of the results of the Epworth sleepiness scale and the multiple sleep latency test. J Psychosomat Res 42:145–155, 1997.

Chervin RD, Kraemer HC, Guilleminault C: Correlates of sleep latency on the multiple sleep latency test in a clinical population. Electromyogr Clin Neurophysiol 95:147–153, 1995.

Cohen AS, Seidel WF, Yost D, et al: Triazolam used in the treatment of jet lag: Effects on sleep and subsequent wakefulness. Sleep Res 20:61, 1991.

Corsi-Cabrera M, Arce C, Del Rio-Portilla IY, et al: Amplitude reduction in visual event-related potentials as a function of sleep deprivation. Sleep 22:181–189, 1999.

Costa G: The problem: Shiftwork. Chronobiol Int 14:89–98, 1997.

Czeisler CA, Johnson MP, Duffy JF, et al: Exposure to bright light and darkness to treat physiologic maladaptation to night work. N Engl J Med 322:1253–1259, 1990.

Czeisler CA, Moore-Ede MC, Coleman RM: Rotating shift work schedules that disrupt sleep are improved by applying circadian principles. Science 217:460–463, 1982.

Dahl RE: The impact of inadequate sleep on children's daytime cognitive function. Sem Pediatr Neurol 3:44–50, 1996.

Dawson D, Reid K: Fatigue, alcohol and performance impairment. Nature 388:235, 1997.

Day R, Gerhardstein R, Lumley A, et al: The behavioral morbidity of obstructive sleep apnea. Prog Cardiovasc Dis 41:341–354, 1999.

Diagnostic Classification Steering Committee, Thorpy MJ, Chairman: International Classification of Sleep Disorders: Diagnostic and Coding Manual. Rochester, MN: American Sleep Disorders Association; 1990.

Dinges DF: Napping patterns and effects in human adults, in Dinges DF, Broughton RJ (eds): Sleeping and Alertness: Chronobiological, Behavioral, and Medical Aspects of Napping. New York: Raven Press, 1989, pp. 171–204.

Dinges DF: Are you awake? Cognitive performance and reverie during the hypnopompic state, in Bootzin RR, Kihlstrom JF, Schacter DL (eds): Sleep and Cognition. Washington, DC: American Psychological Association, 1990, pp. 159–175.

Dinges DF: An overview of sleepiness and accidents. J Sleep Res 4 (Suppl. 2):4–14, 1995.

Dinges DF, Pack F, Williams K, et al: Cumulative sleepiness, mood disturbance, and psychomotor vigilance performance decrements during a week of sleep restricted to 4–5 hours per night. Sleep 20:267–277, 1997.

Doran SM, Van Dongen HPA, Dinges DF: Sustained attention performance during sleep deprivation: Evidence of state instability. Arch Ital Biolog 139:253–276, 2001.

Dorrian J, Lamond N, Dawson D: The ability to self-monitor performance when fatigued. J Sleep Res 9:137–144, 2000.

Edgar DM: Circadian control of sleep/wakefulness: Implications in shiftwork and therapeutic strategies, in Shiraki K, Sagawa S, Yousef MK (eds): Physiological Basis of Occupational Health: Stressful Environments. Amsterdam: SPB Academic Publishing bv, 1996, pp. 253–265.

Edgar DM, Dement WC, Fuller CA: Effect of SCN lesions on sleep in squirrel monkeys: Evidence for opponent process in sleep-wake regulation. J Neurosci 13:1065–1079, 1993.

Everson CA, Gilliland MA, Kushida CA, et al: Sleep deprivation in the rat: IX. Recovery. Sleep 12:60–67, 1989.

Ferrara M, De Gennaro L: The sleep inertia phenomenon during the sleep-wake transition: Theoretical and operational issues. Aviat Space Environ Med 1:843–848, 2000.

Ferrara M, De Gennaro L, Bertini M: Voluntary oculomotor performance upon awakening after total sleep deprivation. Sleep 23:801–811, 2000.

Franken P, Malafosse A, Tafti M: Genetic determinants of sleep regulation in inbred mice. Sleep 22:155–169, 1999.

Gillberg M, Akerstedt T: Sleep loss and performance: No "safe" duration of a monotonous task. Physiol Behav 64:599–604, 1998.

Goldman LS, Genel M, Bexman RJ, Slanetz PJ: Diagnosis and treatment of attention-deficit/hyperactivity disorder in children and adolescents. JAMA 279:1100–1107, 1998.

Guilleminault C: Idiopathic central nervous system hypersomnia, in Kryger MH, Roth T, Dement WC (eds): Principles and Practice of Sleep Medicine, ed 2. Philadelphia: Saunders, 1994a, pp. 562–566.

Guilleminault C: Narcolepsy syndrome, in Kryger MH, Roth T, Dement WC (eds): Principles and Practice of Sleep Medicine, ed 2. Philadelphia: Saunders, 1994b, pp. 549–561.

Harrington JM: Shift work and health—a critical review of the literature on working hours. Ann Acad Med Singapore 23:699–705, 1994.

Harrison Y, Horne JA: Sleep loss impairs short and novel language tasks having a prefrontal focus. J Sleep Res 7:95–100, 1998.

Harrison Y, Horne JA: The impact of sleep deprivation on decision making: A review. J Exper Psychol Appl 6:236–249, 2000.

Hood B, Bruck D: Sleepiness and performance in narcolepsy. J Sleep Res 5:128–134, 1996.

Horne JA: Frontal lobe function and sleep loss. Sleep Res Online 2(Suppl. 1):677, 1999.

Horner RL, Sanford LD, Pack AI, Morrison AR: Activation of a distinct arousal state immediately after spontaneous awakening from sleep. Brain Res 778:127–134, 1997.

Hurd MW, Ralph MR: The significance of circadian organization for longevity in the golden hamster. J Biol Rhythms 13:430–436, 1998.

Institute of Medicine: Sleeping Pills, Insomnia and Medical Practice. Washington, DC: National Academy of Sciences Office of Publications; 1971.

Ito A, Ando K, Hayakawa T, et al: Long-term course of adult patients with delayed sleep phase syndrome. Jpn J Psychiatry Neurol 47:563–567, 1993.

Jahnke B, Aldrich MS: The multiple sleep latency test (MSLT) is not infallible. Sleep Res 19:240, 1990.

Jewett ME, Wyatt JK, Ritz-De Cecco A, et al: Time course of sleep inertia dissipation in human performance and alertness. J Sleep Res 8:1–8, 1999.

Johns MW: A new method for measuring daytime sleepiness. Sleep 14:540–545, 1991.

Johns MW: Daytime sleepiness, snoring, and obstructive sleep apnea. The Epworth sleepiness scale. Chest 103:30–36, 1993.

Johns MW: Sleepiness in different situations measured by the Epworth sleepiness scale. Sleep 17:703–710, 1994.

Jones BE: Basic mechanisms of sleep-wake states, in Kryger MH, Roth T, Dement WC (eds): Principles and Practice of Sleep Medicine, ed 3. Philadelphia: Saunders, 2000, pp. 134–154.

Kas MJH, Edgar DM: Scheduled voluntary wheel running activity modulates free-running circadian body temperature rhythms in Octodon degus. J Biol Rhythms 16:66–75, 2001.

Kavanau JL: Memory, sleep, and the evolution of mechanisms of synaptic efficacy maintenance. Neuroscience 79:7–44, 1997.

Kawachi I, Colditz GA, Stampfer MJ, et al: Prospective study of shift work and risk of coronary heart disease in women. Circulation 92:3178–3182, 1995.

Kim HC, Young T, Matthews CG, et al: Sleep-disordered breathing and neuropsychological deficits: A population-based study. Am J Respir Crit Care Med 156:1813–1819, 1997.

Klarsfeld A, Rouyer F: Effects of circadian mutations and LD periodicity of the life span of Drosophila melanogaster. J Biol Rhythms 13:471–478, 1998.

Knauth P: Changing schedules: Shiftwork. Chronobiol Int 14:159–171, 1997.

Koboyama T, Hori A, Sato T, et al: Changes in cerebral blood flow velocity in healthy young men during overnight sleep and while awake. Electromyogr Clin Neurophysiol 102:125–131, 1997.

Koslowski M, Babkoff H: Meta-analysis of the relationship between total sleep deprivation and performance. Chronobiol Int 9:132–136, 1992.

Krahn LE, Black JL, Silber MH: Narcolepsy: New understanding of irresistible sleep. Mayo Clin Proc 76:185–194, 2001.

Krueger JM, Obal Jr F: A neuronal group theory of sleep function. J Sleep Res 2:63–69, 1993.

Kryger MH: Management of obstructive sleep apnea-hypopnea syndrome, in Kryger MH, Roth T, Dement WC (eds): Principles and Practice of Sleep Medicine, ed 3. Philadelphia: Saunders, 2000, pp. 940–954.

Lahmeyer WH: Sleep in craniopagus twins. Sleep 11:301–306, 1988.

Lavie P, Zvuluni A: The 24-hour sleep propensity function: Experimental bases for somnotypology. Psychophysiology 29:566–575, 1992.

Loat CER, Rhodes EC: Jet-lag and human performance. Sports Med 8:226–238, 1989.

Mahowald MW: Sleep in traumatic brain injury and other acquired CNS conditions, in Culebras A (ed): Sleep Disorders and Neurological Disease. New York: Marcel Dekker, 2000, pp. 365–385.

Mahowald MW, Ettinger MG: Circadian rhythm disorders, in Chokroverty S (ed): Sleep Disorders Medicine: Basic Science, Technical Considerations, and Clinical Aspects, ed 2. Boston: Butterworth Heinemann, 1999, pp. 619–634.

Masel BE, Scheibel RS, Kimbark T, Kuna ST: Excessive daytime sleepiness in adults with brain injuries. Arch Phys Med Rehab 82:1526–1532, 2001.

McCurry SM, Logsdon RG, Teri L, et al: Characteristics of sleep disturbance in community-dwelling Alzheimer's disease patients. J Geriatr Psychiatry Neurol 12:53–59, 1999.

Meier-Ewert K, Broughton RJ: Photomyoclonic response of epileptic and non-epileptic subjects during wakefulness, sleep and arousal. Electromyogr Clin Neurophysiol 23:142–151, 1967.

Mignot E: Pathophysiology of Narcolepsy, in Kryger MH, Roth T, Dement WC (eds): Principles and Practice of Sleep Medicine, ed 3. Philadelphia: Saunders, 2000, pp. 663–675.

Mitchell PJ, Hoese EK, Liu L, et al: Conflicting bright light exposure during night shifts impedes circadian adaptation. J Biol Rhythms 12:5–15, 1997.

Mitler MM, Carskadon MA, Czeisler CA, et al: Catastrophes, sleep, and public policy. Sleep 11:100–109, 1988.

Mitler MM, Carskadon MA, Hirshkowitz M: Evaluating sleepiness, in Kryger MH, Roth T, Dement WC (eds): Principles and Practice of Sleep Medicine, ed 3. Philadelphia: Saunders, 2000, pp. 1251–1257.

Mitler MM, Gujavarty KS, Browman CP: Maintenance of wakefulness test: A polysomnographic technique for evaluating treatment efficacy in patients with excessive somnolence. Electromyogr Clin Neurophysiol 53:568–661, 1982.

Mitler MM, Miller JC: Methods of testing for sleepiness. Behav Med 21:171–183, 1996.

Mitler MM, Walsleben J, Sangal RB, Hirshkowitz M: Sleep latency on the maintenance of wakefulness test (MWT) for 530 patients with narcolepsy while free of psychoactive drugs. Electromyogr Clin Neurophysiol 107:33–38, 1998.

Moe KE, Vitiello MV, Larsen LH, Prinz PN: Sleep/wake patterns in Alzheimer's disease: relationships with cognition and function. J Sleep Res 4:15–20, 1995.

Moldofsky H, Musisi S, Phillipson EA: Treatment of a case of advanced sleep phase syndrome by phase advance chronotherapy. Sleep 9:61–65, 1986.

Monk TH (ed): Sleep, Sleepiness and Performance. Chichester: John Wiley and Sons, 1991.

Monk TH: Shift work, in Kryger MH, Roth T, Dement WC (eds): Principles and Practice of Sleep Medicine, ed 3. Philadelphia: Saunders, 2000a, pp. 600–605.

Monk TH: What can the chronobiologist do to help the shiftworker? J Biol Rhythms 15:86–94, 2000b.

Monk TH, Buysse DJ, Reynolds CFI, Kupfer DJ: Circadian determinants of postlunch dip in performance. Chronobiol Int 13:123–133, 1966.

Moore-Ede M: The Twenty-Four-Hour Society. Reading, MA: Addison-Wesley; 1993.

Moscovitch A, Partinen M, Guilleminault C: The positive diagnosis of narcolepsy and narcolepsy's borderland. Neurology 43:55–60, 1993.

Murphy PJ, Campbell SS: Physiology of the circadian system in animals and humans. J Clin Neurophysiol 13:2–16, 1996.

Naitoh P, Angus RG: Napping and human functioning during prolonged work, in Dinges DF, Broughton RJ (eds): Sleep and Alertness: Chronobiological, Behavioral, and Medical Aspects of Napping. New York: Raven Press, 1989, pp. 221–246.

National Commission on Sleep Disorders Research. Report of the National Commission on Sleep Disorders Research. Washington, DC: Research DHHS Pub. No. 92–XXXX. Supplier of Documents, U. S. Government Printing Office, 1992.

Nicholson AN, Turner C: Intensive and sustained air operations: Potential use of the stimulant, pemoline. Aviat Space Environ Med 69:647–655, 1998.

Nishino S, Mao J, Sampathkumaran B, et al: Increased dopaminergic transmission mediates the wake-promoting effects of CNS stimulants. Sleep Res Online 1:49–61, 1998.

Nishino S, Mignot E: Pharmacological aspects of human and canine narcolepsy. Progr Neurobiol 52:27–78, 1997.

Nobili L, Ferrillo F, Besset A, et al: Ultradian aspects of sleep in narcolepsy. Neurophysiol Clin 26:51–59, 1996.

Partinen M, Hublin C: Epidemiology of sleep disorders. in Kryger MH, Roth T, Dement WC (eds): Principles and Practice of Sleep Medicine, ed 3. Philadelphia: Saunders, 2000, pp. 558–579.

Patten SB, Lauderdale WM: Delayed sleep phase disorder after traumatic brain injury. J Am Acad Child Adolesc Psychiatry 31:100–102, 1992.

Pawluk LK, Hurwitz TD, Schluter JL, et al: Psychiatric morbidity in narcoleptics on chronic high dose methylphenidate therapy. Journal of Nervous and Mental Diseases 183:45–48, 1995.

Petrie K, Dawson AG, Thompson L, Brook R: A double-blind trial of melatonin as a treatment for jet lag in international cabin crew. Biological Psychiatry 33:526–530, 1993.

Pigeau R, Naitoh P, Buguet A, et al: Modafinil, d-amphetamine and placebo during 64 hours of sustained mental work. I. Effects on mood, fatigue, cognitive performance and body temperature. J Sleep Res 4:212–228, 1995.

Pilcher JJ, Huffcutt AI: Effects of sleep deprivation on performance: a meta-analysis. Sleep 19:318–326, 1996.

Pilcher JJ, Walters AS: How sleep deprivation affects psychological variables related to college students' cognitive performance. Journal of American College Health 46:121–126, 1997.

Powell NB, Riley RW, Schechtman KB, Blumen MB, Dinges DF, Guilleminault C: A comparative model: reaction time performance in sleep-disordered breathing versus alcohol-impaired controls. Laryngoscope 109:1648–1654, 1999.

Quera-Salva MA, Defrance R, Claustrat B, De Lattre J, Guilleminault C: Rapid shift in sleep time and acrophase of melatonin secretion in short shift work schedule. Sleep 19:539–543, 1996.

Ralph MR, Foster RG, Davis FC, Menaker M: Transplanted suprachiasmatic nucleus determines circadian period. Science 247:925–978, 1990.

Randazzo AC, Muehlbach MJ, Schweitzer PK, Walsh JK: Cognitive function following acute sleep restriction in children ages 10–14. Sleep 21:861–868, 1998.

Rechtschaffen A: Current perspectives on the function of sleep. Perspectives in Biology and Medicine 41:359–390, 1998.

Redfern P, Minors D, Waterhouse J: Circadian rhythms, jet lag, and chronobiotics: an overview. Chronobiol Int 11:253–265, 1994.

Reed C, Szuba MP, Powell JW, Carlin MM, Dinges DF: Neurobehavioral and somatic complaints during chronic partial sleep deprivation. Sleep 23 (Suppl 2):A242–A243, 2000.

Regestein QR, Monk TH: Delayed sleep phase syndrome; a review of its clinical aspects. American Journal of Psychiatry 152:602–608, 1995a.

Regestein QR, Pavlova M: Treatment of delayed sleep phase syndrome. General Hospital Psychiatry 17:335–345, 1995b.

Reid IC, Dawson D: Comparing performance on a simulated 12 hour shift rotation in young and older subjects. Occup Environ Med 58:58–62, 2001.

Roehrs T, Roth T: Multiple sleep latency test: technical aspects and normal values. Journal of Clinical Neurophysiology 9:63–67, 1992.

Roehrs T, Zorick F, Wittig R, Conway W, Roth T: Predictors of objective level of daytime sleepiness in patients with sleep-related breathing disorders. Chest 95:1202–1206, 1989.

Rosenthal L, Folkerts M, Roehrs T, Zorick F, Roth T: Sleepiness and sleep onset REM periods in the absence of clinical symptomatology. Biological Psychiatry 36:341–343, 1994.

Rosenthal NE, Joseph-Vanderpool JR, Levendosky AA, et al: Phase-shifting effects of bright morning light as treatment for delayed sleep phase syndrome. Sleep 13:354–361, 1990.

Roth B, Nevsimalova S, Sagova V, Paroubkova D, Horakovga A: Neurological, psychological and polygraphic findings in sleep drunkenness. Archives Suisses de Neurologie, Neurochirurgie et de Psychiatrie 129:209–222, 1981.

Roth T, Roehrs TA, Carskadon MA, Dement WC. Daytime sleepiness and alertness. in Kryger MH, Roth T, Dement WC (eds): Principles and Practice of Sleep Medicine, ed 2. Philadelphia: Saunders, 1994, p. 40–49.

Sallinen M, Harma M, Akerstedt T, Rosa R, Lillqvist O: Promoting alertness with a short nap during a night shift. J Sleep Res 7:240–247, 1998.

Samel A, Wegmann H-M, Vejvoda M, Maass H, Gundel A, Schutz M: Influence of melatonin treatment on human circadian rhythmicity before and after a simulated 9-hr time shift. Journal Biological Rhythms 6:235–248, 1991.

Siegel JM: Narcolepsy: a key role for hypocretins (orexins). Cell 98:409–412, 1999.

Tassi P, Muzet A: Sleep inertia. Sleep Medicine Reviews 4:341–353, 2000.

Teran-Santos J, Jimenez-Gomez A, Cordero-Guevara J: The association between sleep apnea and the risk of traffic accidents. N Engl J Med 340:847–851, 1999.

Terman M, Terman JS. Light therapy. in Kryger MH, Roth T, Dement WC (eds): Principles and Practice of Sleep Medicine, ed 3. Philadelphia: Saunders, 2000, p. 1258–1274.

Thomas M, Sing H, Belenky G, et al: Neural basis of alertness and cognitive performance impairments during sleepiness. I. Effects of 24 h of sleep deprivation on waking human regional brain activity. J Sleep Res 9:335–352, 2000.

U. S. Congress Office of Technology Assessment. Biological Rhythms: Implications for the Worker. OTA-BA-463 Washington DC: U. S. Government Printing Office; September, 1991.

Van Dongen HPA, Dinges DF. Circadian rhythms in fatigue, alertness, and performance, in Kryger MH, Roth T, Dement WC (eds): Principles and Practice of Sleep Medicine, ed 3. Philadelphia: Saunders, 2000, pp. 391–399.

VanDongen HPA, Maislin G, Dinges DF: Chronic partial sleep deprivation: Neurobehavioral response and sleep architecture. Sleep Research Online 2(Suppl 1):735, 1999.

Voderholzer U, Backhaus J, Hornyak M, Hohagen F, Berger M, Riemann D: A 19-h spontaneous sleep period in idiopathic central nervous system hypersomnia. J Sleep Res 7:101–103, 1998.

Vogel GW: A review of REM sleep deprivation. Archives of General Psychiatry 32:749–761, 1975.

Wallin MT, Mahowald MW: Blood pressure effects of long-term stimulant use in disorders of hypersomnolence. J Sleep Res 7:209–215, 1998.

Walsh JK, Sugerman JL, Muehlbach MJ, Schweitzer PK: Physiological sleep tendency on a simulated night shift: Adaptation and effects of triazolam. Sleep 11:251–264, 1988.

Weiler JM, Bloomfield JR, Woodworth GG, et al: Effects of fexofenadine, diphenhyramine, and alcohol on driving performance. Ann Intern Med 132:354–363, 2000.

Williamson AM, Feyer A-M: Moderate sleep deprivation produces impairments in cognitive and motor performance equivalent to legally prescribed levels of alcohol intoxication. Occup Environ Med 57:649–655, 2000.

Winter WC, Bliwise DL, Quershi AI: Post sleep reduction in cerebral blood flow velocity is independent of preceding REM vs NREM sleep. Sleep 22 (supplement):S288 (abstract), 1999.

Wright KP, Czeisler CA: The effect of sleep deprivation on cognitive performance upon awakening from sleep. Sleep 22 (supplement):S147 (abstract), 1999.

Young T, Palta M, Dempsey J, et al: The occurrence of sleep-disordered breathing among middle-age adults. N Engl J Med 328:1230–1235, 1993.

Incontinence and Sexual Dysfunction

Karl J. Kreder
Matthew Rizzo
Satish S-C. Rao

Anorgasmia
Biofeedback therapy
Bladder training
Detrusor instability
Drugs
Epidemiology
Erectile dysfunction
Fecal incontinence
Impotence
Incontinence (urge, stress, mixed, overflow, functional)
Klüver-Bucy syndrome

Priapism
Sildenafil
Surgery
TDF (testis determining factor) gene

INTRODUCTION

Peripheral nerve, spinal cord, and cerebral lesions can impair urinary and sexual function and also can cause fecal incontinence. Some patients have neural lesions at more than one level, as in diabetes, alcohol abuse, and multiple sclerosis. Vascular pathology, medication effects, and psychiatric factors further complicate the assessment and treatment of these patients. We approach these issues below in discussions of urinary and fecal incontinence, impotence (the most common sexual impairment caused by neurologic disorders)—and their central nervous system (CNS) substrates.

CENTRAL NERVOUS SYSTEM SUBSTRATES OF GENITOURINARY DYSFUNCTION

Cerebral Substrates

David Ferrier (1876) brought a scientific mind and Victorian sensibility to bear on the neural underpinnings of human sexuality, anticipating later research. He wrote:

> The sexual appetite, those springing from the organic wants of certain glandular structures, centres itself around a certain tactile sensation, which is the reflex key to the gratification of the physiological demand for functional exercise on the part of these organs. The sexual appetite increases only with the development of the generative glands. Its appearance induces considerable perturbation of the other organic functions, and expresses itself subjectively at first in the form of emotional excitability, or obscure longings, morbid desires, or hysterical outbursts. Long before the link between a definite sensation and a definite action for its realization had been established in consciousness, the generative glands may gratify themselves reflexively during sleep, the period, *par excellence*, of reflex excitability.

> As morbid irritation of the generative organs may excite a morbid sexual appetite, so conversely, the sexual appetite may be morbidly excited by pathological irritation of the cerebral paths and cerebral centres of the sensations connected with the exercise of the generative functions. To the former belong the satyriasis or nymphomania occasionally observed in connection with disease of the middle lobe of the cerebellum; to the latter the various morbid exhibitions of the sexual appetite in insanity, where the centres are functionally or organically diseased. From certain facts of experiment, we have seen reason to conclude that the centres of sexual feeling are probably localizable in the regions connecting the occipital lobes with the lower and inner part of the tempero-sphenoidal lobe.

The behaviors that characterize human sexuality are multilayered and complex, ranging from reflexes in the sacral cord that help mediate the mechanisms of sexual intercourse to such complex components of sexual experience as courtship, maternal behavior, gender identity, and the formation of family units. Among the many aspects of human sexuality one can consider such topics as love, jealousy, romance, male and female homosexuality, and premenstrual syndrome, as well as fringe behaviors such as rape, onanism, frotteurism, exhibitionism, nymphomania, pedophilia, zoophilia, coprophilia, sadomasochism, necrophilia, and others. Drugs such as ethanol, marijuana, and methylenedioxymethamphetamine (MDMA, or "Ecstasy") are associated with mental status and behavior changes, memory loss, and "blackouts"; because the prescription sedative Rohypnol (Hoffman-LaRoche) also induces these effects, it is sometimes referred to as the "date rape" drug of choice. The neural substrates underlying these complex biologic and social phenomena are scarcely understood (Halaris, 2003), although research efforts have increased since Masters and Johnson's landmark research and surveys in the 1960s (Masters & Johnson, 1966) and early use of electroencephalogram (EEG) recordings in attempts to correlate pleasure and brain activity during orgasm in humans (Heath, 1972).

In embryonic life females start with two X chromosomes, whereas males have one X and one Y. Y chromosomes have a TDF (testis determining factor) gene, which works on undifferentiated embryonic gonadal tissue to develop the testes. Leydig cells in the testes inhibit formation of female organs from the müllerian duct and produce androgenic hormones that bind receptor molecules in target structures. This leads to further gender differentiation in utero (and through puberty); if not, we would all have female bodies and brains (LeVay, 1993).

Adult sexual and reproductive behavior depend on multilevel interactions between cortical and limbic areas (see Chapter 21), hypothalamus, pituitary, and endorgans. The ovaries, testes, adrenals, and brain produce sexual steroids that affect both the pituitary gland and brain. Cerebral dysfunction, hormone level changes, and drugs may all affect libido, potency, and fertility (Penovich, 2000). These effects vary with changing hormone levels from adolescence throughout the reproductive years and into menopause (estrogen deficiency), andropause (androgen deficiency), and somatopause (growth hormone deficiency) (Lamberts, 2002).

Men's brains are larger than women's, because men have a larger body size. Gender differences in human brain structure are evident in temporoparietal regions, and women may have greater relative volume of the corpus callosum and anterior commissure to connect the hemispheres (see Chapter 19 for details on callosal connections). These differences are thought to depend in part upon effects of sex hormones during embryonic or perinatal sexual differentiation, and might help explain gender differences in language, motor and spatial processes, and even emotional constitution, although specific mechanisms remain elusive, and interpretations are subject to "gender politics" (Fausto-Sterling, 2000). Reported differences between the hypothalamus of homosexuals and heterosexuals undercut the arcane explanatory hypothesis of homosexuality as a casualty of domineering mothers (Levay, 1991), yet have also led to bland pronouncements that brain differences underlie behavior differences, or have been taken to support extreme views of homosexuality as a brain disorder (LeVay, 1993, 1996).

Penfield and Rasmussen (1950) demonstrated the sensory mapping of the genitals on the mesial surface of the hemispheres in the 1940s (see Chapter 14). It is clear that cerebral substrates for genitourinary function comprise multiple limbic system structures, including the cingulate gyrus of the frontal lobe (Brodmann's area 24). These areas communicate through multiple feedback loops with sacral spinal areas that are essential to urinary and sexual function, and with cortical and subcortical brain areas concerned with emotion, hunger, thirst, vegetative functions, and hormone release. Damage to mesial frontal lobe areas can impair bladder control, sexual function, and gait (owing to the proximity of the primary motor leg areas, Brodmann's 3, 1, 2). In normal pressure hydrocephalus (NPH), white matter fibers to these areas are damaged by the expanding ventricles, due to failure to resorb cerebrospinal fluid (see Chapter 29). Additional etiologies of impairment include neurodegenerative disorders, traumatic brain injury, stroke, brain tumor (such as parasagittal meningioma), multiple sclerosis (MS), brain infections, epilepsy, mental retardation, and neurodevelopmental disorders. We review aspects of a few of these conditions below; specific comments on traumatic brain injury are addressed in Chapter 27.

Multiple Sclerosis

In MS sexual dysfunction commonly waxes and wanes with CNS demyelination, depression, and psychological response to disease. Among 41 patients with relapsing-remitting MS (mean age about 35 years old), about half (5 of 9 men and 16 of 32 women) reported at least one sexual disturbance (Barak et al., 1996). The most frequent disturbances affected libido (26.8%) and arousal (19.5%). Women rated their difficulties as more severe. Anorgasmia correlated with brain stem and pyramidal abnormalities and total plaque area on brain magnetic resonance imaging (MRI) scan.

Infections

Infections have various effects on genitourinary function due to destruction of multiple brain areas, as in encephalitis (see Chapter 23), or even due to pain, as in herpes zoster or venereal disease. Several venereal diseases can have serious CNS sequelae (notably, treponemal infection and HIV) including incontinence, impotence, and dementia. Patients with HIV may also have had syphilis or gonorrhea and may develop CNS lesions and behavior changes due to HIV encephalitis or development of an opportunistic CNS infection such as progressive multifocal leukoencephalopathy (PML). Patients with HTLV-1 infections may present with bladder dysfunction to a urologist or gynecologist, or to a genitourinary clinic with impotence or positive treponemal serology, before developing spastic paraparesis (Taylor, 1998). A 58-year-old man with impotence also had progressive peripheral neuropathy, dizziness, unsteady gait, and behavioral changes. Computed tomography (CT) revealed low-density, contrast-enhancing lesions in the right pontine tegmentum and the right medial temporal lobe, and temporal lobe biopsy confirmed CNS infection caused by Whipple disease (Halperin et al., 1982; see section on fecal incontinence).

Klüver-Bucy Syndrome

Incontinence and sexual dysfunction are also seen in human Klüver-Bucy syndrome (KBS) (Lilly et al., 1983), a condition first described in monkeys with bilateral temporal lobectomies (Klüver & Bucy, 1939). These animals showed visual and auditory agnosia, oral proclivities, altered eating habits, emotional blunting, rage, and hypersexuality, including mounting inappropriate objects and species (Klüver & Bucy, 1939). The lesions are typically said to affect the amygdala (see Chapter 21), but the hippocampi, cingulate, orbitofrontal, and insular cortex may also be damaged.

Head injury, heat stroke, herpes encephalitis, neurodegenerative impairments, temporal lobectomy, stroke, shigellosis, psychiatric disease, and even status epilepticus have been associated with KBS in humans (Nakada et al., 1984; Clarke & Brown, 1990; Anson & Kuhlman, 1993; Guedalia et al., 1993; Pitt et al., 1995). Children may be affected as well as adults (Tonsgard et al., 1987; Wong et al., 1991).

Cummings and Duchen (1981) reported KBS in five adults with Pick disease who had severe anterior temporal atrophy, amygdala abnormalities, and Pick bodies. One of the two patients examined with CT showed marked lobar atrophy. Early appearance of KBS syndrome and the late occurrence of amnesia and spatial disorientation identify this presumed Pick disease variant.

Gustafson and colleagues (1992) found non–Alzheimer-type frontal lobe degeneration in about 10% of autopsies in a longitudinal study of several hundred dementia cases (see Chapter 22). Some had KBS, with psychosis and emotional disorders in the context of slowly progressive dementia, personality changes, poor insight, disinhibition, apathy, and aphasia progressing to mutism, but relative sparing of memory, spatial ability, and receptive language. In early stages EEG results were normal, but cerebral blood flow was reduced in frontal areas. Atrophy mainly involved frontal or frontotemporal gray matter, including the insula and anterior cingulate gyrus, without the "knife-blade" atrophy seen in Pick disease. Pathology showed neuronal loss, slight gliosis, and spongiosis, and few senile plaques, tangles, congophilic vessels, or Pick cells, resembling the nonspecific neurodegenerative changes in amyotrophic lateral sclerosis (ALS).

Dickson and colleagues (1986) found KBS in a case of ALS. Autopsy showed extensive limbic system degeneration affecting the entorhinal cortex and subiculum of the medial temporal lobe. Morphometric and biochemical studies suggested damage in small, somatostatinergic cortical neurons. The lobar distribution of cortical atrophy suggested Pick disease, but Pick bodies and ballooned neurons were absent. A 13-year-old boy showed a "partial form" of KBS with hypersexuality, emotional disturbance, recent memory loss, polyphagia, narcolepsy, polydipsia, and polyuria after an encephalopathic illness, but virology studies were negative and frontal lobe biopsy showed Alzheimer type II astrocytosis (Wong et al., 1991). Treatment of symptoms with haloperidol, carbamazepine, serotonin reuptake inhibitors, or leuprolide (a gonadotropin inhibitor often used to treat prostate cancer) has been attempted in some cases (Stewart, 1985; Ott, 1995).

Epilepsy

Epilepsy causes sexual and reproductive dysfunction due to underlying brain lesions, endocrine dysfunction, and antiepileptic drug effects (Fenwick et al., 1985; Jensen et al., 1990; Lundberg and Brattberg, 1992; Duncan et al., 1997, 1999; Jesperson and Nielsen, 1999; Penovich, 2000; see Chapter 34). Antiepileptic drugs may affect hormone binding, reproductive function, and contraceptive hormone efficacy (Penovich, 2000). Changes in progesterone, estrogen, and testosterone levels have neuroendocrine effects that alter seizure frequency throughout life.

Absence seizure status is manifested rarely by compulsive masturbation (Jacome & Risko, 1983), and masturbation can simulate epilepsy (Livingston et al., 1975). Patients with masturbation and self-induced seizures may have idiopathic generalized epilepsy with light or pattern sensitivity. A mentally retarded man triggered his absence seizures by hand waving in association with sexual arousal and erection more than 100 times per day (Newmark & Penry, 1979). A 32-year-old married woman had a strong sense of pleasure with self-induced absence seizures associated with masturbation (Faught et al., 1986). She stood by a window, waved one hand in front of her eyes and masturbated for several hours a day,

neglecting her children and home. EEG results during one episode showed generalized epileptiform activity. She tore down boards that her husband nailed over the windows. When her seizures were treated with clonazepam she became depressed and insisted on stopping the medicine.

URINARY INCONTINENCE

Incidence, Prevalence, and Cost

Urinary incontinence is a common yet underreported problem that affects approximately 13 million Americans at a cost of over $15 billion dollars per year (National Kidney and Urologic Diseases Advisory Board, 1994). Risk factors include delirium, infection, atrophic urethritis, pharmaceuticals, psychological factors, endocrine disorders, restricted mobility, stool impaction, childhood enuresis, and pregnancy (Resnick, 1990; AHCPR, 1992). It affects at least 50% of elderly nursing home residents, 15% to 35% of noninstitutionalized persons over age 60, and women twice as often as men (Burgio et al., 1991; Ouslander, 1991). Toilet training is delayed in developmental disorders (see Chapter 44).

Classification of Urinary Incontinence

Types of acquired urinary incontinence includes urge incontinence, stress incontinence, mixed incontinence, overflow incontinence, and incontinence of other causes.

Urge Incontinence

Urge incontinence is involuntary loss of urine associated with a sudden and strong desire to void. This is usually due to bladder overactivity with abnormal detrusor contractions. When this bladder overactivity is associated with a neurologic lesion it is called detrusor hyperreflexia. In the absence of a neurologic lesion it is called detrusor instability. In elderly patients especially, detrusor overactivity may be accompanied by impaired contractility (DHIC). This type of incontinence may be difficult to diagnose because it can mimic other types of urinary incontinence (Resnick & Yalla, 1987; Abrams et al, 1988).

Stress Incontinence

Stress urinary incontinence is involuntary loss of urine during increased abdominal pressure (as with coughing, straining, or laughing) in the absence of a detrusor contraction. In women, this usually reflects urethral hypermobility or intrinsic sphincter deficiency, two separate conditions which often coexist (Kreder & Austin, 1996). In women with urethral hypermobility, the urethra shifts position due to relaxation of surrounding support structures, and intra-abdominal pressures are not equally transmitted to the urethra during periods of stress; urine loss occurs when intra-abdominal pressure exceeds urethral pressure. Patients with intrinsic sphincter deficiency generally have good support of the urethra but are incontinent because they cannot generate enough pressure to maintain urethral sphincter closure (Staskin et al., 1985). In men, stress urinary incontinence often results from direct trauma to the sphincter following prostate surgery.

Mixed Incontinence

Mixed incontinence refers to co-occurrence of stress incontinence and urge incontinence and is more common in women, but can occur in men after prostatectomy. The most bothersome symptom identifies the main target for diagnostic and therapeutic intervention.

Overflow Incontinence

Overflow incontinence results from bladder overdistention. Patients complain of frequent or constant dribbling incontinence, which may be exacerbated by straining or increased intra-abdominal pressure. Overflow incontinence can be caused by detrusor dysfunction with a noncontractile or hypocontractile detrusor, or by bladder outlet obstruction that leads to bladder overdistention and overflow incontinence. Bladder outlet obstruction in women is rare except in those with prior anti-incontinence surgery or with significant pelvic prolapse. In men, obstruction is commonly caused by benign prostatic hyperplasia. Fecal impaction, neurologic conditions, and diabetes may also cause bladder decompensation.

Unconscious or Reflex Incontinence

Unconscious or reflex incontinence refers to urinary incontinence that occurs without warning or awareness, especially in neurologic patients with paraplegia or quadriplegia.

Functional Incontinence

Functional incontinence refers to urine loss caused by factors such as restricted mobility or cognitive impairment that interfere with the functional ability to use a toilet.

Evaluation of Incontinence

Evaluation of urinary incontinence requires documenting the incontinence, its patterns, triggers, and underlying causes, and determining the need for further diagnostic tests. The basic evaluation should include a history and physical examination, urinalysis, and an estimation of postvoid residual volume. The examiner should ask about the character, duration, and magnitude of incontinence, precipitating factors such as hand washing or bouncing (jumping), recurrent urinary tract infections, and about bladder pain, hematuria, constipation, fecal incontinence, or impotence. The initial evaluation may be expedited if the patient completes a 3-day voiding diary, recording all urinations, voided volumes, fluid intakes, and activity during incontinent episodes. Some patients may be incontinent because of excessive fluid intake, infrequent voiding, or other easily treated factors.

The examiner should perform a neurologic history and physical to assess for stroke, MS, Parkinson disease (PD), Alzheimer disease (AD), and other potential underlying conditions. It is important to test mobility, cognition, and dexterity related to toileting skills. Peripheral edema may help explain nocturia in an elderly patient with a relatively normal bladder (Williams & Gaylord, 1990). An abdominal examination can disclose underlying masses or abdominal tenderness. A rectal examination should assess for perineal sensation, sphincter tone, fecal impaction, and, in men, the size and contour of the prostate gland. In men, a genital examination should also be performed, focusing on any abnormalities of the foreskin, penis, scrotum, or testes. In women, a pelvic exam should address the condition of the perineal skin, presence of genital or vaginal lesions, and presence of pelvic organ prolapse including cystocele, rectocele, enterocele, and uterine or vaginal cuff prolapse. In addition, in women the position and mobility of the urethra at rest and during increased abdominal pressure (as with cough or strain) should be noted. Urine loss with Valsalva maneuver can best be tested in patients who arrive at initial examination with a full bladder. Stress incontinence is a likely diagnosis if instantaneous leakage occurs with cough. Detrusor instability is more likely if leakage is delayed or persists after cough (Kadar, 1988).

A urinalysis or urine culture can rule out any urinary tract infection. Residual urine volume can be determined by performing catheterization or bladder ultrasound within minutes after the patient voids. Postvoid bladder residuals of <100 mL are considered adequate; values of >100 mL are abnormal. AHCPR (Agency for Health Care Policy Research) guidelines (1992) recommend noninvasive (behavioral or pharmacologic) therapy for patients who have urge incontinence with normal urinalysis and postvoid residual volume, and patients who lose urine during physical stress despite no prior anti-incontinence surgeries, normal voiding habits, void residual volumes, and normal neurologic states. Patients with a known neurologic lesion should undergo a urodynamic evaluation (Fig. 32-1).

Patients who show hematuria need follow-up cystoscopy and excretory urography. Those who have

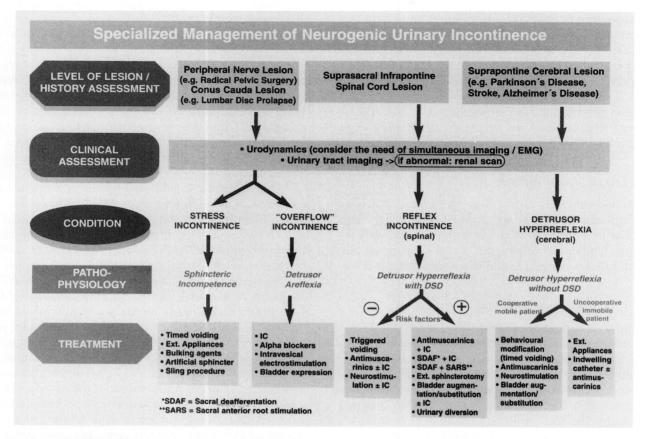

FIGURE 32-1. Algorithm demonstrating the management of neurogenic urinary incontinence. (From Abrams P, Khoury S, Wein A: Incontinence. Plymouth, UK: Health Publication Ltd., 1999.)

painful or irritative voiding symptoms may also be candidates for cystoscopy. Patients who have more complex presentation may be candidates for specialized testing, including urodynamics, voiding cystourethrography, or cystoscopy.

Treatment of Urinary Incontinence

Conservative Management

The two major categories of conservative management of urinary incontinence are behavioral and pharmacologic. Behavioral techniques include bladder training (retraining), habit training (timed voiding), prompted voiding, and pelvic floor muscle–strengthening exercises. Behavioral management can be combined with biofeedback, vaginal cones, and electrical stimulation techniques. Conservative management should be considered prior to any surgery.

Bladder training, also called bladder retraining, relies on education, scheduled voiding, and reinforcement. A bladder retraining program requires the patient to inhibit or delay voiding and to urinate according to a timetable rather than whenever he or she feels the urge to void. Bladder retraining also involves modulating

fluid intake in such a manner that the bladder is subjected to progressively larger volumes and longer intervals between voids. Up to 12% of women who have bladder retraining achieve continence, and 75% decrease their incontinent episodes by at least half (Fantl et al., 1991).

Habit training is scheduled toileting on a planned basis. The patient is told to void at regular intervals chosen to match the patient's natural voiding schedule. This differs from bladder retraining in that there is no effort to resist or delay voiding.

Prompted voiding is effective in patients who are cognitively impaired. Prompted voiding involves regular monitoring to assess dryness and prompting the patient to try to toilet at a predetermined interval.

Pelvic muscle exercises, also known as Kegel exercises, improve the strength of the pelvic floor muscles (periurethral and paravaginal muscles) and help patients with stress incontinence. Patients with urge incontinence also remain dry, because contracting the pelvic floor inhibits unstable detrusor contraction (Nygaard & Kreder, 1996). Pelvic floor muscle exercises must be performed consistently; at least 6 to 8 weeks of consistent exercising are necessary before improvement occurs.

Vaginal cones help patients to perform pelvic floor muscle–strengthening exercises. The sustained contraction required to retain the cone increases the muscle strength. The cones come in various sizes and women start with a cone that is relatively easy to retain and gradually increase the weight as they gain greater strength.

Biofeedback is the use of mechanical or electrical means to feed information back to the patient about bladder activity by auditory or visual means.

The musculature of the pelvic floor and viscera can be stimulated by an anal or vaginal electrode and may help patients who cannot localize or contract their pelvic floor muscles using behavioral techniques, biofeedback, or vaginal cones. The S3 nerve root can be directly simulated by a percutaneous approach, behind the medial malleolus (as part of the posterior tibial nerve) (Govier et al., 2001), or in the sacrum (Siegel et al., 2000).

Pharmacologic Treatment

Urge Incontinence. Anticholinergic agents are a mainstay in treating urge continence. The well-known anticholinergic agent atropine, available in a transdermal form, may be effective. Hyoscyamine is a belladonna alkaloid with anticholinergic effects, with associated adverse effects of tachycardia, drowsiness, constipation, dry mouth, and blurry vision. Oxybutynin has been available for years, has anticholinergic and direct smooth muscle relaxant properties, and is superior to placebo in reducing the frequency of incontinent episodes (Moore et al., 1990). The usual dose of oxybutynin is 5 mg orally three times a day. Adverse effects include dry mouth, dry skin, blurry vision, mental status changes, nausea, and constipation (Tapp et al., 1990). A newer, controlled-release, long-acting form of oxybutynin chloride produces less dry mouth and fosters higher compliance rates than the intermediate-release preparation (Anderson et al., 1999; Versi et al., 2000).

The anticholinergic agent tolterodine acts more selectively on bladder muscle than on salivary glands (Nilvebrant, 2000) and is available in an extended-release form that produces less dry mouth than the immediate-release form. Compared with placebo, both preparations increase the mean voided volume per micturition and reduce the number of incontinent episodes per week, frequency of urination per day, and number of incontinence pads used per day.

Tricyclic agents possess anticholinergic properties and may be helpful in treating urinary incontinence. Imipramine is especially useful for nocturnal incontinence. These agents can be cautiously combined with anticholinergics such as extended-release oxybutynin (Ditropan) or extended-release tolterodine (Detrol LA). Tricyclic side effects include fatigue, dry mouth, dizziness, and blurred vision (Castleden et al., 1986; Lose et al., 1989).

Detrusor instability has been treated with calcium channel blockers, nonsteroidal anti-inflammatory agents, and beta-adrenergic agonists, but efficacy data are limited and these drugs are not used as first-line therapy.

In summary, pharmacologic therapy, at least in short-term trials, seems to benefit patients with detrusor instability. The therapeutic efficacy of these agents has in the past been limited because of the side effects, particularly dry mouth.

Surgical Treatment

Urge Incontinence. Surgical treatments for urge incontinence resulting from detrusor instability or detrusor hyperreflexia are similar in men and women. These include InterStim therapy, bladder autoaugmentation, and augmentation enterocystoplasty. InterStim therapy uses continuous electrical stimulation of the S3 afferent nerve root. The InterStim procedure is performed in two stages. A test stimulation is performed by placing a percutaneous wire near the S3 nerve root. Efficacy of electrical stimulation is determined by comparing pre- and post-stimulation voiding diaries. A successful test stimulation supports implantation of a permanent device, which can then be programmed for maximal effect. The InterStim battery usually must be replaced surgically every 5 to 10 years (Siegel et al., 2000).

Bladder autoaugmentation and augmentation enterocystoplasty procedures are usually limited to patients with incapacitating urinary incontinence who are unresponsive to less invasive treatment. Bladder autoaugmentation involves removal of the detrusor muscle overlying the anterior bladder wall and bladder dome. This preserves the bladder mucosa, creates an iatrogenic diverticulum, and generally lowers bladder storage pressures. The term autoaugmentation indicates that no tissue outside the bladder's own is used (Cartwright & Snow, 1989). Augmentation enterocystoplasty uses a segment of bowel (stomach, ileum, colon) to expand the bladder. The bladder is incised in a longitudinal or sagittal direction and a detubularized section of bowel is incorporated into this incision. Success rates with augmentation enterocystoplasty are high, but complications may include bowel or bladder leaks, excessive mucous production, electrolyte abnormalities, and potential increased chance of malignancy (Smith et al., 1977).

Stress Incontinence. In women, most surgery for urinary stress incontinence aims to treat urethral hypermobility or intrinsic sphincter deficiency. Urethral hypermobility procedures include retropubic and vaginal urethropexies such as the modified Marshall-Marchetti-Kranz (Marshall et al., 1949), Burch

(1961), Stamey (1980), and Pereyra-Raz (Raz, 1981), procedures. Intrinsic sphincter deficiency in women is often a result of surgery for incontinence or radiation therapy and is treated with periurethral collagen injection, artificial urinary sphincter, or sling cystourethropexy. In men, intrinsic sphincter deficiency is often a complication of prostate surgery and can be treated with periurethral injection therapy, artificial urinary sphincter, or a urethral sling procedure.

ERECTILE DYSFUNCTION

Background

Erectile dysfunction (ED) is a common sexual problem and may affect up to 30 million men in the United States (Benet & Melman, 1995). It is defined as the inability to achieve and maintain an erection sufficient to permit sexual intercourse (National Institutes of Health, 1993). Many patients are reluctant to seek treatment or discuss ED because of misconceptions about its etiology and potential treatment, or embarrassment about discussing the condition.

Risk Factors

Aging increases the likelihood of ED, but ED is not an inevitable consequence of aging. ED affects approximately one half the population of diabetic men (Kolodny, et al., 1974a; McCulloch et al., 1980), one third of men with pelvic fracture, 75% of dialysis-dependent men (Korenman, 1998), 40% of men who have had a radical prostatectomy (Quinlan et al., 1991), and 78% of men with MS (Rodriguez et al., 1994). ED may also be due to atherosclerosis, and men with a penile brachial index of <0.65 have a greater risk of myocardial infarction or cerebrovascular accidents than men with a higher index (see Diagnostic Studies section below; Morley et al., 1988). Many men with spinal cord injury have reflex erections only, and approximately 50% have no erections (Aloni et al., 1992). Other risk factors for ED are tobacco, alcohol, and illicit drug use; endocrine abnormalities (such as hyperthyroidism, hypothyroidism, hyperprolactinemia, and hypogonadotropic gonadism); and medication use (Table 32-1) (Kolodny, et al., 1974b; Van Thiel et al., 1983; Johnson & Jarrow, 1992; Mannino et al., 1994; Morgantaler, 1999).

TABLE 32-1. Medications Affecting Sexual Function

Sympatholytics	
Aldomet	ED, ejaculatory dysfunction, and decreased libido
Clonidine	ED, decreased libido
Reserpine	ED and ejaculatory dysfunction
Alpha-adrenergic blockers	
Phentolamine, phenoxybenzamine	Absent seminal emission
Prazocin	ED
Beta-adrenergic blockers	
Propranolol	ED
Antipsychotics	
Thioridazine	Decreased seminal emission, ED, priapism
Chlorpromazine	Ejaculatory dysfunction, priapism
Mesoridazine	Ejaculatory dysfunction
Antidepressants	
Tofranil, amitriptyline	Decreased libido, ED, and ejaculatory dysfunction
Nortriptyline	Ejaculatory dysfunction
Serotonin reuptake inhibitors	Decreased libido, ED
Lithium carbonate	ED
Minor tranquilizers	
Diazepam, chlordiazepoxide, oxazepam	Decreased libido
Miscellaneous agents	
Anticholinergics	ED
Cimetidine	Decreased libido, ED
Colofibiate	Decreased libido, ED
Digoxin	ED

ED, erectile dyfunction.

Anatomy and Physiology of Erection

The penis consists of three components—the paired corpus cavernosum and the corpus spongiosum. Each corpus cavernosum is surrounded by a tough layer of tissue called the tunica albuginea. The corpus cavernosa are filled with spongy tissue, which is made up of vascular space supported by smooth muscle. Arterial inflow is provided by the cavernosum arteries and venous outflow via veins that are just below the tunica albuginea. The penis is innervated by both autonomic and somatic nerves that enter the corpus cavernosa, corpus spongiosum, and glans penis; these veins regulate blood flow during erection and detumescence. Erection occurs as a result of increased arterial blood flow and decreased venous drainage (Figs. 32-2 and 32-3). A number of neurotransmitters have been identified in the physiologic process of tumescence; nitric oxide has been identified as the most likely principal neurotransmitter that mediates penile erection (Fig. 32-4) (Seanz de Tajada et al., 1989; Ignarro et al., 1990). The sacral spinal cord (S2, 3, and 4) is one of the main sites of neural integration of bladder and anal sphincter and sexual function. In addition, cerebral and psychological factors are critical.

Diagnosis of Erectile Dysfunction (ED)

History

It is important to differentiate between true ED and other sexual problems, such as premature ejaculation or diminished libido. In cases of ED, the examiner must distinguish between psychogenic and organic etiologies and consider risk factors such as tobacco, alcohol, and illicit drug use; diabetes; vascular disease; hypertension; cancer or chemotherapy; infection; spinal cord lesions; a variety of neurologic conditions (see section preceding); and penile curvature or pain. Presentations can be varied and complex.

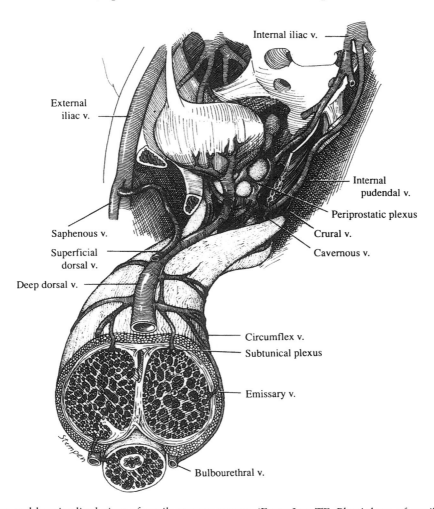

FIGURE 32-2. Transverse and longitudinal view of penile venous return. (From Lue TF: Physiology of penile erection and pathophysiology of erectile dysfunction and priapism, in Walsh PC, Retik AB, Vaughan ED Jr, Wein AJ [eds]: Campbell's Urology. Philadelphia: Saunders, 1998, ed 7, Vol. 2. Used with permission.)

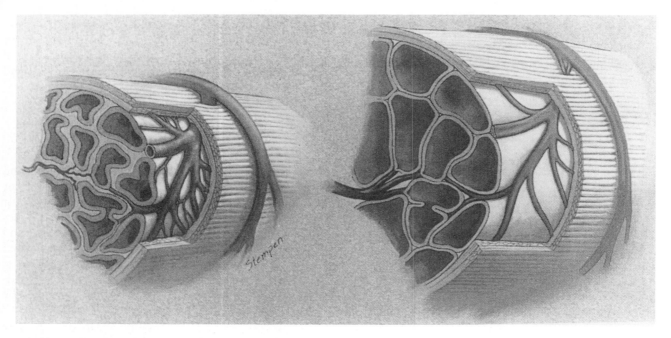

FIGURE 32-3. The mechanism of penile erection. In the flaccid state (*left*), the arteries, arterioles, and sinusoids are contracted. The intersinusoidal and subtunical venular plexuses are wide open, with free flow to the emissary veins. In the erect state (*right*), the muscles of the sinusoidal wall and the arterioles relax, allowing maximal flow to the compliant sinusoidal spaces. Most of the venules are compressed between the expanding sinusoids. Even the larger intermediary venules are sandwiched and flattened by distended sinusoids and the noncompliant tunica albuginea. This process effectively reduces the venous capacity to a minimum. (From Lue TF, Akkus E, Kour NW: Physiology of erectile function and dysfunction. Campbell's Urology Update 12, 1994. Used with permission.)

Physical Examination

After a general physical examination, the examiner should check the penis for abnormal nodules or curvature that indicate Peyronie disease, the testes and prostate (size and consistency) for signs of cancer, and the peripheral pulses for signs of systemic vascular disease. A neurologic exam includes assessment of anal tone, anal wink (puckering of the anal skin to light stroke), and the bulbocavernosus reflex (contraction of the anal sphincter with light pinching of the glans penis).

Diagnostic Studies

Several simple tests can aid the diagnosis of erectile dysfunction. The penile brachial index is a screening test for penile arterial disease that compares penile arterial pressure with systemic arterial pressure. An index of <0.65 is an indicator of vascular disease. Monitoring of nocturnal erections can help distinguish between psychogenic and organic erectile dysfunction. Most men have between three and eight erections each night, and the report of even one adequate nocturnal erection suggests that there are not significant vascular abnormalities (Karacan, 1970). Specialized testing is generally done only after referral to a urologist and may include a penile ultrasonography, cavernosometry, or arteriography. Quantitative study of the sacral reflex can use external stimulation of the dorsal nerve of the penis and recording by a needle electrode in the striated muscle of the anal sphincter or bulbocavernosus muscle. Prolongation of sacral reflex latency correlates with urinary or sexual problems in peripheral neuropathy cases, but is generally normal in patients with CNS disease and psychogenic impotence (Amarenco et al., 1986; Fabra & Porst, 1999).

Treatment

The treatment of ED includes the use of devices, oral or intraurethral agents, intracavernosal agents, or surgery.

Devices

A vacuum constriction device is composed of a plastic cylinder that is placed over the penis and connected to a pump, which creates a vacuum around the penis, thereby drawing blood into the penis and creating rigidity. A constricting band is then placed around the base of the penis to maintain this erection. The device works

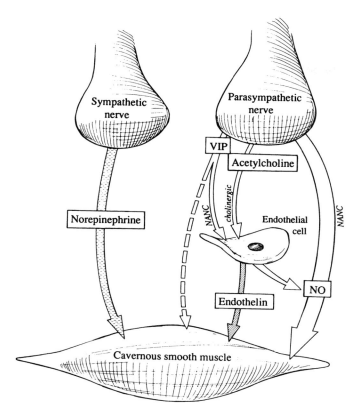

FIGURE 32-4. The interaction among cholinergic, adrenergic, nonadrenergic, and noncholinergic (NANC) influences and their contribution to penile smooth muscle contraction and relaxation (*open arrows*, facilitation of smooth muscle relaxation; *patterned arrows*, smooth muscle contraction; *broken arrow*, vasoactive intestinal polypeptide, controversial effect. NO, nitric oxide. (From Lue TF: Physiology of penile erection and pathophysiology of erectile dysfunction and priapism, in Walsh PC, Retik AB, Vaughan ED Jr, Wein AJ (eds): Campbell's Urology. Philadelphia: Saunders, 1998, ed 7, Vol. 2. Used with permission.)

reasonably well; however, some patients object to either the psychological aspect of using a mechanical device or discomfort from the constricting band.

Oral and Intraurethral Agents

Sildenafil (Viagra). Sildenafil was introduced in 1998 and has changed the approach to ED; now, primary care physicians often treat patients with ED. Sildenafil inhibits phosphodiesterase type 5, the main phosphodiesterase found in the corpus cavernosa (Jeremy et al., 1997; Ballard et al., 1998). Sildenafil has a success rate of approximately 50% in clinical practice (Morgentaler, 1999). Adverse effects include headache, nasal congestion, flushing, dyspepsia, and blue visual tint. Sildenafil should not be used by patients who take nitrates due to the possibility of developing profound hypotension.

Relative contraindications to sildenafil use are medications that prolong its half-life, including erythromycin, cimetidine, and ketoconazole (Cheitlin et al., 1999).

Phentolamine. Oral phentolamine improves erectile function in up to 45% of men with mild to moderate ED but has not been approved by the Food and Drug Administration (FDA) (Goldstein et al., 2001). Potential adverse effects are headache, facial flushing, and nasal congestion.

Apomorphine. Apomorphine has dopaminergic effects and a sublingual formulation. Clinical trials showed that 43% of patients in the treated group were able to engage in sexual intercourse, compared with 27% in the placebo group (Heaton et al., 1995). Adverse effects include nausea, and this preparation has not been approved by the FDA.

Yohimbine. Yohimbine is an alpha-adrenergic antagonist that is more effective than placebo for all types of ED; however, its effects were greatest in patients with nonorganic ED (Lue, 2000).

Transurethral Therapy

Prostaglandin is available in a transurethral form and in a large multicenter trial was demonstrated to be effective in 43% of men with ED. Adverse effects include penile pain and urethral burning (Padma-Nathan et al., 1997).

Intracavernosal Therapy

Papavarine hydrochloride. Papavarine is a phosphodiesterase inhibitor that, when injected into the corpus cavernosum in doses of 15–60 mg, is effective in up to 80% of men with either psychogenic or neurogenic ED. Its major potential adverse effect is priapism (Jeremy et al., 1997).

Prostaglandin. Prostaglandin E_1 is available as an injectable agent. It has been shown to be effective in approximately 70% of men, with a lower incidence of priapism than papavarine. The most common adverse effect is painful erection (Lee et al., 1991).

Combination Therapy. Phentolamine and vasoactive intestinal peptide are agents that are not effective when injected intracavernously. However, when these are combined with either papavarine or prostaglandin, success rates are significantly improved. The most effective combination appears to be a three-drug mixture containing papavarine, phentolamine, and alprostadil (prostaglandin). The response rate of this solution is approximately 90% (Bennett et al., 1991).

Testosterone

Although historically touted as enhancing sexual function, testosterone should be used only in men in whom erectile dysfunction is associated with hypogonadism. Testosterone is available as a topical preparation, deep intramuscular injection, and oral preparation.

Surgical Therapy

Vascular Procedures. Arterial bypass procedures and venous ligation procedures are performed at a few centers around the country, usually for selected patients with a history of traumatic injury.

Penile Prosthesis. Prosthetic surgery has been available for many years. The prosthesis may be semirigid with minimal chance of mechanical malfunction; a more sophisticated device uses fluid-filled cylinders that are inflated via a pump mechanism located in the scrotum. Penile prostheses are reliable and relatively easy to use and yield high satisfaction ratings by patients and partners (Jarow et al., 1996). Complications include infection and device malfunction.

Priapism

Rarely, rather than an inability to achieve erection, there is priapism, a pathologic disorder characterized by spontaneous, prolonged, involuntary erection (Hashmat & Das, 1993) and associated with certain drugs (alpha-2 agonists, androgens, butyrophenones, chlorpromazine, heparin, levodopa, local anesthetics, marijuana, nefazodone, phenothiazines, postganglionic-blocking sympatholytic drugs, trazodone, warfarin), leukemia, pudendal trauma, sickle cell anemia, and other conditions in which relative venous outflow from the penis is reduced. This includes treatment of impotence with intracavernous injections of papaverine, phentolamine, and prostaglandin. Surgical intervention may be required, and impotence may result in patients who were not impotent before.

FECAL INCONTINENCE

Overview

Fecal incontinence is often a major problem for long-term care of patients with Alzheimer disease, and is a deciding factor in placing stroke, head trauma, brain tumor, and multiple sclerosis patients in extended care facilities. Most fecal incontinence cases are chronic unless they follow surgery or trauma (Table 32-2). This costly problem is associated with urinary incontinence, reviewed in a previous section, and with decreased mobility, cognition, dexterity, and self-awareness of impairment. In the section following we summarize current medical, surgical, pharmacologic, and behavioral treatments of fecal incontinence.

Table 32-2. Drugs Causing Fecal Incontinence and Their Mechanism of Action

Drug	Possible mechanism of action
Oxybutynin	Anticholinergic/antispasmodic
Tolterodine tartrate	Muscarinic receptor antagonist
Dantrolene sodium Baclofen Cyclobenzaprine	Centrally acting muscle relaxant
Laxatives Caffeine products	Diarrhea
Antidepressants Amitriptyline Imipramine	Anticholinergic Sensation altering Fecal retention with overflow

Prevalence and Impact on Life

Fecal incontinence is a common, distressing, and embarrassing personal problem that affects people of all ages, but is more prevalent in elderly and institutionalized patients (Rao, 2002). Incontinence affects approximately 1% of younger patients, 4% of the elderly, 25% to 35% of institutionalized patients (Barrett, 1992), and 10% to 25% of hospitalized geriatric patients (Szurszewski et al., 1989), depending on how incontinence is defined and studied (Perry et al., 2002). Although 18% of patients attending a primary care clinic reported incontinence at least once a week, only one third ever discussed the problem with their physician (Johansson & Lafferty, 1996), making this a silent affliction. Fecal incontinence affects 26% of patients in a urogynecology clinic setting (Khullar et al., 1998), is often associated with urinary incontinence in nursing home patients (Nelson et al., 1998; Chiang et al., 2000), and is the second leading cause for placement in nursing homes in the United States (Szurszewski et al., 1989). The problem is compounded by other factors such as cognitive impairment (as in Alzheimer disease), lack of awareness, poor nutrition, paucity of toileting facilities, and lack of assistance for scheduled toileting.

The average annual cost per outpatient, including clinical evaluation, has been estimated at $17,166 (Mellgan et al., 1999). Long-term facility annual cost of caring for a patient with both mixed urinary and fecal incontinence has been estimated at $9,711 (Borrie & Davidson, 1992). Additional costs include emotional distress and reduced quality of life and productivity. The related social stigma often delays presentation and treatment of fecal incontinence for several years.

Pathophysiology and Etiology

Congenital malformations such as anal atresia, anal stenosis, and anorectal malformations can predispose to fecal incontinence in children. Spinal cord abnormalities, including myelomeningocele, spina bifida, and other spinal tumors may also lead to fecal incontinence. Up to one half of patients with Hirschsprung disease have fecal incontinence.

Lesions of the peripheral nerves resulting from alcohol abuse, perineal trauma during childbirth, cauda equina lesions, and diabetic neurotrophy (Schiller et al., 1982; Caruana et al., 1991; Sun et al., 1992) may all cause fecal incontinence. Surgical reconstruction procedures such as ileoanal (Parks & Nicholls, 1978) or coloanal anastomosis (Berger et al., 1992) cause incontinence in up to 40% of patients (Levitt et al., 1994). Muscle disorders such as muscular dystrophy, myasthenia gravis, and a variety of myopathies can impair external and internal anal sphincter function.

In women, the most important predisposing factor for fecal incontinence is obstetric trauma (Sultan et al., 1993; Kamm, 1994; Sultan et al.,1994). Important risk factors include forceps delivery, prolonged second stage of labor, and abnormal fetal presentations (Hill et al., 1994; Engel et al., 1995; Gee & Durdey, 1995). Iatrogenic factors include lateral sphincterotomy (Snooks et al., 1984, 1986; Speakman et al., 1991) and hemorrhoidectomy (Abbsakoor et al., 1998). Incontinence can also be due to internal sphincter degeneration (Vaizey et al., 1997) or to complications of radiation therapy to the pelvic floor (Varma et al., 1986; Rao et al., 2000).

Neurologic disorders may cause incontinence by interfering with perception, motor function, or both, as in multiple sclerosis, strokes, and brain tumors (Caruana et al., 1991, Glickman & Kamm, 1996; Krogh et al., 1997; Brittain et al., 1998). Up to 20% of patients with multiple sclerosis have fecal incontinence (Caruana et al., 1991). In elderly adults and in children with functional fecal incontinence, seepage of liquid stools occurs in the presence of fecal impaction and is associated with impaired rectal sensation and incoordinated or dyssynergic defecation (Read et al., 1985; Rao, et al., 1998a; Rao, et al., 1999b). Normal pressure hydrocephalus causes urinary and fecal incontinence in conjunction with dementia and gait disturbances (see Chapter 29). Whipple disease is a rare infectious condition associated with periodic acid-Schiff–positive (PAS-positive) inclusions in the bowel, which may cause incontinence of liquid stool and dementia due to CNS infection, and which can be successfully treated with antibiotics (Durand et al., 1997).

Clinical Evaluation of Fecal Incontinence

Key steps in the clinical evaluation are to establish a rapport with the patient and to obtain detailed information on the duration and nature of symptoms. Is the patient incontinent of flatus or liquid or solid stool? Can the patient differentiate between formed or unformed stool or gas? What are the effects on quality of life? The history should address obstetric background and coexisting conditions such as diabetes mellitus, spinal cord injury and other neurologic disorders, urinary incontinence, and drug history.

Several clinical systems have been proposed for grading fecal incontinence. The St. Mark's group validated a simple scale (Vaizey et al., 1999) (Table 32-3) that addresses the nature of fecal discharge (solid, liquid, or flatus); effects on lifestyle (Never = 0, Always = 5); and need for pads, antidiarrheal medications, and ability to defer defecation (scores: No = 0, Yes = 2). The total score ranges from 0 (continent) to 24 (severe incontinence). Standard questionnaires may provide useful additional information on psychosocial issues (such as the SCL-90-R) and impact on the quality of life (such as the SF-36).

Few data address the psychosocial effects of fecal incontinence. What are the psychological and psychiatric ramifications of incontinence in an otherwise mentally intact adult? How often is incontinence associated with major psychiatric diseases (schizophrenia, mania, depression) and personality disturbances (e.g., malingering or somatoform disorder)? By what mechanisms do developmental disorders (such as mental retardation and autism) impair acquisition of toileting skills? How are problems in these areas evaluated and treated and by whom? What are optimal patterns of referral? What are the roles of the psychiatrist, psychologist, gastroenterologist (GE), doctor, and nurse in the treatment of these problems? These are all areas for continuing research.

Physical Examination

Because incontinence may be caused by a systemic or neurologic disorder, a detailed physical and neurologic examination is essential. Detailed perineal inspection should note presence of fecal matter or staining, dermatitis, scars, skin excoriation, or gaping anus.

Perianal sensation should be checked. The anocutaneous reflex examines the integrity of the connection between the sensory nerves and the skin, the intermediate neurons in the spinal cord segments S2, S3, and S4 and the motor innervation of the external anal sphincter. This is best assessed by gently stroking the perianal skin with a cotton bud in each of the perianal quadrants. The normal response consists of a brisk contraction of the external anal sphincter (the anal "wink"). Impaired or absent anocutaneous reflex suggests afferent or efferent neuronal injury (Rao, 2002).

A digital rectal examination should assess the resting sphincter tone, length of the anal canal, and the strength of the anal sphincter muscle and puborectalis.

TABLE 32-3. Clinical Grading System for Fecal Incontinence

	Never	Rarely	Sometimes	Weekly	Daily
Incontinence for solid stool	0	1	2	3	4
Incontinence for liquid stool	0	1	2	3	4
Incontinence for gas	0	1	2	3	4
Alteration in lifestyle	0	1	2	3	4

	No	Yes
Need to wear a pad or plug	0	2
Taking constipating medicines	0	2
Unable to defer defecation for 15 minutes	0	4

Never	No episodes in the past 4 weeks
Rarely	One episode in the past 4 weeks
Sometimes	More than one episode in the past 4 weeks but less than one episode a day
Weekly	One or more episodes a week but less than one episode a day
Daily	One or more episode a day

Add one score from each row.
  Minimum score = 0 = perfect continence
  Maximum score = 24 = totally incontinent

Total score = _____

Printed by permission. Vaizey CJ, Carapeti E, Cahill JA, Kamm MA: Prospective comparison of faecal incontinence grading system. Gut 44:77–80, 1999.

The accuracy and positive predictive value of this examination is influenced by the examiner's technique, finger size, and patient cooperation. Rectal examination can identify patients with fecal impaction and overflow, but additional studies are usually needed for accurately diagnosing sphincter dysfunction and therapy (Felt-Bersma et al., 1988; Hill et al., 1994).

Investigations

Many patients mistakenly report diarrhea in the presence of incontinence, and vice versa. Whenever there is coexisting diarrhea, the work-up should include stool studies for infection and luminal examination with a flexible sigmoidoscope or colonoscope. Metabolic tests may reveal thyroid dysfunction or diabetes, and breath tests may identify lactose or fructose intolerance or bacterial overgrowth that can cause diarrhea. Rarely, bile salt malabsorption due to cholecystectomy, ileectomy, or colectomy may present with diarrhea and incontinence. Several specific tests may help identify the underlying pathophysiology if a diarrheal source cannot be identified or other causes of incontinence are suspected (Wald, 1994; Diamant et al., 1999; Rao, et al., 1999a; Rao, 2002). The most useful test is anorectal manometry. Anal endosonography, a balloon expulsion test, and pudendal nerve terminal motor latency can also be useful (Rao & Sun, 1997; Diamant et al., 1999).

Anorectal manometry provides an objective assessment of anal sphincter pressure together with an assessment of rectal sensation, rectoanal reflexes, and rectal compliance. Resting anal sphincter pressure chiefly reflects internal anal sphincter function; voluntary squeeze anal pressure predominately represents external anal sphincter function. Patients with fecal incontinence have low resting and low squeeze sphincter pressures (Read et al., 1979; Felt-Bersma et al., 1988; Read et al., 1989). Impaired rectal sensation can cause fecal incontinence and can be tested by intermittent balloon distention with air or water (Caruana et al., 1991; Sun et al., 1992; Rao & Patel, 1997).

Sampling of rectal contents by the anal mucosa may help to maintain continence (Goligher & Huges, 1951; Duthie & Gaines, 1960; Duthie & Bennett, 1963; Miller et al., 1988). This ability may be assessed using electrical (Rogers, 1992) or thermal (Miller et al., 1987; Rogers, 1992) stimuli, although the role of thermal sensitivity is unclear (Rogers, 1992). A technical review recommended anorectal manometry for evaluating patients with incontinence, because it defines the functional weakness of one or both sphincters and facilitates assessment of patients for biofeedback training (Diamant et al., 1999). The American Motility Society has developed and published standards for manometry testing (Rao et al., 2002).

Anal Endosonography

Anal endosonography is the simplest and most widely available technique for defining structural defects of the anal sphincter and should be considered in all patients with suspected fecal incontinence. It is often performed by placing a 7-MHz rotating transducer into the anorectum, and provides detailed information regarding the thickness and structural integrity of external and internal anal sphincter muscles.

Anal endosonography showed occult sphincter injury in 35% of primipara women after vaginal delivery, and most injuries were not detected clinically (Sultan et al., 1993). Recent studies showed a high agreement between electromyographic (EMG) mapping and anal endosonography in identifying sphincter defects (Tjandra et al., 1993; Enck et al., 1996). Although endosonography is operator-dependent and requires training and experience (Diamant et al., 1999), it is less expensive and less painful than EMG needle insertion, and provides better information on anal sphincter muscle morphology. In the future, newer techniques such as MRI may provide superior imaging with better spatial resolution (Schafer et al., 1994; Bartram, 2001); an endo-anal coil may improve this resolution (DeSouza et al., 1996).

Defecography

Defecography aims to identify patients with suspected rectal prolapse, poor rectal evacuation, or mega rectum. It is usually performed by placing 150 mL of barium-like contrast material into the rectum and asking the subject to squeeze, cough, or expel the contrast material during simultaneous cine video fluoroscopy. However, the functional significance of these defects has been questioned (Muller-Lissner et al., 1998; Diamant et al., 1999).

Balloon Expulsion Test

An artificial stool-like device such as FECOM (Pelsang et al., 1999), or a balloon containing 50 mL water (Rao & Patel, 1997), may serve as a simple bedside test of a patient's ability to evacuate. This is particularly important in elderly patients with fecal seepage and in children with functional fecal incontinence.

Pudendal Nerve Terminal Motor Latency (PNTML)

Measurement of pudendal nerve latency can help distinguish between sphincter muscle injury and nerve injury. A disposable electrode (St. Mark's electrode; Dantec-Medtronics, Minneapolis, MN) is used to measure the latency time (Kiff & Swash, 1984). A prolonged nerve latency time (>2.2 ms) suggests pudendal neuropathy. Women who undergo vaginal delivery may have a prolonged nerve latency (Snooks et al., 1986; Laurberg et al., 1988; Donnelly et al., 1998; Olsen & Rao, 2001). Furthermore, women with obstetric injury

develop fecal incontinence associated with pudendal neuropathy and anal sphincter defects. Two recent reviews of eight uncontrolled studies (Olsen & Rao, 2001; Rothholtz & Wexner, 2001) suggested that patients with pudendal neuropathy have a worse surgical outcome than patients without neuropathy. Normal PNTML does not exclude pudendal neuropathy, because a few intact nerve fibers may generate a normal nerve latency time.

Clinical Utility of Tests for Fecal Incontinence

Physiological tests clearly improve the odds of identifying the underlying mechanisms of fecal incontinence. In a prospective study, history alone could detect an underlying cause of fecal incontinence in only 9 of 80 patients, but physiologic tests revealed an abnormality in 44 patients (55%) (Wexner & Jorge, 1994). In a large retrospective study of 302 patients with fecal incontinence, pathophysiologic abnormalities were identified only after performing anorectal manometry, EMG, and rectal sensory testing (Sun et al., 1992). In a prospective study, a single manometric abnormality was found in 20% of patients, whereas more than one abnormality was found in 80% of patients with fecal incontinence (Rao & Patel, 1997). Because tests alone cannot predict whether a patient is continent or incontinent, an abnormal test result must be interpreted along with the patient's symptoms and other complementary tests.

Management of Patients with Fecal Incontinence

The goal of treatment for patients with fecal incontinence is to restore continence and improve quality of life. Treatment includes providing supportive measures such as avoiding offending foods, ritualizing bowel habits, improving skin hygiene, and instituting lifestyle changes. Caffeine is an important stimulant that enhances gastrocolonic activity (Rao et al., 1998b). Hence, reducing caffeine consumption, particularly after meals, may help to lessen postprandial urgency and diarrhea and fecal incontinence.

Specific Treatments

Supportive therapy. Fecal incontinence is a mortality risk (Chassayre et al., 1999). Managing this problem in the elderly or institutionalized patients depends on having personnel who are experienced in the treatment of fecal incontinence, and includes measures such as timely recognition and immediate cleansing of soiled perianal skin (Gray & Burns, 1996; Leung & Rao, 2001), and changing of undergarments. Wiping the perianal skin with moist tissue paper (baby wipes) rather than with dry toilet paper, and applying barrier creams such as zinc oxide and calamine lotion (Calmoseptine) may prevent skin excoriation (Alvarez & Childs, 1991; Leung & Rao, 2001). Perianal fungal infections should be treated with topical antifungal agents. Stool deodorant (Periwash) can help disguise the smell of feces.

In institutionalized patients, scheduled toileting with a bedpan or bedside commode, dietary intervention, and cognitive training may mitigate fecal incontinence. Other supportive measures can include dietary modifications. Caffeine enhances the gastrocolonic response, colonic motility (Rao, et al., 1998b), and fluid secretion in the small intestine (Wald et al., 1976). Reducing caffeine consumption, particularly after meals, may lessen postprandial urgency and diarrhea. Brisk physical activity just after waking or after meals may precipitate fecal incontinence because these physiologic events are associated with enhanced colonic motility (Bassotti et al., 1995; Rao et al., 1999a; Rao et al., 2001). A food and symptom diary may identify specific dietary factors that cause diarrheal stools and incontinence, as in lactose or fructose malabsorption. Eliminating these food items may prove beneficial (Rao, 1997). Fiber supplements such as psyllium are often advocated in an attempt to increase stool bulk and reduce watery stools; however, there are few data to justify this approach.

Pharmacotherapy. Several drugs have been reported to improve fecal incontinence, but antidiarrheal agents such as loperamide hydrochloride (Imodium) or diphenoxylate/atropine sulfate (Lomotil) remain the mainstay of drug therapy. Placebo-controlled studies have shown that these drugs are effective (Sun & Donnelly, 1997). Cholestyramine, an ion exchange resin, reduces incontinence caused by bile salt malabsorption. A recent open-label trial showed that amitriptyline (20 mg) can be used to treat urinary or fecal incontinence in patients without structural defects or neuropathy (Santoro et al., 1997). Topical phenylephrine gel may increase anal sphincter tone through alpha-2 agonist effects, yet 10% phenylephrine gel did not improve overall symptoms of fecal incontinence in 36 patients (Carapeti et al., 2000).

Biofeedback therapy. Biofeedback therapy utilizes "operant conditioning" techniques for regulating disordered bowel function. The goals are to improve anal sphincter muscle strength and anorectal sensation, and coordination among abdominal, gluteal, and anal sphincter muscles during voluntary squeeze following rectal perception.

Each goal requires specific training techniques and usually relies on verbal feedback or visual feedback from a manometry probe or EMG device (Rao, 1998). When a patient squeezes the anal sphincter, the increase in activity viewable on a video monitor provides instant visual feedback on performance. Patients are taught to selectively squeeze their anal muscles without contracting intra-abdominal and other accessory muscles. The patient learns to perceive balloon distention at lower volumes but with the same intensity. These neuromuscular training techniques are used along with Kegel exercises to improve anal sphincter function. In uncontrolled studies, subjective improvement has been reported in 40% to 85% of patients (MacLeod et al., 1987; Enck, 1993; Glia et al., 1998; Rao, 1998). Objective improvement in anorectal function has been less commonly reported (Wald, 1981; Loening-Baucke, 1990; Miner et al., 1990; Sangwan et al., 1995; Rao et al., 1996). In a recent study of 100 patients, approximately two thirds improved with treatment and those with urge incontinence alone fared better than those with passive incontinence (55% vs. 23%) (Norton & Kamm, 1999). A few authors have argued that therapeutic efficacy of biofeedback training cannot be predicted on the basis of manometric results (Wald, 1981; Loening-Baucke, 1990; Miner et al., 1990).

However, one controlled prospective study showed significantly greater voluntary squeeze pressure, rectoanal coordination, rectal sensation, and capacity to retain saline infusion after 1 year of therapy (Rao et al., 1996). Recent studies provide confirmation and further details (Sangwan et al., 1995; Fynes et al., 1999). Biofeedback therapy is safe, relatively inexpensive, and may improve symptoms and quality of life in patients with fecal incontinence who have failed supportive measures, especially those who are elderly, have comorbid illnesses, pudendal neuropathy, or await reconstructive surgery. Severe fecal incontinence, pudendal neuropathy, and underlying neurologic problems are less amenable to biofeedback therapy (Loening-Baucke et al., 1988; Van Tets et al., 1996; Leroi et al., 1999).

Surgery. Sphincter repair is often effective in treating women with fecal incontinence after obstetric trauma (Parks & McPartlin, 1971). If an internal anal sphincter defect is identified, separate repair of the internal anal sphincter may be undertaken. Symptom improvement in the range of 70% to 80% has been reported (Browning & Motson, 1983; Parks & McPartlin, 1971). The long-term success of this approach is much lower and ranges between 20% and 58% (Rieger et al., 1997). In patients with severe structural damage of the anal sphincter, neosphincter construction has been performed using autologous skeletal muscle (Meehan et al., 1997; Olsen & Rao, 2001) or an artificial bowel sphincter (Baeten et al., 1995; Geerdes et al., 1996; Mander et al., 1997). Dynamic graciloplasty relies on observations that chronic stimulation can transform fast twitch (fatigable) skeletal muscle fibers into slow twitch (nonfatigable) fibers that can sustain tonic sphincter-like contraction. Continuous stimulation is maintained by an implanted pacemaker (Christiansen, 1998; Sielezneff et al., 1999). When the subject has to defecate or expel gas, a magnetically controlled external device temporarily switches off the pacemaker. Clinical improvement rates have ranged from 38% to 90% (Olsen & Rao, 2001). Another approach has been to implant an artificial bowel sphincter that consists of an inflatable cuffed device that is filled with fluid from a subcutaneous reservoir. The cuff is deflated to allow defecation (Lehur et al., 2000). At medium-term follow-up, 50% to 70% of patients have a functioning new sphincter (Vaizey et al., 1998; Lehur et al, 2000; Olsen & Rao, 2001). In one study, the total direct cost of dynamic graciloplasty was estimated to be $31,733, colostomy including stoma care was $71,576, and conventional treatment for fecal incontinence was $12,180 (Adang et al., 1998).

The technique of sacral nerve stimulation appears to be simple, with lower morbidity, and may be worth considering in the management of incontinence. In one study that assessed the short-term effects (Matzel et al., 1995), continence was restored in eight of nine patients. Improvement rates have ranged from 40% to 70% in long-term studies of patients with incontinence caused by spinal cord and obstetric injuries (Kenefick et al., 2002).

Treatment of Patients with Fecal Incontinence and Spinal Cord Injury

Patients with spinal cord injury may develop fecal incontinence due to a cerebral lesion or cauda equina lesions (Sun & Donnelly, 1990; MacDonagh et al., 1992; Sun et al., 1995). In the former group, the sacral neuronal reflex arc is intact and reflex defecation can be triggered by digital stimulation or suppositories. In patients with low spinal cord or cauda equina lesions, digital stimulation may be ineffective, because the defecation reflex is often impaired. Hence, management consists of antidiarrheal agents to prevent continuous soiling, followed by periodic administration of enemas or the use of laxatives (Caruana et al., 1991; Rao 2002). A cecostomy procedure with periodic antegrade enema may allow the patient to better control evacuation (Yang & Stiens, 2000). In some patients colostomy may be the best option (Stone et al., 1990).

CONCLUSION

Fecal and urinary incontinence and genitourinary dysfunction are costly health care problems that can be caused by lesions at several levels of the nervous system, in association with a variety of medical, neurologic, and psychiatric diagnoses. Key symptoms range from incontinence and impotence to sexual aberration. Neural substrates and treatments of these complex biological and psychosocial phenomena are active areas of multidisciplinary research and keen public interest.

■ KEY POINTS

☐ The clinical evaluation of urinary incontinence should include a general examination to detect possible neurologic abnormalities suggestive of stroke, multiple sclerosis, or Parkinson disease.

☐ Erectile dysfunction (ED) is a common problem estimated to affect up to 30 million men in the United States.

☐ In evaluating a male patient for ED it is important to differentiate between true ED and other forms of sexual dysfunction, such as premature ejaculation or diminished libido.

☐ Fecal incontinence is a fairly common symptom, particularly in older individuals, and can often be a deciding factor in placing patients with stroke, head trauma, brain tumor, or multiple sclerosis in care facilities.

☐ Key steps in the clinical evaluation of fecal incontinence are (1) establishing a rapport with the patient and (2) obtaining detailed information on the duration and nature of symptoms.

KEY READINGS

Urinary Incontinence

Abrams P, Blaivas JG, Stanton SL, et al: Standardization of terminology of lower urinary tract function. Neurourol Urodyn 7:403–427, 1988.

AHCPR (Agency for Health Care Policy and Research): Urinary incontinence in adults. Clinical practice guidelines. Washington, DC, 1992.

Burgio KL, Matthews KA, Engel BT: Prevalence, incidence and correlates of urinary incontinence in healthy, middle-aged women. J Urol 146:1255–1259, 1991.

Fantl JA, Wyman JF, McClish DK, et al: Efficacy of bladder training in older women with urinary incontinence. JAMA 265:609–613, 1991.

Govier FE, Litwiller S, Nitti V, et al: Percutaneous afferent neuromodulation: A novel treatment for the refractory overactive bladder. Results of a multicenter study. J Urol 165:1193–1198, 2001.

Erectile Dysfunction

Le Vay S: The Sexual Brain. Cambridge, MA: MIT Press, 1993.

Fecal Incontinence

Diamant NE, Kamm MA, Wald A, et al: AGA technical review on anorectal testing techniques. Gastroenterology 116:735–760, 1999.

Olsen AL, Rao SSC: Clinical neurophysiology and electrodiagnostic testing of the pelvic floor, Gastroenterol Clin North Am 30:33–54, 2001.

Rao SSC: Guidelines for fecal incontinence. Am J Gastroenterol (forthcoming, 2003).

Rao SSC: The technical aspects of biofeedback therapy for defecation. Gastroenterologist 6:96–103, 1998.

Rao SSC, Patel RS: How useful are manometric tests of anorectal function in the management of defecation disorders? Am J Gastroenterol 92:469–475, 1997.

Rothholtz NA, Wexner SD: Surgical treatment of constipation and fecal incontinence. Gastroenterol Clin North Am 30:131–166, 2001.

Sultan AH, Kamm MA, Hudson CN, et al: Anal-sphincter disruption during vaginal delivery. N Engl J Med 329:1905–1911, 1993.

REFERENCES

Abrams P, Blaivas JG, Stanton SL, et al: Standardization of terminology of lower urinary tract function. Neurourol Urodyn 7:403–427, 1988.

Abbsakoor F, Nelson M, Beynon J, et al: Anal endosonography in patients with anorectal symptoms after hemorrhoidectomy. Br J Surg 85:1522–1524, 1998.

Adang EMM, Engel GL, Rutten FFH, et al: Cost-effectiveness of dynamic graciloplasty in patients with fecal incontinence. Dis Colon Rectum 41:725–734, 1998.

AHCPR (Agency for Health Care Policy and Research): Urinary incontinence in adults. Clinical practice guidelines. Washington, DC, 1992.

Alvarez OM, Childs EJ: Pressure ulcers: Physical, supportive, and local aspects of management. Clin Podiatr Med Surg 8:869–890, 1991.

Aloni R, Heller L, Keren O, et al: Non-invasive treatment for erection dysfunction in the neurogenically disabled population. Sex Marital Ther 18:243–249, 1992.

Amarenco G, Ghnassia RT, Chabassol E, et al: Value of evoked sacral potentials in studying bladder sphincter disorders in peripheral neuropathies and central nervous system diseases. A study of 110 cases [in French]. Ann Med Interne (Paris) 137:331–337, 1986.

Anderson RU, Mobley D, Blank B, et al: Once daily controlled versus immediate release oxybutynin chloride for urge urinary incontinence. J Urol 161:1809–1812, 1999.

Anson JA, Kuhlman DT: Post-ictal Klüver-Bucy syndrome after temporal lobectomy. J Neurol Neurosurg Psychiatry 56:311–313, 1993.

Baeten CG, Geerdes BP, Adang EM, et al: Anal dynamic graciloplasty in the treatment of intractable fecal incontinence. New Engl J Med 332:1600–1605, 1995.

Ballard SA, Gingell CJ, Tang K, et al: Effects of sildenafil on the relaxation of human corpus cavernosum tissue in vitro and on the activities of cyclic nucleotide phosphodiesterase isozymes. J Urol 159:2164–2171, 1998.

Barak Y, Achiron A, Elizur A, et al: Sexual dysfunction in relapsing-remitting multiple sclerosis: Magnetic resonance imaging, clinical, and psychological correlates. J Psychiatr Neurosci 21:255–258, 1996.

Barrett JD: Colorectal disorders in elderly people. BMJ 305:764–766, 1992.

Bartram C: Radiological evaluation of anorectal disorders Gastroenterol Clin North Am 30:55–76, 2001.

Bassotti G, Germani U, Morelli A: Human colonic motility: Physiological aspects. Int J Colorectal Dis 10:173–180, 1995.

Benet AE, Melman A: The epidemiology of erectile dysfunction. Urol Clin North Am 22:699–709, 1995.

Bennett AH, Carpenter AJ, Barada JH: An improved vasoactive drug combination for a pharmacological erection program. J Urol 146:1564, 1991.

Berger A, Tiret E, Parc R, et al: Excision of the rectum with colonic J pouch-anal anastomosis for adenocarcinoma of the low and mid rectum. World J Surg 16:470–477, 1992

Borrie MJ, Davidson HA: Incontinence in institutions: Costs and contributing factors. Can Med Assoc J 147:322–328, 1992.

Brittain KR, Peet SM, Castleden CM: Stroke and incontinence. Stroke 1998 29:524–528, 1998.

Browning GGP, Motson RW: Results of Parks operation for faecal incontinence after anal sphincter injury. BMJ (Clin Res Ed) 286:1873–1975, 1983.

Burch JC: Urethrovaginal fixation to Cooper's ligament for correction of stress incontinence and prolapse in females. Am J Obstet Gynecol 81:281–286, 1961.

Burgio KL, Matthews KA, Engel BT: Prevalence, incidence and correlates of urinary incontinence in healthy, middle-aged women. J Urol 146:1255–1259, 1991.

Carapeti EA, Kamm MA, Phillips RK: Randomized controlled trial of topical phenylephrine in the treatment of faecal incontinence. Br J Surg 87:965–966, 2000.

Cartwright PC, Snow BW: Bladder autoaugmentation: Early clinical experience. J Urol 142:505–508, 1989.

Caruana BJ, Wald A, Hinds J, Eidelman B: Anorectal sensory and motor function in neurogenic fecal incontinence: Comparison between multiple sclerosis and diabetes mellitus. Gastroenterology 100:465–470, 1991.

Castleden CM, Duffin HM, Gulati RS: Double-blind study of imipramine and placebo for incontinence due to bladder instability. Age Ageing 15:299–303, 1986.

Chassayre P, Landrin I, Neveu C, et al: Fecal incontinence in the institutionalized elderly: Incidence, risk factors and prognosis. Am J Med 106:185–190, 1999.

Cheitlin MD, Hutter AM Jr., Brindis RG, et al: Use of sildenafil (Viagra) in patients with cardiovascular disease. ACC/AHA expert consensus document. J Am Coll Cardiol 33:273–282, 1999.

Chiang L, Ouslander J, Schnelle J, Reuben DB: Dually incontinent nursing home residents: Clinical characteristics and treatment differences. J Am Geriatr Soc 48:673–676, 2000.

Christiansen J: Modern surgical treatment of anal incontinence. Ann Med 30:273–277, 1998.

Clarke DJ, Brown NS: Klüver-Bucy syndrome and psychiatric illness. Br J Psychiatry 157:439–441, 1990.

Cummings JL, Duchen LW: Klüver-Bucy syndrome in Pick disease: Clinical and pathologic correlations. Neurology 31:1415–1422, 1981.

DeSouza NM, Puni R, Zbar A, et al: MR imaging of the anal sphincter in multiparous women using an endoanal coil: Correlation with in vitro anatomy and appearances in fecal incontinence. Am J Roentgenol 167:1465–1471, 1996.

Diamant NE, Kamm MA, Wald A, et al: AGA technical review on anorectal testing techniques. Gastroenterology 116:735–760, 1999.

Dickson DW, Horoupian DS, Thal LJ, et al: Klüver-Bucy syndrome and amyotrophic lateral sclerosis: A case report with biochemistry, morphometrics, and Golgi study. Neurology 36:1323–1329, 1986.

Donnelly V, Fynes M, Campbell D, et al: Obstetric events leading to anal sphincter damage. Obstet Gynecol 92:955–961, 1998.

Duncan S, Blacklaw J, Beastall GH, et al: Antiepileptic drug therapy and sexual function in men with epilepsy. Epilepsia 40:197–204, 1999.

Duncan S, Blacklaw J, Beastall GH, et al: Sexual function in women with epilepsy. Epilepsia 38:1074–1081, 1997.

Durand DV, Lecomte C, Cathebras P, et al: Whipple disease: Clinical review of 52 cases. The SNFMI Research Group on Whipple Disease. Société Nationale Francaise de Medecine Interne. Medicine 76:170–184, 1997.

Duthie HL, Bennett RC: The relation of sensation in the anal canal to the functional anal sphincter: A possible factor in anal continence. Gut 4:179–182, 1963.

Duthie HL, Gaines FW: Sensory nerve endings and sensation in the anal region of man. Br J Surg 47:585–595, 1960.

Enck P: Biofeedback training in disordered defecation: A critical review. Dig Dis Sci 38:1953–1960, 1993.

Enck P, von Giesen HJ, Schäfer A, et al: Comparison of anal sonography with conventional needle electromyography in the evaluation of anal sphincter defects. Am J Gastroenterol 91:2539–2543, 1996.

Engel AF, Kamm MA, Bartram CI, et al: Relationship of symptoms in fecal incontinence to specific sphincter abnormalities. Int J Colorectal Dis 10:152–155,1995.

Fabra M, Porst H: Bulbocavernosus-reflex latencies and pudendal nerve SSEP compared to penile vascular testing in 669 patients with erectile failure and other sexual dysfunction. Int J Impotence Res 11:167–175, 1999.

Fantl JA, Wyman JF, McClish DK, et al: Efficacy of bladder training in older women with urinary incontinence. JAMA 265:609–613, 1991.

Faught E, Falgout J, Nidiffer FD: Self-induced photosensitive absence seizures with ictal pleasure. Arch Neurol 43:408–410, 1986.

Fausto-Sterling, A: Sexing the Body: Gender Politics and the Construction of Sexuality. New York: Basic Books, 2000.

Felt-Bersma RJ, Klinkenberg-Knol EC, Meuwissen SGM: Investigation of anorectal function. Br J Surg 75:53–55, 1988.

Fenwick PB, Toone BK, Wheeler MJ, et al: Sexual behaviour in a centre for epilepsy. Acta Neurol Scand 71:428–435, 1985.

Ferrier D: The functions of the brain. London: Smith, Elder, 1876, pp. 262–263.

Fynes MM, Marshall K, Cassidy M, et al: A prospective, randomized study comparing the effect of augmented biofeedback with sensory biofeedback alone on fecal incontinence after obstetric trauma. Dis Col Rectum 42:753–761, 1999.

Gee AS, Durdey P: Urge incontinence of faeces is a marker of severe external anal sphincter dysfunction. Br J Surg 82:1179–1182, 1995.

Geerdes BP, Heineman E, Konsten J, et al: Dynamic graciloplasty: Complications and management. Dis Colon Rectum 39:912–917, 1996.

Glia A, Gylin M, Akerlund JE, et al: Biofeedback training in patients with fecal incontinence. Dis Colon Rectum 4:359–364, 1998.

Glickman S, Kamm MA: Bowel dysfunction in spinal-cord-injury patients. Lancet 347:1651–1653, 1996.

Goldstein C, Carson C, Rosen R, Islam A: Vasomax for the treatment of male erectile dysfunction. World J Urol 19:51–56, 2001.

Goligher JC, Huges ESR: Sensibility of the rectum and colon: Its role in the mechanism of anal continence. Lancet 1:543–547, 1951.

Govier FE, Litwiller S, Nitti V, et al: Percutaneous afferent neuromodulation: A novel treatment for the refractory overactive bladder. Results of a multicenter study. J Urol 165:1193–1198, 2001.

Gray M, Burns SM: Continence management. Crit Care Nursing Clin North Am 6:8:29–38, 1996.

Guedalia JSB, Zlotogorski Z, Goren A, et al: A reversible case of Klüver-Bucy syndrome in association with shigellosis. J Child Neurol 8:313–315, 1993.

Gustafson L, Brun A, Passant U: Frontal lobe degeneration of non-Alzheimer type dementia. Baillieres Clin Neurol 1:559–582, 1992.

Halaris A: Introduction: Sexual dysfunction: A neglected area of knowledge. CNS Spectrums 8:178.

Halperin JJ, Landis DM, Kleinman GM: Whipple disease of the nervous system. Neurology 32:612–617, 1982.

Hashmat AI, Das S: The Penis. Philadelphia: Lea and Febiger, 1993.

Heath RG: Pleasure and brain activity in man: Deep and surface EEGs during orgasm. J Nerv Ment Dis 154:3–18, 1972.

Heaton JP, Morales A, Adams MA, et al: Recovery of erectile function by the oral administration of apomorphine. Urology 45:200–206, 1995.

Hill J, Corson RJ, Brandon H, et al: History and examination in the assessment of patients with idiopathic fecal incontinence. Dis Colon Rectum 37:473–477, 1994.

Ignarro LJ, Bush PA, Buga GM, et al: Nitric oxide and cyclic GMP formation upon electrical field stimulation causes relaxation of corpus cavernosum smooth muscle. Biochem Biophys Res Commun 70:845–850, 1990.

Jacome DE, Risko MS: Absence status manifested by compulsive masturbation. Arch Neurol 40:523–524, 1983.

Jarow JP, Nana-Sinkham P, Sabbagh M, Eskew A: Outcome analysis of goal-directed therapy for impotence. J Urol 155:1609–1612, 1996.

Jensen P, Jensen SB, Sorensen PS, et al: Sexual dysfunction in male and female patients with epilepsy: A study of 86 outpatients. Arch Sex Behav 19:1–14, 1990.

Jeremy JY, Ballard SA, Naylor AM, et al: Effects of sildenafil: A type-5 cGMP phosphodiesterase inhibitor, and papaverine on cyclic GMP and cyclic AMP levels in the rabbit corpus cavernosum in vitro. Br J Urol 79:958–963, 1997.

Johansson JF, Lafferty J: Epidemiology of fecal incontinence: The silent affliction. Am J Gastroenterol 91:33–36, 1996.

Johnson AR, Jarow JP: Is routine endocrine testing of impotent men necessary? J Urol 147:1542–1543, 1992.

Kadar N: The value of bladder filling in the clinical detection of urine loss and selection of patients for urodynamic testing. Br J Obstet Gynaecol 95:698–704, 1988.

Kamm MA: Obstetric damage and fecal incontinence. Lancet 344:730–733, 1994.

Karacan I: Clinical value of nocturnal erection in the prognosis and diagnosis of impotence. Med Aspects Hum Sex 4:27–34, 1970.

Kenefick NJ, Vaizey CJ, Cohen RC, et al: Medium-term results of permanent sacral nerve stimulation for faecal incontinence. Br J Surg 89:896–901, 2002.

Khullar V, Damiano R, Toozs-Hobson P, et al: Prevalence of faecal incontinence among women with urinary incontinence. Br J Obstet 105:1211–1213, 1998.

Kiff ES, Swash M: Slowed conduction in the pudendal nerves in idiopathic (neurogenic) faecal incontinence. Br J Surg 71:614–616, 1984.

Klüver H, Bucy PC: Preliminary analysis of functions of the temporal lobes in monkeys. Arch Neurol Psychiatry 42:979–1000, 1939.

Kolodny RC, Kahn CB, Goldstein HH, et al: Sexual dysfunction in diabetic men. Diabetes 23:306–309, 1974a.

Kolodny RC, Masters WH, Kolodner RM, Toro G: Depression of plasma testosterone levels after chronic intensive marihuana use. N Engl J Med 290:872–974, 1974b.

Korenman SG: New insights into erectile dysfunction: A practical approach. Am J Med 105:135–144, 1998.

Kreder KJ, Austin JC: Treatment of stress urinary incontinence in women with urethral hypermobility and intrinsic sphincter deficiency. J Urol 156:1995–1998, 1996.

Krogh K, Nielsen J, Djurhuus JC, et al: Colorectal function in patients with spinal cord lesions. Dis Colon Rectum 40:1233–1239, 1997.

Lamberts, SWJ: The endocrinology of aging and the brain. Arch Neurol 59:1709–1711, 2002.

Laurberg S, Swash M, Henry MM: Delayed external sphincter repair for obstetric tear. Br J Surg 75:786–788, 1988.

Lee LM, Stevenson RW, Szasz G: Prostaglandin E1 versus phentolamine/papaverine for the treatment of erectile impotence: A double-blind comparison. J Urol 141:549–550, 1991.

Lehur PA, Roig JV, Duinslaeger M: Artificial anal sphincter: prospective clinical and manometric evaluation. Dis Colon Rectum 43:1100–1106, 2000.

Leroi AM, Dorival MP, Lecouturier M, et al: Pudendal neuropathy and severity of incontinence but not presence of anal sphincter defect may determine the response to biofeedback therapy in fecal incontinence: Long-term clinical results. Dis Colon Rectum 42:762–769, 1999.

Leung FW, Rao SSC. in Mezey MD, et al (eds): From Treatment of Fecal Incontinence in the Elderly in The Encyclopedia of Elder Care: The Comprehensive Resource on Geriatric and Social Care. New York: Springer, 2001, pp. 261–264.

LeVay S: A difference in hypothalamic structure between heterosexual and homosexual men. Science 253:1034–1037, 1991.

LeVay S: Queer Science: The Use and Abuse of Research into Homosexuality. Cambridge: MIT Press, 1996.

LeVay S: The Sexual Brain. Cambridge: MIT Press, 1993.

Levitt MD, Kamm MA, Van DS, Jr., et al: Ambulatory pouch and anal motility in patients with ileo-anal reservoirs. Int J Colorectal Dis 9:40–41, 1994.

Lilly R, Cummings JL, Benson F, et al: The human Klüver-Bucy syndrome. Neurology 33:1141–1145, 1983.

Livingston S, Berman W, Pauli LL: Masturbation simulating epilepsy. Clin Ped 14:232–234, 1975.

Loening-Baucke V: Efficacy of biofeedback training in improving faecal incontinence and anorectal physiologic function. Gut 31:1395–1402, 1990.

Loening-Baucke V, Desch L, Wolraich M: Biofeedback training for patients with myelomeningocele and fecal incontinence. Dev Med Child Neuro 30:781–790, 1988.

Lose G, Jorgensen L, Thunedborg P: Doxepin in the treatment of female detrusor overactivity: A randomized double-blind crossover study. J Urol 142:1024–1026, 1989.

Lue T: Drug therapy: Erectile dysfunction. N Engl J Med 342:1802–1813, 2000.

Lundberg PO, Brattberg A: Sexual dysfunction in selected neurologic disorders: Hypothalamopituitary disorders, epilepsy, myelopathies, polyneuropathies, and sacral nerve lesions. Sem Neurol 12:115–119, 1992.

MacDonagh R, Sun WM, Thomas DG, et al: Anorectal function in patients with complete supraconal spinal cord lesions. Gut 33:1532–1538, 1992.

MacLeod, JH: Management of anal incontinence by biofeedback. Gastroenterology 93:291–94, 1987.

Mander BJ, Wexner SD, Williams NS, et al: The electrically stimulated gracilis neoanal sphincter. Preliminary results of a multicentre trial. Br J Surg 84:89, 1997.

Mannino DM, Klevens RM, Flanders WD: Cigarette smoking: An independent risk factor for impotence? Am J Epidemiol 140:1003–1008, 1994.

Marshall VF, Marchetti AA, Krantz KE: The correction of stress incontinence by simple retropubic suspension. Surg Gynecol Obstet 88:509–518, 1949.

Masters WH, Johnson VE: Human Sexual Response. Boston: Little, Brown, 1966.

Masters WH, Johnson VE: Human Sexual Inadequacy. Boston: Little, Brown, 1970.

Matzel KE, Stadelmaier U, Hohenfellner M, et al: Electrical stimulation of sacral spinal nerves for treatment of faecal incontinence. Lancet 346:1124–1127, 1995.

McCulloch DK, Campbell IW, Wu FC, et al: The prevalence of diabetic impotence. Diabetologia 18:279–283, 1980.

Meehan JJ, Hardin WD Jr, Georgeson KE: Gluteus maximus augmentation for the treatment of fecal incontinence. J Pediatr Surg 32:1045–1047, 1997.

Mellgan A, Jensen LL, Zetterstrom JP et al: Long-term cost of fecal incontinence secondary to obstetric injuries. Dis Colon Rectum 42:857–865, 1999.

Miller R, Bartolo DC, Cervero F, et al: Anorectal sampling: A comparison of normal and incontinent patients. Br J Surg 75:44–47, 1988.

Miller R, Bartolo DC, Cervero F et al: Anorectal temperature sensation: A comparison of normal and incontinent patients. Br J Surg 74:511–515, 1987.

Miner PB, Donnelly TC, Read NW: Investigation of the mode of action of biofeedback in treatment of fecal incontinence. Dig Dis Sci 35:291–1298, 1990.

Moore KH, Hay DM, Imrie AE, et al: Oxybutynin hydrochloride (3 mg) in the treatment of women with idiopathic detrusor instability. Br J Urol 66:479–485, 1990.

Morgantaler A: Male impotence. Lancet 354:1713–1718, 1999.

Morley JE, Korenman SG, Kaiser FE, et al: Relationship of penile brachial pressure index to myocardial infarction and cerebrovascular accident in older men. Am J Med 84:445–448, 1988.

Muller-Lissner SA, Bartolo DC, Christiansen J. et al: Interobserver agreement in defecography: An international study. Gastroenterology 36:273–279, 1998.

Nakada T, Lee H, Kwee IL, Lerner AM: Epileptic Klüver-Bucy syndrome: Case report. J Clin Psychiat 45:87–88, 1984.

National Institutes of Health: NIH Consensus Conference. Impotence. JAMA 270:83–90, 1993.

National Kidney and Urologic Diseases Advisory Board. Barriers to rehabilitation of persons with end-stage renal disease or chronic urinary incontinence. Workshop summary report. Bethesda, MD, March 7–9, 1994.

Nelson R, Furner S, Jesudason V: Fecal incontinence in Wisconsin nursing homes: Prevalence and associations. Dis Colon Rectum 41:1226–1229, 1998.

Newmark ME, Penry JK: Photosensitivity and epilepsy: A review, in Self-Induced Seizures. Ch. 9. Photosensitivity and Epilepsy: A Review. New York: Raven Press, 1979, p. 115.

Nilvebrant L: The mechanism of action of tolterodine. Rev Contemp Pharmacother 11:13–27, 2000.

Norton C, Kamm MA: Outcome of biofeedback for faecal incontinence. Br J Surg 86:1159–1163, 1999.

Nygaard IE, Kreder KJ: Efficacy of pelvic floor muscle exercises in women with stress, urge, and mixed urinary incontinence. Am J Obstet Gynecol 174:120–125, 1996.

Olsen A.L, Rao SSC: Clinical neurophysiology and electrodiagnostic testing of the pelvic floor. Gastroenterol Clin North Am 30:33–54, 2001.

Ott BR: Leuprolid treatment of sexual aggression in a patient with dementia and the Klüver Bucy syndrome. Clin Neuropharmacol 18:443–447, 1995.

Ouslander JG: Urinary incontinence in the geriatric population. Nippon Ronon Igakkai Zasshi 28:484–492, 1991.

Padma-Nathan H, Hellstrom WJ, Kaiser FE, et al: Treatment of men with erectile dysfunction with transurethral alprostadil. N Engl J Med 336:1–7, 1997.

Parks AG, McPartlin JF: Late repair of injuries of the anal sphincter. Proc Roy Soc Med 64:1187–1189, 1971.

Parks AG, Nicholls FJ: Proctocolectomy without ileostomy for ulcerative colitis. BMJ 2:85–88, 1978.

Pelsang R, Rao SSC, Welcher K: FECOM: A new artificial stool for evaluating defecation. Am J Gastroenterol 94:183–186, 1999.

Penfield W, Rasmussen T: The Cerebral Cortex of Man. New York: MacMillan, 1950.

Penovich PE: The effects of epilepsy and its treatment on sexual and reproductive function. Epilepsia 41(Suppl. 2):S53–S61, 2000.

Perry S, Shaw C, McGrother C, et al: Prevalence of faecal incontinence in adults aged 40 years or more living in a the community. Gut 50:480–484, 2002.

Pitt DC, Kriel RL, Wagner NC, et al: Klüver-Bucy syndrome following heat stroke in a 12-year-old girl. Pediatr Neurol 13:73–76, 1995.

Quinlan DM, Epstein JI, Carter BS, et al: Sexual function following radical prostatectomy: Influence of preservation of neurovascular bundles. J Urol 145:998–1002, 1991.

Rao SSC: Belching, bloating, and flatulence: How to help patients who have troublesome abdominal gas. Postgrad Med 101:263–269, 275–278, 1997.

Rao SSC: The technical aspects of biofeedback therapy for defecation. Gastroenterologist 6:96–103, 1998.

Rao SSC: Guidelines for fecal incontinence. Am J Gastroenterol (forthcoming, 2003).

Rao SSC, Patel RS: How useful are manometric tests of anorectal function in the management of defecation disorders. Am J Gastroenterol 92:469–475, 1997.

Rao SSC, Sun WM: Current techniques of assessing defecation dynamics. Dig Dis 15 (Suppl. 1):64–67, 1997.

Rao SSC, Azpiroz F, Diamant N, et al: Minimum standards of anorectal manometry. Neurogastoroenterol Motil 14:553–559, 2002.

Rao SSC, Beaty J, Chamberlain M, et al: Effects of acute graded exercise on colonic motility. Am J Physiology 276:G1221–G1226, 1999a.

Rao SSC, Happel J, Welcher K: Can biofeedback therapy improve anorectal function in fecal incontinence? Am J Gastroenterol 91:2360–2366, 1996.

Rao SSC, Kempf J, Stessman M: Anal seepage: Sphincter dysfunction or incomplete evacuation? Gastroenterology 114:A824, 1998a.

Rao SSC, Sadeghi P, Beaty J, et al: Ambulatory colonic manometry in healthy humans. Am J Physiol 280:G629–G639, 2001.

Rao SSC, Sood AK, Kempf J, et al: Does radical hysterectomy affect anorectal function? Gastroenterology 118:A.781, 2000.

Rao SSC, Stessman M, Kempf M: Is biofeedback therapy (BT) useful in patients with anal seepage? Gastroenterology 116:G4636, 1999b.

Rao SSC, Stumbo P, Zimmerman B, et al: Is coffee a colonic stimulant? Eur J Gastroenterol Hepatol 10:113–118, 1998b.

Raz S: Modified bladder neck suspension for female stress incontinence. Urology 17:82–85, 1981.

Read NW, Abouzekry L, Read MG, et al: Anorectal function in elderly patients with fecal impaction. Gastroenterology 89:959–966, 1985.

Read NW, Bartollo DC, Read MG: Differences in anal function in patients with incontinence to solids and in patients with incontinence to liquids. Br J Surg 71:39–42, 1989.

Read NW, Harford WF, Schmulen AC, et al: A clinical study of patients with fecal incontinence and diarrhea. Gastroenterology 76:747–756, 1979.

Resnick NM: Initial evaluation of the incontinent patient. J Am Geriatr Soc 38:311–316, 1990.

Resnick NM, Yalla SV: Detrusor hyperactivity with impaired contractile function: An unrecognized but common cause of incontinence in elderly patients. JAMA 257:3076–3081, 1987.

Rieger NA, Sarre RG, Saccone GT, et al: Postanal repair for faecal incontinence: Long-term follow-up. Aust NZ J Surg 67:566–570, 1997.

Rodriguez M, Siva A, Ward J, et al: Impairment, disability, and handicap in multiple sclerosis: A population-based study in Olmstead County, Minnesota. Neurology 44:28–33, 1994.

Rogers J: Anal and rectal sensation, in Henry MM (ed): Baillieres Clinical Gastroenterology. London: Bailliere Tindall, 1992, pp. 179–81.

Rothholtz NA, Wexner SD: Surgical treatment of constipation and fecal incontinence, Gastroenterol Clin North Am 30:131–166, 2001.

Sangwan YP, Coller JA, Barrett RC, et al: Can manometric parameters predict response to biofeedback therapy in fecal incontinence? Dis Colon Rectum 38:1021–1025, 1995.

Santoro GA, Eitan B, Pryde A, et al: Open study of low-dose amitriptyline in the treatment of patients with idiopathic fecal incontinence. Dis Colon Rectum 40:1676–1682, 1997.

Schafer A, Enck P, Furst G, et al: Anatomy of the anal sphincter. Comparison of anal endosonography to magnetic resonance imaging. Dis Colon Rectum 37:777–781, 1994.

Schiller LR, Santa Ana CA, Schmulen AC, et al: Pathogenesis of fecal incontinence in diabetes mellitus: Evidence for internal-anal sphincter dysfunction. N Engl J Med 307:1666–1671, 1982.

Seanz de Tejada I, Goldstein I, Azadzoi K, et al: Impaired neurogenic and endothelium-mediated relaxation of penile smooth muscle from diabetic men with impotence. N Engl J Med 320:1025–1030, 1989.

Siegel SW, Catanzaro F, Dijkema HE, et al: Long-term results of a multicenter study on sacral nerve stimulation for treatment of urinary urge incontinence, urgency-frequency, and retention. Urology 56(Suppl. 1):97–91, 2000.

Sielezneff I, Malouf AJ, Bartolo DC, et al: Dynamic graciloplasty in the treatment of patients with faecal incontinence. Br J Surg 86:61–65, 1999.

Smith RB, van Cangh P, Skinner DG, et al: Augmentation enterocystoplasty: A critical review. J Urol 118:35–39, 1977.

Snooks SJ, Henry MM, Swash M: Faecal incontinence after anal dilatation. Br J Surg 71:617–618, 1984.

Snooks SJ, Swash M, Henry MM, et al: Risk factors in childbirth causing damage to the pelvic floor innervation. Int J Colorectal Dis 1:20–24, 1986.

Speakman CT, Burnett SJ, Kamm MA, et al: Sphincter injury after anal dilatation demonstrated by anal endosonography. Br J Surg 78:1429–1430, 1991.

Stamey TA: Endoscopic suspension of the vesical neck for urinary incontinence in females. Ann Surg 192:465–471, 1980.

Staskin DR, Zimmern PE, Hadley HR, Raz S: The pathophysiology of stress incontinence. Urol Clin North Am 12:271–278, 1985.

Stewart JT: Carbamazepine treatment of a patient with Klüver-Bucy Syndrome. J Clin Psychiatry 46:496–497, 1985.

Stone JM, Wolfe VA, Nino-Murcia M, et al: Colostomy as treatment for complications of spinal cord injury. Arch Phys Med Rehabil 71:514–518, 1990.

Sultan AH, Kamm MA, Hudson CN, Bartram CI: Third degree obstetric anal sphincter tears: Risk factors and outcome of primary repair. Br Med J 308:887–891, 1994.

Sultan AH, Kamm MA, Hudson CN, et al: Anal-sphincter disruption during vaginal delivery. N Engl J Med 329:1905-1911, 1993.

Sun W, Donnelly TC: Anorectal function in incontinent patients with cerebrospinal disease. Gastroenterology 99:1372–1379, 1990.

Sun W, Donnelly TC: Effects of loperamide oxide on gastrointestinal transit time and anorectal function in patients with chronic diarrhea and faecal incontinence. Scand J Gastroenterol 32:34–38, 1997.

Sun W, MacDonagh R, Forster D, et al: Anorectal function in patients with complete spinal transection before and after sacral posterior rhizotomy. Gastroenterology 108:990–998, 1995.

Sun WM, Donnelly TC, Read NW: Utility of a combined test of anorectal manometry, electromyography and sensation in determining the mechanism of 'idiopathic' faecal incontinence. Gut 33:807–813, 1992.

Szurszewski JH, Holt PR, Schuster MM: Proceedings of a workshop entitled "Neuromuscular function and dysfunction of the gastrointestinal tract." Dig Dis Sci 34:1135–1146, 1989.

Tapp AJ, Cardozo LD, Versi E, et al: The treatment of detrusor instability in postmenopausal women with oxybutynin chloride: A
double-blind placebo controlled study. Br J Obstet Gyneacol
97:521–526, 1990.

Taylor GP: Pathogenesis and treatment of HTLV-I associated
myelopathy. Sex Transm Infect 74:316–322, 1998.

Tjandra JJ, Milsom JW, Schroeder T, et al: Endoluminal ultrasound is
preferable to electromyography in mapping anal sphincteric
defects. Dis Colon Rectum 1993 36:689–692.

Tonsgard JH, Harwicke N, Levine SC: Klüver-Bucy syndrome in
children. Pediatr Neurol 3:162–165, 1987.

Vaizey CJ, Carapeti E, Cahill JA, Kamm MA: Prospective comparison
of faecal incontinence grading systems. Gut 44:77–80, 1999.

Vaizey CJ, Kamm MA, Bartram CI: Primary degeneration of the internal anal sphincter as a cause of passive faecal incontinence.
Lancet 349:612–615, 1997.

Vaizey CJ, Kamm MA, Nicholls RJ: Recent advances in the surgical
treatment of faecal incontinence. Br J Surg 85:596–603, 1998.

Van Tets WF, Kuipers JH, Bleijenberg G: Biofeedback treatment is
ineffective in neurogenic fecal incontinence. Dis Colon Rectum
39:992–994, 1996.

Van Thiel DH, Gavaler JS, Sanghri A: Recovery of function in
abstinent alcoholic men. Gastroenterology 84:677–682, 1983.

Varma JS, Smith AN, Busuttil A: Function of the anal sphincters after
chronic radiation injury. Gut 27:528–533, 1986.

Versi E, Appel R, Mobley D, et al: Dry mouth with conventional and
controlled-release oxybutynin in urinary incontinence. Obstet
Gynecol 95:718–721, 2000.

Wald A: Biofeedback therapy for fecal incontinence. Ann Intern Med
95:146–149, 1981.

Wald A: Colonic and anorectal motility testing in clinical practice. Am
J Gastroenterol 789: 2109–2115, 1994.

Wald A, Bock C, Bayless TM: Effect of coffee on the human small
intestine. Gastroenterology 71:738–742, 1976.

Wexner SD, Jorge JM: Colorectal physiological tests: Use or abuse of
technology? Eur J Surg 160:167–174, 1994.

Williams ME, Gaylord SA: Role of functional assessment in the
evaluation of urinary incontinence: National Institutes of
Health Consensus Development Conference on Urinary
Incontinence in Adults. J Am Geriatr Soc 38:296–299, 1990.

Wong VCN, Wong MTH, Ng THK, et al: Unusual case of Klüver-Bucy
syndrome in a Chinese boy. Pediatr Neurol 7:385–388, 1991.

Yang CC, Stiens SA: Antegrade continence enema for the treatment of
neurogenic constipation and fecal incontinence after spinal
cord injury. Arch Phys Med Rehabil 81:683–685, 2000.

Chronic Pain

David J. Hewitt
Stanley L. Chapman

Addiction

Adjuvant analgesic

Goals of care

Incomplete cross-tolerance

Nociception

Opioid phobia

Physical dependence

Suffering

Chronic pain involves much more than the perception of noxious stimuli from an affected body part. The complex nature of chronic pain is due to the over-whelming psychological impact it has on the individual. The successful treatment of chronic pain requires attention to the associated psychological and behavioral factors that can either predate or result from ongoing, unrelieved pain. Also, changes in psychological function, behavior, and cognition can be caused by medications used in the treatment of chronic pain. Importantly, cognitive and behavioral techniques should be included as part of an interdisciplinary, comprehensive approach to the management of patients with chronic pain.

BARRIERS TO PAIN MANAGEMENT

A number of barriers to effective pain management continue to exist. These barriers involve the physician, the patient, family members, the health care system, and regulatory agencies.

Physician Barriers

Lack of physician education remains a significant barrier to adequate pain control (Galer et al., 1999a). Though pain is the number one reason individuals seek medical attention, pain remains inadequately covered by medical school curricula and by residency training programs. In part this fact reflects the limited time available to teach a very large body of information during a relatively brief training period, but it also reflects that only recently has chronic pain been considered a possible chronic disease and not simply a symptom of disease. Indeed, because pain is so ubiquitous and involved in so many conditions, there has been the erroneous assumption that successful management of the primary underlying disease results in resolution of the accompanying pain. The inadequate training in the assessment, diagnosis, and medical management of pain has led to the undertreatment of acute, postoperative, and chronic malignant and nonmalignant pain.

"Opioid-phobia" refers to the fear of opioid analgesic therapy and represents another important barrier to the treatment of chronic pain. Physicians, patients, and society at large often share this fear. Frequently, this fear arises because of concerns over inducing iatrogenic addiction or fear of regulatory scrutiny. There is also the mistaken belief that opioid tolerance will lead to an endless need for dose escalation and that side effects such as sedation and nausea are inevitable and untreatable.

Physicians often wrongly assume that there is a one-to-one correspondence between tissue pathology and the presence of pain. For example, a broken bone causes pain and one might assume the worse the injury, the more severe the pain. Unfortunately, this relationship between the size of the pathologic process and the severity of pain does not always hold for chronic pain. Often, the cause of the pain is not at all clear. Chronic pain commonly occurs even after the underlying pathologic process that initially caused the pain has resolved. For example, surgery may have removed a herniated disk, but pain continues. Chronic pain can also occur when the pathologic process can be identified, but the disease is progressive and adequate treatment is not available to stop or arrest the process. For example, diabetic neuropathy is often progressive, and pain can be a significant and troubling feature of the disease. Sometimes the underlying process producing the pain cannot be detected with the modalities that are currently available. Musculoskeletal pain is very common and yet imaging is often negative or, if positive, may have a questionable association with the symptomatology. Even though most people, including physicians,

have suffered from severe muscular pain that can last weeks, physicians often become skeptical when patients present with a more protracted chronic muscular pain syndrome (e.g., myofascial pain). In addition, many diagnoses given to "explain" the pain, such as osteoarthritis or degenerative disk disease, are more age-related than pain-related (Flor & Turk, 1984). In truth, medical knowledge about the causes of chronic pain is quite limited (Nachemson, 1979; Flor & Turk, 1984).

Lack of education can also lead to the unfortunate and disturbing fact that a physician may prefer not to treat patients with chronic pain. Some physicians may give up when their initial attempts at pain control fail. Others might give up when patient care becomes time consuming. Often, chronic pain patients are unable to work and there are disability and medical/legal issues to be sorted out. Physicians may find themselves trying to determine if the patient's pain is real or if the patient has a secondary motive (e.g., money).

The psychosocial issues that accompany these patients are often complex and require more than the competence of a single physician. This complexity can be daunting to physicians, particularly in combination with time constraints and pressures.

The physician's training and previous life experiences, as well as assessments from previous physicians, may bias him or her toward or against treating the patient with chronic pain. If a previous physician inappropriately labeled a patient as drug-seeking, subsequent physicians may be reluctant to get involved. If litigation or a workers' compensation claim is pending, the physician may be skeptical about the patient's pain, and assume that it is magnified or untreatable, even though evidence does not support the assumption that disability issues prevent successful outcome with treatment. (Dworkin et al., 1985). Because addiction affects about 6% of the population (Reiger et al., 1990), it is not unusual for a physician to have family members or friends or previous patients who may have been addicted to prescription analgesics. Consequently, physicians caring for patients with chronic pain may consider these patients burdensome.

Though the prevalence of addiction has not been shown to be greater in patients with chronic pain compared with the lifetime prevalence of drug addiction in the general population, inducing an addiction disorder in a patient with chronic pain by prescribing an opioid analgesic remains a common concern among physicians. Estimates of addictive disorder among chronic pain patients range from 3% to 19% (Haller & Butler, 1991; Fishbain et al., 1992, 1996), which is similar to the lifetime prevalence rates of addictive disease in the general population, which has been found to range from 6.1% to 16.7% (Reiger et al., 1990).

Physician bias may lead to an overprescribing of opioid analgesics as well. Because the undertreatment of chronic pain is common and has recently been well publicized, physicians may prescribe opioids without regard for the significant side effects associated with opioid analgesia, including the risk of addiction. These physicians may have personal experience with a family member or friend who died a painful death due to inadequate pain management.

Patient Barriers

Inappropriate treatment for pain is common in hospital settings. Patients often are very aware that nurses can grow annoyed by constant requests for pain medication. A patient may learn to endure severe pain in order to be considered a "good patient" by the physicians and nurses. In addition, because pain varies in intensity, patients may inappropriately decrease their dose when the pain lessens and increase it when it worsens. Complex medication regimens can be hard to follow in general but are more of a challenge in the elderly. An altered mental status resulting from the effect of centrally acting medications can also interfere with medication adherence.

Societal Barriers

An important factor leading to the current level of inadequate pain control is the limited number of specialists trained in pain and palliative care. Specialists in the medical management of pain are still not widely available in a number of medical centers and patients and caregivers lack access to these specialists.

Pharmacists contribute to the problem of providing adequate pain management, because they are often undertrained in the area of pain control and more concerned about the regulation of controlled substances than the care of patients with pain. Pharmacists often fail to maintain an adequate opioid supply, particularly in underserved areas (Morrison et al., 2000).

The United States government is aware of the barriers to appropriate pain management and the Joint Commission on Accreditation of Health Care Organizations has mandated that pain be evaluated and treated as routinely as vital signs.

PSYCHOLOGICAL ASPECTS OF CHRONIC PAIN

Patients with chronic pain may or may not have significant psychological and social comorbidities, but it is vitally important to be aware that they may be present and to explore pertinent psychosocial issues. Psychiatric illness associated with chronic pain is common. In their review, Koestler and Doleys (2002) note that most studies report a prevalence rate of depression of between 30% and 60% in the chronic

pain population, and that the occurrence and severity of affective factors have been found to be related to the severity or temporal progression of the pain condition. A premorbid psychological state can adversely affect an individual's ability to cope with pain. Conversely, anxiety and depression may develop in response to chronic pain.

Patients may have social issues that predate the development of chronic pain. For example, patients may be in a maladaptive or stressful relationship with a partner, spouse, child, parent, employer, or a fellow employee. Apart from depression, patients may suffer from a lack of happiness or fun in life. Modern society is filled with multiple stresses. Expectations regarding success, happiness, or one's position in life may not have been achieved. Patients with lives that are seemingly out of control may be unable to cope with the added stress of chronic pain, and a patient's potential disability associated with chronic pain may reinforce focus on pain and complaints. Chronic pain can take an individual out of the "race for success" and provide a good excuse for not having met expectations of one's full potential. Patients may be able to get away from a stressful job or an abusive boss by going on disability.

Chronic pain can allow individuals to develop a semblance of control over their world. For example, a patient's spouse may provide some of the care and nurturing that hadn't been present previously; pain may keep a marriage together because one partner feels a sense of duty to the sick spouse; disobedient children may be more likely to behave if a parent is in chronic severe pain; or teenage rebellion can be tempered.

More commonly, however, chronic pain wreaks havoc on every aspect of the individual's world. Chronic pain can drive away a loving spouse and children. Chronic pain can lead to a loss of control over one's life and lead a previously financially successful individual into poverty.

DEFINING PAIN

Pain, though certainly one of the most universal of human experiences, remains one of the most isolating. It is important to distinguish between pain, nociception, and suffering. *Nociception* has been defined as "the activity produced in the nervous system by potentially tissue damaging stimuli." (IASP, 1979). *Pain*, on the other hand, is a broader term defined as "an unpleasant sensory and emotional experience associated with actual or potential tissue damage or described in terms of such damage" (IASP, 1979). Pain can affect one's emotional state, which, in turn, can also affect one's ability to cope with pain. Consequently, stress, anxiety, and depression can be major determinants in the pain experience. The perceived meaning of the pain is also a major determinant of function and mood (Daut &

Cleeland, 1982). *Suffering* refers to "the global perception of distress engendered by adverse factors that together undermine quality of life" (Cassell, 1982). Suffering is multidimensional. Physical, psychological, social, spiritual, existential, economic, family, and other factors contribute to the individual's suffering. It is important to consider that pain may not be a major component of one's suffering, and because suffering often involves nonmedical issues, it can often be overlooked by the physician.

Because pain and dysfunction are often associated with depression or dysphoria, improvement in either may lead to an improvement in mood.

UNRESPONSIVE PAIN

Sometimes, even with the best efforts of multiple specialists, a patient's pain syndrome may be relatively unresponsive to multiple therapeutic interventions. While unresponsive pain is uncommon, it is important to consider other issues that may be associated with the pain that may be more responsive to psychological, behavioral, and cognitive approaches. These approaches are also important in patients whose pain is a response to treatment.

It is important to consider that the patient's central problem involves many factors besides the patient's pain. Addressing such issues in tandem with needed medication or treatment for pain is essential for treatment success. For example, a woman with a severe chronic daily headache might hate her job or her boss and have a lack of confidence or self-worth that may lead her to feel trapped and unable to leave. Once she is able to realize that the key to resolving her headache lies in changing her job situation, her headaches can resolve or significantly improve. Similar examples may include a person in an abusive or a maladaptive relationship or a patient with chronic anger toward the person who was responsible for the accident or injury that caused the pain.

It is therefore important when assessing patients with chronic intractable pain to understand the context of their life. Interviewing significant others in the patient's life apart from the patient is important, as often a family member or a few family members can be helpful in fleshing out the patient's story. Examples of important information might include the presence of a current or past substance abuse problem, the patient's attitudes and expectations toward treatment, or activity level. In addition, comparing the patient's report with that of the family can provide clues as to whether the patient's self-reports are accurate.

ABUSE OF OPIOID ANALGESICS

Opioids, which have the medical purpose of providing pain relief, can be misused, abused, or even sold to support another addiction. Unfortunately, chronic pain or the claim of chronic pain may be a way for an individual to potentially obtain opioid analgesic drugs for purposes other than pain control. Patients who are intent on obtaining analgesic medications for aberrant purposes will try to deceive the physician who is passionate about providing pain relief for his or her patients. The patient who truly is drug-seeking creates another barrier to the appropriate management of chronic pain. The therapeutic relationship between a doctor and patient is based on trust. The physician who has been intentionally deceived by a patient who has abused pain medication will naturally become more cautious when prescribing opioid analgesics in the future.

While medical schools and residency programs give short shrift to training in pain management (Galer et al., 1999b), the current training in the diagnosis and management of addiction has been inadequate. Confusion regarding the nature of addiction often exists on the part of the patient, family members, and even physicians. Similar to other chronic diseases, addiction is a remitting and relapsing, but treatable disease.

Physical dependence, tolerance, and addiction are often confused and wrongly considered synonymous. Physical dependence and tolerance are physiologic responses to opioid exposure and do not imply aberrant drug use. *Addiction*, on the other hand, refers to a complex of maladaptive behaviors, including using a drug despite the harm that drug is causing in the individual's life, and/or using a drug for purposes other than intended by the treating physician. With addiction, an alteration in central nervous system function occurs that the patient considers desirable. The drug experience produces craving for the drug in order to get this desirable alteration in consciousness. Tolerance to this nonanalgesic effect leads to unsanctioned dose escalations, running out of medication early, and a preoccupation with getting and using the sought-after drug. There is a loss of control over taking the drug and a loss of control over the individual's life. *Physical dependence* is defined by the presence of an abstinence syndrome precipitated by abruptly withdrawing an opioid or administering an opioid antagonist. This results in a syndrome of malaise, yawning, mydriasis, goose flesh, diaphoresis, and anxiety. The abstinence syndrome can be avoided by decreasing the opioid dose slowly. *Tolerance* represents a shift in the dose-response curve: A higher dose of a medication is needed to achieve the same level of analgesia that was present at a previously lower and effective dose. Physical dependence and tolerance develop to other classes of drugs as well, and in some cases the withdrawal syndrome can be very severe.

Pseudoaddiction is a useful term that has gained some level of acceptance and refers to a syndrome of inadequate pain treatment that leads to behaviors that are reminiscent of addiction. These behaviors resolve when appropriate analgesic management leads to adequate pain control (Weissman & Haddox, 1989).

Some behaviors that suggest that addiction be considered include repetitive running out of medications early, getting prescriptions from multiple physicians and pharmacies, and, obviously, forging or altering a prescription. In addition, some patients may request a particular analgesic drug, often an opioid analgesic. While this occurrence does not necessarily mean the patient is drug-seeking, the physician should be vigilant. Meperidine and hydrocodone preparations are commonly sought-after analgesics for abuse. Of the short-acting opioids, tramadol has a low abuse rate, with less than one case per 100,000 individuals during an 18-month period (Cicero et al., 1999).

Because some doctors are uncomfortable prescribing opioid analgesics, they may refer a patient elsewhere for opioid analgesic management. Sometimes, these physicians start patients out on an opioid analgesic, but, because of their own lack of education, become uncomfortable when the dose is escalated past a certain level. In these instances, it may be reasonable to continue the analgesic medication. In other instances, a physician may have very valid concerns that the patient is misusing or abusing the medication. Frequently, a physician may mistakenly decide to stop an opioid analgesic even though it is clearly providing significant pain relief, even in the absence of evidence of aberrant drug use. When physicians are too uncomfortable to prescribe opioid analgesics, they should recognize their limitations and refer patients to physicians who are more knowledgeable. It is very important to communicate with the referring physician by phone to better understand the issues surrounding the patient referral. If addiction is suspected, it is important to make the appropriate referral to a specialist in addiction medicine.

COGNITIVE AND BEHAVIORAL EFFECTS OF ANALGESIC MEDICATIONS

In addition to the effects associated with chronic pain, it is equally important to be aware of the cognitive and behavioral effects associated with the commonly used analgesic medications. *Opioid* analgesics may have a euphoric or a dysphoric effect on mood. Sedation, a "spacy" feeling, and/or various components of a delirium may occur. For example, hallucinations may occur and can be a minor annoyance or truly frightening. Those that occur while waking up are called *hypnopomic* hallucinations, whereas those that occur while falling asleep are called "hypnagogic." Patients may also suffer from illusions and be fully aware of a distortion in their visual reality. A generalized slowing in cognitive function can interfere with the ability to drive and operate heavy machinery. Fortunately, tolerance develops to these psychotomimetic effects of opioids

over a relatively brief period of time. Research has revealed that adverse cognitive effects generally can be demonstrated clearly within a 3- to 7-day period after initiation or increase in the opioid dose and subsequently clears after this time period (Bruera et al., 1989). A review by Chapman, Byas-Smith, and Reed (2002) addresses cognitive effects of opioids in patients with chronic pain.

Special note should be made of the mixed opioid agonist-antagonists as well as the metabolites of meperidine, and propoxyphene. In both instances, significant psychotomimetic effects can occur, including hallucinations and delirium. For unclear reasons, propoxyphene continues to be prescribed in the geriatric population, despite the efforts of specialists in geriatric pain management to curtail its use (AGS, 2002).

A number of the adjuvant analgesics are also known to have an effect on mood. Though the analgesic effects of antidepressants have been demonstrated to be independent of their antidepressant effects (Max et al., 1987), patients with pain who are also depressed may benefit from the dual effect of these drugs. In a similar manner, the anticonvulsants have been appreciated for their mood-stabilizing and antianxiety effects. Less recognized is the potential therapeutic benefit of the opioid analgesics as antidepressant and mood stabilizing agents. Consequently, it is not always clear if the patient using opioid analgesics for the treatment of pain may also be getting positive therapeutic psychological effects.

Other analgesics can also have significant cognitive effects. The tricyclic antidepressants produce confusion and disorientation. Nonsteroidal anti-inflammatories can cause dizziness and drowsiness.

Analgesics from different classes are often combined in an effort to limit the toxicity of the individual drugs and for the additive analgesia that combining medications can provide. Unfortunately, in addition to enhancing analgesic effects, combining medications can create added toxic effects, including cognitive dysfunction.

COGNITIVE AND BEHAVIORAL APPROACHES TO PAIN MANAGEMENT

The current recognition that pain represents not only nociception, but also the associated emotional experience, reflects the central role that cognitive and behavioral therapy should have in the management of pain. As discussed above, pain has been defined as "an unpleasant sensory and emotional experience associated with actual or potential tissue damage, or described in terms of such damage" (IASP, 1979) Functional imaging supports an anatomic basis for division in pain pathways. Pain is distributed within the brain between medial limbic areas subserving the emotional and affective component, and lateral brain areas involved in determining the pain's intensity and localization (Casey et al., 1994; Coghill et al., 1994). Thus, the emotional component directly affects how pain is perceived. Severe pain of limited duration often is tolerated much better than pain that has an unclear etiology and an unknown time course.

Cognitive and behavioral therapies may be the most important component of the interdisciplinary management of chronic pain. Education about the nature of pain is a critical aspect of these therapies, so that patients can have realistic expectations. Patients need to recognize that their pain may never be cured, but that a productive and fulfilling life is possible with appropriate pain management. Because of their efficacy in reducing pain and related problems (Chapman, 1983), relaxation exercises are taught almost universally at multidisciplinary pain centers. Relaxation methods may include meditation, deep breathing, progressive muscle relaxation exercises, and guided imagery. Learning relaxation skills can reduce not only stress associated with chronic pain, but also pain-related muscle tension, and can enhance sleep and improve cognitive function such as memory and concentration. By learning better control over their pain and related problems, many patients can reduce their reliance on medications. The protocol for relaxation therapy often includes having patients practice tape-recorded relaxation methods daily at home. The goal is to learn to relax deeply and quickly, in many situations, so patients can learn to relax during an episode of pain exacerbation.

Many patients find biofeedback, that is, the feeding back of information regarding a biologic process so as to bring it to maximum function and relaxation. Biofeedback can teach patients both discrimination (i.e., detecting the status of the important biologic parameter) and control over that parameter. Research has revealed that biofeedback helps patients in part by increasing their real or perceived control over pain and related problems (Chapman, 1983; Grzesiak & Ciccone, 1988). By providing concrete information regarding progress, it also can motivate patients to work on relaxation and stress management skills.

Given the potential for stress to affect medical problems and quality of life, it is important for patients to increase their management skills. Doing so may necessitate attention not only to modifying stressors, such as a bad marriage or job situation, but also to altering internal reactions. Effective stress management can address time management and schedules of productive activity, rest, enjoyment or "play," social engagements, and exercise. It can also employ techniques for improving communication and assertiveness skills, using humor and positive thinking, and reducing exposure to anxiety-producing events.

Cognition refers to attitudes, thoughts and beliefs. With increased recognition that behavior and emotion are determined largely according to how we construe the world and assign meaning to events, therapy to alter cognition is now recognized as an important aspect of pain management (Turk et al., 1983; Compas et al., 1998). There is a great deal of research showing that pain responses are greater when individuals expect to have more pain, perceive themselves as having little control over it, attend to it closely, and have anxiety-provoking thoughts about it (Turk et al., 1983; Weisenberg, 1977). Indeed, *catastrophization*, which refers to rumination on pain and related problems, exaggeration of the negative aspects and effects of pain, and perceived inability to control pain and related problems, has been found to correlate with higher reports of pain and pain-related emotional distress and disability (Keefe et al., 1989). The basic goals of cognitive therapy include gaining understanding of the role of cognitions in managing pain and related problems and then identifying and replacing one's own maladaptive cognitions (such as those associated with catastrophization) with adaptive ones associated with hope and perceptions of control and self-efficacy (Jensen et al., 1991). Many methods can be used in this process, including discussion of results of cognitively oriented questionnaires such as the Coping Strategies Questionnaire (Rosenstiel & Keefe, 1983), the Multidimensional Health Locus of Control Inventory (Wallston & Wallston, 1978), or the Survey of Pain Attitudes (Jensen et al., 1987), and role-playing and rehearsing adaptive reactions and thoughts.

Adaptive coping with the losses associated with chronic pain often involves an emotional and cognitive acceptance of the limitations in health and function associated with pain, combined with a determination to work at enhanced control over pain and related problems. Elisabeth Kübler-Ross described the stages of coping with loss in her work with terminal cancer patients (1969); her work is applicable also to the losses occurring with chronic pain. Kübler-Ross described a sequence of common reactions to loss, including an initial denial of its reality, anger, "bargaining" (related to anxiety about the loss and its future effects), and depression. This process ideally culminates in "acceptance," associated with an emotional peace about losses, and a focus on the positive quality of life.

Group therapy is ideal for presenting and teaching relaxation methods, teaching stress management and improving cognitive skills, and working on issues of acceptance. Information and education about psychological and behavioral aspects of pain and related problems can be presented efficiently in a group context. Through sharing with other group members, patients often feel less isolated and recognize the commonality of their concerns. Self-esteem and self-acceptance, which often have been compromised greatly with chronic pain and loss of function and/or work can result. In addition, groups can allow patients to receive appropriate feedback and reinforcement for their efforts toward greater control and function. Modeling after successful patients in the group can be powerful in promoting behavior change. A successful group leader will keep the focus of the group on positive steps patients can take toward greater function rather than on how awful pain is.

PHYSICAL THERAPY AND REHABILITATION

The goal of pain management is to optimize analgesia, minimize side effects, and increase function. Achievable goals must be set, and patients should be empowered by their caregivers to take responsibility for themselves and their therapy. Physical therapy and rehabilitative methods are central in improving a patient's ability to function. If too much focus is placed on medication, the patient may consider the benefits of physical therapy to be ancillary. With recent changes in the health care system, reimbursement for multidisciplinary pain management programs may not be available. This short-sightedness drives up medical costs as patients spend more time seeking out physicians who can treat their pain and less time being productive members of society.

PRINCIPLES OF PAIN MANAGEMENT

Pain Assessment

A thorough pain assessment involves a medical and pain history, followed by a directed hypothesis-driven physical and neurologic examination. Pain management involves a dynamic process of assessing and reassessing the pain complaint, identifying possible underlying pain syndromes, making a pain diagnosis, defining the presumed pain pathophysiology, and implementing a comprehensive treatment plan. Defining the presumed pain pathophysiology can prevent needless tests and determine the most effective therapeutic options. Factors such as "total pain" must be considered (Cassell, 1982; Cherny et al., 1994a). This term refers to an overall impairment in quality of life (Saunders, 1984), functional changes, and psychological symptoms (e.g., depression) that must be assessed. Fatigue and psychological distress are particularly common (Ventafridda et al., 1990a, 1990b; Curtis et al., 1991; Portenoy et al., 1994). A flow diagram for pain assessment is given in Figure 33-1.

Believe the Patient When He/She Complains of Pain

Pain is subjective and as such relies on the patient's description of his/her pain. Imaging studies should be used to confirm the etiology, but should never be used to deny that the patient has pain. The lag between a new pain complaint and radiographic evidence of new pathology often leads physicians to doubt the level of pain the patient states he/she is suffering. This lag is particularly common in the management of cancer-related pain, when initial pathologic changes can miss radiographic detection (Hewitt, 1999). Imaging of common pain syndromes such as muscle strain is inadequate. Physicians may wrongly place their faith in the diagnostic studies and not the patient's report of pain (Hewitt, 1999).

Perform a Careful History

The history should concentrate on the area of pain involved and the onset and time course of the painful symptoms. Hypotheses regarding the etiology and presumed pathophysiology should be generated and tested by questioning and by a directed medical and neurologic examination. A number of important pain characteristics should be evaluated, including the temporal pattern of onset, intensity of pain, duration of pain, presence of superimposed breakthrough pain, and the quality of the pain.

Assess Each Pain Separately

Chronic pain often involves multiple areas. It is important to take a careful history of each pain report separately to determine whether different pains share a common etiology and/or pathophysiology.

Assess Previous Episodes of Chronic Pain

One's current experience of pain is influenced by previous experiences with pain, including pain observed in other people. A patient who has watched a family member or loved one go through severe pain (e.g., a painful death resulting from inadequate pain management) may be particularly anxious regarding pain. It is important to discuss these experiences with the patient, and reassure the patient that his/her pain will be treated aggressively.

Assess Previous History of Analgesic Use

The patient's previous experience with analgesic medication, as well as the experiences of people the patient has known, also must be considered. A previous experience of nausea, altered mental state, or an allergic reaction associated with pain medication can influence the patient's willingness to try a similar pain medication in the future. Often previous medications have been prematurely abandoned due to side effects that would have been temporary, whereas the patient perhaps could have

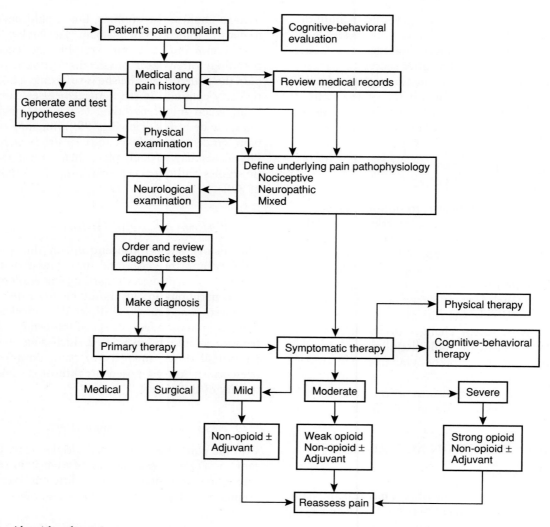

FIGURE 33-1. Algorithm for pain assessment.

been treated with another medication such as an antiemetic. Even in the absence of side effects, a medication might have been abandoned too soon due to the physician's lack of experience with administering it.

An individual with a personal or family history of aberrant drug use may be worried about the risk of addiction. The physician should reassure patients and family members that if issues of aberrant drug use occur, appropriate therapeutic interventions will be employed, including referral to an addiction specialist and possible inpatient detoxification.

Perform a Directed Physical and Neurologic Examination

The physical and neurologic examination tests hypotheses generated from the pain history regarding the cause of the pain. Examinations that are directed by information gained from the history are more likely to yield valuable information than examinations that are com-

prehensive but done without regard to history and the presenting pain complaint.

Review All Pertinent Medical Records

A large stack of medical records often accompanies patients who have chronic disease. Such information can be helpful in preventing repetition of previous studies, but it is important to direct review of the record to the development of the current pain symptom, how the diagnosis was made, past analgesics used, adverse effects from previous attempts at analgesia, and evidence of previous aberrant drug-related behaviors.

Review Relevant Imaging Studies

Radiologists often complain that they do not receive enough clinical information to adequately interpret an imaging study. A collaborative approach with radiologists will allow for a more accurate interpretation of results. Radiologists can help direct a more appropriate diagnostic work-up.

Screen the Patient for Psychosocial and Behavioral Factors Important in Pain

Such screening can occur both through brief psychometric testing as well as interviewing. Psychometric testing has the advantage of providing standardized information about a patient and allows comparison of that patient's responses to those of the normative sample of the test battery. Test results are less likely to depend on the personality or presentation of another person than are results gathered from an interview. In addition, some patients are more willing to disclose information on a written form than to discuss it with a professional.

Two examples of excellent screening batteries are the Multidimensional Pain Inventory (MPI; Kerns et al., 1985) and the Beck Depression Inventory (BDI; Beck et al., 1961). The MPI includes 61 items, each scored on a 0-to-6 scale, requiring about 15 to 20 minutes for the average patient to complete. It has the advantage of having been standardized and specifically devised for patients with chronic pain, and it evaluates those psychosocial and behavioral factors most relevant in determining the nature and comprehensiveness of needed treatment. Scores include measures of perceived pain severity, the degree of perceived interference of pain in activities, overall control over life, emotional distress, and level of interpersonal support related to pain. Separate sections quantify the nature of responses of the spouse or significant other to pain and the extent of participation in activities of daily living (ADLs), including household chores, outdoor work, activities away from home, and social activities. From their pattern of scores, patients can be divided into one of several categories that have been found to be predictive of treatment response (Turk & Rudy, 1988). Those categorized as "adaptive copers" have a high likelihood of responding well to appropriate simple interventions for pain and may not need intensive psychosocial treatment, whereas those categorized as "dysfunctional" often require intensive multidisciplinary rehabilitation for optimal outcome. A third category of patients, "interpersonally distressed," is likely to require close involvement of the spouse or significant other in treatment.

Depression is widely recognized as the most prominent emotion associated with chronic pain (Getto, 1988). Untreated, it can interfere with the success of medical approaches to pain (Block, 1996). A useful screening tool for depression is the short form of the BDI, which includes only 13 questions and is highly correlated with the longer form of the inventory (Beck & Beck, 1972). Each item relates to a particular aspect of depression and includes four statements representing different levels of depression, from which the patient

selects the most applicable. The inventory includes items related to negative affect (such as sadness and dissatisfaction with life), negative cognition (such as guilt and a perception of being a failure in life), and somatic factors (such as low energy, poor appetite, and difficulty getting started). In addition, one item measures suicidal ideation and/or planning. The test is easy to score and interpret and requires only about 5 to 10 minutes for most patients to complete. A high score (approximately 10 or higher on the short form) or the presence of suicidal ideation suggest the need for further psychological evaluation.

Assess Patient's Level of Function—Activity and Work

Reduced physical, social, recreational, and vocational activity frequently accompanies chronic pain. Restriction in activity can affect depression, cognitive abilities, sleep, pain level, and performance of multiple bodily systems (Brena & Chapman, 1985). Many patients with chronic pain are not working, and their loss of work often affects their social, emotional, and financial status. Taking a careful history of the patient's activity level before and after the onset of pain and determining the factors that have led to any restriction in activity can be vital in planning a course of therapy and rehabilitation. A careful work and education history often is critical, and should include measures of the patient's work abilities, transferable skills, work satisfaction and attitudes, belief, interest in the possibilities for future employment, and disability status and income.

Assess Emotional, Social and Behavioral Status and History

A history of the patient's functioning in these areas can help identify factors important in the patient's current level of functioning and areas important for therapeutic intervention. Areas of inquiry should include previous and current problems with depression, anxiety, anger and substance abuse, and the quality and nature of relationships. The attitudes, expectations, and responses of individuals in the patient's support system can be critical in determining the success of treatment, and it often is important to include them in both evaluation and treatment. Relevant individuals may include not only family members, but the patient's attorney, case manager, and other health care professionals.

Assess Goals, Attitudes, and Expectations

Physicians need to understand what the patients and family may be the nature and cause of the patient's pain and what types of treatments or evaluations are relevant in his/her condition. If patients believe that treatments are inappropriate for their conditions or do not address their goals, they likely will not be followed. An example is the patient who believes that pain management is inappropriate unless the medical cause of the pain is found. Furthermore, the patient who has unrealistic expectations, such as that an effective treatment will "cure" the pain, may not adhere to taking medication in the long term, even when it reduces the pain level significantly.

Assess Bodily Functions (Eating, Sleeping, and Sex)

Changes in eating habits may be a symptom of underlying depression, anxiety and frustration, or boredom. Obesity associated with overeating and reduced exercise has the potential to increase pain (Jamison et al., 1990). Sleep status also can provide clues as to underlying medical and/or psychological problems. While early morning awakening frequently accompanies depression, difficulty falling asleep can be symptomatic of anxiety. Important in cognitive and emotional function, sleep loss often can be ameliorated both with medication and with instruction in behavioral methods for controlling sleep. Pain often interferes with sexual function, which can create major relationship problems and accompanying psychological stress. Patients with pain-related sexual dysfunction may benefit from therapy (usually including their partner) designed to help them find alternative methods of sexual activity or the expression of affection, and work through emotional distress regarding sexual dysfunction (see Chapter 32).

Assess Quality of Life

Improving a patient's quality of life is considered one of the most important factors in the overall management of the patient with chronic disease. As discussed above, a number of factors may undermine the quality of life, only one of which is pain. The other factors also can have direct impact on pain perception, and thus need to be explored.

Treat the Patient's Pain to Facilitate the Work-up

Sometimes it is desirable to treat the pain early on in the assessment. Controlling the pain will allow the history, physical examination, and diagnostic work-up to proceed. Intravenous opioid analgesics or placement of an epidural analgesic can be used to gain control of pain quickly.

Define the Goals of Care

The goals of care are defined by what is possible at any particular time in the course of a disease. For example,

in patients with cancer, cure may be the initial goal of care. Later on, if a cure is not possible, goals may include good pain control, increased functional activity, traveling, and/or getting financial concerns in order. The physician and the patient may have very different goals of care. Because these goals might rarely be articulated, discussed, or defined, there often is a large gap between the doctor's and the patient's understanding of the state of the disease and what the options are for cure and further treatment. This gap can lead to significant dissatisfaction for both the patient and physician. The physician must make the state of the disease and the purpose behind therapeutic options clear to the patient. In the cancer population, for example, it is important to distinguish first-line chemotherapy designed to cure from third- or fourth-line chemotherapy designed to keep the tumor under control. Referral to needed hospice care commonly occurs too late, because the goals of care are not defined. For patients with debilitating back pain from arachnoiditis, a goal may be to have a patient spend quality time with family and friends, whereas regaining full employment may be unrealistic.

Determine Appropriate Diagnostic Work-up

Curiosity is not a sufficient reason to perform a diagnostic work-up. Diagnostic investigation should not be performed unless the results of the test would alter therapeutic interventions or provide important prognostic information.

Develop a Therapeutic Regimen

While oral analgesic therapy often provides the cornerstone of any therapeutic regimen, other non-pharmacologic therapies should be employed in cognitive-behavioral therapy or physical therapy. A balance between analgesia and side effects must be reached when medications are used.

Provide Continuity of Care Throughout the Course of Treatment

Patients often complain that they have so many doctors they don't know which one is in charge. Too often, no one is. The patient should be encouraged to select a physician or nurse who will coordinate the activities and information gathered from the various physicians. For patients with nonmalignant pain, it may be difficult to find a physician willing to take on responsibility for continuing care.

Reassess the Patient's Response to Pain Therapy

The success of any analgesic regimen needs to be assessed and reassessed so that the patient obtains good pain relief with minimal side effects. Over the course of time, the pathophysiology and severity of the pain may not remain stable, and analgesic needs may increase or decrease. Dosages may need to be adjusted or medications changed.

Consider Reevaluation and Further Work-up

If new pain develops or there is a change in the location, frequency, duration, or intensity of the pain, further work-up may be required. Pain can also be an important warning of a new pathologic process.

Pain Characteristics

Temporal Pattern

Different temporal patterns may suggest different etiologies and different diagnostic and therapeutic interventions. *Baseline pain* refers to the persistent ongoing nature of chronic pain. *Breakthrough pain* (Portenoy & Hagen, 1990), defined as episodic pain superimposed on baseline pain, may be spontaneous or the result of changes in mechanical stress referred to as *incident pain*. A survey found 64% of 90 patients with cancer pain reported breakthrough pain (Portenoy & Hagen, 1990). In another survey, 51.2% of 164 cancer pain patients had breakthrough pain the previous day. The median number of episodes was 6 per day (range, 1–60) (Portenoy et al., 1999b). A survey of 200 ambulatory patients with cancer found that 90% experienced pain with movement (Banning et al., 1991) or had incident pain. In a study of nonmalignant pain and terminal disease in a hospice, 63% of patients experienced breakthrough pain. The mean number of daily episodes of breakthrough pain was five (range, 1–13) (Zeppetella et al., 2001).

Location of the Pain

The area of pain may not always coincide with the area of pathology. Pain may be referred from a visceral source or result from the compression of a nerve root as in radicular pain (Hewitt, 1999).

Measuring Pain Intensity

Pain intensity is one of the most important characteristics of pain to assess and follow. Verbal rating scales can be very helpful (e.g., "none," "mild," "moderate," or "severe") and are relatively simple to use. Numeric scales are anchored by 0 at one end for no pain and 10 at the other for "worst pain imaginable" or "pain as bad as it could be." Visual analog scales use a straight line with the same anchors and ask the patient to make a mark along the line. Categoric scales use descriptive words to define pain intensity. For the pediatric population, scales can involve a range of faces from happy to very sad. The child is asked which face describes his or her pain experience best. Pain relief can be assessed as a percentage ranging from 0% pain relief to 100% pain relief. Because pain varies over time, it is also helpful to ask about worst pain, least pain, average pain, and pain now over either a 24-hour or 1-week time period. A number of standardized pain assessment tools are available to aid in the evaluation of pain. These include the Brief Pain Inventory, the McGill Pain Questionnaire, and the Memorial Pain Assessment Card. Assessment of pain intensity and relief helps determine the selection of analgesic therapy.

The language used by the patient to describe the pain can provide important information. The McGill Pain Questionnaire (Melzack, 1975) provides a standardized list of words in 20 categories and allows an evaluation of sensory, affective, and evaluative aspects of pain. In addition, the clinician can detect much about the patient by listening to the way that patient describes pain: a dramatized description such as in, "It feels like someone is sticking an ice pick in my back" suggests a strong affective component, in distinction to a description such as "It feels like a deep, dull ache right here."

Exacerbating Factors

It is important to ask patients about activities and situations that are associated with more pain or less pain. For example, a patient with metastatic disease to the hip will avoid standing and walking. Inquiring only about present pain while such a person is lying in a hospital bed and not about its pattern may lead to inappropriate conclusions.

Pain Quality

Because pain is subjective and often poorly correlated with the results from imaging, its assessment often depends on the use of words to describe it. Common descriptors include sharp, stinging, electrical, dull, aching, stabbing, or throbbing. These descriptors may suggest an underlying mechanism and pathophysiology for the pain. For example, burning pain with numbness and tingling, or pain that is electrical or shooting, is often associated with a neuropathic origin, whereas pain that is dull, aching, cramp-like, or throbbing, is often considered nociceptive.

Determination of the Inferred Pain Pathophysiology

The goal of any pain assessment is to define the presumed underlying pain pathophysiology based upon the pain characteristics discussed, findings on the examination (Arner & Meyerson, 1988; McQuay et al., 1992;

TABLE 33-1. Common Nociceptive Pain Syndromes

Low back pain

Osteoarthritis

Fibromyalgia

Myofascial pain

Metastatic bone pain

Pelvic pain

Discogenic pain

Facet pain

Cholecystitis

Pancreatitis

Hepatic abscess

TABLE 33-2. Common Neuropathic Pain Syndromes

Symmetric distal diabetic neuropathy

Postherpetic neuralgia

Trigeminal neuralgia

Sciatica

Radiculopathy

Phantom limb pain

Neuroma

Complex regional pain

Sympathetically maintained pain

Plexopathy

Thalamic pain

Spinal cord injury pain

Cesaro & Ollat, 1997), and diagnostic interventions, such as imaging. Pain has been divided into two predominant mechanisms: *nociceptive* and *neuropathic* (Arner & Meyerson, 1988). Distinguishing between nociceptive and neuropathic pain can be helpful in making a diagnosis and developing an analgesic regimen. Nociceptive pain arises from activation of primary afferent neurons called *nociceptors* following noxious stimuli such as injury to somatic or visceral structures. Nociceptors are present in skin, muscle, connective tissues, and viscera (Mense & Stahnke, 1983; Willis, 1985; Besson & Chaouch, 1987; Wall, 1989; Ness & Ge, 1990) and are normally silent. Somatic nociceptive pain is well localized and described as sharp, aching, throbbing, or pressure-like. Visceral nociceptive pain is more diffuse and described as gnawing or cramping when caused by obstruction of a hollow viscous and aching, sharp, or throbbing when due to involvement of organ capsules or other mesentery. Nociceptive pain is thought to respond to nonopioid and opioid analgesics (Cherny & Foley, 1994; Cherny & Portenoy, 1994; Cherny et al., 1995) and to procedures that denervate the peripheral lesion. Examples of nociceptive pain syndromes are given in Table 33-1.

Neuropathic pain arises from injury to neural structures, creating a site of aberrant somatosensory processing in the peripheral or central nervous system (Portenoy & Coyle, 1991; Portenoy & Kanner, 1996). This aberrant processing leads to unusual sensations called *dysesthesias* that refer to abnormal and unfamiliar pain that occurs in regions of motor, sensory, or autonomic dysfunction (Portenoy & Coyle, 1991). Common descriptors suggestive of neuropathic pain include burning, tingling, sharp, shooting, or electrical.

The first-line drugs for the treatment of neuropathic pain are the adjuvant analgesics, most commonly tricyclic antidepressants and antiepileptic drugs. Neuropathic pain is thought to respond less well to opioid drugs than nociceptive pain (Arner & Meyerson,

1988; Portenoy & Coyle, 1991). Examples of neuropathic pain syndromes are given in Table 33-2.

THERAPEUTIC METHODOLOGY

Though psychological and social issues may play an important role in the overall pain experience, a broad multimodality approach sometimes is not needed. Because pain may vary in its response to analgesic therapy, the breadth of the multimodality approach may also vary according to the specific pain and the patient's needs and goals. For example, a patient with trigeminal neuralgia may need only carbamazepine. If pain becomes well controlled, further therapeutic interventions are not necessary. More frequently, chronic pain syndromes do require a multidimensional approach to treatment. For example, a patient with chronic low back pain will more likely benefit from a combination of medication, physical therapy, and cognitive-behavioral approaches to pain control than from any approach used alone. Education is always an important part of pain management, because understanding basic aspects of pain will help the patient cope better.

The interdisciplinary approach includes the use of physical therapy modalities such as splints, exercises, and teaching proper body mechanics to alleviate pain. Interventional anesthetic and surgical approaches should also be considered whenever analgesic control is hard to obtain or systemic side effects become intolerable. Anesthetic approaches include nerve blocks, epidurals, and intrathecal pumps. Neurosurgical techniques can be helpful in a limited number of cases, though lesions of neural structures can often make pain worse after a period of time. Consequently, these more invasive techniques may be beneficial at the end of life. Neurostimulatory techniques also have a role, and include transcutaneous electrical nerve stimulator (TENS) units as well as spinal cord stimulators.

TABLE 33-3. Weak Opioid Analgesics

	Oral (mg)	IV (mg)	Peak (hr)	Duration (hr)	Half-life (hr)	Available dosages (mg)
Hydrocodone	20	NA	1	4–6	3.8–4.5	Plus acetaminopen: 500/2.5; 500/5; 500/7.5; 500/10; 650/10; 650/7.5
						Elixir 500/7.5 per 15 mL
						Plus aspirin: 500/5
						Plus ibuprofen: 200/7.5
Codeine	200	120	0.5–1	4–6	2.5–3.5	15, 30, 60
						Solution 15 mg/mL; 15/5 mL; 30 mg/mL
Propoxyphene[1]	32–65	NA		4–6	12	50, 65, 100
Meperidine[1]	200–300	75–100	0.5–1.0	3–4	3–4	PO 50, 100
			IM	4–6		IV 50 mg/5 mL
			1–2 PO			
Tramadol	50	NA	0.5		6.7–7.0	37.5 mg with 350 mg acetaminophen

IM, intramuscularly; IV, intravenously; NA, not, applicable; PO, orally.

[1] Contraindicated in patients with renal disease due to accumulation of toxic metabolite.

Involve the Patient in Deciding Treatment Options. Perceptions regarding pain and analgesia will vary among patients, so the approach to improving pain control must be individualized. Similarly, tolerance of therapeutic interventions and the occurrence of side effects will differ. Patients vary in their perceptions and expectations both in what they consider adequate levels of pain relief and what level of side effects are acceptable. Some will be interested in optimizing pain relief and care less about the underlying cause. Still others may be willing to put up with a significant amount of pain so as not to suffer from drug effects such as sedation.

Analgesics

A better understanding of the mechanisms that underlie chronic painful states has increased the effectiveness of treatment options. Analgesics are divided into three distinct classes: opioid analgesics (Tables 33-3 and 33-4), the adjuvant analgesics (Table 33-5), and the nonopioid analgesics (Table 33-6). The opioid drugs are similar to morphine and work by binding to opioid receptors. The availability of long-acting opioid analgesics has made a significant contribution to improving the treatment of chronic pain. The nonopioid analgesics include the nonsteroidal anti-inflammatory drugs (NSAIDs) as well as acetaminophen. One of the most significant advances in pain management is the availability of cyclooxygenase-2 (COX-2) inhibitors with better side effect profiles than the traditional NSAIDs.

The adjuvant analgesics are medications whose initial indications did not include pain control, but were ultimately found to have analgesic properties. The antidepressants and anticonvulsants are two major classes of adjuvant analgesics. The number of adjuvant analgesics has increased recently with newer and safer anticonvulsant drugs and antidepressants. Effective use of all analgesics requires familiarity with pharmacology, dosing and dose titration, and treatment of adverse effects.

Route of Administration

The best way to manage pain is through the least invasive approach possible, which, in most instances, is the oral route of administration. Other routes may be needed when the oral route is not tolerated, but for most malignant and nonmalignant pain the oral route is the preferred because it is effective and safer than more invasive techniques.

The Three-Step Analgesic Ladder of the World Health Organization

The Three-Step Analgesic Ladder of the World Health Organization (WHO) (Ventafridda et al., 1985; WHO, 1990; Foley & Portenoy, 1993; Stjernsward et al., 1996) is the most widely accepted guideline for the treatment of cancer pain. The WHO analgesic ladder provides a good model for non-cancer pain as well. This approach bases the selection of analgesic therapy on the

TABLE 33-4. Strong Opioid Analgesics

	Oral (mg)	IV (mg)	Rectal (mg)	Peak (hr)	Duration (hr)	Half-life (hr)	Available dosages (mg)
Morphine sulfate	30–60	10–15	30	5–1.0 IM 1–1.5 PO	3–5 IM 3–4 PO	2–4	Solution 20 mg/mL; 100 mg/5 mL; 20 mg/5 mL; Tablet 15, 30
Morphine (long-acting)	30–60	NA	90	2.5	8–12	2–4	BID 15, 30, 60, 100 QD 20, 50, 100
Oxycodone	20	NA	NA	1	3–5	2–5	Sol 5 mg/mL, 20 mg/mL Tablet 5 mg, 5 mg/mL, Plus acetaminophen: 325/5; 650/10; 325/2; 500/5; 500/7.5 Plus aspirin 325/4.5
Oxycodone (long-acting)	30	NA		1.5	8–12	Initial 0.6 Secondary 6.2	10, 20, 40, 80, 160
Fentanyl	μ/hr NA	100 mg	NA	0.5	1–2 patch: 3 days	4–21	Patch 25 g/mL, 50 mL, 75 mL, 100 hr OTFC: 200, 400, 600, 800, 1200, 1600
Hydromorphone	7.5	1.5	6	0.5–1.0 IM 1.5–2.0 PO	3–4 IM 4–6 PO	2–3	IV, 1, 2, 4, 10 mg/mL 50 mg/ 5 mL; 500 mg/ 50 mL PO 2; 4; 8
Oxymorphone		1	10	0.5–1.0	3–5	2–3	Numorphan 5 mg suppository
Methadone[1]	20	10	NA	0.5–1.0 IM 1.5–2.0 PO	4–8 IM 4–12 PO	15–30	PO 5, 10 IV 10 mg/mL
Levorphanol[1]	4	2	NA	0.5–1.0 IM 1.5–2.0 PO	4–6 IM 4–7 PO	12–16	2

Table is meant only as a guide. Due to incomplete cross-tolerance the dose calculated from the above chart needs to be decreased by 50%. Special care must be taken when converting to methadone: dose must be decreased by 75%–90% of the calculated dose.

[1] Plasma $T_{1/2}$ much greater than duration of action can lead to drug accumulation.

BID, twice daily; IM, intramuscularly; IV, intravenously; NA, not applicable; OTFC, oral transmucosal fentanyl citrate (Fentanyl Oralet); PO, orally; QD, every day.

severity of pain. The first step of the ladder recommends either an adjuvant analgesic or a nonopioid analgesic, most often an NSAID for the treatment of mild pain. The second level recommends the use of a weak opioid for the treatment of moderate pain. Weak opioids include tramadol, codeine, hydrocodone, oxycodone, and propoxyphene. Combing weak opioids with aspirin, acetaminophen, or ibuprofen potentiates the analgesic effect of the weak opioid and provides analgesia through another mechanism of action. Adding acetaminophen, aspirin, or an NSAID can potentiate the analgesic effect of the opioid, allowing lower doses to be used. This effect is referred to as *opioid sparing*. Aspirin, acetaminophen, and NSAIDs also improve analgesia by working on a separate mechanism of action from the opioid. All have short half-lives and duration of action (3–4 hours). The third tier of the WHO ladder recommends a strong opioid analgesic, such as morphine or hydromorphone, for the treatment of severe pain. Strong opioid analgesics include morphine, hydromorphone, fentanyl, methadone, levorphanol, and oxycodone. On both steps 2 and 3 of the ladder NSAIDs and adjuvant analgesics are also recommended to potentiate the effect of the opioid.

Is the Pain Syndrome Opioid Responsive?

Before initiating opioid analgesic therapy, it is important to consider whether the pain can be expected to be opioid responsive and whether the pain is severe enough

TABLE 33-5. Adjuvant Analgesics

	Starting dose (mg/d)	Effective dose range (mg/d)	Dosing schedule
Anticonvulsants			
Carbamazepine	200	600–1,200	Q6–8h
Clonazepam	0.5	0.5–3	Q8h
Divalproex sodium	500	1,500–3,000	Q8h
Phenytoin PO[1]	300	300	QHS
Phenytoin IV	500–1,000		Loading dose
Topiramate	25 g	100–200	BID
Gabapentin	100	1,800–3,600+	Q8h
Tricyclic antidepressants			
Amitriptyline	10–25	50–150	QHS
Clomipramine	10–25	50–150	QHS
Desipramine	10–25	50–150	QHS
Doxepin	10–25	50–150	QHS
Imipramine	10–25	50–150	QHS
Nortriptyline	10–25	50–150	QHS
New antidepressants[2]			
Fluoxetine	10–20	20–40	QD
Citalopram	10–20	20–60	QD
Venlafaxine	37.5	37.5–75	BID, TID
Paroxetine	20	20–40	QD
Local anesthetics			
Mexiletine	150	900–1,200	Q8h
Lidocaine iv Subcutaneous, IV	2–5 mg/kg	2.5 mg/kg/h	Bolus PRN, infuse over 20–30 minutes Continuous infusion
Lidoderm patch	5%	1–3 patches	QD 12 hours on, 12 hours off
Lidocaine/prilocaine topical cream	2.5/2.5%	Cover the affected area with occlusive dressing.	QID
Others			
Baclofen	15	30–200	Q8h
Calcitonin subcutaneous, IV	25 IU	100–200 IU	QD
Calcitonin nasal spray	200 IU	200–400 IU	QD
Clonidine transdermal	0.1	TTS-1, TTS-2, or TTS-3	Q7 days
Tizanidine hydrochloride	2 mg		Q8h

[1] Can give oral loading dose: 500 mg PO X 2.

[2] Analgesic efficacy less reliable than efficacy of TCAs.

TABLE 33-6. Nonopioid Analgesics

	Recommended starting dose (mg)	Dosing schedule	Maximum oral dose (mg/day)	Peak effect (hr)	Duration (hr)	Half-life (hr)
Acetaminophen	650	Q4–6h	4,000–6,000	0.5–1.0	4–6	0.25
Aspirin	650	Q4–6h	4,000–6,000	2	4–6	1–4
Choline magnesium trisalicylate[1]	500–1,000	Q12h	4,000	0.5–1.0	>12	2–30
Etodolac	200–400	Q6–8h	1,200	2	4–6	6
Diclofenac	25	Q8h	150	1	8	1–2
Diflunisal	200–500	Q12h	1,500	1–2	>12	8–20
Sulindac	150–200	BID	400	1–2	12	7–18
Indomethacin	25–75	BID or QID	200	2	6–8	2–3
Mefenamic acid	500	Q6–8h	1,000	2	2–4	3–4
Ibuprofen[2]	400	Q6h	3,200	1–2	4–6	2
Ketoprofen[3]	25	Q6–8h	300	1–2	6	1–35
Ketorolac	60 IM/IV 30	Single dose Q6h	120	0.5–1	6	5
Ketorolac[4]	10	Q6h	40	<1	6	5
Naproxen	250	Q12h	1,025–1,375	2	8–12	12–15
Oxaprozin	1200	QD		3–6	24	59
Salsalate	500–1,000	Q12h	4,000	0.5–2	3–7	1
Refocoxib[1]	12.5–50[5]	QD	50	2–3	24	17
Celecoxib[1]	100–200	BID, QD	400	2.8	12–24	11.2
Valdecoxib	10	QD	20	3	24	8.1

Group has significant interactions with ACE inhibitors and beta blockers.

[1] No effect on platelet aggregation.

[2] Suspension available.

[3] Rectal and topical gel formulations.

[4] Should not use for more than 5 days.

[5] Should not stay on 50 mg for more than 5 days. h, hour; IM, intramuscularly; IV, intravenously; Q, every.

to start opioid analgesic therapy. Though not all pain is equally responsive to opioid therapy, it is appropriate to try a strong opioid analgesic when pain is severe. The opioid responsiveness of neuropathic pain has been the source of debate, but recent studies clearly demonstrate that it is more appropriate to consider neuropathic pain "relatively" opioid responsive, in that higher doses may be needed to obtain adequate pain relief (Portenoy et al., 1990; Cherny et al., 1994b). Brachial plexopathy from tumor invasion is an example of a severe neuropathic pain syndrome that may respond to an adjuvant analgesic, but an opioid is often helpful as well. On the other hand, trigeminal neuralgia is a very severe neuropathic pain syndrome that often responds well to carbamazepine and is less likely to be effectively treated with an opioid analgesic.

Starting Therapy

Patients who have had limited exposure to opioids should begin at a low dose, starting at the equivalent of 5 to 10 mg of parenteral morphine every 4 hours. Short-acting opioid analgesics should be used first and dosed around the clock. Extra doses of medication should be provided for episodes of breakthrough pain. Once the patient is tolerating the medication, longer-acting preparations should be used. Both morphine and oxycodone come in long-acting formulations lasting 12 hours, and morphine also comes in a 24-hour preparation. Fentanyl has been formulated into a 3-day patch. These long-acting medications should be given on an around-the-clock basis, to avoid the large peaks and troughs that accompany the short-acting opioid analgesics. These long-acting preparations should then be supplemented with short-acting opioids as rescues for breakthrough pain. When patients with chronic pain are given intravenous opioid analgesics, they should receive a baseline infusion supplemented by rescue doses as needed. These doses are frequently given using patient controlled analgesia devices.

The recommended size of the rescue dose ranges from 5% to 15% of the total previous 24-hour opioid dose. It is often given every 2 to 3 hours with oral regimens and every 10 to 15 minutes with intravenous regimens. When more than four rescues are given in a 24-hour period, consideration should be given to increasing the long-acting medication. In such a case, the short-acting rescues should also be increased so that they remain at 5% to 15% of the total 24-hour dose of long-acting opioid. The dose and frequency should be individualized and titrated carefully to achieve a balance between analgesia and side effects. The dose can be increased by calculating the amount of rescue medication given over the previous 24 hours and adding it to the amount of long-acting opioid taken. Once this total 24-hour dose has been calculated, a decision must be made to either increase this dose or keep it unchanged. If the patient's pain is well controlled, but the number of rescues exceeded four in a 24-hour period, it is reasonable to increase the long-acting opioid by the amount of short-acting opioid given and convert the total to the long-acting formulation. On the other hand, if the patient's pain was not well controlled, the total daily dose can be increased by 30% to 50% and provided in a long-acting formulation supplemented by short-acting rescues for breakthrough pain. It is important to increase the rescue medication so it remains at about the same ratio to the long-acting medication.

In the setting of an acute pain crisis, opioid titration can be performed more quickly. Intravenous doses of an opioid can be given every 15 to 20 minutes until pain control is reached. The dose can also be doubled every 20 minutes until analgesia is achieved (Hagen et al., 1997), but care must be taken that patients not become overly sedated and develop respiratory depression. This method of obtaining pain control requires close observation. The hourly infusion rate is calculated by adding up the amount of opioid that was given and dividing by twice the half-life of that medication. For example, if a patient received a 5-mg dose of morphine followed by a 10-mg and a 20-mg dose, the total dose given would be 35 mg of morphine. The half-life of morphine is 3 hours, so the hourly dose could be about 6 mg/hr (35 divided by 6).

Start Low, Go Slow, and Dose to Effect or Side Effect

All analgesic medications should be started at a low dose. Increase the medication by a slow titration so as to avoid or limit side effects. The dose should then be increased gradually until adequate analgesia is obtained or intolerable side effects occur. Slow titration often allows patients to tolerate high doses.

Use Long-Acting Opioid Analgesics Supplemented with Short-Acting Opioids

Many of the long acting opioids have short-acting preparations which can be used with them; the exceptions are levorphanol and methadone, which are by their inherent pharmacology long-acting. It is often convenient, but by no means necessary, to have the long- and short-acting medications be the same.

Controlled-release morphine (Warfield, 1998), controlled release oxycodone (Citron et al., 1998; Kaplan et al., 1998; Parris et al., 1998), and transdermal fentanyl (Sloan et al., 1998) have been shown to be effective in the management of chronic cancer pain and have gained acceptance for the management of non-cancer pain (Roth et al., 2000; Cheville et al., 2001). The transdermal fentanyl patch reaches peak levels within 14 hours and has an elimination half-life that exceeds 24 hours. This patch system is associated with fewer gastrointestinal side effects (nausea, vomiting, and constipation) and better alertness and sleep quality than other long-acting opioid preparations (Payne et al., 1998; Sloan et al., 1998). In one study of 504 cancer patients, those who received transdermal fentanyl were significantly more satisfied overall with their pain medication than those who received sustained-release oral forms of morphine ($P = 0.035$), even though the groups did not differ significantly on pain intensity, sleep adequacy, and other symptoms (Payne et al., 1998).

A new fast-acting analgesic for breakthrough pain is oral transmucosal fentanyl citrate (OTFC), in which the potent synthetic mu-agonist fentanyl is embedded in a sweetened matrix that is dissolved in the mouth. A recent randomized double-blind trial found that this preparation was very effective and had a rapid onset of action (Portenoy et al., 1999a).

No-Ceiling Effect Allows for Ability to Increase Dose

One of the great advantages of opioid analgesic therapy with pure mu-opioid agonists is the absence of a ceiling dose. Nonopioid analgesics have a dose above which no further analgesia is expected to occur, but pure mu-opioids can be increased with the expectation of improved analgesia. The dose can be increased until analgesia is obtained or until analgesia reaches a balance with side effects. Of course, there are some practical issues that prevent titration to infinitely higher doses, including the expense of the medication or the number of pills that can be taken by the oral route.

Unlike the pure mu-agonists, the mixed opioid agonists—antagonists, such as pentazocine, butorphanol, dezocine, and nalbuphine, do have a ceiling effect. When added to pure mu-agonists, they also have the potential to reverse analgesia and cause a physical withdrawal syndrome. These medications should therefore not be used to treat chronic pain syndromes (Portenoy, 1993; Jacox et al., 1994; Portenoy & Lesage, 1999). Meperidine and propoxyphene are popular drugs among patients, and physicians like to prescribe them because they are considered weak opioids and thought to be relatively safe; however, both drugs have a ceiling effect, and chronic use at high doses can lead to an increase to toxic serum levels of their metabolite, normeperidine and norpropoxyphene. Higher doses of meperidine can produce intractable seizures. Similarly, norpropoxyphene has a long half-life and accumulation can lead to adverse side effects, including severe psychotomimetic effects.

Tailor Analgesic Therapy to the Individual Patient

Though a number of guidelines have been published to help manage chronic pain, it is important to individualize therapy. Sometimes creative and unique methods may need to be tried. This need may be present particularly in the elderly, who may have toxic effects from medications at lower doses due to greater sensitivity that occurs with changes in physiology associated with the aging process (Hewitt & Foley, 1996).

Alternate Routes of Administration

While the oral route is generally preferred, a number of factors such as disease progression, intolerance to one route of administration, the need for faster pain relief, and convenience can necessitate a change from the oral to another route of administration (Cherny et al., 1995). Alternative routes to consider include sublingual, transmucosal, transdermal, rectal, intravenous, epidural, intrathecal (Ventafridda et al., 1987c; Devulder et al., 1994; Mercadante & Fulfaro, 1999), and intraventricular. One option for patients with difficulty swallowing is one form of sustained-release morphine (Kadian) that contains polymer-coated pellets that can be sprinkled on a small amount of applesauce and ingested. The pellets

release morphine at a steady state for up to 24 hours, allowing for once-a-day dosing. Transdermal fentanyl would also be reasonable in this setting.

Medications that Work through Transmucosal Absorption

This route is popular in the hospice setting where liquid morphine or hydromorphone is commonly given; however, transmucosal absorption does not work well for these drugs. Fentanyl, buprenorphine, and methadone are better alternatives because they are highly lipophilic and therefore well absorbed through the oral mucosa (Weinberg et al., 1988). The fast onset of action makes the transmucosal route ideal for breakthrough pain (Mercadante & Fulfaro, 1999). The sublingual approach can also be helpful in patients who have trouble swallowing.

The rectal route is commonly employed in the hospice setting and is an effective route of administration. Morphine, hydromorphine, oxymorphone, and controlled-release oral morphine tablets can be administered rectally.

Parenteral administration should be considered for patients who need rapid onset of analgesia, or require doses so high that they cannot be administered conveniently through the oral route. Patients with gastrointestinal obstruction, impaired swallowing, and significant breakthrough and incident pain are candidates for employing the parenteral route. To avoid both the peak dose side effects and trough-related breakthrough pain that occurs with repeated parenteral boluses, a continuous intravenous or subcutaneous infusion should be used. A subcutaneous 25- to 27-gauge butterfly needle can be left in place for up to 1 week (Coyle et al., 1994). Intravenous and indwelling lines can also be placed. Continuous basal rate infusion with rescue doses multiple times per hour can be obtained using patient-controlled analgesic pumps (PCAs).

Management of Common Side Effects

Expertise in the management of chronic pain requires the ability to manage the troubling side effects that can occur as a result of opioid analgesic therapy. Common side effects of opioid analgesic therapy include nausea and vomiting, sedation, cognitive slowing, respiratory depression, pruritus, and myoclonic jerks (sudden movements similar to those sometimes experienced when falling asleep). A troubling and often overlooked side effect is isolated components of a delirium, consisting of vivid dreams or even hallucinations that occur on waking up or falling asleep at night.

These are often easily treated. Psychostimulants such as methylphenidate, modafinil, and a combination product of amphetamine/dextroamphetamine can be used to treat sedation. Nausea can be treated by adding prochlorperazine, metoclopramide, promethazine, trimethobenzamide, or dronabinol. Constipation can be treated using bisacodyl, cascara sagrada, methylcellulose, docusate sodium, senna, glycerin suppositories, polyethylene glycol, lactulose, magnesium citrate, psyllium, mineral oil, and the combination of docusate/casanthranol. Antipsychotic medications such as haloperidol can be used to manage opioid-induced delirium. Myoclonus can be treated using low-dose clonazepam. Naloxone is used to treat respiratory depression, but care must be taken when it is administered to patients on chronic opioid therapy who require much less naloxone than others to reverse sedation and respiratory depression. Consequently, naloxone must be diluted 1:10 and administered slowly.

Side Effects—To Treat or Not to Treat

Tolerance develops to nausea, sedation, respiratory depression, and cognitive slowing, but not to constipation. Because tolerance to most opioid side effects will occur over time, a decision must be made when a side effect is encountered—wait until tolerance develops, treat the side effect, change to another opioid, or change the route of administration. Adding another medication to treat a side effect may make an already burdensome regimen more complicated. Unexpected drug interactions may occur and polypharmacy may interfere with adherence. When side effects are minimal, the patient may elect to keep on the medication for a time until tolerance develops. If the side effects are significant, but the opioid is providing good analgesia, treating the side effect is reasonable.

Importantly, experiencing side effects to one opioid does not mean that the patient will have side effects to all opioids. Consequently, an important option when encountering a side effect is to consider switching to another opioid analgesic.

Sequential trials are often needed in order to find the most effective opioid analgesic with the fewest side effects (Ashby et al., 1999). Also referred to as *opioid rotation*, sequential trials should be considered a routine part of cancer and noncancer pain management. In changing from one opioid to another, one can find the best tolerated drug for the particular individual.

The success of opioid rotation stems in part from the finding that tolerance that occurs with long-term therapy with one opioid analgesic does not lead to an equivalent level of tolerance to other opioids. This incomplete cross-tolerance often allows the dose of the new opioid to be reduced relative to what would have been the equianalgesic dose calculated from commonly used equianalgesic tables. Similarly, tolerance to opioid-related side effects is often incomplete as well (Cherny et al., 1995).

The risk of adhering to the published equianalgesic tables without consideration of incomplete cross-tolerance and without decreasing the calculated dose of the new drug by 50% may lead to significant and potentially dangerous side effects. The equianalgesic dose tables are derived from single dose studies and should provide a rough guide when selecting a starting dose of a drug or when changing the route of administration of a current drug. When switching to another opioid, it is important to calculate the total amount of opioid that was given in the previous 24 hours, calculate the equianalgesic dose, and then, for most opioids, decrease the dose by 30% to 50%. For unclear reasons, methadone is an exception to the 50% rule. Because it has an even greater degree of incomplete cross-tolerance, it is important to decrease the calculated dose of methadone by >90% (Bruera et al., 1996). Ample use of rescue doses when switching from one opioid to another will ensure that conversion to the new opioid does not produce more pain or withdrawal symptoms.

Comparison among Opioids

Because performing sequential trials of opioid analgesics is now commonly accepted practice, a greater understanding of the relative potency of these drugs has developed. While direct comparison of efficacy among the opioids for chronic pain is rare, some recent studies have revealed, for example, that controlled release formulations of oxycodone and morphine showed comparable analgesia at a ratio of 2:3 (Heiskanen & Kalso, 1997).

The unique compound tramadol is a centrally acting analgesic that binds to the mu opioid receptor and inhibits the reuptake of norepinephrine and serotonin. It has been approved for the treatment of moderate to moderately severe pain (Sunshine, 1994; Wilder-Smith et al., 1994), and has been shown to be useful in treating cancer pain (Eisenberg et al., 1994) as well as neuropathic pain (Harati et al., 1998). In one study, a dose of 50 mg tramadol provided similar analgesia to that of 60 mg codeine or 30 mg codeine plus 650 mg acetaminophen in patients with procedure-related pain (Rawal et al., 2001). A combination of tramadol 37.5 mg with acetaminophen 350 mg has recently become available and is well tolerated (Ultracet) (Medve et al., 2001). After oral surgery, two tablets of this compound provided a similar level of analgesia to that provided by a combination of hydrocodone 10 mg and acetaminophen 650 mg with less nausea and vomiting (Fricke, 2002).

Care should also be exercised when converting from other opioids to methadone. In one study (Manfredi et al., 1997), the effective methadone dose converted from hydromorphone was only 3% of the equianalgesic dose calculated from the standard tables of conversion. Comparing rotation from morphine to methadone demonstrated a unified median dose ratio of 11.2:1 in one study (Lawlor et al., 1998), while another found a median ratio of 7.75:1 (Ripamonti et al., 1998). The conversion ratio was strongly dependent on the previous morphine dose, supporting the concept that incomplete cross-tolerance increases at higher opioid doses. Thus chronic opioid exposure changes the equianalgesic ratios and this divergence increases at higher doses, necessitating great care when converting between high-dose chronic morphine and methadone.

One possible explanation for the significant incomplete cross-tolerance associated with conversion from another opioid to methadone is that another analgesic mechanism might be involved (Morley & Makin, 1998; Makin & Ellershaw, 1998). The racemic mixture of methadone demonstrates that the d- and l-isomers of methadone bind to the NMDA receptor (Gormanet al., 1997). The d-isomer is weak or inactive at the opioid receptor, but is antinociceptive for neuropathic pain as an antagonist at the NMDA receptor (Ebert et al., 1995).

Nonopioid Analgesics

Acetaminophen and NSAIDs are helpful in the management of chronic pain (see Table 33-6). They can be used for mild pain and in conjunction with opioid analgesics for moderate to severe chronic pain. An important distinguishing characteristic of acetaminophen and the NSAIDs that sets them apart from the opioid analgesics is that there is a ceiling dose for analgesia. These nonopioids also have a minimum effective dose below which analgesia would not be expected. Importantly, these minimum and maximum doses vary among individuals and produce dose-dependent analgesic effects between these two points.

There is great individual variability among the NSAIDs in both efficacy and side effects. While acetaminophen is analgesic, NSAIDs are both analgesic and anti-inflammatory. The dose of acetaminophen should not exceed 4 gm per day due to the increased risk of liver damage (Jacox et al., 1994; Cherny & Foley, 1996). Because they treat inflammation and have an additive benefit when combined with opioid analgesics, NSAIDs allow lower doses of opioid to be used. NSAIDs should also be considered when treating musculoskeletal, postoperative, and traumatic pain, and headache. NSAIDs have significant gastrointestinal side effects, and can produce renal and hepatic dysfunction and bleeding by interfering with platelet function. They also can interfere with ACE inhibitors and beta blockers and produce problematic edema. The NSAIDs can be very effective, but it may take weeks for the full analgesic effect to occur. A trial of a few different NSAIDs is reasonable, because some may work better than others in particular individuals.

One of the most important advances in the treatment of chronic pain, especially chronic cancer pain, is the more specific COX-2 inhibitors (Moreland & St Clair, 1999). These COX-2 inhibitors have less of an antiplatelet effect and can decrease the risk of gastrointestinal ulcerations (Eisenberg et al., 1994). Currently there are three COX-2 inhibitors on the market: celecoxib, rofecoxib, and valdecoxib. Because low platelet counts and increased risk of hemorrhage can occur from cancer and platelet counts are reduced during chemotherapy, these medications are ideal for the cancer pain population. The nonacetylated salicylates also do not interfere with platelet function and, consequently, also reduce the risk of bleeding. An example is choline magnesium trisalicylate.

Corticosteroids are effective analgesics in a number of diverse nociceptive and neuropathic pain syndromes. Corticosteroids have been used to treat both cancer-related and non-cancer-related pain syndromes (Watanabe & Bruera, 1994). Large infusions of steroids can alleviate severe pain from bone metastasis or compression of a nerve plexus. They then can be discontinued after a rapid taper or reduced to an effective long-term dose (Moore et al., 1994; Tannock et al., 1996). Long-term treatment with steroids is associated with significant adverse effects, such as adrenal suppression, trophic changes, and osteoporosis. As a consequence, the combination of thinning of the mucosal wall with steroids and constipation produced with opioids increase the risk of developing a perforated viscus.

Adjuvant Analgesics

Adjuvant analgesics comprise the third class of analgesics that are important in the treatment of chronic pain (see Table 33-5), defined as medications whose primary indication is for something other than the treatment of pain, but which have been found to have analgesic potential. Though some of the anticonvulsants and the antidepressants are effective analgesics, particularly for the treatment of neuropathic pain, only a relatively small number have been rigorously investigated in randomized, double-blind, placebo-controlled trials. Growing insight into mechanisms that underlie the transmission and encoding of chronic pain has led to investigations of medications that are likely to have analgesic effects. As the name implies, adjuvant drugs are commonly added to other medications to enhance their analgesic effects, but they can also be used as single line therapy for the treatment of some chronic pain syndromes.

The successful use of adjuvant analgesics requires a trial-and-error approach. Medications must be started at a low dose to avoid toxicity and then titrated to analgesic effect or until unacceptable side effects occur.

Determining an appropriate evidence-based algorithm from the available literature is not possible. Most of the few studies that are available are in comparison with placebo rather than other adjuvant analgesics.

The antidepressants (Noyes, 1981; Ventafridda et al., 1987a; Panerai et al., 1991) have demonstrated efficacy in the treatment of lancinating and dysesthetic neuropathic pain and should be used early on in the treatment of chronic pain when the presumed pathophysiology is neuropathic (Portenoy, 1998).

Amitriptyline (Watson, 1994a) is the most commonly used antidepressant for treating neuropathic pain. Doses can be started at 25 mg at night and slowly titrated upward every few days until analgesia is achieved or intolerable side effects occur. In the elderly, therapy should begin with a 10-mg dose. The most troubling side effects include sedation and anticholinergic effects. The secondary amine tricyclics, nortriptyline and desipramine, cause fewer side effects. Doses can be tolerated to as high as 100 to 150 mg nortriptyline or 150 to 300 mg desipramine.

Though the analgesic effect is independent of the antidepressant effect (Max et al., 1987), the latter can be very helpful in treating depression and avoiding polypharmacy. Pain relief occurs faster than the antidepressant effects (Max et al., 1991; Max et al., 1992). Serum levels can be tested to evaluate adherence and to assess whether patients are fast or slow metabolizers. Adjuvant analgesics can be useful in non-neuropathic pain states as well. A comparison of amitriptyline versus nortriptyline demonstrated the latter to be as analgesic and better tolerated (Watson et al., 1998).

The evidence for the use of newer antidepressants is less convincing (Sindrup & Jensen, 1999), but citalopram and paroxetine seem to be effective in some neuropathic pain conditions (Max, 1994). Venlafaxine has been reported to be effective for neuropathic pain (Sumpton & Moulin, 2001) and so has fluoxetine (Theesen & Marsh, 1989), but only from case reports. In double-blind placebo-controlled trials of analgesic efficacy, fluoxetine has shown effectiveness in chronic daily headache (Saper et al., 1994), fibromyalgia (Goldenberg et al., 1996), and rheumatic pain (Rani et al., 1996).

Anticonvulsants

Anticonvulsants are used to manage pain (Kloke et al., 1991; Bhatia, 1992; De Conno et al., 1993; Kenner, 1994; Brant, 1998; Grond et al., 1999). The number of anticonvulsants that are available has increased recently and they are commonly used to treat pain with a presumed neuropathic physiology (Max et al., 1991, 1992), with confirmed utility in diverse neuropathic pain syndromes (Backonja, 2000). The best studied of the newer anticonvulsants for the treatment of neuro-

pathic pain is gabapentin. Double-blind placebo-controlled studies have shown gabapentin to be effective for diabetic neuropathy (Backonja et al., 1998; Gorson et al., 1999) and postherpetic neuralgia (Rowbotham et al., 1998). Similar studies have revealed the effectiveness of lamotrigine in the treatment of central pain (Vestergaard et al., 2001), HIV-associated painful neuropathy (Simpson et al., 2000), trigeminal neuralgia (Zakrzewska et al., 1997), postoperative pain, and other neuropathic pain states (McCleane, 2000). Carbamazepine has been shown to be effective in the treatment of trigeminal neuralgia and diabetic neuropathy (Killian & Fromm, 1968; Nicol, 1969; Rull et al., 1969; Gale et al., 1995), and oxcarbazepine in the treatment of trigeminal neuralgia (Zakrzewska & Patsalos, 1989). Topiramate is also gaining recognition and support as an adjuvant analgesic for the treatment of neuropathic pain (Chong, 2003). Determining which anticonvulsant should be the first-line choice for the treatment of neuropathic pain remains unclear and comparative studies are needed.

Topical Substances

Topical substances can be effective in managing some neuropathic pain syndromes and have the advantage of avoiding systemic side effects. EMLA cream has been used to reduce pain prior to procedures such as venous or arterial catheterization, lumbar puncture, and bone marrow aspiration (Kapelushnik et al., 1990; Miser et al., 1994; Holdsworth et al., 1997). Neuropathic pain may respond well to topical EMLA (Yosipovitch et al., 1999; Fassoulaki et al., 2000). It is recommended that the cream be either applied thickly and covered with an occlusive dressing or applied thinly without a dressing. The Lidoderm patch is a new formulation that can be useful for areas of hyperalgesia (Argoff, 2000; Devers & Galer, 2000). At this time, it is approved for the treatment of postherpetic neuralgia (Rowbotham et al., 1996; Galer et al., 1999b). This patch is convenient and can be cut into small pieces. It is recommended that patients keep the patch on for 12 hours and off for 12 hours. Injections of lidocaine can also be useful (Cherny & Portenoy, 1994). Capsaicin has also been used for the treatment of chronic osteoarthritis pain and neuropathic pain (Rumsfield & West, 1991; Pfeifer et al., 1993; Watson, 1994b). Pretreatment with EMLA can help patients tolerate the burning associated with capsaicin better (Yosipovitch et al., 1999).

Other Adjuvant Analgesics

A number of other medications have been explored for their analgesic potential. The oral local anesthetic mexiletine (Dejgard 1988; Ackerman et al., 1991; Kubota et al., 1991; Wright, 1994) is helpful in some neuropathic pain syndromes, but should be used with caution due to its cardiac effects. Calcitonin is effective in the management of cancer pain associated with bone metastases and nerve compression (Serdengecti et al., 1986; Schiraldi et al., 1987; Miseria et al., 1989; Szanto et al., 1992; Kovcin et al., 1994; Schnur, 1996) and has been used in complex regional pain syndromes I and II (Gobelet et al., 1992; Hamamci et al., 1996; Kingery, 1997) and in phantom limb pain (Kessel & Worz, 1987; Fiddler & Hindman, 1991; Jaeger & Maier, 1992; Wall & Heyneman, 1999). The alpha-2 agonists tizanidine and clonidine are also analgesic in a diverse number of neuropathic pain syndromes as well as headache disorders. Tizanidine was found to be effective in the treatment of trigeminal neuralgia (Fromm et al., 1993), headache (Fogelholm & Murros, 1992), and low back pain (Berry & Hutchinson, 1988a,b).

Antagonists to the NMDA receptor represent a potentially new class of analgesic medications. Ketamine, a commonly used anesthetic, can produce analgesia in subanesthetic doses. Dextromethorphan, a common ingredient in some cough remedies, has been shown to be effective in the treatment of diabetic neuropathy (Nelson et al., 1997). As discussed above, recent studies of methadone suggest that it may provide analgesia as a mu receptor agonist and an NMDA receptor antagonist (Foley & Houde, 1998).

CONCLUSIONS

The successful treatment of chronic pain requires a cognitive-behavioral approach to both diagnosis and treatment. Behavioral issues that impact the total pain must be assessed, and behavioral approaches are often needed if successful control of chronic pain is to be achieved. Analgesics that are commonly used may have their own cognitive and behavioral side effects. A coherent methodology must assess the complaint of pain, determine an appropriate diagnostic work-up, and then develop an analgesic regimen designed to alleviate pain, improve quality of life and limit side effects.

■ KEY POINTS

☐ The successful treatment of chronic pain requires attention to the associated psychological and behavioral factors that can either predate or result from ongoing, unrelieved pain.

☐ Lack of patient education remains the most significant barrier to adequate pain control.

☐ Patients with chronic pain may or may not have significant psychological and social comorbidities, but it is vitally important to be aware that they may be present and to explore pertinent psychosocial issues.

☐ The goal of pain management is to optimize analgesia, minimize side effects, and increase function.

☐ Depression is widely recognized as the most prominent emotion associated with chronic pain. Patients with chronic pain should be screened for symptoms of depression.

☐ An analgesic regimen must be designed to alleviate pain, improve quality of life, and limit side effects.

KEY READINGS

Backonja M, Beydoun A, Edwards KR, et al: Gabapentin for the symptomatic treatment of painful neuropathy in patients with diabetes mellitus: A randomized controlled trial. JAMA 280:1831–1836, 1998.

Casey KL, Minoshima S, Berger KL, et al: Positron emission tomographic analysis of cerebral structures activated specifically by repetitive noxious heat stimuli. J Neurophysiol 71:802–807, 1994.

Cheville A, Chen A, Oster G, et al: A randomized trial of controlled-release oxycodone during inpatient rehabilitation following unilateral total knee arthroplasty. J Bone Joint Surg Am 83:572–576, 2001.

Chong MS, Libretto SE: The rationale and use of topiramate for treating neuropathic pain. Clin J Pain 19:59–68, 2003.

Harati Y, Gooch C, Swenson M, et al: Double-blind randomized trial of tramadol for the treatment of the pain of diabetic neuropathy. Neurology 50:1842–1846, 1998.

Parris WC, Johnson BW Jr, et al: The use of controlled-release oxycodone for the treatment of chronic cancer pain: A randomized, double-blind study. J Pain Symptom Manage 16:205–211, 1998.

Watson CP: Antidepressant drugs as adjuvant analgesics. J Pain Symptom Manage 9:392–405, 1994a.

Zeppetella GCA, O'Doherty, et al: Prevalence and characteristics of breakthrough pain in patients with non-malignant terminal disease admitted to a hospice. Palliat Med 15:243–246, 2001.

REFERENCES

Ackerman WE 3rd, Colclough GW, Juneja MM, Bellinger K: The management of oral mexiletine and intravenous lidocaine to treat chronic painful symmetrical distal diabetic neuropathy. J Kentucky Med Assoc 89):500–501, 1991.

AGS Panel on Persistent Pain in Older Persons: The management of persistent pain in older persons. J Am Geriatric Soc 50:S205–S224, 2002.

Argoff CE: New analgesics for neuropathic pain: The lidocaine patch. Clin J Pain 16(Suppl. 2):S62–S66, 2000.

Arner S, Meyerson BA: Lack of analgesic effect of opioids on neuropathic and idiopathic forms of pain. Pain 33:11–23, 1988.

Ashby MA, Martin P, et al: Opioid substitution to reduce adverse effects in cancer pain management. Med J Aust 170:68–71, 1999.

Backonja M, Beydoun A, et al: (1998). Gabapentin for the symptomatic treatment of painful neuropathy in patients with diabetes mellitus: A randomized controlled trial. JAMA 280:1831–1836, 1998.

Backonja MM: Anticonvulsants (antineuropathics) for neuropathic pain syndromes. Clin J Pain 16(Suppl. 2):S67–S72, 2000.

Banning A, Sjogren P, et al: Treatment outcome in a multidisciplinary cancer pain clinic. Pain 47:129–134; discussion 127–128, 1991.

Beck AT, Beck RW: Screening depressed patients in family practice. Postgrad Med 32:81–85, 1972.

Beck AT, Ward CH, Mendelsohn M, et al: An inventory for measuring depression. Arch Gen Psychiatry 4:561–571, 1961.

Berry H, Hutchinson DR: A multicentre placebo-controlled study in general practice to evaluate the efficacy and safety of tizanidine in acute low-back pain. J Int Med Res 16:75–82, 1988a.

Berry H, Hutchinson DR: Tizanidine and ibuprofen in acute low-back pain: Results of a double-blind multicentre study in general practice. J Intl Med Res 16:83–91, 1988b.

Besson JM, Chaouch A: Peripheral and spinal mechanisms of nociception. Physiol Rev 67:67–186, 1987.

Bhatia MT: Anticonvulsant alone in the relief of cancer pain. J Indian Med Assoc 90:301–302, 1992.

Block AR: Presurgical Psychological Screening in Chronic Pain Syndromes. Mahwah, NJ: Lawrence Erlbaum, 1996.

Brant JM: Cancer-related neuropathic pain. Nurse Pract Forum 9:154–162, 1998.

Brena SF, Chapman SL: Chronic pain: Physiology, diagnosis, management, in JC Leek, ME Gershwin, WM Fowler (eds): Principles of Physical Disease and Rehabilitation in the Musculoskeletal Diseases. Orlando, FL: Grune & Stratton, 1985, pp. 189–217.

Bruera E, Macmillan K, Hanson J, MacDonald J: The cognitive effects of the administration of narcotic analgesics in patients with cancer pain. Pain 39:13–16, 1989.

Bruera E, Pereira J, Watanabe S, et al: Opioid rotation in patients with cancer pain: A retrospective comparison of dose ratios between methadone, hydromorphone, and morphine. Cancer 78:852–857, 1996.

Cassell EJ: The nature of suffering and the goals of medicine. N Engl J Med 306:639–645, 1982.

Cesaro P, Ollat H: Pain and its treatments. Eur Neurol 38:209–215, 1997.

Chapman SL: Relaxation, biofeedback and self-hypnosis, in SF Brena, SL Chapman (eds): Management of Patients with Chronic Pain. New York: SP Medical and Scientific Books, 1983, pp. 161–172.

Chapman SL, Byas-Smith MG, Reed BA: The effects of intermediate- and long-term use of opioids on cognition in patients with low back pain. Clin J Pain 18:583–590, 2002.

Cherny N, Foley K: Current approaches to the management of cancer pain: A review. Ann Acad Med Singapore 23:139–159, 1994.

Cherny NI, Coyle N, Foley KM, et al: Suffering in the advanced cancer patient: A definition and taxonomy. J Palliat Care 10:57–70, 1994a.

Cherny NI, Foley KM: Nonopioid and opioid analgesic pharmacotherapy of cancer pain. Hematol Oncol Clin North Am 10:79–102, 1996.

Cherny NI, Portenoy RK: The management of cancer pain. CA Cancer J Clin 44:263–303, 1994.

Cherny NI, Thaler HT, Friedlander-Klar H, et al: Opioid responsiveness of cancer pain syndromes caused by neuropathic or nociceptive mechanisms: A combined analysis of controlled, single-dose studies. Neurology 44:857–861, 1994b.

Cherny NI, Chang V, Frager G, et al: Opioid pharmacotherapy in the management of cancer pain: A survey of strategies used by pain physicians for the selection of analgesic drugs and routes of administration. Cancer 76:1283–1293, 1995.

Cheville A, Chen A, Oster G, et al: A randomized trial of controlled-release oxycodone during inpatient rehabilitation following unilateral total knee arthroplasty. J Bone Joint Surg Am 83-A:572–576, 2001.

Chong MS, Libretto SE: The rationale and use of topiramate for treating neuropathic pain. Clin J Pain 19:59–68, 2003.

Cicero TJ, Adams EH, Geller A, et al: A postmarketing surveillance program to monitor Ultram (tramadol hydrochloride) abuse in the United States. Drug Alcohol Depend 57:7–22, 1999.

Citron ML, Kaplan R, Parris WC, et al: Long-term administration of controlled-release oxycodone tablets for the treatment of cancer pain. Cancer Invest 16:562–571, 1998.

Coghill CR, Talbot JD, Evans AC, et al: Distributed processing of pain and vibration by the human brain. J Neurosci 14:4095–4108, 1994.

Compas BE, Haaga DAF, Keefe FJ, et al: Sampling of empirically supported psychological treatments from health psychology: Smoking, chronic pain, cancer, and bulimia nervosa. J Consult Clin Psychol 66:89–112, 1998.

Coyle N, Cherny NI, Portenoy RK, et al: Subcutaneous opioid infusions at home. Oncology 8:21–7; discussion 31–32, 1994.

Curtis EB, Krech R, Walsh TD: Common symptoms in patients with advanced cancer. J Palliat Care 7:25–29, 1991.

Daut RL, Cleeland CS: The prevalence and severity of pain in cancer. Cancer 50:1913–1918, 1982.

De Conno F, Caraceni A, Gamba A, et al: Pain measurement in cancer patients: A comparison of six methods. Pain 57:161–166, 1994.

De Conno F, Ripamonti C, Sbanotto A, et al: The pharmacological management of cancer pain. Part 1: The role of non opioid and adjuvant drugs. Ann Oncol 4:187–193, 1993.

Devers A, Galer, BS: Topical lidocaine patch relieves a variety of neuropathic pain conditions: An open-label study. Clin J Pain 16:205–208, 2000.

Devulder J, Ghys L, Dhondt W, et al: Spinal analgesia in terminal care: Risk versus benefit. J Pain Symptom Manage 9:75–81, 1994.

Dworkin RH, Handlin DS, Richlin DM, et al: Unraveling the effects of compensation, litigation, and employment on treatment response in chronic pain. Pain 23:49–59, 1985.

Ebert B, Andersen S, Krosgaard-Larsen P: Ketobemidone, methadone and pethidine are non-competitive N-methyl-D-aspartate (NMDA) antagonists in the rat cortex and spinal cord. Neurosci Lett 187:165–168, 1995.

Eisenberg E, Berkey CS, Carr DB, et al: Efficacy and safety of nonsteroidal antiinflammatory drugs for cancer pain: A meta-analysis. J Clin Oncol 12:2756–2765, 1994.

Fassoulaki A, Sarantopoulos C, Melemeni A, Hogan Q: EMLA reduces acute and chronic pain after breast surgery for cancer. Regional Anesth Pain Med 25:350–355, 2000.

Fiddler DS, Hindman BJ: Intravenous calcitonin alleviates spinal anesthesia-induced phantom limb pain. Anesthesiology 74:187–189, 1991.

Fishbain DA, Rosomoff HL, Rosomoff RS: Detoxification of non-opiate drugs in the chronic pain setting and clonidine opiate detoxification. Clin J Pain 8:191–203, 1992.

Fishbain D: Letter to the editor. Subst Use Misuse 31:945–946, 1996.

Flor H, Turk DC: Etiological theories and treatments for chronic back pain. I. Somatic models and interventions. Pain 19:105–121, 1984.

Fogelholm R, Murros K: Tizanidine in chronic tension-type headache: A placebo controlled double-blind cross-over study. Headache 32:509–513, 1992.

Foley K, Portenoy RK: World Health Organization-International Association for the Study of Pain: Joint initiatives in cancer pain relief. J Pain Symptom Manage 8:335–339, 1993.

Foley KM, Houde RW: Methadone in cancer pain management: Individualize dose and titrate to effect. J Clin Oncol 16:3213–3215, 1998.

Fricke JR, Karim R, Jordan D, Rosenthal N: A double-blind, single-dose comparison of the analgesic efficacy of tramadol/acetaminophen combination tablets, hydrocodone/acetaminophen combination tablets and placebo after oral surgery. Clin Ther 24:1–16, 1999.

Fromm GH, Aumentado D, Terrence CF: A clinical and experimental investigation of the effects of tizanidine in trigeminal neuralgia. Pain 53:265–271, 1993.

Gale D, Prime S, Cambell MJ: Trigeminal neuralgia and multiple sclerosis. A complex diagnosis. Oral Surg Oral Med Oral Pathol Oral Radiol Endod 79:398–401, 1995.

Galer BS, Keran C, Frisinger M: Pain medicine education among American neurologists: A need for improvement. Neurology 52:1710–1712, 1999a.

Galer BS, Rowbotham MC, Perander J, Friedman E: Topical lidocaine patch relieves postherpetic neuralgia more effectively than a vehicle topical patch: Results of an enriched enrollment study. Pain 80:533–538, 1999b.

Getto CJ: Depression, in: Lynch NT, Vasudevan SV (eds): Persistent Pain: Psychosocial Assessment and Intervention. Boston, MA: Kluwer, 1988, pp. 93–101.

Gobelet C, Waldburger M, Meier JL: The effect of adding calcitonin to physical treatment on reflex sympathetic dystrophy. Pain 48:171–175, 1992.

Goldenberg D, Mayskiy M, Mossey C, et al: A randomized, double-blind crossover trial of fluoxetine and amitriptyline in the treatment of fibromyalgia. Arthritis Rheum 39:1852–1859, 1996.

Gorman AL, Elliott KJ, Inturrisi CE, et al: The d- and l-isomers of methadone bind to the non-competitive site on the N-methyl-D-aspartate (NMDA) receptor in rat forebrain and spinal cord. Neurosci Lett 223:5–8, 1997.

Gorson KC, Schott C, Herman R, et al: Gabapentin in the treatment of painful diabetic neuropathy: A placebo controlled, double blind, crossover trial [letter]. J Neurol Neurosurg Psychiatry 66:251–252, 1999.

Grond S, Radbruch L, Meuser T, et al: Assessment and treatment of neuropathic cancer pain following WHO guidelines. Pain 79:15–20, 1999.

Grzesiak R, Ciccone DS: Relaxation, biofeedback, and hypnosis in the management of pain, in Lynch NT, Vasudevan SR (eds): Persistent Pain: Psychosocial Assessment and Intervention. Boston: Kluwer, 1988, pp. 163–188.

Hagen NA, Elwood T, Ernst S: Cancer pain emergencies: A protocol for management. J Pain Symptom Manage 14:45–50, 1997.

Haller D, Butler S: Use and abuse of prescription and recreational drugs by chronic pain patients, in Harris L (ed): Problems of Drug Dependence. Washington DC: Government Printing Office, 1991, pp. 456–457.

Hamamci N, Dursun E, Akbas E, et al: Calcitonin treatment in reflex sympathetic dystrophy: A preliminary study. Br J Clin Prac 50:373–375, 1996.

Harati Y, Gooch C, Swenson M, et al: Double-blind randomized trial of tramadol for the treatment of the pain of diabetic neuropathy. Neurology 50:1842–1846, 1998.

Heiskanen T, Kalso E: Controlled-release oxycodone and morphine in cancer-related pain. Pain 73:37–45, 1997.

Hewitt D: Neuroimaging of pain, in Greenberg J (ed): Neuroimaging: A Companion Book to Adams and Victor's Principles of Neurology. New York: McGraw Hill, 1999. pp. 43–87.

Hewitt D, Foley K: Geriatric pain, in Cassel CK, Levinson D (eds): Geriatric Medicine, ed 3. New York: Springer-Verlag, 1996.

Holdsworth MT, Raisch DW, Winter SS, Chavez CM: Differences among raters evaluating the success of EMLA cream in alleviating procedure-related pain in children with cancer. Pharmacotherapy 17:1017–1022, 1997.

IASP (International Association for the Study of Pain) (Subcommittee on Taxonomy): Pain terms: A list with definitions and notes on usage. Recommended by the IASP Subcommittee on Taxonomy. Pain 6:249, 1979.

Jacox A, Carr DB, Payne R, et al: Management of Cancer Pain: Adults' Quick Reference Guide. No. 9. Rockville, MD: Agency for Health Care Policy and Research, Public Health Service, US Department of Health and Human Services, 1994.

Jaeger H, Maier C: Calcitonin in phantom limb pain: A double-blind study. Pain 48:21–27, 1992.

Jamison RN, Stetson Bl, Sbrocco T, Parris WC: Effects of significant weight gain on chronic pain patients. Clin J Pain 6:47–50, 1990.

Jensen MP, Karoly P, Huger R: The development and preliminary validation of an instrument to assess patients' attitudes toward pain. J Psychosom Res 31:393–400, 1987.

Jensen MP, Turner JA, Romano JM: Self-efficacy and outcome expectancies: Relationship to chronic pain coping strategies and adjustment. Pain 44:263–269, 1991.

Kapelushnik J, Koren G, Jolh H, et al: Evaluating the efficacy of EMLA in alleviating pain associated with lumbar puncture: Comparison of open and double-blinded protocols in children. Pain 42:31–34, 1990.

Kaplan R, Parris WC, Citron ML, et al: Comparison of controlled-release and immediate-release oxycodone tablets in patients with cancer pain. J Clin Oncol 16:3230–3237, 1998.

Keefe FJ, Brown GK, Wallston KA, Caldwell DS: Coping with rheumatoid arthritis pain: Catastrophizing as a maladaptive strategy. Pain 37:51–56, 1989.

Kenner DJ: Pain forum. Part 2. Neuropathic pain. Aust Fam Physician 23:1279–1283, 1994.

Kerns RD, Turk DC, Rudy TE: The West Haven-Yale Multidimensional Personality Inventory. Pain 23:345–356, 1985.

Kessel C, Worz R: Immediate response of phantom limb pain to calcitonin. Pain 30:79–87, 1987.

Killian JM, Fromm GH: Carbamazepine in the treatment of neuralgia: Use of side effects. Arch Neurol 19:129–136, 1968.

Kingery WS: A critical review of controlled clinical trials for peripheral neuropathic pain and complex regional pain syndromes. Pain 73:123–139, 1997.

Kloke M, Hoffken K, Olbrich H, Schmidt CG: Anti-depressants and anti-convulsants for the treatment of neuropathic pain syndromes in cancer patients. Oncology 14:40–43, 1991.

Koestler AJ, Doleys DM: The psychology of pain, in Tollison CD, Satterthwaite JR, Tollison JW (eds): Practical Pain Management, ed 3. Philadelphia, PA: Lippincott, Williams & Wilkins, 2002, pp. 26–39.

Kovcin V, Jelic S, Babovic N, Tomasevic Z: A pilot study to assess the efficacy of salmon calcitonin in the relief of neuropathic pain caused by extraskeletal metastases. Support Care Cancer 2:71–73, 1994.

Kübler-Ross E: On Death and Dying. New York: Macmillan, 1969.

Kubota K, Joshita Y, et al: Relief of severe diabetic truncal pain with mexiletine. J Med 22:307–310, 1991.

Lawlor PG, Turner KS, Hanson J, Bruera ED: Dose ratio between morphine and methadone in patients with cancer pain: A retrospective study. Cancer 82:1167–1173, 1998.

Makin MK, Ellershaw JE: Substitution of another opioid for morphine. Methadone can be used to manage neuropathic pain related to cancer BMJ 317:81, 1998.

Manfredi PL, Borsook D, Chandler SW, Payne R: Intravenous methadone for cancer pain unrelieved by morphine and hydromorphone: Clinical observations. Pain 70:99–101, 1997.

Max, MB: Treatment of post-herpetic neuralgia: Antidepressants. Ann Neurol 35S:S50–S53, 1994.

Max MB, Culnane M, Schafer SC, et al: Amitriptyline relieves diabetic neuropathy pain in patients with normal or depressed mood. Neurology 37:589–596, 1987.

Max MB, Kishore-Kumar R, Schafer SC, et al: Efficacy of desipramine in painful diabetic neuropathy: A placebo-controlled trial. Pain 45:69, 1991.

Max MB, Lynch SA, Muir J, et al: Effects of desipramine, amitriptyline, and fluoxetine on pain in diabetic neuropathy. N Engl J Med 326:1250–1256, 1992.

McCleane GJ: Lamotrigine in the management of neuropathic pain: A review of the literature. Clin J Pain 16:321–326, 2000.

McQuay HJ, Jadad AR, Carroll D, et al: Opioid sensitivity of chronic pain: A patient-controlled analgesia method. Anaesthesia 47:757–767, 1992.

Melzack R: The McGill Pain Questionnaire: Major properties and scoring methods. Pain 1:277–299, 1975.

Medve RA, Wang J, Karim R: Tramadol and acetaminophen tablets for dental pain. Anesth Prog 48:79–81, 2001.

Mense S, Stahnke M: Responses in muscle afferent fibers of slow conduction velocity to contractions and ischemia in the cat. J Physiol 342:343–348, 1983.

Mercadante S, Fulfaro F: Alternatives to oral opioids for cancer pain. Oncology 13:215–220, 1999.

Miser AW, Goh TS, Dose AM, et al: Trial of a topically administered local anesthetic (EMLA cream) for pain relief during central venous port accesses in children with cancer. J Pain Symp Man 9:259–264, 1994.

Miseria S, Torresi U, et al: Analgesia with epidural calcitonin in cancer patients. Tumori 75:183–184, 1989.

Moore MJ, Osoba D, et al: Use of palliative end points to evaluate the effects of mitoxantrone and low-dose prednisone in patients with hormonally resistant prostate cancer. J Clin Oncol 12:689–694, 1994.

Moreland LW, St Clair EW: The use of analgesics in the management of pain in rheumatic diseases. Rheum Dis Clin North Am 25:153–191, 1999.

Morley JS, Makin MK: The use of methadone in cancer pain poorly responsive to other opioids. Pain Rev 5:51–58, 1998.

Morrison RS, Wallenstein S, Natale DK, et al: We don't carry that—failure of pharmacies in predominantly nonwhite neighborhoods to stock opioid analgesics. N Engl J Med 342:1023–1026, 2000.

Nachemson A: A critical look at the treatment of low back pain. Scand J Rehab Med 11:143–149, 1979.

Nelson KA, Park KM, Robinovitz E, et al: High-dose oral dextromethorphan versus placebo in painful diabetic neuropathy and postherpetic neuralgia. Neurology 48:1212–1218, 1997.

Ness TJ, Ge G: Visceral pain: A review of experimental studies. Pain 41:167–234, 1990.

Nicol CF: A four year double-blind study of Tegretol in facial pain. Headache 9:54–57, 1969.

Noyes R Jr: Treatment of cancer pain. Psychosom Med 43:57–70, 1981.

World Health Organization: Cancer Pain Relief and Palliative Care. Geneva, Switzerland: World Health Organization, 1990.

Panerai AE, Bianchi M, Sacerdote P, et al: Antidepressants in cancer pain. J Palliat Care 7:42–4, 1991.

Parris WC, Johnson BW Jr, Croghan MK, et al: The use of controlled-release oxycodone for the treatment of chronic cancer pain: A

randomized, double-blind study. J Pain Symptom Manage 16:205–211, 1998.

Payne R: Factors influencing quality of life in cancer patients: The role of transdermal fentanyl in the management of pain. Semin Oncol 25:47–53, 1998.

Payne RS, Mathias D, Pasta DJ, et al: Quality of life and cancer pain: Satisfaction and side effects with transdermal fentanyl versus oral morphine. J Clin Oncol 16:1588–1593, 1998.

Pfeifer MA, Ross DR, Schrage JP, et al: A highly successful and novel model for treatment of chronic painful diabetic peripheral neuropathy. Diabetes Care 16:1103–1115, 1993.

Portenoy RK: Cancer pain management. Semin Oncol 20:19–35, 1993.

Portenoy RK: Adjuvant analgesics in pain management, in Doyle D, Hanks GW, MacDonald N (eds): Oxford Textbook of Palliative Medicine. New York: Oxford University Press, 1998, pp. 361–390.

Portenoy RK, Kanner RM: Pain management: Theory and practice, in Portenoy RK, Kanner RM (eds): Contemporary Neurology Series, Vol. 48. Philadelphia, PA: Davis, 1996, pp. 199–201, 205–212.

Portenoy RK, Coyle N: Controversies in the long-term management of analgesic therapy in patients with advanced cancer. J Palliat Care 7:13–24, 1991.

Portenoy RK, Foley KM, Inturissi CE, et al: The nature of opioid responsiveness and its implications for neuropathic pain: New hypotheses derived from studies of opioid infusions. Pain 43:273–286, 1990.

Portenoy RK, Hagen NA: Breakthrough pain: Definition, prevalence and characteristics. Pain 41:273–281, 1990.

Portenoy RK, Lesage P: Management of cancer pain. Lancet 353:1695–1700, 1999.

Portenoy RK, Payne R, Coluzzi P, et al: Oral transmucosal fentanyl citrate (OTFC) for the treatment of breakthrough pain in cancer patients: A controlled dose titration study. Pain 79:303–312, 1999a.

Portenoy RK, Payne D, Jacobsen P, et al: Breakthrough pain: Characteristics and impact in patients with cancer pain. Pain 81:129–134, 1999b.

Portenoy RK, Thaler HT, Kornblith AB, et al: Symptom prevalence, characteristics and distress in a cancer population. Qual Life Res 3:183–189, 1994.

Rani PU, Naidu MU, Prasad VB, et al: An evaluation of antidepressants in rheumatic pain conditions. Anesthesia Analgesia 83:371–375, 1996.

Rawal N, Allvin R, Amilon R, et al: Postoperative analgesia at home after ambulatory hand surgery: A controlled comparison of tramadol, metamizol, and paracetamol. Anesthesia Analgesia 92:347–51, 2001.

Reiger DA, Farmer ME, Rae DS, et al: Comorbidity of mental disorders with alcohol and other drug abuse. JAMA 19:2511–2518, 1990.

Ripamonti C, Groff L, Brunelli C, et al: Switching from morphine to oral methadone in treating cancer pain: What is the equianalgesic dose ratio? J Clin Oncol 16:3216–3221, 1998.

Roth SH, Fleischmann RM, Burch FX, et al: Around-the-clock, controlled-release oxycodone therapy for osteoarthritis-related pain: Placebo-controlled trial and long-term evaluation. Arch Intern Med 160:853–860, 2000.

Rowbotham M, Harden N, Stacey B, et al: Gabapentin for the treatment of postherpetic neuralgia: A randomized controlled trial. JAMA 280:1837–1842, 1998.

Rowbotham MC, Davies PS, Verkempinck C, Galer BS: Lidocaine patch: Double-blind controlled study of a new treatment method for post-herpetic neuralgia. Pain 65:39–44, 1996.

Rull JA, Quibrera R, Gonzalez-Millan H, et al: Symptomatic treatment of peripheral diabetic neuropathy with carbamazepine

(Tegretol): Double blind crossover trial. Diabetologia 5:215–218, 1969.

Rumsfield JA, West DP: Topical capsaicin in dermatologic and peripheral pain disorders. Drug Intel Clin Pharmacol 25:381–387, 1991.

Saper JR, Silberstein SD, Lake AE 3rd, Winters ME: Double-blind trial of fluoxetine: Chronic daily headache and migraine. Headache 34:497–502, 1994.

Saunders C: The philosophy of terminal care, in Saunders C (ed): The Management of Terminal Malignant Disease. London, UK: Edward Arnold, 1984, pp. 232–241.

Schiraldi GF, Soresi E, Locicero S, et al: Salmon calcitonin in cancer pain: Comparison between two different treatment schedules. Int J Clin Pharmacol Ther Toxicol 25:229–232, 1987.

Schnur W: Etidronate and calcitonin for cancer bone pain. Am Fam Physician 54:1212, 1996.

Serdengecti S, Serdengecti K, Derman U: Salmon calcitonin in the treatment of bone metastases. Intl J Clin Pharmacol Res 6:151–155, 1986.

Simpson DM, Olney R, McArthur JC, et al: A placebo-controlled trial of lamotrigine for painful HIV-associated neuropathy. Neurology 54:2115–2119, 2000.

Sindrup SH, Jensen TS: Efficacy of pharmacological treatments of neuropathic pain: An update and effect related to mechanism of drug action. Pain 83:389–400, 1999.

Sloan PA, Moulin DE, Hays H: A clinical evaluation of transdermal therapeutic system fentanyl for the treatment of cancer pain. J Pain Symptom Manage 16:102–111, 1998.

Stjernsward J, Colleau SM, Ventafridda V: The World Health Organization Cancer Pain and Palliative Care Program: Past, present, and future. J Pain Symptom Manage 12:65–72, 1996.

Sumpton JE, Moulin DE: Treatment of neuropathic pain with venlafaxine. Ann Pharmacother 35:557–559, 2001.

Sunshine A: New clinical experience with tramadol. Drugs 47 (Suppl. 1):8–18, 1994.

Szanto J, Ady N, Jozsef F: Pain killing with calcitonin nasal spray in patients with malignant tumors. Oncology 49:180–182, 1992.

Tannock IF, Osoba D, Stockler MR, et al: Chemotherapy with mitoxantrone plus prednisone or prednisone alone for symptomatic hormone-resistant prostate cancer: A Canadian randomized trial with palliative end points. J Clin Oncol 14:1756–1764, 1996.

Theesen KA, Marsh WR: Relief of diabetic neuropathy with fluoxetine. Drug Intel Clin Pharmacol 23:572–574, 1989.

Turk DC, Meichenbaum D, Genest M: Pain and Behavioral Medicine: A Cognitive-Behavioral Perspective. New York: Guilford, 1983.

Turk DC, Rudy TE: Toward an empirically derived taxonomy of chronic pain patients: Integration of psychological assessment data. J Consult Clin Psychol 56:233–238, 1988.

Ventafridda V, Bonezzi C, Caraceni A, et al: Antidepressants for cancer pain and other painful syndromes with deafferentation component: Comparison of amitriptyline and trazodone. Ital J Neuro Sci 8:579–587, 1987a.

Ventafridda V, De Conno F, Ripamonti C, et al: Quality-of-life assessment during a palliative care programme. Ann Oncol 1:415–420, 1990a.

Ventafridda V, Ripamonti C, De Conno F, et al: Antidepressants increase bioavailability of morphine in cancer patients [letter]. Lancet 1:1204, 1987b.

Ventafridda V, Ripamonti C, De Conno F, et al: Symptom prevalence and control during cancer patients' last days of life. J Palliat Care 6:7–11, 1990b.

Ventafridda V, Saita L, Ripamonti C, De Conno F: WHO guidelines for the use of analgesics in cancer pain. Intl J Tissue React 7:93–96, 1985.

Ventafridda V, Spoldi E, Caraceni A, De Conno F: Intraspinal morphine for cancer pain. Acta Anaesthesiol Scand Suppl 85: 47–53, 1987c.

Ventafridda V, Stjernsward J: Pain control and the World Health Organization analgesic ladder. JAMA 275:835–836, 1996.

Vestergaard K, Andersen G, Gottrup H, et al: Lamotrigine for central poststroke pain: A randomized controlled trial. Neurology 56:184–190, 2001.

Wall GC, Heyneman CA: Calcitonin in phantom limb pain. Ann Pharmacother 33:499–501, 1999.

Wall PD: Introduction, in Wall PD, Malzack R (eds): Textbook of Pain. Edinburgh, Scotland: Churchill Livingstone, 1989, pp. 1–18.

Wallston KA, Wallston BS: Development of the Multidimensional Health Locus of Control (MHLC) scales. Health Educ Monographs 6:160–170, 1978.

Warfield CA: Controlled-release morphine tablets in patients with chronic cancer pain: A narrative review of controlled clinical trials. Cancer 82:2299–2306, 1998.

Watanabe S, Bruera E: Corticosteroids as adjuvant analgesics. J Pain Symptom Manage 9:442–445, 1994.

Watson CP: Antidepressant drugs as adjuvant analgesics. J Pain Symptom Manage 9:392–405, 1994a.

Watson CP: Topical capsaicin as an adjuvant analgesic. J Pain Symptom Manage 9:425–433, 1994b.

Watson CP, Vernich L, Chipman M, Reed K: Nortriptyline versus amitriptyline in postherpetic neuralgia: A randomized trial. Neurology 51:1166–1171, 1998.

Weinberg DS, Inturrisi CE, et al: Sublingual absorption of selected opioid analgesics. Clin Pharmacol Ther 44:335–342, 1988.

Weisenberg M: Pain and pain control. Psychol Bull 84:1008–1044, 1977.

Weissman D, Haddox J: Opioid pseudoaddiction: An iatrogenic syndrome. Pain 36:363–366.

WHO. World Health Organization Expert Committee: Cancer Pain Relief and Palliative Care, 1989. Geneva, Switzerland: World Health Organization, 1990.

Wilder-Smith CH, Schimke J, Osterwalder B, Senn HJ: Oral tramadol, a mu-opioid agonist and monoamine reuptake-blocker, and morphine for strong cancer-related pain. Ann Oncol 5:141–146, 1994.

Willis WD: The pain system: The neural basis of nociceptive transmission in the mammalian nervous system. Basel, Switzerland: Karger, 1985.

Wright JM: Review of the symptomatic treatment of diabetic neuropathy. Pharmacotherapy 14:689–697, 1994.

Yosipovitch G, Maibach I, Rowbothom MC: Effect of EMLA pretreatment on capsaicin-induced burning and hyperalgesia. Acta Derm Venereol 79:118–121, 1999.

Zakrzewska JM, Chaudhry Z, Nurmikko TJ: Lamotrigine (Lamictal) in refractory trigeminal neuralgia: Results from a double-blind placebo-controlled crossover trial. Pain 73:223–230, 1997.

Zakrzewska JM, Patsalos PN: Oxcarbazepine: A new drug in the management of intractable trigeminal neuralgia. J Neurol Neurosurg Psychiatry 52:472–476, 1989.

Zeppetella GCA, O'Doherty, Collins S: Prevalence and characteristics of breakthrough pain in patients with non-malignant terminal disease admitted to a hospice. Palliat Med 15:243–246, 2001.

Neuropsychiatric Aspects of Epilepsy

Michelle V. Lambert
Pamela J. Thompson
Michael Trimble

Anxiety

Cognitive functions

Depression

Epilepsy

Memory

Psychosis

Seizures

INTRODUCTION

Epilepsy is one of the oldest central nervous system (CNS) disorders described, and is generally considered to be characterized by seizures, the main findings being specific electroencephalographic (EEG) abnormalities, and, in many patients with temporal lobe epilepsy (TLE), pathologic changes in the temporal lobes, namely mesial temporal sclerosis of the hippocampus. Because the most common from of epilepsy is TLE, and the pathologic involvement is in limbic structures, it is not surprising that many patients with epilepsy have behavioral and cognitive problems. The former are the more likely because recurrent seizures represent a devastating social and vocational handicap, and the drugs used to suppress seizures influence neurotransmitter systems that are linked with memory and behavior, namely gamma-aminobutyric acid (GABA) and glutamate.

In this chapter we review the more common behavior and cognitive complications of epilepsy, but for further reviews we recommend Lambert and colleagues (2003), Trimble (1991), and Thompson (2001).

The incidence and prevalence of psychiatric disorders in people with epilepsy is not known. Most studies have been criticized for being retrospective, using nonrepresentative hospital samples, having inadequate or absent controls, and not clearly identifying the seizure and syndrome type. Interpretation and comparison are further complicated by differing methods of determining psychiatric cases, ranging from self-report questionnaires to structured clinical interviews using operational criteria. As a summary, about 30% to 50% of patients with epilepsy appear to experience a psychiatric disorder at some time, usually anxiety or depression. Psychoses are over-represented, and there is a continuing controversy about the type and prevalence of personality disorders.

PSYCHIATRIC DISORDERS IN PATIENTS WITH EPILEPSY

Psychiatric disorders in epilepsy can occur peri- or interictally, the latter being unrelated in time to seizure occurrence. However, in patients with frequent seizures, differentiation may be difficult.

Depression

Prodromal moods of depression or irritability occur hours to days before a seizure and are often relieved by the convulsion. Hughes and colleagues (1993) evaluated 148 adult patients with epilepsy, of whom 128 had partial seizures. A third of the patients with partial seizures reported premonitory symptoms (usually preceding secondarily generalized seizures), compared with none of the patients with primary generalized epilepsy (PGE). Half of the symptoms were "emotional" in nature, usually irritability, depression, fear, elation, or anger, and lasted between 10 minutes and 3 days.

Ictal depression is also well described, but rare. Ictal depression, classically, is of sudden onset and occurs out of context, not related to environmental stimuli. The severity ranges from mild feelings of sadness to profound hopelessness and despair (Devinsky & Bear, 1991).

Interictal depression is common; however, the exact prevalence is not known. Moreover, some studies have reported rates of depressive symptomatology, whereas others reported depressive illness. Mendez and colleagues (1986) found that four times more patients with epilepsy had been hospitalized for depression compared with a control group with similar socioeconomic and disability levels. Other studies have found a history of depression or depressive symptomatology in up to two thirds of patients with medically intractable epilepsy (Standage & Fenton, 1975; Roy, 1979; Victoroff et al., 1990), whereas community studies have demonstrated affective disorder in only a quarter (Edeh & Toone, 1985). Depression tends to occur about 10 years after the onset of epilepsy (Altshuler et al., 1999).

Various causative factors have been proposed for the development of depression in epilepsy, but the etiology is most likely to be multifactorial, in part interlinked with simply having such an unpleasant neurologic disorder.

A family history of depression has been reported by some investigators (Robertson et al., 1987). Many studies have found depression to be more common in patients with complex partial seizures (CPS) (Mendez et al., 1986; Robertson et al., 1987), especially TLE (Altshuler et al., 1999; Schmitz et al., 1999); others, however, suggest that the number of seizure types is correlated with greater risk of psychiatric disorder (Dodrill & Batzel, 1986).

Recent imaging studies have investigated the role of limbic structures in this depression. Quiske and colleagues (2000) found patients with magnetic resonance imaging (MRI)—detected mesial temporal sclerosis to have higher Beck Depression Inventory (BDI) scores than those with circumscribed neocortical temporal lesions. Tebartz van Elst and colleagues (1999) compared amygdala volumes among 48 patients with TLE, 11 of whom had dysthymia, with healthy controls. They found a highly significant enlargement of both amygdalae in the patients with TLE and dysthymia. In addition, none of the patients with dysthymia had amygdala atrophy. Furthermore, they found a positive correlation between left amygdala volumes and depression measured using the BDI. They speculated that enlargement of the amygdala may somehow predispose to the development of depression or that amygdala atrophy might be protective for the development of dysthymia.

The frontal lobes are also involved with this association between TLE and affective states. Hermann and colleagues (1991) found increased perseverative responding on the Wisconsin Card Sorting Test in patients with left TLE and dysphoric mood states. Bromfield and colleagues (1992) confirmed this hypothesis by reporting a bilateral reduction in inferior frontal glucose metabolism in depressed patients with CPS. Schmitz and colleagues (1997), using single photon emission computed tomography (SPECT) scans, noted that in patients with left-sided epilepsy, higher scores on the BDI were associated with contralateral temporal and bilateral frontal hypoperfusion.

The suggestion then emerges that patients with left TLE may be the more susceptible to affective disorders. Although some studies have not confirmed this, most have (Hurwitz et al., 1985, Robertson et al., 1987; Altshuler et al., 1990; Victoroff et al., 1990; Seidenberg et al., 1995). Victoroff and colleagues (1994) found that in patients with CPS, a left-sided ictal onset and cerebral hypometabolism were associated with a history of depression as well as with current depression. However, patients with right-sided hypometabolism also had a history of major depression, suggesting that left-sided ictal onset and degree of hypometabolism were independent risk factors for the development of depression.

Interestingly, several studies have reported a decrease in seizure frequency prior to the onset of a depressive illness (Dongier, 1959–60; Flor-Henry, 1969). Mendez and colleagues (1993) found patients with depression had significantly fewer generalized seizures than those without depression, and they postulated that nonreactive depression may occur when anticonvulsant therapy prevents generalization from an epileptic focus. Others have not found an association (Mendez et al., 1986; Robertson et al., 1987), whereas some researchers have even documented an association with an increase in seizure frequency (Dodrill & Batzel, 1986; Roth et al., 1994). However, interpretation of the data is complicated by diagnostic issues, a confusion between depressive symptoms and major depressive disorder, and the peculiarity of the interictal dysphoric disorder (IDD) (see discussion following). Recent quality of life studies have found frequent seizures to be associated with increased anxiety, depression, and stigma (Baker et al., 1995; Jacoby et al., 1996), as has perceived seizure severity (Baker et al., 1996). Trostle and colleagues (1989) reported fewer psychosocial problems (assessed using the Washington Psychosocial Seizure Inventory, WPSI) in patients who were not taking antiepileptic drugs (AEDs) and had been seizure-free during the preceding year. Patients continuing to experience seizures despite AEDs had the most severe psychosocial problems. Severity of seizures was associated with the severity of self-reported psychosocial problems.

Thus, anticonvulsants play an important role in the etiology of psychiatric comorbidity. Polypharmacy, especially with barbiturates, has been shown to be associated with depression (Fiordelli et al., 1993; Mendez et al., 1993). Other anticonvulsants associated with depression as a treatment-emergent effect include phenytoin and vigabatrin. The AEDs associated least with depression are carbamazepine, valproic acid, lamotrigine, gabapentin, and levetiracetam.

Psychosocial factors are thought to play a major role in the development of depression in patients with epilepsy. Hermann (1979) proposed that the exposure to unpredictable, uncontrollable, aversive events (seizures) might result in depression. This has been developed into the concept of locus of control, a perception of events not being attributable to the patient's own efforts but rather to the effects of fate (Hermann & Wyler, 1989). More recently, a pessimistic attributional style (attributing global difficulties to epilepsy) has been associated with the development of depression in patients with epilepsy (Hermann et al., 1996), and increased stressful life events, poor adjustment to seizures, and financial stress are predictive of increased depression (Hermann & Whitman, 1989).

Compared with patients with depression and no epilepsy, patients with epilepsy and depression tend to have significantly fewer "neurotic" traits such as anxiety, guilt, rumination, hopelessness, low self-esteem, and somatization, and more "psychotic" symptoms such as paranoia, delusions, and persecutory auditory hallucinations. Between episodes of major depression, they tend to be dysthymic with irritability

and humorlessness (Mendez et al., 1986). The concept of the IDD has been revived by Blumer (1991; Blumer et al., 1995). Although he suggested eight core symptoms, the most common were depressive mood, anergia, and irritability. The depressive episodes tended to last up to 12 hours, occurring on average five times a month along with periods of euphoria lasting up to 4 hours, on average three times a month. The outbursts of rage tended to occur in predominantly "good-natured, very ethical, or even deeply religious" individuals and were characteristically followed by remorse. They reported that 57% of 75 patients undergoing neurodiagnostic monitoring for epilepsy surgery had IDD (Blumer et al., 1998), and that patients with a large number of the above symptoms may be at increased risk of sudden unexpected suicide attempts and the development of an interictal psychosis. In fact, he believes that a continuum exists between IDD to a more severe dysphoric disorder with more prolonged and prominent psychosis and that interictal psychosis is invariably preceded by a marked dysphoric disorder (Blumer, 2000).

Treatment of Interictal Depression

Depressive disorders should be treated with supportive therapy provided by trained therapists, social workers, or epilepsy nurse specialists. More severe conditions may require specialized psychotherapy such as cognitive behavioral therapy (Davis et al., 1984). Psychotherapy can also be used to improve coping skills, and this has been shown to improve mild depressive illness and anxiety as well as to reduce seizure frequency (Gillham, 1990).

Patient support groups introduce patients to fellow sufferers who can provide emotional support, which has been shown to modify depression and dysthymia in people with epilepsy (Becú et al., 1993).

In view of the association between polytherapy and certain anticonvulsant drugs and affective disorders, considerable attention should be given to patients' antiepileptic drug prescriptions. Where possible, polytherapy should be reviewed, and treatment with monotherapy attempted. Certain anticonvulsants are more likely to be associated with depression, and are best avoided (see previous discussion).

Approximately 60% to 70% of acute major depressive episodes will respond to antidepressant drug treatment (Klerman, 1990), and early treatment intervention has been shown to reduce the duration of the episode by almost 50% (Kupfer et al., 1989). Choice depends on efficacy, interactions with concomitant medication, and adverse effect profile—in particular, epileptogenic potential. These factors have been reviewed by Lambert and Robertson (1999).

Clinically relevant interactions related to P450 hepatic isoenzymes mainly involve the concomitant use of antidepressants with phenytoin (PHT) and carbamazepine (CBZ). Fluoxetine or fluvoxamine can induce toxic anticonvulsant levels, whereas sertraline, paroxetine, and citalopram should have little effect (Lambert & Robertson, 1999).

The anticonvulsants, phenobarbitone, primidone, PHT, and CBZ are potent liver enzyme inducers (Brodie, 1992), which can result in reduced plasma antidepressant levels (thus reduced efficacy). Clinically significant interactions have been reported with tricyclic antidepressants (TCAs) (Spina et al., 1996) and paroxetine (Boyer & Blumhardt, 1992).

The incidence of seizures in nonepileptic populations occurring with therapeutic doses of antidepressants varies from 0.1% to 4% (Rosenstein et al., 1993), which is not much higher than the annual incidence of first seizures in the general population. Seizures have been found to be more likely to occur during the first week of antidepressant treatment or after an increase in dose, especially following rapid dose escalation (Rosenstein et al., 1993).

The older antidepressants, especially the tricyclic drugs, appear to lower seizure threshold. There is less evidence for such an effect with the newer antidepressants, especially moclobemide and citalopram, and there are no reliable data on newer agents such as mirtazapine and venlafaxine. In practice there have been reports of seizures with all the selective serotonin reuptake inhibitors (SSRIs); however, these have mainly been single case studies and often occur when the SSRI is administered with or shortly after another drug known to lower the seizure threshold, or in association with a withdrawal of a benzodiazepine.

Antidepressants should be introduced at a low dose, gradually increased to therapeutic levels, and they should be continued for at least 6 months after complete clinical recovery to avoid relapse. Electroconvulsive therapy (ECT) is not contraindicated in patients with epilepsy and may be life saving in patients with severe or psychotic depression not responding to antidepressants (Betts, 1981).

There are no data on the treatment of depression in epilepsy with transcranial magnetic stimulation, but early reports suggest that vagal nerve stimulation not only reduces seizures but also improves mood.

Anxiety Disorders

Anxiety can be a reaction to acquiring the label of epilepsy and the accompanying social and family problems (Betts, 1981). A self-reinforcing situation may occur, in which the patient is fearful of leaving the house in case he or she has a seizure, becomes anxious, hyperventilates, and thus increases the likelihood of convulsing. This in turn increases anxiety levels and a phobic anxiety state may ensue (Betts, 1981).

Ictal fear and anxiety have been described (Williams, 1956) and can be mistaken for anxiety or panic attacks, especially when there is a personal or family history of mood disorder. Conversely, anxiety attacks may be misdiagnosed as seizures, especially in people with temporal lobe epileptiform EEG activity or a history of epilepsy. In typical anxiety attacks, the symptoms and sequence may vary from episode to episode. The patients usually recover rapidly but may be tearful following the episode. Conversely, ictal anxiety or fear is usually stereotyped, with rapid onset, and tends to be of shorter duration than panic attacks. Ictal EEG recordings may help determine the diagnosis. Anxiety can also coexist with a depressive disorder, and is particularly common in patients with late-onset epilepsy (Robertson et al., 1987). Treatment of the underlying depression should also alleviate the anxiety.

Treatment of anxiety in epilepsy consists of relaxation training, biofeedback, counseling, behavioral and cognitive therapy, and, if necessary, formal psychotherapy. Minor tranquilizers should be avoided, as most are also anticonvulsants and thus are particularly difficult to withdraw.

Psychoses

When the psychiatric aspects of epilepsy were "rediscovered" in the 1950s and 1960s, American and English authors reported an excess of schizophrenia-like psychoses in epilepsy patients, especially in those suffering from temporal lobe epilepsy (Slater & Beard, 1963).

There is no internationally accepted syndromic classification of psychoses in epilepsy. Psychiatric aspects are not considered in the international classification of epilepsies, and the use of operational diagnostic systems for psychiatric disorders such as the DSM-IV (American Psychiatric Association, 1994) is limited because, if applied strictly, a diagnosis of functional psychosis is not allowed in the context of epilepsy.

Most of the previously proposed classification systems for psychosis in epilepsy are based on a combination of psychopathologic, etiologic, longitudinal, and EEG parameters. Unfortunately, due to a lack of taxonomic studies, our knowledge about regular syndromic associations is still limited. However, it must be recognized that the psychoses of epilepsy represent a separate psychopathologic state, which is subtly different from schizophrenia.

For pragmatic reasons, here psychoses of epilepsy will be grouped according to their temporal relationship to seizures.

Peri-ictal Psychoses

Psychotic symptoms may occur as part of the seizure and can be prolonged in cases of nonconvulsive status epilepticus where concurrent EEG studies may be required to make the diagnosis. Usually, EEG studies performed during generalized (absence) status reveal generalized bilateral synchronous spike and wave activity between 1 and 4 Hz. During complex partial status (epileptic twilight state) the EEG may show focal or bilateral epileptiform patterns with slowed background activity. A wide range of experiential phenomena may occur, including affective, behavioral, and perceptual experiences, often accompanied by automatisms. Consciousness is usually impaired (but not in cases of simple partial status); insight tends to be maintained, but amnesia will often follow.

Nonconvulsive status epilepticus requires immediate treatment with intravenous AEDs. It may closely mimic schizophrenia although atypical features such as eyelid fluttering or myoclonic jerks in absence status or oral automatisms in partial status clarify the diagnosis. However, any suspicion of status merits an EEG, but if unavailable, an intravenous injection of a benzodiazepine may help resolve the diagnosis.

The most common and well-investigated peri-ictal psychosis is that occurring postictally. The incidence and prevalence of postictal psychosis (PIP) is not known; however, rates of up to 18% have been reported in patients with medically intractable focal epilepsy (Kanner et al., 1996).

In 1988, Logsdail and Toone determined operational criteria for the diagnosis of PIP, which have been widely accepted: (1) onset of confusion or psychosis within 1 week of the return of apparently normal mental function; (2) duration of 1 day to 3 months; (3) mental state characterized by (a) clouding of consciousness, disorientation, or delirium; (b) delusions, hallucinations, in clear consciousness; (c) a mixture of (a) and (b); (4) no evidence of factors that may have contributed to the abnormal mental state: (a) anticonvulsant toxicity; (b) a previous history of interictal psychosis; (c) EEG evidence of status epilepticus; (d) recent history of head injury, or alcohol/drug intoxication.

Most patients have complex partial seizures (CPS) with secondary generalization, and develop psychosis after an exacerbation of seizure activity (usually a cluster). Most patients have a lucid interval (usually of 1–2 days) between the restoration of an apparent normal mental state after the seizure and the beginning of the psychosis. The presence of this lucid interval can be confusing diagnostically, and lead to a failure to recognize the behavior disorder as postictal.

The psychosis lasts days to weeks, but tends to recur, and up to 10% of patients go on to develop a chronic psychosis.

The phenomenology of PIP varies widely, abnormal mood, hallucinations, paranoid delusions with mysticism and religious preoccupations being common.

Suicidal ideation and suicide attempts are common, as are aggressive outbursts.

Treatments are related to better epilepsy control, and the use of a benzodiazepine such as clobazam. Antipsychotic drugs can lower the seizure threshold and provoke further seizures, thus prolonging the psychosis, and are best avoided if possible. In a patient with recurrent PIP, their use prophylactically can be important.

Interictal Psychosis

Forced Normalization. This refers to brief episodes of psychosis, characterized by paranoid delusions and auditory hallucinations, which last days to weeks and occur when seizures are infrequent or fully controlled. Such episodes have been reported to alternate with periods of increased seizure activity and may be terminated by a seizure. Landolt (1958) noted that the EEG normalized during such episodes of psychosis, generating the term forced or paradoxical normalization accompanying the alternative psychosis (Tellenbach, 1965). It is now acknowledged that the EEG does not have to fully normalize; however, the interictal disturbances decrease. The EEG abnormalities then return when the psychosis remits.

When patients with habitual seizures have administration of the new antiepileptic drugs abruptly terminated, this clinical picture has been reported frequently. Drugs most implicated include vigabatrin, topiramate, tiagabine, and zonisamide, although the clinical picture has been reported with every known antiepileptic drug.

Chronic Interictal Psychosis: The Schizophrenia-like Psychosis of Epilepsy. In 1963, Slater, Beard, and Glithero described the "schizophrenia-like psychoses of epilepsy." Risk factors for the development of schizophrenia-like psychosis of epilepsy (SLPE) are shown in Table 34-1.

The strongest risk factors for psychosis in epilepsy are those that indicate severity of epilepsy. These are long duration of active epilepsy, multiple seizure types, history of status epilepticus, and poor response to drug treatment. Seizure frequency, however, is reported by most authors to be lower in psychotic epilepsy patients than in nonpsychotic patients (Trimble, 1991). This may represent a variant of forced normalization.

Most authors do not find any evidence for an increased rate of psychiatric disorders in relatives of epilepsy patients with psychoses. The psychosis emerges after the epilepsy has been present for a number of years, and there is a clear excess of temporal lobe epilepsy in almost all case series.

Left lateralization of temporal lobe dysfunction or temporal lobe pathology was originally suggested as a risk factor for the development of schizophreniform psychosis by Flor-Henry (1969). The literature has been

TABLE 34-1. Risk Factors for the Development of Chronic Interictal Psychosis (SLPE)

Age of onset	Before/around puberty (10–14 years before onset of psychosis)
Seizures	Lack of history of febrile convulsions
	Multiple types
	CPS > PGE
	History of status epilepticus
	Medically intractable
Epilepsy syndrome	Localization related—TLE
Seizure frequency	Diminished (especially after temporal lobectomy)
Sex bias	Female > male
Neurology	Sinistrality
Premorbid personality	Normal
Family psychiatric history	None
Electroencephalogram (EEG)	Mesiobasal focus
	Left > right or bilateral
Functional neuroimaging (SPECT)	Left temporal hypoperfusion possibly independent of seizure focus
Pathology	Ganglioglioma/hamartoma

SLPE, schizophrenia-like psychosis of epilepsy; CPS, complex partial seizure; PGE, primary generalized epilepsy; TLE, temporal lobe epilepsy.

summarized by Trimble (1991), and shows a striking bias toward left lateralization, especially in patients with First Rank Symptoms of Schneider. This has been confirmed not only with EEG studies, but also with several imaging studies with SPECT, positron emission tomography (PET), MRI, and magnetic resonance spectroscopy (MRS).

The clinical picture is usually that of a paranoid psychosis, often with a prominence of religious delusions, preservation of affect, and relative lack of negative symptoms (Slater & Beard, 1963). A recent study has compared the phenomenology of interictal psychosis in epilepsy with temporal and frontal lobe foci. Patients with frontal lobe epilepsy tended to show more marked hebephrenic characteristics (emotional withdrawal and blunted affect) compared with patients with TLE (Adachi et al., 2000).

Treatment of Interictal Psychosis. Generally, management of acute psychosis will necessitate treatment with neuroleptic drugs in a calm environment, preferably a ward experienced in managing such neuropsychiatric patients. All neuroleptic medication reduces the seizure threshold to some degree. Generally clozapine, chlorpromazine, and loxapine should be avoided because these drugs would appear to be the most epileptogenic. Of the conventional neuroleptics, haloperidol appears to be relatively safe. If long-term treatment is required, sulpiride, quetiapine, olanzapine, and risperidone have little effect on seizure threshold and have less extrapyramidal adverse effects. Although depot neuroleptics improve compli-

ance, they are more difficult to titrate slowly, and if adverse effects do occur, they will last longer. Thus oral drugs are preferable. When possible, only one neuroleptic drug should be given, starting at the lowest possible dose and gradually increased, while monitoring seizure frequency. In some patients, where there is clear evidence that the psychosis is linked with a reduction of seizures, more proconvulsant drugs can be valuable, including clozapine.

Personality Changes in Epilepsy

Interictal behavioral changes have been documented for centuries. It is generally considered that most patients with epilepsy have a normal personality structure, but many authors agree that some undergo personality alteration. This, in effect, represents a subtle organic personality change.

Waxman and Geschwind (1975) described the interictal behavior syndrome of TLE, consisting of religiosity, hypergraphia, viscosity/stickiness, circumstantiality, and meticulous attention to detail (the Geschwind syndrome). The religiosity is often a part of an increasing sense of mysticism, but ecstatic ictal experiences, in some cases accompanied by visions of a religious nature, have been reported in patients with EEG evidence of temporal lobe discharges (Saver & Rabin, 1997). Patients may explain seizures, especially involving symptoms of depersonalization, derealization, and autoscopy, as religious experiences (attribution theory) (Saver & Rabin, 1997), and sudden religious conversions have been reported in the postictal period.

Waxman and Geschwind (1975) were the first to document the occurrences of hypergraphia, a tendency to excessive and compulsive writing in patients with TLE. They reported meticulous and detailed writing often concerned with moral, ethical, or religious issues. Since then, hypergraphia has been observed in 8% of patients with epilepsy (Hermann et al., 1988).

Sexual dysfunction, predominantly hyposexuality, has also been reported in 22% to 67% of patients with epilepsy. It has been thought to have both a psychological and neurophysiological basis, with factors such as temporal lobe epilepsy and treatment with liver enzyme–inducing anticonvulsants being implicated (for review, see Lambert, 2001).

As a contrast, patients with juvenile myoclonic epilepsy (the Janz syndrome) are said to have an impulsive and immature attitude, which often interferes with their management leading to noncompliance and sleep deprivation. This may relate to subtle frontal lobe changes that are now described in this disorder (Schmitz & Sander, 2000).

NEUROPSYCHOLOGICAL DEFICITS

In the past, cognitive deficits and cognitive decline were considered an integral part of epilepsy. This view was based on observations of biased samples of patients, often those who were living in institutionalized settings. Turner (1907) reported only 14% of 161 residents of a colony for epilepsy were "intact mentally." As the twentieth century progressed, more objective study, involving the assessment of intellect and other cognitive skills, has effectively demonstrated that cognitively, people with epilepsy represent a heterogeneous group.

Cognitive disturbances in epilepsy may be transient and related to seizure occurrence (ictal deficits) and recovery (postictal deficits). Cognitive difficulties, however, may be more stable and persist between seizures (interictal deficits).

Transient Cognitive Deficits

Seizure activity can manifest as a range of cognitive deficits of varying severity.

Transient Cognitive Impairment

Transient cognitive impairment (TCI) is a term used to describe fleeting cognitive disturbances, secondary to brief epileptogenic discharges. Our awareness of this phenomenon has been enhanced as a result of technological developments that have allowed the synchronization of EEG changes with computerized neuropsychological test performance. The length and frequency of the epileptic discharge and the type of cognitive task influence whether cognitive impairments are observed in association with electroencephalographic phenomena. Tasks requiring continuous attention and measures on which speed of response is the performance indicator seem to be particularly sensitive. Material-specific deficits have been reported relating to laterality of the discharge; for instance, disruption of verbal processing with left-sided discharges but not with right-sided discharges. There is some indication that children experiencing such discharges have a greater likelihood of poorer academic achievement, and studies in adults have shown impaired psychomotor performance as a correlate.

Clinical Seizures

Theoretically, any transient cognitive deficit could be the manifestation of epileptic discharges in the brain. Language disturbance, including speech arrest and dysphasic difficulties, can occur with partial seizures arising in the dominant frontal and temporal lobes. A number of cases of ictal amnesia have been reported in the literature defined as recurrent paroxysmal memory loss with no alteration in consciousness (Zeman & Hodges, 2000). During the attack, the person will appear normal, and will continue to engage in activities and conversations appropriately. Cognitive functions other than laying down a memory trace for events during the episode appear unaffected. Such episodes, however, are often reported retrospectively, may be difficult to distinguish from transient global amnesia, and may be misdiagnosed as the onset of a dementing illness in the elderly. Bilateral runs of epileptic discharges from mesial temporal structures may be the physiological bases of pure amnestic seizures.

Nonconvulsive Status

Continuous partial and absence seizures can severely disrupt cognitive processes and may mimic a dementing disorder. However, despite the severity of the symptoms that may present, nonconvulsive status, as a cause of cognitive disturbance, may go undetected and persist for days and months. The risk of misdiagnosis is high if the status occurs in the elderly, in individuals with learning disabilities, and in those without a history of epilepsy (Shorvon, 1994).

During absence status a range of disturbances have been reported, ranging from slight cognitive inefficiency to marked cognitive obtundation. Complex partial status has been associated with a range of deficits, and the presentation is dependent on the cortical regions involved. Prolonged episodes of language disturbance, spatial disorientation, dysgraphia, and perceptual deficits, ranging in severity up to cortical blindness, have been reported.

Postictal Deficits

Recovery from seizures can be variable, and for some individuals neuropsychological assessment undertaken in close proximity to complex partial seizures and generalized attacks may underestimate an individual's potential. Thompson and colleagues (2003) described cases that showed marked fluctuations in their competency on memory tests in relation to the proximity of the testing session to a seizure. Patients assessed as much as 2 days following a bout of complex partial seizures performed significantly less well on tests of learning and memory than 2 weeks following the episode. Performance on other tests of cognitive functioning was unaffected.

Seizure Precipitants

There are a number of case reports in the literature of seizures induced by higher mental activities, including reading, writing, arithmetic, memorizing, and chess and card playing. Anderson and Wallis (1986) report the case of a 34-year-old accountant whose seizures appeared to be activated by difficult mental arithmetic. Written calculation, visualizing numbers, counting, digit span, and other activities involving numerical manipulation had no such effect. Matsuoka and colleagues (2000) describe the findings from a study of 480 patients with epilepsy who underwent a specially devised neuropsychological activation program as part of their routine EEG examination. Eight percent of the sample had epileptic discharges provoked by the mental tasks. Writing and written calculation provoked the most discharges (68% and 55%, respectively).

Interictal Deficits

There is no one cognitive deficit or profile of cognitive functions that characterizes people with epilepsy. The presence and nature of any cognitive problem will be influenced by a variety of factors. The most potent cause is the presence of brain pathology, with the type of cognitive problem being determined by the location, extent, and age of onset of the brain abnormality. Advances in MRI technology have resulted in the identification of brain pathology in an increasing number of cases with intractable epilepsy. Hippocampal sclerosis and cortical dysplasias are among the most common pathologies identified in poorly controlled partial seizure disorders (Sisodiya, 2000). Other factors implicated are drug treatment and psychological causes such as anxiety and depression.

Intelligence

Toward the end of the 19th century, people with epilepsy were regarded as having limited intellectual abilities, which were prone to deteriorate further. Neuropsychological studies over the last 50 years have provided evidence that people with epilepsy encompass the entire range of intellectual abilities, and only a minority deteriorate over time.

In a recent unpublished survey of 100 consecutive outpatients referred for a neuropsychological assessment, we found 40% were of average intellect and a further 15% of above average intelligence. Included in the latter sample was Y.G., a 70-year-old woman with complex partial seizures of temporal lobe origin. Seizures began during her second pregnancy at the age of 34 and have continued at a frequency of two to three episodes per month from that time. When assessed at the age of 61 years, her verbal intellectual quotient (VIQ) was superior (126) and performance quotient (PIQ) was very superior (136). When assessed 9 years later, both VIQ and PIQ fell in the superior ability range (VIQ = 132; PIQ = 142). She was referred due to her complaints that she was experiencing some difficulty retaining mathematical formulae, which was a necessary part of the physics degree she had recently embarked on.

There exist some epilepsy syndromes, however, whose natural history is one of a resultant learning disability. In early infantile epileptic encephalopathy and early myoclonic encephalopathy, seizures develop in the first year of life. Many infants with these disorders die, but those who survive have profound learning disabilities and sensory and motor impairments. In West and Lennox Gastaut syndromes, learning disability is one of the main symptoms. For many individuals there is a slowing of cognitive milestones with a later plateauing.

About 20% of people with learning disabilities have epilepsy; the proportion rises in those with more severe degrees of learning impairment (Coulter, 1993). The learning disability and the seizures are both secondary consequences of underlying cerebral damage or immaturity. For instance, individuals with Down syndrome have a reported 10% risk of developing seizures; for many the epilepsy occurs later in life, and with autism there is a reported incidence in the region of 30%.

Intellectual Deterioration

Intellectual deterioration was once thought to be symptomatic of the epileptic condition. Longitudinal investigations, however, suggest that for adults and children who respond well to drug treatment, the intellectual prognosis is good (Holmes et al., 1998; Neyens et al., 1999). Certainly, intellectual deterioration does occur in a small, but significant, proportion of individuals but this may be related to a variety of factors. Frequent, especially tonic-clonic convulsions and episodes of status epilepticus have been associated with poorer intellectual prognosis. Repeated minor head injuries secondary to tonic and atonic seizures have also been associated with a poor outcome intellectually.

There are a number of rare conditions in which intellectual or cognitive decline is a prominent feature. Rasmussen's encephalitis is one such condition. The onset of epilepsy is usually in mid-childhood, although it can be later. Seizures usually take the form of continuous partial motor seizures, usually in one limb, which gradually progresses to involve the ipsilateral limb. A hemiplegia may result. Repeat MRI scans demonstrate progressive focal atrophy.

Electrical status in slow wave sleep (ESES) describes a condition in which there are continuous periods of abnormal EEG discharges during sleep. It is associated with gross intellectual deterioration and other cognitive and attentional difficulties. Onset is usually in childhood. Seizures usually remit in adolescence and some cognitive improvement can occur at this time, although intellectual and cognitive gains are generally small.

Progressive myoclonic epilepsy refers to a group of rare conditions characterized by a progressive myoclonus, dementia, and motor decline. Lafora body disease and Lundberg's disease are examples of conditions in this group.

There exist a number of other neurologic conditions where epilepsy may be a prominent symptom and also where progressive intellectual decline or some fall in intellectual capacity is expected. Epilepsy can develop following cerebrovascular disease, cerebral infections following severe open head injuries, and in about 20% to 25% of people with Alzheimer disease.

Memory

Patients' complaints of disturbed memory represent the most frequently reported cognitive problem and the most common reason underlying referral for a neuropsychological assessment. In a survey involving 760 people with epilepsy, we found 54% rated their "disturbed" memory as a moderate or severe nuisance. This contrasted to a nuisance rating of 23% in a control group (Thompson & Corcoran, 1992).

Episodic Memory. Deficits of new learning have been the subject of most investigations and are the most common cognitive impairment recorded in patients with temporal lobe epilepsy (Thompson, 1997). The most extreme case of memory disturbance is an amnesic syndrome, which is caused by bilateral pathologic changes in the temporal lobes. The best documented examples have been cases following bilateral resection of the temporal lobes for the surgical relief of epilepsy, or unilateral temporal lobectomy cases where there is pathology in the contralateral temporal lobe (Baxendale, 1998). Individuals with epilepsy secondary to viral encephalitic illnesses may also present with a profound, persisting amnesia.

Cases involving unilateral pathology of the temporal lobes have generally been reported to be associated with material-specific deficits, verbal memory impairments with left temporal lobe lesions, and spatial memory impairment with right temporal lobe lesions. More recent research and clinical experience, however, indicates that these material-specific deficits are more evident following unilateral temporal lobectomy than in preoperative or nonsurgical cases with temporal lobe epilepsy. Several variables have been identified as influencing the presence and severity of memory problems in temporal lobe samples. The nature and age of onset of the underlying pathology are significant factors. Tumors developing in adulthood are more likely to produce material-specific memory problems than earlier onset pathologies. Hippocampal sclerosis is the most common pathologic change identified in patients undergoing temporal lobe surgery, but only a subgroup of cases show material-specific deficits. Hippocampal sclerosis is a cortical dysgenetic lesion that has either developed during embryogenesis, or has arisen secondary to a prolonged febrile convulsion in early infancy. In such cases, the cerebral plasticity of the developing brain may allow for considerable relocation of function to unaffected areas in the ipsilateral hemisphere, or analogous areas in the contralateral hemisphere. Even patients with a severely sclerotic hippocampus may perform within normal limits on memory tests.

Patient Complaints and Memory Test Scores. A clinically common experience is the apparent paradox that patients complaining bitterly of memory problems can perform adequately on formal memory tests. The conclusion often drawn is that the complaints are a reflection of negative perception, secondary to mood disturbance. There is some evidence that elevated levels of anxiety and depression can negatively impact on concentration, and as a consequence, result in memory impairments. Research evidence, however, is accumulating to indicate there are several other explanations for this mismatch between patient complaints and test performance. Conventional memory tests allow for the assessment of memory at intervals up to 1 hour. For some patients, memory performance can be normal when assessed at standardized intervals, and accelerated forgetting is evident only at 24 hours or more.

The clinical assessment of episodic memory is constrained, not only in the timing of delayed recall but also in the type of "experience" that can be assessed. In our own studies we have been striving to develop measures that reflect the retrieval of real-word episodic memories. To this end, we are developing virtual reality paradigms. We hypothesize that, for some individuals who perform adequately on clinical tests, deficits will be revealed on these novel tests which can more readily mimic memory functioning in everyday life.

For other patients, a memory deficit may be something that occurs in proximity to seizures. It is common clinical practice not to embark on a neuropsychological assessment if a patient has had a seizure in the past 24 hours. However, recent evidence suggests that patients assessed following seizures can have material-specific deficits that are not observed interictally. Thus, timing of the assessment may affect whether memory deficits are detected.

Remote Memory. Research into memory functioning in epilepsy has seldom explored for the existence of deficits in other memory systems. We recently assessed memory for past events by administering a specially designed remote memory questionnaire to three groups of patients with epilepsy and a control group without epilepsy (Bergin et al., 2000). The questionnaire assessed knowledge of public events that had occurred between 1980 and 1991. The epilepsy groups comprised patients with temporal lobe epilepsy or extratemporal lobe epilepsy, and individuals with primary generalized epilepsy. Patients with temporal lobe epilepsy performed significantly less well on the questionnaire than all the other groups, but no effect of laterality of temporal lobe disturbance was recorded. Patients with extratemporal or primary generalized epilepsy did not differ in their scores from controls. There was an association with seizure frequency and performance of the questionnaire, with those individuals who had experienced more frequent generalized seizures during the 10-year span of the questionnaire performing more poorly. The fact that extratemporal and primary generalized epilepsy groups performed as well as controls suggested that the occurrence of seizures per se was not sufficient to disrupt the formation and retrieval of remote memories. It seems, rather, that the temporal location of the pathology is the most pertinent variable, and the frequency of the seizures is an indicator of the degree of functional abnormality.

Prospective Memory. Prospective memory refers to the capacity to remember to do things at some future point in time. In our survey of everyday memory problems in epilepsy, it was clear from the replies received that many patients experienced frequent prospective memory errors, including forgetting to take their tablets. Prospective memory is very important but it is seldom tested clinically. This is largely because it is logistically difficult to devise tests to match the complexity of real-life situations. An attempt was made by Bergin and colleagues. They studied 40 patients with intractable temporal lobe seizures who were undergoing a period of video EEG telemetry as part of their presurgical assessment program (Thompson, 1997).

The prospective memory task given to the subjects was to answer a written question regarding the likelihood of a seizure occurring at four predetermined times during the day. Completion of the task was undertaken in full view of the camera, and the videotape was reviewed to determine if and when charts were filled in. Patients with right temporal lobe epilepsy as a group tended to perform more poorly than other patient groups, and this included three patients who failed to complete the task. Patients who reported a weak memory in response to three everyday prospective memory questions tended to perform more poorly on the prospective task described.

Language Functioning

Language functioning has been the subject of less research than memory. Existing evidence, however, suggests deficits may be present that can have a significant impact on academic and social functioning.

Davey and Thompson (1991) reported a high level of language difficulties in adult patients with intractable epilepsy attending a tertiary referral center. Sixty consecutive admissions were administered a range of tests of language competency. The most widespread difficulties were noted on tests of expressive language functioning, with less pronounced difficulties being recorded on tests of comprehension or literacy. It was noteworthy that no patient had ever received a speech therapy evaluation or any intervention, and in several individuals the deficits were clearly contributing to difficulties both occupationally and interpersonally.

An increased incidence of academic underachievement is a long-recognized finding in children with epilepsy. Deficits in reading and spelling seem to be the most marked. In a recent study, Breier and colleagues (2000) indicated that subgroups of adult patients with complex partial seizures have a specific reading and spelling deficit that is not a confound of intellectual level. Individuals with the specific literacy weakness were shown also to have selective verbal processing deficits as measured by tests of word definition, naming ability, and verbal fluency. Other investigators have reported significant relationships between the degree of the pathology in the left temporal lobe and deficits on tests of expressive language ability (Davies et al., 1998).

Acquired Epileptic Aphasia. This condition, also known as Landau-Kleffner syndrome, is a rare disorder in which persisting aphasia develops in association with severe focal EEG abnormalities. It begins in childhood, usually presenting between the ages of 4 to 11 years. Language development prior to the onset is generally normal. The first symptom is usually the experience of receptive language difficulties, and the majority of cases go on to have generalized and partial seizures. In some cases, seizures predate the aphasia. Language deterioration occurs over time and total mutism can result. The EEG recordings are disturbed with multifocal spike and wave, most often seen in temporal and parieto-occipital regions. Although some patients' language functions improve as seizures become less frequent or stop, many individuals are often left with significant language problems.

Language Dominance. Most people have language functions lateralized predominantly to the left cerebral hemisphere. Rates are lower for genetic left-handers. There is an elevated incidence of atypical language dominance in patients with epilepsy. Atypical language dominance refers to language functions lateralized predominantly to the right hemisphere or bilateral representation. Associated factors identified to date include early cerebral insult to the left hemisphere, early onset of recurrent seizures, left- (pathologic) handedness, or weak right-handedness (Springer et al., 1999).

Language laterality is a clinically relevant variable in those undergoing resective surgery. The intracarotid amobarbital (sodium amytal) procedure (IAP) is the gold standard for establishing language dominance. It is an invasive procedure, which involves the temporary anesthetization of one cerebral hemisphere with a short-acting barbiturate, amobarbital sodium. The drug is injected into the carotid artery via catherization of the femoral artery. Following injection, a transient contralateral hemiparesis and EEG changes confirm the drug's unilateral effect. Disruption of language functions, including mutism and dysphasic difficulties, characteristically follows the injection into the language dominant hemisphere. No major difficulties follow the nondominant hemisphere injection, although dysarthria may be a feature. The technique has been used with only minor procedural changes for the past 50 years and there are concerns regarding its reliability and validity. Furthermore, it is an invasive procedure, which carries a risk of physical and psychological morbidity. It is also costly because it necessitates a hospital admission and a specialist team involving a number of professionals (neuropsychologist, neuroradiologist, electro-encephalographic technician, cameraman, radiologic nurse, radiographer, and neurologist). Other measures are being designed in an attempt to replace this procedure, and the greatest promise has been the development of fMRI paradigms (Baxendale, 2000).

Executive Functioning

Executive function is a term covering a range of mental processes that humans employ in situations that require new solutions, strategies, and decision making. The processes encompassed by this term include attention, movement programming, abstract reasoning, mental flexibility, and response inhibition. Impairments of these processes are generally considered to be associated with damage or dysfunction in the frontal brain regions. Faulty operation of these processes can have a profoundly detrimental impact on a person's ability to cope with independent living and to maintain appropriate social behavior. It is therefore surprising, given the importance of such functioning, that there have been few studies exploring whether deficits exist in individuals who have frontal lobe epilepsy. Upton and Thompson (1996a) assessed the test performance of 74 patients with frontal lobe epilepsy on a series of tests tapping executive functioning. Test performance was compared with patients with temporal lobe epilepsy. The measures employed included a number of cognitive and motor tests reported in the research literature to be sensitive to frontal lobe disturbance. Impairments were observed in the frontal lobe group on a number of measures, although the differences between the groups were not great. The left frontal group tended to be most impaired, although the analysis revealed few significant differences between the left and right frontal groups. One explanation is that the frontal brain region acts more as a homologue with less differentiation of functioning than is seen in the temporal brain regions. Furthermore, it is generally accepted that there is rapid propagation of seizure activity within the frontal lobes, such that seizures spread rapidly bilaterally. The investigators went on to analyze whether test performance was affected according to the region of the frontal lobe involved. There were very few significant differences between frontal brain regions, and again it is possible that propagation of seizure spread within the frontal lobe may account for this (Upton & Thompson, 1996b). In a later study the authors reported maximal impairment on a task tapping cognitive reasoning and efficiency in patients with bifrontal pathology. This patient group was clearly limited in their ability to benefit from feedback and their performance contrasted to that of the temporal lobe group and those with more circumscribed frontal lobe lesions (Upton & Thompson, 1999).

Helmstaedter and colleagues (1996) assessed 23 patients with frontal lobe epilepsy on a series of tests, again selected to measure executive and motor functions attributed to the frontal lobes, and compared performance with 38 patients with temporal lobe epilepsy. Significant differences were seen between the frontal and temporal lobe groups on tests tapping response maintenance and inhibition and motor coordination, but not on measures of speed and attention. The authors did not find any effect of lateralization in the frontal group.

Antiepileptic Medication

The number of studies assessing the impact of AEDs on cognition has increased dramatically over the last decade, and yet, despite this potential wealth of data, very little consensus emerges and many findings appear conflicting. On closer inspection, differences in outcome are not surprising because the studies can vary with regard to a number of important parameters. A major factor is the nature of the brain under study. Populations investigated to date include animals (usually rats), healthy volunteers, newly diagnosed patients, chronic epilepsy cases, infants, children, the elderly, the learning disabled, and, more recently, the children of mothers with epilepsy. The reaction to a drug may be expected to be different in an animal versus a human brain, and in a healthy versus an "epileptic" brain. In patients with epilepsy, differences in the impact of a drug may be expected between a developing brain, a cerebrally mature brain, an aging brain, and a severely dysplastic brain. Other sources of variance between studies include drug type and dosage, duration of treatment, and concomitant medication. Additionally, study designs range from prospective, randomized controlled trials to cross-sectional, uncontrolled comparisons. The former are the ideal but on their own may dilute out drug effects if adverse effects occur in only a minority of cases. Furthermore, such studies are costly and logistically difficult, and are generally sponsored by the pharmaceutical industry, which can bring with it another set of biases. Statistical treatment of the data and neuropsychological tests employed are an additional source of variance. Some studies have used a single cognitive measure, whereas others have used extensive batteries.

Problems of interpretation aside, some tentative conclusions can be drawn. Polypharmacy increases the likelihood of adverse cognitive effects, particularly when individuals are using more than two compounds. Certain combinations appear to have particularly potent adverse effects. For instance, phenobarbitone and sodium valproate taken together have long been associated with cognitive slowing. Unfortunately, data are lacking for the majority of drug combinations. There are 15 AEDs available, which results in many varied possible permutations if only duo-therapy combinations are considered. No evidence exists regarding the possible cognitive impact of the combination with other CNS-acting drugs, such as antidepressants and antipsychotic agents.

For individual drugs, it is difficult to rank them in order of cognitive impact—i.e., adverse to positive. However, some consensus exists that phenobarbitone, the oldest AED compound (in use for almost 90 years!), has been associated with more negative cognitive changes. For phenytoin, considerable confusion exists, with some arguing for a slowing in cognitive processing, whereas others have argued that adverse changes have occurred only at toxic levels and that any changes are motor rather than cognitive in nature. Carbamazepine and sodium valproate have been associated with fewer cognitive adverse effects. Both phenytoin and sodium valproate, however, have been associated with cases of reversible encephalopathy. The newer antiepileptic drugs (lamotrigine, tiagabine, and gabapentin) have been much less studied, but available evidence suggests cognitive effects are minimal, or at least no different from carbamazepine and sodium valproate. Controversy, however, surrounds topiramate. Randomized controlled trials have yielded minimal adverse effects, whereas less controlled clinical studies have reported significant cognitive impairment, including reduced attention span, verbal fluency, and impaired verbal learning (Aldenkamp et al., 2000; Thompson et al., 2000).

Clinical experience and available evidence suggests any of the existing AEDs can give rise to adverse cognitive effects. At a clinical level, if patients present with complaints of cognitive decline, even if insidious and not related to drug changes, their antiepileptic drug treatment should be considered as a potential causal factor and the drug hypothesis can be tested out. Neuropsychological assessments can be undertaken before and following drug adjustments.

Surgical Treatment

Temporal lobe resective surgery is the most commonly undertaken procedure (Polkey, 2000a). In such cases, about two thirds of patients are reported to experience complete cessation of seizures postoperatively. Frontal lobe resections are less frequently undertaken, and a seizure-free outcome is less likely with this procedure. A hemispherectomy involves the deactivation of an entire cerebral hemisphere, and this constitutes the most radical resective procedure. In such cases there is extensive evidence of significant atrophy, major structural abnormalities, and limited positive functional capacity in the to-be-resected hemisphere.

Corpus callosotomy and multiple subpial transection (also known as Morrel's procedure) are two surgical procedures in which the aim of surgery is to inhibit the spread of seizure activity by cutting the fibers assessed to be implicated in the transmission. Corpus callosotomy involves complete, or more usually partial, disconnection of the corpus callosum, which joins the two cerebral hemispheres. Multiple subpial transection refers to a procedure in which the neuronal tracts are severed vertically, and it is generally undertaken when the assessed epileptogenic area is known to support important functions, usually those involved in speech or motor functioning, in cases in which resective surgery is not viable.

Temporal Lobe Surgery

If unilateral resection of medial temporal lobe structures is undertaken in a patient whose contralateral temporal lobe is dysfunctional, as mentioned earlier, a severe amnesic syndrome may result. Warrington and Duchenne (1992) reported one such case. Examination of the resected temporal lobe revealed no pathologic changes. When the case later came to autopsy, it was found that the contralateral medial temporal lobe structures were sclerotic. To assess the risk of an amnesic syndrome developing in patients undergoing unilateral temporal lobe surgery, the sodium amytal procedure was modified to allow for memory testing. This was straightforward, because memory is subsequently tested for items initially presented to assess language functions. When the side ipsilateral to the seizure focus is injected, normal memory function is expected. When memory function is impaired, however, the patient would be deemed at risk of developing a postoperative amnesic syndrome and would either not proceed to surgery, or have a more tailored resection (Baxendale, 2000).

Unilateral temporal lobe resection in the presence of an intact contralateral hemisphere is reported to result in material-specific memory losses. The most consistent finding is a decline in verbal memory after surgery on the language-dominant hemisphere. Some reports document changes in nonverbal memory following temporal lobe surgery on the nondominant temporal lobe; however, this has not always been a consistent finding (Baxendale, 1998).

Research studies and clinical experience indicate that although overall memory test scores reveal a decline in memory following temporal lobe resection, such figures mask considerable patient variability. One problem facing the neuropsychologist is the ability to predict which patient may be at risk for memory decline postoperatively. In general, risk factors that have been identified to date for a decline in memory function postoperatively include older age at the time of the operation, dominant temporal lobe resections, and postoperative seizures. The degree of neuronal loss within the resected hippocampus has also been identified with those individuals with less widespread loss in resected structures showing greater decreases in memory (Baxendale, 1998). Furthermore, the functional integrity of the contralateral hemisphere also may influence outcome for memory.

The extent of resection is routinely cited as a relevant factor for memory loss, with larger resections associated with greater impairment postoperatively. Some centers undertake selective operations and spare much of the lateral cortex in an attempt to preserve memory function. Goldstein and Polkey (1993) compared the outcome for memory in 42 patients having either a temporal lobectomy or a smaller resection, a selective amygdalohippocampectomy. Overall, their findings provide some evidence in support of the protective effect for memory for selective operations.

After dominant temporal lobectomy, marked persisting aphasias are rare but declines in naming have been reported. Saykin and colleagues (1992) measured confrontation naming, phonemic and semantic fluency, repetition, comprehension, and reading recognition both before and after surgery. For dominant hemisphere resections a relative decline in naming as well as other language skills was noted, and this occurred particularly in those patients with a later onset of seizures and underlying pathology. Hermann and colleagues (1999) compared changes in naming ability in patients who had the superior temporal gyrus removed versus patients who did not. The nature of the resection did not affect performance on language tests, but older age at onset and absence of hippocampal sclerosis were predictors of a decline in naming skills. This finding supports the view that an early age of onset, which may result in a degree of cerebral reorganization, can be a protective factor regarding deficits after surgery.

There is increasing consensus that decrements in intellectual ability after temporal lobe surgery are minimal and more likely to occur if testing occurs in the early months following surgery. Generally, no marked changes are documented in intellectual functions a year, or more, postoperatively. Indeed, patients may show a substantial gain, particularly those who have become seizure-free.

Frontal Lobe Surgery

Some of the earliest accounts of the impact of frontal lobe surgery come from the Montreal Neurological Institute. These early reports suggest minimal cognitive change, with most difficulties improving over time. In one case, actually the surgeon's sister, it is written that "her sense of humour, memory and insight into the thoughts and feelings of others was altogether unimpaired. She was capable of intelligent conversation and did not talk either more or less than good taste demanded." (Penfield & Evans, 1935) However, reading the report of these early cases there are hints of some executive disturbance. For example, "the capacity to follow instruction was unimpaired but indications and capacity for planned action were clearly defective."

Helmstaedter and colleagues (1998) assessed cognitive functioning in 33 patients before and after frontal lobe surgery. The neuropsychological assessment included tests of speed and attention, motor sequencing and coordination, response maintenance and inhibition, short-term memory, and language. At the 3-month follow-up examination, patients who had undergone a temporal lobectomy showed improved functioning on these tests, whereas patients who had undergone frontal lobe resective surgery showed a mild decline. Those individuals undergoing frontal resections who became seizure-free showed the best cognitive outcome postoperatively.

Hemispherectomy

The cognitive impact of hemispherectomy appears variable. The research literature until recently has indicated that the earlier age of surgery and right hemisphere operations have the most favorable prognosis. There are several reports of positive outcomes following left-sided hemispherectomies. Arzimanoglou and colleagues (2000) reported substantial language gains in four left-sided hemispherectomy cases operated on between the ages of 8 and 30 months. All were rendered seizure-free and all developed some expressive skills, but this was limited to short, syntactically simple sentences. The postoperative outcome appears poorer in individuals with congenitally abnormal cerebral hemispheres than in those with later onset pathologies (de Bode & Curtiss, 2000).

Corpus Callosotomy

The early neuropsychological evaluation of these cases revealed no significant sequelae. A number of studies undertaken in the 1970s on the so-called "split-brain patients" did elicit some cognitive processing abnormalities, but these generally required specialized apparatus such as a tachistoscope. Standard neuropsychological assessment shows little or no persisting negative effect when compared with preoperative level (Polkey, 2000b).

The classic split-brain syndrome had been reported in some cases following complete resection of the colossal fibers. In general, the syndrome is more likely to be evident on manual tasks, but competition is observed between the right and left hands, representing the two halves of the brain. It generally resolves in a few days as the patient uses external cues, although it may still be present on novel tasks requiring bimanual co-operation. There are a few cases documented of persisting deficits.

Anterior resections may be accompanied by transient mutism in the first few days postoperatively, although there are a few cases of persisting language difficulties. These seem to be more prevalent in individuals who have been shown to have abnormal language lateralization. Memory dysfunction has been noted in a minority of patients following partial and complete callosotomy. It is proposed that in these cases it may result from the disconnection of damaged but interdependent hippocampal formation by severing the hippocampal commissure.

NEUROPSYCHOLOGICAL REHABILITATION

Cognitive rehabilitation is an approach generally advocated in the neuropsychological literature. For patients with epilepsy, the main focus of rehabilitation programs has been to reduce the impact of memory problems. Clinical experience suggests such interventions can be effective, with training in the use of external memory aids such as diaries and physical prompts being the most efficacious. Assessment of the effectiveness of such input is limited, and existing studies suggest gains may be small and greatly influenced by motivational factors (Thompson, 1997).

■ KEY POINTS

☐ Psychiatric disorders, usually depression or anxiety, are common in people with epilepsy and the risk tends to increase with severity and frequency of seizures.

☐ Etiologic factors associated with depression include the biological, the psychological, and the iatrogenic: temporal lobe epilepsy especially of left-sided origin, polypharmacy, and treatment with barbiturates, phenytoin, and vigabatrin are commonly implicated. Depression tends to respond to treatment with antidepressant medication, which should be introduced at a low dose, gradually increased, and continued for 6 months after full clinical recovery. Tricyclic drugs are best avoided avoided because of their tendency to lower seizure threshold.

☐ Postictal psychosis may develop in up to 18% of people with medically intractable epilepsy and tends to occur after an exacerbation of seizures. Chronic interictal psychosis tends to develop 10 to 14 years after the onset of seizures and would appear to be associated with severity of epilepsy and a left temporal lobe focus. Long-term neuroleptic medication may be required.

☐ Cognitive disturbance in epilepsy may be transient and be related to the seizure or the recovery period. Chronic cognitive disturbance is most likely to be the result of underlying brain pathology. Memory impairments are the most frequently encountered deficit, and this is a consequence of the increased susceptibility of the temporal lobes for epileptogenesis.

☐ The treatment of epilepsy can result in cognitive impairments. Antiepileptic medications may cause cognitive slowing and other deficits. Of the surgical treatments, the most frequently undertaken is temporal lobectomy, and this can cause exacerbation of underlying memory problems.

KEY READINGS

Lambert MV, Robertson MM: Depression in epilepsy: Etiology, phenomenology, and treatment. Epilepsia 40(Suppl. 10):S21–S47, 1999.

Trimble MR: The Psychoses of Epilepsy. New York: Raven Press, 1991.

Thompson PJ, Shorvon SD, Heaney D: Epilepsy, in Greenwood R, McMillan TM, Barnes MP, Ward CD (eds): Handbook of Neurological Rehabilitation, ed 2. Sussex, UK: Psychology Press, 2001.

REFERENCES

Adachi, N, Onuma, T, Nishiwaki, S, et al: Inter-ictal and post-ictal psychoses in frontal lobe epilepsy: A retrospective comparison with psychoses in temporal lobe. Seizure 9:328–335, 2000.

Aldenkamp AP, Baker G, Mulder OG, et al: A multicenter, randomized clinical study to evaluate the effect on cognitive function of topiramate compared with valproate as add-on therapy to carbamazepine in patients with partial-onset seizures. Epilepsia 41:1167–1178, 2000.

Altshuler LL, Devinsky O, Post RM, et al: Depression, anxiety, and temporal lobe epilepsy: Laterality of focus and symptoms. Arch Neurol 47:284–288, 1990.

Altshuler L, Rausch R, Delrahim S, et al: Temporal lobe epilepsy, temporal lobectomy, and major depression. J Neuropsychiatry Clin Neurosci 11:436–443, 1999.

American Psychiatric Association. Diagnostic and Statistical Manual of Mental Disorders 4th Edition DSM-IV. Washington, DC: APA, 1994.

Anderson NE, Wallis WT: Activation of epileptiform activity by mental arithmetic. Arch Neurol 43:624–626, 1986.

Arzimanoglou AA, Andermann F, Aicardi J, et al: Sturge-Weber syndrome: Indications and results of surgery in patients. Neurology 55:1472–1479, 2000.

Baker GA, Nashef L, van Hout BA: Current issues in the management of epilepsy: The impact of frequent seizures on cost of illness, quality of life and mortality. Epilepsia 38(Suppl. 1):S1–S8, 1995.

Baker GA, Jacoby A, Chadwick DW: The associations of psychopathology in epilepsy: A community study. Epilepsy Res 25:29–39, 1996.

Baxendale SA: Amnesia in temporal lobectomy patients: Historical perspective and review. Seizure 7:15–24, 1998.

Baxendale SA, Van Paesschen W, Thompson PJ, et al: Hippocampal cell loss and gliosis: Relationship to pre-operative and post-operative memory functions. Neuropsychiatry, Neuropsychol Behav Neurol 11:12–21, 1998.

Baxendale SA: Carotid amobarbital testing and other amobarbital procedures, in Oxbury J, Polkey C, Duchowny M (eds): Intractable Focal Epilepsy. London: Saunders, 2000, pp. 627–636.

Becú M, Becú N, Manzur G, Kochen S: Self-help epilepsy groups: An evaluation of effect on depression and schizophrenia. Epilepsia 34:841–845, 1993.

Bergin PS, Thompson PJ, Baxendale SA, et al: Remote memory in epilepsy. Epilepsia 41:231–239, 2000.

Betts TA: Depression, anxiety and epilepsy, in Reynolds EH, Trimble MR (eds): Epilepsy and Psychiatry. Edinburgh, Scotland: Churchill Livingstone, 1981, pp. 60–71.

Blumer D: Epilepsy and disorders of mood, in Smith DB, Treiman DM, Trimble MR (eds): Neurobehavioral Problems in Epilepsy. New York: Raven Press, 1991, pp. 185–195.

Blumer, D: Dysphoric disorders and paroxysmal affects: Recognition and treatment of epilepsy-related psychiatric disorders. Harv Rev Psychiatry 8:8–17, 2000.

Blumer D, Montouris G, Hermann B: Psychiatric morbidity in seizure patients on a neurodiagnostic monitoring unit. J Neuropsychiatry Clin Neurosci 7:445–456, 1995.

Blumer D, Wakhlu S, Davies K, Hermann B: Psychiatric outcome of temporal lobectomy for epilepsy: Incidence and treatment of psychiatric complications. Epilepsia 39:478–486, 1998.

Boyer WF, Blumhardt CL: The safety profile of paroxetine. J Clin Psychiatry 53 (Suppl. 2):61–66, 1992.

Breier JJ, Fletcher JM, Wheless JW, et al: Profiles of cognitive performance associated with reading disability in temporal lobe epilepsy. J Clin Exp Neuropsychol 22:804–816, 2000.

Brodie MJ: Drug interactions in epilepsy. Epilepsia 33(Suppl. 1): S13–S22, 1992.

Bromfield EB, Altshuler L, Leiderman DB, et al: Cerebral metabolism and depression in patients with complex partial seizures. Arch Neurol 49:617–623, 1992.

Coulter DL: Epilepsy and mental retardation: An overview. Am J Ment Retard 98:S1–S11, 1993.

Davey D: Thompson P: Interictal language functioning in chronic epilepsy. J Neurolinguistics 4:381–399, 1991.

Davies KG, Bell BD, Bush AJ, et al: Naming decline after left anterior temporal lobectomy correlates with pathological status of resected hippocampus. Epilepsia 39:407–419, 1998.

Davis GR, Armstrong HE, Donovan DM, Temkin NR: Cognitive-behavioural treatment of depressed affect amongst epileptics: Preliminary findings. J Clin Psychol 4:930–935, 1984.

de Bode S, Curtiss S: Language after hemispherectomy. Brain Cogn 43:135–138, 2000.

Devinsky O, Bear DM: Varieties of depression in epilepsy. Neuropsychiatry Neuropsychol Behav Neurology 4:49–61, 1991.

Dodrill CB, Batzel LW: Inter-ictal behavioural features of patients with epilepsy. Epilepsia 27(Suppl. 2):S64–S76, 1986.

Dongier S: Statistical study of clinical and electroencephalographic manifestations of 536 psychotic episodes occurring in 516 epileptics between clinical seizures. Epilepsia 1:117–142b, 1959–60.

Edeh J, Toone BK: Antiepileptic therapy, folate deficiency and psychiatric morbidity: A general practice survey. Epilepsia 26:434–440, 1985.

Fiordelli E, Beghi E, Bogliun G, Crespi V: Epilepsy and psychiatric disturbance: A cross-sectional study. Br J Psychiatry 163:446–450, 1993.

Flor-Henry P: Psychosis and temporal lobe epilepsy: A controlled investigation. Epilepsia 10:363–395, 1969.

Gillham RA: Refractory epilepsy: An evaluation of psychological methods in outpatient management. Epilepsia 31:427–432, 1990.

Goldstein LH, Polkey C: Short-term cognitive changes after unilateral temporal lobectomy or unilateral amygdalo-hippocampectomy for the relief of temporal lobe epilepsy. J Neurol Neurosurg Psychiatry 56:135–140, 1993.

Helmstaedter C, Kemper B, Elger CE: Neuropsychological aspects of frontal lobe epilepsy. Neuropsychologia 34:399–406, 1998.

Hermann B, Davies K, Foley K, Bell B: Visual confrontation naming outcome after standard left anterior temporal lobectomy with sparing versus resection of the superior temporal gyrus. Epilepsia 40:1070–1076, 1999.

Hermann BP: Psychopathology in epilepsy and learned helplessness. Med Hypotheses 5:723–729, 1979.

Hermann BP, Whitman S: Psychosocial predictors of interictal depression. J Epilepsy 2:231–237, 1989.

Hermann BP, Wyler AR: Depression, locus of control, and the effects of epilepsy surgery. Epilepsia 30:332–338, 1989.

Hermann BP, Seidenberg M, Haltiner A, Wyler AR: Mood state in unilateral temporal lobe epilepsy. Biol Psychiatry 30:1205–1218, 1991.

Hermann BP, Trenerry MR, Colligan RC: Learned helplessness, attributional style and depression in epilepsy. Epilepsia 37:680–686, 1996.

Hermann BP, Whitman S, Wyler AR, et al: The neurological, psychosocial, and demographic correlates of hypergraphia in patients with epilepsy. J Neurol Neurosurg Psychiatry 51:203–208, 1988.

Holmes MD, Dodrill CB, Wilkus RJ, Ojemann GA: Is partial epilepsy progressive? Ten years of EEG and neuropsychological changes in adults with partial seizures. Epilepsia 39:1189–1193, 1998.

Hughes J, Devinsky O, Feldmann E, Bromfield E: Premonitory symptoms in epilepsy. Seizure 2:201–203, 1993.

Hurwitz TA, Wada JA, Kosaka BD, Strauss EH: Cerebral organization of affect suggested by temporal lobe seizures. Neurology 35:1335–1337, 1985.

Jacoby A, Baker GA, Steen N, Potts P, Chadwick DW: The clinical course of epilepsy and its psychosocial correlates: Findings from a U.K. community study. Epilepsia 37:148–161, 1996.

Kanner AM, Stagno S, Kotagal P, Morris HH: Postictal psychiatric events during prolonged video-electroencephalographic monitoring studies. Arch Neurol 53:258–263, 1996.

Klerman GL: Treatment of recurrent unipolar major depressive disorder: Commentary on the Pittsburg Study. Arch Gen Psychiatry 47:1158–1161 1990.

Kupfer DJ, Frank E, Perel JM: The advantage of early treatment intervention in recurrent depression. Arch Gen Psychiatry 46:771–775, 1989.

Lambert MV: Seizures, hormones and sexuality. Seizure 10:319–340, 2001.

Lambert MV, Robertson MM: Depression in epilepsy: Etiology, phenomenology, and treatment. Epilepsia 40(Suppl. 10):S21–S47, 1999.

Lambert MV, Schmitz EB, Ring HA, Trimble M: Neuropsychiatric aspects of epilepsy, in Schiffer RB, Rao SM, Fogel BS (eds): Neuropsychiatry, ed 2. Philadelphia, PA: Lippincott Williams & Wilkins, 2003, pp. 1071–1131.

Landolt H: Serial electroencephalographic investigations during psychotic episodes in epileptic patients and during schizophrenic attacks, in deHass L (ed): Lectures on Epilepsy. London: Elsevier, 1958.

Logsdail SJ, Toone BK: Post-ictal psychosis: A clinical and phenomenological description. Br J Psychiatry 1988:152:246–252.

Matsuoka H, Takahashi T, Sasaki M, et al: Neuropsychological EEG activation in patients with epilepsy. Brain 123:318–330, 2000.

Mendez MF, Cummings JL, Benson DF: Depression in epilepsy: Significance and phenomenology. Arch Neurol 43:766–770, 1986.

Mendez MF, Doss RC, Taylor JL, Salguero P: Depression in epilepsy: Relationship to seizures and anticonvulsant therapy. J Nerv Ment Dis 181:444–447, 1993.

Neyens GJ, Aldenkamp AP. Nardi AM: Prospective follow-up of intellectual development in children with recent onset of epilepsy. Epilepsy Res 34:85–90, 1999.

Penfield W, Evans J: The frontal lobe in man: A clinical study of maximum removals. Brain 63:115–133, 1935.

Polkey CE: Temporal lobe resections, in Oxbury J, Polkey C, Duchowny M (eds): Intractable Focal Epilepsy. London, UK: Saunders, 2000a, pp. 667–696.

Polkey CE: Functional surgery for epilepsy, in Oxbury J, Polkey C, Duchowny M (eds): Intractable Focal Epilepsy. London, UK: Saunders, 2000b, pp. 735–750.

Quiske A, Helmstaedter C, Lux S, et al: Depression in patients with temporal lobe epilepsy is related to mesial temporal sclerosis. Epilepsy Res 39:121–125, 2000.

Robertson MM, Trimble MR, Townsend HRA: Phenomenology of depression in epilepsy. Epilepsia 28:364–372, 1987.

Rosenstein DL, Nelson JC, Jacobs SC: Seizures associated with antidepressants: A review. J Clin Psychiatry 54:289–299, 1993.

Roth DL, Goode KT, Williams VL, Faught E: Physical exercise, stressful life experience, and depression in adults with epilepsy. Epilepsia 35:1248–1255, 1994.

Roy A: Some determinants of affective symptoms in epileptics. Can J Psychiatry 24:554–556, 1979.

Saver, JL, Rabin J: The neural substrates of religious experience. J Neuropsychiatry Clin Neurosci 9:498–510, 1997.

Saykin AJ, Robinson LJ, Stefiniak P, et al: Neuropsychological changes after anterior temporal lobectomy: Acute effects on memory, language and music, in Bennett TL (ed): The Neuropsychology of Epilepsy. New York: Plenum Press, 1992, pp. 263–290.

Schmitz EB, Moriarty J, Costa DC, et al: Psychiatric profiles and patterns of cerebral blood flow in focal epilepsy: Interactions between depression, obsessionality, and perfusion related to the laterality of the epilepsy. J Neurol Neurosurg Psychiatry 62:458–463, 1997.

Schmitz EB, Roberston MM, Trimble MR: Depression and schizophrenia in epilepsy: Social and biological risk factors. Epilepsy Res 35:59–68, 1999.

Schmitz EB, Sander T (eds): Juvenile Myoclonic Epilepsy: The Janz Syndrome. Petersfield, UK: Wrightson Biomedical Publishing, 2000, pp. 101–109.

Seidenberg M, Hermann B, Noe A, Wyler AR: Depression in temporal lobe epilepsy: Interaction between laterality of lesion and Wisconsin Card Sort performance. Neuropsychiatry Neuropsychol Behav Neurol 8:81–87, 1995.

Shorvon SD: Status epilepticus: Its causes and treatment in children and adults. Cambridge, UK: Cambridge University Press, 1994.

Sisodiya SM: Surgery for malformations of cortical development causing epilepsy. Brain 123:1075–1091, 2000.

Slater E, Beard AW: The schizophrenia-like psychoses of epilepsy: Discussion and conclusions. Br J Psychiatry 109:143–150, 1963.

Slater E, Beard AW, Glithero E: The schizophrenia-like psychoses of epilepsy. Br J Psychiatry 109:95–150, 1963.

Spina E, Pisani F, Perucca E: Clinically significant pharmacokinetic drug interactions with carbamazepine: An update. Clin Pharmacokinetics 31:198–214, 1996.

Springer JA, Binder JR, Harmmake TA, et al: Language dominance in neurologically normal and epilepsy patients: A functional MRI study. Brain 122:2033–2046, 1999.

Standage KF, Fenton GW: Psychiatric symptom profiles of patients with epilepsy: A controlled investigation. Psychol Med 5:152–160, 1975.

Tebartz van Elst L, Woermann FG, Lemieux L, Trimble MR: Amygdala enlargement in dysthymia: A volumetric study of patients with temporal lobe epilepsy. Biolog Psychiatry 46:1614–1623, 1999.

Tellenbach H. Epilepsie als Anfallsleiden und als Psychose. Über alternative Psychosen paranoider Praegung bei "forcierter Norma-lisierung" (Landolt) des Elektroencephalogramms Epileptischer. Nervenarzt 36:190–202, 1965.

Thompson PJ, Shorvon S, Heaney D: Epilepsy, in Greenwood R, McMillan TM, Barnes MP, Ward CD (eds): Handbook of Neurological Rehabilitation, ed 2. Sussex, UK: Psychology Press, 2001.

Thompson PJ, Corcoran R: Everyday memory functions in people with epilepsy. Epilepsia 33(Suppl. 6):S18–S20, 1992.

Thompson PJ: Epilepsy and memory, in Cull C, Goldstein L (eds): Epilepsy: A Clinical Psychologists Handbook. London, UK: Routledge, 1997, pp. 35–53.

Thompson PJ, Baxendale SA, Duncan JS, et al: Effects of topiramate on cognitive function. J Neurol Neurosurg Psychiatry 69:636–641, 2000.

Trimble MR: Interictal psychoses of epilepsy, in Smith D, Treiman D, Trimble M (eds): Advances in Neurology. New York: Raven Press, 1991, Vol. 55, pp. 143–152.

Trostle JA, Hauser A, Sharbrough FW: Psychologic and social adjustment to epilepsy in Rochester, Minnesota. Neurology 39:633–637, 1989.

Turner WA: Epilepsy. London, UK: MacMillan Press, 1907.

Upton D, Thompson PJ: General neuropsychological characteristics of frontal lobe epilepsy. Epilepsy Res 23:169–177, 1996a.

Upton D, Thompson PJ: Epilepsy in the frontal lobes: Neuropsychological characteristics. J Epilepsy 9:215–222, 1996b.

Upton D, Thompson PJ: Twenty Questions Task and frontal lobe dysfunction. Arch Clin Neuropsychol 14:203–216, 1999.

Victoroff JI, Benson DF, Engel J Jr, et al: Interictal depression in patients with medically intractable complex partial seizures: Electroencephalography and cerebral metabolic correlates [abstract]. Ann Neurol 28:221, 1990.

Victoroff JI, Benson DF, Grafton ST, et al: Depression in complex partial seizures: Electroencephalography and cerebral metabolic correlates. Arch Neurol 51:155–163, 1994.

Warrington EK, Duchenne LW: A reappraisal of a case of persistent global amnesia following a right temporal lobectomy: A clinicopathological study. Neuropsychologia 24:629–636, 1992.

Waxman SG, Geschwind N: The interictal behaviour syndrome of temporal lobe epilepsy. Arch Gen Psychiatry 32:1580–1586, 1975.

Williams D: The structure of emotions reflected in epileptic experiences. Brain 79:29–67, 1956.

Zeman A, Hodges JR: Transient global amnesia and transient epileptic amnesia, in Berrios G, Hodges JR (eds): Memory Disorders in Psychiatric Practice. Cambridge, UK: Cambridge University Press, 2000, pp. 187–203.

Multiple Sclerosis

Nigel V. Marsh
Ernest W. Willoughby

Beta-interferon

Chronic-progressive

Depression

Expanded Disability Status Scale (EDSS)

Fatigue

Geographic incidence

Lhermitte's symptom

Magnetic resonance imaging

Polygenic inheritance

Pseudobulbar palsy

Relapsing-remitting

White matter disease

Multiple sclerosis (MS) is a complex disorder of the central nervous system (CNS) in which scattered patches of inflammation occur repeatedly over the course of years in the brain and spinal cord, producing damage of variable severity to major motor and sensory pathways. It is the most common disability-producing disease of the CNS in young adults in Europe and North America. The cause is unknown, and the clinical presentation and course are highly variable. This chapter gives an overview of the pathology, epidemiology, effects, assessment, and management of this disease. We conclude by outlining some issues concerning MS, the resolution of which would improve assessment and treatment practices.

PATHOLOGY

Patches of inflammation are most common in the white matter, particularly in the deep periventricular areas, although recent studies have confirmed that the cerebral cortex is also often extensively affected (Kidd et al., 1999). Individual patches or plaques evolve over the course of several weeks, leaving an area of scarring or gliosis. The myelin sheath of axons is particularly vulnerable to the inflammatory process, leading to demyelination with relative sparing of axons—hence the term *demyelinating disease*. However, it has recently been emphasized that there may also be substantial loss of axons in the areas of inflammation at an early stage (Trapp et al., 1999). The inflammatory process is mainly T-cell-mediated, with activation of macrophages, but in some cases antibody-mediated reactions are probably important, and recent studies indicate that there are at least four types of pathologic processes in different patients (Lucchinetti et al., 2000). The trigger for the inflammatory process is widely considered to be autoimmune (largely by analogy with experimental allergic encephalomyelitis in animals), but identification of the putative antigens in the human disease has been inconclusive and controversial. The later gradual loss of cerebral and spinal cord tissue (axons as well as myelin) is clearly responsible for deterioration during the progressive phase of the disease, but the relationship of this degenerative process to the initial and later inflammatory changes remains uncertain.

Magnetic resonance (MR) scanning has provided important insights into the pathology of MS (Figs. 35-1, 35-2, 35-3). Scans clearly show the evolution of acute inflammatory lesions with enhancement with injected gadolinium indicating breakdown of the blood-brain

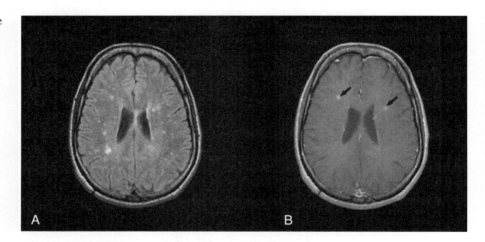

FIGURE 35-1. Axial magnetic resonance brain scans of a 35-year-old man with mild relapsing/remitting multiple sclerosis. *A,* T2-weighted fluid attenuated inversion recovery (FLAIR) image showing several white matter lesions; old scars and new inflammatory lesions are not distinguishable. *B,* T1-weighted image after intravenous gadolinium showing enhancement of two active inflammatory lesions (*arrows*).

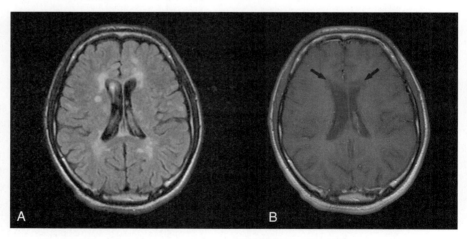

FIGURE 35-2. Axial magnetic resonance brain scans of a 50-year-old man with secondary progressive multiple sclerosis. *A,* T2-weighted fluid attenuated inversion recovery (FLAIR) image showing white matter lesions. *B,* T1-weighted image showing periventricular T1 "black holes (*arrows*)."

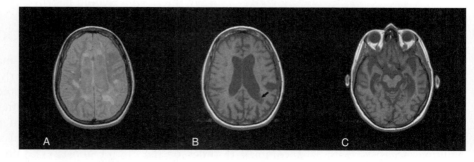

FIGURE 35-3. Axial magnetic resonance brain scans of a 40-year-old woman with secondary progressive multiple sclerosis and substantial cognitive impairment. *A,* proton density T2-weighted image showing periventricular white matter lesions (the cerebral ventricles are also grey). *B* and *C,* T1-weighted images showing extensive cerebral atrophy and moderate enlargement of the cerebral ventricles (*arrow* indicates a T1 "black hole").

barrier initially and later residual scarring or gliosis that persists indefinitely (Filippi, 2000). Most of the acute lesions in the brain occur in clinically "silent" areas and produce no obvious symptoms. Serial scans show the accumulation of white matter scars and also, in many cases, the development of cerebral atrophy reflecting the diffuse loss of brain tissue (Jagust & Noseworthy, 2000). Brain atrophy may occur early in the course of relapsing/remitting MS, and its occurrence is not clearly related to the extent of inflammatory disease (Chard et al., 2002). The complexity of the pathology in MS is also indicated by evidence of subtle changes in the normal-appearing white matter separate from the inflammatory lesions (Barkhof, 2002).

EPIDEMIOLOGY

An understanding of the epidemiologic aspects of MS requires a consideration of the etiology, prevalence, symptoms, and course of the disease. It is the etiology of MS that has caused the greatest debate in this area.

Etiology

Attempts to understand the etiology of MS have focused on genetic, environmental, and immunologic variables. Multicausal theories, which incorporate the effects of both a viral agent and genetic susceptibility, have gained a great deal of popular support. However, evidence of a viral etiology in MS is largely circumstantial, and the transplanting of brain matter from MS patients into nonhuman primates has so far not resulted in transmission of the disease (Granieri et al., 2001).

Genetic explanations focus on the possibility of MS as an autoimmune disease. Evidence supporting genetic explanations is derived from studies of the gender, familial, and racial patterns of MS prevalence. Women are approximately twice as likely to develop the disease as men (Skegg et al., 1987). First-degree relatives of affected individuals have been estimated to be between 6 to 8 times (White et al., 1992) and 20 times (Beatty, 1996) more at risk than the general population, with siblings being most at risk. Monozygotic twins are both affected more frequently than dizygotic twins (White et al., 1992), but the relatively low concordance rate (approximately 25%) in monozygotic twins points to a major environmental influence. Family studies indicate that MS is a polygenic condition (Poser, 1994). Some racial and ethnic groups (e.g., Eskimos, Japanese, Chinese, American Indians, Asian Indians, Australian Aborigines, New Zealand Maoris, Pacific Islanders and Africans) have an extremely low incidence of MS (Knight, 1992; Poser, 1994). These findings suggest at least a partial genetic basis for the disease.

There are other indications that environmental factors are also important. Siblings who develop MS do so in the same calendar year rather than at the same age. More compelling are epidemiologic studies showing that, in general, the prevalence of MS increases as latitude of habitation increases, in both the northern and southern hemispheres (Knight, 1992). It has also been reported that there is a seasonal birth pattern in the development of MS, with such patients tending to be born in the spring (Torrey et al. 2000). Therefore, while genetic differences are evident, they appear to be strongly influenced by environmental variables.

The uncertainty surrounding the etiology of MS is further confounded by migration studies, which have shown that people moving from a high-risk latitude to a low-risk latitude (e.g., Europeans immigrating to South Africa) or vice versa (e.g., African-Asians immigrating to Israel) tend to carry with them the risk of their place of origin, but only if this movement occurs after the age of 15 (Knight, 1992). This suggests that disease acquisition occurs before puberty (Poser, 1994). However, Compston (1990) has pointed out that the increased risk of MS seen in native people moving out of Africa to the United States correlates with the extent to which white genes are introduced into the African-American community.

Recent reviews of the epidemiologic research conducted on MS point to some methodologic problems with studies that have proposed a relationship between the frequency of MS and geographic latitude (Poser, 1994; Rosati, 2001).

Prevalence

Prevalence varies widely throughout the world, with rates being as high as 200 per 100,000 in Canada and Northern Europe. MS currently affects approximately 2.5 million people worldwide. The prevalence of MS is determined by geographic, demographic, and genetic factors.

As noted, geographically the incidence of MS increases as one moves further away from the equator. Disease prevalence can be roughly divided into three zones of frequency: high (30+ per 100,000), medium (5–30 per 100,000) and low (under 5 per 100,000) (Kurtzke, 2000). The high-frequency zone includes northern Europe, Scandinavia, Canada, northern United States, southeastern Australia, and New Zealand. Medium frequency is found in southern Europe and southern United States. Within the low-frequency zones, MS rates range from 1 per 100,000 in equatorial areas such as southeastern Asia, Africa, and northern South America to 5 per 100,000 in Central Asia. Two thirds of patients are diagnosed between the ages of 20 and 40. Onset before age 15 is rare, and late onset (i.e., after age 40) is often characterized by a progressive course from the onset, with or without additional relapses (Beatty, 1996).

Symptoms

The wide variety of symptoms in different MS patients, and in an individual patient over time, reflects the widespread and patchy involvement of major motor and sensory pathways in the white matter. Early symptoms of MS commonly include weakness or clumsiness in one or more limbs (often with difficulty walking), sensory impairment in the limbs or face, visual disturbance (blurring of vision in one eye or double vision), and urinary dysfunction. A number of other symptoms, either singly or together in varying patterns, can also occur in MS, and symptoms include vertigo, seizures, deafness (usually in one ear), facial pain or pain in the trunk or limbs, difficulty speaking or swallowing, and emotional changes (Knight, 1992; White et al., 1992). A common symptom, characteristic of MS but not specific to it, is Lhermitte's symptom, in which neck flexion produces a transient electric shock–like sensation down the spine into the legs (caused by inflammation in the cervical spinal cord). General fatigue, which has both physical and cognitive aspects, is also common. Its severity is not closely related to the amount of physical disability, or to associated depression, and its cause remains obscure.

Physical symptoms have always been seen as the dominant feature of MS. However, it has been recognized over the last 15 years that even during the early stages of the disease, cognitive deficits can be present (Rao, 1986). It is important, therefore, that impairment in cognitive functioning should not be overlooked in cases in which physical disability is not yet advanced (Brassington & Marsh, 1998). MS can affect all aspects of cognitive function, although memory has been found to be particularly susceptible (Thornton & Raz, 1997; Wishart & Sharpe, 1997).

While the physical and cognitive impairments that can result from MS may lead to an understandable state of psychological distress, MS can also be associated with psychiatric illness. Psychosis and bipolar affective disorder (manic episodes) have been reported in conjunction with MS, but it is suggested that the rate of psychosis in MS populations may not exceed chance expectations (Feinstein, 1999). In addition there have been reports of MS presenting initially as a purely psychiatric disorder (Skegg, 1993; Feinstein, 1999), although such cases are rare. Despite the reported occurrence of psychiatric illness, determining the relative contribution of biologic and psychosocial factors to the emotional functioning of a person with MS is very difficult (Gerland & Zis, 1991; Feinstein, 1999).

A particular type of emotional disturbance that may occur in MS (usually in patients with moderately severe disability) is emotional lability with inappropriate and uncontrollable laughter and crying triggered by minor emotional stimuli. This is usually associated with signs of bulbar motor dysfunction of upper motor neuron type (with slurred speech and difficulty coordinating tongue movements: "pseudobulbar palsy") and is the result of damage to pathways involved in involuntary emotional responses.

Course

The usual early course of MS is one of relapses and remissions, with symptoms of a relapse typically increasing over a week or two and then improving over a longer period, either completely or leaving some residual deficit. There may be many years between clinical relapses, with the average being one relapse in 2 years, although MR scans of the brain often show much more inflammatory activity than is apparent clinically. Serial MR scans have shown patches of inflammation occurring up to 5 to 10 times as frequently as clinical attacks.

After a variable number of relapses, over a number of years, about 50% of patients (after 10–15 years) develop a secondary progressive course where there is gradual progressive deterioration, particularly in motor function in the legs and in walking. The development of this phase is insidious and can often be recognized only in retrospect. Many of these patients still have additional acute relapses with partial remissions and the term progressive-relapsing has been used for this course.

While there is wide variation in the course of the disease, a number of attempts have been made to develop terms to allow characterization of particular types. The most fundamental distinction is between a chronic-progressive and relapsing-remitting course (Bennett et al., 1991). Lublin and Reingold (1996) acknowledged that due to the lack of clear biologic markers, there had been no common meaning among clinicians in their use of MS terminology. Following an international survey, they reported that agreement was reached on four different courses of MS: relapsing-remitting, primary-progressive, secondary-progressive, and progressive-relapsing. Although the term relapsing-progressive MS was one of the most frequently used terms, no consensus could be reached on the definition.

In individual cases there is considerable variation in severity that, in the early stages, is difficult to predict (Ebers, 2001). An acute or malignant course is rapidly progressive, leading to significant disability in multiple neurologic systems or death a relatively short time after disease onset. A benign course is comparatively clinically silent, with early relapses resolving without leaving significant disability; the patient remains fully functional in all neurologic systems 10 to 15 years after onset. A working definition of benign MS has been an Expanded Disability Status Scale (EDSS) score of 2.0 or less, 10 years or more after onset. This may apply to 10% to 20% of patients, but the concept of a benign form of relapsing-remitting MS is controversial and recent long-term follow-up studies have shown that up to 50% of patients with a benign course after 10 years develop more significant disability after a further 10 years. Beatty (1996) recently provided working definitions for the taxonomy recommended by Peyser and colleagues (1990), which combines severity and course descrip-

TABLE 35-1. Terminology Used to Describe the Course of Multiple Sclerosis

Bennett et al. (1991)

1. Chronic-progressive: A gradual and steady deterioration.
2. Relapsing-remitting: A stepwise path of degeneration, with periods of exacerbations interspersed with periods of stability or even slight improvements. Accounts for approximately 90% of cases.

Lublin and Reingold (1996)

1. Relapsing-remitting: Relapses with full recovery or with sequelae and residual deficit upon recovery, periods between relapses characterized by lack of disease progression.
2. Primary-progressive: Progression from onset with occasional plateaus and temporary minor improvements allowed.
3. Secondary-progressive: Initial relapsing–remitting disease course followed by progression with or without occasional relapses, minor remissions, and plateaus.
4. Progressive-relapsing: Progressive disease from onset, with clear acute relapses, periods between relapses characterized by continuing progression.

Beatty (1996)

1. Benign sensory: 1 to 2 lifetime episodes consisting mainly of sensory symptoms.
2. Benign relapsing-remitting: Periodic relapses followed by almost complete recovery.
3. Progressive relapsing-remitting: Periodic relapses followed by incomplete recovery.
4. Chronic-progressive: Slow, steady deterioration without substantial recovery.
5. Acute progressive: Rapid deterioration (often leading to death).

tions. The terminology and definitions for these three classification systems are presented in Table 35-1.

There is currently no explanation as to what causes the cycles of relapse and remission or what determines the progression of the disease, but there has been some research into the apparent relationship between stressful life events and exacerbations of the disease (Schwartz et al., 2000). Life expectancy following the onset of MS symptoms is generally estimated to be more than 30 years, and yet, like everything else to do with this disease, this is variable, and a duration of only a few months has been reported in some cases (White et al., 1992).

EFFECTS OF MULTIPLE SCLEROSIS

Due to the highly variable course of the disease, MS can result in a variety of consequences for the physical, cognitive, and psychosocial functioning of the individual.

Physical Consequences

The physical impairments associated with MS can result in significant handicap. Among the many possible physical consequences are visual loss, weakness and clumsiness of the limbs, impaired and altered sensation, ataxia, and urinary dysfunction. Sexual dysfunction is frequently reported (Hatzichristou, 1996); while this may be due to organic factors, it is also possible that the psychosocial impact of having a disabling neurologic disease leads to a decrease in interest, as much as a loss of function.

Cognitive Consequences

Neurocognitive impairment is evident in a substantial proportion of people with MS (Kesselring & Klement, 2001). Two large studies of community-based MS subjects found that, compared with appropriate control groups, the MS groups had a frequency of cognitive impairment of 43% (Rao et al., 1991a) and 46% (McIntosh-Michaelis et al., 1991). As with physical functioning, due to the variable distribution and severity of MS lesions throughout the CNS, there is heterogeneity of cognitive deficits. Attempts to determine whether there is a distinct pattern of neurocognitive deficits for different subtypes of MS, particularly chronic-progressive and relapsing-remitting subtypes, have produced contradictory results (Wishart & Sharpe, 1997; Zakzanis, 2000).

Table 35-2 summarizes the type of cognitive deficits reported in MS, as outlined by three recent major reviews. These studies show that MS can result in impairment across many domains of cognitive function, but deficits in motor speed, speed of information processing, and memory function appear to be the most severe and consistent. In contrast, deficits in intellectual, language, and visuoperceptual functions are less severe. The cognitive domain of executive functions (EF) covers a number of abilities, and impairment is evident in some of these.

The presence of generalized impairment across a variety of cognitive functions begs the question of whether or not the cognitive dysfunctions evident in MS are simply different manifestations of a single underlying

TABLE 35-2. Comparative Findings from Three Recent Reviews of Cognitive Dysfunction in Multiple Sclerosis

Intellectual functioning

Wishart & Sharpe (1997): MS impaired on measures of general cognitive ability. More impaired on Performance IQ than Verbal IQ measures.

Brassington & Marsh (1988): MS shows small but consistent impairment. More impaired on Performance IQ than Verbal IQ measures. Longitudinal studies show small but significant decline over time, with difference between verbal and performance measures being maintained.

Zakzanis (2000): MS shows modest impairment. Impairment more evident on measure of Performance IQ.

Attention/Concentration

Wishart & Sharpe (1997): MS impaired on measures of attention, concentration, and speed of processing.

Brassington & Marsh (1988): MS impaired on a number of measures of visual and auditory attention. Slowed information processing is a major feature of MS.

Zakzanis (2000): MS show consistent but small differences in attention and concentration abilities. Information-processing speed deficits evident.

Memory functioning

Wishart & Sharpe (1997): MS impaired on all aspects of learning, immediate recall, and delayed recall for both verbal and visual tasks, and recognition tasks. Visual and verbal learning more impaired than delayed visual recall and recognition. Immediate verbal recall more impaired than delayed visual recall.

Brassington & Marsh (1988): Memory impairment in the most consistent cognitive impairment in MS. Encoding and storage of information in immediate memory appears to be least affected, while recent and remote memory are frequently found to be impaired. Extent to which faulty retrieval explains memory impairment in MS remains unclear.

Zakzanis (2000): Delayed recall more impaired than immediate recall for both verbal and nonverbal tasks. Verbal recall more impaired than nonverbal recall for both immediate and delayed recall. Recognition memory relatively intact. Impairment evident in remote memory.

Language functioning

Wishart & Sharpe (1997): MS impaired, with impairment more evident in expression than comprehension tasks.

Brassington & Marsh (1988): N/A

Zakzanis (2000): MS shows deficits in verbal fluency, with semantic fluency being more impaired than phonemic fluency. Modest deficits on confrontation naming and comprehension tasks.

Visuospatial/perceptual functioning

Wishart & Sharpe (1997): MS shows deficits in visuoperceptual, visuospatial, and visuoconstructional abilities.

Brassington & Marsh (1988): N/A

Zakzanis (2000): Magnitude of deficits on tests of visuoperceptual and visuospatial processing are minimal or nonexistent.

Motor functioning

Wishart & Sharpe (1997): MS shows impaired motor skills.

Brassington & Marsh (1988): N/A

Zakzanis (2000): Largest deficits for MS evident on tasks of manual dexterity and motor speed. Motor speed more impaired than manual dexterity.

Executive functioning

Wishart & Sharpe (1997): MS impaired on measures of executive and conceptual ability.

Brassington & Marsh (1988): MS impaired on measures of cognitive flexibility, concept formation, and verbal abstract reasoning.

Zakzanis (2000): MS displays moderate impairment on measures of cognitive flexibility and abstraction and conceptual function.

MS, multiple sclerosis or individuals with MS; N/A, not available.

generalized deficit. Wishart and Sharpe (1997) addressed this question and concluded that there is statistical support for viewing the impact of MS on cognitive functioning in terms of its differential impact on discrete cognitive abilities. Further support for a multifunction approach to neuropsychological assessment in MS comes from research that shows that the degree and pattern of cognitive dysfunction is significantly correlated with evidence on MR brain scans of the amount and location of white matter disease in the cerebral hemispheres (Brassington & Marsh, 1998). However the relationship between cognitive impairment and different types of MR brain assessment is complex and conflicting (Benedict et al., 2002; Rovaris et al., 2002).

Limitations in the amount of information able to be processed can make it difficult for an individual with MS to retain and process the information necessary to solve complex tasks efficiently. Impaired memory, attention, and concentration faculties, coupled with fatigue, will have an effect on the individual's personal organization, as well as his or her vocational functioning and normal family role (Rao et al., 1991b). In short, the person with MS will often experience a decrease in psychosocial functioning.

Psychosocial Consequences

Despite the physical and cognitive consequences of MS, there does not appear to be an obvious relationship between the severity of the disease and an individual's psychological reaction. A person who is only mildly affected can be psychologically distraught, whereas someone who is severely handicapped might cope very well. Many factors play a part in determining the individual's response. These include the effect of the disability on the person's normal way of life, his or her personality, and the amount of support received from others (Brassington & Marsh, 1998).

Obviously, the variability and inconsistency of the deficits associated with MS compound the difficulties experienced by the patients and their families. Anxiety can be most prominent in the early stages of the disease, when there is uncertainty about the diagnosis and prognosis (Gordon et al., 1994). Given that the initial symptoms may be confusing to both the patients and their physicians, patients may initially be incorrectly diagnosed as neurotic (White et al., 1992). An incorrect diagnosis of a psychiatric condition may lead to physical symptoms being unnoticed or underestimated, resulting in an unnecessarily long period before a diagnosis of MS is made.

Adjustment can sometimes be more difficult in the early stages, when symptoms are mild. The patients are unsure whether to perceive themselves as normal or handicapped, and may develop a preoccupation with physical symptoms. When physical problems do become more obvious, patients then must come to terms with the stigma of disability (Brassington & Marsh, 1998).

Sleep disorder, sexual dysfunction, and depression are common consequences of MS. Depression is associated with an increased risk of suicide in people with MS, and can also cause patients to perceive their disabilities as greater than objective assessment would indicate (Kleespies et al., 2000; Smith & Young, 2000). The combination of physical and cognitive deficits may result in loss of employment and associated financial difficulties. This, in turn, can lead to a loss of self-esteem, social withdrawal, and deterioration in relationships (Mohr et al., 1999; Hakim et al., 2000; Rumrill et al., 2000). However, it is not only the individual with MS who can experience significant psychosocial problems. Recent studies have demonstrated that their spouses, who, ideally, would be a major source of support, can also experience a decrease in their own well-being (O'Brien, 1993; Knight et al., 1997).

ASSESSMENT

There is no single diagnostic sign or test for MS. Ultimately the diagnosis is made on the basis of clinical assessment supported by a variety of test results. The basic requirement is to show evidence of characteristic lesions in the CNS in different sites occurring at different times, while excluding other disorders that may produce a similar clinical picture.

Depending on the clinical setting, useful investigations include analysis of cerebrospinal fluid, evoked potential studies, and neuroimaging, especially MR scanning, which is very sensitive to the inflammatory lesions of MS. Because the results of these investigations are not specific to MS, they need to be incorporated with other clinical information before a diagnosis can be made. Differential diagnosis includes other multifocal CNS disorders such as acute disseminated encephalomyelitis and cerebral vascular diseases. In patients with complex symptoms but few or no signs on examination, chronic fatigue syndrome (previously called *myalgic encephalomyelitis*) and somatization or conversion disorder may be difficult to distinguish from MS.

The diagnostic criteria for MS established by Poser and colleagues (1983) have been widely adopted for routine clinical use and for most research projects. These criteria set out four diagnostic categories based on the results of a combination of clinical assessment and investigations: clinically definite, clinically probable, laboratory-supported definite, and laboratory-supported probable. Clinically definite MS is defined by the occurrence of two attacks (i.e., characteristic neurologic symptoms and signs), separated by at least a month, each lasting a minimum of 24 hours, and resulting from lesions in two distinct areas of the CNS (e.g., blurred vision and a numb limb). Poser (1994) advocates using only clinically definite and clinically probable MS patients in research, particularly for inclusion in prevalence and incidence studies, due to the fact that laboratory findings are not disease specific and, in some areas detailed investigations may not be available.

The Poser criteria are now clearly outdated because they do not incorporate MR scanning, which is the most useful investigation in confirming a diagnosis of MS and in ruling out other disorders. New criteria established by an international panel and published in 2001 are widely known as the McDonald criteria (McDonald et al., 2001). These new criteria are heavily dependent on MR scanning and simplify the diagnostic criteria by dropping the "laboratory-supported" category. There is continuing discussion on the reliability and sensitivity of the new criteria, particularly for the diagnosis of MS early in the disease course. Once a diagnosis of MS is made, various methods are used for assessing the physical, cognitive, and psychosocial impact of the disease.

Assessment of Physical Disability

The Expanded Disability Status Scale (EDSS; Kurtzke, 1983) was designed to provide an overall rating of disability in MS cases. The scale rates patients on the basis of signs of impairment on neurologic examination, with ambulation being a major component in the upper half of the scale. The EDSS is the standard scale used to rate neurologic disability in MS and is used widely; but, as a measure of neurologic impairment, it fails to give sufficient weight to the cognitive impairment that may accompany MS and has poor reliability. The EDSS, as a measure of impairment, has been combined with the Incapacity Status Scale (measuring disability) and the Environmental Status Scale (handicap) under the aegis of the International Federation of MS Societies (1984), but the latter two measures have not been widely used (Table 35-3). A variety of other scales are also available which assess activities of daily living (ADL) and are predictive of the physical care needs of the MS patient (Brassington & Marsh, 1998).

Assessment of Cognitive Functioning

There is no one pattern of cognitive impairment that can be considered typical in MS, so neuropsychological assessment does not help in the process of differential diagnosis. However, neuropsychological assessment is useful in determining the extent of cognitive impairment, with its implications for social and occupational functioning, and also provides a further measure of change over time (Lezak, 1995). As the extent of cognitive impairment seems unrelated to either neurologic disability or disease duration, neuropsychological assessment is particularly important in those cases where cognitive, not physical, impairment is the prominent consequence of MS. For such people decisions regarding their competence in occupational and other roles need to be made on the basis of their level of cognitive functioning.

The physical impairments that accompany MS may have an impact on the type of tasks that can be used during a neuropsychological assessment. For example, if due care is not given to the choice of a test to assess attentional abilities, the result may be adversely affected by motor problems, even in the absence of any attentional deficits. Visual impairment may affect performance on tests of memory and interpretation requiring recognition of written material. Therefore the neuropsychological assessment of a person with MS can be a highly individualized process. Despite this, recent research has also demonstrated the advantages of undertaking a comprehensive assessment of cognitive ability in MS; as such, assessments can demonstrate the presence of impairment in specific cognitive functions irrespective of the presence of motor or visual difficulties (Wishart & Sharpe, 1997).

In keeping with this general principle, a number of standardized approaches to the neuropsychological

TABLE 35-3. Content of the International Federation of Multiple Sclerosis Societies' (1984) Minimal Record of Disability for Multiple Sclerosis

Functional Systems (impairment)

Eight items covering pyramidal functions, cerebellar functions, brainstem functions, sensory functions, bowel and bladder functions, visual or optic functions, cerebral or mental functions, and spasticity.

Incapacity Status Scale (disability)

Sixteen items covering stair climbing, ambulation, toilet/chair/bed transfer, bowel function, bladder function, bathing, dressing, grooming, feeding, vision, speech and hearing, medical problems, mood and thought disturbances, mentation, fatigability, and sexual function.

Environmental Status Scale (handicap)

Seven items covering actual work status, financial and economic status, place of residence, personal assistance, transportation, community assistance, and social activity.

assessment of people with MS have been recommended. Rao and colleagues (1991a) proposed a brief, 20-minute, screening battery. This battery included a dementia screen and assessed the specific cognitive domains of verbal intelligence; immediate, recent, and remote memory; abstract reasoning; attention/concentration; language; and visuospatial perception. A more comprehensive 2-hour battery was proposed by Peyser et al. (1990). This battery also included a dementia screen and assessed the specific cognitive domains of general knowledge, attention/concentration, memory, language, visuospatial functions, and abstract/conceptual reasoning. Therefore, despite the differences in time required, both batteries advocated assessing the same six cognitive domains of intelligence, attention/concentration, memory, language, visuospatial, and executive functioning.

It is well established that people with MS suffer a significant decrease in speed on motor, information processing, and interhemispheric transfer tasks. However, the nature of the deficits displayed on more complex tasks, such as those assessing memory, language, and EF, continues to be debated. Friend and colleagues (1999) have shown that comprehensive and detailed assessment of language functions in MS provides evidence of deficits in a variety of specific language functions. They found that, relative to normal controls, their MS subjects were impaired on naming, comprehension, and fluency tasks. Similarly, Arnett and colleagues (1997) reported that in addition to the already established executive dysfunctions in conceptual reasoning and set shifting, MS subjects were impaired on semantic encoding and planning, but not temporal ordering tasks.

However it is the nature of the memory impairments in MS that provides the greatest source of debate surrounding the neuropsychological assessment of MS patients. From a clinical perspective, it is apparent that a comprehensive assessment of all aspects of memory function is justified in MS cases. From theoretic and rehabilitation perspectives, the nature of memory impairment in MS has important implications. Thornton and Raz (1997) conducted a review of 36 studies and concluded that MS patients were impaired across all aspects of memory, and that support for a retrieval-based explanation of long-term memory dysfunction could not be justified. They considered that the memory impairment evident in MS was more global in nature than previously thought. In contrast, Zakzanis (2000) reviewed 34 studies and concluded that recognition memory abilities are relatively spared and that there is evidence to support a retrieval-based account of long-term memory impairment in MS.

Assessment of Psychosocial Function

There does not appear to be a consistent relationship between either physical disability or cognitive impairment and emotional distress in MS (Brassington & Marsh, 1998). The high prevalence of depression and its negative impact on the overall function of the MS patient provides strong support for assessing at least this aspect of the MS patients' emotional function. A number of self-administered questionnaires are available to rate the severity of a wide range of emotional and behavioral symptoms (Brassington & Marsh, 1998).

Recent studies have also demonstrated the relationship between stress, social support, coping style, and overall level of psychosocial functioning in MS. Jean and colleagues (1999) have shown that coping style was predictive of psychological distress in MS patients, irrespective of the impact of neuropsychological variables. Similarly, Pakenham (1999) has shown that coping style was a significant predictor of psychosocial adjustment over a 1-year period. The results of these and similar studies demonstrate the usefulness of stress and coping models in explaining individual differences in adjustment to MS. It follows that assessment of relevant variables such as coping style can make valuable contributions to the management plans for individual MS patients.

Dissatisfaction with assessment procedures that have concentrated on the physical status of the MS patient has led to the development of instruments that are now far broader than the traditional scales based on activities of daily living (Brassington & Marsh, 1998). In some ways the International Multiple Sclerosis Societies (1984) Minimal Record of Disability (see Table 35-3) can be seen as a precursor to these new quality-of-life questionnaires. Although still primarily used in a research context, evaluation has found that such measures are also useful in assisting with the clinical management of the individual MS patient (Murrell et al., 1999).

MANAGEMENT

Over the past 10 years there have been substantial developments in the treatment of MS with the appearance and increasing use of new disease-modifying therapies, which reduce the frequency of relapses. However, those therapies are, at best, only partially effective and have no obvious effect in many patients. Apart from the use of high-dose corticosteroids to speed recovery from relapses, the main focus of treatment for many patients, especially those with more physical disability, is a variety of medications and physical therapy to relieve persistent symptoms (Thompson, 2001).

The absence of consistently effective treatment combined with the unpredictable course of the disease commonly causes frustration, if not a feeling of desperation, in MS patients and their familial and professional caregivers. In this setting, the widespread use by MS patients of unproven alternative therapies is not surprising. As Beatty (1996) has noted, the highly unpredictable course of MS not only makes it difficult to demonstrate that a treatment has beneficial effects, but also makes it equally difficult to expose fraud masquerading as therapy.

Disease-Modifying Therapy

Beta-interferon, a genetically engineered natural protein, is the most widely used disease-modifying therapy. It is available in three formulations: Avonex (Biogen), Rebif (Serono)—both type 1a beta-interferons—and Betaseron (Schering)—type 1b. Each must be given by injection once or several times weekly in differing doses and have generally similar effects in reducing the frequency of clinical relapses by about one third, with a more marked reduction in new contrast-enhancing brain lesions on MR scans. There is also reduction in the accumulation of persistent scarring in MR brain scans, but the effect of the treatment in reducing long-term clinical disability is less clear and there is no consistent effect on progressive cerebral atrophy. These features indicate that the treatment has more effect on the acute inflammatory process than on the associated progressive degenerative process (Goodin et al., 2002).

Copaxone (glatiramer acetate) is an alternative treatment that probably has similar, if more modest, effects. It is a polypeptide developed from studies of animal models of CNS inflammatory disease and is given by daily injection (Johnson et al., 1998).

These treatments have complex and incompletely understood immune-modulating actions. Important limiting factors in their use are high cost as well as adverse effects in some patients, especially with beta-interferon. A recent trend has been to encourage treatment earlier in the course of the disease in the belief that reduction in the inflammatory process may reduce late degenerative changes (Comi, 2000).

General immune-suppressing agents have been tried for many years with limited benefit. Azathioprine and methotrexate may have modest effects, and the use of cyclophosphamide is more controversial (Weiner & Cohen, 2002). Recently there has been more interest in mitoxantrone for treatment of aggressive disease, but potential toxicity, particularly on the heart, limits long-term use. Repeated infusions of intravenous immunoglobulin may have some effect in preventing relapses but high cost and restricted availability are major problems in its use (Wiles et al., 2002).

Treatment of Acute Relapses

The mainstay in the treatment of acute relapses in MS is high-dose steroid treatment, which, to a variable degree, speeds up recovery from a relapse, although there is no clear effect on the long-term outcome (Milligan et al.,

1987). Continuing treatment with steroids does not prevent relapses, although recent reports suggest intermittent pulses of steroids may reduce long-term disability. After a short course of high-dose steroids, the benefit of a tailing dose over 3 to 4 weeks is controversial. Plasmapheresis has a limited place for treatment of severe relapses unresponsive to steroids.

Symptomatic Treatment of Physical Symptoms

Spasticity may be eased by medications such as baclofen and tizanidine, although side-effects, especially increased weakness, limit their effectiveness. Low-dose baclofen infused into the spinal cerebrospinal fluid (CSF) by automatic pump may be more effective but is a highly specialized and expensive procedure. Physical therapy also has an important place (Ko Ko, 1999). Urinary dysfunction, especially urgency and frequency, are relieved by anticholinergic agents such as oxybutynin or emepronium. Intermittent self-catheterization is often effective and preferable to an indwelling urethral catheter, but permanent urinary drainage via a suprapubic catheter may be necessary. Acute neuralgic pain resulting from involvement of sensory pathways usually responds to antiepileptic agents such as carbamazepine and chronic pain to low-dose tricyclic antidepressants. Fatigue is difficult to manage, with medications being of limited value. In general, there is evidence supporting the cost effectiveness of a coordinated multidisciplinary team for the provision of rehabilitation services in MS, but it is not clear whether hospital or community-based rehabilitation is most effective (Ko Ko, 1999).

Treatment for Cognitive Dysfunction

Techniques and procedures that are effective in managing cognitive dysfunction following static injuries, for example, traumatic brain injury and stroke, may not be equally effective for a progressive disorder like MS. However the two general approaches to cognitive rehabilitation are applicable across neurologic disorders. These approaches are based on either the restoration of function or the learning of compensatory techniques.

Restorative procedures focus on identifying specific cognitive deficits and providing remedial programs that focus on training particular skills relevant to the identified deficits. The underlying principle is that through training, recovery of function will occur. While gains in the particular skill being trained have been demonstrated, the primary failing of this restorative approach is a failure to demonstrate generalization of the taught skill (Thompson, 1996). For example, MS patients with memory problems may improve their ability to learn a specific list of 15 grocery items but may be unable to show an improvement in their ability to remember a list of 15 items of clothing, unless specifically trained on this task also.

The minimal success of cognitive rehabilitation based on restorative procedures suggests that rehabilitation should focus on compensatory strategies to enable persons with MS to minimize the impact of cognitive deficits on their lives (Bennett et al., 1991). In compensatory techniques, neuropsychological findings regarding deficits are used to both advise the patient and his or her family in areas concerning the patient's cognitive status, and to develop a treatment program so that the patient's cognitive strengths can be used to offset weaknesses. For example, if gist recall is a preserved feature of the memory functioning of an MS patient, then this area of strength can be used in rehabilitation. That is, the patient with MS can be encouraged to encode and retrieve information according to its meaning, as opposed to focusing on irrelevant details (Brassington & Marsh, 1998).

Compensatory approaches focus on maximizing an individual's functional abilities within a naturalistic environment. Training in the use of memory aids such as using lists, record keeping, mnemonics, and other written cues can help to compensate for memory impairment in MS patients. More general organizational strategies that involve careful planning and organization of activities into routines are another form of compensation; this can also benefit energy conservation, a high priority given the prevalence of debilitating fatigue suffered by so many people with MS. Compensatory interventions may also be aimed at modifying environments to minimize the extent to which they place demands on areas of impaired function (Thompson, 1996).

Treatment for Psychosocial Problems

The variable nature of MS means that each patient may be at an individual level of functional independence. Despite this, the need for lifestyle modification and supportive treatment increases for all persons with progression of the disease. Although the physical and cognitive symptoms of MS and the methods of treatment for exacerbations have been the subject of extensive investigations, it is only recently that the unique needs of MS patients for rehabilitative and supportive care in the community have been documented (Brassington & Marsh, 1998). Although the neurologic and neuropsychological deficits caused by the disease frequently lead to inactivity, it is important for people with MS to remain as active as is realistically possible given their current physical and cognitive status. Hence, countering disease-inflicted inactivity is an important component of the treatment for MS (Voss et al., 2002). Early intervention and long-term planning to prepare for possible increased disability may also help to sustain motivation

and desire for employment (Brassington & Marsh, 1998).

Unlike the cognitive impairments that may accompany MS, the affective symptoms are reversible and can be treated using standard management. For those patients who develop a psychiatric illness, appropriate medication can be effective (Knight, 1992). Medication for sleep disturbances may also be appropriate. However for the majority of MS patients, symptoms of emotional distress are an understandable consequence of adjusting to a chronic, unpredictable, and often progressive illness. Given the apparent relationship between stressful events and exacerbations of the disease, psychological interventions aimed at treating distress and depression in MS patients may even have a part to play in slowing the progression of the disease (Schwartz et al., 2000). It has also been suggested that stress reduction techniques and education in the use of more effective coping strategies may prove beneficial for people with MS, regardless of whether the stress precipitates MS exacerbations or vice versa (Brassington & Marsh, 1998).

Recent comprehensive reviews detail the variety of ways in which psychological intervention for psychosocial problems may benefit the MS patient (Mohr & Cox, 2001). Two examples will suffice here; one demonstrates a cost-effective means of treating depression in MS, and the other shows long-term gains from a theoretically derived intervention aimed at teaching coping skills.

Mohr and colleagues (2000) have reported the results of a study examining the efficacy of an 8-week telephone-administered cognitive-behavioral therapy program for the treatment of depression in MS patients. Thirty-two patients with clinically significant levels of depression were randomly assigned to telephone-based treatment or to usual care as control. Depressive symptoms decreased significantly in the treatment group compared with the control group. In addition, at 4-month follow-up, patients from the treatment group had greater adherence to their medical treatment regimen.

It is well established that coping style is a significant and long-term predictor of psychological distress and psychosocial functioning in MS patients (Jean et al., 1999; Pakenham, 1999). Schwartz (1999) has reported on the results from a 2-year randomized trial of 64 MS patients in a coping skills group compared with 68 patients undertaking peer telephone support. In comparing the results between groups, the effects of neurologic disability and gender were controlled for. Although the peer telephone support intervention was effective for those patients with affective problems, the coping skills group showed the greatest overall gains. Patients in the coping skills group showed sustained improvements in psychosocial role performance, coping behavior, and other aspects of well-being.

These examples demonstrate that individual therapy aimed at identifying emotional disturbances and the psychosocial factors that influence them, as well as the teaching of active coping skills, can be beneficial to people with MS. In addition, couple and family therapy may also be necessary, because the changes brought about by MS can cause family and marital stress (Knight et al., 1997). Sexual dysfunction may be an important issue needing to be addressed (Hatzichristou, 1996). Finally, self-help support groups can be therapeutic as they provide social interaction and emotional support, and a venue for the exchange of information and receiving of practical advice for people with MS and their families (Brassington & Marsh, 1998).

CONCLUSIONS

MS is a relatively common inflammatory neurologic disease that usually becomes evident in early adulthood and runs a fluctuating and unpredictable, but usually progressive, course over many years. The cause is unknown but both genetic and environmental factors are important. Diagnosis is based on clinical analysis of symptoms and signs, supported by investigations, especially MR scans of the brain and spinal cord. The most obvious effect of MS is physical neurologic disability, with impairment particularly of visual, motor, and sensory function but cognitive and psychosocial effects are also important and may be the dominant feature. There is no cure but partially effective disease-modifying treatments have been introduced in the past 10 years and there has been increasing interest in the cognitive and psychosocial effects of the disease and their treatment.

Unresolved issues related to the cognitive impairment include the importance of subcortical versus cortical types of involvement. This has implications for management and some of the controversy may be explained by the recent recognition that, in addition to the obvious extensive involvement of subcortical white matter, there are more subtle but nevertheless extensive changes in the cerebral cortex. Characterization of cognitive impairment and its relationship to different types of disease course and severity will always be limited by the somewhat random distribution of inflammatory lesions in the CNS and their uncertain relationship with the secondary, more diffuse degenerative process.

There is a need for better integration of recent knowledge of cognitive changes in MS patients with the diagnostic process and management of physical problems. In particular, the formulation of treatment plans could be improved by a better understanding of the relationship between performance on cognitive tests and performance in real world activities. Attempts to increase our understanding of the relationship between cognitive performance and psychosocial functioning have recently appeared in the literature (Higginson

et al., 2000). This process, known as determining the ecological validity of neuropsychological tests, offers promise for improving the management of this disease and thereby the quality of life for people with MS and their families.

■ KEY POINTS

☐   The early and accurate diagnosis of multiple sclerosis has been greatly improved by the use of magnetic resonance scanning.

☐   Although the evidence is currently inconclusive, autoimmune factors are widely considered to be central to the etiology of multiple sclerosis.

☐   Improved criteria for the diagnosis of multiple sclerosis have recently (2001) been published.

☐   Cognitive deficits are present in approximately 45% of those with multiple sclerosis.

☐   Evidence-based interventions addressing the psychosocial impact of multiple sclerosis have become an established part of the management of the disease.

KEY READINGS

McDonald I, Compston A, Edan G, et al: Recommended diagnostic criteria for multiple sclerosis: Guidelines from the international panel on the diagnosis of multiple sclerosis. Ann Neurol 50:121–127, 2001.

Rosati G: The prevalence of multiple sclerosis in the world: An update. Neurolog Sci 22:117–139, 2001.

Voss WD, Arnett PA, Higginson CI, et al: Contributing factors to depressed mood in multiple sclerosis. Arch Clin Neuropsychol 17:103–115, 2002.

REFERENCES

Arnett PA, Rao SM, Grafman J, et al: Executive functions in multiple sclerosis: An analysis of temporal ordering, semantic encoding, and planning abilities. Neuropsychology 11:535–544, 1997.

Barkhof F: The clinico-pathological paradox in multiple sclerosis revisited. Curr Opin Neurol 15:239–245, 2002.

Beatty WW: Multiple sclerosis, in Adams RL, Parsons OA, Culbertson JL, et al (eds): Neuropsychology for Clinical Practice: Etiology, Assessment, and Treatment of Common Neurological Disorders. Washington DC: American Psychological Association, 1996, pp. 225–242.

Benedict R, Bakshi R, Simon J, et al: Frontal cortex atrophy predicts cognitive impairment in multiple sclerosis. J Neuropsychiat Clin Neurosci 14:44–51, 2002.

Bennett T, Dittmar C, Raubach S: Multiple sclerosis: Cognitive deficits and rehabilitation strategies. Cognitive Rehabil 5:18–23, 1991.

Brassington JC, Marsh NV: Neuropsychological aspects of multiple sclerosis. Neuropsychol Rev 8:43–77, 1998.

Chard D, GriffinC, Parker G, et al: Brain atrophy in clinically early relapsing/remitting multiple sclerosis. Brain 125:327–337, 2002.

Comi G: Why treat early multiple sclerosis patients? Curr Opin Neurol 13:235–240, 2000.

Compston A: Risk factors for multiple sclerosis: Race or place? J Neurol Neurosurg Psychiatry 53:821–823, 1990.

Ebers G: The natural history of multiple sclerosis. J Neurol Neurosurg Psychiatry 71(Suppl. 11):16–19, 2001.

Feinstein A: The Clinical Neuropsychiatry of Multiple Sclerosis. Cambridge, UK: Cambridge University Press, 1999.

Filippi M: Enhanced magnetic resonance imaging in multiple sclerosis. Multiple Sclerosis 6:320–326, 2000.

Friend KB, Rabin BM, Groninger L, et al: Language functions in patients with multiple sclerosis. Clin Neuropsychol 13:78–94, 1999.

Gerland EJ, Zis AP: Multiple sclerosis and affective disorders. Can J Psychiatry 36:112–117, 1991.

Goodin D, Frohman E, Garmany G, et al: Disease-modifying therapies in multiple sclerosis: Report of the Therapeutics and Technology Assessment Subcommittee of the American Academy of Neurology and the MS Council for Clinical Practice Guidelines. Neurology 58(Suppl. 1):169–178, 2002.

Gordon PA, Lewis MD, Wong D: Multiple sclerosis: Strategies for rehabilitation counsellors. J Rehabil 60:34–38, 1994.

Granieri E, Casetta I, Tola M, et al: Multiple sclerosis: Infectious hypothesis. Neurol Sci 22:179–185, 2001.

Hakim EA, Bakheit AMO, Bryant TN, et al: The social impact of multiple sclerosis: A study of 305 patients and their relatives. Disabil Rehabil 22:288–293, 2000.

Hatzichristou DG: Management of voiding, bowel and sexual dysfunction in multiple sclerosis: Towards a holistic approach. Sexuality Disabil 14:3–6, 1996.

Higginson CI, Arnett PA, Voss, WD: The ecological validity of clinical tests of memory and attention in multiple sclerosis. Arch Clin Neuropsychol 15:185–204, 2000.

International Federation of Multiple Sclerosis Societies: The IFMSS Minimal Record of Disability for multiple sclerosis. Acta Neurol Scand 70(Suppl. 101):170–190, 1984.

Jagust W, Noseworthy J: Brain atrophy as a surrogate marker in MS. Neurology 54:782–783, 2000.

Jean VM, Paul RH, Beatty WW: Psychological and neuropsychological predictors of coping patterns by patients with multiple sclerosis. J Clin Psychol 55:21–26, 1999.

Johnson KP, Brooks BR, Cohen JA, et al: Extended use of glatiramer acetate (Copaxone) is well tolerated and maintains its clinical effect on multiple sclerosis relapse rate and degree of disability. Neurology 50:701–708, 1998.

Kesselring J, Klement U: Cognitive and affective disturbances in multiple sclerosis. J Neurol 248:180–183, 2001.

Kidd D, Barkhof F, McConnell R, et al: Cortical lesions in multiple sclerosis. Brain 122:17–26, 1999.

Kleespies PM, Hughes DH, Gallacher FP: Suicide in the medically and terminally ill: Psychological and ethical considerations. J Clin Psychol 56:1153–1171, 2000.

Knight RG: The Neuropsychology of Degenerative Brain Diseases. Hillsdale, NJ: Lawrence Erlbaum Associates, 1992.

Knight RG, Devereux RC, Godfrey HPD: Psychosocial consequences of caring for a spouse with multiple sclerosis. J Clin Exp Neuropsychol 19:7–19, 1997.

Ko Ko C: Effectiveness of rehabilitation for multiple sclerosis. Clin Rehabil 13 (Suppl. 1):33–41, 1999.

Kurtzke JF: Rating neurological impairment in multiple sclerosis: An expanded disability status scale (EDSS). Neurology 33:1444–1452, 1983.

Kurtzke JF: Multiple sclerosis in time and space-geographical clues to cause. J Neurovirol 6 (Suppl. 2):S134–S140, 2000.

Lezak MD: Neuropsychological Assessment, ed 3. New York: Oxford University Press, 1995.

Lublin FD, Reingold SC: Defining the clinical course of multiple sclerosis: Results of an international survey. Neurology 46:907–911, 1996.

Lucchinetti C, Bruck W, Parisi J, et al: Heterogeneity of multiple sclerosis lesions: implications for the pathogenesis of demyelination. Ann Neurol 47:707–717, 2000.

McDonald I, Compston A, Edan G, et al: Recommended diagnostic criteria for multiple sclerosis: Guidelines from the International Panel on the Diagnosis of Multiple Sclerosis. Ann Neurol 50:121–127, 2001.

McIntosh-Michaelis SA, Roberts MH, Wilkinson SM, et al: The prevalence of cognitive impairment in a community survey of multiple sclerosis. Br J Clin Psychol 30:333–348, 1991.

Milligan N, Newcombe R, Compston D: A double-blind controlled trial of high dose methylprednisolone in patients with multiple sclerosis. 1: Clinical effects. J Neurol Neurosurg Psychiatry 50:511–516, 1987.

Mohr DC, Cox D: Multiple sclerosis: Empirical literature for the clinical health psychologist. J Clin Psychol 57:479–499, 2001.

Mohr DC, Dick LP, Russo D, et al: The psychosocial impact of multiple sclerosis: Exploring the patient's perspective. Health Psychol 18:376–382, 1999.

Mohr DC, Likosky W, Bertagnolli A, et al: Telephone-administered cognitive-behavioral therapy for the treatment of depressive symptoms in multiple sclerosis. J Consult Clin Psychol 68:356–361, 2000.

Murrell RC, Kenealy PM, Beaumont JG, et al: Assessing quality of life in persons with severe neurological disability associated with multiple sclerosis: The psychometric evaluation of two quality of life measures. Br J Health Psychol 4:349–362, 1999.

O'Brien MT: Multiple sclerosis: Stressors and coping strategies in spousal caregivers. J Community Health Nurs 10:123–135, 1993.

Pakenham KI: Adjustment to multiple sclerosis: Application of a stress and coping model. Health Psychol 18:383–392, 1999.

Peyser JM, Rao SM, LaRocca NG, et al: Guidelines for neuropsychological research in multiple sclerosis. Arch Neurol 47:94–97, 1990.

Poser CM: The epidemiology of multiple sclerosis: A general overview. Ann Neurol 36(Suppl. 2):180–193, 1994.

Poser CM, Paty DW, Scheinberg L, et al: New diagnostic criteria for multiple sclerosis: Guidelines for research protocols. Ann Neurol 13:227–231, 1983.

Rao S: Neuropsychology of multiple sclerosis: A critical review. J Clin Exp Neuropsychol 8:503–542, 1986.

Rao SM, Leo GJ, Bernardin L, et al: Cognitive dysfunction in multiple sclerosis I: Frequency, patterns, and prediction. Neurology 41:685–691, 1991a.

Rao SM, Leo GJ, Ellington L, et al: Cognitive dysfunction in multiple sclerosis II: Impact on employment and social functioning. Neurology 41:692–696, 1991b.

Rosati G: The prevalence of multiple sclerosis in the world: An update. Neurol Sci 22:117–139, 2001.

Rovaris M, Iannucci G, Falautano M, et al: Cognitive dysfunction in patients with mildly disabling relapsing/remitting multiple sclerosis: An exploratory study with diffusion tensor MR imaging. J Neurol Sci 195:103–109, 2002.

Rumrill PD Jr, Tabor TL, Hennessey ML, et al: Issues in employment and career development for people with multiple sclerosis: Meeting the needs of emerging vocational rehabilitation clientele. J Vocational Rehabil 14:109–117, 2000.

Schwartz CE: Teaching coping skills enhances quality of life more than peer support: Results of a randomized trial with multiple sclerosis patients. Health Psychol 18:211–220, 1999.

Schwartz CE, Foley FW, Rao SM, et al: Stress and course of disease in multiple sclerosis. Behav Med 25:110–116, 2000.

Skegg K: Multiple sclerosis presenting as a purely psychiatric disorder. Psychol Med 23:909–914, 1993.

Skegg DCG, Corwin PA, Craven RS, et al: Occurrence of multiple sclerosis in the north and south of New Zealand. J Neurol Neurosurg Psychiatry 50:134–139, 1987.

Smith SJ, Young CA: The role of affect on the perception of disability in multiple sclerosis. Clin Rehabil 14:50–54, 2000.

Thompson A: Symptomatic management and rehabilitation in multiple sclerosis. J Neurol Neurosug Psychiatry 71(Suppl. 11):22–27, 2001.

Thompson SBN: Providing a neuropsychology service for people with multiple sclerosis in an interdisciplinary rehabilitation unit. Disabil Rehabil 18:348–353, 1996.

Thornton AE, Raz N: Memory impairment in multiple sclerosis: A quantitative review. Neuropsychology 11:357–366, 1997.

Torrey EF, Miller J, Rawlings R, et al: Seasonal birth patterns of neurological disorders. Neuroepidemiology 19:177–185, 2000.

Trapp B, Ransohoff R, Rudick R: Axonal pathology in multiple sclerosis: Relationship to neurologic disability. Curr Opin Neurol 12:295–302, 1999.

Voss WD, Arnett PA, Higginson CI, et al: Contributing factors to depressed mood in multiple sclerosis. Arch Clin Neuropsychol 17:103–115, 2002.

Weiner H, Cohen J: Treatment of multiple sclerosis with cyclophosphamide: Critical review of clinical and immunologic effects. Multiple Sclerosis 8:142–154, 2002.

White RF, Nyenhuis DS, Sax, DS: Multiple sclerosis, in White RF (ed): Clinical Syndromes in Adult Neuropsychology: The Practitioner's Handbook. Amsterdam: Elsevier, 1992, pp. 177–212.

Wiles CM, Brown P, Chapel H, et al: Intravenous immunoglobulin in neurological disease: A specialist review. J Neurol Neurosurg Psychiatry 72:440–448, 2002.

Wishart H, Sharpe D: Neuropsychological aspects of multiple sclerosis: A quantitative review. J Clin Exp Neuropsychol 19:810–824, 1997.

Zakzanis KK: Distinct neurocognitive profiles in multiple sclerosis subtypes. Arch Clin Neuropsychol 15:115–136, 2000.

Aging and the Brain

Karlene K. Ball

David E. Vance

Jerri D. Edwards

Virginia G. Wadley

Cognitive aging
Cognitive decline
Functional performance
Mobility

INTRODUCTION

A number of changes occur in the aging brain. While some of these changes may be noticeable to the affected individual, others are detectable only through fine observations or highly controlled experiments. If intri-cate studies are necessary to discover changes in cognitive abilities, one may ask whether such changes are important. Applied research on normal age-related loss teaches us that even minor changes in areas such as attention or short-term memory can affect a person's ability to function independently, which in turn can affect quality of life (QOL). For example, combined losses in attention and the ability to quickly detect and act upon information may be enough to keep some older adults from driving safely. As the population continues to live longer, more people will be living with functional impairments that can threaten independence, and society may face even greater demands for costly services such as assisted living facilities and nursing home care.

Recent research has indicated that reversing or slowing age-related cognitive declines and augmenting cognitive abilities may improve everyday functioning in older adults. This possibility is linked to the notion that the neural architecture of the aging brain, in the absence of pathology, remains plastic (Kolb & Whishaw, 1998). Neuronal production, migration, and differentiation have been observed in older adults. Processes of neurogenesis in older adults imply that improved functioning is possible (Scharff, 2000). Neural plasticity throughout the lifespan strongly suggests that well-designed cognitive interventions may be able to capitalize on the cognitive underpinnings of certain functional tasks.

This chapter provides an overview of the cognitive/neuropsychological functions that decline with normal aging, how these functions are identified, and the effects of cognitive impairments on everyday functioning (e.g., falling, driving, taking medications, and other instrumental activities of daily living [IADLs]). Theories of age-related cognitive decline, assessment issues, cognitive interventions, and future research directions will also be discussed.

IMPAIRMENTS IN COGNITIVE FUNCTION WITH AGE

Maintenance of cognitive function is important for health, longevity, and QOL. There is a great deal of variability with regard to the cognitive changes that occur with age. Some older adults experience only slight changes in cognitive abilities, while others experience significant declines. Overall, research supports the contention that there are some universal age-related cognitive losses. Generally, changes that occur with age can be organized into areas such as intelligence, executive function (EF), memory and learning, and information processing.

Intelligence

Again, it is important to note that many older adults evidence stable intellectual and cognitive abilities with age, and others may show improvements with age (Schaie, 1996). For the average older adult, declines in intelligence are minimal until a person reaches the eighth decade of life (Schaie, 1996). In some cases, rapid decline in intellectual abilities within the few years before death is observed; this phenomenon is termed terminal drop (Johansson et al., 1992). Severe cognitive decline, however, as occurs with dementia, is not an aspect of ordinary aging. Moderate to severe dementia affects 5.5% to 7% of adults over the age of 65 years

(Di Carlo et al., 2000). Although the incidence of dementia does increase with age, it is not an inevitable outcome of aging even into the tenth decade of life (Anderson-Ranberg et al., 2001).

When declines in intellectual functioning are observed with age, they tend to be specific to the domain of fluid intelligence (Bickley et al., 1995). Fluid intelligence primarily includes active reasoning, logical thought, and solving novel problems (Horn, 1982). Examples of fluid tasks would include selecting unfamiliar rotated figures that match a stimulus figure or inferring a rule to complete a letter series. In contrast, crystallized intelligence involves applying knowledge and rules that are acquired through experience. This type of intelligence relies heavily upon memory, education, and cultural background (Baltes et al., 1995b). Examples of crystallized tasks include checking a simple addition problem or finding a synonym for a stimulus word (Table 36-1). Based on the Seattle Longitudinal Study of Adult Intelligence, Schaie (1994) has reported that fluid abilities may start declining in young adulthood, whereas crystallized abilities increase or remain stable into middle age. Crystallized intelligence declines may occur later in life, but are not dramatic in the course of normal aging.

Several factors, experiences, and strategies are related to maintenance of intelligence. Higher education and continued intellectual activity appear to have protective effects upon intelligence with age (Compton et al., 1997). Extensive experience or expertise in an area also mitigates age-related declines. Hoyer and Rybash (1994) have found that although fluid abilities generally decline with age, these abilities are preserved in areas of expertise. People who have a great deal of experience in a particular area have a strong knowledge base that facilitates their performance. Apparently, information processing and fluid thinking become dedicated to specific knowledge systems and thereby become as resistant to age-related declines as crystallized abilities. Clearly, continued use of one's abilities has the potential to prevent cognitive losses.

Executive Functioning

EF involves the capacity to regulate cognitive behavior, including the ability to plan and sequence actions in order to obtain a goal, to inhibit impulses, to switch attention, and to avoid futile repetitive responses (Malloy & Richardson, 1994; Rabbitt, 1997). Executive functioning is important for maintaining IADLs and functional independence (Grigsby et al., 1998; Cahn-Weiner et al., 2000). Many investigators have demonstrated decline in prefrontal and frontal lobe function, which is responsible for EF, with

TABLE 36-1. Examples of Crystallized and Fluid Intelligence Tests

Questions	Answers	Cognitive ability
Crystallized Intelligence		
1. What is a synonym for the word "difficult"?	1. Hard Arduous Puzzling	Verbal meaning—Recognition and understanding of words
2a. What is 14 x 3? 2b. What is 26 + 46? 2c. What is 51 – 38?	2a. 42 2b. 72 2c. 13	Numerical principles—Applying known numerical principles and concepts
3. What is the opposite of "endure"?	3. Succumb Surrender	Verbal meaning—Recognition and understanding of words
Fluid Intelligence		
1. Match the target figure to the exact copy. A. C. B. D.	1. D	Spatial orientation—Rotating objects mentally in two-dimensional space
2. Complete the following letter series. A B D E G H J K	2. M	Inductive reasoning—Identifying. regularities and inferring principles and rules
3. Police found a man had hung himself from a beam. The man was found hanging 8 feet in the air, there was no furniture in the room, only a puddle of water. How did he position himself to hang?	3. The puddle of water was a block of ice. He stood on the block of ice and as the ice melted, he strangled.	Deductive reasoning—Using facts and principles to determine what happened

normal aging (e.g., Glisky et al., 1995; Parkin & Java, 1999; Souchay et al., 2000; West & Alan, 2000).

Inhibition is one key frontal lobe function that declines with age. The ability to inhibit responses is as important as initiation. Inhibition allows one to access, delete, and restrain cognitive behaviors (Hasher et al., 1999), and fosters access to relevant information by hindering access to irrelevant information. Inhibition facilitates ongoing cognitive processes by deleting extraneous information that is no longer relevant. Restraint functions prevent salient but inappropriate responses from taking over, thereby permitting weaker but correct responses to be made. In essence, inhibition prevents "mental clutter," distraction, and interference and allows the allocation of fuller mental resources to the task at hand. The performance deficits of older adults on tasks that tap executive functioning have been compared to those of younger individuals who have frontal lobe lesions (Moscovitch & Winocur, 1992).

Memory and Learning

Changes in the aging brain also occur in the temporal cortex, hippocampus, and limbic system, all of which are associated with memory (Eustache et al., 1995). Older adults commonly complain about memory loss. Schofield and colleagues (1997) found that 31% of cognitively intact community-residing elders reported memory complaints. Given that there may be declines in metamemory as well (i.e., people forget that they forget), the prevalence of memory declines may be even greater than reported.

One view compartmentalizes memory into three distinct units: sensory memory, short-term memory, and long-term memory. Sensory memory refers to the 1 to 2 seconds in which information is transmitted, perceived, and available visually or audibly. From sensory memory, information is filtered, and relevant information is relayed into short-term memory, sometimes referred to as working memory. At this point, the information is either discarded or encoded and stored in long-term memory. Once in long-term memory, the information can be retrieved and used again. While short-term memory has limited storage capacity (holding only four to nine pieces of information), long-term memory is considered to have unlimited storage capacity (Lovelace, 1990).

It is believed that many age-related changes in memory are due to declines in short-term memory. The phrase "short-term memory" has been used to denote both the immediate recall of information and the function of working memory. Working memory can be described as the ability to both store and use information simultaneously. While the ability to immediately recall relatively simple information remains intact in normal aging, several researchers have noted that working memory declines with age (Foos & Wright, 1992; Salthouse, 1992a). For example, the ability to retain increasingly long strings of digits presented aurally, mentally manipulate those digits so that they are in reverse sequence, and recite them aloud is a classic working memory task (WAIS-III Digit Span) that declines with age. Although normal declines in working memory are expected with age, frank deficits in working memory may be suggestive of dementia and have been associated with early IADL impairments in Alzheimer disease (AD) (Earnst et al., 2001).

Long-term memory consists of two broad classes of memory—declarative (episodic and semantic) and nondeclarative—which are differentially affected by aging. The primary distinction between declarative and nondeclarative memory is that declarative (a.k.a. *explicit recall*) refers to conscious learning and nondeclarative (a.k.a. *procedural memory* or *implicit recall*) refers to unconscious learning. In other words, nondeclarative memory can be described as unintentional, automatic, or without awareness, and relies upon familiarity rather than deliberate study (Kausler, 1994; Smith, 1996). Use of nondeclarative memory occurs when one recalls the procedures needed to perform automatic skills such as twisting a doorknob or flipping a light switch (Poon, 1985; Light & Albertson, 1989). This type of memory includes skills, perceptual learning, motor learning, and classically conditioned responses. Nondeclarative memory remains intact in normal aging as well as in the early stages of Alzheimer disease (Kuzis et al., 1999).

Older adults more often have difficulty with declarative memory as they age, and age-related impairments can be seen in both types of declarative memory: episodic and semantic. Episodic memory involves the recall of temporal and spatial information associated with past personal experiences. Semantic memory involves language and world knowledge. Episodic memory generally becomes impaired with age before

semantic memory. Thus, factual knowledge and language remain resistant to loss longer than episodic memory (Tulving, 1993).

Deficits in long-term memory depend in part upon the manner in which information is retrieved and the complexity of that information. Older adults are more likely to exhibit memory deficits when required to freely recall information, but perform better when they need only recognize information in the presence of cues (Craik & Jennings, 1992). In summary, memory declines with age are not generalized; rather, they are specific to the task at hand and the type of memory employed.

Information Processing

Information processing uses a computer metaphor for understanding how cognition occurs. Simply stated, information is transmitted via the sensory organs, processed in working memory, and stored or erased depending upon its relevance. All pertinent computations are handled by working memory, where most problem solving occurs (Klahr, 1992). Although the computer metaphor is a simplistic representation of very complex phenomena, it has proved helpful for understanding cognition.

With increasing age, adults experience difficulty in processing novel information, especially in the midst of distraction. However, age-related decrements in information processing vary depending upon task complexity (Allen et al., 1995; Fisher et al., 1995; Bashore et al., 1998). Overall, performance decrements with age become more evident as task complexity increases (Mayr & Kliegl, 1993).

In addition to complexity, the amount of distracting information involved in a task can detrimentally impact older adults' information processing performance. Generally, the more distractors that a task involves, the more difficulty older individuals have in comparison with young adults (Dywan & Murphy, 1996). However, older adults' abilities improve when they are provided cues, strategies, and practice (Plude & Hoyer, 1985). For example, Sekuler and Ball (1986) found that brief periods of practice yielded significant and long-lasting improvement in task performance. In sum, older adults have more difficulty processing information when the task is complex, when it involves a great deal of irrelevant information, and when it is unfamiliar; however, such difficulty can be mitigated with practice.

THEORIES OF AGE-RELATED COGNITIVE DECLINE

Several theories have been advanced to explain the age-related declines that are observed in cognition. No

TABLE 36-2. Causal Theories of Age-Related Cognitive Declines

Theory	Definition	Characteristics
Diminished processing speed	Mental processes slow with age, resulting in widespread cognitive declines.	* Slowing of information transmission * Robust across timed tasks
Limited capacity	Brain capacity to process information determines overall cognitive function. Capacity decreases with age.	* Resource allocation model * Cognitive capacity * Cognitive reserve
Frontal aging	Declines in the frontal lobes of the brain result in a loss of executive functioning, which in turn results in widespread cognitive disorganization. Lack of inhibition is most notable.	* Prefrontal areas are more vulnerable to aging. * Executive functioning is associated with frontal and prefrontal areas of the brain. * Metacognition deficits
Activity/disuse	Cognitive decline is a function of disuse and subsequent atrophy of neurons and neural pathways rather than purely age-related.	* Use it or lose it. * Neural plasticity * Training studies support this view.
Cognitive-Perceptual Theories		
Common cause	Cognitive and perceptual declines denote extensive degradation in the central nervous system resulting in systemwide declines.	* Age leads to widespread neural degradation that independently affects both perceptual and cognitive systems.
Sensory deprivation	Sensory declines cause cognitive declines; specifically, prolonged sensory declines lead to neuronal death.	* Deprivation must be prolonged. * Sensory underload

single theory accounts for all age-related cognitive phenomena. Clearly, each explanation spills over into adjacent theories; this spillage hints at the interdependency of the various cognitive systems (Table 36-2). For the sake of brevity, only the most widely cited theories will be discussed in this chapter.

Diminished Speed of Processing

According to the diminished speed of processing theory, (Birren, 1974; Salthouse, 1985), the speed with which older adults can mentally process information slows with age. This diminished speed of processing is due to a generalized slowing that affects information transmission throughout the central nervous system (CNS). Speed of processing declines can occur at all stages of processing, from the speed at which information is encoded to the execution of a response (Cerella & Hale, 1994). Researchers have found that age differences in performance on various cognitive and neuropsychological measures that are indicative of parietal, temporal, and frontal lobe function all can be explained by older individuals' reduced speed of processing (Lindenberger et al., 1993; Schaie, 1994; Salthouse, 1995; Salthouse et al., 1996; Bryan et al., 1997). Lindenberger and

colleagues (1993) found that age-related decrements in fluency, reasoning, and memory were all mediated through differences in speed of processing.

It is important to note, however, that age-related slowing is not necessarily a ubiquitous process. There is a great deal of individual variability in the rate of slowing. Furthermore, speed of processing declines may be specific to a particular aspect of processing such as stimulus encoding rather than generalized slowing. Bashore and colleagues (1998) found that when reaction time alone is measured there is support for the diminished speed of processing theory. However, when both reaction time and event-related brain potentials are examined, there is more evidence for task- and process-specific patterns of cognitive slowing. Decrements in processing speed alone cannot account for all age-related declines in cognitive performance.

Limited Capacity

Another theory proposed to explain age-related cognitive declines is the limited capacity theory. According to this theory, attentional resources peak in young adulthood and decline gradually with age due to reduced or limited processing capacity (Hoyer & Plude, 1982). In other words, there is a surplus of cognitive capacity in young adulthood but as the brain ages and suffers gradual age-related insults (e.g., free radical damage, cerebrovascular or systemic difficulties, chronic hypoxia), the cognitive reservoir slowly diminishes. Researchers have suggested that subtle decrements in processing capacity may result in information processing difficulties in general and working memory declines in particular (Salthouse, 1992b; Kail & Salthouse, 1994).

Frontal Aging

Declines in executive functioning due to deterioration in the neurologic integrity of the frontal lobes, including prefrontal cortical areas, have been proposed to account for age-related declines in several areas including memory (Troyer et al., 1994; Shimamura, 1995) and functional abilities (Grigsby et al., 1998). Support for the frontal lobe theory comes from studies demonstrating that cognitive processes dependent on the prefrontal cortex exhibit age-related declines both earlier and to a greater extent than cognitive processes dependent on nonfrontal regions.

Activity/Disuse

The activity/disuse theory states that cognitive decline is a function of disuse, resulting in neuronal atrophy. Conversely, this theory posits that neurons remain viable when an organism is stimulated and encouraged to use existing abilities. This theory is consistent with research indicating that mental functioning is improved in the presence of stimulating novel events. Research investigating cognitive interventions supports this view. For example, Vance and Porter (2000) found that global cognition was either maintained or improved in adults with AD in adult day care after they were exposed for 3 months to several novel treatment materials. Although the findings were not robust, the presence of an effect even among dementia patients supports the strength of activity/disuse theory. It could be argued that every treatment designed to improve cognitive functioning is predicated upon this theory, implicitly or explicitly, in that treatments are based upon the understanding that cognitive functioning can be augmented through some type of stimulation.

Common Cause

The common cause theory states that age-related cognitive changes are caused by an overall decline in the physiologic integrity of the brain and nervous system. According to this theory, widespread physiologic decline in the nervous system contributes to age-related impairment in motor, sensory, and cognitive functions (Lindenberger & Baltes, 1994). This theory is based on

evidence indicating that declines in mental functioning are related to declines in sensory and motor functioning. For example, researchers have found that after statistically accounting for several confounding variables (e.g., education, health, mood), lower limb strength remained closely associated with age-related variance in reasoning (Anstey et al., 1997). The strength of this association supports the notion that the physiologic integrity of the nervous system affects all neurodependent functions regardless of their seeming dissimilarity.

No single cause of physiologic decline in the nervous system has been identified, but several have been suggested. Possible causes range from speed of processing declines, and frontal lobe declines, to poor nutrition (Gonzalez-Gross et al., 2001) or declines in proteins regulating postsynaptic neuronal plasticity (Hatanpaa et al., 1999).

In conclusion, all of these theories propose mechanisms for observed cognitive changes with age. An examination of the unique and overlapping contributions of these hypotheses can lead to a fuller understanding of cognition and aging.

IMPACT OF COGNITIVE IMPAIRMENTS ON MOBILITY AND EVERYDAY FUNCTIONING

There is substantial evidence that cognitive abilities are important predictors of individual differences in the ability to function in everyday life. The relationship of cognition to mobility is the primary focus of the discussion that follows.

Mobility

Mobility is a functional ability that is important for maintaining QOL and independence with age. Mobility can be defined as a person's intentional movement throughout his or her environment (Owsley et al., 1999) and can be conceptualized on a continuum ranging from bedbound to unrestricted (Stalvey et al., 1999). Mobility also encompasses the ability to move throughout one's environment in order to complete a task or achieve a goal (Owsley et al., 2000).

With increasing age, mobility limitations increase in prevalence and are associated with impairments in sensory, cognitive, and physical functioning (Barberger & Fabrigoule, 1997). In nearly 20% of the 65+ population, mobility restrictions adversely affect QOL by increasing the need for care and decreasing personal independence (Guralnik et al., 1996). Mobility problems have been associated with acute medical conditions (Branch & Meyers, 1987) and depression (Seeman, 1996), and mobility problems also signal the likelihood of further deterioration in functional independence (Manton, 1988).

Mobility can be assessed in many different ways. An individual's ability to perform activities of daily living (ADLs) (e.g., dressing, bathing, and toileting) or instrumental activities of daily living (IADLs) (e.g., handling money, using the phone, and driving) can be examined. Performance of specific maneuvers such as walking or climbing stairs and balance can be observed. The extent to which one travels throughout his or her environment can be quantified. Additionally, adverse mobility outcomes such as automobile crashes or falls may be considered as well. Each of these has been linked to declines in cognitive function.

Activities of Daily Living/Instrumental Activities of Daily Living

There is substantial evidence that cognitive variables are important predictors of individual differences in the ability to perform tasks required in daily living. With age, decline is often noted in the performance of daily activities that rely on cognitive function, referred to as IADLs. Lawton and Brody (1969) described distinct categories of IADLs that are essential to maintaining an independent lifestyle. These categories include abilities such as managing finances, self-administering medications, using the telephone, preparing meals, and housekeeping (Fillenbaum, 1987). Additionally, the inability to independently perform self-care ADLs, such as dressing, feeding oneself, and toileting, has also been linked to cognitive decline and to negative outcomes such as poor nutrition and fatigue (Diehl et al., 1995; Visentin et al., 1998).

It is important to note that the cognitive abilities underlying everyday function are complex (Willis, 1996). The performance of "real-life" tasks relies upon multiple cognitive abilities (Allaire and Marsiske, 1999) as well as an individual's overall health, social skills, and social networks. Even so, the identification of specific cognitive skills that are related to specific functional declines could lead to effective interventions.

In general, everyday performance is more strongly related to fluid intelligence than to crystallized intelligence (Diehl et al., 1995). Specifically, fluid abilities such as memory span and speed of processing appear to affect older adults' performance of IADLs (Willis, 1991). Diehl and colleagues (1995) found that speed of processing best predicted fluid intelligence, which in turn was the strongest predictor of older adults' performance on everyday activities. Limits in the performance of daily activities may also be in part caused by deficits in executive functioning. Royall and colleagues (2000) found that executive function is predictive of IADL impairment and the need for care, even among noninstitutionalized retirees. Even elderly persons without dementia may be at risk with regard to the complex cognitive skills that underlie everyday compe-

tence (Ganguli et al., 1991). Furthermore, older adults who have had lifelong sociocultural disadvantages may be especially at-risk (Willis, 1996).

Falls

Falls are a potentially serious and possibly life-threatening event for older adults. Approximately 20% to 30% of persons over the age of 65 fall at least once each year (Stalenhoef et al., 1999; Bergland et al., 2000). The result can be catastrophic; mobility may be severely limited as a result of a broken hip, and in some cases a fall results in death (Tinetti et al., 1988; Cummings et al., 1995). Falls diminish quality of life by limiting one's ability to ambulate, interfering with the performance of daily activities such as bathing or going to the store, and reducing social activity (Stalenhoef et al., 1999; Tinetti et al., 2000; Sicard-Rosenbaum et al., 2002).

Although some falls have a single obvious cause, many can be linked to cognitive factors (Fuller, 2000). For example, Tinetti and colleagues (1988) found that cognitive decline, excluding dementia, was associated with increased risk for falling. Declines in executive functioning (Nevitt et al., 1991) and attention (Shumway-Cook et al., 1997) have also been associated with increased risk of falls.

Driving

Cognitive losses have been associated with other adverse mobility outcomes such as decreased driving exposure, increased driving avoidance, and crash involvement. Deficiencies in EF, mental status, and memory have been associated with decreased driving exposure, increased avoidance, and increased incidence of crashes among older adults (Foley et al., 1995; Johansson et al., 1996; Ball et al., 1998; Stutts, 1998). Diminished speed of processing (as measured by the Useful Field of View) has also been associated with the avoidance of several types of driving situations (Ball et al., 1998) and has been found to be an excellent predictor of state-recorded motor vehicle crashes in studies using both retrospective and prospective designs (Ball et al., 1990, 1993; Owsley et al., 1998).

Cognitive function is imperative for maintaining mobility and avoiding impairments in ADLs, IADLs, or other adverse events such as falls and crash involvement. Maintaining mobility appears to be vital for sustaining one's quality of life.

ASSESSING AGE-RELATED COGNITIVE DECLINE

Many changes in cognitive abilities occur with age, and several theories to account for these changes have been reviewed. Because impairments in cognitive function are predictive of functional difficulties such as mobility impairments, loss of independence, and decreased QOL, and because the potential exists for reversing or slowing the progression of cognitive declines, it is important to identify those older adults who are at risk by reliably assessing their cognitive abilities.

Age-related cognitive declines can be difficult to determine for several reasons. Individual characteristics such as health, education, and mood state can influence cognitive performance. Lack of baseline cognitive data for a given individual makes it very hard to differentiate between performance that represents, *for that individual*, normal cognition versus cognitive decline. On the other hand, frank cognitive impairment is relatively easy to identify. Issues surrounding the administration of measures and lack of specificity among measures also can cloud interpretation of cognitive assessment.

One test administration issue that has been long debated is the use of self-report versus objective ratings. Self-report assessments can be problematic in that older adults may have trouble accurately estimating their performance (Myers et al., 1993; Diehl et al., 1995). For example, it has been suggested that older adults tend to overestimate their level of everyday competence in comparison with actual performance (Ford et al., 1988). Due to problems such as these, performance-based tests generally are preferred over self-ratings.

Yet another issue to consider is that the time of day that tests are administered may significantly affect performance. Circadian cycles influence arousal patterns, and arousal can influence cognitive performance. Some individuals experience greater arousal in the evenings and others in the mornings. May and Hasher (1998) found that performance of EF tasks was mediated by circadian variations. Older adults performed better during times in which they were more in synchrony with their arousal state.

It is also important to consider the ecological validity of any given assessment measure. Even the most widely used measures of mental status are simply a sampling of one's cognitive ability under artificial circumstances. Although a given instrument may be keen in detecting small variations in certain intellectual abilities, it may be unrelated to everyday function. Furthermore, laboratory assessments of older adults' intellectual functioning often underestimate their ability to function in more familiar everyday situations (Salthouse, 1990).

Additional factors that can create variability in the cognitive assessment of older adults include the influence of prescription medications and interactions among medications. Undesirable medication effects such as psychomotor slowing can result in the appearance of age-related declines. Observed cognitive difficulties are sometimes simply the result of polypharmacy rather than age or early-stage dementia.

Education has repeatedly been shown to complicate the determination of age-related cognitive declines. Education has been found to be an independent predictor of performance among the elderly on measures of language, learning and memory, praxis, and executive functioning (Collie et al., 1999). This link between education and cognitive function can make cognitive performance difficult to interpret.

Mood abnormalities, especially depression, have been widely cited for exerting detrimental effects on cognitive functioning. Severe depression can create a pseudo-dementia that mimics AD. For this reason, clinicians must account for the impact of mood disorders before making a dementia diagnosis (Bassuk et al., 1998). Benedict and colleagues (1999) found that geriatric psychiatry inpatients whose mood improved also exhibited improved cognitive functioning, especially on tests of spatial processing and learning. Considering that depression is a pervasive problem, with about 10% of older adults exhibiting at least some depressive symptoms (Jefferson & Greist, 1993), it must be considered as a potential confound in the assessment process.

Cognitive measures themselves are often subject to cultural and historical biases. Park and colleagues (1999) found that people raised in different cultures process information differently. Historical biases include cohort-specific advantages. For instance, younger adults are more experienced with testing situations, characteristics, and strategies. They have greater sophistication in the areas of computer testing, timed testing, multiple-choice responses, process-of-elimination strategies, and multiprocedure problems. Cognitive tests that use these characteristics may inadvertently place older adults at a disadvantage, artificially lowering their test scores relative to those of younger adults.

Cognitive Assessment Measures

Despite these caveats, current cognitive assessments do provide standardized evaluation of mental functioning and may be helpful for identifying individuals who could benefit from interventions. Below is a list of some of the most widely used cognitive assessments. Such measures are important for research and treatment because they provide global and specific information on one's ability to process information.

Comprehensive assessment is essential for answering questions about the cognitive domains underlying functional performance. Selection of a cognitive battery is guided by the research question at hand; an example of such a battery can be seen in Table 36-3. Consideration also must be given to the amount of time and expertise required for test administration, the availability of individuals qualified to interpret the data (generally neuropsychologists or clinical psychologists with additional training in neuropsychology), and the availability of age-appropriate normative data for each test. A comprehensive battery uses multiple measures of each posited cognitive domain or cognitive construct in order to avoid idiosyncratic, test-specific performance and to more fully represent the construct. As any researcher who has attempted to factor analyze a group's performance on a cognitive battery will fully appreciate, no specific test represents a pure measure of a single domain. Performance on a single test is a minute sample of behavior that at best can only partially represent a given domain. Furthermore, virtually all tests tap more than one domain. The cognitive constructs are interrelated, and many of the measures themselves are also highly related. These complexities necessitate the use of caution in drawing sweeping clinical or research conclusions based upon limited data and imperfect measurement models, whether conceptually or empirically derived.

Having acknowledged the many complexities involved in cognitive assessment, a sample cognitive assessment battery is provided (see Table 36-3) that includes multiple measures of hypothetical cognitive constructs or domains, with some measures appearing under more than one domain—an indication that these measures have been demonstrated to tap multiple constructs. This sample battery is not exhaustive but is one example of many possible assessment batteries. Nevertheless, it may provide the reader with an idea of measures that are generally accepted to represent cognitive domains of interest.

Activities of Daily Living/Instrumental Activities of Daily Living Assessment

In addition to the many measures available for cognitive assessment, there are also a variety of instruments for examining older adults' ability to perform prototypical everyday activities. Although cognitive assessment is often used as an indirect indicator of functional status, an examination of actual performance seems more ecologically valid. Some examples of such measures include the Observed Tasks of Daily Living (Diehl et al., 1995), the Everyday Problems Test (Willis, 1996), the Timed IADL task (Owsley et al., 2001), Barthel Self-Care Rating Scale (Sherwood et al., 1977), the Physical Self-Maintenance Scale (Lawton, 1971), and the Financial Capacity Instrument (Marson et al., 2000).

COGNITIVE INTERVENTIONS

A primary goal of cognitive aging research is to develop interventions that can enhance cognitive function. Cognitive training protocols have been developed for the improvement of memory, reasoning, and speed of processing, among other abilities (Baltes & Willis, 1982; Ball et al., 1988; Baltes et al., 1995a; Hayslip et al., 1995; Kramer et al., 1995; Neely & Bäckman, 1995; Caprio-Prevette & Fry, 1996; Oswald et al., 1996; Mohs et al., 1998; Edwards et al., 2002). These protocols have demonstrated improvement in a designated cognitive skill when training is employed.

Memory training studies have involved a variety of training protocols and often have used a multifactorial approach (Neely & Bäckman, 1995; Caprio-Prevette & Fry, 1996; Mohs et al., 1998). For example, Neely and Bäckman (1995) conducted a memory training study in which they found transfer of training to recall tasks that were similar but not identical to the training tasks. Similarly, Villa and Abeles (2000) used group sessions to help older adults develop prospective memory, using techniques such as memory strategies, internal rehearsal, relaxation techniques, and behavior modification. After seven sessions, participants showed a significant increase in their ability to remember tasks to be done in the future. Similar studies have shown that training can be used to improve memory for names (Schmidt et al., 1999), short-term memory (De Vreese et al., 1998), and facial recognition (Andrewes et al., 1996).

Several reasoning training studies have been conducted using the protocol from the Adult Development and Enrichment Project (ADEPT) (Baltes & Willis, 1982; Schaie & Willis, 1986; Willis et al., 1992; Willis & Schaie, 1994; Hayslip et al., 1995). The ADEPT training protocol consists of two types of training: figural relations training, which involves teaching strategies to facilitate mental rotation of figures; and reasoning training, which involves teaching different rules or strategies to solve letter series, letter sets, and number series problems. Training studies using the ADEPT protocol have generally found that training results in improvement on tasks similar to the training tasks (Willis et al., 1981). However, training effects do not appear to transfer to abilities that were not the focus of training (Willis & Schaie, 1994).

Roenker and colleagues conducted a study examining the effects of speed of processing training upon driving performance (described in Ball & Owsley, 2000; Roenker et al., in press). Individuals who received speed-of-processing training demonstrated significantly faster processing on the Useful Field of View (UFOV) test: a measure of the speed with which a spatial field can be scanned with a single glance; improved stopping time to road signs while in a driving simulator; and fewer dangerous maneuvers on an open road driving test (Ball & Owsley, 2000). A control group received an equivalent amount of training in a standard driver improvement class but did not demonstrate these gains. These findings indicated that speed-of-processing training transfers to similar measures of processing speed as well as to the functional outcome of reacting quickly to

TABLE 36-3. Sample Cognitive Battery

Cognitive domain	Suggested measures
Abstract reasoning (fluid intelligence)	• Mattis Dementia Rating Scale—Conceptualization • WAIS-III Similarities • WAIS Matrix Reasoning
Arithmetic capacity (crystallized intelligence; working memory)	• WRAT-III Arithmetic • WAIS-III Arithmetic
Attention/concentration	• Mattis Dementia Rating Scale—Attention • Trails A • WAIS Digit Symbol Substitution • WMS-III Digit Span • WMS-III Spatial Span • WMS-III Letter-Number Sequencing • Useful Field of View (UFOV®)
Dementia severity	• Mini Mental Status Exam • MOMSSE • Mattis Dementia Rating Scale
Depression	• Beck Depression Inventory • Brief Symptom Inventory—Depression • Geriatric Depression Scale • Hamilton Depression Rating Scale • Center for Epidemiological Studies Depression Scale
Executive function	• Mattis Dementia Rating Scale—Initiation/Perseveration • CLOX 1 (a clock drawing task) • Controlled Oral Word Association Test (COWA) (Letter and Category subtests) • Digit Symbol Substitution • EXIT25 • Trails B • Wisconsin Card Sorting Test
Fine motor function (neural integrity/common cause)	• Halstcad-Reitan Finger Tapping (screening for gross neurologic impairment and/or reduced psychomotor function)
Intellectual function	• WAIS-III VIQ, PIQ, and Full Scale IQ (or prorated IQ) • WAIS-III Processing Speed factor score • WASI Vocabulary and Matrix Reasoning (to form prorated Full Scale IQ)
Language (rule out advance dementia, stroke)	• WAB Auditory Verbal Comprehension • Boston Naming Test • COWA Test (Letter and Category fluency subtests) • WRAT-III Reading
Processing speed	• Useful Field of View (UFOV®) • Letter and Pattern Comparison • Finding As • WAIS Digit Symbol Substitution
Reasoning	• Figural Relations • Letter Series • Raven's Progressive Matrices

TABLE 36-3. Sample Cognitive Battery—cont'd

Cognitive domain	Suggested measures
Verbal memory	• Mattis Dementia Rating Scale—Memory (screening) • California Verbal Learning Test (list learning, recall, recognition, error types) • Hopkins Verbal Learning Test (list learning, recall, recognition, error types) • Rivermead (narrative memory) • WMS-III Logical Memory I (narrative memory) • WMS-III Logical Memory II (narrative memory)
Visual memory	• WMS-III Visual Reproduction I • WMS-III Visual Reproduction II
Visuospatial function (rule out stroke, subcortical dementia)	• Mattis Dementia Rating Scale—Construction • CLOX 2 (a clock drawing task) • WAIS-III Block Design

IQ, Intelligence Quotient; PIQ, Performance Intelligence Quotient; UFOV, Useful Field of View; VIQ, Verbal Intelligence Quotient; WAB, Western Aphasia Battery; WAIS, Wechsler Adult Intelligence Scale; WMS, Wechsler Memory Scale; WRAT, Wide Range Achievement Test.

hazardous situations while driving (Ball & Owsley, 2000). Further research using the speed of processing intervention has replicated the finding of improved UFOV performance and has demonstrated that this training also may transfer to improved performance of timed IADLs (Edwards et al., 2002).

It is now clear that specific cognitive functions can be augmented. However, further investigation is necessary in order to confirm whether interventions that target specific mental abilities transfer to concomitant real-world tasks. To date, many cognitive training studies have indicated that improvements may be limited to performance of tasks similar to those used in training. Given these findings, future interventions must examine ways to improve generalization in order to effectively improve everyday functioning.

CONCLUSIONS

Despite the wide range of individual differences in cognitive changes with aging, in the aggregate there are several areas of cognition that decline with age. In particular, short-term memory, speed of information processing, and executive functioning exhibit robust decrements. No matter how cognitive declines are determined, only global measures and a few specific measures have been shown to directly predict concomitant declines in everyday functioning. This trend stresses two important areas for further study. First, cognitive measures used to predict real-world functioning must be carefully evaluated before determination of risk for certain functional losses can definitively be made. Second, a lack of connection between certain cognitive declines and

everyday functioning is in itself a testament to the compensatory abilities that older adults develop. These compensatory cognitive skills represent a prime area for further investigation and for utilization in protocols designed to help at-risk elders remain autonomous.

Finally, given what is known about cognitive abilities and their impact on specific mobility functions such as driving, additional interventions targeting cognitive skills related to mobility must be developed and tested. Such interventions are the natural outgrowth of cognitive aging research and provide additional meaning to the careful basic research that continues to guide the field.

■ KEY POINTS

☐ Applied research on normal age-related cognitive loss teaches us that even minor changes in areas such as attention or short-term memory can affect a person's ability to function independently, which in turn can affect quality of life.

☐ Despite a great deal of individual variability with regard to the cognitive changes that occur with age, research supports the contention that there are universal age-related losses in executive function, memory, and information processing speed.

☐ With increasing age, mobility limitations increase in prevalence and are associated with impairments in sensory, cognitive, and physical functioning.

☐ Comprehensive cognitive assessment is essential for answering questions about the cognitive domains underlying functional performance. Selection of a cognitive battery is guided by the research question at hand, the amount of time and expertise required for test administration and interpretation, and the availability of age-appropriate normative data for each test. A comprehensive battery uses multiple measures of each posited cognitive domain or cognitive construct in order to more fully represent the construct and to avoid idiosyncratic, test-specific results.

☐   It is now clear that specific cognitive functions can be augmented. However, further investigation is necessary in order to confirm whether interventions that target specific mental abilities transfer to concomitant real-world tasks.

KEY READINGS

Horn JL: The theory of fluid and crystallized intelligence in relation to concepts of cognitive psychology and aging in adulthood, in Craik FIM, Trehub S (eds): Aging and Cognitive Processes, Vol. 8. New York: Plenum, 1982, pp. 237–278.

Lawton MP, Brody E: Assessment of older people: Self-maintaining and instrumental activities of daily living. Gerontologist 9:179–185, 1969.

Schaie KW: The course of adult development. Am Psychologist 49:304–314, 1994.

Willis SL, Jay GM, Diehl M, et al: Longitudinal change and prediction of everyday task competence in the elderly. Res Aging 14:68–91, 1992.

REFERENCES

Allaire JC, Marsiske M: Everyday cognition: Age and intellectual ability correlates. Psychology Aging 14:627–644, 1999.

Allen PA, Madden DJ, Slane S: Visual and word encoding and the effect of adult age and word frequency, in Allen PA, Bashore TR (eds): Age differences in word and language processing. Amsterdam, The Netherlands: North-Holland/Elsevier, 1995, pp. 30–72.

Anderson-Ranberg K, Vasegaard L, Jeune B: Dementia is not inevitable: A population-based study of Danish Centenarians. J Gerontol: Psychol Sci 56B, 152–159, 2001.

Andrewes DG, Kinsella G, Murphy M: Using a memory handbook to improve everyday memory in community-dwelling older adults with memory complaints. Exp Aging Res 22:305–322, 1996.

Anstey KJ, Lord SR, Williams P: Strength in lower limbs, visual contrast sensitivity, and simple reaction time predict cognition in older women. Psychol Aging 12:137–144, 1997.

Ball KK, Roenker DL, Bruni JR: Developmental changes in attention and visual search throughout adulthood, in Enns J (ed): Advances in Psychology, Vol. 69. North Holland, The Netherlands: Elsevier Science, 1990, pp. 489–508.

Ball K, Owsley C: Increasing mobility and reducing accidents of older drivers, in Schaie KW, Pietrucha M (eds): Mobility and Transportation in the Elderly. New York: Springer Publishing Company, 2000, pp. 213–251.

Ball K, Owsley C, Sloane M, et al: Visual attention problems as a predictor of vehicle crashes in older drivers. Invest Ophthalmol Visual Sci 34:3110–3123, 1993.

Ball K, Owsley C, Stalvey B, et al: Driving avoidance and functional impairment in older drivers. Accident Anal Prevent 30:313–322, 1998.

Ball KK, Beard BL, Roenker DL, et al: Age and visual search: Expanding the useful field of view. J Optical Soc Am A-Optics Image Sci 5:2210–2219, 1988.

Baltes MM, Kuhl K, Gutzmann H, et al: Potential of cognitive plasticity as a diagnostic instrument: A cross-validation and extension. Psychol Aging 2:167–172, 1995a.

Baltes PB, Staudinger UM, Maercker A, et al: People nominated as wise: A comparative study of wisdom related knowledge. Psychol Aging 10:155–166, 1995b.

Baltes PB, Willis SL: Plasticity and enhancement of intellectual functioning in old age: Penn State's Adult Development and Enrichment Project (ADEPT), in Craik FIM, Trehub S (eds): Aging and Cognitive Processes. New York: Plenum Press, 1982, pp. 353–390.

Barberger GP, Fabrigoule C: Disability and cognitive impairment in the elderly. Disabil Rehabil 19:175–193, 1997.

Bashore TR, Ridderinkhof KR, Van der Molen WW: The decline of cognitive processing speed in old age. Curr Directions Psychol Sci 6:163–169, 1998.

Bergland A, Pettersen AM, Laake K: Functional status among elderly Norwegian fallers living at home. Physiother Res Int 51:33–45, 2000.

Bassuk SS, Berkman, LF, Wypij D: Depressive symptomatology and incident cognitive decline in an elderly community sample. Arch Gen Psychiatry 55:1073–1081, 1998.

Benedict RH, Dobraski M, Godlstein MZ: A preliminary study of the association between changes in mood and cognition in a mixed geriatric psychiatry sample. J Gerontol Psychol Sci Soc Sci 54:94–99, 1999.

Bickley PG, Keith TZ, Wolfle LM: The three stratum theory of cognitive abilities: Test of the structure of intelligence across the life span. Intelligence 20:309–328, 1995.

Birren JE: Translation in gerontology—from lab to life: Psychophysiology and the speed of response. Am Psychologist 29:808–815, 1974.

Branch LG, Meyers AR: Assessing physical function in the elderly. Clin Geriatr Med 3:29–51, 1987.

Bryan J, Luszcz MA, Crawford, JR: Verbal knowledge and speed of information processing as mediators of age differences in verbal fluency performance among older adults. Psychol Aging 12:473–478, 1997.

Cahn-Weiner DA, Malloy PF, Boyle PA, et al: Prediction of functional status from neuropsychological tests in community-dwelling elderly individuals. Clin Neuropsychologist 14:187–195, 2000.

Caprio-Prevette MD, Fry PS: Memory enhancement program for community-based older adults: Development and evaluation. Exp Aging Res 22:281–303, 1996

Cerella J, Hale S: The rise and fall in information-processing rates over the life span. Acta Psychol 86:109–197, 1994.

Collie A, Shafiq-Antonacci R, Maruff P, et al: Norms and the effects of demographic variables on a neuropsychological battery for use in healthy ageing in Australian populations. Austr N Z J Psychiatry 33:568–578, 1999.

Compton DM, Bachman LD, Logan JA: Aging and intellectual ability in young, middle-aged, and older educated adults: Preliminary results from a sample of college faculty. Psychol Rep 81:79–90, 1997.

Craik FIM, Jennings JM: Human memory, in Craik FIM, Salthouse TA (eds): Handbook of Aging and Cognition. Mahwah, NJ: Erlbaum, 1992, pp. 51–110.

Cummings SR, Nevitt MC, Browner WS, et al: Risk factors for hip fractures in white women. N Engl J Med 332:767–773, 1995.

De Vreese LP, Belloi L, Iacona S, et al: Memory training programs in memory complainers: Efficacy on objective and subjective memory functioning. Arch Gerontol Geriatr 1006:141–154, 1998.

Di Carlo A, Baldereschi M, Amaducci L, et al: Cognitive impairment without dementia in older people: Prevalence, vascular risk factors, impact on disability. The Italian Longitudinal Study on Aging. J Am Geriatr Soc 48:775–782, 2000.

Diehl M, Willis SL, Schaie KW: Everyday problem solving in older adults: Observational assessment and cognitive correlates. Psychol Aging 10:478–490, 1995.

Dywan J, Murphy WE: Aging and inhibitory control in text comprehension. Psychol Aging 11:199–206, 1996.

Earnst K, Wadley V, Aldridge T, et al: Loss of financial capacity in Alzheimer's disease: The role of working memory. Aging Neuropsychol Cogn 8:109–118, 2001.

Edwards JD, Wadley VG, Myers RS, et al: Transfer of a speed of processing intervention to near and far cognitive functions. Gerontology 48:329–340, 2002.

Eustache F, Rioux P, Desgranges B, et al: Healthy aging, memory subsystems and regional cerebral oxygen consumption. Neuropsychologia 33:867–887, 1995.

Fillenbaum GG: Activities of daily living, in Maddox GL (ed): The Encyclopedia of Aging. New York: Springer, 1987, pp. 3–4.

Fisher D L, Fisk AD, Duffy SA: Why latent models are needed to test hypotheses about slowing of word and language processes in older adults, in Allen PA, Bashore TR (eds): Age Differences in Word and Language Processing. Amsterdam, The Netherlands: North-Holland/Elsevier, 1995, pp. 1–29.

Foley DJ, Wallace RB, Eberhard J: Risk factors for motor vehicle crashes among older drivers in a rural community. J Am Geriatr Soc 43:776–781, 1995.

Foos PW, Wright L: Adult age differences in the storage of information in working memory. Exp Aging Res 2:51-57, 1992.

Ford AB, Folmar SJ, Salmon RB, et al: Health and function in the old and very old. J Am Geriatr Soc 36:187–197, 1988.

Fuller GF: Falls in the elderly. Am Fam Physician 61:2159–2168, 2173-2154, 2000.

Ganguli M, Ratcliff G, Huff FJ, et al: Effects of age, gender, and education on cognitive tests in a rural elderly community sample: Norms from the Monongahela Valley Independent Elders. Neuroepidemiology 10:42–52, 1991.

Glisky EL, Polster MR, Routhieaux BC: Double dissociation between item and source memory. Neuropsychology 9:229–235, 1995.

Gonzalez-Gross M, Marcos A, Pietrzik K: Nutrition and cognitive impairment in the elderly. Br J Nutr 86:313–321, 2001.

Grigsby J, Kaye K, Baxter J, et al: Executive cognitive abilities and functional status among community-dwelling older persons in the San Luis Valley Health and Aging Study. J Am Geriatr Soc 46:590–596, 1998.

Guralnik JM, Fried LP, Salive ME: Disability as a public health outcome in the aging population. Annu Rev Public Health 17:25–46, 1996.

Hasher L, Zacks RT, Rahhal TA: Timing, instructions, and inhibitory control: Some missing factors in the age and memory debate. Gerontology 45:355–357, 1999.

Hatanpaa K, Isaacs KR, Shirao T, et al: Loss of proteins regulating synaptic plasticity in normal aging of the human brain and in Alzheimer disease. J Neuropathol Exp Neurol 58:637–643, 1999.

Hayslip B, Maloy RM, Kohl R: Long-term efficacy with fluid ability interventions with older adults. J Gerontol Psychol Sci 50B:141–149, 1995.

Horn JL: The theory of fluid and crystallized intelligence in relation to concepts of cognitive psychology and aging in adulthood, in Craik FIM, Trehub S (eds): Aging and Cognitive Processes, Vol. 8. New York: Plenum, 1982, pp. 237–278.

Hoyer WJ, Plude DJ: Aging and the allocation of attentional resources in visual information processing, in Sekuler R, Kline D, Dismukes K (eds): Aging and Human Visual Function. New York: Liss, 1982, pp. 245–263.

Hoyer WJ, Rybash JM: Characterizing adult cognitive development. J Adult Dev 1:7–12, 1994.

Jefferson JW, Greist JH: Depression and older people: Recognizing hidden signs and taking steps toward recovery. Madison, WI: Pratt Pharmaceuticals, 1993.

Johansson B, Zarit SH, Berg S: Changes in cognitive functioning of the oldest old. J Gerontol Psychol Sci 47:75–80, 1992.

Johansson K, Bronge L, Lundberg C, et al: Can a physician recognize an older driver with increased crash potential? J Am Geriatr Soc 44, 1198–1204, 1996.

Kail R, Salthouse TA: Processing speed as a mental capacity. Acta Psychol 86:199–225, 1994.

Kausler DH: Learning and Memory in Normal Aging. San Diego: Academic Press, 1994.

Klahr D: Information-processing approaches to cognitive development, in Bornstein MH, Lamb ME (eds): Developmental Psychology: An Advanced Textbook, ed 3. Hillsdale, NJ: Lawrence Erlbaum, 1992, pp. 272–336.

Kolb B, Whishaw IQ: Brain plasticity and behavior. Annu Rev Psychol 49:43–64, 1998.

Kramer A, Larish JF, Strayer DL: Training for attentional control in dual task settings: A comparison of young and old adults. J Exp Psychol Appl 1:50–76, 1995.

Kuzis G, Sabe L, Tiberti C, et al: Explicit and implicit learning in patients with Alzheimer disease and Parkinson disease with dementia. Neuropsychiatry Neuropsychol Behav Neurol 12:265–269, 1999.

Lawton MP: The functional assessment of elderly people. J Am Geriatr Soc 19:465–481, 1971.

Lawton MP, Brody E: Assessment of older people: Self-maintaining and instrumental activities of daily living. Gerontologist 9:179–185, 1969.

Light LL, Albertson SA: Direct and indirect tests of memory for category exemplars in young and older adults. Psychol Aging 4:487–492, 1989.

Lindenberger U, Baltes PB: Sensory functioning and intelligence in old age: A strong connection. Psychol Aging 9:339-355, 1994.

Lindenberger U, Mayr U, Kliegl R: Speed and intelligence in old age. Psychol Aging 8:207–220, 1993.

Lovelace EA: Basic concepts in cognition and aging, in Lovelace EA (ed): Aging and Cognition: Mental Processes, Self-Awareness, and Interventions. Amsterdam, The Netherlands: Elsevier, 1990, pp. 1–28.

Malloy PF, Richardson ED: Assessment of frontal lobe functions. J Neuropsychiatry Clin Neurosci 6:399–410, 1994.

Manton KG: A longitudinal study of functional change and mortality in the United States. J Gerontol 43:M5153–M5161, 1988.

Marson DC, Sawrie SM, Snyder S, et al: Assessing financial capacity in patients with Alzheimer disease: A conceptual model and prototype instrument. Arch Neurol 57:877–884, 2000.

May CP, Hasher L: Synchrony effects in inhibitory control over thought and action. J Exp Psychol Human Percept Perform 24:363–379, 1998.

Mayr U, Kliegl R: Sequential and coordinative complexity: Age-based processing limitations in figural transformations. J Exp Psychol Learn Mem Cogn 19:1297–1320, 1993.

Mohs RC, Ashman TA, Jantzen K, et al: A study of the efficacy of a comprehensive enhancement program in healthy elderly persons. Psychiatry Res 77:183–195, 1998.

Moscovitch M, Winocur G: The neuropsychology of memory and aging, in Craik FIM, Salthouse TA (eds): The Handbook of Aging and Cognition. Hillsdale, NJ: Erlbaum, 1992, pp. 315–372.

Myers AM, Holliday PJ, Harvey KA et al: Functional performance measures: Are they superior to self-assessments? J Gerontol Med Sci 48, M196–M206, 1993.

Neely AS, Bäckman L: Effects of multifactorial memory training in old age: Generalizability across tasks and individuals. J Geront Psychol Sci 50B:134–140, 1995.

Nevitt MC, Cummings SR, Hudes ES: Risk factors for injurious falls: A prospective study. J Gerontol Biol Med Sci 46:M164–M170, 1991.

Oswald WD, Rupprecht R, Gunzelmann T, et al: The SIMA-project: Effects of one year cognitive and psychomotor training on cognitive abilities of the elderly. Behav Brain Res 78:67–72, 1996.

Owsley C, Allman RM, Gossman M, et al: Mobility impairment and its consequences in the elderly, in Clarie JM, Allman RM (eds): The Gerontological Prism: Developing Interdisciplinary Bridges. Amityville, NY: Baywood Publishing Co., 2000, pp. 305–310.

Owsley C, Ball K, McGwin G, et al: Visual processing impairment and risk of motor vehicle crash among older adults. JAMA 279:1083–1088, 1998.

Owsley C, McGwin G, Sloane M, et al: Timed instrumental activities of daily living (TIADL) tasks: Relationship to visual function in older adults. Optom Vis Sci 78:350–359, 2001.

Owsley C, Stalvey BT, Wells J, et al: Older drivers and cataract: Driving habits and crash risk. J Gerontol Biol Med Sci 54A:M203–M211, 1999.

Park DC, Nisbett R, Hedden T: Aging, culture, and cognition. J Gerontol Psycholog Sci Soc Sci 54:75–84, 1999.

Parkin AJ, Java RI: Deterioration of frontal lobe function in normal aging: Influences of fluid intelligence versus perceptual speed. Neuropsychology 13:539–545, 1999.

Plude DJ, Hoyer WJ: Attention and performance: Identifying and localizing age deficits, in Charness N (ed): Aging and Human Performance. Chichester, UK: Wiley, 1985, pp. 47–99.

Poon LW: Differences in human memory with aging: Nature, causes, and clinical implications, in Birren J, Schaie KW (eds): Handbook of the Psychology of Aging. New York: Van Nostrand Reinhold, 1985, pp. 427–462.

Rabbitt P: Introduction: Methodologies and models in the study of executive function, in Rabbitt P (ed): Methodology of Frontal and Executive Function. East Sussex, NJ: Psychology Press, 1997, pp. 19–38.

Roenker DL, Cissell GM, Ball K, et al: The effects of speed of processing and driving simulator training on driving performance. Hum Factors, in press.

Royall DR, Chiodo LK, Polk MJ: Correlates of disability among elderly retirees with "subclinical" cognitive impairment. J Gerontol 55:M541–M546, 2000.

Salthouse TA: Speed of behavior and its implications for cognition, in Birren JE, Schaie KW (eds): Handbook of the Psychology of Aging, ed 2. New York: Van Nostrand Reinhold, 1985, pp. 400–426.

Salthouse TA: Cognitive competence and expertise in aging, in Birren JE, Schaie KW (eds): Handbook of the Psychology of Aging, ed 3. San Diego, CA: Academic Press, 1990, pp. 310–319.

Salthouse TA: Influence of processing speed on adult age differences in working memory. Acta Psychologica 79:155–170, 1992a.

Salthouse TA: What do adult age differences in the Digit Symbol Substitution Test reflect? J Gerontol 47:121–128, 1992b.

Salthouse TA: Influence of processing speed on adult age differences in learning. Swiss J Psychol 54:102–112, 1995.

Salthouse TA, Fristoe N, Rhee SH: How localized are age-related effects on neuropsychological measures? Neuropsychology 10:272–285, 1996.

Schaie KW: The course of adult development. Am Psychologist 49:304–314, 1994.

Schaie KW: Intellectual development in adulthood. The Seattle Longitudinal Study. New York: Cambridge University Press, 1996.

Schaie KW, Willis SL: Can decline in intellectual functioning be reversed? Dev Psychol 22:223–232, 1986.

Scharff C: Chasing fate and function of new neurons in adult brains. Curr Opin Neurobiol 10:774–783, 2000.

Schmidt IW, Dijkstra HT, Berg IL, et al: Memory training for remembering names in older adults. Clin Gerontologist 20:57–73, 1999.

Schofield PW, Marder K, Dooneief G, et al: Association of subjective memory complaints with subsequent cognitive decline in community-dwelling elderly individuals with baseline cognitive impairment. Am J Psychiatry 154:609–615, 1997.

Seeman TE: Social ties and health: The benefits of social integration. Ann Epidemiol 6:442–451, 1996.

Sekuler R, Ball K: Visual localization: Age and practice. J Optical Soc Am Optics Image Sci 3:864–867, 1986.

Sherwood SJ, Morris J, Mor V, et al: Compendium of measures for describing and assessing long-term care population. Boston: Hebrew Rehabilitation Center for the Aged, 1977.

Shimamura AP: Memory and frontal lobe function, in Rabbitt P (ed): The Cognitive Neurosciences. Cambridge, MA: MIT Press, 1995, pp. 803–813.

Shumway-Cook A, Woollacott M, Kerns KA, et al: The effects of two types of cognitive tasks on postural stability in older adults with and without a history of falls. J Gerontology Biol Med Sci 52:M232–M240, 1997.

Sicard-Rosenbaum L, Light KE, Behrman AL: Gait, lower extremity strength, and self-assessed mobility after hip arthroplasty. J Gerontol Biol Med Sci 57:M47–M51, 2002.

Smith AD: Memory, in Birren JE, Schaie KW (eds): Handbook of the Psychology of Aging, ed 4. San Diego, CA: Academic Press, 1996, pp. 236–250.

Souchay C, Isingrini M, Espagnet L: Aging, episodic memory feeling-of-knowing, and frontal functioning. Neuropsychology 14:299–309, 2000.

Stalenhoef PA, Diederiks JP, de Witte LP, et al: Impact of gain problems and falls on functioning in independent living persons of 55 years and over: A community survey. Patient Edu Counsel 36:23–31, 1999.

Stalvey BT, Owsley C, Sloane ME, et al: The life space questionnaire: A measure of the extent of mobility of older adults. J Appl Gerontol 18:460–478, 1999.

Stutts JC: Do older drivers with visual cognitive impairments drive less? J Am Geriatr Soc 46:854–861, 1998.

Tinetti ME, Speechley M, Ginter SF: Risk factors for falls among elderly persons living in the community. N Engl J Med 319:1701–1707, 1988.

Tinetti ME, Williams CS, Gill TM: Health, functional, and psychological outcomes among older persons with chronic dizziness. J Am Geriatr Soc 48:417–421, 2000.

Troyer A K, Graves RE, Cullum CM: Executive functioning as a mediator of the relationship between age and episodic memory in healthy aging. Aging Cogn 1:45–53, 1994.

Tulving E: What is episodic memory? Curr Direct Psychol Sci 2:67–60, 1993.

Vance DE, Porter RJ Jr: Cognitive benefits from using Montessori in Alzheimer's day cares. Activities Adaptation Aging 24:1–22, 2000.

Villa KK, Abeles N: Broad spectrum intervention and the remediation of prospective memory declines in the able elderly. Aging Ment Health 4:21–29, 2000.

Visentin P, Scarafiotti C, Marinello R, et al: Symptoms as predictors of functioning in the community-dwelling elderly. Arch Gerontol Geriatr 26:247–255, 1998.

West R, Alan C: Age-related decline in inhibitory control contributes to the increased Stroop effect observed in older adults. Psychophysiology 37:179–189, 2000.

Willis SL: Cognition and everyday competence, in Schaie KW, Lawton MP (eds): Annual Review of Gerontology and Geriatrics, Vol. 11. New York: Springer, 1991, pp. 80–109.

Willis SL: Everyday cognitive competence in elderly persons: Conceptual issues and empirical findings. Gerontologist 36:595–601, 1996.

Willis SL, Bliezner R. Baltes PB: Intellectual training research in aging: Modification of performance on the fluid ability of figural relations. J Edu Psychol 73:41–50, 1981.

Willis SL, Jay GM, Diehl M, et al: Longitudinal change and prediction of everyday task competence in the elderly. Res Aging 14:68–91, 1992.

Willis SL, Schaie KW: Cognitive training in the normal elderly, in Forette F, Christen Y, Boller F (eds): Plasticité cérébrale et stimulation cognitive. Paris, France: Fondation Nationale de Gérontologie, 1994, pp. 91–113.

Nonvasculitic Auto-immune Inflammatory Meningoencephalitis

Richard J. Caselli

Encephalopathy

Hashimoto disease

Hashimoto encephalopathy

Sjogren syndrome

Vasculitis

INTRODUCTION

The differential diagnosis of encephalopathy is extensive and ranges from conditions that are mild, self-limited, and reversible to those which are severe, progressive, and irreversible. Among the least common, but potentially reversible categories of encephalopathy, are the autoimmune inflammatory-mediated forms. The primary and secondary central nervous system vasculitides are the most widely recognized diseases within this broader category. Less well recognized, however, are several autoimmune-mediated meningoencephalitides that have been described under diverse names and pre-sumed etiologies, but collectively reflect a nonvasculitic form of autoimmune-based inflammatory meningo-encephalitis (NAIM) (Caselli et al., 1991; Caselli et al., 1993; Caselli et al., 1999). Presentations of NAIM can be acute, subacute, or chronic, and need to be distinguished from irreversible conditions with a similar temporal and semiologic profiles. NAIM has varied and inconsistent serologic associations, as well as electroencephalographic (EEG) and cerebrospinal fluid (CSF) abnormalities, and there are no diagnostically reliable radiologic signs for NAIM. Ultimately, the diagnosis may require a brain biopsy, but a brief (2-week) course of empiric glucocorticosteroid monotherapy can be a reasonable diagnostic step in many patients.

GENERAL FEATURES

Clinical

The clinical features of encephalopathy reflect wide-spread brain dysfunction. Clinical distinction of encephalopathic cognitive profiles requires sensitivity on the part of the clinician to the specific cognitive and neurologic profiles of more common cognitive disorders.

Alzheimer disease (AD), for example, does not generally produce diffuse hyper-reflexia, impaired level of consciousness, or an unsteady gait. AD impairs memory and naming disproportionately early in its course, with relative sparing of psychomotor speed, motor skills, and alertness. Most AD patients do not develop visual hallucinations early in their course, though a subset with Lewy-body—related forms of dementia often do. Encephalopathic patients, in contrast, will often be somnolent, mildly hyper-reflexic, unsteady or frankly ataxic, agitated, and have widespread cognitive impairment without disproportionately severe impairment of memory and naming. The differences are more relative than absolute, however, and vary widely among patients.

Serologic Features

Three conditions described to produce a steroid responsive acute inflammatory encephalopathy include Hashimoto encephalopathy in patients with autoimmune thyroiditis (Shein et al., 1986; Shaw et al., 1991), idiopathic hypereosinophilic syndrome (Moore et al., 1985; Martin-Gonzalez, et al., 1986), hypereosinophilia associated with L-tryptophan use (Martin et al., 1990; Adair et al., 1992), and Sjogren syndrome (Caselli et al., 1999). Some published examples of acute encephalopathy resulting from Sjogren syndrome, however, have resulted from frank necrotizing cerebral vasculitis that was rapidly fatal and unresponsive to high-dose steroid monotherapy (Alexander et al., 1981; Alexander et al., 1982; Alexander & Alexander, 1983; de la Monte et al., 1983; Sato et al., 1987). Whether Sjogren syndrome represents a pathophysiologic link bridging the cerebral vasculitides and NAIM is uncertain.

Regarding subacute presentations, in several cases Hashimoto encephalopathy has been reported (Brain et al., 1966; Thrush & Boddie, 1974) to cause monophasic as well as relapsing confusional states, as has systemic lupus erythematosus (SLE). In patients with Hashimoto disease, it is important to distinguish the steroid-responsive, autoimmune-mediated meningoencephalitis (which is rare) from the resulting hypothyroidism and consequent metabolic encephalopathy. In patients with central nervous system complications of SLE, autopsy studies have shown a variety of neuropathologic abnormalities, including rare instances of cortical perivascular lymphocytic infiltrates reminiscent of the histologic changes in our patients (Johnson & Richardson, 1968; Gibson & Myers, 1976; Ellis & Verity, 1979). However, no clinically distinguishing features have yet been described that permit identification of this possible subgroup of SLE patients before death. Antiribosomal P protein antibody titers, however, appear to correlate with SLE-related neuropsychiatric manifestations of disease activity (Bonfa & Elkon, 1986; Bonfa et al., 1987; Bluestein, 1987). Other immunologic indices of central nervous system (CNS) autoimmunity in SLE include the presence of anti-neuronal antibodies (Quismorio & Friou, 1972; Seibold et al., 1982; Golombek et al., 1986) and the intrathecal synthesis of the fourth component of complement (Jongen et al., 1990). Despite these indices of autoimmunity, no reliable response to high-dose corticosteroid therapy has yet been observed in patients with SLE-associated neuropsychiatric abnormalities (Gibson & Myers, 1976; Bonfa et al., 1987). Idiopathic hypereosinophilic syndrome has also been associated with subacutely presenting encephalopathy that is steroid responsive (Moore et al., 1985).

Regarding chronic encephalopathy and dementia-like presentations, other cases associated with Sjogren syndrome have been reported (Nishimura et al., 1985; Siller et al., 1995) since our initial reports (Caselli et al., 1991; Caselli et al., 1993). Primary hypereosinophilic syndrome can be associated with a steroid-responsive chronic encephalopathy resembling dementia, and has characteristic CSF and hematologic abnormalities that should facilitate diagnosis (Weaver et al., 1988; Kaplan et al., 1989). Finally, Hashimoto encephalopathy can follow an immunosuppressant-responsive chronic course with or without acute relapses (Henderson et al., 1987).

Electroencephalographic Features

The EEG findings in patients with encephalopathy vary, but typically include diffuse slowing of background rhythms, sometimes with frontally projected paroxysmal high amplitude rhythmic patterns. In NAIM, there is generally an absence of more diagnostically specific morphological patterns (e.g., triphasic waves, periodic complexes) (Caselli et al., 1993), though epileptiform discharges can be seen in NAIM as in any other encephalopathy. More importantly, in a patient with cognitive decline, these nonspecific, generally severe, patterns of slowing are more severe than the typical patient with a degeneratively based dementing illness and should raise suspicion leading to additional diagnostic inquiry. Further, they improve with steroid therapy, and can be used to monitor disease activity (Caselli et al., 1993) (Fig. 37-1).

Cerebrospinal Fluid Examination

The CSF findings are typically subtle and may be overlooked entirely if the correct tests are not pursued. Total protein may be mildly elevated, and glucose is typically normal. There is often little to no lymphocytic pleocytosis, though there are exceptions. Taken together with other routine CSF studies such as the Venereal

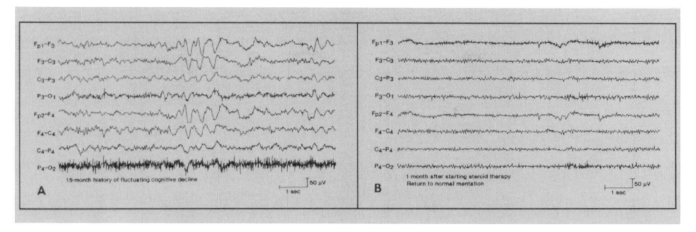

FIGURE 37-1. Electroencephalographic (EEG) demonstration of steroid response in nonvasculitic autoimmune-based inflammatory meningoencephalitis (NAIM). *Panel A*, before treatment, shows slowing of background activity with bursts of frontal intermittent rhythmic delta activity. *Panel B* shows normal EEG pattern after 1 month of oral steroid treatment.

Disease Research Laboratory (VDRL; a test for syphilis) test, microbiologic studies, and cytology, a "routine" CSF exam may be normal or only mildly nonspecifically abnormal, in a fashion often seen in the healthy elderly population. More consistently revealing, however, are the immunologic studies of IgG index, IgG synthesis rate, and oligoclonal bands. These are also nonspecific markers, but elevations generally indicate intrathecal activation of an inflammatory process. In the absence of infection or malignancy, they can reflect an autoimmune process.

Radiologic Features

Despite the unparalleled contributions diagnostic neuroimaging has made to neurologic diagnosis, computed tomography (CT) and magnetic resonance imaging (MRI) studies are typically unaffected by NAIM (Fig. 37-2*A*). There may be meningeal enhancement, but this is inconsistent and its absence does not exclude the diagnosis of NAIM. Cerebral angiography is typically normal in NAIM (Fig. 376-2*B*), unlike in CNS vasculitis. The most useful aspect of neuroimaging is its ability to exclude other causes of encephalopathy such as an acute cerebral infarction or mass lesion.

Histologic Features

The hallmark histologic features of NAIM are nonspecific accumulations of perivenular and periarteriolar lymphocytic infiltrates in leptomeninges and superficial cortical layers (Fig. 3). There is no frank vessel wall invasion or necrosis, and the severity is often described as "mild and nonspecific."

ILLUSTRATIVE CASES

Acute Presentation

An 80-year-old retired school cook was admitted to a psychiatric hospital following a 3-week period of memory loss, paranoid delusions, hallucinations, confusion, and headaches. Before this she had lived alone without difficulty or assistance. On admission, she scored 24 out of 38 on the Kokmen Test of Mental Status (KTMS) (Kokmen et al., 1987). She was mildly hyperreflexic, but there was no tremor. Gait was normal. However, her neurologic status continued to deteriorate. Sixteen days after admission, she was somnolent; her KTMS score was 6, and she could no longer walk without assistance. Serologic abnormalities included elevations in anti-SSA (125.1), antithyroid microsomal antibody (1:400), and antinuclear antibody (ANA) (1:40). A CSF examination showed a mildly elevated total protein (63 mg/dL) with normal glucose (65 mg/dL), and white blood cell (WBC) count (0), but IgG index, synthesis rate, and oligoclonal band OB were not assessed. An MRI of the brain showed a small, chronic-appearing left parietal infarct, and MRI angiography was normal. An EEG showed nonspecific, moderately severe dysrhythmic slowing. A salivary gland biopsy disclosed moderate lymphocytic sialadenitis consistent with Sjogren syndrome. She received a 3-day course of intravenous methylprednisolone (1000 mg daily) followed by oral prednisone (60 mg daily). Delusions and hallucinations improved within 2 days, but her intellectual loss showed little improvement after 2 weeks of therapy. She was then switched to oral methotrexate (7.5 mg weekly), and upon examination 2 months later was greatly improved. She was reading the newspaper daily as well as a lengthy popular novel, doing her own laundry, and preparing her

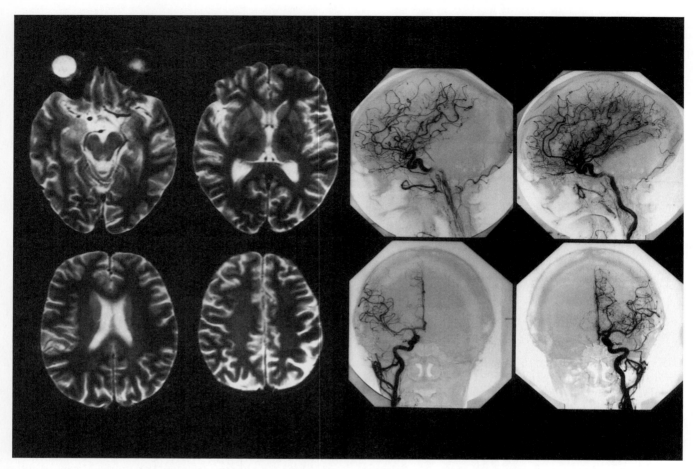

FIGURE 37-2. Radiologic studies in nonvasculitic autoimmune-based inflammatory meningoencephalitis (NAIM) including magnetic resonance imaging (MRI) (*left*) and cerebral angiography (*right*), are normal.

own shopping lists accurately. She scored 25 out of 38 on the Kokmen Short Test of Mental Status (STMS), and over the next few months continued to show modest further clinical, neuropsychological, and electrophysiologic (EEG) improvement.

Subacute Presentation

A 67-year-old college professor became acutely lightheaded and weak after skiing. He was brought to a local emergency room, where he experienced a grand mal seizure followed by transient confusion. He was hospitalized for the next 3 months, during which time he had fluctuating levels of confusion and agitation. He developed bilateral calf deep vein thromboses for which he received warfarin. On some days he was quite bright and lucid, and on such a day, he scored 30 out of 38 on the STMS. On other days he was agitated and severely confused. He often spoke in German, though English was his first language. He was tremulous, mildly hyperreflexic, and mildly unsteady. Serologic abnormalities included an elevated erythrocyte sedimentation rate

(range 40 to 63 mm/hr), elevated anticardiolipin antibody titer (IgG 1:32, IgM 1:32), positive VDRL (1:8 with negative FTA), and low C4. Initial CSF examination was normal with a total protein of 24, WBC count 0, red blood cell (RBC) count 10, IgG index 0.47, IgG synthesis rate of 0, no OB , and a negative VDRL. A second CSF exam 2 weeks later showed an elevated IgG index of 1.5, and IgG synthesis rate of 32. An MRI of the brain was normal, and there was no abnormal enhancement with gadolinium administration. An EEG showed bitemporal (right greater than left) sharp waves and spikes, a 10 to 12 Hz background alpha rhythm, and no focal slowing. A right anterior temporal brain biopsy disclosed lymphocytic perivascular leptomeningeal and intraparenchymal inflammation with both T and B cells present. Minimal gliosis was present in superficial cortical layers. Glucocorticosteroid therapy was initiated (prednisone 60 mg daily) with evident improvement within 2 weeks. By 2 months, his dose was 40 mg daily and he was considered "nearly normal." Upon examination 5 months later, he scored 36 out of 38 on the STMS, and had only mild difficulty

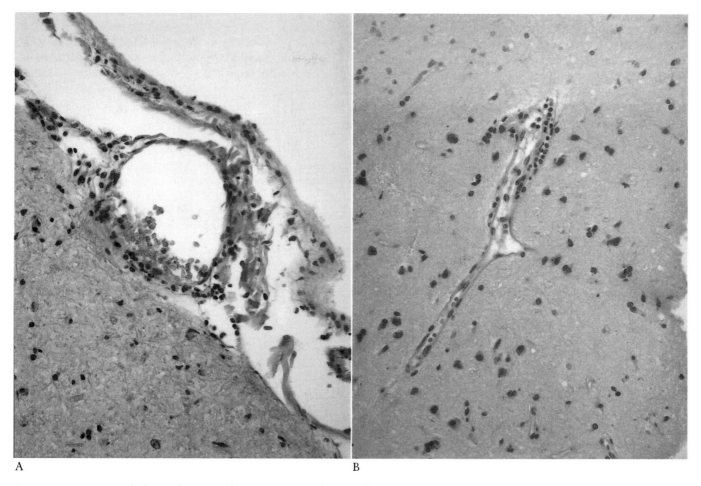

FIGURE 37-3. Histopathology of nonvasculitic autoimmune-based inflammatory meningoencephalitis (NAIM). The leptomeningeal (hematoxylin and eosin × 100) (*A*) and parenchymal perivascular (hematoxylin and eosin × 400) infiltrates (*B*) consist of cytologically benign lymphocytes.

with constructional praxis. Upon examination 8 months later he had normal constructional praxis, and appeared to be back to his normal cognitive state. Two years after diagnosis he had a brief symptomatic relapse when his dose was dropped from 5 mg daily to 2.5 alternating with 5 mg daily. Reinstitution of prednisone 60 mg daily was of minor benefit, prompting institution of intravenous methylprednisolone 1000 mg daily for 3 days. With intravenous steroids he was noticeably improved within a day, and quickly returned to normal. Oral prednisone was reinstituted, and tapered slowly.

Chronic Presentation

A 56-year-old businesswoman had a 16-year history of treated hypothyroidism and Sjogren syndrome. She presented with a 15-month history of fluctuating, progressive cognitive decline, paranoid ideation, and visual hallucinations that had been previously diagnosed as Alzheimer disease. Neurologic examination disclosed

mild hyperreflexia, bilateral Babinski signs, a mild appendicular static and intention tremor, and a normal-based, nonshuffling, unsteady gait. She scored 27 out of 38 on the STMS, and had greater impairment of temporal orientation than recall. Serologic abnormalities included an elevated ESR of 48 mm in 1 hour, the presence of anti-SSA and SSB antibodies, and an increased rheumatoid factor (RF) of 641 IU/mL. CSF examination showed a mildly elevated total protein (66 mg/dL), normal glucose (62 mg/dL with concurrent plasma glucose of 88 mg/dL), WBC count (1.0 per mL), RBC count (0.0 per mL), an IgG index of 0.72 (nL <0.77), an IgG synthesis rate 31.76 mg/24 hr, and 1 oligoclonal band. MRI and cerebral angiography were normal (see Fig. 37-2). EEG performed 6 months after the onset of cognitive decline showed diffuse, nonspecific, severely dysrhythmic slowing. A repeat EEG performed 15 months after onset revealed further deterioration. Right prefrontal brain biopsy (see Fig. 37-3) disclosed lymphocytic perivascular leptomeningeal and, rarely, intraparenchymal inflammation with both T and B cells present. Gliosis was present in superficial cortex, especially in the molecular layer. Corticosteroid therapy was initiated with prednisone 120 mg daily resulting in rapid improvement in mentation, normalization of the ESR, and resolution of preoperative EEG abnormalities (see Fig. 37-1). Improvement was clinically obvious within days. Within 1 month she scored 38 out of 38 on the STMS. Neuropsychological evidence of improvement continued for at least 6 months, and she returned to her normal cognitive state. Upon discontinuation of steroids, she felt worse (despite a score of 38 out of 38 on the STMS), developed severe dysrhythmic slowing on her EEG as well as an elevated ESR once again, all of which resolved with reinstitution of therapy and gradual tapering to a low maintenance dose of prednisone (5 mg daily).

TREATMENT AND COURSE

Treatment should begin with high-dose corticosteroids, and a clinically evident response anticipated within days. Initial treatment can be intravenous or oral, with subsequent oral maintenance. Occasionally other immunosuppressant agents have proven necessary, though generally use of these agents should be guided by histopathologic confirmation of the diagnosis. The dosage can be gradually tapered over the course of months, but a low maintenance dose, typically between 5 and 10 mg of prednisone daily, may be necessary indefinitely. Initial improvement can be striking, but complete improvement, when it occurs, typically requires several weeks to months. ESR, EEG, and clinical cognitive assessment are helpful to monitor a patient's therapeutic course, and care must be taken to distinguish nonspecific steroid reactions of modestly increased wakefulness and alertness from a true therapeutic response with cognitive recovery.

■ KEY POINTS

Nonvasculitic autoimmune inflammatory meningoencephalitis:

☐ Can present as an acute, subacute, or chronic progressive encephalopathy;

☐ Is often associated with any of several autoimmune diseases including but not limited to Sjogren syndrome and Hashimoto disease;

☐ Should be suspected in a patient with serologic and CSF signs of autoimmunity, and further supported by an encephalopathic EEG pattern;

☐ Is most definitively diagnosed by leptomeningeal and brain biopsy; and

☐ Can be reversible with corticosteroid therapy.

KEY READINGS

Caselli RJ, Scheithauer BW, Bowles CA, et al: The treatable dementia of Sjogren's syndrome. Ann Neurol 30:98–101, 1991.

Caselli RJ, Scheithauer BW, O'Duffy JD, et al: Chronic inflammatory meningoencephalitis should not be mistaken for Alzheimer's disease. Mayo Clin Proc 68:846–853, 1993.

Caselli RJ, Boeve BF, Scheithauer BW, et al: Nonvasculitic autoimmune inflammatory meningoencephalitis (NAIM): A reversible form of encephalopathy. Neurology 53:1579–1581, 1999.

Shaw PJ, Walls TJ, Newman PK, et al: Hashimoto's encephalopathy: A steroid responsive disorder associated with high anti-thyroid antibody titers-report of 5 cases. Neurology 41:228–233, 1991.

REFERENCES

Adair JC, Rose JW, Digre KB, et al: Acute encephalopathy associated with the eosinophilia-myalgia syndrome. Neurology 42:461–462, 1992.

Alexander EL, Alexander GE: Aseptic meningoencephalitis in primary Sjogren's syndrome. Neurology 33:593–598, 1983.

Alexander EL, Provost TT, Stevens MB, et al: Neurologic complications of primary Sjogren's syndrome. Medicine 61:247–257, 1982.

Alexander GE, Provost TT, Stevens MB, et al: Sjogren syndrome: Central nervous system complications. Neurology (NY) 31:1391–1396, 1981.

Bluestein HG: Neuropsychiatric manifestations of systemic lupus erythematosus [editorial]. N Engl J Med 317:309–311, 1987.

Bonfa E, Elkon KB: Clinical and serologic associations of the antiribosomal P protein antibody. Arthritis Rheum 29:981–985, 1986.

Bonfa E, Golombek SJ, Kaufman LD, et al: Association between lupus psychosis and anti-ribosomal P protein antibodies. N Engl J Med 317:265–271, 1987.

Brain L, Jellinek EH, Ball K: Hashimoto's disease and encephalopathy. Lancet 2:512–514, 1966.

Caselli RJ, Boeve BF, Scheithauer BW, et al: Nonvasculitic autoimmune inflammatory meningoencephalitis (NAIM): A reversible form of encephalopathy. Neurology 53:1579–1581, 1999.

Caselli RJ, Scheithauer BW, Bowles CA, et al: The treatable dementia of Sjogren's syndrome. Ann Neurol 30:98–101, 1991.

Caselli RJ, Scheithauer BW, O'Duffy JD, et al: Chronic inflammatory meningoencephalitis should not be mistaken for Alzheimer's disease. Mayo Clin Proc 68:846–853, 1993.

de la Monte SM, Hutchins GM, Gupta PK: Polymorphous meningitis with atypical mononuclear cells in Sjogren's syndrome. Ann Neurol 14:455–461, 1983.

Ellis SG, Verity MA: Central nervous system involvement in systemic lupus erythematosus: A review of neuropathologic findings in 57 cases, 1955–1977. Semin Arthritis Rheum 8:212–221, 1979.

Gibson T, Myers AR: Nervous system involvement in systemic lupus erythematosus. Ann Rheum Dis 35:398–406, 1976.

Golombek SJ, Graus F, Elkon KB: Autoantibodies in the cerebrospinal fluid of patients with systemic lupus erythematosus. Arthritis Rheum 29:1090–1097, 1986.

Henderson LM, Behan PO, Aarli J, et al: Hashimoto's encephalopathy: A new neuroimmunological syndrome [abstract]. Ann Neurol 22:140, 1987.

Johnson RT, Richardson EP: The neurological manifestations of systemic lupus erythematosus: A clinico-pathological study of 24 cases and review of the literature. Medicine 47:337–369, 1968.

Jongen PJH, Boerbooms AM, Lamers KJB, et al: Diffuse CNS involvement in systemic lupus erythematosus: Intrathecal synthesis of the 4th component of complement. Neurology 40:1593–1596, 1990.

Kaplan PW, Waterbury L, Kawas C, et al: Reversible dementia with idiopathic hypereosinophilic syndrome. Neurology 39:1388–1391, 1989.

Kokmen E, Naessens JM, Offord KP: A short test of mental status: Description and preliminary results. Mayo Clin Proc 62:281–288, 1987.

Martin RW, Duffy J, Engel AG, et al: The clinical spectrum of the eosinophilia-myalgia syndrome associated with L-tryptophan ingestion. Ann Intern Med 113:124–134, 1990.

Martin-Gonzalez E, Yebra M, Garcia-Merino A, et al: Neurologic dysfunction in the idiopathic hypereosinophilic syndrome. Ann Intern Med 104: 448–449, 1986.

Moore PM, Harley JB, Fauci AS: Neurologic dysfunction in the idiopathic hypereosinophilic syndrome. Ann Intern Med 102:109–114, 1985.

Nishimura H, Tachibana H, Makiura N, et al: Corticosteroid-responsive parkinsonism associated with primary Sjogren's syndrome. Clin Neurol Neurosurg 96:327–331, 1994.

Quismorio FP, Friou GJ: Antibodies reactive with neurons in SLE patients with neuropsychiatric manifestations. Int Arch Allergy 43:740–748, 1972.

Sato K, Miyasaka N, Nishioka K, et al: Primary Sjogren's syndrome associated with systemic necrotizing vasculitis: A fatal case. Arthritis Rheum 30:717–718, 1987.

Seibold JR, Buckingham RB, Medsger TA Jr, et al: Cerebrospinal fluid immune complexes in systemic lupus erythematosus involving the central nervous system. Semin Arthritis Rheum 12:68–76, 1982.

Shaw PJ, Walls TJ, Newman PK, et al: Hashimoto's encephalopathy: A steroid responsive disorder associated with high anti-thyroid antibody titers-report of 5 cases. Neurology 41:228–233, 1991.

Shein M, Apter A, Dickerman Z, et al: Encephalopathy in compensated Hashimoto thyroiditis: A clinical expression of autoimmune cerebral vasculitis. Brain Develop 8:60–64, 1986.

Siller KA, Weinreb HJ, Kimmel SC: The treatable dementia of concurrent Klinefelter's and primary Sjogren's syndromes [abstract]. Ann Neurol 38:292, 1995.

Thrush DC, Boddie HG: Episodic encephalopathy associated with thyroid disorders. J Neurol Neurosurg Psychiatry 37:696–700, 1974.

Weaver DF, Heffernan LP, Purdy RA, et al: Eosinophil-induced neurotoxicity: Axonal neuropathy, cerebral infarction, and dementia. Neurology 38:144–146, 1988.

Neurology and Neuropsychology in Oncology

Jeffrey S. Wefel
Todd J. Janus

Brain tumor
Brachytherapy
Chemotherapy
Glioma
Limbic encephalitis
Paraneoplastic syndrome
Progressive multifocal leukoencephalopathy
Radiation-induced hypersomnia
Radiotherapy

INTRODUCTION

Although brain tumors represent a modest 2% of all cancers, their effect on higher-order cognitive functions such as one's ability to learn, reason, and interact with the world make them especially pernicious to patients so afflicted. Because of the structures they affect, the treatments they require, and the potentially devastating effects these therapies can have on patients' productivity and independence, they are among the most costly cancers to both the individual and society (Kleihues et al., 2002). Brain tumor incidence and mortality estimates have been on the rise, with some authors reporting a 300% increase over the past three decades (Wrensch et al., 2000), and others reporting an increasing incidence of about 1% per year. The incidence of primary brain tumors in the United States has been estimated at 29,000 new cases per year. Most primary brain tumors are glial tumors (approximately 50%), with about a quarter representing meningioma. The reason for this increase is under study as the frequent use of and advances in neuroimaging, improvements in diagnostic histology criteria, and increased immunosuppressive states in the general population do not adequately account for the observed increased incidence of primary brain tumors.

The devastating effects cancer can have on the integrity of the central nervous system (CNS) are well known. Yet, even after diagnosis and treatment, most practitioners fail to obtain comprehensive, standardized, objective assessments of patient's cognitive, emotional, and behavioral functioning through a neuropsychological evaluation to help alleviate patient distress (Meyers, 2000). Cognitive dysfunction may begin insidiously, often discernible only in subtle form to the patient or spouse, and thus clinicians may overlook its significance until the behavioral expression of the disease causes obvious impairments (Cull et al., 1996). An awareness of the changes in a patient's overall functioning during the various stages of therapy can be crucial to the effective multidisciplinary care of cancer patients (Alexander et al., 1993). A comprehensive neuropsychological evaluation can inform the health care team about areas of strengths and weaknesses that will improve the quality of patient care, monitor disease progression or recurrence, monitor treatment-related neurotoxicity, assess the impact of disease on the patient's overall quality of life (QOL), aid the patient and family in developing plans for the future, and assist the patient in securing appropriate rehabilitation services. Neuropsychological evaluations can also assess a patient's ability to provide truly informed consent (Jubelirer et al., 1994) and aid in the determination of disability.

The two most common symptoms in patients with primary brain tumors are headache and alterations in mental status (Snyder et al., 1993; Jaeckle, 1997). The neurologic and neuropsychological effects of primary brain tumors are quite variable and may include general signs of cerebral dysfunction such as accompany increased intracranial pressure (e.g., headache, imbalance) as well as focal signs and symptoms secondary to direct compression or infiltration (e.g., memory loss, superior quadrantanopsia). The clinician evaluating the patient must consider a host of etiologic contributors, including (a) the direct effects of the tumor, which may be infiltrative or noninfiltrative; (b) the presence of secondary damage resulting from edema, hemorrhage, infarction, hydrocephalus, increased ICP, or seizure;

(c) treatment-related neurotoxicity; (d) neuroimmune dysfunction; (e) comorbid neurologic disease (e.g., Alzheimer disease); and (f) affective distress. For example, tumors may create a mass effect that distorts the natural architecture of the brain substance, creating neuronal displacement and associated cognitive dysfunction. Alternatively, cognitive dysfunction may result from diffuse tumor infiltrates that project through the brain parenchyma disconnecting and disrupting neuronal pathways or local blood flow. Either of these processes may produce associated neurologic events such as hemorrhage or seizure. The cytotoxic treatments designed to target both the primary cancer and adjuvant therapies such as glucocorticoids used to treat edema may contribute to cognitive dysfunction. Prolonged use of glucocorticoids can produce symptoms and signs of Cushing syndrome, and even short-term use has been reported to result in memory difficulties (Wolkowitz et al., 1990) and psychiatric symptoms including euphoria, mania, insomnia, restlessness, and increased motor activity (Lewis & Smith, 1983). The occurrence of adverse effects associated with neoadjuvant and adjuvant treatments is an area of great interest and importance. However, the process of examining and understanding the relationship between these treatments and cognitive functioning is in its infancy. The potential adverse effects of emotional distress on cognitive functioning and the incidence of comorbid neurologic disease is likely similar for cancer patients and other groups, with or without CNS disease.

Given that the variables involved in assessing and treating an oncologic population are myriad, this chapter summarizes (1) the classification and treatment of CNS tumors; (2) the cognitive and neurologic effects of primary, metastatic, and non-CNS tumors; (3) the effects of therapies frequently used to treat these cancers; (4) strategies for evaluating cognitive, emotional, and behavioral functioning in these patients; and (5) the effectiveness of rehabilitation programs for these patients. This chapter will attempt to summarize the literature in this burgeoning area of research and clinical practice; however, given space limitations, this review is largely focused on the issues and studies conducted in an adult population. Because of the breadth and complexity inherent in many of the topics addressed in this chapter, it is intended that this serve as an introduction to the many facets involved in working with oncologic populations.

CANCER IN THE CENTRAL NERVOUS SYSTEM

Primary Central Nervous System Malignancies

Several interesting epidemiologic observations have been made concerning the relationship between primary malignant brain tumors and ethnicity, geographic location, age, and gender (Wrensch et al., 2000). In general, areas with a high incidence of brain tumors (e.g., United States and northern Europe) in contrast to areas with lower rates (e.g., India and the Philippines) appear to share either ethnic, cultural, or geographic similarities that may be related to their increased risk. Moreover, these differences are not fully accounted for by differences in access to or quality of medical services. The peak incidence for most primary brain tumors is between the ages of 65 and 75 years with the overall average age of diagnosis occurring at age 53 years. One of the most robust epidemiologic observations is of gender differences in the incidence of glioma and meningioma, with men more frequently diagnosed with glioma, whereas meningioma is more frequently observed in women.

No area of brain parenchyma is a protected site from tumor development; however, certain regions of the brain are more commonly affected. In pediatric populations the vast majority (approximately 70%) of tumors arise in the posterior fossa, whereas supratentorial tumors arise with similar frequency (approximately 70%) in adults. Primary brain tumors are often infiltrative and can wreak havoc within the white matter areas. Case reports have posted examples of tumor seemingly crawling down through white matter tracks into the brainstem. The most common primary nervous system tumors include those involving glial cells (termed *gliomas*) and the surrounding leptomeningeal linings (termed *meningiomas*). Histopathologic examination of tumor tissue is almost always necessary to determine the classification (i.e., tumor type) and grade (i.e., malignancy). The World Health Organization (WHO, 1980, 2002) has developed a system to classify and grade all nervous system tumors (Table 38-1; Kleihues et al., 2002). Within the WHO system, grade I tumors are considered more biologically benign, whereas grade IV tumors are more highly malignant. However, CNS tumor are somewhat unique in that even biologically benign tumors may behave in a clinically malignant fashion via infiltrating large areas of brain tissue, causing neurologic and neuropsychological impairment, and occupying areas not amenable to surgical removal secondary to functional anatomic considerations (De Girolami et al., 1994).

Glioma

Gliomas are infiltrative within the brain, often interdigitating within the various structures of the brain and causing either destruction of neural structures, compression of structures, or secretion of cytokines, leading to biochemical changes in function. Thus, the presentation and clinical course of these tumors provide an almost infinite number of problems, ranging from seizures or stroke to subtle behavioral complaints (Fig. 38-1). The symptom pattern upon initial presenta-

TABLE 38-1. Tumors of Neuroepithelial Origin

Astrocytic tumors
  Diffuse astrocytoma
    Fibrillary astrocytoma
    Protoplasmic astrocytoma
  Anaplastic astrocytoma
  Glioblastoma
    Giant cell glioblastoma
    Gliosarcoma
  Pilocytic astrocytoma
  Pleomorphic xanthoastrocytoma
  Subependymal giant cell astrocytoma
Oligodendroglial tumors
  Oligodendroglioma
  Anaplastic oligoastrocytoma
Mixed gliomas
  Oligoastrocytoma
  Anaplastic oligoastrocytoma
Ependymal tumors
  Ependymoma
    Cellular
    Papillary
    Clear cell
    Tanycytic
  Anaplastic ependymoma
  Myxopapillary ependymoma
  Subependymoma

(From Kleihues P, Louis DN, Scheithauer BW, et al: The WHO classification of tumors of the nervous system. Neuropathol Exp Neurol 2002, 61:215–225.)

tion may be difficult to distinguish from other white matter disease such as multiple sclerosis. In fact, early presentations can provide radiographic appearance more consistent with a demyelinating disease. Episodes of deterioration may be ascribed to more events of demyelination. Further radiographic examinations can appear consistent with these impressions and serve to confirm past errors of diagnosis. In one case known to the authors, a patient with a radiographic reading of multiple sclerosis was rejected for surgical evaluation even after several scans revealed continued growth. Only when mass effect became evident was surgical biopsy performed and glioma (specifically, glioblastoma multiforme) diagnosed. Newer imaging modalities will undoubtedly decrease these errors.

The broad category of glioma includes many different tumors that vary widely in both histopathologic appearance and in overall patient survival (Meyers et al., 2000b). Of the astrocytic lineage, which

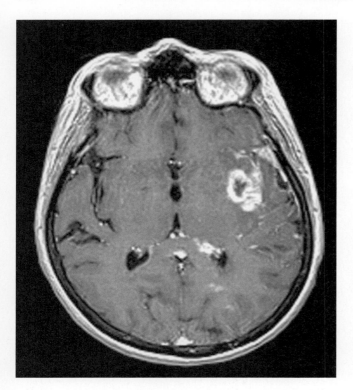

FIGURE 38-1. A 63-year old woman presented with the sudden onset of speech difficulties. Her examination prior to use of steroids demonstrated evidence of an aphasia, finger agnosia, and ideomotor apraxia. She could read numbers but not letters; she could not read numbers that were spelled out. Magnetic resonance imaging with gadolinium infusion revealed multiple lesions in the left hemisphere (*right*). Initially thought to have metastatic disease, biopsy revealed glioblastoma multiforme. Interestingly, her symptoms cleared 24 hours after the administration of high-dose dexamethasone.

TABLE 38-2. Prognostic Factors for Survival in Gliomas

Short duration of symptom
Age less than 40 years
Gross total tumor removal at first surgery
Good performance status
Lower rates of cell division
Oligodendroglioma histology
Received standard radiotherapy
Received chemotherapy

comprises approximately 80% of all gliomas, astrocytomas (low-grade gliomas–grade II) are relatively slow growing and have survival estimates of more than 5 years in younger people. Treatment methods for this tumor are currently debated, with some physicians advocating watchful waiting while others take a more aggressive approach and feel surgical cytoreduction, radiotherapy, or both are indicated. Anaplastic astrocytoma (AA–grade III) and glioblastoma multiforme (GBM–grade IV) are much more aggressive tumors. The primary histopathologic differentiation between GBM and AA includes the presence of tumor necrosis in GBM. Survival estimates for patients with these tumors are usually 3 years and 1 year, respectively. Overall indicators of prognosis for patients with astrocytic tumors are listed in Table 38-2.

The diagnostic criteria of gliomas continue to be one of the most difficult areas of neuro-oncology. As additional genetic and cellular function data are uncovered about the biologic behavior and cellular markers of these tumors, the diagnostic criteria continue to change. The wide use of stereotactic biopsy results in very small tissue samples. These small samples are difficult to examine and may not be representative of the overall histology of the tumor, leading to misdiagnosis or incomplete diagnosis. Finally, histologic interpretation does not necessarily predict biologic behavior in the individual patient. For example, due to new diagnostic pathology categories, tumors once thought to be astrocytomas are now being recategorized and more often newly diagnosed as oligodendrogliomas. Oligodendrogliomas (approximately 5%–15% of gliomas) are derived from the oligodendrocyte, which provides myelin sheathing around neurons within the brain. As a result of this pathologic reclassification, these tumors are becoming more commonly identified, and clinicians are reanalyzing previous survival data to determine whether recent changes in survival estimates in published treatment trials may be caused by contamination of treatment subgroups with heterogeneous pathologic diagnostic sets. Interestingly, oligodendrogliomas are usually diagnosed earlier (owing to a tendency to elicit seizures), are much more amenable to treatment (especially certain chemotherapies), and are associated with longer survival times. Because of their sensitivity to chemotherapeutic intervention and the discovery that this sensitivity is mediated by certain tumor-associated genetic alterations, molecular genetic assessments may become standard diagnostic procedures to help guide treatment selection and anticipate clinical course.

Before the initiation of primary (e.g., surgery) and adjuvant (e.g., radiation, chemotherapy) treatments, cognitive dysfunction tends to correspond to the site of the tumor (Salander et al., 1995). In general, cognitive dysfunction secondary to the tumor itself generally adheres to the principles of brain-behavior relationship that have been more commonly defined on the basis of other pathologic subgroups such as stroke. For example, left hemisphere tumors often produce greater impairments in verbal memory and language abilities, while right-sided lesions are more often associated with visuoconstructive deficits (Meyers, 1986; Tucha et al., 2000). However, Anderson and colleagues (1990) matched tumor patients to stroke patients according to lesion size and location to evaluate the nature and severity of the cognitive and behavioral dysfunction. They found that tumor patients exhibited greater variability in their cognitive functioning and, in general, demonstrated milder cognitive dysfunction than their counterparts with stroke, perhaps owing to differences in the pathophysiology of tumor (i.e., tissue displacement and disconnection via infiltration) and stroke (i.e., tissue destruction).

Recently, efforts have been made to obtain routine preoperative evaluations to document patient problems prior to surgical debulking, which has afforded the opportunity to disentangle the cognitive dysfunction as a result of the tumor itself from that caused by subsequent therapies (e.g., surgery, radiation, and chemotherapy). Preoperative evaluations can also be used to assess overall patient outcome after surgery, which often demonstrates improvements, possibly resulting from removal of mass effects or the cleansing of the brain from untoward cytokines being expressed by the tumor into the brain substance. If persistent problems are confirmed after surgery, further supportive interventions can be planned along with therapies directed towards the tumor. Tucha and colleagues (2000) demonstrated the importance of obtaining a presurgical neuropsychological evaluation for comparison against postsurgical performance results to determine the effects of surgical intervention. They reported on a sample of 139 patients admitted consecutively for neurosurgical management with a primary or metastatic tumor located in either the frontal or temporal lobes who received a presurgical neuropsychological and neurologic assessment. They found that approximately 40% of their sample demonstrated cognitive neurologic deficit before surgery. However, based on neuropsychological assessment, a far greater proportion performed in the impaired range (i.e., less than the 10th percentile based on available normative data) on a variety of cognitive measures. Approximately 78% of these patients showed deficits in executive functioning, 64% exhibited deficits in memory functions, 60% evidenced attentional dysfunction, 50% manifested visuoconstructive disturbance, and 22% displayed language abnormalities. Without this baseline evaluation, the effects of surgery cannot be adequately assessed and postsurgical cognitive dysfunction may be inaccurately assumed to be a consequence of neurosurgical intervention.

Meningioma

Meningiomas are extra-axial tumors of the dura covering surrounding the brain and spinal cord. While considered benign (except for an aggressive anaplastic histologic form that invades the cortex; Fig. 38-2) they can grow to large volumes within the cranial cavity, thereby compressing neural contents and leading to subtle gradual neurocognitive defects. The neurocogni-

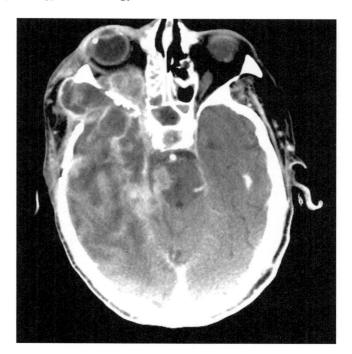

FIGURE 38-2. A 78-year-old man presented initially with a small meningioma of the sphenoid wing. Two years later he was readmitted to the hospital with left-sided weakness and multiple cranial neuropathies. Computed tomography scan of the brain revealed a recurrence of the meningioma in the right face (*left* in the figure) with destruction of the facial bones and encroachment of the left temporal area and brainstem.

tive effects of meningiomas have not been widely studied. The type of cognitive dysfunction is largely dependent on the location. For example, parasagittal or olfactory groove lesions can cause anosmia, dementia, and visual disturbance (Bakay, 1984), whereas meningiomas located over the lateral convexity of the dominant hemisphere can lead to speech abnormalities. Case reports usually identify unusual presenting circumstances or describe the amelioration of symptoms after definitive therapy. These reports range from ascribed cases of pedophilia, depression, panic disorders, or schizophrenia to speech and memory loss. Cognitive dysfunction seems to be more prevalent in convexity tumors, especially tumors located frontally, and in cases receiving radiation therapy (XRT). Most reports "prove" the symptoms were related to the meningioma, because the problems abated after surgical extirpation. Occasionally, reports will try to associate the presence of undiscovered meningiomas in a prison population and attempt to associate the criminality to the presence of the tumor. Usually, these reports only support the conclusion that the presence of meningiomas in the prison population is typical of known societal averages for meningiomas in the general population.

Because of the slow-growing nature of these tumors, patients can often be misdiagnosed with a dementing illness or depression. This can usually be solved by magnetic resonance imaging (MRI) imaging that, while not histologically diagnostic, can demonstrate a "dural tail" that strongly suggests the diagnosis. Companion computed tomography (CT) will often demonstrate hyperostosis of the surrounding bone. Metastatic disease and reactive inflammatory conditions must be ruled out. Differentiation of rare malignant forms from benign forms requires surgical intervention. Depending on location, meningiomas can be completely removed surgically, leading to a virtual cure. Occasionally, only partial removal is possible, such as with sphenoid ridge meningiomas. Follow-up imaging over several years will confirm complete removal or recurrence. The primary decision in the management of these tumors is whether the tumor is the cause of the behavioral or cognitive disturbance and whether operative intervention should be undertaken. Often meningiomas are identified incidentally during imaging for another reason. For those tumors that are inoperable for medical reasons or due to their location, brachytherapy (use of radioactive seed implants) or focused beamed radiotherapy may be feasible. However, radiation damage to the surrounding areas and the resultant diminution of cognitive status over time must be taken into account before proceeding.

Primary Central Nervous System Lymphoma

Primary CNS lymphoma (PCNSL) is a non-Hodgkin variant with presence of lymphoma only in the central nervous system. Since the brain has no lymphatics, how this happens is not yet explained. Perhaps the lymphoma was, in fact, present in other areas of the body but was not found during the routine evaluation of the patient. In about 20% of patients, lymphoma outside the CNS is eventually seen. The diagnosis of PCNSL has increased three- to fivefold during the last 20 years. It is seen more often in men aged 20–64 years owing to the prevalence of HIV infection in this population. While the tumor is commonly associated with immunodeficient states such as that of acquired immune deficiency syndrome (AIDS), organ transplant recipients receiving immunosuppressive therapy, and other genetic immune deficiency states, the rise in cases in the nonimmunosuppressed and in the elderly (over 65 years of age) remains unexplained. In the early 1990s it appeared that the number of cases of PCNSL may exceed that of cases of gliomas, but recently this has been disputed (Kadan-Lottick, et al., 2002).

PCNSL is primarily treated with chemotherapy followed by craniospinal radiotherapy. Intrathecal and systemic therapies with steroids and methotrexate provide the best treatment response in terms of survival time. However, the neurotoxicity associated with these treatments is beginning to be appreciated, producing a difficult clinical decision point. For example, when a reduced fractionated dose of XRT (30 Gy vs. 45 Gy) is used for patients younger than 65 years of age, the overall survival is reduced and the number of patients with disease recurrence appears to be increased, while in those older than 65, cognitive dysfunction and a decrease in overall survival was associated with administration of any dose of radiotherapy (Bessell et al., 2002). Because the number of cases seen per year in the United States is usually less than 700, close study of the neurobehavioral side effects of treatment is difficult. However, both methotrexate and XRT can be neurotoxic individually, and the risk of cognitive dysfunction appears to increase with combined use. The neuropsychologist should be involved as soon as possible in the care of these patients because of the increased incidence of cognitive dysfunction (O'Neill et al., 1999).

NONPRIMARY CENTRAL NERVOUS SYSTEM MALIGNANCIES

Metastatic Malignancies

Metastatic lesions usually result from breast, lung, skin, colon, or renal cell cancers (Schouten et al., 2002). The presence of these tumors in the brain is announced similarly to the symptoms of presentation for primary tumors. However, metastatic lesions commonly present with multiple sites of spread within the brain. Cognitive difficulties can play a role in the initial presentation of these new metastases but prior therapies can also cause dysfunction, including use of prophylactic cranial irradiation (PCI) or systemic chemotherapy (Ahles & Saykin, 2001), thus making attributions about the etiology of cognitive dysfunction difficult. Typically, the area of the lesion will govern the type and severity of cortical impairments. Because these lesions tend to be more expansive, occur in multiple sites, and are less infiltrative than gliomas, disruptions of normal function can occur earlier in the disease course. The noninfiltrative nature of these metastatic tumors also seems to relate to less overall cognitive morbidity in these individuals, because the brain is essentially pushed out of the way as opposed to being destroyed.

Paraneoplastic Syndromes

Paraneoplastic syndromes represent the remote, immune-mediated effects of cancer. Occasionally some cancers will generate an immune response whereby the body directs antibody recognition of the tumor. These antibody recognition sites may be duplicated on normal body cells, especially within the CNS. In turn, this immune response can, unfortunately, recognize key normal physiologic structures. Thus, similar to other neuroimmune diseases, antibodies will be directed towards key brain substrates and lead to neurologic disability. Usually, one area of the brain is predominately affected (such as the cerebellum, limbic, or brainstem areas). In approximately 15% of patients these immune responses predate the discovery of tumor. Even after a careful search for an underlying malignancy, one may not be discovered for many months. Recently, functional imaging (e.g., positron emission tomography [PET]) has been found to help in this diagnostic conundrum.

The most common paraneoplastic syndrome that affects cognition is termed *paraneoplastic limbic encephalitis* (PLE). The majority of patients with PLE are men, more than 60 years of age, and with a diagnosis of small cell carcinoma of the lung. Pathologic studies of brain tissue removed from affected patients have found inflammatory response and neuronal loss. The presence of these histologic changes in various areas of the brain portends a more dramatic and worse outcome. MRI may reveal significant changes on T2-weighted imaging, especially in the mesial temporal lobe. However, case reports have described normal structural imaging findings (i.e., MRI) with abnormal functional imaging findings (i.e. hexamethyl propylene amine oxime single photon emissions computerized tomography [HMPAO SPECT]), and have associated this with better prognosis for recovery after treatment (Bak et al., 2001). Examination of the cerebrospinal fluid (CSF) will show a pleocytosis and an elevated protein with oligoclonal bands. Clinical laboratory testing is commonly used to aid in clinical decision making when a paraneoplastic syndrome is suspected. Antibody studies often show the presence of an antineuronal antibody, anti-Hu, with an epitope directed towards neuronal cells. However, positive antibody findings are not necessary for diagnosis. In fact, preliminary evidence suggests that greater recovery after treatment may be achieved in cases where symptomatic presentation of PLE related to small cell lung cancer occurs with negative anti-Hu antibodies compared to positive antibody findings (Bak et al., 2001). Careful study may also uncover other areas of the nervous system affected, including a sensory neuronopathy.

Symptoms of PLE include anterograde amnesia, although case reports have found evidence of more profound retrograde amnesia in patients with widespread neuronal dysfunction. Patients frequently exhibit psychiatric abnormalities (including hallucination, confusion, agitation), seizures (often complex partial), brainstem abnormalities such as diplopia, and hypothalamic dysregulation (hypersomnia, thermodysregulation, etc.). Symptom onset is usually rapid, developing over a period of weeks to months and in over 10% of patients symptoms of PLE predate a substantiated cancer diagnosis. There is no consensus on the frequency or degree of recovery after treatment of a para-neoplastic syndrome, but there is some evidence that recovery is inversely related to the extent of cortical involvement, degree of retrograde amnesia, and absence of structural abnormalities (Bak et al., 2001).

Leptomeningeal Disease

Leptomeningeal carcinomatosis (or neoplastic meningitis) results from the spread of tumor cells into the area lining and surrounding the brain. This spread occurs either by hematogenous seeding or by direct extension from nearby tumor growths. Seen in approximately 5% of patients with cancer, it most commonly occurs late in the disease of patients with either breast or lung cancer or melanoma. Diagnosis is usually made by the finding of malignant cells in the CSF; malignant cells can be absent in up to 10% of cases. Along with the free-floating tumor cells in the CSF, small nests or nodules of tumor cells are found adherent to nerves within the sack of leptomeninges.

The symptomatic presentation of neoplastic meningitis can range from confusion and memory loss to encephalopathy, although more commonly, cranial or spinal neuropathies are seen, including leg weakness and a loss of bowel or bladder control. Treatments include radiotherapy often combined with intrathecal chemotherapy with Ara-C or methotrexate. Survival ranges from weeks for those declining treatment to months for those aggressively treated. Occasionally, patients will live long enough to experience a leukoencephalopathy from the combined treatments. One of the authors has observed a profound and catastrophic necrotizing leukoencephalopathy resulting from radiotherapy given while methotrexate concentrations in the CSF were exceedingly high.

Progressive Multifocal Leukoencephalopathy

Progressive multifocal leukoencephalopathy (PML) is caused by the JC virus, a human polyomavirus, which becomes activated from its quiescent state within the brain following immunosuppressive therapy. While approximately 80% of all individuals have detectable antibodies to the virus, it usually persists in the kidney and is reactivated after a deficiency in either the cellular or humoral-mediated immune response. Presentation includes cognitive decline usually with focal findings corresponding to the areas of leukoencephalopathy. PML can be confused with disease progression, radiation dementia, or a demyelinating disease such as multiple sclerosis. MRI studies typically reveal patchy white matter lesions, and accurate diagnosis must often be made by brain biopsy and polymerase chain reaction determination from samples of CSF. Although treatment with antiviral agents such as acyclovir is common, prognosis is poor.

COMMON TREATMENT MODALITIES

Surgery

Surgical removal or cytoreduction of neoplasm is often a necessary and optimal treatment to prevent the spread of cancerous processes. Tumor size at diagnosis has not been conclusively demonstrated to play a role in overall survival. However, surgical data suggest that a resection of more than 90% of the tumor evident on radiologic imaging does provide benefit for patients with glioblastoma but less so for less aggressive tumor pathologies (astrocytoma, oligodendroglioma, etc.). In many cases a gross total resection is not possible due to the anatomic location of the lesion. Large resections may remove functioning brain tissue, thus contributing to increased incidence of postoperative cognitive deficit. The use of neuroimaging to confirm removal of tumor is currently the gold standard; however, this is not without potential shortcomings. For example, several studies have found histologic presence of tumor within stereotactic biopsies taken from normal areas of brain that are outside regions of radiographic abnormality. Therefore, specific correlation of known radiologic defects to tissue abnormalities remains problematic and suspect. Procedures using intraoperative cortical mapping and presurgical functional magnetic resonance imaging (fMRI) are being developed and actively investigated to help neurosurgeons delineate the borders between functional brain tissue and tissue that may be resected with a decreased likelihood of consequent cognitive dysfunction.

Few studies have been reported in the literature examining the effects of surgical extirpation of neoplasm on patient's cognitive and emotional functioning. In one of the few methodologically rigorous studies (i.e., studies that included a presurgical baseline neuropsychological assessment) in the neurosurgical literature examining the postsurgical effects of surgery on cognitive functioning, Giorgi and Riva (1994) assessed six pediatric patients before and after stereotactically guided transfrontal surgery for midline intraventricular tumors. The results of their study demonstrated improved neuropsychological function in all of their subjects at 6 months after surgery. Similar investigations with larger samples and longer follow-up periods are necessary to confirm these preliminary findings. Investigations of this nature need to be conducted in the adult population where neural development is complete and the potential for functional reorganization is less pronounced.

Recent work has examined the effect of surgery on overall cognition and QOL in patients with resection for glioma (Klein et al., 2001). When patients with glioma were compared with patients with non–small cell lung cancer (NSCLC) without brain metastases, both groups reported lower QOL than healthy controls. Relative to NSCLC, glioma patients reported greater difficulty with social functioning, visual and motor problems, communication difficulties, headaches, and seizures. Patients with glioma, in comparison with their NSCLC counterparts, were found to exhibit more frequent (100% vs. 52%, respectively) neuropsychological impairment when both groups were compared with healthy controls. When just the two groups with malignancies were compared, glioma patients evidenced greater cognitive deficits in the areas of perception, memory, attention, and executive function. Tumor lateralization affected neuropsychological test performance in the expected fashion, whereas lesion location was not related to QOL.

Radiation Therapy

The use of radiotherapy in the treatment of CNS cancers (whether primary or metastatic) is ubiquitous (Abayomi, 1996). Radiotherapy has well-established palliative and curative efficacy as a primary and adjuvant treatment for primary and secondary brain cancers (Walker et al., 1997), and prophylactic radiotherapy has support for prevention of metastatic disease (Yang & Mathews, 2000). However, there remains considerable debate concerning the relative risks and benefits of radiotherapy, especially in populations such as patients with low-grade glioma (LGG) or small cell lung cancer (SCLC), due to the controversial findings of increased cognitive dysfunction and decreased QOL secondary to radiotherapy (Regime et al., 2001). Radiotherapy given to tumor areas will also affect normal areas of brain that will be present within the field of radiation. Although the tumor, because of its malignant phenotype, can withstand larger doses of irradiation, normal brain is more at risk for damage.

Clinically, XRT can take many forms, including whole brain radiotherapy, partial brain fractionated radiotherapy, stereotactic radiosurgery ("gamma knife"), and implant XRT (brachytherapy). Whole brain radiotherapy is often used prophylactically to bathe the entire neuroaxis in low doses of radiotherapy to attempt to sterilize the brain of any micrometastatic disease that is clinically undetectable or to treat diffusely present metastatic disease. Partial brain radiotherapy is often used to shrink the size of an intracerebral tumor and prevent it from spreading into neighboring tissue. This requires therapeutic doses of radiotherapy to be directed at the tumor bed with decreasing doses of radiotherapy extending outward from the tumor center in a ringlike fashion often several centimeters outside the tumor margins seen on neuroimaging study.

Stereotactic radiosurgery, or gamma knife surgery, is used most frequently with small tumors that are responsive to high-dose radiotherapy. This procedure has the distinct advantage of providing a concentrated dose of radiotherapy to the neoplasm while sparing neighboring tissue. This is achieved by using multiple beams of radiotherapy that enter the cranial vault from different locations, each carrying a low-dose beam of radiation to the primary tumor site that has been mapped via MRI. These beams reach a confluence at the site of the tumor and additively create a large dose of focused radiotherapy to the tumor with little high-dose exposure to the surrounding tissue. Brachytherapy involves the installation of highly radioactive seeds into the brain where the tumor resides and is often used after conventional external beam radiotherapy. The dosage of radiotherapy, measured in Gy (i.e., the amount of energy absorbed—measured as 1 joule of energy absorbed per kilogram of tissue), is partially determined by the histology of the tumor, tumor response (often measured with serial MRI), as well as the number of fractions delivered (i.e., the number of treatments) and patient tolerance of treatment.

The development of neurologic and/or neuropsychological dysfunction is often the greatest dose-limiting factor of radiotherapy (Taylor et al., 1998). Distinguishing neurotoxicity secondary to treatment effects from disease recurrence is critical to providing rapid and appropriate interventions. The occurrence of radiation encephalopathy (Crossen et al., 1994) has been separated into three stages: acute reaction, early delayed reaction, and late delayed reaction (Sheline et al., 1980). Pathologically, autopsy reports have suggested that radiotherapy primarily affects the white matter tracts and cerebral vasculature of the brain via two mechanisms: (1) damaging oligodendrocytes—thereby creating axonal demyelination; and (2) disrupting vascular endothelial cells contributing to coagulative necrosis, vessel wall thickening, and focal mineralization (O'Connor & Mayberg, 2000; Steen et al., 2001). Thus, white matter lesions are more prevalent in follow-up radiologic studies of the brain in patients with cancer; and because of the relative weight of white matter in the frontal and subcortical areas, cognitive impairments consistent with frontal-subcortical dysfunction are common (e.g., executive function [EF] deficits and attentional difficulties).

Acutely affected patients are often asymptomatic or may experience very mild reactions (e.g., hypersomnolence, irritability, decreased appetite), possibly secondary to edema that causes little neurotoxicity. The occurrence of early radiation-induced encephalopathy is now well accepted, although precise estimates of its frequency are still lacking. At this time, it is believed that the early effects of radiotherapy, including nausea and vomiting, lethargy, malaise, alopecia, tinnitus, and dermatologic changes, will usually resolve within the first 2 to 5 months after treatment and are amenable to corticosteroid therapy. A number of cognitive deficits have been found that parallel these changes in physical function. The more methodologically rigorous studies (e.g., those that include a pretreatment baseline assessment

and use sensitive neuropsychological measures of cognitive function) have reported impairments in information processing speed, EF, memory, and motor deficits after radiotherapy (Armstrong et al., 1993, 1995, 2000; Crosson et al., 1994; Vigliani et al., 1996). Pathologically, it appears the observed symptoms represent the effects of demyelinization and remyelinization secondary to radiation damage. Longitudinal studies have demonstrated that the majority of patients experience a "rebound effect" or normalization of their cognitive functioning within approximately 1 year after radiotherapy.

Examination of cognitive functioning in patients surviving more than a year after radiotherapy has yielded conflicting results. A number of studies have failed to find significant late delayed cognitive dysfunction as a result of radiotherapy (Taphoorn et al., 1994; Vigliani et al., 1996; Glosser et al., 1997; Armstrong et al., 2002). Differences in reported radiotherapy-associated cognitive dysfunction (incidence estimates that vary from 0%–86%), may in part be related to the type of radiotherapy administered, the dosage administered (Regine et al., 2001), its use independently or in combination with other treatments (e.g., chemotherapy), the timing of postradiotherapy cognitive testing (i.e., measurement of acute effects vs. late-delayed effects), and the type of cognitive assessment used (e.g., clinician reports or simple mental status exam vs. comprehensive neuropsychological evaluation). In many cases, these studies combine a group of patients with different histologic tumor types, different types of radiotherapy administered, and in some cases, only "radiographic" diagnosis of tumor histology (Armstrong et al., 2002).

For some individuals it appears that there is reason to be concerned about late emerging pathophysiologic dysfunction and the accompanying cognitive decline (Gregor et al., 1996). The late delayed neurologic sequelae of radiotherapy include cranial neuropathies, hormonal disturbance, demyelination, calcification, brain necrosis in the irradiated fields leading to leukoencephalopathy, and even development of tumors or death (Sheline et al., 1980; Martins et al., 1997). Leukoencephalopathy, which is more common in younger patients, begins with increasing confusion and disorientation, memory decline, and later a profound dementia. Personality changes may also be evident. Neuroradiologic imaging reveals changes in the white matter and occasionally a mineralizing microangiopathy (especially in the basal ganglia). These neuropathologic alterations in brain tissue emerge within 6 to 24 months after radiotherapy.

For many brain tumor patients, especially those with low-grade gliomas, among whom approximately 50% will survive for 5 or more years with no signs of tumor progression (North et al., 1990), there is considerable interest in the potential late delayed effects of radiotherapy on cognitive function. For these patients even mild neuropsychological dysfunction can significantly impair their functional status (i.e., ability to work and live independently), emotional function, and QOL. Thus, an understanding of the incidence, severity, and predictors of cognitive dysfunction secondary to radiotherapy is of critical importance in determining the risk-benefit ratio for clinical decision making and in developing novel secondary interventions to either prevent or reduce the impact of these iatrogenic effects (e.g., the development of radiation-sensitizing agents that allow for a smaller dose of radiotherapy to be delivered with similar therapeutic efficacy). This knowledge would also be of great value to patients in assisting them in making plans for the future, developing constructive coping strategies, and seeking appropriate rehabilitation services. As mentioned previously, in evaluating and predicting radiation-induced cognitive decline one must attend to several treatment and assessment variables including the type of radiotherapy administered, dosage (particularly the dose per fraction), its use independently or in combination with other treatments, the timing of postradiotherapy testing, and the sensitivity of the cognitive measures used. Unfortunately, few methodologically rigorous studies to date have been reported in the adult literature on the potential late emerging cognitive deficits in patients who received radiotherapy.

Surma-aho and colleagues (2001) found that LGG patients who were tested on average 7 years after radiotherapy (68% received on average 40-Gy whole brain XRT in 30–33 fractions with a 28-Gy boost to the tumor bed, and 32% received on average 60-Gy partial brain XRT in 28–34 fractions) demonstrated worse memory, motor speed, and visuoconstruction compared with a similar group of subjects who did not receive adjuvant treatment with radiotherapy. Relevant to the interpretation of these findings, 16 of 28 patients who received XRT had tumors located in the right hemisphere and 19 of 28 had tumors located in the anterior aspect of the brain. Patients who received radiotherapy were more likely to manifest signs of leukoencephalopathy on MRI study in the irradiated hemisphere. However, this study failed to include a pre-XRT assessment of cognitive functioning, which would ensure that the observed group differences were caused by the effects of the treatment and were not present before initiation of these therapies.

Meyers and colleagues (2000a) examined a sample of patients with skull base tumors after paranasal sinus radiotherapy (on average 60 Gy, no description of fractionation was provided) to determine the frequency, pattern, and causative factors of late emerging adverse effects (on average 73 months after treatment) of "incidental" radiotherapy on cognitive function. Relative to published normative data, more

than 50% of their sample demonstrated impairments (i.e., performance 1.5 standard deviations or more below the mean) in learning efficiency, 80% showed rapid forgetting of information over time, and approximately one third of the patients demonstrated impairments of visual-motor speed, EF and motor function in the context of preserved general intellectual functioning. A contrast sample of patients with similar disease characteristics assessed before radiotherapy generally performed better than the treated group; however, several patients did perform in the impaired range, demonstrating the importance of obtaining pretreatment baseline evaluations. Examination of treatment and demographic variables found that only the total dose of radiotherapy and the time since treatment were related to the development of cognitive dysfunction, whereas volume of brain irradiated, lateralization of radiation boost, and pretreatment chemotherapy were not associated with symptom development.

The importance of obtaining a pretreatment baseline measurement of cognitive functioning when attempting to characterize the adverse effects of a treatment is further underscored by the results of two studies (Komaki et al., 1995; Meyers et al., 1995) investigating the possible adverse cognitive effects related to SCLC and antineoplastic therapies in a population of patients with no apparent CNS involvement. The use of whole brain prophylactic cranial irradiation (PCI) in patients with newly diagnosed SCLC without radiographic evidence of disease in the brain remains controversial. It is believed that by providing a global radiation dose of 30 Gy to the whole brain the neuroaxis will be sterilized of micro-metastatic disease that is present but clinically undetectable. Advocates state that this practice improves survival for patients receiving the treatments, although no large longitudinal studies have been performed. Others, however, argue that radiation will be given to a brain without disease resulting in no clinical benefit in terms of disease management and an increased risk of iatrogenically induced neurocognitive decline (Cull et al., 1994). Komaki and colleagues (1995) found that after treatment with PCI and chemotherapy, 95% of SCLC patients manifested cognitive dysfunction in the areas of memory and EF. However, a similar proportion of this sample exhibited similar impairments prior to PCI, suggesting that PCI was not the sole etiologic contributor to cognitive dysfunction, at least early after treatment (approximately 6 to 20 months post-PCI). Meyers and colleagues (1995) examined the effects of chemoradiation (i.e., cisplatin, ifosfamide, and etoposide with twice-daily radiation to the chest) in this population by assessing patients either before or after chemoradiation and before PCI. Approximately 70% to 80% of the SCLC patients had memory deficits, 38% had deficits in EF, and 33% had impaired motor coordination both before and after chemotherapy and before PCI, suggesting that the observed cognitive dysfunction initially may be related to the effects of a paraneoplastic syndrome rather than *any* treatment modality.

In general, studies examining the effects of radiotherapy on cognitive functioning suffer from a lack of a prospective design. These studies need to (1) include a pretreatment baseline measure of cognitive function; (2) use a broad and sensitive battery of neuropsychological measures that assess cognitive function, emotional function, and QOL; (3) use a homogeneous population of cancer patients who have received similar treatment; (4) use appropriately timed assessments; (5) include appropriate controls; (6) have adequate sample sizes; and (7) follow patients long enough to accurately determine the potential late emerging effects of radiotherapy. Despite the limitations of the studies published so far and the inconsistent findings of these studies, it is clear that the potential for both early and late emerging cognitive dysfunction exists. Finally, there is an urgent need for integration of neuropsychological services and research within the radiotherapy community.

Chemotherapy

Chemotherapeutic regimens are frequently employed to treat a variety of systemic and CNS malignancies. Although a plethora of reports describe therapeutic gains achieved in a variety of malignancies secondary to the use of chemotherapies, it has been known for many years that these treatments may have adverse effects on the nervous system (Weiss et al., 1974; Keime-Guibert et al., 1998; Lipp, 1999; Fortin et al., 2001). Cognitive changes related to chemotherapy in CNS malignancies have been less well studied secondary to treatment schedules that generally administer chemotherapy after radiation—thereby confounding assessment of the unique effects of chemotherapy on cognitive functioning, the lack of prospective research designs, and limited patient survival in many cases. However, chemotherapy is considered a primary treatment for many cancers outside the CNS when any active disease is detected, which has allowed for study of the unique effects of several agents upon the CNS. A variety of nonspecific neurologic complications associated with chemotherapy have been described. These include (1) an acute encephalopathy characterized by insomnia, confusional state, and often agitation; (2) stroke-like episodes associated with transient motor impairments; (3) chronic encephalopathy characterized by cognitive dysfunction consistent with a "subcortical dementia," incontinence, and gait disturbance; (4) a cerebellar syndrome with symptoms ranging from ataxia to a pancerebellar syndrome; and (5) a variety of peripheral neuropathies (Keime-Guibert et al., 1998, Brezden et al., 2000). The nature and incidence of chemotherapy-induced neuro-

toxicity appears to depend on several important therapeutic variables including the type of chemotherapy, the dosage, the route of administration, administration with other treatments (e.g., radiation), and timing of follow-up studies to assess neurotoxicity (Foster & McLellan, 2000).

As a general rule of thumb, neurotoxicity develops in a dose-related manner for most if not all chemotherapeutic agents, and, because the cortex is bathed in chemotherapy agents, most problems related to these treatments are diffuse rather than focal. For example, paclitaxel (Taxol) when administered in standard doses (<175 mg/m^2) is not thought to cross the bloodbrain barrier and therefore is not believed to be associated with CNS neurotoxicity. However, a recent report (Nieto et al., 1999) described the acute effects of high-dose paclitaxel (>600mg/m^2) with autologous stem cell support administered independently or following whole brain radiation or in combination with cyclophosphamide and cisplatin, or with cyclophosphamide, cisplatin, and carmustine (BCNU). Patients included in this study were heterogeneous in terms of their malignancy, CNS involvement, and treatment history. CNS neurotoxicity occurred in approximately 5% of patients (6/114 patients) and included rapid obtundation and coma (5/6 patients), severe confusion with paranoid ideation (1/6 patients), and death (3/6 patients) within 7 to 23 days after treatment. The authors concluded that, although both radiation and BCNU may have contributed to the observed neurotoxicity, the nature and course of paclitaxel neurotoxicity appears distinct from that reported in the literature for these other treatments alone. Several patients who received paclitaxel alone also experienced a neurotoxic reaction. It is also plausible that bone marrow transplantation itself may have contributed to the observed neurotoxicity in some of these patients (Meyers et al., 1994).

Several studies have attempted to examine the relationship between cognitive function and adjuvant chemotherapy in women with non-CNS cancer (Wienke and Dienst, 1995; van Dam et al., 1998; Schagen et al., 1999; Brezden et al., 2000;). Use of a patient group without CNS involvement has allowed for more rigorous assessment of neurotoxicity due to chemotherapy independent of CNS disease. Each of these studies examined the cognitive effects of standard or high-dose chemotherapeutic regimens (e.g., FAC: cyclophosphamide, doxyrubicin, 5-fluororacil; CMF: cyclophosphamide, methotrexate, 5-fluororacil) in women with breast cancer and concluded that there is significant cognitive impairment associated with chemotherapy. However, methodological limitations (e.g., cross-sectional designs, definitions of "impairment") necessitate cautious interpretation of these conclusions.

Perhaps the most exhaustively studied chemotherapy in terms of its effects on cognitive function is methotrexate (MTX). However, most of this work has been pioneered in the pediatric literature where reports of acute fine motor and perceptual motor disturbance coupled with long-term deficits in intelligence, achievement (math greater than reading), attention, and memory (nonverbal greater than verbal) are frequent long-term sequelae of intrathecal MTX (Moleski, 2000, Riva et al., 2002). In adults, MTX has become a standard component of most treatments for PCNSL (DeAngelis, 1999; Schlegel et al., 1999). MTX has been described as producing a triphasic pattern of neurotoxicity including acute, subacute, and late/chronic effects (Lipp, 1999). Within 24 hours of treatment patients may develop a self-limited (approximately 2 to 3 days) acute neurotoxicity consisting of nausea, emesis, fever, headaches, somnolence, confusion, speech disorder, hemiparesis, seizures, and a stroke-like syndrome (that is frequently reversible) if larger doses are administered. Approximately 1 week after treatment, subacute neurotoxicity develops, possibly secondary to hyperhomocysteinemia and includes affective disturbance, focal neurologic signs, transient paresis, and pseudobulbar palsy. Symptoms of late or chronic neurotoxicity are more likely if administration is intrathecal (IT), intraventricular (IVA), high-dose intravenous (IV), concurrent or subsequent to XRT, or combines more than one modality (i.e., IT MTX and XRT, or IV and IT MTX). Within months cognitive dysfunction, focal seizures, spasticity, ataxia, alterations in consciousness, and personality changes develop. MTX administered concurrent or subsequent to XRT increases the risk of developing a delayed leukoencephalopathy (a year or more later) and resultant dementia. Increased age appears to be another important risk factor in developing a delayed necrotizing leukoencephalopathy. Explanations for the synergistic effect of MTX and XRT are lacking but include potential radiosensitizing properties of MTX and perturbation of the blood-brain barrier via XRT, thereby permitting increased toxicity (Keime-Guibert et al., 1998).

Despite limited research and a variety of methodological limitations, there appears enough evidence that cognitive dysfunction is a potential neurotoxic sequelae of a variety of chemotherapeutic agents to warrant further investigation of these phenomena using more rigorous research designs. As with XRT, future investigations need to incorporate prospective designs; use a broad and sensitive battery of neuropsychological measures; examine homogeneous treatment schedules and a homogeneous population of cancer patients; include appropriate controls; have adequate sample sizes; and follow patients long enough to accurately determine the potential late-emerging effects. Neuropsychological evaluations can contribute important and unique information in clinical trials of new anticancer medications as well as during pharmacologic development of chemoprotective agents.

Biologic/Immunologic Therapy

Use of immunomodulatory therapies such as cytokines (e.g., interleukin-2 [IL-2]; interferon-alpha [IFN-α]) is increasing and has shown promise in treating malignancies (e.g., leukemias), viral infections (e.g., human immunodeficiency virus [HIV]), and neurodegenerative diseases (e.g., multiple sclerosis). The occurrence of treatment-limiting neurotoxicity has been problematic, and our current understanding of the associated cognitive and neuropsychiatric morbidity is limited (Pavol et al., 1995; Valentine et al., 1998, Meyers, 1999b; Lerner et al., 1999; Valentine & Meyers, 2001). It is well known that malignancies can cause increased production of proinflammatory cytokines such as tumor necrosis factor (TNF), interleukin-6 (IL-6), interleukin-1 (IL-1) and IL-2 (Hickie & Lloyd, 1995; Walker et al., 1997). Moreover, Maes and colleagues (1999) have demonstrated that individuals who exhibit increased stress-induced anxiety and depression in the context of a psychological stressor (e.g., academic examination stress) show increased production of the proinflammatory cytokines IFN-γ, IL-6, TNF, and a relatively smaller increase in the anti-inflammatory cytokine IL-10. In contrast, individuals who did not display stress-induced anxiety and depression were best characterized by the opposite pattern: higher anti-inflammatory cytokine activity relative to proinflammatory cytokine activity. Thus, there appear to be multiple causal pathways for increased cytokine activity and potential neurotoxicity.

Cytokines are peptides (i.e., proteins) secreted by a variety of nucleated cells in the human body that manifest their physiological effect locally and are potent in even very small concentrations. Cytokines are involved in maintaining homeostasis in the presence of endogenous and exogenous insults through mediation of local inflammation and the immune response. The mechanism through which cytokines exert their influence is difficult to discern given their overlapping immunologic, hormonal, and inflammatory effects. Cytokines act in cascades, inducing other cytokines and possibly second messengers, any or all of which may contribute to the clinical symptoms of neurotoxicity. This makes the determination about specific effects of an individual cytokine difficult. Whether cytokines are synthesized solely in the brain or are imported from the periphery is still a subject of debate. However, one mechanism by which cytokines are thought to enter the brain from the periphery is via the circumventricular organs, particularly the organum vasculosum of the lamina terminalis (OVLT). This structure is anatomically associated with the hypothalamus, which forms a part of the hypothalamic-pituitary-adrenal (HPA) axis and has connections with the brainstem, frontal cortex, and the limbic system. Not surprisingly, explanations for the observed neurotoxicity include cytokine-induced alterations in neuroendocrine, neurotransmitter, and secondary cytokine systems (Valentine et al., 1998; Meyers, 1999; Murgo et al., 1999).

The cognitive and neuropsychiatric side effects of IFN-α have been reported to include impairments in memory, processing speed, EF, personality, and mood (Pavol et al., 1995; Valentine et al., 1998; Meyers, 1999). Neurotoxicity appears to be associated with dose, duration, route of treatment, and combination with XRT. A 78% incidence of obtundation was reported in a sample of patients treated intraventricularly (dosage ranged from 15 to 54 MIU) after whole brain radiation (Meyers et al., 1991a). Most patients recovered within 3 weeks of treatment cessation, although persistent cognitive dysfunction has been reported years after cessation of IFN-α (Meyers et al., 1991b). In contrast to therapeutic doses, even small doses of IFN-α appear to result in CNS effects. Normal controls given 0.1 MIU of IFN-α reported decreased alertness, and, 10 hours after a single 1.5 MIU dose showed slowed reaction times (Smith et al., 1988). Pavol and colleagues (1995) reported on the cognitive and emotional sequelae of subcutaneous IFN-α therapy (on average 51 MIU for 26 weeks) in patients with chronic myelogenous leukemia (CML). Compared with CML patients not treated with IFN-α, CML patients receiving IFN-α exhibited more frequent impairment in memory, processing speed, executive functioning, and self-reported depressive symptoms suggestive of frontal-subcortical dysfunction in the context of preserved simple attention span, language, visuoperception, and general intellectual function. Surprisingly, the length of IFN-α treatment was associated with cognitive dysfunction, whereas dosage was not.

Patients treated with TNF exhibit dose-dependent toxicity such as decreased attentional abilities, verbal memory deficits, motor coordination impairments, and frontal lobe executive dysfunction. Headache, anorexia, stroke-like events (e.g., transient amnesia), and demyelination in the brain are also found as adverse effects of TNF. Using SPECT, evidence for frontal hypoperfusion has been found in these patients in the absence of structural changes on neuroimaging (e.g., MRI). IL-1 and its receptors are found in many areas of the brain, particularly the hippocampus. IL-1 suppresses the influx of calcium into the hippocampus neurons, possibly suppressing long-term potentiation, which may explain the preponderance of memory impairments in patients with IL-1–associated toxicity. The neurotoxic effects of IL-2 appear to be dose-related and occur in nearly all patients treated with high dosages. The symptoms range from mild agitation, depression, and forgetfulness to frank confusion, dementia, and paranoia. TNF and IL-2 and TNF and IL-1 have been found to be synergistically toxic, with the latter being associated with the development of multiple sclerosis plaques and gliosis (Wollman et al., 1992).

Symptomatic and Palliative Therapies

The majority of patients diagnosed with cancer in the neuroaxis will receive multiple therapies, each capable of contributing independently or interactively to cognitive and/or neuropsychiatric morbidity. Almost all patients will receive anticonvulsants, even in the absence of any seizure, due to the common belief that these patients *appear* to be at a higher risk of seizures, thus necessitating prophylactic use of anticonvulsants. The majority of patients will also be administered glucocorticoids to reduce peritumoral swelling. In many cases steroid therapy will persist long after aggressive debulking of the tumor has occurred. However, it is doubtful that in the presence of a large resection cavity these steroids are needed, and many clinicians believe they should be tapered after surgery. Steroids themselves can cause many cognitive complications, including memory difficulties, mania, weight gain, drug-induced diabetes, and skin striae. Patients with primary gliomas have been shown to have an increased risk for coagulopathy, including deep vein thrombosis and pulmonary embolism, necessitating the use of anticoagulants such as Coumadin. Coumadin and some anticonvulsants have a low therapeutic index, which can result in over- or underdosage and the development of adverse side effects. Using Coumadin, anticonvulsants, and steroids together can lower the therapeutic index even further, thus increasing the risk of developing neurotoxic side effects. Some of these effects can mimic cognitive changes attributed to the tumor or its cell-killing treatments. Clinicians are therefore urged to understand the potential drug interactions and their sequelae when testing a patient for neurocognitive decline. As stated previously, the combination of chemotherapies and radiation therapies frequently leads to cognitive dysfunction as a result of structural damage. Moreover, use of radiotherapies can lead to hormone deficiencies, including thyroid dysfunction, depending on the field and dose administered. Palliative care with medications may also include antidepressants, anxiolytics, and narcotics for pain, some of which may also contribute to cognitive inefficiencies (Strang & Qvarner, 1990). Many palliative pharmacologic agents are employed late in the disease course when neurocognitive decline is usually an accepted part of the late stages of the disease. Unfortunately, there has been little study of therapeutic interventions' effectiveness, whether pharmacologic or psychological in nature, in increasing the overall QOL of the patient and the QOL of the family members and caregivers.

CONSIDERATIONS IN THE NEUROPSYCHOLOGICAL ASSESSMENT OF PATIENTS WITH CANCER

Progressive cognitive decline is an unfortunate consequence for most patients with CNS cancers. In fact, altered mental status is more frequently reported than physical disability in patients with brain tumors (Meyers, 1986, 1994; Meyers & Boake, 1993; Jaeckle, 1997). Moreover, it is clear that patients with CNS and non-CNS cancer may manifest symptoms of cognitive dysfunction secondary to the neoplasm itself, antineoplastic treatments, or affective distress (Meyers & Abbruzzese, 1992). These individuals may also experience alterations in their QOL and ability to carry out their usual activities of daily living (ADL). Despite attempts to develop less neurotoxic therapies, the use of more aggressive treatments that increase patient survival has left in its wake a host of neurologic and neuropsychological deficits that must be balanced against the survival gains achieved. The clinician should also bear in mind that previous treatments can profoundly affect the ability to diagnose subsequent problems. For example, a patient with a dementing illness after prophylactic cranial irradiation could have radiation induced dementia, a dementia of the Alzheimer, type, or both.

Comprehensive evaluations of a patient's performance status must include neuropsychological assessment of cognitive, emotional, and behavioral functioning, which can help to more rapidly identify disease recurrence and lead to earlier diagnostic and therapeutic intervention. For example, Meyers and colleagues (2000b) demonstrated that cognitive decline portends disease progression and deterioration in advance of clinical neurologic and radiographic evidence. In this study, malignant glioma patients were followed with both serial MRI and neuropsychological assessment of cognitive functioning to determine the time-to-tumor-progression (TTP). On average, cognitive decline occurred 30% earlier than neuroimaging evidence of tumor progression. The median TTP on MRI was 93 days, whereas the median time before patients demonstrated declines in cognitive functioning was 64 days. Self-report QOL deteriorated far later, at approximately 149 days, but was confounded by possible comprehension deficits in some of the patients. These findings support the sensitivity of cognitive measures to developing neuropathology and are in accord with neuropathologic reports of histologically confirmed tumor observed in tissue that appears normal on radiologic examination. Meyers and colleagues (2000a) demonstrated that cognitive functioning is a significant prognostic indicator of survival time independent of several other routinely collected clinical variables. Patients with malignant gliomas were studied throughout their participation in either a Phase I or Phase II clinical trial with serial neuropsychological assessments to determine the prognostic value of these assessments in predicting survival. Clinical variables including age, Karnofsky Performance Status, histology, extent of resection, number of recurrences, and time since diagnosis accounted for 34% of the variance in survival time. The addition of nine measures of cognitive functioning accounted for 53% of the variance. with verbal memory, attention span, and graphomotor speed being most significantly related to survival. Thus, serial cognitive assessment of patients with CNS cancer may aid in a more rapid diagnosis of disease regrowth and subsequent implementation of appropriate treatments. Neuropsychological evaluations can also assess the patient's individual strengths and weaknesses and contribute to patient management and rehabilitation planning (Alexander et al., 1993). Neuropsychological evaluations can assess patients' ability to work, drive, participate in medical decision making (Jubelirer et al., 1994), or live independently; provide help in the coordination of disability applications; and assess the efficacy and neurotoxicity of pharmacologic and behavioral interventions.

Multidisciplinary assessment is critical in the oncologic setting. The World Health Organization (WHO, 1980) proposed a model that assists in characterizing the effects of neurologic disease on patient function by measuring the consequences of disease at the organ level (i.e., impairment), the individual level (i.e., disability), and the societal level (i.e., handicap). *Impairment* refers to abnormalities of structure or function at the anatomic level and includes the neurologic (e.g., weakness), cognitive (e.g., impaired retrieval), and emotional (e.g., depression) sequelae caused by a lesion. *Disability* refers to a reduction in the ability to perform "normal" activities secondary to the impairment. For example, a patient with weakness, impaired retrieval, and depression may have associated disabilities such as difficulty walking, requiring a wheelchair; memory impairment; and apathy. However, whether or not these issues result in a handicap is partly determined by factors unique to the individual (e.g., coping styles, social supports) and factors extrinsic to the individual (e.g., environmental supports and access to services). *Handicap* is defined as a "disadvantage for a given individual resulting from an impairment or disability, that limits or prevents the fulfillment of a role that is normal (depending on age, sex, and social and cultural factors) for that individual" (WHO, 1980, p. 183). Thus, a disability may cause a handicap in one individual while another individual in a different environment may experience relatively little handicap. For example, the memory impairment described above may not be a particularly severe handicap for an individual whose occupation involves repetitive activities on an assembly line; however, a stage actor may find himself or herself rapidly unemployed. Thus it is critical to assess all levels of function (i.e., impairment, disability, and handicap) when making determinations regarding patient care and outcome (Meyers, 1997). (See Chapter 50.)

Beyond traditional neurologic exams, neuropsychological assessments can aid in characterizing the

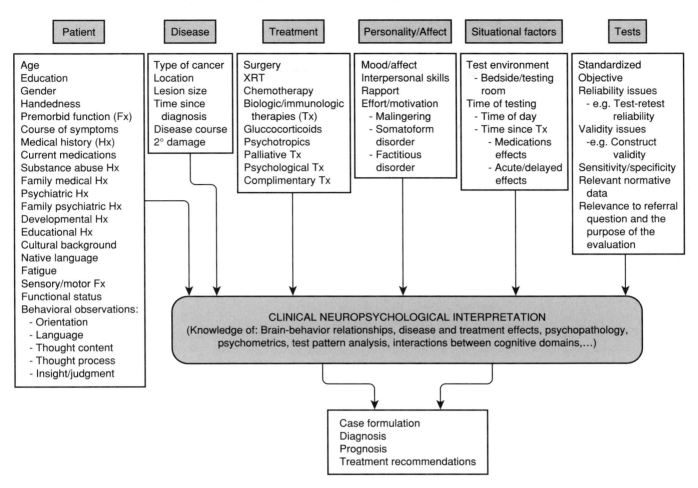

FIGURE 38–3. Key components of a neuropsychological assessment in oncology patients.

nature and extent of a patient's impairment (i.e., neuropsychological test performance), disability (i.e., ability to carry out one's usual ADL), and handicap (i.e., ability to maintain social and occupational roles frequently assessed through subjective QOL measures). Clinical neuropsychological assessment in patients with cancer does not differ substantially from assessment in other neuropathologic groups (see Fig. 38-3). The assessment should include a thorough and informed clinical interview with the patient and, ideally, a caregiver; a flexible and comprehensive assessment of the relevant domains of cognitive and emotional functioning for each patient (both areas of suspected dysfunction and preserved function); and the provision of feedback to the physician and patient to help guide treatment, manage adverse events, and plan for the future (Plumb et al., 1981; Cimino, 2000; Vanderploeg, 2000).

Formal neuropsychological assessments must be sensitive to characteristics of the patient (e.g., age, cultural background), the purpose of the assessment (e.g., designing a test battery to assess strengths and weaknesses of a brain tumor patient to contribute to rehabil-

itation planning *versus* a Phase I treatment trial to examine the neurotoxic effects of a new chemotherapeutic agent), the expected adverse effects of treatments, and the frequency of assessments. While a bedside evaluation of cognitive function such as the Mini-Mental Status Examination (MMSE) can suggest areas of problems, it is *very* insensitive and unreliable. Often patients may score well on the MMSE and still have profound cognitive dysfunction related to the tumor or its treatment; conversely, patients may perform poorly on the MMSE and demonstrate adequate cognitive functioning on more focused assessment. Cullum and colleagues (1993) examined the relationship of a three-word memory paradigm identical to that used on the MMSE with a well-standardized neuropsychological measure of verbal memory (i.e., California Verbal Learning Test [CVLT]) in healthy older adults. In a savvy methodologic manipulation, the authors selected subjects who performed within the average range on the CVLT and subsequently administered two three-word lists to them, one used clinically in an Alzheimer disease research center and another adapted from another mental status screening examination. Results of their study revealed unacceptably high rates of false-positive errors (i.e., presumed cognitive dysfunction) when considering subject performance on three-word memory tasks. The most dramatic portrayal of this testing is evident in one of the three-word tasks (e.g., "brown, tulip, honesty"), where 60% of the sample failed to recall any of the three words and only 10% recalled all three words, whereas all subjects performed within the average range on a much more challenging 16-word list learning task (CVLT). Similarly, assessment of patients' global cognitive functioning via an intelligence quotient (IQ) has been reported to be insensitive to many changes in cognitive function typically seen in oncologic populations (Meyers & Weitzner, 1995). Thus it is essential to obtain a formal comprehensive neuropsychological assessment to adequately identify alterations in cerebral function.

Neuropsychological assessments enjoy the advantage of containing objective and standardized measures of cognitive functioning and standardized measures of neuropsychiatric functioning. This is especially important, considering that several studies have demonstrated a weak or nonexistent relationship between a patient's *self-report* of cognitive difficulties and *objective* findings of cognitive dysfunction through formal neuropsychological evaluation (van Dam et al., 1998; Schagen et al., 1999); there appears to be a positive relationship between self-report of affective distress and self-report of cognitive difficulty. Discrepancy in estimates of cognitive dysfunction may represent a patient's reluctance to acknowledge difficulties, reduced awareness secondary to the neuropathologic destruction of critical areas or general disease progression, or the effects of social desirability bias. Conversely, the exaggeration of deficits may reflect attempts to ensure that a patient's symptom complaints are taken seriously or reflect a patient's affective state or personality structure (e.g., hopelessness secondary to depression or a somatoform disorder).

Besides cognitive dysfunction, many patients experience alterations in their behavioral and personality functioning that can have a negative impact on their cognitive as well as daily activities. These neuropsychiatric alterations include mood changes ranging from mania to depression, thought disorders including hallucinations and delusions, and personality disturbances such as apathy, disinhibition, or poor frustration tolerance. The observed neuropsychiatric disturbance may represent new onset adjustment disorders, maladaptive responses to stress, exacerbations of premorbid psychiatric disorders, tumor-related sequelae, or some combination of these (Weitzner, 1999). The diagnosis of mood disturbance (i.e., depression) apart from apathy can be difficult given their similarity in symptom presentation; however, accurate diagnosis can be critical for effective symptom management via pharmacologic and behavioral interventions. Tumors that disconnect limbic areas

from the rich afferents they receive from heteromodal cortical areas (e.g., frontal or parietal areas) often result in cognitive, emotional, and behavioral apathy or amotivation and has been termed *apathy syndrome*. Clinically, these patients present with decreased energy, flat affect, diminished emotional expressions, and apparent disinterest in most activities. However, the presence of indifference, passivity, and lack of emotional reactivity distinguish the apathy syndrome from depression. Thus, a detailed understanding of each patient's physical, cognitive, behavioral, emotional, and functional well-being is critical to the comprehensive assessment of cancer patients.

Neuropsychological evaluations are also being increasingly incorporated into clinical trials, as estimates of mortality and TTP arguably do not adequately address relevant domains of functioning in populations at risk for developing CNS dysfunction. Net clinical benefit of cancer therapy, as defined by members of the Food and Drug Administration, National Cancer Institute, and the National Cancer Institute Division of Cancer Treatment Board of Scientific Counselors, must demonstrate benefits in (1) survival, (2) time to treatment failure and disease-free survival, (3) complete response rate, (4) response rate, and (5) beneficial effects on disease-related symptoms and/or QOL. Treatments that fail to improve overall survival or response rate but demonstrate an ability to slow or stabilize declines in mental status, given that progressive cognitive deterioration is expected in the case of CNS cancers, may still be considered beneficial (Meyers, 1997). Similarly, it may be that some treatments, while extending the time-honored holy grail of increased survival in cancer patients, may in fact so devastate the patient's abilities to think, speak, and reason, that the treatment would be abandoned for therapies with more modest survival benefits but which provide a longer period of cognitive stability. Eventually cancer researchers must come up with an evaluation that considers overall survival, neurologic function, neuropsychological function, and evaluation of ADL. This may give a more complete sense of the true effect of treatments on any given patient rather than a simple survival advantage.

As more aggressive treatments have lengthened survival time for many cancer patients, it is essential that we recognize the potential adverse effects on the nature and quality of the survival and address these issues directly through psychosocial rehabilitation, pharmacologic management, or surgery. The use of the aforementioned approach to comprehensively evaluate a patient's physical, cognitive, behavioral, emotional, and functional well-being provides the groundwork from which individualized therapies can be initiated that attempt to diminish the effects of the patient's impairments on his or her daily functioning (Sherer et al., 1997).

INTERVENTION STRATEGIES

Beyond diagnosis and treatment of cancers, clinicians have devoted more time to improving the QOL of patients with cancer by adding palliative agents to the list of more standard therapies (i.e., radiotherapy or chemotherapy). Palliative therapies have included multidisciplinary rehabilitation programs, pharmacologic management strategies, and education, counseling, and support groups. These interventions help the patient to understand and cope with the symptoms and psychological impact of the disease and ameliorate some of the side effects of the cancer and its treatment, which can improve patients' QOL and perhaps promote a better response to treatment. It is important to address these subtle and slow changes because interventions with the patient or the caregivers can markedly improve overall functioning of the patient. Even simple adjustments, such as constant monitoring of the patient so there is no wandering off, or provision of assistance when using the stove or bathroom, can maintain overall functioning and prevent accidents.

Multidisciplinary Rehabilitation

Cancer patients frequently are offered a variety of interventions targeting physical difficulties and palliative symptom management (Meyers & Boake, 1993). However, little progress has been made toward designing comprehensive, multidisciplinary rehabilitation programs capable of addressing the cognitive, emotional, behavioral, and functional needs of cancer patients despite the fact that many brain tumor patients may be ideal candidates because they typically manifest milder cognitive dysfunction and less physical disability than many patients commonly referred for such services (e.g., stroke, TBI patients). This remains the case in part due to the relative dearth of programs equipped to provide services for brain tumor patients, the reluctance to recommend rehabilitation for brain tumor patients given their prognosis, and clinician and patient unfamiliarity with such services.

A recent literature review (Spelten et al., 2002) examining return to work in cancer patients found an average return-to-work rate of 62% in a mixed sample of cancer patients. At present, far fewer patients with brain tumors are reported to resume their premorbid activities and level of function. Fobair and colleagues (1990) reported that only 18% of patients return to full-time competitive employment, while another 10% return to part-time employment; many more patients with brain tumors require attendant care provided either by a family member or a hired caregiver. Clearly, the sequelae of cancer, and particularly CNS malignancies, can be costly for the patient, family, and society. Thus, rehabilitation programs that assist the patient to regain independent function and return to productive activities through treatments that restore, develop, or compensate for losses in physical, sensory, or cognitive functions are of significant import. Sherer and colleagues (1997) modified a multidisciplinary outpatient brain injury rehabilitation program designed for TBI patients (Kreutzer & Wehman, 1991; Malec & Basford, 1996) to determine the extent to which brain tumor patients could benefit from such services and to assess the comparative costs of such treatment for brain tumor patients versus TBI patients. Overall, the brain tumor patients demonstrated favorable improvements in independent function and employment status compared with TBI patients. Approximately 85% (11/13) of the brain tumor patients completed the program (two were discharged early due to medical complications) and, on average, brain tumor patients length of treatment (about 2.6 months) was half that of TBI patients. This provides preliminary evidence that brain tumor patients can benefit substantially from multidisciplinary outpatient brain injury programs and may, in fact, require less treatment time and financial resources for comparable outcomes.

Pharmacologic Management

Many drugs are now under investigation for use as palliative medications. For example, erythropoietin might be considered a palliative drug for its use in increasing red blood cell volume to help with cancer-related fatigue, while the more plentiful use of narcotics and new-line medications for pain relief (Stray et al., 1990) adds to patient comfort and ability to tolerate therapies. Comprehensive neuropsychological evaluations may also provide indications for several other palliative therapies for cognitive, behavioral, or mood disturbances.

Patients exhibiting either neurobehavioral slowing or apathy syndrome as a result of the tumor itself or subsequent treatments may benefit from stimulant therapy with methylphenidate (Meyers et al., 1998; Valentine & Meyers, 2001). It is believed that the frontal-brainstem reticular activating system monoamine pathways are disturbed in these patients and that use of a catecholamine agonist such as methylphenidate may help alleviate the neuropsychological and neuropsychiatric disturbances frequently observed (Weitzner et al., 1995). Preliminary evidence supports the use of methylphenidate for amelioration of such neurobehavioral difficulties (Meyers et al., 1998). Methylphenidate therapy was well tolerated in doses of 10 mg twice daily, 20 mg twice daily, and 30 mg twice daily in most patients and appeared to result in both subjective and objective improvements in cognitive, emotional, and daily functioning (Meyers et al., 1998). Specifically, improvements were observed in visual-motor speed, memory, expressive speech, EF, fine motor coordination, subjective mood ratings, gait, stamina, and even bladder control. Remarkably these improvements occurred in the context of expectations for progressive deterioration of function given the nature of primary malignant gliomas. Ongoing investigations are attempting to examine optimal dosing schedules and the effectiveness of sustained-release formulas in treating these disturbances in brain tumor populations. Other "cognition enhancing" medications such as donepezil are also being actively investigated to determine their potential roles as palliative therapies.

Psychotherapy, Education, and Support Groups

Accurate differential diagnosis of apathy syndrome and depression facilitates appropriate therapeutic interventions such as methylphenidate for apathy syndrome and an antidepressant for depression (Kugaya et al., 1999). Many patients with cancer may also develop a range of affective distress that can be appropriately managed with pharmacotherapy, psychotherapy, or both. The most frequently reported mood disorders that arise during diagnosis and treatment in cancer, patients is an adjustment disorder with depressed or anxious mood. However, some degree of emotional distress is present in almost all patients diagnosed with cancer, and many express an interest in receiving supportive interventions for these alterations in their mood even if they have not manifested a clinically diagnosable disorder (e.g., *Diagnostic and Statistic Manual of Mental Disorders* (DSM)-*IV* Major Depressive Disorder). Referral to an appropriately trained mental health professional such as a health psychologist affords patients the opportunity to receive a thorough and comprehensive assessment of their mood and current level of functioning, accurate diagnosis, and intensive psychosocial intervention to alleviate distress coupled with frequent monitoring of alterations in patient mood that may warrant referral for additional interventions such as pharmacologic management. Recommendations for support groups and educational materials that help the patient and family understand the nature of the illness, normalize their reactions, and bolster adaptive coping strategies can substantially improve QOL and even decrease disease recurrence. A provocative review of recent work in psychoneuroimmunology by Turner-Cobb and colleagues (2001) provided the mounting evidence that psychosocial interventions may not only improve subjective quality of life but also have direct effects on immune (e.g., NK-cell activity) and neuroendocrine (e.g., glucocorticoids) mediators of cancer progression and survival as well as improve health-related behaviors (e.g., smoking cessation). Unfortunately, many patients and their families are forced to deal with the knowledge

that their disease may ultimately result in a premature death. Hospice care and end-of-life counseling are paramount in helping the patient and family process the psychological trauma that accompanies this experience.

CASE STUDY

A 46-year-old white woman presented to her physicians with a seizure. Evaluations resulted in the discovery of a left frontal mass lesion. A subtotal resection was accomplished, and the pathology specimen was described as an anaplastic astrocytoma; however, oligodendrocytes and gemistocytes were present, suggesting the tumor may have actually been an oligoastrocytoma. This tumor responds better to chemotherapy than an anaplastic astrocytoma. She underwent radiotherapy with whole brain radiation and a boost to the tumor area. Following radiotherapy she received several courses of chemotherapy with lomustine (CCNU), procarbazine, and vincristine. Seizures were controlled with carbamazepine.

Following therapy completion, she resumed her previous occupation at a large utilities company with her previous supervisor. After another year, she was transferred to a new position with a new supervisor who did not offer much support. The patient felt she had difficulty with learning new job responsibilities. This same year she sustained a generalized seizure after an attempt to taper her anticonvulsant medication. She was also divorced. During this time, her family noted her to have increasing difficulty with forgetfulness, distractibility, and word finding; these difficulties progressed over the ensuing year.

A comprehensive neuropsychological evaluation was requested to evaluate her cognitive complaints in order to assist in differential diagnosis and treatment planning, to assist in evaluating her capacity for return to work, and to establish a baseline for future comparison. At the time of evaluation, the patient was 52 years of age and right-handed, with 12 years of education. She denied any developmental delays or complications during birth. She had been in otherwise good health before the diagnosis of her tumor. After another seizure her position with her former employer was eliminated and she sought permanent disability.

During the evaluation, she was observed to be alert and oriented. Thought processes were organized and goal-directed with no evidence of delusions or hallucinations. Expressive speech was fluent and goal-directed but contained occasional semantic paraphasic errors. No gross motor disturbance was observed. Affect was full-ranging and consistent with thought content. On several occasions throughout the testing she became anxious and frustrated and chastised herself when she perceived she did not know an answer or responded slowly. Both clinical judgment and the results of psychometric measurement indicted adequate cognitive effort.

The results of the evaluation demonstrated that this patient was a woman of average range premorbid intellectual functioning, who exhibited symptoms of frontal-subcortical dysfunction on select aspects of memory, executive function, language, and motor function. Specifically, within tests of verbal memory she performed better when the verbal material was well organized and contained structure rather than when she was required to self-impose structure. In general, she demonstrated encoding inefficiencies for unstructured verbal material with retrieval difficulties and intact consolidation. Her memory for nonverbal material was significant for encoding deficits with intact consolidation for material that was initially learned. Additionally, there was variability in her executive functioning, including mildly impaired abstract verbal and nonverbal reasoning with variable mild inefficiencies in mental flexibility. She manifested variable word-retrieval deficits (mild to profoundly impaired, depending on task demands) in the context of intact comprehension and repetition; diminished strength and dexterity bilaterally; and grossly intact visuoconstructional and simple attentional functioning. Her emotional and personality assessment suggested feelings of isolation and moderate levels of emotional distress, especially symptoms of depression and anxiety.

Etiologic attributions concerning the causal agents for her observed cognitive and emotional dysfunction were difficult to distinguish given the lack of prospective evaluations, including a presurgical baseline assessment. The nature and pattern of her cognitive dysfunction were thought likely to prevent her from returning to her prior occupation. However, from a cognitive standpoint, it was possible that she may secure some form of competitive employment that was well structured, repetitive, required minimal "multi-tasking," and had few changing task demands. Prognosis for long-term success even in a structured and supportive environment was considered guarded. She was referred both to a brain tumor support group and for comprehensive multidisciplinary cognitive rehabilitation including cognitive and psychological interventions, vocational counseling, and job coaching. Consideration of a trial of methylphenidate was recommended.

Acknowledgments

This work was funded by numerous grants to the University of Chicago, the University of Texas M.D. Anderson Cancer Center, and from the Duinick Foundation. We wish to thank Joseph Fink, PhD, and Christina Meyers, PhD, for helpful comments and editorial review.

■ KEY POINTS

☐ As treatments for brain tumors (both primary and metastatic) improve and prolong life, neuropsychological sequelae of these therapies will become increasingly important.

☐ Few prospective studies of the neurocognitive effects have been published. Most current information is largely anecdotal.

☐ A thorough neuropsychological analysis before, during, and after treatment for a a patient with a brain tumor will permit more detailed assistance and rehabilitation for the cancer patient.

KEY READINGS

Baile WF: Neuropsychiatric disorders in cancer patients. Curr Opin Oncol 8:182–187, 1996.

Bernstein M, Berger MS (eds): Neuro-Oncology: The Essentials. New York: Thieme Medical, 2002.

Crossen JR, Garwood D, Glatstein E, et al: Neurobehavioral sequelae of cranial irradiation in adults: A review of radiation-induced encephalopathy. J Clin Oncol 12:627–642, 1994.

Janus TJ, Yung WKA: Primary neoplasms of the brain, in Goetz C (ed): Textbook of Clinical Neurology, ed 2. Philadelphia, PA: Saunders, 2003, p. 1017.

Meyers CA: Issues of quality of life in neuro-oncology, in Vecht CJ (ed): Handbook of Clinical Neurology, Vol. 67. Vinken JP, Bruyn GW (series eds): Neuro-Oncology Part I. New York and Amsterdam: Elsevier Science, 1997, pp. 389–409.

Meyers CA, Hess KR, Yung WK, et al: Cognitive function as a predictor of survival in patients with recurrent malignant glioma. J Clin Oncol 18: 646–650, 2000.

Moleski M: Neuropsychological, neuroanatomical, and neurophysiological consequences of CNS chemotherapy for acute lymphoblastic leukemia. Arch Clin Neuropsychol 15:603–630, 2000.

Regine WF, Scott C, Murray K, et al: Neurocognitive outcome in brain metastases patients treated with accelerated-fractionation vs. accelerated-hyper-fractionated radiotherapy: An analysis from Radiation Therapy Oncology Group Study 91-04. Int J Radiat Oncol Biol Phys 51:711–717, 2001.

Weitzner MA, Meyers CA: Cognitive functioning and quality of life in malignant glioma patients: A review of the literature. Psychooncology 6:169–177, 1997.

REFERENCES

Abayomi OK: Pathogenesis of irradiation-induced cognitive dysfunction. Acta Oncol 35:659–663, 1996.

Ahles TA, Saykin A: Cognitive effects of standard-dose chemotherapy in patients with cancer. Cancer Invest 19:812–820, 2001.

Alexander PJ, Dinesh N, Vidyasagar MS: Psychiatric morbidity among cancer patients and its relationship with awareness of illness and expectations about treatment outcome. Acta Oncol 32:623–626, 1993.

Anderson SW, Damasio H, Tranel D: Neuropsychological impairments associated with lesions caused by tumor or stroke. Arch Neurol 47:397–405, 1990.

Armstrong C, Corn B, Ruffer JE, et al: Radiotherapeutic effects on brain function: Double dissociation of memory systems. Neuropsychiatry, Neuropsychol Behav Neurol 13:101–111, 2000.

Armstrong CL, Hunter JV, Ledakis GE, et al: Late cognitive and radiographic changes related to radiotherapy: Initial prospective findings. Neurology 59:40–48, 2002.

Armstrong C, Mollman J, Corn B, et al: Effects of radiation therapy on adult brain behavior: Evidence for a rebound phenomena in a phase 1 trial. Neurology 43:1961–1965, 1993.

Armstrong C, Ruffer J, Corn B, et al: Biphasic patterns of memory deficits following moderate dose partial brain irradiation: Neuropsychologic outcome and proposed mechanisms. J Clin Oncol 13:263–2271, 1995.

Bak TH, Antoun N, Balan KK, et al: Memory lost, memory regained: Neuropsychological findings and neuroimaging in two cases of paraneoplastic limbic encephalitis with radically different outcomes. J Neurol Neurosurg Psychiatry 71:40–47, 2001.

Bakay L: Olfactory meningiomas: The missed diagnosis. JAMA 251:53–55, 1984.

Bessell EM, Lopez-Guillermo A, Villa S, et al: Importance of radiotherapy in the outcome of patients with primary CNS lymphoma: An analysis of the CHOD/BVAM regimen followed by two different radiotherapy treatments. J Clin Oncol 20:231–236, 2002.

Brezden CB, Phillips KA, Abdolell M, et al: Cognitive function in breast cancer patients receiving adjuvant chemotherapy. J Clin Oncol 18:2695–2701, 2000.

Cimino CR: Principles of neuropsychological interpretation, in Vanderploeg RD (ed): Clinician's Guide to Neuropsychological Assessment, ed 2. Mahwah, NJ: Lawrence Erlbaum Associates, 2000, pp. 69–110.

Crossen JR, Garwood D, Glatstein E, et al: Neurobehavioral sequelae of cranial irradiation in adults: A review of radiation-induced encephalopathy. J Clin Oncol 12:627–642, 1994.

Cull A, Gregor A, Hopwood P, et al: Neurological and cognitive impairment in long-term survivors of small cell lung cancer. Eur J Cancer 30:1067–1074, 1994.

Cull A, Hay C, Love SB, et al: What do cancer patients mean when they complain of concentration and memory problems? Br J Cancer 74:1674–1679, 1996.

Cullum CM, Thompson LL, Smernoff EN: Three-word recall as a measure of memory. J Clin Exp Neuropsychol 15:321–329, 1993.

DeAngelis LM: Primary CNS lymphoma: Treatment with combined chemotherapy and radiotherapy. J Neurooncol 43:249–257, 1999.

De Girolami U, Frosch MP, Anthony DC: The central nervous system, in Cotran RS, Kumar V, Robbins SL, et al (eds): Robbins Pathologic Basis of Disease, ed 5. Philadelphia, PA: Saunders, 1994, pp. 1295–1356.

Fobair P, Mackworth N, Varghese A, et al: Quality of life issues among 200 brain tumor patients treated at the University of California in San Francisco, interviewed 1988. Presented at the Brain Tumor Conference: A Living Source Guide, San Francisco, 1990.

Fortin D, Macdonald DR, Stitt L, et al: PCV for oligodendroglial tumors: In search of prognostic factors for response and survival. Can J Neurol Sci 28:215–223, 2001.

Foster LW, McLellan L: Cognition and the cancer experience: Clinical implications. Cancer Pract 8:25–31, 2000.

Glosser G, McManus P, Munzenrider J, et al: Neuropsychological function in adults after high dose fractionated radiation therapy of skull base tumors. Intl J Radiat Oncol Biol Phys 38:231–239, 1997.

Gregor A, Cull A, Traynor E, et al: Neuropsychometric evaluation of long-term survivors of adult brain tumours: Relationship with tumour and treatment parameters. Radiother Oncol 41:55–59, 1996.

Hickie I, Lloyd A.: Are cytokines associated with neuropsychiatric syndromes in humans? Intl J Immunopharmacol 17:677–683, 1995.

Jaeckle KA: Signs of focal lesions and of increased intracranial pressure in brain tumors, in Vecht CJ (ed): Handbook of Clinical Neurology. Neuro-Oncology Part I, Vol. 67. New York: Elsevier, 1997, pp. 139–165.

Jubelirer SJ, Linton JC, Magnetti SM: Reading versus comprehension: Implications for patient education and consent in an outpatient oncology clinic. J Cancer Educ 9:26–29, 1994.

Kadan-Lottick NS, Skluzacek MC, Gurney JG: Decreasing incidence rates of primary central nervous system lymphoma. Cancer 95:193–202, 2002.

Keime-Guibert F, Napolitano M, Delattre JY: Neurological complications of radiotherapy and chemotherapy. J Neurol 245: 695–708, 1998.

Kleihues P, Louis DN, Scheithauer BW, et al: The WHO classification of tumors of the nervous system. J Neuropathol Exp Neurol 61: 215–225, 2002.

Klein M, Taphoorn MJB, Heimans JJ, et al: Neurobehavioral status and health-related quality of life in newly diagnosed high-grade glioma patients. J Clin Oncol 19:4037–4047, 2001.

Komaki R, Meyers CA, Shin DM, et al: Evaluation of cognitive function in patients with limited small cell lung cancer prior to and shortly following prophylactic cranial irradiation. Int J Radiat Oncol Biol Phys 33:179–182, 1995.

Kugaya A, Akechi T, Nakano T: Successful antidepressant treatment for five terminally ill cancer patients with major depression, suicidal ideation and a desire for death. Support Care Cancer 7:432–436, 1999.

Lerner DM, Stoudemire A, Rosenstein DL: Neuropsychiatric toxicity associated with cytokine therapies. Psychosomatics 40:428–435, 1999.

Lipp HP: Neurotoxicity (including sensory toxicity) induced by cytostatics, in Lipp H-P (ed): Anticancer Drug Toxicity Prevention, Management, and Clinical Pharmacokinetics. New York: Marcel Dekker, 1999, pp. 431–454.

Maes M, Song CA, De Jongh R, et al: in Plotnikoff NP, Faith RE, Murgo AJ, et al. (eds): Cytokines Stress and Immunity. Boca Raton, FL: CRC Press, 1999, pp. 39–50.

Martins AN, Johnston JS, Henry JM, et al: Delayed radiation necrosis of the brain. J Neurosurg 47:336–345, 1997.

Moleski M: Neuropsychological, neuroanatomical, and neurophysiological consequences of CNS chemotherapy for acute lymphoblastic leukemia. Arch Clin Neuropsychol 15:603–630, 2000.

Murgo AJ, Faith RE, Plotnikoff NP: Neuropeptides, cytokines, and cancer- Interrelationships, in Plotnikoff NP, Faith RE, Murgo AJ, et al (eds): Cytokines Stress and Immunity. Boca Raton: CRC Press, 1999, pp. 39–50.

Meyers CA: Issues of quality of life in neuro-oncology, in Vecht CJ (ed): Handbook of Clinical Neurology: Neuro-Oncology Part I, Vol. 67. New York: Elsevier, 1997, pp. 389–409.

Meyers CA: Mood and cognitive disorders in cancer patients receiving cytokine therapy. Adv Exp Med Biol 461:75–81, 1999b.

Meyers CA: Mood and cognitive disorders in cancer patients receiving cytokine therapy, in Dantzer, et al. (eds): Cytokines, Stress, and Depression. New York: Plenum Publishers, 1999a, pp. 75–81.

Meyers CA: Neuropsychological aspects of cancer and cancer treatment, in Grabois M (ed): Physical Medicine and Rehabilitation: State of the Art Reviews. Philadelphia, PA: Hanley and Belfus, 1994, pp. 229–241.

Meyers CA: Neuropsychological deficits in brain tumor patients: Effect of location, chronicity, and treatment. Cancer Bull 38:30–32, 1986.

Meyers CA, Abbruzzese JL: Cognitive functioning in cancer patients: Effect of previous treatment. Neurology 42:434–436, 1992.

Meyers CA, Boake C: Neurobehavioral disorders in brain tumor patients: Rehabilitation strategies. Cancer Bull 45:362–364, 1993.

Meyers CA, Boake C, Levin VA, et al: Symptom management, rehabilitation strategies, and improved quality of life for patients with brain tumors, in Levin VA (ed): Cancer in the Nervous System. New York: Churchill Livingstone, 1996a, pp. 449–462.

Meyers CA, Weitzner MA: Neurobehavioral functioning and quality of life in patients treated for cancer of the central nervous system. Curr Opin Oncol 7:197–200, 1995.

Meyers CA, Byrne KS, Komaki R: Cognitive deficits in patients with small cell lung cancer before and after chemotherapy. Lung Cancer 12:231–235, 1995.

Meyers CA, Gera F, Wong P-F, et al: Neurocognitive effects of therapeutic irradiation for base of skull tumors. Intl J Radiat Oncol Biol Phys 46:51–55, 2000a.

Meyers CA, Grous JJ, Ford KM, et al: Multifaceted models for assessing quality of life in brain cancer therapy trials. Drug Info J 30:856–857, 1996b.

Meyers CA, Hess KR, Yung WK, et al: Cognitive function as a predictor of survival in patients with recurrent malignant glioma. J Clin Oncol 18:646–650, 2000b.

Meyers CA, Obbens EA, Scheibel RS, et al: Neurotoxicity of intraventricularly administered alpha-interferon for leptomeningeal disease. Cancer 68:88–92, 1991a.

Meyers CA, Scheibel RS, Forman AD: Persistent neurotoxicity of systemically administered interferon-alpha. Neurology 41:672–676, 1991b.

Meyers CA, Weitzner M, Byrne K, et al: Evaluation of the neurobehavioral functioning of patients before, during, and after bone marrow transplantation. J Clin Oncol 12:820–826, 1994.

Meyers CA, Weitzner MA, Valentine AD, et al: Methylphenidate therapy improves cognition, mood, and function of brain tumor patients. J Clin Oncol 16:2522–2527, 1998.

Nieto YN, Cagnoni PJ, Bearman SI, et al: Acute encephalopathy: A new toxicity associated with high-dose paclitaxel. Clin Cancer Res 5:501–506, 1999.

O'Connor MM, Mayberg MR: Effects of radiation on cerebral vasculature: A review. Neurosurgery 46:138–151, 2000.

O'Neill BP, Wang CH, O'Fallon JR, et al: The consequences of treatment and disease in patients with primary CNS non-Hodgkin's lymphoma: Cognitive function and performance status. North Central Cancer Treatment Group. J Neurooncol 1:196–203, 1999.

Pavol MA, Meyers CA, Rexer JL, et al: Pattern of neurobehavioral deficits associated with interferon alfa therapy for leukemia. Neurology 45:947–950, 1995.

Plumb M, Holland J: Comparative studies of psychological function in patients with advanced cancer. II. Interviewer-rated current and past psychological symptoms. Psychosom Med 43:243–51, 1981.

Regine WF, Scott C, Murray K, et al: Neurocognitive outcome in brain metastases patients treated with accelerated-fractionation vs. accelerated-hyperfractionated radiotherapy: An analysis from Radiation Therapy Oncology Group Study 91-04. Intl J Radiat Oncol Biol Phys 51: 711–717, 2001.

Riva D, Giorgi C, Nichelli F, et al: Intrathecal methotrexate affects cognitive function in children with medulloblastoma. Neurology 59:48–53, 2002.

Salander P, Karlsson T, Bergenheim T, et al: Long-term memory deficits in patients with malignant gliomas. J Neurooncol 25: 227–238, 1995.

Schagen SB, van Dam FS, Muller MJ, et al: Cognitive deficits after postoperative chemotherapy for breast carcinoma. Cancer 85:640–650, 1999.

Schlegel U, Pels H, Oehring R, et al: Neurologic sequelae of treatment of primary CNS lymphoma. J Neurooncol 43:277–286, 1999.

Schouten LJ, Rutten, J, Huveneers HAM, et al: Incidences of brain metastases in a cohort of patients with carcinoma of the breast, colon, kidney, lung and melanoma. Cancer 94:2698–2705, 2002.

Sheline GE, Wara WM, Smith V: Therapeutic irradiation and brain injury. Intl J Radiat Oncol Biol Phys 6:1215–1228, 1980.

Sherer M, Meyers CA, Bergloff P: Efficacy of postacute brain injury rehabilitation for patients with primary malignant brain tumors. Cancer 80:250–257, 1997.

Smith A, Tyrrell D, Coyle K, et al: Effects of interferon alpha on performance in man: A preliminary study. Psychopharmacology 96:414–416, 1988.

Snyder HK, Robinson D, Shah D, et al: Signs and symptoms of patients with brain tumors presenting to the emergency department. J Emerg Med 11:253–258, 1993.

Spelten ER, Sprangers MAG, Verbeek JH: Factors reported to influence the return to work of cancer survivors: A literature review. Psycho-Oncology 11:124–131, 2002.

Steen RG, Spence D, Wu S, et al: Effect of therapeutic ionizing radiation on the human brain. Ann Neurol 50:787–795, 2001.

Strang P, Qvarner H: Cancer-related pain and its influence on quality of life. Anticancer Res 10:109–112, 1990.

Surma-aho O, Niemelä M, Vilkki J, et al: Adverse long-term effects of brain radiotherapy in adult low-grade glioma patients. Neurology 56:1285–1290, 2001.

Taphoorn MJB, Schiphorst AK, Snoek FJ, et al: Cognitive functions and quality of life in patients with low grade gliomas: The impact of radiotherapy. Ann Neurol 36:48–54, 1994.

Tucha O, Smely C, Preier M, et al: Cognitive deficits before treatment among patients with brain tumors. Neurosurgery 47:324–333, 2000.

Taylor BV, Buckner JC, Cascino TL, et al: Effects of radiation and chemotherapy on cognitive function in patients with high-grade glioma. J Clin Oncol 16:2195–201, 1998.

Turner-Cobb JM, Sephton SE, Spiegel D, et al: Psychosocial effects on immune function and disease progression in cancer: Human studies, in Ader R, Felten DL, Cohen N (eds): Psychoneuroimmunology. San Diego, CA: Academic Press, 2001, pp. 565–582.

Vanderploeg RD: Interview and testing: The data collection phase of neuropsychological evaluations, in: Vanderploeg RD (ed):

Clinician's Guide to Neuropsychological Assessment, ed 2. Mahwah, NJ: Lawrence Erlbaum Associates, 2000, pp 3–38.

Valentine AD, Meyers CA, Kling MA, et al: Mood and cognitive side effects of interferon-alpha therapy. Semin Oncol 25:39–47, 1998.

Valentine AD, Meyers CA: Cognitive and mood disturbance as causes and symptoms of fatigue in cancer patients. Cancer 92:1694–1698, 2001.

van Dam FSAM, Schagen SB, Muller MJ, et al: Impairment of cognitive function in women receiving adjuvant treatment for high-risk breast cancer: High-dose versus standard-dose chemotherapy. J Nat Cancer Inst 90:210–218, 1998.

Vigliani M-C, Sichez N, Poisson M, et al: A prospective study of cognitive functions following conventional radiotherapy for supratentorial gliomas in young adults: 4-year results. Intl J Radiat Oncol Biol Phys 35:527–533, 1996.

Yang GY, Matthews RH: Prophylactic cranial irradiation in small-cell lung cancer. Oncologist 5:293–298, 2000.

Weiss HD, Walker MD, Wiernik PH: Neurotoxicity of commonly used antineoplastic agents. N Engl J Med 291:127–133, 1974.

Weitzner MA, Meyers CA, Valentine AD: Methylphenidate in the treatment of neurobehavioral slowing associated with cancer and cancer treatment. J Neuropsychiatry 7:347–350, 1995.

Weitzner MA: Psychosocial and neuropsychiatric aspects of patients with primary brain tumors. Cancer Invest 17:285–91; 296–297, 1999.

Walker LG, Walker MB, Heys SD, et al: The psychological and psychiatric effects of rIL-2 therapy: A controlled clinical trial. Psychooncology 6:290–301, 1997.

Wollman EE, Kopmels B, Bakalian A, et al: Cytokines and neuronal degeneration, in Rothwell NJ, Dantzer RD (eds): Interleukin-1 in the Brain. New York: Pergamon Press, 1992, pp. 187–203.

World Health Organization (WHO). International Classification of Impairments, Disabilities, and Handicaps. Geneva: WHO, 1980.

World Health Organization (WHO). International Classification of Functioning, Disability and Health (ICF). Geneva: WHO, 2002.

Wrensch MR, Minn Y, Bondy ML: Epidemiology, in Bernstein M, Berger MS (eds): Neuro-Oncology: The Essentials. New York: Thieme Medical, 2000, pp. 2–17.

Pediatric/Developmental Behavioral Neurology and Neuropsychology

Child Neuropsychological Assessment

Mary J. Roman

Adolescents

Assessment

Children

Cognitive

Neuropsychology

Pediatric

Testing

INTRODUCTION

Child neuropsychological assessment examines the neurobehavioral functioning of children from birth through late adolescence. A neuropsychological assessment can be sought when a child is failing to meet developmental expectations in some way, with anomalous brain function being suspected as the cause, or when there is known brain injury but its impact on cognitive functioning is unclear. Family, teachers, physicians, and others involved in the child's care may have concerns about the child's adaptation or progress at home, in school, in his or her social relationships, or in other areas critical to his or her well-being. The assessment aims to address these concerns by providing a broad-based and detailed view of the child's cognitive, emotional, and behavioral functioning through the administration of psychometric tests. Additional relevant information is obtained from medical records, direct observation of the child, and interviews with parents, teachers, and others who might have insights into the child's abilities and skills. This information is integrated into a report that describes the child's cognitive and behavioral profile, relates the findings to the presenting problem, provides a formal diagnosis, and offers recommendations for treatment.

The assessment usually begins with one or more questions posed by parents or referring professionals. They may be quite specific (e.g., "Does this child have a problem learning new information?") or more general (e.g., "Why is my child struggling in school?"). In answering the referral question, the neuropsychologist strives to educate the child, family, and others involved in the child's treatment, about the nature of the difficulties observed (Baron, 2000), with its implications for the child's current and future functioning. Another major goal is to provide a list of recommendations for addressing difficulties and capitalizing on strengths. Ultimately, the assessment should assist the child in attaining the best possible developmental course, so as to achieve independence, productivity, and emotional health as an adult (Bernstein, 2000).

CHILD VERSUS ADULT NEUROPSYCHOLOGICAL ASSESSMENT

Like its adult counterpart, child neuropsychological assessment investigates relationships between the brain and behavior, and it uses similar methods such as psychometric testing to gather information about an individual's abilities. However, it is distinct in a number of regards. Adult assessments are usually conducted on individuals who have received an injury to the brain after a course of normal development, and the question for the neuropsychologist is how the injury has affected previously intact skills and a fully functioning brain. Child assessments, however, must address how an injury or developmental anomaly has affected an immature brain in the process of organizing itself and acquiring a rapidly expanding repertoire of skills. Whereas adults lose and reacquire abilities, many scenarios are possible for children. Partially or fully acquired skills may be lost, with various levels of recovery, and skills that have barely begun to develop may fail to emerge, may be delayed in emergence, or may develop abnormally. Some deficits may not become evident until years after the injury, when the child is challenged with new developmental demands (Rourke et al., 1983; Kolb & Fantie, 1997).

Cognitive functions are localized in an adult brain such that one can often deduce the location of an adult's injury from the functions that are impaired (e.g., language deficits are associated with left brain hemisphere injury, whereas difficulty with certain aspects of visuospatial processing indicates right hemisphere injury). In children, the relationship between brain and behavior is less direct, especially early in development. Some brain regions appear specialized from birth to perform certain

brain functions, with early injuries to those regions resulting in delays or distortions in the acquisition of those functions. For example, children with early (prenatal or perinatal) focal brain lesions in the left hemisphere show greater difficulty developing language skills than those with right hemisphere damage (e.g., Vicari et al., 2000). However, the immature brain appears able to undergo neuronal reorganization, such that when a part of the brain is injured, other uncommitted or partially committed brain regions may assume functions typically localized to the injured area. Thus, children with their entire left brain hemispheres removed may nonetheless develop sufficient language skills to obtain normal-range verbal intelligence scores (Dennis & Whitaker, 1976). Longitudinal research on children with early focal brain injuries has revealed that for some cognitive skills (e.g., language and visuoconstructional or drawing skills), initial periods of impairment are followed by relative normalization of abilities. This suggests that intact brain regions that assume the functions of injured brain regions may eventually become proficient at those functions, and the degree to which the child's neurocognitive profile fits the adult brain-behavior relationship patterns will vary as a function of time after injury (Stiles et al., 1997; Vicari et al., 2000). Interestingly, other cognitive skills may be deficient in such children, suggesting that brain reorganization may come at a cost (Kolb & Fantie, 1997).

Recovery from discrete lesions in childhood may generally be better than is typically observed in adults, but outcomes from diffuse or multifocal conditions are frequently worse. Poorer cognitive outcome is associated with earlier onset in many medical conditions including hydrocephalus, child human immunodeficiency virus (HIV), diabetes, and heart disease (Dennis, 2000). It should be noted that age-related differences in outcomes might in some cases reflect age-related differences in the types of brain insults most commonly experienced (Tramontana & Hooper, 1988).

Problems relating neuropsychological deficits to brain regions in children are compounded by additional factors. When the child's difficulties do not appear to be developmental in origin, but rather begin after a period of presumably normal development, there may be difficulty determining the exact time of onset of dysfunction, and information about premorbid neuropsychological functioning may be lacking. Furthermore, one must factor in the presence of environmental variables that influence cognitive outcomes, such as family stresses or resources (Aylward, 1988; Tramontana & Hooper, 1988; Taylor & Schatschneider, 1992; Max et al., 1999).

Because of these complexities, neuropsychological reports on children will typically emphasize the cognitive and behavioral profiles obtained and their implications for treatment, rather than localization of brain lesion. Exceptions to this may be found in cases of discrete injury in older adolescents, whose postinjury presentation and course may more closely follow the pattern seen in adults. It is also common in child evaluations to find that the neuropsychologist has taken a brain-oriented approach to test selection and analysis of findings, using general principles of functional organization within the adult brain to guide the design and interpretation of their test battery (Bernstein, 2000).

Another distinction between adult and child neuropsychological assessment is that school functioning figures more prominently in the child assessment, whereas employment-related or independent living issues are a focus for adults. With children, skill levels across academic domains are typically examined, as well as the component skills that underlie school achievement, including attention, ability to understand and follow directions, learning of new information, and retrieval of previously learned information. To obtain an appropriately comprehensive view of the child, it is often necessary for the child neuropsychologist to administer academic achievement measures or to integrate educational testing done by other professionals into the neuropsychological report. The neuropsychologist must also be familiar with the educational demands placed on children of different ages and must be able to interact with school personnel to gather information, report back on results, and participate in educational planning.

A methodological difference between adult and child assessments involves the measures used. Child assessment uses tests "normed" specifically for child populations. Unlike adult measures, which are typically intended for use throughout the adult years, children's measures target narrower age ranges such as birth to 1 year or ages 9 through 14. This is essential, because the skills that are important to assess change throughout childhood (e.g., response to sound in infancy versus reasoning and judgment in adolescence). The behavioral repertoires of children evolve over time as well; one cannot assess language comprehension or drawing skill in an infant, for example. By mid-adolescence, neuropsychological test performance is very similar to that of adults (Halstead, 1950), and a test battery for older teens may include adult measures. Child neuropsychologists must be aware of how testing requirements change across the age range of children within their practice, and professionals who conduct child neuropsychological assessments should expect to see a variety of measures used across patients of different ages.

WHEN TO REFER A CHILD FOR NEUROPSYCHOLOGICAL TESTING

It is likely that the number of children who are appropriate candidates for neuropsychological assessment is on the rise. Thanks to advances in medicine, many more children are surviving serious medical disorders, but as a consequence of these disorders or their treatment, they are experiencing neurologic difficulties that need to be identified and addressed. In addition, changes in educational legislation over the past three decades have increased the need for schools to obtain detailed information about the cognitive functioning of children with neurologic and neurodevelopmental disorders to provide them with adequate educational services (Tramontana & Hooper, 1988). According to one estimate extrapolated from pediatricians' reports of their patient base, the average pediatrician will see a child with a neurobehavioral disorder about once every other day (Bigler et al., 1997). Common conditions associated with potential neuropsychological deficits are learning disorders, traumatic brain injury, epilepsy, low birth weight, and hydrocephalus (Hauser & Hesdorffer, 1990; Gaddes & Edgell, 1993; Kraus, 1995; Paneth, 1995; Fletcher et al., 2000). Rarer conditions with possible neuropsychological sequelae include brain tumors, central nervous system (CNS) infections, exposure to neurotoxic substances, HIV, neurofibromatosis, neurodegenerative disorders, and certain metabolic disorders such as phenylketonuria (Hartman, 1995; Berg & Linton, 1997; Welsh & Pennington, 2000). Neuropsychological deficits are also being found in a growing number of medical disorders that are not specifically neurologic, such as sickle cell disease, acute lymphocytic leukemia, diabetes, and end-stage renal disease (Berg & Linton, 1997; Fennell, 2000). Attention-deficit/hyperactivity disorder (ADHD), autism, and other psychiatric disorders are associated with neuropsychological dysfunction as well (Tramontana & Hooper, 1997). (See also Chapters 42 and 43.)

Obtaining a neuropsychological assessment should be considered whenever there are concerns about a child's ability to function cognitively or behaviorally in one or more environments, and it is suspected that the problem is brain-based in origin. The following is a list of circumstances in which one might want to pursue testing. This list is not meant to be comprehensive but rather to suggest some of the more common scenarios in which neuropsychological testing is likely to be helpful.

1. The child has a known neurologic condition that is commonly associated with cognitive deficits, such as severe traumatic brain injury, and either the child has not yet undergone a neuropsychological evaluation or the last evaluation does not provide sufficiently current information for adequate treatment planning. Thus, the disorder's effects on cognitive and behavioral functioning at the present time need to be determined.
2. The child has a disorder that either is not considered neurologic (e.g., sickle cell disease or diabetes) or does not have a well-defined neurologic basis (e.g., a learning disability),

but nonetheless is associated with cognitive difficulties and therefore raises questions regarding the child's neurocognitive or neurobehavioral functioning. There may be no awareness as yet that the child has cognitive difficulties, but the disorder would suggest that the likelihood of deficits is high. Alternatively, cognitive or behavioral deficits may have been observed, but their nature and magnitude remain unknown.

3. The child is having cognitive or behavioral difficulties of unclear etiology and neuropsychological testing is sought to clarify the nature and extent of the problem. For example, a preschooler might be exhibiting delays in the acquisition of motor and language skills, or a school-aged child might be struggling to master basic reading and math skills. Obvious neurologic disease may or may not be present. A neuropsychological evaluation may be particularly helpful when the child's problem is complex and requires consideration of multiple aspects of functioning (e.g., cognitive, emotional, behavioral, adaptive, familial, medical).

4. The child has not yet entered school and school readiness is in question due to a history of neurologic or other risk factors for cognitive difficulties (Hartlage, 1986). Testing may help the child's family and educators time the start of school more appropriately to reduce the likelihood of negative academic outcomes. Interventions to increase the child's school preparedness can also be planned and implemented.

5. The child needs to have a disability formally documented for purposes of obtaining special services (e.g., disability compensation) or academic accommodations (e.g., extended time for standardized testing).

6. The child has previously been evaluated by a non-neuropsychologist (e.g., by a school psychologist in the public schools), and the findings raise questions about cognitive functioning that require further investigation. The child can then undergo a partial neuropsychological evaluation that incorporates the previously obtained test findings but focuses new testing on the cognitive areas in question.

7. The child has been evaluated in the past, but more current information is sought to document changes in the child's condition, to evaluate treatment effectiveness, or to guide adjustments in treatment procedures.

Initial evaluations are often important in determining the presence of a cognitive disorder, documenting its characteristics, and setting in motion a plan of treatment to address the difficulties found. Periodic retesting is frequently a critical part of follow-up because it can identify treatment-related changes in symptom presentation and enables the treatment team to adjust interventions accordingly. Symptoms may also evolve with development, changes in the child's medical condition, or changes in other risk factors such as family stress or emotional status (Dennis, 2000). Retesting may be important even when the child's condition appears to remain stable over time because the child's behaviors and needs evolve over time. Different abilities may need to be investigated across evaluations, depending on developmental expectations and environmental demands.

Several avenues for assessment are often available to children, though what is available varies by state and school district. School-aged children with academic difficulties can undergo assessments of intellectual, academic achievement, and emotional/behavioral functioning through the public schools, at no cost to parents. Alternatively, parents may elect to have their child's aptitude and achievement evaluated privately by a psychologist outside the school system. For some children, standard intellectual and achievement testing may be adequate, but in other cases, a more comprehensive, neuropsychologically oriented look at a child's abilities is necessary to clarify the nature of the problem and to formulate an appropriate treatment plan. When a neuropsychological evaluation follows another type of evaluation, the neuropsychologist may incorporate that prior information into the neuropsychological assessment if the previous tests are relevant and administered within a time frame that permits their utilization. A collaborative evaluation such as this can be an efficient and cost-effective way to obtain important information about a child's developmental needs (Reynolds & Mayfield, 1999).

Research suggests that parents of children with developmental disabilities consider evaluation of their children's difficulties to be an important component of quality health care (Rosenbaum et al., 1992). Parents have reported dissatisfaction when their children's disabilities are not identified early, when they are not given adequate information about the developmental implications of their child's disabilities, or when an effective referral system for treatment is lacking (Fischler & Tancer, 1984; O'Sullivan et al., 1992). However, when treatment includes a referral for in-depth evaluation of their children's difficulties, or when specific suggestions for improving or dealing with the difficulties are provided, parents tend to take a more favorable view of the services they are receiving (Kanoy & Schroeder, 1985).

FINANCIAL CONSIDERATIONS

The cost of a full assessment outside the public schools may exceed $1000, although cost will likely vary depending on the region of the country in which the assessment is being conducted, the complexity of the case, the extent of the evaluation, and the time taken to complete it. There may be extra charges for activities such as feedback sessions, school meetings, consultations with other professionals, and treatment sessions. Screening evaluations may be available for a lesser cost but may need to be followed up with a full evaluation if results suggest possible impairment.

Insurance coverage for neuropsychological testing varies from one plan to another. The family's health insurance will dictate whether their child has access to a neuropsychologist through their plan and how the evaluation should be initiated. For example, a referral may need to come from a primary care physician. Obtaining prior approval for testing may be a necessary and lengthy process; a physician or neuropsychologist may have to justify in writing the medical necessity of the evaluation or to submit for review and prior approval a list of tests to be administered. Academic achievement testing may be excluded from coverage because it is a service provided by schools. If coverage for the remainder of the evaluation is denied, or if a family does not have health insurance, and they nonetheless wish to pursue testing, they can obtain an evaluation from a neuropsychologist on a fee-for-service basis.

RELIABILITY AND VALIDITY OF TESTING

Research into the reliability and validity of child neuropsychological tests investigates how stable and meaningful test results are. This branch of child neuropsychological research needs greater attention and development, but work done thus far has yielded a number of positive findings. A starting point for establishing the reliability and validity of neuropsychological assessment is the battery of tests used. Each test possesses its own psychometric properties, which should be taken into consideration when the neuropsychologist is selecting a group of measures for an assessment. These properties vary across tests, but there are many measures available that are considered psychometrically adequate (e.g., Williams & Boll, 1997; Franzen, 2000). Also of concern are the ability of neuropsychologists to use tests reliably and the relevance of testing for the child's functional adaptation (Yeates & Taylor, 1998). Inter-rater agreement in child neuropsychological test interpretation and diagnosis has been examined, with good to excellent agreement in ratings of patient impairment and diagnosis (Waber et al., 1992; Brown et al.,

1993). Child neuropsychological tests themselves have been found to be sensitive to severity of neurologic impairment and predictive of academic skills, behavioral adjustment, and adaptive functioning in children with a history of neurologic compromise (Taylor & Schatschneider, 1992). A number of neuropsychological measures have been found to predict academic achievement independent of overall intellectual ability (Hartlage & Templer, 1996), which suggests that neuropsychological testing makes a unique contribution to the understanding of a child's school performance.

Such findings support the perception of child neuropsychological assessment as a useful tool for parents, teachers, and health professionals. However, future research will need to examine further whether test results adequately capture children's observed deficiencies outside of the testing environment and can predict a child's later functioning and response to particular treatments. Challenges to attaining this goal include (1) the disparity between the tightly controlled environment of neuropsychological testing and the greater variability and complexity of life outside of testing, (2) possible effects of treatments and environmental accommodations such that children's abilities are constantly changing and their difficulties are obscured, and (3) difficulties in selecting and evaluating outcome measures that capture "real-world" functioning (Silver, 2000). It has been suggested that studies investigating neuropsychological test validity ought to examine a broader range of outcomes rather than focusing on academic achievement, which has been the tendency, and predictive validity research should address whether children with particular cognitive profiles benefit from specific types of interventions (Yeates & Taylor, 1998). As neuropsychological measures become more refined, we will ideally attain greater precision in linking test results to the child's real-world functioning and intervention needs.

TESTING PROCEDURES

Obtaining Background Information

An assessment typically begins by gathering background information that will guide the rest of the evaluation. A typical starting point is a clinical interview with the child and parents. Early in the interview, the neuropsychologist elicits information about the presenting problem, including the timing and characteristics of its onset, symptoms, factors that influence it positively or negatively, and responses to past attempts at treatment. The neuropsychologist will also attempt to determine if the difficulties have always been present or arose following a period of normal development. One might expect different profiles of cognitive functioning from a child who never experienced a period of normalcy versus a child whose injury interrupted the functioning of previously intact brain systems, with the latter child possibly displaying more circumscribed deficits (Rourke et al., 1986).

Other elements of a good clinical history include: (1) information about the child's prenatal, birth, and early developmental history, such as in utero drug or alcohol exposure, birth trauma, and developmental milestones; (2) the child's medical history, with particular attention to factors associated with neuropsychological difficulties, such as neurologic illnesses, malnutrition, head injuries, exposure to toxins such as lead paint, or chronic ear infections; (3) medications currently being taken by the child; (4) psychiatric history; and (5) history of academic progress, including any grade repetitions or special educational assistance. Family history should be reviewed, including family composition, medical, psychiatric, and academic history in immediate and extended family members, and history of significant family stresses or traumas. Indications of familial neuropsychological dysfunction should be noted. Findings of difficulties or anomalies in the child's or family's history increase the likelihood that the presenting problem has a constitutional or neuropsychological basis (Yeates & Taylor, 1998). To gather the necessary historical information, the neuropsychologist may need to interview collateral informants such as teachers, physicians, tutors, and therapists. Their input may also be elicited through the completion of questionnaires or checklists.

Information should be gathered about each environment in which the child functions, which may include home, school, time spent with childcare providers or relatives, and recreational or social time. Inconsistencies across environments in symptom expression are important to note, as they have implications for understanding the cause of the child's problem. For example, a child with significant attentional problems only at school may not have a primary attentional disorder, but rather anxiety-related inattention due to a learning disability or difficulties with peer relationships.

A review of records is an important step in the assessment process. Medical records are typically reviewed if the child has a significant medical history and relevant records can be accessed. Surgical records, neuroimaging results, and electroencephalographic findings provide critical information. Evaluations by speech and language pathologists, physical and occupational therapists, and mental health staff can also be important in shaping the neuropsychological assessment. If the child has been in rehabilitation, records of treatments and outcomes should be examined. Academic records are another rich source of information about the child, including standardized test scores, report cards, reports of past school assessments, records of special educational plans, and samples of academic work. Past psychological reports should be carefully reviewed, unless there is a particular reason for not doing so, as in the case of a family who is seeking an independent second opinion concerning their child's functioning and would like the examiner to be blind to previous examiners' findings.

Assessed formally or informally, mental status and behavioral observations before and during testing are critical pieces of information to gather throughout the evaluation (Rourke et al., 1986). As part of the mental status examination, one must ascertain whether the child is sufficiently awake, alert, oriented, and attentive to participate meaningfully in the examination. Hearing and vision should be checked directly or by obtaining records of recent testing. Affect, frustration tolerance, thought content and process, and the quality of the child's relationship with the examiner may point toward psychological or psychiatric issues that bear on test interpretation. Observations of the child's gait, balance, physical coordination, general appearance, activity level, characteristics of speech, and reasoning and judgment can direct the neuropsychologist toward particular areas of functioning, which may require more in-depth testing. In addition, the child's level of motivation and attitude toward testing must be evaluated by the examiner because they influence the validity of the assessment.

Selection of Tests

With this information in mind, the neuropsychologist selects a test battery to investigate further the difficulties reported. Neuropsychological batteries often consist of many tests covering a wide range of cognitive and behavioral functions and requiring several hours to administer. This is appropriate, because brain injury can be quite variable in its effects, even within a single disorder, and a broad-ranging battery is often needed to capture the many possible outcomes (Tramontana & Hooper, 1988). In some circumstances, it will not be possible to conduct a full examination. For example, the child may be too ill to participate in a lengthy assessment, or the family's insurance may allow only a brief evaluation. In such cases, the neuropsychologist may administer a short screening battery that briefly surveys major domains of functioning for signs of difficulty. This would not be meant to replace a full battery but to indicate if further evaluation were warranted.

Neuropsychologists differ in how they select their test batteries. Some take a "fixed battery approach," administering the same group of tests regardless of the presenting problem. Commonly administered fixed batteries are the Reitan-Indiana Neuropsychological Test Battery for Children for ages 5 to 8 (Reitan, 1969), the Halstead Neuropsychological Test Battery for Children for ages 9 to 14 (Reitan & Wolfson, 1974), the Luria-Nebraska Neuropsychological Battery—Children's

Revision for ages 8 to 12 (Golden, 1986), and the NEPSY for ages 3 to 12 (Korkman et al., 1998). Proponents of the "flexible battery approach" create their own batteries, tailoring their selection of standardized tests to the individual child. More qualitative approaches to assessment focus on *how* the child performs the tasks at hand, gathering useful clinical information from such features as task strategies used and the type and pattern of errors. Qualitative assessment techniques include informal testing procedures and modification of tests to yield more information about why an individual is performing poorly.

There are advantages and disadvantages to each of the above approaches (Tramontana & Hooper, 1988). Some neuropsychologists prefer the fixed battery approach because of psychometric concerns. Unlike flexible batteries, fixed batteries have been validated as a unit, typically to discriminate brain-impaired from non–brain-impaired children. However, no battery covers all cognitive skills, leaving open the possibility that significant cognitive deficits may go undetected. With the flexible battery approach, a neuropsychologist can administer measures that have not as a group been subjected to validation studies, but individually have good psychometric properties. Tests are usually chosen to cover a broad range of skills, and particular areas of cognitive functioning can be examined in greater depth to address a referral question or test a hypothesis about the nature of the child's deficits. Qualitative approaches to assessment lend themselves well to hypothesis testing, but interpretations of findings may be based on clinical judgment rather than standardization data, and administration techniques may be difficult to master for individuals not specifically trained in them (Reynolds & Mayfield, 1999). In practice, it is very common for clinicians to mix approaches, for example, administering a standard battery and augmenting it with additional measures for hypothesis-testing purposes or to examine additional cognitive skills. Because of this, the psychometric properties (e.g., reliability and validity) of the assessment as a whole will likely vary across evaluations.

Within a test battery, it is common for test complexity to vary from purer measures of discrete abilities to more complex or multiskill tasks, which may be more reflective of the child's ability to cope with difficult environmental challenges (Rourke et al., 1986). One test selection strategy is to administer more complex measures that require a range of intact skills; if the child has difficulty on a complex task, additional, simpler tests can be administered to identify the intact and impaired component skills underlying the deficient task performance. It is also common for areas of suspected dysfunction to be investigated in greater depth through the administration of tests targeting individual component skills.

Early Childhood Assessment

There has been a growing interest in infant and early childhood neuropsychological assessment, in part due to the greater survival rates of very-low-birth-weight and premature infants and the need to identify those at risk for later neurobehavioral difficulties. Of necessity, infant assessment measures differ in length and item type from those used with school-aged children. Infants possess limitations in language, motor, and other skills that restrict the range of activities one can use to glean information about cognitive processing. Their participation in a formal assessment may be greatly influenced by more pressing needs for nourishment, sleep, and comforting, and critical neurologic variables such as the quality of their reflexes, habituation to external stimuli, and muscle tone vary as a function of their sleep/wake state (Prechtl, 1977). Clearly, the need for clinical flexibility and familiarity with children in this age range is crucial for a successful testing experience. Not surprisingly, test scores obtained from infants tend to be poor predictors of later functioning (Molfese, 1992). However, assessment can facilitate early diagnosis and problem-focused treatment (Reynolds & Mayfield, 1999).

Infant tests vary in the depth and breadth with which the child's skills are evaluated. Screening measures are generally briefer and easier to administer; they are intended to identify infants at risk who should undergo more in-depth testing. Lengthier measures are also available to evaluate infants with likely neurologic dysfunction. Such measures provide more detailed information about the type and extent of the infant's difficulties and can provide a basis for tracking changes in functioning over time. Some item types found on infant assessment scales include response to stimulation, muscle movement and tone, reflexes, object permanence, social responsiveness, vocalizations, and behaviors such as crying, alertness, and consolability (Molfese, 1992).

Areas of functioning that are typically assessed in children from later infancy through age 2 years include memory and learning, speech and language, motor skills, self-help skills, and social-emotional development. Information about the child is gleaned from parent interviews or questionnaires in combination with direct testing of the child (Spreen et al., 1995). As with infants, tester experience and flexibility can assist in circumventing difficulties that might arise in testing due to attentional, motivational, or temperamental factors. For example, extra time in the assessment may need to be devoted to building rapport, a parent may need to be present during testing, and the evaluation may need to be conducted as a play session with the child. By age 2, the ability of test scores to predict later functioning has become more robust (Hartlage, 1986), possibly due in part to the greater similarity between abilities assessed in 2-year-olds and those examined in older children.

Some of the simpler tests used with older children are also appropriate for use with 2-year-olds.

From ages 3 through 6, the range of behaviors amenable to formal testing greatly expands. In most cases, language skills have advanced to the point that the child can follow commands and use sentences to answer questions, discuss events, and describe objects. Motor and sensory skills permit the child to copy increasingly complex drawings and eventually to identify objects by touch. Verbal logical reasoning skills can usually be assessed by the middle of the child's fifth year (Hartlage, 1986). At 5 or 6 years of age, children without severe deficits are typically able to use the test measures designed for school-aged children.

Aylward (1988) has proposed a classification schema for the components of a neuropsychological assessment during early childhood. Domains of functioning within this system are listed in Table 39-1. According to Aylward's schema, assessment of younger infants focuses on the intactness of neurologic functions, gross motor ability, and mental activity (i.e., activity level and level of consciousness). In later infancy, receptive, expressive, and processing skills such as visual perceptual ability, eye-hand coordination, and object permanency are the focus. There is some continued consideration of mental activity and basic neurologic functions at this age. In the toddler and preschool years, neurologic function and mental activity are deemphasized, but receptive, expressive, and processing skills are examined more thoroughly. For example, object naming, drawing ability, and recall of objects presented visually may be assessed in the preschooler. Table 39-2 lists several measures the child neuropsychologist may use to assess cognitive and motor functioning in children from infancy through the preschool years, with approximate time to complete each measure. Although some of these measures are best known as providing an index of global functioning (e.g., the Stanford-Binet Intelligence Scale or the Wechsler Preschool and Primary Scale of Intelligence-III [WPPSI-III]), their subtests provide information about abilities in more discrete skill areas, which enhances their value to the neuropsychologist.

Assessment of School-Aged Children

By the time children enter school, it is possible to examine the cognitive, behavioral, sensory, and motor domains routinely investigated in adult neuropsychological evaluations. These domains are described below. Table 39-3 provides examples of tests that measure these skills in the school-aged child. The tests chosen are a small subset of the many instruments child neuropsychologists have at their disposal.

Time to complete neuropsychological testing with school-aged children can vary greatly from one assessment to another. Many factors will influence the duration of the evaluation, including the referral question, the child's profile of intact and deficient skills, the tests chosen, and the limitations imposed by the child's health insurance. The child's age, ability level, speed of responding, and compliance will also impact testing time. For example, adolescents will often require more testing time than younger children because they are usually able to complete more test items within a measure and have more cognitive and academic skill areas to evaluate. As another example, children with intact performance on screening measures within a domain may complete the evaluation of that domain in a brief period of time, whereas the time required for adequate domain assessment in a child exhibiting deficiencies may be much longer. Overall intellectual ability, if assessed with measures such as those listed in Table 39-3, will typically take 1 to 1.5 hours to administer. Assessment of the remaining areas of functioning may take 10 to 30 minutes or more depending on the quality of the child's performance and the depth and breadth of information needed to address the referral question. Thus, one should not be surprised to hear of testing times ranging from 2 to 6 hours or more.

TABLE 39-1. Aylward's Classification Schema for Components of an Early Childhood Neuropsychological Assessment

Functional domain	Examples of abilities assessed
Basic neurologic functions	Early reflexes
	Visual tracking skills
	Comparison of left- and right-side motor skills
	Muscle tone
Receptive or sensory processing	Visual perception
	Auditory perception
	Language comprehension
Expressive functions	Oral language
	Drawing ability
	Fine motor skills
	Gross motor skills
Processing	Memory and learning
	Thinking/reasoning
	Problem solving
	Verbal and nonverbal abstracting
Mental activity	Activity level
	Level of consciousness
	Alertness

Note. Data from *Assessment Issues in Child Neuropsychology* (p. 232), by Tramontana MG and Hooper SR (eds.): New York: Plenum Press, 1988.

TABLE 39-2. Examples of Measures Used in Early Childhood Neuropsychological Assessment

Test	Age range	Approximate time to administer*
Bayley Scales of Infant Development-II	1–42 mo	25–35 min for children under 15 mo; up to 1 hr for children over 15 mo
Mullen Scales of Early Learning	Birth to 5 yr 8 mo	15 min to 1 hr, with lengthier assessments for older children
Stanford-Binet Intelligence Scale, ed 5	2 yr to adult	45–60 min for younger children
Differential Ability Scales (DAS)	2 yr 6 mo to 17 yr 11 mo	45–65 min for cognitive portion of battery
Wechsler Preschool and Primary Scale of Intelligence-III (WPPSI-III)	2 yr 6 mo to 7 years 3 mo	30–45 min for ages 2–3; 45–60 min for ages 4–7
NEPSY	3–12 yr	1 hr for ages 3–4; 2 hr for ages 5–12

* According to product information provided by the test publishers.

TABLE 39-3. Examples of Measures Evaluating Neuropsychological Domains in School-Aged Children

Domain	Measures
Intellectual ability	Wechsler Intelligence Scale for Children-IV (WISC IV) Standford-Binet Intelligence Scale, ed 5 Differential Ability Scales Kaufman Assessment Battery for Children
Verbal skills	WISC-IV Vocabulary subtest NEPSY Language Domain subtests Boston Naming Test Peabody Picture Vocabulary Test-III Test of Language Development, ed 3 Comprehensive Test of Phonological Processing Clinical Evaluation of Language Fundamentals, ed 4
Visuoperceptual, visuospatial, and visuomotor skills	WISC-IV Picture Completion, Block Design, and Object Assembly subtests NEPSY Visuospatial Processing Domain subtests Hooper Visual Organization Test Benton Judgment of Line Orientation Test Beery Developmental Test of Visual-Motor Integration, ed 4 Rey-Osterrieth Complex Figure, Copy Condition
Attention	WISC-IV Digit Span subtest NEPSY Auditory Attention and Response Set and Visual Attention subtests Conners' Continuous Performance Test-II Test of Variables of Attention
Learning and memory	NEPSY Memory and Learning Domain subtests Wide Range Assessment of Memory and Learning Test of Memory and Learning Children's Memory Scale California Verbal Learning Test-Children's Version Rey-Osterrieth Complex Figure, Delayed Recall Condition
Motor and psychomotor functioning	Lateral Dominance Examination Right-Left Orientation Test Grip Strength Test Finger Tapping Test Lafayette Grooved Pegboard Test WISC-IV Coding subtest
Sensory-perceptual functioning	Reitan-Kløve Sensory-Perceptual Examination NEPSY Finger Discrimination Subtest

Continued

TABLE 39-3. Examples of Measures Evaluating Neuropsychological Domains in School-Aged Children—cont'd

Domain	Measures
Executive functioning, reasoning, and concept formation	WISC-IV Similarities and Comprehension subtests
	Verbal Fluency Test
	NEPSY Tower, Statue, Design Fluency, Knock and Tap, and Auditory Attention and Response Set subtests
	Children's Category Test
	Wisconsin Card Sorting Test
	Trail Making Test
	Delis-Kaplan Executive Function System
Academic achievement	Wechsler Individual Achievement Test, ed 2
	Wide Range Achievement Test, ed 3
	Peabody Individual Achievement Test-Revised
	Woodcock Johnson III Tests of Achievement
	Woodcock Diagnostic Reading Battery
	Gray Oral Reading Tests, ed 4
	Key Math Test-Revised
Adaptive functioning and psychological status	Vineland Adaptive Behavior Scales
	Achenbach Child Behavior Checklist, Teacher's Report Form, and Youth Self-Report Form
	Conners Rating Scales-Revised
	Children's Depression Inventory
	State-Trait Anxiety Inventory for Children
	Minnesota Multiphasic Personality Inventory (MMPI)-Adolescent

Intellectual Ability

A child neuropsychological assessment usually includes a measure of intellectual function, or an IQ test. The most frequently used IQ tests are comprised of a number of subtests assessing different cognitive abilities. The overall IQ score essentially averages a child's score across subtests and thus indicates the typical level of performance across cognitive domains. In neurologically intact individuals, this score is informative because abilities across domains tend to be similar in the normal population (Matarazzo & Prifitera, 1989). IQ tests are familiar to many non-neuropsychologists, and may therefore provide an accessible introduction to the rest of the evaluation. In addition, IQ scores are often required for children to be considered for special assistance such as disability compensation or special educational services. For example, many schools use a discrepancy formula to determine the presence of a learning disability, whereby a child must have a discrepancy of a certain magnitude between IQ and achievement test scores to be considered learning disabled.

In terms of identifying specific neuropsychological deficits, however, the IQ test has limited value (Lezak, 1995). Averaging scores across subtests to arrive at a general score means losing valuable information about performance in the domains assessed by the subtests. If one were looking for discrete areas of deficit, one would be more likely to get that information from individual subtest scores. Furthermore, when a child has an uneven cognitive profile, an overall IQ score by itself could be misleading. Consider a hypothetical IQ test comprised half of language skills subtests and half of visual skills subtests. A child who excels on language tasks and is severely impaired on visual tasks might obtain an average-range IQ, but that IQ would not reflect the child's performance on either language or visual tasks.

From a neuropsychological perspective, another problem with IQ tests is that they do not assess all abilities that could be affected by neurologic compromise (Yeates & Taylor, 1998). IQ scores can remain remarkably intact in the face of significant brain injury, whereas other skills not assessed, such as learning and memory, organizational skills, or motivation can be seriously impaired. A normal-range IQ score in a child's evaluation should not be taken as an indication that the child is unimpaired. Rather, when neurologic issues are of concern, one must look at individual subtests and other measures administered for evidence of deficiencies, which may in some cases be very focal.

Nonetheless, the convention is to administer a full IQ test, or at least enough subtests to yield an IQ estimate. To obtain information from the IQ test about more specific areas of deficit, one can examine individual subtest scores or summary scores derived from groupings of subtests assessing similar kinds of abilities (e.g., language skills or attention-related abilities).

Verbal Skills

The child's language ability deserves close scrutiny in the neuropsychological evaluation. Language plays a central role in many aspects of development and is often found to be deficient in children with learning disorders and brain injuries (Ewing-Cobbs et al., 1987). Language skill is critical for social interaction, academic achievement, and complex thought (Spreen et al., 1995). It follows that children with deficient language skills may have serious problems relating to peers and family, may experience prolonged and pervasive school failure, and may have difficulty with independent living when they enter adulthood. Identifying these problems and offering early remediation may enable the child to avoid years of difficulty.

Language evaluation may be accomplished through the use of a number of comprehensive test batteries of language development, as well as individual measures assessing more discrete linguistic abilities. Aspects of language to consider in an evaluation include object naming, comprehension of word meanings, the ability to understand grammatical structures of varying complexity and produce grammatical utterances, and comprehension and production of sentences and paragraphs (Spreen & Strauss, 1998). Assessment of phonological awareness, or the appreciation of letter-sound relationships, may be particularly important in evaluation of children with reading disabilities. This may be accomplished through the use of tasks evaluating the ability to segment words into component sounds, to substitute sounds within words, or to rhyme.

Visuoperceptual, Visuospatial, and Visuomotor Skills

The abilities in this category relate to the perception, analysis, manipulation, localization, and organization of visual information such as a picture or a three-dimensional form (Benton & Tranel, 1993). Deficits in this domain may interfere with the ability to find one's way from one place to another, to understand charts and graphs, and to interpret nonverbal cues such as body posture and facial expression. Such deficits have been associated with learning disabilities in mathematics (Rourke, 1989).

Visuoperceptual skill is the ability to perceive and discriminate visual images. It can be assessed by tasks that involve identification of an image or its features. Visuospatial skill allows one to appreciate the spatial configuration of a visually perceived form or the relationship among its parts. Tasks assessing this skill might require the child to arrange blocks to copy a pictorial model or to identify objects from their parts. Visuomotor or visuoconstructional skill is the ability to integrate visual perception and motor skill, and it is typically assessed through building, drawing, or figure-copying tasks. Many tasks assessing abilities in this domain are timed tasks and involve manipulation of materials or use of drawing implements. Interpretation of deficits on such tasks requires one to discriminate among problems with perception, the ability to analyze a form's spatial properties, motor dexterity, and motor or processing speed.

Patterns of spatial, analytic, and visuomotor deficit tend to differ as a function of the side of neurologic insult in the brain. Injury to the left hemisphere in adults tends to interfere with the ability to appreciate and render visual details, whereas right hemisphere injury produces deficits relating to the global form or overall configuration of visual images (Delis et al., 1988). This same distinction is found for a period of time even in children whose lateralized brain insults occurred in infancy (Stiles et al., 1997). Thus, analysis of detail versus configural aspects of children's drawings as well as their errors or task strategies on other spatial tasks can provide clues as to localization of their impairment within the brain.

Attention

The ability to attend is a prerequisite for other nonautomatic, goal-oriented, meaningful cognitive activities such as conversing, creating, and learning. It is a relatively fragile cognitive ability and is among the most commonly reported deficits in cases of brain injury (Reynolds & Mayfield, 1999). Developmentally based attentional dysfunction is also common, with the prevalence of ADHD falling at around 3% to 5% of school-aged children (American Psychiatric Association, 1994). Components of attention that may need to be assessed in an evaluation include attention span, or the quantity of discrete bits of information that can be attended to at once; focused attention, which involves directing one's attention to a stimulus and screening out competing distracting stimuli; sustained attention, which is the maintenance of attentional focus over a lengthy period of time; divided attention, the division of one's attention across two or more tasks that are simultaneously being performed; and shifting of attention from one stimulus to another.

Learning and Memory

Problems with learning and memory are also common in cases of brain injury, with the formation of new memories being particularly vulnerable (Reynolds & Mayfield, 1999). Profound amnesia, such as is observed in adults with Alzheimer disease or Korsakoff syndrome, is rarely seen in children, but particular patterns of memory impairment have been associated with a number of disorders in children (Roman et al., 1998; Mattson & Riley, 1999). Memory deficits can be devastating for children, who spend much of their time in learning activities and who must encode and retain large amounts of new information to meet developmental expectations. Components of memory include characteristics of learning, such as learning capacity and learning strategies used; storage or retention of information over time; and the ability to retrieve stored information at will. Verbal and visual learning modalities can be differentially affected by brain injury and deserve separate consideration in a test battery. Remote memory, or memory for information learned well in the past, is typically resistant to brain damage but may be assessed through formal tests or informal questioning. Other characteristics of the material to be learned, such as meaningfulness and complexity, may affect learning proficiency, and tasks that vary along these dimensions can provide useful information for treatment planning.

Motor and Psychomotor Functioning

In the neuropsychological examination, laterality of motor function, especially hand dominance, is examined. Hand dominance has been associated with a number of neurobehavioral variables including the side of language lateralization in the adult brain, aptitude on visuospatial tasks, and both extremely high and extremely low cognitive functioning (Lezak, 1995). Motor abilities are also typically assessed, including grip strength, fine motor speed, and fine motor dexterity. Motor tasks may require children to insert pegs into holes or to tap their index finger as rapidly as possible. Absolute level of performance is considered, as well as the comparison between right and left hand performance, which could indicate lateralization of brain impairment. Psychomotor test measures are often administered to examine fine motor dexterity or speed in conjunction with a more cognitively complex task. Handwriting may be evaluated for fluency, accuracy, and legibility.

Sensory-Perceptual Functioning

Intact sensory functioning is essential to the learning process because incoming information must be perceived accurately to be learned accurately. Standard tests of sensory-perceptual functioning evaluate tactile, auditory, and visual perception. Tasks may compare perception with and without competing stimuli and may vary the complexity of the stimuli to be perceived. In the visual domain, intactness of the visual fields is often tested. Perception of smell is not routinely tested

but can be evaluated when concerns exist, as is sometimes the case with traumatic brain injuries.

Executive Functioning

Abilities within this domain concern the organization and direction of one's behavior. Lezak (1995) identifies four component skills in this domain, which are (1) volition, which involves awareness of one's own needs and the motivation to pursue those needs; (2) planning, which includes organizational skills and the ability to conceive of and evaluate choices; (3) purposive action, or the ability to initiate, maintain, adjust, and stop one's behavior in an appropriate manner; and (4) effective performance, which requires self-monitoring, self-correction, and self-regulation. These skills do not reach maturity until sometime in adolescence or later, and many executive skills do not become part of a child's behavioral repertoire until adolescence, concurrent with an increase in expectations for youth to direct and organize their own behavior. For example, it is rare to see grade school-aged children purposefully and effectively using specific memorization or recall strategies to improve their performance on memory tasks, but adolescents regularly do so (Delis et al., 1994). In children, motivation and self-monitoring are often evaluated informally, through observation, or from reports of collateral informants. Planning, initiation, and maintenance and shifting of behavior in response to feedback are typically measured with formal tests.

Reasoning and Concept Formation

Activities that fall into this domain involve abstract thinking, logic, judgment, and comprehension of relationships among words, pictures, or other stimuli (Lezak, 1995). Some of the test formats used to tap into these skills include analogy tests, measures in which the child must describe how several things are alike, and tasks requiring the child to explain what they should do when faced with various problems. For many of these skills, visual versus verbal capacities may be compared.

Academic Achievement

For school-aged children, performance on academic tasks is important to examine as part of the overall assessment, if recent achievement testing is not available. Problems with learning may be the reason for the evaluation or may be only one of many problems resulting from a brain injury or disorder. Areas most commonly assessed are reading, written expression, and mathematics. Younger children may be asked to write their name, the alphabet, and numbers from 1 to 10. In older children, reading skills to examine include single-word reading, which reflects the child's word attack skills and sight vocabulary; nonsense word reading, which indicates knowledge of sound-symbol relationships and the ability to sound out novel words; and reading of prose passages, which can provide a view of reading fluency, reading rate, and reading comprehension. Written expression skills can be investigated through the use of single-word spelling tests, which indicate rote memorization of spelling and knowledge of spelling rules, and paragraph- or story-writing tasks, which contribute information about contextual spelling skills and ability to organize written information. Math skills to assess include written and mental calculations, understanding of basic and advanced number concepts, and mathematical reasoning such as is required to set up and solve algebraic equations.

Adaptive Functioning

The neuropsychologist should assess how children are adapting to the various environments in which they function. As noted by Rourke and colleagues (1986) it is critical to examine a child's adaptive behavior within the family, the school, and the community. The quality of a child's relationships with parents, siblings, teachers, and peers may be symptomatic of a particular kind of learning disability or psychiatric disorder or could indicate adjustment difficulties in response to neuropsychological dysfunction. Difficulties with activities of daily living (ADL) such as self-care or participation in household routines could also be diagnostic. When the clinical interview raises questions about adaptive behavior, more formal questionnaires or structured interviews can be administered to investigate how the child's functioning compares to that of neurologically intact peers.

Psychiatric Status

Psychiatric difficulties commonly co-occur with neuropsychological dysfunction. The relationship between psychiatric and neuropsychological status can be difficult to discern, because brain injury can interact with thought processes, mood, and behavior in multiple ways. Emotional or behavioral difficulties could be the direct result of an abnormally functioning brain. Alternatively, they could be a response to the stress of coping with neuropsychological dysfunction or other life stressors in conjunction with neuropsychological dysfunction. Furthermore, as noted above, children whose primary difficulty is a psychiatric disorder have a greater likelihood of neuropsychological dysfunction (Tramontana & Hooper, 1997). Psychiatric problems that result from, co-occur with, or give rise to neuropsychological difficulties may be transient, or may persist over time, waxing and waning in response to developmental transitions, external stressors, or changes in neurologic status.

Examining the child's emotional and behavioral functioning is crucial for diagnosis, for accurate test interpretation, and for understanding the complexity of the difficulties faced by the child so that interventions can be appropriately designed. This should be done through both observation and administration of formal measures such as psychological tests or checklists. Ideally, information will be gathered from multiple environments in which the child functions. Taking a careful history, which includes a timeline of the emergence of different problems and symptoms, can assist in teasing apart direct and indirect effects (Reynolds & Mayfield, 1999).

INTERPRETATION OF TEST RESULTS

At the conclusion of testing, the neuropsychologist compares the child's scores to those obtained by a normative reference group. The child's performance is most often compared to that of children of the same age range or grade. Norms or standardized scores specific to gender, ethnicity, nationality, or other relevant stratifying variables are sometimes available as well. The purpose of this comparison is to enable the clinician to distinguish scores truly reflecting dysfunction from those that fall within the broad range of normal ability. A convention for making this distinction is that scores falling more than 2 standard deviations in the impaired direction from the average score of a normal reference group are taken as evidence of dysfunction (Lezak, 1995).

Interpretation of results involves the integration of all information gathered, including interview data, behavioral observations, test scores, and qualitative aspects of task performance. This integration is necessary because a poor performance on any one test can often be attributed to many different skill deficits. For example, reasons for difficulty with a story recall task include an inability to attend to the story, deficient auditory processing or language comprehension, inadequate verbal expressive skills, poor retention of verbal information, difficulty retrieving information from memory, and lack of motivation to perform the task. Examining other measures assessing attention, language, and memory skills, along with observations of the child's perceived motivation level during testing, could clarify which domains are more or less likely to account for the difficulty. The neuropsychologist will also look for groupings of deficits, or "diagnostic behavior clusters" (Bernstein & Waber, 1990), which indicate particular types of dysfunction and are consistent with current knowledge of brain function and brain-behavior relationships in children. In cases where there is a known neurologic condition, the neuropsychologist will consider the child's profile in relation to the most typical profile for that condition.

Perhaps to the frustration of the referring parties, this analytic process may or may not result in a definitive diagnosis or identification of the problem. When it is not possible or appropriate to select one interpretation of the child's profile, the most logical alternative interpretations should be presented, along with a plan for discriminating among them. For example, consider the hypothetical case of a child referred for testing with a history of moderate traumatic brain injury (TBI) suffered 3 months earlier. The child was briefly hospitalized and was not referred for rehabilitation. Testing indicates significant attentional problems. The child seems depressed and distracted during testing. Parents report that they have recently separated. They recall no attentional difficulties prior to the head injury, but the head injury, their separation, and a worsening of their child's mood and attentional functioning all seemed to occur around the same time. It would be reasonable for the neuropsychologist to present the various scenarios that would explain the results, that is, the child's difficulties stem from the head injury, or from his or her response to family stressors, or from a combination of these. Recommendations can then include a plan for teasing apart the nature of the child's difficulties, so as to arrive at the most effective treatment plan. This might include referrals to a psychiatrist for evaluation and possible treatment of mood difficulties, to individual or family counseling, and to rehabilitation services for assistance with attentional problems. The child could undergo reevaluation of attention and mood after he or she has made some progress in treatment. If it were found that attentional problems persisted after mood problems resolved, it could be inferred that inattention was a consequence of the head injury, which would have implications for further treatment and prognosis.

A major issue in test interpretation is the validity of a child's test results, which should be noted in each report. Invalid test results cannot be interpreted because they do not reflect the child's abilities. It is possible to obtain invalid test results from children who are too ill, cognitively compromised, emotionally troubled, or unwilling to participate meaningfully in testing. When this occurs, testing may be postponed until better participation or cooperation can be achieved. There is the additional issue to consider of whether a child's test performance truly reflects his or her optimal functioning. The neuropsychologist will attempt to structure the testing situation to improve chances for optimal functioning, for example, by providing a testing environment that facilitates good concentration, and by scheduling testing for times when the child is not likely to be fatigued. However, many neurologic disorders are marked by variability in symptoms over time, and this variability may influence test performance significantly, despite the examiner's best efforts to control it. The final test profile may therefore reflect not optimal functioning, but rather one of the possible profiles the child is capable of producing. The report should state in such cases that testing might underestimate the child's potential, with an explanation of the factors that might be influencing test performance.

THE NEUROPSYCHOLOGICAL REPORT

After the results have been scored and interpreted, the family or other referring individuals receive a written report of the evaluation. Most reports provide relevant history, behavioral observations, an analysis of test performance, a summary and interpretation of findings, a clinical diagnosis, and recommendations. The summary should highlight strengths and weaknesses, documenting the problems that need to be fixed or circumvented, as well as the talents and skills that permit the child to excel in some areas and perhaps to circumvent difficulties in others. Utilization of cognitive strengths is critical for the success of rehabilitation or other treatment programs, because interventions need to be based on what works for the child, or what the child is able to do (Williams & Boll, 1997; Reynolds & Mayfield, 1999; Bernstein, 2000). As an example, the rehabilitation of a child with good language skills will probably incorporate verbal instruction and feedback about performance in other, more deficient domains. For children with impaired language skills but intact visuoperceptual and spatial skills, treatment may proceed more smoothly if pictures, signs, and other nonverbal symbols are used for communication.

Presenting strengths along with weaknesses in a report serves other functions. When parents bring their child to be evaluated by a neuropsychologist, the focus is on the child's perceived deficiencies, and there is often grave concern, anxiety, frustration, or hopelessness about things the child cannot do. Providing a balanced view of the child's abilities can positively influence parent's perceptions of the child and attitudes about the potential for improvement (Reynolds & Mayfield, 1999). It also may bolster the child's self-esteem (Baron, 2000) and motivation for treatment.

The summary section of the report may also address potential risks for the child in the future (Bernstein, 2000). These risks may include worsening of difficulties if treatment is not pursued, emergence of new difficulties as the child develops and is expected to master newer, more challenging skills, or exacerbations of difficulties during developmental transitions or other times of greater stress. Children with neuropsychological deficits may also be at risk for developing nonadaptive responses to brain disorders, such as low self-esteem, loss of interest in school, and attraction to negative peer influences. There may be risks associated with changes in the child's neurologic status, and these can be indicated.

When a diagnosis is given to a child, it is meant to serve a clinical purpose. Ideally, it should provide treating professionals with an idea of the symptom cluster experienced by the child, the likely prognosis of the problem, and the most effective treatments to pursue. Unfortunately, current diagnostic systems leave neuropsychologists struggling to select from among inadequate alternatives. However, a diagnosis is often required for insurance or educational purposes, and the diagnostic choice made by the neuropsychologist may represent a clinical compromise. As a rule, the reader of the report should examine the summary of findings for information that clarifies, qualifies, or expands on the diagnosis given.

Treatment recommendations are provided at the end of the report. Recommendations typically address direct remediation or treatment of the child's deficits, development of compensatory strategies for circumventing problems, and modification of the child's environment or environmental demands (Yeates & Taylor, 1998). Each recommendation may target a specific problem identified in the report, and when many problems are identified, the list of recommendations can be lengthy. However, recommendations can be prioritized so that the family and treating professionals can be directed toward more critical issues first, and then can address residual issues as time and resources permit.

Because testing covers a broad range of functions, recommendations may as well. They may include referrals for further evaluation in neurology, psychiatry, speech and language pathology, audiology, physical or occupational therapy, psychology, or social work. Counseling may be suggested for the child or family. Academic recommendations may suggest modifications to the standard program, such as preferential seating in the classroom, extra time on examinations, or tutoring in a particular academic subject. Recommendations for school should be appropriate to the child's grade and classroom curriculum and may include how to use the child's cognitive strengths, manage behavioral difficulties, and keep the child motivated to work on areas of weakness. When a child has an evolving condition, such as a fairly recent brain injury, recommendations can remind treating individuals that the child's cognitive profile may be evolving as well and that the current results may not be an accurate predictor of functioning several months in the future. When this is the case, retesting and adjustment of the child's treatment at some point in the future should be recommended (Reynolds & Mayfield, 1999).

Research on parents' perceptions of their child's neuropsychological assessment has indicated that gaining understanding into their child's strengths and weaknesses and having a set of recommendations for treatment makes a positive difference for the child (Farmer & Brazeal, 1998). Having this information does not appear to increase parents' stress or negative perceptions of the child. Rather, parents report an improvement in school services for their child as a result of the evaluation and an increased awareness of other professionals or groups who can assist them in dealing with their child's difficulties.

THE FEEDBACK SESSION

When the report has been completed, the test findings must be communicated to parents, and when appropriate, to the child who was evaluated. Parents may wish to share the findings with other adults involved in the child's life such as physicians or teachers. This can be done in a feedback session involving all of the interested parties. A key purpose of providing feedback is to educate the family about the child's cognitive profile, including strengths and weaknesses, as well as to share recommendations for dealing with the identified problem(s) and to answer any questions about the evaluation, report content, terminology, diagnoses, or other matters of concern. Explaining test results in terms of real-life behaviors can facilitate the education process. Helping parents to understand their child's abilities and needs is critical because they will be better able to communicate them to others, make appropriate decisions regarding interventions, and lobby for appropriate assistance for their child as roadblocks are encountered (Baron, 2000).

When a child is involved in rehabilitation, it is likely that the neuropsychological report will be shared with the child's treatment team as well as family, and test results and recommendations will be incorporated into the child's treatment. Even when a child is not receiving rehabilitation services, it may be advantageous to take a "treatment team" approach to the feedback session. The neuropsychologist can present recommendations for follow-up to the people present, who then can jointly plan what assistance the child will get, who will be responsible for different aspects of follow-up, and when interventions will be undertaken. Plans for communication among members of this informal treatment team can be established, perhaps including periodic meetings to confer about the child's progress and evolving needs.

The feedback session also provides the opportunity for educating the child about her or his ability profile. Children who are having cognitive difficulties are often aware of this fact on some level. They may remember an accident, a hospitalization, or a series of medical treatments that were stressful or frightening. They may recognize that they are not progressing as well as their peers academically or seem to have to work much harder than their siblings to make the same developmental gains. The experience of the neuropsychological assessment provides an opportunity for discussion in age-appropriate language about their struggles. Such open communication conveys that their problems are not too frightening or shameful to discuss. The neuropsychologist can bolster their self-esteem by identifying tasks on which they performed well. Furthermore, hearing how their family, doctor, or teacher will be helping them in the future can provide children with hope. When appropriate, children can be taught words to describe their difficulties and can practice asking for the assistance they need, taking the first steps toward self-advocacy. Of course, clinical judgment will dictate what can be communicated to the child and in what manner it would best be done. For example, it would not be appropriate to include a young child in a lengthy feedback session in which complicated information is being communicated to adults in adult language. A separate, brief session for the child would be more appropriate, using simpler language and conveying the portion of the assessment results that would be most useful and comprehensible to the child.

MAXIMIZING THE BENEFIT OF AN ASSESSMENT

Meeting the needs of all parties involved in the assessment process can be a challenge at times. Frustration may occur because of a lack of understanding of what neuropsychological assessments are and are not capable of providing. For example, parents may want a definitive diagnosis for their child's difficulties, but this may not be possible due to the complex nature of the problem. Furthermore, the outcomes desired by different participants may conflict, as when school staff recognizes a disability that parents are reluctant to acknowledge, or vice versa. To the extent that individuals are willing to discuss their expectations and needs, communication early in the assessment can help the neuropsychologist to clarify misconceptions and anticipate roadblocks to implementing treatment recommendations. One way to communicate the participants' needs is for the referring individuals to make their referral question as specific to their interests as possible, eschewing broad questions such as, "Does this child have an organic brain disorder?" in favor of more focused ones, such as "Does this child have neuropsychological deficits which could explain her difficulties with math, problem-solving, and social skills?" Whenever there are particular cognitive domains or functions that are of interest, such as learning or sustained attention, this should be stated at the time of the referral.

When there are constraints that will make it difficult for the referring parties to understand or use a report in its usual form, this should be made clear to the neuropsychologist, who has flexibility in how results can be communicated. Parents who have difficulty reading may prefer a report that is explained verbally by the neuropsychologist or is tape-recorded for later review. Feedback sessions can be tape-recorded when it is anticipated that the family will not be able to process all of the information that is being discussed and would benefit from hearing it more than once. To some extent, written reports can be tailored to their intended audience. When a report is to be shared with many people, some of whom should not have access to all of the information collected in the evaluation, the neuropsychologist can exercise judgment in excluding that which is not essential to share.

A neuropsychological report can be useful to parents far beyond the time of the initial assessment. Over the course of the child's years in school, the child will have different teachers and may experience changes in physicians and other treating professionals. In addition, as part of follow-up, the child may need periodic neuropsychological reevaluation, and different neuropsychologists may perform this service. For optimal continuity of educational services, medical treatment, or other therapies, and for maximum benefit from future assessments, it is critical for all individuals new to the child's situation to have access to past test reports. In some cases, physicians, therapists, or schools may retain a copy of the child's neuropsychological report as part of the child's permanent record, but it is not uncommon for past reports to be difficult to locate. It is preferable for the parents to keep a copy and share it when necessary or to request that the assessing neuropsychologist forward a copy to whomever the parents wish, with the parents' written consent. In addition to facilitating transitions of therapeutic and educational services through the school years, documentation of disabilities identified in childhood may be required for access to special services later in life. For example, students with learning disabilities who are applying for academic accommodations in college may need to justify their request by providing a report diagnosing their disability earlier in their school career. Parents should be made aware of the importance of retaining their child's report and of possible situations in which they might need to share it in the future.

CROSS-CULTURAL ISSUES IN CHILD NEUROPSYCHOLOGICAL ASSESSMENT

A fundamental assumption of neuropsychological assessment is that the cognitive functioning of neurologically intact children will tend to be similar to that of age- or grade-matched peers, with deviations from similarity indicating potentially significant cognitive strengths or weaknesses. This assumption, however, presumes a certain similarity between the characteristics of the child being tested and those of the children from whom test norms were gathered. When a child's background differs substantially from that of the majority of children in the normative group, the norms may not be predictive of the child's functioning, even when the child is neurologically intact. Inevitably, given the multiethnic, multicultural nature of the United States, a certain percentage of children referred to neuropsychologists for testing due to brain injuries, neurologic diseases, or developmental disabilities will not be native speakers of American English. Such children present a challenge for the neuropsychologist, who must decide how to conduct the assessment to maximize its chances of being meaningful and useful to parents, educators, and health care providers.

Some of the factors that the neuropsychologist must consider include languages spoken by the family and child, cultural background and level of acculturation, educational background, and socioeconomic status, each of which has been shown to influence performance on psychometric testing (e.g., Puente et al., 1997). Language differences between the neuropsychologist, the child, and the child's family are perhaps the most obvious potential hindrance to a valid neuropsychological assessment. When children are not fully fluent in English, they may not understand interview questions, task instructions, or test questions. Their ability to share their knowledge verbally may be hindered by limited English vocabulary or grammar, which is especially significant considering that neuropsychological tests often require precise responses. Furthermore, when language differences exist, children may feel too timid or uncomfortable in the testing situation to put forth their best verbal effort. If parents are not fluent speakers of English, the neuropsychologist may fail to gather important historical information in the interview (Marlowe, 2000).

To minimize these difficulties, the child would ideally be referred to a neuropsychologist who is fluent in the child's language. Alternatively, the neuropsychologist may use an interpreter to interpret task instructions and questions into the language of the child and family and interpret back their responses. The quality of interpretation can vary tremendously, in part as a function of the level of training received by the interpreter (Brislin, 1988). Even when trained interpreters are used, communications could lack precision, affecting test scores.

Additional psychometric concerns result from using tests written in English with children who are not fluent English speakers (Puente et al., 1997). Psychometric tests have been written in other languages for use with non–English-speaking populations, but their numbers are limited. Direct translations of English language tests into other languages are problematic because words and concepts from one language may not have precise equivalents in another language. If a test can be adequately translated in terms of its language, questions follow about whether the translation has the same psychometric properties (e.g., means, reliability coefficients, internal factor structure) as the original version. An additional question concerns whether appropriate norms are available for the non–English-speaking

children being tested. Not uncommonly, the original norms are used with test translations, but this practice is at best questionable (Puente et al., 1997).

Cultural background may influence test results through such variables as attitude toward education, experience with the concepts and skills being tested, response to time pressure on timed tasks, and comfort with being the sole focus of a professional adult's attention. Culture dictates what information children should learn and the age at which they should learn it, which will determine their skill and knowledge base at different ages (Harris, 1990; Jones, 1991). Children whose educational experiences have differed greatly from that of the mainstream United States school population may enter the testing situation uncomfortable being questioned by an unfamiliar adult, unclear as to how to behave or respond, and unfamiliar with the materials being presented or discussed. Culture can also influence how comfortable a family feels communicating private information to the neuropsychologist and how such information should best be elicited (Marlowe, 2000). Familiarity with a family's background can sensitize the neuropsychologist to potential cultural differences that could undermine the assessment. Understanding a family's background includes awareness of the extent to which family members identify with their culture of origin; families that are more assimilated into the cultural mainstream will take on more of the characteristics and values of the mainstream and will have had more similar experiences.

Wong and colleagues (2000) have offered general guidelines for neuropsychological evaluations of culturally dissimilar patients. Regarding language differences, they strongly discourage the use of untrained, nonprofessional interpreters, especially family members. They recommend instead that whenever possible, patients should be referred to another professional fluent in their language and familiar with their culture, and professional interpreters should be used when an appropriate referral is not possible. It is further recommended that translated tests be avoided unless the translated test interpretations have been validated. If nonvalidated translated tests are used, or if the tests selected were not normed or intended for use with patients from the population in question, they should be used qualitatively only. Rhodes and colleagues (2000) have similarly suggested that test data obtained in a nonstandard manner should be used as a means to examine the child's responses and not as an absolute index of ability. In such cases, reports should not provide normative statistics such as standard scores and should contain statements indicating that the tests administered were not meant for use with the language or cultural group to which the child belongs. In addition, test responses should be interpreted in a conservative fashion, giving the benefit of doubt to the patient, with contextual variables influencing whether the neuropsychologist should favor false-positive or false-negative diagnostic error (Wong et al., 2000).

When cultural or language factors play a role in an assessment, it is essential for individuals receiving neuropsychological services to be sensitized to the issues involved and educated about the nonstandard manner in which tests results were interpreted, documented, and used. For example, the reasons for the report's lack of formal scores should be explained, along with the potential utility of qualitative descriptions of the child's functioning for the family and treating staff. If interventions fail to produce positive results, or if the child's functioning outside of testing is inconsistent with test findings as they are interpreted, retesting or other methods of gathering information about the child's functioning may be required, and the treatment plan would need to be altered. Understanding the abilities and needs of such children must ultimately be a dynamic process involving ongoing hypothesis testing, with frequent communications among treating individuals, the family, and the child, and incorporating data collected from all sources.

SUMMARY

Child neuropsychological assessment makes an important contribution to the evaluation and ongoing care of the child with known or suspected brain impairment. Identification of the specific cognitive deficits that underlie a child's difficulties can help that child avoid years of frustration and failure due to inappropriate interventions or lack of access to treatment or environmental modifications. When neuropsychological findings are provided to families and treating individuals, the child can be linked to needed services, appropriate expectations for the future can be formulated, and the child and family can gain a deeper understanding of the child's struggles. Of equal importance is the knowledge provided about the child's strengths and talents, for these will form the foundation of intervention strategies and can be targeted in efforts to build the child's self-esteem. Ongoing coordination of services among the family, physician, educators, the neuropsychologist, and other intervention specialists can facilitate long-term monitoring of the child's changing needs and adjustment of treatments as necessary. Ideally, future child neuropsychological research will permit a clearer link between test findings and interventions and broaden our understanding of the biologic bases of the child's difficulties.

■ KEY POINTS

☐ Child neuropsychological assessment examines the neurobehavioral functioning of children from birth through late adolescence.

☐ A child neuropsychological assessment provides a detailed view of the child's or adolescent's cognitive, emotional, and behavioral functioning through the administration of psychometric tests, in conjunction with information from medical and academic records, direct observation of the child, and interviews with parents, teachers, and other relevant adults.

☐ Obtaining a neuropsychological assessment should be considered whenever there are concerns about a child's ability to function cognitively or behaviorally in one or more environments, and it is suspected that the problem is brain-based in origin.

☐ Areas to evaluate in a child neuropsychological assessment include language, visual processing skills, attention, learning and memory, motor and sensory ability, reasoning and problem solving, academic achievement, adaptive functioning, and emotional/behavioral functioning.

☐ At the conclusion of the evaluation, the neuropsychologist provides a report describing the child's test results, documenting problems that need to be remediated or circumvented and strengths that can serve as the foundation for intervention efforts. Recommendations are made to direct the family and other involved individuals toward appropriate treatments and environmental accommodations for the child.

KEY READINGS

Rourke BP, Fisk JL, Strang JD: Neuropsychological Assessment of Children: A Treatment-Oriented Approach. New York: Guilford Press, 1986.

Spreen O, Risser AH, Edgell D: Developmental Neuropsychology. New York: Oxford University Press, 1995.

Tramontana MG, Hooper SR (eds): Assessment Issues in Child Neuropsychology. New York: Plenum Press, 1988.

Yeates KO, Ris MD, Taylor HG (eds): Pediatric Neuropsychology: Research, Theory, and Practice. New York: Guilford Press, 2000.

REFERENCES

American Psychiatric Association: Diagnostic and Statistical Manual of Mental Disorders, ed 4. Washington, DC: Author, 1994.

Aylward GP: Infant and early childhood assessment, in Tramontana MG, Hooper SR (eds): Assessment Issues in Child Neuropsychology. New York: Plenum Press, 1988, pp. 225–248.

Baron IS: Clinical implications and practical applications of child neuropsychological evaluations, in Yeates KO, Ris MD, Taylor HG (eds): Pediatric Neuropsychology: Research, Theory, and Practice. New York: Guilford Press, 2000, pp. 439–456.

Benton A, Tranel D: Visuoperceptual, visuospatial, and visuo-constructive disorders, in Heilman KM, Valenstein E (eds): Clinical Neuropsychology, ed 3. New York: Oxford University Press, 1993, pp. 165–213.

Berg RA, Linton JD: Neuropsychological sequelae of chronic medical disorders in children and youth, in Reynolds CR, Fletcher-Janzen E (eds): Handbook of Clinical Child Neuropsychology, ed 2. New York: Plenum Press, 1997, pp. 663–687.

Bernstein JH: Developmental neuropsychological assessment, in Yeates KO, Ris MD, Taylor HG (eds): Pediatric Neuropsychology: Research, Theory, and Practice. New York: Guilford Press, 2000, pp. 405–438.

Bernstein JH, Waber DP: Developmental neuropsychological assessment: The systemic approach, in Boulton AA, Baker GB, Hiscock M (eds): Neuromethods: Neuropsychology. New York: Humana Press, 1990, Vol. 17, pp. 311–371.

Bigler ED, Nussbaum NL, Foley HA: Child neuropsychology in the private medical practice, in Goldstein S, Reynolds CR (eds): Handbook of Neurodevelopmental and Genetic Disorders in Children. New York: Guilford Press, 1997, pp. 726–742.

Brislin RW: Increasing awareness of class, ethnicity, culture, and race by expanding on students' own experiences, in Cohen IS (ed): The G. Stanley Hall Lecture Series. Washington, DC: American Psychological Association, 1988, Vol. 8, pp. 137–180.

Brown G, Del Dotto JE, Fisk JL, et al: Analyzing clinical ratings of performance on pediatric neuropsychology tests. Clin Neuropsychol 7:179–189, 1993.

Delis DC, Kiefner MG, Fridlund AJ: Visuospatial dysfunction following unilateral brain damage: Dissociations in hierarchical and hemispatial analysis. J Clin Neuropsychol 10:421–431, 1988.

Delis DC, Kramer JH, Kaplan E, et al: The California Verbal Learning Test, Children's Version Manual. San Antonio, TX: The Psychological Corporation, 1994.

Dennis M: Childhood medical disorders and cognitive impairment: Biological risk, time, development, and reserve, in Yeates KO, Ris MD, Taylor HG (eds): Pediatric Neuropsychology: Research, Theory, and Practice. New York: Guilford Press, 2000, pp. 3–22.

Dennis M, Whitaker HA: Language acquisition following hemidecortication: Linguistic superiority of the left over the right hemisphere. Brain Lang 3:404–433, 1976.

Ewing-Cobbs L, Levin HS, Eisenberg HM, et al: Language functions following closed-head injury in children and adolescents. J Clin Exp Neuropsychol 9:575–592, 1987.

Farmer JE, Brazeal TJ: Parent perceptions about the process and outcomes of child neuropsychological assessment. Appl Neuropsychol 5:194–201, 1998.

Fennell EB: End-stage renal disease, in Yeates KO, Ris MD, Taylor HG (eds): Pediatric Neuropsychology: Research, Theory, and Practice. New York: Guilford Press, 2000, pp. 366–380.

Fischler R, Tancer M: The primary physician's role in care for developmentally handicapped children. J Fam Pract 18:85–88, 1984.

Fletcher JM, Dennis M, Northrup H: Hydrocephalus, in Yeates KO, Ris MD, Taylor HG (eds): Pediatric Neuropsychology: Research, Theory, and Practice. New York: Guilford, 2000, pp. 25–46.

Franzen MD: Reliability and Validity in Neuropsychological Assessment. New York: Kluwer, 2000.

Gaddes WH, Edgell D: Learning Disabilities and Brain Function, ed 3. New York: Springer, 1993.

Golden CJ: Manual for the Luria-Nebraska Neuropsychological Battery–Children's Revision. Los Angeles, CA: Western Psychological Services, 1986.

Halstead W: Biological intelligence and the frontal lobes. Paper presented at the Cleveland Symposium (Halstead Papers, Box M-187; Archives of the History of Psychology; Bierce Library, University of Akron), December 29, 1950.

Harris JL: Cultural influences on handedness: Historical and contemporary theory and evidence, in Coren S (ed): Left-handedness: Behavioral Implications and Anomalies. Amsterdam, The Netherlands: North-Holland, 1990, pp. 195–258.

Hartlage LC: Pediatric neuropsychology, in Wedding D, Horton AM, Webster J (eds): The Neuropsychology Handbook: Behavioral and Clinical Perspectives. New York: Springer, 1986, pp. 441–455.

Hartlage LC, Templer DI: Ecological issues and child neuropsychological assessment, in Sbordone RJ, Long CJ (eds): Ecological Validity of Neuropsychological Testing. Delray Beach, FL: Gr Press/St. Lucie Press, 1996, pp. 301–313.

Hartman DE: Neuropsychological Toxicology: Identification and Assessment of Human Neurotoxic Syndromes, ed 2. New York: Plenum Press, 1995.

Hauser WA, Hesdorffer DC: Epilepsy: Frequency, Causes, and Consequences. New York: Demos, 1990.

Jones J: Piercing the veil: Bi-cultural strategies for coping with prejudice and racism, in Knopke HJ, Norrell RJ, Rogers RW (eds): Opening Doors: Perspectives on Race Relations in Contemporary America. Tuscaloosa, AL: University of Alabama Press, 1991, pp. 179–197.

Kanoy KW, Schroeder CS: Suggestions to parents about common behavior problems in a pediatric primary care office: Five years of follow-up. J Pediatr Psychol 10:15–30, 1985.

Kolb B, Fantie B: Development of the child's brain and behavior, in Reynolds CR, Fletcher-Janzen E (eds): Handbook of Clinical Child Neuropsychology, ed 2. New York: Plenum Press, 1997, pp. 17–41.

Korkman M, Kirk U, Kemp SL: NEPSY. A Developmental Neuropsychological Assessment. San Antonio, TX: The Psychological Corporation, 1998.

Kraus JF: Epidemiological features of brain injury in children: Occurrence, children at risk, causes and manner of injury, severity, and outcomes, in Broman SH, Michel MD (eds): Traumatic Head Injury in Children. New York: Oxford University Press, 1995, pp. 22–39.

Lezak MD: Neuropsychological Assessment, ed 3. New York: Oxford University Press, 1995.

Marlowe WB: Multicultural perspectives on the neuropsychological assessment of children and adolescents, in Fletcher-Janzen E, Strickland TL, Reynolds CR (eds): Handbook of Cross-Cultural Neuropsychology. New York: Kluwer Academic/Plenum Publishers, 2000, pp. 145–165.

Matarazzo JD, Prifitera A: Subtest scatter and premorbid intelligence: Lessons from the WAIS-R standardization sample. Psychol Assess 1:186–191, 1989.

Mattson SN, Riley EP: Implicit and explicit memory functioning in children with heavy prenatal alcohol exposure. J Int Neuropsychol Soc 5:462–471, 1999.

Max JE, Roberts MA, Koele SL, et al: Cognitive outcome in children and adolescents following severe traumatic brain injury: Influence of psychosocial, psychiatric, and injury-related variables. J Int Neuropsychol Soc 5:58–68, 1999.

Molfese VJ: Neuropsychological assessment in infancy, in Boller F, Grafman J (series eds), Rapin I, Segalowitz SJ (vol eds): Handbook of Neuropsychology: Child Neuropsychology. Amsterdam, The Netherlands: Elsevier, 1992, Vol. 6, pp. 353–376.

O'Sullivan P, Mahoney G, Robinson C: Perceptions of pediatricians' helpfulness: A national study of mothers of young disabled children. Dev Med Child Neurol 34:1064–1071, 1992.

Paneth NS: The problem of low birth weight. Future Child 5:19–34, 1995.

Prechtl H: The Neurological Examination of the Fullterm Newborn Infant. Philadelphia, PA: Lippincott, 1977.

Puente AE, Sol Mora M, Munoz-Cespedes JM: Neuropsychological assessment of Spanish-speaking children and youth, in Reynolds CR, Fletcher-Janzen E (eds): Handbook of Clinical Child Neuropsychology, ed 2. New York: Plenum Press, 1997, pp. 371–383.

Reitan RM: Manual for Administration of Neuropsychological Test Batteries for Adults and Children. Indianapolis, IN: Author, 1969.

Reitan RM, Wolfson D: Clinical Neuropsychology: Current Status and Applications. Washington, DC: Winston, 1974.

Reynolds CR, Mayfield JW: Neuropsychological assessment in genetically linked neurodevelopmental disorders, in Goldstein S, Reynolds CR (eds): Handbook of Neurodevelopmental and Genetic Disorders in Children. New York: Guilford, 1999, pp. 9–37.

Rhodes RL, Kayser H, Hess RS: Neuropsychological differential diagnosis of Spanish-speaking preschool children, in Fletcher-Janzen E, Strickland TL, Reynolds CR (eds): Handbook of Cross-Cultural Neuropsychology. New York: Kluwer Academic/Plenum Publishers, 2000, pp. 317–333.

Roman MJ, Delis DC, Willerman L, et al: The impact of pediatric traumatic brain injury on components of verbal memory. J Clin Exp Neuropsychol 20:245–258, 1998.

Rosenbaum PL, King SM, Cadman DT: Measuring processes of caregiving to physically disabled children and their families. I: Identifying relevant components of care. Dev Med Child Neurol 34:103–114, 1992.

Rourke BP: Nonverbal Learning Disabilities: The Syndrome and the Model. New York: Guilford Press, 1989.

Rourke BP, Bakker DJ, Fisk JL, et al: Child Neuropsychology: An Introduction to Theory, Research, and Clinical Practice. New York: Guilford Press, 1983.

Rourke BP, Fisk JL, Strang J D: Neuropsychological Assessment of Children: A Treatment-Oriented Approach. New York: Guilford Press, 1986.

Silver CH: Ecological validity of neuropsychological assessment in childhood traumatic brain injury. J Head Trauma Rehabil 15:973–988, 2000.

Spreen O, Risser AH, Edgell D: Developmental Neuropsychology. New York: Oxford University Press, 1995.

Spreen O, Strauss E: A Compendium of Neuropsychological Tests: Administration, Norms, and Commentary. New York: Oxford University Press, 1998.

Stiles J, Trauner D, Engel M, Nass R: The development of drawing in children with congenital focal brain injury: Evidence for limited functional recovery. Neuropsychologia 35:299–312, 1997.

Taylor HG, Schatschneider C: Child neuropsychological assessment: A test of basic assumptions. Clin Neuropsychol 6:259–275, 1992.

Tramontana MG, Hooper SR: Child neuropsychological assessment: Overview of current status, in Tramontana MG, Hooper SR (eds): Assessment Issues in Child Neuropsychology. New York: Plenum Press, 1988, pp. 3–38.

Tramontana MG, Hooper SR: Neuropsychology of child psychopathology, in Reynolds CR, Fletcher-Janzen E (eds): Handbook of Clinical Child Neuropsychology, ed 2. New York: Plenum Press, 1997, pp. 120–139.

Vicari S, Albertoni A, Chilosi AM, et al: Plasticity and reorganization during language development in children with early brain injury. Cortex 36:31–46, 2000.

Waber DP, Bernstein JH, Kammerer BL, et al: Neuropsychological diagnostic profiles of children who received CNS treatment for acute lymphoblastic leukemia: The systemic approach to assessment. Dev Neuropsychol 8:1–28, 1992.

Welsh M, Pennington B: Phenylketonuria, in Yeates KO, Ris MD, Taylor HG (eds): Pediatric Neuropsychology: Research, Theory, and Practice. New York: Guilford Press, 2000, pp. 275–299.

Williams MA, Boll TJ: Recent advances in neuropsychological assessment of children, in Goldstein G, Incagnoli TM (eds): Contemporary Approaches to Neuropsychological Assessment. New York: Plenum Press, 1997.

Wong TM, Strickland TL, Fletcher-Janzen E, et al: Theoretical and practical issues in the neuropsychological assessment and treatment of culturally dissimilar patients, in Fletcher-Janzen E, Strickland TL, Reynolds CR (eds): Handbook of Cross-Cultural Neuropsychology. New York: Kluwer Academic/Plenum Publishers, 2000, pp. 3–18.

Yeates KO, Taylor HG: Neuropsychological assessment of older children, in Goldstein G, Nussbaum PD, Beers S (eds): Neuropsychology. Human Brain Function: Assessment and Rehabilitation. New York: Plenum Press, 1998, pp. 35–61.

Pediatric Head Injury

Vicki A. Anderson

Child traumatic brain injury
cognitive predictors
Closed head injury
Glasgow Coma Score
Penetrating head injury
Post-traumatic amnesia

Pediatric traumatic brain injury (TBI) is a frequent cause of acquired disability in childhood. The majority of such injuries are mild, with few, if any, sequelae. However, children sustaining more severe TBIs may suffer permanent physical, cognitive, and behavioral impairment. Clinical reports document residual deficits in a range of skills, particularly information processing speed and efficiency, attention, memory, and learning. These deficits may interfere with the child's ability to function effectively in his or her environment, resulting in lags in the acquisition of skills and knowledge. Secondary deficits may also emerge, relating to family

stress and adjustment difficulties. Treatment of the head-injured child and the child's family is best managed using a multidisciplinary team-based approach, and requires long-term involvement, in which the role of the rehabilitation team is to understand the consequences of the child's injuries; identify potential risk factors within the child's environment; liaise with teachers and schools; design physical, academic, and behavior programs; and provide counseling with respect to adjustment issues for the child and family. This chapter aims to examine these areas, in particular: recovery patterns post-TBI, plotting changes from the acute phase to subacute, and long-term outcome, with respect to physical, cognitive, and psychosocial factors.

EPIDEMIOLOGY

Epidemiologic reports suggest that 250/100,000 children suffer TBI each year. Of these, half will not seek medical care, between 5% and 10% will experience temporary and/or permanent neuropsychological impairment, and 5% to 10% will sustain fatal injuries

(Goldstein & Levin, 1987). Eighty-five percent of head injuries are classified as mild, with 44% having no documented loss of consciousness (Kraus et al., 1986). Examination of data specific to severe TBI shows that the mortality rate is approximately one third—one third of children make a good recovery, and one third exhibit residual disability (Michaud et al., 1992).

The nature of pediatric TBI varies with age. Infants are more likely to suffer injury due to falls or child abuse. For nonaccidental injuries (i.e., child abuse), 61% of such injuries occur in children less than 12 months of age and commonly result in more severe injury and higher mortality and morbidity than accidental injuries (Holloway et al. 1994). The preschool stage is a high-risk period, with the majority of injuries caused by falls and pedestrian accidents, in keeping with the greater mobility and lack of awareness of danger characteristics of this age group (Lehr, 1990). Older children and adolescents are more commonly victims of sporting, cycling, or pedestrian accidents. Boys and girls are not equally at risk of injury. In preschool children, the male-to-female ratio is approximately 1.5:1 (Horowitz et al., 1983; Hayes & Jackson, 1989), whereas in the school-aged group boys are more than twice as likely to suffer TBI (Kraus, 1995). The incidence of TBI increases in boys through childhood and adolescence, with a contrasting decline for girls over this period (Kraus et al., 1986).

Pediatric TBI occurs most frequently on holidays, weekends, and afternoons, when children are involved in leisure pursuits, suggesting that many injuries may result from reckless behaviors, in poorly supervised environments (Chadwick et al., 1981; Dalby & Obrzut, 1991). It has been argued that pediatric TBI is more common in socially disadvantaged families (Klonoff, 1971; Brown et al., 1981; Rivara et al., 1993; Taylor et al., 1995; Anderson et al., 1997) and in children with preexisting learning and behavioral deficits (Craft et al., 1972; Brown et al., 1981; Asarnow et al., 1991). Some researchers argue that postinjury sequelae may merely reflect premorbid cognitive, behavioral, and social disturbances. Although such a view has become well accepted, a number of recent studies have failed to support such findings, arguing that children who sustain injury cannot be differentiated from the general population (Perrot et al., 1991; Prior et al., 1994).

PATHOPHYSIOLOGY

TBI refers to a traumatic insult to the brain, usually due to a blow or wound to the head, sufficient to cause altered consciousness (Begali, 1992). Evidence of alteration of conscious state is often used to distinguish between true TBI and more minor insult. TBI is frequently depicted as a unitary entity; however, the mechanics and underlying pathophysiology associated with these injuries may be substantially different, depending on the cause of injury, and may result in a range of possible outcomes. Consequences of TBI may also be related to various risk factors including (1) force of impact; (2) site of impact; (3) thickness of the scalp and skull; (4) presence or absence of skull fracture; and (5) intracranial vectors of transmitted force (linear, rotational) (Amacher, 1988). The greater the force applied, the more severe the associated damage.

Pathophysiology of TBI may be classified according to characteristics of the insult: (1) *primary impact injuries* occur as a direct result of force to the brain and include fractures, diffuse axonal damage contusions, and lacerations. Such injuries are generally permanent and show little response to early treatment; and (2) *secondary injuries*, such as extradural, subdural, and intracerebral hemorrhage, which may result from the primary injury. Raised intracranial pressure, brain swelling, hypoxia, infection, and metabolic changes, including hypothermia, electrolyte imbalance, and respiratory difficulties may also occur (North, 1984; Pang, 1985; Begali, 1992). Secondary injuries are more amenable to appropriate and timely medical interventions. For children who die as a result of TBI, common findings at autopsy include raised intracranial pressure, brain swelling, contusions, ischemia, cerebral herniation, diffuse axonal damage, and subarachnoid hemorrhage (Bruce et al., 1979; Graham et al., 1989; Michaud et al., 1992; Sharples et al., 1995).

TBI may be classified as penetrating (or open) head injury or closed head injury (CHI). The mechanics, pathophysiology, incidence, and neurobehavioral outcomes for these injuries are quite different.

Penetrating Head Injury

Penetrating injuries account for approximately 10% of all childhood TBIs, and refer to injuries which involve penetration of the skull by some form of "missile." Cerebral pathology tends to be localized around the path of the missile, with additional damage resulting from skull fragments or shattered fragments from the missile itself. Secondary damage may occur as a result of cerebral infection (from the alien object entering the brain), swelling, bleeding, and raised intracranial pressure. While loss of consciousness (LOC) is relatively uncommon following penetrating head injury, neurologic deficits and post-traumatic epilepsy are frequently observed, and are more prevalent after penetrating head injury than in CHI. Neurobehavioral sequelae from penetrating head injury tend to reflect the focal nature of the insult, and children often exhibit specific deficits consistent with the localization of the lesion, with other skills intact.

Closed Head Injury

CHI refers to an insult in which the skull is not penetrated, but rather the brain is shaken within the skull cavity, resulting in multiple injury sites, as well as diffuse axonal damage. This form of injury accounts for the majority of pediatric TBIs, and is a common consequence of motor vehicle accidents and other high-velocity deceleration forces. Damage results from compression and deformation of the skull at the point of impact. The primary pathology includes contusion, or bruising, at point of impact of the blow and at other cerebral sites. Specific areas of the brain are particularly vulnerable to such damage, including the temporal lobes and basal frontal regions (Courville, 1945). In CHI, the brain is shaken backward and forward and rotated, with the extent of this process dependent on the force of the blow. These processes can result in damage to cerebral areas opposite the site of damage and shearing injuries to white matter, as these nerve tracts are bent and torn (Amacher, 1988). Figure 40-1 illustrates the mechanisms that may occur in such a CHI.

Secondary mechanisms, including hematoma, cerebral edema, and raised intracranial pressure, may also occur, and are predictive of poor outcome in children (Quattrocchi et al., 1991). If not treated quickly, usually via surgical intervention, these secondary complications may cause cerebral herniation and ultimately death. Recent investigations have found that secondary damage may also result from neurochemical processes. Elevated levels of excitatory amino acids, such as glutamate and aspartate, have been detected in cerebrospinal fluid (CSF) immediately after TBI and found to persist for several days, causing disruption to cell function and eventual cell death (Yeates, 1999). Presence of high levels of excitatory amino acids has been correlated with greater degree of pathology on computed tomography (CT) scan (Baker et al., 1993). Animal research has suggested that pharmacologic interventions may be successful in minimizing any pathology related to such mechanisms (Novack et al., 1996).

While relatively uncommon, a number of delayed complications may develop in the subacute stages after TBI. Communicating hydrocephalus may occur when there is an obstruction of the flow of CSF, often caused by vascular disruption. Cerebral infections may arise in association with skull fractures, where such infections usually take the form of meningitis or cerebral abscess. Each of these complications may be detected on the basis of increased intracranial pressure and associated late deterioration in function. After CHI, children also

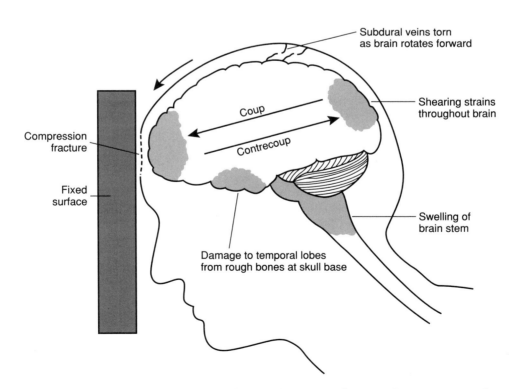

FIGURE 40-1. Brain damage caused by closed head injury, showing the impact of coup and contrecoup insults at the site of impact and directly opposite, as well as shearing and vascular damage. (Reproduced with permission from Begali V: Head Injury in Children and Adolescents, ed 2. Brandon, VT: Clinical Psychology Publishing Co., 1992.)

have increased risk of epilepsy (Jennett, 1979; Raimondi & Hirschauer, 1984; Pang, 1985; Ponsford et al., 1995).

Mechanics, Pathophysiology, and Age at Insult

A range of age-specific injury mechanisms may be acting, depending upon the maturity of the central nervous system (CNS) at the time of injury. First, the etiology of TBI changes during childhood, with infants and toddlers more likely to be injured as a result of falls, and older children more commonly involved in accidents associated with recreational activities or motor vehicles (Kraus, 1995), thus leading to varying injury processes. In addition, the skull and brain develop throughout childhood, resulting in different injury consequences at different developmental stages. For example, the infant has relatively weak neck muscles that do not adequately support a proportionately large head, leading to less resistance to force of impact. Further, the infant and toddler possess a relatively thin skull, easily deformed by a direct blow, that can result in more frequent skull fractures. Studies show that more than one third of children in this age bracket who sustain TBI will have skull fractures. In contrast, contusions, lacerations, and subdural hematomas are extremely rare in infancy (Choux, 1986; Berney et al., 1994; Sharma & Sharma, 1994). This may be due to the flexibility and open sutures present in the infant skull. For older children and adolescents, intracranial mass lesions (hematomas, contusions) are more common, although not as common as in adult samples (Bruce et al., 1978; Berger et al., 1985). Contrecoup lesions are relatively rare in all age groups, but least for young children with a gradual increase through childhood (Berney et al., 1994).

The relative lack of myelination present in the CNS during infancy and early childhood also leads to different consequences in response to TBI. Immature myelination causes the cerebral hemispheres to be relatively soft and pliable, enabling them to absorb the force of impact better than in an older child or adult. However, unmyelinated fibers are particularly vulnerable to shearing effects, rendering the younger child more vulnerable to diffuse axonal injury (DAI) (Zimmerman & Bilaniuk, 1994). Bruce and colleagues (1978) suggest that TBI in children is more likely to result in diffuse cerebral swelling associated with vascular disruptions, with such pathology identified in one third of the children (Jennett et al., 1977; Bruce et al., 1978). Outcomes are also different. Babies and toddlers lose consciousness less frequently than other age groups, however post-traumatic epilepsy is more common after early TBI (Raimondi & Hirschauer, 1984; Berney, Froidevaux et al., 1994). The implica-

tions of these age-related differences are important and argue that pathophysiology, sequelae, recovery, and outcome from childhood TBI cannot easily be extrapolated from adult findings.

DIAGNOSIS AND RECOVERY

Assessment and management of the traumatized child commences at the scene of the injury, where conscious state and neurologic status are evaluated. On admission, a range of data are collected to determine the nature and severity of the injury and the extent of primary and secondary pathology. By the time the child reaches a hospital he or she may have sustained permanent primary impact-related brain injury, which is thought to be relatively insensitive to medical treatment. Secondary effects of insult will also be developing, and these have been shown to be more amenable to medical intervention. Early treatment is very much directed towards the accurate identification of these secondary complications and their rapid treatment (Miller, 1991). A number of parameters are particularly informative for determining injury severity at this early stage: level of consciousness, clinical evidence of skull fracture or cerebral pathology, and neurologic and mental status.

Measuring Injury Severity

Coma Scales

Loss of consciousness (LOC) or coma is defined as a state in which there is no eye opening, even in response to pain, no recognizable verbal response, and an inability to obey commands (Miller, 1991). It usually results from direct damage or dysfunction to the brainstem, or deafferentation through DAI. The Glasgow Coma Scale (GCS) (Teasdale & Jennett, 1974) is employed to indicate level of consciousness after TBI. In the adult version of the Glasgow Coma Scale, a score of 13–15 indicates mild TBI, in which there may be some slight alteration of conscious level (e.g., drowsiness, disorientation). Moderate TBI is defined as a GCS score of 9–12, and severe TBI is reflected by a GCS score of <8. The adult version of the GCS is not appropriate for infants and young children, in whom some motor and verbal responses require a level of development not achieved until late childhood. To address this problem, the GCS has been modified for use with children under 5 years of age (Pediatric Coma Scale: Reilly et al., 1988). The score and severity rating will depend on the age of the child.

The advantage of the GCS, and its adapted pediatric version, is that they provide a universal benchmark for classifying injury severity. However, there are a number of limitations that must be considered when interpreting these scores. First, reliability varies depending upon the experience of the rater, with results from inexperienced raters less consistent than those recorded on and after hospital admission (Rowley & Fielding, 1991). Second, when patients require sedation or undergo surgery, GCS monitoring is interrupted. Further, there is no clear agreement about the optimal time to measure GCS score.

Post-traumatic amnesia (PTA) duration is also employed as an index of injury severity, and has been argued to provide a more reliable indicator of functional outcome than other severity measures (Shores, 1989; Ewing-Cobbs et al., 1990). Clinically, post-traumatic amnesia refers to the period of confusion and disorientation after TBI or emergence from coma, and is generally conceptualized as a disturbance of memory and/or attention. Several standardized measures of PTA have been developed and adapted for children (Westmead Post-Traumatic Amnesia Scale: Shores, 1989; Children's Orientation and Amnesia Test: Ewing-Cobbs et al., 1990). These measures require the child to provide information regarding personal details and temporal orientation as well as completing some basic memory tasks. The measures are serially administered in the days after the injury until the child reaches a criterion level of functioning.

Radiologic Investigations

Structural Imaging Techniques: CT/MRI Scans

Radiologic investigations are conducted where there is evidence of skull fracture, neurologic abnormality, or depressed consciousness. Approximately one half of all comatose TBI patients have evidence of an intracranial bleed on CT, encouraging the use of this medium on admission. CT scans are not sensitive in detecting DAI, and some patients with severe TBI have recorded normal CT results (Zimmerman & Bilaniuk, 1994). MRI scans are more sensitive, particularly for detecting DAI, and have been reported to have greater power for predicting outcome from TBI, particularly when scans are taken after the acute recovery phase (Wilson et al., 1988).

Functional Imaging Techniques: SPECT/PET

Although not routinely used for diagnostic purposes, functional imaging may have a role in delineating more subtle injuries, providing information about areas of the brain where cerebral metabolism may be abnormal due to injury (Newton et al., 1992; Nedd et al., 1993). A number of individual case studies of children with mild TBI have detected such abnormalities on positron emission tomography (PET) scan, consistent with neuropsychological data showing memory impairment (Roberts et al., 1995). However, the utility of these techniques is limited in pediatric populations due to the need to use radioactive agents in the imaging process.

Electrophysiologic Methods: EEG/ Evoked Potentials

In general, electroencephalogram (EEG) testing is thought to have limited diagnostic value following TBI. However, in pediatric samples there is evidence that EEG, used in combination with CT scan, during the acute phase after TBI may be predictive of both neurologic outcome and educational success (Ruijs et al., 1994). Evoked potentials have also been found to be helpful in determining injury severity and prognosis. These measures are able to provide information regarding the integrity of sensory systems in situations where the patient is unresponsive.

Functional Impairment: Neurologic Examination

Neurologic examination is routinely conducted with TBI patients, regardless of injury severity. Assessment of motor power, sensation, and coordination provides an indication of brain function. Presence of hemiparesis or cranial nerve dysfunction may give localizing information, while not excluding the presence of other damage (Miller, 1991).

In pediatric patients a combination of measures is usually employed to determine the severity of the injury, because no single indicator has proven to have sufficient predictive power in isolation (Fletcher et al., 1995). The poor reliability of these injury indicators may reflect the relatively recent development of tools, such as the pediatric versions of the GCS, PTA scales, the range of mechanisms of injury, and the developmental level of the child at time of injury, as well as preinjury factors, including environment and premorbid ability.

The Recovery Process

The stages of recovery after pediatric TBI tend to follow a relatively routine path, depending on injury severity. In the following discussion a distinction is made between the relatively rapid and uncomplicated recovery generally exhibited by children sustaining mild TBI, and the more protracted process associated with moderate and severe TBI.

Mild Injuries

Following mild TBI, there is a short period of altered consciousness, and perhaps a period of PTA, characterized by confusion and disorientation. Children are often observed for a short time and discharged home without hospital admission. Clinically, children may exhibit symptoms of fatigue and irritability. Transient cognitive problems may also occur, including reduced attention, psychomotor slowing, poor memory, and behavioral symptoms (Boll, 1983; Beers, 1992). More significant motor and language deficits are uncommon. Over time, these deficits decline and, while there is ongoing debate with respect to outcome, a good recovery is common, particularly in school-aged children, and where no premorbid problems were present (Polissar et al., 1994; Asarnow et al., 1995; Ponsford et al., 1997).

Moderate and Severe Injuries

Recovery from moderate and severe TBI is more protracted and may be seen as a multiphase process in which there is an interaction among the child's physical recovery and developmental level, the family response, and the reintegration of the child into the wider community. These phases are summarized in Figure 40-2.

Acute Phase

Where TBI is more severe, resulting in a period of unconsciousness, children will spend some time in the hospital. During this stage the child's progress is monitored for evidence of deterioration caused by raised intracranial pressure or hematoma, which may require surgery. Physical rehabilitation commences at this early stage, focusing on maintaining the child's physical strength. This is a period of high anxiety for families, during which the major concern is the child's survival. Additional stressors may include family separation, the need to care for other siblings, injuries sustained by other family members, and financial or employment pressures. Feelings may fluctuate from hope and optimism to devastation and despair. Grief, guilt, and blame can also be central issues for parents and siblings during this period.

Early Rehabilitation

As the child emerges from coma, more active rehabilitation begins. At this stage, the child may be restless, agitated, confused, and disoriented. Some children are difficult to manage at this time. On emergence from PTA, functional impairments will be evident, and more intensive rehabilitation, including physical and speech therapies, will begin. The goal is to work towards an early return home to a familiar environment. Following discharge, the child may continue to receive regular rehabilitation while he or she recovers. Return to school is generally a gradual process, with the child initially attending for short periods, primarily for social contact, with attendance increasing as he or she gains physical strength.

This phase of recovery tends to involve a degree of balancing between rehabilitation goals, social adjustment needs of the child, and school and family resources. It is a stage in which constant communication and liaison are required to ensure that the child's deficits are acknowledged and understood, and the appropriate resources are available. It is a stressful time for the family, who must negotiate and organize the various resources required for the child, as well as adjust to the child's physical and behavioral limitations. Families react in different ways to these stresses, depending upon their own strategies and coping styles (Waaland & Kreutzer, 1988).

FIGURE 40-2. Family response to traumatic brain injury during the acute and postacute stages following a childhood injury. (Reproduced with permission from Ponsford J, Wilmott C, Rothwell A, et al: Cognitive and behavioural outcome following mild traumatic brain injury in children. J Intl Neuropsychol Soc 3:225, 1997.)

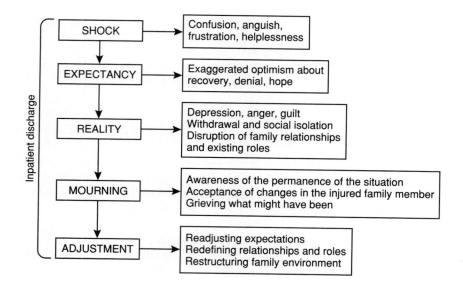

Chronic Phase

Some children sustaining more severe TBI may enjoy a relatively full recovery, with little requirement for professional intervention or support. More commonly, such injuries are associated with ongoing impairments necessitating lifelong medical and rehabilitation involvement. These problems are often most apparent at each developmental transition. At such times the child and family may need support and professional input to negotiate new challenges and enhance the understanding of those working with the child. School entry may emphasize the child's limitations, for example, poor motor coordination may be apparent in diminished sporting ability or writing and drawing difficulties. Communication and attentional difficulties may limit the child's capacity to participate fully in many academic and social activities. Children experiencing these problems may require support additional to that provided within regular school resources. Perhaps the most stressful transition of all is into adolescence, a time when peer pressure and issues of identity are paramount. Adolescents may refuse to accept therapy or intervention, which identifies them as different from their peers. They may become depressed as they begin to fully appreciate the impact that their deficits will have on their future. This pattern of recovery, with its developmental implications, argues that children sustaining moderate and severe TBI require ongoing professional support into adulthood, particularly as they and their families gradually adjust to residual physical, cognitive, and behavioral sequelae, and then at critical developmental transitions.

NEUROPSYCHOLOGICAL CONSEQUENCES OF PEDIATRIC TRAUMATIC BRAIN INJURY

Initially, research into pediatric TBI was directed at identifying long-term sequelae from injuries. The popular view was that, because the child's brain was plastic and able to accommodate the impact of brain insult, the child would experience fewer deficits than an adult. However, even the earliest studies found little support for this view, documenting significant consequences in terms of functional impairments. Later studies focused on injury severity as a predictor of outcome. Results from this endeavor have been less than ideal, showing that, while severity may account for a proportion of the variance in postinjury performance, there is still much unexplained. Such findings have led researchers to seek alternative explanations. Some have argued that the deficits observed reflect premorbid behavioral or learning deficits, or other psychosocial factors such as family dysfunction or low socioeconomic status. Others have investigated age at injury and time since injury, predicting that developmental processes may be largely responsible for variations in outcome. Historically, these variables have been studied separately, and it is only recently that researchers have attempted large scale studies which incorporate measures of preinjury child and family characteristics, age at injury, and recovery over time in a multidimensional model, in an attempt to begin to tease out the complex interactions, and the relative contributions of these various factors to outcome.

Domain-Specific Outcome Studies

Intelligence Quotient

Most studies employ intelligence quotient (IQ) scores either as an outcome measure or as a sample descriptor (Brown et al., 1981; Chadwick, Rutter, Brown, et al., 1981; Chadwick, Rutter, Shaffer, et al., 1981; Rutter et al., 1983; Prior et al., 1994; Anderson & Moore, 1995; Ewing-Cobbs et al., 1997; Ponsford et al., 1997). Results are relatively definitive. Mild TBI is associated with little if any global intellectual deficit, either in acute or chronic stages of recovery. There is ongoing debate as to whether such null findings represent a true lack of impairment, or if IQ measures are unable to detect the subtle deficits occurring as a consequence of mild TBI. In contrast, depressed IQ scores are commonly reported following moderate and severe TBI. Most studies report recovery of IQ scores immediately postinjury, with greatest improvement in the first 6 months and a plateauing effect from that time. Even in the acute stages postinjury, verbal IQ is reported to be relatively unaffected, indicating sparing of established or "crystallized" knowledge, such as general knowledge and word knowledge. Performance IQ scores are more vulnerable, and are consistently reported to be depressed both acutely and in the long term. These findings suggest that more "fluid" skills—problem solving, reasoning, speed of response, and motor coordination—may be specifically impaired in TBI.

Clinically, IQ tests alone are generally considered insufficient to fully demonstrate the range of impairments experienced postinjury. IQ scores may drop over time, as children fail to develop appropriately. However, in the acute stages postinjury, many children, even those with severe TBI, may be able to function within the average range on these tests, despite significant functional impairments, probably using their store of well-learned knowledge and the structure imposed by standardized testing to achieve adequate results. Research suggests that there may be specific neurobehavioral domains that are particularly vulnerable to the impact of TBI—for example, attention, speed of processing, memory, and learning—and the effect of deficiencies in these abilities may not be apparent on IQ testing until sometime after the injury.

Language Skills

Aphasias are rare after childhood TBI. However, clinical reports frequently document communication deficits, including slowed speech, dysfluency, poor logical sequencing of ideas, and word-finding difficulties (Dennis, 1989; Morse et al., 2000). Research findings support such observations, with studies consistently documenting persisting impairments in expressive language skills and writing abilities (Ewing-Cobbs et al., 1987; Campbell & Dolloghan, 1990; Ewing-Cobbs et al., 1997). Not surprisingly, greater deficits are associated with more severe injuries. Further, younger children appear to exhibit more global language difficulties, with additional deficiencies in language comprehension observed when injuries occur in the preschool period (Anderson, Morse, et al., 1997).

Recent research has focussed on the examination of functional language skills, important for day-to-day communication (Dennis & Barnes, 1990; Chapman, 1995; Haritou et al., 1997; Chapman et al., 1998; Ewing-Cobbs et al., 1998a; Didus et al., 2000). These studies have shown that, even when performances on standardized language tests are intact, children with a history of TBI demonstrate functional difficulties, producing less information content and poorer organizational structure on conversational tasks. Haritou and colleagues (1997) document results that indicate that severe TBI may also impact on language development in young children, causing increasing difficulties with time, with the quality of conversation syntactically very simple, and well below the level of complexity expected for age.

Visual and Motor Skills

Severe visual and motor deficits, including hemiparesis, impaired balance, and steadiness, as well as visual field defects, are common in the acute recovery stages, with rapid recovery occurring in the first few months postinjury, and systematic, but nonlinear recovery up to 5 years postinjury (Mahoney et al., 1983; Thompson et al., 1994). It is only when children sustain very severe injuries, or injuries early in life, that such motor deficits persist (Thompson et al., 1994). Subtle deficits, such as visuomotor impairments and reduced eye-hand coordination are more persistent, and may occur even after relatively mild injury (Winogron et al., 1984). Such problems may limit the child's capacity for day-to-day activities such as sport and other physical pursuits and school-based skills including writing, drawing, and copying, with possible secondary implications for self-esteem, socialization, and academic development. Further, as speed requirements increase, children with significant TBI have been found to demonstrate increasing difficulties (Ewing-Cobbs et al., 1989, 1997).

Memory and Learning

Early studies identified memory function as the most likely cognitive domain to show impairment after childhood TBI (Levin & Eisenberg, 1979; Levin et al., 1982; Levin et al., 1988), with greatest impairment and poorest recovery occurring after severe TBI. More recent literature has extended these findings, documenting a consistent trend for children with severe TBI to exhibit generalized deficits in learning, storage, and retrieval. For children with mild/moderate injuries consequences are less clear, but indicate that these children perform closer to normal, with perhaps some mild retrieval problems evident (Jaffe et al., 1992, 1993; Levin et al., 1993, 1994; Jaffe et al., 1995; Yeates et al., 1995; Ong et al., 1998).

The implications of memory impairment in the child are likely to be substantial, given that the day-to-day tasks of childhood largely revolve around acquiring knowledge and learning and perfecting new skills. Memory problems may interfere with this process, resulting in a failure to develop at an age appropriate rate. Kinsella and colleagues (1997) have clearly demonstrated the long-term impact of impaired learning capacity, showing that verbal learning skills are predictive of educational progress at 2 years postinjury, and that children with learning deficits post-TBI are more likely to be in a special school environment or in need of individual remedial intervention.

Attention Skills

Deficits in attention and information processing skills may also impede learning and accumulation of new knowledge, possibly resulting in the global cognitive dysfunction commonly reported in the long term following childhood TBI (Fletcher et al., 1987; Anderson & Moore, 1995; Dennis et al., 1995). In contrast to the specific psychomotor slowing seen after moderate to severe adult TBI, children present with more global attention deficits, with many of these problems persisting beyond the acute recovery stage (Catroppa et al., 1999; Bakker & Anderson, 2000; Catroppa & Anderson, in press). A handful of recent studies have investigated objective indices of attention (Murray et al., 1992; Kaufmann et al., 1993; Dennis et al., 1995; Anderson et al., 1998; Anderson & Pentland, 1998; Ewing-Cobbs, Prasad, et al., 1998b; Fenwick & Anderson, 1999) and have detected attentional problems, specifically for younger, severely injured children. When specific attentional components are localized, results consistently show relatively intact sustained attention capacity, but difficulty with rate of motor execution and with response selection. Further, performances are highly variable within the TBI group, suggesting fluctuating attention, which may be difficult to detect on traditional attention measures.

These more generalized problems may reflect the relatively immature state of attention development at the time of injury. The injury, and its associated pathology, may interrupt ongoing development, so that components of attention which usually emerge and differentiate postinjury, will fail to do so, leading to delayed or deficient performance. Thus, the implications of attention deficits following childhood TBI may be twofold: in addition to the initial injury and associated cognitive impairment, there may be an ongoing impact on cerebral development as well as an inability to acquire new skills. This may lead to increasing lags in knowledge and skills, and a failure in the development and differentiation of cognitive and attentional abilities.

Executive Functions

Deficits in executive functions are commonly reported in children who have suffered TBI, in keeping with the vulnerability of the prefrontal regions in head trauma (Courville, 1945; Walsh, 1978). Despite these observations, there have been few formal studies of executive abilities, though some case descriptions do exist (Passler et al., 1985; Mateer & Williams, 1991; Williams & Mateer, 1992; Dennis et al., 1996). Neuropsychological studies have examined outcomes on a range of traditional executive function tests in children with TBI, showing that performance on executive measures is consistently related to injury severity, with a trend for younger age at injury to be implicated in poorer performances as well (Levin et al., 1994; Garth et al., 1997; Levin et al., 1997; Pentland et al., 1998). Children exhibit poorer reasoning skills, make more errors and use less efficient strategies, and provided ineffective or unworkable planning strategies as a result.

Functional Outcome after Traumatic Brain Injury in Childhood

Children who suffer TBI frequently make a good physical recovery and appear outwardly normal. The expectations of their abilities and behaviors are often determined by this relatively healthy presentation, despite ongoing significant cognitive and behavioral difficulties (Johnson, 1992). In instances of mild TBI, children may perform adequately on neuropsychological testing, but continue to experience problems when faced with the complexities of everyday life, in particular learning and skill acquisition and psychosocial functioning (Asarnow et al., 1991, 1995; Willmott et al., 2000).

Educational Abilities

Academic failure has been argued to be one of the most serious consequences of pediatric TBI (Goldstein & Levin, 1985; Levin et al., 1987; Greenspan & MacKenzie, 1994; Catroppa & Anderson, 2000). Even the early studies identified a relationship between injury severity and educational achievement of childhood TBI were interested in educational outcome, with Klonoff and associates (1977) reporting that one quarter of their sample required remedial classes by 5 years postinjury. More recently, Kinsella and colleagues (1995, 1997) have found that by 2 years postinjury 70% of children with severe injuries, and 40% of those with moderate injuries, were receiving special education. Socioeconomic status, male sex, maladaptive behaviors, reduced verbal learning skills, and slowed psychomotor processing have been identified as predictors of poorer academic achievement postinjury (Donders, 1994; Stalings et al., 1996; Kinsella et al., 1997).

Qualitative analysis of data from these studies suggests that reading skills appear to be relatively resilient following TBI in school-aged children, with arithmetic and comprehension more vulnerable (Berger-Gross & Shackelford, 1985; Kinsella et al., 1997; Barnes et al., 1999; Catroppa & Anderson, 1999a). In contrast, preschool TBI, even of mild degree, has been noted to be associated with school failure. Despite appearing to be fully recovered immediately postinjury, these children are more likely to have reading difficulties and require special education input (Gronwall et al., 1997; Wrightson et al., 1995). Barnes and colleagues (1999) have also addressed the issue of age at injury in association with educational impairment. For reading decoding skills young children achieved poorest results, with older groups performing normally. Reading comprehension was reduced for children sustaining injuries before age nine, but intact for the older group. These findings suggest that the age at injury may interact with the level and complexity of skills previously acquired to determine the outcome.

Behavior and Adaptive Abilities

Debate continues with respect to the etiology of behavioral and adaptive problems after TBI. Some authors claim that these problems reflect premorbid behavioral and family problems, whereas others support an important impact of brain injury (Fletcher et al., 1990; Perrot et al., 1991; Donders, 1992; Prior et al., 1994; Farmer et al., 1996; Wade et al., 1996; Max et al., 1997a, 1997b). Clinical reports frequently describe behavioral change post-TBI, even in the absence of physical disability or cognitive impairment. Problems range from initial symptoms of fatigue and irritability to more persisting deficits such as aggression, poor impulse control, hyperactivity, distractibility, depression, and anxiety (Black et al., 1969; Brink et al., 1980; Brown et al., 1981; Asarnow et al., 1991; Klonoff et al., 1995; Bohnert et al., 1997; Butler et al., 1997; Max et al.,

1997b; Cattelani et al., 1998). Reduced self-esteem and social difficulties may accompany these problems (Bohnert et al., 1997).

Children sustaining mild TBI are least likely to exhibit postinjury behavioral difficulties, whereas those with severe injuries have been found to show a marked increase in psychiatric disturbance, both acutely and in the long term postinjury. Brink and colleagues (1980) report that while only 10% of their sample of severely head-injured children had any persisting neurologic impairment, 46% had severe emotional/behavioral disturbances requiring professional counseling. Brown and colleagues (1981) noted that the rate of new psychiatric disorder was more than doubled in the severely injured group compared with controls. Within this severely injured group, history of preinjury behavioral deficits was predictive of later psychiatric disturbance, with over half of these children developing a disturbance in the 12 months postinjury, in contrast to a figure of 29% for children with no premorbid problems.

A number of studies report increasing problems in behavior, and increased incidence of psychiatric disturbance after TBI (Brink et al., 1980; Brown et al., 1981; Perrot et al., 1991; Cattelani et al., 1998). This pattern may be due to the direct effects of TBI (e.g., increased impulsivity, hyperactivity associated with right frontal damage) or related to secondary factors such as family dysfunction or depression and adjustment difficulties occurring in the process of coming to terms with long-term implications of injury.

A summary of the common consequences of significant TBI in childhood is provided in Table 40-1.

INJURY-RELATED PREDICTORS OF OUTCOME

Following the pioneering work of early researchers such as Klonoff and Rutter, there has been less emphasis on documenting recovery patterns following childhood TBI. The prevailing view has been that children recover better than adults, and usually attain preinjury levels of performance. However, the findings presented in the previous discussion question this position, particularly following serious injury. In reality, recovery after childhood TBI is variable and difficult to predict. As shown in Figure 40-3, neurologic recovery probably stabilizes earliest, with the majority of transient neurologic symptoms abating by about 3 months postinjury. In more severe injuries, neurologic symptoms persist and may indicate permanent impairment. Behavioral recovery is not so clear-cut, with an initial reduction in acute symptoms, such as fatigue and irritability, perhaps reflecting a decrease in the global effects of cerebral injury. Most researchers describe an increase in psychological problems and psychiatric disturbance with time. It is likely that, rather than resulting from physiologic factors,

TABLE 40-1. Consequences of Significant TBI in Childhood

Domain	Deficit
Language	Reduced expressive skills
	Impaired pragmatics
Motor skills	Gross motor problems
	Poor balance
	Fine and visuomotor incoordination
	Slowed speed of motor response
Memory	Reduced earning
	Poor storage skills
	Retrieval problems
Attention	Fluctuating attention
	Impulsivity
Executive functions	Poor planning and organization
	Impaired reasoning
	Reduced self-monitoring
Education	Poor reading comprehension
	Poor mathematics
	Slow, untidy writing
Behavior/social skills	Social difficulties
	Reduced self-esteem
	Irritability
	Low frustration tolerance

these emerging symptoms represent secondary adjustment problems which a child may experience in response to physiologic and cognitive disability.

Intellectual "recovery" has also been documented by a number of authors (Chadwick, Rutter, Brown et al., 1981; Jaffe et al., 1993; Prior et al., 1994), with a range of factors implicated as important for cognitive recovery. Younger age at injury has been noted to be associated with poorer recovery initially, and a failure to maintain developmental progress in the years postinjury (Anderson & Moore, 1995; Anderson et al., 1997; Ewing-Cobbs et al., 1997; Gronwall et al., 1997). Psychosocial parameters including reduced access to rehabilitation services and special education, and significant family dysfunction and psychiatric problems may all impact on future recovery. Nature and degree of injury are also paramount. Recovery has been shown to be more complete in mild injuries (Ponsford et al., 1997), while more compensation for disabilities may be possible in focal injuries, where much brain remains intact.

It is probable that specific factors are predictive of recovery at different stages post-TBI. For example, injury severity is a crucial predictor of function in the

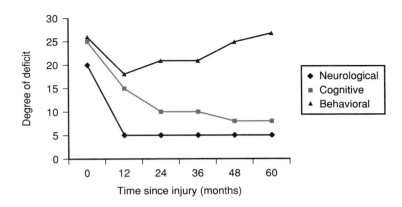

FIGURE 40-3. Schematic representation of differential recovery of neurologic, behavioral, and intellectual functions after traumatic brain injury in children.

acute stages of recovery, but may become less important in the long term. Yeates and colleagues (1997) suggest that premorbid factors may influence outcome, and additionally Rivara and associates (1994) report that better outcome is associated with better family functioning. Other factors, such as the degree of family burden—e.g., financial difficulty, time stress, degree of child disability—will also play a role in determining the functional outcome of the child in the long term post-TBI (Table 40-2). Longitudinal studies are underway (Jaffe et al., 1995; Taylor et al., 1995; Anderson et al., 1997; Ewing-Cobbs et al., 1997; Kinsella et al., 1997) that build on the knowledge of functional impairment gained from past research, but currently there is minimal information regarding outcome after 2 years postinjury.

Injury Severity

As is true for adult TBI, injury severity is an important predictor of outcome from TBI. Studies describe impairments in a range of neuropsychological and functional areas following severe TBI in children. A recent prospective, longitudinal study by Jaffe and colleagues (1995) has investigated the relationship between injury severity, recovery, and outcome by following a cohort of

TABLE 40-2. Predictors of Long-Term Recovery from Childhood TBI

Predictor
Injury severity (mild, moderate, severe)
Nature of injury (closed, penetrating)
Degree of physical disability (e.g., hemiparesis, dysarthria)
Age at injury
Premorbid characteristics (e.g., cognitive abilities, behavioral function)
Family function (e.g., socioeconomic status, family structure and style)
Environmental factors (e.g., access to rehabilitation)

children sustaining TBI, following children for up to 3 years postinjury. This group has examined a variety of cognitive skills including IQ, memory, problem solving, motor performance, academic performance, and daily living skills. They note that severity exerts a significant influence on recovery patterns in the period postinjury. Severe and moderate injury was associated with deficits across the range of domains assessed, suggestive of a consistent dose-response relationship, with severely injured children exhibiting most impaired performances in all areas, and the moderate TBI group exhibiting less severe deficits. Significant recovery was observed in the 12 months postinjury, but performance then plateaued, remaining stable over the following 2 years. For the mild TBI group, the recovery curve was consistently flat across domains, with performance levels age appropriate, suggesting minimal initial impact of injury.

It appears that, while degree of residual deficit may be similar for children and adults, the recovery period may be relatively short in children. This brief recovery phase may suggest differing pathophysiologic processes, perhaps a quicker neuronal recovery reflecting a younger CNS. Alternately, it may represent the additive effects of underlying physiologic recovery, plus the negative impact of cognitive sequelae for ongoing development. While at a superficial level the recovery process for adults and children may appear similar, such an interpretation does not account for the ongoing developmental processes occurring during childhood.

The nature of injury is also relevant to recovery and long-term outcome, with more focal injuries generally thought to lead to better outcome than generalized insults. A number of injury characteristics have been found to be associated with poorer prognosis in children, including depth of lesion (Ommaya & Gennarelli, 1974), presence of secondary damage due to intracranial hematomas (Berger et al., 1985; Walker et al., 1985), DAI (Filley et al., 1987), edema, hypoxia, hemorrhage, and herniation (Gentry et al., 1988). Severity of total injuries has also been identified as a predictive factor (Michaud et al., 1992).

Age at Injury

Contrary to plasticity theories, which argue for the greater capacity for reorganization within the young brain, persisting effects of brain damage in infancy and early childhood are consistently documented. Evidence shows that young children sustaining generalized brain insult are at great risk for long-term cognitive deficits (Ewing-Cobbs et al., 1989; Cousens et al., 1991; Anderson et al., 1994; Anderson, Bond et al., 1997; Gronwall et al., 1997; Taylor & Alden, 1997; Anderson & Taylor, 1999), perhaps due to the vulnerability of the immature brain. Of note, the functional domains most crucial for normal development, such as information processing, memory and executive function, rely on neural substrates particularly vulnerable to the impact of TBI. Deficiencies in these skills are significant for children, because they reduce the ability to learn from the surrounding environment, potentially affecting not only cognitive ability but also social and emotional development (Anderson, 1998).

Early studies detected no relationship between age at injury and neurobehavioural outcome, perhaps because assessment measures were insensitive to affected skills, or because sampling has generally been limited to school-aged children (Klonoff et al., 1977; Chadwick, Rutter, Brown et al., 1981; Tompkins et al., 1990). A small number of studies have identified differences between children sustaining TBI during the preschool years and those injured in later childhood (Lange-Cosack et al., 1979; Ewing-Cobbs et al, 1989; Kriel et al., 1989;), and when younger children are examined, poorer cognitive and motor outcomes have been found (Anderson et al., 1997; Ewing-Cobbs et al., 1997; Gronwall et al., 1997). Recent studies conducted in our laboratory (Anderson & Moore, 1995; Anderson et al., 2000) have investigated children with moderate and severe TBI, and found that, while school-aged children show recovery profiles similar to those seen in adults, preschool groups demonstrate minimal recovery (Fig. 40-4). In contrast to the generally reported trends for IQ, younger age at injury was related to deterioration in verbal IQ scores over time, perhaps indicating a

failure to acquire verbal knowledge from the environment. For performance IQ, a small increase in scores are evident for both age groups, but greater for older children, suggesting "recovery" of performance skills is not so evident for younger injuries.

PREMORBID AND PSYCHOSOCIAL FACTORS

The nature of the link between premorbid characteristics and postinjury function is controversial. Rutter and associates (Brown et al., 1981; Rutter et al., 1983) were the first to describe such a relationship, arguing that children sustaining TBI were at greater risk for developing psychiatric and cognitive sequelae if they had demonstrated such problems premorbidly. They noted that over half of the children in their study with some evidence of preinjury behavioral or psychiatric disorder developed a clinically significant disorder by 12 months postinjury, and none were without symptoms. For those children with no preexisting problems, more than half were symptom-free 12 months postinjury. It appears that when preinjury problems are present, TBI may exacerbate them. Similar findings have been reported in studies which focus on mild TBI, documenting that problems in this group arise only where preinjury risk factors were present (Ponsford et al., 1997).

Premorbid levels of family function have also been found to be predictive of postinjury child behavior and family function. Wade and associates (1996) found that, postinjury, degree of family burden and parental problems was greater in families who reported chronic life stress and maladaptive coping styles. These families reported primary concerns about their child's injuries, interpersonal stresses with other family members, and disruption of family routines and school and work schedules. Yeates and colleagues (1997) extended these results identifying a relationship between injury severity and family/psychosocial factors. They noted that premorbid psychosocial functioning was an important determinant of rate of recovery. In addition, they reported that the impact of severe TBI was buffered by above average social resources and exacerbated by below average

FIGURE 40-4. Comparison of recovery trajectories for children injured before and after 7 years, represented by mental age—chronological age at 4 months and 24 months postinjury. These findings suggest that earlier age at injury is related to poorer recovery postinjury. M.A., Mental Age; C.A., Chronological Age; HI, Head Injury.

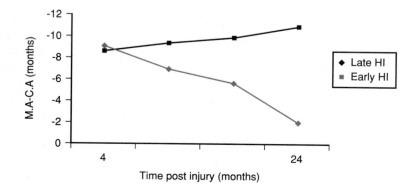

resources. Similarly, Rivara and colleagues (1993, 1994) found that levels of family coping are predictive of child behavior and academic performance.

MANAGEMENT AND INTERVENTION

Pediatric rehabilitation is a multidisciplinary endeavor, incorporating rehabilitation physicians, physical therapists, occupational therapists, speech therapists, play therapists, special educators, and social workers, as well as neuropsychologists. The goals of the rehabilitation process are to promote recovery and help the child compensate for residual deficits, to understand and treat cognitive and behavioral impairments and monitor family and other social factors (Rourke et al., 1983; Ylvisaker, 1985).

General rehabilitation approaches can be divided according to the aim of the intervention: (1) restoration of function: the reestablishment of impaired functions via a range of therapeutic modalities; (2) functional adaptation: intact abilities are used to "re-route" skills that have been disrupted via behavioral training—for example, training a child in visual imagery strategies to compensate for a verbal memory deficit; and (3) environmental modification: alteration of the environment to meet the child's new needs, of particular relevance once the child has returned home to family and school, in the postacute phase. In many centers a combination of these approaches is employed. Currently, there is little research available on the relative efficacy of each of these models.

During the acute recovery phase, rehabilitation is often intense, and focussed on areas of identified deficit. The child with hemiparesis will require daily physical therapy, while speech intervention will be the first priority for the dysarthric child. Input from the neuropsychologist may be sought regarding issues such as emergence from post-traumatic amnesia or appropriate environment for optimal recovery, but by and large these tasks are incorporated into other therapists' roles. During this phase of rapid recovery, appropriate rehabilitation may maximize the child's recovery. However, fatigue is a major issue, and therapies must be balanced with the need for rest. When a multidisciplinary team approach is employed, therapists often combine to provide shorter, more holistic therapeutic techniques. As the child becomes oriented and more robust, more specific treatments become possible and may continue on a regular basis for many months postinjury, according to the child's needs.

The neuropsychologist becomes more central once the child is able to cope with assessment procedures, and an initial evaluation may be conducted to determine early impairment. Neuropsychological findings may then be communicated to therapists, consultants, and parents to guide rehabilitation. The neuropsychologist also has an important role in the school reintegration process, providing appropriate information regarding the child's cognitive strengths and weaknesses, behavioral function and the implications of the child's injuries for the school context. Once full reintegration has occurred, the need for additional educational support may become evident. Teaching aids, to provide individual instruction or tailoring of educational programs, are frequently employed to encourage ongoing development and recovery. The child may continue to receive therapies during this period, either at a rehabilitation facility, or via the school. Regular liaison may be established with school staff, parents, and involved professionals, to ensure that programs are being implemented appropriately and with expected impact. Ongoing assessment of recovery and current levels of functioning is important in order to inform the neuropsychologist of the child's current needs. Results will inform parents and teachers about any recovery that may have occurred or of plateaus in recovery and may provide much needed motivation, or help determine why the child is not progressing, despite enthusiastic input. In addition, such reviews may alert the neuropsychologist to the need for additional therapeutic intervention.

There is also a role for monitoring family function and coping. The added demands of the child's injury, in terms of emotional, financial, and physical resources, may be great. Issues of blame, loss, and grief may need to be addressed. Feelings of hopelessness, being trapped, and ambivalence to the child may also emerge. Even in families that cope well, behavioral difficulties exhibited by the TBI child are often difficult to understand and manage. Treatment of these problems may be best done by the neuropsychologist, perhaps in consultation with a family therapist or individual counselor.

CONCLUSIONS

Consequences of childhood TBI are varied and difficult to predict. Current research suggests that mild TBI may result in few, if any, residual impairments for the normal child. In contrast, children with premorbid vulnerabilities, for example behavioral or learning problems, are more likely to demonstrate continued or increased problems. For moderate-to-severe injuries residual neurobehavioral deficits are common. Crystallized skills (e.g., well-learned skills and knowledge) appear less vulnerable than fluid skills (e.g., planning, reasoning, problem solving), with greatest deficits in attention, memory speed of processing, and high-level language and nonverbal abilities. Further, the consequences of childhood TBI appear to be qualitatively different from those observed following similar damage to the mature CNS. Whereas adult injury may lead to immediate consequences in terms of brain injury, cognitive disability, and behavioral impairment, in the child there is an ongoing interaction among these domains, resulting in cumulative and often global dysfunction. Thus, recovery is less complete, with additional deficits often emerging as the child passes through each developmental stage.

Recent longitudinal research has shown that recovery and ultimate outcome are dependent on a number of biologic, developmental, and psychosocial factors, including nature and severity of injury, premorbid abilities, developmental level at time of injury, time since injury, stability of family unit, and access to resources. The relative importance of each of these parameters, and the possibility that their impact may be greatest at different stages in the recovery process, and their mechanisms of interaction, are still to be determined. While significant gains in knowledge and understanding of childhood TBI have been achieved in recent years, future research needs to address these complexities, in the context of longitudinal, multidimensional research, to plot the natural history of these injuries.

■ KEY POINTS

☐   The nature of pediatric traumatic brain injury varies with age. Infants are more likely to suffer injury due to falls or child abuse, whereas preschoolers are injured in falls and pedestrian accidents. Older children and adolescents are more commonly victims of sporting, cycling, or pedestrian accidents.

☐   Upon hospital admission, the following parameters are particularly important for determining injury severity: level of consciousness, clinical evidence of skull fracture or cerebral pathology, and neurologic and mental status.

☐   Studies suggest that reading skills are relatively resilient after traumatic brain injury in school-aged children, with arithmetic and comprehension more vulnerable.

☐   Better outcome is associated with better family functioning.

☐   For children with no preexisting problems, more than half are symptom-free 12 months after injury. When preinjury problems are present, traumatic brain injury will exacerbate them.

KEY READINGS

Anderson V, Moore C: Age at injury as a predictor of outcome following pediatric head injury. Child Neuropsychol 1:187–202, 1995.

Fletcher J, Ewing-Cobbs L, Francis D, et al: Variability in outcomes after traumatic brain injury in children: a developmental perspective, in Broman SH, Michel ME (eds): Traumatic Head Injury in

Children. New York: Oxford University Press, 1995, pp. 3–21.

Jaffe KM, Polizzar NL, Fay GC, et al: Recovery trends over three years following prediatric traumatic brain injury. Arch Phys Med Rehabil 76:17–26, 1995.

REFERENCES

Amacher AL: Pediatric head injuries. St Louis, MO: Warren H. Green Inc., 1988.

Anderson V: Assessing executive functions in children: Biological, physiological, and developmental considerations. Neuropsychol Rehab 8:319–350, 1998.

Anderson V, Bond L, Catroppa C, et al: Childhood bacterial meningitis: Impact of age at illness and medical complications on long term outcome. J Intl Neuropsychol Soc 3:147–158, 1997.

Anderson V, Catroppa C, Morse S, et al: Recovery of intellectual ability following TBI in childhood: Impact of injury severity and age at injury. Pediatr Neurosurg 32:282–290, 2000.

Anderson V, Fenwick T, Manly T, et al: Attentional skills following traumatic brain injury in childhood: A componential analysis. Brain Inj 12:937–949, 1998.

Anderson V, Moore C: Age at injury as a predictor of outcome following pediatric head injury. Child Neuropsychol 1:187–202, 1995.

Anderson V, Morse SA, Klug G, et al: Predicting recovery from head injury in school-aged children: A prospective analysis. J Intl Neuropsychol Soc 3:568–580, 1997.

Anderson V, Pentland L: Residual attention deficits following childhood head injury. Neuropsychol Rehab 8:283–300, 1998.

Anderson V, Smibert E, Ekert H, et al: Intellectual, educational and behavioral sequelae following cranial irradiation and chemotherapy. Arch Dis Child 70:476–483, 1994.

Anderson V, Taylor HG: Meningitis, in Yeates KO, Ris MD, Taylor HG (eds): Pediatric Neuropsychology: Research, Theory and Practice. New York: Guilford, 1999, pp. 117–148.

Asarnow RF, Satz P, Light R, et al: Behavior problems and adaptive functioning in children with mild and severe closed head injury. J Pediatr Psychol 16:543–555, 1991.

Asarnow RF, Satz P, Light R, et al: The UCLA study of mild head injury in children and adolescents, in Broman SH, Michel ME (eds): Traumatic Head Injury in Children. New York: Oxford University Press, 1995, pp. 117–146.

Baker A, Moulton R, MacMillan V, et al: Excitatory amino acid in cerebrospinal fluid following traumatic brain injury in humans. J Neurosurg 79:369–372, 1993.

Bakker K, Anderson V: Assessment of attention following preschool traumatic brain injury: A behavioural attention measure. Pediatr Rehab 3:149–158, 2000.

Barnes M, Dennis M, Wilkinson M: Reading after closed head injury in childhood: Effects on accuracy, fluency, and comprehension. Devel Neuropsychol 151–124, 1999.

Beers S: Cognitive effects of mild head injury in children and adolescents. Neuropsychol Rev 3:281–319, 1992.

Begali V: Head Injury in Children and Adolescents, ed 2. Brandon, VT: Clinical Psychology Publishing Company, 1992.

Berger MS, Pitts LH, Lovely M, et al: Outcome from severe head injury in children and adolescents. J Neurosurg 62:194–1985, 1985.

Berger-Gross P, Shackelford M: Closed-head injury in children: Neuropsychological and scholastic outcomes. Percept Mot Skills 61:254, 1985.

Berney J, Froidevaux A, Favier J: Pediatric head trauma: Influence of age and sex. II. Biochemical and anatomo-clinical observations. Child Nerv Syst 10:517–523, 1994.

Berney J, Favier J, Froidevaux A: Pediatric head trauma: Influence of age and sex. I. Epidemiology. Child Nerv Syst 10:509–516, 1994.

Black P, Jeffries J, Blumer D, et al: The post-traumatic syndrome in children, in Walker A, Caveness W, Critchley M, et al (eds): The Late Effects of Head Injury. Springfield, IL: Charles C Thomas, 1969, pp. 142–149.

Bohnert A, Parker J, Warschausky S: Friendship and social adjustment following traumatic brain injury: An exploratory investigation. Devel Neuropsychol 13:477–486, 1997.

Boll T : Minor head injury in children—Out of sight but not out of mind. J Clin Child Psychol 12:74–80, 1983.

Brink J, Imbus C, Woo-Sam J: Physical recovery after closed head trauma in children and adolescents. J Pediatr 97:721–727, 1980.

Brown G, Chadwick O, Shaffer D, et al: A prospective study of children with head injuries: II. Psychiatric sequelae. Psychol Med 11:49–62, 1981.

Bruce DA, Raphaely RC, Goldberg AI, et al: Pathophysiology, treatment and outcome following severe head injury in children. Child Brain 2:174–191, 1979.

Bruce DA, Schut L, Bruno LA, et al: Outcome following severe head injury in children. J Neurosurg 48:679–688, 1978.

Butler K, Rourke B, Feurst D, et al: A typology of psychosocial functioning in pediatric closed head injury. Child Neuropsychol 3:98–133, 1997.

Campbell TF, Dollaghan CA: Expressive language recovery in severely brain-injured children and adolescents. J Speech Hearing Dis 55:567–581, 1990.

Catroppa C, Anderson V: Recovery of educational skills following pediatric traumatic head injury. Pediatr Rehab 3:167–175, 2000.

Catroppa C, Anderson V: Attentional skills in the acute phase following pediatric traumatic brain injury. Child Neuropsychol 5:251–264, 1999.

Catroppa C, Anderson V, Stargatt R: A prospective analysis of the recovery of attention following pediatric head injury. J Intl Neuropsychol Soc 5:48–57, 1999.

Cattelani R, Lombardi F, Brianti R, et al: Traumatic brain injury in childhood: Intellectual, behavioral and social outcome into adulthood. Brain Inj 12:283–296, 1998.

Chadwick O, Rutter M, Brown G, et al: A prospective study of children with head injuries: II. Cognitive sequelae. Psychol Med 11:49–61, 1981.

Chadwick O, Rutter M, Shaffer D, et al: A prospective study of children with head injuries: IV. Specific cognitive deficits. J Clin Neuropsychol 2:101–120, 1981.

Chapman S: Discourse as an outcome measure in pediatric head-injured populations, in Broman SH, Michel ME (eds): Traumatic Head Injury in Children. New York: Oxford University Press, 1995, pp. 95–116.

Chapman S, Levin H, Wanek A, et al: Discourse after closed head injury in young children: Relationship of age to outcome. Brain Lang 61:420–449, 1998.

Choux M: Incidence, diagnosis and management of skull fractures, in Raimondi AJ, Choux M, DiRocco C (eds): Head Injuries in the New Born and Infant. New York: Springer-Verlag, 1986, pp. 163–182.

Courville CB: Pathology and the Nervous System. Mountain View, CA: Pacific Press, 1945.

Cousens P, Ungerer JA, Crawford JA, et al: Cognitive effects of childhood leukemia therapy: A case for four specific deficits. J Pediatr Psychol 16:475–488, 1991.

Craft AW, Shaw DA, Cartlidge NE: Head injuries in children. BMJ 4:200–2003, 1972.

Dalby PR, Obrzut JE: Epidemiologic characteristics and sequelae of closed head-injured children and adolescents: A review. Devel Neuropsychol 7:35–68, 1991.

Dennis M: Language and the young damaged brain, in Boll T, Bryant BK (eds): Clinical Neuropsychology and Brain Function: Research, Measurement and Practice. Washington, DC: American Psychological Association, 1989, pp. 85–124.

Dennis M, Barnes M: Knowing the meaning, getting the point, bridging the gap, and carrying the message: Aspects of discourse following closed head injury in childhood and adolescence. Brain Lang 39:428–446, 1990.

Dennis M, Barnes MA, Donnelly RE, et al: Appraising and managing knowledge: Metacognitive skills after childhood head injury. Devel Neuropsychol 12:77–103, 1996.

Dennis M, Wilkinson M, Koski L, et al: Attention deficits in the long term after childhood head injury, in Broman S, Michel ME (eds): Traumatic Head Injury in Children. New York: Oxford University Press, 1995, pp. 165–187.

Didus E, Anderson V, Catroppa C: The development of pragmatic communication skills in head-injured children. Pediatr Rehabil 3:177–186, 2000.

Donders J: Premorbid behavioral and psychosocial adjustment of children with traumatic brain injury. J Abnorm Child Psychol 20:233–246, 1992.

Donders J: Academic placement after traumatic brain injury. J School Psychol 32:53–56, 1994.

Ewing-Cobbs L, Brookshire B, Scott M, et al: Children's narratives following traumatic brain injury: Linguistic structure, cohesion, and thematic recall. Brain Lang 61:395–419, 1998a.

Ewing-Cobbs L, Fletcher J, Levin H, et al: Longitudinal neuropsychological outcome in infants and preschoolers with traumatic brain injury. J Intl Neuropsychol Soc 3:581–591, 1997.

Ewing-Cobbs L, Levin H, Eisenberg H, et al: Language functions following closed head injury in children and adolescents. J Clin Exper Neuropsychol 9:575–592, 1987.

Ewing-Cobbs L, Levin H, Fletcher JM, et al: The Children's Orientation and Amnesia Test: Relationship to severity of acute head injury and to recovery of memory. Neurosurgery 27:683–691, 1990.

Ewing-Cobbs L, Miner ME, Fletcher JM, et al: Intellectual, language and motor sequelae following closed head injury in infants and preschoolers. J Pediatr Psychol 14:531–547, 1989.

Ewing-Cobbs L, Prasad M, Fletcher JM, et al: Attention after pediatric traumatic brain injury: A multidimensional assessment. Child Neuropsychol 4:35–48, 1998b.

Farmer J, Haut J, Williams J, et al: Memory functioning in children with traumatic brain injury and premorbid learning problems. J Intl Neuropsychol Soc 2:38–39, 1996.

Fenwick T, Anderson V: Impairments of attention following childhood traumatic brain injury. Child Neuropsychol 5:213–223, 1999.

Filley CM, Cranberg MD, Alexander MP, et al: Neurobehavioral outcome after closed head injury in childhood and adolescence. Arch Neurol 44:194–198, 1987.

Fletcher J, Ewing-Cobbs L, Francis D, et al: Variability in outcomes after traumatic brain injury in children: A developmental perspective, in Broman SH, Michel ME (eds): Traumatic Head Injury in Children. New York: Oxford University Press, 1995, pp. 3–21.

Fletcher J, Ewing-Cobbs, Miner ME, Levin HS, et al: Behavioral changes after closed head injury in children. J Consult Clin Psychol 58:93–98, 1990.

Fletcher J, Miner M, Ewing-Cobbs L, et al: Age and recovery from head injury in children: Developmental issues, in Levin H, Eisenberg H, Grafman J (eds): Neurobehavioral Recovery from Head Injury. New York: Oxford, 1987, pp. 290–291.

Garth J, Anderson VA, Wrennall J, et al: Executive functions following moderate to severe frontal lobe injury: Impact of injury and age at injury. Pediatr Rehab 1:99–108, 1997.

Gentry L, Godersky J, Thompson B: MR imaging of head trauma: Review of the distribution and radiographic features of traumatic lesions. Arch Neurol 44:194–198, 1988.

Goldstein FC, Levin HS: Epidemiology of pediatric closed head injury: Incidence, clinical characteristics and risk factors. J Learn Disabil 20:518–525, 1987.

Goldstein FC, Levin HS: Intellectual and academic outcome following closed head injury in children and adolescents: Research and empirical findings. Devel Neuropsychol 1:195–214, 1985.

Graham D, Ford I, Adams J, et al: Fatal head injury in children. Clin Pathol 42:18, 1989.

Greenspan A, MacKenzie E: Functional outcome after pediatric head injury. Pediatrics 94:425–432, 1994.

Gronwall D, Wrightson P, McGinn V: Effects of mild head injury during the preschool years. J Intl Neuropsychol Soc 6:592–597, 1997.

Haritou F, Ong K, Morse S, et al: A syntactic and pragmatic analysis of the conversational speech of young head injured children, in Ponsford J, Snow P, Anderson V (eds): Proceedings: 5th International Association for the Study of Traumatic Brain Injury Conference, Melbourne, Australia, 1996. Bowen Hills, Australia: Australian Academic Press, 1997, pp. 187–190.

Hayes HR, Jackson RH: The incidence and prevention of head injuries, in Johnson DA, Uttley D, Wyke MA (eds): Children's Head Injury: Who Cares? London, UK: Taylor & Francis, 1989, pp. 183–193.

Holloway M, Bye A, Moran K: Non-accidental head injury in children. Med J Aust 160:786–789, 1994.

Horowitz I, Costeff H, Sadan N, et al: Childhood head injuries in Israel: Epidemiology and outcome. Intl Rehabil Med 5:32–36, 1983.

Jaffe KM, Polissar NL, Fay GC, et al: Recovery trends over three years following pediatric traumatic brain injury. Arch Phys Med Rehabil 76:17–26, 1995.

Jaffe KM, Fay GC, Polissar NL, Martin KM, et al: Severity of pediatric traumatic brain injury and neurobehavioral recovery at one year—a cohort study. Arch Phys Med Rehabil 74:587–595, 1993.

Jaffe KM, Fay GC, Polissar NL, et al: Severity of pediatric traumatic brain injury and neurobehavioral outcome: A cohort study. Arch Phys Med Rehabil 73:540–547, 1992.

Jennett B: Post-traumatic epilepsy. Adv Neurol 22:137–147, 1979.

Jennett B, Teasdale G, Galbraith S, et al: Severe head injuries in three countries. J Neurol Neurosurg Psychiatry 40:291–298, 1977.

Kaufmann P, Fletcher J, Levin H, et al: Attention disturbance after pediatric closed head injury. J Child Neurol 8:348–353, 1993.

Kinsella G, Prior M, Sawyer M, et al: Neuropsychological deficit and academic performance in children and adolescents following traumatic brain injury. J Pediatr Psychol 20:753–767, 1995.

Kinsella G, Prior M, Sawyer M, et al: Predictors and indicators of academic outcome in children 2 years following traumatic head injury. J Int Neuropsychol Soc 3:608–616, 1997.

Klonoff H: Head injuries in children: Predisposing factors, accident conditions, accident proneness and sequelae. Am J Pub Health 61:2405–2417, 1971.

Klonoff H, Clark C, Klonoff P: Outcome of head injuries from childhood to adulthood: A twenty-three year follow-up study, in Broman SH, Michel ME (eds): Traumatic Head Injury in Children. New York: Oxford University Press, 1995, pp. 219–234.

Klonoff H, Low MD, Clark C: Head injuries in children: A prospective five year follow-up. J Neurol Neurosurg Psychiatry 40:1211–1219, 1977.

Kraus JF: Epidemiological features of brain injury in children, in Broman SH Michel ME (eds): Traumatic Head Injury in Children. New York: Oxford University Press, 1995, pp. 117–146.

Kraus JF, Fife D, Cox P, et al: Incidence, severity, and external causes of pediatric brain injury. Am J Epidemiol 119:186–201, 1986.

Kriel RL, Krach LE, Panser LA: Closed head injury: Comparisons of children younger and older than six years of age. Pediatr Neurol 5:296–300, 1989.

Lange-Cosack H, Wider B, Schlesner HJ, et al: Prognosis of brain injuries in young children (one until five years of age). Neuropaediatrics 10:105–127, 1979.

Lehr E: Psychological Management of Traumatic Brain Injuries in Children and Adolescents. Rockville, MD: Aspen, 1990.

Levin H, Culhane K, Mendelsohn D, et al: Cognition in relation to magnetic resonance imaging in head-injured children and adolescents. Arch Neurol 50:897–905, 1993.

Levin H, Eisenberg H: Neuropsychological impairment after closed head injury in children and adolescents. J Pediatr Psychol 4:389–402, 1979.

Levin H, Eisenberg H, Wigg N, et al: Memory and intellectual ability after head injury in children and adolescents. Neurosurgery 11:668–673, 1982.

Levin H, Grafman J , Eisenberg H: Neurobehavioral recovery from head injury. New York: Oxford University Press, 1987.

Levin H, Mendelsohn D, Lilly M, et al: Tower of London performance in relation to magnetic resonance imaging following closed head injury in children. Neuropsychology 8:171–179, 1994.

Levin H, Song J, Scheibel R, et al: Concept formation and problem solving following closed head injury in children. J Intl Neuropsychol Soc 3:598–607, 1997.

Levin HS, High W, Ewing-Cobbs L, et al: Memory functioning during the first year after closed head injury in children and adolescents. Neurosurgery 22:17–34, 1988.

Levin HS, Kraus MF: The frontal lobes and traumatic brain injury. J Neuropsychiatr 6:443–454, 1994.

Mahoney W, D'Souza B, Haller J, et al: Long-term outcome of children with severe head trauma and prolonged coma. Pediatrics 71:756–762, 1983.

Mateer CA, Williams D: Effects of frontal lobe injury in childhood. Devel Neuropsychol 7:69–86, 1991.

Max J, Smith W, Sato Y, et al: Predictors of family functioning following traumatic brain injury in children and adolescents. J Acad Child Adolesc Psychiatry, 37:83–90, 1997a.

Max J, Smith W, Sato Y, et al: Traumatic brain injury in children and adolescents: Psychiatric disorders in the first three months. J Acad Child Adolesc Psychiatry 36: 94–102, 1997b.

Michaud LJ, Rivara FP, Grady MS, et al: Predictors of survival and severe disability after severe brain injury in children. Neurosurgery 31:254–264, 1992.

Miller JD: Pathophysiology and management of head injury. Neuropsychology 5:235–261, 1991.

Morse S, Haritou F, Ong K, et al: Early effects of traumatic brain injury on young children's language performance: A preliminary analysis. Pediatr Rehabil 3:139–148, 2000.

Murray R, Shum D, McFarland K: Attentional deficits in head-injured children: An information processing analysis. Brain Cogn 18:99–115, 1992.

Nedd K, Sfakianakis G, Ganz W, et al: 99m Tc-HMPAQ SPECT of the brain in mild to moderate traumatic brain injury patients: Compared with CT—a prospective study. Brain Inj 7:469–479, 1993.

Newton M, Greenwood R, Britton K, et al: A study comparing SPECT with CT and MRI after closed head injury. J Neurol Neurosurg Psychiatry 55:92–94, 1992.

North B: Jamieson's First Notebook of Head Injury, ed 3. London, UK: Butterworths, 1984.

Novack T, Dillon M, Jackson W: Neurochemical mechanisms in brain injury and treatment: A review. J Clin Exper Neuropsychol 18685–18706, 1996.

Ommaya A, Gennarelli T: Cerebral concussion and traumatic unconsciousness: Correlation of experimental and clinical observations on blunt head injuries. Brain 97:633–654, 1974.

Ong L, Chandran V, Zasmani S, et al: Outcome of closed head injury in Malaysian children: Neurocognitive and behavioural sequelae. J Pediatr Child Health 34:363–368, 1998.

Pang D: Pathophysiologic correlates of neurobehavioral syndromes following closed head injury, in Ylvisaker M (ed): Head Injury Rehabilitation: Children and Adolescents. London: Taylor & Francis, 1985, pp. 3–70.

Passler MA, Isaac W, Hynd GW: Neuropsychological development of behavior attributed to frontal lobe functioning in children. Dev Neuropsychol 1:349–370, 1985.

Pentland L, Todd JA, Anderson V: The impact of head injury severity on planning ability in adolescence: A functional analysis. Neuropsychol Rehabil 8:301–317, 1998.

Perrott SB, Taylor HG, Montes JL: Neuropsychological sequelae, familial stress, and environmental adaptation following pediatric head injury. Devel Neuropsychol 7:69–86, 1991.

Polissar N, Fay G, Jaffe K, et al: Mild pediatric traumatic brain injury: adjusting significance levels for multiple comparisons. Brain Inj 8:249–264, 1994.

Ponsford J, Sloan S, Snow P: Traumatic brain injury: Rehabilitation for everyday adaptive living. Hove, UK: Lawrence Erlbaum & Associates, 1995.

Ponsford J, Willmott C, Rothwell A, et al: Cognitive and behavioural outcome following mild traumatic brain injury in children. J Intl Neuropsychol Soc 3:225, 1997.

Prior M, Kinsella G, Sawyer M, et al: Cognitive and psychosocial outcomes after head injury in childhood. Austr Psychol 29:116–123, 1994.

Quattrocchi K, Prasad P, Willits N, et al: Quantification of midline shift as a predictor of poor outcome following head injury. Surg Neurol 35:183–188, 1991.

Raimondi A, Hirschauer J: Head injury in the infant and toddler. Child Brain 11 12–35, 1984.

Reilly P, Simpson D, Sprod R, et al: Assessing the conscious level of infants and young children: A pediatric version of the Glasgow Coma Scale. Child Nerv Syst 4:30–33, 1988.

Rivara JB, Jaffe KM, Fay GC, et al: Family functioning and injury severity as predictors of child functioning one year following traumatic brain injury. Arch Phys Med Rehabil 74:1047–1055, 1993.

Rivara JB, Jaffe KM, Polissar NL, et al: Family functioning and children's academic performance and behavior problems in the year following traumatic brain injury. Arch Phys Med Rehabil 75:368–379, 1994.

Roberts M, Manshad F, Bushnell D, et al: Neurobehavioural dysfunction following mild traumatic brain injury in childhood: A case report with positive findings on positron emission tomography (PET). Brain Inj 9: 427–436, 1995.

Rourke BP, Bakker DJ, Fisk JL et al: Child neuropsychology: An introduction to theory, research, and clinical practice. New York: Guilford, 1983.

Rowley G. Fielding K: Reliability and accuracy of the Glasgow Coma Scale with experienced and inexperienced raters. Lancet 337:535–538, 1991.

Ruijs M, Gabreels F, Thijssen H: The utility of electroencephalography and cerebral computed tomography in children with mild and moderately severe closed head injuries. Neuropediatrics 25:73–77, 1994.

Rutter M, Chadwick O, Shaffer D: Head injury, in Rutter M (ed): Developmental Neuropsychiatry. New York: Guilford, 1983, pp. 83–111.

Sharma M, Sharma A: Mode, presentation, CT findings and outcome of pediatric head injury. Indian J Pediatr 31:733–739, 1994.

Sharples P, Stuart A, Matthews D, et al: Cerebral blood flow and metabolism in children with severe head injury. Part I: Relation to age, Glasgow Coma Score, outcome, intracranial pressure, and time after injury. J Neurol Neurosurg Psychiatry 58:145–152, 1995.

Shores AE: Comparison of the Westmead PTA Scale and the Glasgow Coma Scale of predictors of neuropsychological outcome following extremely severe blunt head injury. J Neurol Neurosurg Psychiatry 52:126–127, 1989.

Stallings G, Ewing-Cobbs L, Francis D, et al: Prediction of academic placement after pediatric head injury using neurologic, demographic and neuropsychological variables. J Intl Neuropsychol Soc 1996.

Taylor HG, Alden J: Age-related differences in outcomes following childhood brain insults: An introduction and overview. J Intl Neuropsychol Soc 3:555–567, 1997.

Taylor HG, Drotar D, Wade S, et al: Recovery from traumatic brain injury in children: The importance of the family, in Broman SH, Michel ME (eds): Traumatic Head Injury in Children. New York: Oxford University Press, 1995, pp. 188–218.

Teasdale G, Jennett B: Assessment of coma and impaired consciousness. Lancet 2:81–84, 1974.

Thompson NM, Francis DJ, Stuebing KK, et al: Motor, visuo-spatial, and somatosensory skills after closed head injury in children and adolescents: A study of change. Neuropsychology, 8:333–342, 1994.

Tompkins CA, Holland AL, Ratcliff G, et al: Predicting cognitive recovery from closed head injury in children and adolescents. Brain Cogn 13:86–97, 1990.

Waaland P, Kreutzer J: Family response to childhood traumatic brain injury. J Head Trauma Rehabil 3:51–63, 1988.

Wade S, Taylor HG, Drotar D, et al: Childhood traumatic brain injury: Initial impact on the family. J Learn Disabil 29:652–661, 1996.

Walker M, Mayer T, Storrs B, et al: Pediatric head injury: Factors which influence outcome, in Chapman P (ed): Concepts in Pediatric Neurosurgery, Vol. 6. Basel: Karger, 1985, pp. 84–97.

Walsh KW: Neuropsychology: A Clinical Approach. New York: Churchill Livinstone, 1978.

Williams D, Mateer C: Developmental impact of frontal lobe injury in middle childhood. Brain Cogn 20:96–204, 1992.

Willmott C, Anderson V, Anderson P: Attention following pediatric head injury: A developmental perspective. Devel Neuropsychol 17:361–379, 2000.

Wilson J, Wiedmann K, Hadley D, et al: Early and late magnetic resonance imaging and neuropsychological outcome after head injury. J Neurol Neurosurg Psychiatry 51:391–396, 1988.

Winogron HW, Knights R M, Bawden HN: Neuropsychological deficits following head injury in children. J Clin Neuropsychol 6:269–286, 1984.

Wrightson P, McGinn V, Gronwall D: Mild head injury in preschool children: Evidence that it can be associated with persisting cognitive defect. J Neurol Neurosurg Psychiatry 59:375–380, 1995.

Yeates K: Closed-head injury, in Yeates KO, Ris MD, Taylor HG (eds): Pediatric Neuropsychology: Research, Theory and Practice. New York: Guilford, 1999, pp. 192–218.

Yeates K, Blumstein E, Patterson CM, et al: Verbal memory and learning following pediatric closed head injury. J Intl Neuropsychol Soc 1:78–87, 1995.

Yeates K, Taylor MG, Drotar D et al.: Pre-injury environment as a determinant of recovery from traumatic brain injuries in school-aged children. J Int Neuropsycol Society 3:617–630, 1997.

Zimmerman R, Bilaniuk L: Pediatric head trauma. Pediatr Neuroradiol 4349–366, 1994.

Learning Disabilities: Neurobiologic Foundations and Topographic Manifestations Across the Life Span

Stephen R. Hooper

Evidenced-based treatments
Learning disabilities
Learning disability subtypes
Math disabilities
Dyslexia
Written language disabilities

INTRODUCTION

Learning disabilities represent some of the most prevalent problems affecting children, adolescents, and adults, with this category representing approximately 52% of all students with disabilities (U.S. Department of Education, 2000). In addition to this general group of learning problems being the most frequently identified special education classification in the United States, and perhaps around the world, a large number of other individuals teeter on the edge of this grouping. The developmental outcomes of children identified with learning disabilities also remain a critical problem, with many adults at risk for being underemployed, undereducated, and evidencing relatively higher rates of social-emotional adjustment difficulties (Schonhaut & Satz, 1983). Despite these overarching concerns, the classification of learning disabilities remains a clinical quagmire, with diagnosis being plagued by a variety of issues not the least of which include extreme heterogeneity, definitional issues, and assessment-treatment linkages.

This chapter provides an overview of the field of learning disabilities, with a particular focus on definitional issues, two key conceptual models, and domain-specific information pertaining to epidemiologic findings, academic and social-behavioral comorbidity, neurobiologic underpinnings, and topographic manifestations. Although the bulk of research has tended to focus on reading over the past decade, emergent findings related to written language and arithmetic also are presented. Evidenced-based treatment strategies are described, particularly as they relate to specific types of learning disabilities. The chapter concludes with some suggested guidelines for clinical practice and a discussion of the key issues confronting those working in the field of learning disabilities. Some directions for future clinical and research initiatives are offered.

DEFINITIONAL ISSUES

Definitional issues have confronted the field of learning disabilities since the term entered the vocabulary of professionals working with these children about 40 years ago (Kirk, 1963). Kirk originally described learning disabilities as "unexpected underachievement." This underachievement, by federal definition, should be manifested in one or more of seven core skills: oral expression, listening comprehension, written expression, basic reading skills, reading comprehension, mathematics calculation, and mathematics reasoning. The "unexpected" part of the definition typically relates to some type of ability-achievement discrepancy—even after being provided with learning experiences appropriate to the child's chronological age and ability levels. This aspect of the operationalization of learning disabilities, however, has been highly controversial since its introduction in 1977. Significant concerns have been raised about the utility of such an operationalization, particularly with respect to who actually may be identified as requiring services, the lack of sensitivity to younger children—including preschool children who may be at risk, the limited linkages provided for understanding the underlying problems for the academic underachievement, and the poor relationship to response to treatment.

Unfortunately, despite enormous rhetoric, many of the same issues continue to confront clinicians and researchers (Kavale & Forness, 2000). The earlier

definitions of learning disabilities, such as the one asserted by the Education for All Handicapped Children Act (i.e., Public Law 94-142, U.S. Office of Education, 1977), provided little guidance with respect to operational criteria for identification and diagnosis. These earlier definitions did little to improve our knowledge base with respect to specific outcomes, and they served to hinder communication between professionals—especially professionals representing different disciplines. Unfortunately, the reauthorization of the Individuals with Disabilities Education Act (IDEA) legislation has continued this legacy. The current federal definition of learning disabilities in IDEA, which virtually has remained unchanged since 1977, is as follows:

> The term "specific learning disability" means a disorder in one or more of the basic psychological processes involved in understanding or in using language, spoken or written, that may manifest itself in an imperfect ability to listen, think, speak, read, write, spell, or to do mathematical calculations. This term includes such conditions as perceptual disabilities, brain injury, minimal brain dysfunction, dyslexia, and developmental aphasia. The term does not include children who have learning problems that are primarily the result of visual, hearing, or motor disabilities; or mental retardation, or emotional disturbance, or of environmental, cultural, or economic disadvantage (Federal Regulations, 1997, 34, Subtitle B, Chapter III, Section 300, 2(b)1500).

Despite the difficulties posed by our federal definition of learning disabilities, there have been some notable efforts to improve on the definitional conceptualization of learning disabilities. Specifically, the National Joint Committee on Learning Disabilities (Hammill et al., 1981) and the Interagency Committee on Learning Disabilities (ICLD, 1987) did provide more detailed definitions that acknowledged the generic nature of the term "learning disabilities," the extreme heterogeneity of this population of individuals, and the suspicion of neurologic dysfunction. These definitions also adopted a life span approach to learning problems and permitted concomitant conditions (e.g., social and emotional disturbance) to be present. Even these definitions, however, did not provide operational guidelines for identification strategies and, consequently, they remained definitions of an exclusionary nature.

More recent research evidence has driven the re-emergence of Kirk's original conceptualization of learning disabilities as "unexpected underachievement"; however, an increased emphasis on research-based criteria has been asserted. For example, approximately a decade ago Shaywitz and colleagues (1992) found that reading disability does not represent a "hump" at the lower end of the normal distribution. Rather than a categorical grouping for individuals with reading disabilities, these investigators suggested that reading problems merely represent the lower end of the normal distribution of reading abilities. In fact, their work (Fletcher et al., 1994), and that of others (Siegel & Metsala, 1992), demonstrated that a discrepancy definition of reading disabilities fares no better than simply using a low achievement criterion (e.g., standard score <90 on a standardized achievement test); however, where to draw this cutoff criterion will remain a challenge, particularly with respect to uncovering specific subtypes that might be seen in this population.

These findings also have led to proposed definitions of learning disabilities in terms of domain-specific disabilities. For example, a contemporary definition of dyslexia was developed by an interagency group comprised of representatives from the Orton Dyslexia Society, the National Institute of Child Health and Human Development, and other investigators and advocacy groups. This proposed definition reads as follows (Shaywitz et al., 1995b, p. S55):

> Dyslexia is one of several distinct learning disabilities. It is a specific language based disorder of constitutional origin characterized by difficulties in single word decoding, usually reflecting insufficient phonological processing abilities. These difficulties in single word decoding are often unexpected in relation to age and other cognitive and academic abilities; they are not the result of generalized developmental disability or sensory impairment. Dyslexia is manifest by variable difficulty with different forms of language, often including, in addition to problems reading, a conspicuous problem with acquiring proficiency in writing and spelling (Operational definition of the Orton Dyslexia Society Research Committee, April 18, 1994).

This definition represents a significant improvement over previous definitions of reading disabilities. It is domain specific; addresses the underlying mechanisms for these disorders (i.e., language-based disorders) and, consequently, keeps the door open with respect to specific subtypes; and addresses the issue that this is an "unexpected difficulty in relation to age and other cognitive and academic abilities." Additionally, this proposed definition indirectly argues against the use of discrepancy-type formula in the identification of reading disabilities and, consequently, avoids many of the problems inherent in the current federal definition. Research-based definitions of other domain-specific disorders likely will be forthcoming within the next decade.

Perhaps one of the more hopeful approaches to documenting the presence of a learning disorder is the examination of responsiveness to intervention.

Although this concept has been defined as pertinent to the field of learning disabilities for over 15 years (e.g., Reschly, 1988), it has only been recently that this approach has begun to be operationalized in school-based practice (Lyon et al., 2001). This model stresses the need for a problem-solving approach that is proactive in the identification and intervention processes. This problem-solving approach requires four steps: (1) identification of the severity of the problem and why it is occurring; (2) development of a goal-directed intervention plan; (3) initiation of the intervention with associated monitoring procedures to determine whether the intervention is working—modifications are asserted based on the student's responsiveness to intervention; and (4) examination of the findings to determine future educational interventions. In this way, intervention always is considered in the process of defining the presence of a learning disorder as opposed to current practices wherein there is a dissociation between identification and intervention (Velluntino & Scanlon, 2002). Further, this approach moves away from the necessity to work with one student at a time and has been used in school-wide models that address the learning needs of many different students at the same time (Kame'enui et al., 2000).

These definitional issues are critical to understanding the current quagmire in which the field finds itself. Further, they are highlighted when one considers related assessment issues such as cross-cultural concerns and English-as-second language (ESL) students. Although our educational system proposes to address the needs of all of its students, particularly those with cultural differences, and to provide a "fair" assessment for these children, the literature is not at all clear how to proceed with these students or how current definitional standards or state procedural guidelines should be operationalized. Although it is commonly accepted that if students have problems learning in their primary language, they will be at significant risk for problems in their second language (Berninger & Richards, 2002), there are precious few guidelines for school psychologists, educators, neuropsychologists, or other professionals to follow to facilitate such evaluations. In addition, there is a plethora of measurement issues that plague such evaluations, and it is likely that the learning needs of these children are not being adequately assessed, identified, or treated. All of these issues can prove challenging to the practicing clinician.

CONCEPTUAL MODELS OF LEARNING DISABILITIES

Verbal Learning Disability Model

Reading and writing represent special forms of speech activity. In this regard, auditory-perceptual and language deficits historically have been linked to poor performance in these language-based academic domains. These types of deficits and inefficiencies have been documented by many different investigators for nearly 40 years (e.g., Blank & Bridger, 1964), with case study descriptions extending back even further, and their influence on language-based learning problems continues to be prominent today.

Specific theories have been advanced along these lines wherein functional-anatomic linkages have been asserted in the reading, spelling, and writing process. For example, according to the Wernicke-Geschwind model for dyslexia, the reading process begins with the visual perception and analysis of a grapheme. The grapheme is recoded to its phonemic structure, which subsequently is comprehended. The automaticity of this process varies as a function of development. Thus, during initial stages of reading, all of the fundamental neurologic operations are incorporated in a clear, serial fashion. During later stages, however, graphemes may come to elicit direct comprehension of written words or even entire phrases, essentially eliminating intermediate phonemic analysis and synthesis. Although some supporting evidence for the Wernicke-Geschwind model did emerge (Mayeux & Kandel, 1985), perhaps its greatest contribution was to continue to stimulate work in the phonological processing aspects of spoken language, particularly as it relates to reading.

Phonological Core Deficits Model

At present, the phonological core deficits model represents one of the most evidenced-based theories to account for reading problems (Shapiro, 2001). In fact, it has been estimated that over 80% of individuals, children and adults alike, have an underlying phonological deficit contributing to their reading problems, and that the integrity of these functions predicts later reading achievement better than most other abilities, even in preschool children (Gallagher et al., 2000). Children with phonological reading disabilities also tend to experience problems in other aspects of language including speech perception, speech production, and naming. Further, Olson and colleagues (1994) described that genetic factors account for about 40% of the variance in word recognition deficits, with phonological deficits having a much higher heritability factor than orthographic deficits.

But what is phonological processing? In any alphabetic system, each letter or cluster of letters will be associated directly with a specific sound unit of speech. This speech unit is called a phoneme. To engage in phonological awareness, an individual must have a working understanding that speech can be segmented into specific phonemes or sounds. This becomes a critical aspect in the early stages of reading. Reading requires learning the relationship between graphemes (written letters) and phonemes (sounds), and children with reading problems fail to use the "alphabetic principle" accurately, efficiently, or consistently. In addition to phonological awareness, phonological working memory (i.e., retrieval and manipulation of the phonemes in a reading task) and rapid naming have been included in a broader model of phonological processing. General cognitive abilities and speech perception also have been included in models of phonological processing (McBride-Chang & Manis, 1996), while reading fluency, vocabulary development, and reading comprehension have been included in a broader scientifically based model of reading development. Schatschneider and colleagues (1999) found that phonological awareness could be represented by a single dimension, regardless of how it was measured, but that the actual tasks to tap phonological awareness differed over the course of reading development. Tasks of first blending abilities and rhymes appear best suited for children just learning to read, whereas tasks tapping more complex sound deletion manipulations were better suited for other children with emergent phonological awareness capabilities.

Finally, it is important to note that phonological processing deficits have been uncovered in individuals manifesting ability-achievement discrepancies, variously defined, and those in individuals with general reading problems showing no such discrepancies. In this regard, the importance of intact phonological processing underpinnings in reading acquisition has been well documented. Also, research has demonstrated that without appropriate, directed intervention, individuals with phonologically based reading deficits likely will experience lifelong struggles with reading (Shapiro, 2001).

Nonverbal Learning Disability Model

Although Rourke (1989) has popularized the nonverbal learning disability model, early descriptions by Johnson and Myklebust (1971) approximately 30 years ago provided detailed depictions of these individuals. They stated that individuals with nonverbal learning disabilities typically were unable to comprehend the significance of many aspects of the environment, could not pretend and anticipate, and failed to learn and appreciate the implications of actions such as gestures, facial expressions, and other elements of emotion. Johnson and Myklebust (1971) noted that this disorder constituted a fundamental distortion of the total perceptual experience of the individual. They labeled this a social perception disability, and Myklebust (1975) later coined the term "nonverbal learning disability." These observations were consistent with findings of Borod and colleagues (1983) in their study of adult patients with right brain damage, and Denckla (1983) extended this conceptualization to children in her description of a social (emotional) learning disability.

Rourke (1989) extended this model by applying a developmental perspective to his work in learning disability subtyping, with a focus on nonverbal types of learning problems. Rourke hypothesized that involvement of the white matter of the right hemisphere (i.e., lesioned, excised, or dysfunctional white matter) interacts with developmental parameters, to produce nonverbal learning disabilities. He reasoned that, although a significant lesion in the right hemisphere may be sufficient to produce a nonverbal learning disability, it is the destruction of white matter (i.e., matter associated with rapid information transmission and intermodal functions) that is necessary to produce these types of learning disabilities. Generally, the nonverbal learning disability syndrome would be expected to develop under any circumstance that significantly interferes with the functioning of right hemispheric systems or with access to those systems (e.g., agenesis of the corpus callosum). Functionally, the characteristics of such an individual, which Rourke noted should be observable by approximately ages 7 to 9 years, predict the presence of selected neuropsychological, academic, and social-emotional/ adaptive dysfunctions.

Neuropsychologically, individuals with nonverbal learning disabilities tend to present a distinct profile of strengths and weaknesses. Relative strengths include auditory perception, simple motor functions, and intact rote verbal learning. Selective auditory attention, phonological skills, and auditory-verbal memory also appear intact. Neuropsychological deficits include bilateral tactile-perception problems and motor difficulties that usually are more marked on the left than on the right side of the body, visual-spatial organization problems, and nonverbal problem-solving difficulties. Paralinguistic aspects of language also are impaired (e.g., prosody, pragmatics).

Academically, given their relatively intact core language functions, these individuals evidence adequate word decoding and spelling, with most spelling errors reflecting good phonetic equivalents. Graphomotor skills eventually can be age appropriate, but are delayed early in development. Marked academic deficits tend to be manifested in mechanical arithmetic, mathematical reasoning, and reading comprehension. Academic subject areas, such as science, also tend to be impaired, largely due to reading comprehension deficiencies, deficits in nonverbal problem solving, and problems with the integration of information.

Perhaps one of the most interesting aspects associated with this model is that there appears to be a strong relationship with social-emotional and adaptive behavior deficits. These individuals present great difficulty adapting to novel situations and manifest poor social perception. These difficulties, in turn, result in poor social judgment and social skill deficits. There appears to be a marked tendency for these individuals to engage in social withdrawal and social isolation as age increases and, consequently, they are at risk for internalized forms of psychopathology such as depression and anxiety. In fact, Rourke (1989) and Bigler (1989) noted the increased risk that these individuals have for depression and suicide and that these symptoms may manifest more clearly to the primary care provider.

Rourke proposed this model as an approximation of a developmental neuropsychological model for nonverbal learning disabilities, but the neuropsychiatric manifestations also are of significant interest to clinicians and researchers. Further, this model is noteworthy because it provides another neuropsychologically based conceptualization to account for the wide range of heterogeneity that can be seen in the broader population of individuals with learning problems.

DOMAIN-SPECIFIC BEHAVIORAL MANIFESTATIONS

Reading Learning Disabilities

Epidemiology

Reading disabilities represent some of the most common forms of learning disabilities. Recent research initiatives have found that these disorders account for approximately 80% of children diagnosed with learning disabilities (Flynn & Rabar, 1994; Shaywitz et al., 1990); however, it remains clear that these disabilities represent a heterogeneous group of problems. Related findings also have suggested that boys and girls are equally affected (Flynn & Rabar, 1994; Shaywitz et al., 1990). Although these findings clearly place reading on a continuum, it is still likely that modularity (i.e., separation of specific reading functions/dysfunctions) may exist throughout the continuum.

Academic and Social-Behavioral Comorbidity

Although specific reading disorders can be found to exist in isolation, it is clear that students with reading problems also can manifest associated language disorders and writing problems (Ingalls & Goldstein, 1999). The co-occurrence with math disabilities also has been documented, with Badian (1983) noting a high degree of overlap between reading and arithmetic problems. Specifically, of the total sample of children with reading disabilities, Badian found that approximately 52.5% also showed arithmetic problems.

Many studies also have documented the comorbidity of learning and behavior problems in school-aged children, with a particular focus on the overlap between reading disabilities and attention-deficit/hyperactivity disorder (ADHD; Hinshaw, 1992; Shaywitz et al., 1995b). For example, using an epidemiologic sample, Shaywitz and colleagues (1995b) reported the prevalence of inattention in children with specific reading disability to be about 12% in first grade, and noted that this rate increased to about 24% by ninth grade. In children with inattention, however, specific reading disability was present in about 34% of first graders and increased to approximately 50% for ninth graders. Despite these findings, few other social or behavioral difficulties have been linked directly to reading disorders (Hynd et al., 1995). Reading problems frequently do appear in children diagnosed with a variety of specific genetic (e.g., neurofibromatosis) and neurologic (e.g., seizure disorders) conditions, and the manifestation of learning problems in these disorders should not be overlooked—even if secondary to the medical/genetic disorder.

Neurobiologic Underpinnings

Given the influence of the verbal learning disability models, recent neurobiologic efforts have conceptualized reading primarily as a set of functions that are subserved by specific neurolinguistic abilities and their associated neuroanatomic structures and neurologic processes (Liberman et al., 1989). Neurocognitive functions such as attention and memory, along with specific neurolinguistic functions, such as phonological processing, morphology, semantic knowledge, and syntax, have been investigated as part of a larger neurolinguistic model of reading. Recent findings suggest that children with reading disabilities typically will manifest phonological processing deficits and, to some extent, morphologic deficits (Stanovich et al., 1997). Indeed, children as young as 2 years of age who were born to dyslexic parents have shown delayed development of syntactic and morphologic skills (Scarborough, 1990), and Molfese and colleagues (2002) have used auditory evoked potentials in newborns to predict later language-based problems in preschool and early school-aged children, as well as reading problems, at age 8 years.

Using well marked but undifferentiated groups of children with reading disabilities, recent research also has begun to identify specific neuroanatomic associations for some of these neurolinguistic processes. For example, using postmortem and neuroimaging techniques, a number of neuroanatomic irregularities have begun to be described in individuals with dyslexia. In most individuals, the planum temporale in the left hemisphere (i.e., a triangular region comprising the auditory association cortex and extending into the parietal lobe) tends to be larger than in the right hemisphere (Geschwind & Levitsky, 1968), even in fetuses (Witelson & Pallie, 1973); however, this normal asym-

metry is not typically found in individuals with dyslexia. These individuals tend to show symmetrical plana or reversed asymmetry with the right side being larger than the left (Leonard et al., 1993). These findings have been correlated with linguistic deficits, such as phonological awareness deficiencies (Semrud-Clikeman et al., 1992), and targeted structures have been used to predict dyslexic group membership (Semrud-Clikeman et al., 1996).

Magnetic resonance imaging (MRI) morphometric studies also have shown that individuals with dyslexia have symmetry or reversed asymmetry in the plana (Eckert & Leonard, 2000) and in the parietal-occipital and prefrontal regions (Jernigan et al., 1991), and a smaller or thinner corpus callosum (Hynd et al., 1995). Further, Galaburda and Livingstone (1993) have demonstrated on postmortem examination that cellular layers sensitive to the processing of visual information (i.e., the ventral magnocellular layers in the lateral geniculate) tend to be disorganized and smaller in shape. Using functional MRI (fMRI), Shaywitz and colleagues (2002) found semantic processing in individuals with dyslexia to be associated with widespread brain activity, with overactivity being noted in the bilateral inferior frontal regions and underactivity in the left posterior temporal region, when compared to normal readers. Orthographic and phonological processing abilities also have been associated with extrastriate sites and the inferior frontal gyrus, respectively (Shaywitz et al., 1996), and there appear to be age-related changes in regional brain activation (Simos et al., 2001). Gender differences also have been asserted in terms of how phonological processing and semantic processing are organized in the brain (Shaywitz et al., 1995a), with girls with reading problems showing greater distribution of their neural network for these functions than boys.

These advances in our knowledge of the neurolinguistic components of the reading process and their associated neuroanatomic processes are impressive with respect to increasing our understanding of the neurobiologic underpinnings of reading. Taken together, these advances would also argue strongly for the presence of different reading subtypes. What is not clear, however, is how these neurobiologic mechanisms might be manifested in selected subtypes of reading disabilities and what other neurocognitive processes might be implicated. For example, although phonological processes have received overwhelming support as one of the core deficits in dyslexia, and associated neuroanatomic structures have been linked to various neurolinguistic components of reading, other studies have shown problems with oculomotor movements and latencies (Fischer & Weber, 1990). Further, Eden and colleagues (1994) have shown that several visual tasks may be as good at predicting poor readers as the phonological measures. Eden and colleagues (1995) even combined measures of visual processes and phonological processes to account for nearly 70% of the variance in reading ability. Consequently, it is highly likely that other neurobiologic factors are at play in the developmental aspects of reading acquisition, and specific subtypes may evolve based on their differential manifestations at specific developmental periods.

Current Subtyping Initiatives

Over 40 years ago, Smith and Carrigan (1959) published one of the first studies addressing the existence of reading disability subtypes. Using cluster analysis techniques in a sample of 40 elementary schoolchildren with reading disabilities, and a comprehensive battery of tasks, these investigators identified three reading disability subtypes (i.e., cognitive-association deficits, poor cognitive-perceptual abilities, and undifferentiated pattern) and two superior functioning groups. The innovativeness of this exploration cannot be overstated, because it set the stage for a proliferation of studies attempting to identify learning disability subtypes (for a review, see Hooper, 1996).

Over the next three decades, a large number of models of learning disabilities were presented in the literature. Most of these models were conceptually derived, as opposed to empirically derived, and most used samples of individuals manifesting a myriad of academic problems. For example, Denckla (1972) proposed three syndromes that she had observed via her clinical work (i.e., specific language disabilities, specific visuospatial disabilities, dyscontrol syndrome), and suggested that professionals working with children with learning problems should be able to "split" children into different kinds of learning profiles that more accurately reflected their unique abilities and disabilities; however, a domain-specific approach was not used.

A number of previous subtyping initiatives, however, have attempted to remain within the domain-specific area of reading. For example, Boder (1970) provided one of the first subtyping schemes for dyslexia, in which she described multiple subtypes of reading problems characterized by different information-processing capabilities. Dysphonetic readers were characterized by deficient phonetic decoding strategies, poor letter-sound integration, and weak auditory memory. Consistent with more contemporary findings, Boder suggested that these types of problems were the most prevalent difficulties manifested by poor readers. The dyseidetic readers were characterized by poor visual-perceptual abilities and weak visual memory. These children were described as using phonetic decoding strategies almost exclusively and had limited sight-word vocabularies. Finally, the alexic readers were characterized by a combination of deficits and represented the most severely involved group of readers. Other domain-specific

models evolved during this time period, with some of these models attempting to intimately link treatment strategies to their respective subtypes. The Bakker model is noteworthy in this regard in that it remains contemporary in its evolution, proposes a neurodevelopmental model for reading, and provides a specific evidenced-based treatment strategy for the subtypes derived. More recently, there have been a number of ongoing efforts to uncover specific reading subtypes within a domain-specific framework (Bakker et al., 1995; Morris et al., 1998).

Morris and colleagues (1998) provided a contemporary model of reading subtypes based on the phonological processing model. Using eight measures of cognitive and language functions in a large sample of children, cluster analysis procedures produced nine subtypes that accounted for about 90% of their sample. In addition to two intact reading groups, seven reading-deficient subtypes were identified. Of the seven impaired groups, two were globally and severely impaired across all measures, four manifested primary problems in variance aspects of phonological processing, and one showed problems in general rate of processing verbal and nonverbal materials. At a minimum, this study showcased the multidimensionality of reading problems even within a relatively strong latent trait dimension.

Wolf and Bowers (1999) proposed three different subtypes based on the double dissociation model of dyslexia. Using a comprehensive model of phonological processing, these investigators described a reading subtype deficient for phonological awareness, a second subtype showing deficits in naming speed, and a third subtype evidencing problems within both dimensions. In fact, these investigators argued that processing speed should be considered a second core deficit in dyslexia.

These subtyping efforts clearly have reinforced the notion of heterogeneity within the domain of reading. Based on these subtype findings, as well as the available scientifically based reading research, there appear to be five major components of reading that should be examined: phonological awareness, phonics, reading fluency, vocabulary, and reading comprehension. In addition, given the ongoing work of some investigators (Eden et al., 1994), the orthography of reading remains important to continue to examine as well. Table 41-1 lists these topographic features and suspected neurocognitive dysfunctions.

Evidenced-Based Treatment Efforts

One key reason for determining homogeneous subtypes of reading disabilities and, ultimately, developing a classification system, is the potential for specific intervention plans to be asserted. In general, despite the use of a variety of subtyping strategies, the findings to date

TABLE 41-1. Topographic Features of Specific Reading Disorder(s) and Possible Neurocognitive Dysfunctions

Topographic feature	Possible neurocognitive dysfunctions
Phonological awareness	Attention, auditory-verbal memory
Phonics/alphabetic principle	Verbal working memory, visual memory, visual perception
Reading fluency	Oral-motor coordination
Vocabulary	Receptive language
Reading comprehension	Receptive language, working memory, executive functions
Orthography	Visual perception, visual memory

suggest that specific subtype patterns may exhibit a differential response to treatment, particularly if treatment is designed to accommodate an individual's cognitive processing strengths. Current research initiatives are beginning to examine the efficacy of specific interventions as well as the multitude of variables (e.g., family factors, psycho-social issues, teacher knowledge, environmental constraints) that have an impact on the possible subtype-by-treatment interactions (Lyon et al., 2001).

Although earlier intervention models were largely conceptual, more recent efforts have been based on data. In fact, evidenced-based linkages to phonological training models have proven to be relatively powerful, with current efforts showing short-term gains in phonological decoding and word recognition and long-term gains being relatively maintained (Bus & van IJzendoorn, 1999). Programs designed to address phonological awareness, however, vary extensively in terms of specific content, length of intervention, and the timing of the intervention. Wagner and colleagues (1993) noted that only highly intensive and aggressively sustained phonological awareness training programs will facilitate the development of reading abilities. Over 20 years ago, Ehri (1979) suggested that children might learn much more about phonology when the training is accompanied by actual reading and spelling activities, and these specific differences between reading intervention programs will require ongoing study and verification.

Finally, it is important to note that with what is being uncovered regarding the phenotypic performance of children with reading disabilities, particularly with respect to various nuances of the broader phonological processing model, it is highly likely that prevention intervention may begin to emerge as important for these children wherein services are provided before a youngster experiences profound failure and frustration in the school setting (Lyon et al., 2001). This will demand better identification practices in early childhood and require developmentally appropriate treatment methods.

Written Language Learning Disabilities

Epidemiology

The prevalence rate of writing problems is variably high. In fact, about 25 years ago Lerner (1976) speculated that "poor facility in expressing thoughts through written language is probably the most prevalent disability of the communication skills." In this regard, using an unreferred sample, Berninger and Hart (1992) reported that about 1.3% to 2.7% of 300 primary grade children had problems with handwriting, 3.7% to 4% had problems in spelling, and 1% to 3% had problems with written narratives. Hooper and colleagues (1993) reported significantly higher rates of written language problems in a large epidemiologic sample of middle school students. Using the Test of Written Language-2 Spontaneous Writing Quotient, Hooper and associates reported about 6% to 22% of the middle-school students exhibited significant writing problems (i.e., >2 standard deviations below the test mean) depending on region of the country, gender, and ethnic status. Most recently, the National Center for Education Statistics (NCES, 1999) reported that only about 23% of fourth graders could write at a proficient level or above, 61% wrote at a basic level, and 16% wrote below the basic level. At the fourth grade level, only 1% of students were able to write at an advanced level.

Obviously, the available prevalence rates will vary as a function of the definition of writing problems, how much instruction has been provided to students, and the type of writing that students are being asked to perform. Collectively, however, these prevalence estimates do suggest the importance of studying the various components of the process of written expression.

Academic and Social-Behavioral Comorbidity

Similar to the domain of reading, it should not be surprising that children with writing disorders would be plagued by a number of co-occurring features. In particular, if writing does indeed represent the last language function to develop (Myklebust, 1973), language problems and associated academic problems may be pervasive throughout a child's academic career, and they likely will manifest early in school. When one considers the hypothesized involvement of other kinds of cognitive mechanisms in the writing progress (e.g., attention, memory, executive functions), the chances of a child's experiencing an associated learning problem would appear to increase geometrically. Further, given the convergence of so many cognitive abilities in the development of the writing process, a child's failure to transcribe on paper may represent the "tip of the iceberg" with regard to the functioning of that child's central nervous system and its subsequent manifestation in learning and behavioral functioning. Unfortunately, outside of its association with reading development, the comorbid aspects of written language function and dysfunction are not well understood at this time, particularly with respect to the social-emotional concomitants. Further investigation into these associations is warranted.

Neurobiologic Underpinnings

The study of written expression has lagged well behind the investigation of other academic domains (e.g., reading), particularly with respect to investigation of its neurocognitive and neurobiologic underpinnings. Although discussion of disorders of written expression has been around for well over 100 years (e.g., Ogle, 1867), and models have been evolving since the 1960s (e.g., Ellis, 1983; Hayes, 1996), it has only been in the last two decades that this complex set of skills has begun to be examined in more detail (Hooper, 2002). This is particularly the case with respect to specific neurocognitive underpinnings that influence the writing process.

To date, a number of efforts have been designed to increase our knowledge of the writing process. These efforts have included model development as well as studies examining selected aspects of the written language process. Generally, most models of written expression have conceptualized writing as a problem-solving process whereby writers attempt to produce visible, understandable, and legible language reflecting their declarative knowledge (i.e., knowledge of a topic). The quality of written products is enhanced or constrained by a multitude of documented factors, such as a writer's declarative knowledge, procedural knowledge, and conditional knowledge (Gagne, 1985). For example, in the most recent revision of the Hayes and Flower (1980) model, Hayes (1996) described the processes of planning, translating, and reviewing—functions that require constant monitoring throughout the writing task. There also are reciprocal relationships between variables in the task environment (e.g., the writing task and the generated text at any point in time) and the writer's long-term memory. The Hayes and Flower (1980) model and its revision (Hayes, 1996), along with other conceptual models (e.g., Ellis, 1983), clearly suggest the need for strong problem-solving abilities to be present for competent writing to be generated. In addition to problem-solving capabilities, Hayes (1996) noted that reading and language generation appear to be core contributors to adequate written expression.

A number of studies also have documented the qualities inherent in good or "expert" writers (e.g., Berninger et al., 2002). In general, expert writers are goal directed and tend to move in a recursive fashion from translating ideas to using generated text to plan the next sentence or paragraph. Each of these steps is evaluated with respect to its relevance of meeting proximal or distal goals (or both). Embedded within this recursive process is a keen orchestration of the expert writer's understanding of the goals of the writing assignment, knowledge of the topic, and knowledge of the audience. In addition to this recursive process, expert writers typically generate more ideas and use an abundance of transitional ties (e.g., referential, connective, lexical) to produce more cohesive text and a smooth flow of ideas.

In contrast, poor writers not only show deficits in their strategies during production of written text, but they also are deficient in their acquisition and use of declarative, procedural, and conditional knowledge about writing. In addition, they show clear problems in simply generating text. Poor writers are more likely to produce shorter and less "interesting" essays, and they produce poorly organized text at both the sentence and paragraph levels. Furthermore, they are less likely to revise spelling, punctuation, grammar, or the substantive nature of their text to increase communication clarity.

Despite these findings, the influence of neuropsychological factors (e.g., memory, attention) on the writing process is less well documented. The characteristics describing "expert" versus "poor" writers would suggest the strong influence of selected neuropsychological functions in the development and quality of written expression. Levine and colleagues (1993) suggested the importance of a variety of neuropsychological functions in the writing process. These functions included memory, attention, graphomotor output, sequential processing, higher-order cognition, language, and visual-spatial functions; however, no data were available to support when and to what degree these functions influenced the writing process.

Abbott and Berninger (1993) provided one of the first empirical studies examining these questions. They noted that oral language/verbal reasoning, including such functions as sentence memory, word finding, phonological processing, and reading contributed to composition fluency. Berninger and Rutberg (1992) also described the importance of a finger succession task, an index of early fine-motor planning and control, to the identification of emergent writing problems in early elementary grade children.

One neurocognitive function on which investigators have begun to focus is working memory (Lea & Levy, 1999). The cognitive workspace, or working memory, is important to written expression because it is the function that underlies the active maintenance of multiple ideas, the retrieval of grammatical rules from long-term memory, and the recursive self-monitoring that is required during the act of writing (Kellogg, 1999). Working memory contributes to the management of these simultaneous processes, and a breakdown may well lead to problems with written output (Levy & Marek, 1999). McCutchen (1996) has noted that poor writers typically have reduced working memory capacity when compared to good writers.

Kellogg (1996) also proposed a model of writing that was based on the concept of working memory. This model included three major components: verbal formulation, execution, and monitoring. Planning and translating were considered key subcomponents of the formulation process in writing. The programming and executing functions were key subcomponents of the execution process. Finally, the reading and editing subcomponents were considered critical to the monitoring processes of written expression. These latter subcomponents are important because reading has been positively linked to the development and quality of written language, and this relationship has been expressed in a number of theoretical (Fitzgerald & Shanahan, 2000) and empirical models (Berninger et al., 2002). Kellogg's model provided for a recursive loop between each of these three major processes of writing. Kellogg conceptually linked this system to the working memory model of Baddeley (1986), wherein the visuospatial sketchpad was linked to formulation, the phonological loop to monitoring, and the central executive to the execution processes.

Hooper and colleagues (2002) examined the integrity of selected executive functions across good and poor writers in elementary school. Using a conceptually driven four factor model of executive functions (Denckla, 1996), Hooper and colleagues found that poor writers performed significantly lower in the initiation and set-shifting domains of executive functioning when compared to good writers. Further, they also exhibited poorer sustaining executive function capabilities, although these findings only approached statistical significance. In this regard, although working memory appears to be critical to the writing process, other executive functions would seem to be important to the

writing process as well. Indeed, Graham (1997) even has used selective executive functions in developing writing intervention programs for elementary school students.

Current Subtyping Initiatives

Despite the proliferation of reading subtyping models, there have been very few published studies examining possible written language subtyping models. To date, however, there are several noteworthy efforts.

In one of the first studies to explore this possibility, Sandler and colleagues (1992) attempted to classify the writing disorders in a clinic-referred sample of students (n = 190), aged 9 to 15 years. Teachers responded to a questionnaire about different aspects of student's writing including legibility, mechanics, writing rate, and linguistic sophistication. Ninety-nine cases of writing disorders were found in the sample. Empirically derived subgroups revealed the following clusters: (1) motor and linguistic deficits, (2) visual-spatial deficits, (3) attention and memory deficits, and (4) sequencing deficits. The findings from this study were limited because writing disorders were defined on the basis of a teacher's responses to questionnaires, as opposed to an actual writing sample, and there was no reliability and validity evidence for the cutoff score chosen for a particular subgroup. Evidence for the internal and external validation of the classification model was also limited. Despite these limitations, this study was one of the first efforts to classify writing disorders into more heterogeneous clinical groupings.

Roid (1994) provided a second effort to classify students' writing with a large sample of students in Oregon. Using the State of Oregon writing sample, Roid examined the importance of analytical and holistic scoring strategies for evaluating students' writing. Cluster analyses identified 11 subgroups of students who revealed similar patterns across five writing genres. The results indicated the need for evaluating analytical traits of writing (e.g., ideas, voice, word choice, etc.), in addition to more holistic scoring rubrics.

One final subtyping initiative deserves mention at this juncture. Swartz and associates (2001) examined the presence of specific neurocognitively based subtypes of written language in a sample of fourth and fifth graders. Neurocognitive measures included various measures of attention, motor, language, visual processing, memory, and executive functions. Six empirically derived clusters were retained for examination. These clusters reflected two groups with adequate writing skills and four groups with poor writing skills. The four deficient writing groups were differentiated by (1) combined executive function and expressive language deficits, (2) mild expressive language problems with accompanying reading comprehension deficits, (3) per-

TABLE 41-2. Topographic Features of Specific Writing Disorder(s) and Possible Neurocognitive Dysfunctions

Topographic feature	Possible neurocognitive dysfunctions
Handwriting legibility	Fine-motor control, visual memory, attention
Handwriting fluency	Fine-motor control, fine-motor speed, attention, working memory
Spelling	Attention, working memory, visual perception
Narrative fluency	Executive functions, attention, fine-motor speed
Narrative organization	Executive functions tapping organization, planning, self-monitoring, cognitive flexibility, and problem solving, expressive language, receptive language, language pragmatics

vasive language problems with severe reading comprehension deficits, and (4) a high degree of perseveration with pervasive reading problems. Empirical validation of this model will require further examination.

Although the numbers of writing subtyping efforts have lagged behind those available to reading, the notion of heterogeneity within this academic domain has some emergent support. At present, there appear to be a number of key topographic features that investigators and clinicians should always examine when exploring the various aspects of written language. These include handwriting legibility, handwriting fluency, spelling, narrative fluency, and narrative organization. These topographic features and suspected neurocognitive dysfunctions can be seen in Table 41-2.

Evidenced-Based Treatment Efforts

Studies that have used classification models in combination with specific, well-developed intervention strategies have begun to improve our ability to address educators' questions of how reading difficulties may best be treated, under what instructional conditions, and with what degree of expected improvement in reading (Lyon & Moats, 1997). The development of equally specific interventions designed to prevent or improve writing disorders, however, has lagged behind interventions in reading. To the misfortune of classroom teachers, educational interventionists, and ultimately students who struggle with written output, there is a less well-developed empirical base from which they can make instructional decisions about the nature, intensity, and duration of writing interventions specific to a student's profile of neurocognitive functions or achievement in writing. There have been several efforts to address this concern.

Using the above subtyping model described by Swartz and colleagues (2001), findings have begun to emerge to show the benefits of a subtype-by-treatment approach to intervention for dysfunction in written language. Specifically, Swartz and colleagues used a targeted intervention to address the self-regulation and metacognitive processes involved in writing. All stu-

dents received a total of 20 intervention sessions. Each session comprised 45 minutes of instruction in these selected processes during their daily written language lessons. In this small sample, all of the students showed improvements in their holistic writing scores; however, only the subtypes manifesting weak expressive language skills demonstrated significant changes after treatment.

Mathematics Learning Disabilities

Epidemiology

Problems with mathematics (math) in children have been described as far back as the early 1900s (e.g., Buswell & John, 1926); however, in comparison to the study of reading recognition and, more recently, written expression, the scientific study of math skills remains in its infancy (Fleischner, 1994). Rutter (1978) made this observation over 20 years ago, and this state of the science of math persists into the present. Despite this apparent lack of emphasis, the most recent figures from the U.S. Department of Education (1999) revealed that the rate of identification of learning disabilities is increasing, and math disabilities likely account for many of these cases.

Prevalence estimates of math learning disabilities have hovered around 6% of elementary school children, with some estimates being as low as 3% (Rasanen & Ahonen, 1995). Using the 375 fifth grade children in a small Czechoslovakian town, Kosc (1974) reported a prevalence rate of approximately 6.4% in basic math skills testing. Similarly, using results from a group of achievement tests of reading and math skills for all students in grades 1 though 8 in a small town, Badian (1983) also reported the prevalence rate of math problems to be approximately 6.4%. The use of epidemiologic samples would appear critical to determining such prevalence rates, but how math problems are operationally defined and what measurement procedures are used would also be critical to establishing these rates. Gender differences have also been reported (Geary, 1996), with boys showing better math functions than girls.

Perhaps one of the biggest challenges that confront researchers interested in the prevalence rate of problems with math is how to define the nature of these problems. Currently, most states subscribed to a form of the ability-achievement discrepancy, either in a simple form (e.g., IQ – Math Score > 15 points) or via a regression form; however, there are precious few studies that have compared the similarities and differences between these definitions. In the reading literature these definitions have been compared, with a fair degree of overlap being reported (Fletcher et al., 1994). In one of the few studies examining this question in the math domain, Hooper and Brown (2001) showed virtually no overlap of these definitions in an adolescent sample. Sample differences aside, this latter study challenges the notion that findings from the reading domain can be applied to the domain of mathematics, at least at the adolescent level, and it raises questions as to how such definitions might have an impact on obtaining accurate prevalence rates for mathematics.

Academic and Social-Behavioral Comorbidity

For the math domain, although a variety of comorbid relationships have been proposed, particularly given the commonalities of some of the cognitive underpinnings for both reading and math (Geary, 1993), only a few such data exist. Earlier work by Badian (1983) suggested a high degree of overlap between reading and arithmetic deficits. Specifically, of the total sample with math disabilities, approximately 42.6% of the sample had reading disabilities. White and colleagues (1992) demonstrated a significantly lower rate of comorbidity, with about 10% of their sample showing both reading and arithmetic disabilities. Ackerman and Dykman (1995) showed that students with reading and arithmetic disabilities versus those with reading disabilities only did not differ on phonological processing skills, memory, naming speed, or picture vocabulary. No social-behavioral difficulties were noted between the groups. The two groups did differ on spelling and selected tasks from the Wechsler Intelligence Scale for Children-III (WISC-III) (i.e., Arithmetic and Coding subtests), with the children with arithmetic disabilities falling further behind with increasing age. In addition, a core weakness in processing speed was apparent in the students with arithmetic and reading disabilities.

Perhaps one of the most described associations with math problems has been the purported presence of internalizing problems in this sample of children. For example, students can manifest heightened levels of anxiety when performing math, such as with the observance of math anxiety, and these feelings clearly can overwhelm a student and hinder efficient use of attention, working memory, and related problem-solving functions. Rourke (1989) asserted an association between those students manifesting a specific neuropsychological pattern of disabilities (i.e., nonverbal learning disability), as reflected in visual-perceptual deficits, poor visual attention, poor visual memory, left-sided sensory-motor problems, manifest math deficits, and associated internalizing symptoms. According to Rourke, children showing language-based problems also could evidence social-behavioral problems, but these were more diffuse in their manifestation. White and colleagues (1992) also showed a greater frequency of internalizing psychopathology in students with math disabilities.

Other problems in the social-behavioral realm have been described in children with math-related problems. In a study of nonreferred Israeli fourth grade students, Gross-Tur and colleagues (1996) found that 26% of the children diagnosed with dyscalculia had symptoms of ADHD, using parent and teaching rating scales. Conversely, Zentall and colleagues (1994) found that boys with ADHD experienced greater difficulties with arithmetic, even after controlling for the effects of IQ and reading. More generally, Pearl's (1992) review of much of this literature reported that students with learning disabilities are at risk for social-behavioral difficulties spanning a wide range of problems (e.g., peer relationships, pragmatics, behavior, social motivation, self-esteem); however, the specific contributors to these patterns and the timing of their emergence require further study.

Neurobiologic Underpinnings

What constitutes the various components of math competency has been debated for the past 50 years or more. This debate is compounded by the different kinds of mathematics functions that can be studied (e.g., counting skills, algebra, geometry). An early factor analysis conducted approximately 50 years ago (Barakat, 1951) revealed four key components in mathematics ability: general intelligence, a math factor, a verbal factor, and a visual-spatial factor. In a similar study, Wrigley (1958) noted that when general intelligence is removed from the model, verbal ability seems to have little relationship to math functioning. Over 25 years ago Larsen and Hammill (1975) reviewed more than 600 studies and found that visual discrimination, memory for visual sequences, and visual-motor coordination correlated highest with arithmetic success. Verbal abilities also were highly correlated with success in arithmetic with increasing chronological age. Other investigators have reported an array of problems that contribute to the manifestation of specific arithmetic disabilities.

More recently, Fleischner (1994) reported that most math assessment tasks should tap several key dimensions including conceptual understanding, computational skills, and the ability to apply skills to routine problems. Gaddes and Edgell (1990) described three main underpinnings: language, reading, and spatial imagery. These have included verbal expression, an inability to read numerical symbols, an inability to copy arithmetic problems, difficulty performing arithmetic operations, and disturbances in mental calculation (Kosc, 1981); a variety of memory problems including working memory (Geary, 1993), visual memory (Strang & Rourke, 1985), and verbal memory (Rourke & Finlayson, 1978); abstract reasoning and cognitive flexibility (Strang & Rourke, 1985); inattentive and disorganized (Badian & Ghublikian, 1983); primary reading recognition and reading comprehension problems (Stone & Michals, 1986); and sequential processing (Gaddes & Spellacy, 1977). As can be seen, nearly every major neuropsychological function has been identified with respect to its importance to math skills acquisition and development; however, it is not clear when specific neurocognitive functions become more predictive of overall math functions or more predictive of specific math functions. Their relative predictive weightings also remain unknown in this regard.

From a neurologic perspective, Luria (1980) noted that damage or disruption to temporal-parietal-occipital association areas in the right hemisphere will contribute to spatial-based deficits and, subsequently, contribute to problems with calculations and arithmetic operations; however, it is clear from this list of neuropsychological characteristics that the neurologic origins of problems with math extend beyond a simple notion of right hemisphere dysfunction, with more contemporary neurologic models suggesting that math skills are mediated by both hemispheres (Kahn & Whitaker, 1991). In fact, similar to earlier single-factor theories in dyslexia, there would appear to be strong rationale for supporting a subtype approach to the topographic manifestation of math skills and their respective neurologic underpinnings.

Current Subtyping Initiatives

In this regard, a small number of math subtype models have been proposed; however, some of these have been based on clinical conjecture, small sample sizes, retrospective analyses, and clinic-based samples. None of these has used contemporary methodology, adequate sample sizes, or a school-based sample, nor have the assessment strategies been conducted from a prospective perspective nor has the stability of specific subtype models been tested. With these concerns in mind, however, there have been several key conceptual and empirical efforts to date.

One of the earlier subtyping efforts comes from the work of Rourke and colleagues (Rourke & Finlayson, 1978; Strang & Rourke, 1985). Using the Wide Range Achievement Test, which taps math calculation skills (and not application, reasoning, or word problems), Rourke (1993) described three subgroups of students: Group 1 evidenced deficits in all academic domains, group 2 had higher arithmetic than reading/spelling, and group 3 had higher reading/spelling than arithmetic. Group 3, the arithmetic-deficient group had relatively, intact language-based abilities but deficits in visual-perception, spatial organization, and bilateral tactile perception. This subtype also formed the foundation for the nonverbal learning disability model presented earlier.

Other conceptual models for math subtyping have been proposed. For example, Kosc (1974) proposed a classification model for developmental dyscalculia. These forms of disturbed mathematics included verbal (e.g., naming amounts), practognostic (e.g., poor manipulation of real objects), lexical (e.g., poor reading of math symbols), graphical (e.g., manipulating math symbols in writing), ideognostical (e.g., poor understanding of math ideas), and operational (e.g., "anarithmetia," or the inability to carry out math operations). Using case study methodology, Temple (1991) has provided evidence for some of these subtypes by describing a double dissociation between procedural dyscalculia and number fact dyscalculia. Geary (1993) proposed conceptual subtypes that reflected problems in semantic memory, procedural processes, and visuospatial functions. Geary speculated that the semantic memory subtype, and perhaps the procedural subtype, was associated with left hemisphere dysfunction, whereas the visuospatial subtype was associated with right hemisphere dysfunction.

Another strategy that appears to hold promise for subtyping math problems or inclusion in more comprehensive subtyping efforts is error pattern analysis. Specifically, the notion of examining the kinds of errors that a student makes in math calculations and reasoning processes may provide diagnostic clues as well as avenues for intervention. This strategy for analysis of math problems goes back nearly 100 years to Brown (1906) who described several calculation error patterns for the four basic arithmetic processes. Roberts (1968) described four types of "failure strategies" in the math calculations of children. These included (1) wrong operation, (2) obvious computational error, (3) defective algorithm, and (4) random responses. Engelhardt (1977) also found that impulsive subjects tended to make more errors, although not of a particular type; however, he noted that with more precise testing such a relationship might emerge. Spiers (1987) expanded on the work of Engelhardt and presented a more comprehensive description of error types. These included five types of place-holding errors, four types of digit errors, seven types of borrow and carry errors, two types of basic fact errors, nine types of algorithm errors, and three types of symbol errors. Error pattern models have also been presented by Cohn (1971), Kosc (1981), and Rourke (1993), with the model by Spiers being the most expansive at this time.

Although this strategy for analysis appears to hold promise, few studies have examined its ultimate utility for diagnosis or treatment. One study that does exist showed a similar pattern of errors between normal and school-identified students with math disabilities, with the specific errors of the impaired group resembling those of the younger normal group (Fleischner, 1994). A slightly more recent study (Rasanen & Ahonen, 1995) showed a connection between error types and reading accuracy and speed, particularly with respect to multiplication fact retrieval. Geary (1993) also has attempted to subtype arithmetic disabilities based on their error patterns. Specific subtypes have included a visuospatial subtype, a semantic memory subtype, and a procedural subtype. A recent study by Bryant and colleagues (2000) described characteristic behaviors of students with teacher-identified math deficits. These behaviors included an array of 32 different types of arithmetic errors and related strategy behaviors wherein 9 of them contributed to an accurate prediction of children with math disabilities (e.g., does not remember number words or digits, has difficulty with multistep problems, makes "borrowing" errors). Clearly, these qualitative aspects of math function and dysfunction need to be accounted for when examining the topography of arithmetic problems in elementary schoolchildren.

The numbers of conceptual and empirical subtyping efforts in math have been impressive, particularly when the qualitative error analysis data are considered. Despite this progress, however, the area of mathematics is perhaps one of the largest domain-specific areas to cover. To address calculation skills may require one model, but math functions such as geometry and trigonometry actually may require a different model. Nonetheless, based on math subtype findings to date, several key topographic features should be included in any appraisal of math function. These include fact retrieval, procedural processes, visuospatial functions, understanding of math concepts, and math fluency.

Table 41-3 lists these topographic features and suspected neurocognitive dysfunctions.

Evidenced-Based Treatment Efforts

Consistent with the limited progress to date in the area of written expression, relatively little progress has been made in the area of mathematics. Although a number of treatments abound and evidenced-based treatment initiatives are few and far between, some emergent efforts are worth noting.

Wright and associates (2000) have begun to provide specific intervention strategies for early numeracy in young children. Using a curriculum-based approach to assessment, these investigators have provided a clearly delineated model for targeted intervention. Their Mathematics Recovery Program was designed to address not only calculation skills but math reasoning skills as well. Teaching is problem-based and subsequently contributes to ongoing evaluation of the child's progress. As such, the Math Recovery Program provides a detailed approach to early intervention for emergent math problem. Its relationship to other child-specific variables, such as neurocognitive functions (e.g., memory, attention), and its utility with specific subtypes of mathematics remains to be examined.

SELECTED GUIDELINES FOR CURRENT CLINICAL PRACTICE

Despite the explosion in the amount of literature addressing a wide range of topics in the field of learning disabilities, particularly the domain-specific findings, the current practice of the day-to-day practitioner who must deal with these children and their families is not well articulated. Evidenced-based practices are slowly creeping into clinical practice, such as the understanding that a thorough reading assessment should include measures of phonological awareness, phonics, vocabulary, reading comprehension, and fluency, but how these functions should be measured remains an open debate. Further, conducting such an assessment, which would permit stronger diagnosis and treatment linkages,

TABLE 41-3. Topographic Features of Specific Mathematics Disorder(s) and Possible Neurocognitive Dysfunctions

Topographic feature	Possible neurocognitive dysfunctions
Fact retrieval	Memory, working memory, attention, cognitive fluency
Procedural processes	Attention, working memory, receptive language, executive functions, fine-motor output
Math fluency	Processing speed, visual and verbal memory, working memory
Visuospatial functions	Visual discrimination, visual-spatial abilities, visuoconstructive abilities
Understanding of math concepts	Receptive language, problem solving, organization

stands in stark contrast to the state and federal requirements stating the need to document some type of discrepancy.

Further complicating this situation is the multitude of professionals who lay claim to this field. Although the multidisciplinary input has actually proved to be quite fruitful, particularly with respect to the scientific advancement of the field, how each of the disciplines functions is not necessarily in concert with one another. For example, a pediatrician may approach learning problems from a medical/health perspective, whereas a developmental-behavioral pediatrician may actually engage in specific assessment strategies designed to tap various neurodevelopmental constructs purportedly related to learning. A speech-language pathologist may focus on language-related functions and intervene at that level, whereas an occupational therapist may focus on fine-motor, sensory, and visual-perceptual functions. School psychologists and educators have been classic players, but they have been hamstrung by the state rules and regulations and, frankly, many antiquated training models that primarily focus on simple psychoeducational assessment strategies (e.g., IQ, achievement). Neuropsychologists, pediatric neurologists, psychiatrists, and optometrists also have fallen into the assessment-treatment quagmire, but their approaches also can be as varied and as different as the other professionals. An interdisciplinary approach would clearly address many of these differences in approach by opening up discussions regarding the similarities and differences in findings; however, this is not the typical approach used by schools—even given the presence of school-based teams. Further, given this approach to assessment, the construction of the educational treatment plan, i.e., the Individual Education Plan (IEP), also has the potential to lack an evidenced-based approach to treatment.

Given the current state of clinical practice in the field of learning disabilities, there appear to be some clear guidelines that all clinicians could follow in working with these children and their families:

- Use a domain-specific approach when examining students with suspected learning disabilities. The discussion should not center on whether a child has a learning disability but, rather, what kind of learning problem is present.
- Although it will remain important to provide documentable assessment findings to assist special education classification of a child with a learning disability and to access necessary services, it should be less important than identifying specific learning needs. In what components of a domain (e.g., reading) does the child experience problems?

- Despite evidence to the contrary, the ongoing use of a discrepancy model to classify most children with learning disabilities remains problematic and operationally confusing. In this regard, clinicians should look carefully for the "loopholes" in the special education classification system (e.g., liberally using alternatives to the discrepancy model to advocate for services for at-risk children). The IQ-achievement discrepancy is neither necessary nor sufficient for identifying individuals with learning disabilities and, in fact, may preclude the availability of services to students who do not manifest such a discrepancy, but who may require such services to continue to develop.
- In addition, it will be important for the clinician to identify what specific neurocognitive underpinnings might be contributing to the specific learning problem. By approaching the specific domains in a componential fashion, as illustrated in Tables 41-1, 41-2, and 41-3, assessment hypotheses can be generated that will facilitate closer examination of neurocognitive problems that may be contributory to the learning problems.
- All professionals should strive to conduct their assessments via an interdisciplinary perspective when evaluating students with suspected learning problems. This model should involve closer communication among professionals, with similarities and differences in assessment findings being discussed.
- It will be important for professionals working with students manifesting learning disabilities to attempt to identify such problems much earlier than early to middle elementary school. For example, available data do suggest that we can begin to identify children with reading problems during the preschool years (e.g., by using phonological awareness assessment strategies), and these types of assessment should be incorporated into preschool and prekindergarten screening strategies. The problem-solving approach to identification may be one strategy for addressing the early identification needs of many students.
- Once a learning problem has been identified, it will be important for the assessment findings to assist in the development of intervention plans. In particular, and when available, it will be important for the clinician to be aware of and recommend evidence-based interventions. When such interventions are not available, the clinician should depend on use of "best practices" (i.e., strategies that have theoretical

relationships to the assessment findings). It will be just as important to avoid interventions with little or no documentation as to their potential effectiveness.

- It will remain important for all involved professionals to provide routine monitoring and tracking of a student's learning progress. The once- or twice-per year review required by state and federal law simply may not be frequent enough for some children.
- Learning disabilities reflect lifelong conditions. Although this does not mean that children will underachieve or fail as they progress into adulthood, it does mean that careful attention to secondary and postsecondary educational needs should be carefully modulated so as to increase the chances of a positive learning outcome.

ONGOING ISSUES AND FUTURE DIRECTIONS

This chapter has provided an overview of the critical issues and contemporary findings in the field of learning disabilities. Information pertaining to key issues in the conceptualization and definition of learning disabilities was presented, with a keen focus on domain-specific findings. Three key domain-specific learning problems were reviewed with respect to their epidemiology, academic and social-behavioral comorbidity, neurobiologic underpinnings, subtyping initiatives, and available evidenced-based treatment efforts. Despite the apparent progress noted in each of these academic domains, particularly reading, the field has far to go with respect to improved understanding of the different kinds of learning problems and disabilities that can be manifested across the life span. In addition, many ongoing issues must be addressed, particularly with respect to moving research and clinical practice forward in the 21st century.

Operational Definitions

It will be essential for definitions of learning disabilities to be operationalized in a clear manner and for the samples to be well marked from the time of diagnosis through adulthood. Although the field is moving in the direction of meaningful operational criteria for identifying reading disabilities, it has yet to achieve this goal, and operational definitions for other areas of learning disability require increased attention. Clearly, definitional efforts need to benefit from the mistakes of the past and attempt to become more consistent with emergent evidenced-based models of learning. Alternative definitional models also should be explored, such as those examining specific response-to-treatment approaches (Lyon et al., 2001).

Topographic Manifestations and Subtyping Efforts

The studies addressing the heterogeneous nature of reading disorders attest to the remarkable progress made in the field of learning disability subtyping in a relatively brief amount of time. The elusive "gold ring" is the development of a more refined diagnostic system—one that moves clinicians and researchers beyond global categorizations, such as "learning disabilities," and into an operational and ecologically valid diagnostic system. A system that holds validity with respect to etiology, prognosis, response to treatment and, perhaps, early identification and prevention, will serve the clinical and research communities well. This will require a significant shift in how these children are identified, particularly with respect to long-held assessment traditions such as the use of ability-achievement discrepancies and typical psychoeducational appraisals. Improvement in our assessment strategies will be needed, and diagnosis-treatment connections will need to be given more than token attention, particularly with respect to needed subtype validation.

Progress has been made over the past decade, but we have far to go to attain the golden ring. Some of the current findings do advance the field in a scientific fashion unparalleled in this domain of investigation, particularly with respect to domain-specific classification issues in reading, but many questions remain (e.g., how many subtypes, developmental continuity of specific subtypes, the influence of other endogenous and exogenous factors). Greater appreciation for scientific rigor, including aspects such as the use of longitudinal methodologies, epidemiologic sampling, theoretically driven assessment batteries, and statistical technologies (e.g., growth curve modeling to measure change over time), all will facilitate our movement toward this goal.

Assessment Practices

In tandem with the above, it will be essential for evaluators to be cognizant of different models of learning disabilities, such as the verbal and nonverbal learning disability models, and how these heuristic models explain the manifestations inherent in the various learning disabilities. These models implicate specific underlying processes in a particular learning problem and directly target specific assessment strategies that go way beyond the prototypic IQ and achievement battery. For example, the phonological processing model strongly implicates the need for assessment strategies tapping phonological awareness, phonological/working memory, and rapid naming in any evaluation of reading. Further, a profiling of these phonological processing abilities actually may suggest specific interventions for a particular child. Similarly, the importance of executive functions in the writing process and the need to examine error patterns in arithmetic operations require different types of approaches to the assessment of these types of problems.

Life Span Manifestations and Outcomes

While researchers and clinicians continue to struggle with learning disabilities in the school-age realm, from which the bulk of our research findings have come, the manifestation of learning disabilities across the life span is becoming increasing relevant. Efforts in the adult domain clearly have begun to affect how practitioners address undiagnosed learning problems in this age band, with emergent findings implicating the continuity of phonological processing problems extending into the adult years. Further, given the emergent data indicating a differential social-emotional pattern for the nonverbal learning disability subtype, it will be important for researchers and clinicians to include some means for subtyping their adults presenting with learning problems. From a clinical perspective, it will be important for individuals working with adults with learning disabilities to be sensitive to the psychosocial difficulties as well as the learning differences that can be manifested in this population (Gregg et al., 1996). The treatment issues may be more pervasive in adulthood because the neurocognitive and psychosocial deficits may extend into marriage relationships, parenthood, vocational choices, unemployment/underemployment, and selection of leisure activities (Bender, 1994).

On the other end of the age continuum, recent work has begun to call for increased attention to be directed to the learning problems in preschool children (Lyon et al., 2001). Although this is an extremely challenging age domain, particularly with respect to available measurement, our current knowledge base has only begun to uncover some of the neurocognitive underpinnings that can identified during the preschool years, and, at this point, is largely applied to reading decoding problems. Preschool predictors of later problems in mathematics, written language, listening comprehension, and reading comprehension remain to be determined.

Brain-Behavior Associations

The ongoing examination of the neurobiologic foundations of learning problems will be essential for moving the field forward. Neurologic and neuropsychological deficiencies and dysfunctions have been linked to a variety of learning components and problems, and these linkages will continue to require ongoing study using various imaging strategies, well-marked samples, and groups of individuals from various age ranges across the life span. The linkages of brain-based findings to specific

interventions also remain a fruitful avenue of exploration (e.g., Berninger et al., 2002), particularly with respect to documenting different brain activation patterns following specific types of interventions.

CONCLUSION

The field of learning disabilities has forged ahead significantly in the past decade. The research rigor in the field has been tightened, and this increased rigor has contributed findings that have begun to have an impact on our understanding of the neurobiologic bases of these problems and to influence daily clinical practice. Despite these advances, much remains to be done. While work continues to proliferate in the domain of reading, increased efforts need to be devoted to the other learning problems delineated in our federal law. With the increased scientific rigor that has come to bear on the field, however, it is hoped that findings in these other academic domains will be advanced at a faster rate. In this fashion, the impact on research, clinical practice, and public policy will continue to be more evidenced-based and, consequently, facilitate the learning of all individuals manifesting specific types of learning problems.

Acknowledgments

This chapter was completed with support from grants awarded to the Center for Development and Learning from the Administration on Developmental Disabilities (no. 90DD043003) and the Maternal Child Health Bureau (no. MCJ379154A). Requests for reprints should be directed to Stephen R. Hooper, Ph.D., The Clinical Center for the Study of Development and Learning, CB# 7255, University of North Carolina School of Medicine, Chapel Hill, NC. 27599-7255; e-mail: stephen.hooper@cdl.unc.edu

■ KEY POINTS

☐ Use a domain-specific approach when examining school-aged children and students with suspected learning disabilities.

☐ Assessment findings should help to identify what components of a specific academic domain (e.g., reading) are problematic for a particular child.

☐ The ongoing use of a discrepancy model to classify most children with learning disabilities remains problematic and operationally confusing, and clinicians should look carefully for the "loopholes" in the special education classification system (e.g., liberally using alternatives to the discrepancy model to advocate for services for at-risk children).

☐ The IQ-achievement discrepancy is neither necessary nor sufficient for identifying individuals with learning disabilities and, in fact, may preclude the availability of services to students who do not manifest such a discrepancy, but who may require such services to continue to develop.

☐   All professionals should strive to conduct their assessments via an interdisciplinary perspective when evaluating students with suspected learning problems.

☐   It will be important for professionals working with students manifesting learning disabilities to attempt to identify such problems much earlier than early to middle elementary school (e.g., by using phonological awareness assessment strategies to examine prereading development), and these types of assessment should be incorporated into preschool and prekindergarten screening strategies.

☐   When available, it will be important for the clinician to be aware of and recommend evidence-based interventions. When such interventions are not available, the clinician should depend on the use of "best practices" (i.e., strategies that have theoretical relationships to the assessment findings). It will be just as important to avoid interventions with little or no documentation as to their potential effectiveness.

☐   It will remain important for all involved professionals to provide routine monitoring and tracking of a student's learning progress.

☐   Learning disabilities reflect lifelong conditions. Although this does not mean that children will underachieve or fail as they progress into adulthood, it does mean that careful attention to secondary and postsecondary educational needs should be carefully modulated so as to increase the chances of a positive learning outcome.

KEY READINGS

Berninger VW, Richards TL: Brain Literacy for Educators and Psychologists. New York: Academic Press, 2002.

Flanagan DP, Ortiz SO, Alfonso VC, et al: The Achievement Test Desk Reference. Boston: Allyn & Bacon, 2002.

Geary D: Children's Mathematical Development. Washington, DC: American Psychological Association, 1994.

Hooper SR (guest ed): J Learn Disabil 23, 2002 (special issue on the Disorders of Written Language).

REFERENCES

Abbott RD, Berninger VW: Structural equation modeling of relationships among developmental skills and writing skills in primary- and intermediate-grade writers. J Ed Psychol 85:478–508, 1993.

Ackerman PT, Dykman RA: Reading-disabled students with and without comorbid arithmetic disability. Dev Neuropsychol 11:351–371, 1995.

Baddeley AD: Working Memory. Oxford, United Kingdom: Oxford University Press, 1986.

Badian NA: Dyscalculia and nonverbal disorders of learning, in Myklebust HR (ed): Progress in Learning Disabilities. New York: Grune & Stratton, 1983, Vol. 5, pp. 235–264.

Badian NA, Ghublikian M: The personal-social characteristics of children with poor mathematical computation skills. J Learn Disabil 16:154–157, 1983.

Bakker DJ, Licht R, Kapper EJ: Hemispheric stimulation techniques in children with dyslexia, in Tramontana MG, Hooper SR (eds): Advances in Child Neuropsychology. New York: Springer-Verlag, 1995, Vol. 3, pp. 144–177.

Barakat M: A factorial study of mathematical abilities. Br J Psychol Stat Sec 4:137–156, 1951.

Bender M: Learning disabilities: Beyond the school years, in Capute AJ, Accardo PJ, Shapiro BK (eds): Learning Disabilities Spectrum: ADD, ADHD, and LD. Baltimore: York Press, 1994, pp. 241–253.

Berninger VW, Abbott RD, Abbott SP, et al: Writing and reading: Connections between language by hand and language by eye. J Learn Disabil 35:39–56, 2002.

Berninger VW, Hart T: A developmental neuropsychological perspective for reading and writing acquisition. Ed Psychol 27:415–434, 1992.

Berninger VW, Rutberg J: Relationship of finger function to beginning writing: Application to diagnosis of writing disabilities. Dev Med Child Neurol 34:155–172, 1992.

Bigler ED: On the neuropsychology of suicide. J Learn Disabil 22:180–185, 1989.

Blank M, Bridger WH: Cross-modal transfer in nursery school children. J Comp Physiol Psychol 58:227–282, 1964.

Boder E: Developmental dyslexia: New diagnostic approach based on the identification of three subtypes. J Sch Health 40:289–290, 1970.

Borod JC, Koff E, Caron HS: Right hemispheric specialization for the expression and appreciation of emotions: A focus on the face, in Perecman E (ed): Cognitive Processing in the Right Hemisphere. New York: Academic Press, 1983, pp. 83–110.

Brown CE: The psychology of simple arithmetical processes: A study of certain habits of attention and association. Am J Psychol 17:1–37, 1906.

Bryant D, Bryant BR, Hammill DD: Characteristic behaviors of students with LD who have teacher-identified math weaknesses. J Learn Disabil 33:168–177, 2000.

Bus AG, van IJzendoorn MJ: Phonological awareness and early reading: A meta-analysis of experimental training studies. J Educ Psychol 91:403–414, 1999.

Buswell GT, John L: Fundamental Processes in Arithmetic. Indianapolis, IN: Bobbs-Merrill, 1926.

Cohn R: Arithmetic and learning disabilities, in Myklebust HR (ed): Progress in Learning Disabilities. New York: Grune & Stratton, 1971, Vol. 2, pp. 176–194.

Denckla MB: Clinical syndromes in learning disabilities: The case for "splitting" versus "lumping." J Learn Disabil 5:401–406, 1972.

Denckla MB: The neuropsychology of social-emotional learning disabilities. Arch Neurol 40:461–462, 1983.

Denckla MB: Theory and model of executive function, in Lyon GR, Krasnegor NA (eds): Attention, Memory, and Executive Function. Baltimore: Paul H. Brookes, 1996, pp. 263–278.

Eckert MA, Leonard CM: Structural imaging in dyslexia: The planum temporale. Ment Retard Dev Disabil Res Rev 6:198–206, 2000.

Eden GF, Stein JF, Wood HM, et al: Differences in eye movements and reading problems in dyslexic and normal children. Vision Res 34:1345–1358, 1994.

Eden GF, Stein JF, Wood HM, et al: Verbal and visual problems in reading disability. J Learn Disabil 28:272–290, 1995.

Ehri LC: Linguistic insight: Threshold of reading acquisition, in Waller G, MacKinnon G (eds): Reading Research: Advances in Theory and Practice. New York: Academic Press, 1979, Vol. 1, pp. 63–111.

Ellis AW: Reading, writing, and dyslexia: A cognitive analysis. Hillsdale, NJ: Lawrence Erlbaum Associates, 1983.

Engelhardt JM: Analysis of children's computational errors: A qualitative approach. Br J Educ Psychol 47:149–154, 1977.

Fischer B, Weber H: Saccadic reaction times of dyslexia and age-matched normal subjects. Perception 19:805–818, 1990.

Fitzgerald J, Shanahan T: Reading and writing relationships and their development. Educ Psychol 35:39–50, 2000.

Fleischner JE: Diagnosis and assessment of mathematics learning disabilities, in Lyon GR (ed): Frames of Reference for the Assessment of Learning Disabilities. Baltimore: Paul H. Brookes, 1994, pp. 441–458.

Fletcher JM, Shaywitz SE, Shakweiler DP, et al: Cognitive profiles of reading disability: Comparisons of discrepancy and low achievement definitions. J Educ Psychol 85:1–18, 1994.

Flynn JM, Rabar MH: Prevalence of reading failure in boys compared with girls. Psychol Sch 31:66, 1994.

Gaddes WH, Edgell D: Learning Disabilities and Brain Function: A Neuropsychological Approach, ed 3. New York: Springer-Verlag, 1990.

Gaddes WH, Spellacy FJ: Serial order perceptual and motor performances in children and their relation to academic achievement (research monograph no. 35). Victoria BC, Department of Psychology, University of Victoria, 1977.

Gagne RM: The Conditions of Learning. A Theory of Instruction, ed 4. New York: Holt, Rinehart & Winston, 1985.

Galaburda AM, Livingstone M: Evidence for a magnocellular defect in developmental dyslexia. Ann N Y Acad Sc 682:70–82, 1993.

Gallagher A, Frith U, Snowling MJ: Precursors of literacy delay among children at genetic risk of dyslexia. J Child Psychol Psychiatry 41:203–213, 2000.

Geary DC: Mathematical disabilities: Cognitive, neuropsychological, and genetic components. Psychol Bull 114:345–362, 1993.

Geary DC: Sexual selection and sex differences in mathematical abilities. Behav Brain Sci 19:229–284, 1996.

Geschwind N, Levitsky W: Human brain: Left-right asymmetries in temporal speech region. Science 161:186–187, 1968.

Graham S: Executive control in the revising of students with learning and writing difficulties. J Educ Psychol 89:223–234, 1997.

Gregg N, Hoy C, Gay AF (eds): Adults with Learning Disabilities. Theoretical and Practical Perspectives. New York: Guilford Press, 1996.

Gross-Tsur V, Manor O, Shalev RS: Developmental dyscalculia: Prevalence and demographic features. Dev Med Child Neurol 38:25–33, 1996.

Hammill DD, Leigh J, McNutt G, et al: The new definition of learning disabilities. Learn Disabil Q 4:336–342, 1981.

Hayes JR: A new framework for understanding cognition and affect in writing, in Levy CM, Ransdell S (eds): The Science of Writing: Theories, Methods, Individual Differences, and Applications. Mahwah, NJ: Lawrence Erlbaum Associates, 1996, pp. 1–27.

Hayes JR, Flower LS: Identifying the organization of writing processes, in Gregg LW, Steinbert ER (eds): Cognitive Processes in Writing. Hillsdale, NJ: Lawrence Erlbaum Associates, 1980, pp. 3–30.

Hinshaw, SP: Academic underachievement, attention deficits, and aggression: Comorbidity and implications for intervention. J Consult Clin Psychol 60:893–903, 1992.

Hooper SR: Subtyping specific reading disabilities: Classification approaches, recent advances, and current status. Ment Retard Dev Dis Res Rev 2:14–20, 1996.

Hooper SR: The language of written language: An introduction to the special issue. J Learn Disabil 35:2–6, 2002.

Hooper SR, Brown TT: Neuropsychological profiles of adolescents with arithmetic disabilities using regression based ability-achievement versus low achievement definitional criteria. Manuscript submitted for publication, 2001.

Hooper SR, Swartz CW, Wakely MB, et al: Executive functions in elementary school children with and without problems in written expression. J Learn Disabil 35:57–68, 2002.

Hooper SR, Swartz C, Montgomery J, et al: Prevalence of writing problems across three middle school samples. Sch Psychol Rev 22:608–620, 1993.

Hynd GW, Hall J, Novey ES, Eliopulos D, et al: Dyslexia and corpus callosum morphology. Arch Neurol 52:32–38, 1995.

Interagency Committee on Learning Disabilities: Learning Disabilities: A Report to the U.S. Congress. Bethesda, MD: National Institutes of Health (ERIC Document Reproduction Service No. ED 294 358), 1987.

Hynd GW, Morgan AE, Edmonds JE, et al: Reading disabilities, comorbid psychopathology, and the specificity of neurolinguistic deficits. Dev Neuropsychol 11:311–322, 1995.

Ingalls S, Goldstein S: Learning disabilities. Handbook of Neurodevelopmental and Genetic Disorders in Children. New York: Guilford Press, 1999, pp. 101–153.

Jernigan TL, Hesselink JR, Stowell E, et al: Cerebral structure on magnetic resonance imaging in language- and learning-impaired children. Arch Neurol 48:539–545, 1991.

Johnson DJ, Myklebust HR: Learning Disabilities. New York: Grune & Stratton, 1971.

Kahn HJ, Whitaker HA: Acalculia: An historical review of localization. Brain Cogn 17:102–115, 1991.

Kame'enui EJ, Simmons DC, Coyne MD: Schools as host environmnets: Toward a schoolwide reading improvement model. Ann Dyslexia 50:33–51, 2000.

Kavale KA, Forness SR: What definitions of learning disability say and don't say: A critical analysis. J Learn Disabil 33:239–256, 2000.

Kellogg RT: Components of working memory in text production, in Torrance M, Jeffery G (eds): The Cognitive Demands of Writing. Amsterdam: Amsterdam University Press, 1999, pp. 143–161.

Kirk SA: Behavioral diagnosis and remediation of learning disabilities, in Proceedings of the Conference on Exploration into the Problems of the Perceptually Handicapped Child. Chicago, Perceptually Handicapped Children, 1963.

Kosc L: Developmental dyscalculia. J Learn Disabil 7:165–178, 1974.

Kosc L: Neuropsychological implications of diagnosis and treatment of mathematical learning disabilities. Top Learn Disabil 1:19–30, 1981.

Larsen SC, Hammill DD: The relationship of selected visual-perceptual abilities to school learning. J Spec Educ 9:281–291, 1975.

Lea J, Levy CM: Working memory as a resource in the writing process, in Torrance M, Jeffery G (eds): The Cognitive Demands of Writing. Amsterdam: Amsterdam University Press, 1999, pp. 63–82.

Leonard CM, Voeller KKS, Lombardino LJ, et al: Anomalous cerebral structure in dyslexia revealed with magnetic resonance imaging. Arch Neurol 50:461–469, 1993.

Lerner JW: Children with learning disabilities: Theories, diagnosis, teaching strategies. Boston: Houghton Mifflin, 1976.

Levine MD, Hooper SR, Montgomery JW, et al: Learning disabilities. An interactive developmental paradigm, in Lyon GR, Gray DB, Kavanagh JF, et al (eds): Better Understanding of Learning Disabilities: New Views from Research and Their Implications for Educational and Public Policies. Baltimore: Paul H. Brookes, 1993, pp. 229–250.

Levy CM, Marek, P: Testing components of Kellog's multicomponent model of working memory in writing: The role of the phonological loop, in Torrance M, Jeffrey G (eds): The Cognitive Demands of Writing. Amsterdam: Amsterdam University Press, 1999, pp. 25–41.

Liberman IY, Shankweiler DP, Liberman AM: The alphabetic principle and learning to read, in Shankweiler DP, Liberman IY (eds): Phonology and Reading Disability: Solving the Reading Puzzle (IARLD Monograph Series). Ann Arbor, MI: University of Michigan Press, 1989, pp. 1–33.

Luria AR: Higher Cortical Functions in Man. New York: Basic Books, 1980.

Lyon GR, Fletcher JM, Shaywitz SE, et al: Rethinking learning disabilities, in Finn CE, Rotherham AJ, Hokanson CR (eds): Rethinking Special Education for a New Century. New York: The Thomas B. Fordham Foundation and Progressive Policy Institute, 2001, pp. 259–287.

Lyon GR, Moats LC: Critical conceptual and methodological considerations in reading intervention research. J Learn Disabil 30:578–588, 1997.

Mayeux R, Kandel ER: Natural language, disorders of language, and other localizable disorders of cognitive functioning, in Kandel ER, Schwartz JH (eds): Principles of Neural Science, ed 2. New York: Elsevier, 1985, pp. 688–703.

McBride-Chang C, Manis FR: Structural invariance in the associations of naming speed, phonological awareness, and verbal reasoning in good and poor readers: A test of the double deficit hypothesis. Reading Writing Interdisciplinary J 8:323–339, 1996.

McCutchen D: A capacity theory of writing: Working memory in composition. Educ Psychol Rev 8:299–325, 1996.

Molfese DL, Narter DB, Modglin AA: The relation between language development and brain activity, in Molfese DL, Molfese VJ (eds): Developmental Variations in Learning: Applications to Social, Executive Function, Language, and Reading Skills. Mahwah, NJ: Lawrence Erlbaum Associates, 2002, pp. 187–224.

Morris RD, Stuebing KK, Fletcher JM, et al: Subtypes of reading disability: Variability around a phonological core. J Educ Psychol 90:347–373, 1998.

Myklebust H: Development and Disorders of Written Language: Studies of Normal and Exceptional Children. New York: Grune & Stratton, 1973, Vol. 2.

Myklebust HR: Nonverbal learning disabilities: Assessment and intervention, in Myklebust HR (ed): Progress in Learning Disabilities. New York: Grune & Stratton, 1975, Vol. 3, 85–121.

National Center for Educational Statistics: NAEP 1998 Writing Report Card for the Nation and the States (NCES 1999-462). Washington, DC: Office of Educational Research and Improvement, 1999.

Ogle JW: Aphasia and agraphia. Report of the Medical Research Council of St George's Hosp 2:83–122, 1867.

Olson R, Forsberg H, Wise B, et al: Measurement of word recognition, orthographic, and phonological skills, in Lyon GR (ed): Frames of Reference for the Assessment of Learning Disabilities. Baltimore: Paul H. Brookes, 1994, pp. 243–277.

Pearl R: Psychosocial characteristics of learning disabled students, in Singh NN, Beale IL (eds): Learning Disabilities: Nature, Theory, and Treatment. New York: Springer-Verlag, 1992, pp. 96–125.

Rasanen P, Ahonen T: Arithmetic disabilities with and without reading difficulties: A comparison of arithmetic errors. Dev Neuropsychol 11:275–295, 1995.

Roberts GH: The failure strategies of third grade arithmetic pupils. Arithmetic Teach 15:442–446, 1968.

Reschley DJ: Special education reform: School psychology revolution. Sch Psychol Rev 17:459–475, 1988.

Roid GH: Patterns of writing skills derived from cluster analysis of direct writing assessments. Appl Measure Educ 7:159–170, 1994.

Rourke BP: Nonverbal Learning Disabilities: The Syndrome and the Model. New York: Guilford Press, 1989.

Rourke BP: Arithmetic disabilities, specific and otherwise: A neuropsychological perspective. J Learn Disabil 26:214–226, 1993.

Rourke BP, Finlayson MAJ: Neuropsychological significance of variations in patterns of academic performance: Verbal and visual-spatial abilities. J Abnorm Child Psychol 6:121–133, 1978.

Rutter M: Prevalence and types of dyslexia, in Benton A, Pearl D (eds): Dyslexia: An Appraisal of Current Knowledge. New York: Oxford University Press, 1978, pp. 3–28.

Sandler AD, Watson TE, Footo M, et al: Neurodevelopmental study of writing disorders in middle childhood. J Dev Behav Pediatr 13:17–23, 1992.

Scarborough HS: Very early language deficits in dyslexic children. Child Dev 61:1728–1743, 1990.

Schatschneider C, Francis DJ, Foorman BR, et al: The dimensionality of phonological awareness: An application of item response theory. J Educ Psychol 91:439–449, 1999.

Schonhaut S, Satz P: Prognosis for children with learning disabilities: A review of follow-up studies, in Rutter M (ed): Developmental Neuropsychology. New York: Guilford Press, 1983, pp. 542–563.

Semrud-Clikeman M, Hooper SR, Hynd GW, et al: Prediction of group membership in developmental dyslexia, attention deficit-hyperactivity disorder, and normal controls using brain morphometric analysis of magnetic resonance imaging. Arch Clin Neuropsychol 11:521–528 1996.

Semrud-Clikeman M, Hynd GW, Novey ES, et al: Dyslexia and brain morphology: Relationships between neuroanatomical variation and neurolinguistic tasks. Learn Ind Diff 3:225–242, 1992.

Shapiro BK: Specific reading disability: A multiplanar view. Ment Retard Dev Dis Res Rev 7:13–20, 2001.

Shaywitz BA, Pugh KR, Constable RT, et al: Semantic processing activates bilateral frontal regions during conventional (1.5 Tesla) functional magnetic resonance imaging. Hum Brain Map 2:149–158, 1995a.

Shaywitz BA, Shaywitz SE, Pugh KR, et al: Disruption of posterior brain systems for reading in children with developmental dyslexia. Biol Psychiatry 52:101–110, 2002.

Shaywitz BA, Shaywitz SE, Pugh KR, et al: The neurobiology of developmental reading disorders as viewed through the lens of neuroimaging technology, in Lyon GR, Rumsey J (eds): A Window to the Neurological Foundations of Learning and Behavior. Baltimore: Paul H. Brookes, 1996, pp. 79–94.

Shaywitz SE, Escobar MD, Shaywitz BA, et al: Distribution and temporal stability of dyslexia in an epidemiological sample of 414 children followed longitudinally. N Engl J Med 326:145–150, 1992.

Shaywitz SE, Fletcher JM, Shaywitz BA: Defining and classifying learning disabilities and attention-deficit hyperactivity disorder. J Child Neurol 10:S50–S57, 1995b.

Shaywitz SE, Shaywitz BA, Fletcher JM, et al: Prevalence of reading disability in boys and girls: Results of the Connecticut longitudinal study. JAMA 264:998–1002, 1990.

Siegel LS, Metsala J: An alternative to the food processor approach to subtypes of learning disabilities, in Singh NN, Beale IL (eds):

Learning Disabilities. Nature, Theory, and Treatment. New York: Springer-Verlag, 1992, pp. 44–60.

Simos PG, Breier JI, Fletcher JM, et al: Age-related changes in regional brain activation during phonological decoding and printed word recognition. Dev Neuropsychol 19:191–210, 2001.

Smith DEP, Carrigan PM: The Nature of Reading Disability. New York: Harcourt, Brace, 1959.

Spiers PA: Acalculia revisited: Current issues, in Deloche G, Seron X (eds): Mathematical Disabilities. A Cognitive Neuropsychological Perspective. Hillsdale, NJ: Lawrence Erlbaum Associates, 1987, pp. 1–26.

Stanovich KE, Siegel LS, Gattardo A: Converging evidence for phonological and surface subtypes of reading disability. J Educ Psychol 89:114–128, 1997.

Stone A, Michals D: Problem solving skills in learning-disabled children, in Ceci JJ (ed): Handbook in Cognitive, Social, and Neuropsychological Aspects of Learning Disabilities. Hillsdale, NJ: Lawrence Erlbaum Associates, 1986, pp. 291–315.

Strang JD, Rourke BP: Adaptive behavior of children who exhibit specific arithmetic disabilities and associated neuropsychological abilities and deficits, in Rourke BP (ed): Neuropsychology of Learning Disabilities: Essentials of Subtype Analysis. New York: Guilford Press, 1985, pp. 302–328.

Swartz CW, Wakely MB, Hooper SR, et al: A model of neurocognitive and performance-based subtypes of written expression. Manuscript submitted for publication, 2001.

Temple CM: Procedural dyscalculia and number fact dyscalculia: Double dissociation in developmental dyscalculia. Cogn Neuropsychol 8:155–176, 1991.

U.S. Department of Education: Washington, DC: Author, 1999.

U.S. Office of Education: Public Law 94-142 regulations: Proposed Rulemaking. Fed Reg 41:52404–52407, 1977.

Vellutino FR, Scanlon DM: The interactive strategies approach to reading intervention. Contemp Educ Psychol 27:573–635, 2002.

Wagner RK, Torgesen JK, Laughon P, et al: Development of young readers' phonological processing abilities. J Educ Psychol 85:83–103, 1993.

White JL, Moffitt TE, Silva PA: Neuropsychological and socio-emotional correlates of specific-arithmetic disability. Arch Clin Neuropsychol 7:1–16, 1992.

Witelson SF, Pallie W: Left hemisphere specialization for language in the newborn: Neuroanatomical evidence of asymmetry. Brain 96:641–646, 1973.

Wolf M, Bowers PG: The double-deficit hypothesis for the developmental dyslexias. J Educ Psychol 91:415–438, 1999.

Wright RJ, Martland M, Stafford AK: Early Numeracy. Assessment for Teaching and Intervention. Thousand Oaks, CA: Sage, 2000.

Wrigley J: The factorial nature of ability in elementary mathematics. Br J Educ Psychol 28:61–78, 1958.

Zentall SS, Smith YN, Lee YB, et al: Mathematical outcomes of attention-deficit hyperactivity disorder. J Learn Disabil 27:510–519, 1994.

Attention-Deficit Disorder: An Overview

Jeanette C. Ramer

Attention-deficit disorder

Dopaminergic pathways

Genetics of ADHD

Hyperactivity

Learning disorders

Neurostructural findings

Stimulant medications

INTRODUCTION AND HISTORICAL OVERVIEW

It is highly likely that attention-deficit disorder (ADD) has been a dimension of human behavior for many generations, but, in past, it was easier for people with ADD to blend in with the general population because of a lack of required completion of public school and the prevalence of apprenticeships and other alternative means of learning, and earning, a living. Contemporary accounts of the temperament and personality of Davy Crockett and Daniel Boone suggest that both had significantly short attention spans, impulsivity, physical restlessness, and tendency to engage in risk-taking behaviors. Congressional colleagues of Davy Crockett complained about his frequent absences and missing of crucial votes, often because he was in the hallway conversing, having lost track of time. Many other examples could be given, but there are no collected reviews or studies of individuals with these temperament qualities until the early 20th century, when George Still, an English physician, described 20 children with core symptoms of what would now be termed ADD, combined type. He suggested that they had a "defect in moral control" (Still, 1902). Attribution of cause changed based on observations from the 1920s through the 1940s, noting that encephalitis and other infections, birth trauma, and traumatic brain injury often led to impaired attention focus and physical fidgitiness. Thinking shifted from "moral control" toward "minimal brain damage" as the primary cause of ADD. Lack of demonstrable pathologic changes in brains of affected individuals challenged this attribution, a situation that persists among opponents of classification of ADD as a medical disorder.

The cause-neutral label, "hyperkinetic child syndrome," was used beginning in the 1960s in recognition of one of the core symptoms of ADD. This entity officially entered the mental health catalog of defined disorders in the second edition of the *Diagnostic and Statistical Manual of Mental Disorders* (DSM; 1968) as "hyperkinetic reaction of childhood." Evolution of recognition of the range of symptoms evident associated with this disorder led to identification of failure to sustain attention and distractibility as core traits. In 1980, this led to another change in name as "attention deficit disorder" was born in DSM-III. Research emphasis remained on symptom delineation with Douglas (1983) suggesting four major attributes: (1) poor attention and effort maintenance, (2) poor inhibition of impulsive behavior, (3) inability to appropriately modulate arousal to match the situation (mood lability), and (4) relentless search for immediate gratification. DSM-III also initiated division of the disorder into subtypes, those with and without hyperactivity. Disagreement about the uniqueness of the inattentive subtype remains; no distinct neuropsychological profile or consistent genetic transmission pattern has emerged based on this symptom (Carlson, 1986; Goodyear & Hynd, 1992). This uncertainty was reflected in the reshuffling of subtypes in DSM-III-R in 1987 and their re-emergence with an added "combined" phenotype, representing those individuals with both significant inattention and hyperactivity, in DSM-IV (1994).

The last 15 years have seen parallel studies of ADD from genetic, cognitive, educational, neuroanatomic, and neurofunctional perspectives resulting in a considerable volume of information but no fundamental, unified understanding of the origin or neurology of the disorder. Despite the complexities, the majority of professionals dealing with this disorder find compelling evidence of its neurostructural or neurochemical basis and clinicians from a variety of backgrounds continue to recognize children, adolescents, and, increasingly, adults, with a distinctive and reproducible set of symptoms that lead them to diagnose ADD (Faraone & Biederman, 1998). A minority regard children with symptoms of inattention and high activity level as either "improperly motivated or parented, or as victims of the educational system which finds it easier to label and medicate children who are difficult to teach" (Kohn, 1989, p. 99).

ADD is estimated to occur in 5.8% to 13.6% of school-aged boys and 1.9% to 4.5% of girls of similar age (Wolraich, 1996). The prevalence varies by diagnostic criteria, source of the study population, societal norms in the region of study, and age of the individuals evaluated. The characteristic behaviors vary in intensity but are frequently sufficiently severe to diminish classroom performance, limit ultimate academic achievement, impair social relationships, and negatively affect self-esteem. Adults with ADD may be predisposed to school failure, substance abuse, frequent job changes,

and marital instability. The combination of high prevalence and potentially significant impact on an individual's long-term social function make ADD a major health concern.

In recent years, ADD has entered public consciousness because of the debate over an apparently increasing rate of diagnosis, rapidly rising national usage of stimulant medication in children, including those younger than 5 years, and inclusion of ADD as an educational exceptionality.

DEFINITIONS AND DIAGNOSIS

The most widely used diagnostic criteria for clinical and research purposes are those contained in the *Diagnostic and Statistical Manual for Mental Health Disorders-IV* (DSM-IV). These criteria were developed by the American Psychiatric Association in 1994 and are specifically designed for use with children 6 to 12 years of age (Table 42-1). The American Academy of Pediatrics recently endorsed their use by the primary care physicians (2000). They contain symptom lists that define three subgroups of children with ADD. The primarily inattentive subtype is characterized by difficulty sustaining attention to task, poor organizational skills, easy distractibility, problems following directions, failing to pay attention to details, and avoidance of tasks requiring sustained attention. Criteria for primarily hyperactive-impulsive ADD include figitiness, difficulty remaining seated, physical overactivity inappropriate to the situation, difficulty playing quietly, and excessive talkitiveness as symptoms of hyperactivity. Impulsivity is shown by difficulty taking turns, interrupting others, and blurting out answers before questions are completed. The third category, combined subtype, contains children who meet criteria for both inattentive and hyperactive ADD. For all subtypes, the differences in behavior must reflect core temperament qualities present for at least 6 months and be clearly divergent from age expectations. It is generally agreed that the symptoms must be present in two or more settings and impair daily functioning.

Wolraich applied these criteria to teacher-generated data describing elementary school children in Tennessee in 1996. A prevalence rate of 4.7% for primarily inattentive, 3.4% for primarily hyperactive, and 4.4% for combined type ADD was reported. A study using the same guidelines applied to German children showed rates of 9.0%, 3.9%, and 4.8% for these subtypes (Baumgaertel, 1995).

Gender differences in prevalence have been noted consistently in children referred for clinical services, with male-female ratios as high as 9:1 (Lahey et al., 1994). Epidemiologic studies show ratios of 2:1 to 4:1. The validity of these differences in prevalence has been challenged as a product of cultural bias but may also

TABLE 42.1. Diagnostic Criteria for Attention Deficit Disorder

Criteria are met for **Attention-Deficit Disorder, Predominantly Inattentive Type** *if the individual has six or more of the following symptoms*

Inattention:

1. Poor attention to detail or careless errors, especially in schoolwork, but also may include other activities

2. Frequent difficulty maintaining attention to tasks or play activities

3. Ignores or fails to respond when addressed directly

4. Often fails to follow instructions and is unable to finish schoolwork, chores or at job (not related primarily to oppositional behavior)

5. Poor organizatinal skills

6. Avoidance or dislike for tasks requiring sustained mental effort

7. Frequent loss of materials needed to complete tasks or activities

8. Easily distracted by environmental stimuli

9. Frequently forgetful in daily activities or tasks

Criteria are met for **Attention-Deficit Disorder, Predominantly Hyperactive, Impulsive Type** *if the individual has six or more of the following symptoms*

Hyperectivity and Impulsivity:

1. Fidgety or squirms in seat

2. Frequently gets out of seat in the classroom or in other situations in which remaining seated is expected

3. Often runs or climbs excessively in situations in which it is not appropriate

4. Excessively noisy at play or leisure activities

5. Often "on the go" or acts as if "driven by a motor"

6. Frequently talks excessively

7. Often impulsively blurts out answers before questions have been completed

8. Problems waiting for turn

9. Often interrupts, especially ongoing conversations or intrudes on others activities

Criteria are met for **Attention-Deficit Disorder, Combined Type** *if the individual has six or more symptoms from both the inattention and hyperactivity/impulsivity lists*

These criteria also specify that the symptoms must have been present for at least 6 months to a degree that is maladaptive and unexpected for developmental level, and had onset prior to 7 years of age. The symptoms should be present in two or more settings and present functionally and clinically significant impact on social, academic, or occupational functioning. Finally, the criteria are fulfilled only in the absence of other mental disorders.

Adapted from American Psychiatric Assciation. Diagnostic and Statistical Manual of Mental Disorders: ed 4. Washington, DC: Author, 1994.

reflect sex-influenced expression of ADD symptoms. Girls are over-represented in the inattentive subtype, which may lead to under-referral, especially at young ages, because of reduced recognition of symptoms. It is generally agreed that boys are more likely to be hyperactive or have comorbid oppositional qualities, characteristics likely to provoke greater teacher and parent distress and, thus, earlier recognition and referral for services. In adult samples, the proportion of female patients increases, again supporting a more equal incidence, but differential expression, of ADD (Arcia & Connors, 1998). A higher incidence of cognitive impair-

ment has been thought to characterize girls referred for ADD. Recent studies also challenge this finding, noting similar neuropsychological profiles in boys and girls, suggesting that this observation may reflect a differential referral bias rather than the true nature of ADD in girls (Arcia & Connors, 1998). The issue of gender-related expression is critical to clinicians, but also to genetic researchers who must accurately assign affectedness to both sexes to clearly understand pattern of inheritance and calculate linkage to specific genes or loci.

A second important issue is that of definition of ADD across the age spectrum. DSM-IV criteria are designed for use with children from ages 6 to 12. There is no equivalent, generally accepted, definition for children under age 6, adolescents, and adults, age groups presenting for evaluation with increasing frequency. Several authors (Barkley, 1993; Ward, 1993) have addressed symptoms of ADD in adults. Rating scales have been developed for this age group but controversial issues remain, especially differentiating the extensive crossover in symptoms among oppositional defiant disorder, dysthymia, and other mood disorders and intermittent explosive personality disorder.

Although DSM-IV provides a definition of childhood ADD accepted by most researchers and practitioners, it does not operationalize the definition, nor does it provide norms by which children suspected of having ADD can be compared to their same-age peers. Numerous questionnaires have been developed for research and clinical purposes to quantify intensity of inattention, impulsivity, and hyperactivity and provide comparison norms. However, few precisely replicate, and most predate, the criteria set forth in DSM-IV. This leads to a disconnect in the evaluation process. The Clinical Practice Guidelines of the American Academy of Pediatrics recommend using behavior questionnaires as adjuncts to interviews of parents and teachers. Questionnaires with extensive validation and a close correspondence with DSM-IV definitions include those developed by Conners (Conners Parent and Teacher Rating Scales, 1997) and Swanson (SNAP, IV, 1995; Table 42-2). Other specialized tests, including continuous performance tasks, Wisconsin Card Sorting Task, subtest combinations of the Wechsler Intelligence Scale-III (freedom from distractibility scale), and the Paired Associated Learning Task may add specific information about selected skills, but do not provide sufficient criteria for diagnosis of ADD. Much to the frustration of parents and clinicians, there is still no "diagnostic" questionnaire, test, or scan for ADD (Grodzinsky & Barkley, 1999). Diagnosis remains in the hands of clinicians after information is obtained from several settings (home, school, sports, social), assessment is completed for (uncommon) medical conditions that mimic ADD, and assessment is performed for other neurobehavioral disorders that have an impact on focus and learning. This represents a time-consuming process, which is poorly compensated by most insurers.

TABLE 42.2. Commonly Used Questionnaires to Identify Children at Risk for ADD

Rating Scales Specifically Designed to Detect Symptoms of Attention Deficit Disorder

*Conners' Rating Scales
    Ages 3–17 yr
    Parent and teacher scales
    DSM-IV Scales are keyed to correspond to symptoms set forth in DSM-IV

*ADHD Symptom Checklist-4
    Ages 3–18 yr

*ADD-H Comprehensive Teacher's Rating Scales (ACTeRS)
    Grades kindergarten to 8
    Primarily for teachers, parent scale available

*ADHD Rating Scale IV
    Ages 5–17 yr
    Parent and teacher scales

*Brown Attention-Deficit Disorder Scales (Brown ADD Scales)
    Ages 3 to adult
    Parent and teacher scales

General Behavior Questionnaires with ADHD Sections

*Child Behavior Checklist
    Ages 6–18 yr
    Parent scales
    Newest version keyed to correspond to symptoms set forth in DSM-IV

*Child Symptom Inventory-4
    Ages 5–12 yr
    Parent and teacher scales

THE LIFE CYCLE OF ATTENTION-DEFICIT DISORDER

The majority of studies of symptoms and temperament qualities associated with ADD have focused on the school-aged child. However, if, as most researchers and clinicians believe, ADD is a developmental brain disorder, it would be expected to exert an effect throughout the life span. Age-dependent sequences of temperament traits have been described by several authors (Levine, 1987; Barkley, 1993) and are regularly observed by professionals who evaluate children with ADD. Children with the primarily hyperactive or combined types of the disorder and those with comorbid oppositional-defiant disorder (ODD) are most likely to manifest obvious symptoms from an early age.

Infants later diagnosed with ADD frequently manifest over-reactivity, irritability, "colic," and inability to tolerate a regular schedule for feeding and sleeping. Prolonged crying is a frequent parental complaint as is failure to sleep through the night at the expected age.

By toddler age, high activity level emerges along with short attention span. At this age, the range of "normal" is wide, making it unwise to label a child younger than 3 years as having ADD. Other qualities frequently described include poor safety awareness, mood lability, difficulty remaining entertained without adult intervention, continued sleep disturbance (frequent night-time waking, short duration of naps) and, for some, aggressive interactions with peers. Oppositional qualities may surface in those preschooler children who also have ODD, a combination noted in 30% to 40% of boys with ADD.

In nursery school, the gap in attention-focus skills between typically developing children and those with ADD often becomes more apparent. Distractibility during group activities and social "immaturity" are often reported by parents and teachers. Failure to follow rules or "mind" the parent may prompt a medical or mental health evaluation at this age. Positive qualities can include creativity and good verbal skills.

Entry into a formal school program further stresses ability to focus attention on a directed task and remain seated. Distractibility is often more obvious. Early elementary students with primarily hyperactive or combined type ADD are often described to be out of their seats excessively, to "call out" in class, fail to follow directions, and are forgetful and disruptive of the class. Those with accompanying learning disabilities may begin to struggle academically. Children with primarily inattentive ADD may not be detected at this age; they are much less likely to disturb classmates or teachers. Social interaction may also be problematic for the ADD child with impulsive verbalizations or emotional over-reactivity as the catalysts for avoidance by other students. It is in elementary school that many children with ADD, especially those with hyperactivity, are first evaluated for the disorder.

Homework completion provides another challenge to both attention-focus and organizational skills (forgotten assignments, lost papers). Neatness of work and handwriting are often compromised. Significant variability in quality of work from day to day makes parents and teachers doubt the child's sincerity of effort. Excessive fatigue may be apparent in some children and understandable in view of studies suggesting that individuals with ADD expend 2 to 4 times the mental energy of nonaffected peers to stay focused. This may also explain why homework completion is a major problem, especially if attempted immediately after school.

The persistence of symptoms of ADD into adolescence and adulthood is now recognized. Studies documenting the outcome include a recent one by Mannuzza and Klein (1993) who report the 20-year outcome for 100 individuals with ADD compared to a group matched for socioeconomic status and age. In adolescence, 52% with continued ADD characteristics engaged in substance abuse or criminal behavior. Barkley (1990) documents rates of cigarette and marijuana use that are 1.5 to 2 times the age-matched population rate. These rates were significantly accentuated in adolescents with ADD combined with oppositional-defiant or conduct disorders. Their study did not document increased alcohol or other drug abuse in contrast to the results of several others.

Academically, ADD also exacts a toll with approximately one third of affected children having failed a grade by high school and 30.6% having been suspended (Barkley, 1990). Barkley's study was completed prior to the "zero tolerance" movement and, although no clear documentation is yet available, it is quite likely that this approach differentially penalizes adolescents with ADD. Particularly at risk are those with significant residual impulsivity or comorbid ODD. School dropout rates for adolescents with ADD are noted to range from 10% to 35%. A higher incidence of driving infractions (usually speeding), car accidents, and other types of accidental trauma are documented (Barkley et al., 1996), likely as a result of a general trend toward greater risk taking and disregard for consequences.

By adulthood, 50% to 65% of men with ADD continue to have significant, persistent symptoms. Substance abuse rates remain higher than the general population but with diminishing disparity. Rates of job change, divorce, and number of moves are all increased. On the positive side, a study by Mannuzza and Klein (1993) found that 18% of young adults with ADD owned their own businesses compared to 5% of same age, unaffected peers. Despite this observation, lower socioeconomic status in adulthood was noted for affected men compared to their brothers (Barkley, 1990).

Girls and women with ADD have been less frequently studied, but clear differences are evident in symptom sets between boys/men and girls/women. These also stratify with age. Girls have a lower percentage of comorbid conduct disorder (19% versus 32.9%), but higher rates of phobia/anxiety (47.6% versus 16.4%) and depression (38.1% versus 26.7%; Faraone et al., 1991). Adult women with ADD rate themselves as more impaired in self-control, confidence, concentration, and restlessness than adult men with the disorder (Arcia & Connors, 1998). The prevalence of cognitive differences between affected boys and girls is controversial. Some studies suggest that girls with ADD manifest lower verbal intelligence and academic performance (Berry et al., 1985; Ernst et al., 1994). In contrast, Arcia and Conners (1998) did not report gender-related differences in verbal or performance subscale of intelligence measures.

ETIOLOGY

The definition of ADD and its subtypes has evolved to the current DSM-IV iteration, which has been endorsed by most North American clinicians and researchers. No such consensus exists regarding etiology of the disorder. Strong evidence suggests a genetic component, but no specific gene (or more likely genes) has been implicated nor has the neurobiologic basis been convincingly shown by current technology. Competing cognitive theories have been advanced, which implicate brain systems that may interact to produce the observed symptoms, but there is, as yet, no conjunction between theory and neurobiology.

Genetic Research and Theory

Clinical observations have long suggested familial clustering of ADD, especially the hyperactive subtype. However, the formal study of familial connections began in the 1960s with only five studies published between 1966 and 1986. Thereafter, a plethora of publications have defined an increased risk for the disorder in first- and second-degree relatives of affected children, studied twins, documented familial rates of comorbidity, searched for genetically distinguishable subtypes and, most recently, reported results of genome-wide searches using molecular genetics and linkage or association studies examining specific candidate genes or loci.

It can be reliably concluded that first-degree relatives have a twofold to threefold increased risk of also having the disorder (Biederman et al., 1986; Faraone et al., 1994).Interpretation of these data is complicated by elevated rate of conduct, ODD, and anxiety disorders as well as learning disability observed in close relatives of

children with ADD. Each of these disorders may have independent heritability risks that contribute to apparent transmissibility. Observed familial aggregation could also be explained by shared psychosocial factors or adversity generated by having a child who is difficult to manage. This possibility was examined by Biederman and colleagues in 1990; they found that the occurrence of ADD among first-degree relatives of probands with ADD did not differ based on social class, age of proband, nor family intactness. Families of children referred for other psychiatric disorders did not have an increased risk for ADD, providing evidence that the observed increased risk in ADD families did not arise simply from having a dysfunctional family member. Familiality has also been convincingly documented for female probands (Faraone et al., 1991) and second-degree relatives (Faraone et al., 1994).

Twin studies provide additional confirmation of the heritability of ADD. High concordance rates (mostly in the 0.6 to 0.8 range) are reported for monozygotic twins, who share 100% of their genes in common, compared to 0.2 to 0.35 for dizygotic twins who share 50% of their genes (Tannock, 1998). Heritability estimates range from 0.50 to 0.98, based on these studies, and remain in this range regardless of severity of symptoms or differences in diagnostic criteria among studies.

Thus, it can be concluded that ADD is highly heritable, but no study has convincingly demonstrated a consistent mode of transmission. A single gene with a major effect, often acting in an autosomal dominant pattern, seems the best fit with the current data (Faraone et al., 1992). It also appears likely that at least several, if not multiple, genes produce the ADD phenotype. Investigators have searched for genetically independent subtypes of ADD, which include specific comorbidities or clusters of symptoms. Results are equivocal for a unique phenotype of ADD and reading disorder (Gillis et al., 1992; (Stevenson, 1992). Comorbidity between ADD and ODD and conduct disorders is 42.7% to 93.0% (Jensen et al., 1997) and, also, anxiety disorder co-occurs with ADD more frequently than in the general population (13.0%–50.8%). The former combination is more common in boys, especially those with hyperactivity, whereas depression/anxiety is more likely to occur in girls. Although the co-occurrence of these disorders is well documented, it remains unclear whether either combination is a genetically distinct subtype (Cadoret & Stewart, 1991). This unresolved issue has clear implications for genetic research. Grouping of distinctive subtypes, which might localize to different genetic loci, would obscure true correlation with specific regions if analyzed together.

The most recent genetic effort has been the identification of candidate genes. The first association reported was in 1993 between a very rare autosomal recessive disorder, generalized resistance to thyroid hormone, and clinical ADD, hyperactive subtype in affected family members (Hauser et al., 1993). Although this association with mutations in the thyroid-receptor ß gene is clearly valid in this disorder, it has not been found to be a general defect in the general population of individuals with ADD (Weiss et al., 1993). More recently, genes within the dopamine neurotransmitter system have been proposed as likely candidate for this disorder because of its likely role in mediating response to stimulant medications. Several studies have found an association (as distinct from linkage) between one allele of the dopamine transporter gene and ADD (Cook et al., 1995; Waldman et al., 1996), but the sample sizes are small and further study is required. A second dopamine-related gene, the D4 receptor gene, has shown association with "novelty seeking" behavior (Benjamin et al., 1996) and, in two subsequent studies, with ADD (LaHoste et al., 1996; Sunohara et al., 1997). There are several consortia, both in Europe and the United States, currently engaged in genome-wide searches for genes that link with ADD.

Neurostructural and Neurofunctional Findings

Two categories of brain imaging have been used to study ADD: static studies that evaluate structure and include computed tomography (CT) and magnetic resonance imaging (MRI) and dynamic imaging technique that compares metabolic changes between the static state and during specific tasks. Dynamic imaging techniques include positron emission tomography (PET) scans, single photon emission computed tomography (SPECT) scans, and functional MRI (fMRI). In general, studies using these techniques have had small numbers of subjects, differing ages, and varying diagnostic criteria.

Neurostructural and functional studies do not all implicate the same brain regions, but there are some congruent findings. Anatomic areas most frequently noted to differ between subjects with ADD and comparison individuals include either or both frontal lobes. These areas are found to be smaller than in comparison subjects in the majority of CT- or MRI-based structural studies (Hynd et al., 1991; Filipek et al., 1997). Decreased glucose metabolism in this same region was noted in several PET scanning studies (Lou et al., 1984; Zametkin et al., 1993). Conflicting results have been reported from fMRI studies, with a study by Rubia and colleagues (1997) showing reduced brain activation during an attention task in the right inferior frontal gyrus and right precentral and postcentral gyrus, whereas Vaidya and colleagues (1998) reported greater frontal activation during a response inhibition task.

The majority of studies also demonstrated structural aberrations in the basal ganglia, thalamus, or both. The side preferentially affected and precise nuclear localization differ. Some studies implicate the caudate (Castellanos et al., 1994), whereas others the globus pallidus (Aylward, 1996; Castellanos et al., 1996). Studies of glucose metabolism also found differences in these areas with diminished metabolism in the right thalamus and caudate in one study (Zametkin et al., 1990), but left thalamic dysfunction in another (Zametkin et al., 1993). A recent fMRI study showed diminished blood volume in the putamen during a computerized attention task (Teicher et al., 2000).

A hypothesis connecting these findings suggests that ADD is mediated by dysfunction of the frontostriatal pathways. This correlates well with the known ameliorative effects of medications, especially stimulants, which act on both dopaminergic and noradrenergic pathways that are abundant in these regions. A single study, completed in 1999, has shown an increase in dopamine transporter density in the striatum (Dougherty et al., 1999). In two studies, changes noted by PET scanning in the frontal and basal ganglia regions were partially reversed by methylphenidate treatment (Lou et al., 1994; Vaidya et al., 1998), providing additional support for involvement of the frontostriatal pathways. Clearly, much more needs to be done to strengthen these results because most studies evaluated fewer than 20, and often fewer than 10, subjects of varying ages, both genders and with an admixture of comorbidities.

COGNITIVE THEORIES

The most widely supported and accepted neurocognitive theories of ADD center on a defect of behavioral inhibition and its effects on executive functions. Multiple models have postulated a defect in inhibitory function including those that view it as a conditioning defect (Gray, 1982), as inefficiencies in control processes (Schachar et al., 1993; Logan, 1994), and as response inhibition as a primary inborn neurologic "wiring" deficit (Barkley, 1994, 1996). Barkley's model is probably the best elaborated and most comprehensive.

Behavioral inhibition is conceptualized by Barkley (1996) as inhibition of preprogrammed responses both before and after initiation, allowing a delay in response to an event and the protection of this delay from competing brain functions. Executive functions are designated as working memory (holding information in a way that is accessible while manipulating additional or incoming data), self-regulation of affect, internalization of speech, and use of analysis and synthesis when responding to an event (reconstitution).

Behaviors predicted by this theory include impaired time sense, poor short-term memory, inefficient organizational skills, overexpression of emotions, especially in reaction to an event, social impulsivity, excessive talking, and diminished fluency and logic. These temperament qualities are all frequent in individuals with ADD with the exception of impaired verbal logic and fluency. Studies of cognitive skills show no consistent pattern suggesting stronger visual or constructional aptitudes compared to language, although reading disorder is common.

Direct evaluation of executive functions is difficult because of their complexity, but the majority of studies examining these functions appear to demonstrate abnormalities. Pennington and Ozonoff (1996) summarized 18 controlled studies and reported that 15 of them showed significant deficits in executive functions, with a compiled total of 40 of 60 executive function measures differentiating typical individuals from those with ADD. The most consistent deficits were found in motor task inhibition. Unfortunately, the executive functions are sufficiently complex, imprecisely defined, and functionally linked to one another that it is difficult to be certain whether one or several functions are actually being assessed.

Inhibition dysfunction models less successfully explain inattention, an integral component of ADD. It should be noted that Barkley (1996) specifically excludes primarily inattentive ADD as defined by DSM-IV from his conceptual model.

The next advance in the understanding of ADD will occur with the successful union of cognitive theory and neurobiology. Identifying pathways subserving executive functions may be feasible using fMRI technology if sufficiently specific tasks can be devised to differentiate executive functions in typical individuals from those with ADD.

TREATMENT AND OUTCOME

Effective intervention for children, and especially adolescents, with ADD requires cooperation among the affected child, parents, school personnel, physician and, frequently, therapist. Unfortunately, with so many required participants, coordination of intervention and unity of approach are difficult to achieve. Also, prioritizing services is problematic because there is no clear correlation between specific treatment approaches and outcome. This may be related to the wide variation in intensity and type of symptoms, frequent presence of comorbidities, variability in availability of educational support services, and the social milieu of the patient, each of which exerts independent influence on outcome. Despite the controversy, multimodality intervention remains the recommended approach (Elia et al., 1999; Zametkin & Ernst, 1999).

TREATMENT MODALITIES

Education of Family and Patient

The first priority after a diagnosis of ADD is education of family and, depending on age, the child. It is crucial that they understand that for most affected individuals, the symptoms are not primarily caused by willful misbehavior, but rather have their origin in the neurologic system. It is clear that a "behavioral" component is often built on the neurologic predisposition, but a completely behavioral origin is untenable with the current evidence. This explanation is often of help to families who frequently feel guilty that they have a child with problems and may blame their parenting style. An explanation of what is understood of the genetics and neurology of ADD may alleviate the guilt and allow a family to move ahead with treatment.

There is an abundance of printed material including popular books, websites, and pamphlets written for families, the children themselves, siblings, and education professionals. The approaches advocated may vary widely so each clinician will need to adopt those that best represent his viewpoint. A large, national support group with local chapters, Children and Adults with Attention Deficit Disorder (8181 Professional Pl, Suite 201, Landover, MD; (800) 233–4050; http://www.chadd.ord) is an appropriate initial contact for many families. This resource can provide local contacts, as well as written information designed for families.

Behavior Modification and Other Psychotherapeutic Approaches

Behavioral approaches have been shown to be of greater value in treating ODD and other disruptive behaviors than in modification of core symptoms of ADD (Pelham et al., 1998) but few studies are available and the type of intervention studied was inconsistent. A behavior management approach emphasizing consistent identification of targeted behaviors among caregivers, use of positive reinforcement for younger children, and contracts with adolescents to achieve completion of specific tasks may be of benefit. This is appropriate as a general approach to working with children in a constructive way, but not specifically expected to ameliorate core symptoms of ADD. Enhancement of the child's self-esteem is an important goal of behavioral intervention because of the frequent occurrence of depression in middle school and high school among students with ADD. Supportive family and marital therapy have a role in assisting parents to cope with the stress of dealing with a child who has ADD.

Cognitive therapies using self-monitoring, organizational skill development, and task analysis have not been proven effective in controlled studies (Abikoff,

1991; Douglas, 1980). Nonetheless, if the adolescent patient participates actively in generating problem-solving strategies and education about ADD is also provided, benefit may be realized in allowing the children to better understand their own strengths and weaknesses.

Training in social skills emphasizes techniques to improve peer interaction and is often done with a same age group. Dealing with problem interactions as they arise in the group is an important component to allow the participants practical experience with mediation under supervision of a moderator. As with other psychotherapeutic approaches, studies of outcome are rare and the results inconsistent (Barkley, 1990).

Educational Interventions

Remediation of and accommodation for learning, which are common comorbidities with ADD, is an important component of overall management. However, there is no universal consensus among educators as to how this is most effectively accomplished (Silberberg & Silberberg, 1969). Interventions appear to vary widely even with a given geographic location with little research to support specific approaches. For the practitioner providing care for children with ADD, it will be most important to ensure an adequate evaluation for specific learning disabilities, specifically including written language, a frequent but commonly overlooked problem area for children and adolescents with ADD. Education professionals are responsible for specifying remediation.

The Individuals with Disabilities Education Act (1999) specifically recognized ADD (with and without hyperactivity) as an educational exceptionality included under "other health impaired." Thus children with this diagnosis are legally entitled to services if their disability "adversely affects educational performance." However, specific compensations are not mandated, once again leading to variation from region to region, and sometimes among schools in a district as to how ADD is addressed. Commonly used interventions include preferential seating, use of assignment book initialed by teacher and family, extended time for taking tests, behavior modification programs, counseling, and decreased workload. Educational research validating these interventions is scanty.

Medication Management

Stimulant medications have remained at the forefront of treatment for symptoms of ADD since effectiveness was demonstrated about 65 years ago for children with a combination of cognitive impairment and poor attention focus (Bradley, 1937). Many controlled studies have documented the effectiveness of dextroamphetamine, amphetamine, and methylphenidate in improving on-task behavior and short-term memory, while decreasing motor overactivity and impulsivity (Carlson & Bunner, 1993; Swanson et al., 1993; Spencer et al., 1996). These medications also often enhance academic productivity and improve handwriting. Reduced aggression and confrontation have been reported, especially for amphetamine-based medications (Hinshaw, 1991). Temperament qualities that respond less well, or not at all, include impaired social skills, antisocial or defiant behavior, poor organizational skills, and learning deficits. There is also no direct effect on intelligence test scores or academic achievement, although enhanced concentration may secondarily improve grades by allowing more work to be completed. In clinical practice, it is critical that parents and school personnel understand the expectations and limitations of the effects of stimulant medication. Lack of effect on organizational skills is a particular issue, especially in later elementary grades and middle school. Expectations for manipulation, organization, and retention of complex information often rise rapidly at that time and children with attention-deficit/hyperactivity disorder (ADHD), with or without medication support, often do not have the organizational skill capacity to successfully deal with this increased load.

The rate of response to stimulant medication is generally acknowledged to be around 70% (Swanson et al., 1993), but most studies are of short duration (weeks to several months). Long-term response, without development of tolerance, is less well shown but has recent support in a study by Gillberg and colleagues (1997). There is an impression that children with primarily inattentive ADD, as currently defined in DSM-IV, may respond less well to the stimulants than children in the other subgroups, but greater study is required. Also controversial is equivalency of response between boys and girls. A factor likely influencing this is the relative prevalence of primary inattention in girls. Positive response across the age spectrum, including adulthood, is demonstrated (Spencer et al., 1996).

Stimulants in current use include methylphenidate, dextroamphetamine, and amphetamine, as well as pemoline. Pemoline currently is infrequently prescribed because of the rare association of this medication with potentially severe toxic hepatitis. Methylphenidate and dextroamphetamine preparations are known to affect different components of the dopamine neurotransmitter pathway in brain, but beyond this, their precise mechanism of action remains unknown. They do appear to enhance the "signal-to-noise" ratio and, thus, improve efficiency (Hunt et al., 2001). Observations suggest that children and adolescents commonly have a positive response to either medication, but selected individuals have a marked difference in intensity of response between methylphenidate and dextroamphetamine. Hunt and colleagues (2001) summarize a recent study with 31 adults who participated in a placebo-controlled, crossover study of amphetamine sulfate, dextroamphetamine sulfate, and methylphenidate. In this group, 55% preferred the effect of amphetamine sulfate and 21% chose dextroamphetamine, whereas 23% favored methylphenidate. Of interest was the observation that men generally chose to remain on amphetamine sulfate, but women split equally among the three medications.

A significant difference among the stimulant medications is duration of action. Standard methylphenidate preparations yield a 3- to 4-hour duration of action, whereas dextroamphetamine standard preparations last 6 to 8 hours and fixed combinations of dextroamphetamine and amphetamine salts appear to cover 8 to 10 hours (Pelham et al., 1999). In recent years, more reliable extended-release preparations have been developed for methylphenidate. A preparation of methylphenidate, using a new extended-release system, has increased duration of action up to 12 hours with relatively even release through that time (Swanson et al., 1999). This system also appears to have overcome the lack of reliable initiation of action encountered in the earlier sustained-release preparations. Spectrum of coverage is especially important for adolescents who are frequently reluctant to take medication during school. Also, short-acting stimulants may foster a "peak and valley" effect, with diminished coverage at lunch and recess while producing side effects during peak levels. Age, weight, and intensity of symptoms do not accurately predict the optimal dose of stimulant medication. Therefore, the most prudent course is to begin with a low dose to minimize side effects and increase slowly over a period of weeks using observations from home and school to guide changes. Usual doses of methylphenidate range from 0.25 to 0.75 mg/kg per dose for short-acting preparations; if doses greater than 0.8 mg/kg per dose are needed, other factors affecting performance should be sought (Spencer et al., 1996). For dextroamphetamine, the per-dose range is 0.2 to 0.5 mg/kg for the standard preparation; dose range for the long-acting preparations is not well established.

Side effects of all stimulant medications are similar and can included decreased appetite (up to 80%), insomnia (5%–85%), headache (5%–15%), abdominal pain (*bl5%), dizziness (*bl5%) and irritability, especially as the medication "wears off" (Barkley et al., 1990). Motor or vocal tics are associated with use in approximately 1/150 individuals (Price et al., 1986). It remains controversial as to whether these medications "cause" or simply trigger these movements in predisposed individuals. Dextroamphetamine-based medications may be less likely to trigger tics than methylphenidate. It has been the usual recommendation that stimulants be stopped if tics become evident, but it has been observed in some children that the movements

may subside on their own without removal of the medication. Appetite suppression also tends to diminish over time and may be less intense for amphetamine-containing medications. Sleeplessness can pose a significant problem for families and may require decreasing or stopping the last stimulant dose of the day. For those children who have persistent problems with poor onset of sleep, but good daytime response to stimulants, consideration may be given to use of a second medication. Melatonin, promethazine, diphenhydramine, and, in severe situations, atypical antipsychotic medications can be considered.

Other medications have been used to treat symptoms of ADD with varying response, but none have been as consistently effective as stimulants. Clonidine and guanfacine have been used, both as a primary and secondary medications for hyperactivity and inattention (usually combined with a stimulant), for the last 20 years. They act by decreasing brain noradrenergic activity. Connor and colleagues (1999) reported a meta-analysis, which reviewed 39 studies of the effectiveness of clonidine. It was concluded that this medication had a moderate effect on symptoms of ADD in both children and adolescents. Clinicians note a potentially significant positive effect of clonidine on comorbid symptoms of aggression that suggests considering its use specifically in this situation. Guanfacine has a longer duration of action allowing twice per day dosing compared to three times per day for clonidine. Side effects of these medications include tiredness, which frequently limited ability to increase dose to an effective level, dizziness, and decreased blood pressure. A total of five deaths have been reported in individuals taking a combination of stimulants and clonidine, but no clear causal relationship is apparent (Finichel, 1995; Cantwell, 1996).

Antidepressant medications have been used to treat a variety of neurobehavioral symptoms in children. They are also known to modify levels of dopamine and norepinephrine consistent with current hypotheses of the neurochemical basis of ADD. Tricyclic antidepressants have had the longest use, but are now infrequently prescribed because of potential for cardiac toxicity (especially with desipramine) and relatively low overall efficacy (Popper, 1997). A new medication in this family, tamoxiten, which appears to have a much lower risk of cardiac side effects and higher efficacy, is under study.

Selective serotonin reuptake inhibitors (SSRIs) have not been shown to be effective against the core symptoms of ADD but are of benefit in individuals, especially adolescents, with concomitant irritability, depressed mood, or anxiety. In this situation, they are usually used in combination with a stimulant.

Bupropion has had recent use for symptoms of ADD, especially with comorbid anxiety. A limited number of studies are available to document its effect. A study from 1995, by Barrickman and colleagues, evaluated the response to this medication of 15 children with ADD, ages 7 to 17, and reported equal efficacy of bupropion and methylphenidate. Side effects in this study were minor, but changes in blood pressure, rash, and, rarely, seizure, have been associated with bupropion use for other indications (Johnston, 1991).

It can be safely concluded that stimulant medications remain the most effective and well-tolerated medications for treatment of symptoms of ADD. It is equally true that for most individuals with this disorder, medication alone is insufficient to ameliorate the long-term effects of ADD. Although not fully proven by studies, school-based interventions, education of parents about the nature of ADD, and therapies directed at support of self-esteem and self-monitoring all have a role in the overall well-being of these individuals.

KEY POINTS

☐ The symptoms of attention-deficit/hyperactivity disorder are generally present from early childhood, but the range of behaviors evolves over the life span of the affected individual.

☐ Identification of ADD/ADHD relies on observations from several sources (family, school), exclusion of other medical, learning, and mental health disorders with similar symptoms, and careful evaluation by an experienced clinician. Behavior questionnaires, psychological testing, and continuous performance tests are adjunctive evaluations, but cannot be relied on as independent means of diagnosis.

☐ The neurologic underpinnings of ADD/ADHD remain unclear, but the central dopaminergic system appears to be the prime mediator of medication effect, with input from noradrenergic neurons. Structural studies implicate the basal ganglia and subfrontal regions in the pathology of ADD, but some studies suggest abnormalities in the temporal lobes as well. A genetic predisposition to the disorder is clearly evident, but the pattern of inheritance is yet to be established.

☐ Medication intervention is effective about 70% of the time to ameliorate the attention focus and hyperactivity symptoms of ADD. Stimulant medications are most frequently used and, generally, most effective. Other medications that can be of help include clonidine, bupropion, and tricyclic antidepressants.

☐ The most effective approach to overall treatment of individuals with ADD involves educational interventions, including support for learning problems when present, behavior management by parents, medication when appropriate, and careful monitoring for and treatment of secondary depression or accompanying oppositional behaviors.

KEY READINGS

American Academy of Pediatrics Committee on Quality Improvement, Subcommittee on Attention-Deficit/Hyperactivity Disorder: Clinical practice guideline: Diagnosis and evaluation of the child with attention-deficit/hyperactivity disorder. Pediatrics 105:1158–1170, 2000.

Elia J, Ambrosini PJ, Rapoport JL: Treatment of attention-deficit-hyperactivity disorder. N Eng J Med 340:780–788, 1999.

Faraone SV, Biederman J: Neurobiology of attention-deficit hyperactivity disorder. Biol Psychiatry 44:951–958, 1998.

REFERENCES

Abikoff H: Cognitive training in ADHD children: Less to it than meets the eye. J Learn Disabil 24:205–209, 1991.
American Academy of Pediatrics Committee on Quality Improvement, Subcommittee on Attention-Deficit/ Hyperactivity Disorder: Clinical practice guideline: Diagnosis and evaluation of the child with attention-deficit/hyperactivity disorder. Pediatrics 105:1158–1170, 2000.
American Psychiatric Association: Diagnostic and Statistical Manual of Mental Disorders, ed 2 (DSM). Washington, DC: Author, 1968.
American Psychiatric Association: Diagnostic and Statistical Manual of Mental Disorders, ed 3 (DSM-III). Washington, DC: Author, 1980.
American Psychiatric Association: Diagnostic and Statistical Manual of Mental Disorders, ed 3, revised (DSM-III-R). Washington, DC: Author, 1987.
American Psychiatric Association: Diagnostic and Statistical Manual of Mental Disorders, ed 4 (DSM-IV). Washington, DC: Author, 1994.
Arcia E, Conners CK: Gender Differences in ADHD? Dev Behav Pediatr 19:77–82, 1998.
Aylward EH, Reiss AL, Reader MJ et al: Basal ganglia volumes in children with attention-deficit hyperactivity disorder. J Child Neurol 11:112–115, 1996.
Barkley RA: Developmental course and adult outcome, in Barkley RA (ed): Attention-Deficit Hyperactivity Disorder: A Handbook for Diagnosis and Treatment. New York: Guilford Press, 1990, pp. 107–129.
Barkley RA: Impaired delayed responding: A unified theory of attention deficit hyperactivity disorder, in Routh DK (ed): Disruptive Behavior Disorders: Essays in Honor of Herbert Quay. New York: Plenum Press, 1994, pp. 11–57.
Barkley RA: Attention-deficit/hyperactivity disorder, in Marsh EJ, Barkley RA (eds): Child Psychopatholgy. New York, Guilford Press, 1996, pp. 63–111.
Barkley RA, Guevremont DG, Anastopoulos AD, et al: Driving-related risks and outcomes of attention deficit hyperactivity disorder in adolescents and young adults: A 3-5 year follow-up survey. Pediatrics 92:212–218, 1993.
Barkley RA, McMurray MB, Edelbrock CS, Robbins K: Side effects of methylphenidate in children with attention deficit hyperactivity

disorder: A systemic, placebo-controlled evaluation. Pediatrics 86:184–192, 1990.

Barkley RA, Murphy KR, Kwasnik D: Motor vehicle driving competencies and risks in teens and young adults with attention deficit hyperactivity disorder. Pediatrics 98:1089–1095, 1996.

Barrickman C, Perry PJ, Allen AJ, et al: Bupropion versus methylphenidate in the treatment of attention-deficit hyperactivity disorder. Am Acad Child Adolesc Psychiatry 34:649–657, 1995.

Baumgaertel A: Assessment of German school children using DSM criteria based on teacher report. Paper presented at the Society for Research in Child and Adolescent Psychopathology, London, England, 1994.

Benjamin J, Li L, Patterson C, et al: Population and familial association between the D4 receptor gene and measures of novelty seeking. Nat Genet 12:81–84, 1996.

Berry CA, Shaywitz SE, Shaywitz BA: Girls with attention deficit disorder: A silent minority? A report on behavioral and cognitive characteristics. Pediatrics 76:801–809, 1985.

Biederman J, Munir K, Knee D, et al: A family study of patients with attention deficit disorder and normal controls. J Psychiatr Res 20:263–274, 1986.

Biederman J, Faraone SV, Keenan K, et al: Family-genetic and psychosocial risk factors in DSM-III attention deficit disorder. J Am Acad Child Adolesc Psychiatry 29:526–533, 1990.

Bradley C: The behavior of children receiving benzedrine. Am J Psychiatry 94:577–585, 1937.

Cadoret RJ, Stewart MA: An adoption study of attention deficit/hyperactivity/aggression and their relationship to adult antisocial personality. Compr Psychiatry 32:73–82, 1991.

Cantwell DP: Attention deficit disorder: A review of the past 10 years. J Am Acad Child Adolesc Psychiatry 35:978–986, 1996.

Carlson C: Attention deficit disorder without hyperactivity: A review of preliminary experimental evidence, in Lahey B, Kazdin A (eds): Advances in Clinical Child Psychology. New York: Plenium Press, 1986, Vol. 9, pp. 153–176.

Carlson CL, Bunner MR: Effects of methylphenidate on the academic performance of children with attention-deficit disorder and learning disabilities. Sch Psychol Rev 22:184–198, 1993.

Castellanos FX, Elia J, Kruesi MJP, et al: Cerebrospinal fluid monoamine metabolites in boys with attention-deficit hyperactivity disorder. Psychiatry Res 52:305–316, 1994.

Castellanos FX, Giedd JN, Marsh WL, et al: Quantitative brain magnetic resonance imaging in attention-deficit/hyperactivity disorder. Arch Gen Psychiatry 53:607–616,1996.

Connor DF, Fletcher KE, Swanson JM: A meta-analysis of clonidine for symptoms of attention-deficit hyperactivity disorder. J Am Acad Child Adolesc Psychiatry 38:1551–1559, 1999.

Cook EH Jr, Stein MA, Krasowski MD, et al: Association of attention deficit disorder and the dopamine transporter gene. Am J Hum Genet 56:993–998, 1995.

Dougherty, DD, Vonab AA, Spencer TJ, et al: Dopamine transporter density in patients with attention deficit hyperactivity disorder. Lancet 354:2132–2134, 1999.

Douglas VI: Higher mental processes in hyperactive children: Implications for training, in Knights R, Bakker D (eds): Treatment of Hyperactive and Learning Disordered Children. Baltimore: University Park Press, 1980, pp. 65–92.

Douglas VI: Attention and cognitive problems, in Rutter M (ed): Developmental Neuropsychiatry. New York: Guilford Press, 1983, pp. 280–329.

Elia J, Ambrosini PJ, Rapoport JL: Treatment of attention-deficit-hyperactivity disorder. N Engl J Med 340:780–788, 1999.

Ernst M, Liebenauer IL, King CA, et al: Reduced brain metabolism in hyperactive girls. J Am Acad Child Adolesc Psychiat 33:858–868, 1994.

Faraone SV, Biederman J: Neurobiology of attention-deficit hyperactivity disorder. Biol Psychiatry 44:951–958, 1998.

Faraone SV, Biederman J, Chen WJ, et al: Segregation analysis of attention deficit hyperactivity disorder. Psychiatr Genet 2:257–275, 1992.

Faraone SV, Biederman J, Keenan K, et al: A family-genetic study of girls with DSM-III attention deficit disorder. Am J Psychiatry 148:112–117, 1991.

Faraone SV, Biederman J, Milberger S: An exploratory study of ADHD among second-degree relatives of ADHD children. Biol Psychiatry 35:398–402, 1994.

Filipek PA, Semrud-Clikeman M, Steingerd RJ, et al: Volumetric MRI analysis comparing subjects having attention-deficit hyperactivity disorder with normal controls. Neurology 48:589–601, 1997.

Finichel RR: Combining methylphenidate and clonidine: The role of post-marketing surveillance. J Child Adolesc Psychopharmacol 5:155–156, 1995.

Gillberg C, Melander H, von Knorring AL, et al: Long-term stimulant treatment of children with attention-deficit hyperactivity disorder symptoms: A randomized, double-blind, placebo-controlled trial. Arch Gen Psychiatry 54:857–864, 1997.

Gillis JJ, Gilger JW, Pennington BF, et al: Attention deficit disorder in reading-disabled twins: Evidence for a genetic etiology. J Abnorm Child Psychol 20:303–315, 1992.

Goodyear P, Hynd G: Attention deficit disorder with (ADD/H) and without (ADD/WO) hyperactivity: Behavioral and neuropsychological differentiation. J Clin Child Psychol 21:273–304, 1992.

Gray JA: The Neuropsychology of Anxiety. New York: Oxford Press, 1982, pp. 128–130.

Grodzinsky GM, Barkley RA: Predictive power of frontal lobe tests in the diagnosis of attention deficits hyperactivity disorder. Clin Neuropsychol 13:12–21, 1999.

Hauser P, Zametkin AJ, Martinez P, et al: Attention-deficit-hyperactivity disorder in people with generalized resistance to thyroid hormone. N Engl J Med 328:997–1001, 1993.

Hinshaw SP: Stimulant medication and the treatment of aggression in children with attentional deficits. J Clin Child Psychol 20:301–312, 1991.

Hunt RD, Paguin A, Payton K: An update on assessment and treatment of complex attention-deficit hyperactivity disorder. Pediatr Ann 30:162–172, 2001.

Hynd GW, Semrud-Clikeman M, Lorys AR, et al: Corpus callosum morphology in attention deficit-hyperactivity disorder: Morphometric analysis of MRI. J Learn Disabil 24:141–145, 1991.

Jensen PS, Martin D, Cantwell DP: Comorbidity in ADHD: Implications for research, practice and DSM-V. J Am Acad Child Adolesc Psychiatry 36:1065–1079, 1997.

Johnston JA, Lineberry CG, Ascher JA, et al: A 102-center prospective study of seizures in association with bupropion. J Clin Psychiatry 52:450–456, 1991.

Kohn A: Suffer the restless children. The Atlantic Monthly, 1989, pp. 90–100.

Lahey BB, Applegate B, McBurnett K, et al: DSM-IV field trials for attention deficit/hyperactivity disorder in children and adolescents. J Am Acad Child Adolesc Psychiatry 27:330–325, 1994.

LaHoste GJ, Swanson JM, Wigal SB, et al: Dopamine D4 receptor gene polymorphism is associated with attention deficit hyperactivity disorder. Mol Psychiatry 1:121–124, 1996.

Levine MD: Attention deficit, the diverse effects of weak control systems in childhood. Pediatr Ann 16:117–131, 1987.

Logan GD: On the ability to inhibit thought and action: A user's guide to the stop signal paradigm, in Dagenbach D, Carr TH (eds): Inhibitory Processes in Attention, Memory, and Language. San Diego, CA: Academic Press, 1994, pp. 208–215.

Lou HC, Henriksen L, Bruhn P: Focal cerebral hypoperfusion in children with dysphasia and/or attention deficit disorder. Arch Neurol 41:825–829, 1984.

Mannuzza S, Klein RG, Bessler A, et al: Adult outcome of hyperactive boys: Educational achievement, occupational rank, and psychiatric status. Arch Gen Psychiatry 50:565–576, 1993.

Pelham WE, Gnagy EM, Chronis AM, et al: A comparison of morning-only and morning/late afternoon adderall to morning-only, twice daily, and three time-daily methylphenidate in children with attention-deficit/hyperactivity disorder. Pediatrics 104:1300–1321, 1999.

Pelham WE, Wheeler T, Chronis A. Empirically supported psychosocial treatments for attention deficit hyperactivity disorder. J Clin Child Psychol 27:190–205, 1998.

Pennington BF, Ozonoff S: Executive functions and developmental psychopathology. J Child Psychol Psychiatry 37:51–87, 1996.

Popper CW: Antidepressants in the treatment of attention-deficit/hyperactivity disorder. J Clin Psychiatry 58(suppl 14):14–29, 1997.

Price RA, Leckman JF, Pauls DL, et al: Gilles de la Tourette's syndrome: Tics and central nervous system stimulants in twins and nontwins. Neurology 36:232–237, 1986.

Rubia K, Overmeyer S, Taylor E, et al: Inhibitory control of hyperactive adolescents, using fMRI, in Toga AW, Frackowiak RSJ, Mazziotta JC (eds): Neuroimage, Third International Conference on Functional Mapping of the Human Brain. New York: Academic Press, 1997, A157.

Schachar R, Tannock R. Logan G: Inhibitory control, impulsiveness, and attention deficit hyperactivity disorder. Clin Psychol Rev 13:721–739, 1993.

Silberberg N, Silberberg M: Myths in remedial education. J Learn Disabil 2:158–272, 1969.

Spencer R, Biederman J, Wilens T, et al: Pharmacotherapy of attention-deficit hyperactivity disorder across the life cycle. J Am Acad Child Adolesc Psychiatry 35:409–432, 1996.

Stevenson J: Evidence for a genetic etiology in hyperactivity in children. Behav Genet 22:337–344, 1992.

Still GF: Some abnormal psychical conditions in children. Lancet 1:1008–1012, 1077–1082, 1163–1168, 1902.

Sunohara G, Barr C, Jain U, et al: Association of the D4 receptor gene in individuals with ADHD: 1. A family-based control study of children with ADHD: 2. A case-control study of adults with ADHD. Am J Hum Genet 61(suppl):A296, 1997.

Swanson JM: SNAP-IV Scale. University of California Child Development Center, Irvine, 1995.

Swanson JL, Gupta S, Guinta D, et al: Acute tolerance to methylphenidate in the treatment of attention deficit hyperactivity disorder in children. Clin Pharmacol Ther 66:295–305, 1999.

Swanson JM, McBurnett K, Wigal T, et al. Effect of stimulant mediation on children with attention deficit disorder: A "review of reviews." Except Child 60:154–162, 1993.

Tannock R: Attention deficit hyperactivity disorder: Advances in cognitive, neurobiological, and genetic research. J Child Psychol Psychiatry 39:65–99, 1998.

Teicher MH, Anderson CM, Polcari A, et al: Functional deficits in basal ganglia of children with attention-deficit/hyperactivity disorder shown with functional magnetic resonance imaging relaxometry. Nat Med 6:470–473, 2000.

Vaidya CJ, Austin G, Kirkorian G, et al: Selective effects of methylphenidate in attention deficit hyperactivity disorder: A functional magnetic resonance study. Proc Natl Acad Sci U S A 95:14494–14499, 1998.

Waldman ID, Rowe DC, Abrmowitz A, et al: Association of the dopamine transporter gene (DAT1) and attention deficit hyperactivity disorder in children. Am J Hum Genet Suppl 59:A25.

Ward MF, Wender PH, Reimherr FW: The Wender Utah rating scale: An aid in the retrospective diagnosis of childhood attention deficit hyperactivity disorder. Am J Psychiatry 150:885–890, 1993.

Weiss R, Stein M, Trommer B, et al: Attention-deficit hyperactivity disorder and thyroid function. J Pediatr 123:539–545, 1993.

Wolraich ML, Hanah JN, Pinnock TY, et al: Comparison of diagnostic criteria for attention-deficit hyperactivity disorder in a country-wide sample. J Am Acad Child Adolesc Psychiat 35:319–324, 1996.

Zametkin AJ, Ernst M: Problems in the management of attention-deficit hyperactivity disorder. N Eng J Med 340:40–46, 1999.

Zametkin AJ, Liebnauer LL, Fitzgerald GA, et al: Brain metabolism in teenagers with attention-deficit hyperactivity disorder. Arch Gen Psychiat 50:333–340, 1993.

Zametkin AJ, Nordahl TE, Gross M, et al: Cerebral glucose metabolism in adults with hyperactivity of childhood onset. N Eng J Med 323:1361–1366, 1990.

The Autistic Spectrum Disorders: Disorders of Communication, Sociability, and Range of Interests and Behaviors

Ruth Nass

Fern Leventhal

Cerebral Substrate

Treatment

DISORDERS OF VERBAL AND NONVERBAL COMMUNICATION: SEMANTIC-PRAGMATIC LANGUAGE SYNDROME

Cerebral Substrate

Treatment

SUMMARY AND CONCLUSIONS

Anxiety

Asperger syndrome

Autistic spectrum disorder

Obsessive-compulsive disorder

Tourette syndrome

INTRODUCTION

Robert, aged 4 years, is referred for a multidisciplinary evaluation because of concerns about his failure to develop normal language and display appropriate social behavior. Robert is seen by a pediatric neurologist, a pediatric psychologist, a pediatric psychiatrist, and a speech therapist. At the case conference, the pediatric neurologist proposes that the child has a developmental language disorder based on his poor comprehension and his abnormal expressive language in the context of normal hearing and good nonverbal abilities like copying and doing jigsaw puzzles. He notes that the family history is positive for obsessive-compulsive disorder in the maternal aunt. In addition, the neurologic examination reveals motor and vocal tics ongoing by history for over a year. Therefore the pediatric neurologist diagnoses Tourette syndrome as well. The psychologist, however, thinks that the child is autistic because along with his language problem, his social behavior is poorly developed. He does not play well with other children and lacks warmth in his relationship with his parents. In addition, the child has great difficulty with transitions and engages in repetitive activities with his toys. The psychiatrist argues that the child's social and language abnormalities are not severe enough to warrant a diagnosis of autism. The child does initiate communication with others, makes eye contact, and enjoys rough and tumble play. His social forays tend to be rejected by other children because he wants them to participate in the activities that interest him, while he is insensitive to their needs. Robert can produce long and complicated sentences, but his responses to

questions are often inappropriate. He often asks questions of others, but just as frequently disregards their answers. The psychiatrist suggests a diagnosis of Asperger syndrome. The speech therapist states that an analysis of Robert's language shows that it is phonologically and grammatically normal, but that there are many abnormalities in the way in which language is used, and that comprehension in conversational contexts is poor. She suggests that this is a case of semantic-pragmatic language disorder. The psychologist responds that semantic-pragmatic language disorder is just another name for autism. The visiting professor of psychiatry (who was on the DSM-IV field trial committee) to whom the case is presented diagnoses pervasive developmental disorder not otherwise specified, because the child does not meet criteria for a diagnosis of autism or Asperger syndrome (Bishop, 1989).

The diagnostic dilemmas presented in this clinical vignette are familiar to clinicians and researchers, and raise questions regarding diagnostic criteria common to several related conditions as well as professional perspectives. Public interest in these conditions is rising; the numbers of children diagnosed with these syndromes seem also to be increasing (Gross, 2003). Clarification of ambiguous terminology, diagnostic criteria, and the interrelationship of symptoms is critical to accurate clinical decision making and the formulation of empirical research that addresses natural history, etiology, and treatment approaches.

The aims of this chapter are to describe and summarize the autistic spectrum disorders (ASD). This relatively new term is meant to encompass autism, high functioning autism (HFA), Asperger syndrome (AS), pervasive developmental disorder not otherwise specified (PDD-NOS), and disorders that overlap with one or more of the three cardinal features of the ASD. These include communication impairment (the semantic-pragmatic developmental language disorder); sociability impairment (social anxiety/phobic disorder); and repetitive or restricted range of activities, behaviors, and interests (obsessive-compulsive disorder [OCD], Tourette syndrome [TS]) (Fig. 43-1).

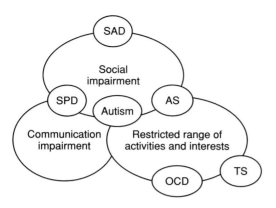

FIGURE 43-1. The relative involvement of language, social skills, and restricted range of behaviors for the several disorders abutting the autistic spectrum are indicated. OCD, obsessive-compulsive disorder; SPD, semantic-pragmatic disorder; SAD, social anxiety disorder; AS, Asperger syndrome; TS, Tourette syndrome.

AUTISTIC SPECTRUM DISORDERS

Definition and Epidemiology

The triad of early-onset symptoms that defines ASD (Rapin, 1997) includes:

1. Impaired verbal and nonverbal communication
2. Impaired sociability
3. A restricted range of activities, behaviors, and interests

Mental retardation is a comorbid feature in about three quarters of ASD children (Fig. 43-2). In the remaining portion, intellect can range from borderline to superior.

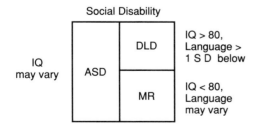

FIGURE 43-2. This diagram shows the distinction between ASD and the developmental language disorders based on the presence or absence of social difficulties. Mental retardation may or may not be present. ASD, autistic spectrum disorders; DLD, developmental language disorders; MR, mental retardation; SD, standard deviation. (Reproduced with permission from Nass R, Ross G: Disorders of Higher Cortical Function in the Preschooler, in David R (ed): Child and Adolescent Neurology. St. Louis: Mosby, 1997.)

The prevalence of ASD is approximately 1 per 2000. The reported prevalence of AS ranges from 1 to as high as 7 per 1000, depending on sampling procedures and diagnostic criteria (Tanguay, 2000; Gillberg, 1998, 2002; Fombonne & Tidmarsh, 2003). It is unclear whether the prevalence of these neurodevelopmental disorders is increasing (Wing & Potter, 2002). A genetic basis is the suspected underlying etiology in many cases. This is supported by data indicating a high concordance of ASD in monozygotic twins, increased risk for recurrence in siblings (4.5%), presence of the so-called "broader autistic phenotype" in families of ASD probands, and the association with a number of single gene disorders such as fragile X syndrome (Cook, 1998; Murphy et al., 2000; Veenstra-Vanderweele et al., 2003).

Clinical Features: The Autistic Spectrum Disorder Triad

Impairment of Verbal and Nonverbal Communication

Language impairment is a cardinal feature of ASD, and degree generally parallels IQ. Low functioning children with ASD tend to have limited comprehension, sometimes to the point of verbal auditory agnosia (see Chapter 13 on the Auditory System and Chapter 17 on Aphasia). Their expressive language is comprised of repetitive, stereotyped phrases, with prominent echolalia. Higher functioning ASD children often talk too much. They talk just to talk, rather than to communicate. They also tend to process language in very literal terms and exhibit weak verbal abstract skills. Hence, these children demonstrate many pragmatic language impairments. For example, they have trouble finding humor in a situation, using appropriate greeting behavior, turn-taking in conversation, and using informal or colloquial speech. Speech can be mechanical, excessively rapid, monotonic, high-pitched, or poorly modulated. Symbolic play, an important form of social communication among children, is either delayed, limited, repetitive, or odd.

Social Impairment

Severity of social dysfunction in ASD children also tends to parallel their general intellectual level. Lower functioning children are often interpersonally aloof and detached even from their parents. For example, they rarely run to greet their parents or seek comfort from them when in pain. Their interest in objects exceeds their interest in people. ASD children with prominent social impairment are most like the traditional notion of the autistic child. Higher functioning ASD children may be more passive than detached. Most do not make social approaches, but accept them when made by others. They engage in some pretend play and join in games, but usually take a passive role. Some children are socially interactive but initiate peculiar social approaches toward others. They tend to talk *at* other people and their persistence may be very annoying. Impairments in empathy, theory of mind, and pragmatic social skills significantly limit the range and variety of their social relationships (Waterhouse et al., 1996). Though classified clinically as social impairments, this domain of symptoms also encompasses underlying emotion-processing deficits that will be important to clearly elucidate.

Restricted Range of Behaviors, Interests, and Activities

The restricted range of behaviors, interests, and activities in lower functioning ASD children consists mainly of repetitive, stereotyped behaviors such as twirling, rocking, flapping, toe walking, banging, and licking. More complex routines can include turning water on and off or opening and closing doors (Krug et al., 1993). Repetitive aggressive and self-injurious behaviors are also frequent. Symptomatic overlap with tic disorders and OCD can be observed in higher functioning ASD children. A small subgroup of ASD individuals demonstrate exceptional and all-consuming artistic talents, and may meet criteria for AS. Others grow up to be single-minded, peculiar, and socially inept, but otherwise independent and successful adults who may be chess players or mathematicians.

Theory and Classification

Critical Features: Deficient Theory of Mind

Some investigators suggest that the critical feature of ASD is the inability to "mind read" (Baron-Cohen et al., 1993). That is, ASD children do not develop "theory of mind" capabilities that allow them to understand how others think and feel. As indicated in Table 43-1, "mind reading" shows a developmental progression. The earliest signs in infancy center around conjoint attention. For example, a child learns to look at and attend to what someone else is focusing on and thereby joins in the experience. Through regular social interactions, toddlers come to understand what other people are thinking and that it can be different from what they are thinking. Thus, they develop understanding of pretending, false beliefs, and deception (i.e., first-order beliefs). Through neurocognitive and social-emotional maturation, older children learn to distinguish what one person thinks about what another person is saying or thinking in specific circumstances (i.e., second-order beliefs). They can recognize a faux pas, deception, and subtle interpersonal conflicts between others. This kind of knowledge becomes more complex when factored into diverse social situations, varying intentions of others, and the range of relationships shared with others. The ability to "mind

TABLE 43-1. Stages of Development of A Theory of Mind

18 months	Joint attention: adult and child look at the toy together
	Protodeclarative pointing: child calls adult's attention to object he wants
18–24 months	Symbolic play
2 years	Understanding desire "I want a hamburger."
3–4 years	First-order TOM: knowing what another person is thinking
	First-Order False Belief Measure:
	Sam wants to find his puppy. Sam's puppy is really in the kitchen. Sam thinks his puppy is in the bathroom. Where will Sam look for the puppy?
	Where is it really?
	Autistic children cannot anticipate that another child in the same situation would make the same mistake.
6–7 yrs	Second-order TOM: knowing what another person thinks another person is thinking; belief about beliefs
	Second-Order false belief Measures: jokes, lies (one person's knowledge about another person's knowledge, what he knows or doesn't know)
9–11 yrs	Second-order False Belief—faux pas
	Someone says something they should not have said not knowing that they should not have said it
	Mike was in one of the bathroom stalls. Joe and Peter were talking at the sink. Joe said "you know that new boy Mike, isn't he weird?" Mike came out of the stall. Peter said "Oh hello Mike, are you going to play football now?"
	Where were Joe and Peter when they were talking?
	Did Joe know that Mike was in the bathroom stall?

TOM, theory of mind.

read" also provides an important basis for development of empathy or sharing in the personal experiences of others. These cognitive and emotion-based processes have been linked to maturation of executive functions, metacognition, and social cognition.

Criteria for Distinguishing Autism, High Functioning Autism, Asperger Syndrome, and Pervasive Developmental Disorder Not Otherwise Specified

Autism

Current debate centers on whether the ASD represent several different disorders or a spectrum of severity within a single disorder. The criteria for diagnosis of autistic disorder is delineated in the Diagnostic and Statistical Manual-Fourth Edition (DSM-IV) (APA, 1994), the gold standard for diagnosis based on the consensus of a panel of experts, primarily psychiatrists. It is viewed as distinct from other pervasive developmental disorders, such as AS and PDD-NOS. Diagnosis of autistic disorder requires impairments in the following three areas: (1) verbal and nonverbal communication, (2) social interaction, and (3) restricted range of behaviors, interests, and activities (Table 43-2 shows criteria). No specific criteria for differentiating HFA from autistic disorder are included in the DSM-IV. According to the DSM-IV, when a child fails to meet all three criteria for autism, a diagnosis of PDD-NOS can be made. Children with AS typically demonstrate impaired social interaction and restricted range of behavior and interests but comparatively normal language development. Hence, they do not meet the DSM-IV criteria for a diagnosis of autism.

High Functioning Autism

Many clinicians and investigators will diagnose HFA if a child with an ASD has an IQ of 70 or greater. Others will diagnose HFA if the child's autistic features are mild (Schopler & Mesibov, 1997). Adding to the confusion, diagnoses of HFA and AS are sometimes made in the same individual at different stages of development.

Asperger Syndrome

More than 50 years ago Hans Asperger, a Viennese pediatrician, reported on a group of children with fluent language but poor conversational skills, marked difficulties in reciprocal social interaction, and unusual and intense interests that interfered with normal development (Table 43-3 shows a summary of criteria for AS). The nosology of AS is still debated today (e.g., Klin et al., 2000; Gillberg, 2002). The frequency of developmental coordination disorders in AS is controversial and requires further empirical research on comorbidity and natural history. Another area of debate concerns the diagnostic criterion of normal language development required by the DSM-IV. Children

---

TABLE 43-2. Criteria for Diagnosis of Autism (Modified from DSM-IV; American Psychiatric Association, 1994)

Six items or more from 1, 2, and 3, with at least 2 from 1, and one each from 2 and 3.

1. Impairment in social interaction
   a. Impaired use of nonverbal behaviors (eye gaze, facial expression)
   b. Poor peer relationships
   c. Impaired sharing of enjoyment, interests, or achievements with others
   d. Lack or social or emotional reciprocity
2. Impaired communication
   a. Delayed language
   b. Impaired ability to sustain conversation
   c. Repetitive or idiosyncratic language
   d. Impaired pretend play
3. Restricted range of behaviors or interests
   a. Encompassing preoccupation
   b. Inflexible adherence to routines
   c. Stereotyped motor mannerisms
   d. Preoccupation with parts of objects
4. Onset prior to age 3 years

TABLE 43-3. Asperger Syndrome Diagnostic Criteria (Modified from DSM-IV; American Psychiatric Association, 1994)

A. Qualitative impairment in social interaction, manifested by at least two of the following:
   1. Impairment in use of nonverbal behaviors to regulate social interaction
   2. Failure to develop peer relationships
   3. Lack of spontaneous seeking to share enjoyments and interests
   4. Lack of social or emotional reciprocity
B. Restricted range of repetitive and stereotyped behaviors, interests and activities, manifested by at least one of the following:
   1. Encompassing preoccupation
   2. Inflexible adherence to non functional routines
   3. Stereotyped and repetitive motor mannerisms
   4. Persistent preoccupation with parts of objects
C. Disturbance causes significant impairment in functioning
D. No clinically significant language delay
E. No clinically significant cognitive deficit
F. Criteria not met for another pervasive developmental disorder diagnosis or schizophrenia

diagnosed with AS cannot have obvious developmental delays in language acquisition. They may even have exceptional vocabulary skills and overly formal pseudosophisticated language. However, children with AS appear to be overly focused on language details, pedantic rules, and semantics (Willey, 1999; Klin et al., 2000). They exhibit impairments in paralinguistic skills such as abstraction, metaphor, discourse, and pragmatics. Ghaziuddin and Gerstein (1996) reported that pedantic use of language was the key feature that discriminated AS from HFA.

The relationship between HFA and AS continues to be evaluated (e.g., Schopler & Mesibov, 1997; Gillberg, 1998; Gillberg & Ehlers, 1998; Klin et al., 2000). Some experts view AS as the highest form of HFA, while others consider it a separate disorder that shares features with the nonverbal learning disabilities (NVLD) (Rourke, 1995; Rourke & Tsatsanis, 2000), as well as with autism. Neuropsychological processes associated with the right hemisphere are commonly impaired in AS and NLVD (Klin et al., 2000). Verbal linguistic skills are superior to visuospatial, nonverbal, and visual-motor skills. Verbal IQ is higher than performance IQ. Communication skills associated with the right hemisphere, such as pragmatics, prosody, narrative, humor, and inference are particularly impaired in AS.

Children diagnosed with NVLD have been reported to show combinations of the following symptoms:

- Emotional and interpersonal difficulties
- Difficulty interpreting the behavior of others (impaired theory of mind)
- Paralinguistic communication problems involving prosody and/or pragmatics
- Impaired visuoperceptual, visuospatial organization, and visuomotor skills
- Visuospatial working memory dysfunction
- Marked slowness of performance
- Tactile perceptual dysfunction
- Both gross and fine motor skill disorders, including dysgraphia and dyspraxia
- Problems with reading comprehension, written expression, and dyscalculia
- Attention-deficit/hyperactivity disorder (ADHD)
- Mood and anxiety disorders
- Executive function impairments in nonverbal problem solving, concept formation, and hypothesis testing; and difficulty in adapting to novel or complex situations

In contrast, NVLD children demonstrate certain very well–developed verbal processing capacities, including extremely well–developed rote verbal memory skills and strong reading decoding skills.

When one steps back to evaluate these many characteristics and clinical symptoms, areas of potential overlap among NVLD, ASD, and AS become clearer. Klin and colleagues (1995) specifically compared children with AS versus children with NVLD. They reported a robust overlap between their neuropsychological profiles, suggesting that from a clinical viewpoint, the groups can appear quite similar. Both NVLD and AS children generate higher verbal and poorer performance IQ scores than children with HFA (Klin et al., 1995; Ehlers et al., 1997). On the other hand, many HFA subjects have lower verbal IQ than performance IQ scores because of their linguistic problems. Even when HFA subjects do not have a clear pattern of performance higher than verbal IQ scores, their comprehension subtest tends to be lower than the block design subtest score (Siegel et al., 1996).

A number of studies emphasize cognitive differences between AS and HFA. Compared with children with ASD (including HFA), children with AS perform adequately or display only mild deficiencies only on theory of mind tasks (Buitelaar, van der Wees, et al., 1999; Baron-Cohen et al., 1997, 1999a). They are somewhat more self-aware, and this awareness is occasionally associated with depression. Some clinicians separate AS from HFA based on earlier language onset and higher verbal mental age in AS (Eisenmajer et al., 1996; Landa, 2000). They also use certain characteristics from language, social, and range of interests domains as well as the Autism Diagnostic Interview-Revised (ADI-R), the Autism Diagnostic Observation Schedule (ADOS), and IQ scores to differentiate AS from HFA (Table 43-4 shows summary of criteria) (Lord & Risi, 1998).

Although motor coordination problems are still viewed by some as critical to the diagnosis of AS, few studies find that motor impairments or clumsiness specifically distinguish AS (Ghaziuddin & Butler, 1998). No major difference between AS and HFA groups was found on a projective test (Rorschach), although AS subjects demonstrated a trend toward greater levels of

TABLE 43-4. Clinical Variables That Distinguish High Functioning Autism Asperger Syndrome

Demonstrate desire for friendship (despite poor grasp of the concept of friendship)
Are more willing/able to join in play with others
Engage with one other who has same circumscribed interest
Exhibit long-winded pedantic speech
Ask repetitive questions/talk on repetitive themes
Collect facts on specific subjects

(Data from Eisenmajer R, Prior M, Leekam S, et al: Comparison of clinical symptoms in autism and Asperger's Syndrome. Child Adolesc Psychiatry 35:1523–1531, 1996)

disorganized thinking compared with the HFA group. AS children are also more likely to be classified as "introversive." This may allude to the clinical perception that AS subjects experience more complex inner lives involving elaborate fantasies and are more focused on their internal experiences (Ghaziuddin et al., 1995).

Pervasive Developmental Disorder Not Otherwise Specified

The nature of PDD-NOS, as well as its relation to the ASD, is also controversial. PDD-NOS is generally diagnosed in a child with social and communication difficulties who fails to meet full DSM-IV diagnostic criteria for autism (Table 43-5). However, Buitelaar and colleagues (1999a) reported that one third of children clinically diagnosed with PDD-NOS also met DSM or ICD criteria for autism. Two DSM-IV items were particularly sensitive and specific in characterizing autism in comparison with PDD-NOS: lack of make-believe play and preoccupation with restricted patterns of interest. Ninety percent of those diagnosed with autism had problems with social interactions, 70% had problems with communication, and 60% had symptoms in the interests and activities domain. Only three items had a sensitivity of greater than 0.6 for PDD-NOS:

- Lack of reciprocity
- Failure to develop peer relations
- Impairment in conversation

Symptoms in the activities and interests domain were infrequently endorsed in the children clinically diagnosed with PDD-NOS, which may help differentiate it from AS.

PDD-NOS appears to be more heterogenous than DSM-IV autistic disorder. PDD-NOS may be a variant of ASD with social interaction impairments as the crucial variable. The prototypic PDD-NOS child has early onset social interaction problems or communication delay. Thereafter, the child continues to have problems with peer relationships. Alternatively, PDD-NOS children may share social and communication problems with ASD children, but have additional impairments in other areas (anxiety, thought disorder, aggressivity) as a distinguishing feature (Buitelaar et al., 1999b).

Further empirical research in natural history, functional brain imaging, and cognitive-behavioral parameters should help eventually delineate the most reliable characteristics that distinguish among autism, HFA, AS, and PDD-NOS.

Evaluation of the Child with Autistic Spectrum Disorders

Neurologic and Neuropsychological Evaluation and Diagnosis

A detailed developmental and psychosocial history is essential for the accurate diagnosis of ASD. Reports from parents, teachers, and other caretakers are important in establishing reliable behavioral data because children's behavior may vary considerably in different settings. Direct observation of the child in the clinic as well as in his or her familiar environment is also informative. Although the behavior of lower functioning autistic children will not differ much, HFA and AS children may behave quite differently when in structured versus unstructured settings and when they are alone versus within a group of children.

If the diagnosis remains uncertain or degree of severity needs to be determined, a number of different assessment tools are available for use by specialists in pediatric neurology, behavioral pediatrics, psychiatry, and psychology (Lord & Risi, 1998) (Table 43-6 shows a summary of clinical instruments). In general these diagnostic instruments cover the same ground as the DSM-IV, although psychiatrists and psychologists tend to put more emphasis on the DSM criteria for diagnosis than do pediatric neurologists and developmental pediatricians.

Behavioral checklists and questionnaires completed by parents are quite helpful, especially when the child is not cooperative with teachers (Gilliam, 2001a,b). Some are particularly useful for teasing apart the effects of IQ variations versus autistic features (Krug et al., 1993) (Fig. 43-3).

In addition, measures based on parent interview such as the Vineland Adaptive Behavior Scales (Sparrow et al., 1984) can be administered to specifically assess a child's ability to cope with the activities of daily living. New questionnaires have become available, such as the Autism Spectrum Screening Questionnaire (ASSQ) (Table 43-7), that focus on the

---

TABLE 43-5. Diagnostic Criteria for PDD-NOS (Modified from DSM-IV; American Psychiatric Association, 1994)

Severe and pervasive impairment in the development of reciprocal social interaction, or severe and pervasive impairment in verbal and nonverbal communication skills, or when stereotyped behavior, interests, and activities are present, but the criteria are not met for a specific pervasive development disorder, schizophrenia, schizotypal personality disorder, or avoidant personality disorder.

For example, this category includes "atypical autism"—presentations that do not meet the criteria for autistic disorder because of late age at onset, atypical symptomatology, or subthreshold symptomatology, or all of these.

TABLE 43-6. Clinical Instruments for the Diagnosis of Autistic Spectrum Disorders

Measure	Special features
Checklist for Autism in Toddlers (CHAT) (Charman et al., 2002)	Screening measure; administered in the office; intended for early diagnosis at 18–36 months.
Chilhood Autism Rating Scale (CARS) (Schopler et al., 1988)	Combines parent report and direct observation; useful for clinicians in the office; provides a measure of severity, but may be less helpful with milder forms of ASD.
Autism Behavior Checklist (ABC) (Krug et al., 1993)	Questionnaire completed by parent or teacher; intended for children above age 3 years; more useful for low functioning children, distinguishing them from MR children; breaks deficits down into five categories, see Figure 43-3.
Vineland Adaptive Behavior Scales (Sparrow et al., 1984)	Primarily for low functioning children; scores based on parent interviews; provides separate scales for communication, socialization, daily living skills, and motor skills (Szatmari et al., 2002).
Gilliam Autism Rating Scale (Gilliam, 2001b)	Completed by parents of low functioning children; good screening tool for office use; derived from the DSM.
Autism Screening Questionnaire (Berument et al., 1999)	Questionnaire for caregiver validated against ADI, useful for both verbal and nonverbal patients.
Gilliam Asperger Disorder Scale (Gilliam, 2001a)	Completed by parents of high functioning children; good screening tool for office use.
Children's Social Behavior Questionnaire (Luteijn et al., 2000)	Questionnaire for caregiver of higher functioning children. 5 factors: acting out, social contact problems, social insight problems, anxious/rigid, stereotypical.
Asperger Syndrome Screening Questionnaire (ASSQ) (Ehlers et al., 1999)	Checklist completed by parent or teacher; intended for children or adolescents with normal IQ or mild mental retardation; oriented toward higher functioning autistic spectrum disorders.
Diagnostic Interview for Social and Communication Disorders (DISCO) (Leekam et al., 2002)	This is a structured interview coordinated with the ICD 9 diagnosis of PDD. It Is appropriate throughout childhood and at all levels of function. Assesses for broader autistic phenotype.
Child Behavior Checklist (Achenbach & Rescorla, 2001)	A commonly used behavior checklist with parent and teacher versions as well as a youth self-report for 11–18 year olds. Although not designed to diagnose autistic spectrum disorders, ASD children score high on the scales measuring attention problems, social problems, and thought problems and low on the scale for somatic complaints (Boelte et al., 1999; Luteijin, et al., 2000b).
Autism Diagnostic Interview Revised (ADI-R) (Lord & Risi, 1998)	Semistructured parent interview that is used primarily for children 3–5 years of age; in-depth assessment administered by trained professional.
Autism Diagnostic Observation Scale (ADOS) (Lord & Risi, 1998)	In-depth, standardized assessment instrument to be administered by trained professional; primarily a research tool, but can also be used clinically to diagnosis and evaluate social, communicative, and play behaviors in verbal and nonverbal children, adolescents, and adults.

ADI, Autism Diagnostic Interview; ASD, Autistic spectrum disorder; MR, mental retardation; PDD, pervasive developmental disorder.

more subtle characteristics required for the diagnosis of AS (Attwood, 1998; Ehlers et al., 1999). Some questionnaires for older high functioning individuals evaluate responses to questions about the acceptability of social behaviors (e.g., Dewey, 1991) (Table 43-8).

Neuropsychological assessment can be extremely important, not only to confirm diagnosis, but also to explore the child's specific strengths and weaknesses so that appropriate treatment and school planning can take place. Due to behavioral difficulties, some severely impaired autistic children can be difficult to assess in the standard manner. Less behaviorally disruptive and higher functioning autistic children and adolescents will have little trouble cooperating with structured, formal testing. Assessment typically includes measures of general intellectual functioning, attention, learning and memory, gross and fine motor skills, visuospatial abilities, language skills, problem solving and executive functioning, and academic achievement levels. AS and HFA youngsters generally possess good semantic and grammatical language skills, but pragmatic aspects of language pose a problem. Traditional receptive and

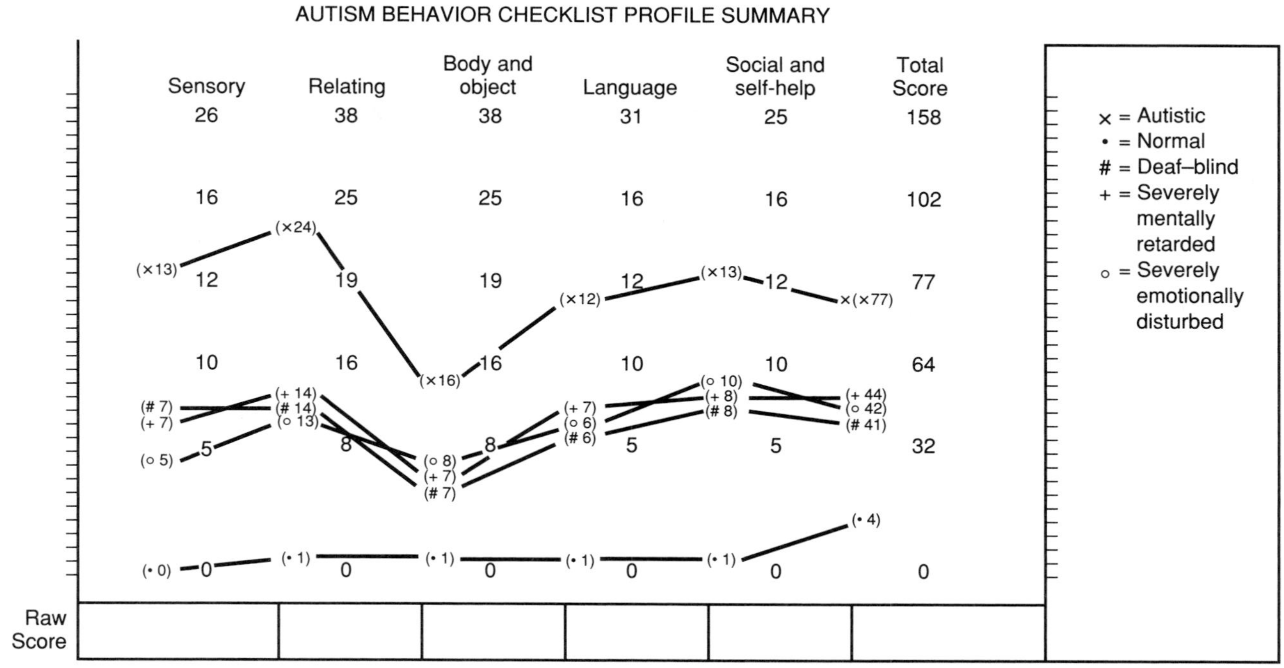

AUTISM BEHAVIOR CHECKLIST PROFILE SUMMARY

Sensory	Relating	Body and object	Language	Social and self-help	Total Score	
26	38	38	31	25	158	x = Autistic
16	25	25	16	16	102	• = Normal
(×13) 12	(×24) 19	19	(×12) 12 (×13) 12	12 x (×77)	77	# = Deaf–blind + = Severely mentally retarded
10 (# 7) (+ 7) (○ 5) 5	16 (+ 14) (# 14) (○ 13) 8	(×16) 16 (○ 8) (+ 7) (# 7) 8	10 (+ 7) (○ 6) (# 6) 5	10 (○ 10) (+ 8) (# 8) 5	64 (+ 44) (○ 42) (# 41) 32	○ = Severely emotionally disturbed
(• 0) 0	(• 1) 0	(• 1) 0	(• 1) 0	(• 1) 0 (• 4)	0	

Raw Score

FIGURE 43-3. The Autism Behavior Checklist allows the clinician to distinguish mental retardation from the autistic spectrum disorders and to look at specific areas of function for strengths and weaknesses. (Reproduced with permission from Krug D, Arisk J, Almond P: Autism Screening Instrument for Educational Planning. Austin, TX: Pro-Ed).

expressive language assessment tends to miss these communication deficits. Therefore, it is helpful to employ standardized measures of pragmatic language and pragmatic language checklists.

Medical Evaluation

Neurologic examination in ASD children is generally normal. The skin should be carefully examined because the neurocutaneous disorder, tuberous sclerosis, is among the most common definable causes of autism. Hearing impairment should be excluded by formal audiologic assessment. Epilepsy occurs in up to one third of patients with autism by early adulthood. A standard electroencephalogram (EEG), overnight video-EEG monitoring, and even magnetoencephalography (MEG) may help identify subclinical seizures, especially when language comprehension is very impaired or a regression has occurred (Tuchman, 1997; Lewine et al., 1999). Brain imaging is not usually clinically remarkable, although a number of research studies have suggested a variety of subtle abnormalities. Further metabolic and genetic work-up depends on clinical suspicions.

Natural History and Outcome

The natural history of ASD is highly variable, as would be expected. About one third of autistic children regress between the ages of 1 and 3 years and are at highest risk for poor outcome. Scholastic success is best predicted by overall intelligence level and by language facility. Some autistic toddlers and preschoolers improve greatly by school age, but may still seem socially odd and have peculiarities of language prosody and pragmatics. Many of these children have tics. ASD can evolve into prominent symptoms of NVLD, ADHD, and OCD in the middle school years. Long-term outcome studies suggest that about one third of ASD children improve and one third deteriorate during adolescence (Table 43-9). Onset of seizures or mood disorders, especially depression, can underlie adolescent decline and should be evaluated carefully. About two thirds of ASD adults have limited independence and almost one half require institutionalized care. Adult outcomes are fair to good in 15% to 30%, but only about 5% become competitively employed, lead independent lives, marry, and raise families. Psychiatric problems are common even in this group. Some adults, including family members who share phenotypic characteristics of an autistic proband, may go undiagnosed in childhood and adolescence, and function in the mainstream (Nass, 1998a). This is exemplified by the broader autistic phenotype seen in families of an autistic proband (Piven, 2001).

The natural history of AS is less clear. Because early language development is normal, the diagnosis is often delayed until elementary school age,

TABLE 43-7. Screening Questionnaire for Aspergers Syndrome and Other High Functioning Autistic Spectrum Disorders (ASSQ)

- Is old-fashioned and precocious
- Is regarded as an eccentric professor by other children
- Lives somewhat in a world of his own with restricted idiosyncratic intellectual interests
- Accumulates facts on certain subjects (good rote memory) but does not really understand the meaning
- Has a literal understanding of ambiguous and metaphorical language*
- Has a deviant style of communication with a formal fussy old-fashioned or robotic language*
- Invents idiosyncratic words and expression*
- Has a different speech or voice*
- Expresses sounds involuntarily, clears throat, grunts
- Is surprisingly good at some things and poor at others
- Uses language freely but fails to make adjustments to fit social contexts or the needs of different listeners*
- Lacks empathy
- Makes naive or embarrassing remarks*
- Has a deviant style of gaze
- Wishes to be sociable but fails to make relationships with peers
- Can be with other children but only on his own terms
- Lacks best friend
- Lacks common sense
- Is poor at games, has no idea of cooperating in a team "scores own goals"
- Has clumsy ill coordinated ungainly awkward movements or gestures
- Has involuntary facial or body movements
- Has difficulties completing simple daily activities because of compulsory repetition of certain thought or ideas
- Has special routines insists on no change
- Shows idiosyncratic attachment to objects
- Is bullied by other children
- Has markedly unusual facial expression
- Has markedly unusual posture

Each item is scored 0, 1, or 2. The goal of the questionnaire is to distinguish Asperger Syndrome (AS) from other psychiatric disorders. In a control cohort a parent score of 19 produced a 62% true positive rate and a 10% false positive rate relative to traditionally diagnosed AS. A teacher score of 22 resulted in a 70% true positive rate and a 9% false positive rate. When the ASSQ scores were used for validation of an AS sample a parent score of 19 yielded 82% true positives and a teacher score of 22 yielded 65% true positives.

* Items in Table 7 are examples of language prosody and pragmatics.

(Reprinted with permission from Ehlers S, Gillberg C, Wing L: A screening questionnaire for Aspergers syndrome and other high-functioning autism spectrum disorders in school age children. J Autism Dev Dis 29:129–141, 1999.)

TABLE 43-8. Adult Understanding of Typical and Atypical Behaviors

In the following stories some parts are _underlined and in italics_. Immediately following there is a pair of brackets ( ). Rate the behavior which is illustrated by the portion in italics according to how you think most people would judge that behavior if they witnessed it. Use this scale.

Fairly normal behavior in that situation	(A)
Rather strange behavior in that situation	(B)
Very eccentric behavior in that situation	(C)
Shocking behavior in that situation	(D)

In the airplane

Emily, age 19, overslept on the morning of her airplane trip. When she woke up, there was just enough time to dress and get to the airport, _so she skipped her breakfast._ ( )

At noon, the stewardess came around with lunch, but Emily was so hungry by then that one portion did not satisfy her. She watched a little girl across the aisle toy with her food, complaining, "I can't eat it." Apparently, the father didn't want any more, because he told the child to just leave it. _Emily leaned across the aisle and said, "If your little girl doesn't want her tray, can you pass it over for me?"_ ( )

(Reprinted with permission from Dewey M: Living with Asperger's disorder, in Frith Uta (ed): Autism and Asperger Syndrome. Cambridge, UK: Cambridge University Press, 1991).

TABLE 43-9. Adolescent Complications of Autism

Complication	Frequency	Examples/comments
Epilepsy	20%–30%, F>M	Partial complex and generalized
Deterioration	12%–22%, 40% F>M	Not necessarily related epilepsy; some recover
Aggravation of symptoms	35–50	Often periodic, not correlated with deterioration; consists of stereotypies, hyperactivity, self-destructive or unmanageable behavior
Problems associated with sexual maturation	35%, M>>>F	Public masturbation
Depression	22%–44%	Often highest functioning patients

F, female; M, male.

(Reprinted with permission from Nass R: Long-term outcome of autism, in Gilchrist E (ed): Prognosis in Neurology. Boston: Butterworth-Heinemann, 1998.)

adolescence, or even adulthood. NVLD, ADHD, and OCD, or social isolation may be the main complaints during the early elementary and middle school years. Many individuals with AS may fit within the broader autistic phenotype, functioning independently until life circumstances lend themselves to an evaluation. Eminent philosophers, mathematicians, physicists, artists, and musicians such as Wittgenstein, Bartok, and Kandinsky are thought to have perhaps had AS (Gillberg, 2002).

Cerebral Substrate

Several medical disorders can produce an ASD phenotype (Nass & Ross, 1997; Table 43-10). Neuropsychological measures suggest relatively diffuse cerebral dysfunction in autism, with lateralized right hemisphere dysfunction, particularly in AS. Patients who have prominent theory of mind impairments may have frontal lobe dysfunction. Structural abnormalities reported predominantly in research studies of autism (Hendren et al., 2000; Tsatsanis et al., 2003) include:

TABLE 43-10. Medical Disorders That May Be Associated with Autism

Prenatal
  First and second trimester bleeding
  "Suboptimality"
  Congenital infections

Congenital
  Cornelia de Lange
  Dandy Walker syndrome
  Goldenhar syndrome
  Hydrocephalus
  Hypomelanosis of Ito
  Microcephaly
  Moebius syndrome
  Noonan syndrome
  Oculocutaneous albinism
  Tuberous sclerosis
  Neurofibromatosis
  Duchenne muscular dystrophy

Metabolic
  Adenylosuccinate lyase deficiency
  Addison disease
  Adrenoleukodystrophy
  Celiac disease
  Histidinemia
  Hurler syndrome
  Hyperthyroidism

  Hyperuricosuria
  Lead encephalopathy
  Lipidosis
  Phenylketonuria
  Hypothyroidism
  Lactic acidosis
  Purine, pyrimidine

Chromosomal
  Trisomy 21, maternally inherited duplications of chromosome 15q11–13, 2q37, 7q, 22q13, 18q-, 18 long dupl, 18 short deletion
  Fragile X
  Marker chromosome syndrome
  Sex chromosome abnormalities (XYY, XXX)
  Rett mutation

Epilepsy
  Infantile spasms
  Landau-Kleffner variant

Vascular

Infection
  Meningitis
  Herpes encephalitis

Trauma

(Data from Nass R, Ross G: Disorders of higher cortical function in the preschooler, in David R (ed): Child and Adolescent Neurology. St. Louis, MO: Mosby, 1997.)

- Increased whole brain, ventricular, and white matter volume
- Reduced thalamic volume
- Hypoplastic corpus callosum, parietal lobes, and cerebellum (vermian lobules VI and VII)
- Abnormalities in right cingulate gyrus, hippocampus, and amygdala
- Hyperplastic cerebellum

Most metabolic imaging studies in autism reveal hypometabolism in frontal and temporal regions (Rumsey & Ernst, 2000). Some show metabolic abnormalities in the amygdala (particularly when processing emotional facial expressions) (see Haxby et al., 2002) and cingulate gyrus (Haznedar et al., 1997). Recent studies reveal even further detail and relate findings to specific cognitive dysfunctions. General decreases in regional cerebral blood flow (rCBF) in autistic patients compared with controls were identified in the bilateral insula and superior temporal gyri and left prefrontal cortices. Impairments in communication and social interaction (putatively related to deficits in the theory of mind) were associated with altered perfusion in the medial prefrontal cortex and anterior cingulate gyrus. An obsessive desire for sameness was associated with altered perfusion in the right medial temporal lobe (Ohnishi et al., 2000).

Few brain imaging studies have specifically addressed AS. Cortical dysplasia has been described in both right and left hemisphere as well as bilaterally. When Tourette syndrome (TS) co-occurred with AS, 70% of the sample showed abnormalities in the opercular/perisylvian region versus 11% in those with TS only (Berthier et al., 1993). Some AS patients have hypoperfusion in the right hemisphere and cerebellum (McElvey et al., 1995), whereas others show reduced metabolism in the cingulate. A recent positron emission tomography (PET) study demonstrated that young men with AS failed to activate the left frontal region during a theory of mind task (Gillberg, 2002). AS patients also did not activate the brain areas implicated in processing facial emotions (Critchley et al., 2000), similar to patients with autism.

Treatment

General Recommendations

Early intervention offers the best opportunity for mitigating the developmental abnormalities in ASD and related developmental disorders. In many states, children younger than 3 years who have a diagnosed disability or developmental delay are eligible for state-financed early intervention programs. It is recommended that toddlers and preschool children with a diagnosis of ASD and PDD-NOS receive special education services in a therapeutic nursery or in a home-based behavioral modifi-cation program. Several university centers throughout the country (i.e., TEACCH, University of North Carolina, or Young Autism Program, UCLA) have exceptional programs for ASD children. They also have excellent referral resources and provide access to therapeutic materials that can be used at home as well as at local schools.

When ASD children enter elementary school, level of intellectual functioning and degree of maladaptive and disruptive behavior largely determine their placement in mainstream or special education classes. Regardless of placement, the setting must provide a small enough student-to-teacher ratio so that opportunities for individualized attention are consistently available. Children with ASD generally perform best in highly structured classrooms with routinized or academically driven curricula. Higher functioning children placed in mainstream classrooms may, however, require a "shadow" or assistant to help them develop more appropriate problem-solving skills and learn new ways to handle troublesome situations, facilitate peer interactions, or manage frustration. A disruptive child in a class full of typical children requires much attention and resources, or he or she can affect the education of the entire group.

Language

Communication deficits are a core feature of ASD. Interventions are aimed at improving receptive and expressive language skills as well as paralinguistic aspects of communication. Various techniques address the issue of enhancing spontaneous language in ASD children. Lower functioning autistic children with minimal communication must be taught enough language to communicate basic needs. Pragmatic aspects of language in particular must be addressed in children with AS. Learning how to initiate and maintain conversation, shift topics and take conversational turns, modify vocabulary and grammar for the setting, or sustain eye contact are just some of the pragmatic skills needed to optimize their chances for success in social, academic, and vocational settings.

Social Skills Deficits

Because of the significant social interaction deficits in the ASD, behavioral intervention techniques to improve social skills are a vital component of any therapeutic program (Kransny et al., 2003). It is fundamentally important to concentrate on the young child's ability to initiate interactions and to respond appropriately to others.

Because ASD children resist social interaction, social skill-building entails learning to tolerate the presence of other people. Whereas cooperative play may not be a realistic goal, parallel play may be. Treatment efforts in AS can take advantage of a child's intact verbal abilities, and verbal techniques can be used to teach important social and communication skills. Social awareness should be encouraged at every opportunity (Klin & Volkmar, 2000) and can be highlighted in daily routine interactions and specialized social skills groups. Emphasis on appropriate perception of social cues from others and the self-monitoring of communication are essential.

Visual-Motor Skills

For children with fine motor difficulties that limit handwriting capacities, computer assistive technology can help a child to communicate potentially good verbal ideas in a neat, legible fashion, while improving his or her organizational skills (Klin & Volkmar, 2000). Computers can also provide a mechanism for training these socially inept children to interact with others in a concrete way (i.e., e-mail). Occupational therapy can provide important instruction and guidance in many functional living skills.

Psychotherapy

Children with ASD lack insight and empathy, abilities that are needed to succeed in traditional dynamic psychotherapy. Psychological interventions using more targeted cognitive-behavioral approaches may help mitigate some conduct problems, interpersonal difficulties, and self-image/self-esteem concerns. Most importantly, families need strong support to cope with the chronic stress of caregiver burden, academic issues, and psychosocial concerns of children with ASD, AS, and PDD-NOS. Developing a relationship with a professional who is knowledgeable about individual concerns and family dynamics can be helpful for acute situations and long-term care (Ruberman, 2002; Kabot et al., 2003).

Psychopharmacology

In some low-functioning ASD children, medication can be helpful in targeting the most prominent behavior problems (Gilman & Tuchman, 1995; Martin et al., 2000; Table 43-11 shows summary). Psychopharmacologic treatment of AS generally focuses on reducing rituals, obsessions, and compulsions; attentional problems; and mood disorders.

TOURETTE SYNDROME

Definition and Epidemiology

Tourette syndrome (TS) is characterized by multiple motor and one or more vocal tics, present for at least 1 year, which vary in type and frequency over time. The prevalence of tics ranges from 1% to 20% in normal school-aged children and as high as 30% in children in special education (Mason et al., 1998; Kadesjo &

Gillberg, 2000). Boys are more commonly affected. The frequency of TS is 0.1% to 2.9% in general populations (Banerjee et al., 1998; Kadesjo & Gillberg, 2000) and as high as 10% in special education populations (Eapen et al., 1997b). TS appears to be hereditary, with variable manifestations within families. Chronic motor tics and/or OCD have been hypothesized to reflect the expression of a TS gene (see section following).

Evaluation and Diagnosis

The diagnosis of TS is made by history, clinical examination, and physical examination. A number of severity rating scales for clinicians, parents, and for self-report are available, such as the Yale Global Tic Severity Scale (Leckman et al., 1989).

Clinical Features

In TS, simple and complex tics occur, including blinking, shoulder shrugging, facial grimacing, coughing, touching, and licking and sniffing objects (Robertson, 2000). Tics may be abrupt in onset, and may be fast and brief or slow and sustained (dystonic tics). Sensory tics are common. Coprolalia (inappropriate involuntary uttering of obscenities) occurs in about one third of severe TS patients, but in few children with mild disorders (Robertson, 2000), and usually manifests by age 15 years. Copropraxia (inappropriate involuntary obscene gestures), echolalia (repeating the speech of others), echopraxia (imitation of actions of others), and palilalia (repeating one's own speech) also occur in as many as one third of severely involved TS patients.

A number of neuropsychological disorders are reported in children with TS (Comings, 1994; Comings & Comings, 1987). These include OCD and obsessive-compulsive behavior (OCB); ADHD; anxiety disorders; disorders of empathy/autistic spectrum problems (Comings & Comings, 1991); disorders of attention, motor function, and perception (DAMP); and various learning disabilities (Brookshire et al., 1994; Kadesjo & Gillberg, 2000; Robertson, 2000). Kadesjo and Gillberg (2000) identified 5 subgroups in their 58-patient TS cohort:

1. Tics only (20%)
2. Tics + ADHD/DAMP (17%)
3. Tics + ADHD/DAMP + empathy/autism spectrum problems + mild compulsions (25%)
4. Tics + ADHD/DAMP + empathy/autism spectrum problems + severe compulsions (25%)
5. Other (n = 13%)

Groups 3 and 4 were the most impaired and showed a complicated clinical picture requiring multidisciplinary intervention. Groups 3 and 4 accounted for 50% of all TS cases.

TABLE 43-11. Medication Options in the Treatment of Autism

Hyperactivity impulsivity	Anxiety
Methylphenidate (Ritalin)	Buspirone (Buspar)
Methylphenidate (Focalin)	Clonazapam (Klonipin)
d-amphetamine (Dexedrine)	SSRIs
Adderall and Adderall XR (Adderall)	Mood stabilizer
Long-acting forms of methylphenidate (Concerta, Ritalin SR and LA, Metadate CD)	Valproate (Depakote)
Atomoxetine (Straitera)	Carbamazepine (Tegretol)
Clonidine (Catapres)	Gabapentin (Neurontin)
Guanfacine (Tenex)	Topiramate (Topamax)
Obsessive-compulsive behaviors	Self-Mutilation
Clomipramine (Anafranil)	Naloxone (Narcan)
Fluoxetine (Prozac)	Propranolol (Inderal)
Sertraline (Zoloft)	Fluoxetine (Prozac)
Paroxetine (Paxil)	Clomipramine (Anafranil)
Fluvoxamine (Luvox)	Lithium (Lithium)
Risperidone (Risperdal)	Psychosis
Aggressive behaviors	Neuroleptics
Carbamazepine (Tegretol) and oxcarbazepine (Trileptal)	Haloperidol (Haldol)
Valproate (Depakote)	Risperidone (Risperdal)
Topiramate (Topamax)	Olanzapine (Zyprexa)
Clonidine (Catapres)	Ziprasidone (Geodon)
Propranolol (Inderal)	Older phenothiazines
Buspirone (Buspar)	Sleep problems
Lithium (Lithium)	Clonidine (Catapres)
Neuroleptics	Melatonin
Depression	Antihistamines
Tricyclics	Others
SSRIs	ACTH and analogues, prednisone
Bupropion (Wellbutrin)	Multi B vitamins
Venlafaxine (Effexor)	

(Data from Gilman J, Tuchman R: Autism and associated behavioral disorders: Pharmacologic intervention. Ann Psychopharmacolo, 29:47–56, 1995, and Martin A, Patzer D, Volkmar F: Psychopharmacologic treatment of higher functioning PDD, in Klin A, Volkmar F, Sparrow S (eds): Asperger Syndrome. New York; Guilford Press, 2000, pp. 210–228.) Towbin, 2003; McDougle, et al. 2002A

Tourette Syndrome/Obsessive-Compulsive Disorder Overlap

The reported frequency of OCD and OCB in TS populations ranges from 11% to as high as 80% (Steingard & Dillon-Stout, 1992; Eapenet al., 1997a; Zohar et al., 1997; Robertson, 2000). Some investigators believe that an individual inherits a vulnerability to a spectrum disorder that includes both TS and OCB (Eapenet al., 1997a). The obsessions in OCD and TS may differ (Miguel et al., 1997). In TS, obsessions have more to do with sex, violence, religion, and aggression; compulsions have to do with checking, ordering, counting, repeating, forced touching, symmetry ("evening up"), getting things "just right," self-damage, or socially inappropriate behaviors (SIB). By contrast, obsessions in isolated OCD are related predominantly to contamination,

dirt, germs, being neat and clean, fear of something going wrong or bad happening, or the fear of becoming ill; compulsions in isolated OCD have mainly to do with cleaning and washing. The OCD/OCB in TS appears to be egosyntonic (personally comfortable), rather than the egodystonic (subjectively uncomfortable), as in typical OCD.

Nonobscene, complex, and socially inappropriate behaviors such as insulting others (e.g., aspersions on weight, height, intelligence) are considered by many investigators to be a specific type of compulsion, peculiar to TS (Kurlan et al., 1996). Despite attempts to suppress these behaviors, social difficulties commonly result, including verbal arguments, school problems, fist fights, job problems, removal from a public place, legal trouble, or even arrest. Nonobscene complex socially inappropriate behaviors are more common in young boys and often co-occur with ADHD and conduct disorder. Other obsessive-compulsive behaviors do not necessarily co-occur. Some investigators, therefore, suggest that non-obscene complex socially inappropriate behaviors are part of a more general disorder of impulse control in TS (Kurlan et al., 1996). Such socially inappropriate behaviors represent another way in which TS fits into ASD.

Tourett Syndrome/Autistic Spectrum Disorders Overlap

The link between TS and ASD is highlighted by the co-occurrence of TS with ASD and with AS (Nass & Gutman, 1997; Baron-Cohen et al., 1999b; Ringman & Jankovic, 2000). In this context TS can be considered as a type of stereotyped behavior. The largest scale study to date (Baron-Cohen et al., 1999b) examined 447 children with autism. Definite TS was confirmed in 19 children, giving a prevalence rate of 4%; 10 more children were diagnosed as having probable TS (2.2%). Many others (34%) showed tics on observation (but not both motor and vocal tics). TS was not related to the severity of the ASD in these youngsters. In a Swedish population study (Gillberg, 2002) 80% with definite AS and 60% with definite or suspected AS had tics. At least 1 in 10, perhaps 1 in 5 children with definite AS, had TS. Consistent with a genetic link, family members with autism and PDD are reported in TS families (Baron-Cohen et al., 1999b; Murphy et al., 2000).

The development of TS may be a good prognostic sign in patients with PDD (Burd et al., 1987; Kano et al., 1987). Homozygosity for the TS gene may give rise to autism with or without TS (Comings & Comings, 1991). Patients with TS alone are less impaired than patients with co-occurring TS and AS. Visuospatial difficulties were present in 10 patients with AS. Visuospatial and language difficulties were present in 7 patients with co-occurring TS and AS (Marriage et al., 1993). The two cohorts of Berthier and colleagues (1993) (TS plus AS, and TS only) did not differ in degree of tics, obsessiveness, depression, anxiety, intelligence, memory, and language function. However, those with co-occurring TS and AS had more psychiatric hospitalizations, worse academic achievement, more neurologic soft signs, more seizure diagnosis, and appeared to perform worse on complex problem-solving and spatial tasks.

Disorders of empathy/social emotional problems and full-blown ASD are second in frequency only to ADHD as comorbid conditions in TS (Baron-Cohen, 1998; Kadesjo & Gillberg, 2000). Two thirds of TS patients in a recent study scored above the cutoff for suspected AS or HFA on a screening measures (the ASSQ; Kadesjo & Gillberg, 2000).

Tourette Syndrome/Anxiety Disorder Overlap

Anxiety disorders occur in 20% to 80% of TS patients, a much higher rate than the 1% to 6% reported in the control population (Pliszka & Olvera, 1999). Twenty-six percent of TS patients have more than three phobias, in contrast to 8.5% of controls. Fourteen percent of TS patients and only 4.2% of controls have both panic attacks and phobias (Comings & Comings, 1987).

Natural History and Outcome

TS typically emerges in early elementary school (mean age 7 years), although preschool onset can be observed. TS disappears with age; most children with TS can expect to have few or no tics by adulthood, regardless of tic severity in childhood.

Cerebral Substrate

Many neural circuits (e.g., frontal-subcortical; basal ganglia-thalamocortical, nucleus accumbens-limbic system) have been implicated in the pathogenesis of TS. Neurotransmitter systems implicated include catecholamines (dopamine and noradrenaline); tryptophan and its metabolites (serotonin, kynurenine, tryptamine), acetylcholine, the GABA amino acids (glutamate, phenylalanine, p-tyrosine), trace amines (e.g., tyramine), opioid peptides (e.g., dynorphin), the second messenger (cyclic AMP), and androgenic hormones (Robertson, 2000). Imaging studies demonstrate that basal ganglia nuclei may show atypical right-left asymmetry patterns. The corpus callosum is reported to be reduced in size (Bigler et al., 1999). T2 signal abnormalities in frontal lobe, basal ganglia, red nucleus, and amygdala have been described. Reduced metabolism in frontal, cingulate, and insular cortices, as well as in the basal ganglia, is reported in dynamic imaging studies (Brody et al., 1998; Buitelaar et al., 1998; Bigler et al., 1999). These research findings have not yet translated to reliable clinical tests or diagnostic criteria.

Treatment

Management of TS begins with education for parents, patients, teachers, and other care providers. Behavioral modification methods and reassurance may suffice in cases with mild symptoms. Clonidine (Catapres) and clonazepam (Klonopin) are the most frequently used medications for treating mild tics, and may have potential therapeutic overlap with comorbid disorders like ADHD and anxiety disorder. More severe motor and vocal tics are generally treated with dopamine antagonists—haloperidol and pimozide. Risperidone is being more frequently used, in part because of the lesser risk of tardive dyskinesias compared with older neuroleptics. A number of other drugs including nicotinic agents, baclofen Lioresal (Lioresal), and antiandrogenic agents have been reported to work in some cases. In patients who are recalcitrant to medical management, TS can be quite disruptive to their lives and social interactions.

OBSESSIVE-COMPULSIVE DISORDER

Definition and Epidemiology

Obsessions are recurrent, intrusive, senseless thoughts, and are egodystonic (internally uncomfortable); compulsions are repetitive and seemingly purposeful behaviors performed according to certain rules or in a stereotyped fashion. Patients with OCD are distressed by both and show personal and social problems (DSM-IV). The most common obsessions in children (and adults) are related to fear of dirt and contamination, something terrible happening, and harming a loved one. The most common compulsions are washing fixations, and checking behavior and rituals (including mental rituals) (Thomson, 2000). OCD has a lifetime prevalence rate of between 1.9% and 4% (Thomson, 1993). The prevalence in a large epidemiologic sample of adolescents of OCD and OCB is 3% and 19%, respectively. Major depressive disorder (45%), anxiety disorders (34%–76%), dysthymia (29%), suicidal ideation (15%), and phobia (8%) frequently accompany OCD. Three subtypes of OCD are (1) familial related to tic disorders/TS; (2) familial unrelated to tics; and (3) nonfamilial (Alsobrook et al., 1995).

Obsessive-Compulsive Disorder/Tourette Syndrome Overlap

TS is relatively common in OCD probands and 11% to 80% of individuals with TS have OCD (Zohar et al., 1997). In TS cohorts, obsessive-compulsive symptoms are common and often accompany empathy/autism spectrum problems (Kadesjo & Gillberg, 2000).

Obsessive-Compulsive Disorder/Asperger Syndrome Overlap

OCD clearly resemble AS in terms of overfocus on particular activities, and the distinction between AS and OCD is sometimes unclear (Gillberg, 1998). However, the rituals and compulsive behaviors of children with AS are not experienced as egodystonic or alien, as they are in OCD. Rather, in AS they are self-stimulatory and soothing.

Obsessive-Compulsive Disorder/Anxiety Disorder Overlap

Anxiety disorders are common in patients with OCD (Steketee et al., 1999). Anxiety and panic may precede or follow the obsessive and compulsive behaviors.

Natural History and Outcome

The only factor that appears to predict a poor outcome, defined as the presence of OCD in adulthood, is severity of OCD in childhood, indexed by the duration of the obsessive-compulsive symptoms. Age of onset does not predict the long-term course of OCD.

Cerebral Substrate

Failure of gabaminergic inhibition of glutaminergic, dopaminergic, and serotonergic pathways between frontal cortex and basal ganglia are involved in OCD (Brody et al., 1998). OCD symptoms are mediated by hyperactivity in orbitofrontal-subcortical circuits, perhaps due to an imbalance of tone between direct and indirect striato-pallidal pathways (Saxena et al., 1998). Functional neuroimaging indicates that OCD symptoms are associated with increased activity in orbitofrontal cortex, caudate nucleus, thalamus, and anterior cingulate gyrus (Garreau, 1998).

Treatment

Cognitive-behavioral therapies are an important treatment modality. Exposure and response prevention are the major behavioral intervention methods (King et al., 1998). Selective serotonin reuptake inhibitors (SSRIs), particularly fluvoxamine maleate (Luvox), are the mainstay of treatment. Clomipramine (Anafranil), a tricyclic with some SRI, is also frequently therapeutic. In partial responders, these drugs can be augmented by a neuroleptic or atypical neuroleptic, another SRI (e.g., using clomipramine and an SSRI together), or clonazepam (Rapaport & Inoff, 2000). Ritalin is not recommended because it may increase OCD symptoms.

SOCIAL DYSFUNCTION SPECTRUM DISORDERS: SOCIAL PHOBIA/SOCIAL ANXIETY DISORDER

Definition and Epidemiology

Anxiety disorders are subdivided in DSM-IV as panic disorder, agoraphobia, separation anxiety disorder, social phobia, OCD, generalized anxiety disorder, and specific phobia. The different anxiety disorders frequently co-occur—e.g., in the same cohort 10% had generalized anxiety disorder and 25% had phobias. Anxiety disorders are relatively common, but infrequently associated with serious impairment in functioning and often go unreported by families (Vasey & Ollendick, 2000). In large epidemiologic samples generalized anxiety disorder occurs in 2.6% to 6.3% and social phobia/social anxiety disorder occurs in 1% to 3% (Pliszka & Olvera, 1999). Common settings for social fears are parties, school, and situations necessitating speaking, eating, or writing.

There may be a genetic component to anxiety disorders; relatives of child probands and children of adult probands show an increased incidence of anxiety disorders compared with controls. Panic disorders have the strongest genetic component and phobias the weakest. Environmental factors are often suspected of contributing to social anxiety disorder. Social phobia can be observed as one of the characteristics of the broader autistic phenotype described in families of probands with ASD (Murphy et al., 2000).

A number of parent and self-report rating scales are available to assess anxiety in children (Chorpita et al., 1996; Reynolds & Richmond, 2000). Notably, parent-child inter-rater reliability is poor when anxiety is the trait in question.

Anxiety Disorder/Autistic Spectrum Disorder Overlap

Anxiety disorders appear to be relatively common among children with ASD, particularly those who are high functioning (Muris et al., 1998; Gillott et al., 2001). In one sample almost two thirds of the ASD children had simple phobias, one quarter separation anxiety disorder, and one fifth overanxious disorder.

Natural History and Outcome

Social anxiety disorder has a peak age of onset in adolescence. Early onset predicts a poor prognosis. Early diagnosis and treatment may improve long-term outcome (Beidel, 1998).

Cerebral Substrate

Few data are available about the pathophysiology of social phobia. A single photon emission tomography (SPECT) study with Tc-99m HMPAO suggested that treatment with an SSRI led to significantly reduced activity in the anterior and lateral part of the left temporal cortex; the anterior, lateral, and posterior part of the left mid frontal cortex; and the left cingulate gyrus. Nonresponders had higher activity at baseline in the ante-rior and lateral part of the left temporal cortex and the lateral part of the left mid frontal regions compared with responders (Van der Linden et al., 2000).

Treatment

Treatment of social dysfunction spectrum disorders includes cognitive behavioral therapy with or without pharmacologic therapy. Despite voluminous data on treatment in adults there are relatively few data on efficacy of medicines in children (Pliszka & Olvera, 1999). SSRIs are the current mainstay of medical treatment. Tricyclics have proven effective, but are used less frequently now than in the 1970s, when they were tested, because of adverse effects (including drowsiness), and anticholinergic effects. Benzodiazepines, beta blockers, buspirone (BuSpar) have also been used.

DISORDERS OF VERBAL AND NONVERBAL COMMUNICATION: SEMANTIC-PRAGMATIC LANGUAGE SYNDROME

Children with the semantic-pragmatic language syndrome (SPS) speak fluently and may even be verbose. Vocabulary is often large, somewhat formal, and sometimes highly specialized (e.g., many dinosaur names). Parents often believe that their child's large vocabulary indicates superior verbal and cognitive skills. In fact, these children fall short in the basic semantic and pragmatic skills required for meaningful conversation and informative exchange of ideas. They talk to talk. Phonological and syntactic skills are generally intact, but comprehension is impaired to varying degrees. For example, they may answer a different "wh" question than the one being asked, provide a tangential response, or be too literal in their interpretation of a query. Further, they have not learned pragmatic rules and skills that govern conversational exchanges, e.g., turn-taking, topic maintenance, varying style (e.g., when talking to a child versus an adult, knowing when to interrupt and when to repeat [rather than to echo], and understanding social gaze cues and the appropriateness of physical contact). These children tend to provide the listener with too much or too little information (Bishop 1989; Rapin, 1996) and often show deficits in prosody. Their speech can have a monotonous, mechanical, or sing-song quality that prevents them from conveying emotion or indicating by tone of voice that they are asking a question. Children with SPS also have difficulty using prosody to enhance comprehension (Bishop, 1989; Rapin, 1996). In AS, verbal IQ (VIQ) tends to be better than performance IQ (PIQ), but the opposite is true in children with SPS.

SPS is often seen in higher functioning, more verbal ASD children, but also occurs apart from ASD. SPS is also seen in children with hydrocephalus (where it has been called the cocktail party syndrome), in agenesis of the corpus callosum, and in children with Williams syndrome, who are hypersocial (Nass, 1998b).

Cerebral Substrate

In general, imaging research of children with developmental language disorders has shown abnormalities in the left temporal region and atypical planum temporale asymmetry patterns. SPS has not been specifically investigated (Semrud-Clikeman, 1997).

Treatment

Treatment of children with SPS focuses on the underlying cognitive deficits and specific language difficulties. These children have difficulty identifying the main theme, subtopics, and lower level details (the hierarchical structure of language) of what they are trying to discuss and hear (or read). Relevant therapy promotes more varied speech, appropriate use of learned forms and cohesive devices, conversational turn-taking, and topic maintenance (Dunn, 1997). Children with SPS, like others with developmental language disorders, are at-risk for later language-related reading and learning disabilities; their progress should be monitored even after the original language disorder has been seemingly remediated.

SUMMARY AND CONCLUSIONS

ASD is characterized by three cardinal features that overlap with several related neurodevelopmental conditions. These features are (1) impaired verbal and nonverbal communication, (2) deficient sociability, and (3) restricted range of activities, behaviors, and interests. Comprehensive history, interview, examination, and neuropsychological assessment are essential to diagnosis. Debates on taxonomy, classification, and operational definitions abound, and diagnostic confusion is common. Specific characteristics define the different disorders subsumed by the term ASD, but nonspecific social dysfunction and subtle pragmatic language deficits are a common source of overlap. Further research must focus on clarifying diagnostic criteria, natural history, intervention outcomes, and developing measures aimed at specific impairments such as poor topic maintenance in communication and poor eye contact. Results of neuroimaging studies have yet to be incorporated into diagnostic criteria, although they may in some circumstances identify an underlying medical disorder (such as tuberous sclerosis). Clinical genetic tests are another topic for further research. Psychopharmacological intervention has eased some of the primary and secondary effects of ASD, yet these disorders continue to put children at risk for ridicule and social isolation as well as academic and vocational underachievement. Low functioning autistic children may be oblivious to the environment. Higher functioning children (with repetitive behaviors, poor language skills, or social dysfunction) are more sensitive to social and environmental circumstances, and may suffer rejection by their peers, anxiety, and depression. Long-term medical and psychological follow-up for these children is crucial.

■ KEY POINTS

☐   An autistic spectrum disorder exists when language, social skills, and flexibility and range of behaviors are affected to varying degrees. This chapter discusses the degree to which Asperger disorder, Tourette syndrome, obsessive-compusive disorder, and social anxiety disorder are examples of autistic spectrum disorders.

KEY READINGS

Robertson M: Tourette syndrome, associated conditions and the complexities of treatment. Brain 123: 425–462, 2000.

Gillberg C, Coleman M: Autistic Spectrum Disorders. New York: Cambridge University Press, 2000.

Klin A, Volkmar F, Sparrow S (eds): Asperger Syndrome. New York: Guilford Press, 2000.

REFERENCES

Achenbach TM: Assessment and Taxonomy of Child and Adolescent Psychopathology. Newbury Park, CA: Sage Publications, 1985.

Achenbach TM: Manual for the Child Behavior Checklist 6–18 years. Burlington, VT: University of Vermont Department of Psychiatry, 2002.

Alsobrook JP 2nd, Goodman W, Rasmussen S, et al: A family study of obsessive-compulsive disorder. Am J Psychiatry 152:76–84, 1995.

American Psychiatric Association (APA): Diagnostic and Statistical Manual of Mental Disorders, 4th ed. DSM-IV. Washington, DC: American Psychiatric Association, 1994.

Attwood T: Asperger Syndrome. London, UK: Jessica Kingsley Publishers, 1998.

Banerjee S, Mason A, Eapen V, et al: Prevalence of Tourette syndrome in a mainstream school population. Dev Med Child Neurol 40:817–818, 1998.

Baron-Cohen S: Modularity in developmental cognitive neuropsychology: Evidence from autism and TS, in Burack J, Hodapp R, Zigler E (eds): Handbook of Mental Retardation and Development. New York: Cambridge University Press, 1998, pp. 334–348.

Baron-Cohen S, Jolliffe T, Mortimore C, et al: Another advanced test of theory of mind: Evidence from very high functioning adults with autism or Asperger Syndrome. J Child Psychol Psychiatry 38:813–822, 1997.

Baron-Cohen S, O'Riordan M, Stone V, et al: Recognition of faux pas by normally developing children with Asperger syndrome or high-functioning autism. J Autism Dev Dis 29:407–418, 1999a.

Baron-Cohen S, Scahill VL, Izaguirre J, et al: The prevalence of Gilles de la Tourette syndrome in children and adolescents with autism: A large scale study. Psychol Med 29:1151–1159, 1999b.

Baron-Cohen S, Tager-Flusberg H, Cohen D: Understanding Other Minds: Perspectives from Autism. Oxford, UK: Oxford University Press, 1993.

Beidel D: Social anxiety disorder: Etiology and early clinical presentation. J Clin Psychiatry 59(Suppl. 17):27–31, 1998.

Berthier ML, Bayes A, Tolosa ES: Magnetic resonance imaging in patients with concurrent Tourette disorder and Asperger syndrome. J Am Acad Child Adolesc Psychiatry 32:633–639, 1993.

Berument S, Rutter M, Lord C, et al: Autism screening questionnaire: Diagnostic validity. Br J Psychiatry 175:444–451, 1999.

Bigler E, Nielsen D, Wilde E, et al: Neuroimaging and genetic disorders, in Goldstein S, Reynolds C (eds): Handbook of Neurodevelopmental and Genetic Disorders in Children. New York: Guilford Press, 1999, pp. 61–80.

Bishop DVM: Autism, Asperger's syndrome and semantic-pragmatic disorder: Where are the boundaries? Br J Dis Commun 24:107–121, 1989.

Boelte S, Boelte S, Dickhut H, et al: Patterns of parent-reported problems indicative in autism. Psychopathology 32:93–97, 1999.

Brody SS, Schwartz AL, Baxter LR: Neuroimaging and frontal cortical circuitry in obsessive compulsive disorder. Br J Psychiatry 35:26–37, 1998.

Brookshire BL, Butler I, Ewing-Cobb L, et al: Neuropsychological characteristics in children with Tourette's syndrome. J Clin Exp Neuropsychol 16:289–302, 1994.

Buitelaar JK, De Bruin WI, van Rijk PP: SPECT studies in Tourette syndrome, in Garreau B (ed): Neuroimaging in Child Neuropsychiatric Disorders. Berlin, Germany: Springer-Verlag, 1998, pp. 133–139.

Buitelaar J, Van der Gaag R, Klin A, et al: Exploring the boundaries of pervasive developmental disorder not otherwise specified: Analyses of data from the DSM-IV Autistic Disorder Field Trial. J Autism Dev Dis 29:33–44, 1999a.

Buitelaar JK, van der Wees M, Swaab-Barneveld HJ, et al: Verbal memory and performance IQ predict theory of mind and emotion recognition ability in children with autistic spectrum disorders and in psychiatric control children. J Child Psychol Psychiatry 40:869–881, 1999b.

Burd L, Fisher W, Kerbeshian J, et al: Is the development of Tourette's syndrome a marker for improvement in patients with autism and other pervasive developmental disorders? J Am Acad Child Adolesc Psychiatry 26:162–165, 1987.

Charman T, Baron-Cohen S, Baird G, et al: Is 18 months too early for the CHAT? J Am Acad Child Adolesc Psychiatry 41:235–236, 2002.

Chorpita BF, Albano AM, Barlow D: Child anxiety sensitivity index. J Clin Child Psychol 25:77–82, 1996.

Comings DE: Tourette syndrome: A hereditary neuropsychiatric spectrum disorder. Ann Clin Psychiatry 6:235–247, 1994.

Comings DE, Comings BG: A controlled study of Tourette syndrome. I. attention deficit disorder, learning disorders, and school problems. Am J Hum Genet 41:701–741, 1987.

Comings DE, Comings BG: Clinical and genetic relationships between autism-pervasive developmental disorder and Tourette syndrome: A study of 19 cases. Am J Med Genet 39:180–191, 1991.

Cook E: Genetics of autism. Ment Retard Dev Dis 4:113–120, 1998.

Critchley HD, Daly E, Bullmore E, et al: The functional neuroanatomy of social behaviour: Changes in cerebral blood flow when people with autistic disorder process facial expressions. Brain 123:2203–2212, 2000.

Dewey M: Living with Asperger's disorder, in Frith, U (ed): Autism and Asperger Syndrome. Cambridge, UK: Cambridge University Press, 1991.

Dunn M: Remediation of developmental language disorders, in Nass R, Rapin I (eds): Seminars in Pediatric Neurology, Language Disorders in Children. Philadelphia, PA: Saunders, 1997, pp. 127–134.

Eapen V, Robertson MM, Alsobrook JP 2nd, et al: Obsessive compulsive symptoms in Gilles de la Tourette syndrome and obsessive compulsive disorder: Differences by diagnosis and family history. Am J Med Genet 74:432–438, 1997a.

Eapen V, Robertson MM, Zeitlin H, et al: Gilles de la Tourette syndrome in special education schools: A United Kingdom study. J Neurol 244:378–382, 1997b.

Ehlers S, Nyden A, Gillberg C, et al: Asperger syndrome, autism and attention disorders: A comparative study of the cognitive profiles of 120 children. J Child Psychol Psychiatry 38:207–217, 1997.

Ehlers S, Gillberg C, Wing L: A screening questionnaire for Aspergers syndrome and other high-functioning autism spectrum disorders in school age children. J Autism Dev Dis 29:129–141, 1999.

Eisenmajer R, Prior M, Leekam S, et al: Comparison of clinical symptoms in autism and Asperger's disorder. J Am Acad Child Adolesc Psychiatry 35:1523–1531, 1996.

Fombonne E, Tidmarsh L: Epidemiologic data on Asperger disorder. Child Adolesc Psychiatr Clin North Am 12:15–21, 2003.

Garreau B (ed): Neuroimaging in child neuropsychiatric disorders. Berlin: Springer-Verlag, 1998.

Ghaziuddin M, Butler E: Clumsiness in autism and Asperger syndrome: A further report. J Intellect Dis Res 42:43–48, 1998.

Ghaziuddin M, Gerstein L: Pedantic speaking style differentiates Asperger syndrome from high-functioning autism. J Autism Dev Dis 26:585–595, 1996.

Ghaziuddin M, Leininger L, Tsai L: Brief report: Thought disorder in Asperger syndrome: Comparison with high-functioning autism. J Autism Develop Dis 25:311–317, 1995.

Gillberg C: A Guide to Asperger Syndrome. New York: Cambridge University Press, 2002.

Gillberg C: Asperger syndrome and high-functioning autism. Br J Psychiatry 172:200–209, 1998.

Gillberg C, Ehlers S: High functioning people with autism and Asperger syndrome: A literature review, in Schopler E, Mesibov GB, Kunce LJ (eds): Asperger Syndrome or High-Functioning Autism? New York: Plenum Press, 1998, pp. 79–106.

Gilliam S: Asperger's Disorder Scale. Austin, TX: Pro-Ed, 2001a.

Gilliam S: Autism Rating Scale. Austin, TX: Pro-Ed, 2001b.

Gillott A, Furniss F, Walter A: Anxiety in high-functioning children with autism. Autism 5:277–286, 2001.

Gilman J, Tuchman R: Autism and associated behavioral disorders: Pharmacologic intervention. Ann Psychopharmacol 29:47–56, 1995.

Gross J: Learning with disabilities: An answer to autism. The New York Times. April 13, 2003: Section 4A, pp. 27–28, 32–33.

Haxby J, Hoffman E, Gobbini M: Human neural systems for face recognition and social communication. Biol Psychiatry 51:59–67, 2002.

Haznedar M, Buchsbaum MS, Metzger M, et al: Anterior cingulate gyrus volume and glucose metabolism in autistic disorder. Am J Psychiatry 154:1047–1050, 1997.

Hendren RL, De Backer I, Pandina GJ: Review of neuroimaging studies of child and adolescent psychiatric disorders from the past 10 years. J Am Acad Child Adolesc Psychiatry 39:815–828, 2000.

Kabot S, Masi W, Segal M: Advances in the diagnosis and treatment of autism spectrum disorders. Prof Psychol Res Pract 34:26–33, 2003.

Kadesjo B, Gillberg C: Tourette's disorder: Epidemiology and comorbidity in primary school children. J Am Acad Child Adolesc Psychiatry 39:548–555, 2000.

Kano Y, Ohta M, Nagia Y: Two case reports of autistic boys developing Tourette's syndrome: Indications of improvement? J Am Acad Child Adolesc Psychiatry 26:937–938, 1987.

King R, Leonard H, March J: Summary of the practice parameters for the assessment and treatment of children and adolescents with obsessive-compulsive disorder. J Am Acad Child Adolesc Psychiatry 37:1110–1116, 1998.

Klin A, Volkmar F: Treatment and intervention guidelines for individuals with Asperger syndrome, in Klin A, Volkmar F, Sparrow S (eds): Asperger Syndrome. New York: Guilford Press, 2000, pp. 340–366.

Klin A Volkmar F, Sparrow S (eds): Asperger Syndrome. New York: Guilford Press, 2000.

Klin A, Volkmar FR, Sparrow SS, et al: Validity and neuropsychological characterization of Asperger syndrome: Convergence with nonverbal learning disabilities syndrome. J Child Psychol Psychiatry 36:1127–1140, 1995.

Kransny L, Williams BJ, Provencal S, et al: Social skills interventions for the autism spectrum: Essential ingredients and a model curriculum. Child Adolesc Psychiatr Clin North Am 12:107–122, 2003.

Krug D, Arisk J, Almond P: Autism Screening Instrument for Educational Planning. Austin, TX: Pro-Ed, 1993.

Kurlan R, Daragjati C, Como PG, et al: Non-obscene complex socially inappropriate behavior in Tourette's syndrome. J Neuropsychiatry Clin Neurosci 8:311–317, 1996.

Landa R: Social language use in asperger syndrome and high-functioning autism, in Klin A, Volkmar F, Sparrow S (eds): Asperger Syndrome. New York: Guilford Press, 2000, pp. 125–155.

Leckman JF, Riddle MA, Hardin MT, et al: The Yale Global Tic Severity Scale: Initial testing of a clinician-rated scale of tic severity. J Am Acad Child Adolesc Psychiatry 28:566–573, 1989.

Leekam SR, Libby SJ, Wing L, et al: The diagnostic interview for social and communication disorders: Algorithms for ICD-10 childhood autism and Wing and Gould autistic spectrum disorder. J Child Psychol Psychiatry 43:310–314, 2002.

Lewine J, Andrews R, Chez M, et al: Magnetoencephalographic patterns of epileptiform activity in children with regressive autistic spectrum disorders. Pediatrics 104:405–418, 1999.

Lord C, Risi S: Frameworks and methods in diagnosing ASD. Ment Retard Dev Dis 4:90–96, 1998.

Luteijn E, Luteijn F, Jackson S, et al: The Children's Social Behavior Questionnaire for milder variants of PDD problems: Evaluation of the psychometric characteristics. J Autism Dev Dis 30:317–330, 2000.

Luteijn EF, Serra M, Jackson S, et al: How unspecified are disorders of children with a pervasive developmental disorder not otherwise specified? A study of social problems in children with PDD-NOS and ADHD. Eur Child Adolesc Psychiatry 9:168–179, 2000.

Marriage K, Miles T, Stokes D, et al: Clinical and research implications of the co-occurrence of Asperger's disorders and Tourette's syndrome. Aust N Z J Psychiatry 27:666–672, 1993.

Martin A, Patzer D, Volkmar F: Psychopharmacologic treatment of higher functioning PDD, in Klin A, Volkmar F, Sparrow S (eds): Asperger Syndrome. New York: Guilford Press, 2000, pp. 210–228.

Mason A, Banerjee S, Eapen V, et al: The prevalence of Tourette syndrome in a mainstream school population. Dev Med Child Neurol 40:292–296, 1998.

McDougle CJ, Posey D, Lombroso PJ (eds): Genetics of childhood disorders: XLIV. Autism, part 3: Psychopharmacology of autism. J Am Acad Child Adolesc Psychiatry 41:1380–1383, 2002.

McElvey J, Lambert R, Mottron L, et al: Right hemisphere dysfunction in Asperger's syndrome. J Child Neurol 10:310–314, 1995.

Miguel EC, Baer L, Coffey BJ, et al: Phenomenological differences appearing with repetitive behaviours in obsessive-compulsive disorder and Gilles de la Tourette's syndrome. Br J Psychiatry 170:140–145, 1997.

Muris P, Steerneman P, Merckelbach H, et al: Comorbid anxiety symptoms in children with pervasive developmental disorders. J Anxiety Disord 12:387–393, 1998.

Murphy M: Bolton PF, Pickles A, et al: Personality traits of the relatives of autistic probands. Psycholog Med 30:1411–1424, 2000.

Nass R: Developmental language disorders, in Berg B (ed): Principles of Child Neurology, 2nd ed. New York: McGraw-Hill, 1998a, pp. 397–410.

Nass R: Long term outcome of autism, in Gilchrist E (ed): Prognosis in Neurology. Boston, MA: Butterworth-Heinemann, 1998b, pp. 110–115.

Nass R, Gutman R: Asperger's syndrome: superior verbal intelligence with tics. Dev Med Child Neurol 39:691–695, 1997.

Nass R, Ross G: Disorders of higher cortical function in the preschooler, in David R (ed): Child and Adolescent Neurology. St. Louis, MO: Mosby, 1997, pp. 21–27.

Ohnishi T, Matsuda H, Hashimoto H, et al: Abnormal regional cerebral blood flow in childhood autism. Brain 123: 1838–1844, 2000.

Piven J: The broad autism phenotype: A complementary strategy for molecular genetic studies of autism. Am J Med Genet 105:34–35, 2001.

Pliszka S, Olvera R: Anxiety disorders, in Goldstein S, Reynolds C (eds): Handbook of Neurodevelopmental and Genetic Disorders in Children. New York: Guilford Press, 1999, pp. 216–246.

Rapin I (ed): Preschool Children with Inadequate Communication: Developmental Language Disorders, Autism, Low IQ. No. 139 of Clinics in Developmental Medicine. London: Mac Keith Press, 1996.

Rapin I: Autism. N Engl J Med 337:97–104, 1997.

Reynolds C, Richmond B: 2000 Revised Children's Manifest Anxiety Scales. Lutz, FL: Psychological Assessment Resources, 2000.

Ringman J, Jankovic J: Occurrence of tics in Asperger syndrome and autistic disorder. J Child Neurol 15:394–400, 2000.

Robertson M: Tourette syndrome, associated conditions and the complexities of treatment. Brain 123:425–462, 2000.

Rourke B: Non verbal learning disabilities. New York: Guilford Press, 1995.

Rourke B, Tsatsanis K: Non verbal learning disabilities and Aspergers syndrome, in Klin A, Volkmar F, Sparrow S (eds): Asperger Syndrome. New York: Guilford Press, 2000, pp. 231–253.

Ruberman L: Psychotherapy of children with pervasive developmental disorders. Am J Psychother 56:262–274, 2002.

Rumsey J, Ernst M: Functional neuroimaging of autistic disorders. Ment Retard Dev Dis Res Rev 6:171–179, 2000.

Saxena S, Brody AL, Schwartz JM, et al: Neuroimaging and frontal-subcortical circuitry in obsessive-compulsive disorder. Br J Psychiatry 35(Suppl.):26-37, 1998.

Schopler E, Mesibov GB (eds): High Functioning Individuals with Autism. New York: Plenum Press, 1997.

Schopler E, Reichler R, Renner B: Childhood Autism Rating Scale—CARS. Los Angeles, CA: Western Psychological Services, 1988.

Semrud-Clikeman M: Imaging in developmental language disorders, in Nass R, Rapin I (eds): Seminars in Pediatric Neurology, Language Disorders in Children. Philadelphia, PA: Saunders, 1997, pp. 96–101.

Siegel D, Minshew N, Goldstein S: Wechsler IQ profiles in diagnosis of high functioning autism. J Autism Dev Dis 26:389–406, 1996.

Sparrow S, Balla D, Cicchetti D: Vineland Adaptive Behavior Scales. Circle Pines, MN: American Guidance Services, 1984.

Steingard R, Dillon-Stout D: Tourette's syndrome and obsessive compulsive disorder. Psychiatr Clin North Am 15:849–860, 1992.

Steketee G, Eisen J, Dyck I, et al: Predictors of course in obsessive compulsive disorder. Psychiatry Res 89:229–238, 1999.

Szatmari P, Merette C, Bryson S, et al: Quantifying dimensions in autism: A factor-analytic study. J Am Acad Child Adolesc Psychiatry 41:467–474, 2002.

Tanguay P: Pervasive developmental disorders: A 10-year review. J Am Acad Child Adolesc Psychiatry 39:1079–1095, 2000.

Towbin, KE: Strategies for pharmacologic treatment of high functioning autism and Asperger syndrome. Child Adolesc Psychiatr Clin North Am 12:23–45, 2003.

Tuchman R: Epileptic aphasia: Seminars in Neurology. Philadelphia, PA: Saunders, 1997, pp. 76–84.

Van der Linden G, van Heerden B, Warwick J, et al: Functional brain imaging and pharmacotherapy in social phobia: Single photon emission computed tomography before and after treatment with the selective serotonin reuptake inhibitor citalopram. Prog Neuro-Psychopharmacol Biolog Psychiatry 24:419–438, 2000.

Vasey M, Ollendick T: Anxiety, in Sameroff A (ed): Handbook of Developmental Psychopathology. New York: Plenum Press, 2000, pp. 201–211.

Veenstra-Vanderweele J, Cook EH: Genetics of childhood disorders: XLVI. Autism, part 5: Genetics of autism. J Am Acad Child Adolesc Psychiatry 42:116–118, 2003.

Tsatsanis KD, Rourke BP, Klin A, et al: Reduced thalamic volume in high-functioning individuals with autism. Biol Psychiatry 53:121–129, 2003.

Waterhouse L, Morris R, Allen D, et al: Diagnosis and classification of autism. J Autism Dev Disord 26:59–86, 1996

Willey LH: Pretending to be Normal: Living with Asperger's Syndrome. London, UK: Jessica Kingsley Publishers, 1999.

Wing L, Potter D: The epidemiology of autistic spectrum disorders: Is the prevalence rising? Ment Retard Dev Dis Res Rev 8:151–161, 2002.

Zohar AH, Pauls DL, Ratzoni G, et al: Obsessive-compulsive disorder with and without tics in an epidemiological sample of adolescents. Am J Psychiatry 154:274–276, 1997.

Developmental Disabilities: Mental Retardation and Cerebral Palsy

Ruth Nass

Gail Ross

Cerebral palsy
Choreoathetosis
Down syndrome (DS)
Fragile X syndrome (FXS)
Hemiplegia
Hypoxic–ischemic encephalopathy
Mental retardation
Prader-Willi syndrome (PWS)
Williams syndrome (WS)

INTRODUCTION

Two common neurodevelopmental disorders are discussed in this chapter: mental retardation (MR) and cerebral palsy (CP). Though MR and CP may co-occur, each is associated with a wide range of medical causes and conditions. Recent research in MR has focused on genetic advances, defining developmental trajectories, and delineating specific cognitive and behavioral impairments in specific genetically determined MR syndromes (Burack et al., 1998; Howlin, 2002). Current investigations are beginning to address the complex interplay of genes, brain development, and behavior. Several of the better studied genetic disorders associated with MR (Down syndrome, Williams syndrome, Prader-Willi syndrome, fragile X syndrome) will be reviewed in order to highlight the cognitive, behavioral, social, and adaptive variability that occurs in MR. Contemporary research in CP has emphasized its changing epidemiology, risk factors, and etiologic mechanisms in the pre- and perinatal periods (Hagberg et al., 2001; Drummond & Colver, 2002; du Plessiss & Volpe, 2002; Winter et al., 2002). This chapter summarizes recent advances and the specific cognitive and behavioral profile documented in hemiplegic CP (Nass & Stiles, 1996).

MENTAL RETARDATION

Definition

According to the American Association of Mental Retardation (AAMR) (Luckasson et al., 1992), MR has multiple etiologies and serves as a broad construct that assists in educational planning and determining daily living needs of intellectually impaired individuals. MR is defined by two main criteria: (1) an intellectual quotient (IQ) that is less than 70 (or 2 standard deviations below the mean), and (2) difficulties in at least two areas of adaptive functioning that can include communication, self-care, home living, social skills, community involvement, self-direction, health and safety, functional academics, leisure, and work. The AAMR definition links degree of MR severity to the degree of community support that persons require to achieve optimal independence. In this context, mild MR generally implies the need for intermittent support, moderate MR for limited support, severe MR for extensive support, and profound MR for pervasive support. The term minimally conscious state has been recently proposed as a diagnostic category for patients who demonstrate inconsistent but discernible evidence of consciousness (see Chapter 30). Thus, they are neither in a persistent vegetative state, nor are they sufficiently aware to be considered profoundly retarded (Giacino et al., 2002).

The judgment capacity of the MR patient has been an area of contemporary public interest (see Chapters in Section VII, especially Chapter 52). Gudjonsson and colleagues (2000) reported that 75% of a group with MR ranging from mild to severe were able to complete an assessment of their capacity to be interviewed for judicial purposes. The assessment included evaluations of their intellectual ability, memory, acquiescence, suggestibility, and ability to explain concepts relating to an oath to tell the truth. Most of those with a full-scale IQ score above 60 had a basic understanding of the oath, compared with only one third of those with IQ scores between 50 and 59, and none of those with IQ scores

less than 50. Nevertheless, some participants who were unable to understand the oath did understand the words *truth* and *lie*, especially in relation to concrete examples. Wong and colleagues (2000) investigated the capacity to make a valid decision about a clinically required medical test, specifically a blood test. This study included diverse persons with a "mental disability" (i.e., schizophrenia, mental retardation, and dementia). Results indicated that, compared with the general population, MR individuals were significantly more impaired in the capacity to make such a decision. Similar findings were evident in the dementia group, but the schizophrenia group was not impaired. All three groups benefited from simplification of the task, such that answering did not tax subjects' limited expressive language skills.

The degree of mental retardation can be gauged by IQ scores. Standardized IQ tests are psychometrically designed to have a mean score of 100 and a standard deviation of 15. On this quantitative basis, mild MR is defined by an IQ score between 55 and 70; moderate MR by an IQ score between 35 and 50; severe MR by an IQ score between 20 and 35; and profound MR by an IQ score less than 20 (American Psychiatric Association, 2000). There is wide variability in the level of adaptive functioning shown by children with IQs around 70. About one half require special education and one half attend regular school with learning support services. Those who require special education are more likely to have a personal or family history of language delay (Rutter et al., 1996). Such differences in functional level of children with similar IQ highlight the need to carefully examine the specific cognitive and behavioral profile of those with MR, as described in the section following.

Epidemiology

Prevalence of MR in industrialized countries is reported to be 1% to 3%, with mild MR predominating (75%–80%) (Roeleveld et al., 1997). Individuals with severe MR are more likely to have an identifiable biologic cause. Children with mild MR tend to come from socially disadvantaged backgrounds (Roeleveld et al., 1997; Stromme & Magnus, 2000). Attendant risk factors include:

- Poverty
- New immigrant status
- Language and cultural barriers
- Suboptimal or poor living conditions
- Child neglect and abuse
- Poor intellectual stimulation
- Prenatal risk factors, including smoking and suboptimal perinatal care
- Nutritional deficiencies
- Parental psychopathology and bias to labeling children as mentally retarded

Children with MR often have a family history of borderline IQ or mild retardation. The risk of familial recurrence of severe MR is 3% to 10% and of mild MR 5% to 40% (Hodgson, 1998). With advanced technology, deletions in the subtelomeric chromosomal regions have been found to underlie about 3.5% of previously undiagnosed cases of MR (Leonard & Wen, 2002).

More boys than girls (1.4:1) are diagnosed with MR, primarily in the mild range. Males predominate among MR patients with autism, nonsyndromal mental retardation (Opitz, 2000) (in contrast to specific syndromes like Russell Silver or Treacher Collins, for example), and X-linked monogenic disorders. More than 150 known mental retardation syndromes show an X-linked inheritance pattern (Partington et al., 2000). Within the last 5 years, specific X-linked gene abnormalities have been identified in 15 syndromes causing severe MR and in 8 syndromes causing moderate MR (Leonard & Wen, 2002). Fragile X syndrome (FXS) has been considered the most frequent X-linked disorder known to occur among the moderately handicapped. It is thought to occur with even higher frequency in mild MR. Nonspecific X-linked MR (XLMR) refers to conditions in which genetic etiology remains unknown. These occur with a prevalence of 2.5/10,000, which is three times greater than FXS. Diagnosis of XLMR may be difficult because most males with XLMR do not yet have specifiable phenotypic, neurologic, or biochemical features. Advances in genetic technology should continue to clarify these ambiguities.

Associated Conditions

Sensory deficits such as blindness or deafness are estimated to occur in 2% of mild MR individuals and 11% of the severe MR. Cerebral palsy (described in more detail in the section following) occurs in 6% to 8% of the mildly retarded and as many as 30% of the severely retarded.

Epilepsy is an important comorbid feature of MR. Its frequency varies according to the severity and the cause of the retardation as well as the presence of additional disabilities (see Chapter 45 on Pediatric Epilepsy). In one large epidemiologic study, one fifth of MR children were diagnosed with epilepsy by 10 years of age (Airaksinen et al., 2000). As many as 35% of those with severe MR are diagnosed with epilepsy, in comparison with 7% of those with mild MR. Postnatal causes of mental retardation (like infection or trauma) or associated CP also increase the risk for epilepsy, especially in mild MR. When these risk factors were not present, children with mild MR had only a 3% risk for epilepsy.

Diagnosis

A large number of diagnostic instruments are available to aid in the assessment of children's general intellectual level in different age groups, with additional physical disabilities (e.g., blindness, deafness, cerebral palsy) and with specific cognitive impairments such as severe language disorders (Table 44-1 shows summary).

TABLE 44-1. Standardized Instruments for Intellectual, Sensory, Language, and Motor Assessment in Mental Retardation

Name of test	Age range	Description
General intelligence		
Brigance Diagnostic Inventory of Early Development	0–7 yr	Diagnoses developmental delays
Battele Developmental Inventory	0–8 yr	Examines developmental strengths/weaknesses
Bayley Scales of Infant Development II (BSID II)	1 mo–42 mo	Measures cognitive and motor development
Kaufman Infant & Preschool Scale	1 mo–4 yr	Measures cognitive processes
Cattell Infant Intelligence Scale	3–30 mo	Measures development progress
Stanford-Binet Scale of Intelligence	2 yr–adult	Intelligence and cognitive ability
McCarthy Scales of Children's Abilities	2.5–8.5 yr	Intelligence and motor development
First Step	2.9–6.2 yr	Identifies preschoolers at risk for delays, can be administered to a group
Miler Assessment for Preschoolers	2.9–5.8 yr	Assess development delays
Wechsler Preschool and Primary Scales of Intelligence—R (WPPSI)	3–7.3 yr	Intelligence in young children
Wechsler Intelligence Scale for Children—3 (WISC)	6–16 yr	Intelligence in children
Hammill Multiability Intelligence Test	6–17 yr	Measure of general intelligence
Kaufman Adolescent & Adult Intelligence Test	11–85 yr	General intelligence
Wechsler Adult Intelligence Scale (WAIS)	16–74 yr	Adolescent and adult intelligence

Continued

TABLE 44-1. Standardized Instruments for Intellectual, Sensory, Language, and Motor Assessment in Mental Retardation—cont'd

Name of test	Age range	Description
Hearing impairment		
Kahn Intelligence Test	All ages	Measures intelligence in special group—blind, deaf
Naglieri Nonverbal Ability Test	Grades K–12	Screens nonverbal ability; unbiased for children with hearing, motor, or color vision impairment
Snyders-Oomen Nonverbal Intelligence Test-R	2.5–7 yr	Used with children with impaired hearing or who are deaf
Stoellting Brief Nonverbal Intelligence Test	6–20 yr	Measures intelligence, aptitude, nonverbal reasoning; used for individual with communication or thinking disorders (aphasia, deafness, autism, CP)
Language impairment		
Porteus Mazes	All ages	Measures nonverbal mental ability
Cognitive Ability Scale	2–3 yr	Measures cognitive/development problems
		Good for children with poor articulation or who are nonverbal
Leiter International Performance Scale	2–12 yr	Measures general intelligence; untimed
		Good for nonverbal or non–English speaking individuals
Snyders-Oomen Nonverbal Intelligence Test-R	2.5–7 yr	Used with children with impaired hearing or who are deaf
Culture Fair Intelligence Test	4–yr	Measures intelligence without influence of verbal fluency, culture, or education
Stoellting Brief Nonverbal Intelligence Test	6–20 yr	Measures intelligence, aptitude, nonverbal reasoning; used for people with communication or thinking disorders (aphasia, deafness, autism, CP)
Comprehensive Test of Nonverbal Intelligence	6–90 yr	Good for individuals with language and fine motor problem; bilingual or low SES individuals
Test of Nonverbal Intelligence—3rd edition	6–90 yr	Language-free, motor reduced intelligence measure; 15–20-min administration time
SES (low)		
Kaufman Assessment Battery for Children (K ABC)	2.5–12.5 yr	Good for low SES persons
Comprehensive Test of Nonverbal Intelligence	6–90 yr	Good for people with language and fine-motor problem; bilingual or low SES individuals
Short administration time		
Kaufman Brief Intelligence Test	4–90 yr	Short administration time (15–30 min)
Slosson Full Range Intelligence Test	5–21 yr	15–30 min to administer
Test of Nonverbal Intelligence—3rd edition	6–90 yr	Language-free, motor reduced intelligence measure; 15–20-min administration time
Wechsler Abbreviated Scale of intelligence (WASI)	6–89 yr	15–30-min administration time
Visual impairment		
Kahn Intelligence Test	All ages	Measures intelligence in special groups—blind, deaf
Reynell-Zinkin Developmental Scales for Young Children with Visual Impairments	0–5 yr	Good for visually handicapped, but no standardization or reliability
Fine motor		
Comprehensive Test of Nonverbal Intelligence	6–90 yr	Good for individuals with language and fine-motor problems; bilingual or low SES individuals

CP, cerebral palsy; SES, socioeconomic status.

Instruments used to assess the severely cognitively impaired are generally based on parent interview and emphasize everyday living and adaptive skills.

Natural History

Until recently, children with mild to moderate MR were assumed to show delays in all areas of development and to progress slowly to their ultimate level of cognitive and adaptive functioning. The "typical child" with MR was thought to gain skills at about one half the normal rate, plateauing developmentally at the level of a 6- or 7-year-old child. Children with IQs over 55 generally can acquire basic conversational language skills and some develop rudimentary reading skills. In comparison with children with autistic spectrum disorders (ASD), children with MR are more sociable and their language abilities are more aligned with their intelligence (see Chapter 43 on Autistic Spectrum Disorders). Children with profound MR do not progress beyond a newborn's level, including alerting to sound, perhaps recognizing mother, and smiling.

Psychopathology

There is an increased prevalence of psychopathology and maladaptive behavior among children with intellectual disability. In the epidemiologic study of Stromme and Diseth (2000), it was estimated that almost 40% of the total MR population were affected with dual psychiatric diagnoses. These occurred in 42% of those with severe MR and 33% of those with mild MR. The most common comorbidities were hyperactivity and autism. Autistic features have been reported in 9% to 15% of mild MR cases and 12% to 20% of severe MR cases. Table 44-2 provides a summary of specific psychopathology and behavioral problems commonly observed in a number of genetically defined MR syndromes (several are discussed in more detail in later sections).

The increased prevalence of psychopathology in MR has been attributed to several factors. Psychologically, children with MR may have an unrealistic or negative self-image associated with repeated exposure to failure, loss of confidence, "learned helplessness," depression, and related problems. Certain personality and coping styles (e.g., social wariness, disinhibition, and low expectancy or enjoyment of success) may also be associated with psychopathology. These can be expressed as low self-esteem, distrust of self, sadness, depression, dependency, withdrawal, helplessness, and impulsivity (Dykens, 2000). Additional external factors such as degree of familial support and nurturance, parental adjustment and knowledge, and perception of impairment will affect the child's development, range of

TABLE 44-2. Maladaptive Vulnerabilities in Children with Specific Genetic Syndromes

Down syndrome. Noncompliance, stubbornness, inattention, overactivity, argumentative, withdrawn (depression and dementia among adults).

Williams syndrome. Anxiety, fears, phobias, inattention, hyperactivity, social disinhibition, hypersocial, indiscriminate relating, sensitive, emphatic.

Prader-Willi Syndrome. Hyperphagia, non–food obsessions and compulsions, skin-picking, temper tantrums, lability, perseveration, stubbornness, underactivity.

Fragile X syndrome. Social anxiety, shyness, gaze aversion, perseveration, autism/PDD, inattention, hyperactivity, sadness/depression (primarily females).

Smith-Magenis Syndrome. Inattention, hyperactivity, aggression, attention-seeking, self-injury, stereotypies (often with mouth, self-hugging, flip and lick), sleep disturbance.

Cri du chat syndrome. Infantile high-pitched catlike cry, hyperactivity, inattention, stereotypies, self-injury, social, interests in communicating.

FS syndrome. Affability, hyperactivity, socially oriented, attention-seeking behaviors, excessive talkativeness.

Smith Lemli Opitz. Sensory hypersensitivity, irritability, aggression, sleep disturbances, self-injurious behaviors, stereotypies (opisthokinesis 50%), autistic features (50%).

Velocardiofacial syndrome. Withdrawn, socially isolated, extremes of behavior ranging from very shy to disinhibited, aggressive; bland affect; often described as bland, uncommunicative, fearful, phobic, ADHD, adult schizophrenia, schizoaffective disorder, and bipolar disorder (often rapid cycling).

ADHD, attention-deficit/hyperactivity disorder; PDD, pervasive developmental disorder.

behavior skills, and interactions. Social problems within or outside the family may also foster psychopathology. Children and adults with intellectual disability are at greater risk for exploitation, physical and emotional abuse, peer rejection, and ostracism. Associated medical conditions described throughout this chapter may also contribute to family and patient stress, caregiver burden, financial pressures, and many other difficulties that affect the child's development and adjustment.

Specific Mental Retardation Syndromes

Down Syndrome

Chromosomal abnormalities are a common cause of severe mental retardation (Jones, 1994). Down syndrome (DS) (trisomy 21) is the most common chromosomal disorder associated with moderate to severe MR. It accounts for one third of cases and occurs at a rate of 1.5 per 1000 live births (Carr, 2002). A small region in the distal part of the long arm of chromosome 21 appears to be the critical locus for DS, but other regions also contribute to the full phenotype.

DS causes characteristic dysmorphic features that are generally recognizable at birth. These include flat face, upslanting palpebral fissures, epicanthal folds, small nose with low nasal bridge, anomalous ears, and simian creases. Major organ systems can be affected as well in DS, especially the heart (40% of cases). Atrial ventricular communication cushion defects are particularly common (Jones, 1994). DS children have also been reported to have moya-moya syndrome—basal ganglia telangiectasia (de Borchgrave et al., 2002).

Mental age in DS does not keep pace with chronologic age. By adulthood, IQ is generally in the moderate-to-severe MR range (mean IQ, 50; range, 30–70) and mental age is about 7 years. Relative to IQ and other children of similar IQ, the social adaptive skills of children with MR are comparatively strong (Table 44-3).

TABLE 44-3. Vineland Adaptive Behaviors Scale

Syndrome	Communication	Social	Daily living
Down syndrome	↓↓	↑↑	↓
Williams syndrome	↑↑	↑↑↑	↓↓
Fragile X syndrome	↓↓↓	↓	↑↑↑
Pervasive developmental disorder	↓↓	↓↓↓	↓
FG syndrome	↓	↑↑↑	↓↓
Smith-Magenis syndrome	↓↓	↓↓	↓↓

Arrows indicate relative strength (↑) or weakness (↓) of communication, social and daily living skills in comparison with general intellectual ability.

Spatial skills are generally commensurate with IQ, and nonverbal cognition is superior to language skills (Fowler, 1998; Tager-Flusberg & Sullivan, 1998). Babbling is delayed; articulation, phonology, and expressive grammar are relatively weak; and longer sentences do not contain complex grammar. Verbal short-term memory in DS lags behind mental age and may underlie some speech and language problems because affected children are less able to rehearse speech acts. Despite verbal weaknesses, vocabulary is on par with IQ, and pragmatic conversational abilities are a relative strength. Children with DS can stay on topic and take turns (Chapman & Hesketh, 2000).

Children with DS tend to show fewer maladaptive behaviors and less serious psychopathology than many other children with MR (Dykens & Kasari, 1997; Dykens, 2000) (Table 44-4; see also Tables 44-2 and 44-3). Their relatively preserved social graces may be related to the stereotypic friendly, outgoing, and "Prince Charming" personality, the greater availability of parent support groups, and general public knowledge about DS. The syndrome's characteristic "babyface" may also be protective, because baby-faced persons are generally considered to be warm, kind, naive, honest, cuddly, and compliant (Dykens, 1998). However, children with DS are not problem-free: at least 15% of children and 20% to 40% of adolescents with DS show behavioral or psychiatric difficulties, including disruptive disorders (such as attention-deficit/hyperactivity disorder [ADHD] and conduct disorders), oppositional behavior, anxiety disorders, withdrawn behaviors, executive dysfunction, including problems with impulse control and perseverative behaviors, and, rarely, autism (Dykens & Kasari, 1997; Ghaziuddin, 1997). These traits may increase with advancing age and predict depression in adulthood. There is an increased risk of Alzheimer dementia in DS due to excess amyloid precursor protein production resulting from having trisomy 21. Most adults over 40 years of age have amyloid plaques and neurofibrillary tangles. About one half of those over 50 years show symptoms of dementia (see Chapter 22).

Neuroimaging studies in DS have reported reduced whole brain and grey matter volumes, especially in the frontal lobe. The cerebellum is also reduced in size (Aylward et al., 1997; Bigler et al., 1999), a finding that correlates with reduced motor functioning, but not with autistic features (see following section). Brain perfusion is generally normal, although unilateral hypoperfusion and reduced interaction between frontal and parietal lobes has been reported (Gokcora et al., 1999).

Williams Syndrome

Williams syndrome (WS) is a multisystem neurodevelopmental disorder that occurs in 1/20,000 births. It is usually caused by a 1.5Mb deletion involving at least

TABLE 44-4. Achenbach's Child Behavior Checklist Scores in Various Mental Retardation (MR) Syndromes

Syndrome and characteristics	Internalizing (percentile)	Externalizing (percentile)	Total behavior score (percentile)	Attention (percentile)
Down syndrome (DS) (IQ 48) moderate MR	55	50	70	84
Williams syndrome (WS) (IQ 66) mild–moderate MR	70	80	96	>98
Prader-Willi syndrome (PWS) (IQ 69) MR	68	90	93	96
Prader-Willi syndrome (IQ 63) deletion	>98	96	96	
Prader-Willi syndrome (IQ 71) UPD	84	80	68	
SM (IQ 50) moderate MR*	84	>98	>98	>98
FG moderate MR	<50	54	80	90
Mixed MR (IQ 60) moderate MR	51	80	82	96

* Often misdiagnosed as PW

The 50th percentile is the basal score for normal children ages 5 to 18 years. The 96th to 98 percentile is considered the grey zone for problems. Greater than the 98th percentile is a problem area. Attention is an issue in WS, PWS, SM, Mixed MR. Internalizing behaviors (e.g., anxiety, somatic complaints) are special issues in PWS. Externalizing behaviors (e.g., hyperactivity, aggression) are special issues in PWS and SM. Behavioral problems, in general, are issues in WS, PWS, and SM.

16 genes on chromosome 7 (7q11.23). Findings in several kindreds with smaller deletions suggest that the gene for LIM kinase 1 may correlate with visuospatial constructional ability in WS. The lower IQ of a few patients with larger deletions suggests that some genes responsible for cognitive functioning are located close to the classic WS deletion (Morris & Mervis, 2000).

Facial features in WS are characteristically "elfin-like," with full cheeks and lips, a bulbous nose and long philtrum, and small, widely spaced teeth. Cardiac anomalies are relatively common, particularly supravalvular aortic stenosis.

Seventy-five percent of children with WS have MR, which varies between mild and moderate (mean IQ 66). Range of adaptive behaviors are generally commensurate with overall IQ. Communication and social skills tend to be better developed than independent living skills (see Table 44-3). Individuals with WS show variable patterns of cognitive development and decline. For example, some WS individuals show good numeric judgment and poor language skills at any early age, but show the reverse pattern of abilities and disabilities in adulthood (Paterson, 1999). These findings underscore the dynamic interactions among genes, brain, and behavioral development. More specifically, different genetic disorders have diverse effects on cognitive domains that can change further throughout development.

There are many other cognitive aspects in WS. Language is often superior to and develops faster than nonverbal cognition (Jarrold et al., 1998). This pattern is opposite that in DS. Although language development in WS is delayed, expressive and (to a lesser degree) receptive vocabulary ultimately exceed mental age expectation. While individuals with WS achieve adult-level

grammatical systems, some studies suggest that grammatical difficulties exceed those in other MR syndromes, and resemble bilingual non-native speakers (Karmiloff-Smith et al., 1998). Pragmatics and conversational abilities are areas of strength in WS (Tager-Flusberg & Sullivan, 2000), although extreme loquaciousness may be a disadvantage. Evoked-response potential (ERP) studies have demonstrated that despite spared verbal skills, cerebral organization for language is atypical (as can be the case in bilingual persons) and not fully localized to the left hemisphere (Mills et al., 2000).

Individuals with WS show marked visuospatial, visuoconstructional, and global processing deficits. By contrast, they tend to perform well on face recognition tasks from the outset and show continuing improvement with age. However, ERP studies indicate that neurophysiologic markers of facial recognition are atypical (Mills et al., 2000). WS subjects may not show the same responses as controls to upright versus inverted faces. Consistent with their hypersocial behavior, they rate approachability based on facial expressions excessively positively (Bellugi et al., 1999).

Individuals with WS show relatively strong auditory verbal memory skills. Procedural memory and visuospatial short-term memory are areas of deficit (in contrast to DS, where verbal short-term memory is impaired). Executive function deficits have also been reported, such as difficulty staying on task. Performance on theory of mind tasks, however, is relatively spared (Baron-Cohen, 1998; Bellugi et al., 1999) (see Chapter 43 on Autism Spectrum Disorders). In this respect their abilities are more advanced than individuals with Prader-Willi syndrome (see later section) and with nonspecified MR. However, the individuals with WS tend to perform poorly in other areas of social cognition (e.g., on tasks that probe detection of false belief, irony), suggesting that distinct cognitive modules may underlie different components of theory of mind (Tager-Flusberg & Sullivan, 2000).

The behavior of WS children is typically charming, outgoing, friendly, and empathetic (Dykens & Rosner, 1999). They may even show hypersociability beginning at an early age; toddlers with WS rarely show stranger anxiety. Individuals with WS are apt to draw attention to themselves, relate indiscriminately to others, and yet maintain fewer friends than their IQ-matched counterparts. They risk exploitation and abuse as a result of their social disinhibition (Dykens & Rosner, 1999). Despite their highly sociable nature, 60% to 70% of individuals with WS have high total problem scores on the Child Behavior Checklist (see Table 44-4). This is especially evident on the attention scale. Many children are described as hyperactive. Anxiety becomes more of a problem, with 50% eventually showing generalized or anticipatory anxiety (Dykens & Rosner, 1999). When combined with fears, worries, and phobias, these behavioral and emotional characteristics may contribute to the difficult temperament sometimes ascribed to WS. Personality characteristics in WS may change over time. Adults become less lively, determined, and active, as well as more restless, tearful, aggressive, quarrelsome, impertinent, and overly friendly. Adolescents and adults are often assessed as being better balanced than children, despite being more withdrawn and having more depressive symptoms than children (Gosch & Pankau, 1997).

Brain imaging and autopsy findings are compatible with the overall behavioral and cognitive profile. Some structures considered to be related to social behaviors (frontal and limbic regions) are relatively spared (Galaburda & Bellugi, 2000). However, abnormalities in the amygdala have been reported. This subcortical region is responsible for the perception of emotional facial expressions. WS patients can appreciate emotional facial expressions, but, like patients with bilateral amygdala damage, they give abnormally positive ratings to facial expressions (Bellugi et al., 1999). Autistic patients show decreased metabolic activity in the amygdala when they attempt unsuccessfully to process facial expressions. The cerebellum, another area reported to be abnormal in autism (see Chapter 25), has been found to be abnormal in some studies of WS patients, but not in others (e.g., Radda et al., 1998; Galaburda & Bellugi, 2000). Various absolute and relative abnormalities of the parietal and occipital regions have been described (Reiss et al., 2000) and could relate to the visuospatial processing deficits characteristic of WS.

Prader-Willi Syndrome

Prader-Willi syndrome (PWS) has an incidence of about 1 in 12,000 live births. Most cases (70%) are caused by a paternally inherited deletion on chromosome 15 (15q11-q13). Some cases are due to a maternal uniparental disomy (UPD), in which both copies of chromosome 15 are of maternal origin. In typical PWS, the abnormal paternally donated chromosome expresses (imprints) multiple abnormal genes in the PWS region, while the maternal chromosome is largely silent. In maternal UPD the genes in the PWS region are not expressed from either chromosome. As a result, despite the presence of two intact chromosomes, there is a functional abnormality that is largely equivalent to the structural abnormality found in the more common 15q11-q13 deletion. The importance of imprinting is further highlighted by the existence of a genetic "mirror image" syndrome to PWS, described as Angelman syndrome. Here, the abnormality is on the maternal chromosome. The latter syndrome is characterized by severe to profound MR, and microcephaly, seizures, ataxic gait, and bouts of inappropriate laughter. Abnormalities of the small nuclear ribonucleoprotein associated polypeptide N (involved in protein splicing throughout the brain) may play a role in PWS. Genes regulating subunits of GABA receptors are probably located in the deleted region of chromosome 15 as well (State & Dykens, 2000).

Individuals with PWS have characteristic facial features (upslanting almond-shaped palpebral fissures, light skin and hair, and blue eyes), hypotonia, short stature, small hands and feet, and hypogonadism.

MR is generally mild to moderate in PWS, with a mean IQ of 70, which is high relative to other genetic mental retardation syndromes. There is, however, a wide range of IQs from profoundly retarded to average. Those with deletions have lower IQs (mean 63) than those with UPD (mean 71) (Dykens et al., 1999). Adaptively (see Table 44-3), however, even those with normal IQ rarely function at a level commensurate with their IQ, usually because of their compulsive eating and other behavioral problems (see text following). IQ remains stable with advancing age.

Individuals with PWS have oral motor dysfunction. Expressive vocabulary is a relative strength, but a specific language profile has not been described. Individuals with PWS have a particular interest in word search puzzles.

Weaknesses have commonly been noted in sequential processing (Akefeldt et al., 1997). In sharp contrast to WS, individuals with PWS have relative strengths in spatial-perceptual organization, visuospatial integration, and visual processing. An unusual interest in jigsaw puzzles is common in PWS (Dykens, 1999). Individuals with PWS show weaknesses in short-term memory tasks, particularly those involving motor and auditory modalities. Relative strengths are observed in visual long-term memory.

Children and adults with PWS suffer from a number of behavioral and psychiatric problems. Severe temper tantrums, impulsivity, and stubbornness are common. They have more internalizing symptoms (e.g., withdrawn, somatic complaints, anxious/depressed), externalizing problems (delinquent and aggressive behaviors), and a higher total problem behavior score than most other patients with MR (see Table 44-4). Individuals with PWS differed from other groups (e.g., DS and nonspecific MR groups) in several Child Behavior Checklist (CBCL) items, including skin picking, excessive arguing, obsessing, underactivity, overeating, talking too much, sleeping excessively, obesity, fatigue, compulsions, stealing, and getting teased (Dykens, 1999, 2000) (Table 44-5).

PWS is best known for abnormalities of hyperphagia and intense food preoccupation. PWS individuals appear to lack satiation and to display incessant food-seeking behavior. The eating disorder is usually apparent by 2 years of age, and obesity can quickly ensue. Eating behaviors can be odd, and include choosing unappealing foods such as a stick of butter or even garbage. Compared with WS and obese controls, individuals with PWS switch from food to food less often, and ritualized eating behaviors are more prominent. More than 60% of cases show obsessive-compulsive symptoms with moderate to severe levels of symptom-related distress and adaptive impairment. Symptoms are of similar type and severity to those found in nonretarded individuals with obsessive-compulsive disorders (OCD), and include hoarding, arranging, needing to tell or ask, and counting, as well as repetitive self-injurious behaviors like skin-picking (33%–97%). Both OCD and self-injurious behaviors are more frequent in those with deletions than with UPD (Dykens et al., 1999). On rare occasions PWS is associated with autism, generally co-occurring with a relatively low IQ. This is in contrast to the frequent association of autism with fragile X syndrome (see discussion following).

PWS is associated with a combination of abnormal food intake regulation, delayed sexual development, sleep irregularities, difficulties with thermoregulation, and growth hormone problems that all point to the hypothalamus as key region of pathophysiology (Dimiropoulos et al., 2000). Magnetic resonance imaging (MRI) studies in PWS suggest functional abnormalities in the hypothalamus.

Fragile X Syndrome

Fragile X syndrome (FXS) is generally considered the most common currently known cause of inherited mental retardation, occurring in 1/1000 males and 1/2000 females. The FXS gene (FMR-1) contains an excessive number of triplet repeats. Approximately 5 to 50 triplet repeats occur normally. In premutations (pM), which are not associated with symptoms, triplet repeats number from 50 to between 200 and 500. In the full mutation (fM), the triplet repeats expand up to 3000 repeats and result in mental retardation in more than 95% of males and nearly one half of females. The triplet repeat area is unstable and repeats numbering in the premutation range tend to increase with each generation. Disease severity generally parallels number of repeats. Thus, succeeding generations are more likely to have more severe disease, a process known as generational anticipation. While chromosome studies can detect males with FXS, DNA studies may be required to detect female heterozygotes.

Characteristic facial features in FXS include a long, narrow face, hypoplastic midface, enlarged protuberant ears; macro-orchidism is commonly present after puberty.

Moderate to severe mental retardation is common in males with FXS, affecting up to 80% of cases. IQ ranges from 20 to 50, with an average of about 35. Mild to moderate MR is the modal presentation in affected females. There are interactive effects of age and IQ (Bailey et al., 1998). Boys with FXS tend to have a stable IQ in the mildly retarded range until puberty, when IQ declines. Many boys with FXS demonstrate relative strengths in adaptive functioning, but these too decline after puberty. Girls with FXS do not show as much IQ decline (Fisch et al., 1999). Fully methylated individuals are more likely to show a decline. Approximately 10% of affected males develop seizures, which may also contribute to declining IQ.

Boys with FXS have particular problems with articulation and with rate and fluency of speech production

TABLE 44-5. Behavioral Characteristics That Differentiate Three Mental Retardation (MR) Syndromes

Behavior	Prader-Willi syndrome	Down syndrome	Mixed MR
Skin-picking	High	Low	Low
Excessive fatigue	High	Low	Low
Obsessions	High	Low	Low
Impulsive behavior	High	Low	High
Speech problems	High	High	Low
Excessive talking	High	Low	Low/high
Hyperactivity	Low	Low	High

Data from Achenbach TM, Rescurla L: Child Behavior Checklist. Burlington, VT: University of Vermont, 2001.

that result in cluttering, a form of verbal dyspraxia. These problems do not correlate with mental age or IQ (Tager-Flusberg & Sullivan, 1998). Receptive and expressive vocabulary are strengths, but word retrieval difficulties may underlie their tendency toward perseveration (Fowler, 1998). Syntactic development is delayed, and longer utterances are not paralleled by more complex grammar. Like autistic children, those with FXS may use words idiosyncratically; pragmatics and conversational abilities are relatively weak.

Males with FXS tend to show task-specific rather than global deficits in spatial abilities, with visuoconstructive and visuomotor skills most vulnerable. Interestingly, performance on tasks with a visuoperceptual component correlate negatively with expansion of triplet repeat size (Cornish et al., 1999). Recognition of emotional facial expression is normal, similar to WS but unlike autism (Turk & Cornish, 1998).

Males with FXS score poorly on short-term memory tasks that require repetition of sentences and bead patterns, but not on tasks measuring memory for objects. Long-term verbal memory is a relative strength, as in autistic children. Individuals with FXS often show deficits in attention and executive function (e.g., formulating a multistep plan and shifting cognitive sets) (Hagerman & Hagerman, 2002).

The cognitive deficits in females with FXS are similar to affected males but less pronounced. Most heterozygotic females with the full fragile X mutation who are not mentally retarded have nonverbal learning disabilities, compromising executive function and spatial memory. Autism in females affected with FXS is rare (Mazzocco et al., 1997).

There is a wide range of behavioral problems reported in males with FXS. These include ADHD, impulsivity, aggressivity, general anxiety, social anxiety, depression, social disabilities with poor eye contact, shyness, and social withdrawal, poor transitioning, and stereotypies (Mazzocco, 2000). FXS is currently the most commonly known genetic syndrome associated with autism. However, the Rett syndrome mutation (MECP2), now being found in males, is almost equal in frequency (Leonard & Wen, 2002). The majority of males with FXS have some autistic features, and approximately 10% meet criteria for a dual diagnosis of autism. In children diagnosed with autism, 0% to 16% or greater have FXS (Howlin, 2002).

The relationship between triplet repeats and the loss of expression of the fragile X mental retardation protein (FMRP) is thought to be due to methylation, which results in reduced transcription. Morphologic studies raise the possibility that a failure of synapse maturation process occurs in FXS, possibly a failure of synapse elimination. These findings, together with evidence of (1) neurotransmitter activation of the synthesis of FMRP at synapses in vitro, (2) behaviorally induced

FMRP expression in vivo, and (3) the apparent role for FMRP in regulating the synthesis of other proteins, suggest that FMRP serves as an "immediate early protein" at the synapse that orchestrates aspects of synaptic development and plasticity (Irwin et al., 2000). FMR-1 is maximally expressed in the hippocampus, cerebellum, cortex, and nucleus basalis magnocellularis. Number of triplet repeats and level of FMRP correlate with IQ (Menon et al., 2000). Three distinct patterns of FMRP immunoreactivity (-ir) are found in fragile X, as follows:

- FMRP activity (-ir) in individuals with normal and pM alleles as well as most females with fM show the highest levels with multiple approximately 70–80 kDa FMRP-ir bands.
- Males with the fM have only a 70 kDa FMRP-ir band and have the lowest levels of FMRP.
- Females with mosaicism and some females with fM display a doublet with equal amounts of the highest and lowest molecular weight FMRP-ir bands.

Both the FMRP-ir level and the presence of a typical ratio correlated with IQ (Kaufmann et al., 1999). There is a correlation between left hippocampal volume and performance on delayed memory tests observed in pM subjects, but not in fM subjects. Hippocampal volume does not appear to differ between fM and pM groups (Jakala et al., 1997). Neuroanatomical abnormalities that have been reported include decreased size of cerebellum (Mostofsky et al., 1998) and superior temporal gyri, and atypical grey white matter ratio, particularly subcortically and in the context of developmental changes (Eliez et al., 2001). Posterior cerebellar vermis area correlates not only with number of triplet repeats, but with measures of communication and stereotypic/restricted behaviors (Mazzocco, 2000), providing a link with the pathophysiology of autism. By contrast the thalamus, hippocampus, and caudate are enlarged.

Etiology and Evaluation

The diagnostic evaluation of a child with MR may often be unrevealing, although more than 500 genetic diseases are currently known to be associated with MR (Table 44-6). The likelihood of finding a specific diagnosis is inversely related to the degree of retardation. About 70% of children with an IQ less than 50 will have a definable cause of retardation, whereas only about 25% of those with an IQ between 50 and 70 will have a definable cause. Therefore, diagnostic workup should be dictated by individual findings in mild MR children and be more comprehensive the more severe the MR (Murphy et al., 1998). Recognizable syndromes are associated with MR (Jones, 1994), particularly in those who are severely retarded, where about one third have

TABLE 44-6. Causes of Mental Retardation

Prenatal
  Genetic
    Chromosomal (Down syndrome, trisomy 18)
    Syndromic nonchromosomal (Treacher Collins,
      Smith-Opitz)
    Neurocutaneous syndromes (tuberous sclerosis)
  Metabolic
    Amino and organic acidopathies (phenylketonuria
      untreated, maple syrup urine)
    Mitochondrial disorders with lactic acidosis
    Mucopolysaccharidosis and mucolipidosis
    Sialidosis
    Carbohydrate-deficient glycoprotein syndromes
    Hypothyroidism (untreated)
  Malformations (lissencephaly, holoprosencephaly)
  Congenital infections (cytomegalic virus, syphilis,
    toxoplasmosis, rubella, HIV)
  Teratogens and toxins (fetal alcohol syndrome, fetal
    hydantoin syndrome)
  Intrauterine growth retardation (placental insufficiency,
    preeclampsia)
Perinatal
  Infections (herpes, HIV)
  Prematurity
Postnatal
  Trauma
  Infection (meningitis, encephalitis)
  Epileptic encephalopathy (Lennox Gastaut)
  Environmental (malnutrition, lead encephalopathy)
  Psychosocial disorder

Data from Fenichel GM: in Clinical Pediatric Neurology: A Signs
and Symptoms Approach, ed 4. Philadelphia: Saunders, 2001,
pp. 117–147.

an identifiable syndrome. Brain imaging may show nonspecific abnormalities; dysplastic brain malformations are being increasingly described as the resolution of neuroimaging improves. At the molecular level, a model of genotype to neurologic phenotype pathway in MR has been postulated, centered in dendritic abnormalities (Table 44-7) (Kaufman & Moser, 2000).

A recent position paper recommended the following guidelines for several practice parameters (Shevell et al., 2003):

- Routine metabolic screening for inborn errors of metabolism was not considered indicated in the initial evaluation of a child with global developmental delay, provided that universal newborn screening had been performed and the results are available for review (given the low yield of about 1%).
- Routine cytogenetic testing (yield of 3.7%) was considered indicated.
- Testing for fragile X (yield of 2.6%), particularly in the presence of a family history of developmental delay, could be considered.
- Screening for Rett syndrome should be considered in females with unexplained moderate to severe mental retardation.
- In children with unexplained moderate or severe developmental delay, additional testing using newer molecular techniques (e.g., FISH, microsatellite markers) to assess for subtelomeric chromosomal rearrangements (yield 6.6%) may be considered.
- Audiologic and ophthalmologic screening was recommended in all children with global developmental delay.
- Imaging studies are indicated in the face of their relatively high, albeit sometimes nonspecific, yield.

Treatment

Medical treatment focuses mainly on the management of behavioral problems (Matson et al., 2000). Some patients need neuroleptic medications to manage maladaptive behavior. Treatment with selective serotonin reuptake inhibitors (SSRIs) helps curb impulsive, compulsive, and aggressive behaviors. PWS patients in particular need in that regard. Some MR patients, however, may become disinhibited when taking SSRIs. Hence, dosing should be conservative and increased under careful follow-up observation. Stimulants are sometimes useful in the treatment of behavioral symptoms of hyperactivity and aggressivity. Other classes of antidepressants may be

TABLE 44-7. Cerebral Substrate of Mental Retardation: Different Dendritic Abnormalities

Syndrome	Laminar distribution	Packing density	Dendrite length	Spine dysgenesis
Down syndrome	Yes	No	Yes	Yes
Williams syndrome	Yes	Yes	?	?
Fragile X syndrome	No	No	No	Yes
Rett syndrome	No	Yes	Yes	Yes

Data from Kaufmann WE, Moser HW: Dendritic anomalies in disorders associated with mental retardation. Cereb Cortex 10:981–991, 2000.

necessary at certain times in some patients. Obesity in PWS is optimally managed by behavioral modification, although stimulants may prove useful supplements. When social behavior is problematic, behaviorally based social skills training and social support systems can be considered. These interventions can help those who are hypersocial (WS) as well as those who are hyposocial. Other nonmedical treatments focus on finding the appropriate educational setting, delineating learning support services, and vocational training for mild and moderate MR individuals. The most pressing issue for severe and profound MR individuals is determining home/institutional care. From a medical perspective, prevention is also increasingly possible via prenatal genetic diagnosis and counseling (Leonard & Wen, 2002).

It is important to note that individuals with MR may develop medical disorders apart from MR and be unable to articulate their symptoms, understand tests, and evaluate treatments. For example, individuals with DS and WS sometimes have cardiac defects that require continuous monitoring. Careful assessment is important in these individuals who cannot advocate for themselves.

In summary, MR refers to diverse neurodevelopmental disorders that are characterized by intellectual deficiencies and a wide range of symptoms and causes. Recent studies have identified a number of MR syndromes that have differing cognitive, behavioral, and developmental profiles. Delineating the cause of MR in any given child is currently more likely to be unknown, but rapid advances in genetics are expected to improve diagnostic capabilities. Treatment services are multifaceted and can include pharmacologic, behavioral, rehabilitative (e.g., physical, occupational, speech, and cognitive therapies), and educational options that are designed to target specific symptoms.

CEREBRAL PALSY

Definition

Cerebral palsy (CP) is an umbrella term that refers to nonprogressive motor system impairments resulting from central nervous system injuries. Any simple definition of CP is difficult, because the disorder has diverse causes and the motor symptoms take many forms. Although some describe postnatal injury during infancy and in early childhood as CP, we will focus on cases occurring in utero or around the time of birth (perinatal period). Although the underlying brain damage is static, the symptoms of the motor impairment may change as the child develops and motor demands increase.

Classification

The most commonly used classifications of CP are: spastic, extrapyramidal or choreoathetoid (also called dyskinetic), and ataxic. Some children are diagnosed with a mixed picture of clinical deficits that are usually a combination of spastic and athetoid characteristics (Table 44-8).

Spastic CP, the most common form, results from dysfunction of the corticospinal tracts, which leads to increased muscle tone, hyperreflexia, and the prolonged persistence of primitive reflexes (e.g., Moro reflex, tonic neck reflex), which in the normal child disappear during the first few months. As a result of increased tone, contractures may develop. Spastic CP is further divided into three types—diplegia, hemiplegia, and quadriplegia, based on the areas of the body that are most affected. These types occur with about equal frequency, although the etiologies differ (see text following) (Niswander & Gordon, 1972; Hagberg et al., 2001).

TABLE 44-8. Classification of Cerebral Palsy

Type	Incidence (%)	Description	Area of lesion
Spastic	70	Muscles are stiff and contractures may occur	Corticospinal tracts
Diplegia			
Hemiplegia			
Quadriplegia			
Extrapyramidal (choreoathetoid)	10–15	Slow, writhing can be punctuated by jerky movements	Basal ganglia damage
Ataxic	5–10	Poor balance and depth perception; poor coordination; difficulty in performing precise movements; intention tremor	Cerebellar damage
Mixed	15	Most often a combination of spastic and athetoid movements	Varied

Spastic diplegia is characterized by bilateral spasticity with more involvement of the legs than the arms. In infancy the legs are straight with the feet extended, adducted, and crossed over each other (scissoring). When individuals with diplegia walk, their legs move stiffly and nearly touch at the knees, resulting in a characteristic gait. Spastic diplegia is generally the result of preterm birth; periventricular leukomalacia (PVL) is the most frequent underlying pathology (Bracewell & Marlow, 2002).

Spastic hemiplegia involves unilateral spasticity of the arm, leg, and face, with the arm involved more than the leg. The face is often spared. The involved limbs are often slightly atrophic. A less broad thumb nail bed is characteristic. The affected leg, especially the heel cord, is shortened, resulting in toe walking. Individuals with spastic hemiplegia show early hand preference, since they cannot use to varying degrees and/or neglect the hand contralateral to the lesion. In some instances late onset dystonia develops in the spastic limbs (Nardocci et al., 1996). Synkinesis (involuntary movements of muscles or limbs following voluntary movements) in both the involved and uninvolved limbs is also common during precision movements (Nass, 1985). Spastic hemiparesis in the term infant is generally the result of an infarction in the middle cerebral artery territory. In the preterm infant it is often the result of a grade 4 intraventricular hemorrhage with focal white matter infarction.

Spastic quadriparesis involves all four limbs, generally in a symmetric fashion. Often the child is not ambulatory. Hand function may be sufficiently compromised to necessitate feeding by others or gastrostomy tube feedings. Spastic quadriparesis is generally the result of a severe hypoxic ischemic insult or a congenital brain malformation or a metabolic abnormality. Cognitive impairments are frequently associated with spastic quadriparesis.

Extrapyramidal (dyskinetic) or choreoathetoid CP is characterized by involuntary writhing (athetosis) of the face, tongue, hands, and feet, that can be punctuated and overridden by chorea (jerking movements) of the trunk, arms, and legs. Choreoathetosis interferes with both gross and fine motor activity, as well as with maintaining posture. The classic, although now rare, cause is kernicterus, in which high bilirubin levels in jaundiced infants result in toxic damage to the basal ganglia. The auditory pathways are also susceptible to damage, and thus hearing impairments often are seen in this type of CP. Hypoxic ischemic insults can also cause choreoathetoid CP (Volpe, 2000).

Ataxic CP, which occurs rarely, affects balance and depth perception. Individuals with this form of CP often have poor coordination, walk unsteadily with a wide-based gait, show difficulty in performing quick or precise movements, and may have an intention tremor.

Metabolic and hereditary causes are the most common etiologies of ataxic CP.

Mixed forms are generally combinations of spastic and choreoathetoid CP. They represent the most extensive form of central nervous system injury. Some children who ultimately develop spastic or ataxic CP are hypotonic in infancy.

Like many other neurodevelopmental disorders, CP is often classified as mild, moderate, or severe. Some authors have classified CP based on functional disability (disabling vs. nondisabling CP). For example, one group (Pinto-Martin et al., 1995) bases the diagnosis of disabling CP on the presence of any one of the following criteria:

1. Inability to walk five steps unaided by 2 years of age
2. Psychomotor development index more than one standard deviation less than the mental development index
3. Physical therapy or surgery for motor disability
4. Use of braces or other assisting devices

It is sometimes difficult to distinguish mild or nondisabling CP from neurologic "soft signs" or delayed motor development (Touwen, 1979). Hence, it has been argued that the term *CP* should be limited to children whose motor findings are severe enough to cause true interference with normal functioning (O' Shea et al., 1998).

Epidemiology

CP is estimated to occur in from 1.5 to 3 in 1000 live births (Topp et al., 2001; Hagberg et al., 2001; Drummond & Colver, 2002; Winter et al., 2002). Although low birthweight infants (<2500 g) account for approximately 7% of all births, they currently comprise one third to one half of all CP cases (Pharoah et al., 1996). In a population-based study (Hagberg et al., 1996), the specific prevalence per 1000 was 57 for infants with birth weights <1000 g; 68 for infants with birth weights between 1000 and 1499 g; 14 for those with birth weights between 1500 and 2499 g; and 1.4 for infants with birth weights greater than or equal to 2500 g. Spastic hemiplegic, diplegic, and quadriplegic syndromes accounted for 22%, 66%, and 7% of CP in preterm infants; and 44%, 29%, and 10% of that in term infants. Thus, diplegic CP is most commonly found in preterm infants, and hemiplegic CP in term infants.

Despite improved pre- and perinatal care with resulting decreases in perinatal deaths and hypoxic ischemic insults (as measured by low Apgar scores), there has been no apparent decline over the past two decades in the occurrence of CP among term infants (Blair, 2001; Hagberg et al., 2001). Indeed, some population-based studies suggest an increasing incidence of CP over the past 25 years. The incidence of CP increased from 1.7 to 2.0 per 1000 children during the period from 1975 to 1991 in a population-based study in Atlanta, GA (Winter et al., 2002). This increase in CP was attributable to a modest rise in CP in infants of normal birth weight from 17% in 1975 to 1977 to 39% in 1986 to 1991. For children with birth weights less than 1500 g, the proportion of children with spastic diplegia increased over time from 7% of the cases in 1975 through 1988 to 36% in 1985 to 1988, and 32% in 1986 to 1991. Another population based study in northeast England found an increase from 1.6 to 2.3 per 1000 in the periods from 1970 to 1975 to 1990 to 1994 (Drummond & Colver, 2002). While there was little change in the rate of CP in term infants, in premature infants (<37 weeks gestational age), it rose from 5.5 to 16.8 per 1000. The rises occurred in three gestational age groups: less than 28, 28 to 31 weeks, and 32 to 36 weeks, with the greatest rise in the less than 28-week group. Presumably, extremely preterm infants are surviving more often, but are left with significant neurologic residua (O'Shea et al., 1998).

Associated Conditions

MR and epilepsy are the conditions commonly associated with CP, and their frequency increases with level of the motoric involvement. Estimates of the frequency of MR (defined as IQ scores of 69 or below), range from 10% to 75% and depend on type of CP as well as degree of severity. MR occurs in less than 10% of children with choreoathetosis 25% with diplegia, 25% to 50% with hemiplegia (depending on etiology), and as many as 75% with quadriplegia. Approximately one third of children with CP have epilepsy (Senbil et al., 2002), either generalized or partial (see Chapter 45). CP may also be associated with other developmental problems, including failure to thrive, hyperactivity, learning disabilities, dysarthria, and hearing impairments. Visual impairments, such as strabismus and hemianopia in children with hemiplegia are common (Guzzetta et al., 2001). If left untreated, strabismus can lead to poor vision in one eye and can interfere with certain visual skills, such as depth perception. Children with severe CP may also have problems with drooling (Blasco, 2002), eating and swallowing, and incontinence, due to poor muscle control. Of the 1649 cases of cerebral palsy registered in the late 1980s in England and Scotland, 550 (33.4%) were nonambulatory, 390 (23.7%) had severe manual disability (incapable of feeding or dressing unaided), 381 (23.1%) were mentally retarded (IQ <50), 146 (8.9%) had severe visual disability (vision <6/60 in the better eye), and 12 had severe hearing disability (>70 dB loss) (Pharoah et al., 1998). Children who are immobile and who require feeding through a gastrostomy tube have severely curtailed life expectancy (Strauss et al., 1997).

Diagnosis and Natural History

Identifying cases of CP may be problematic because examiners sometimes disagree on the degree of deficit required (see previous discussion). In addition, there are changes in clinical findings over time, due to developmental changes in the nervous system during infancy and early childhood.

Diagnosis of CP is based on a history of delays in attainment of motor milestones coupled with the appropriate findings on physical examination. Often, children who are later definitively diagnosed with CP have abnormal muscle tone in infancy, either hypotonia or hypertonia. In some cases, hypotonia progresses to hypertonia after the first several months of life. In addition, infants with CP often show persistence of primitive reflexes that should have diminished or disappeared earlier (Capute et al., 1997). In a recent prospective study, infants who later became dyskinetic displayed a poor repertoire of general movements, "arm movements in circles" and finger spreading during the first 2 months (as monitored on videotape). Abnormal arm and finger movements remained until at least 5 months and were then concurrent with a lack of arm and leg movements toward the midline. Later dyskinetic infants share with later spastic infants the absence of fidgety movements, a spontaneous movement pattern that is normally present from 3 to 5 months (Einspieler et al., 2002). Several neurologic examinations have been developed for use primarily during the first year of life (Amiel-Tison & Grenier, 1986; Ellison, 1990; Dubowitz et al., 2002) (Fig. 44-1). Assessments of primitive reflexes, muscle tone (e.g., assessed by observing posture), clonus, and body angles can help to identify infants who are at risk for or who have cerebral palsy.

Examinations during the first several months of life can identify most cases of severe CP, but a normal examination during the first 6 months of life does not exclude the possibility of later mild or moderately severe CP. At least one third of infants who develop CP are not identified by examination during the first 4 months of life (Coolman et al., 1985). Children with hemiplegic CP do not typically evidence a hemiparesis or even a reflex asymmetry until 6 to 9 months of age, when they begin to be expected to use the involved extremities. Although the basal ganglia damage usually occurs at birth, choreoathetosis may not be evident until children are 2 years of age, at which time they should have developed stable walking and fine motor skills.

On the other hand, an abnormal examination during the first 6 months does not always predict CP. Approximately 25% of premature infants evidence transient neurologic symptoms, such as increased extensor muscle tone and persistence of primitive reflexes, which may resemble spastic CP, but typically resolve by 12 months of age (post-term) (Sommerfelt et al., 1996). Abnormalities of motor tone or movement in the first

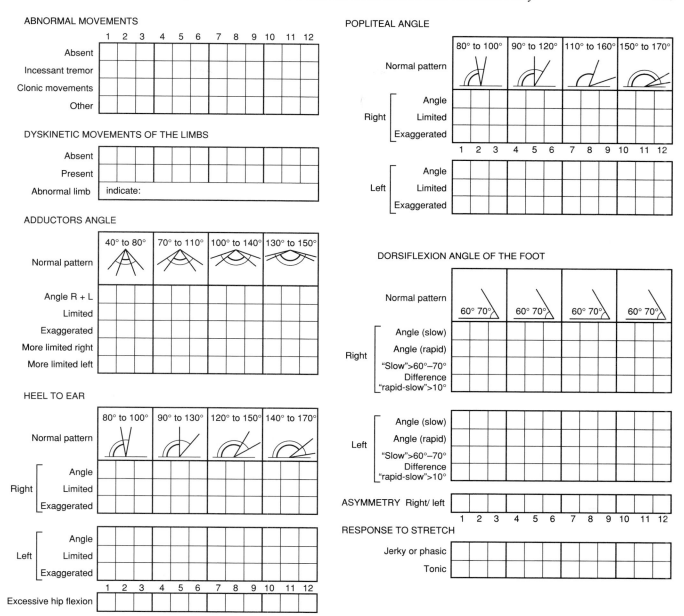

FIGURE 44-1. Features of the early neurologic examination. (Reproduced with permission from Amiel-Tison C, Grenier A: Neurological Assessment During the First Year of Life. New York: Oxford University Press, 1986.)

several weeks or months after birth may gradually improve, especially during the first year. Furthermore, CP diagnosed in the first 2 years of life may resolve during early childhood, especially when the functional impairment is mild (Nelson & Ellenberg, 1982; Ross et al., 1985). Of 229 children diagnosed with CP in the National Collaborative Perinatal Project (NCPP)*, over 50%

reportedly "outgrew" CP by 7 years of age (Niswander & Gordon, 1972; Nelson & Ellenberg, 1982) (Fig. 44-2). Children with mild CP at 1 year of age were more likely to be free of motor deficit at 7 years of age than children with moderate or severe CP at 1 year of age. Furthermore, children with dyskinetic/ataxic CP and children with spastic diplegia "outgrew" CP more often than children with hemiplegia and quadriplegia; children with mixed CP (spasticity with dyskinesia or ataxia) did not show resolution of CP.

It is important to note that children in the NCPP who "outgrew" CP were more likely than the general controls to have developmental disabilities. While 3%

_____

*The National Collaborative Perinatal Project was a National Institutes of Health–supervised project (involving a number of major medical centers) prospectively following over 50,000 pregnancies occurring from 1959 to 1965 and the children born thereof through 7 years of age.

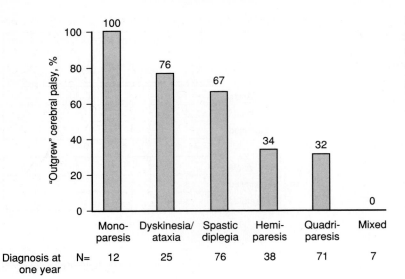

FIGURE 44-2. Percentage of children who were free of cerebral palsy at 7 years of age, according to type of cerebral palsy diagnosed when they were 1 year old. (Reproduced with permission from Nelson KB, Ellenberg JH: Children who "outgrew" cerebral palsy. Pediatrics 69:529–536, 1982.)

of children who were never diagnosed with CP were mentally retarded, 22% of children who had outgrown CP had IQs less than 70. Children who outgrew CP also were more likely than children considered normal at 1 year of age to have hyperactivity, nonfebrile seizures, speech articulation problems, and visual and visuomotor abnormalities. It appears that initial damage to brain areas serving motor and cognitive functions in some children with suspected CP may recover, with improvement of motor function, but with residual effects on vision, cognition, and behavior.

In summary, a diagnosis of CP should not be assigned too early in an infant with suspicious neurologic features, unless the motor abnormality is very severe. Some clinicians recommend withholding the diagnosis until children are 2 years of age (Kyllerman et al., 1982). Conversely, relatively nonspecific motor signs, such as hypotonia or abnormal persistence of primitive reflexes within the first few months of life, may develop over the first year into spasticity or extrapyramidal abnormalities. Myelination of axons and maturation of neurons in the basal ganglia may be required before spasticity, dystonia, and athetosis are apparent.

Etiology

Etiology reflects both the timing of the brain insult (prenatal, perinatal, postnatal) and gestational age of the infant (preterm vs. term infant). In the most recent Swedish population-based study, probable etiology was identified in 73% of preterm and 86% of term children. Among preterm children it was considered prenatal in 12%, peri/neonatal in 61%, and unclassifiable in 27%, whereas it was 51%, 36%, and 14%, respectively, among term children (Hagberg et al., 2001).

Timing of Insult

The multiple causes of CP in relationship to timing of insult are enumerated in Table 44-9. Prenatal conditions associated with CP that are subjects of current investigations include:

- History of spontaneous abortions and stillbirth (Gilstrap & Ramin, 2000)
- Suboptimality of pregnancy, including excessive stress (Mulder et al., 2002)
- Multiple gestation (see text following) (Pharoah, 2001)
- Maternal infections (Walstab et al., 2002)
- Intrauterine growth retardation (Doctor et al., 2001; Becroft et al., 2002)
- Placental insufficiency (Redline et al., 1998)
- Genetic causes, including those underlying brain malformations
- Maternal drug use—e.g., smoking (Walstab et al., 2002), alcohol (Thackray & Tifft, 2001), and cocaine (Frank et al., 2002)

Perinatal conditions associated with CP that are subjects of current investigations include hypoxic ischemic encephalopathy (du Plessis & Volpe, 2002), breech delivery (Nelson & Ellenberg, 1986), chorioamnionitis during labor (Grether & Nelson, 1999; Gilstrap & Ramin, 2000), hypothyroidism, particularly in the preterm (Rapaport et al., 2001), preterm birth (with associated intraventricular hemorrhage [IVH] and PVL) (O'Shea et al., 1998), and kernicterus. Recurrent neonatal seizures appear to be a risk factor for development of CP (whether associated with hypoxic ischemic encephalopathy [HIE] or not), but likely reflect the underlying processes that lead to CP rather than being the direct cause of the CP (Kuban & Leviton, 1994).

TABLE 44-9. Potential Causes of Cerebral Palsy

Congenital/genetic (acquired in utero)
    Infectious (rubella, toxoplasmosis, cytomegalic virus, herpes
      simplex, HIV, or other infections, possibly urinary tract
      infections)
    Maternal anoxia (e.g., carbon monoxide poisoning,
      strangulation)
    Maternal hypotension/hypovolemia (e.g., maternal
      hemorrhage)
    Intrauterine growth retardation
    Placental insufficiency, placental infarcts, placental abruption
    Brain malformations
    Toxins and drugs
    Twin gestation, twin-twin transfusion
Perinatal
    Hypoxic-ischemic insult
    Prematurity
    Trauma
    Postmaturity
    Hyperbilirubinemia with kernicterus
    Peripartum infection
    Infection (meningitis, encephalitis)
    Metabolic
Postnatal (infancy)
    Trauma
    Infections (meningitis, encephalitis, brain abscess)
    Vascular events (ischemic stroke, hemorrhage)
    Anoxia (carbon monoxide poisoning, strangulation)
    Metabolic (hypoglycemia)

Postnatal causes of CP that are currently under investigation include infections and trauma.

Gestational Age

The Term Infant. Results of the NCPP suggested that in the term infant prenatal factors are better predictors of CP than the events of labor and delivery (Nelson & Ellenberg, 1986). Breech presentation, a malformation of any organ system, and maternal mental retardation are risk factors for CP. HIE can cause CP. However, clear evidence of such an insult must be reflected in depressed Apgar scores and neonatal encephalopathy (lethargy, hypotonia, seizures). Even then many term infants do not develop CP. Recent studies suggest that disorders of coagulation and intrauterine exposure to infection or inflammation are associated with risk of CP, and that both can be accompanied by signs of neonatal encephalopathy, the best available predictor of CP in term neonates (Nelson, 2002). Perinatal strokes, generally manifesting as hemiplegic CP (Sreenan et al., 2000), may be due to prenatal events, or such perinatal events as placental thrombi (Kraus, 1997) or protothrombotic

disorders, such as factor V Leiden deficiency (Mecuri et al., 2001). Brain malformations are also a cause of CP in the term infant (Croen et al., 2001; Decoufle et al., 2001). Among term infants, multiple gestation is associated with an increased risk of CP (Peterson et al., 1993; Pharoah, 2001). The major factor associated with CP in twins of normal birth weight is the death of one of the twins in utero, particularly if the twins are of the same sex (Pharoah, 2001).

Combinations of risk factors increase the likelihood of CP in term infants. Thus, in one study, potentially asphyxiating events and markers of infection, considered singly, were associated with moderate increase in risk of CP, but a combination of the two types of risk factors significantly increased the chances of having CP (Nelson & Grether, 1998).

The Preterm Infant. PVL is the most common pathology in premature infants with CP (Kuban & Leviton, 1994; Paneth, 1990). Posthemorrhagic hydrocephalus with or without porencephaly secondary to white matter infarction is also seen (Levitan & Gilles, 1999).

Cerebral white matter damage that results in CP in low-birth-weight infants is probably the result of three major factors, which may occur independently or concurrently: (1) pathologic decreases in blood flow (ischemia) to the brain; (2) perinatal infection and inflammation; and (3) insufficient levels of substances (e.g., cytokines, thyroid hormone) that protect the brain from injury (O'Shea, 2002).

Preterm infants are likely to have pathologic decreases of blood flow to the brain, both because of events leading to decreased systemic blood pressure and lack of cerebral autoregulation to compensate for those decreases. Although no research has demonstrated a direct relationship between measures of cerebral perfusion and CP, there are a number of findings that indicate that brain ischemia can cause white matter damage and increase the risk of CP in very preterm infants. History of hypotension has been associated with a modest increase in white matter abnormalities (Perlman et al., 1996) and of CP (Murphy et al., 1997a,b) in preterm infants. Neonatal complications, such as respiratory distress syndrome, sepsis, and pneumothorax, all of which can cause hypotension, have all been associated with increased risk of CP.

Metabolic acidemia, which often is due to tissue ischemia and lactic acid accumulation, has been associated with CP (Volpe, 2000), as has hypocarbia (abnormally low carbon dioxide), which can cause a decrease in cerebral blood flow and has been associated with increased white matter damage (Dammann et al., 2001) and CP (Solokorpi et al., 1999). In addition, maternal obstetric complications associated with a decrease in blood pressure, such as placental abruption and chorioamnionitis, are considered risk factors. By contrast, factors related to increased neonatal blood pressure, such as antenatal use of glucocorticoid (Gray et al., 2001; O'Shea & Doyle, 2001) and maternal preeclampsia, may actually decrease the risk of CP.

A number of studies have suggested that infection and inflammation play a major role in the development of PVL and CP. In addition, maternal chorioamnionitis is associated with an increase in the risk of both periventricular echolucency on cranial ultrasound and CP (Wu & Colford, 2000). Neonatal sepsis has been related to a twofold increase in CP, even when controlling for the potentially confounding effect of chorioamnionitis (Murphy et al., 1997a,b; Wilson-Costello et al., 1998).

Cytokines, particularly tumor necrosis factor, may mediate harmful effects of sepsis (Leviton, 1993), and have been found to be elevated in amniotic fluid, umbilical cords, and brains of infants with white matter damage and cerebral palsy. On the other hand, there is some indication that specific molecules, such as glucocorticoids and thyroxine, may protect the brain from white matter damage (O'Shea & Doyle, 2001).

Finally, it appears that kernicterus, once nearly nonexistent, is an increasing cause of CP. This is especially evident in preterm infants who develop kernicterus at relatively low levels of bilirubin compared with term infants (Johnson & Bhutani, 1998; Johnson & Brown, 1999).

Medical Evaluation

History

As with any disorder the personal and family histories are important to determining the case of CP in a particular child.

Assessment of Vision and Hearing

Because both vision and hearing impairments are relatively common in children with CP, routine screening is appropriate. The preterm infant is at particular risk for hearing difficulties and any delay in language acquisition should be a signal for formal testing.

Neuroimaging Evaluation

Neuroimaging has proved an important tool for defining etiology and prognosticating in the child with CP. Early cranial ultrasonography provides information about the occurrence of germinal matrix and intraventricular hemorrhage. Early echolucencies may be the forerunner of focal PVL. Echogenicity may resolve or evolve into cystic PVL (deVries & Groenendaal, 2002). Patchy relatively persistent echogenicity is more likely to lead to transient dystonia or spastic diplegia (Pierrat et al., 2001). Infants with cystic PVL are at considerable risk of developing CP (deVries & Groenendaal, 2002).

Preterm infants with uncomplicated nursery courses and normal ultrasounds may have CP, but it is mild and nondisabling (Pinto-Martin et al., 1995).

Brain malformations documented on MRI scans are the most common finding in the term infant with CP, whereas PVL is the common finding in the preterm infant (Barkovich, 2002). Asymmetry of myelination of the posterior limb of the internal capsule at 40 weeks corrected age as demonstrated on MRI is predictive of hemiparetic CP (deVries & Groenendaal, 2002). In a recent study of thalamic and basal ganglia abnormalities, MRI findings correlated significantly with the severity of both cognitive and motor impairment and type of CP. Normal cognitive development and mild motor delay were related to the mild pattern of lesions. All children developed CP. Purely dyskinetic CP was observed only with the mild pattern, whereas the dyskinetic-spastic or spastic CP types could be associated with all three lesion patterns (i.e., dyskinetic-spastic CP was more related to the moderate, and purely spastic CP was more related to the severe pattern in the child with CP secondary to birth asphyxia) (Krageloh-Mann et al., 2002). MRI findings at the posteromedial border of the globus pallidus in patients with athetotic cerebral palsy are strong evidence of brain damage caused by kernicterus (Sugama et al., 2001). Brain single photon emission computed tomography (SPECT) regional cerebral blood flow (rCBF) in thalamus and cerebellum predicted gross-motor development as well as cognitive and motor performance variables in children with CP (Yin et al., 2000). Poor performance by preterm infants on tasks requiring spatial and visuoperceptual abilities was associated with the finding of PVL on MRI, especially with posterior ventricular enlargement (Olsen et al., 1998). Structural MRI and, increasingly, functional magnetic resonance imaging (fMRI), can thus be used to define the areas of brain injury, improving our understanding of structure-function correlations.

Metabolic/Genetic Evaluation

There are a number of genetic disorders with a phenotype that may suggest/mimic a diagnosis of CP (Table 44-10). Although they ultimately result in progressive disability, some remain static for years. For example, a small proportion of bilateral spastic CP appears to have a genetic basis (McHale et al., 1999). Genetic predisposition to thrombosis and embolism, as well as polymorphism related to cytokine expression and inflammatory pathologies, may increase risk for CP. Ataxic CP, cognitive dysfunction that appears more severe than motor dysfunction, and a history of other affected family members should flag some patients for metabolic or genetic evaluation, because these attributes suggest that CP may be the result of specific disorders that may ultimately be treatable. Dopamine-responsive dystonia is a prime example (Furukawa & Kish, 1999).

TABLE 44-10. Genetic Syndromes That May Mimic Cerebral Palsy (CP)

Ataxia-telangiectasia (progressive by second decade)

Behr syndrome

Dopamine-responsive dystonia

Familial spastic paraplegia (progressive by second or third decade)

Glutaric aciduria (like dyskinetic CP)

Hereditary microcephaly

Krabbe disease (akin to spastic diplegia)

Leigh disease

Lesch-Nyhan disease

Marinescu-Sjögren syndrome

Metachromatic leukodystrophy

Phenylketonuria

Sjögren-Larsson syndrome

Subacute sclerosing panencephalitis (like ataxic CP)

Cognitive Evaluation

Hemiplegic CP has been better studied than other forms of CP because it allows a comparison between the effects of a unilateral lesion on the immature versus the mature nervous system. Overall intelligence at school age is often normal. Size of lesion plays a role (Levine et al., 1987). Most children with a left hemisphere lesion have higher verbal than performance IQ scores; most children with right hemisphere lesions have equal verbal and performance IQ scores (Nass et al., 1989). Teuber (1974) interpreted the verbal IQ superiority in patients with left hemisphere lesions as evidence of a "crowding effect"—i.e., when resources are decreased, language processes take priority over functions ordinarily mediated by the right hemisphere. Overall, the IQ of CP patients with congenital right hemisphere lesions tends to be lower than patients with left hemisphere lesions. IQ in CP patients with focal lesions seems to decline over time, more so with right hemisphere lesions (Banich et al., 1990).

Cognitive demands associated with increasing age may tax the resources and "plasticity" (ability to compensate for lost neural tissue or function) of the developing brain. Children with brain lesions at an earlier age may show better outcome because a less mature hemisphere may be more plastic. Other potential factors in outcomes of CP are differential maturation rates of the right and left hemispheres and changing representation of function in the normal maturing brain.

Several factors should be considered in assessing the intelligence of a child with CP in whom sensorimotor handicaps can lead to underestimates of intellect.

The overall IQ score reflects both verbal and performance (visuomotor or nonverbal) abilities. Children with CP may be unable to execute tasks that require motor coordination (e.g., assembling puzzle pieces, tracing mazes), producing low scores despite normal verbal abilities and intellect. Incoordination of facial muscles affecting language production may also lower the child's score on tests that require elaborated verbal responses. Sensory impairment (visual and hearing deficits) must also be taken into account in evaluating a child's cognitive ability.

The neuropsychological assessment should include:

- Visual attention
- Visual–motor functioning
- Auditory processing
- Fine-motor coordination
- Executive functioning (planning, impulse control)
- Memory
- Language
- Academic achievement (reading, writing, mathematics)

Results that identify the child's strengths and weaknesses will allow for more effective educational planning and prediction of outcomes.

Language

Younger children with CP appear to have greater language difficulties than school-aged children. Toddlers and preschoolers with both congenital left and right hemisphere lesions may show mild to moderate delays in language acquisition. Between the ages of 1 and 2 years, children with right hemisphere lesions show more delays in word comprehension and communicative gesture. Children with left temporal lobe involvement show greater delays in expressive vocabulary and grammar acquisition through age 5 years (Reilly et al., 1995; Bates et al., 1997; Bates & Roe, 2001). Children of school age with left hemisphere lesions have more problems with language-based academic skills than those with right hemisphere lesions, but the problems are subtle in both groups (Eisele et al., 1998; Bates & Roe, 2001). School-aged children with congenital right hemisphere lesions have difficulties with comprehension and expression of affective prosody and (to a lesser extent) linguistic prosody; those with left hemisphere pathology have more difficulty than controls on measures of linguistic prosody (Trauner et al., 1996).

Language development in brain-damaged children with CP depends on innate specialization of the left hemisphere for language, intrahemispheric language specialization that evolves over time, and right hemisphere contributions to verbal cognition and language acquisition, particularly semantics. Language deficits appear to diminish after damage to either hemisphere with increasing age, suggesting that alternative routes to language acquisition can evolve (Reilly et al., 1998; Bates & Roe, 2001).

Visuoperceptual Skills

Children who have CP associated with left hemisphere lesions may show a delay in the development of a specific spatial skill, but generally recover over time. Those with right hemisphere lesions show deficits that recover only incompletely. Residual impairments are especially evident when task complexity is increased. Early lesions of the right hemisphere are generally associated with recovery of language functions with advancing age; however, visuospatial and visuomotor functions are apt never to recover fully (Stiles, 2001).

Children with early left and right focal lesions in various locations examined on a range of face recognition tasks (famous faces, emotional expression, identity, sex, divided visual field presentation of unfamiliar faces) showed different strengths and weaknesses, suggesting that various skills involved in facial processing develop independently and have different interhemispheric and intrahemispheric locations (Ballantyne & Trauner, 1999).

Behavior

Infants with right hemisphere lesions show more negativity; for example, it is difficult to elicit smiling behavior (Reilly et al., 1995). Studies of temperament in children with CP from preschool to school age also suggest more negative behaviors (Nass & Koch, 1991). Psychiatric interviews indicate that as many as 50% of hemiplegic children show behavioral or psychiatric problems (including hyperactivity, conduct disorders, aggression, and oppositional behaviors) (Goodman, 2002). Longitudinal testing indicates that the psychiatric problems are present early in life (often during preschool years) and persist into the school years (Goodman, 2002). Based on the results of a parent questionnaire (Child Behavior Checklist), school-aged children with CP have social and attention problems. Social problems tend to increase over time, posing a potential risk in adulthood. Children with left hemisphere lesions have more abnormal scores on the checklist (Trauner et al., 2001).

Pathophysiology of Reorganization and Recovery in Hemiplegic Cerebral Palsy

More information is available about the pathophysiologic changes after early unilateral lesions—i.e., in hemiplegic CP—than in other forms of CP. Extent of reorganization varies for different skill domains. Homotopic interhemispheric reorganization potential in the language domain is greater than in the motor domain, compatible with more apparent motor than language deficits (Muller et al., 1997; Muller et al., 1998d). Compensatory allocation for movement of the weak hand may occur in the frontal and insular cortices and the supplementary motor area in the unaffected hemisphere and bilateral cerebellum (Muller et al., 1998c). Movement of the hemiparetic hand is associated with activation in the supplementary motor area bilaterally and in the contralesional premotor cortex. Blood flow increase in the ipsilesional temporal lobe adjacent to an area of extensive encephalomalacia suggested possible atypical motor function in the temporal lobe (Muller et al., 1998b).

Postlesional reorganization of language appears to reflect "additive" and "subtractive" effects—i.e., activation in some regions that are not normally involved in language processing (in basal ganglia) and lack of activation in other (undamaged) regions that are normally activated by language tasks (Muller et al., 1998a, 1999a). Thus, a rightward shift of language activations occurs in patients with early left perisylvian and temporoparietal lesions. Intrahemispheric reorganization after late childhood lesions is relatively minimal (Muller et al., 1999a, 1999b).

Prevention

Several causes of CP are preventable. Kernicterus can be prevented by treating neonatal jaundice with phototherapy or exchange transfusion, if necessary, and minimizing complications of Rh incompatibility through RhoGAM antibody treatments during the pregnancies of RH-negative women. Rubella can be prevented by vaccinating women before they become pregnant.

Current research has suggested a number of new approaches to preventing CP after birth. Because perinatal infection and inflammation appear to be risk factors for CP, it has been suggested that aggressive antibiotic treatment of mothers with intrauterine infection is a logical strategy for preventing CP (O'Shea, 2002). Since low-birth-weight infants are 25 to 30 times more likely to have CP than other infants, prevention of low birth weight may diminish the number of children with CP. Ongoing research on the causes of prematurity, drugs that safely delay premature labor, and development of new techniques for the medical treatment of premature infants may reduce the prevalence of prematurity and diminish the incidence and severity of CP in low-birth-weight infants. Most recently, the use of progesterone has been reported to prevent prematurity, and thereby potentially lessen the prevalence of CP in future years. A large study found that weekly injections of progesterone lowered the rate of premature births by more than a third among women who were at high risk because they had histories of giving birth early (Grady, 2003). Prenatal treatment with glucocorticoids (betamethasone, dexamethasone), used to improve lung function and therefore survival among preterm infants, appears to reduce risk for cerebral white matter damage (Leviton et al., 2000) and CP (O'Shea & Doyle, 2001). For example, a single course of prenatal glucocorticoids was found to be associated with a 50% reduction in risk of brain hemorrhage and a 30% reduction in the risk of CP in premature infants (O'Shea & Doyle, 2001). Although controversial (Wilson-Costello et al., 1998), magnesium sulfate (used to treat preeclampsia or preterm labor) has been reported to reduce the risk of CP by 7- to 10-fold in preterm infants when administered to their mothers prenatally (Nelson & Grether, 1995; Schendel et al., 1996; Kirschbaum, 2002), suggesting that magnesium protects against bleeding in the brains of very premature infants. Also, because recent reports have suggested a higher risk of CP among preterm infants with low thyroxine levels, it is possible that thyroid hormone might promote normal brain myelination and reduce risk of white matter damage (Leviton et al., 1999; Rapaport et al., 2001).

Treatment

Physical therapy

Physical therapy in CP is used to decrease muscle tone, increase muscle strength, and improve motor control (Goldsmith, 2001). A neurodevelopmental method (NDT) (Bobath & Bobath, 1972) teaches the child to compensate for abnormal movements and maintain equilibrium in space. It is different from other physical therapies because it relies on active participation of the child, rather than on passive movement of the child's affected limbs. Studies assessing the benefits of physical therapy on the outcome of CP generally show that early physical therapy helps parents and children cope better and may improve postural control, but that it does not appear to reduce spasticity or diminish primitive reflexes (Bower et al., 2000).

Surgery

Surgical procedures in CP are sometimes performed to lengthen muscles and tendons and eliminate contractures. Dorsal rhizotomy is a surgical procedure in which some of the lumbar–sacral dorsal nerve roots are severed to disrupt the overactive stretch reflex circuitry and reduce spasticity. It is important to determine whether a child has spasticity or dystonia before surgery because children with dystonic posturing will not benefit from the procedure. A report of 208 patients who received selective posterior rhizotomy between 1990 and 1999 showed an overall improvement (over 95%) in spasticity, passive range of motion, and gait pattern (Kim et al., 2001). Studies have indicated that rhizotomy has lessened spasticity

in lower extremities; in addition, there is evidence that the procedure can result in improvements in upper extremity functions, such as grasping, hand use, eye-hand coordination, and manual dexterity (Mittal et al., 2002).

Pharmacologic Agents

The armamentarium of medications available to treat the behavioral problems of the child with CP overlap those used to treat similar problems in other children with neurologic disorders (see Chapter 43). Numerous medications have been used to treat abnormal muscle tone, including antiadrenergic, dopaminergic, and antidopaminergic drugs, anticonvulsants, antidepressants, and antispasticity agents. The most common side effect is drowsiness. Localized treatments to reduce spasticity at specific times, including neuromuscular blocks, such as Botulinum toxin (Botox) (Komman et al., 2000; Boyd & Hays, 2001; Baker et al., 2002) and local anesthetics have been used. Baclofen (an antispasticity drug) has been given orally and through intrathecal injections to reduce diffuse spasticity and generalized dystonia (Murphy et al., 2002). In addition, researchers are also exploring the use of tiny implanted pumps that deliver a constant supply of antispasticity drugs into the spinal fluid, in hopes of improving drug effectiveness and reducing side effects (Goldstein, 2001).

Team Approach

CP has wide ranging effects on children's development and functional adaptation. In order to address physical, language, cognitive, educational, visual, psychological, social-emotional, and functional deficits, a team of rehabilitation professionals is often needed to manage the care of CP children (see Table 44-11).

CONCLUSION

CP is one of the more common neurologic disorders of childhood. It is highly associated with MR and epilepsy. Despite declines in neonatal mortality, the prevalence of CP generally has not decreased during the past two decades. Contemporary studies have made progress in identifying the pathogenesis of CP in both term and preterm infants, linking it to infection and inflammation, decreased blood flow and infarcts that result in white matter damage, and specific endogenous molecules, such as cytokines, thyroid hormone, and magnesium sulfate that may mediate brain injury. These discoveries may lead to more effective means of preventing CP. Although there currently are no cures, comprehensive treatments and services can ameliorate some of the symptoms.

TABLE 44-11. Multidisciplinary Team for Managing Cerebral Palsy

Pediatrician, pediatric neurologist, or pediatric psychiatrist	Manages overall plan, implements medical treatment, follows the child's development, plans work-up. Manages self-esteem, behavioral issues.
Orthopedist	Diagnoses or treats muscle problems.
Physical therapist	Implements exercise programs to facilitate the child's movement and strengthen muscles.
Occupational therapist	Helps patients with fine-motor and adaptive skills.
Psychologist	Educates children and their parents on the nature of the child's cerebral palsy and how best to cope with the disorder.
Social worker	Helps the family find appropriate services in the community (e.g., special schools; therapy programs; support groups).
Educator	Remediates cognitive or learning disorders the child with cerebral palsy is found to have.
Ophthalmologist	Diagnoses and treat any visual or eye problems associated with cerebral palsy.

■   KEY POINTS

☐   Mental retardation can be gauged by IQ scores. Standardized IQ tests are psychometrically designed with 100 as the mean and 15 as the standard deviation: children with mild MR have an IQ of 55 to 70; children with moderate MR have an IQ of 35 to 50; children with severe MR have an IQ of 20 to 35; and children with profound MR have an IQ under 20 (DSM-IV). There is high variability in the level of functioning of children with IQs around 70; about half require special education and half attend regular school.

☐   In Down syndrome (DS), chromosomal abnormalities are a common cause of severe mental retardation. DS (trisomy 21), the most common chromosomal disorder, is the single most common cause of moderate to severe retardation (one third), occurring at a rate of 1.5 per 1000 live births. A small region in the distal part of the long arm of chromosome 21 appears to be critical to DS, but other regions also contribute to the full phenotype.

☐   Williams syndrome (WS) is a multisystem disorder occurring in 1/20,000, which is usually caused by a 1.5Mb deletion involving at least 16 genes on chromosome 7 (7q11.23). Findings in several kindreds with smaller deletions suggest that the gene for LIM kinase 1 may be important to visuospatial constructional ability. Seventy-five percent of children with WS have MR, which is generally mild to moderate (mean IQ 66). Adaptive behaviors are generally commensurate with overall IQ. Communication and social skills tend to be better developed than daily living skills. Visuospatial, but not face recognition, skills are most impaired.

☐   Prader-Willi syndrome (PWS) has an incidence of about 1/12,000 live births. Most cases (70%) are caused by a paternally inherited deletion on chromosome 15 (15q11-q13). MR is generally mild to moderate, with a mean IQ of 70. There is, however, a wide range of IQs, from profoundly retarded to average. Adaptively, however, even those with normal IQ rarely function at a level commensurate with their IQ, usually because their compulsive eating and other behavioral problems interfere.

☐   Fragile X syndrome (FXS) is generally considered the most common currently known cause of inherited mental retardation, occurring in 1/1000 males and 1/2000 females. The FXS gene (FMR-1) contains an excessive number of triplet repeats. Moderate to severe mental retardation is common in males with FXS, with 80% in the 20 to 50 IQ range and an average IQ of around 35. Mild to moderate retardation is the norm in affected females. Autistic features are common.

☐   Cerebral palsy (CP) is one of the more common neurologic disorders of childhood. It is highly associated with MR and epilepsy. Despite declines in neonatal mortality, the prevalence of CP generally has not decreased during the past two decades. Numerous recent studies have made progress in identifying the pathogenesis of CP in both term and preterm infants, linking it to infection and inflammation, decreased blood flow and infarcts that result in white matter damage, and specific endogenous molecules, such as cytokines, thyroid hormone, and magnesium sulfate that may mediate brain injury. This information may lead to means of preventing CP.

KEY READINGS

Howlin P, Udwin O (eds): Outcomes in Neurodevelopmental and Genetic Disorders. New York: Cambridge University Press, 2002. [reviews of retardation syndromes]

Volpe JJ: Neurology of the Newborn, ed 4. Philadelphia: Saunders, 2000. [References for etiology of CP are found in this source.]

References for Population-Based Epidemiology

Hagberg B, Hagberg H, Beckung E, et al: Changing panorama of cerebral palsy in Sweden. VIII. Prevalence and origin in the birth year period 1991–1994. Acta Pediatr 90:271–277, 2001.

O'Shea TM: Cerebral palsy in very preterm infants: New epidemiological insights. Ment Retard Dev Disabil Res Rev 8:135–145, 2002.

Nelson KB: The epidemiology of cerebral palsy in term infants. Ment Retard Dev Disabil Res Rev 8:146–150, 2002. [review of risk factors for CP]

REFERENCES

Achenbach TM, Rescurla L: Child Behavior Checklist. Burlington, VT: University of Vermont, 2001.

Airaksinen EM, Matilainen R, Mononen T, et al: A population-based study on epilepsy in mentally retarded children. Epilepsia 41:1214–1220, 2000.

Akefeldt A, Akefeldt B, Gillberg C: Voice, speech and language characteristics of children with Prader-Willi syndrome. J Intellect Disabil Res 41:302–311, 1997.

American Psychiatric Association: Diagnostic and Statistical Manual of Mental Disorders, ed 4. Washington: American Psychiatric Association, 2000, pp. 41–49.

Amiel-Tison C, Grenier A: Neurological assessment during the first year of life. New York: Oxford University Press, 1986.

Aylward EH, Habbak R, Warren AC, et al: Cerebellar volume in adults with Down's syndrome. Arch Neurol 54:209–212, 1997.

Aylward G: Cognitive and neuropsychological outcomes: More than IQ scores. Ment Retard Dev Disabil Res Rev 8:234–240, 2002.

Bailey DB, Hatton D, Skinner M: Early developmental trajectories of males with fragile X syndrome. Am J Ment Retard 1:29–39, 1998.

Baker R, Jasinski M, Maciag-Tymecka I, et al: Botulinum toxin treatment of spasticity in diplegic cerebral palsy: A randomized, double-blind, placebo-controlled, dose-ranging study. Dev Med Child Neurol 44:666–675, 2002

Ballantyne AO, Trauner DA: Facial recognition in children after perinatal stroke. Neuropsychiatry Neuropsychol Behav Neurol 12:82–87, 1999.

Banich M, Levine S, Kim H, et al: The effects of developmental factors on IQ in hemiplegic children. Neuropsychologia 28:35–45, 1990.

Barkovich AJ: Magnetic resonance imaging: Role in the understanding of cerebral malformations. Brain Devel 24:2–12, 2002.

Baron-Cohen S: Modularity in developmental cognitive neuropsychology: Evidence from autism and Tourettes syndrome, in Burack J, Hodapp R, Zigler E (eds): Handbook of Mental Retardation and Development. New York: Cambridge University Press, 1998, pp. 334–348.

Bates E, Roe K: Language development in children with unilateral brain damage, in Nelson C, Luciana M (eds): Handbook of Developmental Cognitive Neuroscience. Cambridge, MA: MIT Press, 2001, pp. 281–308.

Bates E, Thal D, Aram D, et al: Language acquisition—from first words to grammar—after congenital focal lesion. Devel Psychol 13:275–343, 1997.

Becroft DM, Thompson JM, Mitchell EA: The epidemiology of placental infarction at term. Placenta 23:343–351, 2002.

Bellugi U, Adolphs R, Cassady C, et al: Towards the neural basis for hypersocialability in a genetic syndrome. Neuroreport 10:1653–1657, 1999.

Bigler E, Nielsen D, Wilde E, et al: Neuroimaging and genetic disorders, in Goldstein S, Reynolds C (eds): Handbook of Neurodevelopmental and Genetic Disorders in Children. New York: Guilford Press, 1999, pp. 61–80.

Blair E: Trends in cerebral palsy. Ind J Pediatr 68:433–437, 2001.

Blasco PA: Management of drooling: 10 years after the Consortium on Drooling. Dev Med Child Neurol 44:778–781, 1990.

Bobath K, Bobath B: The neurodevelopmental approach to treatment, in Pearson PH, Williams CE (eds): Physical Therapy Services in the Developmental Disabilities. Springfield, IL: Charles C Thomas, 1972, pp. 31–104.

Bower E, Michell D, Burnett M: Randomized controlled trial of physiotherapy in 56 children with cerebral palsy followed for 18 months. Dev Med Child Neurol 43:4–15, 2000.

Boyd RN, Hays RM: Outcome measurement of effectiveness of botulinum toxin type A in children with cerebral palsy: An ICIDH-2 approach. Eur J Neurol 5:167–177, 2001.

Bracewell M, Marlow N: Patterns of motor disability in very preterm children. Ment Retard Dev Disabil Res Rev 4:241–248, 2002.

Burack J, Hodapp R, Zigler E: Handbook of Mental Retardation and Development. New York: Cambridge University Press, 1998, pp. 80–114.

Capute AJ, Aiccardi PJ, Vining EPG: Abnormal Persistence of Primitive Reflex Profile. Baltimore: University Park Press, 1997.

Carr J: Downs syndrome, in Howlin P, Udwin O (eds): Outcomes in Neurodevelopmental and Genetic Disorders. New York: Cambridge University Press, 2002, pp. 169–197.

Chapman R, Hesketh L: Downs syndrome. Ment Retard Dev Disabil Res Rev 6:84–95, 2000.

Coolman RB, Bennett FC, Sells CJ, et al: Neurodevelopment of graduates of the neonatal intensive care unit: Patterns encountered in the first years of life. Dev Behav Pediatr 5:327–333, 1985.

Cornish KM, Munir F, Cross G: Spatial cognition in males with fragile-X syndrome: Evidence for a neuropsychological phenotype. Cortex 35:263–271, 1999.

Croen LA, Grether JK, Curry CJ, et al: Congenital abnormalities among children with cerebral palsy: More evidence for prenatal antecedents. J Pediatr 138:804–810, 2001.

Dammann O, Alfred EN, Kuban KCK, et al: Hypocarbia during the first 24-postnatal hours and white matter echolucencies in new-borns <28 weeks gestation. Pediatr Res 49:388–393, 2001.

de Borchgrave V, Saussu F, Depre A: Moyamoya disease and Down syndrome: Case report and review of the literature. Acta Neurol Belg 102:63–66, 2002.

Decoufle P, Boyle CA, Palozzi LJ, et al: Increased risk for developmental disabilities in children who have major birth defects: A population-based study. Pediatrics 108:728–734, 2001.

deVries L, Groenendaal F: Neuroimaging in the preterm infant. Ment Retard Dev Disabil Res Rev 8:273–280, 2002.

Dimiropoulos A, Feurer I, Roof E, et al: Appetitive behavior, compulsivity, and neurochemistry in Prader Willi Syndrome. Ment Retard Dev Dis Res Rev 6:125–130, 2000.

Doctor BA, O'Riordan MA, Kirchner HL, et al: Perinatal correlates and neonatal outcomes of small for gestational age infants born at term gestation. Am J Obstet Gynecol 185:652–659, 2001.

Drummond PM, Colver AF: Analysis by gestational age of cerebral palsy in singleton births in north-east England 1970–1994. Paediatr Perinatal Epidemiol 16:172, 2002.

Dubowitz LMS, Dubowitz V, Mercuri M: The Neurological Assessment of the Preterm and Full-term Newborn Infant. New York: Cambridge University Press, 2002.

du Plessis AJ, Volpe JJ: Perinatal brain injury in the preterm and term newborn. Curr Opin Neurol 15:151–157, 2002.

Dykens E: Maladaptive behavior and dual diagnosis in persons with mental retardation, in Burack J, Hodapp R, Zigler E (eds): Handbook of Mental Retardation and Development. New York: Cambridge University Press, 1998, pp. 542–562.

Dykens EM: Annotation: Psychopathology in children with intellectual disability. J Child Psychol Psychiatry Allied Disc 41: 407–417, 2000.

Dykens EM: Prader Willi Syndrome: Towards a behavioral phenotype, in Tager-Flusberg H (ed): Neurodevelopmental Disorders. Cambridge, MA: MIT Press, 1999.

Dykens E, Cassidy S, King BH: Maladaptive behavior differences in Prader Willi Syndrome due to paternal deletion versus uni parental disomy. Am J Ment Retard 104:67–77, 1999.

Dykens EM, Goldstein S, Reynolds C (eds): Handbook of Neurodevelopmental and Genetic Disorders in Children. New York, Guilford Press, 1999, pp. 81–90.

Dykens EM, Kasari C: Maladaptive behavior in children with Prader-Willi syndrome, Down syndrome, and nonspecific mental retardation. Am J Ment Retard 102:228–237, 1997.

Dykens EM, Rosner BA: Refining behavioral phenotypes: Personality-motivation in Williams and Prader-Willi syndromes. Am J Ment Retard 104:158–169, 1999.

Einspieler C, Cioni G, Paolicelli PB: The early markers for later dyskinetic cerebral palsy are different from those for spastic cerebral palsy. Neuropediatrics 33:73–78, 2002.

Eisele JA, Lust B, Aram DM: Presupposition and implication of truth: Linguistic deficits following early brain lesions. Brain Lang 61:376–394, 1998.

Eliez S, Blasey C, Freund L, et al: Brain anatomy, gender and IQ in children and adolescents with fragile X syndrome. Brain 124: 1610–1618, 2001.

Ellison P: The infant neurological examination. Adv Dev Behav Pediatr 9:75–138, 1990.

Fenichel GM: Clinical Pediatric Neurology: A Signs and Symptoms Approach, ed 4. Philadelphia, PA: Saunders, 2001, pp. 117–147.

Fisch GS, Carpenter N, Holden JJ, et al: Longitudinal changes in cognitive and adaptive behavior in fragile X females: A prospective multicenter analysis. Am J Med Genet 83:308–312, 1999.

Fowler A: Language in mental retardation, in Burack J, Hodapp R, Zigler E (eds): Handbook of Mental Retardation and Development. New York: Cambridge University Press, 1998, pp. 290–333.

Frank DA, Jacobs RR, Beeghly M, et al: Level of prenatal cocaine exposure and scores on the Bayley Scales of Infant Development: Modifying effects of caregiver, early intervention, and birth weight. Pediatrics 110:1143–1152, 2002.

Furukawa Y, Kish SJ: Dopa responsive dystonia: Recent advances and remaining issues to be addressed. Mov Disord 14:709–715, 1999.

Galaburda AM, Bellugi UV: Multi-level analysis of cortical neuroanatomy in Williams's syndrome. J Cogn Neurosci 12:74–88, 2000.

Ghaziuddin M: Autism in Down's syndrome: Family history correlates. J Intellect Disabil Res 41:87–91, 1997.

Giacino JT, Ashwal S, Childs N, et al: The minimally conscious state. Neurology 58:349–353, 2002.

Gilstrap LC, Ramin SM: Infection and cerebral palsy. Semin Perinatol 24:200–203, 2000.

Gokcora N, Atasever T, Karabacak NI, et al: Tc-99m HMPAO brain perfusion imaging in young Down's syndrome patients. Brain Dev 21:107–112, 1999.

Goldstein EM: Spasticity management: An overview. J Child Neurol 16:16–23, 2001.

Goodman R: Hemiplegic CP, in Howlin P, Udwin O (eds): Outcomes in Neurodevelopmental and Genetic Disorders. New York: Cambridge University Press, 2002, pp. 112–136.

Gosch A, Pankau R: Personality and behavior of WS at different ages. Dev Med Child Neurol 39:527–33, 1997.

Grady, D: Hormone cuts risk of premature birth, researchers report. New York Times, February 7, 2003, p. 1.

Gray PH, Jones P, O'Callaghan MJ: Maternal antecedents for cerebral palsy in extremely preterm babies: A case-control study. Dev Med Child Neurol 43:580–585, 2001.

Grether JK, Nelson KB: Maternal infection and risk of cerebral palsy in infants of normal birthweight. JAMA 278:207–211, 1999.

Gudjonsson GH, Murphy GH, Clare IC: Assessing the capacity of people with intellectual disabilities to be witnesses in court. Psychol Med 30:307–314, 2000.

Hagberg B, Hagberg H, Beckung E, et al: Changing panorama of cerebral palsy in Sweden. VIII. Prevalence and origin in the birth year period 1991–1994. Acta Pediatr 90:271–277, 2001.

Hagberg G, Olow I, Van Wendt L: The changing panorama of cerebral palsy in Sweden. VII. Prevalence and origin in the birth year period 1987–1990. Acta Pediatr Scand 85:954–960, 1996.

Hagerman, R, Hagerman J: Fragile X, in Howlin P, Udwin O (eds): Outcomes in Neurodevelopmental and Genetic Disorders. New York: Cambridge University Press, 2002, pp. 198–210.

Hodgson S: The genetics of learning disabilities/ mental retardation. Dev Med Child Neurol 40:137–141, 1998.

Howlin P: Autism, in Howlin P, Udwin O (eds): Outcomes in Neurodevelopmental and Genetic Disorders. New York: Cambridge University Press, 2002, pp. 136–168.

Irwin S, Galvez R, Greenough W: Dendritic spine structural anomalies in Fragile-X mental retardation syndrome. Cereb Cortex 10:1038–1044, 2000.

Jakala P, Hanninen T, Ryynanen M, et al: Fragile-X: neuropsychological test performance, CGG triplet repeat lengths, and hippocampal volumes. J Clin Invest 100:331–338, 1997.

Jarrold C, Baddeley AD, Hewes AK: Verbal and nonverbal abilities in the syndrome phenotype: evidence for diverging developmental trajectories. J Child Psychol Psychiatry 39:511–523, 1998.

Johnson L, Bhutani VK: Guidelines for management of the jaundiced term and near-term infant. Current Controversies in Perinatal Care III. Clin Perinatol 25:555–573, 1998.

Johnson L, Brown AK: A pilot registry for acute and chronic kernicterus in term and near-term infants. Pediatrics 104:736, 1999.

Jones K: Smith's Recognizable Patterns of Human Malformations. Philadelphia, PA: Saunders, 1994.

Karmiloff-Smith A, Tyler LK, Voice K, et al: Linguistic dissociations in Williams's syndrome: Evaluating receptive syntax in on-line and off-line tasks. Neuropsychologia 36:343–351, 1998.

Kaufmann W, Abrams MT, Chen W, et al: Genotype, molecular phenotype, and cognitive phenotype: Correlations in fragile X syndrome. Am J Med Gen 83:286–295, 1999.

Kaufmann, WE, Moser HW: Dendritic anomalies in disorders associated with mental retardation. Cereb Cortex 10:981–991, 2000.

Kim DS, Choi JU, Yang KH, et al: Selective posterior rhizotomy in children with cerebral palsy: A 10-year experience. Child Nerv Sys 17:556–562, 2001.

Kirschbaum TH: Magnesium sulfate and prematurity. J Soc Gynecol Invest 9:58–59, 2002.

Krageloh-Mann I, Helber A, Mader I, et al: Bilateral lesions of thalamus and basal ganglia: Origin and outcome. Dev Med Child Neurol 44:477–484, 2002.

Kraus FT: Cerebral palsy and thromi in placental vessels of the fetus: Insights from litigation. Hum Pathol 28:246–248, 1997.

Kuban KCK, Leviton A: Cerebral palsy. N Engl J Med 330:188–191, 1994.

Kyllerman M, Baber B, Bille B: Dyskinetic cerebral palsy. Acta Pediatr Scand 71:543–550, 1982.

Leonard H, Wen X: The epidemiology of mental retardation: Challenges and opportunities in the new millennium. Ment Retard Dev Disabil Res Rev 8:117–134, 2002.

Levine S, Huttenlocher P, Banich M, et al: Factors affecting cognitive functioning of hemiplegic children. Dev Med Child Neurol 29:27–35, 1987.

Leviton A: Preterm birth and cerebral palsy: Is tumor necrosis the missing link? Dev Med Child Neurol 35:553–558, 1993.

Leviton A, Dammann O, Allred EN: Antenatal corticosteroids and cranial ultrasound abnormalities. Am J Obstet Gynecol 181:1007–1017, 2000.

Leviton A, Gilles F: Ventriculomegaly, delayed myelination, white matter hypoplasia and periventricular leukomalacia: How are they related? Pediatr Neurol 15:127–136, 1999.

Leviton A, Paneth N, Reuss ML, et al: Hypothyroxinemia of prematurity and the risk of cerebral white matter damage. J Pediatr 134:706–711, 1999.

Luckasson R, Coulter D, Polloway E: Mental retardation: Definition, classification and system support. Washington, DC: American Association of Mental Retardation, 1992.

Matson JL, Bamburg JW, Mayville EA, et al: Psychopharmacology and mental retardation: A 10 year review (1990–1999). Res Dev Disabil 21:263–296, 2000.

Mazzocco M: Advances in research on the fragile X syndrome. Ment Retard Dev Disabil Res Rev 6:96–106, 2000.

Mazzocco MM, Kates WR, Baumgardner TL: Autistic behaviors among girls with fragile X syndrome. J Autism Dev Disord 24:415–435, 1997.

McHale DP, Mitchell S, Bundey S, et al: A gene for autosomal recessive symmetrical spastic cerebral palsy maps to chromosome 2q24-25. Am J Hum Genet 64:526–532, 1999.

Menon V, Kwon H, Eliez S, et al: Functional brain activation during cognition is related to FMR1 gene expression. Brain Res 877:367–370, 2000.

Mercuri E, Cowan F, Gupte G, et al: Prothrombotic disorders and abnormal neurodevelopmental outcome in infants with neonatal cerebral infarction. Pediatrics 107:1400–1404, 2001.

Mervis C, Klein-Tasman B: WS. Ment Retard Dev Disabil Res Rev 6:148–158, 2000.

Mills DL, Alvarez TD, St George M, et al: Electrophysiological studies of face processing in Williams syndrome. J Cogn Neurosci 12:47–64, 2000.

Mittal S, Farmer JP, Al-Atassi B, et al: Impact of selective posterior rhizotomy on fine motor skills: Long-term results using a validated evaluative measure. Pediatr Neurosurg 36:133–141, 2002.

Morris C, Mervis C: WS. Ann Rev Genomics Hum Genet 1:461–484, 2000.

Mostofsky SH, Mazzocco MM, Aakalu G, et al: Decreased cerebellar posterior vermis size in fragile X syndrome: Correlation with neurocognitive performance. Neurology 50:121–130, 1998.

Mulder E, Robles de Medina PG, Huizink A: Prenatal stress: Effects on pregnancy and the unborn child. Early Hum Dev 70:3–14, 2002.

Muller RA, Behen ME, Rothermel RD, et al: Brain organization for language in children, adolescents, and adults with left hemisphere lesion: A PET study. Prog NeuroPsychopharmacol Biol Psychiatry 23:657–668, 1999a.

Muller RA, Chugani HT, Muzik O, et al: Brain organization of motor and language functions following hemispherectomy: A [(15)O]-water positron emission tomography study. J Child Neurol 13:16–22, 1998a.

Muller RA, Rothermel RD, Behen ME, et al: Language organization in patients with early and late left-hemisphere lesion: A PET study. Neuropsychologia 37:545–557, 1999b.

Muller RA, Rothermel RD, Behen ME, et al: Plasticity of motor organization in children and adults. Neuroreport 8:3103–3108, 1997.

Muller RA, Rothermel RD, Behen ME, et al: Brain organization of language after early unilateral lesion: A PET study. Brain Lang 62:422–451, 1998b.

Muller RA, Rothermel RD, Behen ME, et al: Differential patterns of language and motor reorganization following early left hemisphere lesion: A PET study. Arch Neurol 55:1113–1119, 1998c.

Muller RA, Watson CE, Muzik O, et al: Motor organization after early middle cerebral artery stroke: A PET study. Pediatr Neurol 19:294–298, 1998.

Murphy C, Boyle C, Schendel D, et al: Epidemiology of mental retardation. Ment Retard Dev Disabil Res Rev 4:6–13, 1998d.

Murphy DJ, Hope PL, Johnson A: Neonatal risk factors for cerebral palsy in very preterm babies: Case–control study. Br Med J 314:404–408, 1997b.

Murphy DJ, Sellers S, MacKenzie IZ, et al: Case-control study of antenatal and intrapartum risk factors for cerebral palsy in very preterm singleton babies. Lancet 346:1449–1454, 1997a.

Murphy NA, Irwin MC, Hoff C: Intrathecal baclofen therapy in children with cerebral palsy: Efficacy and complication. Arch Phys Med Rehabil 83:1721–1725, 2002.

Nardocci N, Zorzi G, Grisoli M, et al: Acquired hemidystonia in childhood: A clinical and neuroradiological study of thirteen patients. Pediatr Neurol 15:108–113, 1996.

Nass R: Mirror movement asymmetries after congenital unilateral brain injury. Neurology 35:1059–1062, 1985.

Nass R, Koch D: Specialization for emotion: Temperament after congenital unilateral injury, in Amir N, Rapin I (eds): Pediatric Neurology: Behavior and Cognition of the Child with Brain Dysfunction. Basel, Switzerland: Karger, 1991, pp. 1–17.

Nass R, Peterson H, Koch D: Differential effects of early left versus right brain injury on intelligence. Brain Cogn 9:258–266, 1989.

Nass R, Stiles J: Cognitive complications of the perinatum: Congenital focal lesions, in Frank Y (ed): Pediatric Behavioral Neurology. Boca Raton, FL: CRC Press, 1996, pp. 45–59.

Nelson KB: The epidemiology of cerebral palsy in term infants. Ment Retard Dev Disabil Res Rev 8:146–150, 2002.

Nelson K, Ellenberg JH: Antecedents of cerebral palsy: Multivariate analysis of risk. N Engl J Med 315:81–86, 1986.

Nelson KB, Ellenberg JH: Children who outgrew cerebral palsy. Pediatrics 69:529–536, 1982.

Nelson KB, Grether JK: Can magnesium sulfate reduce the risk of cerebral palsy in very low birth weight infants? Pediatrics 95:263–269, 1995.

Nelson KB, Grether JK: Potentially asphyxiating conditions and spastic cerebral palsy in infants of normal birth weight. Am J Obstet Gynecol 179:507–513, 1998.

Niswander KR, Gordon M: The Women and Their Pregnancies. Philadelphia, PA: Saunders, 1972.

Olsen P, Vainionpaa L, Paakko E, et al: Psychological findings in preterm children related to neurologic status and magnetic resonance imaging. Pediatrics 102:329–336, 1998.

Opitz JM: Vision and insight in the search for gene mutations causing nonsyndromal mental deficiency. Neurology 55:328–330, 2000.

O'Shea TM: Cerebral palsy in very preterm infants: New epidemiological insights. Ment Retard Dev Disabil Res Rev 8:135–145, 2002.

O'Shea TM, Doyle IW: Perinatal glucocorticoid therapy and neurodevelopmental outcome: An epidemiologic perspective. Semin Neonatal 6:299–307, 2001.

O'Shea TM, Klinepeter KL, Dillard RG: Prenatal events and the risk of cerebral palsy in very low birth weight infants. Am J Epidemiol 147:362–369, 1998.

Paneth N: Classifying brain damage in preterm infants. J Pediatr 134:527–530, 1990.

Partington M, Mowat D, Einfeld S, et al: Genes on the X chromosome are important in undiagnosed mental retardation. Am J Med Genet 92:57–61, 2000.

Paterson SJ: Cognitive modularity and genetic disorders. Science 286:2355–2356, 1999.

Perlman JM, Risser R, Broyles S: Bilateral cystic periventricular leukomalacia in the premature infant: Associated risk factors. Pediatrics 97:823–827, 1996.

Pharoah PO: Twins and cerebral palsy. Acta Paediatr Suppl 90:6–10, 2001.

Pharoah PO, Cooke T, Johnson MA, et al:. Epidemiology of cerebral palsy in England and Scotland, 1984-9. Arch Dis Child Fetal Neonat Ed 79:21–25, 1998.

Pharoah PO, Platt MJ, Cooke T: The changing epidemiology of cerebral palsy. Arch Dis Child Fetal Neonat Ed 75:169–173, 1996.

Pierrat V, Duqennoy C, van Haastert IC: Ultrasound diagnosis and neurodevelopmental outcome of localized and extensive cystic PVL. Arch Dis Child Neonatal Ed 84:151–156, 2001.

Pinto-Martin JA, Riolo S, Cnaan A, et al: Cranial ultrasound prediction of disabling and nondisabling cerebral palsy at age two in a low birth weight population. Pediatrics 95:249–254, 1995.

Radda GK: Brain biochemistry in Williams syndrome: Evidence for a role of the cerebellum in cognition? Neurology 51:8–9, 1998. Comment in Neurology 51:33–40, 1998; Neurology 52: 898–899, 1999.

Rapaport R, Rose SR, Freemark M: Hypothyroxinemia in the preterm infant: The benefits and risks of thyroxine treatment. J Pediatr 139:182–188, 2001.

Redline RW, Wilson-Costello D, Borawski E, et al: Placental lesions associated with neurologic impairment and cerebral palsy in very low-birth-weight infants. Arch Pathol Lab Med 122:1091–1098, 1998.

Reilly J, Stiles J, Larsen J, et al: Affective facial expression in infants with focal brain damage. Neuropsychologia 33:83–99, 1995.

Reilly JS, Bates E, Marchman V: Narrative discourse in children with early focal brain injury. Brain Lang 61:335–375, 1998.

Reiss AL, Eliez S, Schmitt JE, et al: IV. Neuroanatomy of Williams syndrome: A high-resolution MRI study. J Cogn Neurosci 1:65–73, 2000.

Roeleveld N, Zielhuis GA, Gabreels F: The prevalence of mental retardation: A critical review of recent literature. Dev Med Child Neurol 39:125–132, 1997.

Ross G, Lipper EG, Auld PAM: Consistency and change in the development of premature infants weighing less than 1,500 grams at birth. Pediatrics 76:885–891, 1985.

Rutter M, Simonoff E, Plomin R: Genetic influences on mild mental retardation: Concepts, findings and research implications. J Biosoc Sci 28:509–526, 1996.

Schendel DE, Berg CJ, Yeargin-Allsop M, et al: Prenatal magnesium sulfate exposure and the risk for cerebral palsy or mental retardation among very low birth weight children aged 3 to 5 years. JAMA 276:1805–1810, 1996.

Senbil N, Sonel B, Aydin OF, et al: Epileptic and non-epileptic cerebral palsy: EEG and cranial imaging findings. Brain Dev 24:166–169, 2002.

Shevell M, Ashwal S, Donley D, et al: Practice parameter: Evaluation of the child with global developmental delay. Neurology 60:367–380, 2003.

Smith A, Dykens E, Greenberg F: Behavioral phenotype of Smith Magenis. Am J Med Genet 81:179–185, 1998.

Sommerfelt K, Pedersen S, Ellertsen B, et al: Transient dystonia in non-handicapped low-birth weight infants and later development. Acta Paed Scand 85:1445–1449, 1996.

Sparrow S, Balla D, Cicchetti D: Vineland Adaptive Behavior Scales. Circle Pines, MN: American Guidance Services, 1984.

Sreenan C, Bhargava R, Robertson CMT: Cerebral infarction in the term newborn: Clinical presentation and long-term outcome. J Pediatr 137:351–355, 2000.

State MW, Dykens EM: Genetics of childhood disorders: XV. Prader-Willi syndrome: Genes, brain, and behavior. J Am Acad Child Adoles Psychiatry 39:797–800, 2000.

Stiles J: Spatial cognitive development, in Nelson C, Luciana M (eds): Handbook of Developmental Cognitive Neuroscience. Cambridge, MA: MIT Press, 2001, pp. 399–414.

Strauss D, Ashwal S, Shavelle R, et al: Prognosis for survival and improvement in function in children with severe developmental disabilities. J Pediatr 131:712–717, 1997.

Stromme P, Diseth TH: Prevalence of psychiatric diagnoses in children with mental retardation: Data from a population-based study. Dev Med Child Neurol 42:266–270, 2000.

Stromme P, Magnus P: Correlations between socioeconomic status, IQ and aetiology in mental retardation: A population-based study of Norwegian children. Soc Psychiatry Psychiatr Epidemiol 35:12–18, 2000.

Sugama S, Soeda A, Eto Y: Magnetic resonance imaging in three children with kernicterus. Pediatr Neurol 25:328–331, 2001.

Tager-Flusberg H, Sullivan K: A component view of theory of mind: Evidence from Williams syndrome. Cognition 76:59–90, 2000.

Tager-Flusberg H, Sullivan K: Early language development in children with mental retardation, in Burack J, Hodapp R, Zigler E (eds): Handbook of Mental Retardation and Development. New York: Cambridge University Press, 1998, pp. 208–239.

Teuber H: Why two brains? in Schmitt F, Worden F (eds): The Neurosciences: Third Study Program. Cambridge, MA: MIT Press, 1974, pp. 127–133.

Thackray H, Tifft C: Fetal alcohol syndrome. Pediatr Rev 22:47–55, 2001.

Topp M, Udall P, Greisen: Cerebral palsy births in eastern Denmark, 1987–1990: Implications for neonatal care. Paediatr Perinat Epidemiol 15: 271–277, 2001.

Touwen B: Examination of the child with minor neurologic dysfunction. London, UK: Spastics International Medical Publications, 1979.

Trauner DA, Ballantyne A, Friedland S, et al: Disorders of affective and linguistic prosody in children after early unilateral brain damage. Ann Neurol 39:361–367, 1996.

Trauner DA, Nass R, Ballantyne A: Behavioral profiles of children and adolescents after pre- or perinatal unilateral brain damage. Brain 124:995–1002, 2001.

Turk J, Cornish K: Face recognition and emotion perception in boys with fragile-X syndrome. J Intellect Disabil Res 42:490–499, 1998.

Volpe JJ: Neurology of the Newborn, ed 4. Philadelphia, PA: Saunders, 2000.

Walstab J, Bell R, Reddihough D, et al: Antenatal and intrapartum antecedents of cerebral palsy: A case-control study. Austr N Z J Obstet Gynaecol 42:138–146, 2002.

Wilson-Costello D, Botawski E, Friedman H, et al: Perinatal correlates of cerebral palsy and other neurologic impairment among very low birth weight children. Pediatrics 102: 315–322, 1998.

Winter S, Autry A, Boyle C, et al: Trends in the prevalence of cerebral palsy in a population-based study. Pediatrics 110:1220–1225, 2002.

Wong JG, Clare CH, Holland AJ, et al: The capacity of people with a "mental disability" to make a health care decision. Psychol Med 30:295–306, 2000.

Wu YW, Colford JM: Chorioamnionitis as a risk factor for cerebral palsy. JAMA 284:1417–1424, 2000.

Pediatric Epilepsy

Philip S. Fastenau
David W. Dunn
Joan K. Austin

Anticonvulsants
Child
Cognition
Epilepsy
Mental disorders
Neuropsychology
Psychiatry
Psychology

CLASSIFICATION AND EPIDEMIOLOGY

Definitions

Seizures are the result of sudden, transient, excessive discharges from neurons in the central nervous system (CNS). The clinical manifestation of the seizure is determined by the spread of the discharge from the epileptogenic focus to normal pathways within the CNS. *Epilepsy* is defined as recurrent seizures. Seizures and epilepsy are common neurologic problems in children.

Up to 10% of children may have a seizure at some time during the first two decades of life. Fever, head trauma, metabolic derangement, drugs, or toxins provoke most of these. Roughly 1% of children will develop epilepsy by 20 years of age (Hauser, 1994).

Classification

The Commission on Classification and Terminology of the International League Against Epilepsy (ILAE) has developed classifications for both seizures and epilepsy (Commission on Terminology and Classification of the ILAE, 1981, 1989). Classification of seizures requires a description of the event and, in most cases, results of an electroencephalogram (EEG). Epilepsies or epileptic syndromes are defined by age of onset, seizure manifestation, EEG data, and presumed etiology. Definition of the epileptic syndrome is necessary for decisions on appropriate therapy and counseling concerning the expected natural history.

Seizure Types

Epileptic seizures are divided into partial and generalized seizures. The partial seizures, also called focal or local seizures, begin within a cluster of neurons within one hemisphere. The EEG typically shows an interictal spike focus originating in the involved area of the CNS. Partial seizures are subdivided into simple, complex, and partial with secondary generalization. *Simple partial seizures* have motor, sensory, or psychic symptoms without impairment of consciousness. *Complex partial seizures,* previously called psychomotor seizures, always result in some alteration in consciousness. The *partial seizures with secondary generalization* begin as simple or complex partial seizures and then spread to affect both hemispheres resulting in a generalized tonic-clonic seizure. *Generalized seizures* are defined by discharges involving both cerebral hemispheres at the onset of the attack. Generalized seizures include absence (previously called petit mal), myoclonic, atonic, tonic, clonic, and tonic-clonic (previously grand mal) seizures (Commission on Terminology and Classification of the ILAE, 1981).

Figure 45-1 provides a flow chart to help guide the practitioner in the classification of seizure types. Classification of seizure types begins with a description of the episode. Start by asking the child and parents to describe the events preceding the episode. In particular, ask about the "aura" (or warning sign) that may occur immediately before a seizure. Next, obtain a detailed description of the episode, or ictus, asking about movements, automatisms, sensations, and alteration in contact with the environment. Finally, have the child and witnesses describe the postictal period, or time immediately following a seizure.

If there is no alteration of consciousness, the episode may be a simple partial seizure or a myoclonic seizure. Myoclonic seizures consist of a sudden brief contraction of one or more muscle groups. Alteration of consciousness occurs in complex partial seizures, partial seizures with secondary generalization, absence, tonic, atonic, and tonic-clonic seizures. With atonic seizures there is a sudden loss of muscle tone, and with tonic seizures, a sudden increase in tone. With both absence and partial complex seizures there may be a brief loss of consciousness. There is no aura or postictal period with absence seizures, whereas with partial complex seizures there is usually a brief period of confusion following the episode. Multiple motor, sensory, or psychic phenomena may accompany the partial complex seizures. Partial seizures with secondary generalization may look very much like a tonic-clonic seizure. At times there may be a focal component immediately preceding the episode in partial seizures with secondary generalization. An EEG is often necessary to differentiate absence seizures from complex partial seizures and to differentiate tonic-clonic seizures from partial seizures with secondary generalization.

FIGURE 45-1. Decision tree for classification of seizures (Sz).

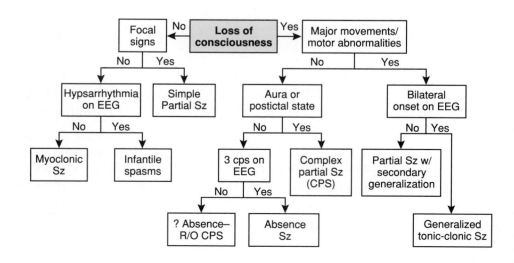

Epileptic Syndromes

Epileptic syndromes are first divided into localization-related epilepsies, generalized epilepsies, epilepsies undetermined whether focal or generalized, and special syndromes. The *localization-related epilepsies* (or "focal epilepsies") are manifested by partial seizures. These syndromes are subdivided into idiopathic epilepsies (no known cause), symptomatic (due to an identifiable cause), or cryptogenic epilepsies (due to a presumed but unidentified cause). The idiopathic focal epilepsies are usually familial disorders such as benign childhood epilepsy with centrotemporal spikes. The symptomatic focal epilepsies have a presumed site of localized dysfunction. They are labeled according to the site of origin as frontal, temporal, parietal, or occipital epilepsies. The *generalized epilepsies* are also subdivided into idiopathic and cryptogenic or symptomatic epilepsies. The idiopathic generalized epilepsies are familial and include benign neonatal familial convulsions, childhood absence epilepsy, and juvenile myoclonic epilepsy. The cryptogenic generalized epilepsies are severe disorders. The seizures are often intractable and the children have both cognitive and behavioral impairment. Examples are the Lennox-Gastaut syndrome and infantile spasms. If there is no clear focal or generalized origin to the discharges, the epileptic syndrome is placed in a separate category of *special syndromes*. Examples are epilepsy with continuous spike-wave discharges during slow-wave sleep and acquired epileptic aphasia (Landau-Kleffner syndrome). Febrile convulsions, seizures triggered by toxins or metabolic derangement, and isolated seizures are also special syndromes (Commission on Terminology and Classification of the ILAE, 1989).

Adverse Psychosocial Outcomes

As a group, children with epilepsy show two adverse psychosocial outcomes: academic underachievement and behavior problems. These outcomes are critical to quality of life and especially to success in relationships, school, and vocation. The factors contributing to the outcomes are complex, but identifying the factors that place some children at risk is essential for ameliorating these outcomes or preventing them altogether. A discussion of these follows. In addition, we are in the process of empirically testing the model illustrated in Figure 45-2. We include this diagram to help organize the many complex relationships among risk factors and outcomes and to help identify potential points of intervention to illustrate how different interventions can help address different contributing factors and possibly minimize the "cascade" effect of epileptiform activity on neuropsychological, academic, and behavioral outcomes.

ACADEMIC UNDERACHIEVEMENT

Extent and Nature of Underachievement

Children with epilepsy do not perform optimally in the classroom. They are at greater risk for academic difficulties compared with many other chronic illnesses of childhood (Fowler et al., 1985; Westbrook et al., 1991; Austin et al., 1998). Boys with severe epilepsy are at heightened risk (Austin et al., 1998). This has been demonstrated in the form of lower grades (Westbrook et al., 1991), lower achievement test scores (Farwell et al., 1985; Seidenberg et al., 1986; Mitchell et al., 1991), greater frequency of repeating one or more school years (Farwell et al., 1985), greater frequency of

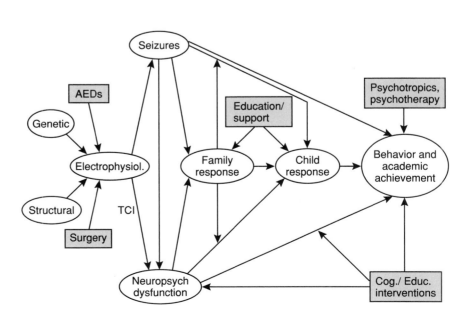

FIGURE 45-2. Conceptual model of behavioral and academic outcomes in pediatric epilepsy. AEDs, antiepileptic drugs.

learning disability diagnoses (Westbrook et al., 1991), and greater frequency of special education placements (Farwell et al., 1985; Westbrook et al., 1991). Furthermore, children with epilepsy are less successful than peers without epilepsy at obtaining gainful employment as adults (Dodrill & Clemmons, 1984).

Risk Factors for Underachievement

Five broad categories of variables (Table 45-1) appear to contribute to these academic problems: (1) neurologic abnormalities, (2) seizures, (3) neuropsychological dysfunction, (4) side effects of medication, and (5) poor child and family response to the seizure disorder. These factors are often interrelated. For example, it is likely that severe neurologic dysfunction would be associated with more frequent and severe seizures. Moreover, more frequent seizures can lead to treatment with higher levels of antiepileptic drugs (AEDs) and, therefore, more side effects. Finally, worse seizure control carries the burden of more stress and, as a result, worse adaptation.

TABLE 45–1. Risk Factors for Academic and Behavioral Problems in Pediatric Epilepsy

Neurologic dysfunction
  EEG abnormalities, especially slow-wave activity
  Structural abnormalities on CT or MRI
  Mental retardation (an indicator of global neural involvement)
  Severe epileptic syndromes (often associated with mental retardation)

Seizure variables
  Early age of onset
  Long seizure duration
  High seizure frequency
  Multiple seizure types
  Prior unrecognized seizures

Neuropsychological dysfunction
  Mental retardation
  Language
  Attention
  Psychomotor speed
  Memory and learning
  Problem solving

Side effects of medication

Poor child and family response to the epilepsy condition
  Family stress
  Low family adaptive resources
  Negative perceptions or attitudes
  Maladaptive coping behaviors
  External locus of control
  Child's satisfaction with family relationships

CT, computed tomography; MRI, magnetic resonance imaging.

Neurologic Abnormalities and Seizure Variables

Cognitive delays, a contributing factor to underachievement, have been associated with neurologic and seizure variables. Cortical dysplasias (especially if bilateral or diffuse) are associated with more severe epilepsy and more severe developmental delays (Whiting & Duchowny, 1999). More severe epileptic syndromes (e.g., neonatal seizures, infantile spasms, Lennox-Gastaut) are associated with mental retardation or severe language deficits.

Even in children without mental retardation, neurologic and seizure variables account for some of the academic outcomes. Age of seizure onset correlates with reading; age of onset, seizure severity, and type of epileptic syndrome correlate with arithmetic (Seidenberg et al., 1986). Austin and her colleagues found a robust effect for seizure severity on group achievement tests, but only in boys (Austin et al., 1998). Earlier age of onset, generalized seizures, and frequent episodes of status epilepticus are also associated with cognitive delays in children (Dam, 1990).

Slow-wave activity on the EEG correlated with attention and memory deficits in children (Koop et al., 2001). This was evident in children with chronic epilepsy but not in children with recent onset; in addition, children with chronic epilepsy showed greater neuropsychological impairment with longer duration of the condition. These findings suggest that abnormal electrical activity may have a progressive impact on cognitive function in children.

Neuropsychological Functioning

Intellectual Deficits. A relatively small proportion of children with epilepsy (those with severe and chronic epilepsy) have been shown to experience slower cognitive development and even cognitive regression. Some of this appears attributable to structural brain lesions, some to the severity and frequency of seizures, and some to the use of polytherapy with strong AEDs (e.g., Lesser et al., 1986; Rodin et al., 1986). For the majority of children, however, intellectual abilities are stable and broadly within the normal range; specific cognitive deficits (rather than global deterioration) appear to be responsible for their underachievement.

Specific Cognitive Deficits. Attention and psychomotor skills (eye-hand coordination and speed) very likely contribute to poor academic outcomes. Among children with epilepsy but without mental retardation, Fastenau and colleagues (1999a) found that attention, processing speed, and manual dexterity were one to two standard deviations below the mean for healthy children. Others, too, have reported slowed reaction time, inattention, variability, and cognitive fatigue in these children, even in children with strong intellectual abilities and even when unmedicated; these deficiencies are not necessarily related to any seizure history variables (Mitchell et al., 1992; Deonna, 1993; Williams et al., 1998b; Semrud-Clikeman & Wical, 1999). Children diagnosed with benign epilepsy have shown attentional deficiencies despite having a normal neurologic and neuroradiologic exam, having normal intellectual abilities, being unmedicated, and being free of clinical seizures for 6 months prior to the neuropsychological test (Piccirilli et al., 1994).

Memory is typically affected. Memory deficiencies can be specific to either the verbal or visual-spatial modality, corresponding with predominantly left or right cerebral discharges, respectively. Memory disturbances are observed even in high-functioning children (e.g., Seidenberg, 1989; Aldenkamp et al., 1993). In a sample that excluded children with intellectual impairments, Fastenau and his colleagues reported that children with epilepsy scored approximately one standard deviation below the mean for healthy children on a standardized battery of memory tests (Fastenau et al., 1999a).

Language disturbances exist. These can be profound in certain syndromes such as Landau-Kleffner syndrome (Soprano et al., 1994), but they are not limited to severe syndromes. In one study of children without intellectual delays (Fastenau et al., 1999a), both receptive language and expressive language were well below normal. In that sample and in similar heterogeneous samples, linguistic functioning discriminated between successful and unsuccessful achievers in school (Dodrill & Clemmons, 1984; Seidenberg, 1989; Fastenau et al., 1999a).

Executive functioning (e.g., mental flexibility, abstract reasoning, ability to generate ideas and solutions) also has been affected in children with epilepsy. Fastenau and colleagues (Fastenau et al., 1999a) found that executive functioning was close to one standard deviation below normal. Furthermore, these deficiencies were highly correlated with academic achievement.

Transient Cognitive Impairment as a Model. Binnie (1993) hypothesized that ongoing subclinical interictal epileptiform discharges produce transient cognitive impairment (TCI), which in turn leads to psychosocial dysfunction. There is some support for this model. During recording of abnormal EEG discharges, impaired cognitive performances have been observed for reading and arithmetic achievement (Kasteleijn-Nolst Trenité et al., 1988) and for neuropsychological skills such as abstraction/reasoning, paired associate learning, visual perception, and fine-motor skills (Siebelink et al., 1988). As further support for the model, aggressive pharmaceutical treatment reduced

EEG abnormalities, which resulted in improved cognitive and emotional-behavioral functioning (Marston et al., 1993).

Based on the TCI model, one would expect neuropsychological deficiencies to be apparent at or near the onset of the seizure disorder. Recent studies have provided such support. Austin and colleagues (2001) found that children with new-onset seizures had more attention problems than their healthy siblings, based on parent- and teacher-reported scales. Using standardized neuropsychological tests, Fastenau and colleagues (1999b) confirmed this in children with recent onset of seizures. Compared to their siblings, children with epilepsy showed deficits in attention, mental processing speed, memory and learning, and receptive language. Individual neuropsychological functions (excluding IQ) explained up to 50% of the variance in academic achievement (Fastenau et al., 1999a) and up to 36% of the variance in behavior problems (Fastenau et al., 2000).

Side Effects of Antiepileptic Drugs

The AEDs have been implicated in some of the adverse cognitive changes. However, in a review of 90 studies, Vermeulen and Aldenkamp (1995) identified the many methodological issues that place constraints on interpretations. After considering these factors they concluded, "Still, the tentative overall picture emerging from the crème de la crème of research on cognitive AED effects is that differences in cognitive profiles may not be *very* large" (p. 89, emphasis in original text). Others have reached a similar conclusion (Dodrill, 1992; Nichols et al., 1993; Bourgeois, 1998). In children, phenobarbital is associated with greater cognitive deficits; bromide and benzodiazepines may also carry adverse effects. For other AEDs, effects on cognition appear to be minimal when used as monotherapy in the therapeutic range (Nichols et al., 1993; Vermeulen & Aldenkamp, 1995). A recent prospective study with children using a sensitive neuropsychological battery and a matched control group with newly diagnosed diabetes found no effects of AEDs on cognitive functioning (Williams et al., 1998a).

Child and Family Response

Child and family factors in academic underachievement have been explored by Austin and her colleagues (Austin et al., 1998). Children's attitudes toward their epilepsy condition predicted achievement scores on standardized group tests. This suggests that how well children adapt to their medical condition affects academic performance. Thus, educating children about their condition could help optimize academic outcomes.

BEHAVIORAL AND PSYCHIATRIC FUNCTIONING

Extent of Behavior Problems

Children with epilepsy have higher than expected rates of behavioral maladjustment. Epidemiologic studies indicate that they are five to nine times more likely to have behavioral problems than children in the general population (Rutter et al., 1970; McDermott et al., 1995). Epilepsy results in higher rates of behavior problems than do other chronic health conditions without neurologic involvement. In a major epidemiologic study, the prevalence of psychiatric disturbance was 6.6% in children in the general population, 11.6% in children with chronic conditions without CNS involvement, 28.6% in children with idiopathic epilepsy, 37.5% in children with neurologic damage, and 58.3% in children with both seizures and neurologic damage (Rutter et al., 1970). In another epidemiologic study, psychiatric problems were found in 8.5% of children in the control group, in 21% of children with cardiac problems, and in 31% of children with epilepsy (McDermott et al., 1995). Thus, children with epilepsy are at risk for behavioral problems both because of their chronic physical condition and because of CNS involvement.

Nature of Behavior Problems

In general, reviews of literature on adjustment in children with chronic conditions show that these children are vulnerable to internalizing problems such as depression and social withdrawal (Boekaerts & Roder, 1999). Adjustment problems experienced by children with epilepsy, however, vary widely and range from minor problems in daily living to psychosis. In a study comparing quality of life in children with either epilepsy or asthma, Austin and colleagues (Austin et al., 1994) found children with epilepsy to have relatively more negative attitudes toward their condition, more self-anxiety, less happiness and satisfaction with self, and more internalizing (e.g., depression, anxiety) and externalizing behavior problems (e.g., hyperactivity, aggression). When compared to children with diabetes, children with epilepsy have poorer self-concepts (Matthews et al., 1982) and more psychiatric disturbances (Hoare, 1984).

Risk Factors for Behavior Problems

Factors accounting for these high rates of behavioral maladjustment in children with epilepsy are not well delineated. However, the five broad categories of variables implicated in academic underachievement (see Table 45-1) appear to contribute to behavior problems as well.

Neurologic Abnormalities

There is substantial evidence that neurologic dysfunction is associated with behavioral maladjustment. Empirical studies show that children with epilepsy and accompanying neurologic deficits have higher than expected rates of behavioral maladjustment (Hermann, 1981, 1982; Rutter, 1981). Among children with both epilepsy and mental retardation (implicating neurologic dysfunction), over half have abnormally high rates of behavioral maladjustment (Steffenburg et al., 1996). Even when IQ is low (low average, borderline, and very mildly impaired) but without diagnosable mental retardation, children with epilepsy showed elevated rates of behavior problems compared to children with epilepsy who had higher cognitive functioning, despite equal distributions of seizure type across IQ groups (Buelow et al., in press).

Cortical dysplasias (especially those with bilateral or diffuse involvement) are associated with more severe epilepsy and more severe developmental delays (Whiting & Duchowny, 1999), which are associated with worse behavioral adjustment. Tuberous sclerosis, in particular, is associated with high rates of behavioral and psychiatric disorders (Hunt & Dennis, 1987; Smalley, 1998). Koop and colleagues (2001) found a relationship between slow-wave activity on EEG and behavior problems among children with epilepsy, after excluding those with mental retardation. Certain epileptic syndromes and types also carry a high risk of behavioral disorders. These include infantile spasms (West syndrome), Lennox-Gastaut syndrome, and acquired aphasias associated with epilepsy such as Landau-Kleffner syndrome (Aicardi, 1996).

Neurologic factors that place children at risk for seizures (possibly subclinical epileptiform activity) may contribute to behavior problems. Hoare (1984) found that 45% of children with new-onset epilepsy had a psychiatric disturbance. More recently, Dunn and colleagues (1997) found that 24% of children with new-onset seizures had behavior problem scores on the Child Behavior Checklist (CBCL; Achenbach, 1991) in the at-risk range in the months preceding the first recognized seizure.

Seizure Variables

Little is known about the effect of seizures on behavioral maladjustment. Early age of onset, long seizure duration, high seizure frequency, and multiple seizure types are associated with greater behavioral maladjustment (Hoare, 1984; Hermann et al., 1989; Austin et al., 1992, 1994). In addition, some seizure types and syndromes (e.g., minor motor seizures, atypical absences, and infantile spasms) are related to mental health problems, but this relationship probably reflects mental retardation associated with these syndromes (Dunn & Austin, 1999).

In the otherwise neurologically intact child (with IQ in the normal range), however, seizure type and epileptic syndrome have not been consistent predictors of behavioral maladjustment. Although complex partial seizures have been associated with adjustment problems in adults, this relationship has not been consistently supported in pediatric populations.

Neuropsychological Functioning

Papero and colleagues (1992) propose that neurologic abnormalities lead to deficits in neuropsychological functioning and that these deficits, in turn, lead to mental health problems. When mental retardation is present in children with epilepsy, over half of the children have abnormally high rates of behavioral maladjustment (Steffenburg et al., 1996). Even among children without mental retardation, cognitive functioning is related to behavior and emotional adjustment. Fastenau and colleagues (2000) reported that all domains of neuropsychological functioning (especially attention, psychomotor speed, and verbal learning) were related to behavioral problems, explaining as much as 36% of the variance.

Side Effects of Antiepileptic Drugs

Although side effects of antiepileptic drugs are related to emotional and behavior disorders in some people with epilepsy (Reynolds, 1991), this relationship is probably not strong. Prospective studies of behavior change associated with initiation of antiepileptic medication in children with newly diagnosed epilepsy suggest that AEDs affect cognitive and behavioral functioning only minimally. For example, Mandelbaum and Burack (1997) found no significant deterioration in behavioral performance over a 12-month period of AED treatment. In another antiepileptic medication initiation study (Williams et al., 1998a), behavioral disruptions over a 6-month period in children with epilepsy were not significantly higher than in controls. Minimal differences in behavior also were found in a recent antiepileptic medication withdrawal study. After drug withdrawal, children reported improvements in only one area (tiredness) out of eight areas studied (Aldenkamp et al., 1998). In this same study, parents reported that their children improved in areas of activation (e.g., alertness, drowsiness, and concentration disorders) but not in adjustment (e.g., depression and aggressiveness).

Child and Family Response

Consistent with family stress theory, Austin and colleagues (1992) found higher levels of family stress, lower levels of family adaptive resources, and high seizure frequency to be associated with child behavior problems. Lower socioeconomic status has also been associated with child behavioral maladjustment (Hoare & Kerley, 1991). Because recent studies of children with new-onset seizures show behavior problems to occur very early (Dunn et al., 1997; Austin et al., 2001), it is difficult to determine if negative family responses precede or follow the behavioral problems in the child.

Child responses to epilepsy have been associated with a variety of adjustment outcomes. In adolescents with chronic epilepsy (Dunn et al., 1999), four child variables (negative attitudes about having seizures, external locus of control, negative coping strategies, and satisfaction with family relationships) predicted depression.

ASSESSMENT

Table 45-2 lists assessment procedures that should be considered in the evaluation of seizures. Selection of specific procedures depends on the presentation of the child with seizures.

Laboratory Tests

The physician should check standard metabolic screens such as glucose, calcium, and electrolytes on all children with new-onset seizures. If the child is developmentally delayed, serum and urine screens for inborn errors of metabolism are obtained.

Electroencephalography

The EEG is an essential part of the evaluation of seizures, with the exception of febrile seizures and seizures that are clearly due to metabolic derangements, trauma, or infection. EEG assists in ruling out nonepileptic phenomena such as breath-holding spells, movement disorders, syncope and cardiac arrhythmias, sleep disorders, migraine, and various psychiatric syndromes that may mimic epilepsy in children. Also, EEG provides valuable information for classifying epileptic syndromes, which guide treatment decisions and inform practitioners and families of prognosis. Finally, EEG can identify subclinical and nonconvulsive seizures and AED toxicity (Nordli & Pedley, 2001). Although it has been argued that EEG carries limited information in predicting seizure recurrence (Gilbert & Buncher, 2000), its utility in differential diagnosis and prognosis is critical, even after the first unprovoked seizure (Berg et al., 2000; Dlugos, 2000).

Epileptiform activity (spikes, sharp waves, or spike-wave discharges) is fairly specific to epilepsy and is largely diagnostic. The false-positive rate is relatively small (spikes or spike-wave complexes observed in 2%–9% of children without neurologic disorders). The false-negative

TABLE 45-2. Assessment and Treatment of Pediatric Epilepsy

Assessment
Laboratory tests
EEG
Neuroimaging (MRI unless acute hemorrhage suspected)
Neuropsychological assessment
Psychiatric consultation
Sleep study

Treatment
Control the Seizures
AEDs (monotherapy, followed by polytherapy if required)
Consultation with epilepsy surgery team and/or ketogenic diet specialist if seizures are medically refractory and disabling
Optimize Learning
Obtain neuropsychological evaluation
Implement classroom supports for attentional deficits
Implement speech/language therapy for language delays
Implement occupational therapy for handwriting and fine-motor skills
Coordinate with school for specific learning interventions (e.g., for learning disabilities)
Manage Behavior
Psychotherapy
Psychopharmacologic therapy
Education and Support for the Child and Family
Provide brochures, pamphlets, and videos describing epilepsy, its course, its treatment, and seizure first aid
Provide contact information for nearest support group
Provide contact information for the National Epilepsy Foundation

rate, on the other hand, can be as high as 70% following a single routine EEG (Aicardi, 1996). This failure to detect epileptiform activity can be reduced to 10% to 30% with repeat EEGs, activation procedures (sleep deprivation, hyperventilation, and photic stimulation), and long-term monitoring (Kim, 1991; Aicardi, 1996; Nordli & Pedley, 2001). Adding sleep recordings to a routine EEG greatly increases sensitivity with little extra time or cost. The success of sleep recordings is doubled for young children (ages 2–8) and tripled for older children (ages 8 and older) when using partial sleep deprivation the night before the EEG instead of using hypnotic agents during the exam (Liamsuwan et al., 2000).

Nonepileptiform activity (e.g., slow-wave activity) is not specific to epilepsy. Nonetheless, nonepileptiform patterns can be very useful for identifying encephalopathies, focal lesions, or progressive syndromes (Nordli & Pedley, 2001). In addition, slow-wave activity in children with epilepsy seems to be a predictor of neuropsychological dysfunction (Koop et al., 2000) and behavioral problems (Koop et al., 2001), even in children without mental retardation.

Neuroimaging

Neuroimaging should be performed in all children with partial seizures and recurrent generalized seizures. At onset of the seizures, structural imaging can help to characterize the source of seizures (e.g., agenesis of the corpus callosum, tuberous sclerosis, cortical dysplasia) and to rule out an acute treatable cause (e.g., intracranial hemorrhage or neoplasm). Structural magnetic resonance imaging (MRI) is the tool of choice in most applications, except when acute hemorrhage or hydrocephalus is a concern or when urgency precludes immediate access to a magnet for MRI. Established functional exams (positron emission tomography [PET], single photon emission computed tomography [SPECT]) are generally reserved for presurgical evaluations; functional MRI (fMRI), magnetic resonance spectroscopy (MRS), and magnetic resonance relaxometry (MRR) hold some promise for the future but are currently considered experimental (Kuzniecky, 2001). Neuroimaging may not be necessary in all children. For example, well-defined idiopathic generalized syndromes such as childhood absence epilepsy (with a characteristic semiology and EEG profile) generally do not warrant imaging.

Neuropsychological Assessment

Neuropsychological consultation can be invaluable in the evaluation of a child with seizures. Many subtle neuropsychological deficiencies (especially in language and memory processes) will be evident only with comprehensive neuropsychological testing. Formal assessment can identify specific deficits that might impede cognitive development and skill acquisition. The assessment can also identify strengths that can be used in retraining or in compensatory strategies. Using these data, the neuropsychologist can design specific rehabilitation strategies, make recommendations to the teachers and educational specialists at the child's school (e.g., instructional strategies and classroom accommodations), coordinate the efforts of other health care and rehabilitation specialists (e.g., speech-language pathologists or occupational therapists), and provide follow-up assessment to monitor progress. Children with any risk factors in Table 45-1 would be especially good candidates for a neuropsychological examination.

Psychiatric Consultation

Psychiatric consultation should be obtained for those children with epilepsy who develop symptoms of disruptive behavior disorders, depression, anxiety, or psychosis. Children with any risk factors highlighted in Table 45-1, in particular, should be considered for a psychiatric consultation to rule out formal psychiatric disorders and behavior problems that may warrant brief intervention or monitoring. The psychiatrist or psychologist will confirm the presence of symptoms and determine appropriate diagnosis. Psychiatric consultation will include assessment of risk factors for emotional or behavioral problems other than epilepsy, such as family history of illness, stresses within the family, or preexisting psychiatric problems. The psychiatrist or psychologist can help assess the effect of AEDs, seizure origin, and seizure severity on the child's behavior and the impact of illness on the child and family.

Sleep Study

Sleep problems are common in children with epilepsy (Stores et al., 1998; Cortesi et al., 1999). Bourgeois (1996) points out that there is a reciprocal relationship between sleep and epilepsy. Epilepsy (particularly when it involves primarily or secondarily generalized seizures) can affect sleep, decreasing rapid eye movement (REM) sleep by 41% to 50%. Conversely, sleep deprivation increases the occurrence of epileptiform activity on EEG and increases the frequency of overt seizures. Finally, some sleep disorders can be misdiagnosed as epilepsy, and some forms of epilepsy can be misdiagnosed as sleep disorders in children (Bourgeois, 1996). Furthermore, sleep problems are associated with greater behavior problems in children with idiopathic epilepsy (Stores et al., 1998; Cortesi et al., 1999). Consequently, an informal inquiry into sleep habits and sleep disturbances should be a routine part of the epilepsy evalua-

tion. A formal sleep study may be beneficial in those children with restless sleep, daytime lethargy, or known nocturnal seizures.

TREATMENT

Control the Seizures

Antiepileptic Drugs

Description and Indications. Appropriate treatment of most epileptic syndromes requires AEDs. If a child has a single seizure, febrile seizures, seizures provoked by a reversible cause, or benign idiopathic localization-related epilepsy, AEDs may not be warranted. For almost all other epileptic syndromes, the child will be started on an AED chosen on the basis of the syndrome and the potential side effects of the AED. With the exception of ethosuximide, most AEDs are effective against partial seizures and primary generalized tonic-clonic seizures. Childhood absence epilepsy may respond to ethosuximide, valproate, and lamotrigine. Infantile spasms are difficult to control. The AEDs most often used for infantile spasms are corticosteroids, valproate, lamotrigine, topiramate, tiagabine, and, in Europe, vigabatrin. Lennox-Gastaut syndrome is also very difficult to control, but may respond to valproate, topiramate, lamotrigine, or felbamate.

Adverse Effects. A decision on first-choice agent depends on expected effectiveness of the agent and potential side effects. Behavior and cognitive problems are most often associated with phenobarbital, benzodiazepines, topiramate, and tiagabine. Aplastic anemia may occur with felbamate, hepatic dysfunction with felbamate and valproate, and skin rash with many agents, but more commonly with lamotrigine and phenytoin. Vigabatrin is available in Europe and Canada and has caused visual field constriction and psychiatric symptoms (Pellock, 1998; Browne & Holmes, 2000).

Cost-Benefit Analysis. The lifetime monetary cost of treatment (direct cost) for AED-responsive pediatric epilepsy (recurrent seizures) is estimated at $3600 (Annegers & Begley, 2001). In addition to monetary costs, adverse effects range from emotionally distressing changes (e.g., acne, weight gain, hair loss) to physical discomfort (e.g., nausea, diarrhea, abdominal pain) to iatrogenic morbidities (e.g., osteoporosis, aplastic anemia, hepatic failure); however, many of these symptoms can be controlled or minimized by careful monitoring of drug levels and by dietary supplements (Willmore et al., 2001). Although these costs are not negligible, about 50% of children will achieve seizure remission for 5 years or more on AEDs (Hauser et al., 1995; Cockerell et al., 1997). By comparison, the costs of uncontrolled seizures include decreased quality of life, limited educational and vocational opportunities, cognitive deterioration, risk of injury during a seizure, and even risk of death from accidents during a seizure, from status epilepticus, or from sudden epileptic death. Table 45-3 lists established and newer AEDs for pediatric populations, together with their indications (by seizure type), recommended dosing procedures, and adverse effects (Zupanc, 1996; Pellock, 1999).

Specific Treatment Guidelines. Empirically based guidelines have emerged for several common treatment decisions: treating the first seizure, withdrawing medications after the child is seizure free, and treating febrile seizures. For treating the first seizure, Shinnar and O'Dell (2001) delineate the risk factors of having a second, defining seizure. These include an abnormal EEG (epileptiform more predictive than nonepileptiform, but both are risk factors), prior nonacute brain injury, and seizure during sleep (versus wakefulness); prior history of febrile seizures and Todd's paresis may increase the risk, as well. Shinnar and O'Dell (2001) advocate that the provider and family jointly weigh the risks of treatment against risks of recurrence in making a decision.

Similarly, withdrawing AEDs requires consideration of the risks of chronic treatment versus the risks of withdrawal (Shinnar & O'Dell, 2001). After 2 years of being seizure-free on medications, 60% to 70% of children will remain seizure-free after AEDs are withdrawn; prior to 2 years, risks of recurrence are significant. Primary risk factors that predict recurrence after withdrawal include abnormal EEG at time of withdrawal, prior neurologic insult, and age of onset past 12 years; long duration of epilepsy and multiple seizure types may increase the risk as well. Again, the provider and family should jointly weigh the risks of treatment against risks of recurrence in making a decision (Shinnar & O'Dell, 2001).

Current guidelines stipulate that simple febrile seizures do not require medication (Baumann & Duffner, 2000). However, families of children experiencing febrile seizures still require treatment in the form of support, reassurance, and education (Freeman & Vining, 1995).

Optimizing AED Adherence. Although AEDs are effective in managing seizures in the vast majority of children with epilepsy, adherence among children and adolescents is far from optimal. Ventura and colleagues (2000) reviewed the literature on medication adherence in childhood epilepsy and in other childhood conditions. Estimates of nonadherence to AEDs range from 25% to 75% among children with epilepsy (Leppik, 1988; Shope, 1988; Hazzard et al., 1990; Buck et al., 1997). Nonadherence was more common in older children than in younger children (Shope, 1988), probably because parents oversee medications in younger children. Older children and adolescents are very self-conscious; they

often feel stigmatized when they must take medication in front of their peers. Consequently, morning and evening dosing may lead to better adherence in children. Side effects play a significant role; acne, weight gain, hair loss, and cognitive slowing can be devastating for anyone, but especially for older children and adolescents.

Low parental education and modest family income (which are not independent factors) are associated with lower adherence. Although affordability of drugs seems like the most obvious barrier to families with modest economic resources, other barriers may play an even greater role. For example, without ready access to a telephone, scheduling of medical appointments and calling in prescriptions becomes more tedious; similarly, lack of convenient or consistent transportation can impede follow-through on medical appointments and retrieval of prescriptions. Attitudes toward health care, toward the treating physician, and toward medication can interfere with AED adherence, as can treatment complexity (e.g., polytherapy versus monotherapy).

The treating professional plays an important role in promoting medication adherence and thereby seizure control. Developing rapport with the younger patient is a critical step; this can be achieved, in part, by acknowledging the difficulties of living with epilepsy, the stigma of taking medications, and the discomfort and embarrassment of side effects. Collaborating to identify a medication that has an acceptable tradeoff between seizure control and side effects in the child's eyes can be very beneficial. Finally, breakthrough seizures may not occur for days after the child misses a dose or stops taking AEDs; thus, children and adolescents may not appreciate the causal relationship without the empathic tutelage of a caring provider.

Surgery

Seizure surgery is considered for the child with difficult-to-control seizures. Surgery is usually considered if the child's seizures have failed to respond to three AEDs and if the seizure is focal and in a location that can be removed without significant functional impairment. Three types of surgery have been used: cortical resection, callosotomy, and hemispherectomy. Cortical resection is most likely to be effective if there is a discrete focus in the temporal lobe (Wyllie et al., 1998). In children with lateralized but diffuse epileptic foci that are rapidly generalizing, corpus callosotomy or hemispherectomy may be considered (Carmant & Holmes, 1994).

In addition to these three surgical procedures, vagus nerve stimulation is emerging as a new surgical option and is approved by the Food and Drug Administration (FDA) for adults and adolescents over 12 years of age (Cyberonics, 2001). No subcortical tracts are severed or cortical tissue removed; instead, a

TABLE 45-3. Established and Newer Antiepileptic Drugs and Their Treatment Profiles for Pediatric Epilepsy

Drug	FDA-Approved indications	Maintenance dose	Adverse effects
Established Antiepileptic Drugs for Children*			
Phenytoin	Generalized; partial	5–7 mg/kg/d	Ataxia, incoordination, diplopia, nystagmus, gingival hyperplasia, hirsutism, coarsening of facial features, lupus syndrome, hepatic enzyme increases, megaloblastic anemia
Carbamazepine	Partial; generalized	10–20 mg/kg/d in 2–3 divided doses	Ataxia, incoordination, diplopia, nystagmus, nausea, leukopenia or other bone marrow abnormalities, syndrome of inappropriate antidiuretic hormone secretion
Valproic Acid (or divalproex sodium)	Mixed (absence & GTC); GTC; Partial with secondary generalization	20–60 mg/kg/d in 3–4 divided doses	Ataxia, incoordination, diplopia, nystagmus, nausea, weight gain, pancreatitis, hepatic enzyme increases, liver failure, amenorrhea, alopecia, thrombocytopenia
Ethosuximide	Absence	15–40 mg/kg/d	Ataxia, incoordination, diplopia, nystagmus, nausea, vomiting, leukopenia or other bone marrow abnormalities
Phenobarbital	Childhood GTC; partial	3–5 mg/kg/d	Ataxia, incoordination, diplopia, nystagmus, sedation, cognitive dysfunction, hyperactivity, sleep disturbance, aggression, poor attention and concentration
Newer Drugs			
Felbamate [†]	Adjunctive for partial and generalized in Lennox-Gastaut syndrome	15–>75 mg/kg/d	Anorexia, aplastic anemia, gait abnormalities, hepatotoxicity, insomnia, nausea, somnolence, vomiting, weight loss
Gabapentin [†]	(Adults only)	30–>90 mg/kg/d	Ataxia, behavioral changes, dizziness, fatigue, nystagmus, somnolence, weight gain
Lamotrigine [†]	Adjunctive for generalized in Lennox-Gastaut syndrome	1–>15 mg/kg/d	Ataxia, diplopia, dizziness, headache, nausea, rash (potentially Stevens-Johnson syndrome), somnolence, vomiting
Tiagabine [†]	Adjunctive for partial	32–56 mg/d	Dizziness, headache, somnolence, twilight state
Topiramate [†]	(Adults only)	3–>10 mg/kg/d	Abnormal thinking, ataxia, confusion, diplopia, dizziness, fatigue, headache, impaired concentration, nystagmus, paresthesia, psychomotor slowing, somnolence, speech difficulties
Oxcarbazepine	Partial seizures in children ages 4–16 yr	20–50 mg/kg/d	Sedation, dizziness, headache, nausea, unsteadiness, double vision, hyponatremia, rash, hepatotoxicity
Levetiracetam	(Adults only)	Child doses not established	Lethargy, nervousness, dizziness, headache
Zonisamide	(Adults only)	4–8 mg/kg/d	Poor concentration, agitation, lethargy, headache, nausea, anorexia, renal stones, rash, hepatotoxicity

The dose ranges provided do not take into account individual patient characteristics or possible drug interactions. The practitioner should always consult current recommendations from the manufacturer and the most recent published studies and guidelines.

GTC, generalized tonic-clonic.

* Adapted from Zupane ML: Update on epilepsy in pediatric patients. Mayo Clin Proc 71:899–916, 1996

† Adapted from Pellock JM: Managing pediatric epilepsy syndromes with new antiepileptic drugs. Pediatrics 104:1106–1116, 1999.

device is implanted to stimulate the vagus nerve at regular intervals to prevent seizures and to abort a seizure at its onset. Evidence for its efficacy is mounting in adults; although trials with children are still in early stages, preliminary evidence appears promising (Amar et al., 2001).

Epilepsy surgery is much more costly than AEDs, with lifetime direct costs of surgery and presurgical evaluations averaging between $18,000 and $45,000 (Annegers & Begley, 2001). Also, surgery carries some risk of morbidity and mortality. Thus, surgery is reserved for seizure conditions that are sufficiently severe and disabling.

Ketogenic Diet

The ketogenic diet (a high-fat, low-protein, low-carbohydrate diet) has provided an alternative to surgery for medically refractory seizures in children for 80 years. Swink and colleagues (1997) recently reviewed the literature on this diet. Several forms of the diet exist, but a comparative trial showed no differences in their effectiveness to treat seizures. Representative studies dating back to 1925 have shown very similar outcomes. Secondary analysis of eight studies presented in the Swink and colleagues (1997) review showed that 37% of all patients experienced more than 90% reduction in seizures; 31% experienced less than 50% reduction in seizures. A recent multicenter study and a prospective study at Johns Hopkins showed similar results at three months (>90% reduction in 26% and 38%, respectively; <50% reduction in 43% and 33%, respectively). However, significant dropout rates inflated the rates of good response somewhat. Success rate is reported to be equivalent across most seizure types and etiologies (Swink et al., 1997). The ketogenic diet has very few monetary costs, particularly beyond the initial stages of implementing the diet and monitoring reactions; however, side effects can include elevated serum lipid levels, constipation, water-soluble vitamin deficiency, renal stones, growth inhibition, and acidosis and excess ketosis during illness (Swink et al., 1997).

Optimize Learning and Adaptation

Interventions to enhance learning and adaptation in children with epilepsy typically are implemented in the school. The neuropsychological evaluation will identify specific functions that are compromised and should provide specific recommendations tailored to the individual's profile of strengths and weaknesses (e.g., McCoy et al., 1997; Teeter, 1997; Ylvisaker, 1998). The neuropsychological consultation is most effective when the neuropsychologist communicates directly with staff at the child's school and can monitor progress as

various interventions are implemented. In addition, teachers and educational specialists have resources for addressing subject-specific skills (e.g., Mather, 1991; Mather & Jaffe, 1992). Rehabilitation specialists will have other techniques for the management of physical and sensory handicaps associated with more severe forms of epilepsy (Molnar & Alexander, 1999).

Manage Behavior Problems

Clinical interventions are needed to address the behavioral adjustment problems commonly found in children with epilepsy. Recent findings showing higher than expected rates of behavior problems in children with new-onset seizures (Austin et al., 2001; Dunn et al., 1997) strongly indicate that these intervention programs are needed early in the course of the disorder to prevent or reduce problems. Minimally, children's behavior needs to be routinely assessed so that treatment can be initiated. Children who are experiencing adjustment problems should be referred for mental health counseling. In addition, assessment of sleep problems is especially important to managing behavior problems in children who have epilepsy (Cortesi et al., 1999).

Psychopharmacologic interventions may be necessary for behavioral problems causing significant impairment. The effectiveness of psychotropic agents for children with epilepsy and behavioral problems is probably the same as seen in children with isolated behavioral difficulties. Two questions to be considered are the effect of psychotropic drugs on seizure threshold and drug interactions between antiepileptic and psychotropic medications. Stimulants such as methylphenidate and dextroamphetamines for attention-deficit/hyperactivity disorder and the serotonin reuptake inhibitors for depression and anxiety have not led to an increase in number of seizures. Drugs with higher risk of lowering seizure threshold are clozapine, chlorpromazine, clomipramine, and bupropion. Most drug interactions occur due to effects on the cytochrome P-450 enzyme system. Barbiturates are inducers that cause a drop in drug levels and several of the serotonin reuptake agents are inhibitors that may cause an increase in drug levels. In general, AED levels should be monitored after the addition of psychotropic agents (Alldridge, 1999).

Educate the Child and Family

Research suggests that seizures in children are stressful for families and children with new-onset epilepsy and their families have many concerns and fears related to seizures. Children report that they feel helpless, scared, and different from others (Brown, 1994; McNelis et al., 1998; Austin, 2000). Parents report fears of death, brain damage, cognitive deterioration, and brain tumors. Parents also are worried about possible side effects of antiepileptic medications such as addiction (Ward & Bower, 1978; Shore et al., 1998).

Psychoeducational interventions that provide information about the condition and skills training on adaptive coping should be helpful in reducing stress. Families often have incomplete or inaccurate information about epilepsy that could be addressed in such an intervention. Moreover, studies indicate that many parents are not satisfied with explanations given to them and desire more information about their child's seizures (Shore et al., 1998; Webb et al., 1998). Psychoeducational interventions could help address these problems also.

Few studies assessing psychosocial educational interventions for children with epilepsy have been conducted. A group psychosocial educational program was successful in increasing parents' knowledge, reducing parents' anxiety, and improving children's social competence (Lewis et al., 1990, 1991). Recently, Austin and colleagues (2002) completed a feasibility study of a psychoeducational intervention tailored to address the individual concerns and fears of each child with epilepsy and each of their parents. Preliminary results show increases in knowledge and reductions in need for information and support for both parents and children. Children also had fewer concerns and more satisfaction with family relationships after the intervention. More intervention research with the goal of reducing behavioral maladjustment is sorely needed.

The Epilepsy Foundation (EF; formerly known as Epilepsy Foundation of America) is an excellent resource for children and teens who have epilepsy and their families. EF is a consumer organization that is well informed by continuous input from a professional advisory board and by scholarly research activity. EF maintains a website (http://www.efa.org/) that contains news and updates relevant to living with epilepsy (e.g., state laws on driving, updates on medications). The site also provides contact information on state support groups. EF maintains a catalog of invaluable educational resources (pamphlets, brochures, books, and videos) for children with epilepsy and their families. Families can also reach EF by phone (301-459-3700) or by mail (4351 Garden City Drive, Landover, MD 20785).

PROGNOSIS

The prognosis for most children with seizures or epilepsy is good. In general, approximately 90% of children with epilepsy will experience a 1-year remission and at least 50% will experience a 5-year remission of seizures (Hauser & Hesdorffer, 1990; Hauser et al., 1995; Cockerell et al., 1997). Factors associated with increased risk of poor outcome are: age of onset less than 2 years, neurologic impairment or mental handicap, seizures that are initially difficult to control, and multiple seizure types. The idiopathic partial epilepsies and the idiopathic generalized epilepsies on average have the best prognosis and the cryptogenic generalized epilepsies the worst outcome (Aicardi, 1994).

CONTROVERSIES AND EMERGING ISSUES

Monotherapy versus Polytherapy

Animal studies suggest that AEDs have additive or supra-additive effects on antiepileptic properties but only additive or even infra-additive effects on neurotoxicity. Therefore, low-dose combination therapies may prove superior to high-dose monotherapy, but there are too few systematic comparisons in humans to endorse this concept at this time (Bourgeois, 2001). Given the interactions among AEDs (Gilman, 2001), monotherapy is currently preferred to polytherapy.

"Treating the EEG"

As described earlier, suppressing epileptiform activity on the EEG reduces cognitive dysfunction and improves psychosocial functioning. The concept of "treating the EEG" in the absence of clinical seizures has been met with increasing receptiveness (e.g., Mantovani, 2000). It is not without its precedent in current practice. In fact, consensus guidelines for treatment of neonatal seizures specify treating the EEG in the absence of clinical seizures (Mizrahi & Kellaway, 2001). In addition, in some cases where cognitive and behavioral regression is imminent, the tradeoffs are easily reconciled (e.g., Marescaux et al., 1990). A recent carefully controlled study with children demonstrated the effectiveness of low-dose clonazepam to mute epileptiform activity on EEG, with concomitant reduction in seizure activity (Dahlin et al., 2000). For treating cognitive deficits, however, the potential benefits do not appear to outweigh the risks of adverse reactions and neurotoxicity. Binnie (1993) argues that the only drugs that have proven to suppress interictal discharges are valproate, ethosuximide, and benzodiazepines, all of which appear to produce cognitive side effects. Although not feasible now, newer AEDs may hold promise in the near future for higher titrations that would suppress interictal epileptiform activity, resulting in better cognitive and behavioral functioning.

CASE STUDY: "TIM"

Identifying Information and Developmental/Medical History

Tim is a 13½-year-old, right-handed, white male who was referred from a psychiatric inpatient facility with explosive outbursts and with problems in math, expressive language, and writing. He was delivered vaginally at full term with the use of forceps at 7 pounds 10 ounces. He attained developmental milestones in timely fashion. He sustained a stroke at 10 months of age and began having seizures at that time (treated with phenytoin); his last recognized seizure was around 2 years of age. Recent EEG showed epileptiform activity in the right posterior temporal region; recent MRI showed asymmetry in the left hippocampal body suggestive of heterotopia, but possibly cortical dysplasia or low-grade neoplasm.

Family History

Tim lives with his mother and 11-year-old sister. There are two siblings who are much older (24 and 25) who do not live at home. Tim's father has not been in the home since Tim was an infant. The family is living on limited financial resources. There is a family history of depression, substance abuse, attention-deficit/hyperactivity disorder (ADHD), diabetes, hypertension, heart disease, and stroke.

Psychiatric, Psychosocial, and Educational History

Tim has been in a classroom for children with emotional handicaps full time since kindergarten; he repeated that grade. Tim was diagnosed with ADHD in grade 1 and was placed on methylphenidate, but reportedly without benefit. He was diagnosed with a learning disability in written expression in grade 3 (at age 8). He started becoming disruptive and more impulsive beginning around age 9, and repeated grade 4. Just before he turned 11 years old, emotional lability and "out of control" behavior led to his first psychiatric hospitalization.

Just before turning 13 years old, Tim became increasingly aggressive; he assaulted his teacher (twice), his mother, and her roommate. He set fires, urinated and defecated on the floor, and engaged in lying and stealing. Within months, he developed daily mood swings and threatened suicide. These behaviors led to four more psychiatric hospitalizations in rapid succession (within 6 months of one another), including the present one. There is no history of substance abuse. Over the course of his history, Tim has completed trials on methylphenidate, dextroamphetamine, gabapentin, clonidine, sertraline, risperidone, chlorpromazine, and olanzapine.

Assessment and Consultations

At the time of admission to the hospital, Tim was prescribed only dextroamphetamine. On admission, a multidisciplinary psychiatric team (psychiatrist, psychologist, social worker, nurse, recreational therapist, educational specialist, nutritionist, and clergy) evaluated Tim. Admitting diagnoses were conduct disorder, ADHD, and major depression; other diagnoses under consideration (to be ruled out) included bipolar disorder, personality syndrome secondary to a medical disorder, and psychosis. Neurologic consultation and neuropsychological evaluation were requested from two authors of this chapter (D.W.D. and P.S.F., respectively). The neurologic examination was normal. Head circumference was at the 25th percentile.

As part of the neuropsychological consultation, past academic test results were reviewed. In addition to a diagnosis of learning disability and two repeated grades documented in his history above, over the previous 2 years Tim showed declining achievement scores in reading and in math. On formal neuropsychological testing, Tim showed relative weaknesses in attention, mental processing speed, receptive and expressive language (18-point discrepancy from IQ), rapid automatic naming (a linguistic competency that contributes to reading development), and academic achievement in math (16- to 22-point discrepancy from IQ). These findings (together with history and behavioral observations) met criteria for DSM-IV (American Psychiatric Association, 1994) diagnoses of Mathematics Disorder (DSM-IV 315.1), Mixed Receptive-Expressive Language Disorder (DSM-IV 315.31), and Attention-Deficit/Hyperactivity Disorder, Combined Type (DSM-IV 314.01).

Treatment

Over the course of his hospitalization, Tim began individual therapy, group therapy with other children his age, and family therapy. In addition, educational interventions and accommodations were implemented in the classroom. During this time, the attending psychiatrist at the hospital, with input from the consulting neurologist, monitored Tim and adjusted the medication regime on the hospital unit. Drug therapies addressed the underlying epileptiform activity with valproic acid, depression with trazodone, and attentional deficits with dextroamphetamine.

In addition to pharmacologic management, various cognitive and educational interventions were prescribed. Given that the many tasks that face Tim in the next several years (and for the rest of his life) rely heavily on language (e.g., academic work, social interactions/relationships, psychotherapy), aggressive language therapy was identified as a high priority to remediate his language skills and to enable him to keep pace with peers in all areas. In addition, to minimize the impact of language limitations on everyday activities in Tim's life, parents, teachers, therapists, and unit staff were advised to use brief and direct statements when talking with him, to conduct frequent comprehension checks (e.g., have Tim repeat back what was said to ensure understanding), and to repeat information several times (and ask him to repeat it back several times). Supplementing verbal insights, homework, and instructions with written instructions was another strategy to help allow Tim to compensate for deficiencies in language comprehension. Finally, psychotherapeutic interventions to address Tim's aggressive behavior were couched in an explanation that takes verbal limitations into consideration, emphasizing that we all need to express our thoughts and emotions somehow, and when we have difficulty saying what we feel we may act out physically.

Exercises to enhance rapid naming were recommended, either by Tim's teachers or by a speech-language pathologist. A deficiency in rapid automatic naming can interfere with the development of automaticity in reading and hinder speed of reading. This can add increasing challenges later in school as well, when the curriculum requires more and more independent reading (especially in high school).

Accommodations in the classroom were identified to help to circumvent attentional problems. These included breaking long tasks into much smaller units, using small-group activity, having Tim sit at the front of the classroom to minimize any distraction during class, and providing one-on-one time with a teacher's aide to review important concepts and assignments. Given Tim's slower speed of mental processing, teachers were asked to consider untimed assignments and tests. Finally, teachers were advised to provide additional support, intervention, and monitoring for addressing Tim's declining academic skills in the area of math.

Discussion of Case Study

Tim's case illustrates numerous principles about pediatric epilepsy discussed in this chapter:

- Neuropsychological deficiencies are common, especially attention deficits (which may not respond to stimulant therapy), slowed mental processing speed, and language delays.
- Behavior problems (especially depression) are common and undermine many areas of living. These problems can be debilitating.
- Academic underachievement is common, as manifested by diagnoses of learning disabilities, repeated grade levels, and declining performance at different junctures of schooling.
- Certain factors increase the risk of both academic and behavioral problems. In Tim's case, he had EEG abnormalities, structural abnormalities on MRI, early age of onset, neuropsychological deficits, family stress, low family adaptive resources, and maladaptive coping behaviors.
- A multidisciplinary approach to assessment and management (especially with neurologic, psychiatric, neuropsychological, and educational input) is critical. This will typically include pharmacologic therapies to address the underlying epileptiform activity, psychiatric symptoms, and attentional deficits; psychotherapy to promote healthy perceptions, thought patterns, and lifestyle changes; and cognitive and educational interventions to address specific cognitive limitations.

SUMMARY

Our understanding of pediatric epilepsy is progressing, and this knowledge has implications for treatment. Health care professionals working with this population need to identify risk factors for adverse psychosocial outcomes (i.e., academic underachievement and behavioral maladjustment), which can lead to a rational approach to assessment procedures. The results of such assessment will be critical for informing treatment decisions. Perhaps the most important implication of the literature reviewed in this chapter is that pediatric epilepsy is a multifactorial disorder that requires multiple approaches to treatment. Controlling seizures is the first and critical step. AEDs will be the treatment of choice for most children. Health care professionals must be alert to the high rates of nonadherence in this population; developing rapport with the younger patient and acknowledging the difficulties of living with epilepsy will be important in promoting treatment adherence. In addition to medications, specific attention must be directed toward minimizing the impact of neuropsychological deficits on school success, managing behavior problems, and educating the child and family about the seizure disorder and about resources that are available to them (e.g., literature and support groups). With this multifactorial approach to treatment, prognosis (not only for seizure control but also for quality of life) can be expected to be very good for most children.

■ KEY POINTS

☐ Seizures and epilepsy are common neurologic problems in children; up to 10% of children may have a seizure at some time during the first two decades of life, and roughly 1% of children will develop epilepsy (recurrent unprovoked seizures) by 20 years of age (Hauser, 1994).

☐ Children with epilepsy, as a group, show two adverse psychosocial outcomes: academic underachievement and behavior problems.

☐ Risk factors for academic and behavior problems fall under five broad categories: (1) neurologic abnormalities, (2) seizures, (3) neuropsychological dysfunction, (4) side effects of medication, and (5) poor child and family response to the seizure disorder.

☐ Assessment strategies should include neurologic evaluation at onset of seizures and ongoing monitoring for neuropsychological, behavioral, and academic problems.

☐ Treatment strategies are fourfold: (1) control the seizures, (2) optimize learning, (3) manage behavior, and (4) provide education and support to the child and family.

KEY READINGS

Austin JK, Huberty TJ, Huster GA, Dunn DW: Academic achievement in children with epilepsy or asthma. Dev Med Child Neurol 40:248–255, 1998.

Dunn DW, Austin JK: Behavioral issues in pediatric epilepsy. Neurology 53(Suppl. 2):S96–S100, 1999.

Pellock JM, Dodson WE, Bourgeois BFD (eds): Pediatric Epilepsy: Diagnosis and Therapy. New York: Demos Medical Publishing, 2001, pp. 291–300.

REFERENCES

Achenbach TM: Manual for the Child Behavior Checklist/4–18 and 1991 profile. Burlington, VT: University of Vermont Department of Psychiatry, 1991.

Aicardi J: Epilepsy in Children, ed 2. Philadelphia, PA: Lippincott-Raven, 1996.

Aldenkamp AP, Alpherts WCJ, Blennow G, et al: Withdrawal of antiepileptic medication in children—effects on cognitive function: The multicenter Holmfrid study. Neurology 43:41–50, 1993.

Aldenkamp AP, Alpherts WCJ, Sandstedt P, et al: Antiepileptic drug-related cognitive complaints in seizure-free children with epilepsy before and after drug discontinuation. Epilepsia 39:1070–1074, 1998.

Alldridge BK: Seizure risk associated with psychotropic drugs: Clinical and pharmacokinetic considerations. Neurology 53(Suppl 2):S68–S75, 1999.

Amar AP, Levy ML, McComb JG, et al: Vagus nerve stimulation for control of intractable seizures in childhood. Pediatr Neurosurg 34:218–223, 2001.

American Psychiatric Association: Diagnostic and Statistical Manual of Mental Disorders, 4th ed. Washington, DC: American Psychiatric Association, 1994.

Annegers JF, Begley CE: Costs of pediatric epilepsy, in Pellock JM, Dodson WE, Bourgeois BFD (eds): Pediatric Epilepsy: Diagnosis and Therapy. New York: Demos Medical Publishing, 2001, pp. 569–574.

Austin JK: Impact of epilepsy in children. Epilepsy Behav 1(Suppl. 1):S9–S11, 2000.

Austin JK, Harezlak J, Dunn DW, et al: Behavior problems in children before first recognized seizures. Pediatrics 107:115–122, 2001.

Austin JK, Huberty TJ, Huster GA, et al: Academic achievement in children with epilepsy or asthma. Dev Med Child Neurol 40:248–255, 1998.

Austin JK, McNelis AM, Shore CP, et al: A feasibility study of a family seizure management program: Be seizure smart. J Neurosci Nurs 34:30–37, 2002.

Austin JK, Risinger MW, Beckett L: Correlates of behavior problems in children with epilepsy. Epilepsia 33:1115–1122, 1992.

Austin JK, Smith MS, Risinger MW, et al: Childhood epilepsy and asthma: Comparison of quality of life. Epilepsia 35:608–615, 1994.

Baumann RJ, Duffner PK: Treatment of children with simple febrile seizures: The AAP practice parameter. Pediatr Neurol 23:11–17, 2000.

Berg AT, Arts W, Boulloche J, et al: An EEG should not be obtained routinely after first unprovoked seizure in childhood [comment]. Neurology 55:898–899, 2000.

Binnie CD: Significance and management of transitory cognitive impairment due to subclinical EEG discharges in children. Brain Dev 15:23–30, 1993.

Boekaerts M, Roder I: Stress, coping, and adjustment in children with a chronic disease: A review of the literature. Disabil Rehabil 21:311–337, 1999.

Bourgeois B: The relationship between sleep and epilepsy in children. Semin Pediatr Neurol 3:29–35, 1996.

Bourgeois B: Antiepileptic drugs, learning, and behavior in childhood epilepsy. Epilepsia 39:913–921, 1998.

Bourgeois BFD: Combination drug therapy (monotherapy versus polytherapy), in Pellock JM, Dodson WE, Bourgeois BFD (eds): Pediatric Epilepsy: Diagnosis and Therapy. New York: Demos Medical Publishing, 2001, pp. 563–568.

Brown SW: Quality of life: A view from the playground. Seizure 3:11–15, 1994.

Browne TR, Holmes GL: Handbook of Epilepsy, ed 2. Philadelphia, PA: Lippincott Williams & Wilkins, 2000.

Buck D, Jacoby A, Baker GA, et al: Factors influencing compliance with antiepileptic drug regimes. Seizure 6:87–93, 1997.

Buelow JM, Perkins SM, Austin JK, et al: Behavior and mental health problems of children with epilepsy and low IQ. Dev Med Child Neurol, in press.

Carmant L, Holmes GL: Commissurotomies in children. J Child Neurol 9(Suppl. 2):2S50–2S60, 1994.

Cockerell OC, Johnson AL, Sander JW, et al: Prognosis of epilepsy: A review and further analysis of the first nine years of the British national general practice study of epilepsy, a prospective population-based study. Epilepsia 38:31–46, 1997.

Commission on Terminology and Classification of the International League against Epilepsy: Proposal for revised clinical and electroencephalographic classification of epileptic seizures. Epilepsia 22:489–501, 1981.

Commission on Terminology and Classification of the International League against Epilepsy: Proposal for revised classification of epilepsies and epileptic syndromes. Epilepsia 30:389–399, 1989.

Cortesi F, Giannoti F, Ottaviano S: Sleep problems and daytime behavior in childhood idiopathic epilepsy. Epilepsia 40:1557–1565, 1999

Cyberonics, Inc: Physician's Manual: NeuroCybernetic Prosthesis System—NCP Pulse Generator Models 100 and 101. Houston, TX: Cyberonics, Inc, 2001.

Dahlin M, Knutsson E, Åmark P, et al: Reduction of epileptiform activity in response to low-dose clonazepam in children with epilepsy: A randomized double-blind study. Epilepsia 41:308–315, 2000.

Dam M: Children with epilepsy: The effect of seizures, syndromes, and etiological factors on cognitive functioning. Epilepsia 31(Suppl. 4):S26–S29, 1990.

Deonna T: Annotation: Cognitive and behavioural correlates of epileptic activity in children. J Child Psychol Psychiatry 34:611–620, 1993.

Dlugos DJ: An EEG should not be obtained routinely after first unprovoked seizure in childhood [comment]. Neurology 55:898–899, 2000.

Dodrill CB: Problems in the assessment of cognitive effects of antiepileptic drugs. Epilepsia 33:S29–S32, 1992.

Dodrill CB, Clemmons D: Use of neuropsychological tests to identify high school students with epilepsy who later demonstrate inadequate performances in life. J Consult Clin Psychol 52:520–527, 1984.

Dunn DW, Austin JK: Behavioral issues in pediatric epilepsy. Neurology 53(Suppl. 2):S96–S100, 1999.

Dunn DW, Austin JK, Huster GA: Behaviour problems in children with new-onset epilepsy. Seizure 6:283–287, 1997.

Dunn DW, Austin JK, Huster GA: Symptoms of depression in adolescents with epilepsy. J Am Acad Child Adolesc Psychiatry 38:1132–1138, 1999.

Farwell JR, Dodrill CB, Batzel LW: Neuropsychological abilities of children with epilepsy. Epilepsia 26:395–400, 1985.

Fastenau PS, Austin JK, Dunn DW, et al: The role of neuropsychological dysfunction in academic underachievement among children with chronic epilepsy. Epilepsia 40:43, 1999a.

Fastenau PS, Austin JK, Dunn DW, et al: Relationship between neuropsychological functioning and behavior problems in chronic epilepsy. J Int Neuropsychol Soc 6:228, 2000.

Fastenau PS, Tansinsin SL, Koop JI, et al: Neuropsychological impairments in children with new-onset epilepsy. Clin Neuropsychol 13:225, 1999b.

Fowler MG, Johnson MP, Atkinson SS: School achievement and absence in children with chronic health conditions. J Pediatr 106:683–687, 1985.

Freeman JM, Vining EP: Febrile Seizures: A decision-making analysis. Am Fam Physician 52:1401–1406, 1995.

Gilbert DL, Buncher CR: An EEG should not be obtained routinely after first unprovoked seizure in childhood. Neurology 54:635–641, 2000.

Gilman JT: Drug interactions, in Pellock JM, Dodson WE, Bourgeois BFD (eds): Pediatric Epilepsy: Diagnosis and Therapy. New York: Demos Medical Publishing, 2001, pp. 555–562.

Hauser E, Freilinger M, Seidl R, et al: Prognosis of childhood epilepsy in newly referred patients. J Child Neurol 11:201–204, 1995.

Hauser WA: The prevalence and incidence of convulsive disorders in children. Epilepsia 25(Suppl. 2):S1–S6, 1994.

Hauser WA, Hesdorffer DC: Epilepsy: Frequency, Causes, and Consequences. New York: Demos Publications, 1990.

Hazzard A, Hutchinson SJ, Krawiecki N: Factors related to adherence to medication regimens in pediatric seizure patients. J Pediatr Psychol 15:543–555, 1990.

Hermann BP: Deficits in neuropsychological functioning and psychopathology in persons with epilepsy: A rejected hypothesis revisited. Epilepsia 22:161–167, 1981.

Hermann BP: Neurological functioning and psychopathology in children with epilepsy. Epilepsia 22:703–710, 1982.

Hermann BP, Whitman S, Dell J: Correlates of behavior problems and social competence in children with epilepsy, aged 6–11, in Hermann B, Seidenberg M (eds): Childhood Epilepsies: Neuropsychological, Psychosocial and Intervention Aspects, New York: Wiley, 143–157, 1989.

Hoare P: The development of psychiatric disorder among schoolchildren with epilepsy. Dev Med Child Neurol 26:3–13, 1984.

Hoare P, Kerley S: Psychosocial adjustment of children with chronic epilepsy and their families. Dev Med Child Neurol 33:201–215, 1991.

Kasteleijn-Nolst Trenité DGA, Bakker DJ, Binnie CD, et al: Psychological effects of subclinical epileptiform discharges: Scholastic skills. Epilepsy Res 2:111–116, 1988.

Kim WJ: Psychiatric aspects of epileptic children and adolescents. J Am Acad Child Adolesc Psychiatry 30:874–886, 1991.

Koop JI, Fastenau PS, Austin JK, et al: Behavioral correlates of electroencephalograms in children with epilepsy [abstract]. Epilepsia 42(Suppl. 7):160, 2001.

Koop JI, Fastenau PS, Dunn DW, et al: Neuropsychological correlates of electroencephalograms in children with epilepsy [abstract]. I Int Neuropsychol Soc 6:227, 2000.

Kuzniecky RI: Neuroimaging in pediatric epilepsy, in Pellock JM, Dodson WE, Bourgeois BFD (eds): Pediatric Epilepsy: Diagnosis and Therapy. New York: Demos Medical Publishing, 2001, pp. 133–143.

Leppik IE: Compliance during treatment of epilepsy. Epilepsia 29(Suppl. 2):S79–S84, 1988.

Lesser RP, Luders H, Wyllie E, et al: Mental deterioration in epilepsy. Epilepsia 27(Suppl. 2):S105–S123, 1986.

Lewis MA, Hatton CL, Salas I, et al: Impact of the children's epilepsy program on parents. Epilepsia 32:365–374, 1991.

Lewis MA, Salas I, de la Soto A, et al: Randomized trial of a program to enhance the competencies of children with epilepsy. Epilepsia 31:101–109, 1990.

Liamsuwan S, Grattan-Smith P, Fagan E, et al: The value of partial sleep deprivation as a routine measure in pediatric electroencephalography. J Child Neurol 15:26–29, 2000.

Mandelbaum DE, Burack GD: The effect of seizure type and medication on cognitive and behavioral functioning in children with idiopathic epilepsy. Dev Med Child Neurol 39:731–735, 1997.

Mantovani J: "Treat the patient, not the EEG"? Dev Med Child Neurol 42:579, 2000.

Marescaux C, Hirsch E, Finck S, et al: Landau-Kleffner syndrome: A pharmacologic study of five cases. Epilepsia 31:768–777, 1990.

Marston D, Besag F, Binnie CD, et al: Effects of transitory cognitive impairment on psychosocial functioning in children with epilepsy: A therapeutic trial. Dev Med Child Neurol 35:574–581, 1993.

Mather N: Instructional Guide to the WJ-R. Allen, TX: DLM Teaching Resources, 1991.

Mather N, Jaffe LE: WJ-R Recommendations and Reports. Allen, TX: DLM Teaching Resources, 1992.

Matthews WS, Barabas G, Ferrari M: Emotional concomitants of childhood epilepsy. Epilepsia 23:671–681, 1982.

McCoy KD, Gelder BC, van Horn RE, et al: Approaches to the cognitive rehabilitation of children with neuropsychological impairment, in Reynolds CR, Fletcher-Janzen E (eds): Handbook of Clinical Child Neuropsychology, ed 2. New York: Plenum Press, 1997, pp. 439–451.

McDermott S, Mani S, Krishnaswami S: A population-based analysis of specific behavior problems associated with childhood seizures. J Epilepsy 8:110–118, 1995.

McNelis A, Musick B, Austin J, et al: Psychosocial care needs of children with new-onset seizures. J Neurosci Nurs 30:161–165, 1998.

Mitchell WG, Chavez JM, Lee H, et al: Academic underachievement in children with epilepsy. J Child Neurol 6:65–72, 1991.

Mitchell WG, Zhou Y, Chavez JM, et al: Reaction time, attention, and impulsivity in epilepsy. Pediatr Epilepsy 8:19–24, 1992.

Mizrahi EM, Kellaway P: Neonatal seizures, in Pellock JM, Dodson WE, Bourgeois BFD (eds): Pediatric Epilepsy: Diagnosis and Therapy. New York: Demos Medical Publishing, 2001, pp. 145–161.

Molnar GE, Alexander MA: Pediatric Rehabilitation, ed 3. Philadelphia: Hanley & Belfus, 1999.

Nichols ME, Meador KJ, Loring DW: Neuropsychological effects of antiepileptic drugs: A current perspective. Clin Neuropharmacol 16:471–484, 1993.

Nordli DR Jr., Pedley TA: The use of electroencephalography in the diagnosis of epilepsy in childhood, in Pellock JM, Dodson WE, Bourgeois BFD (eds): Pediatric Epilepsy: Diagnosis and Therapy. New York: Demos Medical Publishing, 2001, pp. 117–132.

Papero PH, Howe GW, Reiss D: Neuropsychological function and psychosocial deficit in adolescents with chronic neurological impairment. J Dev Phys Disabil 4:317–340, 1992.

Pellock JM: Treatment of seizures and epilepsy in children and adolescents. Neurology 51(Suppl. 4):S8–S14, 1998.

Pellock JM: Managing pediatric epilepsy syndromes with new antiepileptic drugs. Pediatrics 104:1106–1116, 1999.

Piccirilli M, D'Alessandro P, Sciarma T, et al: Attention problems in epilepsy: Possible significance of epileptogenic focus. Epilepsia 35:1091–1096, 1994.

Reynolds EH: Interictal psychiatric disorders: Neurochemical aspects, in Smith DB, Treiman DM, Trimble MR (eds): Advances in Neurology. New York: Raven Press, 1991, Vol. 55, pp. 47–58.

Rodin EA, Schmaltz S, Twitty G: Intellectual functions of patients with childhood-onset epilepsy. Dev Med Child Neurol 28:25–33, 1986.

Rutter M: Psychological sequelae of brain damage in children. Am J Psychiatry 138:1533–1544, 1981.

Rutter M, Graham P, Yule W: A neuropsychiatric study in childhood. Philadelphia: JB Lippincott, 1970.

Seidenberg M: Academic achievement and school performance of children with epilepsy, in Hermann BP, Seidenberg M (eds): Childhood Epilepsies: Neuropsychological, Psychosocial and Intervention Aspects. New York: Wiley, 1989, pp. 105–118.

Seidenberg M, Beck N, Geisser M, et al: Academic achievement of children with epilepsy. Epilepsia 27:753–759, 1986.

Semrud-Clikeman M, Wical B: Components of attention in children with complex partial seizures with and without ADHD. Epilepsia 40:211–215, 1999.

Shinnar S, O'Dell C: Treatment decisions in childhood seizures, in Pellock JM, Dodson WE, Bourgeois BFD (eds): Pediatric Epilepsy: Diagnosis and Therapy. New York: Demos Medical Publishing, 2001, pp. 291–300.

Shope JT: Compliance in children and adults: Review of studies. Epilepsy Res 2(Suppl. 1):23–47, 1988.

Shore C, Austin J, Musick B, et al: Psychosocial care needs of parents of children with new-onset seizures. J Neurosci Nurs 30:169–174, 1998.

Siebelink BM, Bakker DJ, Binnie CD, et al: Psychological effects of subclinical epileptiform discharges: General intelligence tests. Epilepsy Res 2:117–121, 1988.

Soprano AM, Garcia EF, Caraballo R, et al: Acquired epileptic aphasia: Neuropsychologic follow-up of 12 patients. Pediatr Neurol 11:230–235, 1994.

Steffenburg S, Gillberg C, Steffenburg U: Psychiatric disorders in children and adolescents with mental retardation and active epilepsy. Arch Neurol 53:904–912, 1996.

Stores G, Wiggs L, Campling G: Sleep disorders and their relationship to psychological disturbance in children with epilepsy. Child Care, Health, Dev 24:5–19, 1998.

Swink TD, Vining EP, Freeman JM: The Ketogenic Diet: 1997. Adv Pediatr 44:297–329, 1997.

Teeter PA: Neurocognitive interventions for childhood and adolescent disorders: A transactional model, in Reynolds CR, Fletcher-Janzen E (eds): Handbook of Clinical Child Neuropsychology, ed 2. New York: Plenum Press, 1997, pp. 387–417.

Ventura TG, Fastenau PS, Austin JK, et al: Sociodemographic factors in treatment adherence for pediatric epilepsy. J Int Neuropsychol Soc 6:228, 2000.

Vermeulen J, Aldenkamp AP: Cognitive side-effects of chronic antiepileptic drug treatment: A review of 25 years of research. Epilepsy Res 22:65–95, 1995.

Ward F, Bower BD: A study of certain social aspects of epilepsy in childhood. Dev Med Child Neurol 20(Suppl. 39):1–63, 1978.

Webb DW, Coleman H, Fielder A, et al: An audit of pediatric epilepsy care. Arch Dis Child 79:145–148, 1998.

Westbrook LE, Silver EJ, Coupey SM, et al: Social characteristics of adolescents with idiopathic epilepsy: A comparison to chronically ill and nonchronically ill peers. J Epilepsy 4:87–94, 1991.

Whiting S, Duchowny M: Clinical spectrum of cortical dysplasia in childhood: Diagnosis and treatment issues. J Child Neurol 14:759–771, 1999.

Williams J, Bates S, Griebel ML, et al: Does short-term antiepileptic drug treatment in children result in cognitive or behavioral changes? Epilepsia 39:1064–1069, 1998a.

Williams J, Griebel ML, Dykman RA: Neuropsychological patterns in pediatric epilepsy. Seizure 7:223–228, 1998b.

Willmore LJ, Wheless JW, Pellock JM: Adverse effects of antiepileptic drugs, in Pellock JM, Dodson WE, Bourgeois BFD (eds): Pediatric Epilepsy: Diagnosis and Therapy. New York: Demos Medical Publishing, 2001, pp. 343–355.

Wyllie E, Comair YG, Kotagal P, et al: Seizure outcome after epilepsy surgery in children and adolescents. Ann Neurol 44:740–748, 1998.

Ylvisaker M (ed): Traumatic Brain Injury Rehabilitation: Children and Adolescents, ed 2. Boston, MA: Butterworth-Heinermann, 1998.

Zupanc ML: Update on epilepsy in pediatric patients. Mayo Clinic Proc 71:899–916, 1996.

C H A P T E R

46

Chronic Diseases in Childhood

Lawrence Charnas

Richard Ziegler

Elsa G. Shapiro

Chromosomal abnormalities

Congenital heart disease

Diabetes

Duchenne muscular dystrophy

Human Immunodeficiency Virus (HIV)

Inborn errors of metabolism

Meningitis and encephalitis

Neurotoxin—lead exposure

PANDAS

Pediatric brain tumors

Sickle cell disease

Thyroid

INTRODUCTION

Advances in medical care of young children have improved survival, but in some cases have converted an acute process into a chronic illness. Initial outcome measures focused on survival and paid little attention to the survivor's quality of life, cognitive function, and disability. Recognition that neurocognitive function is a critical outcome measure has accelerated research on the behavioral and cognitive profiles of children with chronic disease. The paradigm for measuring outcome in childhood, particularly for disease processes early in childhood, differs dramatically from the adult model. Adults reach a stable plateau that is generally known as a premorbid function prior to injury. Because a child's ability is a moving target with expected but unachieved goals in the future, there is no measure of premorbid function. Childhood outcomes must recognize the pace of acquisition of cognitive, behavioral, and physical skills over time, rather than a single measurement, to define a child's developmental trajectory. The neurocognitive outcome of an illness is a complex interaction of disease pathophysiology; the timing, efficacy, and complications of treatment; and the child's age, genetic endowment, and environment and psychosocial background. Traditional medical approaches to treatment have focused on early diagnosis and changes in treatment with some acknowledgement of the child's age. More recent advances in human genomics have led to the emergence of genetic factors in directing therapy and predicting outcome. There has been much less appreciation of the large contributions of a child's environmental and psychosocial background to disease outcomes.

Disease processes and their treatment identify a child at risk for a decreased rate of the child's developmental trajectory. The impact that an illness has on the child must be considered in the context of the child's pre-existing biologic and psychosocial background, as well as the specific changes in the child's environment that occur as a result of the illness. This chapter will focus on selected diseases that are illustrative of the interaction between an illness, its treatment, and the neurologic and neuropsychological outcome. When known, the impact of the psychosocial environment on outcome will be discussed. It is our hope that recognition of the importance of psychosocial environment on neurocognitive outcome in chronic diseases will lead to interventions directed to conditions that can be improved.

Previously common diseases, such as subacute sclerosing panencephalitis (SSPE) and tubercular meningitis, are rare in the United States, but prevalent in developing countries. They deserve mention because of the changing demographics, with immigration of people with childhood exposure to measles, and of the epidemic of children infected with human immunodeficiency virus (HIV) who are prone to tubercular meningitis.

INFECTIONS/INFLAMMATORY PROCESSES

Changes in behavior and cognition as late effects of infectious processes in the brain were first described in 1934. Eugene Kahn and Louis Cohen (1934) described hyperactive and impulsive behavior, which they called "organic driveness" in people who had been affected by the encephalitis epidemic of 1917–1918. They made a connection between an infectious disease process and a behavioral syndrome not unlike attention-deficit/hyperactive disorder (ADHD). Since that time, we have become increasingly aware that infectious and inflammatory processes can result in chronic alteration in behavior and cognition.

Acute Infections of the Central Nervous System

Three general types of acute infections of the central nervous system (CNS) are recognized: meningitis (infection of the lining around the brain), encephalitis (brain infection), and meningoencephalitis (infection of the meninges and brain). The most common infectious agents are bacteria and viruses. Outcomes vary with the infectious agent, effectiveness of treatment, age at infection, and overall health status of the child, including the psychosocial environment. Cases of bacterial meningitis, formerly common in neonates and young children, have dropped precipitously with the introduction of *Haemophilus influenzae* type B (Hib) vaccine and obstetric screening and treatment for streptococcus type B. The efficacy of vaccinations and public health measures of antibiotic prophylaxis in outbreaks has also reduced meningococcal meningitis. Tubercular meningitis remains a serious problem in developing countries and in children with HIV.

The long-term behavioral and cognitive outcomes of CNS infections are quite variable, ranging from normal outcome to profound injury. Early recognition and effective treatment of bacterial meningitis has produced surprisingly good outcomes. Hearing loss remains a common sequela of bacterial meningitis. In a study in Great Britain, 25% of children with bacterial meningitis only were left with a cognitive or behavioral disability in long-term follow-up (Grimwood et al., 2000). More severe outcomes were seen in children with streptococcus pneumonia as the source of the meningitis, delayed diagnosis, age younger than 1 year, and neurologic deficits including seizures, stroke, and impaired level of consciousness (Grimwood et al., 1996). Social adversity may have contributed to delay in diagnosis or treatment of streptococcal pneumonia, whereas outcomes such as learning difficulties where not associated with late diagnosis or neurologic dysfunction in the hospital.

Similarly, Taylor and colleagues (1998) found the majority of children with *H. influenzae* meningitis had no sequelae. Of the 126 children, 53 had adverse educational outcomes that were associated with persistent neurologic deficits and bilateral hearing loss, seizures, coma, and hemiparesis. Neurologic complications at the initial stages of infection were a substantial risk factor for poorer cognitive growth as these children were followed (Taylor et al., 2000). Lower socioeconomic status of the child's family was associated with a disproportionate share of poorer outcomes. *H. influenzae* meningitis in Navajo Indian children resulted in more neurologic, cognitive, and school-related disability (D'Angio et al., 1995) than was seen in Taylor's group, reflecting the recurring themes that diffuse early brain insults lead to poorer outcomes and health outcomes are related to social status. It bears mention that not all childhood infections have bad outcomes. Children with Lyme meningoencephalitis who are properly treated have an excellent prognosis for normal cognitive functioning (Adams et al., 1999) and may even do better than adults with the identical infection.

A number of acute viral infections of the CNS pose serious risks for neurodevelopment. Congenital infection with cytomegalovirus (CMV) is estimated to occur in up to 1% of all pregnancies and is the most common congenital infection. Nevertheless, neurologic injury occurs in less than 5% of all exposed children. CMV infections in older immunocompetent children produce a flulike illness with no neurologic component.

Herpes simplex infections have a much greater likelihood of severe injury, although the clinical course varies depending on the age of the child. Congenital herpes infections are usually acquired following an initial infection of the neonate from exposure in the birth canal or active herpetic lesions in adult caretakers. The encephalitis is diffuse, rapidly progressive, and associated with hemorrhagic necrosis and seizures. In contrast, in older children and adults, herpes encephalitis is caused by a reactivation of herpes virus from a dormant state in the nucleus of sensory neurons. In some undetermined manner, the herpes virus is able to get into the brain. Once there it localizes initially in the temporal and frontal lobes, but will show the same destructive pathology as is seen in neonates. As expected from a process localizing to the limbic system, personality and behavior changes, as well as language difficulties, are the earliest symptoms of the infection. Early treatment with acyclovir reduces mortality and morbidity, but about half of survivors are left with serious neurologic and neuropsychological deficits. Medial temporal and inferior frontal lobe injury are commonly seen on magnetic resonance imaging (MRI), and are consistent with cognitive sequelae of inability to recognize words or speak (auditory agnosia or aphasia). Typical residual behavioral abnormalities include hyperactivity, difficulties in emotional regula-

tion, and a Klüver-Bucy–like state with hyperorality. Unlike adult survivors, the long-term outcomes of children surviving herpes encephalitis have not been systematically studied, but reports of long-term serious behavioral and cognitive impairments are frequent. Epstein-Barr virus, the causative agent in mononucleosis, is another herpes group virus, which can cause encephalitis. Although rare in children, the encephalitis can have serious long-term consequences, with both global and specific cognitive impairments, behavioral and psychiatric abnormalities, seizures, autistic-like behaviors, and paresis (Caruso et al., 2000).

A large number of viruses cause CNS infection without the severe destructive capabilities of the herpes group. For example, the mosquito-borne La Crosse encephalitis, endemic in the upper Midwestern United States is seen in children playing near mosquito-breeding areas. There is no specific treatment for this virus, although survival is typical with only a small minority of children, roughly 12%, having cognitive deficits 10 to 18 months after the encephalitis episode (McJunkin et al., 2001). Viral meningitis, in contrast, is not usually associated with any neurologic residua.

As with all infectious diseases, early treatment is associated with better outcomes to avoid or minimize the potential for significant cognitive and behavioral difficulties. After any CNS infection, neuropsychological evaluation is necessary to identify areas of cognitive difficulties to provide appropriate school support services. Serial neuropsychological monitoring is mandatory to identify more subtle learning disorders that will not become apparent until the children are older and develop more complex cognitive processes. Language difficulties in severe cases (especially in those children with mild hearing difficulties) require special educational interventions including speech and language therapy. Impaired math and social skills in the milder cases also require school interventions. Attention/behavioral problems with hyperactivity and poor emotional self-regulation are common sequelae and may exist independently of any learning difficulties. If present, medical management with stimulants should be considered along with rigorous behavioral treatment, parental education, and school support services.

Human Immunodeficiency Virus

Of all the chronic illness in childhood, none has as much social influence and as many social confounding factors as HIV infection. Despite being a relative newcomer in infectious disease, it is a significant source of anxiety for society. Fortunately, the impact of pediatric HIV in the developed countries is attenuating because of more successful prevention and better treatment. The association of pediatric HIV infection with poverty and its noxious teammates poor medical resources, psychosocial stress, and poor social support add additional complexity to the research study and clinical care of these children with HIV.

The child's biologic and psychosocial environments are major factors in the behavioral and neurocognitive outcomes and recovery from illness. Low birth weight, prenatal exposures, neurotoxic exposures such as lead poisoning, poor nutrition, and maternal stress, among others (McLellan, 2002), contribute to the adverse effects of poverty on many illnesses, including HIV. The long-term effects of any of these factors cannot be easily separated from other problems associated with poverty. The impact of these factors may not be simply additive but multiplicative with respect to their cumulative adverse effects. Several studies have found that adverse events may contribute more than HIV to negative behavioral and cognitive outcomes.

HIV may be acquired horizontally through contaminated blood or blood products (such as in hemophilia) or vertically (most commonly at birth from the infected mother). With better surveillance techniques to ensure the safety of the blood supply, and since the introduction of maternal zidovudine (ZDV) use in 1994, a dramatic drop in vertical transmission of the virus has occurred.

Children with HIV are at risk for significant neurologic and neuropsychological problems. Although the presence of CNS disease varies in severity, children with earlier onset of disease, neurologic findings, MRI abnormalities, cognitive delay, and increased viral load have poorer outcomes. Children with HIV encephalopathy have the most impaired brain growth, show decline in cognitive performance and behavioral problems, have serious motor/neurologic problems, and the highest risk for death (Brouwers et al., 1995).

Neurologic findings such as motor dysfunction and increased tone are present in many children with HIV and are related to poorer neuropsychological function. Imaging findings include cortical atrophy, increased ventricular size, basal ganglia calcifications, and increased white matter signal with greater viral load related to cortical atrophy.

Impaired language development is a specific and consistent neuropsychological finding in childhood HIV. Such impaired language findings have been confirmed even in the absence of neurologic abnormalities (Coplan et al., 1998). Expressive language can be more impaired than receptive language and continues to decline despite antiretroviral therapy (ART) that improves overall outcome (Wolters et al., 1995). Motor development is also impaired in children with HIV.

In children who ultimately die from HIV, more had adverse life events and a more virulent course (Moss et al., 1998) and had more behavioral and social problems (Bose et al., 1994). Behavioral and psychiatric problems in children with HIV are due to both CNS disease and problems in the social environment. Lower activity levels, poorer motor and verbal skills, and lack of responsivity are seen in infants severely affected by HIV. The impact of social adversity is best demonstrated in boys with hemophilia and blood product HIV transmission. They have psychological resilience and are more prone to cognitive but not behavioral difficulties. School absenteeism contributes to poor academic achievement, as does immune compromise; these children do more poorly, similar to children with vertically acquired HIV (Nichols et al., 2000).

The effectiveness of ARTs in children is gratifying. Combinations, for example, ZDV and didanosine (ddI), offer better medical outcomes than monotherapy (McKinney et al., 1998), with benefits to cognitive and behavioral development. Morbidity (negative developmental outcomes) and mortality rates are dropping with more effective combinations of ARTs. Due to decreased mortality and morbidity with treatment, HIV is becoming a chronic rather than acute disorder of childhood. Most children with HIV have significant need for social support, adequate medical intervention, and decreased stress; such interventions have a major positive impact in improving prognosis and are a major component of providing optimal care for children with HIV.

Indirect Effects of Bacterial Infection: Streptococcal-Related Disorders

Sydenham chorea, like rheumatic fever, is a postinfectious autoimmune disorder complicating some streptococcal infections. Neurologic symptoms include involuntary movements, hypotonia, dysarthria, and tics, with behavioral changes that include obsessions and compulsions. Recent evidence suggests that with recurrent episodes, obsessive-compulsive symptoms increase due to changes in the caudate and putamen, and possibly the thalamus. Penicillin is the treatment of choice for prevention of recurrent infections.

Several other neuropsychiatric disorders have been proposed to be associated with group A β-hemolytic streptococcal (GABHS) infections similar to Sydenham chorea, but without the involuntary movements (Leonard & Swedo, 2001). Pediatric autoimmune neuropsychiatric disorders associated with streptococcal infections (PANDAS) include infection-triggered obsessive-compulsive disorder (OCD) or tics or both. Some cases of anorexia nervosa have also been purported to be associated with streptococcal infections. About 11% of abrupt onset of tic disorders were found to be associated with streptococcal infections (Singer et al., 2000). On MRI scans, increased size of the basal ganglia has been noted in both PANDAS and Sydenham chorea (Giedd et al., 2000).

However, the validity of the PANDAS syndrome is controversial and some think it should be a subcategory of Sydenham chorea (Murphy et al., 2000). Singer (1999) cautions that the studies do not confirm a causal relationship and that the evidence continues to be circumstantial. Penicillin prophylactic treatment has not been effective. Plasma exchange is ineffective in non-PANDAS OCD.

Children who present for OCD or tic disorders including Tourette syndrome require a careful history of the onset of the disorder. Two characteristics may identify the child with PANDAS: sudden onset or exacerbation of previous symptoms associated with a GABHS infection and frequent waxing and waning of signs and symptoms. Treatments for PANDAS may include antibiotics, plasma exchange, or neuroimmunomodulatory drugs as well as medication and the same behavioral interventions as for non-PANDAS OCD and tic disorders. However, the clinician must be extremely cautious because the majority of children with tic disorders and OCD do not have PANDAS. The treatments for PANDAS are not benign.

Subacute Sclerosing Panencephalitis

SSPE, a progressive neurodegenerative disease due to late complications of infections with measles virus, is rare in developed countries because of effective vaccination programs. Measles still occurs in other parts of the world and poses a risk for development of SSPE in immigrant children and international children who are adopted (Bonthius et al., 2000). SSPE presents with variable symptoms, including personality change, psychiatric symptoms, and loss of cognitive skills months to years after the measles infection. The specific cause of SSPE is unclear although it is most likely due to the host's abnormal immune response after infection by the common wild-type virus and a subsequent mutation of the virus. The disease progresses with seizures, myoclonus, and spasticity. Cognitive deterioration is relentless, with a 1- to 3-year survival after disease onset. Antiviral agents have slowed the course of the disease, but only infrequently arrested the deterioration and have not shown improvement in function. The response to antiviral therapy depends on the stage of the disease when the antiviral agent is administered and the previous pace of the neurologic decline (Park & Kohl, 1999).

EXPOSURE TO NEUROTOXINS

Exposure to neurotoxins at high levels has devastating effects on the developing fetus and child. Exposure to lead, mercury, polychlorinated biphenyls (PCBs), pesticides, and solvents have effects on the developing fetus as well as effects on the developed nervous system. Food contamination (mercury, PCBs), chemical abuse (sol-vents), ingestion of inedible substances (lead), and industrial exposure cause encephalopathy and sometimes death in high-level exposures.

The subtle effects of low-level exposure for most neurotoxins are often controversial and embedded in a background of confounding factors. Although children from all socioeconomic groups can be exposed to a variety of neurotoxins, inner-city children are known to be specifically at risk for health problems from higher exposure to environmental pollutants. They may be more susceptible to the adverse effects from these toxins as well. As indicated, this chapter's recurring theme of the adverse effects of poverty on brain development of young children is most salient due to the confluence of many factors, only one of which is neurotoxic exposure. The relative contributions of the neurotoxic effects of an unhealthy psychological environment, substance use in family members, poor nutrition, poor health care, and stress confound and may multiply the effects of exogenous chemical neurotoxin exposure. The impact of the child's total neurotoxic burden is unexplored.

Lead Exposure

Lead is a ubiquitous element in the environment and has been an essential component of the development of western civilization for over two millennia. Blood lead level exceeding the Centers for Disease Control and Prevention (CDC) threshold of concern of 10 µg/dL is estimated to affect 1 in every 12 children younger than 6 years of age in the United States. Lead overburden refers to elevated lead levels; lead poisoning refers to high levels causing symptoms. Elevated lead levels primarily derive from lead paint chips and dust in old or poorly maintained housing. Residues of leaded gasoline also affect soil, especially in urban areas with high traffic. The effects of low to moderate lead levels on children's cognitive and behavioral functioning continue to be unresolved. Extreme positions have been taken on both sides of the issue. Because lead overburden, like other neurotoxic exposures, is associated with social disadvantage, the cause of cognitive deficits has been in question. Few studies have been able to account for all confounding factors that coexist with elevated lead levels. However, the effects of lead overburden, though likely real, are small. Summing across research relating elevated lead levels and IQ, a relationship has been calculated on the order of a 2.6-point deficit in IQ for an increase of lifetime average lead overburden from 10 to 20 µg/dL (Dietrich, 2000). Behavioral findings have generally included hyperactivity, irritability, emotional/aggressive over-reactivity, and delinquent behavior with similar difficulty in teasing confounding factors away from lead exposure.

Cross-sectional studies using tests of visuospatial skills, executive functions, motor skills, attention, and memory (Dietrich, 2000) demonstrate that lead-burdened children tend to perform worse on these tasks, but often these differences do not reach significance when social factors are considered. Performance deficits on visual motor tasks are often the only robust finding. Several researchers have suggested that different deficit patterns emerge depending on the age of the child at the time of first or highest lead levels, without consistent findings across studies. A window of vulnerability to effects on the brain has been hypothesized for the 12- to 36-month age range, with little effect on cognition if exposure is later than 5 years of age. In addition, duration of exposure and repeated exposures are hypothesized to produce cognitive and behavioral deficits.

In dealing clinically with the individual child, social and other environmental factors have larger effects on the child's behavior than lead overburden in most cases. This is underscored by a very interesting study indicating that enriched environments can protect against the effects of lead on spatial learning as well as neurochemical toxicity in male rats (Schneider et al., 2001). Bellinger has pointed out that environmental factors may serve to protect or to intensify the effects of lead on the nervous system (Bellinger, 1995).

Clinicians should be cautious about applying research group results of low-level lead exposure in the clinical setting to the individual child's development (Ruff, 1999). The very small effect of lead compared to other factors makes it very difficult to ferret out causal relationships. Attributing behavioral abnormality to low-level lead exposure can often divert attention from bigger and possibly more solvable problems. Preventive measures such as abatement are very expensive and may re-expose the child during the abatement process when not done carefully. Short-term educational interventions have a small effect; a recently completed published study of intensive educational intervention suggests a positive benefit in reducing low-level exposure but not sufficient alone to prevent lead burden (Jordan, 2003).

Lead poisoning in children with very high blood lead levels, greater than 70 µg/dL, can cause lead encephalopathy, which can be fatal. Symptoms are nonspecific such as lethargy, vomiting, ataxia, coma, and seizures. Prompt chelation to rapidly reduce blood lead levels is required. Permanent brain damage can be the result in surviving children. Symptomatic treatment to address specific sequelae might include social, behavioral, and educational interventions. Often, stimulant medication or other behavioral medications are appropriate. Most importantly, the child should be removed from the source of the lead poisoning, and parents should be educated to prevent recurrence. Low-intensity oral chelation therapy in asymptomatic children with lead levels between 20 and 45 µg/dL is ineffective in altering cognitive outcomes (Rogan et al., 2001).

Other Neurotoxins

The neurotoxic effects of lead, PCBs, and mercury are well documented, whereas new studies of the impact of volatile organic compounds and pesticides on pediatric cognitive development are in process. High mercury exposure produces devastating effects on the developing nervous system. Low-level mercury exposure occurs from ingestion of contaminated fish, but the threshold of effects is not known. Acute toxicity from high levels of PCBs, pesticides, and volatile organic compounds are recognized, but the impacts of lower asymptomatic exposures are being actively studied. Knowledge regarding dose-response relationships and low-dose exposures is sparse. Addressing the total burden and interaction effects of neurotoxins as well as the concomitant health and social variables in the inner-city child remains the challenge.

INBORN ERRORS OF METABOLISM

Inborn errors of metabolism are diseases caused by genetic defects producing alterations in biochemical processes. The altered biochemical pathways may lead to toxic accumulation of compounds or deficiency of necessary precursor compounds that produce injury to specific organs of the body. Such diseases are individually rare, but in aggregate affect 1/5000 births. Diagnosis of these disorders depends on the health care professional being alert to the possibility of such diagnoses.

Age of onset is often related to the sufficient accumulation of toxic substances to cause symptoms, or on the deficiency of the substrate. Environmental factors can affect onset. Disorders of carbohydrate or protein metabolism often present very early and are rapidly progressive. In general, children with later onset of a metabolic disease have a less rapid course, although the outcome is the same.

With better understanding of the genetics and pathophysiology of these disorders, new treatments including dietary treatments, enzyme replacements, hematopoietic stem cell transplant (HSCT; includes bone marrow and cord blood transplants) have been developed. It is hoped that in the future, gene therapy will be added to this list. The effectiveness of many interventions is often difficult to assess because the natural history of cognitive losses in these diseases was not well studied before treatments were available. Prior to effective treatment, involved children died or were considered as hopeless. When treatments are costly and dangerous, such as in bone marrow and cord blood transplants, precise calculation of the risks and benefits of treatment are mandatory. Dietary treatments for some disorders produce early dramatic improvements but are followed by gradual cognitive developmental arrest. The causes of these deficits are complex and not completely known. Developmental growth curves for longitudinal monitoring are critical in assessing treatments of childhood neurodegenerative disorders.

Shapiro and Balthazor (2000) offer a more comprehensive discussion of the neurologic and neuropsychological characteristics of inborn errors. We discuss two different leukodystrophies (adrenoleukodystrophy and metachromatic leukodystrophy), a mucopolysaccharidosis, phenylketonuria, and galactosemia as representative metabolic disorders with different treatments and outcomes.

All of these diseases have dementia and death without treatment. Dementia in childhood is very difficult to assess, because, unlike adults with a known premorbid level of functioning, children may never have been normal. The child's function is the result of the two vectors of normal development and of disease (Shapiro & Balthazor, 2000). As a result of disease, mental development first slows, then levels off with a plateau in learning, and finally, as in the adult model, frank loss of skills occurs. Treatment after the child reaches the plateau stage is ineffective because the child is no longer able to learn the new information required for continuing development. Many childhood neurodegenerative diseases affect the white matter or connectivity of the brain. The behavioral and cognitive effects of white matter disease are dependent on the age of the child.

Adrenoleukodystrophy

Adrenoleukodystrophy (ALD) was made popular by the movie "Lorenzo's Oil," which dramatically presented a parent's efforts to convince the experts that a dietary supplement would alter the course of the disease. Unfortunately, this treatment has been shown to be ineffective to prevent the relentless, downhill course associated with the cerebral form of this disease (Aubourg et al., 1993). ALD is an X-linked disorder mapping to Xq28, which is diagnosed by elevated plasma, very-long-chain fatty acids (VLCFAs), and is characterized by defective peroxisomal β-oxidation of VLCFAs that accumulate in plasma, brain, and adrenal cortex.

ALD has several phenotypes. The most lethal form is the cerebral form of ALD, occurring in more than 40% of cases. Cerebral ALD is a rapid demyelination of the brain that frequently results in death within several years. The most frequent age of onset is 5 to 7 years, but it can occur at any age. Generally, the later the onset, the slower the downhill course of the disease (Shapiro et al., 1995). Early manifestations are gradual loss of visual processing ability, leading to visual agnosia, and then to cortical blindness. This occurs in about 80% of cases with characteristic posterior demyelination on MRI. In 20% of cases, the onset is anterior and the symptoms are behavioral including inattention, poor self-regulation, and other behaviors associated with frontal lobe damage. Often these chil-

dren are incorrectly diagnosed with ADHD (Shapiro & Balthazor, 2000).

Several treatments have been tried in ALD. The first specific therapy was Lorenzo's oil. It is a mixture of erucic and oleic acids along with a low-fat diet. This treatment is successful in lowering the VLCFAs in plasma to normal levels but is ineffective in stopping cerebral disease once it has evolved. Lorenzo's oil has also been used to prevent onset of cerebral disease without clear benefit. Agents that increase the number of marginal peroxisomes in theory could produce enough enzymatic activity to meet the VLCFA oxidative demands. Both lovastatin and 4-phenylbutyrate cause peroxisomal proliferation. Lovastatin has been demonstrated to be unhelpful in ALD treatment. 4-Phenylbutyrate, also a peroxisomal proliferator, produces better in vitro activity and is being considered for a multicenter trial.

The only effective treatment for cerebral ALD is HSCT, either bone marrow or cord blood (Shapiro et al., 2000). These treatments have a 30% mortality rate. Children who have lost more than a standard deviation of IQ points (usually an IQ < 80) do not benefit from current techniques. In such children, the treatment exacerbates the course of the disease. In children who have been identified early through careful monitoring with MRI and neuropsychological testing, HSCT is effective in halting the disease. However, some deterioration is often seen soon after transplantation because it often takes 6 months before the disease is halted. Many of the children with ALD who have had early transplants are leading normal lives with good quality of life. Worldwide, about 126 boys with ALD have had transplants (Peters et al., 2000). Understanding the factors that differentiate those who develop cerebral disease from those who do not will be critical in developing a less risky treatment for this disease.

HSCT is high risk and should not be offered to children with the biochemical defect only and no cerebral disease. Children who are clinically symptomatic with cerebral ALD are too far along in their disease process to benefit from HSCT as it is currently done. Therefore, management of children with ALD requires monitoring boys at risk with MRI and neuropsychological testing every 6 months between the ages of 5 years to adolescence to identify the earliest manifestations of CNS demyelination without clinical symptoms. This subgroup has the best outcome for HSCT. In addition, adrenal function also needs to be monitored by an endocrinologist familiar with the disorder. At the first indication of cerebral disease, further detailed imaging and neuropsychological and neurological evaluation are necessary.

The diagnosis of ALD should be considered in boys with new onset of ADHD after age 7, those with ADHD for whom no treatment is effective, and boys with new onset of visual, auditory, or motor difficulties.

The degree of impairment must be evaluated in boys presenting with symptoms to determine if HCST is appropriate.

Metachromatic Leukodystrophy

Metachromatic leukodystrophy (MLD) is also a leukodystrophy or demyelinating disease. It is an autosomal recessive gene localized to 22q13. Arylsulfatase activity is diminished and as a result cerebroside sulfate is stored in brain and other tissues. Sulfatides appear in the urine, which aid in diagnosis. MRI scans invariably show increased signal in the white matter, more in anterior than posterior regions.

MLD is invariably fatal in children and young adults, although its course is slower in adults than children. In the late infantile form with onset around 2 to 6 years of age, both peripheral and CNS deterioration occur, with tremor and weakness preceding cognitive decline. In the late-onset juvenile or adult form (after age 6), the CNS decline is invariable with or without later peripheral involvement. The late infantile form of the disease is often mistaken for cerebral palsy. Children present with increasing motor difficulties and spasticity (Shapiro & Balthazor, 2000). The juvenile form with an onset in children between 6 and 12 years often presents with attention-deficit disorder (ADD). Children may be treated with stimulant medications, but they are ineffective and the child is unable to learn and ultimately loses milestones. In adolescence and adulthood, the presentation is psychiatric. The frontal dementia that is associated with the disease often masquerades initially as depression, schizophrenia, or personality disorder (Shapiro et al., 1994). Loss of mental function usually prompts an MRI, which demonstrates demyelination, and the diagnosis follows with a biochemical test.

MLD is fascinating because the behavioral phenotype differs by age of onset even though the MRI frontal findings are identical. Motor abnormalities in the youngest children, attentional problems in school-aged children, and psychiatric problems in adolescents and adults are associated with the same MRI patterns and biochemical abnormality (Shapiro et al., 1995). The neuropsychological profiles are quite different, with severe abnormalities in adolescents and adults in tests of executive function. These findings are a reminder that brain-behavior relationships are not the same across human development.

The effectiveness of HSCT is still undecided in younger children with MLD, although it has halted the dementia in some cases (Krivit et al., 1990). Those individuals with the late infantile form usually do poorly and continue to show motor deterioration. It is clear the HSCT does not halt the course of the peripheral disease, but it does seem to benefit the cerebral disease. In adults, HSCT has been quite effective in halting the course of the disease and is usually recommended (Navarro et al., 1996). However, most adult patients with MLD have advanced disease when the diagnosis is made because they have been invariably misdiagnosed with psychiatric disorder. As a result, their quality of life after treatment is marginal. Many MLD patients behave like, and have difficulties that are similar to, individuals with closed-head injuries. Treatment is often best in rehabilitation settings familiar with frontal lobe injury where problems such as disinhibition, poor behavioral initiation, and memory difficulties can be addressed.

Earlier diagnosis will lead to more effective treatment of children and adults with MLD, averting these cognitive and behavioral impairments. Efforts are underway to develop gene therapies as well as to develop a neonatal screening for MLD. Then the dilemma will be when, not whether, to treat.

Mucopolysaccharidosis I (Hurler Syndrome)

The mucopolysaccharidoses are a group of diseases in which abnormal material is stored in all of the cells of the body. In contrast to the leukodystrophies described above, physical abnormalities make diagnosis easier. Although there are six types of mucopolysaccharidoses, we will discuss only Hurler disease, because it is the most common. More information regarding the other mucopolysaccharide disorders can be found in Shapiro and Balthazor (2000).

Hurler syndrome is an autosomal recessive disease (gene locus 4p16.3) present at birth, which results from deficiency of α-iduronadase and subsequent deposition of heparan and dermatan sulfate in most organs and cells in the body. Disordered function of the skeletal system, heart, liver, spleen, and lungs results. Both hearing and vision can be affected. Most importantly, these children have cognitive decline that starts in the second year of life. Most children with Hurler syndrome have normal developmental quotients until 1 year of life. Then they begin to slow in development, and by age 2 most are below average, and by age 3, retarded (Peters et al., 1996, 1998). The mean age of death, usually from respiratory and cardiac problems, is 5 years of age.

Children with Hurler syndrome usually have differentially affected language, especially expressive language. Interestingly, their social and emotional development is relatively normal and behavioral abnormalities are rare. It has been noted in the past, and other clinicians working with children with Hurler syndrome have noticed that intensive cognitive intervention, especially in language development, does improve clinical outcomes before and after treatment. Further research is needed in this area.

Neurologic signs, other than occasional hydrocephalus, are not present. MRIs are abnormal with enlarged perivascular spaces (Virchow Robin spaces), increased periventricular white matter signal, and increased ventricle size and atrophy. Mental or language development is unrelated to any MRI variable except atrophy in late stages of the disease. There is no storage of abnormal material in the neuron. Thus, the dilemma is: What causes the dementia observed in this disease? We do not understand the pathophysiology of the dementia, but we know HSCT can be effective in preventing further deterioration.

HSCT works to halt the course of the disease and prevent further mental deterioration. Research suggests that it is most effective and outcomes are better when done when the child is under the age of 2 years and with a Bayley Mental Development Index of at least 70 (Peters et al., 1996, 1998). Unfortunately, skeletal problems are not resolved after HSCT, leading to multiple surgeries and poorer post-treatment quality of life. In addition, problems with engraftment and the high risk of HSCT lead one to other treatment. Enzyme replacement is in initial trials (Kakkis et al., 2001), but although it is likely effective in the peripheral organs, it will not likely have benefit for cognitive function. Some combination of treatments may be the most effective intervention.

Managing the child with Hurler syndrome requires a medical team consisting of specialists in genetics, neurology, neuropsychology, audiology, cardiology, ophthalmology, orthopedics, and pulmonology to name just a few. Often with the life-threatening and overwhelming physical problems of children with Hurler syndrome, parents overlook normal developmental needs. In addition to obtaining treatment for the disease, parents often need simple redirection to attend to these needs.

Phenylketonuria

Phenylketonuria (PKU) is a relatively frequent inborn error of metabolism (1/14,000 to 1/18,000). Universal screening now identifies these children at birth. Immediately after birth, no abnormalities can be detected, but serious decline in the first year of life is noted in untreated children with resultant severe mental retardation, microcephaly, and seizures. The genetic mutation (gene locus is 12q.24.1) results in absent phenylalanine hydroxylase causing accumulation of toxic metabolites and interference with production of normal neurotransmitters. Treatment consists of a low-phenylalanine diet.

In children with PKU treated early and who are compliant with the diet may still be at risk for neuropsychological difficulties (Welsh & Pennington, 2000). A number of studies have been done examining cognitive outcomes in children with early dietary intervention, which suggest that intellectual function is normal. In a

sample of children who discontinued the diet, they did no worse on IQ tests than those on the diet. However, later analysis showed that these children were more discrepant in IQ from siblings than those who did not discontinue. Poor dietary control before the age of 6 resulted in lower IQs. In some children, declining mental abilities were related to phenylalanine elevations due to poor dietary control. However, despite findings of normal IQ levels in most children, problems with attention, impulse control, and other signs and symptoms of mild ADHD have been found in several studies. Executive functions have also found to be impaired in several studies of children with PKU treated early with difficulty in spatial representations and behavioral inhibition (Welsh & Pennington, 2000). These executive function problems and ADHD-like symptoms have been thought to be consistent with problems in dopamine synthesis that have been found to be affected by this disorder (Welsh & Pennington, 2000). In contrast to these findings, a few studies have found no evidence for executive dysfunction, but instead spatial cognitive abnormalities have been found (Griffiths et al., 2000), which are consistent with the findings of defective myelination and periventricular increased signal that have been found on imaging studies.

Dietary compliance, phenylalanine levels, and genotypes have been hypothesized to account for the variability in cognitive and behavioral outcomes. Weglage and colleagues (2000) found that blood-brain barrier phenylalanine transport characteristics and the resultant brain phenylalanine levels seem to be causative factors for the individual clinical outcome in PKU. Genotype might be useful in predicting the likelihood of intellectual change in patients with PKU whose diet is relaxed after the age of 8 years. Neuropsychological research conducted so far on treatment factors in PKU suggests that dietary cessation at age 6 is too early (Griffiths, 2000). However, continuation of diet until age 10 appears to provide protection in the domains of perception, memory, and motor skills if concentrations remain at least below 1200 μmol/L thereafter. Overall, in addition to continuation of the diet until at least age 10, management of PKU involves appropriate medications for the ADHD, psychological and educational support, and help with compliance issues around the diet, especially during adolescence. Most clinicians strongly recommend lifelong dietary compliance.

Galactosemia

Galactosemia is an autosomal-recessive (gene locus at 9p13) inborn error of carbohydrate metabolism in which a toxic response results from exposure to galactose through milk. Damage occurs to the liver, CNS, and other body organs. Infants show failure to thrive, cataracts, and enlarged liver and spleen. Growth is poor both physically and mentally, with major speech problems. Early treatment with a strict lactose-free diet results in rapid improvement. However, simple dietary treatment does not result in resolution of CNS problems. It appears that intellectual development is more related to genetic factors than to dietary and metabolic control.

Longitudinal evidence points to continuing and progressive disease with poor myelin development despite dietary restrictions in galactosemia. Intellectual deficits are present over time even in treated children, and a very specific verbal apraxia is present (Nelson, 1995; Hansen et al., 1996). These children are unable to plan motor sequences and are therefore unable to develop articulate speech. Verbal deficits predominate in most neuropsychological studies of these children. MRI abnormalities include atrophy of cerebrum and cerebellum as well as multiple hyperintense white matter lesions. Ataxia, tremor, dysarthria, and hypotonia are common neurologic findings. Decreased IQ appears to be related to having a specific genetic mutation (Gln188Arg) but is not related to enzyme levels (Tyfield, 2000). Genetic mutations appear to have differing frequencies in different ethnicities. In studies of children with galactosemia, variability of cognitive function is due to different mutations. From a management perspective, in addition to diet, early speech and language therapy is indicated, although the efficacy of such treatment is not yet established. Parents must be counseled so that they do not expect that dietary intervention will be curative.

CHROMOSOMAL ABNORMALITIES

People have 46 chromosomes, with two sex chromosomes, either XY or XX. Each parent contributes one half of the total genetic material. Any change in the number, organization, parental origin, or amount of genetic material transferred has the potential to cause problems. Those problems of interest are those in which the chromosomal abnormality is compatible with intrauterine and postuterine survival.

The most common abnormalities are disorders of sex chromosome number, trisomies, and partial deletions. Sex chromosome disorders (Turner 45, XO, Klinefelter 47, XXY, XYY syndrome, and XXX syndrome) are the most frequently encountered. All of these disorders have a higher incidence of learning disabilities and executive dysfunction than is found in the general population. Turner syndrome, without treatment of the estrogen deficiency, is associated with a nonverbal learning disability. Klinefelter syndrome has both speech and language-based difficulties, whereas XYY syndrome has a slightly increased risk of antisocial behavior. XXX syndrome is associated with a slightly lower IQ than the general population. People with XYY

and XXX syndromes have normal fertility, unlike Turner and Klinefelter syndromes.

Many disorders have specific names because of the well-recognized clinical features (Down syndrome [DS], Prader-Willi syndrome [PWS], Williams syndrome [WS], velocardiofacial or DiGeorge syndrome). Of the five trisomies that are compatible with extrauterine life, trisomy 21 (Down syndrome) is the most common and causes mental retardation in the moderate range. There is no consistent neuropsychological profile identified that is specific to Down syndrome.

Deletion syndromes produce a wide variety of medical and neuropsychological findings and depend on the specific deletion location and size (Korf, 1999). The most common is 22q11, causing velocardiofacial or DiGeorge syndrome. These have a characteristic neuropsychological profile of attentional deficits, low-normal IQ, and nonverbal learning disabilities (Woodin et al., 2001). There is a higher incidence of serious psychiatric pathology, such as schizophrenia, than in the general population. WS, due to a deletion of 7q11.2, is characterized by deficits in visuospatial function and executive function, with relative preservation of language skills. Many have particular ability in musical skills. PWS, due to a loss of the maternal region of 15q11.3, is characterized by variable degrees of cognitive difficulties, with obesity due to absent hypothalamic satiety control. Skin-picking and fire-setting behaviors are also seen. Smith Magenis syndrome, a deletion in the 17q11.2 region, is characterized by hoarse voice, speech delay, developmental delay, and self-injurious behaviors, including insertion of foreign bodies into the ears (Greenberg et al., 1991).

Many other chromosomal abnormalities exist and are associated with cognitive dysfunction of variable degrees but in general do not have the specificity of findings of these named syndromes. In cases of identified chromosomal abnormalities, genetic counseling, supportive symptom-oriented treatments, and educational interventions are appropriate. Psychotropic medications may be useful in children with behavioral dysregulation.

MUSCLE DISEASE—DUCHENNE MUSCULAR DYSTROPHY

Myopathies encompass a large variety of diseases, with most being quite rare in childhood. Duchenne muscular dystrophy (DMD) is the most common inherited muscle disease of early childhood with an incidence of 1/3300 male births. It is a fatal X-linked recessive disorder due to mutation in the dystrophic gene, which maps to chromosome Xp21 region. Children with DMD suffer from progressive muscle weakness and degeneration. In classic DMD, dystrophin is absent from skeletal muscle. In Becker muscular dystrophy, a milder form of muscular dystrophin, the dystrophin molecule size and quantity are reduced.

DMD follows a fairly predictable course. The disease can be detected in infancy using muscle biopsy findings and high serum creatine kinase levels although the diagnosis is currently usually made with molecular genetic testing. The clinical manifestations may not be recognized until 3 to 5 years of age, starting with gait abnormalities or late development of walking. There is progressive loss of muscle strength with replacement of muscle by scar, producing hypertrophic-appearing calf muscles. The loss of strength is continuous with most boys being wheelchair bound by 12 years of age. Intercurrent disease or surgical immobilization (such as tendon releases requiring splints or casts) can accelerate deterioration in strength and balance. Adolescent patients show increased weakness and are often unable to perform routine daily tasks with their arms, hands, and fingers. Pulmonary function is profoundly compromised because of kyphoscoliosis and advancing weakness of the intercostal and diaphragmatic muscles. Cardiomyopathy is common and chronic heart failure may affect 50% of patients. Death usually occurs between 10 and 29 years of age. A subgroup of children, whose course is somewhat more prolonged, may survive to the fourth decade of life (Smith & Swaiman, 1999).

Although DMD was originally thought to be associated with progressive mental retardation, this has not been supported by research. However, studies have indicated the risk for mental retardation is high, affecting 20% to 60% of patients with DMD. Overall, IQ scores of patients with DMD have been described as averaging one standard deviation below the mean, although some dispute the sensitivity of IQ tests in this population (Cotton et al., 2001).

Children with DMD have variable neurocognitive presentation ranging from normal to learning disabled and mentally retarded. Deficits are noted in attention, verbal working memory, and academic achievement (Cotton et al., 1998). Psychosocial adjustment and family stress factors correlate among boys with DMD and speak to the need for psychological support (Reid & Renwick, 2001).

There are no specific treatments for DMD. Gene therapy with retroviral vectors has been unsuccessful in correcting the genetic defect. Myoblast transfer treatments have also been unsuccessful. Several clinical trials are in progress. Treatment in late stages should be directed to symptom relief and improving quality of life.

CHILDHOOD CANCER—PEDIATRIC BRAIN TUMORS

Acute lymphocytic leukemia is the most common childhood cancer that affects the CNS. Neurocognitive late effects are significant but milder in severity than that of CNS cancers. CNS solid tumors are the second most common childhood cancer. Although the incidence rates of pediatric brain tumors have increased from 1975 to 1995, this is likely the result of improved diagnosis. Although pediatric patients have a better prognosis than do adults with CNS tumors, the morbidity resulting from these tumors is significant and consists of an interaction between the effects of tumor location, size, histology, and treatment. Mortality rates for CNS cancers have declined by 20% from 1975 to 1995 (Linet et al., 1999). As a result, understanding the long-term effects of pediatric brain tumor survival is crucial to appropriate medical treatment (Anderson et al., 2001).

Location of the CNS tumor is a crucial factor determining the type and severity of late effects. Pediatric brain tumors are classified as either infratentorial, that is, in the brainstem or cerebellum, or supratentorial involving the remaining portions of the brain. In adults the majority of tumors arise above the tentorium. In children the majority of tumors arise below the tentorium with supratentorial tumors resulting in greater morbidity than infratentorial tumors.

The classification of brain tumors is based on the microscopic histology and histochemical markers. Common examples are primitive neuroectodermal tumors (medulloblastoma is the most common), ependymoma, astrocyte-derived tumors, oligodendrogliomas, and many other cell types. Of these, gliomas are the most common, accounting for over half of all pediatric CNS tumors. Because survival and treatments vary among tumor types, histology plays a strong indirect role in determining the occurrence of late effects.

The primary treatment of most pediatric brain tumors is surgical (Anderson et al., 2001). Resection reduces tumor size and gives a histologic diagnosis. Low-grade gliomas respond well to surgery alone. Radiotherapy is a major treatment for pediatric brain tumors. Treatments tend to be delivered either to the tumor itself (i.e., stereotactic radiosurgery) or to the whole brain and spinal cord with a boost to the tumor site. The use of radiotherapy in children under the age of 3 is generally contraindicated due to the heightened radiosensitivity of children's brains. Radiotherapy damages healthy cells, resulting in a significant proportion of undesirable long-term neurocognitive effects. Treatment with chemotherapy is based on tumor sensitivity to such agents. Chemotherapeutic efficacy has been demonstrated in primitive neuroectodermal tumors (PNETs) and low- and high-grade gliomas (Prados & Russo, 1998). In children younger than age 3, chemotherapy is the standard treatment in preference to radiotherapy (Duffner et al., 1993). Pediatric brain tumor survivors suffer greater long-term effects than other childhood cancer survivors.

Neuropsychological late effects in survivors are common and highly debilitating (Anderson et al.,

2001). Deficits have frequently been noted in intellectual ability, academic achievement, memory, attention, visual perceptual ability, and language (Ris & Noll, 1994). Most of the studies examining neuropsychological functioning in survivors of pediatric brain tumors have focused on the sequelae of radiotherapy. Risk factors for poor neuropsychological outcomes include the age of the patient and treatment. Children younger than age 7 treated with whole brain radiation have greater cognitive decline. Infants and toddlers have the highest risk for intellectual and neuropsychological difficulties. The younger a child at the time of treatment the greater is the risk for poor neuropsychological outcomes later.

Tumor location plays a role in long-term outcomes. Supratentorial tumors have greater cognitive impairment than infratentorial tumors when treatment did not include whole brain radiation. Hemispheric localization results in specific cognitive impairment with left hemisphere lesions associated with language-based deficits and right hemisphere lesions with visual perceptual deficits. Although children with brain tumors often suffer from hydrocephalus, obstructive hydrocephalus is not necessarily a risk factor for increased cognitive deficits if managed well. Other factors such as family stress, socioeconomic status, and behavioral problems are important predictors of neurocognitive outcomes (Anderson et al., 2001).

Neurologic sequelae can be significant in childhood brain tumors (Anderson et al., 2001). These can include difficulties with gross- and fine-motor functioning, ambulation, seizures, and sensory loss (vision and hearing). Young age at treatment appears to be a risk factor for all neurologic late effects. Tumor location appears to be a risk for more specific late effects. Seizures have been strongly associated with supratentorial tumors, as well as hand-eye coordination deficits and hemiplegia. Infratentorial tumors may be more frequently associated with ataxia and balance problems.

Neuroendocrine complications caused by damage to the hypothalamus (e.g., growth hormone deficiency) as well as damage to specific organs (thyroid, ovaries, and testicles) are common. Growth hormone deficiency is the most frequent endocrine problem in long-term survivors of CNS tumors. Risk factors for growth hormone deficiency appear to be most strongly related to radiotherapy. Total dose of radiation strongly correlates with the development of growth hormone deficiency. Thyroid dysfunction also occurs in a substantial portion of children treated for CNS tumors. Gonadal disorders may occur in brain tumor survivors, but may not become apparent until children enter puberty or adulthood, making their incidence more difficult to quantify (Anderson et al., 2001).

The management of brain tumors poses a challenge due to the many factors the clinician must keep in mind such as tumor type, localization of the tumor, treatment type, age of the child, and family factors and their interactions, and the effect of these factors on medical, neuropsychological, and quality-of-life outcomes.

VASCULAR DISEASE—SICKLE CELL DISEASE

Disorders causing stroke in children are rare. However, children with sickle cell disease (SCD) carry a significant risk for stroke. Whether the stroke is recognized through clear signs of motor or other dysfunction or even if the stroke is silent, such vascular events can have a significant impact on short- and long-term cognitive and behavioral function (Ris & Grueneich, 2000). SCD is an autosomal recessive disorder that occurs in 1/600 African American newborns and 1/1000 to 1400 Hispanic Americans. The "sickling" of red blood cells from the normal biconcave disk form to the sickle form causes SCD. Sickling increases blood viscosity that in turn increases the formation of masses of red blood cells that may occlude small blood vessels.

Although fetal hemoglobin protects newborns with SCD, symptoms such as anemia, colic, and feeding problems are often manifested by the second month of life. A major risk factor in infancy is infection with *Steptococcus pneumoniae,* which can cause septicemia and meningitis. Throughout the first decade of life, periods of normal health are interrupted by acute illness and pain episodes in association with many types of physical stress. The frequency and duration of pain episodes increase with age. In early and middle childhood there is a significant risk of neurologic and neuropsychological dysfunction in association with CNS blood vessel disease and associated infarctions. Disease management becomes crucial in late adolescence and adulthood with chronic damage to most organ systems.

Neuropsychological studies have demonstrated both cognitive decline and focal deficits in association with both clinical and subclinical strokes. As a result, children with SCD are at risk for academic deficits, especially in reading development. Children with SCD are also at risk for social-emotional adjustment problems. Quality-of-life studies of children with SCD found difficulties in emotion, general physical function, motor function, and independent daily functioning (Ris & Grueneich, 2000). Further, the issue of pain in SCD can play a central role in the perception of quality of life, with sickle pain resulting in over seven times increased risk of not attending school and negatively affecting social and recreational activities (Fuggle et al., 1996).

Children with SCD are often socioeconomically disadvantaged, and these environmental factors amplify the effects of SCD on neuropsychological function. Understanding the impact of adversity in SCD is essential to appropriate care to ensure access to appropriate medical, psychological, and rehabilitative evaluation and treatment (Fuggle et al., 1996).

Transfusion therapy is the main treatment for SCD. It significantly reduces the rate of stroke recurrence. The only cure that corrects the genetic defect is HSCT. However, many patients are ineligible for HSCT due to the difficulty finding compatible donors. Moreover, the effects of the conditioning regimens on children with SCD are often devastating. The development of a nonmyeloablative conditioning regimen holds the promise of treating SCD without the stringent HLA-typing demands and the risk of early death from regimen-related side effects.

COMMON MEDICAL CONDITIONS

Diabetes Mellitus

Diabetes mellitus is an impairment in the regulation of blood sugar (glucose) leading to elevated levels of glucose (hyperglycemia). Impaired regulation is caused by either the absence of insulin (type 1 or juvenile diabetes) or resistance to the effect of insulin on glucose uptake into cells (type 2 or adult-onset diabetes). Type 1 management requires insulin injection, is subject to both high and low swings of blood glucose, and carries a risk for ketoacidosis. Type 1 diabetes exists in both children and adults. Type 2 diabetes is uncommon in children, but has reached epidemic proportions in adults due to obesity.

The neurologic and neuropsychological impact of diabetes on the developing nervous system depends on the timing of exposure. Hyperglycemia early in pregnancy is associated with severe fetal malformations, including holoprosencephaly, a brain malformation associated with severe mental retardation and neural tube, cardiac, and caudal defects (Barr et al., 1983). Gestational diabetes alone is a risk factor for congenital malformations. The syndrome of infant of a diabetic mother (IDM) is associated with poor diabetic control and causes large babies and neonatal hypoglycemia with cardiac and pulmonary dysfunction. If untreated, the low blood sugar and impaired oxygenation can lead to permanent brain injury, although the neonatal brain is relatively protected from hypoglycemia compared to the adult brain (Volpe, 1995). An increasing body of evidence suggests that long-term cognitive outcome is impaired following in utero exposure to hyperglycemia. Outcome measures include lower IQ, impaired attention and fine-motor control, and poorer academic achievement scores (Ornoy et al., 1998). Some investigators suggest that the impairment in iron transport to the developing hippocampus that has been found in rodent hyperglycemic models is a model for impaired attention and memory in IDM.

Intensive glycemic control "tight" in children and adults significantly reduces the risk of late complications of diabetes of retinal and kidney failure, but is associated with a substantially increased risk of hypoglycemic episodes and complications of hypoglycemia, such as seizures (Diabetes Control and Complications Trial [DCCT], 1993). Recurrent hypoglycemic episodes appear to cause deficits in IQ, memory, executive function, attention, and speed of processing. The latter three are particularly prevalent in children with disease onset younger than 4 years of age. Full-scale and verbal IQ appear to be more directly affected with more severe hypoglycemic episodes and hypoglycemic seizures (Northam et al., 2001). Intensive insulin therapy with more frequent hypoglycemic episodes is associated with poorer memory function. The role of hyperglycemia in producing these deficits is not clearly understood.

Diabetic control worsens with adolescence compared with childhood due to the developmental need in adolescence for independence leading to the decreased regimen adherence without fully understanding the long-term consequences (Johnson, 1995). Management of type 1 diabetes is a delicate balancing act between too little insulin, leading to hyperglycemia and risk of ketoacidosis, and too much insulin, with the risk of hypoglycemia.

Thyroid Disease

Congenital hypothyroidism is the most common condition detected in newborn screening, occurring with an incidence between 1/3000 and 1/4000 live births across most countries and ethnic groups studied with a twofold increase in girls compared with boys. Most causes are sporadic, with thyroid gland dysgenesis (ectopic thyroid tissue) being slightly more common than the absence of thyroid tissue. Biochemical abnormalities in production of thyroid hormone represent about 15% of congenital hypothyroidism. Failure to treat congenital hypothyroidism can lead to cretinism, a severe mental retardation form with growth retardation, constipation, and lethargy; but even milder cases of hypothyroidism, if untreated, are associated with adverse cognitive outcomes. Attentional difficulties and visual spatial difficulties are also related to hypothyroidism (Leneman et al., 2001; Rovet & Hepworth, 2001). Recent evidence suggests that unrecognized maternal hypothyroidism during pregnancy causes an IQ loss of up to 10 points in their offspring (Klein et al., 2001).

Congenital Heart Disease

Congenital heart defects are among the most common birth defects identified, with an incidence between 6 and 9/1000. The most common form is ventricular septal defect, which has a high frequency of resolving without invasive intervention. Neurologic and neuropsychological consequences of congenital heart disease may be due to cause of the congenital heart disease, the altered physiologic consequence of the heart defect, or the treatment of the defect. Toxins, with recognized neurocognitive sequelae (i.e., ethanol, antiepileptic medication), nutrient deficiencies, chromosomal disorders, recognized syndromes, and single gene defects can cause congenital heart defects. Trisomy 21, DiGeorge syndrome, and hypoplastic left heart syndrome are associated with specific risks of cognitive impairment unrelated to the cardiac pathology.

The abnormal physiology from congenital heart defects also puts the brain at additional risk for injury. The physiologic deficits from congenital heart defects can be roughly divided into those that cause impaired pump function, with risks of hypoperfusion and acidosis, and those associated with right-to-left shunt. A right-to-left cardiac shunt bypasses the pulmonary circulation and produces low oxygenation states. These shunts also eliminate the lung's capillary system as a filter of small blood clots that arise in the venous system. These small emboli entering the arterial systemic circulation explain the associated high risk of stroke and brain abscess in right-to-left shunt. In addition, structural cardiac defects associated with impaired pump function predispose to endocarditis and the complication of septic emboli.

The procedures used to repair congenital heart disease place the children at further risk for neurologic and cognitive injury. Cardiac bypass use is associated with subtle neuropsychological deficits in adults and children. The use of deep hypothermic cardiac arrest is also associated with neuropsychological sequelae (Mahle, 2001) and the risk of postoperative complications, including low flow states and clots, puts the brain at significant risk for hypoperfusion injuries.

SUMMARY

The adverse effects of chronic disease on neurologic and neuropsychological development reflect a combination of the physiology of the disorders affecting brain development, the effects of specific treatment for the condition on the CNS, and the social and psychological milieu of the child. Each of these factors alone cannot entirely account for the medical, psychological, and quality-of-life outcomes and pose a daunting challenge to the clinician to integrate all of these factors in management. The clinician should keep in mind that although the developing child is more vulnerable to the effects of these factors, the child is also more responsive to intervention due to neurodevelopmental flexibility. Every effort must be made to provide the environment and treatment necessary to enable development to be accelerated.

■ KEY POINTS

☐   Childhood outcomes of chronic disease are measured by examining the developmental trajectory or rate of acquisition of cognitive, behavior, and physical skills over time.

☐   Disease physiology, the child's age at onset, genetic endowment, environmental supports and adversities, and the timing, effectiveness, and complications of treatment interact to produce neurocognitive and neurobehavioral outcomes.

☐   Outcomes of infectious diseases vary with the agent, the effectiveness of treatment, the age at infection, the health status of the child, and the psychosocial environment. Early treatment is better.

☐   To detect subtle learning disorders resulting from infectious processes that only become apparent as the child ages and develops more complex abilities, serial neuropsychological monitoring is necessary.

☐   For many diseases such as HIV and sickle cell disease (SCD), the effect of the child's psychosocial environment is a major factor in behavioral and neurocognitive outcomes and recovery. Problems associated with poverty and adversity cannot be easily separated out from disease-specific factors.

☐   HIV is becoming a chronic rather than acute disorder of childhood due to treatment.

☐   Some diseases that have diminished in importance, such as subacute sclerosing panencephalitis (SSPE), which are more common in third world countries, still require attention due to increased numbers of immigrant children and international adoptees who may have contracted measles elsewhere.

☐   In most cases, social, health, and environmental factors associated with poverty have a larger effect on children's behavior and learning than does low-level lead burden.

☐   Identifying children who will benefit from high-risk treatment such as bone marrow transplantation for inborn errors of metabolism will depend on knowing the natural history of the disease and early ascertainment before the disease has irreversible effects.

☐   Some diseases such as metachromatic leukodystrophy (MLD) have differing clinical and neuropsychological phenotypes depending on age of onset even though MRI and biochemical abnormalities are identical at all ages.

☐   Despite dietary treatment, children with phenylketonuria (PKU) and galactosemia often have cognitive abnormalities.

☐ Although motor function deteriorates in Duchenne muscular dystrophy (DMD), cognitive abnormalities appear to be static.

☐ More infratentorial brain tumors are found in children compared to adults.

☐ Long-term neuropsychological and neurobehavioral late effects of brain tumors in children are common and debilitating. Radiation is especially devastating to the young child.

☐ Pain is very important in sickle cell disease, adversely affecting perception of quality of life, school attendance, and social development.

☐ Diabetic control and PKU dietary compliance worsen with adolescence due to the developmental need in adolescence for independence, which may result in decreased regimen adherence without fully understanding the long-term consequences.

☐ Although the developing child may be more vulnerable to insults to the brain, the child is more responsive to intervention due to brain and behavioral plasticity.

KEY READINGS

Anderson DM, Rennie KM, Ziegler RS, et al: Medical and neurocognitive late effects among survivors of childhood central nervous system tumors. Cancer 92:2709–2719, 2001.

Anderson VA, Taylor HG: Meningitis, in Yeates KO, Ris MD, Taylor HG (eds): Pediatric Neuropsychology: Research, Theory, and Practice. The Science and Practice of Neuropsychology. New York: Guilford Press, 2000, pp. 117–148.

Bale JF Jr: Human herpesviruses and neurological disorders of childhood. Semin Pediatr Neurol 6:278–287, 1999.

Diabetes Control and Complications Trial (DCCT): The effect of intensive treatment of diabetes on the development and progression of long-term complications in insulin dependent diabetes mellitus. N Engl J Med 329:977–986, 1993.

Dietrich KN: Environmental neurotoxicants and psychological development, in Yeates KO, Ris MD, Taylor HG (eds): Pediatric Neuropsychology: Research, Theory, and Practice. New York: Guilford Press, 2000, pp. 206–234.

Mahle WT: Neurologic and cognitive outcomes in children with congenital heart disease. Curr Opin Pediatr 13:482–486, 2001.

Shapiro E, Balthazor M: Metabolic and neurodegenerative disorders, in Yeates KO, Ris MD, Taylor HG (eds): Pediatric Neuropsychology: Research, Theory, and Practice. New York: Guilford Press, 2000, pp. 171–205.

Smith SA, Swaiman KF: Progressive muscular dystrophies, in Swaiman KF, Ashwal S (eds): Pediatric Neurology: Principles and Practice, ed 3. St. Louis, MO: CV Mosby, 1999, pp. 1139–1149.

Wolters PL, Brouwers P, Perez LA: Pediatric HIV infection, in Brown RT (ed): Cognitive Aspects of Chronic Illness in Children. New York: Guilford Press, 1999, pp. 105–141.

REFERENCES

Adams WV, Rose CD Eppes SC, Klein JD: Cognitive effects of Lyme disease in children: A 4 year followup study. J Rheumatol 26:1190–1194, 1999.

Anderson DM, Rennie KM, Ziegler RS, et al: Medical and neurocognitive late effects among survivors of childhood central nervous system tumors. Cancer. 92:2709–2719, 2001.

Aubourg P, Adamsbaum C, Lavallard-Rousseau MC, et al: A two-year trial of oleic and erucic acids ("Lorenzo's oil") as treatment for adrenomyeloneuropathy [see comments]. N Engl J Med 329:745–752, 1993.

Barr M Jr, Hanson JW, Curry K, et al: Holoprosencephaly in infants of diabetic mothers. J Pediatr 102:565–568, 1983.

Bellinger D: Interpreting the literature on lead and child development: The neglected role of the "experimental system." Neurotoxicol Teratol 17:201–212, 1995.

Bonthius DJ, Stanek N, Grose C, et al: Subacute sclerosing panencephalitis, a measles complication, in an internationally adopted child. Emerg Infect Dis 6:377–381, 2000.

Bose S, Moss H, Brouwers P, et al: Psychologic adjustment of human immunodeficiency virus-infected school-age children. J Dev Behav Pediatr 15:S26–S33, 1994.

Brouwers P, Tudor-Williams G, DeCarli C, et al: Relation between stage of disease and neurobehavioral measures in children with symptomatic HIV disease. AIDS 9:713–720, 1995.

Caruso JM, Tung GA, Gascon GC, et al: Persistent preceding focal neurologic deficits in children with chronic Epstein-Barr virus encephalitis. J Child Neurol 15:791–796, 2000.

Coplan J, Contello KA, Cunningham CA, et al: Early language development in children exposed to or infected with human immunodeficiency virus. Pediatrics 102:e8, 1998.

Cotton S, Crowe SF, Voudouris N, et al: Neuropsychological profile of Duchenne muscular dystrophy. Child Neuropsychol 4:110–117, 1998.

Cotton S, Voudouris NJ, Greenwood KM, et al: Intelligence and Duchenne muscular dystrophy: Full-scale, verbal, and performance intelligence quotients. Dev MedChild Neurol 43:497–501, 2001.

D'Angio CT, Froehlke RG, Plank G, et al: Long-term outcome of *Haemophilus influenzae* meningitis in Navajo Indian children. Archives of Pediatrics & Adolescent Medicine 149: 1001–1008, 1995.

Diabetes Control and Complications Trial (DCCT): The effect of intensive treatment of diabetes on the development and progression of long-term complications in insulin dependent diabetes mellitus. N Engl J Med 329:977–986, 1993.

Dietrich KN: Environmental neurotoxicants and psychological development, in Yeates KO, Ris MD, Taylor HG (eds): Pediatric Neuropsychology: Research, Theory, and Practice. New York: Guilford Press, 2000, pp. 206–234.

Duffner PK, Horowitz ME, Krischer J, et al: Postoperative chemotherapy and delayed radiation in children less than three years of age with malignant brain tumors. N Engl J Med 328:1725–1731, 1993.

Fuggle P, Shand PA, et al: Pain, quality of life, and coping in sickle cell disease. Arch Dis Child 75:199–203, 1996.

Giedd JN, Rapoport JL, et al: MRI assessment of children with obsessive-compulsive disorder or tics associated with streptococcal infection. Am J Psychiatry 157:281–283, 2000.

Greenberg F, Guzzetta V, et al: Molecular analysis of the Smith-Magenis syndrome: A possible contiguous-gene syndrome associated with del(17)(p11.2). Am J Hum Genet 49:1207–1218, 1991.

Griffiths P: Neuropsychological approaches to treatment policy issues in phenylketonuria. Eur J Pediatr 159(Suppl.):S82–S86, 2000.

Griffiths PV, Demellweek C, et al: Wechsler subscale IQ and subtest profile in early treated phenylketonuria. Arch Dis Child 82:209–215, 2000.

Grimwood K, Anderson P, et al: Twelve year outcomes following bacterial meningitis: Further evidence for persisting effects. Arch Dis Child 83:111–116, 2000.

Grimwood K, Nolan TM, et al: Risk factors for adverse outcomes of bacterial meningitis. J Paediatr Child Health 32:457–462, 1996.

Hansen TW, Henrichsen B, et al: Neuropsychological and linguistic follow-up studies of children with galactosaemia from an unscreened population. Acta Paediatr 85:1197–1201, 1996.

Johnson SB: Managing insulin-dependent diabetes mellitus in adolescence: A developmental perspective, in Wallander JL, Sieger LJ (eds): Advances in Pediatric Psychology Adolescent Health Problems: Behavioral Perspectives. New York: Guilford Press, 1995, pp. 265–288.

Jordan CM, Yust BL, Robison LL, Hannan P, and Deinard AS: A randomized trial of education to prevent lead burden in high risk children: Efficacy as measured by blood lead monitoring. Environmental Health Perspectives, 2003, in press.

Kahn E, Cohen LH: Organic drivenness: A brain-stem syndrome and an experience. N Engl J Med 210:748–756, 1934.

Kakkis ED, Muenzer J, Tiller GE, et al: Enzyme-replacement therapy in mucopolysaccharidosis I. N Engl J Med 344:182–188, 2001.

Klein RZ Sargent JD, Larsen PR, et al: Relation of severity of maternal hypothyroidism to cognitive development of offspring. J Med Screen 8:18–20, 2001.

Korf BR: Chromosomes and chromosomal abnormalities, in Swaiman KF, Ashwal S (eds): Pediatric Neurology: Principals and Practice. St. Louis, MO: CV Mosby, 1999, pp. 354–376.

Krivit W, Shapiro E, Kennedy W, et al: Effective treatment of late infantile metachromatic leukodystrophy by bone marrow transplantation. N Engl J Med 322:28–32, 1990.

Leneman M, Buchanan L, Rovet J: Where and what visuospatial processing in adolescents with congenital hypothyroidism. J Int Neuropsychol Soc 7:556–562, 2001.

Leonard HL, Swedo SE: Pediatric autoimmune neuropsychiatric disorders associated with streptococcal infection (PANDAS). Int J Neuropsychopharmacol 4:191–198, 2001.

Linet MS, Ries LA, Smith MA, et al: Cancer surveillance series: Recent trends in childhood cancer incidence and mortality in the United States. J Natl Cancer Inst 91:1051–1058, 1999.

Mahle WT: Neurologic and cognitive outcomes in children with congenital heart disease. Curr Opin Pediatr 13:482–486, 2001.

McJunkin JE, de los Reyes EC, Irazuzta JE, et al: La Crosse encephalitis in children. N Engl J Med 344:801–807, 2001.

McKinney RE Jr, Johnson GM, Stanley K, et al: A randomized study of combined zidovudine-lamivudine versus didanosine monotherapy in children with symptomatic therapy-naive HIV-1 infection. The Pediatric AIDS Clinical Trials Group Protocol 300 Study Team. J Pediatr 133:50–508, 1998.

McLellan F: Countering poverty's hindrance of neurodevelopment. Lancet 359:236, 2002.

Moss H, Bose S, Wolters P, Brouwers P, et al: A preliminary study of factors associated with psychological adjustment and disease course in school-age children infected with the human immunodeficiency virus. J Dev Behav Pediatr 19:18–25, 1998.

Murphy TK, Goodman WK, Ayoube M, et al: On defining Sydenham's chorea: Where do we draw the line? Biol Psychiatry 47:851–857, 2000.

Navarro C, Fernandez JM, Dominguez C, et al: Late juvenile metachromatic leukodystrophy treated with bone marrow transplantation: A 4-year follow-up study. Neurology 46:254–256, 1996.

Nelson D: Verbal dyspraxia in children with galactosemia. Eur J Pediatr 154:S6–S7, 1995.

Nichols S, Mahoney EM, Sirois P, et al: HIV-associated changes in adaptive, emotional, and behavioral functioning in children and adolescents with hemophilia: Results from the Hemophilia Growth and Development Study. J Pediatr Psychol 25:545–556, 2000.

Northam EA, Anderson PJ, Jacobs R, Warne GL: Neuropsychological profiles of children with type 1 diabetes 6 years after disease onset. Diabetes Care 24:1541–1546, 2001.

Ornoy A, Ratzon N, Greenbaum C, et al: Neurobehaviour of school age children born to diabetic mothers. Arch Dis Child Fetal Neonatal Ed 79:F94–F99, 1998.

Park SY, Kohl S: Subacute sclerosing panencephalitis in an identical twin [review]. Pediatrics 104:1390–1394, 1999.

Peters C, Abel S, Defor TE, et al: The Worldwide Hematopoietic Cell Transplantation Experience for Childhood Onset Cerebral X-linked Adrenoleukodystrophy. Tampa, FL: International Society for Experimental Hematology, 2000.

Peters C, Balthazor M, Shapiro EG, et al: Outcome of unrelated donor bone marrow transplantation in forty children with Hurler syndrome. Blood 87:4894–4902, 1996.

Peters C, Shapiro E, Anderson J: Hurler syndrome. II. Outcome of HLA-genotypically identical sibling and HLA-haploidentical related donor bone marrow transplantation in fifty-four children. Blood 91:2601–2608, 1998.

Prados MD, Russo C: Chemotherapy of brain tumors. Semin Surg Oncol 14:88–95, 1998.

Reid DT, Renwick RM: Relating familial stress to the psychosocial adjustment of adolescents with Duchenne muscular dystrophy. Int J Rehabil Res 24:83–93, 2001.

Ris MD, Grueneich R: Sickle cell disease, in Yeates KO, Ris MD, Taylor HG (eds): Pediatric Neuropsychology: Research, Theory and Practice. New York: Guilford Press, 2000, pp. 320–335.

Ris MD, Noll RB: Long-term neurobehavioral outcome in pediatric brain-tumor patients: Review and methodological critique. J Clin Exp Neuropsychol 16:21–42, 1994.

Rogan WJ, Dietrich KN, Ware JH: The effect of chelation therapy with succimer on neuropsychological development in children exposed to lead. N Engl J Med 344:1421–1426, 2001.

Rovet JF, Hepworth S: Attention problems in adolescents with congenital hypothyroidism: A multicomponential analysis. J Int Neuropsychol Soc 7:734–744, 2001.

Ruff HA: Population-based data and the development of individual children: The case of low to moderate lead levels and intelligence. J Dev Behav Pediatr 20:42–49, 1999.

Schneider JS, Lee MH, Anderson DW, et al: Enriched environment during development is protective against lead-induced neurotoxicity. Brain Res 896:48–55, 2001.

Shapiro E, Balthazor M: Metabolic and neurodegenerative disorders, in Yeates KO, Ris MD, Taylor, HG (eds): Pediatric Neuropsychology: Research, Theory, and Practice. New York: Guilford Press, 2000, pp. 171–205.

Shapiro E, Krivit W, Lockman L, et al: Long-term effect of bone-marrow transplantation for childhood-onset cerebral X-linked adrenoleukodystrophy. Lancet 356:713–718, 2000.

Shapiro E, Lockman L, Balthazor M, Krivit W: Neuropsychological outcomes of several storage diseases with and without bone marrow transplantation. J Inherit Metab Dis 18:413–429, 1995.

Shapiro EG, Lockman LA, Knopman D, Krivit W: Characteristics of the dementia in late-onset metachromatic leukodystrophy. Neurology 44:662–665, 1994.

Singer HS: PANDAS and immunomodulatory therapy. Lancet 354:1137–1138, 1999.

Singer HS, Giuliano JD, Zimmerman AM, et al: Infection: A stimulus for tic disorders. Pediatr Neurol 22:380–383, 2000.

Smith SA, Swaiman KF: Progressive muscular dystrophies, in Swaiman KF, Ashwal S (eds): Pediatric Neurology: Principles and Practice, ed 3. St. Louis, MO: CV Mosby, 1999, pp. 1139–1149.

Taylor HG, Schatschneider C, Minich VM: Longitudinal outcomes of *Haemophilus influenzae* meningitis in school-age children. Neuropsychology 14:509–518, 2000.

Taylor HG, Schatschneider C, Watters GV, et al: Acute-phase neurologic complications of *Haemophilus influenzae* type b meningitis: Association with developmental problems at school age. J Child Neurol 13:113–119, 1998.

Tyfield LA: Galactosaemia and allelic variation at the galactose-1-phosphate uridyltransferase gene: A complex relationship between genotype and phenotype. Eur J Pediatr 159(Suppl. 3):2204–2207, 2000.

Volpe JJ: Neurology of the Newborn. Philadelphia: Saunders, 1995.

Weglage J, Grenzebach M, Pietsch M, et al: Behavioural and emotional problems in early-treated adolescents with phenylketonuria in comparison with diabetic patients and healthy controls. J Inherit Metab Dis 23:487–496, 2000.

Welsh M, Pennington B: Phenylketonuria, in Yeates KO, Ris MD, Taylor HG (eds): Pediatric Neuropsychology: Research, Theory and Practice. New York: Guilford Press, 2000, pp. 275–299.

Wolters PL, Brouwers P, Moss HA, Pizzo PA, et al: Differential receptive and expressive language functioning of children with symptomatic HIV disease and relation to CT scan brain abnormalities. Pediatrics 95:112–119, 1995.

Woodin M, Wang P, Aleman D, et al: Neuropsychological profile of children and adolescents with the 22q11.2 microdeletion. Genet Med 3:34–39, 2001.

Rehabilitation and Treatment

Overview of Rehabilitation and Treatment

Michael Weinrich

INTRODUCTION

Disability because of neurologic injury and disease remains a major health problem for the United States and other industrialized nations. Stroke is the single largest cause of acquired disability among adults, with over 3 million Americans currently disabled because of it. Although the incidence of stroke has been declining, the "graying" of the populations in industrialized nations has resulted in a nearly constant prevalence of stroke. Approximately 600,000 individuals in the United States suffer a stroke annually (American Heart Association, 2001). Traumatic brain injury affects over 1 million individuals in the United States annually. Approximately 80,000 individuals in the United States survive hospitalization for traumatic brain injury annually, but are left with disabilities; 5.3 million Americans are living today with disabilities related to traumatic brain injury (Centers for Disease Control and Prevention, 2000). New spinal cord injuries affect approximately 10,000 individuals in the United States annually. The number of individuals in the United States with disabilities related to spinal cord injury is estimated at approximately 200,000 (National Spinal Cord Injury Statistical Center, 2001). Statistics from Western Europe vary somewhat but are not qualitatively dissimilar (Engberg & Teasdale, 1998; Martins et al., 1998; Thorvaldsen et al., 1999; MacDonald et al., 2000).

Although the goal of preventive and acute care medicine is to minimize neurologic damage, it is the task of rehabilitation to aid patients in recovery and to help restore their functioning as persons within society. Improving rehabilitation and community reintegration for individuals who have suffered neurologic illness or injury can be viewed as economic imperatives, given the projected expansion of need and costs for long-term care as the "baby boom" generation ages (Stuart & Weinrich, 2001).

All material in this chapter is in the public domain, with the exception of any borrowed figures or tables.

HISTORICAL OVERVIEW OF REHABILITATION

The major expansion of rehabilitation services in the United States occurred after World War II. Advances in emergency treatment and transportation improved the survival of severely injured soldiers. The determination of clinicians such as Howard Rusk and advocates such as Mary Switzer, coupled with the much larger number of individuals requiring rehabilitation, created a separate clinical identity and research enterprise for rehabilitation medicine and associated disciplines. The experimental studies of Karl Lashley (1963) and the neuropsychological studies of Alexander Luria (1965) and Norman Geschwind (1965), among others, provided an exciting scientific foundation for neurorehabilitation. However, the tremendous expansion in acute care medicine and the paucity of scientific tools available to study the difficult problems of neurologic recovery soon relegated rehabilitation to a backstage. The institution of diagnosis-related group (DRG) payment for acute hospitalizations for Medicare beneficiaries in 1983 exempted rehabilitation units and hospitals. Within a few years the number of beds in freestanding rehabilitation hospitals and rehabilitation units in acute care facilities increased enormously. In this expansion, however, existing rehabilitation practice became frozen into reimbursement rules. Perhaps the most famous of these, the so-called 3-hour rule, was actually developed as an empirical distinction between rehabilitation hospitals and nursing homes, but has become the standard of care for inpatient rehabilitation.

It is not my intention to criticize the field of rehabilitation or to imply that other fields in medicine are scientifically more rigorous. Advocates for the emerging dogma of evidence-based medicine agree that much of routine clinical practice throughout medicine has not been rigorously evaluated. My purpose here is to highlight assumptions and routine operating principles in rehabilitation together with the evidence supporting them. To divulge the conclusion in advance, these assumptions, stated as research hypotheses, are fertile ground for experimental and clinical investigations. Indeed, these investigations are vital to enhancing the practice of rehabilitation and to its survival in an increasingly competitive (and one hopes) data-driven medical marketplace.

BASIC ASSUMPTIONS/RESEARCH HYPOTHESES

Rehabilitation therapists often assume that patients' neurologic systems are arranged in modular fashion, that is, that different systems function more or less autonomously and deficits can be isolated and treated independently. Fodor made this assumption explicit in his influential monograph, *Modularity of Mind* (Fodor, 1983). Neuropsychologists have constructed elegant models of the psychological processes underlying reading, writing, and other cognitive processes, using precise analyses of the deficits of patients with neurologic damage. Although the striking syndromes of apparently focal functional deficits (e.g., alexia without agraphia) and the numerous examples of well-defined double dissociations of functional deficits give great intuitive appeal to the notion of modular brain organization, distributed (neural net) models can also exhibit such phenomena (Plaut, 1995). More recent investigations emphasize the demands of different cognitive and perceptual tasks on attentional and central processing resources. This should not, however, be taken to imply that brain regions do not perform specialized tasks. A large body of literature using functional imaging clearly demonstrates that many regions of the brain are preferentially activated during the performance of certain tasks (see discussion below). However, patients who have recovered from focal neurological damage may be unusually sensitive to the imposition of additional processing or attentional demands; for example, patients who have recovered from aphasia may have difficulty in understanding speech when multiple people are talking in a crowded room. These observations suggest that recovery is mediated, at least in part, by reliance on general processing abilities of the brain. In other words, specialized functions, such as language, which may function autonomously, and certainly unconsciously in normal individuals, may be performed in patients who have suffered neurological damage, but at the expense of general processing resources normally used for other tasks.

These considerations lead directly to a second assumption—that specific deficits are remediable through practice or therapy. Certainly, a proportion of patients with focal neurologic deficits improve, and evidence indicates that rehabilitation improves outcomes for a variety of conditions, including stroke. At least with motor disorders, we have solid physiological evidence that repeated practice can change the representations in the sensorimotor cortex. Jenkins and colleagues (1990) demonstrated that repeated stimulation of a monkey's digit expanded the portion of the sensory cortex responding to its stimulation. Nudo and Milliken (1996) found that regions of monkey cortex adjacent to an experimental lesion in the hand representation took on the representation of the hand and arm if and only if the monkey engaged in repetitive practice using the arm and hand contralateral to the experimental lesion. Ziemann and colleagues (1998) used transcortical magnetic stimulation to noninvasively map human motor cortex. They found adaptation within minutes to temporary deafferentation and evidence for long-lasting modifications of the motor map with repeated practice. Serial functional imaging studies of patients with a variety of neurological deficits demonstrate recruitment of new areas of brain activation for patients who demonstrate functional improvement over time. Certainly, there do appear to be limits on the extent of brain plasticity to compensate for motor deficits. Patients with large lesions are less likely to recover, as are patients with complete flaccid hemiparesis secondary to internal capsule lesions. Moreover, although early mobilization and exercise after injury and illness are widely thought to improve outcomes, few controlled studies are available to support the practice of specific physical therapy interventions. The few well-controlled studies that have been accomplished generally do not demonstrate any convincing superiority of one therapeutic approach over another (Law et al., 1997; Palmer et al., 1998; Langhammer & Stanghelle, 2000). Despite initial encouraging reports (Taub et al., 1999), studies on the most recent approach developed, constraint-induced movement therapy, are not yet conclusive (Dromerick et al., 2000), and a randomized multicenter clinical trial is under way.

The demonstration of therapeutic effects of practiced exercise becomes more problematic as we move from motor behaviors to sensation and cognition. Although patients may adapt to focal field defects and even hemianopia, there is no evidence that any form of visual practice is helpful in diminishing the extent of the field deficits (but see below for positive results in treating visual neglect). Speech therapy for new-onset aphasia probably does confer some modest benefit (Robey, 1994); however, there is certainly a wide heterogeneity in patient outcomes, with the most severely aphasic patients often demonstrating the least improvements in communicative function (Kertesz & McCabe, 1977). Language therapies based on a detailed cognitive neuropsychological analysis of patients' deficits have been attempted. Focal deficits identified in a few patients (e.g., deficits in mapping grammatical constructs onto sentence structures) have been addressed with targeted treatments by a number of investigators (Haendiges et al., 1996). While striking improvements have been evident on laboratory tasks after specific treatments (sometimes extending into functional tasks such as reading) (Conway et al., 1998), it is not clear that these have translated into significant improvements in real-world language function for a large number of patients. Patients can be taught a variety of compensatory strategies to improve their performance on memory tasks, if they can remember to use them! However, no amount of memory training appears to restore patients' short-term or working memory as measured in formal laboratory testing. More recently, clinicians and basic scientists have elaborated conceptual schemes for other cognitive functions that may lead to the development of more effective therapies for cognitive disorders (Stuss & Alexander, 2000). An understanding of the precise

nature of complex deficits such as intentional neglect (Schwartz et al., 1999) and inattention (Whyte et al., 2000) in individual patients appears necessary to design effective intervention strategies. When appropriately applied, treatments for neglect may improve a patient's function not only in the laboratory (Robertson et al., 1995; Robertson, 1999), but also in daily life (Atonucci et al., 1995). Few well-controlled studies are available to document the efficacy of treatments for disorders of executive function.

In this era of cost containment one obvious strategy for payers to control costs is to limit the quantity of therapy provided to patients. Providers respond that this strategy withholds benefit from patients. Is more therapy better? As mentioned above, the 3-hour rule is an arbitrary guideline that developed for historical reasons. Rehabilitation professionals often assume that the greater number of hours in therapy, the greater the benefit to the patient. Certainly, evidence from human performance training indicates that performance on skilled motor tasks improves with increased practice. However, the schedule of practice is important. For most skilled activities, 5 hours of practice distributed over a week is superior to 5 hours concentrated in a single day. Once individuals become fatigued, practice may become less effective. Optimal schedules of practice for patients with neurological deficits are not known. Patients with different thresholds for fatigue may well require different therapy schedules for maximum benefit. Patients with different neurological lesions may also require different schedules to optimize reorganization. How long should therapy be continued? Current practice continues therapy until the patients reach a plateau of function, that is, until we do not have therapies that improve their performance. However, it is not clear that patients will remain at optimal levels of performance when therapy is withdrawn. Sunderland and colleagues (1994) demonstrated in a randomized controlled trial of 97 stroke patients that patients who received "enhanced" therapy for arm function had better functional use of their arms, but that the improvement diminished to a nonsignificant difference as compared with controls at 1 year after therapy was discontinued. Kwakkel and colleagues (1997), in a meta-analysis, found minor differences in outcomes of stroke patients as a result of increased intensity of rehabilitation. However, in a well-controlled study, Lincoln and associates (1999) found no evidence of increased benefit to stroke patients with increased therapy intensity. Results from my own laboratory on providing therapy to severely aphasic patients suggest that performance decays after therapy is withdrawn and that multiple "boosts" of refresher therapy may be necessary to maintain performance (Boser et al., 2000).

Is earlier intervention better? Rehabilitation providers often assume that this is the case. Intuitively, it does make sense to intervene early after injury when the brain appears to be more plastic. The conventional wisdom is that patients with acute neurological injuries will improve far more than those with chronic deficits. However, recent data on aerobic and strength training in chronic stroke patients demonstrate that remarkable improvement is possible in these individuals (Macko et al., 2001). A randomized, controlled study of speech therapy provided to patients either immediately after stroke or delayed by 12 weeks showed no difference in language function between the two groups at the end of the study (Wertz et al., 1986). Bland and colleagues (2000) demonstrated in a rat model that very early mobilization actually increased the extent of the lesion in motor cortex. Again, it is likely that patients with lesions of different neurological locations and types (ischemic, traumatic, demyelinating, etc.) will have different optimal times to begin therapy interventions.

Are interdisciplinary treatment plans better than single-discipline treatment plans? Again, it is intuitively obvious that different professionals sharing information and different perspectives about patients will arrive at a more balanced and holistic plan. However, in today's pressured health care environment it is not clear how much genuine information is transmitted and shared during team meetings, nor is it clear that this information actually changes practice or is translated into measurably better patient outcomes.

Lastly, rehabilitation professionals measure patients' functional deficits, that is, problems in performing tasks of daily living, such as walking, dressing, bathing, and eating, and measure their impairments, such as weakness, incoordination, and sensory loss. Treatment is usually focused on the impairment with specific exercises. The assumption is made that an improvement at the impairment level (e.g., strength) will result in a more or less linear improvement at the functional level. This is certainly a gross oversimplification. Patients adapt quickly to neurological impairment. The characteristic circumduction gait evident in hemiparetic stoke patients is an adaptation to weakness in hip flexors and foot dorsiflexors, just as the wide-based gait is an adaptation to position-sense loss or cerebellar dysfunction. Thus, measured function always includes both the effect of the impairment and adaptation. Adaptations may be quite successful within a given range of impairment, only to fail when a certain threshold is reached. This threshold may be quite different for different individuals depending on premorbid physical activity, education, economic resources, and life situation. The crucial issue here is that rehabilitation interventions must ultimately be measured by the difference that they make to the patient.

This brief overview of common assumptions in the field of rehabilitation will, I hope, set the stage for what I view as the crucial research problems to advance the practice of rehabilitation. These problems include precise measurement of impairments, function, disabilities, and community integration; elucidation of the temporal and causal relationships between specific therapies and measured performance; development of a quantification scheme for therapies; development and use of clinical trials designed to provide meaningful results despite the unique logistical and ethical problems in rehabilitation; quantification of the confounding factors of motivation and socioeconomic status; and, of course, development of more effective therapies.

CRUCIAL RESEARCH PROBLEMS

Measurement of Impairments

Clinicians usually measure impairment with simple manual tests, either at the bedside or in the therapy gym. Although there may be substantial variability between clinicians, with specific training and feedback, clinical investigators can achieve consistency and reliability using such measures. However, the effort required to initially calibrate clinical staff and maintain calibration can be quite substantial. Clinicians have justifiably resisted the use of more advanced measurements in the absence of demonstrated benefit to patients. Many computerized programs for neuropsychological evaluation have simply transferred paper-and-pencil tests to a new medium. However, a new generation of tests may allow for rapid quantification of patient performance while retaining test-retest reliability (Bleiberg et al., 1997; Kiscanin et al., 2000). Use of anatomically accurate biomechanical computer models (Kepple et al., 1998) now allows for the analysis of patient movements that can inform clinicians of the underlying deficits causing abnormalities (Bastian et al., 2000; Arnols et al., 2001). Ultimately, these methods may lead to the development of new therapeutic interventions based on enhanced understanding of pathophysiology.

Absolutely essential is that the tests used address the impairments being treated. A recent study of therapies for social problem-solving deficits in individuals with traumatic brain injuries, for example, demonstrated that conventional neuropsychological test data were not sensitive to treatment gains seen on social problem-solving measures (Rath et al., 2000). Also critical is assurance that improvement on test measures reflects recovery of function rather than practice on tests (Wilson et al., 2000).

Rehabilitation was among the first medical fields to seriously address measurement of patient function. Simple and reliable measures such as the Barthel Index (BI) and the Functional Independence Measure (FIM), among others, are routinely used to measure patient progress at the functional level. Unfortunately, these scales also require calibration of raters to achieve reliability, are subject to bias, and have psychometric properties that are less than ideal. For example, the Expanded Disability Status Scale (EDSS), commonly used in clinical trials for patients with multiple sclerosis, is relatively insensitive to changes in patient function, whereas the FIM has limited content validity (Sharrach et al., 1999). These shortcomings highlight a grave difficulty with all of the commonly used scales—none are related to impairments in any meaningful, causal way. Thus, measurement of function using these scales provides no guidance to clinicians in which therapeutic approach to use for an individual patient. Measurement of disability and community integration relies chiefly on patient and family self-report. Although much work has been accomplished in developing reliable measures with appropriate psychometric properties for the general population, valid measures for populations with specific neurologic problems, for example, spinal cord injury, stroke, and traumatic brain injury, may require the development of specialized assessment tools that reflect the unique challenges that face these individuals.

Quantification Schemes for Therapies

How do we begin to establish the relationships between specific therapeutic interventions and patient improvement? We have already alluded to the issues in measuring patient outcomes, but the other side of the issue is quantification of the therapy interventions. Many current studies measure therapies solely by the time therapists spend with patients. Clearly, exactly what is done, how it is done, and who does it are equally important aspects (Ballinger et al., 1999). An immediate difficulty is that measurement on this scale requires an explicit protocol for therapy treatments. This need not require that all patients receive exactly the same treatment, but at least that an explicit algorithm to assign patients to specific treatments be followed. Rehabilitation professionals should make use of the lessons learned in other fields regarding teaching motor and cognitive skills. Teaching techniques established in cognitive psychological explorations of intact individuals, such as the method of vanishing cues (Hunkin & Parkin, 1995) and errorless learning (Clare et al., 2000), are just beginning to make their way into controlled studies of rehabilitation techniques.

Design of Clinical Trials

Adequate trial design is crucial to advancing knowledge in rehabilitation, but clinical trials in rehabilitation pose some unique challenges. Single-subject design can provide valuable information regarding the utility of therapeutic interventions in the context of normal clinical practice; however, adequate and stable baselines must be obtained. In addition, some designs that are useful in other areas of research, such as ABAB and crossover designs, may be impractical because patients do not return to baseline after a treatment is withdrawn. Ultimately, randomized blinded studies are required to test the efficacy of specific treatments. Patient populations for the proposed studies must be chosen so that they are likely to benefit from the interventions. Although all patients enrolled in a clinical trial should have the potential of receiving benefit from participation, withholding therapies is not unethical if they have not been proven effective. The task of constructing a control group may not be simple when families and staff believe that an established clinical practice has value. Comparison of alternative therapies, delayed treatment trials, and newer trial designs (Jadad, 1998) may be helpful in ensuring that everyone benefits optimally from participation in a clinical trial. Although studies to determine optimal therapies and therapy schedules will be time consuming and arduous, the potential benefits to patients and the economic benefits to the health care system may be enormous. A national program of research on reading and reading disabilities in children, sponsored by the National Institute of Child Health and Human Development, has surmounted similar organizational difficulties and firmly established the role of instruction in phonics and phonological awareness skills as essential components of remedial reading education programs (Fletcher & Lyon, 2000).

Pharmacologic manipulation of synaptic plasticity may potentiate the effect of physical and cognitive rehabilitation interventions. Feeney and colleagues (1982) demonstrated that administration of amphetamine to rats with motor cortex lesions, in combination with physical practice, improved their ability to walk across a narrow beam. These findings have now been extended to observations in humans following stroke (Goldstein, 2000), and clinical trials to establish dose size and timing are in progress. Patients with traumatic brain injury and diminished attention due to slow mental processing may benefit from administration of methylphenidate (Whyte et al., 1997). Clinicians should be aware, however, that pharmacologic stimulation of receptors is not always beneficial. Dopamine agonist therapy, though it may be helpful for patients with diminished arousal, may also worsen neglect (Barrett et al., 1999). The rapid advance of our understanding of neuropharmacology, aided in large measure by powerful methods from molecular biology (Dubnau & Tully, 1998), will surely increase both the number of potential pharmacologic targets for manipulation as well as the specificity of the agents.

Computerized aids to cognition have had limited success. A large number of computerized programs for cognitive rehabilitation have been developed, but randomized, controlled studies have not yet demonstrated convincing evidence that such programs improve patient function outside the laboratory (Hoffmann et al., 1996; Chen et al., 1997; Dirette et al., 1999). This is not to imply that such efforts should be abandoned. On the contrary, programs developed with an understanding of patients' neuropsychological deficits and that take advantage of the unique properties of the computer medium may well make substantial contributions to our therapeutics for cognitive disorders. The treatments for neglect represent a promising beginning. The advent of powerful portable processors and new tools, such as global positioning sensors, make possible a new range of devices for cuing and aiding patients with cognitive disorders.

No discussion of future developments in rehabilitation would be complete without a discussion of tissue engineering or stem cell (Haji & Leiden, 2001) transplantation for recovery of brain functions. Contrary to previous dogma, we now know that the subventricular zone of the brain is a germinal zone in mature animals containing cells that continually renew themselves and produce new neurons and glia (Alavrez-Buylla et al., 2000). These new cells have the potential to migrate to damaged areas. In adult animals, neurogenesis is most apparent in the hippocampus and olfactory system and appears to be dependent on the level of activity (Kempermann et al., 2000). Transplantation of cultured human neural cells has already been attempted as treatments for Parkinson disease (Bjorkland & Lindvall, 2000) and stroke (Kondiolka et al., 2000). The recent demonstration that transplanted bone marrow cells have the potential to migrate into the central nervous system and differentiate into neural cells (Mezey et al., 2000) provides the prospect of a readily available source for obtaining autologous stem cells available for repair of central nervous system injury. However, to replace damaged cognitive functions, such as language, we will not only have to understand and master the sequences of neurotrophic factors that will permit reconstitution of normal brain tissue from stem cells, but also the sequences necessary to integrate this tissue into biologically meaningful connections with existing brain structures. Almost certainly this will involve not only pharmacologic manipulations but also the presentation of specific behavioral experiences to induce neuronal activations that will sculpt synaptic connections of the new tissue.

Direct coupling of the brain to computers is currently limited to information transfer rates of about 25 bits/min. Approaches to obtaining useful output control signals from the brain include the use of evoked potentials, slow cortical potentials, mu and beta rhythms, and cortical neuronal activity from implanted electrodes. Thus, brain-computer interfaces are currently useful only for individuals with nearly complete paralysis, such as individuals "locked-in" secondary to brainstem stroke, amyotrophic lateral sclerosis, and high cervical spinal cord injury (Wolpaw et al., 2000). Applications of brain-computer interfaces for the enhancement of cognitive function or treatment of behavioral disorders await far more sophisticated interfaces. Simple electrical stimulation of deep brain structures does not appear to enhance cognition. Deep-brain stimulation can provide effective symptomatic relief for some of the motor symptoms of Parkinson disease; however, its effects on cognition appear to be deleterious or minimal rather than positive (Dujardin et al., 2000). Further study on this issue is under way (Morrison et al., 2000).

On the other hand, computer modulation of the environment, also known as "virtual reality," provides the opportunity to transmit considerable information into the brain through existing sensory channels. Such approaches have already demonstrated utility in pain control (Hoffman et al., 2000), and applications in education and rehabilitation are under active investigation. Preliminary investigations with virtual environments for individuals with traumatic brain injury have demonstrated that such individuals can tolerate virtual environments (Christiansen et al., 1998), and that exercises in a virtual environment can produce measurable gains in performance (Grealy et al., 1999). Virtual dialogues with experienced amputees, implemented through voice-controlled, interactive video, have been developed for use by new amputees and their families (Harless, 2003). This technology provides patients with an educational and personal connection to a large number of individuals who have dealt with similar problems. Much work remains to be done to determine the appropriate roles for these new technologies for different populations of patients in the various stages of the rehabilitation process.

SUMMARY

It is appropriate to end this brief overview with the observation that medical interventions play only a limited role in determining patient outcomes. In their classic study of health outcomes in the British Civil Service, Marmot and colleagues (1991) noted that mortality rates were inversely related to socioeconomic status. This relationship between socioeconomic class and health outcomes has been replicated in a variety of studies, for example, physical function in the elderly population of Sweden (Parker et al., 1994). Such factors may play major roles in determining commonly used but causally complex measures such as return to work (Lawrence et al., 1996). The level of resources and the social support networks available to patients are very important in determining whether they will be able to return to the community after severe neurological trauma and illness. Of all the different physical and social factors that may affect recovery from illness, most rehabilitation clinicians place special emphasis on individual motivation. Certainly, all of us in clinical practice have witnessed remarkable recoveries in patients with devastating injuries—recoveries that seemed impossible and were achieved only with remarkable determination. Equally impressive are those individuals with very severe residual impairments who, nonetheless, live productive and satisfying lives. However, motivation may be affected by neurological injuries that produce depression, abulia, inattention, and difficulty with initiation. Clinicians and families must take care not to blame patients for slow recoveries. Patients' impairments may not recover despite their best efforts, and some patients' apparently poor motivation in therapy may be an integral part of their neurological injuries. Measurement of patient motivation, in conjunction with appropriate neuropsychological evaluations, may be useful in predicting long-term outcomes (Grahn et al., 1999).

■ KEY POINTS

☐ Clinical assumptions can be fruitful research hypotheses.

☐ Appropriate intensity, timing, and duration for most rehabilitation interventions are not yet established by empirical evidence.

☐ Well-controlled clinical trials are essential to establishing a sound evidence base for clinical practice in rehabilitation.

☐ A wide variety of emerging technologies that may be useful in rehabilitation are becoming available.

☐ The practice and measurement of rehabilitation interventions and their effects must remain person-centered but must also link more closely with improved understanding of pathophysiology and the physiology of recovery.

KEY READINGS

Jadad AR: Randomized Clinical Trials. London: BMJ Books, 1998.

Kaji EH, Leiden JM: Gene and stem cell therapies. JAMA 285:545–550, 2001

Nudo RJ, Milliken GW: Reorganization of movement representations in primary motor cortex following focal ischemic infarcts in adult squirrel monkeys. J Neurophysiol 75:2144–2149, 1996.

REFERENCES

Alavrez-Buyulla A, Herrera DG, Wichterle H: The subventricular zone: Source of neuronal precursors for brain repair. Prog Brain Res 127:1–11, 2000.

American Heart Association: 2002 Heart and Stroke Statistical Update. Retrieved from the World Wide Web at http://www.americanheart.org/statistics/stroke/html on 2/18/01.

Arnols AS, Blemker SS, Delp SL: Evaluation of a deformable musculoskeletal model for estimating muscle-tendon lengths during crouch gait. Ann Biomed Eng 29:263–274, 2001.

Atonucci G, Guariglia C, Judica A, et al: Effectiveness of neglect rehabilitation in a randomized group study. J Clin Exp Neuropsychol 17:383–389, 1995.

Ballinger C, Ashburn A, Low J, et al: Unpacking the black box of therapy: A pilot study to describe occupational therapy and physiotherapy interventions for people with stroke. Clin Rehabil 13:301–309, 1999.

Barrett AM, Crucian GP, Scwartz RL, et al: Adverse effect of dopamine agonist therapy in a patient with motor-intentional neglect. Arch Phys Med Rehabil 80:600–603, 1999.

Bastian AJ, Zackowski KM, Thach WT: Cerebellar ataxia: Torque deficiency or torque mismatch between joints? J Neurophysiol 83:3019–3030, 2000.

Bjorkland A, Lindvall O: Cell replacement therapies for central nervous system disorders. Nat Neuroscience 3:537–544, 2000.

Bland ST, Schallert T, Strong R, et al: Early exclusive use of the affected forelimb after moderate transient focal ischemia in rats: Functional and anatomic outcome. Stroke 31:1144–1152, 2000.

Bleiberg J, Garmoe WS, Halpern EL, et al: Consistency of within-day and across-day performance after mild traumatic brain injury. Neuropsychiatry Neuropsychol Behav Neurol 10:247–253, 1997.

Boser K, Weinrich M, McCall D: Maintenance of oral production in agrammatic aphasia: Verb tense morphology training. Neurorehabil Neural Repair 14:105–118, 2000.

Centers for Disease Control and Prevention: Epidemiology of traumatic brain injury in the United States. Retrieved from the World Wide Web at http://www.cdc.gov/ncipc/dacrrdp/tbi.htm on 5/19/00.

Chen SH, Thomas JD, Glueckauf RL, et al: The effectiveness of computer-assisted cognitive rehabilitation for persons with traumatic brain injury. Brain Inj 11:197–209, 1997.

Christiansen C, Abreu B, Ottenbacher K, et al: Task performance in virtual environments for cognitive rehabilitation after traumatic brain injury. Arch Phys Med Rehabil 79:888–892, 1998.

Clare L, Wilson BA, Carter G: Intervening with everyday memory problems in dementia of Alzheimer type: An errorless learning approach. J Clin Exp Neuropsychol 22:132–146, 2000.

Conway TW, Heilman P, Rothi LJ, et al: Treatment of a case of phonological agraphia using the Auditory Discrimination in Dept program. J Int Neuropsychol Soc 4:608–620, 1998.

Dirette DK, Hinojosa J, Carnevale GJ: Comparison of remedial and compensatory interventions for adults with acquired brain injuries. J Head Trauma Rehabil 14:595–601, 1999.

Dromerick AW, Edwards, Hahn M: Does the application of constraint-induced movement therapy during acute rehabilitation reduce arm impairment after ischemic stroke? Stroke 31:29844–29888, 2000.

Dubnau J, Tully T: Gene discovery in *Drosophila*: New insights for learning and memory. Ann Rev Neurosci 21:407–444, 1998.

Dujardin K, Krystkowiak P, Defebvre L, et al: A case of severe dysexecutive syndrome consecutive to chronic bilateral pallidal stimulation. Neuropsychologia 38:1305–1315, 2000.

Engberg A, Teasdale TW: Traumatic brain injury in children in Denmark: A national 15-year study. Eur J Epidemiol 14:165–173, 1998.

Feeney DM, Gonzalez A, Law WA: Amphetamine, haloperidol and experience interact to affect the rate of recovery after motor cortex injury. Science 217:855–857, 1982.

Fletcher JM, Lyon GR: Reading: A research based approach, in Evers W (ed): What's Gone Wrong in America's Classrooms. Stanford, CA: Hoover Institution Press, 1998, pp. 49–90.

Fodor JA: The Modularity of Mind: An Essay on Faculty Psychology. Cambridge, MA: MIT Press, 1983.

Geschwind N: Disconnexion syndromes in animals and man II. Brain 88:585–644, 1965.

Goldstein LB: Effects of amphetamines and small related molecules on recovery after stroke in animals and man. Neuropharmacology 39:952–859, 2000.

Grahn B, Stigmar K, Ekdahl C: Motivation for change in patients with prolonged musculoskeletal disorders: A qualitative two-year follow-up study. Physiother Res Int 4:170–189, 1999.

Grealy MA, Johnson DA, Rushton SK: Improving cognitive function after brain injury: The use of exercise and virtual reality. Arch Phys Med Rehabil 80:661–667, 1999.

Haendiges AN, Berndt RS, Mitchum CC: Assessing the elements and contributing to a "mapping" deficit: A targeted treatment study. Brain Lang 52:276–302, 1996.

Harless WG: Interactive drama. Information available at http://www.idrama.com/AmputeeSeries.htm. 2003.

Hoffman HG, Doctor JN, Patterson DR, et al: Use of virtual reality for adjunctive treatment of adult burn pain during physical therapy: A controlled study. Pain 85:305–309, 2000.

Hofmann M, Hock C, Kuhler A, et al: Interactive computer-based cognitive training in patients with Alzheimer's disease. Psychiatr Res 30:493–501, 1996.

Hunkin NM, Parkin AJ: The method of vanishing cues: An evaluation of its effectiveness in teaching memory-impaired individuals. Neuropsychologia 33:1255–1279, 1995.

Jadad AR: Randomized Clinical Trials. London: BMJ Books, 1998.

Jenkins WM, Merzenich MM, Ochs MT, et al: Functional reorganization of primary somatosensory cortex in adult owl monkeys after behaviorally controlled tactile stimulation. J Neurophysiol 63:82–104, 1990.

Kaji EH, Leiden JM: Gene and stem cell therapies. JAMA 285:545–550, 2001.

Kempermann G, van Pragg K, Gage FH: Activity-dependent regulation of neuronal plasticity and self-repair. Prog Brain Res 127:35–48, 2000.

Kepple TM, Sommer HJ, Lohmann SK, et al: A three-dimensional musculoskeletal database for the lower extremities. J Biomech 31:77–80, 1998.

Kertesz A, McCabe P: Recovery patterns and prognosis in aphasia. Brain 100:1–18, 1977.

Kisacanin B, Agarwal GC, Taber J, et al: Computerized evaluation of cognitive and motor function. Med Biol Eng Compu 38:68–73, 2000.

Kondiolka D, Wechsler L, Goldstein S, et al: Transplantation of cultured neuronal cells for patients with stroke. Neurology 55:565–569, 2000.

Kwakkel G, Wagenaar RC, Koelman TW, et al: Effects of intensity of rehabilitation after stroke: A research synthesis. Stroke 28:1550–1556, 1997.

Langhammer B, Stanghelle JK: Bobath or motor relearning programme? A comparison of two different approaches of physiotherapy in stroke rehabilitation: A randomized controlled study. Clin Rehabil 14:361–369, 2000.

Lashley HS: Brain Mechanisms and Intelligence: A Quantitative Study of Injuries to the Brain. New York: Dover, 1963.

Law M, Russell D, Pollock N, et al: A comparison of intensive neurodevelopmental therapy plus casting and a regular occupational therapy program for children with cerebral palsy. Dev Med Child Neurol 39:664–670, 1997.

Lawrence K, Doll H, McWhinnie D: Relationship between health status and postoperative return to work. J Public Health Med 18:49–53, 1996.

Lincoln NB, Parry RH, Vass CD: Randomized, controlled trial to evaluate increased intensity of physiotherapy treatment of arm function after stroke. Stroke 30:573–579, 1999.

Luria AR: Aspects of aphasia. J Neurol Sci 2:278–287, 1965.

MacDonald BK, Cockerell OC, Sander WAS, et al: The incidence and lifetime prevalence of neurologic disorders in a prospective community-based study in the UK. Brain 123:665–676, 2000.

Macko RF, Smith GV, Dobrovolny CL, et al: Treadmill training improves fitness reserve in chronic stroke patients. Res Phys Med Rehabil 82:879–884, 2001.

Marmot MG, Smith GD, Stansfeld S, et al: Health inequities among British civil servants: The Whitehall II Study. Lancet 337:1387–1392, 1991.

Martins F, Freitas F, Martins L, et al: Spinal cord injuries: Epidemiology in Portugal's central region. Spinal Cord 36:574–578, 1998.

Mezey E, Chandross KJ, Harta G, et al: Turning blood into brain: Cells bearing neuronal antigens generated in vivo from bone marrow. Science 290:1779–1782, 2000.

Morrison CE, Borod JC, Brin MF, et al: A program for neuropsychological investigation of deep brain stimulation (PNIDBS) in movement disorder patients: Development, feasibility, and preliminary data. Neuropsychiatry Neuropsychol Behav Neurol 13:204–219, 2000.

National Spinal Cord Injury Statistical Center: Facts and Figures at a Glance—June 2000. Retrieved from the World Wide Web at http://www.spinalcord.uab.edu/show.asp?durki=21446 on 2/8/01.

Nudo RJ, Milliken GW: Reorganization of movement representations in primary motor cortex following focal ischemic infarcts in adult squirrel monkeys. J Neurophysiol 75:2144–2149, 1996.

Palmer FB, Shapiro BK, Wachtel RC, et al: The effects of physical therapy on cerebral diplegia: A controlled trial in infants with spastic diplegia. N Engl J Med 318:803–808, 1998.

Parker MG, Thorslund M, Lundberg O: Physical function and social class among Swedish oldest old. J Gerontol 49:S196–S201, 1994.

Plaut DC: Double dissociation without modularity: Evidence from connectionist neuropsychology. J Clin Exp Neuropsychol 17:291–321, 1995.

Rath JF, Simon D, Langenbahn DM, et al: Measurement of problem-solving deficits in adults with acquired brain damage. J Head Trauma Rehabil 15:724–733, 2000.

Robertson IH: Cognitive rehabilitation: Attention and neglect. Trends Cogn Sci 3:385–393, 1999.

Robertson IH, Tegner R, Tham K, et al: Sustained attention training for unilateral neglect: Theoretical and rehabilitation implications. J Clin Exp Neuropsychol 17:416–430, 1995.

Robey RR: The efficacy of treatment for aphasic persons: A meta-analysis. Brain Lang 47:582–608, 1994.

Schwartz RL, Barrett AM, Kim M, et al: Ipsilateral intentional neglect and the effect of cueing. Neurology 53:2017–2022, 1999.

Sharrack B, Highes RA, Soundain S, et al: The psychometric properties of clinical rating scales used in multiple sclerosis. Brain 122:141–159, 1999.

Stuart M, Weinrich M: Home- and community-based long-term care: Lessons from Denmark. Gerontologist 41:474–480, 2001.

Stuss DT, Alexander MP: Executive functions and the frontal lobes: A conceptual view. Psychol Res 63:289–298, 2000.

Sunderland A, Fletcher D, Bradley L, et al: Enhanced physical therapy for arm function after stroke: A one year follow up study. J Neurol Neurosurg Psychiatry 57:856–858, 1994.

Taub E, Uswatte G, Pidikiti R: Constraint-induced movement therapy: A new family of techniques with broad application to physical rehabilitation—a clinical review. J Rehabil Res Dev 36:237–251, 1999.

Thorvaldsen P, Davidsen M, Bronnum-Hansen H, et al: Stable stroke occurrence despite incidence reduction in an aging population: Stroke trends in the Danish monitoring trends and determinants in cardiovascular disease (MONICA) population. Stroke 30:2529–2534, 1999.

Wertz RT, Weiss DG, Brookshire RH, et al: Comparison of clinic, home, and deferred language treatment for aphasia: A Veterans Administration Cooperative Study. Arch Neurol 43:653–658, 1986.

Whyte J, Hart T, Schuster K, et al: Effects of methylphenidate on attentional function after traumatic brain injury. Am J Phys Med Rehabil 75:440–450, 1997.

Whyte J, Schuster K, Polansky M, et al: Frequency and duration of inattentive behavior after traumatic brain injury: Effects of distraction, task, and practice. J Int Neuropsychol Soc 6:1–11, 2000.

Wilson BA, Watson PC, Baddley AD, et al: Improvement or simply practice? The effects of twenty repeated assessments on people with and without brain injury. J Int Neuropsych Soc 6:469–479, 2000.

Wolpaw JR, Birbaumer N, Heetderkss WJ, et al: Brain-computer interface technology: A review of the first international meeting. IEEE Trans Rehab Engin 8:164–173, 2000.

Ziemann U, Corwell B, Choen LG: Modulation of plasticity in human motor cortex after forearm ischemic nerve block. J Neurosci 18:115–123, 1998.

Rehabilitation Strategies for Individuals with Acquired Cognitive Impairment

Catherine A. Mateer

Attention
Cognitive rehabilitation
Compensatory strategies
Disability
Executive functions
Functional outcomes
Memory
Treatment efficacy

HISTORY OF COGNITIVE REHABILITATION

The rehabilitation of individuals who have suffered neurologic disease or trauma has received increasing interest in the last decade. Several factors have contributed to this. Survival rates from even very severe neurologic injury have been increasing since the mid-1970s with greater understanding of the effects of trauma and the advent of more responsive emergency care and sophisti-

cated diagnosis of acute intracranial injury. Coupled with this growing population of "survivors" of neurologic injury is a much more optimistic view with respect to the potential for reorganization and recovery of function than had been previously held (Kolb, 1996; Robertson & Murre, 1999). Considerable experience-dependent neuroplasticity, particularly at the level of the synapse, has been demonstrated in adult mammalian brains. Finally, advances in cognitive neuroscience have increased our understanding of cognitive processes and the nature of acquired cognitive impairments. These developments have occurred in the context of medical care and management systems that emphasize functional outcomes and the use of empirically validated approaches to treatment and intervention. Recent comprehensive reviews of literature on the rehabilitation of individuals with acquired brain injury have led to position papers identifying particular interventions that have shown efficacy (Cicerone & Giacino, 1992; Carney et al., 1999; National Institutes of Health Consensus Panel, 1999). This chapter reviews some of the basic tenets and primary approaches used in the rehabilitation of individuals with cognitive impairments.

The field of rehabilitation has a long history. The first rehabilitation "specialists" appear to have been neurologists who worked closely with young soldiers injured in World Wars I and II in Germany, Russia, and England. Prominent early figures in neurology such as Kurt Goldstein, Alexander Luria, Richie Russell, Henry Head, and Henri Hecaen wrote extensively about their experiences with wounded soldiers. Their observations of individuals with focal brain injuries contributed greatly to our understanding of acquired disorders of language, perception, memory, and executive functions (Luria, 1996). They also left a legacy in rehabilitation in which recovery was not viewed simply in physical terms, but in a social context. It was not enough to assist individuals in being able to walk, talk, and care for their immediate physical needs. Rather, rehabilitation was seen as involving families, communities, and the ability to integrate into home, school, and work. (For a review of rehabilitation's early history, the reader is referred to *Neuropsychological Rehabilitation*, Vol. 6, 1996).

DEFINITION OF COGNITIVE REHABILITATION

Consistent with this early perspective, rehabilitation can be defined as the application of techniques and procedures, and the implementation of supports, to allow individuals to function as independently as possible in their environment (Mill et al., 1997; Rosenthal et al., 1999). Although physical therapy aimed at restoring or improving postural stability, balance, and mobility is a key element of most rehabilitation programs, this chapter primarily focuses on interventions designed to address acquired impairments in cognitive abilities and concomitant alterations in behavior, mood, and emotional regulation. Impairments in these domains can negatively affect a wide range of adaptive abilities, including the ability to care for one's own needs, to maintain personal and social relationships, to achieve in school, or to engage in gainful employment (Sohlberg & Mateer, 1989a, 2001).

The cognitive skills that are most commonly observed following diffuse or frontal brain injury are problems with attention and concentration, speed of processing new information, memory and new learning, and the executive skills of initiating, selecting goals, planning, organizing, and self-monitoring. Individuals with focal brain injury may also demonstrate impairments in speech and language expression and comprehension, object or face recognition, spatial abilities, and the expression and appreciation of emotional signals. The nature and extent of changes in someone's functioning may or may not be apparent to the person. Indeed,

limitations in awareness and insight are a common consequence of many forms of neurologic injury (Prigatano, 1991; Stuss, 1991; Sohlberg & Mateer, 2001). The changes are, however, usually evident and of concern to family members, friends, and colleagues.

WORLD HEALTH ORGANIZATION MODEL OF DISABILITY

The World Health Organization has defined five levels (domains) that need to be considered in working with individuals who are challenged by disability. The first level, *pathophysiology*, refers to the underlying disruption of physical functioning (e.g., a tumor or stroke). The second level, *impairment*, refers to the specific losses or alterations relative to normal functioning that occur as a result of the pathophysiologic injury or disease (e.g., loss of ability to speak or to remember new information). The third level, *activity/functional limitation*, refers to changes in routine or daily functioning that occur as a result of the *impairment* (e.g., inability to communicate with others, inability to drive or take public transportation). The fourth level, *participation*, refers to the effect of activity and functional limitations on the person's ability to engage in age-appropriate social activities and roles (e.g., working, parenting, ability to live independently). The fifth level, *environmental factors*, refers to social support and technological and societal variables that can serve to either mitigate functional limitation and participation or further contribute to marginalization and disability in these areas. Although rehabilitation is not traditionally viewed as altering the underlying pathophysiology, it seeks to improve areas of impairment or implement compensations for impairments, so as to reduce functional limitations and increase and normalize participation. Many individuals who have even severe physical and cognitive impairments can live well-adjusted and productive lives with appropriate supports and assistance, hence the emphasis on the importance of larger environmental factors and societal attitudes. Table 48-1 provides some examples within each of the five domains.

Consistent with this model, effective rehabilitation planning for individuals with cognitive impairment requires information about a number of critical elements. The rehabilitation team needs to gain:

- An understanding of the underlying disease process or injury and its natural course.
- An appreciation of premorbid strengths, weaknesses, and lifestyle.
- A comprehensive assessment of cognitive and behavioral strengths and weaknesses.
- An assessment of current and projected living environment, including the

TABLE 48-1. World Health Organization Model of Disability

Domain	Examples within the domain
Pathophysiology	Stroke
	Brain injury
	Multiple sclerosis
	Neoplasm
	Parkinson disease
Impairment	Hemiplegia
	Hemianopsia
	Amnesia
	Aphasia
	Impaired self-awareness
Activity/functional limitation	Impaired communication
	Reduced capacity for self-care
	Reduced mobility
	Impaired ability to learn new skills
	Altered interpersonal skills
Participation	Ability to maintain relationships
	Ability to access the community
	Capacity for school achievement
	Ability to maintain employment
	Capability of home and financial management
	Ability to parent
Environmental factors	Supportive relationships
	Available products and technologies
	Societal attitudes
	Social services and policies

demands on the individual and supports available.

- An assessment of the individual's awareness of his or her situation and the ability to regulate behavior and emotions.
- An assessment of the individual's ability to learn and an appreciation of teaching strategies to which the person is likely to best respond.

Acute Interventions for Individuals with Moderate to Severe Neurologic Insult

During the initial period of coma and medical instability, efforts are directed toward preventing further secondary injury where possible, monitoring signs of neurologic improvement or decline, maintaining any necessary life support, providing nutrition, guarding the integrity of skin and corneas, and preventing contractures. A percentage of individuals in coma recover spontaneous eye opening and sleep-wake cycles, and may begin to show orienting or tracking responses to visual or auditory stimuli. This stage, termed persistent vegetative state

(PVS), does not necessarily imply any conscious awareness of the world but rather the recovery of brainstem systems involved in arousal and orienting. Although some controversy exists with regard to the potential efficacy of any rehabilitative efforts in such individuals, no convincing experimental evidence supports extensive "coma stimulation" exercises.

More commonly, following severe traumatic brain injuries, individuals emerge from a period of coma or unresponsiveness and begin to respond to the environment. However, they often display marked disturbances in behavior. The individual may appear confused, impulsive, restless, easily agitated, and become quickly fatigued. These behavioral abnormalities usually occur in the context of markedly impaired cognitive function and diminished awareness. The severe anterograde amnesia often observed during this period is termed post-traumatic amnesia (PTA) (see also Chapter 27). Attention, moment-to-moment retention of information, learning capacity, problem solving, and judgment might all be significantly compromised. Such individuals appear easily overwhelmed by complex or stimulating environments and are easily distracted. Rehabilitation efforts at this stage focus on monitoring medical and nutritional status, preventing contractures, ensuring safety, developing consistent communication, and beginning to encourage and shape responses to simple cognitive tasks and functional activities. During this period, attempts are made to limit or reduce potentially distracting or confusing stimuli. Structuring sensory input to reduce extraneous noise or visual stimuli is often helpful in decreasing agitation and confusion. Confusion and disorientation can also be reduced by providing familiar objects and family pictures and by the presence of family members. Patients in this acute stage are also quickly overwhelmed by task demands. Rehabilitation staff members are trained to be sensitive to signs of escalating distress and fatigue, and, in such circumstances, to modify tasks to make them easier or shorter (Alderman & Burgess, 1990; Sohlberg & Mateer, 2001).

This period of agitation and postinjury confusion is often bewildering to families. They may have waited hours, days, or weeks for their loved one to "wake up," but now the injured individual behaves in ways that are unusual, unexpected, and frightening. Information about the common stages of recovery after injury is helpful, as is emotional support and assistance with dealing with legal and financial matters. Table 48-2 provides an overview of the common stages of recovery from severe diffuse brain injury.

Acute Interventions for Individuals with Mild Injuries

There is little dispute with respect to how individuals with severe injury should be managed and treated from

TABLE 48-2. Stages of Recovery from Diffuse Brain Injury

Stage of recovery	Common clinical features
Coma	Unresponsive, eyes closed
Vegetative state	No cognitive response, presence of sleep-wake cycles
Minimally conscious state	Wakefulness, some response to commands, often mute
Confusional state	Amnesic (PTA), severe attention problems, agitation
Postconfusional state	Cognitive improvement, resolution of PTA, gains in ADLs
Return to home and community	Gains in social interaction and personal independence

ADLs, activities of daily living; PTA, post-traumatic amnesia.

a rehabilitation perspective in the early stages. There is considerably more controversy with respect to best practices in the later stages of rehabilitation with individuals with severe injuries. There is also a great deal of disagreement about the best course of action to take with respect to acute management of individuals with mild head trauma who are not admitted to the hospital.

Individuals with cerebral concussion or mild traumatic brain injury (MTBI) are subjects of great debate within the medical and neuropsychological community. Large-scale prospective studies of individuals who have been diagnosed with concussion or MTBI in the emergency room have indicated that 85% to 90% of such individuals go on to have a full or at least unremarkable recovery and return to their regular routine by 6 months to a year after injury. Nevertheless, across a number of studies, 10% to 15% of individuals with MTBI go on to report a significant number of symptoms and may demonstrate substantial disruption of everyday activities (Kraus & Nourjah, 1998). The controversy surrounding such individuals generally focuses on trying to identify whether there are injury-related variables, premorbid personality characteristics, and medicolegal/compensation issues that might account for the lack of full recovery in this groups of individuals with MTBI (Raskin & Mateer, 2000).

Regardless of underlying causes, the conventional wisdom has seemed to lean toward providing individuals with concussion little in the way of information beyond reassurance they will be fine and a head injury discharge sheet directed at detecting acute complications such as undetected intracranial bleeds. It is apparently believed by many that more detailed information about possible consequences or the suggestion they may have suffered a brain injury will result in iatrogenic symptom development, particularly in suggestible or vulnerable individuals. However, the results of research

addressing this question suggest quite the opposite. In a number of studies, providing information about the typical course of recovery; common physical, cognitive, and emotional sequelae; and recommendation for a gradual return to full activities has been shown to actually reduce the number and severity of symptoms measured weeks and months later (Minderhoud et al., 1980; Gronwall, 1986). In a carefully controlled study (Mittenberg et al., 1996), one group of subjects was given a handout shortly after concussion listing common symptoms experienced by some people after concussion, stress reduction techniques, and advice with respect to rest and gradual return to a full range of regular activities. Also stressed was the fact that the great majority of individuals with mild head injuries or concussions make a full recovery. The control group was provided only with standard emergency room care but no additional information. When followed up 6 months after injury, symptom rates differed significantly. A much smaller percentage of patients who received additional information continued to report headache, fatigue, memory difficulties, problems with concentration, anxiety, depression, and dizziness compared with the control group (Table 48-3).

These findings strongly suggest that information provided at the time of injury, which normalizes common symptoms that may occur and provides advice, support, and encouragement about the resolution of these symptoms, has a very positive impact on overall reduction of symptom frequency and severity. Without this information, the experience of symptoms may create fear, anxiety, and distress and result in poor long-term adjustment.

TABLE 48-3. Percentage of Initially Symptomatic Patients Seen for Mild Traumatic Brain Injury or Concussion Who Continued to Report Specific Symptoms 6 Months Postinjury

Symptom	% Reporting symptom in control group	% Reporting symptom in information group
Headache	86	44
Fatigue	82	47
Memory	80	38
Concentration	80	29
Anxiety	58	38
Depression	56	27
Dizziness	50	36

From Mittenberg W, Inemont M, Zielinki RE, et al: Cognitive-behavioral prevention of postconcussive syndrome. Arch Clin Neuropsychol 11:139–146, 1996.

TABLE 48-4. Commonly Used Approaches to Working with Individuals with Cognitive Impairment

Approach	Brief description
Environmental modifications	Altering or providing cues in the individual's environment to prompt and support more adaptive behavior
Adoption of specialized learning and teaching techniques	Using techniques derived from learning theory to optimize attempts to train new skills or learn new information
Implementation of compensatory strategies	Teaching individuals to use internal or external mnemonic strategies or devices to alleviate the impact of memory impairment
Restorative approaches	Providing systematic training and practice on various skills and cognitive abilities so as to improve or restore functioning
Education and awareness training	Providing didactic and experiential information to facilitate an accurate appraisal of strengths and weaknesses
Counseling and emotional support	Providing therapeutic support to foster hope, decrease fear and uncertainty, combat depression and isolation, and facilitate adjustment

Postacute Rehabilitation

In the postacute stage of rehabilitation, the patient is usually medically stable, though it is important to monitor for the development of seizure disorders and reduce risk factors for further injury. In most cases, florid post-traumatic amnesia has cleared, although the person may be left with a significant decrement in the ability to learn and remember new information. Marked difficulty may also be evident in the patient's ability to attend and concentrate, to understand and process information, and to initiate, plan, and organize activity toward purposeful ends. There may be problems with the production and comprehension of speech and language. The individual may also have a great deal of difficulty controlling emotions and responses. Irritability, emotional lability, quickness to anger, and decreased frustration tolerance may result in behavioral outbursts, sometimes putting the individual or others at risk. The individual may react to others and to situations in profoundly different ways than before injury, which can be a source of confusion to family, friends, and even the patient. Given the wide range and somewhat unique pattern of each patient's premorbid and postmorbid strengths and difficulties, effective interventions must be tailored to the individual and the circumstances. At this stage patients may be seen in inpatient rehabilitation, as outpatients, in day treatment programs, in community-based care centers, or in assisted living environments.

Many approaches to working with cognitively impaired adults and children have been articulated. Cicerone and colleagues (2000) provide a detailed review of the evidence for efficacy of specific interventions in the most commonly targeted cognitive domains. Ideally, specific interventions are selected to meet specific functional goals that are developed in collaboration among the patient, family, and rehabilitation team (Webb & Glueckauf, 1994). Most comprehensive rehabilitation programs will use an eclectic array of strategies and approaches. Commonly described categories of intervention are listed and defined in Table 48-4.

Environmental Interventions

Environmental modifications involve changing aspects of the injured individual's environment to reduce behavioral and functional impairments. Different modifications are typically engaged in the early stage following injury versus in the more chronic stage of disability. In the acute stage after injury, most environmental interventions are designed to keep the person safe (e.g., locked doors to stairwells, temperature controls on taps) and to minimize overstimulation. Bright lights, noisy environments, and rapidly changing scenes can cause further confusion and distress. Attention is paid to limiting fatigue and monitoring the level of demand during tasks. Rehabilitation specialists are trained to be alert to signs of escalating distress and to redirect the individual, often averting outbursts or decompensation in the situation.

In the more chronic stage, environmental modifications are tailored to areas of specific functional impact. For example, individuals with significant memory deficits may be provided with labels on cupboards and calendars to monitor passage of days and activities. Those with significant problems with self-monitoring, planning, and organization may be provided with checklists for dressing or grooming routines, doing the laundry, and simple meal preparation.

Although such aids can be thought of as environmental supports, the injured person most always needs to be trained to orient to the aids and must be provided with training and practice to use them appropriately.

New technological advances designed mainly for use by the general public have opened up new opportunities for people with disabilities. For example, some pharmacies provide electronic reminders that patients wear to remind them to take medications. Alarms on watches can also provide reminders. Some watches (e.g., the Timex Data Link) interface with personal computers via simple programs and a bar code reader on the watch to provide detailed information about scheduled appointments, medication reminders, and the like. Alphanumeric pagers can interface with either telephone or computer programs, allowing individuals to be reminded about things to do (Wilson et al., 1997). A number of Internet websites offer customized paging and notification systems that interface with pagers, cell phones, and personal organizers. Rehabilitation specialists can review available or potential systems with the injured individual and family. Such factors as initial and ongoing cost, ease and flexibility of programming, and type of notification (auditory or vibratory) must be considered. Even more important is an analysis of what sort of supports the injured person needs, who is available for ongoing support if it is needed, and how the person will be trained to use the system effectively. Some environmental interventions can be considered quite passive and not under the control of the injured individual, whereas others involve more initiative and control.

Adoption of Specialized Learning and Teaching Techniques

Of necessity, the process of rehabilitation usually involves teaching the individual new information or skills or redeveloping old ones. For example, learning to safely use and navigate a wheelchair in the hospital, at home, and on city streets requires a new set of knowledge, skills, and behaviors. Learning to use a compensatory memory or organizational system to manage one's daily life often may also require a new set of information and the establishment of new habits. In addition, many individuals must be able to acquire and retain new information if they are to succeed at school or work. These demands for new learning pose particular challenges given the learning and memory difficulties that are extremely common after many forms of brain injury and disease.

Memory difficulties are certainly among the most common consequences of traumatic brain injury (Sohlberg & Mateer, 2001), as well as anoxic/hypoxic episodes (cardiac arrest, near drowning, asphyxiation; Mill et al., 1997). Memory problems are also frequent following stroke, after cranial radiation therapy for tumors, in multiple sclerosis, and in many other acquired neurologic disorders.

From a rehabilitation perspective, memory disorders differ significantly according to the particular brain structures affected. Many different components are involved in memory, and different aspects of memory ability are distributed across many brain systems. One approach to thinking about memory is as a series of information-processing stages.

- First, the individual must attend to incoming information. Attention can be affected by arousal, alertness, ability to sustain attention, the ability to screen out and inhibit responding to distraction, and overall speed of processing. Attention can be affected by injury to widely distributed systems in the brainstem, thalamus, and frontal lobes. For these individuals, increasing arousal and improving attentional skills may have a major impact on memory performance. The individual is taught to focus on information to be learned and to avoid distractions when attempting to learn.

- Second, individuals must understand the information they see or hear. And those who have primary language, auditory, visual, or other perceptual disorders due to posterior cortical damage may not remember accurately, because they are unable to interpret information correctly. Speech and language therapy may have a positive impact on memory performance.

- Third, the memory and information processing system must be able to store new information in some form for later retrieval. The medial temporal lobes, including structures of the amygdala and hippocampi, are critical in the ability to store new information (even though the information is not stored in those structures per se). The medial temporal lobes and related subcortical structures are preferentially affected by anoxia/hypoxia, by certain infectious processes (e.g., herpes simplex encephalitis), and by vascular accidents involving the anterior communicating arteries. Individuals with damage to these areas will have great difficulty holding on to any new information because there are no known procedures to improve memory storage, and therapeutic interventions typically focus strongly on training in the use of compensatory memory aids and systems.

- Fourth, the system must be able to initiate and monitor retrieval of information from memory storage. It must also place memories in time and place so that memories are organized. Increasingly, it has been recognized that the frontal lobes are critical in these so-called "meta-memory functions." Retrieval of information from memory that is not linked to time and place and is poorly monitored with respect to accuracy is considered to be a form of confabulation, and is frequently observed in association with frontal injury. Individuals with frontal lobe injury often will not spontaneously act on intentions or information in memory unless prompted or cued. This kind of memory is called prospective memory, and failures of prospective memory are among the most common sorts of functional memory impairments. Individuals with frontal lobe injury also have difficulty accurately remembering the source of information or the order in which events occurred. Thus, memory interventions for individuals with frontal lobe injury often focus on helping them to initiate and follow through on intentions through a variety of cueing techniques and devices.

A number of other distinctions in memory can be capitalized on in memory rehabilitation. One distinction is between *semantic memory*, memory for information and facts, and *episodic memory*, which is memory for personally experienced events. Knowing that the colors of the American flag are red, white, and blue is something one learns, but where or when it was learned is not certain, and is an example of semantic memory. Knowing where you sat on the bus this morning (or even that you were on a bus) is an example of episodic memory. In many cases of acquired brain injury, the learning of new semantic information is slow and inefficient but possible, whereas new episodic memories remain very elusive.

Various training strategies can be used to teach new information. Commonly recognized ones include repetition of information, obtaining the information from multiple sources (e.g., reading it as well as hearing it), engaging in strategies that encourage deeper encoding of information, training first at simpler levels and moving to more complex, and providing distributed versus massed practice. For many individuals with brain injuries, such approaches are helpful and an important part of rehabilitation treatment planning.

However, some other forms of learning that may be effective for individuals with intact nervous systems are either ineffective or harmful to learning in individuals with memory impairment. One example of this is trial-and-error learning. Although this approach can be effective for unimpaired individuals, making errors can actually disrupt later recall in an individual with moderate to severe memory impairment. For example, if you

ask an individual with a memory impairment to remember your name, and if he cannot, to "take a guess," he is more likely to recall his incorrect guess the next time he is asked, even though the correct name is provided immediately after he guessed incorrectly. Similarly, in trying to recall a list of words, the individual is likely to keep recalling incorrect words that he or she generates, even after being told the word is incorrect. It is as if the word generated (incorrectly) becomes *primed* in memory and is, as a result, more accessible and likely to be recalled in later recall attempts. This phenomenon can be demonstrated in normal aging but is particularly pronounced in individuals with amnesia. To avoid this confusion, a technique called "errorless learning" has been described (Wilson et al., 1994). When using this technique, correct answers or strong cues for correct answers are provided to memory-impaired individuals until they establish the new information (Evans et al., 2000). By avoiding incorrect guesses (errors), confusion in memory is reduced while the new information is consolidated and stored. Errorless learning techniques have been shown to be superior to trial-and-error learning of name and face associations, orientation information, short sequences of behavior (such as entering information into a memory device or organizer), and routes around a hospital. Such approaches do not in any way change or correct deficiencies in the memory system, but they allow individuals with impaired memory systems to more efficiently learn new information. This technique has also been shown to be useful in working with children with memory difficulties in the learning of academic information and skills such as spelling and math. Errorless learning techniques also tend to reduce stress and frustration in learning new skills and information, as frustrating errors are decreased.

Another distinction in memory relates to the conscious or unconscious nature of "memories." Conscious recall of information involves the medial temporal, thalamic, and frontal systems described above. Recall of biographical information, word lists or stories, discussions with friends or family, television shows, and books one reads are all examples of explicit, conscious recollections, or what is termed *declarative memory*. Traditional neurologic and neuropsychological tests typically sample this kind of memory for which we are consciously aware. However, there are other ways to demonstrate that one has been affected by experience, and some kinds of learning are considered unconscious or implicit. Sometimes referred to as *procedural memory*, this kind of memory typically involves learning that occurs over time with repeated exposure to a task. For example, the widely described case of amnesia, H.M., demonstrated very little retention of any new information that he was told. Nevertheless, after repeatedly engaging in a pursuit rotor motor learning task over many days, he demonstrated consistent improvements on the task. Although he improved on the task, however, he did not have any conscious recollection of having done the task from session to session.

This kind of procedural learning seems to have a different neurologic substrate, perhaps involving the basal ganglia. Importantly for rehabilitation, this kind of learning is often relatively spared, and its potential effectiveness can be used to train new skills and procedures in individuals with otherwise very impaired new semantic learning ability (Kime et al., 1996).

Another aspect of this form of "implicit" or unconscious learning versus the more commonly recognized "explicit" or conscious learning is the potential to "prime" new information. Backward chaining is a teaching procedure in which the individual is first given all of the information needed to respond correctly. Then, a small part of the information or cue is taken away. Cues are continuously reduced until the person can perform without cueing. An adaptation of backward chaining, called the "method of vanishing cues," has been used to train individuals with severe memory impairments to learn new skills such as entering data into a computer or using a memory organizer (Glisky, 1995). Somewhat akin to errorless learning, in that the provision of effective cues throughout learning reduces the likelihood of errors, this technique is often used in the rehabilitation of individuals with memory impairment.

Implementation of Compensatory Devices and Strategies

A major focus of rehabilitation is the development and implementation of compensatory devices and strategies. These are objects, devices, or behaviors that will help the person to function more effectively despite physical and cognitive limitations or impairments. Corrective lenses and hearing aids are commonly used compensatory devices for physical limitations used by the general public. Computers, cell phones, pagers, and electronic organizers can be thought of as cognitive prosthetics widely used in the culture.

Within the brain-injured population physical compensations may involve wheelchairs, splints, specially designed utensils and tools, adapted living spaces, alarms, specially designed vehicles, and adaptive sporting equipment. There are a wide variety of manual and electronic communication devices to assist individuals who are unable to make themselves understood through speaking, signing, or gesturing. Increasingly sophisticated devices allow for speech synthesis and complex interfacing with computers and other devices. All of these devices make the individual more independent and able to affect and interact with the environment.

Within the realm of cognitive rehabilitation, compensatory aids may take many forms. Probably the most effort has gone into the study of compensatory memory devices. As indicated earlier, compensatory memory aids, in the form of calendars, alarms, watches with the date, memory books or organizers, and personal computers, are widely used by many people who are not injured. The complexity of daily life often simply requires assists for retaining information and detail that could not otherwise be managed. For individuals with any decrement in new learning and memory, such aids can be invaluable and are often essential to daily functioning (Sohlberg & Mateer, 1989b; Freeman et al., 1992; Burke et al., 1994; Schmitter-Edgecombe et al., 1995; Squires et al., 1996).

Before selecting an appropriate memory system, the rehabilitation specialist should understand the person's cognitive strengths and weaknesses. How is the person's semantic memory? Is he or she able to write? Will she be able to initiate use of the system independently? One must then ask what the demands of memory will be and in what environment it will be used? The person's premorbid use of aids should be considered, and the cost of devices may be a factor. Also relevant are the potential sources of support for using the system.

An individual with a significant impairment in episodic memory and in executive functions, for example, might require a system with a *calendar* to keep track of the current date and schedule and to look forward to and anticipate scheduled events, a *diary* section to record hourly events and thereby supplement episodic memory loss, a *things to do* section to record intended tasks and indicate when they have been completed, and an *information* section to record phone numbers, addresses, contacts, and so forth.

Once the sections of a memory book or organizer are determined, the person must be acquainted with the system, learn its parts, learn how to record in the system, practice referring to the system, and demonstrate its use in everyday functional environments. In someone with a mild injury, this may take just a few sessions over several days or weeks. However, for someone with a severe memory deficit, learning to use a memory system may require intensive work with therapists over months.

One 23-year-old man with whom we worked sustained a severe injury in a dockyard accident, when he was hit on the head by a shipping container. He was in a coma for almost 2 weeks. Subsequently, he demonstrated good physical and speech recovery, but he continued to have a profound amnesia. He had been living in a nursing home for the 2 years prior to entering active rehabilitation. After becoming involved in rehabilitation, it took him approximately 3 weeks of daily therapy to learn the names and sections of his memory notebook. It took an additional 2 months of daily therapy to learn to write in his book each time his watch alarm sounded or he changed activities, as well as to refer consistently to the book throughout the day. It took an additional 2 months of therapy to use the system flexibly to undertake activities in the community. The training was long, arduous, and costly. However, at the end of the training, he was able to live independently in an apartment, with some support for money management, and take public transportation to a volunteer worksite and recreational activities. As a society we must weigh the costs and benefits of maximizing independence and quality of life in our most vulnerable members.

Pager systems can also provide valuable cues and prompts to individuals who have initiation problems (adynamia). For those with executive function problems affecting their ability to plan and organize their behavior, external cueing and organizing systems can be used to facilitate dressing, grooming, housekeeping, and simple work-related tasks like photocopying or sorting mail, or to prompt a variety of activities including communication and activities of daily living (ADL) (Sohlberg et al., 1988; 1993b; Sohlberg & Mateer, 2001). Typically, tasks are analyzed, a list of critical steps is constructed, and the person is trained to use the list to carry out a sequence of behavior. Vocational counselors often take this approach in evaluating a job site and position. Supported work programs, which involve providing cues and supports by people in the workplace, have shown good success for many brain-injured individuals.

Restorative Approaches

Another approach to working with cognitive problems is to engage the person in systematic activities that are designed to improve some underlying cognitive capacity. The cognitive ability that has probably received the most attention in this regard is attention. Attention is a multifaceted capacity that underlies many other aspects of cognitive functioning. For example, limited attention can result in poor learning or memory of new information, difficulty following a conversation or movie, and ineffective problem solving. Underlying this approach is a belief that systematic practice and exercise of certain cognitive skills will result in a strengthening of those skills.

Attention can be conceived of as having multiple components. From a clinical perspective, it is common to talk about sustained attention or vigilance, selective attention, and divided attention. Individuals with brain injury commonly describe problems maintaining attention to task, difficulty dealing with distraction, and problems paying attention to or doing more than one thing at once. Deficits in these areas are borne out in studies of the cognitive consequences of brain injury.

Many individuals with traumatic brain injury have been shown to benefit substantially from exercise and training of attentional skills. Indeed, some of the earliest work in cognitive rehabilitation demonstrating

positive findings involved systematic intervention with the attentional system (Diller et al., 1974; Kewman et al., 1985; Ben-Yishay et al., 1987; Sohlberg & Mateer, 1987; Wood & Fussey, 1987; Sohlberg et al., 1993a;). There is now substantial literature on the rehabilitation of attention following traumatic brain injury, although a review of research in this area reveals a variety of methodological challenges in determining which approaches are the most efficacious.

The major premise of direct intervention approaches to the treatment of attentional impairments is that attentional abilities can be improved by providing opportunities for exercising a particular aspect or aspects of attention. Treatment has usually involved having patients engage in a series of repetitive drills or exercises, designed to provide opportunities for practice on tasks with increasingly greater attentional demands. Repeated activation and stimulation of attentional systems is hypothesized to facilitate changes in cognitive capacity.

Although a wide variety of tasks have been used in experimental studies of attention training, the Attention Process Training (APT) and Attention Process Training II (APT II) materials developed by Sohlberg and Mateer have been widely used in clinical settings and will be discussed in more detail here. The APT materials are a group of hierarchically organized tasks designed to exercise sustained, selective, alternating, and divided attention. APT II was developed for individuals with higher-level attentional abilities and provides more complex and demanding tasks. In both programs, tasks make increasingly greater demands on complex attentional control and working memory. Examples of tasks include listening for descending number sequences, shifting set on calculation tasks and a series of Stroop-like activities, alphabetizing words in sentences, detecting targets under noise conditions, and dividing attention between tasks (e.g., card sorting by suit and letter, combined auditory target detection and visual cancellation). In one study (Sohlberg & Mateer, 1987), multiple baseline designs revealed improvements on a complex measure of attention (i.e., the Paced Auditory Serial Addition Test [PASAT]) after training, but no evidence of improvement on an unrelated visuospatial task. This latter finding argued against a generalized effect related to stimulation. Similar changes in attention have been demonstrated by a number of other researchers using a variety of either paper and pencil, auditory, or computer-based training exercises (Ben-Yishay et al., 1987; Ethier et al., 1989; Gray & Robertson, 1989; Gray et al., 1992; Sturm et al., 1993; Sturm et al., 1997).

If attention actually improves following such training, one would expect to see changes in other cognitive abilities dependent on attention, such as memory, as well as on functional skills dependent on attention. Another level of evaluation of efficacy involves measurement of changes on tasks of cognitive ability, which are somewhat different from, yet dependent on attentional capacity. In a series of studies (Mateer & Sohlberg, 1988; Mateer et al., 1990; Mateer, 1992), we reported improved scores following attention training not only on measures of attention, but also on measures of memory and learning in patients who had sustained moderate to severe traumatic brain injury. On the basis of these studies, it was concluded that some patients with brain injury who experienced memory failures secondary to impairments in attention demonstrated improved attention and memory function following attention training. Similar findings of improved memory ability following attention training were reported by Niemann and colleagues (1990).

Another line of research has focused on determining whether there are underlying changes in brain activity associated with such training. Several researchers have now shown changes in the amplitude and latency of evoked potential components (N200 and P300 waves) following systematic attention training (Baribeau et al., 1989). These components of the evoked potential response are believed to be an index of attentional processing, and changes in them suggest differences in the way the brain is processing information after training.

Another area in which process-oriented or restorative training has been addressed is in the area of impaired executive functions. Difficulties with problem solving and reasoning are often apparent in individuals with acquired brain injury. Some of the difficulty in these domains may be due to more basic problems with attention, working memory, or learning and information retrieval, and interventions in these domains might help alleviate some of the higher-order functions. Nevertheless, a number of researchers have addressed the potential to improve skills necessary for problem solving, reasoning, and accurate decision making through exercise, feedback, and practice (Cicerone & Wood, 1987; Burke et al., 1991; Von Cramon et al, 1991; Cicerone & Giacino, 1992; Mateer, 1997).

In one study, a doctor who had sustained a traumatic brain injury was taught to generate hypotheses, make diagnoses, and write histopathology reports (Von Cramon et al., 1991). For 2 to 3 hours a week over 12 months, he was trained to look for all available information, describe pathologic features, look up observations in a book, generate hypotheses (including the pros and cons of every diagnosis), and render a decision and a report. He was provided with detailed feedback from a supervising pathologist. Following the intervention, there was an increase in correct diagnoses and the physician was able to work with support in the department of pathology. However, he did not show any generalization of problem-solving abilities to tasks different from the one on which he was trained. In addition, his awareness of his difficulties remained unchanged, and he continued to overestimate his abilities. Nevertheless, he demonstrated functional gains in the area of ability targeted by the treatment plan.

Generalization of Training

Although a few studies have described improvements in such practical functions as cooking and driving, a major concern with regard to the use of process-oriented training exercises has been the limited demonstration of generalization. Strictly *restorative* approaches focus on the systematic "drill and practice" retraining of component cognitive processes (i.e., attention, executive skills, etc.), whereas *functional* approaches emphasize the stepwise training of observable behaviors, skills, and ADL. The restorative approach places as the primary objective, retraining individuals to *process information more effectively*, in the belief that improved cognitive processing will generalize to many practical skills, whereas the primary emphasis of the functional approach is on teaching individuals how to *actually perform* a specific functional task or activity. There have been many attempts to marry these techniques, and attention-training protocols typically include generalization exercises and protocols. Nevertheless, training in a wide variety of functional contexts is difficult, and it has not proved easy to demonstrate generalization, due to problems with transfer of gains from the training environment to new settings.

For many functions, therapy is clearly most effective when the patient practices skills in the manner and setting in which they will be used. Redevelopment of basic eating, dressing, and grooming abilities in more severely injured individuals relies heavily on repetitive practice of these abilities in as natural a context as possible. However, simply engaging an individual in a "naturalistic" activity may not be sufficient to address the specific higher-level cognitive deficits, which are disrupting performance. Most naturalistic activities (e.g., cooking, money management, driving) are multidimensional and depend on many different cognitive processes (e.g., reasoning, visuoperceptual processing, executive functions, and attention), and hence may not directly target the underlying impairments in attentional control. However, process-oriented techniques can be paired with generalization activities, which represent functional activities that have been carefully graded in terms of difficulty and task demand.

One exciting new area of rehabilitation research involves use of new technologies such as virtual reality to allow practice of skills in virtual environments that closely mimic real-world environments. Virtual reality environments, for example, can mimic a classroom, office setting, or grocery store, allow the individual to interact with the virtual environment, and have the potential to provide systematic *restorative* training within the context of *functionally* relevant, ecologically valid simulated environments. Virtual reality technology can allow systematic, theoretically based interventions that could be carefully graded to increase in difficulty and complexity as a person's skills increase and optimize the degree of transfer of training to the person's real-world environment as skills. It is increasingly recognized as a useful tool for the assessment and rehabilitation of cognitive processes and functional abilities (Grealy & Heffernan, 2001; Schultheis & Rizzo, 2001).

Education, Emotional Support, and Awareness Training

A major role played by rehabilitation specialists is providers of information about brain injury and its effects. Families are often puzzled by or misinterpret common symptoms of brain injury. Adynamic syndromes in which the injured individual shows limited spontaneous activity can appear to others as a lack of motivation or interest, when in fact the disorder is one of impaired behavioral initiation. Reframing this disorder can allow better understanding and management of the condition. Similarly, families are often confused by day-to-day variability in function, whereby the individual can perform a task one day but not the next. This can appear to be volitional or motivational in nature, whereas it may actually reflect variability in skills or factors related to fatigue or changes in cueing or support to do the activity. Problems with irritability and anger can be particularly difficult for family members to cope with and guidance with respect to managing challenging behaviors is critical.

Acquired injuries resulting in permanent alterations in an individual's functioning commonly cause significant emotional disruption. Depression, feelings of loss, anxiety, fear about the future, guilt, and feelings of helplessness are often seen during the weeks, months, and years following injury. Family members and the injured person will experience emotional reactions that vary over time. Rehabilitation psychologists play an important role in providing support, increasing motivation, and combating fear and hopelessness.

Traumatic brain injury is often associated with somewhat paradoxical effects with respect to awareness. Awareness refers to recognizing ways in which one's abilities and behavior have changed and appreciating the impact of those changes on one's future activities. Individuals with significant injury, particularly to the frontal lobe, often display very limited or blunted awareness with respect to the effects of the injury and its consequences. Without such insight and awareness there is often limited motivation to participate in rehabilitation or to use compensatory techniques and strategies. Part of the treatment involves increasing awareness through education and experiential exercises.

Awareness training is also a critical component of many cognitive and behavioral interventions in which the goal is to facilitate self-regulation of cognitive and emotional difficulties. With increased awareness of the nature of their difficulties, injured individuals can learn to minimize distractions, use compensatory memory aids, and gain skill in self-regulation of depression, anxiety, irritability, and anger.

As indicated earlier, a somewhat paradoxical finding is that individuals with apparently much more mild injuries and better preserved cognition often become acutely aware of and concerned about even subtle changes in their abilities. Indeed, individuals with persistent postconcussive complaints are often very focused on and distressed about perceived changes in their cognitive ability. For some individuals, these changes and the frustration, fear, and anxiety that accompany them trigger a profound loss of self-perception. Rehabilitation is aimed at decreasing emotional response to perceived cognitive failures, increasing the person's sense of self-control and self-efficacy, and normalizing expectations for performance.

Indeed, recent developments in attention training programs have emphasized not only practice on attention tasks, but activities that require the person to monitor and evaluate attentional failures and successes as a way of improving awareness. They also focus on assisting the individual to become more knowledgeable and active in managing situations such as to enhance the capacity to attend (Sohlberg et al., 1993a). This reflects a shift to techniques which not only increase self-awareness but also enhance a sense of self-control and mastery over cognitive weaknesses.

SUMMARY AND CONCLUSIONS

The rehabilitation of individuals with cognitive impairments is broad in scope. Advances in medical science and cognitive neuroscience have prompted more interest and research in this field, and there is substantial progress in translating new knowledge into new theory-driven rehabilitation practice. Rehabilitation covers the life span, and new interventions originally designed for children and adults with acquired neurologic injury have been adapted and used with children with developmental disabilities, and with aging adults. Rehabilitation is best delivered in a transdisciplinary approach by rehabilitation professionals with a broad range of expertise. Effective rehabilitation is best conceptualized as a treatment that is delivered as a partnership forged between an injured person, the family, and the rehabilitation team. Interventions are wide ranging and eclectic. Goals must be framed in functional terms, and outcomes need to be examined to continue to identify the most efficacious rehabilitation practices. The primary goals of therapy are to assist individuals and their families to maximize independence, adjustment, quality of life, and the capacity for self-direction and self-regulation.

■ KEY POINTS

☐   Cognitive interventions must be tailored to the individual, taking into account the individual's strengths, weaknesses, background, and current and future circumstances.

☐   Cognitive interventions are most effectively viewed as a collaborative effort between the patient, the patient's family or caregivers, and the therapist.

☐   Cognitive intervention should be focused on mutually set and functionally relevant goals. Evaluation of efficacy and outcome should incorporate and capture changes in everyday functional abilities.

☐   Most successful cognitive interventions are eclectic and involve multiple approaches, including compensatory strategies, skills training, and specialized instructional techniques.

☐   Behavioral interventions, brain injury education, and the development of insight and self-regulation may be integral components of treatment.

☐   Interventions must address the affective and emotional components of cognitive loss or inefficiency and resulting disability.

☐   Interventions should be self-evaluative and build in both generalization activities and measures to guide treatment and ensure efficacy.

KEY READINGS

Cicerone KD, Dahlberg C, Kalmar K, et al: Evidence-based cognitive rehabilitation: Recommendations for clinical practice. Arch Phys Med Rehabil 81:1596–1615, 2000.

National Institutes of Health Consensus Development Panel on Rehabilitation of Persons with Traumatic Brain Injury: Rehabilitation of persons with traumatic brain injury. JAMA 282:974–983, 1999.

Ponsford J, Sloan S, Snow P: Traumatic Brain Injury: Rehabilitation for Everyday Adaptive Living. Hove, UK: Lawrence Erlbaum Associates, 1995.

Rosenthal M, Griffith ER, Kreutzer JS, et al (eds): Rehabilitation of the Adult and Child with Traumatic Brain Injury. Philadelphia: F.A. Davis, 1999.

Sohlberg MM, Mateer CA: Cognitive Rehabilitation: An Integrated Neuropsychological Approach. New York: Guilford Press, 2001.

REFERENCES

Alderman N, Burgess PW: Integrating cognition and behaviour: A pragmatic approach to brain injury rehabilitation, in Wood RL, Fussey I (eds): Cognitive Rehabilitation in Perspective. Basingstoke, UK: Taylor & Francis, 1990, pp. 204–228.

Baribeau J, Ethier M, Braun C: A neurophysiological assessment of attention before and after cognitive remediation in patients with severe closed head injury. J Neurol Rehabil 3:71–92, 1989.

Ben-Yishay Y, Piasetsky EB, Rattock J: A systematic method for ameliorating disorders in basic attention, in Meyer MJ, Benton AL, Diller L (eds): Neuropsychological Rehabilitation. New York: Guilford Press, 1987, pp. 165–181.

Burke J, Danick J, Bemis B, et al: A process approach to memory book training for neurological patients. Brain Inj 8:71–81, 1994.

Burke WH, Zenicus AH, Wesolowski MD, et al: Improving executive function disorders in brain-injured clients. Brain Inj 5:25–28, 1991.

Carney N, Chetnut RM, Maynard H, et al: Effect of cognitive rehabilitation on outcomes for persons with traumatic brain injury: A systematic review. J Head Trauma Rehabil 14:277–307, 1999.

Cicerone KD, Giacino JT: Remediation of executive function deficits after traumatic brain injury. Neuropsychol Rehabil 2:12–22, 1992.

Cicerone KD, Dahlberg C, Kalmar K, et al: Evidence-based cognitive rehabilitation: Recommendations for clinical practice. Arch Phys Med Rehabil 81:1596–1615, 2000.

Cicerone KD, Wood JC: Planning disorder after closed head injury: A case study. Arch Phys Med Rehabil 68:111–115, 1987.

Diller L, Ben-Yishay Y, Gerstmann LJ, et al: Studies of Cognition and Rehabilitation in Hemiplegia (Rehabilitation Monograph No. 50). New York: New York University Medical Center, 1974.

Ethier M, Baribeau JMC, Braun CMJ: Computer-dispensed cognitive-perceptual training of closed head injury patients after spontaneous recovery. Study 2: Non-speeded tasks. Can J Rehabil 3:7–16, 1989.

Evans JJ, Wilson BA, Schuri U, et al: A comparison of "errorless" and "trial-and-error" learning methods for teaching individuals with acquired memory deficits. Neuropsychol Rehabil 10:67–101, 2000.

Freeman MR, Mittenberg W, DiCowden M, et al: Executive and compensatory memory retraining in traumatic brain injury. Brain Inj 6:65–70, 1992.

Glisky EL: Acquisition and transfer of word processing skills by an amnesic patient. Neuropsychol Rehabil 5:299–318, 1995.

Gray JM, Robertson I: Remediation of attentional difficulties following brain injury: Three experimental single case designs. Brain Inj 3:163–170, 1989.

Gray JM, Robertson I, Pentland B, et al: Microcomputer-based attentional retraining after brain damage: A randomised group controlled trial. Neuropsychol Rehabil 2:97–115, 1992.

Grealy MA, Heffernan D: The rehabilitation of brain injured children: The case for including physical exercise and virtual reality. Pediatr Rehabil 4:41–49, 2001.

Gronwall D: Rehabilitation programs for patients with mild head injury: Components, problems and evaluation. J Head Trauma Rehabil 1:53–62, 1986.

Kewman DG, Seigerman C, Kinter H, et al: Stimulation and training of psychomotor skills: Teaching the brain-injured to drive. Rehabil Psychol 30:11–27, 1985.

Kime S, Lamb D, Wilson G: Use of a comprehensive programme of external cueing to enhance procedural memory in a patient with dense amnesia. Brain Inj 10:17–25, 1996.

Kolb B: Brain plasticity and behavior. Hillsdale, NJ: Erlbaum Associates, 1996.

Kraus JF, Nourjah P: The epidemiology of mild uncomplicated head injury. Trauma 28:1637–1643, 1998.

Luria AR: Higher Cortical Functions in Man. London, UK: Tavistock, 1966.

Mateer CA: Systems of care for post-concussive syndrome, in Horn LJ, Zasler ND (eds): Rehabilitation of Post-Concussive Disorders. Philadelphia: Henley & Belfus, 1992, pp. 143–160.

Mateer CA: Rehabilitation of individuals with frontal lobe impairment, in Jose Leon-Carrion (ed): Neuropsychological Rehabilitation: Fundamentals, Innovations and Directions. Delray Beach, FL: GR/St. Lucie Press, 1997, pp. 285–300.

Mateer CA, Sohlberg MM: A paradigm shift in memory rehabilitation, in Whitaker H (ed): Neuropsychological Studies of Nonfocal Brain Injury: Dementia and Closed Head Injury. New York: Springer-Verlag, 1988, pp. 202–225.

Mateer CA, Sohlberg MM, Youngman P: The management of acquired attentional and memory disorders following mild closed head injury, in Wood R (ed): Cognitive Rehabilitation in Perspective. London, UK: Taylor & Francis, 1990, pp. 68–95.

Mill VM, Cassidy JW, Katz DI: Neurologic Rehabilitation: A Guide to Diagnosis, Prognosis, and Treatment Planning. Malden, MA: Blackwell Science, 1997.

Minderhoud JM, Boelens ME, Huizenga J, et al: Treatment of minor head injuries. Clin Neurol Neurosurg 82:127–140, 1980.

Mittenberg W, Tremont G, Zielinski RE, et al: Cognitive-behavioral prevention of postconcussive syndrome. Arch Clin Neuropsychol 11:139–146, 1996.

National Institutes of Health Consensus Development Panel on Rehabilitation of Persons with Traumatic Brain Injury: Rehabilitation of persons with traumatic brain injury. JAMA 282:974–983, 1999.

Niemann H, Ruff RM, Baser CA: Computer assisted attention training in head injured individuals: A controlled efficacy study of an outpatient program. J Clin Consult Psychol 58:811–817, 1990.

Penkman LC: Rehabilitation of attention deficits in traumatic brain injury. Unpublished doctoral dissertation. University of Victoria, 2001.

Prigatano GP: Disturbances of self-awareness of deficit after traumatic brain injury, in Prigatano GP, Schacter DL (eds): Awareness of Deficit after Brain Injury: Clinical and Theoretical Perspectives. New York: Oxford University Press, 1991, pp. 111–126.

Raskin SA, Mateer CA: Neuropsychological Management of Mild Traumatic Brain Injury. New York: Oxford University Press, 2000.

Robertson IH, Murre JMJ: Rehabilitation of brain damage: Brain plasticity and principles of guided recovery. Psychol Bull 125:544–575, 1999.

Rosenthal M, Griffith ER, Kreutzer JS, et al (eds): Rehabilitation of the Adult and Child with Traumatic Brain Injury. Philadelphia: F.A. Davis, 1999.

Schmitter-Edgecombe M, Fahy J, Whelan J, et al: Memory remediation after severe closed head injury: Notebook training versus supportive therapy. J Consult Clin Psychol 63:484–489, 1995.

Schultheis MT, Rizzo AA: The application of virtual reality technology in rehabilitation. Rehabil Psychol 46:296–311, 2001.

Sohlberg MM, Johnson L, Paule L, et al: Attention Process Training-II: A Program to Address Attentional Deficits for Persons with Mild Cognitive Dysfunction. Wake Forest, NC: Lash, 1993a.

Sohlberg MM, Mateer CA: Effectiveness of an attention training program. J Clin Exp Neuropsychol 19:117–130, 1987.

Sohlberg MM, Mateer CA: Introduction to Cognitive Rehabilitation: Theory and Practice. New York: Guilford Press, 1989a.

Sohlberg MM, Mateer CA: Training use of compensatory memory books: A three stage behavioral approach. J Clin Exp Neuropsychol 11:871–891, 1989b.

Sohlberg MM, Mateer CA: Cognitive Rehabilitation: An Integrated Neuropsychological Approach. New York: Guilford Press, 2001.

Sohlberg MM, Mateer CA, Stuss DT: Contemporary approaches to the management of executive control dysfunction. J Head Trauma Rehabil 8:45–58, 1993b.

Sohlberg MM, Sprunk H, Metzelaar K: Efficacy of an external cuing system in an individual with severe frontal lobe damage. Cogn Rehabil 6:36–40, 1988.

Squires EJ, Hunkin NM, Parkin AJ: Memory notebook training in a case of severe amnesia: Generalization from paired associate learning to real life. Neuropsychol Rehabil 6:55–65, 1996.

Sturm W, Hartje W, Orgass B, et al: Computer-assisted rehabilitation of attention impairments, in Stachowiak FJ, De Blesser R, Deloche G, et al (eds): Developments in the Assessment and Rehabilitation of Brain-Damaged Patients: Perspectives from a European Concerted Action. Tübingen, Germany: Guenter Narr Verlag, 1993, pp. 49–54.

Sturm W, Willmes K, Orgass B, et al: Do specific attention deficits need specific training? Neuropsychol Rehabil 7:81–103, 1997.

Stuss DT: Self, awareness, and the frontal lobes: A neuropsychological perspective, in Strauss J, Goethals GR (eds): The Self: An Interdisciplinary Approach . New York: Springer-Verlag, 1991, pp. 255–278.

Von Cramon DY, Matthes-von Cramon G, Mai N: Problem solving deficits in brain injured patients: A therapeutic approach. Neuropsychol Rehabil 1:45–64, 1991.

Webb PM, Glueckauf RL: The effects of direct involvement in goal setting on rehabilitation outcome for persons with traumatic brain injuries. Rehabil Psychol 39:179–188, 1994.

Wilson BA, Baddeley AD, Evans E, et al: Errorless learning in the rehabilitation of memory impaired people. Neuropsychol Rehabil 4:307–326, 1994.

Wilson BA, Evans JJ, Emslie H, et al: Evaluation of NeuroPage: A new memory aid. J Neurol Neurosurg Psychiatry 63:113–115, 1997.

Wood RL, Fussey I: Computer-based cognitive retraining: A controlled study. Int Disability Stud 9:149–154, 1987.

C H A P T E R

49

Speech and Language Rehabilitation

Jacqueline J. Hinckley

INTRODUCTION

The Effectiveness of Speech and Language Rehabilitation

The World Health Organization's Framework for Rehabilitation

General Principles of Speech-Language Rehabilitation

TREATMENT APPROACHES

Which Treatment for Which Outcome?

Treatment for Speech Disorders

Treatment for Language Disorders

Speech-Language Pathologists and Family Education and Counseling

SUMMARY

Aphasia

Apraxia

Dementia

Dysarthria

Dysphagia

Right hemisphere disorder

Traumatic brain injury

Voice disorders

This chapter outlines the scientific evidence for the efficacy of speech-language interventions for individuals with neurologic impairments and provides an overview of typical speech-language rehabilitation approaches for the range of communication impairments encountered in medical settings. An introduction addresses the effectiveness of speech-language rehabilitation and its basis on general principles of learning and plasticity. Treatment for each type of speech and language disorder is reviewed, with an emphasis on treatment outcomes.

INTRODUCTION

Speech-language pathologists first became involved in medical rehabilitation during World War II, when there was a need for clinicians to provide services to soldiers with gunshot wounds and other head injuries (Shewan, 1986). Since that time speech-language pathologists have played a fundamental role in all aspects of rehabilitation (see Appendix: Training and Scope of Practice). A comprehensive literature on assessing and treating speech and language disorders that arise as a result of neurologic etiologies of all kinds exists and establishes the foundation on which speech-language pathologists base their work.

The Effectiveness of Speech and Language Rehabilitation

Speech and language rehabilitation has been subjected to various types of evaluation to determine efficacy. We can evaluate the effects of any given treatment through a number of levels of evidence. At the weakest level are case studies and other single-study designs. Retrospective, nonrandomized studies provide a somewhat more convincing case and can be strengthened by randomizing subjects to the treatment and control groups. Prospective nonrandomized and randomized studies with control conditions provide the strongest level of evidence for the effectiveness of any given treatment.

A meta-analysis is another persuasive tool for determining the effectiveness of a treatment for which a body of literature already exists. In this procedure, a number of studies are identified that investigate the effects of a particular treatment. Such meta-analyses include studies with both positive and negative results. The findings of all of these studies are subjected to statistical analysis, which can answer questions about the overall efficacy of any treatment procedure or type.

Meta-analyses for the treatment of various neurogenic speech and language disorders are available. Robey (1994, 1998) has shown that aphasia therapy is effective, both in the acute and chronic stages, but the degree to which the treatment is effective is greater in the acute stages. The meta-analysis of Whurr and colleagues (1992) agrees with the conclusion that aphasia therapy has been effective when analysis of all available treatment research studies is completed.

Comprehensive literature syntheses are another route to examining the overall effectiveness of rehabilitation. Such syntheses are available for speech-language rehabilitation among patients with speech disorders (Pearson, 1995; Yorkston, 1996), swallowing disorders (Logemann, 1999), cognitive-linguistic disorders (Coelho et al., 1996), and aphasia (Holland et al., 1996) and show the overall effectiveness of speech-language rehabilitation in addressing these communication disorders. Taking these meta-analyses and literature syntheses together, we have a firm foundation on which to base our work in treating individuals with neurogenic speech and language disorders.

The World Health Organization's Framework for Rehabilitation

The World Health Organization (WHO) has established a framework describing the goals and desirable levels of outcomes for rehabilitation. The goal of rehabilitation is to return the individual to the appropriate level of participation based on the person's age, gender, and social role. This goal is delineated in the International Classification of Functioning, Disability and Health (ICF), most recently revised in its 2001 version. The WHO framework provides an important basis on which all rehabilitation practitioners can communicate, so that the patient's needs are central and a common vocabulary is applied across all disciplines. All aspects of an individual's life can be described within this framework, so that we can ensure that we are meeting all of the needs of an individual in rehabilitation.

Definitions

The ICF classification system helps clinicians to identify the outcomes of their intervention by describing three basic levels. The first of these is the impairment level,

defined as the aspect or component of the cognitive, linguistic, or physical system in which the deficit has occurred. At this level, we are interested in physiologic and behavioral signs and symptoms and measure their specific change over the course of rehabilitation. For example, tongue strength and range of motion are specific components of dysarthria, and change in tongue strength is an impairment level outcome of intervention.

The activity level of the framework is concerned with the activities that have been affected as a result of the impairment. Making a phone call independently and ordering in a restaurant are examples of activities that might be affected by a communication disorder. At this level, the same activity can be affected due to different impairments. For example, placing phone calls may be affected by either a speech disorder such as dysarthria or by a language disorder like aphasia. In any case, we are still interested in the individual's ability to perform such activities as independently as possible.

Thirdly, the participation level reveals the social effects of the impairment, by describing the person's level of productivity and ability to participate in normal social roles. Participation in life is the return of the individual to functioning in appropriate social roles, including economic, family, and community participation. Life participation means that the individual returns to some level of productivity, including gainful or volunteer employment; that the individual fulfills social roles in a manner comparable to that prior to rehabilitation with friends and family; and that the individual participates as a citizen of the community. This participation is observed through return to work, participation in meaningful hobbies and interests with others, development and maintenance of friendships and other relationships, and participation in civic activities such as voting or other community-related events. Various impairments can affect any given social role; relationships with families and friends can be changed due to either speech or language impairments.

Measuring Treatment Outcomes

The way in which we measure these outcomes demonstrates our understanding of what we believe fit in these categories. Examples of assessment tools typically used by speech-language pathologists for each of the three types of outcomes are listed in Table 49-1. Impairment-level outcomes are typically measured by the administration of tests that address the basic components of a disorder. Among speech disorders, a variety of oral-motor assessments will help to quantify changes in strength, range, and rate of movement of the articulators. For patients with language disorders, standardized aphasia batteries will accomplish the same goal. Other assessment tools, focused on specific aspects of attention, memory, executive function, or other cognitive

TABLE 49-1. Examples of Commonly Used Assessment Measures, Pertaining to the WHO ICF Framework

WHO ICF Framework		
Impairment	**Activity**	**Participation**
Oral-motor abilities	ASHA-FACS	Wellness questionnaires
Standardized aphasia batteries	Communication Effectiveness Index (CETI)	Life satisfaction measures
Specific cognitive tests		Voice Handicap Index
	Communication Abilities in Daily Living	Community Integration Questionnaire

ASHA, American Speech-Language-Hearing Association; FACS, Functional Assessment of Communication Skills.

abilities, will measure impairment-related outcomes for individuals with a predominant cognitive disorder.

A common tool for assessing activity-level outcomes is the American Speech-Language-Hearing Association's Functional Assessment of Communication Skills (ASHA-FACS) (Frattali et al., 1995). The ASHA-FACS was designed for use with adults with a variety of neurogenic communication impairments and is particularly appropriate for use in hospitals and clinics. This rating scale is designed to measure change related to treatment on a variety of social communication, reading and writing, and daily activity tasks. Examples of items include ratings of the independence and quality of the completion of tasks such as following a map, participating in conversations, requesting help, making money transactions, and telling time.

Activities such as eating in public, understandability of speech, and normalcy of diet, which may be affected by head and neck cancer treatment, are rated from total incapacity to full function on one scale (List et al., 1990). A similar rating scale for persons with language disorder is the Communicative Effectiveness Index (CET) (Lomas et al., 1989). This instrument also provides a range of activities, and the caregiver rates each one according to a scale of "as able as before stroke" or "unable." Rating scales like these provide not only a measure of activity-level outcomes but also a measure of the social validity of changes made in treatment.

Another useful tool is the Communicative Abilities in Daily Living task (CADL-2) (Holland et al., 1999). This assessment measure uses role-play as a primary form of observing functional communication abilities. For example, the test includes a role-play of going to a doctor's office, including filling out a personal information form and communicating with the physi-

cian. Other scenarios include shopping and requesting assistance, ordering in a restaurant, and reading a bus schedule. An advantage of this kind of assessment is that it provides a more objective measure of activity-level outcomes, compared to clinician or caregiver rating scales.

Measurement of life participation can occur in several ways. Wellness questionnaires, perceived quality of life and life satisfaction scales, and community integration questionnaires including family adjustment measures are the primary sources of information regarding the effects of treatment on life participation. Wellness questionnaires such as Ryff's (1989) ask participants to respond to items regarding self-acceptance, autonomy, environmental mastery, purpose in life, and personal growth.

Quality of life and life satisfaction scales can range from long questionnaires to short, four-item questions that are more easily understood by those with cognitive-linguistic disorders (Diener et al., 1985). Other communication disorder–specific quality of life tools have been developed, designed to address the specific impact of a communication disorder on perceived quality of life. For example, the Voice Handicap Index (Jacobson et al., 1997) measures life participation by assessing an individual's self-perceptions about the physical, emotional, and functional effects of a voice disorder. Finally, the Community Integration Questionnaire (Willer et al., 1993) has been used extensively in the population with traumatic brain injuries (TBI) to address issues of social, home, and community integration, including productivity, by asking about specific activities and whether they are completed independently, with someone else, or not at all. All of these measures emphasize the perceptions of the patient and significant others as sources for determining perceived quality of life and the reestablishment of social roles.

General Principles of Speech-Language Rehabilitation

Speech-language pathologists base their work on the plentiful literature and understanding of human learning and behavior change, as well as on detailed knowledge of cognitive-linguistic functions, sensory pathways, motor pathways and motor control, anatomy and physiology, and disease- and injury-specific processes. Assessment provides the clinician with test results and a sample of the patient's speech, language, and cognitive abilities so that a proper communication diagnosis can be made. This diagnosis is separate from the medical diagnosis and will relate to the best treatment choice. However, rehabilitation will have to be planned specifically for the strengths and weaknesses of a particular individual. As a result, a competent speech-language pathologist may not use the same particular treatment procedure with all patients with the same communication diagnosis.

Typically, individualized treatment goals are developed based on the results of the initial assessment, injury and disease factors, social support, and goals for living situation. Because so many critical factors that affect the development of treatment goals vary among individuals, it is necessary to develop individualized goals. These goals will be addressed in the context of particular treatment approaches and procedures that have been tested and their effectiveness reported in the clinical literature.

One pervasive approach to speech-language rehabilitation is stimulation-facilitation (Schuell et al., 1964). In this approach, clinicians devise tasks that require the person to respond within a targeted domain area, using strong, controlled, intensive stimulation (Duffy, 1994). The underlying principle is that continued practice with a variety of exemplars will improve the speech, language, or cognitive process that is fundamental to the task performance. The goal of the clinician is to elicit responses that will maximize the reorganization of the language system. This approach is often chosen in situations when direct remediation of a particular cognitive or language component is desirable, for example, during periods of spontaneous recovery.

The development of compensatory strategies that accommodate for an anticipated chronic loss, or as a temporary measure to enable communication while specific speech-language skills improve, is also an important approach in speech-language rehabilitation. In this approach, the clinician provides mechanisms by which individuals can accomplish tasks via alternative means, thereby increasing their functional level as well as facilitating other social and personal benefits (Holland & Beeson, 1993).

Finally, management of the environment is an appropriate approach in many situations and involves training caregivers and others to use communication techniques that facilitate the patient's participation, as well as the general management of other activities or procedures in the environment that will maximize the person's performance. Environmental management is particularly appropriate for those who have progressive communication disorders and for whom an improvement in ability cannot be expected.

The communication diagnosis and the individualized potential for behavior change or behavior facilitation must be combined with an understanding of the underlying disease processes and plasticity mechanisms. Speech-language rehabilitation is best deferred until disease management occurs in some cases, whereas in others, maximizing recovery during the period of spontaneous recovery will be the most beneficial intervention.

During these various phases of acute, postacute, and long-term recovery, various frequencies of treatment and treatment duration may be appropriate. In general, more treatment results in better outcomes; this is true for every stage of recovery in aphasia (Robey, 1998). However, not every patient is a potential candidate for maximal treatment rates. Medical status, psychological status, cognitive endurance, motivation, and financial ability to pay must typically be considered when making recommendations about treatment rate. The interaction between these individual factors and various treatment rate options needs to be further researched, so that clinical decisions about these matters can rest more firmly on empirical evidence. This is also true for the duration of treatment. At present, the overwhelming force in determining total amount and duration of treatment is financial ability, including insurance benefits. Many individuals have the potential to benefit from additional treatment but are not accorded benefits for speech-language services by their health insurance carrier. In the future, scientific evidence about treatment rate and duration should be a more powerful determinant of these important clinical decisions.

Desired outcomes can also be addressed through treatment format, such as making choices between individual and group therapy. Group therapy is an effective and cost-efficient model for improving the impairments, functional activities, and social integration of patients with all kinds of neurogenic communication disorders (Elman, 1999). Groups have the advantage of providing peer modeling, cooperative learning, and social support opportunities that are rarely if ever available in individual, clinician-to-patient treatment. Incorporation of modeling techniques enables clinicians to demonstrate effective communication behaviors. Perhaps more importantly, linking several patients and families together who are experiencing similar communication challenges provides them with peer examples of solutions and coping strategies. Again, the timing of the delivery of such services must be carefully considered in relation to the patient's needs and abilities.

TREATMENT APPROACHES

Which Treatment for Which Outcome?

Any particular treatment approach may have impairment, activity, and participation outcomes. The impairment that underlies the activities can be targeted, with the hope that improving the cognitive, linguistic, and speech components that contribute to the accomplishment of a particular activity will improve the independence level of the activity. Alternatively, the activity itself can be targeted for direct intervention through a functional approach that incorporates role-playing, scripting, and the development of context-specific compensatory strategies, which may in turn improve the underlying impairment and also the social role

TABLE 49-2. Examples of General Treatment Approaches Used in Speech-Language Rehabilitation

Treatment example	Brief description or examples
Stimulation-facilitation	Intensive stimulation of a particular skill or ability
Specific treatments for specific impairments	Syntactic training for agrammatical patients; direct remediation for memory impairments
Compensatory strategies	Use of assistive/alternative communication; pacing and timing compensations for dysarthria; use of a memory notebook for cognitively impaired patients
Computer-assisted treatment	Practice on specific skills, like reading comprehension or writing; use of speech input or output to compensate for communication difficulties; use of specialized word processing programs
Environmental management	Family education and development of specific communication strategies among family members; establishing procedures within the environment that facilitate communication and cognitive performances

functioning of the individual. Finally, the social aspects of a communication disorder can be foregrounded through facilitation of lifestyle changes, and caregiver, volunteer, and public education, with probable related changes to activities, and possibly impairments, as the patient becomes more mentally and physically active. Examples of various treatment approaches are listed in Table 49-2.

As an example, Hinckley and colleagues (2001) investigated the differential outcomes of two different treatment approaches for aphasia. One treatment focused on the component skills required for a task, and the other treatment focused on the compensatory strategies required to perform the functional task. Subjects in the skill-based treatment improved on measures of activity (CADL-2), and subjects in the context-based treatment improved on an impairment-level measure of oral naming. This study confirms the multiple level outcomes of any particular treatment regimen.

We must be cautious, however, about assuming that an impairment-based treatment will have effects on desired communication activities. Although some impairment-based treatment procedures have been shown to generalize to communication activities, others have not. The issue of generalization is a critical one to any treatment approach. Because treatment cannot focus on every context in which a specific communication ability is going to be used, an effective treatment will be one in which generalization to desired contexts occurs. The critical action related to generalization patterns among different treatment approaches probably lies in the process of the treatment and how it corresponds to underlying mechanisms.

For example, some theoretically based treatments do affect activities without specifically targeting those contexts. Movement therapy for agrammatic aphasics

(Thompson et al., 1997), which targets the specific grammatical impairment, has an effect on conversational and narrative discourse, certainly a desirable activity-level outcome. Improvement of speech production among dysarthric patients through a physiologic treatment approach can have effects on a wide range of communication activities, including communicating with family members and friends, speaking on the phone, and other critical communication activities. Swallowing management, when focused on the specific physiologic impairment, can also affect independence in eating.

However, some impairment-level treatments may not always generalize to communication activities. This may occur when too few exemplars or contexts are used in the training. If one specific treatment activity is seen to improve a particular cognitive or linguistic mechanism, and that activity is repeated, then, intuitively, the underlying cognitive/linguistic processes should improve. Ylvisaker and Feeney (1998) describe this as the "Fallacy of Decontextualized Training" and recommend that training, particularly that which is focused on patients with various cognitive disorders, should be incorporated into natural contexts.

Computer-assisted interventions can easily fall into this trap because it is convenient for clinicians to have patients work on computer-based activities each day; yet the outcome, particularly if the computer activities are not chosen well or varied appropriately, may be an improvement in the single task completed on the computer with no generalization to other activities. One young man with TBI explained his experience with such a situation this way: "If I went to the video arcade every day and played the same game, my score would improve. And that's what I think I'm doing in therapy."

Many computer-based interventions for cognitive, linguistic, and speech disorders have been shown to be effective (Katz & Wertz, 1997). However, in each of these successful cases, a battery of exercises was used in an appropriate hierarchy, and participants were not simply repeating the same kind of task or game without clinician-directed integration across multiple modalities and tasks.

Because of the desire to affect as many levels of outcomes as possible, many clinicians use a well-chosen blend of treatment procedures. More traditional, stimulation-type treatment may be administered along with functional training of performance within specific activities and accompanied by caregiver education or other interventions that provide social reintegration. The point at which rehabilitation occurs will also play a significant factor in choosing a treatment approach; the more acute, the more likely a traditional treatment that emphasizes the physiologic, speech, and language components of the disorder will be selected; the more chronic, the more likely that compensatory strategies and social approaches to rehabilitation will be chosen.

In the next section, examples of treatment approaches for neurogenic speech, swallowing, and language disorders are reviewed. A listing of each of the major speech and language disorders, specific types of each of the disorders, and a brief definition are given in Table 49-3.

Treatment for Speech Disorders

Dysarthria

Dysarthria, also known as motor speech disorder, is the motor-based impairment that affects the speech musculature. Dysarthria-causing lesions may originate in the cortex or the cerebellum, along the upper motor

TABLE 49-3. Definitions of Major Speech and Language Disorders

Speech or language disorders	Specific types	Brief definition
Dysarthria	Disorders of speech mechanism: flaccid; spastic; ataxic; mixed	Speech disorder due to impairment of the speech musculature
Neurogenic voice disorders	Disorders of the vocal folds: unilateral/bilateral; adduction/abduction; spastic/paralytic	Voice disorder due to a neurologic impairment of control or function of the vocal folds and vocal mechanism
Dysphagia	Disorders of the swallowing mechanism: oral preparatory phase/oral phase/pharyngeal phase; poor bolus control; delayed swallow response	Swallowing disorder due to impairment of the oral and/or pharyngeal mechanism, which can be due to neurologic control of the involved structures
Apraxia of speech	Disorders of motor speech programming; in addition to speech, apraxia can affect use of limbs and production of communicative gestures; specific types of apraxia can include ideomotor, ideational, conduction	Speech disorder due to impairment of motor programming ability pertaining to the speech mechanism
Aphasia	Fluent/nonfluent; receptive/expressive: classic syndromes: Broca's aphasia, Wernicke's aphasia, conduction aphasia, global aphasia, transcortical aphasia, anomic aphasia; related syndromes include alexia, agraphia	Language disorder affecting auditory comprehension, spoken language production, reading, and writing due to brain injury
Cognitive-linguistic impairment	Specific types usually described in terms of the nature of the cognitive impairment (memory disorder, executive dysfunction) and their relationships to language	Language disorder associated with cognitive impairments, all of which are due to brain injury
Language of generalized intellectual impairment	Specific types usually described in terms of the nature of the cognitive impairment (memory disorder, executive dysfunction) and their relationships to language	Language disorder associated with cognitive impairments, usually due to degenerative disease of the brain

neuron (UMN) or lower motor neuron (LMN) or at the myoneural junction. Perceptual analysis of the patient's speech characteristics, in conjunction with knowledge about the underlying medical disorder, will aid the speech-language pathologist in making an appropriate speech diagnosis and determining the type of dysarthria. A traditional framework of dysarthria types includes spastic, ataxic, flaccid, and mixed dysarthrias (Duffy, 1995). Spastic dysarthrias are typically associated with lesions in the UMN, whereas flaccid dysarthrias come from a lesion of the LMN. Cerebellar involvement is indicated by ataxic dysarthria. Various disorders such as amyotrophic lateral sclerosis (ALS), multiple sclerosis, cerebral palsy, and Wilson disease have characteristic mixed dysarthrias.

A common approach to dysarthria will target the underlying physiologic problem through particular oral-motor and speech exercises. Respiration, phonation, and aspects of articulation including tongue and lip movements must be assessed and the nature of the deficit will lead to an appropriate treatment. For example, patients with spastic dysarthria display hypertonicity, weakness, and exaggerated reflexes. Treatment that combines tone reduction exercises with a specific hierarchy of the production of sounds, words, and phrases may be one of the best impairment-based treatments. For the flaccid dysarthrias, exercises that increase strength will be appropriate, along with practice in speech production.

Augmentative and alternative communication approaches are also appropriate for some people with severe dysarthria that cannot be remediated to a point that allows for comprehensibility. Both low- and high-technology solutions may offer individuals with dysarthria the opportunity to function more independently. Low-tech solutions include letter boards, with which the person points to the first letter of the spoken word, to aid listener comprehension. High-tech solutions include various devices that provide speech output with typed or other button-press input. These devices can allow individuals with dysarthric speech to be understandable in many social contexts, including on the telephone.

Dysarthria often occurs along with other speech, language, and cognitive disorders and affects not only the ability of the individuals to make themselves understood, but may also relate to swallowing ability and management of drooling/saliva. Improving speech and saliva management can make these individuals more socially acceptable, thus increasing social relationships and interactions, with an ultimate effect on perceived quality of life. In this regard, the education of caregivers and important others regarding the nature of the disorder, and tips and techniques for facilitating communication, will also go a long way toward improving social integration.

Neurogenic Voice Disorders

Like the dysarthrias, neurogenic voice disorders can be related to lesions of the UMN, LMN, cerebellum, extrapyramidal motor systems, or the myoneural junction. Patients who have had cortical or subcortical strokes, or who suffer from pseudobulbar/supranuclear palsy will display a voice disorder related to the functioning of the UMN, with a spastic harshness/hoarseness quality.

Damage to the peripheral nerves or the brainstem may produce voice disorders associated with the LMN, which are characterized by breathiness, hoarseness, and diplophonia. Voice therapy targets the overadduction of the normal vocal fold and minimizes maladaptive vocal behaviors such as muscular tension or ventricular fold adduction.

Parkinson disease (PD) provides an example for the voice disorders that may result from involvement of the extrapyramidal system. The Lee Silverman Voice Treatment (Ramig et al., 1996) focuses on the patient's relatively intact volitional abilities to modify loudness and pitch. Recent data have also shown that patients with PD treated with this technique show additional improvements in articulation, facial expression, and swallowing.

Lesions of the cerebellum usually result in a dyscoordination between vocalization and other aspects of the speech process, including respiration and articulation. Treatment typically focuses on the timing of phonation and its coordination with respiration.

Myasthenia gravis attacks the myoneural junction and results in vocal fatigue over prolonged usage. Treatment is typically symptomatic and will emphasize compensatory strategies for managing the vocal problems of this disease.

A physiologic voice therapy approach is the most appropriate for addressing the needs of individuals who have voice disorders due to some underlying neurologic disease process (Jacobson et al., 1998). In this approach, techniques and exercises are used to alter the physiology of the vocal mechanism. Respiration, laryngeal musculature, and the coordination of these two processes must be intact for adequate voice production. Vocal function exercises, resonant voice therapy, and the accent method are examples of the holistic exercises derived from the physiologic approach.

Situation-specific training, involving the practice of vocal techniques in specific contexts, may be helpful in facilitating transfer and generalization. Caregiver education, as in all the communication disorders, is an important means to facilitate social relationships.

Dysphagia

Dysphagia, also known as swallowing disorder and disorder of deglutition, can occur as a result of lesions in the peripheral nerves, brainstem, or cortex. Swallowing is an important issue in medical settings because of its relationship to proper nutrition and hydration and the feeding implications that are an important part of any discharge or care plan.

The cranial nerves V, VII, IX, X, XI, and XII are all involved in the movements and responses required for adequate swallowing. They contribute to maintenance and manipulation of the bolus in the oral cavity and the initiation of the swallow response, as well as affecting airway protection during swallowing. Brainstem involvement due to ALS, tumors, trauma, or bulbar palsy may affect hyoid-laryngeal elevation or cricopharyngeal relaxation, resulting in pharyngeal residue and subsequent aspiration. Cortical involvement may have a variety of effects on swallowing. Unilateral hemispheric lesions have the least likely affect on swallowing, whereas bilateral lesions or multiple infarcts, such as in vascular dementia, will have the greatest effect on swallowing. Unilateral left hemispheric strokes are most likely to affect the oral phase of the swallow, whereas right hemispheric lesions are more likely to affect the pharyngeal aspects of the swallow (Musson, 1998).

Treatment of dysphagia is based on a combination of swallowing exercises and maneuvers, compensatory positioning and techniques, and diet management (Logemann, 1999). In those patients for whom the swallowing response is delayed, a program of swallowing stimulation may be effective in enhancing and improving the swallow response. Others who have underlying weakness of various aspects of the swallowing mechanism will benefit from the implementation of specific postures and techniques during eating. For example, positioning the head and neck in specific ways may facilitate airway protection and complete swallows without pooling or residual. Furthermore, appropriate assessments such as the videofluoroscopic assessment of swallowing can demonstrate that the management of the thickness of liquids and the consistency of solid foods can help to ensure eating safety for the individual. The outcomes of these management techniques are critical because they bear on hydration, nutrition, and prevention of aspiration.

Apraxia of Speech

Apraxia of speech (AOS; motor programming impairment, apraxia, impairment of praxis) is the loss of motor programming that enables the individual to produce the articulatory gestures needed for speech. AOS is usually associated with lesions of the frontal and prefrontal regions of the left hemisphere, as well as subcortical structures and connections. Groping for positions for specific sounds, inconsistent articulation errors, and phonetic errors are the hallmarks of AOS.

AOS can be treated with a systematic targeting of speech sounds, while taking into account the placement, voicing, and manner characteristics of the various speech sounds. Many treatment procedures for AOS exist and target either the articulatory-kinematic aspects at the syllable level or focus on the sequencing of multisyllabic productions. For example, a classic AOS treatment is the eight-step continuum, involving modeling, imitation, integral stimulation, and repetition with auditory and visual cues (Rosenbek et al., 1973). Other approaches use minimal contrast pairs, focused on postural shaping, with positive outcomes. Treatment manipulations of rhythm, rate, and stress to facilitate motor speech control can also have important positive outcomes (McNeil et al., 2000).

Augmentative and alternative communication approaches can also be fruitful for those with severe AOS. These patients may not be able to produce any usable speech, and as a result benefit from low- or high-tech devices that can provide a means of communication. Like those individuals with dysarthria, many functional tasks such as using the phone and accomplishing errands in the community can be handled when the individual makes use of a low- or high-tech augmentative device, which aids them in communicating the message.

Apraxia of speech, like other speech disorders, can occur with language or cognitive disorders, depending on the etiology. In many cases, the left hemispheric, frontal lobe, and subcortical lesions that can produce AOS may also produce a concomitant aphasia, or language disorder. The type of aphasia that usually relates to frontal lobe, and the corresponding subcortical regions, is a nonfluent-type aphasia, which produces its own language symptoms affecting auditory comprehension, spoken production, reading, and writing. AOS specifically refers to the motor aspects of speech programming, whereas the frequently co-occurring aphasia that may also result from similar lesions refers to the language symptoms that result. We turn now to a description of these and other language disorders.

Treatment for Language Disorders

Aphasia

Aphasia (language disorder due to focal injury of the dominant hemisphere, dysphasia) is an impairment of all aspects of language including understanding speech, speaking, reading, and writing due to a brain injury. Although most cases of aphasia are caused by focal lesion to language areas of the dominant hemisphere such as stroke or gunshot wound, occasionally aphasia can occur after more diffuse injuries, such as those associated with closed head injury.

Different types and severities of aphasia, interacting with an individual's unique experiences and cognitive profiles, and the nature of the etiology, result in a wide variety of specific language profiles and recovery patterns. Bilingual and multilingual individuals with aphasia present various profiles; occasionally one language is much more preserved than the other, or one language may recover more than another, and these recovery patterns are not necessarily related to whether the language in question was the native language. These factors must be considered by the clinician who is selecting the appropriate treatment.

Auditory comprehension is a concern for persons with all types of aphasia, but it is a particular problem for those with posterior aphasias, such as Wernicke's aphasia. Depending on the severity of the deficit, clinicians may apply procedures that target abilities ranging from single word identification to comprehending sentences and paragraphs. For example, Treatment for Wernicke's Aphasia (TWA) (Helm-Estabrooks & Albert, 1991) focuses on the comprehension needs of these patients. In this treatment, a hierarchy beginning with matching written words to pictures progresses based on established criteria up through spoken word-picture matching.

Reading comprehension can also be a particular impairment for those with posterior aphasias. Deficits can range from alexia with or without agraphia to various types of dyslexia, such as phonological or surface dyslexia, to the deep dyslexia that is usually associated with aphasia. Treatment for these reading disorders must target the specific process underlying the disorder. For example, retraining sound-letter correspondences may aid the person in improving overall reading skills. This can be accomplished in a stimulation approach or by a more didactic training, and for some patients, it can be a long and tedious process. Alternatively, training a visual recognition vocabulary of particularly important functional words may also be useful and can be accomplished with picture cues. Computerized approaches can be particularly helpful for reading disorders and provide useful home practice opportunities (Katz & Wertz, 1997). In addition, computer-based practice may generalize to other specific language improvements, such as oral naming.

Written language skills are also impaired in the aphasias and typically parallel the nature of the spoken language output deficit. As in reading treatments, writing rehabilitation can focus on sound-letter correspondences or on training a particular functional vocabulary of certain words. Patients with aphasia can often be trained to make use of various technological assists for writing, such as spelling and grammar prediction and checkers. Many of these specialized software programs also provide speech output so that patients can rely on other modalities for checking their own work.

Finally, many individuals with severe writing disorders can compensate by using speech recognition software to dictate written documents including e-mail.

Spoken language rehabilitation focuses on two general aspects of language production—naming and grammar. This is different from the kind of treatment provided to those with speech disorders, such as apraxia or dysarthria. In treatment of speech production, the movement of the articulators is targeted, along with motor planning abilities that relate to the production of specific kinds of speech sounds. For example, "b" and "p" are articulated similarly because the lips must come together to produce both sounds (bilabials). This is quite different from the way in which a "z" is articulated. The characteristics of sounds are a focus in treatment of speech disorders, whereas the characteristics of language are an emphasis in aphasia and other language treatment. So, recalling a word is not only reliant on one's ability to produce sounds, but it is also reliant on one's ability to retrieve the semantic information about a word. It is the approaches concerned with semantics, phonology, and grammar that make up the foundation for language intervention approaches.

All patients with aphasia have some level of anomia, or an impairment of word retrieval. Various semantic and phonological cueing systems have been developed to aid those with word retrieval problems. Phonological naming treatment often consists of a hierarchy of rhyming cues, phonemic cues, and repetition. Semantic-based naming treatment focuses on the activation of word meanings and associated concepts to facilitate retrieval of words. For example, semantic feature training incorporates a feature analysis chart including cues for various conceptual aspects of an object, such as function, location, or size/color characteristics (Lowell et al., 1995).

Grammar has been a focus of rehabilitation especially designed for anterior aphasics, especially Broca's aphasia. Mapping treatment and movement therapy are probably two of the most popular current approaches to treating grammar in spoken language production. The underlying principle of mapping therapy is that agrammatic patients have difficulty with the thematic role relationships within sentences (Byng, 1988). Sentences are read or printed and the person points to or underlines the agent, action, and recipient, often with the use of a color-coding system for each of the sentence roles.

Movement therapy is based on the Chomsky Government and Binding Theory. Using cue cards with written words that correspond to a sentence that describes a picture, the patient moves the words from one sentence type to the corresponding wh- question type. This training procedure is meant to embody the underlying theory about linguistic movement of sentence structure. Results of research investigating the effectiveness of this treatment have shown that generalization from one trained type of wh- question to untrained items is consistent with theoretical predictions (Thompson et al., 1997).

Situation-specific training is an approach that begins with the selection of a specific activity that is important and meaningful to the participant. Then, in a role-play and dialogue format, training focuses on the exact communication needs of the identified situation. Hopper and Holland (1998) showed that this approach could be applied successfully to the training of making emergency phone calls among aphasic adults, and Hinckley and coworkers (2001) have also shown that adults with aphasia can be trained to do a catalog-ordering task in a similar way.

Conversational and discourse-based treatments also build in strategy use for accomplishing functional communication. Promoting Aphasics' Communicative Effectiveness (PACE) (Davis & Wilcox, 1985), Response Elaboration Training (RET) (Kearns, 1985), and Hierarchical Discourse Therapy (Penn et al., 1997) are examples of conversationally based approaches in which the clinician works through a hierarchy that is based on the natural and spontaneous conversation of the patient.

Some patients with language impairments will also benefit from various augmentative and alternative communication approaches. Those with aphasia can be trained to use drawing, gesture, or other alternative modalities as primary communication modes in effective ways. Low-tech augmentative aids, such as communication notebooks or boards, provide an organized collection of pictures and words that can be used to aid comprehension, by having the speaker point to key words/pictures in the notebook, and can also provide an opportunity for the expression of information that could not otherwise be communicated. Speech-output devices are also appropriate for individuals with aphasia, and in some cases may be more desirable, because they are more likely to be positively perceived by others in the social environment, and because the speech-output function provides for the accomplishment of certain tasks such as telephone usage (Lasker & Beukelman, 1999).

Facilitating the participation of individuals with aphasia into conversation, community and family life, and civic events is another treatment approach for those with chronic communication disorders. Volunteer training in techniques of supported conversation, conversational coaching (Hopper et al., 2002), and communication partners (Lyon et al., 1997) all share an emphasis on the training of caregivers, volunteers, or important others in communication strategies and facilitation of the patient with aphasia into activities of interest.

Primary progressive aphasia (PPA) is a focal progressive neuropathology of the left perisylvian area. It typically begins with naming problems and a slowness and effortfulness of speech. Some authors have included only nonfluent case presentations as true cases of PPA and have excluded the fluent aphasia that may be more likely associated with ultimate dementia. The progressive loss of language abilities can occur over several years, and speech-language pathologists can be instrumental in aiding patients to develop compensatory strategies that help them and their families to cope with the communication problem. Communication books, electronic systems, and other augmentative communication devices are important tools to provide individuals with progressive speech or language loss.

Cognitive-Linguistic Impairment

Cognitive-linguistic impairment refers to cognitive impairment or cognitive and language impairment due to traumatic brain injury or injury to the nondominant hemisphere. Lesions of the minor hemisphere will produce communicative impairments associated with the cognitive skills subserved by this hemisphere. Attention, memory, and affective processing disorders are common, and relate to a variety of communication impairments, such as lack of relevance, coherence, and listener sensitivity. Verbosity and perseveration are often commonly observed among individuals with right hemisphere lesions. Pragmatic disorders, or the social use of language, are commonly observed in this population. This can include the inability to process metaphor and social inferencing, use and appreciation of humor, and production and comprehension of facial expressions. Furthermore, the prosody or intonation associated with indirect and emotional meanings and associated gestures may be impaired. Reading and writing impairments are also observed and usually associated with underlying visuospatial disorders or neglect (Tompkins, 1995).

Patients with diffuse injuries, which extend to both hemispheres, are likely to show some combination of signs. These injuries may be caused by closed head injury, encephalopathy, or other diffuse traumatic injuries. Attention and memory impairments will relate to a variety of pragmatic and discourse difficulties and impair the processing of verbal information. Executive function (EF) abilities, such as self-monitoring, planning, and sequencing, may be impaired when damage has occurred to the frontal lobes and its extended cortical-subcortical networks, and will affect a wide variety of functional communication activities.

Because these cognitive disorders often affect the ability to perform important communication tasks and abilities, the speech-language pathologist takes an active role in providing rehabilitation for both cognitive and linguistic disorders. Attention-training programs can be effective in improving the overall attention and cognitive abilities of some individuals. In these programs a variety of tasks that require focused, divided, or selective attention are presented in a hierarchy moving from simple and successful to more challenging (Sohlberg & Mateer, 1987). Tasks such as visual or auditory scanning and tracking, selecting a target from an array of distractors, focusing on a specific verbal task are typical for this kind of approach. Typically, the speech-language pathologist would address this kind of deficit as it pertains to the use of verbal information.

Similarly, working memory is often impaired in patients with more diffuse brain injuries, and a variety of approaches have been used in an attempt to improve general memory function, particularly for verbal information. Environmental adaptation, new learning, and implementation of new technology are all common forms of rehabilitation (Wilson, 1999). One effective training technique is Spaced Retrieval, which has been used to train a variety of types of information to patients with memory disorders due to stroke or dementia (Brush & Camp, 1998). In this technique, a specific piece of critical information, such as room number, birth date, or even a strategy such as checking a memory notebook, is trained by asking the patients to retrieve the information at progressively longer intervals. Fading cues is another effective technique for training specific procedural information to patients with memory impairments. Here, the patient is provided with the support needed to complete the task, and gradually these assists are faded until the behavior is embedded in the desired context (Wilson, 1999). Prospective memory training, an organized approach to handling some memory impairments, has also been shown to be effective (Raskin & Sohlberg, 1996)

EFs such as self-monitoring, evaluating future consequences, planning, and sequencing are also often impaired in these patients. These deficits are manifested both in activities of daily life (ADL) and in communication. For example, those with cognitive-linguistic impairment often display difficulties sequencing verbal information, accomplishing verbal problem solving, social appropriateness in conversation, initiating and maintaining conversational topics, and providing cohesion in discourse. Providing informative feedback about social skills including discourse and specifically targeting these various social communication skills are important goals in rehabilitation. Indeed, attention process training, focusing on prospective skills, and brain injury education, focusing on EF abilities, have important positive outcomes among patients with TBI (Sohlberg et al., 2000).

An approach that is more highly contextualized is Positive Everyday Routines (Ylvisaker & Feeney, 1998). In this approach, the patient is trained to use specific strategies during the course of normal activities. For example, persons with executive function impairment may be trained to use a plan-do-check strategy with the support of the clinician and external visual aids.

Individuals with attention or sequencing disorders that affect their narrative and procedural discourse abilities may benefit from strategies that address the appropriate, sequenced parts of such discourse styles. A pictograph-based visual chart showing the beginning, middle, end, and key information about a story can aid such a patient in producing more cohesive and appropriate discourse. Conversationally based treatment also provides the opportunity to target other pragmatic behaviors, such as appropriate turn-taking, relevancy, cohesiveness, and topic management behaviors. A variety of compensatory techniques may be fruitful in the redevelopment of these skills among patients with cognitive impairments. Colored markers can be passed from one person to the next to work on turn-taking, informative feedback may improve relevancy, and visual and written cues and charts can be helpful in facilitating topic management.

Language of Generalized Intellectual Impairment

Generalized intellectual impairment refers to cognitive and language impairments due to dementia. Individuals with dementia have communication difficulties that include word-finding problems, vocabulary reduction, pragmatic impairments, and disordered written and oral discourse. For these individuals, who will have progressive loss of communication and cognitive abilities, management focuses on the environment and caregivers, and these types of interventions are generally effective (Bourgeois, 1991). In this population, we do not expect nor do we generally look for intervention outcomes at the impairment level. However, speech-language pathologists can help to maintain functional abilities and social participation of adults with progressive loss of language and cognition through a variety of different interventions (Ripich & Ziol, 1998).

Environmental manipulations such as rearranging furniture; adding plants, pictures, and personal items; providing conversational partners; and offering recreational activities increase opportunities for communication. Posting orientation information and personally relevant information, such as name, date, and season, can provide natural opportunities for the individual to check basic orientation information.

External memory aids, such as memory wallets containing personally relevant verbal information and pictures, can aid in appropriate conversation. Similarly, memory notebooks or wallets, when placed strategically in a patient's room, will often be looked at, further reinforcing and maintaining relevant information.

Speech-Language Pathologists and Family Education and Counseling

Family education and counseling are important aspects of any intervention program and can be critical in changing the perceptions and views of important others in the lives of those with communication disorders. Dynamics in family relationships change, and appropriate education about the nature of the communication disorder can significantly improve perceptions of relationships, including marital satisfaction (for an example pertaining to aphasia, see Williams, 1993). Ongoing family education for years is also important because of changing needs over time.

It is within the scope of practice for speech-language pathologists to provide education and counseling regarding communication disorders. When a neurogenic speech or language disorder has been diagnosed, it usually has a significant impact on basic communication between family members and friends. Not only is the communication of basic needs affected, but also the communication that was the means for relationship bonding has been changed for the worse. This then will have implications for family wellness and functioning.

First, families and other support persons need to understand the nature of the particular disorder. Communication impairments are often mistaken by laypersons for either a lack of motivation to communicate, a lack of a desire to communicate, or some other emotional response by the patient. Furthermore, certain speech or language disorders, when they occur without concomitant cognitive disorders, are sometimes interpreted as a loss of general intellect, and this perception, when untrue, is particularly detrimental both to the patients and their families and friends. So, information about the nature of the disorder is a critical first step.

Second, family members must be educated about how best to cope with the communication disorder. Caregivers need to be trained to be good communication partners; it is not sufficient to provide a list of communication suggestions without practice, feedback, and mastery opportunities. This will provide the means for continued family communication during a time when other health and social matters are also demanding the family's attention and resources.

Social support is a significant, positive factor in prognosis, so family members who are given the means and information that will help them to participate in the rehabilitation process, and to communicate effectively with the patient, will have an important role in recovery. Family members should participate in the rehabilitation process as much as is feasible.

In regard to specific practice activities, occasionally family members can provide encouragement to a patient to engage in home practice. However, this additional role of the family member must be carefully broached by the speech-language pathologist. Spouses, children, sibling, and important others have already established roles with the patient and these roles may not include the additional role of "teacher" or "therapist." Indeed, in some cases, spouses who take on the role of "trainer" or "therapist" at home may be creating a dynamic that is difficult to escape. There are exceptions, and some individuals and their partners will be comfortable with this kind of role. But this needs to be addressed with sensitivity, keeping in mind that spouses of adults with communication disorders perceive a high degree of burden. Indeed, the rate of divorce among adults with aphasia and their spouses is significantly higher than the rate of divorce among other adults who have had stroke without aphasia.

Developing the communication and coping strategies of caregivers is critical to maintaining the social participation of the patient, as well as facilitating the health and well-being of the caregiver. When family members and friends understand how best to communicate with the patient with a communication disorder, they will be able to facilitate that person's return to household and community activities. This is perhaps the most important role of family and friends, which will extend throughout the length of the individual's impairment—for some patients, this will be the rest of their life. Finally, community resources such as respite care and support groups help to ease the caregiver's burden, and speech-language pathologists should provide caregivers with information about these resources.

SUMMARY

Speech-language rehabilitation is effective for many neurogenic communication disorders, and a firm basis of evidence for clinical practice is available for the practicing clinician. Treatments for neurogenic speech, language, and cognitive disorders yield impairment-, activity-, and participation-level outcomes. Direct training of specific speech, language, or cognitive skills; the development of compensatory strategies; a focus on functional tasks; and the redevelopment of life participation with an emphasis on caregiver, volunteer, and family education and training are approaches that can be combined by the competent speech-language pathologist for the desired outcome.

■ KEY POINTS

☐   The scope of practice for speech-language pathologists includes the identification, assessment, and rehabilitation of neurogenic communication disorders such as motor speech impairments, language impairments, swallowing disorders, and cognitive-linguistic impairments. Speech-language pathologists are also charged with family education and counseling for those with communication impairments.

☐ Speech-language rehabilitation is based on principles of learning and behavior change, within the constraints of the neurologic disease, injury, and recovery processes.

☐ The WHO model of classification provides a framework that describes all of the areas in which treatment approaches, processes, and outcomes are addressed in speech and language rehabilitation.

☐ Specific treatment approaches have various targeted outcomes and different patterns of generalization and transfer. Because the success of various treatment procedures depends on the interaction of the treatment with a variety of individual factors and characteristics, treatment plan, durations, and frequencies are highly individualized.

☐ The role of the family and support system is important to outcomes in speech and language rehabilitation. Because psychological and social adjustment to disability is often accomplished through communication, the treatment of communication is critical to the ultimate health and social success of the individual.

Acknowledgments

This project was supported in part by a grant from the James S. McDonnell Foundation, JSMF 97-44, Pilot Studies in Cognitive Rehabilitation Research, and by a Research and Creative Scholarship Grant from the University of South Florida.

KEY READINGS

Coelho, CM, DeRuyter F, Stein M: Treatment efficacy: Cognitive-communicative disorders resulting from traumatic brain injury in adults. J Speech Lang Hear Res 39:S5–S17, 1996.

Duffy JR: Motor Speech Disorders: Substrates, Differential Diagnosis, and Management. St. Louis: Mosby Year Book, 1995.

Robey RR: A meta-analysis of clinical outcomes in the treatment of aphasia. J Speech Lang Hear Res 41:172–187, 1998.

REFERENCES

Bourgeois M: Communication treatment for adults with dementia. J Speech Lang Hear Res 34:831–844, 1991.

Brush JA, Camp CJ: Using spaced retrieval as an intervention during speech-language therapy. Clin Gerontol 19:51–64, 1998.

Byng S: Sentence processing deficits: Theory and therapy. Cogn Neuropsychol 5:629–676, 1988.

Coelho, CM, DeRuyter F, Stein M: Treatment efficacy: Cognitive-communicative disorders resulting from traumatic brain injury in adults. J Speech Lang Hear Res 39:S5–S17, 1996.

Davis GA, Wilcox MJ: Adult Aphasia Rehabilitation: Applied Pragmatics. San Diego, CA: Singular Press, 1985.

Diener E, Emmons RA, Larsen RJ, et al: The Satisfaction with Life Scale. J Pers Assess 49:71–75, 1985.

Duffy JR: Motor Speech Disorders: Substrates, Differential Diagnosis, and Management. St. Louis, MO: Mosby Year Book, 1995.

Duffy JR: Schuell's stimulation approach to rehabilitation, in Chapey R (ed): Language Intervention Strategies for Adult Aphasia. Baltimore: Williams & Wilkins, 1994, pp. 146–174.

Elman R: Group Treatment of Neurogenic Communication Disorders: The Expert Clinician's Approach. Boston, MA: Butterworth-Heineman, 1999.

Frattali C, Thompson C, Holland A, et al: American Speech-Language-Hearing Association Functional Assessment of Communication Skills for Adults. Rockville, MD: ASHA, 1995.

Helm-Estabrooks N, Albert ML: Manual of Aphasia Therapy. Austin, TX: Pro-Ed, 1991.

Hinckley JJ, Patterson JP, Carr TH: Differential outcomes of skill-based and context-based treatment in aphasia: Preliminary findings. Aphasiology 15:463–476, 2001.

Holland AL, Beeson PM: Finding a new sense of self: What the clinician can do to help. Aphasiology 7:581–584, 1993.

Holland AL, Frattali CM, Fromm D: Communicative Abilities in Daily Living-Revised. Austin, TX: Pro-Ed, 1999.

Holland AL, Fromm DS, De Ruyter F, et al: Treatment efficacy: Aphasia. J Speech Lang Hear Res 39:S27–S36, 1996.

Hopper T, Holland AL: Situation-specific training for adults with aphasia: An example. Aphasiology 12:933–944, 1998.

Hopper T, Holland A, Rewega M: Conversational coaching: Treatment of outcomes and future directions. Aphasiology 16:745–761, 2002.

ICF: International Classification of Functioning, Disability, and Health. Geneva, Switzerland: World Health Organization, 2001.

Jacobson BH, Johnson A, Grywalski C, et al: The voice handicap index (VHI): Development and validation. Am J Speech Lang Pathol 6:66–70, 1997.

Jacobson BH, Stemple JC, Glaze LE, et al: Assessment and management of voice disorders in adults, in Johnson AF, Jacobson BH (eds): Medical Speech-Language Pathology: A Practitioner's Guide. New York: Thieme, 1998, pp. 529–562.

Katz RC, Wertz RT: The efficacy of computer-provided reading treatment for chronic aphasic adults. J Lang Speech Hear Res 40:493–507, 1997.

Kearns K: Response elaboration training for patient initiated utterances, in Brookshire RH (ed): Clinical Aphasiology. Minneapolis, MN: BRK, 1985, Vol. 15, pp. 196–204, 1985.

Lasker J, Beukelman D: Peers' perceptions of storytelling by an adult with aphasia. Aphasiology 13:219–224, 1999.

List MA, Ritter-Sterr C, Lansky SB: A performance status scale for head and neck cancer patients. Cancer 66:564–569, 1990.

Logemann JA: Behavioral management for oropharyngeal dysphagia. Folia Phoniatr Logop 51:199–212, 1999.

Lomas J, Pickard L, Bester S, et al: The Communicative Effectiveness Index: Development and psychometric evaluation of a functional communication measure for adults. J Speech Hearing Disord 54:113–124, 1989.

Lowell S, Beeson PM, Holland AL: The efficacy of a semantic cueing procedure on naming performance of adults with aphasia. Am J Speech Lang Pathol 4:109–114, 1995.

Lyon JG, Cariski D, Keisler L, Rosenbek J, et al: Communication partners: Enhancing participation in life and communication for adults with aphasia in natural settings. Aphasiology 11:693–708, 1997.

McNeil MR, Doyle PJ, Wambaugh J: Apraxia of speech: A treatable disorder of motor planning and programming, in Nadeau SE, Gonzalez Rothi LJ, Crosson B (eds): Aphasia and Language: Theory to Practice. New York: Guilford Press, 2000, pp. 221–266.

Musson N: An introduction to neurogenic swallowing disorders, in Johnson AF, Jacobson BH (eds): Medical Speech-Language Pathology: A Practitioner's Guide. New York: Thieme, 1998, pp. 354–389.

Pearson VAH: Speech and language therapy: Is it effective? Public Health 109:143–153, 1995.

Penn C, Jones D, Joffe V: Hierarchical discourse therapy: A method for the mild patient. Aphasiology 11:601–613, 1997.

Ramig LO, Countryman S, O'Brien C, et al: Intensive speech treatment for patients with Parkinson disease: Short and long-term comparison of two techniques. Neurology 47:1496–1504, 1996.

Raskin SA, Sohlberg MM: The efficacy of prospective memory training in two adults with brain injury. J Head Trauma Rehabil 11:32–51, 1996.

Ripich DN, Ziol E: Dementia: A review for the speech-language pathologist, in Johnson AF, Jacobson BH (eds): Medical Speech-Language Pathology: A Practitioner's Guide. New York: Thieme, 1998, pp. 467–494.

Robey RR: The efficacy of treatment for aphasic persons: A meta-analysis. Brain Lang 47:585–608, 1994.

Robey RR: A meta-analysis of clinical outcomes in the treatment of aphasia. J Speech Lang Hear Res 41:172–187, 1998.

Rosenbek JC, Lemme ML, Ahern, MB, et al: A treatment for apraxia of speech in adults. J Speech Hear Disord 38:462–472, 1973.

Ryff C: Scales of psychological well-being (short form). J Pers Social Psychol 57:1069–1081, 1989.

Schuell H, Jenkins JJ, Jimenez-Pabon E: Aphasia in Adults. New York: Harper & Row, 1964.

Shewan CM: The history and efficacy of aphasia treatment, in Chapey R (ed): Language Intervention Strategies for Adult Aphasia. Baltimore, MD: Williams & Wilkins, 1986, pp. 28–43.

Sohlberg MM, Mateer CA: Effectiveness of an attention training program. J Clin Exp Neuropsychol 9:117–130, 1987.

Sohlberg MM, McLaughlin KA, Pavese A, et al: Evaluation of attention process training and brain injury education in persons with acquired brain injury. J Clin Exp Neuropsychol 22:656–676, 2000.

Thompson CK, Shapiro LP, Ballard KJ, et al: Training and generalized production of wh- and NP-movement structures in agrammatic aphasia. J Speech Lang Hear Res 40:228–244, 1997.

Tompkins CA: Right Hemisphere Communication Disorders: Theory and Management. San Diego, CA: Singular, 1995.

Whurr R, Lorch MP, Nye C: A meta-analysis of studies carried out between 1946 and 1988 concerned with the efficacy of speech and language therapy treatment for aphasic patients. Eur J Disord Commun 27:1–17, 1992.

Willer B, Rosenthal M., Kreutzer JS, et al: Assessment of community integration following rehabilitation for traumatic brain injury. J Head Trauma Rehabil 8:75–87, 1993.

Williams SE: The impact of aphasia on marital satisfaction. Arch Phys Med Rehabil 74:361–367, 1993.

Wilson BA: Memory rehabilitation in brain-injured people, in Stuss DT, Winocur G (eds): Cognitive Neurorehabilitation. New York: Cambridge University Press, 1999, pp. 333–346.

Ylvisaker M, Feeney TJ: Collaborative Brain Injury Intervention: Positive Everyday Routines. Boston: Butterworth-Heineman, 1998.

Yorkston KM: Treatment efficacy in dysarthria. J Speech Lang Hear Res 39:S46–S57, 1996.

Appendix

TRAINING AND SCOPE OF PRACTICE FOR SPEECH-LANGUAGE PATHOLOGISTS

Training and Credentials

A competent speech-language pathologist holds a minimum of a Master's degree in speech-language pathology, and will also hold the Certificate of Clinical Competence in Speech-Language Pathology (CCC-SLP) from the American Speech-Language-Hearing Association (ASHA). The Certificate of Clinical Competence is earned by satisfactorily completing a 9-month post-Master's fellowship with clinical supervision and by passing a national examination. Board Certification in Neurogenic Communication Disorders (BC-NCD) is also available to experienced clinicians who pass an examination and an in-depth case presentation to a review panel. Board Certification is available through the Academy of Neurologic Communication Disorders and Sciences. Some speech-language pathologists hold a doctorate, and these individuals are especially trained in research principles and practice, in addition to having an even deeper knowledge base about communication disorders. Speech-Language Pathology Assistants usually hold an associate's (2-year) or bachelor's (4-year) degree with no other certification. Speech-Language Pathology Assistants aid the certified speech-language pathologist in completing routine tasks such as filing, oral-motor exercises, or other repetitive tasks. Supervision of Speech-Language Pathology Assistants must adhere to national guidelines (ASHA). Assistants cannot provide diagnosis or develop treatment plans. State licensure for speech-language pathologists and assistants is required in most states, and most states require documentation of continuing education for license renewal.

Scope of Practice

Speech-language pathologists are prepared to provide assessment and treatment for speech, language, cognitive, and swallowing disorders, including selection and training of augmentative communication devices and general education and specific counseling related to communication disorders. The ASHA describes the scope of practice for speech-language pathologists as follows.

The practice of speech-language pathology includes: prevention, diagnosis, habilitation, and rehabilitation of communication, swallowing, or other upper aerodigestive disorders; elective modification of communication behaviors; and enhancement of communication. This practice includes the services that address the dimensions of body structure and function, activity, and/or participation as proposed by the World Health Organization model. (I-22c/2001)

Impairment and Disability Evaluation

Nathan D. Zasler

Michael F. Martelli

Disability

Employability

**Guidelines to Evaluation of
Permanent Impairment (GEPI)**

Impairment

Pain

Response bias

Symptom validity tests

INTRODUCTION

Evaluation of impairment and disability is probably one
of the more confounding and misunderstood areas of
health care–related work as it applies to caring for
persons with injury residua or functional limitations
due to disease. Traditionally, impairment and disability
evaluation has not been taught as part of the medical
school curriculum, nor is it typically included in any
neuroscience-related residency program.

The task of making determinations regarding
impairment and disability in persons with brain-related
disorders (BRDs) is fraught with potential obstacles and
confounding issues. This is due to the sometimes subtle,
yet complex, nature of the deficits involved, as well as
the lack of formal "rating systems" for many of the
observed deficits.

Additionally, multiple medical specialties are
often called on to perform impairment and disability

evaluation and debate continues regarding ethical, legal, and clinical boundaries between these different medical disciplines, whether neurology, neuropsychiatry, neurosurgery, psychiatry, or other specialty areas. These same debates apply as well to clinical management of persons with BRDs.

Clearly, there exists a need for appreciating the interface of biologic, social, and psychological factors that have an impact on impairment presentation as well as disability adaptation. Holistic assessment tends to provide the best means of accomplishing meaningful impairment and disability evaluations. Within that context, functionally based assessments with emphasis on ecologically valid instruments have been shown to yield the most salient results.

NOMENCLATURE ISSUES

Within the field of neurorehabilitation and disability, a historical problem relating to a lack of a common language existed prior to the publication of a system for classifying consequences of disease (World Health Organization [WHO], 1980). WHO developed this taxonomy, known as the International Classification of Impairments, Disabilities, and Handicaps (ICIDH), to assist with structuring of a comprehensive model of illness. Probably the most important concept introduced by the model proposed by WHO was that any illness can be represented at four levels, namely, pathology, impairment, disability, and handicap. The term *illness* is generally used to refer to all the consequences of any disease as well as its social implications. The term *disease* is more restrictive and refers to a specific diagnosis or pathology. Appropriate distinctions must be made between the aforementioned WHO classification categories for clinical, research, and disability administrative purposes.

An understanding of this terminology is important in the sense that health care interventions including rehabilitation may have an impact on one level and not another. For example, a person with short-term memory deficits following a mild traumatic brain injury (TBI) may demonstrate functional memory and executive skill problems in the real world, yet may show no impairments on neuropsychological tests. This aforementioned problem addresses the issue of what has been termed the ecological validity of neuropsychological testing (Sbordone, 1996). It is also critical to not "bundle" terms as often happens in the real world; that is, a physician performs a "whole person impairment rating" using the American Medical Association Guidelines for Evaluation of Permanent Impairment (GEPI) (Cocchiarella & Andersson, 2001) and states in his report that he has done a disability evaluation. In the context of disability evaluation, it is crucial to differentiate between an examinee and a patient for both ethical and medicolegal purposes.

Pathology refers to the perturbation in function occurring within an organ or organ system in the body. Pathology has traditionally been the focus of medical care in our society both from a clinical as well as an administrative perspective. The International Classification of Diseases (ICD), for example, focuses primarily on pathologies, not impairments, disabilities, or handicap.

Impairments are the direct and indirect neuroanatomic and neurophysiologic consequences of the underlying pathology. The types of impairments germane to assessing persons with postconcussive disorders include diplopia, hearing loss, olfactory dysfunction, balance dysfunction, and cognitive deficits, among others. Psychological aberrations would also be classified as impairments according to the ICIDH definition. Importantly, certain pathologic entities including trauma, multiple sclerosis, and stroke may produce no measurable impairment. In contrast, some entities, such as conversion disorders, factitious disorders, and other "nonorganic" conditions (Ruff et al., 1993), produce functional difficulties despite the absence of an obvious anatomic lesion. Lastly, impairment evaluation does not take into account a person's vocational, avocational, sociocultural, or educational background.

Disability can be thought of as the functional loss the individual suffers and how that loss interacts with the environment due to the result of the impairment. This disability can be viewed as a behavioral manifestation of the disease under a specific set of circumstances. In the case of an individual with a brain-based disorder, this may be reflected in a decreased ability to work, drive, or pursue hobbies. Psychological issues and the local milieu may significantly affect the manner in which a disability is manifested relative to severity and nature. Examiners should also realize that there is not generally a "one-to-one" correlation between impairment and disability. That is, an individual can be mildly impaired but severely functionally disabled just as another examinee may be significantly impaired by examination but have little consequential functional disability.

Handicap is the expression of the impact of a given pathology, impairment, or disability on an individual's specific social roles and activities. In this situation, normality is defined relative to the individual's own social context. Variables that may dictate what is "normal" for an examinee include age, gender, and social and cultural factors. Importantly, there may arise situations in which the degree of handicap correlates poorly with the degree of functional disability. Handicap is shaped by environmental factors such as social expectations, legal stipulations, family network, financial solvency, and community physical barriers. The term *social disadvantage* is a valuable near synonym for handicap (National Institutes of Health [NIH], 1993).

WHO recently finalized an update of its seminal 1980 document, entitled "International Classification of Functioning, Disability and Health," also referred to as ICIDH-2, which was endorsed at the 54th World Health Assembly in May 2001 (WHO, 2001). The overall aim of this document is to provide a unified and standard language and framework for the description of health and health-related states. The major domains are described from body, individual, and societal perspectives based on "body functions and structures" and "activities and participation." ICIDH-2 is touted as a "components of health" classification as opposed to the older version, which was seen as a "consequence of disease" classification.

ICIDH-2 encompasses all aspects of human health and some health-relevant components of well-being, describing them as health domains and health-related domains. It is a universal system that does not only apply to persons with disabilities. ICIDH-2 organizes information into two parts: (1) functioning and disability and (2) contextual factors. The components of "functioning and disability" include the "body" and "activities and participation." The "body" component is comprised of two classifications: body systems and body structures. The "activities and participation" component covers the complete range of domains denoting aspects of functioning from both individual and societal perspectives. Contextual factors include "environmental factors" and "personal factors."

The new nomenclature is much more cumbersome than the older, more simplified WHO language, the latter having become entrenched in the impairment and disability literature. Time will tell if the "weighty" methodology proposed in ICIDH-2 will be espoused by practitioners in the field of impairment and disability assessment. For most practitioners, we suspect that the system will be considered overly cumbersome and time consuming.

PRACTICAL CONSEQUENCES OF THE ICIDH MODEL

The focus of clinical intervention should evolve over time from concentration on making a pathologic diagnosis to assessment and treatment of the resultant disability, to reducing handicap. In practical terms, this requires the clinician to spend adequate time inquiring as to the functional difficulties. Consequently, the examiner must also include assessment of functional abilities during the physical examination as opposed to purely "clinical signs." Our evolving health care system, driven by health care reform, has not given adequate consideration to the aforementioned aspects of clinical care with models such as diagnosis-related groups (DRGs). This has led to little or no consideration of such factors when considering trends in hospital usage. Additionally, our general model of health care has historically been curative, not amelio-

rative. That is, we tend to focus, as a health care system, on management of acute illness, which is viewed to be self-limiting and to occur within a social vacuum, without much heed being given to potential resultant functional disability or handicap. Lastly, multidisciplinary medical management allows for the most effective methodologies to be instituted relative to treating the breadth of neurologic disease from pathology to handicap (Ragnarsson et al., 1993).

Impairments must be measured to understand and prescribe appropriate treatment. Impairment measures allow the examiner to determine whether the outcome is due to neurologic recovery processes, environmental alterations, or compensatory adaptations. Measures of clinical disability or functional limitations can tell us whether function is improving in a manner that will be meaningful for the person. Real-world disability measures give information regarding whether the individual in fact used the skill. Handicap measures tell us if the interventions as a whole correlate with outcomes valued by most of society (Johnston et al., 1993).

MEASUREMENT ISSUES IN NEUROLOGIC ASSESSMENT: AN OVERVIEW

It is critical for clinicians and in particular those who formally evaluate impairment and disability to be familiar with currently available measurement techniques applicable to neurologic conditions due to brain disorders. Quantification of an observation in an objective fashion is essential if such evaluations are to serve as the basis for administrative decisions regarding disability determination. Practitioners should become familiar with standardized measures for cognitive, behavioral, and physical impairment. Reasons for using objective measurement tools include establishment of diagnosis, prognosis, severity, and outcome. Clinicians should also be aware of whether or not the measure can be generalized from one population to another; specifically, a measure of affective status used in stroke populations may not be transferable to a person with depression following concussion. Additionally, it is critical to remain aware of both the false-negative and false-positive rates with any particular measure for the population in question. One must also be familiar with the variety of levels of measurement including nominal, ordinal, interval, and ratio (Wade, 1992).

There are significant differences between these levels of measurement that have an impact on the utility of the data generated and how they are interpreted. Lastly, measure construction can be of three types. The simplest involves simple description. Multi-item indices such as the Barthel Activities of Daily Living Index are one such example (Wade, 1992). True ratio measurements probably give the most absolute data such as measuring the speed of gait, stride length, and so forth.

There is significant consensus in medical rehabilitation that functional assessment needs to be improved and standardized. Some clinicians have espoused specific criteria to guide selection of rehabilitation-related standards (Johnston et al., 1992). Issues regarding validity, both predictive and construct, and reliability must be analyzed carefully. Ceiling and floor limitations of existing functional measures must be kept in mind. Most of the functional assessment measures used in the field of medical rehabilitation require clinician training prior to clinical use.

The aforementioned approach is juxtaposed in contradistinction to the more traditional method used by physicians in the evaluation of impairment such as the *Guidelines to the Evaluation of Permanent Impairment* (GEPI) published by the American Medical Association (Cocchiarella & Andersson, 2001). It is this author's opinion that the "Guides" has significant limitations when used in the evaluation of brain-based impairments, particularly in cases of mild neural insult such as with postconcussive disorders. There are no scientific studies establishing predictive validity of the guidelines for its common applications nor are there any scientific data demonstrating a link between level of impairment and potential for the affected person to return to work, school, or other activities including independent living. There are no published data in the guidelines, or elsewhere for that matter, which demonstrate reliability of the recommended impairment ratings.

We know that human work performance is a multifaceted interaction of strengths as well as weaknesses that are determined by many other factors aside from impairments per se. These factors include community barriers, job demands, and willingness of the employer to work together with the person to facilitate job re-entry. Clinicians *and* administrators are generally not in a position to judge adequately the summation of these factors relative to traditional methodologies used to determine impairment and disability as germane to decisions regarding work re-entry potential. If we are to provide responsible opinions on disability status, we are obliged to evaluate not only impairment but also the resultant disability and handicap. Evaluation of disability and handicap is a time-consuming process. Lengthy inquiries regarding the functional implications, if any, of the examinee's impairments are paramount to this process. Additionally, a thorough understanding of the examinee's work and community environment is essential. Community-based issues that need to be clarified include availability of transportation, mobility barriers, accessibility issues, and need for workplace modifications, whether cognitive, behavioral, or physical (Wehman & Kreutzer, 1990).

RESPONSE BIAS ISSUES IN IMPAIRMENT AND DISABILITY EVALUATION

The effects of response bias as a critical element in the conduct of impairment and disability evaluations, particularly in the medicolegal context, cannot be ignored. *Response bias*, as used here, refers to a class of behaviors that reflect less than fully truthful, accurate, or valid symptom report and presentation, whether conscious or unconscious. Given the frequent, highly desirable incentives to distort performance, patient or examinee motivation to provide a truthful report and full effort is an extremely important prerequisite to valid assessment. Valid assessment is required for provision of (1) accurate diagnosis, (2) appropriate and timely treatment to promote optimal recovery, (3) prevention of iatrogenic impairment and disability reinforcement and promulgation of unnecessary health care costs, and (4) appropriate legal compensation decisions based on causality and level of damages suffered (Blau, 1992). In the context of impairment and disability evaluations, or insurance-related evaluations, reports demonstrating high prevalence rates of response bias in examinees are proliferating (Rohling & Binder, 1995; Youngjohn et al., 1995; Binder & Rohling, 1996; Larabee, 2000; Rohling, 2000; Green et al., 2001).

Although most studies focus on exaggeration of impairments, incentives also exist for minimizing deficits (i.e., simulation behavior). Another often neglected area of response bias is examiner response bias (Johnson et al., 2000). After a review of response bias issues, recommendations for enhancing objectivity in medicolegal evaluations are offered.

Attribution and Bias

A brief review of important sources of bias seen during evaluation of physical, neurocognitive, or psychological impairments follows (Ruff et al., 1993; Martelli et al., 1999). Examinee attribution biases that may confound accurate diagnosis include mistaking clinical conditions like depression and sleep disorders and associated sequelae for neurologic injury and sequelae. This can occur due to misattribution, overattribution, illusory correlation, or heightened vigilance to benign problems (Lees-Haley, 1997).

Avoidance of parallel examiner misattribution requires careful differential diagnosis of sequelae secondary to brain dysfunction from other neurologic impairments, cranial/cranial adnexal and cervical trauma impairments, chronic pain symptoms, psychological sequelae, and motivational factors, among others. When "abnormal" neurocognitive findings and nonspecific somatic complaints are obtained, "overdiagnosis" of neurologic disorders such as mild TBI can be avoided only through careful differential diagnosis. For example, brain injury specialists sensitized to neurologic symptoms might interpret chronic pain sequelae as postconcussive symptoms. Of note, such examiner attribution bias may be of concern in any health care specialty, reflecting the fact that we see what we look for, or, in other words, we see what we have been trained to see.

Examinee Response Bias

Although the incidence of response bias in various medical or psychological problems can only be estimated, it is increasingly evident that compensation is an important issue affecting presentation (Binder & Rohling, 1996). Numerous reports demonstrate high prevalence rates of response bias with significant impact on symptom report and test performance in medicolegal evaluations (Rohling & Binder, 1995; Youngjohn et al., 1995; Binder & Rohling, 1996; Larabee, 2000; Rohling, 2000; Green et al., 2001). For example, Green and colleagues report on cross-validated findings of poor effort measured by response bias testing in more than 40% in some examinee groups (i.e., worker's compensation evaluations). Further, poor effort was found to have a stronger effect on neuropsychological test scores than did severity of brain injury or neurologic disease (Rohling, 2000; Green et al., 2001). These findings imply that failure to control for effort level may lead to false conclusions, not only for individual clinical diagnoses, but also for group data from which we derive clinical diagnostic and prognostic information.

Although response bias is most commonly conceptualized as deliberate exaggeration of difficulty (e.g., symptom magnification, malingering), a continuum exists that extends from denial or unawareness of impairments through symptom minimization, normal or average symptom presentation, sensitization to subtle or benign symptoms or problems, exaggeration or symptom magnification, and finally, malingering. This one-dimensional conceptualization likely represents an oversimplification that obscures the subtleties of a wide range of response biases that may be demonstrated, but nonetheless serves as a useful framework.

Malingering reflects deliberate symptom production for purposes of secondary gain. In the medicolegal evaluation, it is often reflected by responses biased in the direction of false symptom reports or managed effort to produce poor performance on tests. Administration measures of this type of response bias should always be considered in cases of medicolegal presentation and where there is suspicion of any disincentive to exert full effort, or suspicion of sociopathic personality disorder (American Psychiatric Association [APA], 1994).

Response bias represents an especially important threat to validity of disability assessments, particularly when in a medicolegal or worker's compensation context. Because assessments include and usually begin with an interview about self-reported symptoms and rely heavily on measures of performance on standardized tests, the validity of the results requires the veracity, cooperation, and motivation of the patient. However, patients seen for presumptive brain-related impairments may over-report pre-injury functional status in regard to certain symptoms that often appear with similar frequency in the general population (Lees-Haley, 1997; Lees-Haley et al., 1997). Further, the ability of neuropsychologists to accurately detect malingering in routine test protocols has been less than impressive (e.g., see Martelli et al., 2001a).

Table 50-1 lists hallmark signs of response bias and provides an overview of the various instruments, techniques, and strategies that have shown at least some utility in detecting response bias to estimate validity and increase confidence in assessment findings.

Table 50-2 includes a compendium of suggested response bias detection tests and strategies with estimates and signs of suspicious performance and qualitative variables with potential utility for detecting response bias.

Table 50-3 includes qualitative variables with potential utility for detecting response bias.

In a review of the literature, Martelli and colleagues (1999) found the following vulnerability factors associated with increased likelihood of maladaptive postinjury adjustment and response bias: anger, resentment, or perceived mistreatment; fear of failure or rejection (e.g., being fired after injury); loss of self-efficacy; external locus of control; irrational fear of injury extension, reinjury, or pain; limits in usual coping style (e.g., highly physically active person who has a back injury); insufficient residual coping resources and skills; prolonged inactivity resulting in disuse atrophy; fear of losing disability status, benefits, or safety net; high compensability for injury; pre-injury job dissatisfaction; sociopathic or manipulative personality traits; collateral injuries (especially if "silent"); retention of an attorney; reinforcement for "illness" versus "wellness" behavior; inadequate or inaccurate medical information; misdiagnosis, late diagnosis, or delays in instituting treatment; and insurance resistance or delays in authorizing treatment or paying bills.

With regard to external factors affecting outcome following injury, several important studies demonstrate a negative impact associated with an adversarial medicolegal system (Binder et al., 1991; Evans, 1994; Mendelson, 1995; Cassidy et al., 2000).

It should be emphasized that "failure" on one measure of response bias or malingering does not mean

Text continues on page 1050.

TABLE 50–1. Hallmark Signs of Response Bias

I. Inconsistencies within and between the following:

   1. Reported symptoms

   2. Examination/test performance

   3. Clinical presentation

   4. Known diagnostic patterns

   5. Observed behavior (in another setting)

   6. Reported symptoms and exam/test performance

   7. Measures of similar abilities (intertest scatter)

   8. Similar tasks or items within the same exam or test (intratest scatter)—especially when difficult tasks are performed more easily than easy ones

   9. Different testing sessions

(Of note, the potential contributions of significant psychiatric, attentional, comprehension, or other factors that often involve inconsistent presentations should also be considered.)

II. Overly impaired performance (versus what would normally be expected)

   1. Very poor performance on easy tasks presented as difficult

   2. Failing tasks that all but those with severe impairment perform easily

   3. Poorer performance than normative data for similar injury/illness

   4. Below chance-level performance

III. Lack of specific diagnostic signs of impairment

IV. Specific signs of response bias on psychological or neuropsychological tests

   1. MMPI scale: F, F-K

   2. MMPI-2 "Fake Bad"

   3. Malingering detection tests

   4. Actuarial formulas for clinical neuropsychological tests (e.g., WCST, CVLT)

V. Interview evidence

   1. Atypical temporal relationship of symptoms to injury

   2. Psychological symptoms, or symptoms which are improbable, absurd, overly specific, or of unusual frequency or severity (e.g., triple vision)

   3. Disparate examinee history or complaints across interviews or examiners

   4. Disparate corroboratory interview data versus examinee report

VI. Physical exam findings

   1. Nonorganic sensory findings

   2. Nonorganic motor findings

   3. Pseudoneurologic findings in the absence of anticipated associated pathologic findings

   4. Inconsistent exam findings

   5. Failure on physical exam procedures designed to specifically assess malingering

CVLT, California Verbal Learning Test; MMPI, Minnesota Multiphasic Personality Inventory; WCST, Wisconsin Card Sorting Task.
(Adapted from Rogers R [ed]: Clinical Assessment of Malingering and Deception, ed 2. New York: Guilford Press, 1997.)

TABLE 50–2. Response Bias Detection Measures and Strategies

Pain assessment measures with built-in response bias indicators	
Pain Assessment Battery (PAB)-in Research Edition:	I. Symptom Magnification Frequency (SMF) > 40%
Proposed clinical hypothesis procedure evaluating:	II. Extreme Beliefs Frequency (EBF) > 35%
	III. Four other "validity" indicators (i.e., alienation, rating percent of max, percent extreme ratings [2 scales])
Millon Behavioral Health Inventory (MBHI)	Elevations on 3-item validity scale
Hendler (i.e., Mensana Clinic) Back Pain Test	Scores of 21–31 (exaggerating)
	Scores > 31 (primary psychological influence)
Medical indicators	
Hoover test	Test for malingered lower extremity weakness associated with normal crossed extensor response
Astasia abasia	"Drunken-type" gait with near falls but no actual falls to ground
Nonorganic sensory loss	Patchy sensory loss, midline sensory loss, large scotoma in visual field, tunnel vision
Nonorganic upper extremity drift	Long tract involvement results in pronator type drift. Proximal shoulder girdle weakness and malingering typically present with downward drift while in supination.
Stenger test	Test for malingered hearing loss during audiologic evaluation
Gait discrepancies when observed versus not observed	If organic, should be consistent regardless of whether observed or not
Gait discrepancies relative to direction of requested ambulation	Gait for a patient with hemiparesis should present similarly in all directions; malingerers do not as a rule practice a feigned gait in all directions.
Forearm pronation, hand-clasping and forearm supination test for digit/finger sensory loss	Malingered finger sensory loss is difficult to maintain in this perceptually confusing, intertwined hand/finger position.
Pain versus temperature discrepancies	Due to the fact that both sensory modalities run in the spinothalamic tract, they should be commensurately impaired contralateral to the side of the CNS lesion.
Lack of atrophy in a chronically paretic/paralytic limb	Lack of atrophy in a paralyzed/paretic limb suggests the limb is being used or is getting regular electrical stimulation to maintain mass.
Impairment diminishes under influence of sodium amytal, hypnosis, or lack of observation	All these observations are most consistent with nonorganic presentations including consideration of malingering or conversion disorder.
Incongruence between neuroanatomic imaging and neurologic examination	Lack of any static imaging findings on brain computed tomography or magnetic resonance imaging in the presence of a dense motor or sensory deficit suggests nonorganicity.
Arm drop test	An aware patient malingering profound alteration in consciousness or significant arm paresis will not let his or her own hand, when held over his head, drop onto his face.
Presence of ipsilateral findings when implied neuroanatomy would dictate contralateral findings	An examinee claiming severe right brain damage who claims right eye blindness and right-sided weakness and sensory loss
Tell me "when I'm not touching" responses	An examinee with claimed sensory loss who endorses that he does not feel you touch him when you ask him to tell you "if you do not feel this."
Lack of shoe wear in presence of gait disturbance	An examinee with claimed longer-term gait deviation due to orthopedic or neurologic causes should demonstrate commensurate wear on shoes (if worn with any frequency).

TABLE 50–2. Response Bias Detection Measures and Strategies—cont'd

Calluses on hands in "totally disabled" examinee	An examinee who is unable to work should not present with signs of ongoing evidence of physical labor.
Assistive device "wear and tear" signs	In any examinee using assistive devices for any period of time (e.g. cane, crutches) there should be commensurate wear on the device consistent with his or her claimed impairment and disability.
Mankopf maneuver	Increase in heart rate commensurate with nociceptive stimulation during exam (there is some controversy on whether this always occurs).
Lack of atrophy in a limb that is claimed to be significantly impaired	If side-to-side measurements and/or inspection do not bear out atrophy, consider other causes aside from one being claimed.
Sudden motor give-away or ratchetiness on manual strength testing	Considered to normally be a sign of incomplete effort or symptom exaggeration
Weakness on manual muscle testing without commensurate asymmetry of deep tendon reflexes or muscle bulk.	Suggests simulated muscle weakness if long-standing
Toe test for simulated low back pain	Flexion of hip and knee with movement only of toes should not produce an increase in low back pain.
Magnuson test	Have examinee point to area several times over period of examination; inconsistencies suggest increased potential for nonorganicity.
Delayed response sign	Pain reaction temporally delayed relative to application of perceived nociceptive stimulus
Wrist drop test	In an examinee with claimed wrist extensor loss, have her pronate forearm, extend elbow, and flex shoulder . . . if on making a fist in this position she also extends wrist, then nonorganicity should be suspected.
Object drop test	Examinee claims inability to bend down yet does so to pick up a light object "inadvertently" dropped by examiner.
Hip adductor test	Test for claimed paralysis of lower extremity, similar to Hoover test yet looks for crossed adductor response
Disparity between tested range of motion (ROM) and observed ROM of any joint	When ROM under testing is significantly disparate (e.g., less) from observed, spontaneous ROM, suspect functional contributors.
Straight leg raise (SLR) disparities dependent on examinee positioning	Differences in SLR between sitting, standing, or bending may suggest a functional overlay to low back complaints.
Grip strength testing via dynamometer	Three repetitions at any given setting should not vary more than 20%, or bell-shaped curve should be generated if all 5 positions are tested.
Sensory "flip" test	Sensory findings should be the same if testing upper extremity in supination or pronation or lower extremity in internal versus external rotation. Differences may suggest a functional overlay.
Pinch test for low back pain	Pinching the lumbar fat pad should not reproduce pain due to axial structure involvement; if test is positive, suspect a functional overlay.

Psychoemotional instruments with built-in response bias designs

Personality Assessment Inventory (PAI)	• Inconsistency (INC), Infrequency (INF), Positive Impression Management (PIM), and Negative Impression Management (NIM) scales

TABLE 50–2. Response Bias Detection Measures and Strategies—cont'd

Psychoemotional instruments with built-in response bias designs	
Personality Assessment Inventory (PAI)	• 8 score patterns thought to comprise a "Malingering Index" (Morey, 1996) • >2 patterns malingering suspected • >4 patterns likely malingering
Minnesota Multiphasic Personality Inventory (MMPI-2)	• Validity indices (L, F, Fb, Fp, Ds, K, VRIN, TRIN, F-K 54) • The Fake Bad Scale (Lees-Haley, 1991) • Compare subtle to obvious items (tentative) • Fp Scale • Rogers et al. (1994) – cutoff scores: Liberal: (1) F-Scale raw score > 23 (2) F-Scale T-Score > 81 (3) F-K Index > 10 (4) Obvious – subtle score > 83 Conservative: (1) F-scale raw > 30 (2) F-K index > 25 (3) Obvious – subtle score > 190

Other domain specific measures with built-in response bias designs	
Trauma Symptom Inventory (TSI)	• 3 validity scales (response level, atypical, inconsistent)

Cognitive effort measures: *Performance patterns on existing psychological/neuropsychological tests*	
Full-scale IQ	Low versus expected or predicted IQ
Arithmetic, orientation	"Near-miss" (Ganser errors)
WMS-R Malingering Index: Attention/Concentration Index versus Memory Index	Attention-Concentration Index Score < General Memory Index (AC-GMI)
Grip strength	Usually low without gross motor deficit
Recognition memory: California Verbal Learning Test	<13
Rey Complex Figure Recognition Trial	Atypical recognition errors (≤2); recognition failure errors
Haltstead or Luria Nebraska Battery Formulas	Several formulas are available.*

Specific cognitive effort/response bias measures	
Any symptom validity testing (SVT)	<50%, chance responding or below cutoff
Computer Assessment of Response Bias (CARB)	<89% raises suspicion
Dot Counting Test (DCT)	Correct/incorrect responses; time on group v ungrouped
Hiscock Forced Choice Test	<50% chance level responding or below cutoff
Portland Digit Recognition Test	<50% chance level responding or below cutoff
Pritchard Tests of Neuropsychological Malingering	<50% chance level responding or below cutoff
Rey Memory for 15 Items Test (MFIT)	<3 complete sets, <9 items
Test of Memory Malingering (TOMM)	<50% chance level responding or below cutoff
Validity Indicator Profile	<50% chance level responding or below cutoff
Victoria Symptom Validity Test	<50% chance level responding or below cutoff
Word Completion Memory Test (WCMT); any implicit memory word stem priming task	R < 9 or Inclusion <15; poor or unusual performance
Word Memory Test (WMT)	<50%, chance responding or below cutoff

*McKinzey RK, Podd MH, Krehbiel, et al.: Detection of malingering on the Luria-Nebraska Neuropsychological Battery: An initial and cross-validation. Arch Clin Neuropsychology 12:505–512, 1997.
*McKinzey RK, Russell EW: Detection of malingering on the Halstead-Reitan Battery: A cross-validation. Arch Clin Neuropsychology 12:585–590, 1997.
(Adapted from Martelli MF, Zasler ND, Pickett T: Motivation and Response Bias during Evaluations following ABI: An Assessment Model. Presented at the 25th Annual Williamsburg Brain Injury International Conference, Williamsburg, VA, June 7, 2001, poster 30.)

TABLE 50–3. Qualitative Variables in Assessing Response Bias

Time/response latency comparisons across similar tasks	Inconsistencies across tasks
Performance on easy tasks presented as hard	Low scores or unusual errors
Remote memory report	Difficulties, especially if < recent memory, or severely impaired in absence of gross amnesia
Personal information	Very poor personal information in absence of gross amnesia
Comparison between test performance and behavioral observations	Discrepancies
Inconsistencies in history or complaints, performance	Inconsistencies across time, setting, interviewer, etc.
Comparisons for inconsistencies within testing session (quantitative & qualitative):	A. Within tasks (e.g., easy versus hard items) B. Between tasks (e.g., easy versus hard) C. Across repetitions of same/parallel tasks (R/O fatigue) D. Across similar tasks under different motivational sets
Comparisons across testing sessions (qualitative, quantitative)	Poorer/inconsistent performance on retesting
Symptom self-report: complaints	High frequency, severity of complaints and severity versus significant other report or other collaborative report
Main & Spanswick, 1995 • Failure to comply with reasonable treatment • Report of severe pain with no associated psychological effects • Marked inconsistencies in effects of pain on general activities • Poor work record and history of persistent appeals against awards • Previous litigation	
Symptom self report: early/acute versus late/chronic Symptom complaint	Early symptoms reported late or acute symptoms reported as chronic
Response to typically helpful pain interventions	1. Failure to show any pain relief to at least one of the following: biofeedback, hypnosis, mild analgesics, psychotherapy, relaxation exercises, heat and ice, mild exercise 2. Failure to show any pain relief in response to TENS
Genuine versus malingered post-traumatic stress disorder (Resnick, 1995)	Stress initiator minimized versus emphasized, blame self versus other: helpless versus grandiose dreams, deny versus emphasize emotional impact, reluctant versus easy memory elicitation, specific versus general guilt, more versus less stress-associated environmental avoidance, helpless versus directed anger.

that the entire set of complaints is biased. Ethical guidelines of psychologists caution against overzealous interpretation of limited test data, as they should for physicians. Unfortunately, the recent increase in attention to response bias assessment has been accompanied by frequently overzealous application of poorly validated detection procedures with resultant potential for questionable opinions regarding malingering. Although these instruments and procedures vary in terms of utility and empirical support, virtually all have identifiable limitations (Hayes et al., 1999; Williams, 2000; Senior & Douglas, 2001; Vanderploeg & Curtiss, 2001).

General weaknesses of symptom validity tests (SVTs) include: (1) psychometric shortcomings (i.e., test construction issues such as inadequate reliability and validity data and not meeting professional standards for educational and psychological tests [Williams, 2000]); (2) limited ability to generalize from findings on simulated malingerers (i.e., analogue research) to real malingerers; (3) limited ability to generalize from one SVT to other SVTs or clinical tests in a battery; (4) differential subtlety of measures; (5) wide variability in research sample characteristics; (6) confounding of exaggeration and real disorder in clinical groups; (7) limited validation research on "effort" as a construct; (8) unknown specificity with regard to effects of fatigue, pain, disinterest, nonattended (computer) administration, and so on; and (9) frequently high misclassification rates (i.e.,

TABLE 50–4. Diagnostic Complexities

Genuine pathology	Residual functional impairments	Residual impairments on examination testing
1. Yes	1. Yes and exaggerated	1. Yes and not exaggerated
2. Mixed	2. Yes and not exaggerated	2. Yes and exaggerated
3. Indeterminate	3. No and exaggerated	3. No and exaggerated
4. No	4. No and not exaggerated	4. No and not exaggerated

false positives or false negatives), both experimentally and when tested clinically (Senior & Douglas, 2001; Vanderploeg & Curtiss, 2001).

This summary of shortcomings of current procedures is offered to emphasize: (1) the need for caution in interpretation; (2) the importance of using multiple data sources and making thoughtful inferences only after integrating behavioral observations, interview data, tests results, and collateral sources of information; (3) the complexity of potential diagnostic situations; and (4) the need for further research. Table 50-4 includes a tabular representation of the complexity and range of diagnostic possibilities with regard to injury-related presentations.

Examiner Response Bias

Examiner bias/misattribution also occurs and may be an equally problematic source of error. Clinicians sensitized to the signs and symptoms of their particular specialty may misdiagnose or overdiagnose problems, with inadequate attention to competing explanations. Chapman and Elstein (2000) have discussed how biases can occur in the face of uncertainty in medical decision making. Examiners may also display response bias by tendencies to doubt the sincerity of complaints or disregard their veracity (Lees-Haley, 1997; McBeath, 2000). The other extreme is blind acceptance of complaints at face value without introspection or further inquiry. Finally, there is increasing recognition of bias in arbitrators' case perceptions and award recommendations (Eylon et al., 2000).

We have reported preliminary data regarding the common suspicion that examiner bias is influenced by compensation issues (Martelli et al., 2000b). Compelling evidence of perceived expert witness bias comes from a recent report from a study sanctioned by the Federal Judiciary Committee (Krafka et al., 2002) involving a large sample of active federal judges and the lead plaintiff and defense attorneys who presented the

docket cases before them. Findings, based on compliance-enhanced return rates of 51% for judges and 66% for attorneys, were consistent from 1991 to 1998 in revealing that the primary problem with expert testimony was experts who "abandon objectivity and become advocates for the side that hired them (p. 5)." On a 1 (very infrequent) to 5 (very frequent) Likert scale of this problem, the mean response was 3.69 for judges and 3.72 for attorneys.

Recommendations for Enhancing Validity in Impairment and Disability Assessments

The following recommendations are offered to promote objectivity and validity of impairment and disability assessments. These suggestions become even more relevant in the context of potential secondary gain issues. Examiners should always assess response bias (including malingering) and make efforts to guard against motivational deficiencies as a threat to evaluation validity. They should emphasize the importance of accurate report on all interview questions and full effort on tests to produce valid profiles that permit comparison with known symptom patterns. Examiners should use standardized, validated, and well-normed procedures and tests and use only appropriate normative data for comparisons. They should take into account symptom base rates (i.e., how frequently the symptoms occur in the general population and in the absence of the injury for which they are being evaluated), other explanatory factors for symptoms (e.g., medications, sleep disturbance, depression, pain, post-traumatic stress disorder), symptoms typical for the medical condition (e.g., inherent somatic complaints of disorders like multiple sclerosis, Parkinson disease, and chronic pain), relevant situational variables (e.g., attention fluctuation due to chronic pain conditions, fatigue, insomnia/sleep deprivation, chronic stress), sociocultural factors (e.g., rural impoverished backgrounds), and other contextual factors and considerations.

One should avoid joining the attorney-client "team," respect role boundaries (e.g., treating doctor, expert, trial consultant), and emphasize objectivity. Clinicians involved in impairment and disability evaluation should arrive at opinions only after review of all available evidence. Examiners should monitor excessive favoritism to the side of the retaining party. Objective opinions should vary in the same manner that truth varies. Balanced opinions are characterized by elements that are favorable to each side in the medicolegal context, both in terms of findings in any one case and for the sample of cases represented (Martelli et al., 2001a). Notably, Brodsky (1991) and Martelli and colleagues (2000a) have attempted to offer very preliminary guidelines regarding the expected rates of disagreement in diagnostic conclusions (e.g., 25%).

One should dispute the opinion of other experts only in the context of a complete and accurate representation of the other expert's findings, inferential reasoning, and conclusions. Examiners should spend sufficient time evaluating and treating the patient population that one is offering testimony about. Clinicians should attempt to devise and use a system that allows them to monitor the validity of diagnostic and prognostic statements against external criteria (i.e., actual social and occupational functioning). Ideally, but maybe idealistically, one should also develop a mechanism that facilitates feedback from peers on quality and objectivity.

It is also important to recognize the limitations of medical and neuropsychological opinions because few findings and symptoms are black or white, that is, attributable to a single event (e.g., Ockam's Razor). As much as possible, assessment of motivational issues should integrate information from a variety of sources rather than rely on individual indicators. Although there are many techniques to assess response bias, the methodology is still developing. At present, determination of response bias largely relies on clinical skill and judgment, without recourse to any simple tests and decision-making algorithms. The more challenging problems include ferreting out mixtures of exaggeration and true symptomatology, understanding what aspects of response bias are consciously versus unconsciously determined, and appreciating which symptoms and signs may be modified by psychosocial or biomedical factors.

THE GUIDES TO EVALUATION OF PERMANENT IMPAIRMENT

First published in 1971, the AMA guidelines provide information to assist clinicians in rating *permanent* impairment, not disability. The "Guides" is presently in its fifth edition and provides comprehensive rating systems for all types of impairments and organ systems except for those germane to psychological and psychiatric disease. The GEPI is divided into four main sections: (1) concepts of impairment evaluation; (2) records and reports; (3) definitive evaluation protocols for evaluation of a particular body part, function, or system; and (4) reference tables keyed to evaluation protocols. The examiner must describe the specific clinical findings related to each impairment noted as well as document any absent data or inability to obtain specific relevant data. Each impairment rated should be referenced to the appropriate section of the GEPI with an explanation of the percent rating assigned. All impairment ratings should be subsequently listed in summary fashion prior to determining a whole person impairment rating.

As per the GEPI, the evaluating clinician should include a narrative history; results of the most recent clinical evaluation; assessment of current clinical status; plans for future treatment, including rehabilitation and reevaluation, diagnosis, and clinical impressions; and an estimate of time for full or partial recovery. The clinician must also analyze the findings relative to explanation of the impact of the medical condition(s) on life activities, static or stabilized nature of the medical condition, or chance of sudden or subtle incapacitation as a result of the medical condition. The risk of injury, harm, or further impairment with activity needed to meet personal, social, or occupational demands must also be addressed. The clinician should also elaborate on any restrictions or accommodations regarding required activities to meet life demands. The medical condition in question must be stable before permanency can be established and rated. The GEPI lists four criteria that must be met before a medical condition may be considered stable: (1) the clinical condition is stabilized and not likely to improve with surgical intervention or active medical treatment, and medical maintenance care only is warranted; (2) the degree of impairment is not likely to change by more than 3% within the next year; (3) employability is not likely to improve with surgical intervention or active medical treatment; and (4) the individual is not likely to suffer sudden or subtle incapacitation. If the aforementioned conditions are unmet, then impairment evaluation should be deferred.

It should also be realized that the concept and definition of permanency might differ between the GEPI and other disability determination systems or programs. Additionally, examiners should be fully aware of the fact that the GEPI was developed in an attempt to produce a system that enabled clinicians to predict disability level by evaluation of simple physical organ system impairments. This basic tenet flaw mistakenly analogizes the task of impairment rating with determination of disability status. This error is not only a grave mistake, but it is potentially a significant disservice to the person with the disability, to society, and to the administrative disability determination system.

When an individual presents with brain disease or damage, the impairments may involve several parts of the body as well as several parts of the nervous system, for example, the brain, spinal cord, or peripheral nerves. The fifth edition revisions include addition of an impairment evaluation summary at the end of Chapter 13 (the central and peripheral nervous system), section 13.10, to "allow easy access to the neurologic impairment in question," description of ancillary tests with some of their indications, greater guidance in the assessment of several impairment categories, and additional illustrative cases.

Individual impairments should be separately calculated and their whole person values combined using the "combined values chart" in the GEPI. In general, only the medical condition causing the greatest impairment should be evaluated. The GEPI also divides the assessment of the most severe central nervous system (CNS) impairment, based on neurologic evaluation and relevant clinical investigations into four categories: state of consciousness and level of awareness (whether permanent or episodic), mental status evaluation and integrative functioning, use and understanding of language, and influence of behavior and mood on cerebral function. The most severe of the aforementioned impairments is then combined with any of the following impairments, as applicable, using the Combined Values Chart: cranial nerve impairments; station, gait, and movement disorders; extremity disorders related to central impairment; chronic pain; spinal cord impairments; and, lastly, peripheral nerve, motor, and sensory impairments.

As per the GEPI, the evaluation of sensory and motor impairments due to cerebral disorders should be based on the examinee's ability to perform activities of daily living (ADL) (again bringing up the concern of analogizing impairment and disability rating in the process of what should otherwise be only an impairment rating system). Sensory disturbances may be related to thalamic pain, phantom limb pain, complex regional pain syndrome (causalgia), disorders of stereognosis, and disturbances of two-point and position sense. Motor disturbances may occur with or without associated weakness. The nonparetic motor deficits may include movement disorders, tonal aberrations, and restrictions in expression of motor behavior such as in bradykinesia and ataxia.

Impairments due to aphasia or dysphasia are based on gradations of impairment severity and on the results of specific language/communication-based testing. Some of the objective assessment strategies include naming objects by sight or describing them after reading about them, repeating speech, following oral and written commands, reading and comprehending, writing, spelling, and demonstrating the use of an object (a test for aphasia). As with other impairments, the combined values chart should be used to calculate the whole person impairment.

Mental status and integrative functions are determined based on bedside assessment. Ten "traditional" measures of cognitive function are used: (1) orientation to time, person, and place; (2) recent recall; (3) ability to remember and repeat a series of digits and repeat them in reverse order; (4) ability to perform serial subtraction of 7s from 100 or 3s from 20; (5) ability to do other simple calculations; (6) ability to repeat three unrelated words; (7) ability to spell a word forward and backward (e.g., world); (8) ability to repeat a short paragraph; (9) ability to understand and explain proverbs or abstract thought; and (10) judgment. These tests of cognitive function can be performed only in the absence of significant aphasia. In the presence of a significant communication disturbance and a disturb-

ance of mental status, the greater of the two impairments should be used as the impairment estimate. The methodology for bedside mental status testing may underestimate the extent of more subtle albeit functionally significant cognitive deficits in patients with milder cognitive impairment due to brain injury or disease. The fifth edition recommends that examiners consider using the Clinical Dementia Rating (CDR) scale in conjunction with a standardized mental status test such as the Mini-Mental State Exam. Once again, the GEPI requires the examiner to grade mental status impairment based on ability to do activities of daily living, thereby confounding impairment and disability assessment procedures.

Emotional and behavioral disturbances are again rated based on the relative degree of impairment in "daily functions" ranging from mild to severe. The disorders that may fall under this category of impairments include depression, emotional lability, mania, pathologic laughing or crying, psychosis, disinhibited behavior, and others. As with many other impairment measures, there is a significant degree of subjectivity within each category of impairment relative to the percent impairment assigned.

Disturbances in the level of consciousness and awareness are rated based on ability to care for self relative to the overall level of altered consciousness with persistent vegetative state or irreversible coma correlating with a 70% to 90% impairment rating. Brief repetitive or persisting alterations in one's state of consciousness, limiting the ability to perform usual activities, correlate with an impairment rating of 0% to 14%. The impairment criteria for disturbances in consciousness and awareness do not apply to seizure disorders, syncope (neurogenic or cardiogenic), or sleep-wake cycle disturbances.

Episodic neurologic disorders include three main subcategories: syncope with alteration in awareness, convulsive disorders, and sleep and arousal disorders. Because these disorders may relate to other organ systems outside the CNS, the impairments should be combined. If a disorder is expected to change to a moderate or greater degree within the next year, then the impairment should not be rated, because it is not permanent. This class of disorders should be described relative to onset, duration, associated symptoms, and impact on daily function. Even in the worst-case scenario, the highest level of impairment would be 70% (whole person) for this class of disorders.

The forebrain assessment should also include cranial nerves I and II. All too often, examiners neglect to assess cranial nerve I, which is responsible for olfactory function. Taste may be perceived by the examinee to be altered when in fact only the sense of smell has been perturbed. Olfactory impairment may be partial or complete. Additionally, dysosmia may occur in the form of parosmias or cacosmias, which need to be considered in the impairment rating. The maximum impairment rating for loss of smell is 5% of the whole person. Optic nerve impairments relative to decreased visual acuity should be combined with any other visual system impairment. The GEPI provides a table to assist in rating impairment due to visual field loss.

The remaining GEPI-rated CNS structures include the midbrain, pons, medulla, and spinal cord. Midbrain injury resulting in extraocular muscle dysfunction related to cranial nerves III, IV, and VI may produce diplopia. The extent of diplopia in the various directions of gaze is determined in an arc perimeter at 33 cm, or with a bowl perimeter. Pontine dysfunction may result in vestibulocochlear nerve aberrations. Tinnitus in the presence of unilateral hearing loss may impair speech discrimination and adversely influence the patient's ability to conduct daily activities. Up to 5% may be added because of tinnitus to an impairment estimate for severe unilateral hearing loss. Vestibular dysfunction may be unilateral or bilateral. Vertigo is rated as a single entity, without reference to its many potential associated symptoms. Impairment ratings range from 1% to 70% of the whole person. Disorders of station and gait may result from a variety of conditions involving the CNS as well as the peripheral nervous system. Whole person impairments for gait disturbance range from 1% to 60%. Altered libido can be rated under sexual impairment criteria and receives a whole person impairment rating from 1% to 9%.

The aforementioned information on the GEPI is at best a brief introduction to its utility, as well as limitations, for rating permanent impairments in persons with brain-based injury or disease. The presenting symptoms of brain injury or disease must be differentiated from other conditions including but not limited to mental disorders. Concurrent unrelated as well as related neuropsychiatric diagnoses must be considered. Clinical psychological and psychiatric conditions such as depression (reactive or organic or both), pain disorders, somatoform and factitious disorders as well as posttraumatic stress disorder need to be appropriately considered in both litigating and nonlitigating individuals. Less commonly, clinicians may encounter malingering examinees. A diagnosis of malingering should be considered in the differential diagnosis of any individual where history, symptoms, and signs are a mismatch, particularly when there is identifiable secondary gain such as litigation or worker's compensation (Martelli et al., 2000a).

DISABILITY EVALUATION UNDER WORKERS' COMPENSATION

Workers' compensation typically defines three categories of payments for persons unable to work due to injury or illness (Cocchiarella & Andersson, 2001). Financial compensation may be for lost wages due to temporary total disability, payment for medical bills, or for permanent disability, partial or total. Temporary total disability as defined by most workers' compensation boards is met when a claimant is unable to earn wages, return to work is expected, and the medical condition has not yet stabilized. On the other hand, temporary partial disability implies that the claimant has returned to work but is earning a lower wage than previously. Regarding permanent disability, workers' compensation awards are normally independent of work capacity. Rather, financial remuneration depends on the economic loss associated with the permanent medical impairment. Benefits are normally paid based on an average weekly wage with a capped payment schedule. A rating of partial permanent disability is necessary when the loss of use or loss of the body part, function, or system is less than total. No formulas exist that incorporate physician-determined impairment ratings with other factors to determine the percentage by which the industrial use of the employee's body is impaired (Cocchiarella & Andersson, 2001). The final determination regarding work capacity status is made by an agency representative based on available medical and nonmedical information of the claimant's ability to meet personal, social, or occupational demands or to meet statutory or regulatory requirements (LaForge & Harrison, 1987).

DISABILITY EVALUATION UNDER SOCIAL SECURITY

The Social Security Administration (SSA) defines disability as the "inability to engage in *any* substantial gainful activity by reason of a medically determinable physical or mental impairment(s) which can be expected to result in death or which has lasted or can be expected to last for a continuous period of not less than 12 months" (SSA, 2001, p. 2). The latest disability evaluation guidelines (also known as "the blue book") were published by the SSA in January 2001. There are two sections, one for adults and one for children, each divided into 13 sections. Adults are classified based on chronological age greater than 18 years of age. If an applicant's impairment is established by medical evidence consisting of symptoms, signs, and laboratory findings, a presumption is made in the absence of work that the applicant meets Social Security requirements for disability. Reliance on the individual's statement of symptoms alone is insufficient to meet criteria for "medically determinable impairment."

Social Security presently has two programs for disability, title II and title XVI, the Social Security Disability Insurance Program and the Supplemental Security Income Program, respectively. The definitions for disability are essentially the same under both programs; specifically, an individual must have a "medically determinable impairment." This translates to impairment with medically demonstrable anatomic, physiologic, or psychological abnormalities. Such abnormalities are medically determinable if they manifest themselves as signs or laboratory findings apart from symptoms. Abnormalities that manifest only as symptoms are not medically determinable.

The Title II program is provided through a trust fund contributed into by workers through FICA tax on their earnings. There are three basic categories under Title II. Title XVI provides Supplemental Security Income (SSI) to individuals who meet specific financial criteria, are 65 years of age or older, or are blind. As per Social Security Disability Income (SSDI) criteria, the examiner must stipulate both degree and duration modifiers. Specifically, degree of impairment modifiers include "partial" or "total,"; whereas, duration modifiers include "temporary" or "permanent." This is in contradistinction to the AMA GEPI, which is used only for assessment of permanent impairment. Examiners should also be aware of "presumptive disability" determinations, which allow a person with a disability to receive disability benefits prior to the required normal duration stipulated by the SSA if the person is expected to persist with a level of disability that is severe enough and anticipated to last at least 1 year from the date of disability onset (Olsheski & Growick, 1994).

As per the 2001 guidelines, the health care professional may take on any of the following roles: treating physician, consultative examiner, full- or part-time consultant reviewer of claims, or medical expert who testifies at administrative law judge hearings. Medical reports should include medical history, clinical findings, laboratory results, diagnoses, treatment prescribed with response and prognosis, and a statement providing an opinion regarding what the individual can still do despite the impairments. In developing evidence of the impact of symptoms on claimant functional abilities, various factors are considered including but not limited to daily activities; location, duration, frequency, and intensity of the symptom; precipitating and aggravating factors; the type dosage, effectiveness, and side effects of any treatment including medications; the treatments used for symptom relief; claimant measures to modulate symptoms; and other factors germane to the claimant's functional limitations due to pain or other symptoms.

EMPLOYABILITY: MANAGEMENT AND ADMINISTRATIVE CONSIDERATIONS

One of the major issues relative to the administrative determination of work capability of a claimant is whether or not the claimant can work with or without accommodation. Employability determinations depend on several variables including capacity to travel to and from work, to perform assigned tasks and duties at work or related to work, and ability to be at work (Cailliet, 1969). Employability determination also depends on ongoing reassessment of work performance through monitoring of attendance, work quality, and conduct. From a medical standpoint, the initial burden of proof typically lies with the claimant. The medical evaluation protocol relative to any employment determination should remain independent of the person's motivation to work. In practical terms, however, there are common financial and other disincentives to return to work once "out on disability," which are inextricably intertwined with other difficult-to-quantify potential obstacles to work re-entry. Some of these include disability adaptation, illness behavior, and learned helplessness, among other factors.

Medical determination of employability should include developing an understanding of the job specifics, assessing available medical documentation, and demonstrating a causal relationship between the medical condition and the employment deficiency. Inquiries should be made regarding job specifics including performance, physical activity requirements, reliability, availability, productivity, and "useful service life" (Koppenhoefer, 1988).

PAIN ISSUES IN IMPAIRMENT AND DISABILITY EVALUATION

The examiner should attempt to quantify any pain complaint, including that of headache, and the impact on functional skills as part of the evaluation. The GEPI contains a section (i.e., 13.8) on impairment evaluation of pain in the chapter on nervous system impairment rating, which focuses on causalgia, post-traumatic neuralgia, and reflex sympathetic dystrophy. Chapter 18, on pain rating, is entirely revised and updated in the fifth edition. The need for assessing the "eight Ds" is crucial: duration, dramatization, diagnostic dilemma, drugs, dependence, depression, disuse, and dysfunction. If the pain condition is to be rated it must be stable and unlikely to change in the future despite therapy.

Methods for measurement of overt motor behaviors include direct behavioral observations, automated measurement devices such as "uptime" recorders, self-monitored observations such as daily diaries, and self-report of functional disability using such standardized methods as the Sickness Impact Profile (SIP; Bergner et al., 1981; Gonzales et al., 2000). Although measurement of overt motor behaviors is a very practical approach by which to assess the impact of pain on physical functioning, it is limited by patient initiation of behavior change due to the assessment procedure itself as well as the lack of information provided to the examiner regarding affective and sensory components of the pain experience.

The area of pain assessment that has received the most attention is by far the measurement of affective responses to pain. The earliest affective responses to pain typically are driven by the autonomic nervous system and produce symptoms of anxiety. Chronic pain, on the other hand, tends to produce vegetative signs of depression and hypochondriasis. Multiple psychometric measures have been used to evaluate "chronic pain behavior" and associated affective status including the Minnesota Multiphasic Personality Inventory (MMPI), Illness Behavior Questionnaire, pain drawing, Symptom Checklist-90 and Millon Behavioral Health Inventory (Martelli et al., 1999). The examiner must be aware of the limitations of such testing and the anticipated "deviations from the norm" when administered to persons with brain-based disorders. Not uncommonly, persons with neurologic disease will produce elevations on primary MMPI-2 scales 1, 2, 3, 7, and 8, similar to chronic pain examinees.

Several methods of assessing cognitive distortions and coping strategies related to pain have been developed. Several questionnaires measure cognitive distortions concerning general life experiences and pain-related problems. Several pain assessment techniques have been developed that rely on subjective judgments including category scales, visual analogue scales, McGill Pain Questionnaire, and ratio scales of verbal pain descriptors. The examiner should also establish how pain has affected spousal relationships and family interactions where applicable (Bradley et al., 1989; Gonzales et al., 2000).

Although not commonly used for "objectification" of pain complaints, measurement of physiologic variables may provide additional information regarding subjective pain complaints. Some of the methods used include electromyographic techniques, particularly with surface electrodes; use of pressure algometers or "dolorimeters" to assess myofascial trigger point sensitivity; galvanic skin response; and skin surface temperature (including thermographic evaluation) with the latter remaining the most controversial (Masterson, 1998).

Given the frequency of pain complaints in behavioral neurologic practice and neurorehabilitation, examiners should be aware of the aforementioned assessment techniques as well as the AMA GEPI section on pain impairment evaluation (Chapter 18 in fifth edition). The latest edition provides a "worksheet" for calculating the "total pain-related impairment score" based on a qualitative six-step process, the score of which is then converted into an impairment class of five categorizations. Psychogenic pain and malingering are also discussed in this chapter. Obviously, pain issues need to be integrated, when present, with the other observed impairments, and overall impairment rating determinations made only once this is accomplished (Zasler & Martelli, 1998).

PRACTICAL CONSEQUENCES OF CURRENT DISABILITY ASSESSMENT METHODOLOGIES

Tradition has dictated that disability determination remain within the purview of administrators. Clinician advocates may have an ethical dilemma leaving "disability determination" to administrative personnel given the latter party's lack of medical and disability training. Presently, most administrative bodies making such decisions do so based on general criteria relative to the person's ability to perform prior duties based on education, training, and experience and ability to perform *any* competitive employment (McBride, 1963).

Administrative personnel make such decisions based on available medical and paramedical documentation including impairment ratings, insurance company impairment forms, and "functional capacity" evaluation (FCE) forms, which are all typically completed by the treating physician. In most cases, however, there is only an estimation of functional capabilities and no true functional assessment is completed. This practice is viewed by some to be irresponsible and even unfair, to both the person being evaluated and society at large. Physicians either should have an FCE performed or document that the FCE forms cannot be filled out due to lack of objective, standardized information. Bedside assessment of impairment may not necessarily correlate particularly well with a person's general level of functional disability and handicap. To an even greater extent, there are concerns regarding how such impairment ratings correlate with specific job responsibilities and work environment. Just as significantly, there exist concerns regarding the predictive validity of FCEs to assess work re-entry readiness and, more importantly, the ability to sustain long-term employment.

CONCLUSIONS

Evaluation of impairment and disability is by no means a simple undertaking for any clinician regardless of specialty. Clinicians must take the time to familiarize themselves with the variety of disability and impairment evaluation protocols and understand their limitations relative to the specific clinical condition being assessed. Presently, there is no ideal system for rating impairment and disability associated with brain-based disorders (Hinnant & Tollison, 1994). A thorough understanding of the underlying disease process as well as associated illness or injury, as applicable, is paramount for optimal evaluation and reliable neurologic and vocational re-entry prognosis.

■ KEY POINTS

☐ Appropriate use of nomenclature is paramount to performance of impairment and disability evaluations.

☐ The *Guidelines to the Evaluation of Permanent Impairment* (GEPI), although serving as a guidepost for the CNS impairment assessment, is fraught with limitations including but not limited to the admixture of impairment and disability criteria for calculating ratings, lack of validity and reliability studies, and lack of correlation between impairment ratings and functional disability.

☐ In the context of impairment and disability evaluation, examiners must recognize the potential for examinee, as well as examiner, response bias and the various forms that bias may take in this context.

☐ Examiners should be aware of how they can optimize the validity of their assessments by taking into consideration motivational factors, symptom base rates, alternative explanations for signs or symptoms, situational variables, sociocultural factors, numerous input data points (e.g., records, interview with examinee, corroboratory information), and the context of the evaluation, among other important points.

☐ Disability determination is generally an administrative determination based on the individual's ability to meet personal, social, or occupational demands or to meet statutory or regulatory requirements.

KEY READINGS

Martelli MF, Zasler ND, Johnson-Greene D: Promoting ethical and objective practice in the medico-legal arena of disability evaluation. Phys Med Rehabil Clin North Am 12:571–586, 2001.

Zasler ND: Psychiatric assessment in traumatic brain injury, in Rosenthal M, Griffith ER, Kreutzer JS, et al (eds): Rehabilitation of the Adult and Child with Traumatic Brain Injury, ed 3. Philadelphia: Davis, 1999, pp 117–130.

Zasler ND, Martelli MF: Assessing mild traumatic brain injury. AMA Guides Newsletter, November/December, 1–5, 1998.

REFERENCES

American Psychiatric Association: Diagnostic and Statistical Manual of Mental Disorders, ed 4. Washington, DC: Author 1994.

Bergner M, Bobbitt RA, Carter WB, et al: The Sickness Impact Profile: Development and final revision of a health status measure. Med Care 19:787–805, 1981.

Binder LM, Rohling ML: Money matters: A meta-analytic review of the effects of financial incentives on recovery after closed-head injury. Am J Psychiatry 153:7–10, 1996.

Binder RL, Trimble MR, McNiel DE: The course of psychological symptoms after resolution of lawsuits. J Psychiatry 148:1073–1075, 1991.

Blau T: The Psychologist as Expert Witness. Presented at the National Academy of Neuropsychology annual meeting, Reno, Nevada, 1992.

Bradley LA: Psychological Testing, in Tollison CD, Kriegel ML (eds): Interdisciplinary Rehabilitation of Low Back Pain. Baltimore, MD: Williams & Wilkins, 1989, pp 30–50.

Brodsky SL: Testifying in court: Guidelines and maxims for the expert witnesses. Washington, DC: American Psychological Association, 1991.

Cailliet R: Disability evaluation: A physiatric method. South Med J 62:1380–1382, 1969.

Cassidy JD, Carroll LJ, Coye P, et al: Effect of elimination compensation for pain and suffering on the outcome of insurance claims for whiplash injury. N Engl J Med 342:1179–1186, 2000.

Chapman GB, Elstein AS: Cognitive processes and biases in medical decision making, in Chapman GB, Sonnenberg FA et al (eds): Decision Making in Health Care: Theory, Psychology, and Applications. Cambridge Series on Judgment and Decision Making. New York: Cambridge University Press, 2000, pp 183–210.

Cocchiarella L, Andersson GBJ (eds): Guides to the Evaluation of Permanent Impairment, ed 5. Chicago: AMA Press, 2001.

Evans RW: The effects of litigation on treatment outcome with personal injury patients. Am J Forensic Psychol 12:19–34, 1994.

Eylon D, Giacalone RA, Pollard HG: Beyond contractual interpretation: Bias in arbitrators' case perceptions and award recommendations. J Organizational Behav 21:513–524, 2000.

Gonzales VA, Martelli MF, Baker JM: Psychological assessment of persons with chronic pain. Neurorehabilitation 14:69–83, 2000.

Green P, Rohling ML, Lees-Haley PR, et al: Effort has a greater effect on test scores than severe brain injury in compensation claimants. Brain Inj 15:1045–1060, 2001.

Hayes JS, Hilsabeck RC, Gouvier WD: Malingering traumatic brain injury: Current issues and caveats in assessment and classification, in Varney NR, Roberts RJ (eds): The Evaluation and Treatment of Mild Traumatic Brain Injury. Mahwah, NJ: Lawrence Erlbaum Associates, 1999, pp 249–290.

Hinnant D, Tollison CD: Impairment and disability associated with mild head injury: Medical and legal aspects. Semin Neurol 14:84–89, 1994.

Johnston MV, Keith RA, Hinderer S: Measurement standards for interdisciplinary medical rehabiliation. Arch Phys Med Rehabil 73(Suppl):S6–S23, 1992.

Johnston MV, Wilkerson DL, Maney M: Evaluation of the quality and outcomes of medial rehabilitation programs, in DeLisa JA, Currie DM, Gans BM, et al (eds): Rehabilitation Medicine: Principles and Practice. Philadelphia: Lippincott, 1993.

Koppenhoefer RM: Disability Evaluation, in Delissa JA, Currie DM, Gans BM et al (eds): Rehabilitation Medicine: Principles and Practice. Philadelphia: Lippincott, 1988, pp 140–144.

Krafka C, Dunn MA, Johnson MT, et al.: Judge and attorney experiences, practices, and concerns regarding expert testimony in federal civil trials. Psychology, Public Policy, and Law. 8:309–332, 2002.

LaForge J, Harrison D: Limited and unlimited workers' compensation wage replacement benefits and rehabilitation outcomes. J Appl Rehabil Counsel 18:3–5, 1987.

Larrabee GJ: Neuropsychology in personal injury litigation. J Clin Exp Neuropsychol 22:702–707, 2000.

Lees-Haley PR: Challenges to validity and reliability in neurotoxic assessment of mass injuries. Presentation at the National Academy of Neuropsychology annual meeting, Las Vegas, NV, 1997.

Lees-Haley PR, Williams CW, Zasler ND, et al: Response bias in plaintiff's histories. Brain Injury 11:791–799, 1997.

Martelli MF, Zasler ND, Bush S: Assessment of response bias in impairment and disability evaluations following brain injury, in Carrion JL, Zitnay G (eds): Practices in Brain Injury. Philadelphia: Hanley and Belfus, in press.

Martelli MF, Zasler ND, Grayson R: Ethics and medicolegal evaluation of impairment after brain injury, in Schiffman M (ed): Attorney's Guide to Ethics in Forensic Science and Medicine. Springfield, IL: Charles C Thomas, 2000a.

Martelli MF, Zasler ND, LeFever F: Preliminary consumer guidelines to choosing a well suited neuropsychologist for assessment and rehabilitation of acquired brain injury. Brain Injury Source 4:36–39, 2000b.

Martelli MF, Zasler ND, Mancini AM, et al: Psychological assessment and applications in impairment and disability evaluations, in May RV, Martelli MF (eds): Guide to Functional Capacity Evaluation with Impairment Rating Applications. Richmond, VA: NADEP Publications, 1999, Ch. 3, pp. 1–84.

Martelli MF, Zasler ND, Nicholson K, et al: Masquerades of brain injury. Part II: Response bias in medicolegal examinees and examiners. J Controversial Med Claims 8:13–23, 2001a.

Martelli MF, Zasler ND, Pickett T: Motivation and Response Bias During Evaluations Following ABI: An Assessment Model. Presented at the Annual Williamsburg Traumatic Brain Injury International Conference, Williamsburg, VA, 2001b.

Masterson RZ: Techniques for assessing and diagnosing pain, in Weiner RB (ed): Pain Management: A Practical Guide for Clinicians. Boca Raton, FL: St. Lucie Press, 1998, pp. 45–58.

McBeath JG: Labelling of postconcussion patients as malingering and litigious: A common practice in need of criticism. Headache 40:609–610, 2000.

McBride ED: Disability Evaluation and Principles of Treatment of Compensable Injuries. Philadelphia: Lippincott, 1963.

Mendelson G: Compensation neurosis revisited: Outcome studies of the effects of litigation. J Psychosom Res 39:695–706, 1995.

National Institutes of Health, National Institute of Child Health and Human Development (U.S. Department of Health and Human Services, Public Health Service). Research Plan for the National Center for Medical Rehabilitation Research. NIH Publication No. 93-3509. Rockville, MD: National Institutes of Health, March, 1993.

Olsheski JA, Growick B: The Social Security disability system and rehabilitation in review. NARPPS J 8:143–156, 1994.

Ragnarsson KT, Thomas JP, Zasler ND: Model system of care for individuals with traumatic brain injury. J Head Trauma Rehabil 8:1–11, 1993.

Rogers R (ed): Clinical Assessment of Malingering and Deception, ed 2. New York: Guilford Press, 1997.

Rohling ML, Binder LM: Money matters: A meta-analytic review of the association between financial compensation and the experience and treatment of chronic pain. Health Psychol 14:537–545, 1995.

Rohling M: Effect sizes of impairment associated with symptom exaggeration versus definite traumatic brain injury. Arch Clin Neuropsychol 15:843–852, 2000.

Ruff RM, Wylie T, Tennant W: Malingering and malingering-like aspects of mild closed head injury. J Head Trauma Rehabil 8:60–73, 1993.

Sbordone RJ: The Ecological Validity of Neuropsychological Testing. Delray Beach, FL: St. Lucie Press, 1996.

Senior G, Douglas L: Misconceptions and misuse of the MMPI-2 in assessing personal injury claimants. Neurorehabilitation 16:203–213, 2001.

Social Security Administration: Disability Evaluation under Social Security: Medical Criteria for Evaluating Social Security Disability Claims. Washington, DC: Author, January 2001.

Vanderploeg RD, Curtiss G: Malingering assessment: Evaluation of validity of performance. Neurorehabilitation 16:245–252, 2001.

Wade DT: Measurement in Neurological Rehabilitation. New York: Oxford University Press, 1992.

Wehman P, Kreutzer JS (eds): Vocational Rehabilitation for Persons with Traumatic Brain Injury. Rockville, MD: Aspen Publishers, 1990.

Williams AD: Psychometric concerns in neuropsychological assessment. Brain Injury Source 4:41–47, 2000.

World Health Organization: International Classification of Impairments, Disabilities and Handicaps. Geneva, Switzerland, 1980.

World Health Organization: International Classification of Functioning, Disability and Health. Geneva, Switzerland, 2001.

Youngjohn JR, Burrows L, Erdal K: Brain damage or compensation neurosis? The controversial post-concussion syndrome. Clin Neuropsychol 9:112–117, 1995.

Zasler ND, Martelli MF: Assessing mild traumatic brain injury. AMA Guides Newsletter, November/December, 1–5, 1998.

Occupational Therapy and Rehabilitation Counseling

Debora A. Davidson

Linda Hunt

Lance W. Carluccio

Assistive technology

Disability

Functional capacity

Inclusion

Independent living

Occupational performance

Quality of life

Rehabilitation

INTRODUCTION

The field of rehabilitation has experienced and continues to experience rapid developments that reflect changes in medical science, technology, and society. The past 30 years have brought significantly improved rates of survival and increased life spans for persons with neurologic injuries and disorders. During this time, persons with disabilities have increasingly sought full inclusion in society, together with the freedom to pursue careers, relationships, and creative self-expression.

Significant gains have been made toward achieving this end. Through federal legislation, computer technology, and biomedical engineering it is possible for persons with severely limited sensory and motor abilities to communicate, control their environments, and achieve functional mobility. These powerful factors have increased the potential for persons with disabilities to live productive, satisfying lives. Occupational therapists and rehabilitation counselors provide expertise to help individuals with disabilities formulate and achieve meaningful lifestyles made possible by the many opportunities that are available though the advances in medicine, technology, and society.

The community of professionals who subscribe to a rehabilitation philosophy and the citizens who comprise the independent living movement have worked together with legislators to craft and promote the passage of laws that both reflect and facilitate the ongoing movement toward an inclusive society. Achievement of true and full integration of any disadvantaged minority group is a long process that requires continuous vigilance and effort on the parts of all concerned. The mere passage of legislation does not automatically result in its enactment for specific communities or individuals; this must be pursued one situation at a time and at every level. For this reason it is imperative that medical and rehabilitation practitioners be aware of the laws pertaining to the rights of persons with disabilities, so that all may participate as effective advocates and patient educators. These laws have had a significant impact on the practices of rehabilitation counseling and occupational therapy as they support three of the major goals of rehabilitation: work, independent living, and inclusion.

Table 51-1 outlines the key features of U.S. legislation relating to disability rights since 1973.

Occupational therapy and rehabilitation counseling are professions that help people regain, develop, and improve skills that are necessary for independent functioning, health, well-being, security, informed choice, and happiness. These practitioners work with people of all ages who, due to illness, injury, or developmental or psychological impairment, need specialized assistance in learning skills and habits that enable them to achieve their goals for quality of life and independence. Occupational therapy and rehabilitation counseling promote independent functioning in individuals who may otherwise require institutionalization or lifelong public assistance. These points of agreement result in effective teamwork between occupational therapists and rehabilitation counselors.

Although many aspects of their philosophies are congruent, occupational therapy and rehabilitation counseling remain distinct professions. Occupational therapists view an individual's daily activities and routines, or occupations, as central to quality of life and strive to facilitate a person's participation in all valued roles. These practitioners approach evaluation and intervention from a biopsychosocial perspective and may address a patient's needs through individualized combinations of physical, interpersonal, and environmental means. Rehabilitation counselors are oriented toward helping people focus on their functional capacities while keeping disability in perspective, effect change in their environment, and attain or regain participation in careers. They approach evaluation and intervention through counseling, situational and standardized assessment, case management, and advocacy. Table 51-2 summarizes some of the key concerns of each profession in the context of patient capabilities. Further clarification of the two professions may be gained through understanding their academic preparation and scholarly pursuits.

OCCUPATIONAL THERAPY EDUCATION AND RESEARCH

Occupational therapy practitioners are graduates of master's, bachelor's, or associate's degree programs and may be designated as registered occupational therapists (OTRs) or certified occupational therapy assistants (COTAs). Beginning in 2007, all entering OTRs will have master's degrees; COTAs will continue with the associate's degree. Occupational therapy educational programs are accredited by the American Occupational Therapy Association (AOTA) and certification is regulated by the National Board of Occupational Therapy Examination. Most states license occupational therapy practitioners and may require passage of an examination or other evidence of continuing competency to obtain and maintain the right to practice.

OTRs have passed curricula that include basic arts and sciences; human anatomy, physiology, and neurology; kinesiology; human growth and development;

Table 51-1. U.S. Federal Legislation That Has Affected Rehabilitation

Legislation	Summary
Rehabilitation Act of 1973	Prohibits discrimination on the basis of handicap under any program or activity receiving federal financial assistance
Education for All Handicapped Children Act (PL 94-142); 1975	Mandates that all children receive a free, appropriate public education in the least restrictive environment possible, regardless of the level or severity of their disability; provides funds to assist states in the education of students with disabilities and requires that states make sure that these students receive an individualized education program based on their unique needs
Handicapped Infants and Toddlers Act (PL 99-457); 1986	Extended PL 94-142 to infants and to ages 3–5 yr; calls for a coordinated, interagency, multidisciplinary approach
Amendments to the Rehabilitation Act of 1973 (PL 99-506); 1986	Requires all states to include provision for assistive technology services and mandates equal access to electronic office equipment for all federal employees
Americans with Disabilities Act (ADA) (PL 101-336); 1990	Civil rights act for disabled citizens in terms of public accommodation, private employment, transportation, and telecommunications
Individuals with Disabilities Education Act (PL 101-476); 1991	Continues the mandates initiated in PL 94-142; adds assistive technology and transition planning for post–high school work, educational and lifestyle decisions

TABLE 51-2. Patient Capabilities Contributing to Success in Rehabilitation Counseling and Occupational Therapy*

Patient capabilities	Rehabilitation counseling	Occupational therapy
Language skills: verbal, written or signing	×	
Potential for supported or competitive work	×	
Potential for engagement in assisted or independent self-care, productive activity, or leisure, now or in the future		×
Able to benefit from a program of experiences and/or environmental modifications designed to increase orientation to the environment and progress toward occupational performance in the areas of self-care, productive activity, and/or leisure		×
Patient or patient's guardian/identified advocate is able to identify occupational performance goals that are considered to be attainable by the patient.		×

*This table is intended as a general guideline for making decisions about referrals for rehabilitation services. Occupational therapy and rehabilitation counseling practitioners should be consulted when making decisions about referral for individual patients.

basic and abnormal psychology; occupational therapy theory; occupational therapy intervention; and research. Many educational programs also emphasize health care management, community intervention, interpersonal communication, program development and evaluation, and research skills. All graduates have passed 24 weeks of full-time internship before they can take the national certification examination.

Occupational therapy as a profession has, over the past decade, experienced rapid development and a paradigm shift related to changes in health care and society in general. These changes reflect not so much a radical departure from earlier values, but a recommitment to the founding values of the profession (Meyer, 1922; Royeen, 1995). A central theme has been a deliberate and concerted movement toward ensuring that intervention results in improved performance in activities that are valued by the patient (Wood et al., 2000) and that intervention methods themselves be meaningful and purposeful to the patient (Gray, 1998; AOTA, 1999; Pierce, 2001). Contemporary occupational therapists consider not only the patient as an individual, but also the patient's social, cultural, physical, economic, and political environments as key aspects of the clinical formulation (Dunn et al., 1994; Letts et al., 1994). This multifaceted approach is evident in evaluation and intervention processes that consider factors related not only to the person's pathology and disability, but also the person's strengths, values and interests, personal priorities, resources, and environmental barriers (Moyers, 1999). The goal of intervention is often to improve the environment's ability to support the individual toward meeting personal goals, rather than to change the patient. To do this, occupational therapy evaluation and intervention are increasingly being delivered in homes,

schools, childcare centers, homeless shelters, businesses, and other community settings. This is illustrated in the case examples that follow later in this chapter.

Research in occupational therapy reflects many of the trends evident throughout health care and society. These trends include an increased desire for evidence of the effectiveness of various assessments and interventions (Chakerian & Larson, 1993; Holm, 2000; Shu-Kei Cheng, 2000), an emphasis on patients' rights and responsibilities as directors of their care teams (Law, 1998), the promotion of health and wellness (Larson & Fanchiang, 1996; Clark et al., 1997), and the consideration of life satisfaction as a key measure of therapeutic success (Burleigh et al., 1998). In addition to empirical designs, qualitative research methods have become more widely used and accepted as legitimate ways of gaining knowledge that is crucial to understanding patients' experiences of disability and intervention (Bedell, 2000; Tham et al., 2000), and practitioners' experiences and ways of reasoning (Fleming & Mattingly, 1994; Velde, 2000). Another source of relevant research comes from the realm of occupational science, a scholarly discipline that has grown from a melding of academic occupational therapy and anthropology (Yerxa et al., 1989). Such studies include investigations of the forms and meanings of human occupation in persons with and without disabilities.

REHABILITATION COUNSELING EDUCATION AND RESEARCH

In 1954, the federal government recognized the need to capture, to the fullest extent possible, the resources found in people with disabilities. The 1954 Vocational Rehabilitation Act amendments provided for research grants to develop knowledge in vocational rehabilitation and gave federal fellowships to students who chose to enter a master's degree program in rehabilitation counseling. Through the 1954 amendments the federal government gave impetus for the professionalization of rehabilitation counseling (Parker & Syzmanski, 1998; Rubin & Roessler, 2001).

The standard for education for the professional rehabilitation counselor is a master's degree in rehabilitation counseling with a minimum of 48 graduate credits. Students complete a 600-hour supervised internship in the field as part of the graduate program. The Council on Rehabilitation Education (CORE) defines the standards of professional graduate education (CORE, 2000). Rehabilitation counselors receive advanced education in the following areas: counseling, advocacy, group and family dynamics, comprehensive assessment, medical aspects of disability, the psychosocial dynamics of disabling conditions, the functional requirements for work and independent living, benefits analysis, career development, work requirements, vocational evaluation, the job placement process, and the total system for rehabilitation services, including understanding the roles of various other rehabilitation professionals. With successful completion of a master's degree from a CORE-accredited program, the graduate meets the educational requirement for national certification as a rehabilitation counselor (CRC) and state licensing for those states that require it.

Universities and colleges have shaped the profession of rehabilitation counseling by offering graduate education with a solid clinical counseling foundation and the practical knowledge and skills needed to assist individuals with disabilities in achieving their goals. Rehabilitation counselors are prepared to work in a variety of settings, including state agencies, private for-profit rehabilitation agencies, nonprofit social service and rehabilitation agencies, hospitals, psychiatric rehabilitation centers, school systems, colleges and universities, correctional facilities, probation programs, substance abuse programs, corporations and businesses, and in private practice. Through the counseling relationship, the rehabilitation counselor creates a working alliance with the individual. The goals in rehabilitation counseling are for the person to gain important knowledge of self, the environment, resources, and skills necessary for achievement of rehabilitation goals in the areas of work, independent living, and inclusion.

Current research initiatives in rehabilitation counseling include: (1) exploration of the critical factors for engaging persons of diverse cultural background in maintaining rehabilitation efforts (Harley, 2000; Middleton et al., 2000; Marini, 2001), (2) effective intervention strategies (Patterson et al., 2000; Currier et al., 2001;), (3) worker expectations (Chase et al., 2000; Roessler, 2001;), (4) employer-worker relationships

(Habeck et al., 1998; Balser et al., 2000; Gilbride et al., 2000; Hernandez et al., 2000), (5) worker-worker relationships (Kirsh, 2000), (6) psychosocial aspects of the workplace (Merz et al., 2001), (7) attitudes toward disability (Garske & Stewart, 1999; Williams et al., 2000; Wilson, 2000; Wolf-Branigin et al., 2000), (8) self-perception of the individual with disability (Marty et al., 2000; McReynolds, 2001), (9) benefits analysis and work (Marini & Reid, 2001), (10) effective use of assistive technology (Denson, 2000; Holmes et al., 2000; Patterson, 2000, Riemer-Reiss, 2000), and (11) the functional roles of the rehabilitation counselor (Scully et al., 1999; Bolton, 2001; Thielson & Leahy, 2001).

CASE DISCUSSIONS

The following case examples have been designed to illustrate and clarify some of the ways that occupational therapists and rehabilitation counselors assist persons with neurologic impairments. They are intended to reflect issues that present at various points in the life span and some of the ways that evaluation and intervention may be approached.

DEVELOPMENTAL DISORDER IN A SOCIALLY DISADVANTAGED FAMILY: CASE EXAMPLE

Sami is a 27-month-old girl who has been hospitalized repeatedly for health complications that include a history of failure to thrive. Recently, she was evaluated by a pediatric neurologist, who diagnosed autistic spectrum disorder.

Sami is a restless, active toddler who prefers interacting with objects to interacting with people. She arches her back and cries when lifted and cuddled and avoids looking at peoples' faces. Her affect is flat unless she is intruded on by an adult. She eats inefficiently and derives little enjoyment from food. When left to her own devices, Sami sits and rocks herself in a remote corner of the room, briefly touching objects but not exploring or playing with anything. She does not vocalize or respond to verbal communication, but she does approach her mother when her mother sings favorite songs.

Sami's mother, Lydia, is a 17-year-old who has a severe learning disability and left high school in her junior year. She lived with Sami's father for a time, but moved into her own place because he beat her while she was pregnant with Sami. Lydia has no family support and few friends. She currently receives welfare funding but wants very much to be self-supporting.

Occupational Therapy Intervention

The American Association of Pediatric Neurology and Child Neurology Society has stated that occupational therapy should be involved in evaluating and treating children with autistic spectrum disorders who evidence deficits in sensory processing or daily living skills (American Academy of Pediatrics, 2001). The occupational therapist might come into contact with this family within the hospital system or through government-funded early childhood intervention (ECI) services. By taking a person-environment-occupation approach (Letts et al., 1994) to this case, the therapist would note that concerns about Sami include her problems with social interaction, eating, and playing, and an inability to self-regulate in a manner that allows her to engage in these activities. Assessments that could help to answer questions as to the nature of these problems include the Hawaii Early Learning Profile (Furuno et al., 1997), the Bayley Scales of Infant Development-II (Bayley, 1993), the Peabody Developmental Motor Scales-II (Folio & Fewell, 2000), or the Test of Sensory Function in Infants (DeGangi, 1988). Clinical observations of Sami's eating behaviors, responses to various sensations, and movement patterns would also be made, and Lydia would be asked to describe Sami's general routines and behaviors.

Lydia is a very young, inexperienced mother who has no natural social support system and has a child with special needs. She is the most influential aspect of Sami's environment, and her competence and motivation determine Sami's safety and quality of life. From an ECI perspective, Lydia is a patient in her own right, because ECI is designed to take a family-centered approach to care (Stephens & Tauber, 2001). Lydia's and Sami's interactions related to feeding, interpersonal relating, and the tasks that comprise infant care could be evaluated through naturalistic observation. In addition, Lydia's occupational health and satisfaction could be explored using the second edition of the Canadian Occupational Performance Measure (Law et al., 1994) or the Occupational Performance History Interview-II (Kielhofner et al., 1998).

Occupational therapy intervention for Sami and Lydia would focus on the identified areas of need. The practitioner might work directly with Sami to establish how to best position her for eating, social interaction, and play. Lydia might benefit from parenting education regarding what to expect from Sami, considering her developmental level, ways to feed her effectively, and why and how to engage Sami in social interaction and play.

Techniques to help Sami become more behaviorally organized, calm, and purposeful would be established and taught to Lydia. After learning about Lydia's interests and lifestyle the occupational therapist might conclude that she would benefit from engagement in paid work; this would best be achieved by referring her to resources for adults who need job preparation and placement, such as vocational rehabilitation. Lydia would also benefit from increased social support and interaction. This might be achieved through discussion with the therapist regarding resources that are available to all community members, such as parenting support groups, churches, and social clubs. If Lydia has special needs that affect her ability to initiate or participate in community activities she would benefit from referral to counseling or other social services.

Rehabilitation Counseling Intervention

Sami, at 27 months old, would not be engaged in a traditional counseling relationship. Behavioral and developmental assessments and interventions would be provided by neurologists, neuropsychologists, developmental psychologists, or occupational therapists. However, the skills and knowledge of a rehabilitation counselor can provide important resources for this family system. Lydia's diagnosis of learning disability would qualify her for rehabilitation counseling services through her state's Department of Vocational Rehabilitation. Alternatively, a rehabilitation counselor might work with Lydia via the hospital or a community-based social service agency.

Lydia has expressed the desire to work. A benefits analysis can be undertaken, giving Lydia important information regarding her present financial support system and the implications for her return to work. At the time when it is feasible, a vocational assessment through interviewing, job history analysis, possible interest testing and evaluation of abilities through standardized testing, or situational assessments could help to identify vocational opportunities for Lydia. She could be encouraged to complete her general equivalency diploma from high school, and training could be provided through actual on-the-job experience or further formal education. As needed, resources for child day care would be identified.

In addition to addressing vocational needs, a rehabilitation counselor could provide basic short-term counseling intervention to help assess Lydia's psychological readiness to deal with her current situation. Lydia is a candidate for a counseling relationship that helps her focus on her reactions to the health issues of her child, her history with abuse and the traumatic effects of the abuse by Sami's father, her isolation, and her plans for the future. If long-term counseling were needed, the rehabilitation counselor would most likely refer her to a therapist for individual or group counseling. When appropriate, the rehabilitation counselor can facilitate Lydia's exploration of community resources to reduce the sense of isolation.

Case Summary

Families often have complex needs that span medical, social, and economic issues, as the case illustrates. Many times the social and economic concerns have a direct and deleterious effect on the patient's medical condition and must be addressed if wellness is to be achieved. By involving rehabilitation professionals such as occupational therapists and vocational rehabilitation counselors in the care process, these needs can be approached in a concerted effort.

TRAUMATIC BRAIN INJURY IN YOUNG ADULTHOOD: CASE EXAMPLE

John is a 21-year-old man who is entering a transitional living center for persons who are recovering from traumatic brain injuries (TBIs). One year ago John fell from a second-story balcony during a party. He sustained injuries affecting frontal, prefrontal, and occipital areas. He was hospitalized for a few days and then released to home with outpatient medical follow-up and prophylactic antiseizure medication.

John is the oldest of four sons and the first in his family to attend college. He grew up working on his family's farm, but left for college with aspirations of becoming an architect. He earned high grades in college, even while holding down a part-time job. He enjoyed dating and hoped to "find the right girl" before too long. His leisure time consisted of playing video games, playing softball, and listening to popular music.

John has been unable to return to college due to persisting problems. He does not take care of personal hygiene and grooming without firm directives from family members. He spends his days watching television and eating junk food. John expresses a desire to return to college but has done nothing toward enrolling in classes. He is extremely irritable and has punched holes in the walls of his room. Each time friends have visited or called he has chatted only briefly, then returned to watching television. When reading he often rubs his eyes and quickly loses interest. John's parents are disappointed, perplexed, and wondering what they have done wrong to have such a wayward child. When asked about his plans for the future John mumbled, "I'm going to be an architect, butthead!"

Rehabilitation Counseling Intervention

John is a candidate for rehabilitation counseling services through the state Office of Vocational Rehabilitation. John has a disability that interferes with functioning for work and independent living. It is assumed that John will be able to work, given appropriate assistance. It is also possible that John should be seen by a rehabilitation counselor at the transitional living center with similar goals.

John's current reactions suggest the need for a full assessment of the emotional and neuropsychological actors affecting his adaptation and performance. Referral for a neuropsychological assessment would seem appropriate with specific attention to understanding functional capacity, depressive symptoms, and irritability. An eye and vision assessment is recommended to determine the presence of visual acuity or perception deficits and whether corrective intervention is possible.

Traditionally, the rehabilitation counselor in a state vocational rehabilitation office would work with John regarding his education and career plans. Although John holds firm to becoming an architect, he needs to take part in an assessment process to help him examine his current level of functioning and the implications for his present career goals. The rehabilitation counselor and John need to examine John's reasons for choosing architecture as a career goal, his work history, current functional capacity, and general interests. If it becomes evident that John should change career goals he will be helped to look at realistic alternatives that fit his interests. If he is able to pursue being an architect, John will need appropriate accommodations and coping skills to handle the limitations caused by his disability. Once a realistic career goal is established, the rehabilitation counselor can assist John with obtaining training and education, situational internship/work experiences, and appropriate ongoing support for work.

Loss is a major part of John's current experience as he adjusts to his disability. Counseling is recommended to assist him in examining his reactions, expressing his anger, and dealing with his apparent depression. John will benefit from working with a counselor who actively listens and who can provide him with a sense of hope that his life can continue in a productive way and in a manner that allows him to have important relationships. Depending on the job role of the rehabilitation counselor, John may see the rehabilitation counselor for this or he could be referred to another, more long-term counselor.

Occupational Therapy Intervention

Occupational therapy intervention would begin by evaluating John's current lifestyle and comparing this with his hopes and wishes. Interviews and observations would help the practitioner and John develop a sense of how he is spending his time and how satisfying and functional this is for him and his family. By reviewing the evaluations of the neurologists, neuropsychologists, and optometrists, the occupational therapist could estimate the contribution of cognitive and visual deficits to John's current behavior. John's past and present interests could be identified through checklist tools or structured interviews, such as the Occupational Performance History Interview II (Kielhofner et al., 1998). Motor control and cognitive skills needed for complex task performance could be measured with standardized tools, such as the Assessment of Motor and Processing Skills (Fisher, 1997). Fine- and gross-motor skills, sensory processing, and functional cognition would be evaluated as indicated, possibly as part of a driving assessment.

The resultant information would be shared with John in a collaborative effort to develop intervention goals and methods that fit his priorities and life circumstances. Intervention would focus on John's learning and practicing needed skills in a variety of natural contexts and with assistive devices or modifications as appropriate. For example, John might use an occupational therapy session to make a wall chart that provides visual cues regarding the sequence of tasks for his morning grooming and dressing routine, if evaluation indicated that cognitive deficits were a cause of his ineffective self-care. On the other hand, if John's problem appeared to be more emotional or motivational than cognitive, the occupational therapy practitioner might take another approach. For example, if John indicated that he would like to go to a sporting event or out for a meal, the practitioner would help him strategize the logistics of doing this and encourage appropriate self-care as a part of such an activity. The occupational therapist would observe John for signs and symptoms of mental disorders such as clinical depression or chemical abuse and would report such concerns to the referring physician.

Case Summary

The complex problems presented by this type of patient require responses at multiple levels if he is to achieve the quality of life that he wants and of which he is capable. The patient, rehabilitation counselor, occupational therapist, physician, and family each play unique and essential roles in determining the kind of lifestyle that John will have. The difference between failure and success in doing this is as vast as that between living an indigent existence and functioning as a respected and productive member of the community.

AGING, HEALTH, AND QUALITY OF LIFE

A great challenge for health care providers and researchers is how to ensure that the quality of life is expanded into the aging process. As capabilities change due to illness, aging, or decreasing interest in activities, older adults may require interventions in lifestyle redesign to prevent depression and further decline in activities of daily living (eating, bathing, and dressing) and instrumental activities of daily living (community activities). Neurologists may hear concerns from caregivers that an individual recovering from a neurologic condition seems depressed. Complicating psychosocial factors coupled with physical pathology may result in symptoms in common with clinical depression. Often, depression medication may be prescribed without addressing environmental and psychological factors, such as social isolation or decreasing abilities, which may contribute significantly to the problem. Barkin and colleagues (2000) report that antidepressant pharmacotherapy combined with cognitive and behavioral therapy appears to offer the most benefit to the patient.

Clark and colleagues (1997) used a process of occupational self-analysis and occupational redesign in the Well Elderly Research Study as an intervention for older adults. Through this program older adults learned how the quality of their daily occupations contributed to health and life satisfaction. This knowledge, together with the reflective skills needed to analyze their own occupational patterns, prepared the elders to identify how what one does during the day contributes to perceived quality of life. This approach showed a significantly positive effect on mental health in this study sample and may be useful to older adults who have chronic neurologic disease in preventing depression.

Another approach to enhancing quality of life in older adults is through education in the uses of technology. Technology may compensate for loss of ability and enable the older adult to return to active participation in meaningful occupations, such as self-care, independent driving, reading through low-vision aids, engagement in recreation and leisure activities, household management, and paid or volunteer work. Consider the following case study that illustrates the concepts discussed in this section.

REHABILITATION AFTER A CEREBROVASCULAR ACCIDENT: CASE EXAMPLE

Mrs. King is an African American woman aged 68 years; she was discharged from the hospital after a minor stroke, which left her with weakness and reduced fine-motor coordination in her left hand. Before her stroke she lived alone, drove, and worked as an office manager for a small construction company. Although her employer has expressed concerns about her ability to safely come back to the office, Mrs. King is determined to return to her job.

Rehabilitation Counseling Intervention

The hospital social worker referred Mrs. King to a rehabilitation counselor to help define an appropriate discharge plan. The rehabilitation counselor interviewed Mrs. King alone and with her daughter to determine her living and work history. Given Mrs. King's permission, the rehabilitation counselor also contacted her employer to evaluate the potential for Mrs. King to return to her previous job. During this contact the rehabilitation counselor answered questions that the employer had about the law as it is outlined in the Americans with Disabilities Act. Based on the ensuing information, the rehabilitation counselor determined that the work environment should be assessed to determine what modifications or accommodations were necessary. This was referred to an occupational therapist. The rehabilitation counselor and occupational therapist then worked together to effect the necessary changes for work and living.

Occupational Therapy Intervention

The occupational therapist working with Mrs. King evaluated her motor and cognitive abilities and determined their degree of fit with her environments and daily tasks. To continue working, Mrs. King needed a speaker-phone, built-up writing utensils, and adaptations to her computer, which she used to enter data on a spreadsheet and type business letters. These adaptations included specialized software to compensate for her inability to release the keys quickly enough to prevent them repeating and her tendency to accidentally hit the wrong keys.

Despite her successful return to work, Mrs. King became despondent and discouraged. Her daughter accompanied her to a follow-up medical visit and expressed her concerns. Through the interview process, it was discovered that

Mrs. King was upset by her inability to participate in her usual social activities because she lacked transportation. The roads around her home had undergone major rerouting and construction and she was fearful of venturing out independently. The physician gave Mrs. King a referral for an occupational driving evaluation, the results of which reflected problems with strength, control, and anxiety. Mrs. King attended 6 hours of training, during which she learned to drive with a spinner knob to compensate for her loss of hand strength. Mrs. King conquered her anxiety about driving on the newly designed roads by repeatedly driving with the occupational therapist to the various destinations that Mrs. King desired to frequent. By the end of training, Mrs. King was able to take herself to work and her social activities and reported feeling "my old self again."

Case Summary

In this case both a successful return to work and satisfactory social and community mobility levels were essential to achievement of full rehabilitation. Older adults may ask family and friends for transportation to work, church, and medical appointments, yet they may not ask for rides to leisure and social activities because they view them as nonessential luxuries. They feel that this assistance with community mobility may be too burdensome for family and friends to provide. Health care providers must use a patient-centered evaluation process to identify those activities that are key to each individual's quality of life.

CONCLUSION

The rehabilitation professions of occupational therapy and rehabilitation counseling represent part of the continuum of care that begins with the physician and medical team. Just as the lifesaving and sustaining efforts of the medical team are essential to life, so are the skills and knowledge of rehabilitation professions essential to achievement of quality and purpose in life. The physician team leader who understands the roles and expertise of these professionals is ideally positioned to identify when patients can benefit from rehabilitation counseling or occupational therapy and to facilitate their access to these valuable services.

■ KEY POINTS

☐ Through advances in technology, social evolution, and legislative progress, persons with disabilities can become active members of the community.

☐ Occupational therapists and rehabilitation counselors represent unique professions that work together to promote the full inclusion and participation of individuals with disabilities.

☐ Occupational therapists and rehabilitation counselors engage in processes of clinical reasoning that begin with the patient's goals and wishes and consider the complex interactions of multiple factors in planning outcomes and interventions.

☐ The primary focus of occupational therapy is the attainment of levels of occupational performance that are satisfactory to the patient and his significant others. This includes participation in self-care, productive activities such as paid work, childcare, household responsibilities, and leisure.

☐ The primary goals of rehabilitation counseling are inclusion, independent living, and work.

KEY READINGS

Case-Smith J (ed): Occupational Therapy for Children, ed 4. St. Louis: Mosby, 2001.

Trombly CA, Vining Radomski M (eds): Occupational Therapy for Physical Dysfunction. Baltimore: Lippincott Williams & Wilkins, 2002.

Rumrill PD Jr, Bellini JL, Koch LC: Emerging Issues in Rehabilitation Counseling: Perspectives on the New Millennium. Springfield, IL: Charles C Thomas, 2001.

REFERENCES

American Academy of Pediatrics, Committee on Children With Disabilities: Technical report: The pediatrician's role in the diagnosis and management of autistic spectrum disorder in children. Pediatrics 107:1221–1226, 2001.

American Occupational Therapy Association: Definition of OT Practice for the AOTA Model Practice Act. Am J Occup Ther 53:608, 1999.

Balser RM, Hagner D, Hornby H: Partnership with the business community: The Mental Health Employer Consortium. J Appl Rehabil Counsel 31:47–53, 2000.

Barkin RL, Schwer WA, Barkin SJ: Recognition and management of depression in primary care: A focus on the elderly. A pharmacotherapeutic overview of the selection process among the traditional and new antidepressants. Am J Ther 7:205–226, 2000.

Bayley N: Bayley Scales of Infant Development, ed 2. San Antonio, TX: The Psychological Corporation, 1993.

Bedell G: Daily lie for eight urban gay men with HIV/AIDS. Am J Occup Ther 54:197–206, 2000.

Bolton B: Measuring rehabilitation outcomes. Rehabil Counsel Bull 44:67–75, 2001.

Burleigh S, Farber R, Gillard M: Community integration and life satisfaction after traumatic brain injury: Long-term findings. Am J Occup Ther 52:45–52, 1998.

Chakarian D, Larson M: Effects of upper-extremity weight-bearing on hand-opening and prehension patterns in children with cerebral palsy. Dev Med Child Neurol 35:216–229, 1993.

Chase BW, Corville TA, English RW: Life satisfaction among persons with spinal cord injuries. J Rehabil 66:14–20, 2000.

Clark F, Azen S, Zemke R, et al: Occupational therapy for independent-living older adults: A randomized controlled trial. JAMA 278:1321–1326, 1997.

Council on Rehabilitation Education: Standards for rehabilitation counselor education programs. March 20, 2000. Retrieved August 20, 2001 from http://www.core-rehab.org/manual/manual.html#standardsRCEP.

Currier KF, Chan F, Berven NL, et al: Functions and knowledge domains for disability management practice: A Delphi study. Rehabil Counsel Bull 44:133–143, 2001.

DeGangi G: Test of Sensory Function in Infants. Los Angeles: Western Psychological Services, 1998.

Denson CR: Public sector transportation for people with disabilities: A satisfaction survey. J Rehabil 66:29–37, 2000.

Dunn W, Brown C, McGuigan A: The ecology of human performance: A framework for considering the effect of context. Am J Occup Ther 48:595–607, 1994.

Fisher A: Assessment of Motor and Process Skills, ed 3. Fort Collins, CO: Three Star Press, 1999.

Fleming M, Mattingly C: Clinical Reasoning: Forms of Inquiry in a Therapeutic Practice. Philadelphia, PA: F.A. Davis, 1994.

Folio M, Fewell R: Peabody Developmental Motor Scales. Austin, TX: Pro-Ed, 2000.

Furuno S, O'Reilly K, Hosaka C, et al: The Hawaii Early Learning Profile. Palo Alto, CA: Vort, 1997.

Garske GG, Stewart JR: Stigmatic and mythical thinking: Barriers of vocational rehabilitation service for persons with severe mental illness. J Rehabil 65:4–8, 1999.

Gilbride D, Stensrud R, Ehlers C, et al: Employers' attitudes toward hiring persons with disabilities and vocational rehabilitation services. J Rehabil 66:17–23, 2000.

Gray JM: Putting occupation into practice: Occupation as ends, occupation as means. Am J Occup Ther 52:354–364, 1998.

Habeck RV, Scully SM, VanTol B, et al: Successful employer strategies for preventing and managing disability. Rehabil Counsel Bull 42:144–161, 1998.

Harley D (ed): Cultural diversity [special issue]. J Appl Rehabil Counsel 31, 2000.

Hernandez B, Keys C, Balcazar F: Employer attitudes toward workers with disabilities and their ADA employment rights: A literature review. J Rehabil 66:4–16, 2000.

Holm M: Our mandate for the new millennium: Evidence-based practice. Am J Occup Ther 54:575–597, 2000.

Holmes AE, Kaplan HS, Saxon JP: Assistive listening devices and systems: Amplification technology for consumers with hearing loss. J Rehabil 66:56–62, 2000.

Kielhofner G, Mallinson T, Crawford C, et al: The Occupational Performance History Interview, Version 2.0. Chicago: University of Illinois, 1998.

Kirsh B: Work, workers and workplaces: A qualitative analysis of narratives of mental health consumers. J Rehabil 66:24–30, 2000.

Larson E, Fanchiang S-P: Nationally speaking: Life history and narrative research: Generating a human knowledge base for occupational therapy. Am J Occup Ther 50:247–250, 1996.

Law M (ed): Client-Centred Occupational Therapy. Thorofare, NJ: Slack, 1998.

Law M, Baptiste S, Carswell A, et al: Canadian Occupational Performance Measure, ed 2. Ottawa, Ontario: Canadian Association of Occupational Therapists, 1994.

Letts L, Law M, Rigby P, et al: Person-environment assessments in occupational therapy. Am J Occup Ther 48:608–618, 1994.

Marini I: Cross cultural counseling issues of males who sustain a disability. J Appl Rehabil Counsel 32:36–44, 2001.

Marini I, Reid CR: A survey of rehabilitation professionals as alternative provider contractors with Social Security: Problems and solutions. J Rehabil 67:36–41, 2001.

Marty E, Livneh H, Turpin J: Locus of control orientation and acceptance of disability. J Appl Rehabil Counsel 31:14–21, 2000.

McReynolds CJ: The meaning of work in the lives of people living with HIV disease and AIDS. Rehabil Counsel Bull 44: 104–115, 2001.

Merz MA, Bricourt J, Koch LC, et al: Psychosocial characteristics of the new American workplace: Implications for job development and placement, in Rumrill PD Jr, Bellini JL, Koch LC (eds): Emerging Issues in Rehabilitation Counseling: Perspectives in the New Millennium. Springfield, IL: Charles C Thomas, 2001, pp. 127–147.

Meyer A: The philosophy of occupational therapy. Arch Occup Ther 1:1–10, 1922.

Middleton RA, Rollins CW, Sanderson PL, et al: Endorsement of professional multicultural rehabilitation competencies and standards: A call to action. Rehabil Counsel Bull 43: 219–240, 2000.

Moyers P: The guide to occupational therapy practice. Am J Occup Ther 53:247–297, 1999.

Parker RM, Szymanski EM (eds): Rehabilitation Counseling: Basics and Beyond. Austin, TX: Pro-Ed, 1998.

Patterson JB: Using the Internet to facilitate the rehabilitation process. J Rehabil 66:4–10, 2000.

Patterson JB, Allen TB, Parnell L, et al: Equitable treatment in the rehabilitation process: Implications for future investigations related to ethnicity. J Rehabil 66:14–18, 2000.

Pierce D: Occupation by design: Dimensions, therapeutic power, and creative process. Am J Occup Ther 55:249–259, 2001.

Riemer-Reiss ML: Factors associated with assistive technology discontinuance among individuals with disabilities. J Rehabil 66:44–50, 2000.

Roessler RT: Job retention services for employees with spinal cord injuries: A critical need in vocational rehabilitation. J Appl Rehabil Counsel 32:3–9, 2001.

Royeen C (ed): The Practice of the Future: Putting Occupation Back into Therapy. Bethesda, MD: American Occupational Therapy Association, 1999.

Rubin SE, Roessler RT: Foundations of the Vocational Rehabilitation Process, ed 5. Austin, TX: Pro-Ed, 2001.

Scully SM, Habeck RV, Leahy MJ: Knowledge and skill areas associated with disability management practice for rehabilitation counselors. Rehabil Counsel Bull 43:20–29, 1999.

Shu-Kei Cheng A: Use of early tactile stimulation in rehabilitation of digital nerve injuries. Am J Occup Ther 54:159–165, 2000.

Stephens L, Tauber S: Early intervention, in Case-Smith J (ed): Occupational Therapy for Children, ed 4. St. Louis: Mosby, 2001, pp. 708–730.

Tham K, Borell L, Gustavasson A: The discovery of disability: A phenomenological study of unilateral neglect. Am J Occup Ther 55:398–406, 2000.

Thielson VA, Leahy MJ: Essential knowledge and skills for effective clinical supervision in rehabilitation counseling. Rehabil Counsel Bull 44:196–208, 2001.

Velde B: The experience of being an occupational therapist with a disability. Am J Occup Ther 54:183–188, 2000.

Williams DT, Hershenson DB, Fabian ES: Causal attributions of disabilities and the choice of rehabilitation approach. Rehabil Counsel Bull 43:106–113, 2000.

Wilson KB: Predicting vocational rehabilitation acceptance based on race, education, work status and source of support. Rehabil Counsel Bull 43:97–105, 2000.

Wolf-Branigin M, Daeschlein M, Cardinal B, et al: Differing priorities of counselors and customers to a consumer choice model in rehabilitation. J Rehabil 66:18–22, 2000.

Wood W, Nielson C, Humphry R, et al: A curricular renaissance, graduate education centered on occupation. Am J Occup Ther 54:586–597, 2000.

Yerxa E, Clark F, Frank G, et al: An introduction to occupational science: A foundation for occupational therapy. Occup Ther Health Care 6:1–18, 1989.

VII

Forensics, Competence, Legal Issues

Competency, Power of Attorney, Informed Consent, Wills

Edward David

Capacity

Competency

Consent

Directive

Will

INTRODUCTION

Many neurologic conditions raise the question of patients' ability to conduct legal activities of daily living. This chapter looks at the issues of competency and capacity and how these concepts affect making decisions in several areas. These are areas in which a physician/health care provider may be asked to give an opinion or advise the patient or family on a certain course of action.

COMPETENCY AND CAPACITY

The law requires that an individual be competent for that individual's actions to hold force. Similarly, to be held accountable, a person must be found to be competent.

Legal definitions of competency tend to be vague. Individuals are considered *competent* when they possess "the requisite natural or legal qualifications" to "under-

stand the general nature and extent" of the issues before them (Black's Law Dictionary, 1979, p. 257). The definition is purposefully vague because competency as a concept is used in many different legal areas. Depending on the area, requirements may vary greatly.

The law strives to allow individuals their autonomy in decision-making efforts. Therefore, adequate cognitive or mental activity must be present to perform the particular legal task. This must not be confused with credibility. Competency refers to the personal qualifications of an individual, whereas credibility speaks to his or her truthfulness. A competent individual may make incredible demands or statements. Conversely, an incompetent individual's statements and demands may appear perfectly credible.

Another legal concept that is frequently mistaken or interchanged with competency is capacity. *Capacity* refers to "legal qualification" including "competency, power or fitness." It is the individual's ability to "understand the nature and effect of one's acts" (Black's Law Dictionary, 1979, p. 188). Capacity is legally defined for many human activities. As an example, to make a will, an individual must "know the natural objects of his bounty, comprehend the kind and character of his property, the nature and effect of his act, and make a disposition of his property according to some plan formed in his mind" (Am. Jur. 2d, §71, 1962). An individual who fails this test of capacity can then be termed incompetent. A person considered legally incompetent is considered by the law to be mentally incapable of performing the act for which he or she lacks capacity. Thus, a finding of incompetence is specific to the subject or tasks under review. Someone incompetent to make a will could be found competent to testify in a court proceeding.

A diagnosis of psychiatric or organic mental disease is not synonymous with incompetence. One cannot presume lack of capacity or incompetence based on diagnosis, treatment for mental illness, or institutionalization (*Rennie v Klein*, 1978). Significant mental illness, even acute psychosis, does not render an individual incompetent in all areas of functioning. An assessment must be made to determine solely whether the person is incapable of deciding or performing the particular task at hand (see Chapters 2 and 3). Individual autonomy demands that a person be allowed to make any decision for which he or she is capable even when seriously mentally ill (*Schloendorff v Society of New York Hospital*, 1914). A person with a mental illness may not lose the same legal power as adults who are not mentally ill until judicially declared incompetent.

A person accused of committing a crime might sometimes lack competency or capacity. For a discussion of these issues and relevant legal rules (e.g., the M'Naghten, or McNaughton, Rule), see Chapters 54 and 55.

INFORMED CONSENT

Informed consent is a legal principle first spelled out by the courts in the case of *Canterbury v Spence* (1972). The doctrine holds that a physician must disclose sufficient information to enable an intelligent choice. It implies joint decision making between the health care provider and the patient. The patient needs not only to be informed but also educated as to the nature of his or her condition and the various treatment options. The patient must be given all relevant information necessary to make an informed decision regarding treatment (Ad Hoc Committee on Medical Ethics, 1984). The doctrine further recognizes that patients have a right to know presumptive diagnoses, differential diagnoses, purposes of tests, treatment options, risks associated with treatment, alternatives to treatment, and the relative prognoses and expectations (*Canterbury v Spence*, 1972).

There are two types of risks of which the physician will be aware. The first is the "inherent risk." This is purely a medical concept and embodies any number of known adverse effects that may result from a diagnostic procedure, drug therapy, or surgical operation (*Sard v Hardy*, 1977).

The second type of risk and the one of significance in the doctrine of informed consent is "material" risk. A material risk is also an inherent risk, but it is one that a reasonable person would consider a significant factor in deciding whether or not to undergo a procedure or treatment (*Sard v Hardy*, 1977). The physician must disclose those inherent risks that are material, not all risks. The patient needs to know only what is material in making an informed choice.

The doctrine of informed consent presumes that the patient is competent and has the capacity to make the necessary decisions. Physical or mental incapacitation leading to incompetence presents the physician with a person unable to understand the nature and consequences of his or her actions and therefore unable to give valid informed consent. The mere fact, however, that the patient has a diagnosis of mental illness or even transitory episodes of nonlucidity may not mean that capacity to consent is absent. Similarly, the fact that the patient refuses what the physician feels is in his or her best interest does not equate with a lack of capacity and therefore incompetence.

Emergency care presents a specific situation where the courts recognize it may be impossible to obtain express informed consent. The courts also recognize that no surrogate decision maker or, in the case of a minor, parent, may be available within the time constraint of the emergency. Courts therefore assume that were the patient competent, he or she would consent to lifesaving treatment. The emergency must be documented. Treatment given must be for the patient's benefit and essential at that time. Treatment that could be medically advisable or even essential at some further time does not fall under the emergency exception.

Some patients with neurologic problems become subjects in clinical research studies and must be informed clearly of the risks and benefits of the proposed research, in written documents reviewed by a local human subjects review committee (an institutional review board [IRB]), and authorized to operate under the U.S. Department of Health and Human Services.

Informed consent as it relates to human subjects of biomedical research is governed by federal law found in Title 45 of the Code of Federal Regulations (CFR), Part 46, Protection of Human Subjects (45 CFR, Part 46). Section 46.116 says in part that "no investigator may involve a human being as a subject in research covered by this policy unless the investigator has obtained the legally effective informed consent of the subject or the subject's legal authorized representative."

Much of the current law surrounding medical research and informed consent grew out of the abuses discovered after World War II. It was discovered that Nazi doctors had performed horrific experiments on prisoners in concentration camps. Abuses, however, were also found in this country, most notably the Tuskegee experiment using black men as subjects to research the course of untreated syphilis.

Various codes, commissions, and declarations have dealt with the issue of biomedical research and informed consent since the Nuremberg trials. The first of these is the Nuremberg Code. It provides for voluntary consent as an absolute essential for experiments designed to yield results for the good of society based on prior animal experimentation. Experiments should be conducted so as to avoid any unnecessary physical or mental suffering and injury (Wecht, 2001)

The Declaration of Helsinki includes principles regarding the necessity of informed consent. This document has been modified many times by the world medical associations, beginning in 1975 and continuing to the present.

The IRBs are mandated by federal law and must examine closely issues of informed consent. Section 116(a) of the U.S. Code lays out eight elements of informed consent that must be adhered to in any biomedical research setting (45 CFR, Part 46). These are:

1. A statement that the study involves research, along with an explanation of the purposes of that research and the expected duration of the participation. There should be a description of the procedures to be followed and identification of those that are experimental.
2. A description of reasonably foreseeable risks.
3. A description of reasonably expected benefits, both to the subject and to others.
4. Disclosure of alternative procedures with courses of treatment, particularly those that might be advantageous to the subject.
5. Statements regarding confidentiality and how it will be protected in the records.
6. Issues of compensation or medical treatments if injury occurs resulting from involvement in the research project.
7. How to contact someone to answer questions regarding the research, the subject's rights, and any research-related injury.
8. A statement making it clear that the subject's participation is voluntary and that refusing to participate will have no retaliatory features, such as penalty or loss of benefits. There should also be a statement regarding discontinuation of participation, again without any retaliatory features.

Often an IRB may require in the informed consent document information on the number of subjects, any cost that a subject may incur because of participation, and the possible consequences to the project should the subject withdraw.

IRBs are required to deal with the issue of "vulnerable populations." These include children, pregnant women, prisoners, mentally disabled individuals, and those who are economically or educationally disadvantaged. These individuals are required to be given special consideration. Issues surrounding children are quite particular and extensive.

The U.S. Department of Health and Human Services realizes that emergency services present particular problems. An individual in a life-threatening or emergency situation would not understand or be able to consent to the various points that must be included in the research informed consent document. A waiver of the informed consent requirement for this particular situation is allowed. However, it must be shown that the research could not occur if the consent were required and that there are sufficient preclinical studies to support a direct benefit to the subject (Wecht, 2001).

When an individual lacks capacity, someone else becomes his or her decision maker. This individual is considered a surrogate and gives substituted consent. Such persons may be the closest known relative, a court-appointed guardian, or a person empowered to act on behalf of the patient under the terms of a written power of attorney.

There are problems associated with substituted consent. Consent implies the right not to consent. The right of refusal, however, has been restricted by the courts. The physician or institution can seek court authorization to proceed with treatment. Generally, the courts will consider two issues. The first is whether the treatment constitutes an emergency, and whether a demonstrable need to proceed exists before one can expect the patient to regain capacity. The second issue is whether the proposed treatment is appropriate for the patient's condition (*Superintendent of Belchertown State School v Saikewicz*, 1977).

Still more difficulty may arise if disagreement develops among the next of kin. This is particularly troublesome when those disagreeing have some standing, for example, both parents or among children. The greatest caution must be taken by the physician in these circumstances. Occasionally an individual felt to be incompetent by providers and family may still make a decision. Family members may view this as a demonstration of competency and capacity.

The best way to avoid these risks is to place the entire matter before a court. Most states have statutes allowing adult citizens of that state, including a relative, to petition the court for the establishment of a guardianship for the patient (18-A MRSA §5-506). The process is generally straightforward, with little cost involved. The court will weigh conflicts of interest in appointing the guardian.

POWER OF ATTORNEY

A durable power of attorney (DPOA) is one form of an advanced directive. Advanced directives were an outgrowth of the changing definition of death brought about by advances in medical technology. During the late 1950s and early 1960s, medicine became aware that some cases of cardiac arrest represented electrical dysfunction of the heart, particularly ventricular tachyarrhythmias. Maintenance of an airway and conversion of these rhythms could therefore return an individual from "death" to sentient existence. At the same time, however, a growing number of individuals were having successful resuscitation of cardiac or pulmonary function alone, without any return to consciousness. Testing revealed that in many of these individuals all brain function had ceased.

At the same time, great strides were being made in the field of organ transplantation. There was recognition that a new definition of death was needed both to prevent a charge of homicide in the community of health care providers and to allow the harvest of viable organs from "dead" individuals.

An ad hoc committee at the Harvard Medical School was the first to address this issue. The committee put forward a definition of brain death and criteria by which to determine it (Beecher, 1968). This work was followed by the appointment of a blue ribbon commission made up of health care researchers and practitioners, ethicists, attorneys, and public representatives (Report of the President's Commission, 1981). The commission urged all states to accept a Uniform Determination of Death Act. This would provide physicians with the necessary guidelines and protections to determine death on the basis of irreversible cessation of all functions of the entire brain.

Unfortunately, as resuscitative technology and life support technology improved, ever more ill and infirm individuals were being resuscitated where no hope of survival really existed. Most of these resuscitated individuals did not return to a cognitive state. Many individuals remained on ventilators because the criteria for brain death were not met and support could not be removed.

The right of an individual to refuse treatment had been accepted since Schloendorff (*Schloendorff v Society of New York Hospital*, 1914). These rights were grounded in the common law right of self-determination or the constitutional rights of privacy and liberty. What was necessary was an extension of these rights to the situation in which the withholding or withdrawing of treatment meant death.

The Cruzan case (*Cruzan v Director, Missouri Department of Health*, 1990) gave constitutional recognition to the right of a patient with capacity to refuse unwanted medical treatment. The court characterized the right as a protected liberty interest in refusing unwanted medical treatment.

The right of a competent individual to refuse life-sustaining treatment, even when not terminally ill, was upheld in the case of Elizabeth Boubia (*Elizabeth Boubia v Riverside General Hospital*, 1983). In this case, a young woman with so little use of voluntary muscles as to be unable to take her own life was allowed by the court to discontinue artificial feeding and so to die from lack of nutrition and hydration.

Legal theory supported an extension of the right of a competent individual to refuse treatment to the incompetent patient. However, exercising that right presented problems. Patients without capacity might be unable to express any treatment decision. Others, though able to verbalize, might be expressing preferences that were not really what they meant. This set of circumstances has led to the concept of the surrogate decision maker.

Surrogate decision making can be through a Living Will, Durable Power of Attorney, Appointment of Health Care Proxy, or any other legal device allowing a competent person to give directions concerning medical treatment to be given if they become incompetent (Robertson, 1991). The Patient Self-Determination Act was enacted by the United States in 1990. The act mandated health care institutions receiving federal funds to provide patients with written information regarding their rights under law to participate in the medical decision-making process and to execute an advanced directive.

The simplest and most direct of advanced directives is the living will. This document, however, is quite limiting. It takes effect only when the decision maker is terminally ill with no expectancy of recovery. It authorizes only the withdrawal or withholding of treatment in that circumstance. As such, it can only allow an individual to state that they do not wish heroic measures, including cardiopulmonary resuscitation, and it can allow for the removal of ventilators and other heroic measures that are merely prolonging life. There is no ability for the living will to function outside these limited circumstances. The DPOA for health care is a significantly more flexible document. A competent adult may appoint a surrogate decision maker. This individual is empowered to make health care decisions when the patient is unable to express his or her own wishes. It is legally enforceable and functions not only when the issue of life support or heroic measures arises, but in all treatment situations where the patient is unable to decide or communicate. The individual holding the DPOA can speak for the patient in accordance with the patient's instructions or previously expressed sentiments. If there is no guidance, however, the durable power may still be guided by the patient's best interests (Medicolegal Primer, 1991).

WILLS

It is an unfortunate aspect of the human condition that persons feel wronged when a will does not reward them as they would wish. Frequently the challenge brought is based on testamentary capacity. The physicians who were treating the deceased at the time that the will was made may find that their assessment of the individual's ability to make that will becomes critical information.

Four requirements are necessary in the formation of a valid will. These are testamentary intent; testamentary capacity; the absence of fraud, duress, undue influence, or mistake; and execution of the document in compliance with statutory finalities. The competency and capacity of the testator are crucial for a determination of intent and capacity.

An individual is said to have testamentary intent when the words executed are intended to operate as a will (*Re Kemp's Will*, 1936). There are three elements to testamentary intent. First, the maker of the document must have intended to dispose of his or her property. Secondly, the disposition of this property was to occur only on death. Finally, the individual must have intended that the writing in question accomplished that end (*Meek v Bledsoe*, 1953). Requisite intent is a question of fact. Examination of both the testator and the will are necessary. If the writing does not contain the requisite formalities of a will, the inquiry will go no further (*Estate of Pagel*, 1942).

Where the formalities of execution are present, it is up to the person seeking to prove otherwise to show that the testator lacked the necessary intent at the time an otherwise valid document was executed. The principal evidence relied on in this regard is the statements of the testator before and after execution. The statements are the strongest evidence to show that an individual did indeed regard the document as a will (*Estate of Sargavak*, 1950).

The mental condition of the testator is more frequently called into question in the matter of testamentary capacity. Competency to execute a will relates to specific legal requirements associated with the making of a will. A lack of testamentary capacity will result in a will being invalidated at probate. If a will is found to have no legal effect because of lack of testamentary capacity, state-specific statutory provisions will guide the division of a testator's estate. If present, a prior will guides distribution. Lacking a prior will, intestate succession will govern distribution as long as there are immediate family members. Where immediate family is lacking, the estate may escheat (revert) to the state itself.

Despite the passage of time and the increasing complexities of society, the elements of testamentary capacity for the majority of jurisdictions in the United States remain those found in the English case of *Banks v Goodfellow* (1879). The Banks tests have five parts. First, to make a valid will, one must be of sound mind, though he or she need not possess superior or even average mentality. One is of sound mind for testamentary purposes only when he or she can understand and carry in his or her mind in a general way: (1) the nature and extent of his or her property, (2) the persons who are the natural objects of his or her bounty, and (3) the disposition that he or she is making of his or her property. He or she must also be capable of: (4) appreciating these elements in relation to one another, and (5) forming an orderly desire as to the vivid disposition of his or her property.

The presence of a disability, mental illness, or addiction does not by itself invalidate testamentary capacity (Am. Jur. 2d, §§77–101). Absolute soundness of mind and memory in every respect is not essential. The law recognizes that there are degrees of mental unsoundness and that not every one of these is sufficient to destroy testamentary capacity (Am. Jur. 2d, §75). Testamentary capacity differs from the capacity necessary to transact ordinary business, execute a deed, or execute a contract

Testamentary capacity—indeed, the definition of capacity in any civil situation—differs from that used in criminal cases. The criminal law tests of capacity rely heavily on the defendant's power to distinguish right from wrong. The question of distinguishing right from wrong is not a salient issue when testing the validity of a will (*Slaughter v Heath*, 1907).

The presence of knowledge as to the actual size of one's estate may be the basis of questioning a will. Courts have concluded that the testator need not have all necessary information in his or her mind at any one time. It is sufficient that the testator retain facts long enough to have the will prepared and executed. This is a task that may take several days or weeks and many meetings with the preparer (attorney) (Am. Jur. 2d, §72). A testator who is mistaken as to how many nieces, nephews, or similar relatives he or she has may still be deemed to have a capacity. There are cases that conclude that an inability to name all of one's children in a will or failure to devise anything to them likewise shows no want of testamentary capacity (Am. Jur. 2d, §72).

Issues of the complexity and size of one's estate have led to diverse results regarding testamentary capacity. Some courts have been of the opinion that it requires less capacity to make a simple will than one containing complicated provisions. These authorities find that the capacity necessary to comprehend a few details is insufficient when dealing with a large estate or a will complicated by multiple provisions (*Campbell v Campbell*). Others, however, are of the view that testamentary capacity relates to the capacity to make a will regardless of its size or complexity (*Dilman v McDanel*).

Failure of memory by itself does not equate to testamentary incapacity. Although it is true that testamentary capacity requires sufficient memory to collect and hold in one's mind the particulars of one's bounty and to form a judgment as to their disposal, intermittent forgetfulness does not necessarily prevent one from making a will. In fact, an individual can be forgetful, unable to recognize persons and places, and at times have delusions, but if he or she knows what his or her property consists of and how he or she wants to dispose of it, he or she has capacity (*Hall v Perry*, 1895).

CONCLUSION

Patients with neurobehavioral impairments such as those outlined in Part IV of this book may not be competent; that is, they may lack the ability to understand the legal issues before them. These patients may be unable to make informed decisions relevant to their health care, research participation, financial contracts, or creation of a will. A patient's incapacities can be operationally defined in forensic assessments aimed at tests of cognition and executive functions. A patient's advanced directive may help guide care decisions when emergency treatment decisions are required, in combination with a family member or legal assistant who has the power-of-attorney. The behavioral neurologist or neuropsychologist must be prepared to help, especially when the patient's wishes are not known.

■ KEY POINTS

☐   Competency varies according to the capacity needed for a specific action.

☐   Informed consent requires a physician to disclose sufficient information for a patient to make an intelligent choice.

☐   Various types of substituted consent can be used where competency to decide health care issues does not exist.

☐   Testamentary intent and capacity are required for a valid will.

☐   There are five parts to the test for determining testamentary capacity.

KEY READINGS

45 CFR Part 46. Section 46.116, Code of Federal Regulations, URL: http://ohrp.osophs.dhhs.gov/humansubjects/guidance/45cfr46.htm

McDonald MG, Meyer KC, Essig B: Healthcare Law: A Practical Guide. New York: Matthew Bender, 1991.

Sanbar SS, Gibofsky A, Firestone M, et al: Legal Medicine. Philadelphia: Mosby, 2001.

Wadlington W, Waltz JR, Dworkin RB: Law and Medicine: Cases and Materials. Mineola, NY: Foundation Press, 1980.

REFERENCES

Cases Cited

Banks v Goodfellow, 5 QB 549 (1879).
Campbell v Campbell, 130 Ill 46.
Canterbury v Spence, 464 F 2d 772 DC Cir. (1972).
Cruzan v Director, Missouri Department of Health, 110 SCt 2851 (1990).
Dilman v McDanel, 222 Ill 276.
Elizabeth Boubia v Riverside General Hospital, Mo 159780 Riverside Co, Cal Supr Ct (Dec. 19, 1983).
Estate of Pagel, 52 Cal App 2b 38. *In re* Pagel's Estate (1942).
Estate of Sargavak, 35 Cal 2d 93. *In re* Sargavak's Estate (1950).
Hall v Perry, 87 Me 569 (1895).
Meek v Bledsoe, 221 Ark 395, 253 SW 2d (1953).
In re Kemp's Will, 37 Del 514, 186 (1936).
Rennie v Klein, 462 F Supp 11, 11–31 DNJ (1978).
Sard v Hardy, 379 A 2d 1014 MD (1977).
Schloendorff v Society of New York Hospital, 105 NE 92 NY (1914).
Slaughter v Heath, 127 Ga 747, 57 SE 69 (1907).
Superintendent of Belchertown State School v Saikewicz, 373 Mass 728, 370 NE 2d 417 (1977).

References Cited

Ad Hoc Committee on Medical Ethics: American College of Physicians' Ethics Manual. Ann Intern Med 101:121–137, 1984.
American Jurisprudence 2d: Wills. 79:§§71; 72; 75; 77–101, 1962.
Beecher A: A definition of irreversible coma: Report of the Ad Hoc Committee of the Harvard Medical School to examine the definition of death. JAMA 205:337–340, 1968.
Black's Law Dictionary, ed 5. St. Paul, MN: West Group, 1979.
45 Code of Federal Regulations, C.F.R., Part 46.
18-A MRSA §5-506.
Medicolegal Primer. Pittsburgh: American College of Legal Medicine Foundation, 1991.
Report of the President's Commission for the Study of Ethical Problems in Medicine and Biomedical and Behavioral Research: Defining Death: Medical, Legal, and Ethical Issues in the Determination of Death, 1981.
Robertson JA: Second thoughts on living wills. Hastings Cent Rep 21(6):6–9, 1991.
Wecht CH: Human experimentation and research in legal medicine, in Sanbar SS, Gibofsky A, Firestone M, et al. (eds). Legal Medicine, ed 5. Philadelphia, PA: Mosby, 592–607, 2001.

Evaluation of Malingered Neurocognitive Disorders

Scott R. Millis

Brain injuries
Evidence-based medicine
Forensic psychiatry
Malingering
Models, statistical
Neuropsychological tests
Psychometrics
Psychophysiologic disorders

"What we observe is not nature itself but nature exposed to our method of questioning."
Heisenberg (1958, p. 58)

INTRODUCTION

The meaning and significance of patients' symptoms are not necessarily self-evident. Many symptoms are not diagnostically specific to a single disorder. For example, a patient's report of memory impairment could be caused by a traumatic brain injury (TBI) . On the other hand, the subjective report of a decline in memory might be a symptom of a major depressive disorder. Alternatively,

the patient may complain of memory impairment to obtain financial compensation. Symptom reporting occurs within a social context and influences human interactions. Individuals can obtain needed attention and care for illnesses by reporting their symptoms to family members and health care providers. However, symptom reporting and illness behaviors more broadly are not necessarily confined to medical disorders. People can use illness behavior to resolve personal, financial, and social problems in the absence of medical disorders, particularly when coping skills are limited or when the social support system is perceived to be inadequate (Ford, 1983). Children learn at an early age that reporting a stomach ache is a socially acceptable way to avoid taking a test at school. Hence, it is not surprising that the association between subjective symptoms and tissue pathology is complex. In clinical practice, 30% to 80% of patients consulting a physician have conditions for which no physiologic cause can be found (Wilson & Cleary, 1995). Medically unexplained symptoms appear to be common among neurologic complaints (Reid et al., 2001).

The diagnostic meaning of cognitive symptoms can be particularly ambiguous in the context of litigation and disability determination. The cognitive symptoms might indeed reflect an injury or illness involving the brain. Yet, financial and other environmental incentives apart from any brain injury may elicit and reinforce symptom report and illness behavior in these cases. Alternative diagnoses need to be considered, including malingering. This chapter presents one approach to the evaluation of malingered neurocognitive complaints. Malingering can be defined as ". . . the volitional exaggeration or fabrication of cognitive dysfunction for the purpose of obtaining substantial material gain, or avoiding or escaping formal duty or responsibility" (Slick et al., 1999, p. 552). No single test in isolation can detect malingering. Evaluation of malingering involves the collection and integration of several types of information.

For the purposes of illustrating the application of this approach, a specific disorder will be selected: traumatic brain injury (TBI). There are numerous reasons for selecting TBI as a focus:

- Clinicians will frequently encounter patients who present with cognitive complaints that are attributed to TBI. Based on hospitalization and mortality data from 12 states collected during 1995 to 1996, the Centers for Disease Control and Prevention (Thurman et al., 1995) found the average TBI incidence rate to be 95/100,000 population. One million people are treated and released from hospital emergency departments (Guerrero et al., 2000) and 230,000 people are hospitalized and survive (Thurman & Guerrero, 1999).
- Litigation involving TBI is not uncommon. The leading cause of TBI is the motor vehicle crash. Analysis by Jury Verdict Research (2000) found that brain injury claims accounted for 6% of total plaintiff verdicts in vehicular accidents. Neurologists and neuropsychologists often provide testimony in these cases either as expert witnesses or as treating doctors.
- Jury awards in brain injury cases are not insubstantial. In an analysis of compensatory awards for plaintiffs with mild and moderate brain injury claims for the years 1993 through 1999, Jury Verdict Research (2000) found that the overall median award was $434,200 with an interquartile range of $65,000 to $1,500,000. The anticipation of this level of compensation can be a powerful incentive for illness behavior.
- In a meta-analysis of 1277 subjects, Binder and Rohling (1996) found a strong statistical association between financial incentives and recovery following mild head injury, as indicated by a moderate effect size (e.g., Hedges's $g = 0.53$).
- A Rand study (Carroll et al., 1995) found that about 42% of costs related to auto accidents in the United States in 1993 were associated with staged or nonexistent accidents, nonexistent injuries, or inflated claims from actual injuries.
- The median number of months from accident date to trial date in vehicular liability cases in 1999 was 37 months (Jury Verdict Research, 2000). During this time, most litigants will have been examined by many health care providers, given depositions, recounted their accident and symptoms hundreds of times, and undergone extensive treatment with a wide variety of practitioners. It is not inconceivable that this long process of dispute resolution could perpetuate illness behavior.
- Many litigated TBI cases involve injuries at the mild end of the severity spectrum. Typically, the neurologic exam and neuroimaging studies are unremarkable. The primary symptoms are cognitive that are diagnostically nonspecific. The primary methods to investigate mild TBI cases are the history and physical and neuropsychological testing. Both require patient cooperation and are subject to conscious manipulation by the patient.
- Given the relative ubiquity of litigated TBI cases in comparison with other neurologic disorders, research on malingering has tended to focus on this diagnostic group. Consequently, most tests and indexes designed to detect malingering or response bias have been developed and normed on TBI samples.
- The methods used to evaluate malingered neurocognitive dysfunction in the TBI case can often be generalized to other disorders.

ASSESSING INJURY-RELATED VARIABLES

A starting point in the assessment of malingering in the TBI case is to obtain sufficient information regarding injury parameters:

- Initial injury severity and level of neuropsychological impairment
- Time after injury and expected outcome
- Findings from neuroimaging
- Injuries to other body systems

Initial Injury Severity and Level of Neuropsychological Impairment

The patient's initial injury severity is crucial in determining the likely cognitive and functional outcome following brain injury. Initial injury severity can be established by measures that assess alteration in consciousness, including the Glasgow Coma Scale, Revised Trauma Score, time-to-follow commands (derived from the motor score on the Glasgow Coma Scale), or length of posttraumatic amnesia as determined by the Galveston Orientation and Amnesia Scale. There is a "dose-response" relationship between initial TBI injury severity (as measured by length of coma) and the degree of associated cognitive impairment (Dikmen et al., 1995). That is, neuropsychological impairment tends to increase in a near linear fashion as the severity of brain injury increases (Rohling, 2000). In short, one would not expect to see severe, chronic neuropsychological impairment associated with mild TBI. It would be unusual for a patient with a mild TBI at 1 year after injury to obtain a poor score on Trailmaking B, a common neuropsychological test. For example, if that patient required 300 seconds to complete Trailmaking B, questions should be raised regarding the validity of that score. Based on a representative sample of TBI patients (Dikmen et al., 1995), Trailmaking B scores this poor might be expected among TBI patients with coma histories of 1 month but not in mild TBI cases. In summarizing their findings from their study of outcome following TBI, Dikmen and colleagues (1995) note that ". . . significant neuropsychological impairment due to a mild head injury is as unlikely as is escaping an impairment in the case of a very severe head injury" (p. 87). From the broader perspective of a meta-analysis of 11 studies involving 622 subjects, Binder and colleagues (1997) found a small effect of mild TBI on cognitive functioning (Hedges's $g = 0.07$).

Although excessively poor neuropsychological test scores alone cannot establish a diagnosis of malingering in the litigated mild TBI case, they do represent aberrant findings in need of explanation. Inclusion of malingering in the differential diagnosis is warranted because numerous studies have found that people without brain dysfunction are able to intentionally produce impaired neuropsychological test scores (Coleman et al., 1998; Iverson & Franzen, 1998). Neurologists and neuropsychologists often have neuropsychological test scores available in the litigated mild TBI case. A useful starting point in the evaluation of malingering is to determine if a panel of test results deviates significantly from expected patterns of outcome. Several studies that provide data on typical neuropsychological test performances of persons from different backgrounds with varying levels of TBI severity include Levin and associates (1987); Kreutzer and colleagues (1993); Dikmen and colleagues (1995); Ponsford and colleagues (2000); and Millis and colleagues (2001). These data can assist the clinician in determining whether an individual's neuropsychological test profile is atypical.

In the atypical case, the clinician can combine the psychometric test findings with other information, as discussed in the Integration of Findings section. In this process of information integration, discrepancies are identified between test data and (1) known patterns of brain functioning, (2) observed behavior, (3) information from other observers or records, and (4) documented background history (Slick et al., 1999). A similar approach can be used when the question of malingering arises in the differential diagnosis of other neurologic disorders. Information regarding the relationship between illness severity and associated neuropsychological test patterns is often available, which can assist the clinician in determining whether a given patient's presentation is atypical. For example, the Recognition Memory Test (Warrington, 1984) has been used to detect memory impairment in a broad range of neurologic and psychiatric disorders, including probable Alzheimer-type dementia, cerebral vascular disease, Parkinson disease, neurosyphilis, herpes encephalitis, seizure disorders, aneurysms, TBI, tumors, and various psychiatric illnesses in North America and Europe (Diesfeldt, 1990; Millis & Dijkers, 1993; Naugle et al., 1994; Rapcsak et al., 1994; Hermann et al., 1995; Morris et al., 1995; Aggleton & Shaw, 1996; Bigler et al., 1996; Kelly et al., 1996; Baxendale, 1997; Kneeborn et al., 1997; Soukup et al., 1999; Sweet et al., 2000a).

Time after Injury and Expected Outcome

Although measurable cognitive impairment may occur within days of mild TBI, the preponderance of empirical evidence has failed to find an association between chronic, disabling handicap and uncomplicated mild TBI. Studies of mild TBI that have included appropriate control groups have found resolution of cognitive deficits to occur within 1 to 3 months after injury (McLean et al., 1983; Gentilini et al., 1985; Dikmen et al., 1986; Levin et al., 1987; Newcombe et al., 1994; Maddocks & Saling, 1996; Hinton-Bayre et al., 1997; Ponsford et al., 2000). In one study, Ponsford and colleagues (2000) recruited consecutive admissions to an emergency department with mild TBI along with a trauma control group without head injury. At 1 month, the mild TBI group showed slowed information processing on neuropsychological measures compared to the trauma controls. At 3 months, the deficits were not evident. In a separate study, Dikmen and colleagues (1995), at 1 year after injury, found no significant differences in neuropsychological outcome between their mild TBI group and trauma control group despite large sample sizes and use of a comprehensive test battery.

Studies that have purported to find persistent impairment in mild TBI have been hampered by a number of methodological flaws, including inconsistency or inaccuracy in the classification of brain injury severity, enrollment of participants on the basis of symptoms rather than history of brain injury, failure to control for preexisting conditions, or lack of appropriate control groups (Dikmen & Levin, 1993). In an often-cited study, Rimel and colleagues (1981) reported cognitive impairment persisting beyond 3 months following mild TBI in a subset of their sample. However, over one third of their sample had excessive blood alcohol levels at the time of the accident and about one third gave a history of previous head injury. Leininger and associates (1990) purported to find "measurable neuropsychological deficits" following mild TBI. However, 59% of their "mild concussion" group and 81% of their "concussion" group were pursuing compensation claims, suggesting that these groups were highly unrepresentative of persons with mild TBI.

The patient with a history of mild TBI who presents with complaints of concentration and memory problems and headaches at 3 days after injury is not usual. However, a patient with a mild TBI who reports disabling symptoms at 1 year is atypical. This is not to imply that the patient is malingering but factors other than the mild TBI need to be considered in the differential diagnosis, as outlined in the section Integration of Findings. Discrepancies are identified between self-reported symptoms and history and (1) documented history, (2) known patterns of brain functioning, (3) behavioral observations, and (4) information obtained from informants (Slick et al., 1999). Similarly, in the non-TBI context, the natural course of many neurologic disorders is well known. Departure from the typical course in the individual case may raise the question of malingering when substantial external incentives for illness behavior are present.

Findings from Neuroimaging

It is important to make the distinction between "complicated" and "uncomplicated" mild TBI. Complicated mild TBI is defined by a Glasgow Coma Scale score of 13 to 15 with intracranial pathology, that is, parenchymal contusion or hematoma or with subdural or epidural hematoma. Williams and colleagues (1990) found that patients with complicated mild TBI tended to have neurobehavioral sequelae similar to persons with moderate head injury. In addition, complications occasionally occur subsequent to what was initially a mild brain injury. Neurosurgical interventions for mass lesions, nonreactive pupils, and occurrence of cardiac arrest have been related strongly to poorer outcome (Dikmen et al., 1995). Hence, clinicians need to adjust their expectations accordingly regarding outcome when evaluating this subgroup of patients with mild TBI.

Injuries to Other Body Systems

In TBI cases, orthopedic injuries and injuries to systems other than the brain can have a major impact on the ability to return to work and the resumption of other daily activities (Dikmen et al., 1986; Dacey et al., 1991). Consideration of other system injuries is particularly important in the mild TBI case. Dikmen and colleagues

(1986) found that 9 of 11 patients with both mild TBI and additional injuries were not working or going to school at 1 month after injury, whereas 1 of 8 patients with mild TBI alone had not returned to work. Hence, the evaluation of disability claims following mild TBI is not based on making a binary diagnostic decision of brain injury versus malingering. Nonbrain injuries need to be considered in the differential diagnosis. As will be discussed in the following section, psychiatric and psychosocial factors must also be considered.

ASSESSING PSYCHOSOCIAL VARIABLES

In taking the history following mild TBI, some patients will report various symptoms such as anxiety, dizziness, headache, memory and concentration problems, fatigue, irritability, depression, and noise sensitivity (Alexander, 1995), often referred to as "postconcussion symptoms." By 1 year after injury, the vast majority of patients will report recovery, but some investigators have found that 10% to 15% of patients with mild TBI continue to be symptomatic (Rutherford et al., 1978; Alves, 1992). Yet, this set of somatic, psychological, and cognitive complaints typically attributed to mild TBI is not specific to the disorder. Endorsement of these symptoms is actually quite common in the normal population as well as in individuals with medical or psychological problems (Gouvier et al., 1988; Lees-Haley & Brown, 1993; Fox et al., 1995; Sawchyn et al., 1999; Lees-Haley et al., 2001; Trahan et al., 2001). For example, Kellner and Sheffield (1973) found that 90% of healthy individuals in their sample reported various somatic symptoms during a 1-week period. The most commonly endorsed symptoms were headaches, fatigue, muscle pains, and irritability. In a symptom survey of individuals seeking outpatient psychotherapy from a large southern California health maintenance organization, Fox and colleagues (1995) found high rates of mild TBI symptom endorsement: headache (52%), memory problems (31%), dizziness (30%), concentration problems (45%), fatigue (55%), and irritability (55%).

In addition to the high prevalence of postconcussive symptoms in a wide range of normal and clinical groups, increasing evidence indicates a strong association between persisting symptoms following mild TBI and preexisting emotional stress, chronic social difficulties, or mental disorders (Fenton et al., 1993; Klonoff & Lamb, 1998; Ponsford et al., 2000). Trahan and colleagues (2001) found that their mild TBI group reported minimally higher scores on a postconcussion symptom checklist than their normal control group. However, their clinical depression group without head injury had a statistically higher rate of symptom endorsement than the normal control and mild TBI groups.

This pattern of findings suggests that the clinician needs to carefully evaluate the role of premorbid mental disorders in the litigated mild TBI case. The prevalence of mental disorders in the United States is high. Two epidemiologic surveys, the Epidemiologic Catchment Survey (ECA; Robins & Regier, 1991) and the National Comorbidity Survey (NCS; Kessler, 1994), estimate that about 20% of the U.S. population are affected by mental disorders during a given year, including anxiety, mood, somatoform, and schizophrenic disorders. Overall, 19% have a mental disorder alone, 3% have both mental and addictive disorders, and 6% have addictive disorders alone. Table 53-1 presents additional descriptive data. It should be noted that the ECA data might underestimate the true prevalence of somatoform disorders due to the limitations of the Diagnostic Interview Schedule used in the survey. It has been estimated that up to 3 of every 50 patients seen by primary care providers may have a somatoform disorder or a subsyndromal form of somatization (NIMH, 1990).

Postconcussion symptoms that could easily be attributed to a mild TBI might actually be related to a preinjury mental disorder such as a somatoform disorder. Cursory screening for preexisting psychopathology is likely to be insufficient (Butler et al., 1993). Along with a thorough history, standardized personality assessment instruments like the Minnesota Multiphasic Personality Inventory-2 (MMPI-2; Butcher et al., 1989) or the Personality Assessment Inventory (Morley, 1991) are useful in examining psychosocial factors in the litigated mild TBI case.

INTEGRATION OF FINDINGS

Slick and colleagues (1999) have proposed a set of diagnostic criteria for what they have termed malingered neurocognitive dysfunction. These criteria can assist clinicians in the evaluation of malingering by organizing and integrating information from multiple sources. This author has converted these criteria with slight modifications into a decision-tree format (Fig. 53-1). As discussed in the previous sections of this chapter, the clinician collects information on the initial injury severity and level of neuropsychological impairment, time after injury and expected outcome, findings from neuroimaging and neuropsychological assessment, injuries to other body systems, and psychosocial variables. This information is then applied to the decision-tree analysis. The

diagnosis of malingering is not a binary decision; there are different levels of certainty regarding the diagnosis in any given case. Some investigators, such as Slick and colleagues (1999), have argued that, short of an individual's confession, one cannot establish with 100% certainty that a person is malingering. Yet, few if any disorders can be diagnosed with this level of accuracy. Short of autopsy, it is difficult to make the diagnosis of Alzheimer disease with absolute certainty. Although one may dispute the criteria, the goal is to make the diagnostic decision-making process explicit and transparent.

As Figure 53-1 illustrates, a starting point is to determine whether substantial external incentive is present. Slick and colleagues (1999) have proposed that such incentives may take several forms, such as obtaining material gain or avoiding or escaping formal duty or responsibility:

> Substantial material gain includes money, goods, or services of nontrivial values (e.g., financial compensation for personal injury). Formal duties are actions that people are legally obligated to perform (e.g., prison, military, or public service, or child support payments or other financial obligations). Formal responsibilities are those that involve accountability or liability in legal proceedings (e.g., competency to stand trial). (p. 552)

If substantial external incentives are not present, then other disorders need to be considered. Patients typically come to the attention of the clinician because their neurobehavioral outcome is atypical, for example, protracted symptomatology, excessively impaired neuropsychological test scores, and claimed vocational disability. As noted earlier, the primary disorders to be considered when substantial external incentives are absent include somatoform, factitious, mood, anxiety, and personality disorders. In the somatoform disorders, the behavior may be reinforced and maintained because it effectively regulates and controls interpersonal relationships (Ford, 1983). In addition, somatization is a frequent comorbidity in major depression (55%), anxiety disorders (34%), and personality disorders (61%) (Martin & Yutzy, 1997) and, hence, these disorders need to be considered in the differential diagnosis.

TABLE 53-1. Estimated 1-yr Prevalence Rates Based on Epidemiologic Catchment Area (ECA) Study and National Comorbidity Study (NCS)

	ECA prevalence (%)	NCS prevalence (%)
Any anxiety disorder	13.1	18.7
Any mood disorder	7.1	11.1
Schizophrenia	1.3	—
Somatization	0.2	—
Any disorder	19.5	23.4

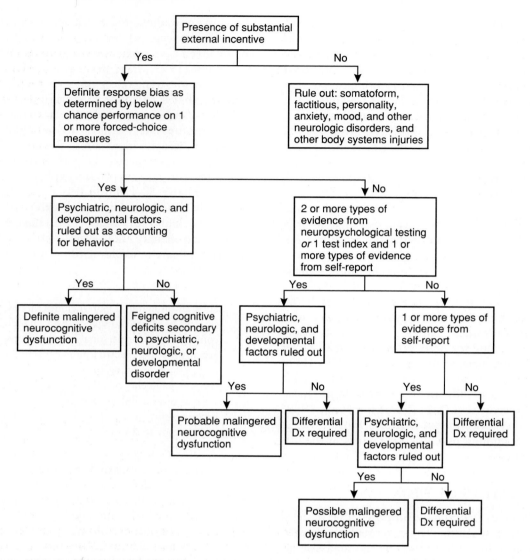

FIGURE 53-1. Diagnostic decision tree. Dx, diagnosis. (Adapted from Slick DJ, Sherman EMS, Iverson GL: Diagnostic criteria for malingered neurocognitive dysfunction: Proposed standards for clinical practices and research. Clin Neuropsychol 13:545–561, 1999.)

In factitious disorder, illness behavior is thought to be motivated by the person's desire to assume the sick role absent of external incentives (American Psychiatric Association, 1994). Of course, the patient may have injuries to other body systems or medical disorders not related to the accident in question, which need to be considered.

At this point, specialized psychometric measures need to be used to determine whether response bias is present, that is, the patient is intentionally performing the psychometric tests poorly so as to appear impaired. As Figure 53-1 indicates, definite response bias is established if the patient obtains a score that is significantly below chance on one or more forced-choice tests (FCTs), as described in the following section. It is also recommended that FCTs and related measures be used in the assessment of response bias even when substantial external incentives are absent.

Definite Response Bias: Definite Malingered Neurocognitive Dysfunction

The FCTs, also known as symptom validity tests (SVTs), are among the most extensively evaluated tests for the detection of response bias (Slick et al., 1999). A target stimulus is presented and is then followed by a two-choice recognition task with the original target item paired with a distractor item not presented. The individual is then asked to identify the target item that was presented during the acquisition trial. The delay between the exposure and recognition trials varies across tests, ranging from essentially no delay to a delay of several minutes. A wide variety of stimuli have been used in this test paradigm, including words, digits, photographs, line drawings, and tasks modified from the sensory-perceptual examination (e.g., fingertip number writing and tactile finger recognition).

An individual who has not been exposed to the target items and, thus, having no prior knowledge or memory of the stimuli, would perform at chance level during the recognition trial. That is, with two choices, the person has a 50% chance of choosing the correct item. A performance that is significantly below chance from a statistical perspective (e.g., $P < .05$) would imply that an individual did, indeed, remember the target items. Pankratz and Erickson (1990) described a significantly below chance performance on an FCT as "motivated wrong answering," which, in turn, is the "smoking gun of intent." As Bianchini and colleagues (2001) note, "Below-chance performance is indication that the patient does recognize the correct stimulus and is responding with bias against this item" (p. 21).

The normal approximation to the binomial distribution (Altman, 1999) can be used to determine the probability of obtaining a given score on a dichotomous FCT, where x is the observed score and n is the total number of items:

$$z = \frac{|x - (0.5 \times n)| - 0.5}{\sqrt{0.25 \times n}}$$

For example, the probability of obtaining a score of less than 19 on a test containing 50 items is 0.03. The digit recognition tests are perhaps the most widely used and empirically evaluated of the FCTs (Fig. 53-2). Of the digit recognition FCTs, the Hiscock Forced-Choice Procedure (HFCP; Hiscock & Hiscock, 1989) and Portland Digit Recognition Test (PDRT; Binder & Willis, 1991) have the greatest empirical support to date. In addition to being able to calculate the probability of obtaining a specific score, the digit recognition tests tend to be easy for persons with psychiatric disorders or brain dysfunction. Mean scores for clinical groups range from 84% to 99% correct on the PDRT or HFCP (Binder, 1993; Guilmette et al., 1993; Prigatano & Amin, 1993; Guilmette et al., 1994). Other digit recognition FCTs include the Computerized Assessment of Response Bias (CARB; Conder et al., 1992) and the Victoria Symptom Validity Test (VSVT; Slick et al., 1997; Doss et al., 1999).

The Test of Memory Malingering (TOMM; Tombaugh, 1997; Rees et al., 1998) is a modification of the digit recognition FCT paradigm; it is a visual recognition task that uses 50 drawings of common objects rather than numbers. Although not originally designed as tests for the assessment of malingering, some conventional neuropsychological measures use a forced-choice response format. Subsequent research has shown

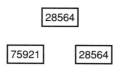

FIGURE 53-2. Example of a prototypical forced-choice digit recognition test.

several of these tests to be useful in detecting feigned cognitive impairment as well: Warrington's Recognition Memory Test (Millis, 1992, 1994; Iverson & Franzen, 1994; Millis & Putnam, 1994; Iverson & Franzen, 1998), Seashore Rhythm Test, and Speech-Sounds Perception Test (Heaton et al., 1978; Goebel, 1983; Trueblood & Schmidt, 1993; Millis et al., 1996; Mittenberg et al., 1996; Gfeller & Cradock, 1998).

Designed to be used as a bedside screening tool, the "coin-in-the-hand" test (Narinder, 1994) is another type of FCT in which the examiner shows the patient a coin in one hand for 2 seconds and then the patient is asked to close his or her eyes and count backward from 10. Next, the patient is asked to open his or her eyes and indicate which clenched fist contains the coin (Fig. 53-3). In its original form, the coin-in-the-hand test was very short, that is, 10 trials. However, it may be difficult to evaluate a patient's performance because with 10 trials, only the score of one correct response is significantly below chance. This author recommends that an FCT use a minimum of 25 trials and preferably 50. Table 53-2 contains an example of a random stimulus presentation order that can be used with the coin-in-the hand test. A score of 18 or less is significantly below chance ($P < .05$).

As Figure 53-1 indicates, a diagnosis of definite malingered neurocognitive dysfunction is made when the patient shows definite response bias on one or more FCTs, and neurologic, psychiatric, and developmental disorders are ruled out as causal factors. As Slick and colleagues (1999) advise, "In cases where psychiatric, developmental, or neurological disorders are the primary cause of feigned cognitive deficits, then a diagnosis of 'feigned cognitive deficits secondary to [specify psychiatric/developmental/neurological disorder]' may be considered" (p. 555).

Although significantly below chance performance on an FCT is persuasive evidence of response bias, the majority of malingerers will not perform below chance. In studies of subjects who were instructed to malinger cognitive deficits, Hiscock and colleagues (1994) found that fewer than one third of subjects performed below chance. The mean scores of groups of clinical subjects suspected of malingering tend to be above chance, that is, 56% to 74% correct on the PDRT or HFCP (Binder, 1993; Prigatano & Amin, 1993; Greiffenstein et al., 1994). One response to these findings has been to select cutoff scores for

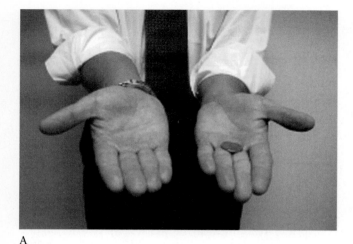

A

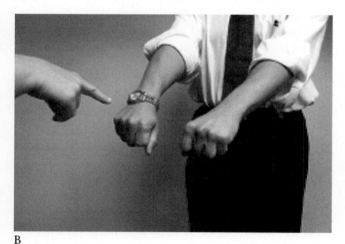

B

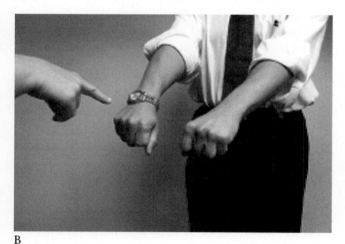

C

FIGURE 53-3. "Coin-in-the-hand" test.

TABLE 53-2. Example of Random Stimulus Presentation Order

1	A	21	B	41	B
2	B	22	B	42	B
3	A	23	A	43	A
4	B	24	A	44	B
5	B	25	B	45	B
6	A	26	B	46	A
7	B	27	B	47	B
8	A	28	A	48	B
9	B	29	A	49	A
10	A	30	B	50	A
11	B	31	B		
12	A	32	A		
13	A	33	B		
14	B	34	A		
15	B	35	A		
16	A	36	B		
17	B	37	B		
18	A	38	A		
19	A	39	A		
20	A	40	A		

few, if any, persons with brain dysfunction score. For example, scores less than 54% to 63% correct on the PDRT may indicate response bias (Binder, 1993; Greiffenstein et al., 1994), whereas a cutoff of 90% or less has been used with the HFCP (e.g., Guilmette et al., 1994). The PDRT and HFCT have been reported to accurately classify 89% to 100% of persons with TBI and 75% to 90% of suspected clinical malingerers or analogue simulators using the modified cutoff scores.

Although this level of diagnostic efficiency is often acceptable in a wide variety of clinical settings, it is more difficult to infer the degree of intent when scores are above chance. In the absence of definite response bias as established by an FCT, the clinician needs to consider other diagnostic categories. Slick and colleagues (1999) have suggested "probable" and "possible malingered neurocognitive dysfunction." In these cases, additional diagnostic information is needed, to which we now turn.

Probable and Possible Malingered Neurocognitive Dysfunction

Evidence from Neuropsychological Testing

In addition to FCTs, several psychometric tests and test indices have been developed to specifically detect exaggerated or feigned cognitive deficits. Use of these test indicators is indicated in the assessment of patients who do not show evidence of definite response bias, that is, significantly below chance performance on FCTs.

FCTs that are above chance but scores that still maintain acceptable levels of diagnostic efficiency based on test score distributions of persons with brain dysfunction. A cutoff score is selected below which

Easy Tests. By design, FCTs are simple for patients to complete, even for patients with marked cognitive impairment or significant brain dysfunction. As discussed in the previous section, FCTs can provide useful diagnostic information even when patients do not perform significantly below chance. If an FCT score is above chance but below an empirically derived cutoff (e.g., <90% correct on the HFCP), diagnoses of probable or possible malingered neurocognitive disorder need to be considered if there is additional evidence from well-validated test indices or evidence from self-report. Other cognitive tasks that are relatively preserved even in the presence of brain dysfunction have been found useful in detecting exaggerated cognitive impairment. For example, forward digit span is often relatively intact in a variety of neurologic disorders. In contrast, a strikingly poor forward span may be associated with malingering (Binder & Willis, 1991; Trueblood & Schmidt, 1993; Greiffenstein et al., 1994; Iverson & Franzen, 1994; Trueblood, 1994; Greiffenstein et al., 1995; Mittenberg et al., 1995; Meyers & Volbrecht, 1998). The Digit Span (DS) subtest from the Wechsler Adult Intelligence Scale-Revised (WAIS-R) or Wechsler Memory Scale-Revised has been used most frequently in these studies. Greiffenstein and colleagues (1994) developed an index, termed Reliable Digit Span (RDS), to detect malingering; the longest numbers of digits repeated accurately on both trials of DS (Forward and Backward trials) are summed. A cutoff score of 7 or less was derived. Meyers and Volbrecht (1998), in a cross-validation study, found that 96% of their nonlitigating TBI participants were correctly classified. Of their litigating mild TBI participants who failed a separate FCT, 78% were correctly classified by the RDS.

Performance Patterns. Malingering tests that are easy or simple to perform run the risk of being insensitive to feigned impairment. The purpose of such tests may be transparent to the examinee; that is, some FCTs are so easy, why would someone fail them unless he or she was trying to act impaired? Examinees might believe that a grossly impaired performance on an FCT would be blatantly obvious and unconvincing to an examiner. Litigants can also be coached to spot these tests, particularly some of the popular FCTs. Rather than depending on FCTs alone, some investigators have attempted to determine whether malingering is associated with specific patterns of performance on neuropsychological tests. The rationale is that persons with TBI perform neuropsychological tests in ways that are quantitatively and qualitatively different from persons feigning impairment. For example, it has been observed that malingering is sometimes associated with disproportionately impaired performances on finger tapping, fingertip number writing, and finger localization (Binder & Willis, 1991). The issue of motivation to perform

poorly should be raised in the litigated mild TBI case if finger-tapping scores drop below a mean of 30 taps per 10-second period (Binder, 1990).

A more sophisticated and rigorous approach to pattern analysis has been the derivation of multivariable statistical functions to differentiate brain dysfunction from malingering using standard cognitive measures. Discriminant function analysis and logistic regression have been used to develop the statistical functions to predict malingering. The diagnostic efficiency of these functions can be evaluated directly: each test variable is assigned a specific coefficient or weight, a composite score is obtained, and a classificatory decision is made. The statistical function can then be replicated on new samples to determine its generalizability. Test or index redundancy or multicollinearity can also be identified so that optimal sets of functions can be derived. In logistic regression, a constant (α) is added the sum of the products of regression coefficients and predictor variables ($\beta_1 x_1 + \beta_2 x_1$). In the derivation of the logistic regression function, the outcome of interest or the group to be predicted is coded "1." The probability of the outcome of interest or group membership is given by the following formula:

$$p = \frac{e^{\alpha + \beta_1 x_1 + \beta_2 x_2}}{1 + e^{\alpha + \beta_1 x_1 + \beta_2 x_2}}$$

Generally, the cutoff for p is .50, but it can be adjusted depending on the sample or the relative costs of making either a false-positive or false-negative error in a given situation. Mittenberg and colleagues (1995) developed a discriminant function composed of seven subtests from the WAIS-R that accurately classified 79% of TBI patients and normal subjects instructed to malinger. Similar to a logistic regression function, the age-corrected scaled score from the WAIS-R are multiplied by coefficients and summed in the discriminant function. Malingering is implicated when the composite score exceeds a cutoff score derived by Mittenberg and associates (1995). In separate studies, Millis and colleagues (1998) and Axelrod and Rawlings (1999) essentially replicated these findings with this discriminant function on independent samples. Other multivariable functions developed to detect feigned impairment have included variables from the California Verbal Learning Test (Millis et al., 1995; Coleman et al., 1998; Baker et al., 2000; Sweet et al., 2000b), Halstead-Reitan Neuropsychological Test Battery (Heaton et al., 1978; Goebel, 1983; Mittenberg et al., 1996; McKinzey & Russell, 1997), and Rey Auditory Verbal Learning Test (Bernard, 1991; Binder et al., 1993; Suhr et al., 1997).

Combining the Neuropsychological Test Data with Other Data. In addition to considering specific psychometric tests of malingering, Slick and colleagues

(1999, pp. 553–554) have proposed that standard neuropsychological tests be used in the assessment of malingering evidence:

- *"Discrepancy between test data and known patterns of brain functioning"* (e.g., patient performs in the profoundly impaired range on measures of attention but within normal limits on memory measures)
- *"Discrepancy between test data and observed behavior"* (e.g., patient is unable to perform confrontation naming test but has no visuoperceptual deficits and spontaneous speech is fluent and without paraphasic errors)
- *"Discrepancy between test data and reliable collateral reports"* (e.g., patient handles financial affairs like balancing checkbook but is unable to perform simple arithmetic problems in the clinical examination)
- *"Discrepancy between test data and documented background history"* (e.g., patient with history of mild TBI who obtains memory test scores in the profoundly impaired range)

If, in a given case, there are two or more types of evidence from neuropsychological testing (i.e., well-validated test indices of malingering or discrepancies between test data and behavior), excluding a significantly below chance performance on an FCT, and psychiatric, neurologic, and developmental disorders are ruled out as causal factors, a diagnosis of probable malingered neurocognitive dysfunction is made. If only one type of psychometric evidence is present, it is necessary to consider evidence from self-report.

Evidence from Self-Report

Slick and colleagues (1999) have proposed that the following behaviors may be associated with malingering. The presence of one or more of these behaviors is insufficient to make the diagnosis of definite malingered neurocognitive dysfunction but may be supportive of the alternative diagnoses of probable or possible malingered neurocognitive dysfunction:

- *"Self-reported history is discrepant with documented history"* (e.g., patient reports an exaggerated length of loss of consciousness)
- *"Self-reported symptoms are discrepant with known patterns of brain functioning"* (e.g., patient claims inability to recall own birth date and address following mild TBI)
- *"Self-reported symptoms are discrepant with behavioral observations"* (e.g., patient reports severe cognitive impairment yet lives independently, manages own financial affairs, and drives self to office)

- *"Self-reported symptoms are discrepant with information obtained from collateral informants"* (e.g., patient acts cognitively impaired, but spouse or job supervisor reports that patient experiences no functional difficulties)
- *"Evidence of exaggerated or fabricated psychological dysfunction"* (e.g., validity scales from the MMPI-2 or Personality Assessment Inventory indicate "fake bad" profile) (Slick et al., 1999, p. 554)

Hence, two or more types of evidence from neuropsychological testing, or one type of neuropsychological evidence combined with one or more types of evidence from self-report are sufficient for a diagnosis of probable malingered neurocognitive dysfunction. In the absence of psychometric evidence, one or more types of evidence from self-report warrant consideration of possible malingered neurocognitive dysfunction when psychiatric, neurologic, and developmental disorders are ruled out as causal factors.

CONCLUSIONS

Broshek and Barth (2000) have advised neuropsychologists to "... tell patients prior to testing that it is important for them to put forth their best effort and explain that the tests are sensitive to any deficits they might be experiencing, so it is not necessary for them to exaggerate their difficulties" (p. 229). However, even warning patients that malingering behavior can be detected apparently is ineffective as a deterrent (Sullivan et al., 2001). By the time patients in litigation come to examination, the roles and behaviors that they have assumed are often well practiced and reinforced by powerful environmental contingencies. Assessment for malingered neurocognitive dysfunction needs to be a routine part of the evaluation. Yet, clinical judgment alone is likely to be insufficient. Our capacity as humans to accurately and efficiently process complex diagnostic information is limited: we tend to ignore prevalence rates, assign nonoptimal weights to variables, disregard regression toward the mean, improperly assess covariation, and overweigh some types of data (Grove et al., 2000). In their meta-analysis, Grove and colleagues (2000) found that statistical prediction significantly outperformed clinical prediction in 33% to 47% of 136 studies surveyed. Clinical judgment is helpful in generating hypotheses, which then are best used in a systematic decision-making process like the one presented in this chapter.

■ KEY POINTS

☐ Evaluation for malingered cognitive disorders needs to be conducted when patients present with cognitive complaints in the presence of substantial external incentives for impairment.

☐ The evaluation involves the integration of multiple sources of data: injury or illness related variables, psychosocial variables, psychometric test data, and knowledge of the natural course of disorders.

☐ Specialized psychometric data from symptom validity tests and test pattern analysis can assist the clinician in detecting malingering behavior.

☐ Discrepancies between psychometric test data and known patterns of brain functioning, observed behavior, collateral reports, and documented background history are also helpful in this evaluation.

☐ Diagnosis of malingered cognitive disorder should not be viewed as a binary decision process, that is, as present or absent. There are different levels of certainty regarding the diagnosis in any given case based on the data at hand. Levels of certainty can be translated into diagnostic impressions, for example, definite, probable, or possible malingered neurocognitive disorder.

KEY READINGS

Binder LM, Rohling ML, Larrabee GJ: A review of mild head trauma. Part I: Meta-analysis review of neuropsychological studies. J Clin Exp Neuropsychol 19:421–431, 1997.

Sackett DL, Straus SE, Richardson WS, et al: Evidence-Based Medicine, ed 2. New York: Churchill Livingstone, 2000.

Slick DJ, Sherman EMS, Iverson GL: Diagnostic criteria for malingered neurocognitive dysfunction: Proposed standards for clinical practice and research. Clin Neuropsychol 13:545–561, 1999.

REFERENCES

Aggleton JP, Shaw C: Amnesia and recognition memory: A re-analysis of psychometric data. Neuropsychologia, 34:51–62, 1996.

Alexander MP: Mild traumatic brain injury: Pathophysiology, natural history, and clinical management. Neurology 45:1253–1260, 1995.

Altman DG: Practical Statistics for Medical Research. Boca Raton, FL: Chapman and Hall/CRC, 1999.

Alves WM: Natural history of post-concussive signs and symptoms. Phys Med Rehabil 6:21–32, 1992.

American Psychiatric Association: Diagnostic and Statistical Manual of Mental Disorders, ed 4. Washington, DC: American Psychiatric Association Press, 1994.

Axelrod BN, Rawlings DB: Clinical utility of incomplete effort WAIS-R formulas: A longitudinal examination of individuals with traumatic brain injuries. J Forensic Neuropsychol 1:15–27, 1999.

Baker R, Donders J, Thompson E: Assessment of incomplete effort with the California Verbal Learning Test. Appl Neuropsychol 7:111–114, 2000.

Baxendale SA: The role of the hippocampus in recognition memory. Neuropsychologia 35:591–598, 1997.

Bernard LC: The detection of faked deficits on the Rey Auditory Verbal Learning Test: The effect of serial position. Arch Clin Neuropsychol 6:81–88, 1991.

Bianchini KJ, Mathias CW, Greve KW: Symptom validity testing: A critical review. Clin Neuropsychol 15:19–45, 2001.

Bigler ED, Johnson SC, Anderson CV, et al: Traumatic brain injury and memory: The role of hippocampal atrophy. Neuropsychology 10:333–342, 1996.

Binder LM: Malingering following minor head trauma. Clin Neuropsychol 4:25–36, 1990.

Binder LM: Assessment of malingering after mild head trauma with the Portland Digit Recognition Test. J Clin Exp Neuropsychol 15:170–182, 1993.

Binder LM, Rohling ML: Money matters: A meta-analytic review of the effect of financial incentives on recovery after closed head injury. Am J Psychiatry 153:7–10, 1996.

Binder LM, Rohling ML, Larrabee GJ: A review of mild head trauma. Part I: Meta-analysis review of neuropsychological studies. J Clin Exp Neuropsychol 19:421–431, 1997.

Binder LM, Villanueva MR, Howieson D, et al: The Rey AVT recognition memory task measures motivational impairment after mild head trauma. Arch Clin Neuropsychol 8:137–147, 1993.

Binder LM, Willis SC: Assessment of motivation after financially compensable minor head injury. Psychol Assess 3:175–181, 1991.

Broshek DK, Barth JT: The Halstead-Reitan Neuropsychological Test Battery, in Groth-Marnat G (ed): Neuropsychological assessment in clinical practice. New York: Wiley, 2000, pp. 223–262.

Butcher JN, Dahlstrom WG, Graham JR, et al: Minnesota Multiphasic Personality Inventory (MMPI-2): Manual for administration and scoring. Minneapolis: University of Minnesota Press, 1989.

Butler RW, Jenkins MA, Braff DL: The abnormality of normal comparison groups: The identification of psychosis proneness and substance abuse in putatively normal research subjects. Am J Psychiatry 150:1386–1391, 1993.

Carroll SJ, Abrahamse AF, Vaiana ME: The Costs of Excess Medical Claims for Automobile Personal Injuries. Santa Monica, CA: Rand, 1995.

Coleman R, Rapport L, Millis S, et al: Effects of coaching on the detection of malingering on the California Verbal Learning Test: An analog study of malingered head injury. Clin Neuropsychol 20:201–210, 1998.

Conder R, Allen L, Cox D: Computerized Assessment of Response Bias Test Manual. Durham, NC: Cognisyst, 1992.

Dacey R, Dikmen S, Temkin N, et al: Relative effects of brain and non-brain injuries on neuropsychological and psychosocial outcome. J Trauma 31:217–222, 1991.

Deisfeldt HFA: Recognition memory for words and faces in primary degenerative dementia of the Alzheimer type and normal old age. J Clin Exp Neuropsychol 12:931–945, 1990.

Dikmen SS, Levin HS: Methodological issues in the study of mild head injury. J Head Trauma Rehab 8:30–37, 1993.

Dikmen SS, Machamer JE, Winn HR, et al: Neuropsychological outcome at one-year post head injury. Neuropsychology 9:80–90, 1995.

Dikmen SS, McLean A, Temkin N: Neuropsychological and psychosocial consequences of minor head injury. J Neurol Neurosurg Psychiatry 49:1227–1232, 1986.

Doss RC, Chelune GJ, Naugle RI: Victoria Symptom Validity Test: Compensation-seeking vs. non-compensation-seeking patients in a general clinical setting. J Forensic Neuropsychol 1:5–20, 1999.

Fenton G, McClelland R, Montgomery A, et al: The postconcussional syndrome: Social antecedents and psychological sequelae. Br J Psychol 162:493–497, 1993.

Ford CV: The Somatizing Disorders: Illness as a Way of Life. New York: Elsevier Biomedical, 1983.

Fox DD, Lees-Haley PR, Earnest K, et al: Base rates of post-concussive symptoms in health maintenance organization patients and controls. Neuropsychology 9:606–611, 1995.

Gentilini M, Nichelli P, Schoenhuber R, et al: Neuropsychological evaluation of mild head injury. J Neurol Neurosurg Psychiatry 48:137–140, 1985.

Gfeller JD, Cradock MM: Detecting feigned neuropsychological impairment with the Seashore Rhythm Test. J Clin Psychol 54:431–438, 1998.

Goebel RA: Detection of faking on the Halstead-Reitan Neuropsychological Test Battery. J Clin Psychology 39:731–742, 1983.

Gouvier WD, Uddo-Crane M, Brown LM: Base rates of post-concussional symptoms. Arch Clin Neuropsychol 3:273–278, 1988.

Greiffenstein MF, Baker WJ, Gola T: Validation of malingered amnesia measures with a large clinical sample. Psychol Assess 6:218–224, 1994.

Greiffenstein MF, Gola T, Baker WJ: MMPI-2 validity scales versus domain specific measures in the detection of factitious traumatic brain injury. Clin Neuropsychol 9:218–224, 1995.

Grove WM, Zald DH, Lebow BS, et al: Clinical versus mechanical prediction: A meta-analysis. Psychol Assess 12:19–30, 2000.

Guerrero JL, Thurman DJ, Sniezek, JE: Emergency visits associated with traumatic brain injury: United States, 1995–1996. Brain Inj 14:181–186, 2000.

Guilmette TJ, Hart KJ, Giuliano AJ: Malingering detection: The use of a forced-choice method in identifying organic versus simulated memory impairment. Clin Neuropsychol 7:59 –69, 1993.

Guilmette TJ, Hart KJ, Giuliano AJ, et al: Detecting simulated memory impairment: Comparison of the Rey Fifteen-Item Test and the Hiscock Forced-Choice Procedure. Clin Neuropsychol 8:283–294, 1994.

Heaton RK, Smith HH, Lehman RAW, et al: Prospects for faking believable deficits on neuropsychological testing. J Consult Clin Psychol 46:892–900, 1978.

Hermann BP, Connell B, Barr WB, et al: The utility of the Warrington Recognition Memory Test for temporal lobe epilepsy: Pre- and postoperative results. J Epilepsy 8:139–145, 1995.

Heisenberg W: Physics and Philosophy: The Revolution in Model Science. New York: Harper, 1958.

Hinton-Bayre AD, Geffen G, McFarland K: Mild head injury and speed of information processing: A prospective study of professional rugby players. J Clin Exp Neuropsychol 19:275–289, 1997.

Hiscock CK, Branham JD, Hiscock M: Detection of feigned cognitive impairment: The two-alternative forced-choice method compared with selected conventional tests. J Psychopathol Behav 16:95–110, 1994.

Hiscock M, Hiscock CK: Refining the forced-choice method for the detection of malingering. J Clin Exp Neuropsychol 11: 967–974, 1989.

Iverson GL, Franzen MD: Detecting malingered memory deficits with the Recognition Memory Test. Brain Inj 12:275–282, 1998.

Iverson GL, Franzen MD: The Recognition Memory Test, Digit Span, and Knox Cube Test as markers of malingered memory impairment. Assessment 1:323–334, 1994.

Jury Verdict Research: 2000 Current Award Trends in Personal Injury. Horsham, PA: LRP Publications, 2000.

Kelly MP, Johnson CT, Govern JM: Recognition memory test: Validity in diffuse traumatic brain injury. Appl Neuropsychol 3/4:147–154, 1996.

Kellner R, Sheffield BF: The one-week prevalence of symptoms in neurotic patients and normals. Am J Psychiatry 130:102–105, 1973.

Kessler RC, McGonagle KA, Zhao S, et al: Lifetime and 12-month prevalence of DSM-III-R psychiatric disorders in the United States: Results from the National Comorbidity Survey. Arch Gen Psychiatry 51:8–19, 1994.

Klonoff PS, Lamb DG: Mild head injury, significant impairment on neuropsychological test scores, and psychiatric disability. Clin Neuropsychol 12:31–42, 1998.

Kneeborn AC, Chelune GJ, Luders HO: Individual patient prediction of seizure lateralization in temporal lobe epilepsy: A comparison between neuropsychological memory measures and the intracarotid amobarbitol procedure. J Int Neuropsychol Soc 3:159–168, 1997.

Kreutzer JS, Gordon WA, Rosenthal M, et al: Neuropsychological characteristics of patients with brain injury: Preliminary findings from a multicenter investigation. J Head Trauma Rehabil 8:47–59, 1993.

Lees-Haley PR, Brown RS: Neuropsychological complaint base rates of 170 personal injury claimants. Arch Clin Neuropsychol 8:203–209, 1993.

Lees-Haley PR, Fox DD, Courtney JC: A comparison of complaints by mild injury claimants and other claimants describing subjective experiences immediately following their injury. Arch Clin Neuropsychol 16:689–695, 2001.

Leininger BE, Gramling SE, Farrell AD, et al: Neuropsychological deficits in symptomatic minor head injury patients after concussion and mild concussion. J Neurol Neurosurg Psychiatry 53:293–296, 1990.

Levin HS, Mattis S, Ruff RM, et al: Neurobehavioral outcome following minor head injury: A 3-center study. J Neurosurg 66:234–243, 1987.

Maddocks D, Saling M: Neuropsychological deficits following concussion. Brain Injury 10:99–104, 1996.

Martin RL, Yutzy SH: Somatoform disorders, in Tasman AK, Kay J, Lieberman JA (eds): Psychiatry. Philadelphia, PA: Saunders, 1997, pp. 1119–1155.

McKinzey RK, Russell EW: Detection of malingering on the Halstead-Reitan Battery: A cross-validation. Arch Clin Neuropsychol 12:585–589, 1997.

McLean,A Jr, Temkin NR, Dikmen S, et al: The behavioral sequelae of head injury. J Clin Neuropsychol 5:361–376, 1983.

Meyers JE, Volbrecht M: Validation of reliable digits for detection of malingering. Assessment 5:303–307, 1998.

Millis SR: Assessment of motivation and memory with the Recognition Memory Test after financially compensable mild head injury. J Clin Psychol 50:601–605, 1994.

Millis SR: The Recognition Memory Test in the detection of malingered and exaggerated memory deficits. Clin Neuropsychol 6:406–414, 1992.

Millis SR, Dijkers M: Use of the Recognition Memory Test in traumatic brain injury. Brain Inj 7:53–58, 1993.

Millis SR, Putnam SH: The Recognition Memory Test in the assessment of memory impairment after financially compensable mild head injury: A replication. Percept Mot Skills 79:384–386, 1994.

Millis SR, Putnam SH, Adams KM: Speech-Sounds Perception Test and Seashore Rhythm Test as validity indicators in the neuropsychological evaluation of mild head injury [abstract]. Arch Clin Neuropsychol 11:425, 1996.

Millis SR, Putnam SH, Adams KM, et al: The California Verbal Learning Test in the detection of incomplete effort in neuropsychological evaluation. Psychol Assess 7:463–471, 1995.

Millis SR, Rosenthal M, Novack TA, et al: Long-term neuropsychological outcome following traumatic brain injury. J Head Trauma Rehabil 16:343–355, 2001.

Millis SR, Ross SR, Ricker JH: Detection of incomplete effort on the Wechsler Adult Intelligence Scale-Revised: A cross-validation. J Clin Exp Neuropsychol 20:167–173, 1998.

Mittenberg W, Rotholc A, Russell E, et al: Identification of malingered head injury on the Halstead-Reitan Battery. Arch Clin Neuropsychol 11:271–281, 1996.

Mittenberg W, Theroux-Fichera S, Zielinski RE, et al: Identification of malingered head injury on the Wechsler Adult Intelligence

Scale-Revised. Professional Psychol Res Pract 26:491–498, 1995.

Morris RG, Abrahams S, Polkey CE: Recognition memory for words and faces following unilateral temporal lobectomy. Br J Clin Psychol 34:571–576, 1995.

Morley LC: Personality Assessment Inventory. Odessa, FL: Personality Assessment Resources, 1991.

Narinder K: The coin-in-the-hand test: A new "beside" test for the detection of malingering in patients with suspected memory disorder. J Neurol Neurosurg Psychiatry 57:385–386, 1994.

National Institute of Mental Health: Somatization Disorder in the Medical Setting (DHHS Publication No. ADM 90–1631). Washington, DC: U.S. Government Printing Office, 1990.

Naugle RI, Chelune GJ, Schuster J, et al: Recognition memory for words and faces before and after temporal lobectomy. Assessment 1:373–381, 1994.

Newcombe F, Rabbitt P, Briggs M: Minor head injury: Pathophysiological or iatrogenic sequelae? J Neurol Neurosurg Psychiatry 57:709–716, 1994.

Pankratz L, Erickson RC: Two view of malingering. Clin Neuropsychol 4:379–389, 1990.

Ponsford J, Willmot C, Rothwell A, et al: Factors influencing outcome following mild traumatic brain injury in adults. J Int Neuropsychol Soc 6:568–570, 2000.

Prigatano GP, Amin K: Digit Memory Test: Unequivocal cerebral dysfunction and suspected malingering. J Clin Exp Neuropsychol 15:537–546, 1993.

Rapscak SZ, Polster MR, Comer JF, et al: False recognition and misidentification of faces following right hemisphere damage. Cortex 30:565–583, 1994.

Rees LM, Tombaugh TN, Gansler DA, et al: Five validation experiments of memory malingering (TOMM). Psychol Assess 10:10–20.

Reid S, Wessely S, Crayford T, et al: Medically unexplained symptoms in frequent attenders of secondary health care: Retrospective cohort study. BMJ 322:767–769, 2001.

Rimel RW, Giordani B, Barth JT, et al: Disability caused by minor head injury. Neurosurgery 9:221–228, 1981.

Robins LN, Regier DA: Psychiatric Disorders in America: The Epidemiologic Catchment Area Study. New York: Free Press, 1991.

Rohling ML: Generating a linear function for residual impairment for TBI: A comparison of the HRB and a flexible battery approach. Arch Clin Neuropsychol 15:821–822, 2000.

Rutherford WH, Merrett JD, McDonald JR: Symptoms at one year following concussion from minor head injuries. Injury 10:225–230, 1978.

Sawchyn JM, Brulot MM, Strauss E: Note on use of the Postconcussion Syndrome Checklist. Arch Clin Neuropsychol 15:1–8, 1999.

Slick DJ, Hopp G, Strauss E, et al: Victoria Symptom Validity Test: Professional Manual. Odessa, FL: Psychological Assessment Resources, 1997.

Slick DJ, Sherman EMS, Iverson GL: Diagnostic criteria for malingered neurocognitive dysfunction: Proposed standards for clinical practice and research. Clin Neuropsychol 13:545–561, 1999.

Soukup VM, Bimbela A, Scheiss MC: Recognition Memory for Faces: Reliability and validity of the Warrington Recognition Memory Test (RMT) in a neurological sample. J Clin Psychol 6:287–293, 1999.

Suhr J, Tranel D, Wefel J, et al: Memory performance after head injury: Contributions of malingering, litigation status, psychological factors, and medication use. J Clin Exp Neuropsychol 19:500–514, 1997.

Sullivan K, Keane B, Deffenti C: Malingering on the RAVLT Part I: Deterrence strategies. Arch Clin Neuropsychol 16:627–641, 2001.

Sweet JJ, Demakis GJ, Ricker JH, et al: Diagnostic efficiency and materiel specificity of the Warrington Recognition Memory Test: A collaborative multisite investigation. Arch Clin Neuropsychol 15:301–309, 2000a.

Sweet JJ, Wolf P, Sattlberger E, et al: Further investigation of traumatic brain injury versus insufficient effort with the California Verbal Learning Test. Arch Clin Neuropsychol 15:105–113, 2000b.

Thurman DJ, Guerrero J: Trends in hospitalization associated with traumatic brain injury. JAMA 282:954–957, 1999.

Thurman DJ, Sniezek JE, Johnson D, et al: Guidelines for Surveillance of Central Nervous System Injury. Atlanta: Centers for Disease Control and Prevention, 1995.

Tombaugh TN: The Test of Memory Malingering (TOMM): Normative data from cognitively intact and cognitively impaired individuals. Psychol Assess 9:260–268, 1997.

Trahan DE, Ross CE, Trahan SL: Relationships among postconcussional-type symptoms, depression, and anxiety in neurologically normal young adults and victims of mild brain injury. Arch Clin Neuropsychol 16:435–445, 2001.

Trueblood W: Qualitative and quantitative characteristics of malingered and other invalid WAIS-R and clinical memory data. J Clin Exp Neuropsychol 16:597–607, 1994.

Trueblood W, Schmidt M: Malingering and other validity considerations in the neuropsychological evaluation of mild head injury. J Clin Exp Neuropsychol 15:578–590, 1993.

Warrington EK: Recognition Memory Test. Windsor, UK: NFER-Nelson, 1984.

Williams DH, Levin HS, Eisenberg HM: Mild head injury classification. Neurosurgery 27:422–428, 1990.

Wilson IB, Cleary PD: Linking clinical variables with health-related quality of life. JAMA 273:59–65, 1995.

C H A P T E R

54

Violent Crime

Jonathan H. Pincus

Abuse

Brain damage

Paranoia

Experience-dependent neural activity

Trauma

Violent crimes, including mass murder, serial murder, murder for profit, and other homicides, are actually rare events committed by only a small number of individuals, each of whom is not violent all the time. Less than 6% of the population commit up to 70% of the violent crimes (Wolfgang, 1975). In consideration of its rarity, violence is almost abnormal by definition. Certainly one is justified in asking the question, "What is wrong with this (violent) person? Could there be something wrong with his/her brain?" I have had the opportunity to examine a significant number of murderers and less violent adults and delinquents. This experience has led to a hypothesis of the potential causes of violent behavior.

The data that arise from studying seriously violent offenders indicate that three factors frequently influence the expression of violence:

(1) Abuse: The experience of severe, daily, physical and/or sexual abuse in childhood. This abuse has often been sustained for years and is of such a quality that it legitimately makes the child fear for his/her life and corporeal integrity.

(2) Brain damage: This frequently derives from prenatal, perinatal, and neonatal insults such as maternal alcohol or drug use or other maternal toxic exposures, complicated deliveries, accidental head trauma, sometimes sustained through parental abuse, exposure to toxins, or any of the other myriad causes of brain damage. It is often very difficult to determine which of the many factors that could have caused brain deficits have been the most destructive in an individual patient, and it is often impossible to date and place the damage within the central nervous system.

(3) Paranoia: This can be the result of mental illness, drugs, brain damage, or environmental factors.

All three factors have been present in about two thirds of violent juveniles (Lewis et al., 1979) and in murderers (Feldman et al., 1986; Lewis et al., 1986; Blake et al., 1995). No violent individual whom I have examined has been free of all three of these factors.

I think it likely that these correlates of violence play an important role in the causation of violence even though the majority of people with only a single one of these factors (abuse, brain damage, or paranoid thinking) are not violent. It is also likely that many individuals who manifest all three factors are not violent. Indeed, even the most violent individuals are not violent most of the time. According to the theory I have evolved with Dr. Dorothy O. Lewis, precipitating factors that would ordinarily not be sufficient to result in violence

1091

are sufficient only in those individuals who carry these vulnerabilities.

The concordance of neurologic damage, abuse, and paranoid thinking was particularly striking in a relatively unselected population of 14 young men who were awaiting execution for crimes committed before they were 18 years old. The 14 men comprised the entire population of murderers of that age in four states and represented 38% of the entire population of condemned juvenile murderers in the United States at that time. All but one had been physically and/or sexually abused. Sixty-four percent had major neurologic impairments and only two had full-scale IQ scores over 90. Ten were paranoid, and the remainder had mood disorders and bizarre behavior. Half had actually been psychotic, with psychiatric hospitalizations before commission of the capital crime (Lewis et al., 1988).

Of 15 other death row inmates, evaluated only because of the imminence of their execution dates, not because of supposed intrinsic brain vulnerability, 13 had suffered severe physical abuse and/or sexual abuse by parents (Feldman et al., 1986). Twelve had neurologic deficits and had sustained concussions or worse. Six were chronically psychotic; three had been episodically psychotic; two others had bipolar mood disorder. Nine of the 15 subjects suffered psychiatric symptoms during childhood severe enough for consultation. Four had attempted suicide in childhood. Eight expressed paranoid ideas at the time of examination (Lewis et al., 1986).

How do neurologic deficits, paranoia, and the experience of abuse relate to the etiology of violence? A follow-up study of 95 delinquent 15-year-old boys 7 years after initial evaluation suggested that paranoid thinking, neurologic dysfunction, and abuse were not merely additive, but that these vulnerabilities interacted to increase the risk and severity of adult violent criminality. The presence of the three variables in delinquents predicted violence over a 7-year period in 85%. The absence of these variables at age 15 also predicted future nonviolent behavior 85% of the time (Lewis et al., 1989).

ABUSE DAMAGES THE DEVELOPING BRAIN

Emotional neglect of institutionalized infants in the first years of life causes long-lasting behavioral/cognitive changes (Spitz & Cobliner, 1966; Provence, 1967; Rutter, 1998). The early isolation of immature monkeys also induces long-lasting behavioral changes (Harlow et al., 1971). These responses of the immature mammalian brain may be analogous to the imprinting experience of newly hatched goslings (Lorenz, 1970). Physical and sexual abuse of infants and children, however, have much greater destructive potential than neglect.

Child abuse has devastating consequences for children and for the adults they become. Abuse early in life correlates with conduct disorder oppositional defiant disorder in children (Ford et al., 1999). Later on it is linked to depression, aggression, anxiety, suicide (Fergusson et al., 1996; Levitan et al., 1998), impulsivity, antisocial personality disorder (Luntz & Widom, 1994), borderline personality disorder (Paris et al., 1994a,b; Gudzer et al., 1999), post-traumatic stress disorder (PTSD) (Famularo et al., 1996), and conversion disorders (Wyllie et al., 1999).

There is a growing perception that prolonged child abuse permanently changes the anatomy and function of the child's brain. Child abuse has thus moved away from the purely sociologic and psychological realm of interest and into the neurologic sphere. Abuse can potentially damage the brain by direct trauma. More insidiously and pervasively, abuse alters the basic developmental anatomy, physiology, and functioning of the brain.

What the brain registers through its sensory systems about the surrounding environment is increasingly recognized as a critical factor that permanently changes the brain by altering its connections. There is an exuberant development of synaptic connections between nerve cells in the first months and years of life, and this connectivity is "pared down" by experience. The changes in synaptic function that occur normally with maturity have been correlated with studies of cerebral glucose utilization, using positron emission tomography (PET) (Chugani, 1998).

Connections that are not used at critical times are lost forever (Huttenlocher & Dabholkar, 1997). The synaptic connections that occur in infancy may form the anatomic substrate for neural plasticity and for early learning as well as for the superior reorganizational capacity of the immature brain after injury (Cao et al., 1994.)

Experience is critical for the functional and structural maturation of connections in the mammalian cortex. Through experience, immature circuits are "sculpted." Experience-dependent neural activity endows the brain with an ongoing ability to accommodate to changing inputs during development and throughout life (Katz & Shatz, 1996). When the brain is deprived of early experience or presented with an abnormal experience during its early development, the functioning of the cortex is disrupted.

The visual system provides a model of the early sensitivity to the environment shown by the connections of brain nerve cells. If an infant is born with a cataract, the cataract must be removed early because, if it is not, vision will never develop in the formerly visually deprived eye. This is not true of adults. If dense cataracts are removed from the sightless eye of an adult, blind for years, vision can be restored.

The development of amblyopia ex anopsia describes permanent blindness in a child, which has developed from strabismus. This form of blindness occurs only in childhood. The development of amblyopia in humans (Grigg et al., 1996; Sengpiel & Blakemore, 1996) illustrates the obliteration of a genetic endowment, present at birth, by abnormal environmental stimulation. Similar permanent changes in the cerebral cortex can occur in other sensory and motor systems (Singer, 1995). Hearing, somatosensory systems, and motor development can all be permanently affected by early experience (Huntley, 1997), including emotional experience (Joseph, 1998). Physical abuse can alter the quantitative electroencephalogram (EEG) results (Teicher et al., 1997; Ito et al., 1998) and the magnetic resonance imaging (MRI) scan results (Bremner & Narayan, 1998), as well as behavior (George et al., 1979).

The vulnerability of the immature nervous system to permanent, irreversible changes as the result of sensory stimulation deprivation or manipulation probably underlies the common observation that children learn quickly and that youth is impressionable. Obviously, the psychosensory environment can cause permanent changes in the brains of children for either good or bad.

Early experiences have dramatic effects on the development of the immature brain. Major depression and other mental conditions follow child abuse (De Bellis et al., 1999; Kaufman et al., 2000).

Unbearable early stress that has been induced by severe corporal and sexual torture might induce changes in a number of different ways. Stress can alter the development of the hypothalamic-pituitary-adrenal axis. In preclinical studies corticotropin-releasing factor (CRF) is a vector of destructive brain changes. CRF hypersecretion throughout life is a consequence of severe abuse in childhood and this could underlie the psychopathology that follows abuse (Heim et al., 2000). Physiologic correlates of abuse lead to a state of chronic hyperarousal (Kendall-Tackett, 2000), and relatively specific neurochemical changes occur in the brains of abused children. For example, there are high levels of excitatory amino acid concentrations in the ventricular cerebrospinal fluid of badly abused children and this could be a source of excitotoxic damage (Ruppel et al., 2001). A low ratio of N-acetylaspartate/creatine, implying a loss of neural integrity, has been described in the anterior cingulate of 11 young victims of abuse who had PTSD, compared with age- and gender-matched controls (De Bellis et al., 2000). The memory loss of dissociative amnesia that has been induced by psychological stress may be the result of the toxic action of high, prolonged levels of glucosteroids on the hippocampus, a region of the brain that is involved with the storage and retrieval of memories (Joseph, 1999). Quantitative MRI studies of the brain in abused populations reveal decreased brain volumes (Bremner et al., 1997; Driessen et al., 2000). PET studies

of sexually abused women with and without PTSD correlated PTSD with dysfunction of the medial premotor cortex, hippocampus, and visual association cortex (Bremner et al., 1999; Shin et al., 1999).

The changes seen clinically and on imaging tests may be the result of developmental and neurochemical factors as indicated above, or simple physical injury to the brain. The temporal and frontal poles, especially the undersurfaces, are the most likely sites of contusion after traumatic brain injury (TBI). Repeated concussions, defined as brain injuries that cause temporary cognitive changes, can cause permanent effects even when each is not severe enough to cause bleeding that is detectable on CT scans (see Chapter 27). Presumably this is the result of the shearing effect of injuries upon the axonal nerve processes (Pearl, 1998). The damage caused by shaking babies, as well as other induced traumatic brain injuries, produce widespread axonal damage (Shannon et al., 1998) with beta-amyloid precursor protein described by immunohistochemistry. The extent of changes induced by trauma is comparable to the changes induced by severe hypoxia (Gleckman, 1999).

Whatever the source of injury, it is not possible to argue that abuse is without long-lasting clinical behavioral, neuropathologic, neurochemical, and neurophysiological effects.

Estimates of the prevalence of previous physical and sexual abuse among incarcerated violent juvenile delinquents have reached up to 80% (Lewis et al., 1979). In prisoners held on death row who have been convicted of homicide, both juveniles (Lewis et al., 1988) and adults (Feldman, 1986; Blake et al., 1995) have prevalence rates of prior sexual and/or physical abuse in their childhood that have approached 100%. Among nondelinquents matched with delinquents for gender, age, race, and socioeconomic level, the prevalence rate of abuse is much lower (13%) (Lewis et al., 1987). The amount of abuse has seldom been quantified. It seems reasonable to postulate that severity, frequency, duration of episodes, and years of exposure could vary, and that the worst abuse would be the most harmful (McClellan et al., 1995).

Despite the high prevalence of abuse amongst violent criminals, the causal role of abuse in violent behavior must be complex because only a minority of abused children become violent criminals. Follow-up studies of children who have been subjected to abuse have described increased levels of aggressive behavior compared with controls, but most previously abused children appear to be neither disturbed nor aggressive. In only a minority of families in which abuse was severe enough to lead to outside intervention is there child abuse in the next generation (Widom, 1989). Even if underreporting of abuse seriously reduced the apparent rate of intergenerational abuse, it is very clear that abuse does not always generate abuse, let alone other violent crimes. Abuse alone is not enough to produce a violent criminal under most circumstances.

The capacity of some abused people to lead relatively normal lives is a testament to the resilience of the human spirit (i.e., the plasticity of the human brain), yet a large number of formerly abused people do become violent and dangerous to society, and there is a direct link between the experience of abuse and later violence (Oliver, 1993).

It may take enormous energy and an intact nervous system, one that is unimpaired by neurologic or psychiatric symptoms, to overcome the tendency to violence that is engendered by consistent, long-term abuse experienced at a tender age. Thus, abused individuals who have become violent may have other vulnerabilities, such as neurologic deficits and paranoia. The concordance of these three factors in violent individuals could be explained if the three interacted to create a violent criminal.

BRAIN DAMAGE

Trauma

Many violent individuals have histories of head injuries, and this may be a common source of neurologic deficits among the violent. Mild concussions can have a cumulative effect. In a study of high school football players who were tested before playing and then after apparent recovery from brain injury sustained in the game, mild concussions caused clinically detectable deficits (McCrea et al., 1997). Athletes who have suffered concussions and who have recovered are more at risk to be detectably and permanently brain damaged by subsequent head injuries than those who have never had a concussion. Repeated mild brain injuries occurring over months or years can result in cumulative neurologic and cognitive defects. This is now called the second impact syndrome (CDC-MMWR, 1997). This finding has provided the basis for a position statement of the American Academy of Neurology on the management of closed head injuries among athletes, limiting their return to the sport after concussion to prevent serious brain damage (Kelly & Rosenberg, 1998). Cognitive dysfunction is not only a short-term consequence of concussion but is also a predisposing risk factor for brain damage from future concussion (Teasdale & Engberg, 1997). Despite the general agreement about the hazards of repeated mild TBIs, it is not possible to determine the exact site of injury in every case nor to define the exact role of each episode in damaging the brain (Kelly & Rosenberg, 1998).

Brain injury, especially inflicted trauma (child abuse), can have devastating effects on children because the inflicted injuries are usually recurrent. Ewing-Cobbs and colleagues (1998) reported that single episodes of inflicted TBI, though comparable in severity to noninflicted TBI, were significantly more likely to impair the cognitive function of the victim, even when the TBI did not cause prolonged impairment of consciousness. Mental deficiency was present in 45% of the inflicted and 5% of the noninflicted TBI groups. The effects of TBI are, thus, linked with previous abuse and neglect.

There is no doubt that frontal lobe injuries can affect violent behavior. In a study of Vietnam War veterans who sustained penetrating brain injuries, those with frontal lobe damage were significantly more likely to be violent in the succeeding years than the veterans who sustained penetrating injuries elsewhere in the brain. Sustaining frontal lobe injury does not guarantee violence; the majority of the frontally injured veterans had not acted violently at follow-up (Grafman et al., 1996).

Episodic Dyscontrol

The concept that episodic dyscontrol, outbursts of rage and violence that seem to be motiveless, arises from an epileptic-like discharge that originates in a sensitive part of the brain (often the temporal lobe) and can be controlled with anticonvulsants, is a concept that we once thought to be likely, but does not provide a comprehensive explanation for more than a few isolated instances of violence. Only a third of murderers show evidence of temporal lobe abnormality (Blake et al., 1995), and only 5 of 97 incarcerated juvenile delinquents seemed to have an episode of violence that could have been the direct result of a complex partial seizure (Lewis et al., 1982). All five of these individuals had other episodes of violence that were clearly not caused by seizures. Any benefit derived from the use of anticonvulsants in treating people with episodic violent behavior may be related to the stabilization of their mood rather than the control of putative epilepsy.

Violent behavior in patients with irritative lesions of the limbic system secondary to temporolimbic epilepsy (Devinsky & Bear, 1984) and focal lesions elsewhere—e.g., a patient with a hamartoma of the ventromedial thalamus (Reeves & Plum, 1969)—seems to support the concept that violent behavior can directly arise from cerebral stimulation or destruction. There is, however, an alternate explanation for these cases: Because limbic circuits and limbic impulses are dampened by the frontal lobe, especially the orbitofrontal cortices, the loss of the frontal lobe, its projections to the basal ganglia and diencephalon, and its inhibiting effect on behavior may allow expression of unacceptable limbic impulses. The case of Phineas Gage has been interpreted this way (Damasio et al., 1994). Patients with orbitofrontal injuries have been found to display disinhibition, impulsivity, and lack of empathy that have justified the appellation "acquired sociopathy" (Tranel, 1994).

It is impossible to make a one-to-one correlation between violence and specific forms of neurologic dysfunction or the brain regions involved. There is no "violence center" in the brain that, when stimulated, always produces violent behavior, though occasional case reports of such a sequence exist (Mark & Ervin, 1970). There is no region of the brain identified on PET or other imaging techniques whose abnormal activity allows doctors to predict that the individual whose brain is abnormal will be violent. The relationship between neurologic dysfunction of the brain and the propensity to violence is more complex.

Brain damage, including epilepsy, mental retardation, and alcohol intoxication, impairs executive functioning and leads to the disinhibition of impulses, irritability, and poor judgment in planning. If the impulses to violence are already encoded in the brain by years of child abuse and/or mental illness, brain damage can unleash violence by limiting the patient's ability to plan wisely, to sequence events, to see the outcome of particular acts, to care about this outcome, or to delay the gratification of impulses. In other words, factors besides frontal dysfunction must also be operative for frontal lobe damage to produce violence. The other vulnerabilities, according to the model I endorse, are abuse and mental illness (Lewis et al., 1979).

Indicia of Damage

The demonstration of brain damage in violent criminals relies on a variety of testing procedures. Unfortunately, no single test infallibly provides a touchstone to determine the presence of brain damage or brain dysfunction. The history, the physical examination, neuropsychological tests, the EEG, and imaging tests individually may fail to identify brain dysfunction that is manifest on another test. The abnormal test is definitive. MRI is a very reliable indicator of gross structural disturbances of the brain (tumors, strokes, multiple sclerosis), but seldom provides useful information with regard to epilepsy, retardation, dementia, intoxication, learning disorders, clumsiness, and movement disorders. EEG testing is better than MRI testing for diagnosing epilepsy. Psychological tests are best for retardation, dementia, and learning disorders. The physical examination is best for clumsiness and movement disorders. Each test of brain function can appear normal in patients with moderate to severe brain disorders that have been revealed in other test(s). In combination, these tests have virtually always revealed evidence of brain dysfunction in violent individuals (Blake et al., 1995). PET scans, especially when they are performed during activation and compared with controls, are very valuable in defining dysfunctional portions of the brain (Raine et al., 1994, 1997).

Antisocial Personality and the Frontal Lobe

There is a tendency to categorize repeatedly violent behavior as the result of "antisocial personality disorder." Though there is no doubt that murderers have acted antisocially, this diagnosis does not provide an understanding of their antisocial behavior. All behavior must be of cerebral origin, and the list of symptoms that describes antisocial personality disorder is very similar to a list of symptoms that might describe patients with frontal lobe damage (e.g., failure to conform to social norms, impulsivity, irritability, recklessness, irresponsibility, lack of remorse, and indifference).

Quantitative analysis of MRI scans has shown deficient volume of the frontal lobes in people with antisocial personality disorder compared with normal controls and drug abusers who did not have antisocial personality disorder (Raine et al., 2000). Raine and colleagues (1994, 1997) have compared PET scans of 41 murderers who pleaded "not guilty by reason of insanity" (NGRI) with 41 controls during a continuous performance test. This visual test activates the frontal region of the brain because it requires focused attention and mental vigilance for a prolonged period. The premotor frontal cortex in the murderers failed to activate. No deficit was found in the temporal or occipital cortex. Murderers tended to show less activation in the left subcortical regions (amygdala, hippocampus, and thalamus) but higher activation than controls in the homologous regions of the right hemisphere (Raine et al., 1994, 1997). The frontal lobes project to the corpus striatum, the pallidum, the dorsomedial nucleus of the thalamus, and elsewhere. Dysfunction in these regions can give rise to disinhibited "frontal"-type behavior, even though these regions are not in the frontal lobe.

Intoxication

The temporary encephalopathy of intoxication also provides a neurologic basis for disinhibition. More than half of all homicides are committed by intoxicated individuals (Yarvis, 1994). The extent of encephalopathy caused by intoxicants like alcohol can be assessed with clinical testing and with blood and urine levels at the time of intoxication. All tests of brain structure and function and body fluids are likely to be normal after the intoxicant has been metabolized. Cocaine and amphetamines are especially likely to result in violence because these drugs induce a sense of invulnerability, akin to mania. This powerful disinhibiting effect is especially sought out by depressed individuals who are treating themselves with street drugs. Prolonged use of these stimulants induces paranoid delusions and a mental state that is indistinguishable from paranoid schizophrenia, except that it ultimately clears after the drug has been fully metabolized. Stimulants thus induce disinhibition and paranoia, two of the main vulnerabilities to violence. The prevalence of the use of cocaine correlates with the rise and fall of violent crime in cities in the United States (Golub & Johnson, 1994; Blumstein et al., 2000).

MENTAL ILLNESS AND VIOLENCE

There is overwhelming evidence to support a causal connection between paranoid delusions and violence (Taylor, 1985). The degree of schizophrenic symptoms is a predictor of dangerousness in hospitalized schizophrenics (Yesavage, 1984). Among men convicted of homicide and arson, a high proportion were considered definitely to have been driven by psychotic symptoms to commit offenses. Our own findings, which indicated a very high rate of paranoid thinking among violent individuals—adults and juveniles incarcerated on death row in the United States—are consistent with these reports. Variability over the course of time in the intensity of paranoia is quite characteristic of depression, mania, schizophrenia, and drug intoxication, and may determine the timing of acts of violence. Of 500 British murderers whose psychiatric reports were reviewed, 44% had a lifetime history of mental illness, and 14% had mental symptoms at the time of the homicide (Shaw et al., 1999). In Sweden, 63% of murderers had prior psychiatric care, 16% committed suicide, and 70% were intoxicated at the time of the homicide (Lindquist, 1986). Major mental disorder is an important factor in violence, especially when comorbid with the encephalopathy of substance abuse (Rasanen et al., 1998; Steadman et al., 1998; Wallace et al., 1998).

There is a strong link between mood disorder and violent crime. Homicide and depression are closely connected, along with the experience of child abuse (Rosenbaum & Bennett, 1986). Unipolar depression causes irritability and anger (Fava, 1998) and bipolar affective disorder can also cause anger and aggression (Oquendo et al., 2000). Male and female adolescents and adults are more likely to be aggressive when they are clinically depressed (Knox et al., 2000). Intrafamilial violence directed at spouses or children also has been linked to depression (Bourget et al., 2000) and to excessive suspiciousness (Rosenbaum & Bennett, 1986).

Paranoia exists on a spectrum ranging from mild to severe. At the most severe end are delusions. Paranoid delusions are very dramatic but very nonspecific symptoms. The diseases that can give rise to paranoid delusions and less severe forms of paranoid thinking vary considerably, falling often within the traditional scope of psychiatric practice, and include schizophrenia, mania, and depression. Neurologic conditions can also cause paranoia. Among these conditions are drug intoxication and many organic condi-

tions of the brain, including virtually anything that can cause cognitive impairment.

Despite the strong correlation of paranoid thinking with violence, how can we explain the fact that most paranoid individuals and most mentally ill individuals are not violent? This question is quite similar to the one asked about neurologic damage and abuse, and the answer is the same. Violent individuals may bring vulnerabilities to their mental symptoms that result in violence. Neurologic dysfunction and the experience of abuse may be the most important of these.

RESPONSIBILITY

If violence comes from the brain, is anyone responsible for his or her acts? Specific behaviors have been associated with specific genetic and chromosomal disorders, implying that abnormal behavior and the urges that drive them are encoded in the brain by genes. Yet violence is very clearly not genetic (Mednick et al., 1984).

Behavior can be conceived as the result of free will that is expressed through brain activity, as a symphony is expressed by an orchestra. If the performance is deficient and the instruments on which the orchestra has played are found to be broken, the fault for the defective performance may not lie with the conception of the composer but with the broken instruments on which that idea was expressed. We speak of the "mind" and "psychological factors" and "volition" as though these terms refer to something outside or above the brain, but it is the brain that expresses them. Even those individuals who do not want to accept biology as the sole determinant of morality must admit that it is one of the determinants. Free will is constrained by disease of the brain. Violence is a behavior that can be understood as the vector of some potentially mitigating influences over which many perpetrators have no control: abuse, neurologic damage, and mental illness.

■ KEY POINTS

☐   Three factors frequently influence the expression of violence: abuse, brain damage, and paranoia.

☐   Emotional neglect of institutionalized infants in the first years of life causes long-lasting behavioral/cognitive changes.

☐   Abuse early in life correlates with conduct disorder and oppositional defiant disorder in children. Later on it is linked to depression, aggression, anxiety, suicide, impulsivity, antisocial personality disorder, borderline personality disorder, and conversion disorders.

☐   Many violent individuals have histories of head injuries, and this may be a common source of neurologic deficits among the violent.

☐   There is a strong link between mood disorder and violent crime. Homicide and depression are closely linked, along with the experience of child abuse.

☐   Free will is constrained by disease of the brain.

KEY READINGS

Bremner JD, et al: Magnetic resonance imaging-based measurement of hippocampal volume in post-traumatic stress disorder related to childhood physical and sexual abuse. Biol Psychiatry 41:23, 1997.

Driessen M, Herrmann J, Stahl K, et al: Magnetic resonance imaging volumes of the hippocampus and the amygdala in women with borderline personality disorder and early traumatization. Arch Gen Psychiatry 57:1115–1122, 2000.

Fergusson DM, Horwood LJ, Lynskey MT: Childhood sexual abuse and psychiatric disorder in young adulthood: II. Psychiatric outcomes of childhood sexual abuse. J Am Acad Child Adolesc Psychiatry 35:1365–1374, 1996.

Harlow HF, Harlow MK, Suomi SJ: From thought to therapy: Lessons from a primate laboratory. How investigation of the learning capability of rhesus monkeys has led to the study of their behavioral abnormalities and rehabilitation. Am Scien 59:538, 1971.

Ruppell RA, Kochanek PM, Adelson PD, et al: Excitatory amino acid concentrations in ventricular cerebrospinal fluid after severe traumatic brain injury in infants and children: The role of child abuse. J Pediatr 138:18–25, 2001.

REFERENCES

Blake PY, Pincus JH, Buckner G: Neurologic abnormalities in murderers. Neurology 45:1641, 1995.

Blumstein A, Rivera FP, Rosenfeld R: The rise and decline of homicide and why. Ann Rev Public Health 21:505–541, 2000.

Bourget D, Gagne P, Moami J: Spousal homicide and suicide in Quebec. J Am Acad Psychiatry Law 28:179–182, 2000.

Bremner JD, Randall P, Vermetten E, et al: Magnetic resonance imaging–based measurement of hippocampal volume in post-traumatic stress disorder related to childhood physical and sexual abuse. Biol Psychiatry 41:23–32, 1997.

Bremner JD, Naryan M: The effects of stress on memory and the hippocampus throughout the life cycle: Implications for childhood development and aging. Dev Psychopathol 10:871–885, 1998.

Bremner JD, Narayan M, Staib LH, et al: Neural correlates of memories of childhood sexual abuse in women with and without posttraumatic stress disorder. Am J Psychiatry 156:1787–1795, 1999.

Cao Y, Vikingstad EM, Huttenlocher PR, et al: Functional magnetic resonance studies of the reorganization of the sensorimotor area after unilateral brain injury in the perinatal period. Proc Natl Acad Sci 91:9612, 1994.

Centers for Disease Control [and Prevention] (CDC): Sports-related recurrent brain injuries—United States. MMWR 46:224–227, 1997.

Chugani HT: A critical period of brain development: Studies of cerebral glucose utilization with PET. Prev Med 27:184, 1998.

Damasio H, Grabowski T, Frank R: The return of Phineas Gage: Clues about the brain from the skull of a famous patient. Science 264:1102, 1994.

De Bellis MD, Keshaven MS, Clark DB, et al: Developmental traumatology. Part II. Brain development. Biol Psychiatry 45:1271–1284, 1999.

De Bellis MD, Keshaven MS, Spencer S, et al: N-Acetylaspartate concentration in the anterior cingulated of maltreated children and adolescents with PTSD. Am J Psychiatry 157:1175–1177, 2000.

Driessen M, Herrmann J, Stahl K, et al: Magnetic resonance imaging volumes of the hippocampus and the amygdala in women with borderline personality disorder and early traumatization. Arch Gen Psychiatry 57:1115–1122, 2000.

Ewing-Cobbs L, Kramer L, M Prasad, et al: Neuroimaging, physical, and developmental findings after inflicted and noninflicted traumatic brain injury in young children. Pediatrics 102:300, 1998.

Famularo R, Fenton T, Kinscherff R, et al: Psychiatric comorbidity in childhood post traumatic stress disorder. Child Abuse Negl 20:953–961, 1996.

Fava M: Depression with anger attacks. J Clin Psychiatry 18:18–22, 1998.

Feldman M, Malhoun K, Lewis DO: Filicidal abuse in the histories of fifteen condemned murderers. Bull Am Acad Psychiatry Law 14:345, 1986.

Fergusson DM, Horwood LJ, Lynskey MT: Childhood sexual abuse and psychiatric disorder in young adulthood: II. Psychiatric outcomes of childhood sexual abuse. J Am Acad Child Adolesc Psychiatry 35:1365–1374, 1996.

Ford JD, Racusin R, Davis WB, et al: Trauma exposure among children with oppositional defiant disorder and attention deficit-hyperactive disorder. J Consult Clin Psychol 67:786–789, 1999.

George C, et al: Social interactions of young abused children: Approach, avoidance, and aggression. Child Dev 50:306, 1979.

Gleckman AM: Diffuse axonal injury in infants with nonaccidental craniocerebral trauma: Enhanced detection by beta-amyloid precursor protein immunohistochemical staining. Arch Pathol Lab Med 123:146–151, 1999.

Golub A, Johnson BD: A recent decline in cocaine use among youthful arrestees in Manhattan 1987 through 1993. Am J Public Health 84:1250–1254, 1994.

Grafman J, Schwab K, Warden D, et al: Frontal lobe injuries, violence, and aggression: A report of the Vietnam Head Injury Study. Neurology 46:1231, 1996.

Grigg J, Thomas R, Billson F: Neuronal basis of amblyopia: A review. Indian J Ophthalmol 44:69, 1996.

Gudzer J, Paris J, Zelkowitz P, et al: Psychological risk factors for borderline pathology in school-aged children. J Am Acad Child Adolesc Psychiatry 38:206, 1999.

Harlow HF, Harlow MK, Suomi SJ: From thought to therapy: Lessons from a primate laboratory. How investigation of the learning capability of rhesus monkeys has led to the study of their behavioral abnormalities and rehabilitation. Am Scien 59:538, 1971.

Heim C, Newport DJ, Heit S, et al: Pituitary-adrenal and autonomic responses to stress in women after sexual and physical abuse in childhood. JAMA 284:592–597, 2000.

Huntley GW: Differential effects of abnormal tactile experience on shaping representation patterns in developing and adult motor cortex. J Neurosci 17:9220, 1997.

Huttenlocher PR, Dabholkar AS: Regional differences in synaptogenesis in human cerebral cortex, J Comp Neurol 387:167, 1997.

Ito Y, Teicher MH, Glod CA, et al: Preliminary evidence for aberrant cortical development in abused children: A quantitative EEG study. J Neuropsychiatry Clin Neurosci 10:298, 1998.

Joseph R: Traumatic amnesia, repression, and hippocampus injury due to emotional stress, corticosteroids, and enkephalins. Child Psychiatry Hum Dev 29:169, 1998.

Joseph R: The neurology of traumatic "dissociative" amnesia: Commentary and literature review. Child Abuse Negl 23:715–727, 1999.

Katz LC, Shatz A: Synaptic activity and the construction of cortical circuits. Science 4:1133, 1996.

Kaufman J, Plotsky PM, Nemeroff CB, et al: Effects of early adverse experiences on brain structure and function: Clinical implications. Biol Psychiatry 48:778–790, 2000.

Kelly JP, Rosenberg JH: The development of guidelines for the management of concussion in sports. J Head Trauma Rehabil 13:53, 1998.

Kendall-Tacket KA: Physiological correlates of childhood abuse: Chronic hyperarousal in PTSD, depression, and irritable bowel syndrome. Child Abuse Negl 24:799–810, 2000.

Knox M, King C, Hanna GL, et al: Aggressive behavior in clinically depressed adolescents. J Am Acad Child Adolesc Psychiatry 39:611–618, 2000.

Levitan RD, Parikh SV, Lesage AD, et al: Major depression in individuals with a history of childhood physical or sexual abuse: Relationship to neurovegetative features, mania, and gender. Am J Psychiatry 155:1746, 1998.

Lewis DO, Lovely R, Yeager C, et al: Toward a theory of the genesis of violence: A followup study of delinquents. J Am Acad Child Adolesc Psychiatry. 28:431, 1989.

Lewis DO, Pincus JH, Bard B, et al: Neuropsychiatric, psychoeducational and family characteristics of fourteen juveniles condemned to death in the United States. Am J Psychiatry 145:584, 1988.

Lewis DO, Pincus JH, Feldman M, et al: Psychiatric, neurological, and psychoeducational characteristics of 15 death row inmates in the United States. Am J Psychiatry 143:838, 1986.

Lewis DO, Pincus JH, Lovely R, et al: Biosocial characteristics of matched samples of delinquents and non-delinquents. J Am Acad Child Adolesc Psychiatry 26:744, 1987.

Lewis DO, Pincus JH, Shanok SS, et al: Psychomotor epilepsy and violence in a group of incarcerated adolescent boys. Am J Psychiatry 139:882, 1982.

Lewis DO, Shanok SS, Pincus JH, et al: Violent juvenile delinquents: Psychiatric, neurological, psychological, and abuse factors. J Am Acad Child Psychiatry 18:307, 1979.

Lindquist P: Criminal homicide in northern Sweden 1970–1981: Alcohol intoxication, alcohol abuse, and mental disease. Int J Psychiatry 8:19, 1986.

Lorenz K: Studies in Animal and Human Behavior, Vol. 1. Robert Martin, trans. London: Methuen, 1970.

Luntz BK, Widom CS: Antisocial personality disorder in abused and neglected children grown up. Am J Psychiatry151:670, 1994.

Mark VH, Ervin FR: Violence and the Brain. New York: Harper and Row, 1970.

McClellan J, Adams J, Douglas D, et al: Clinical characteristics related to severity of sexual abuse: A study of seriously mentally ill youth. Child Abuse Negl 10:1245, 1995.

McCrea M, Kelly JP, Kluge J, et al: Standardized assessment of concussion in football players. Neurology 48:586, 1997.

Mednick SA, Gabrielli Jr. WF, Hutchings B: Genetic influences in criminal convictions: Evidence from an adoption cohort. Science 224:891, 1984.

Oliver JE: Intergenerational transmission of child abuse: Rates research and clinical implications. Am J Psychiatry 150:1351, 1993.

Oquendo MA, Waternaux C, Brodsky B, et al: Suicidal behavior in bipolar mood disorder: Clinical characteristics of attempters and nonattempters. J Affect Disord 59:107–117, 2000.

Paris JH, Zweig-Frank, Gudzer J: Psychological risk factors for borderline personality disorder in female patients. Compr Psychiatry 35:301–305, 1994a.

Paris JH, Zweig-Frank, Gudzer J: Risk factors for borderline personality in male outpatients. J Nerv Ment Dis 182:375–380, 1994b.

Pearl GS: Traumatic neuropathology. Clin Lab Med 18:39, 1998.

Provence S: Infants in Institutions: A Comparison of Their Development Through the First Year of Life with Family Reared Children. New York: International Universities Press, 1967.

Raine A, Buchsbaum MS LaCasse: Brain abnormalities in murderers indicated by positron emission tomography. Biol Psychiatry 42:495, 1997.

Raine A, Buchsbaum MS, Stanley J, et al: Selective reductions in prefrontal glucose metabolism in murderers. Biol Psychiatry 36:365, 1994.

Raine A, Lencz T, Bihrle S, et al: Reduced frontal prefrontal gray matter volume and reduced automatic activity in antisocial personality disorder. Arch Gen Psychiatry 57:119, 2000.

Rasanen P, Tiihonen J, Isohanni M, et al: Schizophrenia, alcohol abuse, and violent behavior: A 26-year follow-up study of an unselected birth cohort. Schizophr Bull 24:432, 1998.

Reeves AG, Plum F: Hyperphagia, rage, and dementia accompanying a ventromedial hypothalamic neoplasm. Arch Neurol 20:616, 1969.

Rosenbaum M, Bennett B: Homicide and depression. Am J Psychiatry 143:367–370, 1986.

Ruppell RA, Kochanek PM, Adelson PD, et al: Excitatory amino acid concentrations in ventricular cerebrospinal fluid after severe traumatic brain injury in infants and children: The role of child abuse. J Pediatr 138:18–25, 2001.

Rutter M: Developmental catch-up and deficit following adoption after severe global, early privation: English and Romanian Adoptees (ERA) Study Team. J Child Psychol Psychiatry 39:405, 1998.

Sengpiel F, Blakemore C: The neural basis of suppression and amblyopia in strabismus. Eye 10:250, 1996.

Shannon P, Smith CR, Deck J, et al: Axonal injury and the neuropathology of shaken baby syndrome. Acta Neuropathol 95:625–631, 1998.

Shaw J, Appleby L Amos T, et al: Mental disorder and clinical care in people convicted of homicide: National clinical survey. BMJ 318:1240, 1999.

Shin LM, McNally RJ, Kosslyn SM, et al: Regional cerebral blood flow during script-driven imagery in childhood sexual abuse-related PTSD: A PET investigation. Am J Psychiatry 156:575–584, 1999.

Singer W, Development and plasticity of cortical processing architectures. Science 270:758, 1995.

Spitz R, Cobliner G: First Year of Life: A Psychoanalytic Study of Normal and Deviant Development of Objective Relations. New York: International Universities Press, 1966.

Steadman HJ, Mulvey EP, Monahan J, et al: Violence by people discharged from acute psychiatric inpatient facilities and by others in the same neighborhoods. Arch Gen Psychiatry 55:393, 1998.

Taylor PJ: Motives for offending among violent and psychotic men. Br J Psychiatry 147:491–498, 1985.

Taylor PJ, Gunn J: Violence and psychosis. I. Risk of violence among psychotic men. BMJ 288:1945, 1984.

Teasdale TW, Engberg A: Duration of cognitive dysfunction after concussion and cognitive dysfunction as a risk factor: A population study of young men. BMJ 315:569, 1997.

Teicher MH, et al: Preliminary evidence for abnormal cortical development in physically and sexually abused children using EEG coherence and MRI. Ann N Y Acad Sci 821:160, 1997.

Tranel D: Acquired sociopathy: The development of sociopathic behavior following focal brain damage, in Fowles, DC, Sutker P, Goodman SH (eds): Progress in Experimental Personality and Psychopathology Research. New York: Springer, 1994.

Wallace C, Muller P, Burgess P, et al: Serious criminal offending and mental disorder case linkage study. Br J Psychiatry 172:477, 1998.

Widom CS: The cycle of violence. Science 244:160, 1989.

Wolfgang M: Delinquency and violence from the viewpoint of - criminality, in Fields WS, Sweet WH (eds): Neural Bases of Violence and Aggression. St. Louis, MO: Warren Green, 1975, pp. 456–469.

Wyllie E, Glazer JP, Benbadis S, et al: Psychiatric features of children and adolescents with pseudoseizures. Arch Pediatr Adolesc Med 153:244–248, 1999.

Yarvis RM: Patterns of substance abuse and intoxication among murderers. Bull Am Acad Psychiatry Law 22:133, 1994.

Yesavage JA: Correlates of dangerous behavior by schizophrenics in a hospital. J Psychiatr Res 18:225, 1984.

Behavioral Evidence in Legal Proceedings

H. Richard Beresford

Admissibility of evidence

Behavioral evidence

***Daubert* factors**

Exclusion of evidence

Expert testimony

***Frye* test**

Judicial gatekeeping

Relevance

Reliability

INTRODUCTION

Evidence relating to cognition, affective state, and behavior can determine or influence the outcome of legal disputes. Such evidence takes several forms. It can range from completion of a simple disability form to protracted and vigorously contested oral testimony in court. Complements to courtroom testimony may include charts, diagrams, videos, electronic presentations, and other demonstrative evidence. The source of the evidence will ordinarily be clinicians with expertise in neurology, neuropsychology, or psychiatry. But legal tribunals will sometimes accept testimony from other witnesses whom the tribunals find are qualified to offer helpful information. This chapter addresses the use of what will be generically called behavioral evidence in various types of legal proceedings. The term will encompass all forms of testimony relating to mental status, emotions, and actual or predicted conduct.

Part I considers rules controlling admissibility and use of behavioral evidence in legal proceedings. It includes a summary of federal evidentiary rules with respect to scientific, technical, and other specialized testimony. Although these rules formally apply only in federal courts, they also serve as models for many state evidentiary codes. Part I also discusses three recent Supreme Court rulings that attempt to spell out how trial courts should apply these evidentiary rules in evaluating the reliability of expert testimony on scientific or clinical issues. Part II describes the role of behavioral evidence in different sorts of legal proceedings. The goals here are to outline the particular legal context in which the evidence is offered, to illustrate how behavioral evidence can affect adjudications and dispositions of legal matters, and to suggest ways in which behavioral evidence can best serve the needs of legal decision makers.

BEHAVIORAL EVIDENCE: ADMISSIBILITY IN LEGAL PROCEEDINGS

Nature of Behavioral Evidence

A threshold question concerning any sort of behavioral evidence is whether it is reliable enough for a court or other legal tribunal to use in resolving a legal issue (Graham, 2000). In weighing reliability, a tribunal will take into account the qualifications of the person who has collected or assembled the evidence, the methods by which the evidence was obtained, its coherence to the legal decision maker, and its level of acceptance within the relevant scientific, technical, or clinical discipline. Behavioral evidence poses certain problems in these respects. The persons offering such evidence may vary widely in training and experience, ranging from seasoned academic behavioral neurologists, neuropsychologists, and psychiatrists to newly minted clinical psychologists or nonspecialist physicians. Also, the data used to support clinical opinions may be difficult to quantify or objectify, resting almost entirely on subjective accounts of symptoms and observations by families or other laypersons. And opinions and interpretations offered by examiners may be quite tentative or contestable.

Legal tribunals may thus find themselves in a quandary. They must choose between admitting into evidence data or opinions of questionable validity or foregoing reliance on the only relevant evidence that is offered. In the interests of resolving a legal dispute, the tribunal may simply decide to take the evidence into account for whatever it is worth. Put in a more legalistic way, it may allow the evidence to be heard—a decision for admissibility—and leave assessment of its weight—a decision as to credibility—to the jury (if there is one) or to the wisdom of the judge. Such a judicial choice risks unfair prejudice to one party to the litigation or reversal of the ruling by an appellate court on the grounds of abuse of judicial discretion. But, in the end, the tribunal may view this risk as less problematic than an outright refusal to hear evidence that could provide a rationale for deciding a case (Imwinkelried, 1999).

"Fact" and "Expert" Testimony

As a general rule, witnesses in legal proceedings are permitted to testify only as to what they have observed. They are not allowed to offer interpretations or opinions about the legal significance of their observations. Thus, an eyewitness to an automobile accident can testify that one driver was driving at a high rate of speed but is not permitted to venture the legal opinion that the speeding driver was therefore acting negligently. The issue of negligence is for judge and jury to determine. Nor can a family physician testify that a neurosurgeon was careless in how he or she operated on a patient's intracranial aneurysm. Such a witness lacks the training and experience to venture an opinion on the standard of surgical care exercised by a neurosurgeon—unless, of course, the patient did not, in fact, have an aneurysm. In these situations, neither the lay eyewitness nor the family physician possesses the qualifications to address what lawyers call the "ultimate issue," the determination as to whether a particular litigant behaved negligently.

When witnesses demonstrably possess specialized knowledge that can aid a court in resolving the "ultimate issue," a legal tribunal may permit them to offer opinions on the legal significance of their observations (Americans with Disabilities Act, 1995). Thus, a specialist in accident reconstruction might be permitted to testify that a driver was driving at an unreasonable rate of speed given existing road conditions. And a neurosurgeon might be allowed to express an opinion that another neurosurgeon acted negligently while operating on an aneurysm. But before these putative "experts" are allowed to testify, courts must be satisfied that they are indeed qualified to offer opinions and that their proffered testimony is both relevant and reliable. Flashy credentials alone will not suffice. There must be a showing of expertise that pertains to the matter at hand.

Rules of Evidence

Rules governing the admissibility of evidence in the federal courts, the *Federal Rules of Evidence* (1975; hereinafter FRE), have been incorporated into many state evidentiary codes. Thus, the following discussion of the FRE will serve to illustrate how most—but certainly not all—legal tribunals can be expected to handle questions relating to whether testimony by purported behavioral experts should be heard. How the FRE and its state analogues are applied to behavioral evidence is pivotal where such evidence goes to the core of a legal claim. For example, if a court excludes behavioral evidence with respect to the neuropsychological consequences of a closed head injury (CHI), a claimant may recover only a nominal amount of monetary damages. If, on the other hand, the court admits such evidence, it may serve as the basis for a large jury award for injury-related cognitive impairment. Accordingly, the outcome of legal arguments about the application of "technical" evidentiary rules may be enormously consequential for litigants—and for the experts they have retained. The following rules from the FRE are especially pertinent to the use of behavioral expert testimony in legal proceedings:

Rule 702 empowers courts to admit expert testimony with respect to scientific or other specialized knowledge if the testimony "will assist the trier of fact to understand the evidence or to determine a fact in issue. To qualify as an expert under this rule, a witness must be qualified "by knowledge, skill, experience, training or education." This language gives trial courts considerable leeway with respect to admitting expert testimony since the threshold of helpfulness of testimony does not appear particularly high. Moreover, it permits courts to accept testimony from witnesses whose expertise derives from experience rather than specialized training.

Rule 703 allows an expert to offer an opinion based on facts or data "perceived by or made known to him at or before the hearing." These data, moreover, need not themselves be admissible into evidence (e.g., hearsay) if "of a type reasonably relied upon by experts in the particular field in forming opinions or inferences upon the subject." In other words, an expert can base an opinion about the behavioral consequences of a head injury on data from sources other than a personal examination of the injured. Clinicians customarily rely on reports of examinations by other clinicians or on reviews of clinical records. Accordingly, they can use these data to formulate an opinion, whether or not they have actually examined the injured person. An opinion of this sort might not carry as much weight as one based on a personal examination, but would still be admissible as evidence.

Rule 704 specifically permits experts in civil trials to offer an opinion on the "ultimate issue to be decided by the trier of fact." Thus, if a crucial issue in a personal injury action is whether a closed head injury caused major cognitive impairment, a qualified expert would be allowed to express an opinion on this "ultimate" issue. This obviously does not mean that a court must abdicate its responsibility as "trier of fact" and defer to whatever testifying experts say. But it does mean that the experts can express themselves on how the court ought to decide the issue to which their testimony pertains and affords an opportunity for an especially charismatic witness to determine how a jury views a particular issue.

Rule 705 allows an expert witness to offer an opinion "without prior disclosure of the underlying facts or data, unless the court requires otherwise." One purpose of such a rule is to expedite trials by allowing experts to express their opinions before relevant data have been introduced into evidence. Thus, the rule lets experts answer hypothetical questions that incorporate evidence that will come before the court later. The rule is not intended to allow experts to avoid rationalizing their opinions. Thus, Rule 705 goes on to say that the expert "may in any event be required to disclose the underlying facts or data on cross-examination."

Rule 403 empowers courts to exclude relevant testimony by a qualified expert if, in the opinion of the trial judge, the "probative" value of the testimony is "substantially outweighed by the danger of unfair prejudice, confusion of the issues, or misleading the jury." In other words, notwithstanding the rather expansive approach to admissibility of expert testimony that inheres in Rules 702 to 705, a court has, under Rule 403, discretion to keep certain expert testimony from being heard by a jury if it determines that it would undermine the integrity of the decisional process.

Rule 706 affords courts another remedy when confronted with confusing or complex expert testimony, or a contentious "battle of the experts." It empowers trial judges to appoint their own experts to provide testimony designed to help resolve contested issues of fact or interpretation. Such court-appointed experts are subject to cross-examination by lawyers for any litigant.

Rulings by trial courts based on applications of these rules are ordinarily subject to appeal to higher courts. Appellate courts tend to defer to rulings of trial courts on evidentiary matters. It is generally assumed that trial judges are better situated than appellate judges to evaluate qualifications and credibility of witnesses and the reliability of proffered expert testimony. The rationale is that trial judges have had the opportunity to actually listen to and observe the behavior of putative expert witnesses, and to question them about the basis of their opinions. But if an appellate court determines that a trial court made an incorrect legal interpretation of a particular rule of evidence or clearly abused its discretion with respect to a particular ruling, the higher court may step in. It can order a new trial or can direct the lower court judge to apply what it views as the correct legal interpretation of an evidentiary rule. Indeed, as will be seen, decisions by appellate courts can provide important guidance to trial courts confronted with a decision on whether to admit expert testimony that is being vigorously challenged and that may have a substantial impact on the outcome of a legal dispute.

Supreme Court Rulings

In recent years, the U.S. Supreme Court has decided three major cases relating to how the FRE ought to be applied by trial courts that are confronted with challenges to the admissibility of potentially crucial expert testimony. There is much debate about how helpful these rulings of the Court have been for trial courts and litigants. But it is generally agreed that one effect of the rulings is to underscore the duty of trial courts to make a good faith effort to assess the reliability of expert testimony on scientific or clinical issues *before* admitting it into evidence (Graham, 2000; Navigating uncertainty, 2000).

Daubert v Merrell Dow Pharmaceuticals (1993)

At issue in this case was the admissibility of expert testimony purporting to show that a pharmaceutical company's prescription antinausea drug, Bendectin, was teratogenic. Claimants included children with birth defects whose mothers had taken the drug during pregnancy. Two types of expert testimony were proffered. The first incorporated findings from in vitro and animal studies suggesting that Bendectin was a potential teratogen. The second was a "reanalysis" of several published human epidemiologic studies that had failed to link Bendectin and birth defects. The claimants' expert planned to testify that, when reinterpreted using his own methodology, the data in these studies in fact indicated such a link. The trial court refused to admit testimony of either type. The first type was rejected on the ground that animal and tissue culture studies were not relevant to the issue of human teratogenesis. As to the expert's "reanalysis," the trial court emphasized that the methodology did not rely on published principles of interpretation and had not been subjected to scientific peer review. The court then dismissed claimants' suit. A federal appeals court sustained this ruling, citing the so-called "Frye test." This rule of evidence was derived from an old federal appellate case holding that "general acceptance" within the relevant scientific discipline is the touchstone of admissibility for expert testimony (*Frye v United States*, 1923). The claimants then appealed to the Supreme Court. They argued that the "Frye test" was superseded by the FRE and that, under these rules, the expert's "reanalysis" should be admitted as evidence of a link between Bendectin and birth defects.

The Supreme Court unanimously reversed the decision of the appellate court and remanded the case for resolution under the FRE. The high Court found that the "Frye test" was no longer applicable once the FRE were enacted, and that the trial court must look to the FRE in determining the relevance and reliability of proffered expert testimony. The Court stressed that, despite the liberal tone of the FRE, trial courts must take their role as "gatekeepers" seriously with respect to scientific testimony. In an effort to provide guidance in the exercise of this responsibility, the Court formulated four questions that trial courts should answer before deciding to admit expert scientific testimony: (1) Is it derived from empirical data? (2) Has it been subjected to peer review and publication? (3) Has it used methodology with a known and low rate of error? (4) And, finally, is it generally accepted by the scientific community?

The Court was mindful of concerns that abandoning the Frye test might result in juries being confronted with "absurd and irrational pseudoscientific assertions." As an antidote, the Court pointed out that a mix of vigorous cross-examination, testimony by opposing experts, and careful judicial instructions can reduce the risk that such "assertions" will be inappropriately credited. The Court further observed that trial courts have an inherent power to override the findings of a jury if they conclude that the jury improperly relied on flawed expert testimony. The Court also briefly addressed the concern that its ruling might cause trial courts to become overly conservative and admit only orthodox scientific evidence, thereby depriving litigants of an opportunity to challenge dogmas that might in truth be unsound. The Court conceded the desirability of open debate in both law and science. But it also stressed the importance of "finally and quickly" resolving legal disputes and avoiding the waste of judicial time inherent in evaluating conjectures that are "probably wrong."

After the case was remanded to the court of appeals, that court determined that, even under the liberal criteria of the FRE, the expert's "reanalysis" should be excluded from evidence (*Daubert v Merrell Dow Pharmaceuticals, Inc.*, 1995). It found that the "reanalysis" was not "scientific knowledge" within the meaning of the FRE because it was not based on prelitigation research, it had not been subjected to peer review, and it was not supported by objective published studies.

General Electric v Joiner (1997)

In this case, the high Court addressed the question of what is the proper legal standard for an appellate court to apply in evaluating a trial court's exercise of its gatekeeper's role. The clinical and scientific issue was whether claimant's small cell carcinoma of the lung was "promoted" by work-related exposure to polychlorinated biphenyls (PCBs). As in *Daubert*, two sorts of expert testimony were subject to challenge. One was testimony that infant mice given large intraperitoneal doses of PCBs developed pulmonary adenomas. The second comprised studies of four groups of factory workers. Three of the groups had been exposed to PCBs and in them there was a modest but statistically insignificant excess mortality from lung cancer. The trial court had determined that relying on these data to support a causal link between claimant's cancer and exposure to PCB amounted to "subjective belief or unsupported speculation." Accordingly, it awarded summary judgment to the claimant's employer and the manufacturers of the equipment that contained PCBs.

In reversing the trial court's decision, a federal appeals court emphasized that the FRE establish a preference for free admissibility of expert testimony and concluded that its role should be to stringently scrutinize lower court rulings that exclude such testimony. Relying on this rationale, the appellate court decided that the trial court had overstepped its discretion. It characterized the trial court's ruling as essentially a disagreement with the claimant's experts about the strength of the evidence of a causal link between claimant's exposure to PCB and his lung cancer.

In reversing the appeals court, the Supreme Court held that the proper standard for an appeals court to apply is whether the trial court abused its discretion. The Court found no such abuse. It emphasized the dissimilarity between the situation of the claimant and the mice that had received PCBs experimentally, both with respect to route and amount of exposure and the type of neoplasm that developed. It also underscored the failure of the epidemiologic studies to demonstrate a convincing association between exposure to PCB and later lung cancer. Under these circumstances, it decided that it was a permissible exercise of discretion for the trial court to conclude that "there is simply too great an analytical gap between the data and the opinion proffered."

In a concurring opinion, Justice Breyer addressed the problem trial courts face when asked to rule on admissibility of complex scientific evidence. He emphasized that they should not forsake their gatekeepers' role because evidence is complex. Rather they should seek the help of court-appointed experts, relying on advice from reputable scientific organizations to identify such experts. In a partial dissent, Justice Stevens suggested that it was not intrinsically unscientific to accept the opinions of experts who applied a "weight of the evidence" approach to a mix of animal and human studies. Thus, it would not have amounted to an abuse of discretion if the trial court had admitted, rather than excluded, the testimony of claimant's experts.

Kumho v Carmichael Tire Company (1999)

In the third case of the triad, the Supreme Court was asked to clarify whether its ruling in *Daubert* applies with respect to expert testimony that is specialized or technical but not, strictly speaking, scientific in character. This is a particularly important issue concerning much of the testimony that clinicians might proffer (Navigating uncertainty, 2000). Such testimony may derive from a mix of accumulated clinical experience and intuition, anecdotal reports, readings from pertinent clinical literature, and deductions that other clinicians would find plausible in light of the available information. The evidence might not be of the quality to support a practice guideline or other benchmark, but it might be of the type that clinicians rely on in their everyday professional activities.

Kumho involved a challenge to expert testimony from an engineer who intended to testify that a defect in a tire manufactured by the defendant was the cause of a blowout that led to a claimant's injury. Invoking *Daubert,* the defendant contended that the engineer's testimony was not reliable in the context of Rule 702 of the FRE and therefore should be excluded from evidence. After assessing the methodology of the engineer's testimony in light of the reliability factors set forth in *Daubert* (i.e., testing, peer review, error rates, general acceptance), the trial court granted the motion to exclude the testimony and awarded summary judgment to defendant. Claimants then asked the trial court to reconsider, arguing that the court's ruling was based on an "inflexible" application of *Daubert.* Although agreeing that *Daubert* should be applied flexibly, the trial court found the scientific basis for the expert's tire failure analysis to be inadequate and reaffirmed its earlier ruling.

The federal appeals court for the 11th Circuit reversed the trial court's ruling. It reasoned that *Daubert* applies only where an expert relies on "application of scientific principles," rather than "on skill- or experience-based observation," and that the engineer's experience-based opinions fell outside the scope of *Daubert.* It thereupon remanded the case to the trial court for a non-*Daubert* analysis under Rule 702.

The defendant manufacturer then asked the Supreme Court to determine if a trial court may consider the *Daubert* factors when ruling on whether to admit testimony of the sort challenged here.

In an opinion authored by Justice Breyer, the Court held that *Daubert* applies to all expert testimony that involves scientific, technical, or other specialized knowledge. The Court noted that it "would prove difficult, if not impossible, for judges to administer evidentiary rules under which a gatekeeping obligation turned on a distinction between 'scientific' knowledge and 'technical' or 'other specialized knowledge.'" It went on to emphasize how important it is for trial courts to "make certain that an expert, whether basing testimony upon professional studies or personal experience, employs in the courtroom the same level of intellectual rigor that characterized the practice of an expert in the relevant field." Against this backdrop, and after a review of the expert's methodology, the Court concluded that the trial court had not abused its discretion in excluding the engineer's testimony as unreliable under Rule 702 and reversed the decision of the 11th Circuit. The effect of this was to reinstate the trial court's summary judgment for the defendant manufacturer.

Taken together these three Supreme Court decisions send several clear signals to trial judges, litigants, and potential expert witnesses. First, they admonish trial courts to take seriously their role as gatekeepers under Rule 702 (or its state analogues). Second, they remind litigants how important it is for them to secure experts whose qualifications and methodology can withstand rigorous substantive challenges. Third, they remind potential experts of the high desirability of proffering only those opinions they would dare before a group of professional peers. Fourth, they indicate to appellate judges that they should defer to the rulings of trial courts that reflect a conscientious exercise of the gatekeeping function.

Clear as these signals may seem, they hardly ensure that expert testimony will be generally reliable or that trial courts will only admit reliable testimony and only exclude unreliable testimony (Graham, 2000). High stakes cases, zealous lawyers, venal experts, inexperienced judges or lawyers, and overburdened court dockets are factors that may compromise assessments of proffered expert testimony and generate erroneous rulings on admissibility. Still, potential experts would be wise to assume that their opinions will be vigorously challenged and prepare themselves accordingly. The challenges may come both before and after opinions are admitted into evidence, and will be most pointed where the opinions bear on pivotal legal issues or on the amount of monetary damages to be awarded.

BEHAVIORAL EVIDENCE: USE IN PARTICULAR LEGAL PROCEEDINGS

Behavioral evidence is relevant in a variety of legal settings, ranging from bitterly contested murder cases in criminal courts to essentially nonadversarial guardianship proceedings in probate courts. Procedures and standards of proof can differ considerably among these settings. Accordingly, it can be helpful for those who provide behavioral evidence to appreciate the pertinent ground rules and how they may have an impact on testimony. No attempt is made here to catalogue every type of legal proceeding in which behavioral evidence might be offered or to consider the full range of such evidence. Instead the focus is on distinctive features of certain sorts of legal proceedings and how these features may affect the admissibility and use of behavioral evidence.

Civil Litigation: Personal Injuries

Claims arising out of personal injuries crowd the dockets of most civil courts. The injuries may stem from automobile crashes, slips and falls, assaults, and alleged medical malpractice, and many claims assert neurologic or psychological harms. The primary litigants are injured claimants and alleged wrongdoers (both individual and corporate). Often defendants are insured with respect to the claims involved, and the insurers may finance defense of the claims, including the payment of lawyers' and expert witness fees, but the insurers are usually not actual parties to the lawsuits. The crux of a personal injury claim is usually that a defendant wrongfully, either intentionally or negligently (unreasonably), caused harm to a claimant that is quantifiable in monetary terms.

The burden of proving an actionable harm is on a claimant. To satisfy this burden, the claimant must ordinarily show by a preponderance of evidence (>50% probability) that the defendant caused the harm and its associated economic consequences. Most personal injury claims are settled before the claims are actually tried in court. But the course of settlement negotiations is very much influenced by the contending lawyers' assessments as to whether claimants can meet their burden of proof. An important element of the calculus is a weighing of the persuasiveness of expert testimony that may be forthcoming. Thus, even though the odds of a personal injury case actually going to trial are small, the relative merits or demerits of anticipated expert testimony incorporating behavioral or other evidence can do much to determine how a case is resolved.

A defendant will typically challenge a claimant's evidence with respect to causation and damages and will develop evidence designed to show absence of wrongful conduct or to show that the claimant has not been harmed as much as asserted. Personal injury cases are usually, although not invariably, heard by juries. Whether or not a jury is involved, the legal outcome is an adjudication as to liability and a determination of monetary damages, if any. These damages include economic losses attributable to the wrongful harm, and so-called "noneconomic" damages, such as awards for pain and suffering and, occasionally, punitive damages.

Behavioral evidence in personal injury litigation usually pertains to damage claims. For example, a claimant who sustained a head injury in an automobile crash can be expected to produce expert testimony as to the behavioral consequences of the head injury. This testimony will include a description of the residual neurologic impairments and the impact of these impairments on the claimant's cognition, mood, and behavior (including social and vocational aspects). Where a claim for pain and suffering has been asserted, the testimony will also include an opinion as to the quantum of the pain and suffering and its relationship to the head injury. Occasionally behavioral evidence may bear on the issue of causation as well. For example, where a claimant alleges severe cognitive impairment after an ostensibly minor CHI, she or he will try to produce expert testimony designed to explain to a court how a seemingly trivial injury could produce such profound effects. The defendant will predictably counter with testimony to the effect that the CHI could not plausibly produce the degree of asserted neurologic impairment.

An attack on expert testimony proffered by a claimant may take various forms. The qualification of a witness as an "expert" may be questioned with respect to credentials, experience, and knowledge about the specific injury at issue. The matter of potential bias may be addressed through inquiries about previous testimony in comparable cases, about fees, or about the amount of time spent testifying in court. The accuracy of the observations on which testimony is founded may be challenged on methodological or other grounds, as might conclusions about the extent of the asserted impairments, their impact on claimant's life, or the amount of pain and suffering the claimant is actually experiencing. The attacks may occur in the form of a motion to the court to exclude the proffered testimony (citing *Daubert* and *Kumho)*, through zealous cross-examination, or by means of testimony by defendant's experts to the effect that the behavioral consequences of a claimant's injury are not as claimed.

Once testimony of behavioral experts is admitted into evidence, the court (including any empaneled jury) will assess its weight and credibility. At this stage, the court will consider how the evidence stands up to attempts to discredit it through cross-examination and the opinions of defendant's experts. Trial courts' determinations as to weight and credibility of testimonial evidence are usually upheld by reviewing judges. The exception is where the reviewing court concludes that a trial court has clearly abused its discretion (*General Electric v Joiner*).

Civil Litigation: Statutory Claims

The personal injury claims discussed above are of a "common law" character. They derive from the idea that law ought to provide a remedy for persons who suffer harm at the hands of wrongdoers, even if the alleged wrongdoing does not violate a criminal statute or other legislative enactment. As noted before, to succeed in a claim, an injured person must ordinarily establish that a defendant acted unreasonably, that is, by violating some generally accepted but unwritten norm of prudent conduct. In recent years, however, federal and state legislatures have increasingly undertaken to codify certain socially desirable standards of conduct and to permit individuals to bring damage claims against persons (including corporate persons) who violate statutory standards. Examples include various civil rights and fair employment laws, the Emergency Medical Treatment and Active Labor Act (1986), and the Americans with Disabilities Act (ADA; 1995). These laws typically place caps on recoveries of monetary damages or may limit remedies to restoration of wrongfully denied benefits or status.

The ADA is a particularly fruitful source of statutory civil claims (Zylan, 2000). Two sorts of ADA-based claims will be used to illustrate the role behavioral evidence may play under such legislation.

Consider first a claim under the ADA alleging discrimination by an employer against a mentally ill employee. To prevail, the employee must establish that he or she (1) is "disabled" as defined by the law, (2) is qualified to perform the "essential functions" of the job at issue, with or without a "reasonable accommodation," and (3) has been discriminated against on the basis of the asserted disability. Thus, the employee must show that, despite a disabling mental illness, he or she is nevertheless able to handle the job at issue and that the employer has used this disability as a basis for discriminating against the employee.

Behavioral evidence would clearly be relevant to establish the disability of mental illness, to show that, despite such disability, the employee can perform the job at issue, and to indicate the nature of any appropriate "reasonable accommodation." An employer defending against such an ADA claim would predictably respond with behavioral evidence to the effect that the employee's mental illness is either not a disability or is so severe that, even with a "reasonable accommodation," it renders the employee unqualified to perform "essential functions" of the job. It will then be up to a court or administrative tribunal to determine if the behavioral evidence proves that the employee has a qualifying disability and can nevertheless perform the job if reasonably accommodated.

Under the ADA, a person is "disabled" if he or she has a "physical or mental impairment that substantially limits one or more major life activities," has a "record" of such impairment, or is "regarded as having such an impairment." Thus, a mentally ill employee can qualify as disabled by proving current mental illness, previous treatment for such illness, or a perception by an employer or others that he or she is mentally ill currently. Although this definition of disability is expansive, it is also imprecise. Moreover, mentally ill employees who pursue an ADA claim must meet the rather contradictory evidentiary burden of showing that their illness has now or once had a substantial impact on their lives but nevertheless does not undercut their ability to work. If they seek a "reasonable accommodation" from their employers so as to enable them to work despite their disability, employers can defeat this effort by proving that a requested accommodation would impose an "undue hardship" on the employers or by showing that an employee poses a "direct threat" to others in the workplace that can not be eliminated by a "reasonable accommodation" (Guiduli, 1998).

In this rather bewildering statutory context, behavioral evidence that meets the reliability standards discussed in the first part of this chapter takes on considerable importance. But even if high-quality behavioral evidence is forthcoming, a court may face a daunting task in deciding whether an employer has, explicitly or implicitly, discriminated against a mentally ill employee solely because of the employee's illness. It should come as no surprise, therefore, that employees who invoke the ADA to remedy discrimination based on their mental illness succeed but infrequently (Guiduli, 1998; Zylan, 2000).

A second type of mental illness–related ADA claim involves efforts to ensure that mentally ill persons are subjected to no greater restraints than are necessary to protect their welfare. The recent Supreme Court decision in *Olmstead v Zimring* (1999) is illustrative. The claimants were two mentally retarded and mentally ill women who were confined to state mental hospitals in Georgia. They contended that Title II of the ADA required that they be placed in the most appropriate integrated community setting and that the state was violating the ADA by keeping them confined to a mental hospital. Their psychiatric treatment teams had determined that they were suitable for community placement, but the state asserted that it lacked appropriate community facilities in which they could be placed. Both a federal district court and the 11th Circuit Court of Appeals decided that unnecessary hospitalization of the mentally disabled would violate Title II of the ADA. But the appellate court remanded the case for a determination of whether caring for the claimants in a community setting would require a fundamental alteration of the state's community treatment programs and thus excuse the state from an obligation to provide claimants care in a community setting.

The Supreme Court agreed with the two lower courts that unnecessary hospitalization could amount to disability-based discrimination. However, three conditions must exist before this conclusion can be reached: (1) state mental health professionals must concur that community placement is appropriate, (2) the disabled persons must not object to community placement, and (3) it ought not be "inequitable" to provide the requested community placement. Accordingly, the Court remanded the case for a determination of whether, given available resources, prompt community placement would be inequitable in light of the state's ongoing efforts to provide care to a large and varied population of persons with mental disabilities.

The *Olmstead* case is of considerable interest in several respects. For example, it interprets the ADA in a way that furthers mainstreaming of the mentally ill and puts state governments on notice that they may be called on to task for failure to provide adequate community mental health services. But for purposes of this chapter, *Olmstead* underscores the importance of behavioral evidence in resolving questions about what level of care is appropriate for mentally ill persons. To be helpful for decision makers in this context, behavioral evidence must focus less on diagnosis and conventional modes of therapy and more on functional capacities. For mentally ill persons who have spent much time in traditional mental health facilities, predicting capacity to function safely under lower levels of supervision or observation could be daunting. And for mentally ill persons who, as a general proposition, seem suited for community care, it may be difficult to decide whether the sort of community care that is actually available or reasonably attainable is in fact appropriate.

Civil Commitment

Laws of every state authorize involuntary judicial commitment of mentally ill persons. Criteria for commitment differ in some respects from state to state, but at a minimum there must be proof of both mental illness and danger to self or others. Some states, in addition, permit involuntary commitments of a mentally ill person on proof of an urgent need for psychiatric treatment. Because commitments represent a substantial deprivation of liberty, the Supreme Court has held that the federal constitution requires "clear and convincing" proof of mental illness and dangerousness before involuntary civil detention can occur (*Addington v Texas*, 1979). This standard of proof is higher than the preponderance of evidence standard that ordinarily applies in civil litigation, and lower than the beyond reasonable doubt standard that ordinarily applies in criminal proceedings. More precise quantification is difficult. But courts generally interpret the "clear and convincing" standard to require evidence that is so compelling as to be invulnerable to serious challenge. For practical purposes, this means that testifying experts must substantially agree that a potential detainee is both mentally ill and dangerous before a court will order commitment.

Proving mental illness is ordinarily less taxing than proving danger to self or others. Expert witnesses for potential detainees may not dispute the presence of mental illness, even though they may believe that the illness is less severe than asserted by those who favor commitment. For example, an expert for a potential detainee may not quibble over whether schizoaffective disorder is a more accurate diagnosis than paranoid schizophrenia. But such an expert may vigorously contest allegations that the potential detainee is a danger to self or others. To support this view, the expert can cite data indicating that predictions of dangerous behaviors are unreliable. Unless a potential detainee has recently engaged in violent behavior or has made recent credible threats of violent or suicidal conduct, a court might well conclude that the evidence of danger is not "clear and convincing" enough to support commitment. Indeed some state statutes require proof that mentally ill persons have recently engaged in dangerous behavior before commitment will be authorized.

To satisfy the "clear and convincing" standard of proof, behavioral evidence of mental illness and dangerousness should be based on rigorous evaluation. This entails a detailed clinical history, a current neuropsychiatric assessment that probes into any violent or suicidal ideation, and inquiries of family, friends, coworkers, and other social contacts. A less complete assessment could be challenged as methodologically inadequate and therefore so unreliable as to be excludable from evidence under a *Daubert* rationale. Alternatively, counsel for a potential detainee could argue that such a deficient assessment is entitled to as little weight in a court's deliberations as to whether to order commitment. The way in which behavioral evidence is presented can also affect its utility. If a witness avoids use of jargon and carefully distinguishes between facts and speculations, a court will be reassured that it has an accurate appreciation of a potential detainee's mental status. It is difficult to know how often high-quality behavioral evidence is provided to courts weighing involuntary commitment. Some commitment proceedings are adversarial in form only. Clinicians, family, and legal counsel may all essentially agree that commitment is appropriate. But where commitment is being contested, courts are constitutionally empowered to require compelling behavioral evidence of dangerousness or urgent need for treatment before overriding the objections of a mentally ill person.

Once a mentally ill person has been detained, danger to self and others may abate because of effective treatment or remission of illness. When this situation arises, the person is, under the Supreme Court decision in *O'Connor v Donaldson* (1975), constitutionally entitled to release from hospitalization. This is true even if diagnosable mental illness persists and treating clinicians believe that further inpatient confinement offers therapeutic advantages.

If an involuntary detainee's mental illness remits, but clinicians believe that he or she presents danger to self or others, a state may seek to continue the detention. This would, however, raise a major constitutional issue, one that was addressed by the Supreme Court in *Foucha v Louisiana* (1992). The claimant in that case had been confined in a state mental hospital because of violent behavior associated with a drug-induced psychosis. When the psychosis cleared, he was no longer deemed mentally ill. But his treating clinicians believed that he had an antisocial personality and could be a danger to others in the future. Accordingly, the state, without providing him procedural due process, detained him in the mental hospital. In a sharply divided 5 to 4 decision, the Court held that forced hospitalization of one who is no longer mentally ill violates constitutional due process standards and ordered his release. The majority opinion stressed that the claimant's diagnosed personality disorder would not support an involuntary civil commitment under state law, and that there was no justification for punishing him through further detention because he had not been convicted of a crime.

Criminal Proceedings

The need for behavioral evidence permeates the criminal justice system. At virtually every stage of the criminal process, the mental competency of a defendant may become an issue. Courts are often asked to consider how probable it is that a defendant will engage in criminal or antisocial behavior in the future. Questions of this sort emerge in the context of a legal process that is designed to ensure that criminal defendants are given every opportunity to challenge allegations of criminality. Thus, before a criminal defendant can be lawfully convicted, a federal, state, or local prosecutor must prove criminal conduct beyond a reasonable doubt.

This high burden of proof—akin to moral certainty—applies with respect to every element of an alleged crime, including both criminal state of mind (so-called *mens rea*) and criminal act (so-called *actus reus*). The elements of a crime are ordinarily spelled out in statutes, and many an indictment has been dismissed because a prosecutor failed to tailor allegations of criminality to specific statutory requirements. To use a simple example, an indictment for murder that does not include an allegation that the defendant acted willfully, knowingly, or with a depraved state of mind could be dismissed for failure to allege the essential element of *mens rea*. Even if a criminal indictment is legally sufficient and the prosecution offers a substantial amount of evidence with respect to *mens rea* and *actus reus*, a criminal defendant can avoid conviction by planting a seed of doubt in the minds of jurors as to whether he or she intended to do wrong or was indifferent to the consequences of his or her behavior. A defendant can also avoid liability by proving insanity at the time the alleged crime was committed. In either situation, behavioral evidence is relevant. It may address doubts about a defendant's motivation to do wrong or about his or her capacity to understand that the allegedly criminal act was the wrong thing to do.

Behavioral evidence may emerge as important in diverse contexts other than formal adjudications of criminality. At the street level, a police officer's decision whether to arrest an unruly person or to take him or her to a hospital for psychiatric evaluation may turn on a more or less informed assessment of the person's mental condition. A judge's or magistrate's decision whether to allow bail to a criminal dependent may be influenced, in part, by a prosecutor's contentions that the defendant would endanger others if not confined in advance of trial. Once a defendant has been formally charged with a crime, questions may be raised as to competency to stand trial. After a defendant has been convicted, a court may take mental condition into account in determining the nature of the sentence. A mentally ill prisoner may allege violations of constitutional or other rights to appropriate psychiatric assessment and treatment. And a defendant who has completed a criminal sentence may be targeted for later civil detention because of an allegedly dangerous mental disorder. Thus, whether used in formal or informal ways, behavioral evidence has considerable potential to influence how the criminal justice system operates. Rather than addressing the gamut of possibilities, the emphasis here will be on the use of behavioral evidence in four circumstances: determinations of competency to stand trial; adjudications of criminal responsibility (including applications of the insanity defense); setting of criminal sentences (including capital punishment); and in post-conviction civil commitment proceedings.

Competency to Stand Trial

Criminal defendants are ordinarily presumed to be competent to stand trial. But once a criminal charge has been filed, defense counsel, the prosecution, or the criminal court on its own initiative can raise the issue of whether a defendant is competent for trial. Indeed conviction of a criminal defendant who was incompetent when tried would be invalid as a violation of constitutional due process (*Medina v California*, 1992). Under rulings of the Supreme Court, legal competency for trial has two dimensions: a rational capacity to understand the criminal charges and the ability to rationally assist counsel in defending against these charges (*Dusky v United States*, 1960). If a defendant lacks either of these capabilities, the prosecution must be abated until legal competency is restored. The burden is on a defendant to overcome the presumption of competency. However, a defendant need establish incompetence only by a preponderance of evidence (*Cooper v Oklahoma*, 1996). The Supreme Court has held unconstitutional a state statute that set a more stringent "clear and convincing" standard of proof (*M'Naghtens Case*, 1843). The Court has also held that forced administration of antipsychotic drugs for the sole purpose of rendering an incompetent defendant competent to stand trial unconstitutionally infringes the right to a fair trial (*Riggins v Nevada*, 1992).

Once a defendant is found incompetent for trial, the prosecution will ordinarily initiate civil commitment proceedings under standards described previously. In this circumstance, providing proof of dangerousness should be easier than in the usual civil commitment proceeding. The state will already have amassed evidence of the defendant's violent or threatening behaviors. As to the proof of mental illness needed to satisfy the second requirement of the civil commitment standard, defense counsel would be hard-pressed to argue that a client who is too mentally ill to be tried for a crime is not mentally ill enough for civil commitment. If treatment renders a defendant legally competent for trial, or if a defendant's mental illness remits enough to allow a determination of competency for trial, the defendant can then be brought to trial on the original charges. For a defendant who never regains legal competency, a potential irony is that the duration of involuntary civil commitment may turn out to far exceed the

confinement that would have been imposed had the defendant been tried and convicted of a crime.

A clinician who is retained to provide behavioral evidence relevant to competency for trial must appreciate the importance of addressing the specific legal standards. It may not be enough to testify that a defendant has a mental condition that impairs memory, executive functions, thinking, or the ability to process information. These data may assist a court in deciding how to rule on the competency issue and, if the defendant is severely disorganized and delusional psychotic, may suffice. But what a court would most appreciate is evidence that specifically addresses whether it is more probable than not that the defendant can understand the nature and specificity of the criminal charges, the consequences of a conviction on these charges, the manner in which the trial will be conducted, the role of judge and jury, and the importance of communicating with defense counsel on trial tactics and strategies. Accordingly, a behavioral assessment of competency should systematically probe the extent to which a defendant does or does not posses these trial-specific cognitive abilities. Where malingering is a serious consideration, a behavioral expert must be prepared to provide data to support whatever conclusion is drawn about this possibility. As noted, the defendant's burden of proof is not high here, and the prosecution may be quite willing to defer prosecution of a mentally ill defendant. But whatever proof of incompetence is offered, it should be enough to persuade the court that proceeding to trial would be unfair to the defendant.

Criminal Responsibility

A legally competent criminal defendant may invoke mental illness or disturbed cognition to escape or limit criminal responsibility. One strategy is the so-called "insanity defense," which, if successful, may enable a defendant to completely avoid criminal responsibility. This defense is seldom asserted and seldom successful (*United States v Lyons*, 1984). But it merits attention because of the compelling legal and moral issues it raises. A more mundane legal strategy is to try to introduce behavioral evidence to explain or account for criminal conduct. The aim is usually not to achieve full exculpation but to demonstrate that the conduct was unintended or at least less blameworthy than alleged by the prosecution. Even if a court admits behavioral evidence of this sort, it can be difficult to assess its impact on judge and jury. Still, the behavioral evidence may, by making a criminal defendant a little more human or understandable than the unmitigated villain portrayed by the prosecution, have an impact. It could, for example, influence a jury to convict on a lesser charge than that sought by the prosecution, or could result in a less severe sentence than might otherwise have been imposed.

The "Insanity Defense." Federal law and laws of all but a few states allow defendants to plead insanity as a defense to criminal charges. Generally speaking, insanity is an "affirmative" defense. This means that the burden is on the defendant to prove that he or she was insane when the alleged crime was committed, and not on the prosecution to prove that he or she was sane then. The formal burden of proof is, depending on the particular law involved, either the low stringency preponderance of evidence standard or the more demanding "clear and convincing" standard. To satisfy this evidentiary burden, a defendant must produce behavioral evidence of insanity. Because "insanity" is a legal construct, the evidence must be cast in terms of the relevant statutory definition.

The Model Penal Code (MPC; 1955), a template for some state laws, excuses a defendant from criminal responsibility if, as a result of mental disease or defect, he lacked at the time of the alleged crime "substantial capacity either to appreciate the criminality of his conduct or to conform his conduct to the requirements of law." In part, this definition represents a modernized version of the venerable *M'Naghten Rule*. It defines legal insanity as the inability to know the nature and quality of an allegedly criminal act, or to know that the act was wrong, thus emphasizing the cognitive dimension of criminal behavior. The MPC adds a volitional prong, however, excusing conduct that a mentally ill defendant cannot control. This addition incorporates the old "irresistible impulse" test and ostensibly allows defendants who were aware their conduct is unlawful to escape criminal responsibility by showing that they could not control their behavior.

After John Hinckley was acquitted of criminal charges stemming from his attempt to assassinate President Reagan under a version of the MPC, federal and many state lawmakers undertook to eliminate the volitional prong and otherwise limit the scope of the insanity defense. Thus, the federal Insanity Defense Reform Act (IDRA; 1988) specifies that the burden of proving insanity is on the defendant by "clear and convincing" evidence, that a qualifying mental illness must be "severe," and that the illness must be the cause of the incapacity to appreciate criminality. In addition, the IDRA contains no volitional prong and bars experts from offering an opinion on the "ultimate issue" of a defendant's insanity.

These legal and attitudinal responses have important implications for behavioral experts in criminal trials where a defendant's mental status at the time of an alleged crime is relevant. First, such experts must steer clear of venturing opinions that could be construed as addressing the "ultimate" issue of a defendant's legal capacity to engage in criminal conduct. An expert can describe a defendant's psychopathology in a factual way and perhaps describe its impact on the general cognitive capacity to comprehend laws. But the same expert would be barred from offering an opinion about the causal relationship between the defendant's psychopathology and the alleged crime. Second, a behavioral expert should have strong factual support for an opinion that a defendant is mentally ill. This not only means that the assessment of a defendant must be rigorous. It also means that the criteria for diagnosis of severe mental illness must be specified and demonstrably satisfied. Third, testimony that addresses a defendant's ability to control his or her behavior is likely to be excluded as irrelevant.

The *mens rea* Defense. Rather than trying to mount a full-scale insanity defense, defendant and counsel might attempt to introduce behavioral evidence designed to show diminished criminality. For example, a cognitively impaired defendant may try to show that he or she was incapable of the sort of deliberation and planning that would support a first-degree murder charge. Or a defendant with post-traumatic stress disorder (PTSD) may attempt to show that a violent outburst occurred in the context of a flashback or what was misinterpreted as threatening behavior on the part of a victim. Or a defendant with bipolar disease may attempt to explain an elaborate securities fraud as a manifestation of mania.

Prosecutors can of course be expected to ask a trial court to limit or exclude such testimony. It will then fall to the court to decide whether the proffered testimony is both relevant to the specific criminal charge and reliable enough to be heard by a jury. The court may also consider at this juncture whether a defendant is attempting a covert insanity defense. If a court decides that this is what is going on, it can instruct the jury that the burden is now on the defendant to prove insanity and that the behavioral evidence must be considered in this framework. This would relieve the prosecution of proving that the defendant was capable of deliberation or planning or that his or her behavior was not influenced by PTSD or by his or her mood disorder. Experts called to offer behavioral evidence with respect to *mens rea* should be attuned to these nuances. This will help them understand the limits that may be placed on use of their testimony and prepare them for the verbal sparring that may occur among counsel and judges over what testimony can be heard and on whether insanity defense instructions should be given to a jury.

Criminal Sentencing

Once a legally competent defendant has been tried and found guilty in a fair trial, the court must determine punishment. Criminal statutes generally specify a range of penalties for particular crimes. These may include probation, fines, and imprisonment; for major crimes, such as murder, rape, and treason, capital punishment may be an option. Historically, appellate courts have allowed trial courts considerable discretion in sentencing, so long as the sentences fall within the range of statutory maximums and minimums. This afforded trial courts leeway to take behavioral evidence into account in setting terms and conditions of confinement.

Concerns over wide disparities in sentences for comparable crimes and a growing loss of confidence in the parole system have fueled efforts to reduce the exercise of judicial discretion in sentencing. A result has been the growing use of so-called determinate sentencing for crimes. The epitome of determinate sentencing is the federal sentencing guidelines (Hill, 1998). Under these guidelines, a numerical base level is established for each offense. This number is then adjusted upward or downward by aggravating or mitigating factors, each of which is assigned a numerical value. The final number, which is the sum of the base offense value and upward and downward departures, is then placed on a sentencing grid. The location on the grid indicates the sentencing range (e.g., 24–36 months, 3–5 years, etc.). An appeals court will ordinarily uphold a sentence in the specified range. Federal trial courts can depart from these guidelines if they identify aggravating or mitigating circumstances but may be overruled if an appellate court finds the justifications for departure to be inadequate. Criminal laws of various states also limit the discretion of trial courts to depart from statutory guidelines. However, if sentencing guidelines allow a wide range of sentences for particular crimes (e.g., no less than 3 to no more than 20 years), trial courts will have an opportunity to consider behavioral evidence in arriving at a sentence.

Noncapital Sentencing. A recent federal appellate case, *United States v McBroom* (1997), illustrates how behavioral evidence can be used to mitigate the impact of determinate sentencing. The defendant, a lawyer, pled guilty to a charge of violating federal law by possessing child pornography he had obtained and shared via the Internet. Under the federal sentencing guidelines, the base offense level was 13. This was adjusted upward by two points because the minor involved was under 12 years of age, and downward by two points because he accepted responsibility for his crime, yielding a total offense level of 13. This was further adjusted upward by two "criminal history points" for three prior convictions for driving while intoxicated. On the sentencing grid, a sentence of 15 to 21 months' imprisonment was specified. At the presentencing hearing, he offered evidence of repeated childhood sexual abuse by his father and compulsive use of alcohol and cocaine as an adult. He also submitted reports from two psychiatrists expressing opinions that his compulsive behaviors (including viewing child pornography) were linked to his experience of sexual abuse as a child. He contended that this evidence demonstrated a reduced capacity to

conform his behavior to the law and justified a reduction in sentence. The trial court disagreed, determining that he was capable of absorbing information in a normal way and of exercising the power of reason.

The 4th Circuit Court of Appeals reversed the trial court's ruling and remanded the case for resentencing. The appellate court found that the offense of which the defendant was convicted was not a crime of violence, and that, under the federal sentencing guidelines, the trial court should therefore have addressed the issue of whether he had a significantly reduced mental capacity at the time of the offense. This would entail considering whether the defendant had a "volitional impairment" that affected his capacity to conform to the law penalizing possession of child pornography. The appeals court rejected the prosecution argument that, because volitional impairment is no longer a ground for raising an insanity defense under the IDRA, it should not be considered in criminal sentencing. The court, however, interpreted the sentencing guidelines as explicitly permitting sentencing courts to weigh the extent to which a defendant's reduced mental capacity contributed to the commission of an offense. In other words, behavioral evidence that neither supports an insanity defense nor negates *mens rea* might, under some circumstances, be considered by a court in determining punishment (Hill, 1998).

Capital Sentencing. Some defendants who have been convicted of capital crimes have demonstrable neurologic or psychological impairments (Blake et al., 1995). If the impairments antedated the crimes, they may have been unsuccessfully asserted to support an insanity defense or to negate *mens rea*. If the impairments developed later, they can be cited in petitions for clemency or motions to reduce a capital sentence to life imprisonment. If the impairments are severe, they may stand as a bar to execution. Thus, in *Ford v Wainwright* (1986), the Supreme Court held that the constitutional prohibition against cruel and unusual punishment (Eighth Amendment) bars execution of an incompetent criminal defendant. Precisely what constitutes incompetence for execution is not clear from the Court's opinion. But, at a minimum, it appears that there must be proof the defendant comprehends that he or she is to be executed and why. In this context, relevant behavioral evidence would address whether a defendant understands that he or she is to be killed and the reasons why this is happening. This is obviously a minimal level of competency and allows for execution of persons with substantial cognitive impairments.

For some psychotic defendants who are incompetent for execution, treatment with antipsychotic drugs may result in the requisite level of competency. But unless a defendant or a lawful proxy gives an informed consent to treatment, serious constitutional problems emerge. In *State v Perry* (1992), the leading case on this issue, the Louisiana Supreme Court held that the state constitution forbids coercive administration of antipsychotic drugs to a capital defendant for the purpose of achieving competency for execution. This decision was reached after the U.S. Supreme Court, acting on an earlier appeal, remanded the case to the Louisiana court for consideration in light of the high Court's ruling in *Washington v Harper* (1990). This ruling permitted state prison officials to forcefully medicate a violent psychotic prisoner where it could be shown that the treatment served important penal goals and was medically beneficial to the prisoner. The Louisiana court determined that the *Harper* case was distinguishable and did not rely on it in reaching its decision.

The South Carolina Supreme Court has also ruled in *Singleton v State* (1993) that forced medication to achieve competency for execution would violate its state constitution. The Louisiana and South Carolina rulings notwithstanding, the Arkansas Supreme Court has recently decided in *Singleton v Norris* (1999) that coercive administration of antipsychotic drugs that rendered a capital defendant competent for execution was permissible under the state constitution where the medication had initially been administered for the defendant's medical benefit. In any case, whether or not a capital defendant is receiving antipsychotic drugs, the questions a behavioral expert should be prepared to answer with respect to competency include:

- Does the capital defendant understand the nature of the criminal process?
- Does he or she know what offense he or she was tried for?
- Does he or she know the reasons why he or she is being punished?
- Does he or she appreciate the nature of the punishment itself?

The answers to these questions should enable an expert to offer an opinion that meets the needs of judicial decision makers.

Postconviction Detention

Mentally ill defendants are subject to civil commitment on completion of their criminal sentences if they have a qualifying mental illness and are a danger to self or others. If the mental illness is a personality disorder (e.g., antisocial, impulse control), it may not be deemed severe enough to justify civil commitment. However, in recent years state legislatures have enacted laws that enable civil commitment of certain types of offenders whose mental disorders do not meet traditional criteria for commitment.

In *Kansas v Hendricks* (1997), the Supreme Court addressed the constitutionality of one such law. The Kansas Sexually Violent Predator Act provides for civil commitment of persons who, due to a "mental abnormality" or "personality disorder," are likely to engage in "predatory acts of sexual violence." Under this Act, the state sought to commit Hendricks on completion of his criminal sentence for the most recent of many acts of child sexual abuse. Although conceding that he was a pedophile and harbored continuing sexual desires toward children, he challenged the constitutionality of the Act on the ground that his "mental abnormality" was not of sufficient severity to justify civil commitment. After a trial in which the jury determined he was a sexually violent predator, the trial court ordered him committed and he appealed to the state supreme court. It agreed with his contention that the precommitment condition of "mental abnormality" did not satisfy the mental illness requirement for involuntary civil commitment. The state thereupon appealed to the U.S. Supreme Court.

The high Court decided that the Act passed constitutional muster. It regarded the "mental abnormality" at issue here as a qualifying mental illness because of the statutory requirement that it be shown to produce a volitional impairment that renders persons dangerous beyond their control. The Court rejected arguments that the Act was in effect a criminal statute because of its punitive dimensions, stressing that a detainee could gain immediate release on a showing he was no longer dangerous. Aside from validating laws permitting postconviction detention of certain sex offenders, this ruling appears to open the door for legislation targeting persons with other personality disorders of a sort that seriously impair behavioral controls and for which treatment is unsatisfactory. Implementing laws of this sort will necessitate behavioral evidence that addresses both the accuracy of diagnosis and the potential dangerousness of afflicted persons.

Other Proceedings

Behavioral evidence may be called for in various other legal proceedings, some of which will be briefly considered.

Administrative Hearings. Social welfare legislation permits qualifying claimants to obtain specified benefits through administrative proceedings. These proceedings are less formal than those in court, rules of evidence are not stringently applied, there are no juries, involvement of lawyers may be limited, and decisions may be rendered on the basis of reports rather than oral testimony. Despite the relative informality, it is important for behavioral experts to prepare reports or testimony that responds to the specific requirements of the particular administrative scheme.

Two of the more common administrative proceedings are workers' compensation hearings and Social

Security disability determinations. In workers' compensation proceedings, workers who establish job-related medical or psychological injuries may obtain defined disability or other benefits. Here behavioral evidence may be relevant in establishing a causal relationship between neurologic or psychological impairment and particular work or in characterizing the extent and prognosis of the impairment. In Social Security disability proceedings, claimants are entitled to benefits on proof they cannot engage in "substantial gainful activity" by reason of a "medically determined physical or mental impairment," which is expected to result in death or to persist for 12 months or more (United States Code). Objective proof is ordinarily required in these proceedings. Accordingly, a behavioral expert must be prepared to substantiate an opinion about cognitive or behavioral impairments with the most quantitative measures available (see Chapter 50).

Family Courts. Much of the business of family courts involves decisions about custody or visitation rights with respect to children. Most courts apply some version of the "best interests of the child" standard in making decisions about custody and visitation (Shulman, 1986). Although their role is not well defined and courts have abundant discretion, behavioral experts may provide considerable input. Ideally, opinions offered in court should be based on evaluations of parents and child that include mental status examinations and careful psychological assessments. In general, these opinions should address the nature of the attachment between parent and child, the child's needs, parental fitness, and family dynamics.

Probate and Guardianship Proceedings. Issues of cognitive capacity are central to legal decisions about competency to make a will (testamentary capacity), capacity to contract, and the need for guardianship or conservatorship (see Chapter 52). Accordingly, behavioral evidence is necessary to help resolve will contests or to determine the extent to which alleged incompetents are capable of managing their persons or their property. Testamentary capacity entails knowing the nature and extent of the property to be distributed, understanding how a will accomplishes this distribution, and knowing the identity of the beneficiaries (*Kerr v O'Donovan*, 1957). Contractual capacity requires understanding of the nature and consequences of the transaction at issue (*Krueger v Zoch*, 1969). The need for guardianship or conservatorship turns on whether a person has sufficient capacity to make or communicate responsible decisions about person or property (Uniform Probate Code, 1983). Although these various standards of competency are quite general, they should alert potential behavioral experts to the elements of cognition that concern legal decision makers. They also suggest a need to couple formal mental status examinations with determinations of relevant functional capacities (such as knowing what one owns or what it may cost to buy a particular item).

■ KEY POINTS

☐ Behavioral evidence can determine or influence outcome of legal disputes.

☐ Admissibility of behavioral evidence in legal proceedings ordinarily turns on its relevance and reliability.

☐ Recent decisions of the Supreme Court encourage trial judges to evaluate reliability of proffered behavioral evidence before admitting it.

☐ Otherwise reliable evidence can be excluded if it risks unfair prejudice, confusion of the issues, or misleading of jurors.

☐ Clinicians and scientists who offer behavioral evidence in legal proceedings should scrupulously respect prevailing professional norms of accuracy and objectivity.

KEY READINGS

Beresford HR: Neurologist as expert witness. Neurol Clin 10:1059–1071, 1992.

Goodwin RJ: The hidden significance of *Kumho Tire Co. v Carmichael*: A compass for problems of definition and procedure created by *Daubert v Merrell Dow Pharmaceuticals, Inc.* Baylor Law Rev 52:603–646, 2000.

Graham MH: The expert witness predicament: Determining "reliable" under the gatekeeping test of Daubert, Kumho, and proposed amended Rule 702 of the Federal Rules of Evidence. Univ Miami Law Rev 54:317–357, 2000.

Imwinkelried EJ: Should the courts incorporate a best evidence rule into the standard determining the admissibility of scientific testimony? Enough is enough even when it is not the best. Case Western Law Rev 50:19–51, 1999.

REFERENCES

Cases Cited

Addington v Texas, 441 US 418 (1979).
Cooper v Oklahoma, 116 S Ct 1373 (1996).
Daubert v Merrell Dow Pharmaceuticals, Inc., 125 S Ct 469 (1993).
Daubert v Merrell Dow Pharmaceuticals, Inc., 43 F 3d 1311 (9th Cir 1995).
Dusky v United States, 362 US 402 (1960).
Ford v Wainwright, 477 US 399 (1986).
Foucha v Louisiana, 112 S Ct 1780 (1992).
Frye v United States, 293 F 1013 (DC Cir 1923).

General Electric v Joiner, 118 S Ct 512 (1997).
Kansas v Hendricks, 117 S Ct 2072 (1997).
Kerr v O'Donovan, 134 A 2d 213 (PA S Ct 1957).
Krueger v Zoch, 173 NW 2d 18 (MN S Ct 1969).
Kumho Tire Company v Carmichael, 119 S Ct 1167 (1999).
Medina v California, 112 S Ct 2572 (1992).
M'Naghtens Case, 8 Eng Rep 718 (HL 1843).
O'Connor v Donaldson, 422 US 563 (1975).
Olmstead v Zimring, 119 S Ct 2176 (1999).
Riggins v Nevada, 112 S Ct 1810 (1992).
Singleton v Norris, 992 SW 2d 768 (AR S Ct 1999).
Singleton v State, 437 SE 2d 53 (SC S Ct 1993).
State v Perry, 610 So 2d 746 (LA S Ct 1992).
United States v Lyons, 739 F 2d 994 (5th Cir 1984).
United States v McBroom, 124 F 3d 533 (1997).
Washington v Harper, 494 US 210 (1990).

References Cited

Americans with Disabilities Act. United States Code, Title 42, section 12101, 1995.

Blake PY, Pincus JH, Buckner C: Neurologic abnormalities in murderers. Neurology 45:1641–1647, 1995

Emergency Medical Treatment and Active Labor Act. United States Code, Title 41, section 1395dd, 1986.

Federal Rules of Evidence, Pub Law 93-595, 89 Stat 1926, 1975.

Graham MH: The expert witness predicament: Determining "reliable" under the gatekeeping test of Daubert, Kumho, and proposed amended Rule 702 of the Federal Rules of Evidence. Univ Miami Law Rev 54:317–357, 2000.

Guiduli KA: Challenges for the mentally ill: The "threat to safety" defense standard and the use of psychotropic medication under Title I of the Americans with Disabilities Act of 1990. Univ Pennsylvania Law Rev 144:1149–1187, 1998.

Hill RA: Character, choice and "aberrant behavior": Aligning criminal sentencing with concepts of moral blame. Univ Chicago Law Rev 65:975–991, 1998.

Imwinkelried EJ: Should the courts incorporate a best evidence rule into the standard determining the admissibility of scientific testimony? Enough is enough even when it is not the best. Case Western Law Rev 50:19–51, 1999.

Insanity Defense Reform Act, US Code, Title 18, section 17, 1988.

Model Penal Code, section 4.01(1) (Tent Draft No 4, 1955).

Navigating uncertainty: Gatekeeping in the absence of hard science. Harvard Law Rev 13:1467–1484, 2000.

Shuman DW: Psychiatric and Psychological Evidence. Colorado Springs, CO: Shepard's/McGraw-Hill, 1986, pp 301–310.

Uniform Probate Code, 5-103(7), 1983.

United States Code, Title 42, section 423(d)(1)(A).

Zylan KD: Legislation that drives us crazy: An overview of "mental disability" under the Americans with Disabilities Act. Cumberland Law Rev 31:79–107, 2000.

Glossary

This glossary contains definitions of terms that are relevant to one or more of the chapters in this book. It is not intended as an exhaustive dictionary of behavioral terms.

Abulia (Adynamia, Amotivation, Bradyphrenia). Loss or slowing of initiation, drive, and motivation that can affect behavior, speech, and/or cognition, often with blunted or flattened emotional expression.

Academic Underachievement. Performing below one's expected level in academic functioning.

Acalculia. Loss of ability to calculate, either mentally or with paper and pencil.

Accommodation. In reference to disability, any alteration in the environment or in the manner of performing a task that allows an individual with a disability to experience equal opportunity.

Acquired Alexia. Loss of reading proficiency. This contrasts with dyslexia, which is a failure to develop normal reading ability.

Acquired Sociopathy. Impairment of social behavior, decision making, empathy, and self-regulation after cerebral damage, often involving the orbitofrontal region.

Activities of Daily Living (ADLs). Basic self-care activities necessary for autonomous functioning; examples are bathing, dressing, and feeding oneself.

Acute Confusional State. A rapidly evolving disorder of behavior that may present as a hypoaroused (lethargic) or hyperaroused (agitated) state (see Delirium).

Acute Vestibular Syndrome. Vertigo, oscillopsia, imbalance, and nausea/vomiting, with acute, asymmetrical vestibular dysfunction. The symptoms are generally transient and last only a few days.

Adaptive Functioning. Personal and social skills (e.g., ability to feed, clothe, and clean oneself; to communicate with others; or to get along with others).

Addiction. A complex of maladaptive behaviors, including using a drug despite the harm the drug is causing or using the drug for purposes other than those intended by the treating physician.

Adjuvant Treatments. Use of additional therapy after the majority of a tumor has been removed. The therapy is thought to be more beneficial when used against small amounts of tumor.

Advanced Sleep Phase Syndrome. A primary disorder of the biologic clock characterized by an earlier than desired sleep onset and sleep offset time. Individuals with this condition often find it impossible to stay up past early evening hours and awaken very early in the morning.

Adynamia. A lack of initiative or drive, often seen in some aspects of behavior or thought processes after frontal lobe injury. It can range from a severe inability to initiate any action without prompting, to less severe forms that present as a lack of spontaneity, to a tendency to appear passive and disinterested, with a limited range of activity.

Affect. A mood or feeling state, used in the context of defining emotional health, and involved in psychiatric disorders that alter personality and behavior. May be heightened, depressed, or blunted.

Ageusia.   A complete loss of taste that may involve part or all of the tongue. Ageusia may affect detection of one (partial or specific), some, or all (total) of the four basic taste qualities (salty, sweet, sour, bitter).

Agnosia (also called associative agnosia).   Inability to recognize (and consequently to name) previously familiar objects (retrograde agnosia) or to learn the identity of new objects (an anterograde defect) despite adequate perception. Associative agnosia is a defect of knowing, not of naming; objects are effectively stripped of their meanings. Specific forms of agnosia include visual agnosia (and the restricted form, prosopagnosia), auditory agnosia, and tactile agnosia.

Agraphia.   Acquired disorder of writing due to brain disease. May occur with alexia (see Angular Gyrus Syndrome).

Akinesia-Mutism.   Profound loss of initiative and sustained goal-directed behavior in a patient who is otherwise awake and alert; frequently associated with bilateral damage to the superior medial frontal lobes.

Akinetopsia.   Impaired perception of visual motion.

Alexia.   Acquired inability to read after cerebral damage despite intact visual abilities in individuals previously able to read (pure alexia); sometimes associated with agraphia (alexia with agraphia) as a component of aphasia.

Alternative Communication.   Use of a different communication modality, like writing or gesturing, when speech functions are not sufficient for normal communication.

Alzheimer Disease (AD).   A chronic, age-related dementing disorder associated with abnormal β-amyloid and τ protein accumulation in the brain. AD is the most common degenerative cause of dementia in adults.

Amblyopia.   Vision impairment without any known organic lesion in the eye.

Amnesia.   Clinical condition of memory loss sufficient to interfere with independent functioning. Specific etiology can be highly variable and either transient, progressive, or static.

Amnestic Dementia.   Class of cognitive disorders exemplified by Alzheimer disease in which disturbances of memory predominate among the initial symptoms.

Amusia.   Designates an acquired deficit in musical abilities occurring after brain damage. The term encompasses all modalities of musical behavior, such as recognizing, playing, composing, and writing. There are several subtypes of amusia that have been described including musical agraphia, musical agnosia, and motor amusia.

Amygdala.   From the Greek *amygdala*, meaning "almond." Collection of nuclei located deep in the medial temporal lobe bilaterally. Extensively connected with cerebral cortex, it projects also to hypothalamus and brainstem nuclei.

Anaplastic Astrocytoma.   Malignant tumor originating from glial cells within the brain. It has features of nuclear atypia, endothelial cell proliferation, and mitoses. Average survival is usually around 2 to 3 years.

Angular Gyrus Syndrome.   Combined deficits of anomia, fluent aphasia, alexia, agraphia, acalculia, right-left disorientation, finger agnosia, and constructional apraxia.

Anorgasmia.   Inability to achieve an orgasm due to psychological factors, vascular dysfunction, peripheral nervous system lesions, or CNS lesions affecting the spinal cord or cerebrum.

Anosmia.   Complete loss of olfactory sensation and perception. Etiologies are highly variable and include congenital conditions, traumatic injuries, environmental exposures, medications side effects, and neurologic diseases.

Anterograde Amnesia.   Loss of ability to retain new information and experiences since onset of a brain lesion.

Anticipation.   A genetic condition that shows earlier onset and greater severity as the causative gene moves from one generation to the next.

Anxiety Disorder.   Excessive anxiety and worry about events or activities recurring more days than not for at least 6 months.

Apathy.   Absence of feeling, emotion, interest, or concern.

Aphasia.   Acquired disorders of speech and language secondary to cerebral damage. The term encompasses multiple aphasia subtypes with distinctive features (e.g., Broca's, Wernicke's, conduction) and lesion localization.

Apperceptive Agnosia.   Failure to identify previously familiar objects due to impaired perception.

Apraxia.   Acquired disorders of skilled movements after cerebral damage that are not caused by sensory or motor deficits. Subtypes include buccofacial, ideomotor, ideational, dressing, and constructional (the latter in spatial problem-solving tasks).

Apraxia of Speech (AOS).   Speech disorder due to impairment of motor programming ability pertaining to the speech mechanism.

Area Measurements.   Evaluation of the size of a central nervous system region by its cross-sectional area. It is the oldest morphometric approach.

Arousal.   The waking state of an individual, determined by the activity of the ascending reticular activating system and its thalamocortical connections.

Arteriovenous Malformation. Abnormal connection between arterial and venous blood vessels, often a "tangle" of blood vessels.

Arthropod-Borne Viral Infection. An infection acquired through the bite of a mosquito.

Assistive Technology. Any item, piece of equipment, or product system (off-the-shelf, modified, or custom-made) that is used to increase, maintain, or improve functional capabilities of disabled individuals.

Association Area. Regions of the cerebral cortex that process information from multiple afferent sources, both exteroceptive and interoceptive, that are linked with other higher order cortical and subcortical regions, and that subserve high level cognitive processing.

Associative Tactile Agnosia. Inability to attribute meaning to objects that are adequately tactually perceived and explored.

Astereognosis. Refers to two terms: *ahylognosis*, which is the inability to tactually perceive texture (e.g., roughness, density, weight), and *amorphognosis*, which is the inability to tactually perceive shape (e.g., size, length).

Asynchrony. Nonsimultaneous electroencephalographic activities over the same or opposite side of the head.

Attention. The capacity to select behaviorally relevant elements of sensory experience for cognitive processing while simultaneously excluding others from consciousness. Attention problems include difficulty sustaining attention over time, a tendency to be easily distracted from a task by noise or competing information, and difficulty dividing one's attention to be able to perform more than one task at a time.

Augmentative Communication. Use of a communication system that supplements residual communication skills. This can be as simple as a pointing board or communication notebook or as complex as a computerized system.

Autotopagnosia. Inability to locate body parts on one's own or on someone else's body, upon verbal or nonverbal command, despite preserved knowledge of their locations and the ability to name them.

Awareness. Ability to appreciate and report changes in one's abilities or functioning and to demonstrate an understanding of the probable impact of those changes on current and future capabilities.

Axonal Shearing. Axons (in white matter) stretched or torn by rotational forces associated with acceleration-deceleration injuries.

Balint Syndrome (or Bálint Syndrome). Loose triad of defects in visuospatial processing, including simul-

tanagnosia, optic ataxia, and ocular motor apraxia.

Basic Emotions. Limited set (usually six) of emotions thought to be primary, exhibited and recognized cross-culturally and observed early in human development. The standard list of basic emotions is: anger, fear, sadness, happiness, disgust, and surprise.

Binding Problem. Difficulty determining which elementary visual features, such as color, shape, or size, belong to the same stimulus. Spatial attention allows elementary features to be bound or grouped together.

Blindsight. Residual visual ability in hemianopic or cortically blind regions of the visual field in some patients, despite their professed lack of awareness of stimuli in the defective visual region.

Block Design. In reference to neuroimaging, a paradigm of stimulation or task performance in which extended periods of stimulation (typically 20 to 30 seconds) are alternated with periods of rest, or different stimulation. Images (e.g., fMRI) acquired during different "blocks" may be subtracted to reveal differential signal.

Blood Oxygenation Level Dependent (BOLD) Contrast. The most widely used MRI contrast mechanism for identification of brain function in fMRI. It exploits the dynamic changes in the regional balance of oxyhemoglobin to deoxyhemoglobin in the capillary bed adjacent to active neurons.

Brachytherapy. Use of radioactive seeds temporarily implanted within the area of a brain tumor to increase the local radiation dose.

Brain at Risk. Individuals with vascular risk factors in isolation or clinically silent cerebrovascular disease at risk for dementia.

Brain Attack. Acute stroke.

Brain Death. Irreversible condition of complete absence of brain function, including brainstem function. Cranial nerve function and brainstem reflexes are absent but there may be some preservation of spinal cord reflex activity.

Burst. In electroencephalography, a group of waves that appear and disappear abruptly and are distinguishable from the background by differences in frequency, waveform, and/or amplitude.

Burst-Suppression. An electroencephalographic pattern characterized by bursts of theta, delta, and, at times, faster activity, interspersed between periods of relative low voltage.

Callosotomy. Transection of the corpus callosum; can be either complete or partial; usually referring to a surgical transection, often for treatment of refractory epilepsy.

Candidate Gene(s). Specific genetic loci, identified either by their function or by location, as determined by linkage studies, as likely to be causative of a particular disorder. For attention-deficit/hyperactivity disorder, potential candidate genes include those that specify the central dopamine synthesis and especially receptor pathways. Less convincingly, genes regulating adrenergic pathways are also under scrutiny.

Cataplexy. Sudden loss of muscle tone triggered by emotionally laden events such as laughter, anger, surprise, or delight. This symptom is pathognomonic of narcolepsy and represents the sudden, inappropriate intrusion of one element of REM sleep (muscle paralysis) into wakefulness.

Cerebellar Agenesis. Congenital absence of the cerebellum, in whole or in part.

Cerebellar Cognitive Affective Syndrome. Clinical constellation resulting from cerebellar lesions characterized by impairments in executive function, spatial cognition, linguistic processing, and emotional control. Affective disturbances occur with lesions of the cerebellar vermis; cognitive deficits follow lesions of the posterior cerebellar hemispheres.

Cerebellar Cortex. Three-layered cortex with essentially uniform appearance throughout. Purkinje cells are the only outflow neuron of the cerebellar cortex. They lie in a single cell layer separating the densely populated granule cell layer below from the molecular layer above that contains Purkinje cell dendrites, granule cell axons, and inhibitory interneurons.

Cerebellar Nucleus. There are four paired deep cerebellar nuclei. The midline fastigial nucleus is anatomically linked with the vermis. The globose and emboliform nuclei lie between the fastigial nucleus and the laterally situated dentate nucleus. The dentate has a phylogenetically older dorsal region linked with motor areas of cerebral cortex and an evolutionarily newer ventral part linked with cerebral association areas.

Cerebral Dyschromatopsia. Impaired color vision as a consequence of cerebral damage. This contrasts with congenital dyschromatopsia, which is poor color vision due to abnormalities of retinal cone pigments.

Cerebral Leukoariosis. Refers to the nonspecific appearance of white matter lesions on magnetic resonance imaging scans that does not imply its underlying etiologic basis.

Cerebral Palsy (CP). Nonprogressive motor system impairments resulting from central nervous system injuries.

Cerebrocerebellar system. Anatomic circuit that links the cerebellum with the cerebral cortex. Consists of two-stage feedforward limb (cerebral cortex projects to neurons in the base of the pons;

pontine neurons project to cerebellar cortex), and a two-stage feedback limb (deep cerebellar nuclei project to thalamic nuclei; thalamus projects back to cerebral cortical areas from which the feedforward limb was derived). The inferior olivary nucleus has strong projections to the cerebellum through the climbing fiber system but is not directly involved in the circuits governing cognition and emotion.

Cerebrospinal Fluid (CSF). Filtrate and secretion of the choroid plexus that supports and nourishes the brain and spinal cord.

Chelation Therapy. A treatment that lowers lead burden in children. This therapy improves outcomes only in children with lead levels above 40 µg/dL.

Chromosome Deletion Syndromes. Syndromes caused by deletion of a known portion of the chromosome that result in specific physical and central nervous system effects. These syndromes may be inherited or can occur sporadically as spontaneous mutations.

Circadian Cycles. Fluctuations in physiologic activity that occur over the course of 24 hours; example is arousal states.

Circadian Rhythm Disorders. Disorders of the circadian timing system, resulting in sleep onset and sleep offset times that are out of synchronization with the environment. In individuals with the disorders there is nothing abnormal about the sleep per se, but the timing of the sleep period is undesirable and uncontrollable.

Clinical Interview. In child neuropsychological assessment, an interview conducted by the neuropsychologist with the child and parents to elicit information about the presenting problem and background information relevant to it.

Closed Head Injury. Head injury in which the skull is not penetrated.

Cognitive Assessment. Inferring specific and global cognitive abilities through an individual's performance on a fixed or flexible battery of standardized cognitive/neuropsychological tests.

Cognitive Therapy. Behavioral approach to treatment of specific symptoms (impaired organizational skills, poor eye contact, test-taking phobia) using observations of the responses of the affected individuals in the problematic situation with analysis of behaviors that either positively or negatively correlate with resolution of the situation. Frequently, videotaping is used to allow individuals to view and critique their own behavior with prompting from the therapist. This represents a way of actively engaging the individuals' analytical skills to take ownership and pose solutions acceptable to them.

Cognitive-Linguistic Impairment. Language disorder associated with cognitive impairments, all of which are due to brain injury.

Color Anomia. Inability to name colors despite the preserved ability to distinguish hues.

Color Constancy. The stability of hue appearance despite changes in lighting, a phenomenon that depends on cortical color mechanisms.

Coma. State of impaired consciousness without capacity for arousal or signs of wakefulness. The eyes of the patients in coma remain closed, and the patients lack any sign of spontaneous or stimulus-induced arousal.

Commissurotomy. Transection of a commissure or white matter tract, which may or may not cross the midline.

Comorbidity. Co-occurrence of two or more disorders that may or may not have a causal linkage or other specific association.

Compensatory Memory Strategies. Refers to a variety of different approaches or aids that work around memory problems and decrease their impact on everyday functioning. An example of an internal aid is mental imagery; an example of an external aid is a memory book or wristwatch alarm.

Compulsions. Repetitive and seemingly purposeful behaviors performed according to certain rules and/or in a stereotypic fashion.

Computed Tomography (CT). Procedure in which a beam of x-rays is passed through the patient with the amount of transmission depending on the tissue properties. Computer software produces a three-dimensional map from measured attenuations of the brain and surrounding structures.

Conceptual Apraxia. Defective concepts relevant to gestures and actions. May be accompanied by evidence of ideomotor limb apraxia or may occur independently.

Concrete Thinking. Difficulties in forming or dealing with abstract concepts and a tendency to focus on specific, concrete aspects of a situation or conversation, failing to generalize from an experience or to distill the essence of a problem.

Concussion. Self-limited group of cognitive, emotional, and somatic symptoms that often follow head trauma associated with brief loss or alteration of consciousness.

Confusion. Inability to maintain a coherent line of thought despite adequate arousal and language function.

Confusional State. Condition of global cognitive impairment related primarily to a deficit in attention. Delirium is another commonly used term for this condition.

Congruity. Degree to which hemifield defects present in both eyes resemble each other. High congruity is typical of striate lesions.

Consolidation. Neurophysiologic processes that underlie retention of learned information over time. Extended interactions between medial temporal lobe structures and cortical association areas permit the long-term retention of knowledge independently of the medial temporal lobe.

Content Errors. In limb praxis assessment, a pantomimed gesture that is recognizable but communicates incorrect subject matter (e.g., a hammering gesture for ice pick).

Continuous Performance Test. Task designed to evaluate an individual's ability to maintain attention to task, inhibit impulsive responses, and screen out distractions over an extended period of time; often used to evaluate attentional and neurodevelopmental disorders.

Contrecoup Injury. Injury to the brain opposite the site of impact after head injury.

Convolution. Process of temporal blurring by which an instantaneous "event" becomes a more extended "measured response"; of interest in fMRI, the reliance on a hemodynamic reporting mechanism to exploit the blood oxygen level dependent effect introduces a hemodynamic convolution, yielding a measured response that is the convolution of the event itself and a characteristic hemodynamic response function (hrf). If the hrf is known, the reverse process of deconvolution, in principle, allows extraction of the underlying "event" of interest from the observed "response."

Corpus Callosum. Arched white matter tract, crossing the midline and connecting both cerebral hemispheres.

Corticobasal Degeneration. Neurodegenerative disorder affecting the basal ganglia and cortex, which shows some overlap in symptomology with other disorders such as Parkinson disease, progressive supranuclear palsy, Pick disease, and Alzheimer disease.

Corticonuclear Microcomplex. Tight interrelationship between zones of the cerebellar cortex and focal regions within the deep cerebellar nuclei. Considered to be the functional unit of the cerebellum.

Corticopontine. Anatomic projection from cerebral cortex to neurons in the basis pontis, the first step in the two-stage feedforward limb of the cerebro-cerebellar circuit.

Coup Injury. Injury to the brain beneath the site of impact after head injury.

Craniectomy. Surgical removal of a portion of the skull.

Cytokine. Low-molecular-weight protein secreted by one cell to alter the function of other close-by cells.

Data Standardization. Process by which MRI images are fit into a standard framework. One of the most widely used is the Talairach method, in which images are aligned according to certain landmarks and transformed to fit into a stereotactic (atlas) coordinate system.

Deafferentation. Loss of sensory input to a region of the brain. For example, a section of the posterior spinal cervical roots will cause deafferentation of the arm representation in the cerebral cortex.

Decision Noise Reduction. Uncertainty associated with reporting the identity of a stimulus reduced by attention.

Declarative Memory. Conscious recollection of facts, knowledge, experiences, and events. This system mediates the general, specific, and personal aspects of declarative knowledge that are acquired through learning and is highly sensitive to acquired brain damage.

Defecography. Method used to identify patients with rectal prolapse, poor rectal evacuation, or mega rectum.

Degenerative Disorders (Neurodegenerative, Central Nervous System Degenerative). Intrinsic diseases of nerve tissue that progressively disrupt the structural integrity of the nervous system and compromise one or more aspect of nervous function.

Delayed Sleep Phase Syndrome. Primary disorder of the biologic clock characterized by an inability to fall asleep until much later than desired and a tendency to sleep very late in the morning. Those afflicted with this condition find it difficult, if not impossible, to awaken at conventional times.

Delirium. Agitated acute confusional state with disturbance of consciousness, characterized by attentional deficits, delusions, and hallucinations.

Dementia. Acquired and persistent impairment of intellect and behavior affecting multiple domains of cognition and emotion and sufficient to interfere with everyday functions. Common causes are neurodegenerative impairments including Alzheimer disease and related disorders including frontotemporal dementia, Lewy body disease, and Parkinson disease; cerebrovascular disease; trauma; and central nervous system infections.

Depression. Disorder of mood that likely results from central neurotransmitter dysfunction and can often be confused with acute confusional state and dementia.

Desynchronization. Attenuation of electroencephalographic activity due to loss of simultaneously occurring waves.

Developmental Growth Curves. Repeated measurements in any domain that can be tracked over time to examine a child's growth, allowing examination of how disease and treatments affect rate of development.

Diaschisis. Physiologic concept introduced by the University of Zurich neurologist Constantin von Monakow in 1911 to describe dynamic changes in metabolic activity and consequently in altered blood flow that can occur in a normal brain region that is anatomically interconnected with a lesioned brain area.

Diffusion-Weighted Imaging (DWI). Magnetic resonance imaging technique based on the principle that water diffusion in the white matter occurs in a restricted and directional way (anisotropy), which is determined by the axonal fibers and their myelin sheaths. DWI can provide information about white matter architecture and integrity.

Disability. Functional limitation resulting from an impairment. A disability is considered a handicap when it entails the inability to perform an activity required for a recognized social role or occupation.

Disconnection Syndrome. Clinical phenomenon resulting from disruption of fiber pathways linking cortical areas with other cortical regions or with subcortical structures.

Discriminant Function Analysis. Multivariate statistical technique that can be used to classify persons into known groups, based on their profile of test scores. Logistic regression analysis can be used in a similar manner. Discriminant analysis, however, has more restrictive statistical assumptions underlying its use than does logistic regression.

Distributed Neural Circuit. System of anatomical locations (nodes) distributed throughout the brain and linked together by anatomical connections that together function as an integrated unit to subserve all neurological function.

Dopaminergic Neurotransmitter System. Principal pathways that use dopamine as a transmitter include the nigrostriatal (from the substantia nigra to the caudate nucleus), mesolimbic (from the ventral tegmental area to the nucleus accumbens), mesocortical (from the ventral tegmental area to the suprarhinal cortex), and tuberohypophysial (from the arcuate nucleus to the median eminence) tracts. These regions have frequently been implicated in neurostructural and neurochemical studies as abnormal in individuals with attention-deficit/hyperactivity disorder.

Dorsal Rhizotomy. Surgical procedure in which some of the lumbar-sacral dorsal nerve roots are severed to disrupt the overactive stretch reflex circuitry and reduce spasticity.

Dorsolateral Frontal Lobe. Region of the prefrontal cortex associated with diverse cognitive processes including working memory, organization of behavior, planning, and other aspects of executive functions.

Double Dissociation. Classical paradigm used in neuropsychology to determine whether functions are independent, both functionally and neuroanatomically.

Driving Simulator. Device that replicates aspects of the road environment to assess driver performance. Simulator studies provide the only means to replicate exactly the experimental road conditions under which driving comparisons are made and have none of the safety risks of the road. Simulator fidelity, scenario-design, and test validity are key issues.

Dysarthria. Speech disorder due to motor impairment.

Dysexecutive Syndrome. Clinical term meant to describe the various impairments of executive functions, typically associated with real-life deficits in social, vocational, and independent living skills.

Dysgeusia. Perceptual distortions in taste quality that most patients describe as an unpleasant salty, bitter, or metallic sensation.

Dyslexia. Learning disability that involves reading, spelling, and/or writing. It is a specific language-based problem of constitutional origin characterized by difficulties in single-word decoding, usually reflecting insufficient phonological processing abilities.

Dysmetria. Greek term implying disturbance of rhythm; used since Gordon Holmes (e.g., 1917) to denote the pattern of disturbance of voluntary movements following cerebellar lesions, characterized by abnormalities of rate, rhythm, and force. As used in the dysmetria of thought hypothesis, the term is expanded to include the aberrations of mental function (as in the cerebellar cognitive affective syndrome) that occur following lesions of cerebellar regions concerned with the regulation of cognition and affect.

Dysmetria of Thought. Hypothesis that holds that the cerebellum impairs high-level processing in a manner similar to the observed motor impairments following anterior lobe lesions. Dysmetria of movement manifests as uncoordinated motor performance or ataxia, whereas dysmetria of thought results in the different manifestations of the cerebellar cognitive affective syndrome.

Dysosmia. Altered olfactory experiences including parosmia (distortions) and phantosmia (olfactory hallucinations).

Dysphagia. Swallowing disorder due to impairment of the oral and/or pharyngeal mechanism, which can be due to neurologic control of the involved structures.

Dysthymic Disorder. Depressed mood for most of the day, for more days than not for at least 2 years.

Dystrophin. Protein that is absent or reduced in quantity in the muscle of boys with muscular dystrophy.

Ecological Validity. Relationship between performance on measures of cognitive functioning and performance in real world tasks; usually in reference to neuropsychological assessment.

Effect Size. Standardized estimate of the effect of a treatment, intervention, or other condition. One example of an effect size is the difference between two sample means divided by the pooled standard deviation.

Emotional Reaction. The physiologic components of an emotion, including but not limited to changes in heart rate, blood pressure, and piloerection.

Encephalitis. Acute infection of brain parenchyma that presents with fever, headache, and an altered level of consciousness.

Encephalopathy. Clinical syndrome caused by any disorder of the brain.

Entorhinal Cortex. Region in the medial temporal lobe that is consistent with Brodmann area 28, forming a large part of the parahippocampal gyrus. This region is important for input and output pathways of the hippocampus.

Epilepsy. Group of neurologic conditions characterized by recurrent epileptic seizures (repetitive seizures separated by more than 24 hours) and caused by various disorders that involve disturbed electrical rhythms of the brain.

Epileptic Seizure. Transient abnormal electrical discharge from the neurons in the brain. Seizures may involve motor, sensory, psychic, or autonomic disturbances, and their manifestation will depend on the regions of the brain involved.

Episodic Memory. Long-term memory system for storing time- and context-specific episodes or events that are personally experienced.

Erectile Dysfunction (ED). Inability to achieve or maintain an erection sufficient to permit sexual intercourse. Risk factors include use of tobacco, alcohol, or illicit drug use, diabetes, vascular disease, hypertension, cancer or chemotherapy, infection, spinal cord lesions, neurological conditions, and penile curvature or pain.

Errorless Learning. Approach to teaching/training individuals with severe memory impairment that emphasizes limiting the production of incorrect guesses or errors so as to improve accurate recall and decrease the likelihood of reinforcing incorrect responses.

Executive Control. Attentional processes closely associated with the frontal lobe appear to involve controlling lower-level perceptual systems. This executive control permits some stimuli to be selected over others on the basis of the relevance of that stimulus to the task currently being performed.

Executive Functions (EF). Neuropsychological term meant to describe the diverse higher cognitive functions that underlie planning, organization, goal-directed behavior, and the integration of cognitive and emotional processing in decision-making and adaptation.

Extrapyramidal (Dyskinetic or Choreoathetoid) Cerebral Palsy. Involuntary writhing movements (athetosis) of the face, tongue, hands, and feet that are punctuated and overridden by chorea (jerking movements) of the trunk, arms, and legs.

FDG [¹⁸F]fluorodeoxyglucose. Radiotracer that is an analog of glucose, labeled with 18 F, and used in positron emission computed tomography to measure regional cerebral glucose metabolism.

Feedback Session. Meeting of a psychologist with recipients of psychological assessment services and other interested parties to discuss assessment findings and recommendations for treatment.

Feeling. Subjective experience of emotion.

Fiber Pathway. White matter system in the brain consisting of axons linking cortical areas with other cortical and subcortical regions.

Flavor. Sensations conveyed by the gustatory, olfactory, and trigeminal nerves that fuse into a single percept.

Forced Normalization. Brief episodes of psychosis that occur when seizures become infrequent or fully controlled.

Frontal Dementia. Cognitive and behavioral loss characterized by a decrease in attention, judgment, self-regulatory processes, and organized behavior associated with abnormalities in the frontal lobe.

Frontotemporal Dementia. Class of dementing illnesses exemplified by Pick disease and tau pathophysiology. Subtypes include primary progressive aphasia, semantic dementia, and behavioral disorder-dysexecutive, with varying involvement of frontal and temporal lobes.

Functional Capacity. Potential for functioning after appropriate accommodation and assistive technology are provided.

Functional MRI (fMRI). Use of a specific contrast mechanism in magnetic resonance imaging to identify brain regions that respond to a particular stimulus or during performance of a particular task.

Functional Neurosurgery. Subspecialty within neurosurgery that focuses on treating movement disorders, pain, and spasticity.

Functional Organization. Model of how a system (e.g., auditory or visual) works, according to the processing components (in contrast to anatomy or physiology) of the structures involved.

Functional Performance. Purposeful activity; includes Activities of Daily Living (ADLs) and Instrumental Activities of Daily Living (IADLs).

Gamma Ray. Electromagnetic radiation emitted from the nucleus of certain radioactive atoms during the process of radioactive decay or produced by the annihilation of a positron-electron pair.

Gender-Specific Expression. Behaviors or traits within a phenotype that differ in intensity or frequency based on the gender of the gene carrier. For attention-deficit/hyperactivity disorder, the primary differences based on gender are the higher frequency of hyperactivity and comorbid oppositional-defiant disorder in boys and the greater occurrence of anxiety/depression in girls.

Gerstmann Syndrome. Five deficits associated with left parietal lesions: agraphia, right-left confusion, disorientation, acalculia, and finger agnosia.

Glasgow Coma Scale. Rating scale commonly used to estimate level of responsiveness after acute head trauma (score range 3–15). The maximum score of 15 depends on intact motor functions, verbal output, and eye opening responses. The lower the score, the lower the level of responsiveness.

Glioma. Infiltrative tumors within the brain often interdigitating within the various structures of the brain causing either destruction of neural structures, compression of structures, or secretion of proteins that leads to biochemical changes in cognitive functioning of the brain.

Glioblastoma Multiforme. Most malignant type of primary brain tumor. It is distinguished from other tumors by the presence of necrosis. Overall survival is often less than a year.

Graphesthesia. Inability to tactually recognize and name numbers written on the hand or skin.

"Guides to the Evaluation to Permanent Impairment" (GEPI). Published by the American Medical Association, now in its fifth edition.

Hallucinations. Sensory perceptions in the absence of identifiable external stimuli.

Handicap. Expression of the impact of a given pathology, impairment, or disability on an individual's specific social roles and activities.

Heinrich's Triangle. Relationships between different performance factors and safety errors represented by an imaginary triangle. In automobile driving, for example, crash events resulting in fatality or serious injury are most infrequent and are represented toward the apex of the triangle. Events that result in property damage only, or in no crash, are far more common, and are represented toward the base of the triangle. As the frequency of events increases, the relevance to serious driver safety errors and crashes decreases.

Hematoma. Abnormal collection of blood outside of the vascular system

Hematopoietic Stem Cell Transplantation (HSCT). Transfer of hematopoietic stem cells either through donor bone marrow or donor cord blood to treat inborn errors of metabolism, sickle cell disease, and other disorders affecting the child's central nervous system development.

Hemianopia (or Hemianopsia, or Homonymous Hemianopia). Visual field defect that occupies both the upper and lower visual portions of the same hemifield of both eyes

Heritability. Proportion of variation in a set of symptoms or physical traits that is due to genotypic differences in affected individuals.

Heterotopic Connection. Interhemispheric connection linking different anatomic cortical areas, which serve a similar function.

Hippocampus. Medial temporal lobe structure named after its appearance (like a seahorse) and consisting of a folded tube of cell layers, namely, CA1, CA2, CA3, CA4, and the dentate gyrus. Definitions of the hippocampus vary from study to study and may include the hippocampus proper (above) and the subiculum and entorhinal cortex.

Homotopic Connection. Interhemispheric connection linking corresponding cortical areas from one hemisphere to another.

Hydrocephalus. Abnormal accumulation of cerebrospinal fluid within the ventricular system and/or subarachnoid space.

Hypogeusia. Diminution of taste intensity for one or more of the gustatory stimuli that may involve part or all of the oral cavity. Total, partial, or specific hypogeusias have been reported.

Hyposmia. Reduction in olfactory sensation and perception. Does not imply a single, specific etiology but may be associated with environmental exposures, aging, brain diseases, medications, and metabolic conditions.

Hypoxic-Ischemic Encephalopathy (HIE). Pathologic decreases in blood flow of oxygen that cause damage to the brain.

Hysteria. Sensory and motor symptoms and signs that cannot be attributed to organic pathology, but resemble a neurologic cause.

Ideomotor Limb Apraxia. Limb apraxia caused defective time-space-movement representations or their connections to motor output, rather than defective concepts relevant to gestures and actions.

Idiopathic Central Nervous System Hypersomnia. Neurologic condition characterized by the tendency to fall asleep during the day when not actively stimulated despite a normal night's sleep. This condition is similar to narcolepsy but lacks the ancillary symptom of cataplexy.

Infant of Diabetic Mother (IDM). Syndrome includes increased birth weight and neonatal size, transient hypoglycemia, and associated risk of cardiac and pulmonary problems and high risk for brain injury if untreated.

Impairment. Direct and indirect neuroanatomic and neurophysiologic consequences of an underlying pathology.

Impotence. Complaint, most often encountered in men, expressed as erectile dysfunction.

Imprinting. Some genes are expressed depending on their maternal versus paternal origin. Differing phenotypes of some genetically transmitted syndromes depend on the parent from whom the mutant allele is inherited. In a paternally expressed gene, a maternal uniparental disomy will result in the disorder in question.

Incidence. Rate of occurrence in a specific population.

Inclusion. Result of individuals with disabilities having full access to and participation in all activities.

Incontinence. Inability to voluntarily control fecal or urinary excretory functions. Subtypes of urinary incontinence include urge, stress, mixed, overflow, unconscious or reflex, and functional.

Independent Living. Freedom of choice to have full access to the utilization of resources that allows for community living.

Independent Living Movement. Civil rights agenda based on the premise that the barriers that confront people with disabilities are less related to individual impairment than to barriers created by societal attitudes, interpretations of disability, and architectural, legal, and educational limitations.

Insanity Defense Reform Act. A federal act that specifies that the burden of proving insanity is on the defendant by "clear and convincing" evidence, that a qualifying mental illness must be "severe," and that the illness must be the cause of the incapacity to appreciate criminality.

Instrumental Activities of Daily Living (IADLs). Daily activities that depend on a number of intact cognitive abilities and that are instrumental in achieving a goal; examples are grocery shopping, handling finances, cooking a meal, using the telephone, and paying bills.

Instrumental and Goal-Directed Behavior. Intentional cognition and action of an individual that acts on the environment and others to achieve goals.

Inter-ictal. Period of time between seizures.

Interrater Agreement. Extent to which there is stability in the test scores assigned to patients by different examiners.

Intransitive Gesture. Pantomimed movement that does not require the use of an object. Many of these gestures are more abstract representational hand/arm movements or commands, such as saluting, "go away," "goodbye" and "be quiet."

Kernicterus. Encephalopathy in newborns due to high levels of bilirubin.

Klüver-Bucy Syndrome. Condition characterized by incontinence and sexual dysfunction. In humans, it may be associated with head injury, heat stroke, herpes encephalitis, neurodegenerative impairments, temporal lobectomy, stroke, shigellosis, psychiatric disease, and status epilepticus.

Labyrinth. Collection of fluid filled tubes and sacs in the inner ear that comprise the vestibular endorgan. It consists of three semicircular canals and two otolith organs. The canals are responsive to angular movements. The otolith organ consists of two parts, the utricle and the saccule. They are responsive to linear movement and head tilt. The area that houses the two otolith organs is called the vestibule.

Language. The manipulation of symbols in the production and comprehension of communicative symbols.

Language Dominance. Refers to the cerebral hemisphere where language functions predominate. This is usually the left hemisphere, although for left-handers and people with epilepsy there is an increased crossed dominance, that is, language functions in the right hemisphere.

Language of Generalized Intellectual Impairment. Language disorder associated with cognitive impairments, usually due to degenerative disease of the brain.

Latency. Refers to the time in milliseconds from the stimulus to the peak of the wave of interest in evoked potential recordings.

Lateropulsion/Ipsipulsion. Lateropulsion describes the sensation of being pulled to the ground to one side. It occurs mainly with lesions in the vestibular nuclei but is also present in lesions from the labyrinth to the thalamus. This is accompanied by ocular lateropulsion. With ipsipulsion the eyes drift toward the side of the lesion when the patient is asked to look upward with the eyes open; the body sway is also toward the side of the lesion.

Leptomeningeal Carcinomatosis. Spread of tumor cells into the area lining and surrounding the brain. This spread occurs either by hematogenous seeding or by direct extension from nearby tumor growths.

Leukoencephalopathy. Syndrome of structural involvement of the cerebral white matter from a wide range of disorders.

Limb apraxia. Disorder of learned skilled purposive movement not caused by elemental neurologic dysfunction such as weakness, sensory impairment, abnormal posture, tone or movement, or lack of understanding/cooperation.

Limbic. General term used to describe brain structures or behaviors concerned with motivation, emotion, and drive, such as the cingulate gyrus, fornix, septum, amygdala, and hippocampus. The concept of the limbic system has been expanded to include paralimbic structures such as supramodal regions in the posterior parahippocampal, posterior parietal, superior temporal, and orbital frontal cortices, limbic thalamic nuclei, and the extended limbic system, including the nucleus accumbens and the basal forebrain. The cerebellar vermis may be limbic as well.

Limbic Encephalitis. Paraneoplastic syndrome characterized by retrograde amnesia, psychiatric abnormalities, seizures, brainstem abnormalities, and hypothalamic dysregulation

Locked-in Syndrome. Condition of loss of voluntary motor control in the setting of preserved consciousness.

Logistic Regression. Type of regression analysis used when the dependent variable is binary.

Magnetic Resonance Imaging (MRI). Process in which a scanner containing a large magnet induces magnetized protons, then a radio frequency pulse causes the protons in differing states (e.g., water, proteins, and lipids) to emit different radio frequency signals. The signal data are converted to an image, and three-dimensional data sets can be created for volumetric assessment.

Magnetic Resonance Spectroscopy (MRS). Method that can detect and measure the concentration of important neurometabolites. In addition to spectra, MRS can lead to images depicting compound concentrations in different central nervous system regions.

Magnetic Source Imaging (MSI). Fusion of the modeled source of the magnetoencephalographic recording with an anatomic, tomographic image, derived from computed tomography or conventional magnetic resonance imaging.

Magnetoencephalography (MEG). Recording of extracranial magnetic fields associated with intracranial electrical activity.

Malingering. Intentional fabrication or faking of impairment or disability based on subjective report or by exam presentation, for identifiable secondary gain (e.g., legal settlement, avoidance of work).

Manic Episode. Distinct period characterized by persistently elevated, expansive, or irritable mood, lasting at least 1 week.

Manual Delineation. Process by which a central nervous system region is outlined in contiguous magnetic resonance imaging slices. It is the method of choice for measuring the volume of small or complex shape structures or for preserving individual subject's features, usually altered by standardization procedures.

Medial Temporal Lobe. Allocortex (phylogenetically one of the oldest parts of the cerebral cortex) in the anteromedial part of the temporal lobe, which includes the hippocampus, entorhinal cortex, parahippocampal gyrus, and amygdala.

Meninges. Protective lining of the central nervous system, including the pia mater, arachnoid, and dura mater.

Meningioma. Tumor originating from the fibrous lining surrounding the brain. It is more common in older individuals. While considered benign such tumors can grow to large volumes within the cranial cavity, thereby compressing neural contents and leading to subtle gradual neurocognitive defects.

Meningoencephalitis. Syndrome that most literally translated means inflammation of the leptomeninges and brain, for which there are numerous causes.

Mental Status Screening Tests. Brief question and answer tests used to quickly evaluate cognitive impairment.

Meta-Analysis. Statistical technique that combines the results of two or more studies in order to calculate an overall effect of a treatment, intervention, or other condition. Statistical power is increased when samples from several studies are combined.

Metabolic Dysfunction. Disturbance of normal homeostasis by any disorder of metabolism.

Metamemory. Awareness of one's own memory—its capacity, strengths, and limits—as well as awareness of one's use of memory strategies.

Metastatic Brain Tumor. Tumor growing within the brain that migrated from another site within the body, probably through hematogenous spread.

Mild Cognitive Impairment (MCI). Prodromal or transitional state between normal cognition in older individuals and early dementia, usually of the Alzheimer type. This state is characterized primarily by short-term or recent-memory deficits and otherwise intact cognition and behavior.

Minimally Conscious State. Condition of severely altered consciousness in which minimal but definite behavioral evidence of self or environmental awareness is demonstrated.

Mobility. Intentional movement throughout the environment; the capacity to move throughout one's environment in order to complete a task or achieve a goal.

Model Penal Code (MPC). Template for some state laws that excuses a defendant from criminal responsibility if, as a result of mental disease or defect, he lacked "substantial capacity either to appreciate the criminality of his conduct or to conform his conduct to the requirements of law" at the time of the alleged crime.

Mood Disorder. Prominent and persistent disturbance in mood, characterized by depressed mood or loss of interest, or elevated or irritable mood.

Morphometric. Measurement of specific brain regions using static neuroimaging techniques such as magnetic resonance imaging.

Multifocal Brain Disorders. Brain disorders associated with multiple sites of cerebral dysfunction or injury.

Multi-Infarct Dementia. Cognitive loss due to multiple large strokes or recurrent lacunar strokes.

Multiple Sclerosis. Inflammatory demyelinating disease of the central nervous system.

Multiple Sleep Latency Test. Objective measurement of the tendency to fall asleep during normal waking hours. The test consists of 4 or 5 20-minute nap opportunities at 2-hour intervals during the day. Normal well-rested adults will fall asleep in an average of 15 minutes across the nap series. Those with narcolepsy or idiopathic hypersomnia often fall asleep in an average of less than 5 minutes, and those with narcolepsy may have REM sleep on multiple naps.

Musical Hallucinations. Phantom auditory perception of music heard in the head. The four possible etiologies are ear pathology, brain disease, psychopathology, and toxic states.

Narcolepsy. Neurologic condition characterized by excessive daytime sleepiness without explanation. Many people with narcolepsy also experience cataplexy.

Neglect (also Extinction). Disorder of attention most often associated with posterior parietal lobe damage. Patients with neglect (also called hemineglect) fail to attend to stimuli on the side of body or within the visual hemifields opposite to the side of the brain lesion. As patients recover, they may only demonstrate extinction to double simultaneous stimulation of both visual hemifields or of both sides of the body.

Neoplastic Meningitis. See Leptomeningeal Carcinomatosis.

Neural Net. Type of computer program in which idealized "neurons" are connected together. The strength of their interconnections changes dependent on their experience, that is, the inputs to the system.

Neural Networks. Multifocal, distributed systems of neuronal ensembles in the brain that subserve various neurobehavioral domains.

Neural Plasticity. Notion that, in the absence of pathology, neurons possess and retain the capacity for alteration and growth.

Neurobehavioral (Neurocognitive, Neuropsychological). Pertains to the broad range of human behaviors and the mediating brain structures responsible for them.

Neurodegenerative Disease. Any progressive neurologic disorder in which the underlying problem is assumed to be related to failure of cellular metabolic systems, for example, Alzheimer disease, Parkinson disease, diffuse Lewy body disease, corticobasal ganglionic degeneration, or progressive supranuclear palsy.

Neurodevelopmental Treatment (NDT). Physical therapy that relies on the child's active participation to learn to compensate for abnormal movements and maintain equilibrium in space.

Neuroergonomics. Study of human-machine-systems interactions in health and disease states. Examples include the study of human errors that contribute to motor vehicle crashes and the effects of health-care worker fatigue on errors in patient care.

Neuropsychological Testing. Clinical application of standardized psychological tests to assess the integrity of cognitive and behavioral processes and their underlying neural substrate.

Nociception. Activity produced in the nervous system by potential tissue damaging stimuli.

Nonconvulsive Status. Refers to almost continuous partial or absence seizures. During such episodes cognitive processes and behavior may be severely disrupted.

Nonsyndromal Mental Retardation. Mental retardation not associated with a recognized syndrome.

Nonverbal Learning Disability. Group of learning disabilities that typically involves nonverbal problems that have an impact on learning and social-emotional functions. White matter damage or dysfunction has been hypothesized as being contributory to these types of problems.

Nystagmus. Repetitive eye movements with slow and fast components; a common sign in vestibular disorders.

Object-Based Attention. Those attentional processes that select a stimulus based on the shape or structure of that stimulus. Many forms of object-based attention appear to involve selecting regions of space that have been grouped together by perceptual grouping processes.

Obsessions. Recurrent, intrusive senseless thoughts that are internally uncomfortable.

Occupational Performance. Accomplishment of tasks related to self-care/self-maintenance, work/education, play/leisure, and rest/relaxation.

Ocular Motor Apraxia. Impaired ability to generate volitional saccades to a target, despite intact range of eye movements with vestibular-ocular reflexes or even spontaneous saccades.

Ocular Tilt Reaction. Ocular cyclorotation, head tilt, and skew deviation. This reaction occurs in peripheral as well as central vestibular system lesions. Lesions caudal to the pons cause the head tilt to be ipsilesional, and in those rostral to the pons the tilt is contralesional. The most rostral site is the rostral interstitial nucleus of the medial longitudinal fasciculus and interstitial nucleus of the Cajal area.

Oligodendroglioma. Malignant tumor of the brain originating from oligodendrocytes. It appears to be more responsive to treatment than other primary tumors of the brain.

Opioid Phobia. Fear of opioid analgesic therapy on the part of physicians, patients, or others.

Optic Ataxia. Defective reaching for objects under visual guidance.

Orbitofrontal Cortex. Inferior region of the frontal lobe that mediates diverse associative processing involving emotion, social cognition, empathy, and aspects of personality.

Organic Personality Disorder. Disturbance characterized by a reduced ability to persevere with goal-directed activities, emotional changes, disinhibited and impulsive behaviors, and cognitive deficits.

Orthography. A method of representing the sounds of a language by written or printed symbols.

Pain. Unpleasant sensory and emotional experience associated with actual or potential tissue damage or described in terms of such damage.

PANDAS. Pediatric autoimmune neuropsychiatric disorders associated with streptococcal infections including tics and obsessive-compulsive disorder.

Panic Attack. Sudden episode of discrete or intense fear or discomfort that reaches a maximum within a few minutes and lasts at least some minutes.

Paraneoplastic Syndrome. Set of symptoms originating from secretion of proteins by the tumor that affects structures in the brain. These symptoms typically involve immune system reactions to brain proteins that resemble tumor antigens.

Parcellation. Process by which central nervous system magnetic resonance imaging images are divided into discrete anatomic regions (e.g., caudate).

Parkinson Disease. A movement disorder characterized by the presence of a pill-rolling resting tremor, rigidity, and bradykinesia (slowed voluntary motor movements).

Parosmia. Alterations and distortions in olfactory sensation and perception.

Paroxysmal. Characteristic of an electroencephalographic pattern (e.g., burst) to have an abrupt onset, a rapid attainment of maximum amplitude, followed by sudden termination. This pattern should be easily distinguished from the background activity.

Periaqueductal Gray Matter (PAG). Several columns of cells in the midbrain, surrounding the aqueduct.

Periodic Discharges. In electroencephalography, waves or complexes occurring in series at approximately regular intervals (typically 1 to several seconds).

Periventricular Leukomalacia (PVL). White matter damage around the ventricles of the brain, often associated with cerebral palsy in preterm infants and with other conditions in adults.

Phantom Limb Phenomena. Perceptual experience that an amputated limb is still present (phantom limb perception), or experience of pain in the amputated limb (phantom limb pain).

Phantosmia. Olfactory hallucinations associated with certain seizures (olfactory aura), brain tumors, or psychotic conditions.

Phoneme. Basic unit of speech that links each letter or cluster of letters to a specific sound.

Phonological Processing. Working understanding that speech can be segmented into specific phonemes or sounds.

Physical Dependence. Abstinence syndrome precipitated by abruptly withdrawing an opioid or administering an opioid antagonist.

Plasticity. Ability to compensate for lost neural tissue or function of the developing brain.

Polymerase Chain Reaction (PCR). Amplifies nucleic acid sequences specific for the microorganism that is suspected to be the infecting agent.

Positron. Subatomic particle with the same mass as an electron but with a positive electrical charge.

Positron Emission Computed Tomography (PET). A nuclear medicine technique that provides cross-sectional images of the distribution in the body of radiotracers labeled with radioactive atoms that emit positrons from their nuclei.

Postconcussive Syndrome. Persistent concussion-like symptoms after head trauma.

Posterior Fossa Syndrome. Clinical phenomenon observed in children within days following midline cerebellar surgery, characterized by mutism, oral motor apraxia, hypotonia, and marked fluctuations in behavior and affect.

Post-ictal. Transient clinical abnormality of central nervous system function that appears or becomes accentuated when clinical signs of the seizure have ended.

Postsynaptic Potentials. Transmembrane potentials measured at the neuronal cell body with a typical intracellular voltage of –60 to –70 mV.

Post-Traumatic Amnesia (PTA). Amnesia for events following head injury. The amnesia ends when "continuous" memory returns.

Pragmatic Language. The method by which language is used to communicate, rather than the content of what is said.

Predictive Validity. Extent to which test scores obtained at one point in time predict a relevant criterion variable at a later point in time.

Prefrontal Cortex. Most rostral neocortical region of brain, comprising the part of the frontal lobe that mediates complex, adaptive behavior including many aspects of executive functions, personality, and the integration of cognition and emotion.

Premotor Cortex. Neocortical region closely associated with the primary motor cortex. It mediates motor planning, skilled motor movement, and aspects of sensory-motor transformations.

Prevalence. Number of people who have a disorder at a given point in time (also known as the base rate or prior probability).

Primary Brain Tumor. Tumor originating from cells within the brain.

Primary Progressive Aphasia. Focal degenerative disorder that typically affects the inferior lateral frontal and anterior frontal cortex of the language-dominant hemisphere, resulting in a progressive decline in language function.

Primary-Progressive Multiple Sclerosis. Disease course characterized by progression from onset with occasional plateaus and temporary minor improvements allowed.

Prion. Infectious agent with protein-like properties.

Procedural Memory. Refers to sensory-motor and skill-based learning (e.g., knowledge of how to ride a bike, play the piano) that is not necessarily accessible to conscious experience. Procedural memory does not require explicit recollection of past experiences to access and implement related aspects of those memories.

Prodrome. Sensation, usually unpleasant, that heralds the onset of an epileptic seizure but does not form a part of it.

Progressive Multifocal Leukoencephalopathy. Activation of the ubiquitous JC virus from its quiescent state within the brain following immunosuppressive therapy, resulting in white matter lesion and cognitive decline.

Progressive-Relapsing Multiple Sclerosis. Disease course characterized by a progressive disease from onset, with clear acute relapses, periods between relapses characterized by continuing progression.

Progressive Supranuclear Palsy. Disorder characterized by bradykinesia, postural instability, rigidity (most notably in the neck and trunk), and visual disturbances due to vertical gaze paresis. It is commonly misdiagnosed for Parkinson disease.

Prophylactic Cranial Irradiation. Radiation administered to sterilize the brain from small tumor deposits thought present but not clinically or radiographically evident. This controversial treatment can lead to cognitive dysfunction with prolonged patient survival.

Prosopagnosia. Subjective loss of familiarity or recognition for faces previously known to the patient.

Psychometrics. Empirical basis underlying the development and administration of quantifiable "measures to measure" individual differences in psychological functioning.

Psychophysical Testing. Quantitative testing of sensory thresholds, detection, and identification. Psychophysical data can also include verbal reports of a subject's sensory experience.

Psychosocial. Behavioral, emotional, and social aspects of a person's functioning. Usually excludes consideration of physical and cognitive aspects of functioning.

Quadrantanopia (Quadrantanopsia). Visual field defect restricted to the upper or lower quadrant of a hemifield. A lesion below the calcarine fissure results in an upper (superior) quadrantanopia; a lesion above it causes a lower (inferior) quadrantanopia.

Quality of Life (QOL). Finding reward and satisfaction in life, which may include finding a sense of meaning, performing expected work/social roles, enjoying relationships, and pursuing education.

Quantitative Magnetic Resonance Imaging (MRI). Use of MRI-generated images (i.e., electronic data) to measure the size (i.e., area, volume), shape, or tissue characteristics (i.e., iron concentration) of central nervous system structures.

Raccoon Eyes. Discoloration around the eyes due to seepage of blood into periorbital tissues, resulting from basilar skull fracture.

Radioactive Decay. Spontaneous transformation of a radioactive atom to an atom of a different element, with the emission from the atomic nucleus of an alpha particle, electron, positron, or gamma ray.

Radiofrequency Spoiled Gradient Echo (SPGR). Most frequently used MRI sequence for morphometric studies, particularly volumetric measures. It receives other terms depending on the MR scanner manufacturer. It has the advantages of fast three-dimensional acquisition and high spatial resolution (thin slices).

Radiotracer. Compound labeled with a radioactive atom, used to trace or follow a physiologic or biochemical process. It is administered in very small amounts so as not to interfere with the process being studied.

Rasmussen's Encephalitis. Onset in childhood, slowly progressive, usually unilateral brain atrophy with intractable focal seizures, paralysis, and cognitive decline that has the histopathologic appearance of chronic encephalitis.

Regional Cerebral Blood Flow (rCBF). Local perfusion of brain tissue by blood; the volume of blood flowing through a particular volume or weight of brain tissue per unit time, in units of milliliters per minute per milliliter or gram of tissue.

Regional Cerebral Metabolic Rate of Glucose (RCMRglc). Speed at which glucose is used by a particular volume or weight of brain tissue, in units or grams of glucose per minute per milliliter or gram of tissue.

Regulatory Neurobehavioral States. Fundamental neural and cognitive processes that subserve wakefulness, attention, inhibition, motor activation, and orientation and permit the conscious experience of the self and the environment.

Rehabilitation. Diverse therapeutic approaches to restore functional capacities of individuals with neurologic deficits.

Relapsing-Remitting Multiple Sclerosis. Disease course characterized by relapses with full recovery or with sequelae and residual deficit upon recovery. Periods between relapses are characterized by lack of disease progression.

Relaxation. Process by which atomic (nuclear) spins return to their original position after being initially aligned by a strong magnetic field property and then excited by radiofrequency (RF) pulses. The process of recording by an RF coil (applied to subject), this phenomenon is termed *resonance*. Tissue components contribute differentially to the relaxation process. T1 and T2 represent the longitudinal and transverse relaxation times, respectively.

Remote Memory. System involved with our ability to recollect information from the past.

Resolution. In nuclear imaging, the minimum distance in space (spatial resolution) or time (temporal resolution) by which two points of radioactivity must be separated to be perceived independently in the reconstructed image.

Response Bias. Class of behaviors that reflects less than accurate or valid symptom report (i.e., under- or over-reporting) and presentation, whether conscious or unconscious.

Response Inhibition. Response inhibition occurs when the brain selectively delays or blocks an action in response to specific learned rules. As an example, during a specific continuous performance test, the test taker must inhibit the button-pushing response until a specific symbol appears on the screen.

Retrograde Amnesia. Loss of ability to retrieve and otherwise access information and experiences acquired prior to onset of cerebral damage.

Rhythmicity. Characteristic of electroencephalographic activity to show waves of approximately equal frequency.

Road Rage. Term used by the media for aggressive, and often criminal, behavior directed toward other drivers. Often associated with drugs, alcohol, stress, emotional disturbances, and personality disorders.

Road Test. "Gold standard" of driver fitness. An expert grades driver performance on several standard driving tasks to calculate a cutoff score to designate a driver as safe or unsafe for licensure. Neuropsychological tests, driving simulators, and instrumented vehicles can provide information on driver fitness that is not available in a standard road test.

Schizophrenia. Form of psychosis characterized by thought disorder, hallucinations and delusions, and disorganized behavior. Subtypes include paranoid, disorganized, catatonic, undifferentiated, and residual.

Secondary-Progressive Multiple Sclerosis. Disease course characterized by an initial relapsing-remitting phase followed by progression with or without occasional relapses, minor remissions, and plateaus.

Sectoranopia. Wedge-shaped visual field defect straddling the horizontal meridian in both eyes that may occur with an infarct of the part of the lateral geniculate nucleus supplied by the lateral posterior choroidal artery.

Seizure. Clinical manifestation of abnormal and excessive activity of a set of cortical neurons.

Semantic Dementia. Form of frontotemporal dementia characterized by progressive loss of semantic memory and knowledge.

Semantic Memory. Long-term memory system that subserves general knowledge about objects and the meaning of words and concepts. This type of knowledge is not temporally related to distinct episodes.

Sensitivity. Conditional probability of a positive test result, given that the disorder is present.

Sildenaphil (Viagra). Medication that treats erectile dysfunction by inhibiting phosphodiesterase type 5. Side effects include headache, nasal congestion, flushing, dyspepsia, and blue visual tint.

Simulator Adaptation Syndrome (SAS). Autonomic symptoms including nausea and sweating in a simulator. The discomfort is thought to be due to a mismatch between visual cues of movement, which are plentiful, and inertial cues, which are lacking or imperfect, even in simulators with a motion base. Related symptoms occur in IMAX theaters and below deck in ships.

Simultanagnosia. Inability to interpret a complex scene with multiple interrelated elements despite intact perception of individual elements.

Six-weeks Rule. Empirical rule proposed by C. M. Fisher stating that transient ischemia attacks/strokes have not been reported to be the cause of isolated dizziness if the dizziness has been recurrent for more than 6 weeks. However, recently cases have been reported with such recurrence for months.

Sleep Inertia. Period of impaired performance and reduced vigilance following awakening from the regular sleep episode or from a nap.

Social Emotions. Set of emotions, thought to exist only in social species, in which emotional states are elicited by specific social situations and require for their experience some awareness of other individuals. Social emotions include embarrassment, pride, and guilt.

Somnotype. Basic level of sleepiness/alertness in a given individual; genetically influenced and stable over time. Some people are inherently sleepier or more alert than others, resulting in two somnotypes: alert and sleepy.

Space and Motion Discomfort (SMD). Constellation of symptoms that may develop in patients who have residual vestibular system dysfunction. Patients tend to complain of dizziness on exposure to complex environment or stimuli.

Spastic Diplegia. Bilateral spasticity in which the legs are affected more than the arms.

Spastic Hemiplegia. Unilateral spasticity of the face, arm, and leg, generally with greater involvement of the arm.

Spatial Attention. Attentional processes that involve selecting a stimulus on the basis of the location that the stimulus occupies.

Spatial Cognition. Awareness of personal and extrapersonal space and the ability to use this information to navigate in space both conceptually and in practice.

Spatial Errors. In limb praxis assessment, a pantomimed gesture in which the characteristic movements are disturbed; for example, while pantomiming the use of a screwdriver, the wrist bends when it should be stable.

Specific Learning Disability. Disorder in one or more of the basic psychological processes involved in understanding or in using language, spoken or written, which may manifest itself in an imperfect ability to listen, speak, read, write, spell, or perform mathematical calculations.

Specificity. Conditional probability of a negative test result, given that the disorder is absent.

Single Photon Emission Computed Tomography (SPECT). Nuclear medicine technique that provides cross-sectional images of the distribution in the body of radiotracers labeled with radioactive atoms that emit gamma rays or single photons.

Speech. Articulation of language.

Speed of Processing. Rate with which information available to the senses is processed by higher order cognitive functions.

Spongiform Encephalopathy. Class of degenerative diseases exemplified by Creutzfeldt-Jakob Disease, in which inheritance or exposure to abnormal prions (small proteinaceous infectious particles) leads to a rapidly progressive and fatal form of dementia associated with sponge-like microscopic holes in brain issue.

Stereotactic Radiation. Directed radiotherapy using multiple angles of administration so as to maximize dose to the tumor and minimize dose to the surrounding brain.

Stereotypic Behaviors. Repetitive behaviors (like hand flapping) that may be self-stimulatory. Tics may be a subset.

Stroke. Neurologic attack originating from pathology in the cerebral vascular system. This includes thrombotic or embolic arterial occlusion resulting in interruption of blood flow to, and death of, a given portion of the brain (also known as cerebrovascular accident). Strokes can also be hemorrhagic as in hypertensive hemorrhage, subarachnoid hemorrhage, and cerebral venous thrombosis.

Structural Neuroimaging. Radiologic procedures in which brain injuries can be viewed in vivo. The principal structural imaging methods currently used include magnetic resonance imaging and computed tomography.

Stupor. State of unresponsiveness from which the individual can be aroused only by repeated or vigorous stimulation.

Subacute Sclerosing Panencephalitis. Inflammatory and degenerative central nervous system disease caused by the measles virus.

Suffering. Global perception of distress engendered by adverse factors that together undermine quality of life.

Suprachiasmatic Nuclei. Small groups of cells in the hypothalamus that drive the various circadian rhythms. These nuclei possess inherent rhythmicity and are entrained by the external light/dark cycle.

Symptom Exaggeration or Magnification. Embellishment (conscious or unconscious), either by subjective report or by exam presentation, of a real/organic sign or symptom for either primary or secondary gain.

Symptom Validity Tests. Measures designed to examine the validity of an examinee's complaints by measuring his or her motivation to perform well on testing procedures.

Synaptic Plasticity. Ability of neurons to change the number, direction, and strength of their connections (synapses) with other neurons.

Tactile Apraxia. Inability to explore tactually objects to achieve tactile object recognition despite adequate perception and motor function.

Tactile Hallucination. Somatosensory perceptual experiences in the absence of stimuli. These experiences can be simple (e.g., paresthesia) or complex (e.g., being touched or having an object put in one's hands).

Tactile Neglect. Inability to attend to unilateral tactile stimuli despite adequate somatosensory perception, often best demonstrated with brief simultaneous tactile stimulation of both sides of the body.

Task Analysis. Technique used in cognitive therapy in which the patient carefully examines the steps of a task that was successfully completed to better understand the principles of planning. The approach used is then generalized to other similar situations. This approach is used to teach organizational skills to adolescents with attention-deficit/hyperactivity disorder.

Taste. Salty, sweet, sour, and bitter sensations evoked by chemical stimuli applied to the tongue.

Taste Buds. Microscopic goblet-shaped multicellular structures in which taste transduction occurs. Taste buds are embedded within specialized papillae or within the surface epithelium of the tongue.

Taste Papillae. Macroscopic structures located on the dorsum and lateral edges of the tongue that contain taste buds.

Temporal Errors. In limb praxis assessment, a pantomimed gesture in which the typical timing, speed, or sequencing required to make the movements is disturbed; for example, irregular cycling of the spoon while pantomiming stirring coffee.

Tentorium Cerebelli. A fold of the dura mater that separates the cerebellum from the cerebrum. In neuro-oncology, supratentorial refers to cerebral tumors above this fold, whereas infratentorial refers to tumors of the cerebellum, brainstem, and other structures below the cerebrum. Brain tumors in children are mostly infratentorial.

Test Reliability. Statistical analysis of how repeatable or similar the results of a test are over time (test-retest), over test items (inter-item and split-half), and between different examiners (inter-rater).

Test Validity. Statistical analysis of how well a test measures what it is purported to measure (construct validity), how a test relates to other existing measures in the same area (concurrent validity), whether a test provides more information than available through other measures (incremental validity), and the test's predictive accuracy for everyday, real life tasks (ecological validity).

Thalamic Nucleus. A subdivision of the thalamus defined by characteristic cytoarchitecture, staining properties, connectional relationships, physiologic properties, and putative functional role.

Theory of Mind. Ability to understand what another is thinking and feeling.

Tinnitus. Phantom auditory perception of a basic continuous sound (often permanent) in the head or ears. There is not yet a unanimous explanation, but tinnitus may involve peripheral and central auditory mechanisms.

Tissue Segmentation. Process by which each volumetric unit (voxel) is assigned to one of the three CNS tissue classes: gray matter, white matter, and cerebrospinal fluid.

Topographagnosia. Inability to orient oneself in familiar surroundings.

Topography. Amplitude distribution of electroencephalographic activities over the surface of the head.

Tourette Syndrome. Inherited neuropsychiatric disorder characterized by motor and phonic tics.

Toxin. Chemical agent with the capacity to produce functional or structural damage to tissue.

Transient Cognitive Impairment. Transient changes in cognitive and behavioral functioning occurring with subclinical inter-ictal epileptiform discharges.

Transitive Gesture. Pantomimed movement that involves manipulating an object, often a tool, for example, using a saw to cut wood or a bowling ball to knock down pins.

Trauma. Physical injury or psychological or emotional damage.

Triphasic Waves. Periodic waves consisting of three components alternating around the baseline. These discharges are commonly seen in the EEG of patients with toxic-metabolic encephalopathies and in Creutzfeldt-Jakob disease.

Uniparental Disomy. A genetic situation in which both copies of a person's chromosome come from the same parent.

Universal Cerebellar Transform (UCT)/ Impairment (UCI). The UCT concept is that the essentially uniform architecture of the cerebellar cortex imbues the cerebellum with the ability to perform a single process of physiological and functional significance. This transform is applied to the topographically arranged information to which the cerebellum has access through the cerebrocerebellar system. The notion of the UCI is that when the cerebellum is lesioned, the loss of the UCT produces a constant impairment, namely dysmetria. The manifestations differ, according to where in the cerebellum the lesion is located, and consequently which anatomic circuits are interrupted.

Valence. Pleasant or unpleasant aspect of an emotional feeling.

Vascular Cognitive Impairment (VCI). Cognitive, behavioral, and emotional deficits that are caused by cerebrovascular disease.

Vegetative State (Arousable Unconsciousness). Condition of unconsciousness with the capacity for spontaneous or stimulus-induced arousal and sleep–wake cycles.

Ventral Striatum. Components of the basal ganglia, including the nucleus accumbens septi, ventral parts of the caudate nucleus, and the putamen. These structures receive input from areas including amygdala and orbitofrontal cortex and project to ventral globus pallidus (which projects via other structures back to amygdala and orbitofrontal cortex).

Verbal Apraxia. Brain-related inability to translate linguistic ideas into sequences of motor movements that produce speech.

Verbal Learning Disability. Group of learning disabilities that typically involve auditory-verbal problems that affect learning and language-based functions. Left hemisphere dysfunction has been hypothesized as being contributory to these types of problems.

Vermis. Midline region of the cerebellum. It is an anatomically identifiable structure in the posterior lobe, but an ill-defined region at the superior aspect of the cerebellum.

Vertically Acquired HIV. HIV in the child acquired perinatally from the infected mother.

Vestibular Cortex. Collectively describes the cortical areas that receive vestibular input. The locations are mainly in the superior temporal and inferior parietal lobes.

Vestibular System. Includes the inner ear labyrinthine structures, the vestibular nerve, and nuclei and their connections to the other brainstem structures and to the cerebellum, thalamus, and cortex. During locomotion this system helps stabilize the eyes with respect to the head, head on body, and body in space.

Vestibulo-Ocular Reflex (VOR). Helps maintain eyes in focus on a target during ambulation and depends on connections between the vestibular and ocular motor nuclei.

Visual Agnosia.   Loss of knowledge about objects perceived visually, usually manifests as a failure to both name and recognize objects.

Visual Search.   Process used to find a visual target (i.e., how you find what you're looking for). Both the elementary visual features of a stimulus (e.g., color, shape, or size) and focal visual attention combine to guide the search for a target.

Working Memory.   Encompasses the representational processes that allow us to keep information active or "in mind" for various periods of time. It involves both temporary storage and processing operations that are critical to comprehension, problem solving, or learning.

z-score.   Standardized score that is obtained when the mean of the distribution of scores is subtracted from a given score and divided by the standard deviation of the distribution. The z-score indicates how many standard deviations a given score falls away from the mean.

Index

Note: Page numbers followed by f indicate figures; those followed by t indicate tables.

DATE DUE

Demco, Inc. 38-293

DEPAUL UNIVERSITY LIBRARY

3 0511 00875 1000